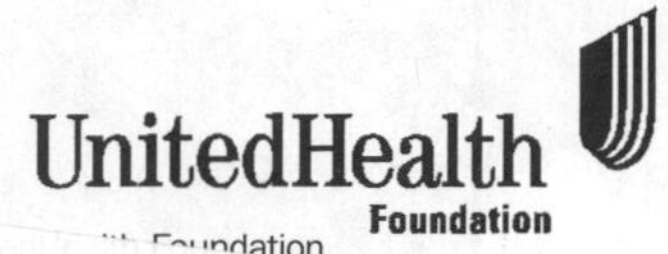

January, 2003

Dear Colleague,

We at UnitedHealth Foundation are once again pleased to provide you a complimentary copy of the BMJ Publishing Group's increasingly relevant publication, *Clinical Evidence*. This eighth edition continues to demonstrate that *Clinical Evidence* is the international resource of the best available evidence for effective health care. We are proud that *Clinical Evidence* benefits from considerable input by leading clinical experts from the United States.

Our nation's healthcare professionals, and their patients, benefit from the continuous development of new clinically relevant knowledge. The challenge for busy clinicians is to keep up with the best and most relevant of this new information. As such, it is our pleasure to provide you with this most recent edition in the hope that it will make a tangible contribution to advancing your own clinical decisions.

In addition to this print version, you are entitled to free access to CE-Online. To make use of this feature go to www.clinicalevidence.com. Once there, register as a recipient of the UHF distribution program.

Our goal at the UnitedHealth Foundation is to support you in enhancing the health of your patients through evidence-based decision making. We hope the integration of *Clinical Evidence* into your daily practice is of benefit to you.

Sincerely,

Bill McGuire

William W. McGuire, M.D.
Chairman
UnitedHealth Foundation

8 ISSUE
DECEMBER 2002

clinical evidence

The international source of the best available evidence for effective health care

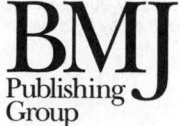

Editorial Office

BMJ Publishing Group, BMA House, Tavistock Square, London, WC1H 9JR, United Kingdom.
Tel: +44 (0)20 7387 4499 • Fax: +44 (0)20 7383 6242 • www.bmjpg.com

Subscription prices for *Clinical Evidence*

Clinical Evidence and *Clinical Evidence Concise* (with companion CD-ROM) are both published six monthly (June/December) by the BMJ Publishing Group. The annual subscription rates for both publications (December, Issue 8, and June, Issue 9) are:

Personal: £85 • €135 • US$135 • Can$200
Institutional: £175 • €280 • US$280 • Can$420
Student/nurse: £40 • €65 • US$65 • Can$95

The above rates are for either the full print or the concise formats. The combined rates, for both formats, are:

Personal £120 • €190 • US$190 • Can$285
Institutional £235 • €375 • US$375 • Can$560
Student/nurse £65 • €105 • US$105 • Can$155

All individual subscriptions (personal, student, nurse) include online access at no additional cost. Institutional subscriptions are for full print/concise version only. Institutions may purchase online site licences separately. For further subscription information please visit the subscription pages of our website www.clinicalevidence.com or email us at CEsubscriptions@bmjgroup.com (UK and ROW) or clinevid@pmds.com (Americas). You may also telephone us or fax us on the following numbers:

UK and ROW Tel: +44 (0)20 7383 6270 • Fax: +44 (0)20 7383 6402
Americas Tel: +1 800 373 2897/240 646 7000 • Fax: +1 240 646 7005

Bulk subscriptions for societies and organisations

The Publishers offer discounts for any society or organisation buying bulk quantities for their members/specific groups. Please contact Miranda Lonsdale, Sales Manager (UK) at mlonsdale@bmjgroup.com or Diane McCabe, Sales and Marketing Manager (USA) at dmccabe@bmjgroup.com.

Contributors

If you are interested in becoming a contributor to *Clinical Evidence* please contact us at clinicalevidence@bmjgroup.com.

Rights

For information on translation rights, please contact Daniel Raymond-Barker at draymond-barker@bmjgroup.com.

Copyright

British Library Cataloguing in Publication Data. A catalogue record for this book is available from the British Library. ISSN 1462-3846 ISBN 0-7279-15649

Permission to reproduce

Please contact Josephine Woodcock at jwoodcock@bmjgroup.com when requesting permission to reprint all or part of any contribution in *Clinical Evidence*.

Legal Disclaimer

Care has been taken to confirm the accuracy of the information presented and to describe generally accepted practices. However, the authors, editors, and publishers are not responsible for errors or omissions or for any consequences from application of the information in this book and make no warranty, express or implied, with respect to the contents of the publication.

Categories presented in *Clinical Evidence* indicate a judgement about the strength of the evidence available and the relative importance of benefits and harms. The categories do not indicate whether a particular treatment is generally appropriate or whether it is suitable for individuals.

Printed by Quebecor World, Kingsport, USA
Designed by Pete Wilder, The Designers Collective Limited, London UK

Team and Advisors

Editor Giselle Jones **Clinical Editors** Mike Bedford, Luis Gabriel Cuervo Amore, Anjana Patel, Charles Young **Quality Assurance Editor** James Woodcock **Content Editor** Karen Pettersen **Assistant Content Editor** Polly Brown **Consulting Editor** Stuart Barton **North American Editor** David Goldmann **Managing Editor** Josephine Woodcock **Production Editors** Samantha Bedser, Alan Thomas **Editorial/Production Assistants** Claire Folkes, Rachael Kriefman **Freelance Editors** Bazian Ltd **Technical Editors** Andy Baker, Melissa Dodd, Anne Lawson, Pamela Morley, Andrea Porter, Jane Tozer **Indexer** Angela Cottingham **Digital Production** Cassara Burgess, Karen Caillé, Kourosh Mojar, BMJ Electronic Production **Print Production** Charlotte Pestridge **Information Specialists** Olwen Beaven, Sarah Greenley, Jane McHugh, Paul Miller, Sam Vincent **Administrator** Varsha Mistry **Business Manager** Paula McQuillan (maternity leave cover for Lisette Cleyndert) **New Product Development Manager** Maysoon Nasser **Knowledge Systems Manager** Jonathan Fistein **Department Administrator** Hannah Lawrence **Marketing and Sales (UK)** Jaspal Chaggar, Diane Harris, Miranda Lonsdale, Daniel Raymond-Barker **Marketing and Sales (USA)** Diane McCabe

SECTION ADVISORS

Cardiovascular disorders Nick Hicks, UK **Child health** Mary Rudolf, UK and Virginia Moyer, USA **Digestive system disorders** David Cave, USA, John McDonald, Canada and David Metz, USA **Ear, nose, and throat disorders** George Browning, UK **Endocrine disorders** Shereen Ezzat, Canada **Eye disorders** Andrew Dick and Liam Smeeth, UK **Infectious diseases** Paul Garner, UK **Kidney disorders** Fred Coe and Michael Coulin, USA **Men's health** Peter Schlegal, USA and Robyn Webber, UK **Mental health** John Geddes, UK **Musculoskeletal disorders** Troels Mork Hansen, Denmark and John Stothard, UK **Neurological disorders** Tony Marson, UK **Oral health** Aubrey Sheiham, UK **Perioperative care** Andrew Smith, UK and Valarie Palda, USA **Poisoning** Robin Ferner and Allister Vale, UK **Pregnancy and childbirth** Metin Gulmezoglu, Switzerland **Respiratory disorders** John Cunnington, Canada **Sexual health** George Schmid, USA **Skin disorders** Hywel Williams and Jane McGregor, UK **Sleep disorders** Michael Hensley, Australia **Women's health** Mike Dixon, UK **Wounds** Nicky Cullum, UK

Acknowledgements

The BMJ Publishing Group thanks the following people and organisations for their advice and support: The Cochrane Collaboration, and especially Iain Chalmers, Mike Clarke, Phil Alderson, Peter Langhorne, and Carol Lefebvre; the National Health Service (NHS) Centre for Reviews and Dissemination, and especially Jos Kleijnen and Julie Glanville; the NHS, and especially Tom Mann, Sir John Patteson, Ron Stamp, Veronica Fraser, Muir Gray, Nick Rosen, and Ben Toth; the British National Formulary, and especially Dinesh Mehta, Eric Connor, and John Martin; Martindale: The Complete Drug Reference, and especially Sean Sweetman; the Health Information Research Unit at McMaster University, and especially Brian Haynes and Ann McKibbon; the UnitedHealth Foundation (UHF), and especially Dr Reed Tuckson and Yvette Krantz; the clinicians, epidemiologists, and members of patient support groups who have acted as peer reviewers.

The BMJ Publishing Group values the ongoing support it has received from the global medical community for *Clinical Evidence*. In addition to others, we wish to acknowledge the efforts of the UHF and the NHS who have provided educational funding to support the wide dissemination of this valuable resource to many physicians and health professionals in the USA (UHF) and UK (NHS). We are grateful to the clinicians and patients who spare time to take part in focus groups, which are crucial to the development of *Clinical Evidence*. Finally, we would like to acknowledge the readers who have taken the time to send us their comments and suggestions.

Contents

Welcome to Issue 8

Welcome to Issue 8 of *Clinical Evidence*, the continuously updated international source of evidence on the effects of clinical interventions. *Clinical Evidence* summarises the current state of knowledge and uncertainty about the prevention and treatment of clinical conditions, based on thorough searches and appraisal of the literature. It is neither a textbook of medicine nor a set of guidelines. It describes the best available evidence, and if there is no good evidence it says so.

WHAT'S NEW IN ISSUE 8?

Issue 8 contains 163 topics, six of which are new: Acute organophosphorus poisoning, Absence seizures in children, Herniated lumbar disc, Leprosy, Tennis elbow (lateral epicondylitis), and Ovarian cancer. Of the remaining 157 topics, 108 have been updated. The most recent search date for inclusion in this issue was August 2002. Updated and new topics completed since September will be posted on to the *Clinical Evidence* website as soon as they become available.

INTEGRATED AND UP TO DATE

Clinical Evidence topics are synopses of the best evidence from the world's literature. The aim is to minimise the interval between literature searching and publication of the updated topic. The contributors of each topic perform a complete revision of the text every 8 months. When contributors stand down, or if there are difficulties that prevent updating, then replacement contributors are commissioned as soon as possible. If we are unable to do this before the next update is due, the topic is updated by a temporary contributor (see temporary contributors below) in the interim period.

Usually, topics that have not been updated in the year before our collection date are removed. This means that there are only three of 163 topics with a search date before September 2001. Stress incontinence has been removed from this issue while we restructure the content around revised questions, and will be published as soon as possible to the website.

The figure below shows a distribution of the search dates for each topic published in this issue of *Clinical Evidence*.

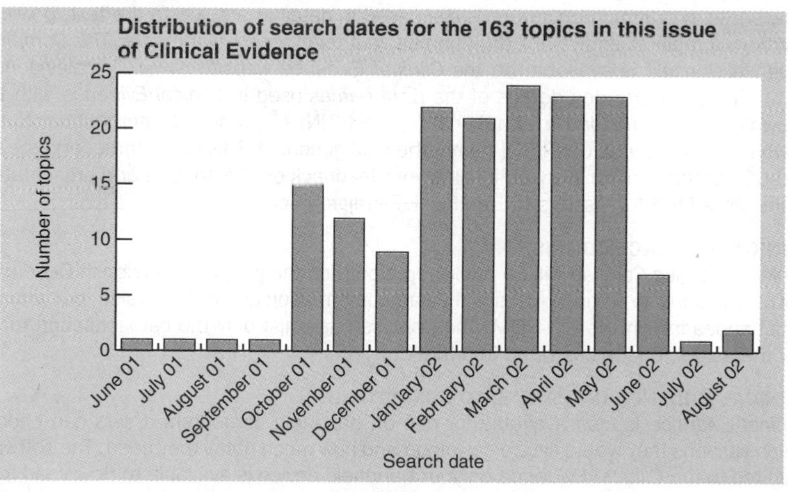

CLINICAL EVIDENCE WEBSITE

The content published in *Clinical Evidence* Issue 8 is a snapshot of the most up to date content available on the *Clinical Evidence* website in September 2002. *Clinical Evidence* topics are now updated continuously and posted to the website every month. We encourage readers to access the site regularly (www.clinicalevidence.com) to see what's new.

Old paper or CD-ROM issues of *Clinical Evidence* should be discarded or treated as a historical curiosity.

TEMPORARY CONTRIBUTORS

It is inevitable that from time to time contributors will stand down from updating their topic and replacement contributors will need to be commissioned. Where it is not possible to find a replacement contributor before the next update is due, the topic is updated by a temporary contributor, for example Bazian Ltd. In this issue, seven topics have been updated by temporary contributors, all of which were subsequently approved for publication by the original contributors. On the first page of these topics the original contributors are cited, followed by the temporary contributors e.g. Bazian Ltd (temporary contributors).

KEY MESSAGES FORMAT

To improve the consistency between the full text version of *Clinical Evidence* and *Clinical Evidence Concise*, and to promote easy access to key information, we have slightly modified the format of the key messages at the beginning of each topic. Each key message is now preceded by a bold intervention heading, which corresponds to the list of interventions in the categorisation table. The key messages are listed alphabetically by intervention, making navigation much easier. Numbers needed to treat (NNTs) with 95% confidence intervals, which were originally only included in *Concise Clinical Evidence*, are now also included in the full text version.

DRUG NAMES

Clinical Evidence aims to present information in a format that is relevant for an international audience. We are aware that difficulties in accessing relevant information about a therapeutic drug can arise when different names for the same drug are used in different parts of the world. The approach used in *Clinical Evidence* for dealing with the differences in drug nomenclature is discussed in detail in A guide to the text, p xvii. In addition, a table of equivalent drug names, put together by *Martindale: The Complete Drug Reference*,[1] is available on the *Clinical Evidence* website (www.clinicalevidence.com). The table provides details of the drug names used in *Clinical Evidence* with the equivalent recommended International Name (rINN) or proposed International Name (pINN), the UK generic (BAN/BP) name, the USA generic (USAN/USP) name, and the UK and USA brand names. We would value your feedback on the content and presentation of the table for future issues (CEfeedback@bmjgroup.com).

CLINICAL EVIDENCE CONCISE

Clinical Evidence Concise will be published alongside the full paper version in December 2002. The *Concise* edition contains the same information as the full version, but with the detail appearing on the CD-ROM. The *Concise* pages list only the categorisation table, key messages, and background information.

CLINICAL EVIDENCE ON HANDHELD COMPUTERS

Clinical Evidence is also available for use on handheld computers. Users can choose which sections they would like to download and how much detail they need. The software required to run *Clinical Evidence* on your handheld device is available to download from the website (www.clinicalevidence.com).

NEW TRANSLATIONS OF CLINICAL EVIDENCE

A Japanese translation of *Clinical Evidence*[2] and a French translation of *Clinical Evidence Concise*[3] (with CD-ROM in English) are now available in addition to the Spanish, Russian, German, Italian and French translations of the full version already available. For more information about these, and other local editions, please visit www.clinicalevidence.com.

FREE ACCESS FOR DEVELOPING COUNTRIES

Clinical Evidence online is now available free to developing countries as part of an initiative spearheaded by the World Health Organization and the BMJ Publishing Group. Details of those countries that qualify, and how they can obtain access, are available from the *Clinical Evidence* website (www.clinicalevidence.com).

CLINICAL EVIDENCE FOR EVERYONE IN ENGLAND

Health professionals in England received paper copies of issues 4–6 of *Clinical Evidence* and online access (www.nelh.nhs.uk) courtesy of the National Health Service. This access has been extended for a further 3 years, with health professionals in England receiving *Clinical Evidence Concise* and having access to the website. This means that patients can now access the same information as their doctors, following the launch of open online access to *Clinical Evidence* and the Cochrane Library through the National electronic Library for Health website (www.nelh.nhs.uk).

FEEDBACK

If you disagree with any of the material, think that important evidence has been missed, or if you have suggestions for new questions or improvements then please let us know. You can contact us at CEfeedback@bmjgroup.com. Many thanks to all of you who have already sent in suggestions.

REFERENCES

1. Sweetman SC (Ed). *Martindale: The Complete Drug Reference*. 33rd ed. London: Pharmaceutical Press, 2002. http://www.pharmpress.com (last accessed 10 October 2002) or contact martindale@rpsgb.org.uk.
2. *Clinical Evidence* (Japanese edition). Tokyo, Japan: Nikkei Medical, 2002.
3. Décider pour traiter abrégé. *Clinical Evidence Concise* (édition française). Paris, France: RanD, 2002.

NEW TRANSLATIONS OF CLINICAL EVIDENCE

A Japanese translation of *Clinical Evidence*[2] and a French translation of *Clinical Evidence Concise*[3] (with CD-ROM in English) are now available in addition to the Spanish, Russian, German, Italian and French translations of the full version already available. For more information about these, and other local editions, please visit www.clinicalevidence.com.

FREE ACCESS FOR DEVELOPING COUNTRIES

Clinical Evidence online is now available free to developing countries, as part of an initiative spearheaded by the World Health Organization and the BMJ Publishing Group. Details of those countries that qualify, and how users can obtain access, are available from the *Clinical Evidence* website (www.clinicalevidence.com).

CLINICAL EVIDENCE FOR EVERYONE IN ENGLAND

Health professionals in England received paper copies of Issues 4–6 of *Clinical Evidence* and online access (www.nelh.nhs.uk) courtesy of the National Health Service. This access has been extended for a further 3 years, to health professionals in England receiving *Clinical Evidence Concise* and having access to the website. This means that patients can now access the same information as their doctors, following the launch of free online access to *Clinical Evidence* and the Cochrane Library through the National electronic Library for Health website (www.nelh.nhs.uk).

FEEDBACK

If you disagree with any of the material, think that important evidence has been missed or if you have suggestions for new questions or improvements, then please let us know. You can contact us at CEfeedback@bmjgroup.com. Many thanks to all of you who have already sent in suggestions.

REFERENCES

1. [illegible]
2. [illegible]
3. [illegible]

About Clinical Evidence

The inspiration for *Clinical Evidence* came in a phone call in 1995. Tom Mann and his colleagues at the NHS Executive asked the BMJ Publishing Group to explore the possibility of developing an evidence "formulary" along the lines of the *British National Formulary*. They recognised that clinicians were under increasing pressure to keep up to date and to base their practice more firmly on evidence, but that few had the necessary time or skills to do this. Their idea was to provide a pocket book containing concise and regularly updated summaries of the best available evidence on clinical interventions. However, they didn't think that the NHS could develop such a formulary itself. "It would be marvellous", said Tom Mann, "if somebody would just do it." A small team at the BMJ set to work to produce a pilot version of what was then called the *Clinical Effectiveness Directory*.

Since that pilot, a great deal has changed. In collaboration with the American College of Physicians–American Society of Internal Medicine, we convened an international advisory board, held focus groups of clinicians, talked to patient support groups, and adopted countless good ideas from early drafts by our contributors. Throughout we have kept in mind an equation set out by Slawson et al.[1] This states that the usefulness of any source of information is equal to its relevance, multiplied by its validity, divided by the work required to extract the information. In order to be as useful as possible, we aimed for high relevance, high validity, and low work in terms of the reader's time and effort. We also kept in mind principles of transparency and explicitness. Readers needed to understand where our information came from and how it was assembled.

A UNIQUE RESOURCE

Clinical Evidence joins a growing number of sources of evidence based information for clinicians. But it has several features that make it unique.

- Its contents are driven by questions rather than by the availability of research evidence. Rather than start with the evidence and summarise what is there, we have tried to identify important clinical questions, and then to search for and summarise the best available evidence to answer them.
- It identifies but does not try to fill important gaps in the evidence. In a phrase used by Jerry Osheroff, who has led much of the recent research on clinicians' information needs,[2] *Clinical Evidence* presents the dark as well as the light side of the moon. We feel that it will be helpful for clinicians to know when their uncertainty stems from gaps in the evidence rather than gaps in their own knowledge.
- It is updated every 6 months in print and monthly online. *Clinical Evidence Concise* is also available with companion CD-ROM.
- It specifically aims not to make recommendations. We feel that simply summarising the evidence will make it more widely useful. The experience of the clinical practice guideline movement has shown that it is nearly impossible to make recommendations that are appropriate in every situation. Differences in individual patients' baseline risks and preferences, and in the local availability of interventions, will always mean that the evidence must be individually interpreted rather than applied across the board. *Clinical Evidence* provides the raw material for developing locally applicable clinical practice guidelines, and for clinicians and patients to make up their own minds on the best course of action. We supply the evidence, you make the decisions.

COMPLEMENTARY BUT DIFFERENT

We are often asked how *Clinical Evidence* differs from two other high quality sources of evidence-based information: The *Cochrane Library*; and the evidence-based journals *ACP Journal Club, Evidence-Based Medicine, Evidence-Based Mental Health,* and *Evidence-Based Nursing*.

Clinical Evidence is complementary to but different from the work of the Cochrane Collaboration, which produces and publishes high quality systematic reviews of controlled trials.[3] *Clinical Evidence* has been called the friendly front end of the *Cochrane Library*, because it takes this and other high quality information and pulls it together in one place in a concise format. Many of our advisors and contributors are active members of the Cochrane Collaboration, and we are exploring closer ties between *Clinical Evidence* and the Collaboration in the way the evidence is searched for, summarised, and accessed by users.

Clinical Evidence is also complementary to but different from the evidence-based journals, which select and abstract the best and most clinically relevant articles as they appear in the world's medical literature. Together these journals form a growing archive of high quality abstracts of individual articles. *Clinical Evidence* takes a different approach. It begins not with the journals but with clinical questions. It is able to answer some. For others it simply reports that no good evidence was found.

A WORK IN PROGRESS

Clinical Evidence is an evolving project. We knew before we started that we were undertaking an enormous task, but the more we worked the more we realised its enormity. We recognise that there is some mismatch between what we aim eventually to achieve and what we have achieved so far. Although we have made every effort to ensure that the searches are thorough and that the appraisals of studies are objective (see Searching and Appraising the literature), we will inevitably have missed some important studies. In order not to make unjustified claims about the accuracy of the information, we use phrases such as "we found no systematic review" rather than "there is no systematic review". In order to be as explicit as possible about the methods used for each contribution, we have asked each set of contributors to provide a brief methods section, describing the searches that were performed and how individual studies were selected.

UPDATING AND EXPANDING CLINICAL EVIDENCE

Our expectation is that *Clinical Evidence* will evolve rapidly in its early years. Indeed, it is already becoming a family of products, appearing in different formats and languages for different audiences. In particular, *Clinical Evidence* will evolve in response to the needs of clinicians. We have tried hard to anticipate those needs (not least by involving clinicians at every stage), but it is only when people begin to use *Clinical Evidence* in daily practice that we can know how best to develop it. That's why your feedback is so important to us, and we are arranging for various ways to evaluate the product.

REFERENCES

1. Slawson DC, Shaughnessy AF, Bennett JH. Becoming a medical information master: feeling good about not knowing everything. *J Fam Pract* 1994;38:505–513.
2. Ely JW, Osheroff JA, Ebell MJ, et al. Analysis of questions asked by family doctors regarding patient care. *BMJ* 1999;319:358–361.
3. Cochrane Collaboration. http://www.cochrane.org (last accessed 8 Oct 2002).

A guide to the text

SUMMARY PAGE

The summary page for each topic presents the questions addressed, some key messages, and a list of the interventions covered, categorised according to whether they have been found to be effective or not. We have developed the categories of effectiveness from one of the Cochrane Collaboration's first and most popular products, *A guide to effective care in pregnancy and childbirth*.[1] The categories we now use are explained in the table below:

TABLE Categorisation of treatment effects in *Clinical Evidence*

Beneficial	Interventions for which effectiveness has been demonstrated by clear evidence from RCTs, and for which expectation of harms is small compared with the benefits.
Likely to be beneficial	Interventions for which effectiveness is less well established than for those listed under "beneficial".
Trade off between benefits and harms	Interventions for which clinicians and patients should weigh up the beneficial and harmful effects according to individual circumstances and priorities.
Unknown effectiveness	Interventions for which there are currently insufficient data or data of inadequate quality.
Unlikely to be beneficial	Interventions for which lack of effectiveness is less well established than for those listed under "likely to be ineffective or harmful".
Likely to be ineffective or harmful	Interventions for which ineffectiveness or harmfulness has been demonstrated by clear evidence.

Fitting interventions into these categories is not always straightforward. For one thing, the categories represent a mix of several hierarchies: the level of benefit (or harm), the level of evidence (RCT or observational data), and the level of certainty around the finding (represented by the confidence interval). Another problem is that much of the evidence that is most relevant to clinical decisions relates to comparisons between different interventions rather than to comparison with placebo or no intervention. Where necessary, we have indicated the comparisons in brackets. A third problem is that interventions may have been tested, or found to be effective, in only one group of people, such as those at high risk of an outcome. Again, we have indicated this where possible. But perhaps most difficult of all has been trying to maintain consistency across different topics. We are working on refining the criteria for putting interventions under each category.

Interventions that cannot be tested in an RCT (perhaps because of ethical or practical reasons) are sometimes cited in the categorisation table, but they are always identified clearly with an asterix (for example, oxygen in severe acute asthma).

NEGATIVE FINDINGS

A surprisingly hard aspect to get right is the reporting of negative findings. As we have had to keep reminding ourselves, saying that there is no good evidence that a treatment works is not the same as saying that the treatment doesn't work. In trying to get this right, we may have erred too much on the side of caution; when in doubt we have changed summary phrases from, for example, "the review found no difference", to "the review found no evidence of a difference". We recognise that to get this right, we need a better handle on the power of individual systematic reviews and trials to demonstrate statistically significant differences between groups, and better information on what constitutes clinically important differences in the major outcomes for each intervention. In the meantime, we hope that the text makes a clear distinction between lack of benefit and lack of evidence of benefit.

OUTCOMES

Clinical Evidence focuses on outcomes that matter to patients, meaning those that patients themselves are aware of, such as symptom severity, quality of life, survival, disability, walking distance, and live birth rate. We are less interested in proxy outcomes such as blood lipid concentrations, blood pressure, or ovulation rates. Each topic includes a list of the main patient oriented outcomes, and where possible describes how these are measured. We have for the moment decided not to address the vexed question of what constitutes a clinically important change in an outcome, but we would welcome any suggestions.

EFFECTS, NOT EFFECTIVENESS

A key aim of *Clinical Evidence* is to emphasise the important trade offs between advantages and disadvantages of different treatment options. We therefore talk about the effects of interventions, both positive and negative, rather than the effectiveness, and for each question or intervention option we present data on benefits and harms under separate headings.

HARMS

Information about harms is often more difficult to integrate than information about benefits.[2] Most controlled trials are designed to investigate benefits. Many either fail to document harms or present the information in a form that is difficult to analyse or interpret. When drugs are licensed they may have been used clinically in only a few thousand people; the absence of documented harms is not strong evidence that harms will not be discovered in the years after licensing.

Clinical Evidence recognises that the evidence about harms is often weaker than that about benefits. In an attempt to correct for this bias, *Clinical Evidence* has lowered the threshold for evidence to be included in the harms section. The policy is to include reports of harms that are included in the systematic reviews (or in individual RCTs if there is no systematic review) in the benefits section. *Clinical Evidence* cross refers to evidence about harms in other populations of people, on the assumption that harms are more likely than benefits to generalise across different subgroups of people. Much of the evidence for harms comes from observational studies ranging from prospective controlled cohort studies to case reports, and these are included when the harm is serious or when there is good corroborating evidence that the harm can be attributed to the treatment.

DRUG INFORMATION

Clinical Evidence aims to present information on therapeutic drugs in a format that is relevant for an international audience. Only the generic or non-proprietary names of drugs rather than the brand names of drugs are used in *Clinical Evidence*, with a few exceptions where the brand name has become the commonly used name in clinical practice, for example EMLA cream (lidocaine-prilocaine). Difficulties arise when different names for the same drug are used in different parts of the world. The recommended International Name (rINN) or proposed International Name (pINN) is used where possible. Where an international name for a therapeutic drug is not available (e.g. aspirin), the most common name has been used.

INFORMATION ON COST

We have decided not to include information on the cost or cost effectiveness of interventions. This is not because we believe cost to be unimportant, but because the question of what constitutes good evidence on cost is much disputed and because costs vary greatly both within and between countries. However, we believe that it will become increasingly untenable for clinicians to act without paying attention to resources. Future companion publications of *Clinical Evidence* may provide relevant information on costs.

NUMERICAL DATA

Whenever possible, data are presented in the same form as in the original studies. However, sometimes we have changed the units or type of information in an attempt to present the results in a systematic and easily interpretable form.

AN INTERNATIONAL APPROACH TO THE EVIDENCE

Clinical Evidence takes an international approach to the evidence. This means including drugs that are not licensed in some countries. It also means keeping in mind the practicalities of treating people in rich as well as poorer countries, by covering interventions even if they have been superseded (for example, single drug treatment for HIV infection as opposed to three drug treatment).

COMPETING INTERESTS

In line with the *BMJ*'s policy,[3] our aim is not to try to eliminate conflicts of interest but to make them explicit so that readers can judge for themselves what influence, if any, these may have had on the contributors' interpretation of the evidence. We therefore ask all contributors to let us know about any potential competing interests, and we append any that are declared to the end of the contribution. Where the contributor gives no competing interests, we record "none declared".

CHANGES SINCE THE LAST UPDATE

The text has been edited and updated. Substantive changes since the last update are listed at the end of each topic. These are defined as:

- Presentation of additional evidence that either confirms or alters the conclusions
- Re-evaluation of the evidence
- Correction of an important error

HOW TO USE THE INFORMATION IN CLINICAL EVIDENCE

The type of information contained in *Clinical Evidence* is necessary but not sufficient for the provision of effective, high quality health care. It is intended as an aid to clinical decision making, to be used in conjunction with other important sources of information. These other sources include estimates of people's baseline risk of a condition or outcome based on history, physical examination and clinical investigations; individual preferences; economic arguments; availability of treatments; and local expertise.

Some guidance on how to apply research evidence in practice is available on our website (www.clinicalevidence.com) and in appendix 3.

REFERENCES

1. Enkin M, Keirse M, Renfrew M, et al. *A guide to effective care in pregnancy and childbirth*. Oxford: Oxford University Press, 1998.
2. Derry S, Loke YK, Aronson JK. Incomplete evidence: the inadequacy of databases in tracing published adverse drug reactions in clinical trials. *BMC Medical Research Methodology* 2001;1:7. http://www.biomedcentral.com/1471-2288/1/7 (last accessed 10 October 2002).
3. Smith R. Beyond conflict of interest. *BMJ* 1998;317:219–292.

How Clinical Evidence is put together

The summaries in *Clinical Evidence* result from a rigorous process aimed at ensuring that the information they contain is both reliable and relevant to clinical practice.

SELECTING TOPICS

Clinical Evidence aims to cover common or important clinical conditions seen in primary and hospital care. To decide which conditions to cover in the first few issues, we reviewed national data on consultation rates, morbidity and mortality, and took advice from generalist clinicians and patient groups. Our website (www.clinicalevidence.com) provides a list of conditions that we are planning to cover in future issues. Further suggestions are welcome.

SELECTING THE QUESTIONS

The questions in *Clinical Evidence* concern the benefits and harms of preventative and therapeutic interventions, with emphasis on outcomes that matter to patients. Questions are selected for their relevance to clinical practice by section advisors and contributors, in collaboration with primary care clinicians and patient groups. Each new issue of *Clinical Evidence* will include new questions as well as updates of existing questions. Readers can suggest new clinical questions using the feedback slips to be found at the back of the book and on the *Clinical Evidence* website (www.clinicalevidence.com), or by writing directly to *Clinical Evidence*.

SEARCHING AND APPRAISING THE LITERATURE

For each question, the literature is searched using the Cochrane Library, Medline, Embase and, occasionally, other electronic databases, looking first for good systematic reviews of RCTs; then for good RCTs published since the search date of the review. Where we find no good recent systematic reviews, we search for individual RCTs. The date of the search is recorded in the methods section for each topic. Of the studies that are identified in the search, we select and summarise only a small proportion. The selection is done by critically appraising the abstracts of the studies identified in the search, a task performed independently by information scientists using validated criteria similar to those of Sackett et al[1] and Jadad.[2] [3] Where the search identifies more than one or two good reviews or trials, we select those we judge to be the most robust or relevant, using the full text of the article. Where we identify few or no good reviews or trials, we include other studies but highlight their limitations. Contributors, who are chosen for their expertise in the field and their skills in epidemiology, are asked to review our selection of studies, and to justify any additions or exclusions they wish to make.

Our search strategy and critical appraisal criteria are available on our website (www.clinicalevidence.com).

SUMMARISING THE EVIDENCE, PEER REVIEW, AND EDITING

The contributors summarise the evidence relating to each question. Each topic is then peer reviewed by the section advisors and by at least three external expert clinicians. The revised text is then extensively edited by editors with clinical and epidemiological training, and data are checked against the original study reports.

REFERENCES

1. Sackett DL, Haynes RB, Guyatt GH, et al. *Clinical Epidemiology: A basic science for clinical medicine*. 2nd ed. Boston: Little Brown, 1991.
2. Jadad A. Assessing the quality of RCTs: Why, what, how and by whom? In: Jadad A, ed. *Randomised Controlled Trials*. London: BMJ Books, 1998:45–60.
3. Jadad AR, Moore RA, Carroll D, et al. Assessing the quality of reports of randomized clinical trials: is blinding necessary? *Control Clin Trials* 1996;17:1–12.

Feedback and Error Correction

Despite the extensive peer review and quality checks, the text may contain some errors and/or inconsistencies. Please let us know if you find any errors, either by using the comment card at the back of the book or by emailing us at CEfeedback@bmjgroup.com.

Errors are graded as minor, moderate, and major based on an assessment of their potential impact. Major and moderate errors are immediately corrected, and minor errors are corrected in the next update.

If you wish to be notified automatically by e-mail of any corrections and updates, then register for the *Clinical Evidence* alerting service on our website. If you are using the information in *Clinical Evidence* to guide your clinical practice then it is essential to register so that you can remain as up to date as possible.

Glossary

Absolute risk (AR) The probability that an individual will experience the specified outcome during a specified period. It lies in the range 0 to 1, or is expressed as a percentage. In contrast to common usage, the word "risk" may refer to adverse events (such as myocardial infarction) or desirable events (such as cure).

Absolute risk increase (ARI) The absolute difference in risk between the experimental and control groups in a trial. It is used when the risk in the experimental group exceeds the risk in the control group, and is calculated by subtracting the AR in the control group from the AR in the experimental group. This figure does not give any idea of the proportional increase between the two groups: for this, relative risk (RR) is needed (see below).

Absolute risk reduction (ARR) The absolute difference in risk between the experimental and control groups in a trial. It is used when the risk in the control group exceeds the risk in the experimental group, and is calculated by subtracting the AR in the experimental group from the AR in the control group. This figure does not give any idea of the proportional reduction between the two groups: for this, relative risk (RR) is needed (see below).

Allocation concealment A method used to prevent selection bias by concealing the allocation sequence from those assigning participants to intervention groups. Allocation concealment prevents researchers from (unconsciously or otherwise) influencing which intervention group each participant is assigned to.

Applicability The application of the results from clinical trials to individual people. A randomised trial only provides direct evidence of causality within that specific trial. It takes an additional logical step to apply this result to a specific individual. Individual characteristics will affect the outcome for this person.

Baseline risk The risk of the event occurring without the active treatment. Estimated by the baseline risk in the control group.

Bias Systematic deviation of study results from the true results, because of the way(s) in which the study is conducted.

Blinding/blinded A trial is fully blinded if all the people involved are unaware of the treatment group to which trial participants are allocated until after the interpretation of results. This includes trial participants and everyone involved in administering treatment or recording trial results.

Block randomisation Randomisation by a pattern to produce the required number of people in each group.

Case control study A study design that examines a group of people who have experienced an event (usually an adverse event) and a group of people who have not experienced the same event, and looks at how exposure to suspect (usually noxious) agents differed between the two groups. This type of study design is most useful for trying to ascertain the cause of rare events, such as rare cancers.

Case series Analysis of series of people with the disease (there is no comparison group in case series).

Clinically significant A finding that is clinically important. Here, "significant" takes its everyday meaning of "important" (compared with statistically significant; see below). Where the word "significant" or "significance" is used without qualification in the text, it is being used in its statistical sense.

Cluster randomisation A cluster randomised study is one in which a group of participants are randomised to the same intervention together. Examples of cluster randomisation include allocating together people in the same village, hospital, or school. If the results are then analysed by individuals rather than the group as a whole bias can occur.

Cohort study A non-experimental study design that follows a group of people (a cohort), and then looks at how events differ among people within the group. A study that examines a cohort, which differs in respect to exposure to some suspected risk factor (e.g. smoking), is useful for trying to ascertain whether exposure is likely to cause specified events (e.g. lung cancer). Prospective cohort studies (which track participants forward in time) are more reliable than retrospective cohort studies.

Completer analysis Analysis of data from only those participants who remained at the end of the study. Compare with intention to treat analysis, which uses data from all participants who enrolled (see below).

Confidence interval (CI) The 95% confidence interval (or 95% confidence limits) would include 95% of results from studies of the same size and design in the same population. This is close but not identical to saying that the true size of the effect (never exactly known) has a 95% chance of falling within the confidence interval. If the 95% confidence interval for a relative risk (RR) or an odds ratio (OR) crosses 1, then this is taken as no evidence of an effect. The practical advantages of a confidence interval (rather than a P value) is that they present the range of likely effects.

Controls In a randomised controlled trial (RCT), controls refer to the participants in its comparison group. They are allocated either to placebo, no treatment, or a standard treatment.

Crossover randomised trial A trial in which participants receive one treatment and have outcomes measured, and then receive an alternative treatment and have outcomes measured again. The order of treatments is randomly assigned. Sometimes a period of no treatment is used before the trial starts and in between the treatments (washout periods) to minimise interference between the treatments (carry over effects). Interpretation of the results from crossover randomised controlled trials (RCTs) can be complex.

Cross sectional study A study design that involves surveying a population about an exposure, or condition, or both, at one point in time. It can be used for assessing prevalence of a condition in the population.

Effect size (standardised mean differences) In the medical literature, effect size is used to refer to a variety of measures of treatment effect. In *Clinical Evidence* it refers to a standardised mean difference: a statistic for combining continuous variables (such as pain scores or height), from different scales, by dividing the difference between two means by an estimate of the within group standard deviation.

Event The occurrence of a dichotomous outcome that is being sought in the study (such as myocardial infarction, death, or a four-point improvement in pain score).

Experimental study A study in which the investigator studies the effect of intentionally altering one or more factors under controlled conditions.

Factorial design A factorial design attempts to evaluate more than one intervention compared with control in a single trial, by means of multiple randomisations.

False negative A person with the target condition (defined by the gold standard) who has a negative test result.

False positive A person without the target condition (defined by the gold standard) who has a positive test result.

Fixed effects The "fixed effects" model of meta-analysis assumes, often unreasonably, that the variability between the studies is exclusively because of a random sampling variation around a fixed effect (see random effects below).

Hazard ratio (HR) Broadly equivalent to relative risk (RR); useful when the risk is not constant with respect to time. It uses information collected at different times. The term is typically used in the context of survival over time. If the HR is 0.5 then the relative risk of dying in one group is half the risk of dying in the other group.

Heterogeneity In the context of meta-analysis, heterogeneity means dissimilarity between studies. It can be because of the use of different statistical methods (statistical heterogeneity), or evaluation of people with different characteristics, treatments or outcomes (clinical heterogeneity). Heterogeneity may render pooling of data in meta-analysis unreliable or inappropriate.

Homogeneity Similarity (see heterogeneity above).

Incidence The number of new cases of a condition occurring in a population over a specified period of time.

Intention to treat analysis Analysis of data for all participants based on the group to which they were randomised and not based on the actual treatment they received.

Likelihood ratio The ratio of the probability that an individual with the target condition has a specified test result to the probability that an individual without the target condition has the same specified test result.

Meta-analysis A statistical technique that summarises the results of several studies in a single weighted estimate, in which more weight is given to results of studies with more events and sometimes to studies of higher quality.

Morbidity Rate of illness but not death.

Mortality Rate of death.

Negative likelihood ratio (NLR) The ratio of the probability that an individual with the target condition has a negative test result to the probability that an individual without the target condition has a negative test result. This is the same as the ratio (1-sensitivity/specificity).

Negative predictive value (NPV) The chance of not having a disease given a negative test result (not to be confused with specificity, which is the other way round; see below).

Not significant/non-significant (NS) In *Clinical Evidence*, not significant means that the observed difference, or a larger difference, could have arisen by chance with a probability of more than 1/20 (i.e. 5%), assuming that there is no underlying difference. This is not the same as saying there is no effect, just that this experiment does not provide convincing evidence of an effect. This could be because the trial was not powered to detect an effect that does exist, because there was no effect, or because of the play of chance.

Number needed to harm (NNH) One measure of treatment harm. It is the average number of people from a defined population you would need to treat with a specific intervention for a given period of time to cause one additional adverse outcome. NNH can be calculated as 1/ARI. In *Clinical Evidence*, these are usually rounded downwards.

Number needed to treat (NNT) One measure of treatment effectiveness. It is the number of people you would on average need to treat with a specific intervention for a given period of time to prevent one additional adverse outcome or achieve one additional beneficial outcome. NNT can be calculated as 1/ARR (see appendix 2). In *Clinical Evidence*, NNTs are usually rounded upwards.

NNT for a meta-analysis Absolute measures are useful at describing the effort required to obtain a benefit, but are limited because they are influenced by both the treatment and also by the baseline risk of the individual. If a meta-analysis includes individuals with a range of baseline risks, then no single NNT will be applicable to the people in that meta-analysis, but a single relative measure (odds ratio or relative risk) may be applicable if there is no heterogeneity. In *Clinical Evidence*, an NNT is provided for meta-analysis, based on a combination of the summary odds ratio (OR) and the mean baseline risk observed in average of the control groups.

Odds The odds of an event happening is defined as the probability that an event will occur, expressed as a proportion of the probability that the event will not occur.

Odds ratio (OR) One measure of treatment effectiveness. It is the odds of an event happening in the experimental group expressed as a proportion of the odds of an event happening in the control group. The closer the OR is to one, the smaller the difference in effect between the experimental intervention and the control intervention. If the OR is greater (or less) than one, then the effects of the treatment are more (or less) than those of the control treatment. Note that the effects being measured may be adverse (e.g. death or disability) or desirable (e.g. survival). When events are rare the OR is analagous to the relative risk (RR), but as event rates increase the OR and RR diverge.

Odds reduction The complement of odds ratio (1-OR), similar to the relative risk reduction (RRR) when events are rare.

Placebo A substance given in the control group of a clinical trial, which is ideally identical in appearance and taste or feel to the experimental treatment and believed to lack any disease specific effects. In the context of non-pharmacological interventions, placebo is usually referred to as sham treatments (see sham treatment below).

Positive likelihood ratio (LR+) The ratio of the probability that an individual with the target condition has a positive test result to the probability that an individual without the target condition has a positive test result. This is the same as the ratio (sensitivity/1-specificity).

Positive predictive value (PPV) The chance of having a disease given a positive test result (not to be confused with sensitivity, which is the other way round; see below).

Power A study has adequate power if it can reliably detect a clinically important difference (i.e. between two treatments) if one actually exists. The power of a study is increased when it includes more events or when its measurement of outcomes is more precise.

Pragmatic study An RCT designed to provide results that are directly applicable to normal practice (compared with explanatory trials that are intended to clarify efficacy under ideal conditions). Pragmatic RCTs recruit a population that is representative of those who are normally treated, allow normal compliance with instructions (by avoiding incentives and by using oral instructions with advice to follow manufacturers instructions), and analyse results by "intention to treat" rather than by "on treatment" methods.

Prevalence The proportion of people with a finding or disease in a given population at a given time.

Publication bias Occurs when the likelihood of a study being published varies with the results it finds. Usually, this occurs when studies that find a significant effect are more likely to be published than studies that do not find a significant effect, so making it appear from surveys of the published literature that treatments are more effective than is truly the case.

P value The probability that an observed or greater difference occurred by chance, if it is assumed that there is in fact no real difference between the effects of the interventions. If this probability is less than 1/20 (which is when the P value is less than 0.05), then the result is conventionally regarded as being "statistically significant".

Quasi randomised A trial using a method of allocating participants to different forms of care that is not truly random; for example, allocation by date of birth, day of the week, medical record number, month of the year, or the order in which participants are included in the study (e.g. alternation).

Random effects The "random effects" model assumes a different underlying effect for each study and takes this into consideration as an additional source of variation, which leads to somewhat wider confidence intervals than the fixed effects model. Effects are assumed to be randomly distributed, and the central point of this distribution is the focus of the combined effect estimate (see fixed effects above).

Randomised controlled trial (RCT) A trial in which participants are randomly assigned to two or more groups: at least one (the experimental group) receiving an intervention that is being tested and an other (the comparison or control group) receiving an alternative treatment or placebo. This design allows assessment of the relative effects of interventions.

Regression analysis Given data on a dependent variable and one or more independent variables, regression analysis involves finding the "best" mathematical model to describe or predict the dependent variable as a function of the independent variable(s). There are several regression models that suit different needs. Common forms are linear, logistic, and proportional hazards.

Relative risk (RR) The number of times more likely (RR > 1) or less likely (RR < 1) an event is to happen in one group compared with another. It is the ratio of the absolute risk (AR) for each group. It is analogous to the odds ratio (OR) when events are rare.

Relative risk increase (RRI) The proportional increase in risk between experimental and control participants in a trial.

Relative risk reduction (RRR) The proportional reduction in risk between experimental and control participants in a trial. It is the complement of the relative risk (1-RR).

Sensitivity The chance of having a positive test result given that you have a disease (not to be confused with positive predictive value [PPV], which is the other way around; see above).

Sensitivity analysis Analysis to test if results from meta-analysis are sensitive to restrictions on the data included. Common examples are large trials only, higher quality trials only, and more recent trials only. If results are consistent this provides stronger evidence of an effect and of generalisability.

Sham treatment An intervention given in the control group of a clinical trial, which is ideally identical in appearance and feel to the experimental treatment and believed to lack any disease specific effects (e.g. detuned ultrasound or random biofeedback).

Significant By convention, taken to mean statistically significant at the 5% level (see statistically significant below). This is the same as a 95% confidence interval not including the value corresponding to no effect.

Specificity The chance of having a negative test result given that you do not have a disease (not to be confused with negative predictive value [NPV], which is the other way around; see above).

Standardised mean difference (SMD) A measure of effect size used when outcomes are continuous (such as height, weight, or symptom scores) rather than dichotomous (such as death or myocardial infarction). The mean differences in outcome between the groups being studied are standardised to account for differences in scoring methods (such as pain scores). The measure is a ratio; therefore, it has no units.

Statistically significant Means that the findings of a study are unlikely to have arisen because of chance. Significance at the commonly cited 5% level ($P < 0.05$) means that the observed difference or greater difference would occur by chance in only 1/20 similar cases. Where the word "significant" or "significance" is used without qualification in the text, it is being used in this statistical sense.

Subgroup analysis Analysis of a part of the trial/meta-analysis population in which it is thought the effect may differ from the mean effect.

Systematic review A review in which specified and appropriate methods have been used to identify, appraise, and summarise studies addressing a defined question. It can, but need not, involve meta-analysis (see meta-analysis). In *Clinical Evidence*, the term systematic review refers to a systematic review of RCTs unless specified otherwise.

True negative A person without the target condition (defined by a gold standard) who has a negative test result.

True positive A person with the target condition (defined by a gold standard) who also has a positive test result.

Validity The soundness or rigour of a study. A study is internally valid if the way it is designed and carried out means that the results are unbiased and it gives you an accurate estimate of the effect that is being measured. A study is externally valid if its results are applicable to people encountered in regular clinical practice.

Weighted mean difference (WMD) A measure of effect size used when outcomes are continuous (such as symptom scores or height) rather than dichotomous (such as death or myocardial infarction). The mean differences in outcome between the groups being studied are weighted to account for different sample sizes and differing precision between studies. The WMD is an absolute figure and so takes the units of the original outcome measure.

Acute atrial fibrillation

Search date October 2001

Gregory Y H Lip, Sridhar Kamath, and Bethan Freestone

QUESTIONS

INTERVENTIONS

To be covered in future updates
Quinidine, procainamide, disopyramide, flecainide, propafenone, amiodarone, sotalol, ibutilide, dofeltilide

Covered elsewhere in *Clinical Evidence*
Stroke prevention (see Stroke prevention, p 184)

See glossary, p 8.

Key Messages

Heart rate control

- **Digoxin** Two RCTs found that digoxin versus placebo significantly reduced ventricular rate after 30 minutes or 18 hours in people with atrial fibrillation.
- **Diltiazem** One RCT in people with atrial fibrillation or atrial flutter found that intravenous diltiazem (a calcium channel blocker) versus placebo significantly reduced heart rate over 15 minutes. Another RCT in people with acute atrial fibrillation or atrial flutter found that intravenous diltiazem versus intravenous digoxin significantly reduced heart rate within 5 minutes.
- **Timolol** One small RCT in people with atrial fibrillation found that intravenous timolol (a β blocker) versus placebo significantly reduced ventricular rate within 20 minutes.
- **Verapamil** Two RCTs found that intravenous verapamil (a calcium channel blocker) versus placebo significantly reduced heart rate at 10 or 30 minutes in people with atrial fibrillation or atrial flutter. One RCT found no significant difference in rate control or measures of systolic function with intravenous verapamil versus intravenous diltiazem in people with atrial fibrillation or atrial flutter, but verapamil caused hypotension in some people.

Conversion to sinus rhythm

- **DC cardioversion** We found no RCTs of DC cardioversion in acute atrial fibrillation. It may be unethical to conduct RCTs.

- **Digoxin** Three RCTs found no significant difference in conversion to sinus rhythm with digoxin versus placebo in people with atrial fibrillation.
- **Timolol** One small RCT found that intravenous timolol (a β blocker) versus placebo increased conversion to sinus rhythm in people with atrial fibrillation, but the difference was not significant.

Prevention of embolism

- **Antithrombotic treatment prior to cardioversion** We found no RCTs of aspirin, heparin, or warfarin as thromboprophylaxis prior to cardioversion in acute atrial fibrillation.

DEFINITION Acute atrial fibrillation is the sudden onset of rapid, irregular, and chaotic atrial activity, and the 48 hours after that onset. It includes both the first symptomatic onset of persistent atrial fibrillation (see glossary, p 9) and episodes of paroxysmal atrial fibrillation (see glossary, p 9). It is sometimes difficult to distinguish episodes of new onset atrial fibrillation from newly diagnosed atrial fibrillation. Atrial fibrillation within 72 hours of onset is sometimes called recent onset atrial fibrillation. By contrast, chronic atrial fibrillation (see glossary, p 8) is a more sustained form of atrial fibrillation, which in turn can be described as paroxysmal, persistent, or permanent atrial fibrillation (see glossary, p 9). If the atrial fibrillation recurs intermittently, with sinus rhythm between recurrences and with spontaneous recurrences/termination, then it is designated as paroxysmal atrial fibrillation. More sustained atrial fibrillation, which can be successfully reverted back to sinus rhythm (cardioversion), is designated persistent atrial fibrillation. If cardioversion is inappropriate, then atrial fibrillation is designated as permanent atrial fibrillation. In this review we have excluded episodes of atrial fibrillation that arise during or soon after cardiac surgery, and we have excluded the management of chronic atrial fibrillation.

INCIDENCE/ PREVALENCE We found limited evidence of the incidence or prevalence of acute atrial fibrillation. Extrapolation from the Framingham study[1] suggests an incidence in men of 3/1000 person years at age 55 years, rising to 38/1000 person years at 94 years. In women, the incidence was 2/1000 person years at age 55 years and 32.5/1000 person years at 94 years. The prevalence of atrial fibrillation ranged from 0.5% for people aged 50–59 years to 9% in people aged 80–89 years. Among acute emergency medical admissions in the UK, 3–6% have atrial fibrillation and about 40% were newly diagnosed.[2,3] Among acute hospital admissions in New Zealand, 10% (95% CI 9% to 12%) had documented atrial fibrillation.[4]

AETIOLOGY/ RISK FACTORS Paroxysms of atrial fibrillation are more common in athletes.[5] Age increases the risk of developing acute atrial fibrillation. Men are more likely to develop atrial fibrillation than women (38 years' follow up from the Framingham Study, RR after adjustment for age and known predisposing conditions 1.5).[6] Atrial fibrillation can occur in association with underlying disease (both cardiac and non-cardiac) or can arise in the absence of any other condition. Epidemiological surveys have found that risk factors for the development of acute atrial fibrillation include ischaemic heart disease, hypertension, heart failure, valve disease, diabetes, alcohol abuse, thyroid disorders, and disorders of the lung and pleura.[1] In a UK survey of acute hospital admissions with atrial fibrillation, a history of ischaemic heart disease was present in 33%, heart failure in 24%, hypertension in 26%, and rheumatic heart disease in 7%.[3] In some populations, the acute effects of alcohol explain a large proportion of the incidence of acute atrial fibrillation.

PROGNOSIS We found no evidence about the proportion of people with acute atrial fibrillation who develop more chronic forms of atrial fibrillation (e.g. paroxysmal, persistent, or permanent atrial fibrillation). Observational studies and placebo arms of RCTs have found that more than 50% of people with acute atrial fibrillation revert spontaneously within 24–48 hours, especially atrial fibrillation associated with an identifiable precipitant such as alcohol or myocardial infarction. We found little evidence about the effects on mortality and morbidity of acute atrial fibrillation where no underlying cause is found. Acute atrial fibrillation during myocardial infarction is an independent predictor of both short term and long term mortality.[7] Onset of atrial fibrillation reduces cardiac output by 10–20% irrespective of the underlying ventricular rate[8,9] and can contribute to heart failure. People with acute atrial fibrillation who present with heart failure have worse prognosis. Acute atrial fibrillation is associated with a risk of imminent stroke.[10–13] One case series used transoesophageal echocardiography in people who had developed acute atrial fibrillation within the preceding 48 hours; it found that 15% had atrial thrombi.[14] An ischaemic stroke associated with atrial fibrillation is more likely to be fatal, have a recurrence, and leave a serious functional deficit among survivors, than a stroke not associated with atrial fibrillation.[15]

AIMS To reduce symptoms, morbidity, and mortality, with minimum adverse effects.

OUTCOMES Major outcomes include measures of symptoms, recurrent stroke or transient ischaemic attack, thromboembolism, mortality, and major bleeding. Proxy measures include heart rhythm, ventricular rate, and timing to restoration of sinus rhythm. Frequent spontaneous reversion to sinus rhythm makes it difficult to interpret short term studies of rhythm; treatments may accelerate restoration of sinus rhythm without increasing the proportion of people who eventually convert. The clinical importance of changes in mean heart rate is also unclear.

METHODS *Clinical Evidence* search and appraisal October 2001. Current Contents, textbooks, review articles, and recent abstracts were reviewed. Many studies were not solely in people with acute atrial fibrillation. The text indicates where results have been extrapolated from studies of paroxysmal, persistent, or permanent atrial fibrillation. Atrial fibrillation that follows coronary surgery has been excluded.

QUESTION **What are the effects of treatments for acute atrial fibrillation?**

OPTION **ANTITHROMBOTIC TREATMENT PRIOR TO CARDIOVERSION**

We found no RCTs on use of aspirin, heparin, or warfarin as thromboprophylaxis prior to cardioversion in acute atrial fibrillation.

Benefits: We found no RCTs on use of aspirin, heparin, or warfarin as thromboprophylaxis prior to cardioversion in acute atrial fibrillation.

Harms: We found no RCTs.

Comment: For acute atrial fibrillation, there is consensus to give heparin to people undergoing cardioversion within 48 hours of arrhythmia onset.[16] Warfarin is not used as an anticoagulant in acute atrial fibrillation because of its slow onset of action. One transoesophageal echocardiography study in people with a recent embolic event found left atrial thrombus in 15% of people with acute atrial fibrillation of less than 3 days' duration.[14] This would suggest that people with atrial fibrillation of less than 3 days' duration may benefit from formal anticoagulation or require evaluation by transoesophageal echocardiography before safe cardioversion. One ongoing trial comparing low molecular weight and unfractionated heparin in people with atrial fibrillation of more than 2 days duration undergoing transoesophageal echocardiographically guided early electrical or chemical cardioversion, will recruit 200 people to assess the feasibility and effects of such a strategy.[17]

OPTION **DC CARDIOVERSION**

We found no RCTs on use of DC cardioversion in acute atrial fibrillation. It may be unethical to conduct RCTs of DC cardioversion in people with acute atrial fibrillation and haemodynamic compromise.

Benefits: We found no RCTs on use of DC cardioversion in acute atrial fibrillation. It may be unethical to conduct RCTs on use of DC cardioversion in people with acute atrial fibrillation and haemodynamic compromise.

Harms: We found no RCTs on use of DC cardioversion in acute atrial fibrillation. Adverse events from synchronised DC cardioversion include those associated with a general anaesthetic, generation of a more serious arrhythmia, superficial burns, and thromboembolism. Cardioversion may be unsuccessful. The atrial fibrillation may recur.

Comment: It may be unethical to conduct RCTs on the use of DC cardioversion in people with acute atrial fibrillation and haemodynamic compromise. The evidence for DC cardioversion in acute atrial fibrillation can only be extrapolated from its use in chronic atrial fibrillation (see glossary, p 8). DC cardioversion has been used for the treatment of atrial fibrillation since the 1960s.[18] There is a consensus[16] that immediate DC cardioversion for acute atrial fibrillation should be attempted only if there are signs of haemodynamic compromise.

Otherwise full anticoagulation is recommended (warfarin for 3 weeks prior to and 4 weeks following cardioversion) to reduce the risk of thromboembolism in people with acute atrial fibrilation of more than 48 hours' duration.[16] We found no clear evidence on whether cardioversion or rate control is superior for acute atrial fibrillation.

OPTION DIGOXIN

Three RCTs found no significant difference in conversion to sinus rhythm with digoxin versus placebo in people with atrial fibrillation. Two RCTs found that digoxin versus placebo significantly reduced ventricular rate after 30 minutes and 18 hours in people with atrial fibrillation.

Benefits: We found no systematic review but found three RCTs.[19–21] **Versus placebo:** One RCT (239 people within 7 days of onset of atrial fibrillation, mean age 66 years, mean ventricular rate 122 beats/min) found that intravenous digoxin (mean 0.88 mg) versus placebo did not increase the restoration of sinus rhythm by 16 hours (51% with digoxin *v* 46% with placebo).[19] It found a rapid and clinically important reduction in ventricular rate at 2 hours (to 105 beats/min with digoxin *v* 117 beats/min with placebo; $P = 0.0001$). The second RCT (40 people within 7 days of the onset of atrial fibrillation, mean age 64 years, 23 men) compared high dose intravenous digoxin (1.25 mg) versus placebo. Restoration to sinus rhythm was not significantly different (9/19 [47%] with digoxin *v* 8/20 [40%] with placebo; $P = 0.6$). The ventricular rate after 30 minutes was significantly lower with digoxin versus placebo ($P < 0.02$).[20] The third RCT (36 people within 7 days of the onset of atrial fibrillation) compared oral digoxin (doses of 0.6, 0.4, 0.2, and 0.2 mg at 0, 4, 8, and 14 h, or until conversion to sinus rhythm, whichever occurred first) versus placebo. Conversion to sinus rhythm by 18 hours was not significantly different (50% with digoxin *v* 44% with placebo; ARR +6%, 95% CI −11% to +22%).[21]

Harms: In one RCT some people developed asymptomatic bradycardia and one person with previously undiagnosed hypertrophic cardiomyopathy suffered circulatory distress.[19] In the second RCT, two people developed bradyarrhythmias.[20] No adverse effects were stated in the third RCT.[21] Digoxin at toxic doses may result in visual, gastrointestinal, and neurological symptoms; heart block; and arrhythmias.

Comment: The peak action of digoxin is delayed: taking 6–12 hours to reduce mean ventricular rate below 100 beats/minute. We found one systematic review and RCTs of digoxin versus placebo in people with chronic atrial fibrillation (see glossary, p 8), which found that control of the ventricular rate during exercise was poor unless a β blocker or rate limiting calcium channel blocker (verapamil or diltiazem) was used in combination.[22–24] The evidence suggests that digoxin is no better than placebo at restoring sinus rhythm in people with recent onset atrial fibrillation.

OPTION DILTIAZEM

One RCT found that intravenous diltiazem (a calcium channel blocker) versus placebo significantly reduced heart rate in people with atrial fibrillation or atrial flutter. One RCT found that intravenous diltiazem versus intravenous digoxin significantly reduced heart rate within 5 minutes in people with acute atrial fibrillation and atrial flutter.

Benefits: We found no systematic review but found three RCTs.[25–27] **Versus placebo:** One RCT (113 people; 89 with atrial fibrillation and 24 with [atrial flutter — see glossary, p 8]; ventricular rate > 120 beats/min; systolic blood pressure ≥ 90 mm Hg without severe heart failure; 108 people with at least one underlying condition that may explain atrial arrhythmia; mean age 64 years) compared intravenous diltiazem (a calcium channel blocker) versus placebo.[25] Following randomisation, a dose of intravenous diltiazem (or equivalent placebo) 0.25 mg/kg every 2 minutes was given; if the first dose had no effect after 15 minutes, then the code was broken and diltiazem 0.35 mg/kg every 2 minutes was given regardless of randomisation. The RCT found that intravenous diltiazem versus placebo significantly decreased heart rate during a 15 minute observation period (ventricular rate below 100 beats/min 42/56 [75%] with diltiazem *v* 4/57 [7%] with placebo; $P < 0.001$; average decrease in heart rate, 22% with diltiazem *v* 3% with placebo; median time from start of drug infusion to maximal decrease in heart rate 4.3 min, mean rate decreased from 139 to 114 beats/min with diltiazem).[25] The RCT found no difference in response rate to diltiazem in people with atrial fibrillation versus those with atrial flutter. **Versus digoxin:** One RCT (30 consecutive people, 10 men, mean age 72 years, 26 with acute atrial fibrillation, 4 with atrial flutter, unspecified duration) compared intravenous diltiazem versus intravenous digoxin versus both given on admission to the Accident and Emergency Department.[26] Heart rate control was defined as a ventricular rate of less than 100 beats/minute. Intravenous digoxin (0.25 mg given as a bolus at 0 and 30 min) and intravenous diltiazem (initially 0.25 mg/kg over the first 2 min, followed by 0.35 mg/kg at 15 min and then a titratable infusion at a rate of 10–20 mg/h) were given to maintain heart rate control. The dosing regimens were the same whether the drugs were given alone or in combination. The RCT found that diltiazem versus digoxin significantly decreased ventricular heart rate within 5 minutes ($P = 0.0006$; mean rates 111 beats/min with diltiazem *v* 144 beats/min with digoxin). The decrease in heart rate achieved with digoxin did not reach statistical significance until 180 minutes ($P = 0.01$; mean rates 90 beats/min with diltiazem *v* 117 beats/min with digoxin). No additional benefit was found with the combination of digoxin and diltiazem. **Versus verapamil:** See text, p 7.

Harms: In one RCT, in the diltiazem treated group, seven people developed asymptomatic hypotension (systolic blood pressure < 90 mm Hg), three developed flushing, three developed itching, and one developed nausea and vomiting; these were not significantly different from placebo.[25] The second RCT was not large enough to adequately assess adverse effects, and none were apparent.[26] Rate limiting calcium channel blockers may exacerbate heart failure and hypotension.

Comment: The evidence suggests that rate limiting calcium channel blockers such as verapamil and diltiazem reduce ventricular rate in acute or recent onset atrial fibrillation, but they are probably no better than placebo in restoring sinus rhythm. We found no studies of the effect of rate limiting calcium channel blockers on exercise tolerance in people with acute or recent onset atrial fibrillation, but studies in people with chronic atrial fibrillation (see glossary, p 8) have found improved exercise tolerance.

OPTION TIMOLOL

One small RCT found that timolol (a β blocker) versus placebo significantly reduced ventricular rate within 20 minutes and found a non-significant increase in conversion to sinus rhythm in people with atrial fibrillation of unspecified duration.

Benefits: We found no systematic review. **Versus placebo:** We found one RCT (61 people with atrial fibrillation of unspecified duration, ventricular rate > 120 beats/min) that compared intravenous timolol (a β blocker) (1 mg) versus intravenous placebo given immediately and repeated twice at 20 minute intervals if sinus rhythm was not achieved.[28] It found that 20 minutes after the last injection, intravenous timolol versus placebo significantly increased the proportion of people who had a ventricular rate below 100 beats/minute (41% with timolol *v* 3% with placebo; $P < 0.01$), and increased the proportion of people who converted to sinus rhythm, although the increase was not significant (5/29 [17%] *v* 2/32 [6%]; $P = 0.18$).

Harms: In the RCT, the most common adverse effects were bradycardia (2%) and hypotension (9%).[28] β Blockers may exacerbate heart failure and hypotension in acute atrial fibrillation. β Blockers plus rate limiting calcium channel blockers (diltiazem, verapamil) may increase the risk of asystole and sinus arrest.[29–31] β Blockers can precipitate bronchospasm.[32]

Comment: In addition to the evidence from people with acute atrial fibrillation, we found one systematic review of β blockers versus placebo in people with either acute or chronic atrial fibrillation (see glossary, p 8).[22] It found that in 7/12 comparisons at rest and in all during exercise, β blockers reduced ventricular rate compared with placebo. We found no RCTs that reported quality of life, functional capacity, or mortality.

OPTION VERAPAMIL

Two RCTs found that intravenous verapamil (a calcium channel blocker) versus placebo significantly reduced heart rate at 10 or 30 minutes in people with atrial fibrillation or atrial flutter. One RCT found no significant difference with intravenous verapamil versus intravenous diltiazem (both calcium channel blockers) in rate control or measures of systolic function in people with atrial fibrillation or atrial flutter, but verapamil caused hypotension in some people.

Benefits: We found no systematic review in people with acute atrial fibrillation. **Versus placebo:** We found two RCTs.[33,34] The first RCT (21 men with atrial fibrillation and a rapid ventricular rate, age 37–70 years) was a crossover comparison of intravenous verapamil versus placebo (saline).[33] It found that intravenous verapamil versus placebo reduced ventricular rate within 10 minutes (reduction > 15% of the initial rate 17/20 [85%] with verapamil *v* 2/14 [14%] with saline). It also found that three people converted to sinus rhythm, but it is not clear from the results whether these effects can be attributed to verapamil or saline. The second RCT (double blind, crossover study of 20 people with atrial fibrillation or [atrial flutter — see glossary, p 8] for 2 h to 2 years) compared intravenous low dose verapamil (0.075 mg/kg) versus placebo.[34] A positive response was defined as conversion to sinus rhythm or a decrease of the ventricular response to less than 100 beats/minute, or by more than 20% of the initial rate. If a positive response did not occur within 10 minutes, then a second bolus injection was given (placebo for people who initially received verapamil, verapamil for people who initially received placebo). It found no significant difference between low dose verapamil (0.075 mg/kg) versus placebo. With the first bolus injection, verapamil versus placebo significantly reduced ventricular rate (mean heart rate 118 beats/min with verapamil *v* 138 beats/min with placebo), and more people converted to sinus rhythm within 30 minutes but the difference was not significant (3/20 [15%] with verapamil *v* 0/15 with placebo; P = 0.12). **Versus diltiazem:** We found one small double blind, crossover RCT (17 men, 5 with acute atrial fibrillation, 10 with atrial flutter, and 2 with combination of atrial fibrillation and atrial flutter; ventricular rate ≥ 120 beats/min, systolic blood pressure > 100 mm Hg) compared intravenous verapamil versus intravenous diltiazem.[27] It found no significant differences in rate control or measures of systolic function.

Harms: One RCT reported that intravenous verapamil caused a transient drop in systolic and diastolic blood pressure greater than with placebo (saline), which did not require treatment, but did not state the number of people affected.[33] The second RCT reported development of 1:1 flutter in one person with Wolff Parkinson White syndrome (see glossary, p 9) and 2:1 flutter.[34] In the third RCT, comparing verapamil versus diltiazem, 3/17 (18%) of people receiving verapamil as the first drug developed symptomatic hypotension and were withdrawn from the study before crossover.[27] Two people recovered, but the episode in the third person was considered to be life threatening. In people with Wolff Parkinson White syndrome, verapamil may increase the ventricular rate and can cause ventricular arrhythmias.[35] Rate limiting calcium channel blockers may exacerbate heart failure and hypotension.

Comment: See comment, p 7

GLOSSARY

Atrial flutter A similar arrhythmia to atrial fibrillation but the atrial electrical activity is less chaotic and has a characteristic saw tooth appearance on an electrocardiogram.

Chronic atrial fibrillation Refers to more sustained or recurrent forms of atrial fibrillation, which can be subdivided into paroxysmal, persistent, or permanent atrial fibrillation.

Paroxysmal atrial fibrillation If the atrial fibrillation recurs intermittently with sinus rhythm, with spontaneous recurrences/termination, it is designated as "paroxysmal", and the objective of management is suppression of paroxysms and maintenance of sinus rhythm.

Permanent atrial fibrillation If cardioversion is inappropriate, and has not been indicated or attempted, atrial fibrillation is designated as "permanent", where the objective of management is rate control and antithrombotic treatment.

Persistent atrial fibrillation When atrial fibrillation is more sustained, atrial fibrillation is designated "persistent", necessitating termination with pharmacological treatment or electrical cardioversion.

Wolff Parkinson White syndrome Occurs when an additional electrical pathway exists between the atria and ventricles as a result of anomalous embryonic development. The extra pathway may cause rapid arrhythmias. Worldwide it affects about 0.2% of the general population. In people with Wolff Parkinson White syndrome, β blockers, calcium channel blockers, and digoxin can increase the ventricular rate and cause ventricular arrhythmias.

REFERENCES

1. Benjamin EJ, Wolf PA, Kannel WA. The epidemiology of atrial fibrillation. In: Falk RH, Podrid P, eds. *Atrial fibrillation: mechanisms and management*. 2nd ed. Philadelphia: Lippincott-Raven Publishers, 1997:1–22.
2. Lip GYH, Tean KN, Dunn FG. Treatment of atrial fibrillation in a district general hospital. *Br Heart J* 1994;71:92–95.
3. Zarifis J, Beevers DG, Lip GYH. Acute admissions with atrial fibrillation in a British multiracial hospital population. *Br J Clin Pract* 1997;51:91–96.
4. Stewart FM, Singh Y, Persson S, Gamble GD, Braatvedt GD. Atrial fibrillation: prevalence and management in an acute general medical unit. *Aust N Z J Med* 1999;29:51–58.
5. Furlanello F, Bertoldi A, Dallago M, et al. Atrial fibrillation in elite athletes. *J Cardiovasc Electrophysiol* 1998;9(8 suppl):63–68.
6. Kannel WB, Wolf PA, Benjamin EJ, Levy D. Prevalence, incidence, prognosis, and predisposing conditions for atrial fibrillation: population-based estimates. *Am J Cardiol* 1998;82:2N–9N.
7. Pedersen OD, Bagger H, Kober L, Torp-Pedersen C. The occurrence and prognostic significance of atrial fibrillation/flutter following acute myocardial infarction. TRACE Study group. TRAndolapril Cardiac Evaluation. *Eur Heart J* 1999;20:748–754.
8. Clark DM, Plumb VJ, Epstein AE, Kay GN. Hemodynamic effects of an irregular sequence of ventricular cycle lengths during atrial fibrillation. *J Am Coll Cardiol* 1997;30:1039–1045.
9. Schumacher B, Luderitz B. Rate issues in atrial fibrillation: consequences of tachycardia and therapy for rate control. *Am J Cardiol* 1998;82:29N–36N.
10. Peterson P, Godfredson J. Embolic complications in paroxysmal atrial fibrillation. *Stroke* 1986;17:622–626.
11. Sherman DG, Goldman L, Whiting RB, Jurgensen K, Kaste M, Easton JD. Thromboembolism in patients with atrial fibrillation. *Arch Neurol* 1984;41:708–710.
12. Wolf PA, Kannel WB, McGee DL, Meeks SL, Bharucha NE, McNamara PM. Duration of atrial fibrillation and imminence of stroke: the Framingham study. *Stroke* 1983;14:664–667.
13. Corbalan R, Arriagada D, Braun S, et al. Risk factors for systemic embolism in patients with paroxysmal atrial fibrillation. *Am Heart J* 1992;124:149–153.
14. Stoddard ME, Dawkins PR, Prince CR, Ammash NM. Left atrial appendage thrombus is not uncommon in patients with acute atrial fibrillation and a recent embolic event: a transesophageal echocardiographic study. *J Am Coll Cardiol* 1995;25:452–459.
15. Lin HJ, Wolf PA, Kelly-Hayes M, et al. Stroke severity in atrial fibrillation. The Framingham Study. *Stroke* 1996;27:1760–1764.
16. Fuster V, Ryden LE, Asinger RW, et al. ACC/AHA/ESC Guidelines for the management of patients with atrial fibrillation: Executive summary. *Circulation* 2001;104:2118–2150.
17. Murray RD, Shah A, Jasper SE, et al. Transoesophageal echocardiography guided enoxaparin antithrombotic strategy for cardioversion of atrial fibrillation: the ACUTE II pilot study. *Am Heart J* 2000;139:1–7.
18. Lown B, Amarasingham R, Neuman J. Landmark article Nov 3, 1962: New method for terminating cardiac arrhythmias. Use of synchronised capacitator discharge. *JAMA* 1986:256;621–627.
19. DAAF trial group. Intravenous digoxin in acute atrial fibrillation. Results of a randomized, placebo-controlled multicentre trial in 239 patients. The Digitalis in Acute AF (DAAF) Trial Group. *Eur Heart J* 1997;18:649–654.
20. Jordaens L, Trouerbach J, Calle P, et al. Conversion of atrial fibrillation to sinus rhythm and rate control by digoxin in comparison to placebo. *Eur Heart J* 1997;18:643–648.
21. Falk RH, Knowlton AA, Bernard SA, Gotlieb NE, Battinelli NJ. Digoxin for converting recent-onset atrial fibrillation to sinus rhythm. *Ann Intern Med* 1987;106:503–506.
22. McNamara RL, Bass EB, Miller MR, et al. Management of new onset atrial fibrillation. Evidence Report/Technology Assessment No. 12 (prepared by the John Hopkins University Evidence-based Practice centre in Baltimore, MD, under contract no. 290–97–0006). AHRQ publication number 01-E026. Rockville, MD: Agency for Healthcare Research and Quality. January 2001. Search date 1998; primary sources The Cochrane Library, Medline, Pubmed's "related links" feature, reviews of Cochrane hand

search results, and handsearches of reference lists and scanning of tables of contents from relevant journals.

23. Farshi R, Kistner D, Sarma JS, Longmate JA, Singh BN. Ventricular rate control in chronic atrial fibrillation during daily activity and programmed exercise: a crossover open-label study of five drug regimens. *J Am Coll Cardiol* 1999;33:304–310.
24. Klein HO, Pauzner H, Di Segni E, David D, Kaplinsky E. The beneficial effects of verapamil in chronic atrial fibrillation. *Arch Intern Med* 1979;139:747–749.
25. Salerno DM, Dias VC, Kleiger RE, et al. Efficacy and safety of intravenous diltiazem for treatment of atrial fibrillation and atrial flutter: the Diltiazem-Atrial Fibrillation/Flutter Study Group. *Am J Cardiol* 1989;63:1046–1051.
26. Schreck DM, Rivera AR, Tricarico VJ. Emergency management of atrial fibrillation and flutter: intravenous diltiazem versus intravenous digoxin *Ann Emerg Med* 1997;29:135–140.
27. Phillips BG, Gandhi AJ, Sanoski CA, Just VL, Bauman JL. Comparison of intravenous diltiazem and verapamil for the acute treatment of atrial fibrillation and atrial flutter. *Pharmacotherapy* 1997;17:1238–1245.
28. Sweany AE, Moncloa F, Vickers FF, Zupkis RV, Rahway NJ. Antiarrhythmic effects of intravenous timolol in supraventricular arrhythmias. *Clin Pharmacol Ther* 1985;37:124–127.
29. Lee TH, Salomon DR, Rayment CM, Antman EM. Hypotension and sinus arrest with exercise-induced hyperkalemia and combined verapamil/propranolol therapy. *Am J Med* 1986;80:1203–1204.
30. Misra M, Thakur R, Bhandari K. Sinus arrest caused by atenolol-verapamil combination. *Clin Cardiol* 1987;10:365–367.
31. Yeh SJ, Yamamoto T, Lin FC, Wang CC, Wu D. Repetitive sinoatrial exit block as the major mechanism of drug-provoked long sinus or atrial pause. *J Am Coll Cardiol* 1991;18:587–595.
32. Doshan HD, Rosenthal RR, Brown R, Slutsky A, Applin WJ, Caruso FS. Celiprolol, atenolol and propranolol: a comparison of pulmonary effects in asthmatic patients. *J Cardiovasc Pharmacol* 1986;8(suppl 4):105–108.
33. Aronow WS, Ferlinz J. Verapamil versus placebo in atrial fibrillation and atrial flutter. *Clin Invest Med* 1980;3:35–39.
34. Waxman HL, Myerburg RJ, Appel R, Sung RJ. Verapamil for control of ventricular rate in paroxysmal supraventricular tachycardia and atrial fibrillation or flutter: a double-blind randomized cross-over study. *Ann Intern Med* 1981;94:1–6.
35. Strasberg B, Sagie A, Rechavia E, et al. Deleterious effects of intravenous verapamil in Wolff-Parkinson-White patients and atrial fibrillation. *Cardiovasc Drugs Ther* 1989;2:801–806.

Bethan Freestone
Research Fellow
Haemostasis Thrombosis and Vascular Biology Unit University Department of Medicine City Hospital
Birmingham
UK

Sridhar Kamath
Research Fellow
Haemostasis Thrombosis and Vascular Biology Unit University Department of Medicine City Hospital
Birmingham
UK

Gregory Lip
Professor of Cardiovascular Medicine
Haemostasis Thrombosis and Vascular Biology Unit University Department of Medicine City Hospital
Birmingham
UK

Competing interests: GL is UK principal investigator for the ERAFT Trial (Knoll) and has been reimbursed by various pharmaceutical companies for attending several conferences, and running educational programmes and research projects. SK, none declared. BF, none declared.

Acute myocardial infarction

Search date October 2001

Nicolas Danchin, Edoardo De Benedetti, and Philip Urban

QUESTIONS

INTERVENTIONS

See glossary, p 27

Key Messages

Improving outcomes in acute myocardial infarction

- **Angiotensin converting enzyme inhibitors** One overview and one systematic review in people within 36 hours of acute myocardial infarction have found that angiotensin converting enzyme inhibitors versus placebo significantly reduce mortality at 30 days. The overview also found that angiotensin converting enzyme inhibitors significantly increase persistent hypotension and renal dysfunction. The question of whether angiotensin converting enzyme inhibitors should be offered to everyone presenting with acute myocardial infarction or only to people with signs of heart failure remains unresolved.
- **Aspirin** One systematic review in people with acute myocardial infarction has found that aspirin versus placebo significantly reduces mortality (NNT 41, 95% CI 31 to 62), non-fatal reinfarction (NNT 84, 95% CI 71 to 109), and non-fatal stroke (NNT 413, 95% CI 273 to 2025) at 1 month.

Acute myocardial infarction

- **β Blockers** Two systematic reviews and one subsequent RCT have found that β blockers versus control given within hours of infarction significantly reduce both mortality and reinfarction. One RCT in people receiving thrombolytic treatment found that immediate versus delayed treatment with metoprolol significantly reduced rates of reinfarction and recurrent chest pain at 6 days, but had no significant effect on mortality in the short term or at 1 year. One RCT comparing carvedilol versus placebo in people with recent myocardial infarction and left ejection fraction ≤40% receiving thrombolytic treatment found no significant difference in the combined endpoint of all cause mortality and hospital admission for any cardiovascular event after a median of 1.3 years, although mortality, and recurrent non fatal myocardial infarction were significantly lower with carvedilol.
- **Calcium channel blockers** RCTs in people within the first few days of an acute myocardial infarction have found that calcium channel blockers versus placebo do not reduce mortality, and in the subgroup of people with left ventricular dysfunction calcium channel blockers versus placebo may increase mortality.
- **Nitrates** One systematic review (prior to the introduction of thrombolysis) has found that nitrates versus placebo significantly reduced the risk of mortality. Two RCTs (after the introduction of thrombolysis) comparing nitrates versus placebo found no significant difference in mortality.
- **Primary percutaneous transluminal coronary angioplasty versus thrombolysis (performed in specialist centres)** Two systematic reviews have found that primary percutaneous transluminal coronary angioplasty versus primary thrombolysis significantly reduces mortality and reinfarction at 30 days. However, the trials were conducted mainly in specialist centres and the effectiveness of percutaneous transluminal coronary angioplasty versus thrombolysis in less specialist centres remains to be defined.
- **Thrombolysis** One overview of RCTs in people with acute myocardial infarction and ST elevation or bundle branch block on their initial electrocardiogram has found that prompt thrombolytic treatment (within 6 h and perhaps up to 12 h and longer after the onset of symptoms) versus placebo significantly reduces short term mortality. The overview found that thrombolytic treatment versus control significantly increased the risk of stroke or major bleeding. Meta-analysis of RCTs comparing different types of thrombolytic agents versus each other have found no significant difference in mortality.

Cardiogenic shock after acute myocardial infarction

- **Early invasive cardiac revascularisation** One RCT has found that early invasive cardiac revascularisation versus initial medical treatment alone significantly reduces mortality after 6 months (NNT 8, 95% CI 5 to 68) and 12 months (NNT 8, 95% CI 5 to 61). A second RCT found similar results, although the difference was not significant.
- **Intra-aortic balloon counterpulsation** One abstract of an RCT comparing intra-aortic balloon counterpulsation plus thrombolysis versus thrombolysis alone found no significant difference in mortality after 6 months.
- **Thrombolysis** Subgroup analysis of people with cardiogenic shock after acute myocardial infarction from one RCT comparing thrombolysis versus no thrombolysis found no significant difference in mortality after 21 days.
- **Early cardiac surgery; positive inotropes and vasodilators; pulmonary artery catheterisation; ventricular assistance devices and cardiac transplantation** We found no evidence from RCTs about the effects of these interventions.

DEFINITION **Acute myocardial infarction:** The sudden occlusion of a coronary artery leading to myocardial cell death. **Cardiogenic shock:** Defined clinically as a poor cardiac output plus evidence of tissue hypoxia that is not improved by correction of reduced intravascular volume.[1] When a pulmonary artery catheter is used, cardiogenic shock may be defined as a cardiac index (see glossary, p 27) below 2.2 litres/minute/m^2 despite an elevated pulmonary capillary wedge pressure ($\geq$ 15 mm Hg).[1–3]

INCIDENCE/ PREVALENCE **Acute myocardial infarction:** One of the most common causes of mortality in both developed and developing nations. In 1990, ischaemic heart disease was the leading cause of death worldwide, accounting for about 6.3 million deaths. The age standardised incidence varies among and within countries.[4] Each year, about 900 000 people in the USA experience an acute myocardial infarction and about 225 000 of them die. About half of these people die within 1 hour of symptoms and before reaching a hospital emergency room.[5] Event rates increase with age for both sexes and are higher in men than in women, and in poorer than richer people at all ages. The incidence of death from acute myocardial infarction has fallen in many Western countries over the past 20 years. **Cardiogenic shock:** Cardiogenic shock occurs in about 7% of people admitted to hospital with acute myocardial infarction.[6] Of these, about half have established cardiogenic shock at the time of admission to hospital, and most of the others develop it during the first 24–48 hours of their admission.[7]

AETIOLOGY/ RISK FACTORS **Acute myocardial infarction (AMI):** See aetiology/risk factors under primary prevention, p 95. The immediate mechanism of acute myocardial infarction is rupture of an atheromatous plaque causing thrombosis and occlusion of coronary arteries and myocardial cell death. Factors that may convert a stable plaque into an unstable plaque (the "active plaque") have yet to be fully elucidated; however, shear stresses, inflammation, and autoimmunity have been proposed. The changing rates of coronary heart disease in different populations are only partly explained by changes in the standard risk factors for ischaemic heart disease (particularly fall in blood pressure and smoking). **Cardiogenic shock:** Cardiogenic shock after acute myocardial infarction usually follows a reduction in functional ventricular myocardium, and is caused by left ventricular infarction (79% of people with cardiogenic shock) more often than by right ventricular infarction (3% of people with cardiogenic shock).[8] Cardiogenic shock after acute myocardial infarction may also be caused by cardiac structural defects, such as mitral valve regurgitation due to papillary muscle dysfunction (7% of people with cardiogenic shock), ventricular septal rupture (4% of people with cardiogenic shock), or cardiac tamponade following free cardiac wall rupture (1% of people with cardiogenic shock). Major risk factors for cardiogenic shock after acute myocardial infarction are previous myocardial infarction, diabetes mellitus, advanced age, hypotension, tachycardia or bradycardia, congestive heart failure with Killip class (see glossary, p 27) II–III, and low left ventricular ejection fraction (ejection fraction < 35%).[7,8]

PROGNOSIS **Acute myocardial infarction:** May lead to a host of mechanical and cardiac electrical complications, including death, ventricular dysfunction, congestive heart failure, fatal and non-fatal arrhythmias, valvular dysfunction, myocardial rupture, and cardiogenic shock. **Cardiogenic shock:** Mortality rates for people in hospital with cardiogenic shock after acute myocardial infarction vary between 50–80%.[2,3,6,7] Most deaths occur within 48 hours of the onset of shock (see figure 1, p 34). People surviving until discharge from hospital have a reasonable long term prognosis (88% survival at 1 year).[10]

AIMS To relieve pain; to restore blood supply to heart muscle; to reduce incidence of complications (such as congestive heart failure, myocardial rupture, valvular dysfunction, fatal and non-fatal arrhythmia); to prevent recurrent ischaemia and infarction; and to decrease mortality with minimal adverse effects of treatments.

OUTCOMES **Efficacy outcomes:** Rates of major cardiovascular events, including death, recurrent acute myocardial infarction, refractory ischaemia, and stroke. **Safety outcomes:** Rates of major bleeding and intracranial haemorrhage.

METHODS *Clinical Evidence* search and appraisal October 2001.

QUESTION Which treatments improve outcomes in acute myocardial infarction?

Nicolas Danchin

OPTION ASPIRIN

One systematic review in people with acute myocardial infarction has found that aspirin versus placebo significantly reduces mortality, reinfarction, and stroke at one month.

Benefits: **Aspirin versus placebo:** We found one systematic review (search date 1990, 9 RCTs, 18 773 people), which compared antiplatelet agents versus placebo started soon after the onset of acute myocardial infarction (AMI) and for a period of at least 1 month afterwards.[11] The absolute and relative benefits found in the systematic review are shown in figure 2, p 35. The largest of the RCTs identified by the review (17 187 people with suspected AMI) compared placebo versus aspirin (162.6 mg) chewed and swallowed on the day of AMI and continued daily for 1 month.[12] In subsequent long term follow up, the mortality benefit was maintained for up to 4 years.[13] In the systematic review, the most widely tested aspirin regimens were 75–325 mg daily.[11] Doses throughout this range seemed similarly effective, with no evidence that "higher" doses were more effective (500–1500 mg aspirin daily *v* placebo; odds reduction 21%, 95% CI 14% to 27%) than "medium" doses (160–325 mg aspirin daily *v* placebo; odds reduction 28%, 95% CI 22% to 33%), or "lower" doses (75–160 mg aspirin daily *v* placebo; odds reduction 26%, 95% CI 5% to 42%). The review found insufficient evidence for efficacy of doses below 75 mg daily. One RCT identified by the review found that administering a loading dose of 160–325 mg daily achieved a prompt antiplatelet effect.[14]

Harms: The largest RCT identified by the review found no significant difference between aspirin versus placebo in rates of cerebral haemorrhage or bleeds requiring transfusion (0.4% on aspirin and placebo).[12] It also found a small absolute excess of "minor" bleeding (ARI 0.6%, 95% CI not provided; P < 0.01).

Comment: None.

OPTION THROMBOLYSIS

One overview of RCTs and one non-systematic review in people with acute myocardial infarction and ST elevation or bundle branch block on their initial electrocardiogram have found that prompt thrombolytic treatment (within 6 h and perhaps up to 12 h and longer after the onset of symptoms) versus placebo significantly reduces mortality. RCTs comparing different types of thrombolytic agents versus each other have found no significant difference in mortality. The overview found that thrombolytic treatment versus control significantly increased the risk of stroke or major bleeding. The overview and review have also found that intracranial haemorrhage is more common in people of advanced age and low body weight, those with hypertension on admission, and those given tissue plasminogen activator rather than another thrombolytic agent. One meta-analysis has found conflicting results of bolus treatment versus infusion of thrombolytic agents on intracerebral haemorrhage.

Benefits: **Versus placebo:** We found one overview (9 RCTs, 58 600 people with suspected acute myocardial infarction [AMI]) comparing thrombolysis versus placebo.[15] Baseline electrocardiograms showed ST segment elevation in 68% of people, and ST segment depression, T wave abnormalities, or no abnormality in the rest. The overview found that thrombolysis versus placebo significantly reduced short term mortality (9.6% with thrombolysis *v* 11.5% with placebo; ARR 1.9%; RR 0.82, 95% CI 0.77 to 0.87; NNT 56). The greatest benefit was found in the large subgroup of people presenting with ST elevation (RR 0.79) or bundle branch block (RR 0.75). Reduced rates of death were seen in people with all types of infarction, but the benefit was several times greater in those with anterior infarction (ARR 3.7%) compared with those with inferior infarction (ARR 0.8%) or infarctions in other zones (ARR 2.7%). One of the RCTs included in the overview found that thrombolysis versus placebo significantly reduced mortality after 12 years (36/107 [34%] dead with thrombolysis *v* 55/112 [49%] with placebo; ARR 15%, 95% CI 2.4% to 29%; RR 0.69, 95% CI 0.49 to 0.95; NNT 7).[16] **Timing of treatment:** The overview found that the earlier thrombolytic treatment was given (with respect to the onset of symptoms), the greater the absolute benefit of treatment (see figure 3, p 36).[15,17] For each hour of delay in thrombolytic treatment, the absolute risk reduction for death decreased by 0.16% (ARR for death if given within 6 h of symptoms 3%; ARR for death if given 7–12 h after onset of symptoms 2%).[15,17] Too few people in the overview received treatment more than 12 hours after the onset of symptoms to determine whether the benefits of thrombolytic treatment given after 12 hours would outweigh the risks (see comment below).

Streptokinase versus tissue plasminogen activator: We found one non-systematic review (3 RCTs;[18–20] see table 1, p 31)[17] comparing streptokinase versus tissue plasminogen activator (tPA). The first RCT, in people with ST elevation and symptoms of AMI for less than 6 hours, was unblinded.[18] People were first randomised to intravenous tPA 100 mg over 3 hours or streptokinase 1.5 MU over 1 hour, and then further randomised to subcutaneous heparin 12 500 U twice daily beginning 12 hours later, or no heparin. It found no significant difference between thrombolysis plus heparin versus thrombolysis plus no heparin in mortality (AR of death in hospital 8.5% with thrombolysis plus heparin *v* 8.9% with thrombolysis plus no heparin; RRR 0.05, 95% CI –0.04 to +0.14). In the second RCT, people with suspected AMI presenting within 24 hours of symptoms were first randomised to receive either streptokinase 1.5 MU over 1 hour, tPA 0.6 MU/kg every 4 hours, or anisoylated plasminogen streptokinase activator complex (APSAC) 30 U every 3 minutes, and then further randomised to subcutaneous heparin 12 500 U starting at 7 hours and continued for 7 days, or no heparin.[19] All people received aspirin on admission. The RCT found no significant difference between thrombolytic agents in mortality (streptokinase 10.6%, APSAC 10.5%, tPA 10.3%), and no significant difference with thrombolysis plus heparin versus thrombolysis plus no heparin in mortality (AR of death 10.3% with thrombolysis plus heparin *v* 10.6% with thrombolysis plus no heparin) after 35 days. The third RCT was unblinded and in people with ST segment elevation presenting within 6 hours of symptom onset.[20] People were randomised to one of four regimens: streptokinase 1.5 MU over 1 hour plus subcutaneous heparin 12 500 U twice daily starting 4 hours after thrombolytic treatment; streptokinase 1.5 MU over 1 hour plus intravenous heparin 5000 U bolus followed by 1000 U every hour; accelerated tPA 15 mg bolus then 0.75 mg/kg over 30 minutes followed by 0.50 mg/kg over 60 minutes, plus intravenous heparin 5000 U bolus then 1000 U every hour; or tPA 1.0 mg/kg over 60 minutes, 10% given as a bolus, plus streptokinase 1.0 MU over 60 minutes.[20] Meta-analysis of the three trials, weighted by sample size, found no significant difference between treatments in the combined outcome of any stroke or death (ARs 9.4% for streptokinase only regimens *v* 9.2% for tPA based regimens, including the combined tPA and streptokinase arm in the third trial; ARR for tPA *v* streptokinase 0.2%, 95% CI –0.2% to +0.5%; RRR 2.1%).[17]
Comparison of other thrombolytic agents: We found two RCTs in people with AMI receiving concomitant treatment with aspirin and heparin, which compared tPA versus other thrombolytic agents.[21,22] The first RCT (15 059 people from 20 different countries with AMI evolving for < 6 h, with ST segment elevation or with the appearance of a new left bundle branch block on their electrocardiogram) compared tPA (accelerated iv administration according to the GUSTO regimen) versus reteplase (recombinant plasminogen activator; two 10 MU iv boluses, 30 min apart) and found no significant difference in mortality after 30 days (OR 1.03, 95% CI 0.91 to 1.18).[21] The second RCT (16 949 people; see comment below) compared tPA (accelerated iv administration)

versus tenecteplase (a genetically engineered variant of tPA; 30–50 mg iv according to body weight as a single bolus).[22] It found no significant difference between treatments in total mortality after 30 days (6% with tenecteplase *v* 6% with tPA; RR 1.0, 95% CI 0.91 to 1.10).

Harms: **Stroke/intracerebral haemorrhage:** The overview found that thrombolytic treatment versus control significantly increased the risk of stroke (ARI 0.4%, 95% CI 0.2% to 0.5%; NNH 250).[15] In the third RCT comparing streptokinase versus tPA, the overall incidence of intracerebral haemorrhage was 0.7% and of stroke 1.4%, of which 31% were severely disabling and 50% were intracerebral haemorrhages.[20] The RCT also found that tPA versus streptokinase plus subcutaneous heparin or streptokinase plus intravenous heparin significantly increased the risk of haemorrhagic stroke (AR 0.54%; P = 0.03 for tPA compared with combined streptokinase arms). The RCT comparing reteplase versus tPA found that the incidence of stroke was similar with both treatments, and the odds ratio for the incidence of death or disabling stroke was 1.0.[21] The RCT comparing tenecteplase versus tPA found no significant difference between treatments in the rate of stroke or death (7% with tenecteplase *v* 7% with tPA; RR 1.01, 95% CI 0.91 to 1.13).[22] We found one meta-analysis which compared bolus thrombolytic treatment versus infusion treatment.[23] Meta-analysis of nine phase II trials (3956 people) found that bolus treatment significantly reduced the risk of intracerebral haemorrhage (OR 0.53, 95% CI 0.27 to 1.01). However, meta-analysis of six phase III trials (62 673 people) found that bolus treatment significantly increased the risk of intracerebral haemorrhage (OR 1.25, 95% CI 1.06 to 1.49). **Predictive factors for stroke/intracranial haemorrhage:** Multivariate analysis of data from a large database of people who experienced intracerebral haemorrhage after thrombolytic treatment identified four independent predictors of increased risk of intracerebral haemorrhage: age 65 years or older (OR 2.2, 95% CI 1.4 to 3.5); weight less than 70 kg (OR 2.1, 95% CI 1.3 to 3.2); hypertension on admission (OR 2.0, 95% CI 1.2 to 3.2); and use of tPA rather than another thrombolytic agent (OR 1.6, 95% CI 1.0 to 2.5).[21] Absolute risk of intracranial haemorrhage was 0.26% on streptokinase in the absence of risk factors, and 0.96%, 1.32%, and 2.17% in people with one, two, or three risk factors.[24] Analysis of 592 strokes in 41 021 people from the trials found seven factors to be predictors of intracerebral haemorrhage: advanced age, lower weight, history of cerebrovascular disease, history of hypertension, higher systolic or diastolic pressure on presentation, and use of tPA rather than streptokinase.[25,26] **Major bleeding:** The overview also found that thrombolytic treatment versus placebo significantly increased the risk of major bleeding (ARI 0.7%, 95% CI 0.6% to 0.9%; NNH 143).[15] Bleeding was most common in people undergoing procedures (coronary artery bypass grafting or percutaneous transluminal coronary angioplasty). Spontaneous bleeds were observed most often in the gastrointestinal tract.[20]

Comment: Extrapolation of the data from the overview (see figure 3, p 36) suggests that, at least for people suspected of having an acute myocardial infarction and with ST elevation on their electrocardiogram, there may be some net benefit of treatment between

12–18 hours after symptom onset (ARR for death 1%).[15] The evidence from the RCT comparing reteplase versus tPA is consistent with a similar efficacy for both treatments, although formal equivalence cannot be established because the trial was designed as a superiority trial.[21] Regarding this RCT's end point of overall mortality, the 95% confidence interval exceeded the 1% difference that might have been considered acceptable for defining equivalence; however, for the combined end point of mortality and disabling stroke (a secondary end point of the trial), the 95% confidence interval was less than 1%. The RCT comparing tPA versus tenecteplase was designed as an equivalence trial, accepting that tenecteplase would be equivalent to tPA if both the absolute risk of death with tenecteplase was not more than 1% higher than that with tPA and that the relative risk of mortality at 30 days would not exceed 14%.[22] The results confirmed equivalence between the two thrombolytics. The evidence suggests that it is far more important to administer prompt thrombolytic treatment than to debate which thrombolytic agent should be used. A strategy of rapid use of any thrombolytic in a broad population is likely to lead to the greatest impact on mortality. When the results of RCTs are taken together, tPA based regimens do not seem to confer a significant advantage over streptokinase in the combined outcome of any stroke and death (unrelated to stroke). The legitimacy of combining the results of the three trials can be questioned, as the selection criteria and protocols differed in important aspects (see review for arguments to justify combining the results of these trials despite their apparent differences).[17]

OPTION β BLOCKERS

Two systematic reviews and one subsequent RCT have found that β blockers versus control given within hours of infarction significantly reduce both mortality and reinfarction. One RCT in people receiving thrombolytic treatment found that immediate versus delayed treatment with metoprolol significantly reduced rates of reinfarction and recurrent chest pain at 6 days, but had no significant effect on mortality in the short term or at 1 year. One RCT comparing carvedilol versus placebo in people with recent myocardial infarction and left ejection fraction ≤ 40% receiving thrombolytic treatment found no significant difference in the combined endpoint of all cause mortality and hospital admission for any cardiovascular event after a median of 1.3 years, although mortality, and recurrent non fatal myocardial infarction were significantly lower with carvedilol.

Benefits: **Given within hours of infarction:** We found two systematic reviews (search dates 1997[27] and not stated[28]) and one overview[29] investigating the early use of β blockers in people suffering acute myocardial infarction (AMI). The older reviews identified 27 RCTs and found that, within 1 week of treatment, β blockers significantly reduced the risk of death and major vascular events (for the combined outcome of death, non-fatal cardiac arrest, or non-fatal reinfarction: 1110 events *v* 1298 events; RR 0.84, 95% CI not provided; P < 0.001).[28,29] The largest of the RCTs identified by the review (16 027 people with AMI) compared atenolol (5–10 mg given iv immediately, followed by 100 mg orally given daily for 7 days) versus standard treatment (no β blocker).[30] The RCT found that atenolol significantly reduced vascular mortality after 7 days (3.9% with atenolol *v* 4.6% with standard treatment; ARR 0.7%; RR 0.85, 95% CI 0.73 to 0.88; NNT 147). The RCT found more benefit in people with electrocardiogram evidence of AMI at entry (in people with electrocardiogram suggesting anterior infarction, inferior infarction, both, or bundle branch block, AR of death: 5.33% with atenolol *v* 6.49% with control; ARR 1.16%; NNT 86, 95% CI not provided), and that people older than 65 years and those with large infarcts had the most benefit.[30] The more recent systematic review (82 RCTs, 54 234 people) separately analysed 51 short term RCTs (people with AMI up to 6 wk after the onset of pain) and 31 long term RCTs.[27] Most of the RCTs did not include thrombolysis. In the short term studies, seven RCTs reported no deaths and many reported only a few. Meta-analysis of the short term RCTs reporting at least one death found that β blockers versus placebo reduced mortality, but that the reduction was not significant (ARR 0.4%; OR 0.96, 95% CI 0.85 to 1.08). In the longer term RCTs, β blockers versus placebo significantly reduced mortality over 6 months to 4 years (OR 0.77, 95% CI 0.69 to 0.85). No significant difference in effectiveness was found between different types of β blocker (based on cardioselectivity or intrinsic sympathomimetic activity). Most evidence was obtained with propranolol, timolol, and metoprolol. **In people receiving thrombolytic treatment:** We found two RCTs.[31,32] The first RCT (1434 people with AMI who had received tissue plasminogen activator thrombolysis) compared early versus delayed metoprolol treatment.[31] Early treatment began on day 1 (iv then oral) and delayed treatment on day 6 (oral). It found that early treatment significantly reduced rates of reinfarction (AR 2.7% with early treatment *v* 5.1% with delayed treatment, 95% CI not provided; P = 0.02), and recurrent chest pain (AR 18.8% with early treatment *v* 24.1% with delayed treatment; P < 0.02) after 6 days. There were no early (6 days) or late (1 year) differences observed in mortality or left ventricular ejection fraction between the two groups. The second RCT (1959 people within 3–21 days of AMI and with left ventricular dysfunction; 46% of people had received thrombolysis or percutaneous transluminal coronary angioplasty at the acute stage of their infarction, and 97% of people received angiotensin converting enzyme inhibitors) compared carvedilol (6.25 mg increased to a maximum of 25 mg over 4–6 wk) versus placebo.[32] It found that carvedilol significantly reduced mortality (12% with carvedilol *v* 15% with placebo; HR 0.77, 95% CI 0.60 to 0.90) and non-fatal AMI (HR 0.59, 95% CI 0.39 to 0.90), but found no significant difference between treatments in the combined end point of total mortality and hospital admission for any cardiovascular event (HR 0.92, 95% CI 0.80 to 1.07) after a median of 1.3 years. **Long term use:** See β blockers under secondary prevention of ischaemic cardiac events, p 129.

Harms: People with asthma or severe congestive cardiac failure were excluded from most trials. One RCT found that in people given immediate versus delayed β blockers following tissue plasminogen activator, there was a non-significant increased frequency of heart failure during the initial admission to hospital (15.3% with immediate *v* 12.2% with delayed; P = 0.10).[31] The presence of first degree heart block and bundle branch block was associated with an increased frequency of adverse events.

Comment: Until recently trials involving the use of β blockers in AMI were mostly conducted in people considered to be of low risk (because of the supposed deleterious effect of β blockers on left ventricular function), and many of these trials took place in the prethrombolytic era. β Blockers may reduce rates of cardiac rupture and ventricular fibrillation. This may explain why people older than 65 years and those with large infarcts benefited most, as they also have higher rates of these complications. The trial comparing early versus delayed β blockade after thrombolysis was too small to rule out an effect on mortality of β blockers when added to thrombolysis.[31]

OPTION ANGIOTENSIN CONVERTING ENZYME INHIBITORS

One overview and one systematic review in people within 36 hours of acute myocardial infarction have found that angiotensin converting enzyme inhibitors versus placebo significantly reduce mortality. The overview also found that angiotensin converting enzyme inhibitors versus control significantly increase persistent hypotension and renal dysfunction. The question of whether angiotensin converting enzyme inhibitors should be offered to everyone presenting with acute myocardial infarction or only to people with signs of heart failure remains unresolved.

Benefits: **In all people after an acute myocardial infarction (AMI):** We found one overview[33] and one systematic review (search date 1997)[34] of angiotensin converting enzyme (ACE) inhibitors versus placebo after AMI. The overview (4 large RCTs, 98 496 people irrespective of clinical heart failure or left ventricular dysfunction, within 36 h of the onset of symptoms of AMI) compared ACE inhibitors versus placebo.[33] It found that ACE inhibitors significantly reduced mortality after 30 days (7.1% with ACE inhibitors *v* 7.6% with placebo; RR 0.93, 95% CI 0.89 to 0.98; NNT 200). The absolute benefit was larger in some high risk subgroups: people in Killip class (see glossary, p 27) II–III (clinically moderate to severe heart failure at first presentation; RR 0.91; NNT 71, 99% CI 36 to 10 000), people with heart rates greater than 100 beats a minute at entry (RR 0.86; NNT 44, 99% CI 25 to 185), and people with an anterior AMI (RR 0.87; NNT 94, 99% CI 56 to 303). The overview also found that ACE inhibitors significantly reduced the incidence of non-fatal cardiac failure (AR 14.6% *v* 15.2%, 95% CI not provided; P = 0.01). The systematic review (search date 1997, 15 RCTs, 15 104 people) found similar results.[34] **In selected people after an AMI:** A selective strategy was tested in three RCTs.[35–37] Treatment was restricted to people with clinical heart failure, objective evidence of left ventricular dysfunction, or both, and was started a few days after AMI (about 6000 people). These RCTs found consistently that long term treatment with ACE inhibitors in this selected population significantly reduced mortality and reinfarction

(RRRs from 1 trial:[33] for cardiovascular death 21%, 95% CI 5% to 35%; for development of severe heart failure 37%, 95% CI 20% to 50%; for congestive heart failure requiring admission to hospital 22%, 95% CI 4% to 37%; and for recurrent AMI 25%, 95% CI 5% to 40%).

Harms: The overview found that ACE inhibitors versus control significantly increased persistent hypotension (AR 17.6% with ACE inhibitor *v* 9.3% with control, 95% CI for difference not provided; $P < 0.01$) and renal dysfunction (AR 1.3% *v* 0.6%; $P < 0.01$).[33] The relative and absolute risks of these adverse effects were uniformly distributed across both the high and lower cardiovascular risk groups.

Comment: The largest benefits of ACE inhibitors in people with AMI are seen when treatment is started within 24 hours. The evidence does not answer the question of which people with an AMI should be offered ACE inhibitors, and for how long after AMI it remains beneficial to start treatment with an ACE inhibitor. We found one systematic review (search date not stated; based on individual data from about 100 000 people in RCTs of ACE inhibitors), which found that people receiving both aspirin and ACE inhibitors had the same relative risk reduction as those receiving ACE inhibitors alone (i.e. there was no evidence of a clinically relevant interaction between ACE inhibitors and aspirin).[38]

OPTION NITRATES

One systematic review (prior to the introduction of thrombolysis) has found that nitrates versus placebo significantly reduce the risk of mortality. Two RCTs (after the introduction of thrombolysis) compared nitrates versus placebo and found no significant difference in mortality.

Benefits: **Without thrombolysis:** We found one systematic review (search date not stated, 10 RCTs, 2000 people with acute myocardial infarction [AMI]), which compared intravenous glyceryl trinitrate or sodium nitroprusside versus placebo.[39] The trials were all conducted in the prethrombolytic era. The review found that nitrates significantly reduced mortality (RRR 35%, 95% CI 16% to 55%). **With aspirin/thrombolysis:** We found two large RCTs (58 050 people with AMI,[40] 17 817 people with AMI;[41] 90% received aspirin and about 70% received thrombolytic treatment), which compared nitrates (given acutely) versus placebo. In one RCT, people received oral controlled release isosorbide mononitrate 30–60 mg/day.[40] In the other RCT, people received intravenous glyceryl trinitrate for 24 hours followed by transdermal glyceryl trinitrate 10 mg daily.[41] Neither trial found a significant difference in mortality, either in the total sample or in subgroups of people at different risks of death. Nitrates were a useful adjunctive treatment to help control symptoms in people with AMI.

Harms: The systematic review and the large RCTs found no significant harm associated with routine use of nitrates.[39–41]

Comment: The two large RCTs had features that may have caused them not to find a benefit even if one exists: a large proportion of people took nitrates outside the study; there was a high rate of concurrent use of other hypotensive agents; people were relatively low risk; and nitrates were not titrated to blood pressure and heart rate.[40,41]

OPTION CALCIUM CHANNEL BLOCKERS

RCTs in people within the first few days of an acute myocardial infarction have found that calcium channel blockers versus placebo do not reduce mortality, and in the subgroup of people with left ventricular dysfunction calcium channel blockers versus placebo may increase mortality.

Benefits: **Dihydropyridine calcium channel blockers:** We found one non-systematic review (2 large RCTs)[42] in people treated within the first few days of acute myocardial infarction (AMI), which compared short acting nifedipine versus placebo.[43,44] One RCT was terminated prematurely because of lack of efficacy.[44] It found that nifedipine versus placebo increased mortality by 33%, although the increase did not reach statistical significance. We found insufficient evidence about sustained release nifedipine, amlodipine, or felodipine in this setting. **Verapamil:** We found one systematic review (search date 1997, 7 RCTs, 6527 people with AMI),[45] which found that verapamil versus placebo had no significant effect on mortality (RR 0.86, 95% CI 0.71 to 1.04).

Harms: Two systematic reviews (search dates not stated; including both randomised and observational trials) in people with AMI investigating the use of calcium channel blockers found a non-significant increase in mortality of about 4% and 6%.[46,47] One RCT (2466 people with AMI) compared diltiazem (60 mg orally 4 times daily starting 3–15 days after AMI) versus placebo.[48] It found that overall there was no significant difference in total mortality or reinfarction. Subgroup analysis in people with congestive heart failure found that diltiazem significantly increased death or reinfarction (RRI 1.41, 95% CI 1.01 to 1.96).

Comment: None.

OPTION PRIMARY PERCUTANEOUS TRANSLUMINAL CORONARY ANGIOPLASTY VERSUS THROMBOLYSIS

Two systematic reviews have found that primary percutaneous transluminal coronary angioplasty versus primary thrombolysis significantly reduces mortality and reinfarction. However, the trials were conducted mainly in specialist centres and the effectiveness of percutaneous transluminal coronary angioplasty versus thrombolysis in less specialist centres remains to be defined.

Benefits: We found two systematic reviews in people with acute myocardial infarction, which compared primary percutaneous transluminal coronary angioplasty (PTCA) versus primary thrombolysis.[49,50] The first systematic review (search date 1996, 10 RCTs, 2606 people) found that primary PTCA versus primary thrombolysis significantly reduced mortality at 30 days after intervention (4.4% with primary PTCA *v* 6.5% with primary thrombolysis; ARR 2.1%; OR 0.66, 95% CI 0.46 to 0.94; NNT 48).[49] It found that the effect was similar regardless of which thrombolysis regimen was used. The review also found that PTCA significantly reduced the combined end point of death and reinfarction (OR 0.58, 95% CI 0.44 to 0.76). The largest single RCT (1138 people, ST elevation on electrocardiogram within 12 h of symptom onset) included in the review found less favourable results. It compared primary PTCA versus thrombolysis with accelerated tissue plasminogen activator and found no significant difference in mortality after 30 days (5.7% with PTCA v 7.0% with thrombolysis).[51] It also found that primary PTCA significantly reduced the primary end point of death, non-fatal acute myocardial infarction, or non-fatal disabling stroke (9.6% with PTCA v 13.7% with thrombolysis; OR 0.67, 95% CI 0.47 to 0.97). The RCT found that this effect was substantially attenuated after 6 months. A second RCT included in the review has reported long term follow up; it found that primary PTCA versus primary thrombolysis significantly improves mortality after 5 years (25/194 [13%] with PCTA v 48/201 [24%] with streptokinase; RR 0.54, 95% CI 0.36 to 0.87).[52] The second systematic review (search date 1998, 10 RCTs, 2573 people) found overall similar results, with significant reductions in mortality and in reinfarction.[50]

Harms: **Stroke:** The review found that PTCA versus thrombolysis significantly reduced the risk of all types of stroke (0.7% with PTCA v 2.0% with thrombolysis) and haemorrhagic stroke (0.1% with PTCA v 1.1% with thrombolysis).[49]

Comment: Although collectively the trials found an overall short term reduction in deaths with PTCA compared with thrombolysis, there were several pitfalls common to individual RCTs, most of which may have inflated the benefit of PTCA.[53] RCTs comparing PTCA with thrombolysis could not be easily blinded, and ascertainment of end points that required some judgement, such as reinfarction or stroke, may have been influenced by the investigators' knowledge of the treatment allocation (only 1 trial had a blinded adjudication events committee). Also, people allocated to PTCA were discharged 1–2 days earlier than those allocated to thrombolysis, which favoured PTCA by reducing the time for detection of in hospital events. In addition, the RCTs conducted before the largest RCT in the first review[51] should be viewed as hypothesis generating, in that the composite outcome (death, reinfarction, and stroke) was not prospectively defined, and attention was only placed on these end points after there seemed to be some benefit on post hoc analysis. The results are also based on short term outcomes only and do not provide information on collective long term benefit. For example, in the largest RCT the composite end point was significant at 30 days but with a wide degree of uncertainty, and this was substantially attenuated to a non-significant difference by 6 months.[51] The lower mortality and reinfarction rates reported with primary PTCA are promising but not conclusive, and the real benefits may well be smaller. Only in a minority of centres that perform a high volume of PTCA, and in the hands of experienced interventionists, may primary PTCA be clearly superior to thrombolytic treatment. Elsewhere, primary PTCA may be of greatest benefit in people with contraindications to thrombolysis, in people in cardiogenic shock, or in people where the mortality reduction with thrombolysis is modest and the risk of intracranial haemorrhage is increased, for example, elderly people.[54] The value of PTCA over thrombolysis in people presenting to hospital more than 12 hours after onset of chest pain remains to be tested. In the largest RCT included in the first systematic review, the collective rate of haemorrhagic stroke in people given thrombolysis was 1.1%, substantially higher than that observed in trials comparing thrombolysis with placebo.[51] This may have been because the trials summarised above were in older people and used tissue plasminogen activator. However, the lower rates of haemorrhagic stroke with primary PTCA were consistent across almost all trials, and this may be the major advantage of PTCA over thrombolysis.

QUESTION **Which treatments improve outcomes for cardiogenic shock after acute myocardial infarction**

Edoardo De Benedetti and Philip Urban

OPTION EARLY INVASIVE CARDIAC REVASCULARISATION

One RCT found that early invasive cardiac revascularisation versus initial medical treatment alone significantly reduces mortality after 6 and 12 months. A second RCT found similar results, although the difference was not significant.

Benefits: We found no systematic review. We found two RCTs in people with cardiogenic shock within 48 hours of acute myocardial infarction comparing early invasive cardiac revascularisation (see glossary, p 27) versus initial medical treatment alone (see comment below).[2,3,55] The first RCT (302 people) found that early invasive cardiac revascularisation significantly reduced mortality after 6 and 12 months (see table 2, p 33).[2,55] The second RCT (55 people) found that early invasive cardiac revascularisation reduced mortality after 30 days and at 12 months, although the difference was not significant (see table 2, p 33). **Percutaneous transluminal coronary angioplasty versus coronary artery bypass graft:** We found no RCTs in people with cardiogenic shock after acute myocardial infarction comparing percutaneous transluminal coronary angioplasty versus coronary bypass grafting.

Harms: The first RCT (56 people aged ≥ 75 years) found that there was a non-significant increase in 30 day mortality with early invasive cardiac revascularisation (18/24 [75%] with early invasive cardiac revascularisation *v* 17/32 [53%] with medical treatment alone; RR 1.41, 95% CI 0.95 to 2.11).[2,55] The first RCT also found that acute renal failure (defined as a serum creatinine level > 265 μmol/L) was significantly more common in the medical treatment alone group versus the early cardiac revascularisation group (36/150 [24%] *v* 20/152 [13%]; RR 1.82, 95% CI 1.1 to 3.0; NNH 9, 95% CI 5 to 48). Other harms reported by the RCT included major haemorrhage, sepsis, and peripheral vascular occlusion, although comparative data between groups for these harms were not provided. The second RCT did not report harms.[3]

Comment: In the first RCT, medical treatment included intra-aortic balloon counterpulsation (see glossary, p 27) and thrombolytic treatment.[2,55] In the second RCT, medical treatment was not defined.[3] The second RCT was stopped prematurely because of difficulties with recruitment. Both RCTs were conducted in centres with expertise in early invasive cardiac revascularisation and their results may not be reproducible in other settings.[2,3,55]

OPTION THROMBOLYSIS

Subgroup analysis of people with cardiogenic shock after acute myocardial infarction from one RCT comparing thrombolysis versus no thrombolysis found no significant difference in mortality after 21 days.

Benefits: We found no systematic review. We found one RCT (11 806 people within 12 h of acute myocardial infarction), which compared thrombolysis using streptokinase versus no thrombolysis (see comment below).[56] Subgroup analysis of people with cardiogenic shock found no significant difference in inpatient mortality after 21 days (280 people; 102/146 [69%] with thrombolysis *v* 94/134 [70%] with no thrombolysis; RR 1.0, 95% CI 0.85 to 1.16).

Harms: The RCT did not report harms specifically in the subgroup of people with cardiogenic shock.[56] Overall, adverse reactions attributed to streptokinase were found in 705/5860 (12%) people either during or after streptokinase infusion. These adverse reactions included minor and major bleeding (3.7%), allergic reactions (2.4%), hypotension (3.0%), anaphylactic shock (0.1%), shivering/fever (1.0%), ventricular arrhythmias (1.2%), and stroke (0.2%).

Comment: The RCT was not blinded.[56] Data presented are from a retrospective subgroup analysis and randomisation was not stratified by the presence of cardiogenic shock.

OPTION POSITIVE INOTROPES (DOBUTAMINE, DOPAMINE, ADRENALINE [EPINEPHRINE], NORADRENALINE [NOREPINEPHRINE], AMRINONE) AND VASODILATORS (ANGIOTENSIN CONVERTING ENZYME INHIBITORS, NITRATES)

We found no RCTs comparing inotropes versus placebo or comparing vasodilators versus placebo.

Benefits: **Positive inotropes:** We found no systematic review or RCTs. We found three non-systematic reviews,[1,57,58] which identified no RCTs evaluating the use of positive inotropes in people with cardiogenic shock after acute myocardial infarction. **Vasodilators:** We found no systematic review or RCTs.

Harms: Positive inotropes may worsen cardiac ischaemia and induce ventricular arrhythmias.[1,57,58] We found no studies of harms specifically in people with cardiogenic shock after acute myocardial infarction (see harms of positive inotropic drugs and vasodilators under heart failure, p 60).

Comment: There is consensus that positive inotropes are beneficial in cardiogenic shock after acute myocardial infarction. We found no evidence to confirm or reject this view. The risk of worsening hypotension has led to concern about the use of any vasodilator to treat acute cardiogenic shock.[58]

OPTION PULMONARY ARTERY CATHETERISATION

We found no RCTs comparing pulmonary artery catheterisation versus no catheterisation.

Benefits: We found no systematic review and no RCTs.

Harms: Observational studies have found an association between pulmonary artery catheterisation and increased morbidity and mortality, but it is unclear whether this arises from an adverse effect of the catheterisation or because people with a poor prognosis were selected for catheterisation.[59] Harms such as major arrhythmias, injury to the lung, thromboembolism (see thromboembolism, p 209), and sepsis occur in 0.1–0.5% of people undergoing pulmonary artery catheterisation.[59]

Comment: Pulmonary artery catheterisation helps to diagnose cardiogenic shock, guide correction of hypovolaemia, optimise filling pressures for both the left and right sides of the heart, and adjust doses of inotropic drugs.[1] There is consensus that pulmonary artery catheterisation is beneficial in patients with cardiogenic shock after acute myocardial infarction,[60,61] although we found no evidence to confirm or reject this view.

OPTION INTRA-AORTIC BALLOON COUNTERPULSATION

One abstract of an RCT compared intra-aortic balloon counterpulsation plus thrombolysis versus thrombolysis alone and found no significant difference in mortality after 6 months.

Benefits: We found no systematic review. We found one abstract of an RCT (57 people), which compared intra-aortic balloon counterpulsation (see glossary, p 27) plus thrombolysis versus thrombolysis alone (see comment below).[62] The RCT found no significant difference in mortality after 6 months (22/57 [39%] with thrombolysis plus balloon counterpulsation *v* 25/57 [43%] with thrombolysis alone; RR 0.9, 95% CI 0.57 to 1.37; P = 0.3).

Harms: Harms were not reported in the abstract of the RCT.[62]

Comment: The abstract did not describe detailed methods for the trial, making interpretation of the results difficult.[58] We also found two additional small RCTs (30 people[63] and 20 people[64]), which compared intra-aortic balloon counterpulsation versus standard treatment in people after acute myocardial infarction. Neither RCT specifically recruited, or identified data from, people with cardiogenic shock after acute myocardial infarction. Neither RCT found a reduction in mortality with intra-aortic balloon counterpulsation. There is consensus that intra-aortic balloon counterpulsation is beneficial in people with cardiogenic shock after acute myocardial infarction. We found no evidence to confirm or reject this view.

OPTION VENTRICULAR ASSISTANCE DEVICES AND CARDIAC TRANSPLANTATION

We found no RCTs evaluating either ventricular assistance devices or cardiac transplantation.

Benefits: We found no systematic review and no RCTs.

Harms: We found no evidence of harms specifically associated with the use of ventricular assistance devices (see glossary, p 27) or cardiac transplantation in people with cardiogenic shock after acute myocardial infarction.

Comment: Reviews of observational studies[1,58,65] and retrospective reports,[66,67] have suggested that ventricular assistance devices may improve outcomes in selected people when used alone or as a bridge to cardiac transplantation. The availability of ventricular assistance devices and cardiac transplantation is limited to a few specialised centres, and results may not bc applicable to other settings.

OPTION EARLY CARDIAC SURGERY

We found no RCTs evaluating early surgical intervention for ventricular septal rupture, free wall rupture, or mitral valve regurgitation complicated by cardiogenic shock after acute myocardial infarction.

Benefits: We found no systematic review and no RCTs.

Harms: We found no evidence about the harms of surgery in people with cardiogenic shock caused by cardiac structural defects after acute myocardial infarction.

Comment: Non-systematic reviews of observational studies have suggested that death is inevitable following free wall rupture without early surgical intervention, and that surgery for both mitral valve regurgitation and ventricular septal rupture is more effective when carried out within 24–48 hours.[1,58]

GLOSSARY

Cardiac index A measure of cardiac output derived from the formula: cardiac output/unit time divided by body surface area (L/min/m^2).

Intra-aortic balloon counterpulsation A technique in which a balloon is placed in the aorta and inflated during diastole and deflated just before systole.

Invasive cardiac revascularisation A term used to describe either percutaneous transluminal coronary angioplasty or coronary artery bypass grafting.

Killip class A categorisation of the severity of heart failure based on easily obtained clinical signs. The main clinical features are Class I: no heart failure; Class II: crackles audible half way up the chest; Class III: crackles heard in all the lung fields; Class IV: cardiogenic shock.

Ventricular assistance device A mechanical device placed in parallel to a failing cardiac ventricle that pumps blood in an attempt to maintain cardiac output. Because of the risk of mechanical failure, thrombosis, and haemolysis they are normally used for short term support while preparing for a heart transplant.

REFERENCES

1. Califf RM, Bengtson JR. Cardiogenic shock. *N Engl J Med* 1994;330:1724–1730.
2. Hochman JS, Sleeper LA, Webb JG, et al, for the SHOCK investigators. Early revascularization in acute myocardial infarction complicated by cardiogenic shock. *N Engl J Med* 1999;341:625–634.
3. Urban P, Stauffer JC, Khatchatrian N, et al. A randomized evaluation of early revascularization to treat shock complicating acute myocardial infarction. The (Swiss) Multicenter Trial of Angioplasty SHOCK - (S)MASH. *Eur Heart Journal* 1999;20:1030–1038.
4. Murray C, Lopez A. Mortality by cause for eight regions of the world: global burden of disease study. *Lancet* 1997;349:1269–1276.
5. National Heart, Lung, and Blood Institute. *Morbidity and mortality: chartbook on cardiovascular, lung, and blood diseases*. Bethesda, Maryland: US Department of Health and Human Services, Public Health Service, National Institutes of Health; May 1992.
6. Goldberg RJ, Samad NA, Yarzebski J, Gurwitz J, Bigelow C, Gore JM. Temporal trends in cardiogenic shock complicating acute myocardial infarction. *N Engl J Med* 1999;340:1162–1168.
7. Hasdai D, Califf RM, Thompson TD, et al. Predictors of cardiogenic shock after thrombolytic therapy for acute myocardial infarction. *J Am Coll Cardiol* 2000;35:136–143.
8. Hochman JS, Buller CE, Sleeper LA, et al. Cardiogenic shock complicating acute myocardial infarction – etiology, management and outcome: a report from the SHOCK trial registry. *J Am Coll Cardiol* 2000;36:1063–1070.
9. Urban P, Bernstein M, Costanza M, Simon R, Frey R, Erne P. An internet-based registry of acute myocardial infarction in Switzerland. *Kardiovasculaäre Medizin* 2000;3:430–441.
10. Berger PB, Tuttle RH, Holmes DR, et al. One year survival among patients with acute myocardial infarction complicated by cardiogenic shock, and its relation to early revascularisation: results of the GUSTO-1 trial. *Circulation* 1999;99:873–878.
11. Antiplatelet Trialists' Collaboration. Collaborative overview of randomised trials of antiplatelet therapy I: prevention of death, myocardial infarction, and stroke by prolonged antiplatelet therapy in various categories of people. *BMJ* 1994;308:81–106. Search date 1990; primary sources Medline and Current Contents.
12. Second International Study of Infarct Survival (ISIS-2) Collaborative Group. Randomized trial of intravenous streptokinase, oral aspirin, both or neither among 17–187 cases of suspected acute myocardial infarction. *Lancet* 1988;ii:349–360.
13. Baigent BM, Collins R. ISIS-2: four year mortality of 17 187 patients after fibrinolytic and antiplatelet therapy in suspected acute myocardial infarction study [abstract]. *Circulation* 1993;88(suppl I):I–291–I–292.
14. Patrignani P, Filabozzi P, Patrono C. Selective cumulative inhibition of platelet thromboxane production by low-dose aspirin in healthy subjects. *J Clin Invest* 1982;69:1366–1372.
15. Fibrinolytic Therapy Trialists' (FTT) Collaborative Group. Indications for fibrinolytic therapy in suspected acute myocardial infarction: collaborative overview of early mortality and major morbidity results of all randomized trials of more than 1000 patients. *Lancet* 1994;343:311–322.
16. French JK, Hyde TA, Patel H, et al. Survival 12 years after randomization to streptokinase: the influence of thrombolysis in myocardial infarction flow at three to four weeks. *J Am Coll Cardiol* 1999;34:62–69.
17. Collins R, Peto R, Baigent BM, Sleight DM. Aspirin, heparin and fibrinolytic therapy in suspected acute myocardial infarction. *N Engl J Med* 1997;336:847–860.
18. Gruppo Italiano per lo studio della streptochinasi nell'infarto miocardico (GISSI). GISSI-2: a factorial randomised trial of alteplase versus streptokinase and heparin versus no heparin among 12–490 patients with acute myocardial infarction. *Lancet* 1990;336:65–71.
19. Third International Study of Infarct Survival (ISIS-3) Collaborative Group. ISIS-3: a randomised comparison of streptokinase vs tissue plasminogen activator vs anistreplase and of aspirin plus heparin vs aspirin alone among 41–299 cases of suspected acute myocardial infarction. *Lancet* 1992;339:753–770.
20. The GUSTO Investigators. An international randomized trial comparing four thrombolytic strategies for acute myocardial infarction. *N Engl J Med* 1993;329:673–682.
21. The Global Use of Strategies to Open Occluded Coronary Arteries (GUSTO III) investigators. A comparison of reteplase with alteplase for acute myocardial infarction. *N Engl J Med* 1997;337:1118–1123.
22. Assessment of the Safety and Efficacy of a New Thrombolytic (ASSENT-2) investigators. Single bolus tenecteplase compared to front-loaded alteplase in acute myocardial infarction: the ASSENT-2 double-blind randomised trial. *Lancet* 1999;354:716–722.
23. Eikelboom JW, Mehta SR, Pogue J, Yusuf S. Safety outcomes in meta-analyses of phase 2 vs phase 3 randomized trials: intracranial hemorrhage in trials of bolus fibrinolytic therapy. *JAMA* 2001;285:444–450.
24. Simoons MI, Maggioni AP, Knatterud G, et al. Individual risk assessment for intracranial hemorrhage during thrombolytic therapy. *Lancet* 1993;342:523–528.
25. Gore JM, Granger CB, Simoons MI, et al. Stroke after thrombolysis: mortality and functional outcomes in the GUSTO-1 trial. *Circulation* 1995;92:2811–2818.
26. Berkowitz SD, Granger CB, Pieper KS, et al. Incidence and predictors of bleeding after contemporary thrombolytic therapy for myocardial infarction. *Circulation* 1997;95:2508–2516.
27. Freemantle N, Cleland J, Young P, Mason J, Harrison J. Beta blockade after myocardial infarction: systematic review and meta regression analysis. *BMJ* 1999;318:1730–1737. Search date 1997; primary sources Medline, Embase, Biosis, Healthstar, Sigle, IHTA, Derwent drug file, dissertation abstracts, Pascal, international pharmaceutical abstracts, science citation index, and hand searches of reference lists.
28. Yusuf S, Peto R, Lewis S, et al. Beta-blockade during and after myocardial infarction: an overview of the randomized trials. *Prog Cardiovasc Dis* 1985;27:355–371. Search date not stated; primary sources computer-aided search of the literature, manual search of reference lists, and enquiries to colleagues about relevant papers.
29. Sleight P for the ISIS Study Group. Beta blockade early in acute myocardial infarction. *Am J Cardiol* 1987;60:6A–12A.
30. First International Study of Infarct Survival (ISIS-1) Collaborative Group. Randomised trial of

intravenous atenolol among 16 027 cases of suspected acute myocardial infarction. *Lancet*. 1986;2(8498):57–66.

31. Roberts R, Rogers WJ, Mueller HS, et al. Immediate versus deferred beta-blockade following thrombolytic therapy in patients with acute myocardial infarction: results of the thrombolysis in myocardial infarction (TIMI) II-B study. *Circulation* 1991;83:422–437.
32. The CAPRICORN investigators. Effect of carvedilol on outcome after myocardial infarction in patients with left-ventricular dysfunction: the CAPRICORN randomized trial. *Lancet* 2001;357:1385–1390.
33. ACE Inhibitor Myocardial Infarction Collaborative Group. Indications for ACE inhibitors in the early treatment of acute myocardial infarction: systematic overview of individual data from 100 000 patients in randomised trials. *Circulation* 1998;97:2202–2212. Search date not stated; primary source collaboration group of principal investigators of all randomised trials who collated individual patient data.
34. Domanski MJ, Exner DV, Borkowf CB, Geller NL, Rosenberg Y, Pfeffer MA. Effect of angiotensin converting enzyme inhibition on sudden cardiac death in patients following acute myocardial infarction. A meta-analysis of randomized clinical trials. *J Am Coll Cardiol* 1999;33:598–604. Search date 1997; primary sources Medline and hand searches of reference lists.
35. Pfeffer MA, Braunwald E, Moye LA, et al. Effect of captopril on mortality and morbidity in patients with left ventricular dysfunction after myocardial infarction. *N Engl J Med* 1992;327:669–677.
36. The Acute Infarction Ramipril Efficacy (AIRE) Study Investigators. Effect of ramipril on mortality and morbidity of survivors of acute myocardial infarction with clinical evidence of heart failure. *Lancet* 1993;342:821–828.
37. The Trandolapril Cardiac Evaluation (TRACE) Study Group. A clinical trial of the angiotensin-converting-enzyme inhibitor trandolapril in patients with left ventricular dysfunction after myocardial infarction. *N Engl J Med* 1995;333:1670–1676.
38. Latini R, Tognoni G, Maggioni AP, et al. Clinical effects of early angiotensin converting enzyme inhibitor treatment for acute myocardial infarction are similar in the presence and absence of aspirin. Systematic overview of individual data from 96 712 randomized patients. *J Am Coll Cardiol* 2000;35:1801–1807. Search date not stated; primary source individual patient data on all trials involving more than 1000 patients.
39. Yusuf S, Collins R, MacMahon S, Peto R. Effect of intravenous nitrates on mortality in acute myocardial infarction: an overview of the randomised trials. *Lancet* 1988;1:1088–1092. Search date not stated; primary sources literature, colleagues, investigators, and pharmaceutical companies.
40. Fourth International Study of Infarct Survival (ISIS-4) Collaborative Group. ISIS-4: a randomised factorial trial assessing early oral captopril, oral mononitrate, and intravenous magnesium sulphate in 58 050 patients with suspected acute myocardial infarction. *Lancet* 1995;345:669–685.
41. Gruppo Italiano per lo studio della streptochinasi nell'infarto miocardico (GISSI). GISSI-3: effects of lisinopril and transdermal glyceryl trinitrate singly and together on 6-week mortality and ventricular function after acute myocardial infarction. *Lancet* 1994;343:1115–1122.
42. Opie LH, Yusuf S, Kubler W. Current status of safety and efficacy of calcium channel blockers in cardiovascular diseases: a critical analysis based on 100 studies. *Prog Cardiovasc Dis* 2000;43:171–196.
43. Wilcox RG, Hampton JR, Banks DC, et al. Early nifedipine in acute myocardial infarction: the TRENT study. *BMJ* 1986;293:1204–1208.
44. Goldbourt U, Behar S, Reicher-Reiss H, et al. Early administration of nifedipine in suspected acute myocardial infarction: the secondary prevention reinfarction Israel nifedipine trial 2 study. *Arch Intern Med* 1993;153:345–353.
45. Pepine CJ, Faich G, Makuch R. Verapamil use in patients with cardiovascular disease: an overview of randomized trials. *Clin Cardiol* 1998;21:633–641. Search date 1997; primary sources Medline, Science Citation Index, Current Contents, and hand searches of reference lists.
46. Yusuf S, Furberg CD. Effects of calcium channel blockers on survival after myocardial infarction. *Cardiovasc Drugs Ther* 1987;1:343–344. Search dates not stated and primary sources not stated.
47. Teo KK, Yusuf S, Furberg CD. Effects of prophylactic antiarrhythmic drug therapy in acute myocardial infarction: an overview of results from randomized controlled trials. *JAMA* 1993;270:1589–1595. Search date not stated; primary sources Medline and correspondence with investigators and pharmaceutical companies.
48. The Multicenter Diltiazem Post Infarction Trial Research Group. The effect of diltiazem on mortality and reinfarction after myocardial infarction. *N Engl J Med* 1988;319:385–392.
49. Weaver WD, Simes RJ, Betriu A, et al. Comparison of primary coronary angioplasty and intravenous thrombolytic therapy for acute myocardial infarction: a quantitative review. *JAMA* 1997;278:2093–2098. Search date 1996; primary sources Medline and scientific session abstracts of stated journals.
50. Cucherat M, Bonnefoy E, Tremeau G. Primary angioplasty versus intravenous thrombolysis for acute myocardial infarction. In: The Cochrane Library, Issue 1, 2001. Oxford: Update Software. Search date 1998; primary sources The Cochrane Library, Medline, and references from reviews and experts.
51. The GUSTO IIb Angioplasty Substudy Investigators. A clinical trial comparing primary coronary angioplasty with tissue plasminogen activator for acute myocardial infarction. *N Engl J Med* 1997;336:1621–1628.
52. Zijlstra F, Hoorntje JC, de Boer MJ, et al. Long-term benefit of primary angioplasty as compared with thrombolytic therapy for acute myocardial infarction. *N Engl J Med* 1999 341:1413–1419.
53. Yusuf S, Pogue J. Primary angioplasty compared to thrombolytic therapy for acute myocardial infarction [editorial]. *JAMA* 1997;278:2110–2111.
54. Van de Werf F, Topol EJ, Lee KL, et al. Variations in patient management and outcomes for acute myocardial infarction in the United States and other countries: results from the GUSTO trial. *JAMA* 1995;273:1586–1591.
55. Hochman JS, Sleeper LA, White HD et al. One year survival following early revascularization for cardiogenic shock. *JAMA* 2001;285:190–192.
56. GISSI-1. Effectiveness of intravenous thrombolytic treatment in acute myocardial infarction. *Lancet* 1986;1:397–401.
57. Herbert P, Tinker J. Inotropic drugs in acute circulatory failure. *Intensive Care Med* 1980;6:101–111.
58. Hollenberg SM, Kavinsky CJ, Parrillo JE. Cardiogenic shock. *Ann Int Med*

1999;131:47–59. Search date 1998; primary sources Medline and hand searches of bibliographies of relevant papers.

59. Bernard GR, Sopko G, Cerra F, et al. Pulmonary artery catheterization and clinical outcomes. *JAMA* 2000;283:2568–2562.
60. Hollenberg SM, Hoyt J. Pulmonary artery catheters in cardiovascular disease. *New Horiz* 1977;5:207–213. Search date 1996; primary sources not stated.
61. Participants. Pulmonary artery catheter consensus conference: consensus statement. *Crit Care Med* 1997;25:910–925.
62. Ohman EM, Nanas J, Stomel R, et al. Thrombolysis and counterpulsation to improve cardiogenic shock survival (Tactics): results of a prospective randomized trial [abstract]. *Circulation* 2000;102(suppl II):II-600.
63. O'Rourke, MF, Norris RM, Campbell TJ, Chang VP, Sammel NL. Randomized controlled trial of intraaortic balloon counterpulsation in early myocardial infarction with acute heart failure. *Am J Cardiol* 1981;47:815–820.
64. Flaherty JT, Becker LC, Weiss JL, et al. Results of a randomized prospective trial of intraaortic balloon counterpulsation and intravenous nitroglycerin in patients with acute myocardial infarction. *J Am Coll Cardiol* 1985;6:434–446.
65. Frazier OH. Future directions of cardiac assistance. *Semin Thorac Cardiovasc Surg* 2000;12:251–258.
66. Pagani FD, Lynch W, Swaniker F, et al. Extracorporal life support to left ventricular assist device bridge to cardiac transplantation. *Circulation* 1999;100(suppl 19):II206–210.
67. Mavroidis D, Sun BC, Pae WE. Bridge to transplantation: the Penn State experience. *Ann Thorac Surg* 1999;68:684–687.

Nicolas Danchin
Professor of Medicine Université Paris VI
Hôpital Européen Georges Pompidou
Paris
France

Philip Urban
Director, Interventional Cardiology
Hôpital de la Tour
Meyrin-Geneva
Switzerland

Edoardo De Benedetti
Cardiologist
C.H.U.V.
Lausanne
Switzerland

Competing interests: PU has received funds for research and public speaking from a variety of pharmaceutical and device companies, both related and unrelated to products discussed here. EdB and ND none declared.

TABLE 1 **Direct randomised comparisons of the standard streptokinase regimen with various tPA based fibrinolytic regimens in patients with suspected AMI in the GISSI-2, ISIS-3, and GUSTO-1 trials (see text, p 15).[18–20]**

Trial and treatment	Number of participants randomised	Any stroke Absolute number (%)	Any death Absolute number (%)	Death not related to stroke* Absolute number (%)	Stroke or death Absolute number (%)
GISSI-2†[18]					
Streptokinase	10 396	98 (0.9)	958 (9.2)	916 (8.8)	1014 (9.8)
t-PA	10 372	136 (1.3)	993 (9.6)	931 (9.0)	1067 (10.3)
Effect/1000 people treated with t-PA instead of streptokinase		3.7 ± 1.5 more	3.6 ± 4.0 more	1.7 ± 4.0 more	5.3 ± 4.2 more
ISIS-3‡[19]					
Streptokinase	13 780	141 (1.0)	1455 (10.6)	1389 (10.1)	1530 (11.1)
t-PA	13 746	188 (1.4)	1418 (10.3)	1325 (9.6)	1513 (11.0)
Effect/1000 people treated with t-PA instead of streptokinase		3.5 ± 1.3 more	2.4 ± 3.7 fewer	4.4 ± 3.6 fewer	1.0 ± 3.8 fewer
GUSTO-1§[20]					
Streptokinase (sc heparin)	9841	117 (1.2)	712 (7.3)	666 (6.8)	783 (8.0)
Streptokinase (iv heparin)	10 410	144 (1.4)	763 (7.4)	709 (6.8)	853 (8.2)
t-PA alone	10 396	161 (1.6)	653 (6.3)	585 (5.6)	746 (7.2)
t-PA plus streptokinase	10 374	170 (1.6)	723 (7.0)	647 (6.2)	817 (7.9)
Effect/1000 people treated with t-PA-based regimens instead of streptinokinase		3.0 ± 1.2 more	6.6 ± 2.5 fewer	8.6 ± 2.4 fewer	5.5 ± 2.6 fewer

TABLE 1 continued

$\chi^2/2$ heterogeneity of effects between 3 trials	0.7	5.6	7.0	5.4
P value	0.3	0.06	0.03	0.07
Weighted average of all 3 trials¶				
Effect/1000 patient treated with t-PA-based regimens instead of streptokinase	3.3 ± 0.8 more	2.9 ± 1.9 fewer	4.9 ± 1.8 fewer	1.6 ± 1.9 fewer
P value	< 0.001	> 0.1	0.01	0.4

Values are numbers (%). This table should not be used to make direct non-randomised comparisons between the absolute event rates in different trials, because the patient populations may have differed substantially in age and other characteristics. Deaths recorded throughout the first 35 days are included for GISSI-2 and ISIS-3 and throughout the first 30 days for GUSTO-1. Numbers randomised and numbers with follow up are from the ISIS-3 report[19] and GUSTO-1[20] (supplemented with revised GUSTO-1 data from the National Auxiliary Publications Service), and numbers with events and the percentages (based on participants with follow up) are from the ISIS-3 report[19] and Van de Werf, et al.[54] Plus-minus values are ± standard deviation. In all three trials, streptokinase was given in intravenous infusions of 1.5 MU over a period of 1 hour. AMI, acute myocardial infarction; iv, intravenous; t-PA, tissue plasminogen activator; sc, subcutaneous.

*Death not related to stroke was defined as death without recorded stroke.

†In the GISSI-2 trial, the t-PA regimen involved an initial bolus of 10 mg, followed by 50 mg in the first hour and 20 mg in each of the second and third hours.

‡In the ISIS-3 trial, the t-PA regimen involved 40 000 clot-lysis units/kg of body weight as an initial bolus, followed by 360 000 units/kg in the first hour and 67 000 units/kg in each of the next 3 hours.

§In the GUSTO-1 trial, the t-PA alone regimen involved an initial bolus of 15 mg, followed by 0.75 mg/kg (up to 50 mg) in the first 30 minutes and 0.5 mg/kg (up to 35 mg) in the next hour; in the GUSTO-1 trial the other t-PA based regimen involved 0.1 mg of t-PA/kg (up to 9 mg) as an initial bolus and 0.9 mg/kg (up to 81 mg) in the remainder of the first hour, plus 1 MU of streptokinase in the first hour.

¶The weights are proportional to the sample sizes of the trials, so this average gives most weight to the GUSTO-1 trial and least to the GISSI-2 trials.[17]

Reproduced from Collins R, Peto R, Baigent BM, Sleight DM. Aspirin, heparin and fibrinolytic therapy in suspected AMI. *N Engl J Med* 1997;336:847–860.

TABLE 2 **Comparison of early invasive cardiac revascularisation versus initial medical treatment on mortality at 30 days, 6 months, and 12 months (see text, p 24).[2,3,55]**

Time after AMI	Mortality in early invasive cardiac revascularisation group Number dead/total number (%)	Mortality in medical treatment alone group Number dead/total number (%)	ARR (95% CI)	RR (95% CI)	NNT (95% CI)
SHOCK study[2,55]					
30 days	71/152 (47)	84/150 (56)	9.3% (–2 to +20.2)	0.83 (0.67 to 1.04)	NA
6 months	76/152 (50)	94/150 (63)	12.7% (1.5 to 23.4)	0.80 (0.65 to 0.98)	8 (5 to 68)
12 months	81/152 (53)	99/150 (66)	12.7% (1.6 to 23.3)	0.80 (0.67 to 0.97)	8 (5 to 61)
SMASH study[3]					
30 days	22/32 (69)	18/23 (78)	9.5% (–14.6 to +30.6)	0.88 (0.64 to 1.2)	NA
12 months	23/32 (74)	19/23 (83)	10.7% (–12.7 to +30.9)	0.87 (0.65 to 1.16)	NA

AMI, acute myocardial infarction; NA, not applicable.

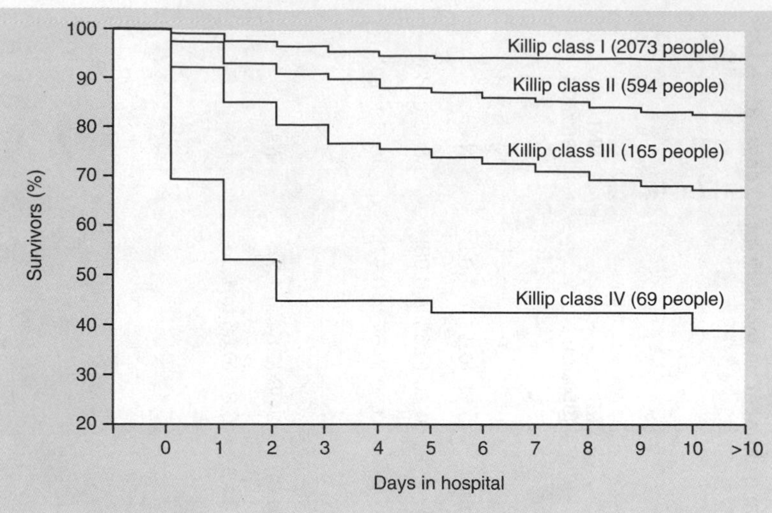

FIGURE 1 **The AMIS registry Kaplan–Meier survival curves as a function of Killip class at hospital admission for 3138 people admitted in 50 Swiss hospitals between 1977 and 1998. Published with permission (see text, p 14).[9]**

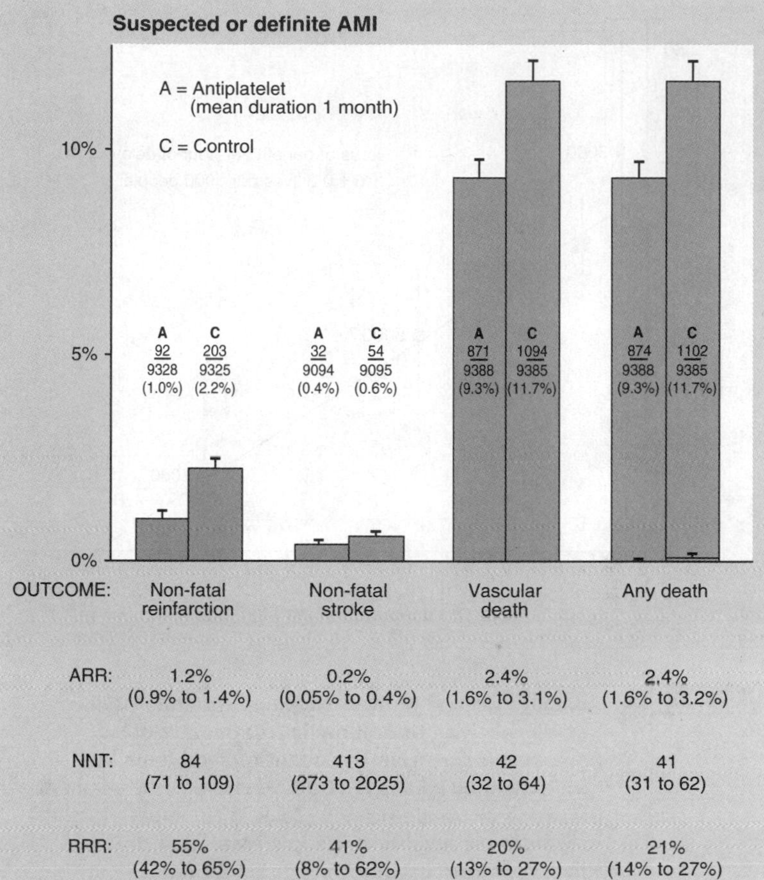

OUTCOME:	Non-fatal reinfarction	Non-fatal stroke	Vascular death	Any death
ARR:	1.2% (0.9% to 1.4%)	0.2% (0.05% to 0.4%)	2.4% (1.6% to 3.1%)	2.4% (1.6% to 3.2%)
NNT:	84 (71 to 109)	413 (273 to 2025)	42 (32 to 64)	41 (31 to 62)
RRR:	55% (42% to 65%)	41% (8% to 62%)	20% (13% to 27%)	21% (14% to 27%)

FIGURE 2 **Absolute effects of antiplatelet treatment on various outcomes in people with a prior suspected or definite acute myocardial infarction (AMI).[11] The columns show the absolute risks over 1 month for each category; the error bars are the upper 95% confidence interval. In "any death" column, non-vascular deaths are represented by lower horizontal lines. The table displays for each outcome the absolute risk reduction (ARR), the number of people needing treatment for 1 month to avoid one additional event (NNT), and the relative risk reduction (RRR), with their 95% CIs (see text, p 14). Published with permission.[11]**

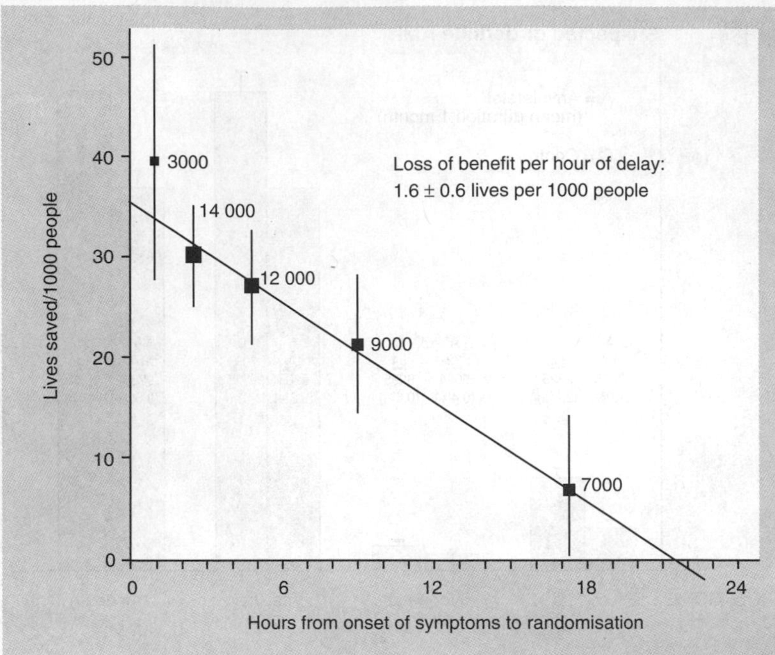

FIGURE 3 **Absolute number of lives saved at 1 month/1000 people receiving thrombolytic treatment plotted against the time from the onset of symptoms to randomisation among 45 000 people with ST segment elevation or bundle branch block.[15] Numbers along the curve are the number of people treated at different times (see text, p 15). Copyright © 1997 Massachusetts Medical Society. All rights reserved.[17]**

We are pleased to provide you with this copy of *Clinical Evidence*.

We at UnitedHealth Foundation support you in your efforts to provide the best quality of health care for your patients.

For more information on UnitedHealth Foundation, please visit our website at

www.unitedhealthfoundation.org.

To continue receiving *Clinical Evidence*......

We hope that you enjoy receiving this **complimentary** copy of *Clinical Evidence*.
The UnitedHealth Foundation is pleased to be able to provide you with this copy and has made a commitment to provide copies of the next Issue **of *Clinical Evidence Concise*.**

In order to receive the next Issue, please provide us with the information requested below or visit our website at www.unitedhealthfoundation.org.

Sincerely,
William W. McGuire, M.D.

Chairman
UnitedHealth Foundation

Name..

Address..

....

City/State/Zip ....

Specialty ....

e-mail address: ....

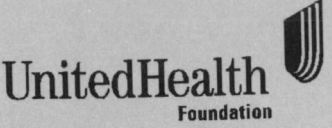

P.O. Box 1459
Minneapolis, Minnesota 55440
www.unitedhealthfoundation.org
e-mail: ce@unitedhealthfoundation.org

UnitedHealth Foundation
MN008-T500
P.O. Box 1459
Minneapolis, MN 55440

Please add Postage for Mailing

*To continue receiving your complimentary issue of **Clinical Evidence** please send to:*

UnitedHealth Foundation
Clinical Evidence
MN008-T500
P.O. Box 1459
Minneapolis, MN 55440-1459

Changing behaviour

Search date May 2002

Margaret Thorogood, Melvyn Hillsdon, and Carolyn Summerbell

QUESTIONS

INTERVENTIONS

*In terms of producing the intended behavioural change

See glossary, p 55

Changing behaviour

Key Messages

- **Acupuncture for smoking cessation** One systematic review has found no significant difference in rates of smoking cessation at 1 year with acupuncture versus control.
- **Advice from nurses to quit smoking** One systematic review has found that advice to quit smoking versus no advice significantly increased the rate of quitting at 1 year.
- **Advice from physicians and trained counsellors to quit smoking** Systematic reviews have found that simple, one off advice from a physician during a routine consultation is associated with 2% of smokers quitting smoking and not relapsing for 1 year. Advice from trained counsellors (who are neither doctors nor nurses) increases quit rates compared with minimal intervention.
- **Advice on cholesterol lowering diet** Systematic reviews have found that advice on cholesterol lowering diet (i.e. advice to lower total fat intake or increase the ratio of polyunsaturated to saturated fatty acid) leads to a small reduction in blood cholesterol concentrations in the long term (≥ 6 months).
- **Advice on diet and exercise supported by behavioural therapy for the encouragement of weight loss** Systematic reviews and subsequent RCTs have found that a combination of advice on diet and exercise supported by behavioural therapy is probably more effective than either diet or exercise advice alone in the treatment of obesity, and might lead to sustained weight loss.
- **Advice on reducing sodium intake to reduce blood pressure** Systematic reviews have found that salt restriction significantly reduces blood pressure in people with hypertension, and have found limited evidence that salt restriction is effective in preventing hypertension. One RCT found limited evidence that advice on restricting salt intake was less effective than advice on weight reduction in preventing hypertension.
- **Anxiolytics for smoking cessation** One systematic review found no significant difference in quit rates with anxiolytics versus control.
- **Bupropion as part of a smoking cessation programme** One systematic review of antidepressants used as part of a smoking cessation programme has found that bupropion increases quit rates at 1 year.
- **Counselling people at high risk of disease to quit smoking** Systematic reviews and subsequent RCTs have found that antismoking advice improves smoking cessation in people at higher risk of smoking related disease.
- **Counselling pregnant women to quit smoking** Two systematic reviews have found that antismoking interventions in pregnant women increase abstinence rates during pregnancy and reduce the risk of low birthweight babies. Interventions without nicotine replacement were as effective as nicotine replacement in healthy non-pregnant women.
- **Counselling sedentary people to increase physical activity** We found weak evidence from systematic reviews and subsequent RCTs that counselling sedentary people increases physical activity compared with no intervention. Limited evidence from RCTs suggests that consultation with an exercise specialist rather than a physician may increase physical activity at 1 year.

- **Exercise advice to women over 80 years** One RCT found that exercise advice delivered in the home by physiotherapists increased physical activity and reduced the risk of falling in women over 80 years.
- **Nicotine replacement in smokers who smoke at least 10 cigarettes daily** One systematic review and one subsequent RCT have found that nicotine replacement is an effective additional component of cessation strategies in smokers who smoke at least 10 cigarettes daily. We found no clear evidence that any method of delivery of nicotine is more effective than others. We found limited evidence from three RCTs with follow up of 2–6 years that the additional benefit of nicotine replacement treatment on quit rates reduced with time.
- **Physical exercise to aid smoking cessation** One systematic review found very limited evidence that exercise might increase smoking cessation.
- **Self help materials for people who want to stop smoking** One systematic review found that self help materials slightly improve smoking cessation compared with no intervention. It found that individually tailored materials were more effective than standard or stage based materials and that telephone counselling increased the effectiveness of postal self help materials.
- **Training health professionals to give advice on smoking cessation** One systematic review has found that training professionals increases the frequency of antismoking interventions being offered, but found no good evidence that antismoking interventions are more effective if the health professionals delivering the interventions received training. One RCT found that a structured intervention delivered by trained community pharmacists increased smoking cessation rates compared to usual care delivered by untrained community pharmacists.

DEFINITION Cigarette smoking, diet, and level of physical activity are important in the aetiology of many chronic diseases. Individual change in behaviour has the potential to decrease the burden of chronic disease, particularly cardiovascular disease. This topic focuses on the evidence that specific interventions lead to changed behaviour.

INCIDENCE/ PREVALENCE In the developed world, the decline in smoking has slowed and the prevalence of regular smoking is increasing in young people. A sedentary lifestyle is becoming increasingly common and the prevalence of obesity is increasing rapidly.

AIMS To encourage individuals to reduce or abandon unhealthy behaviours and to take up healthy behaviours; to support the maintenance of these changes in the long term.

OUTCOMES Ideal outcomes are clinical, and relate to the underlying conditions (longevity, quality of life, and rate of stroke or myocardial infarction). However, the focus of this topic and the outcomes reported by most studies are proxy outcomes, such as the proportion of people changing behaviour (e.g. stopping smoking) in a specified period.

METHODS *Clinical Evidence* update search and appraisal May 2002.

QUESTION **Which interventions reduce cigarette smoking?**

OPTION **ADVICE TO QUIT SMOKING**

Systematic reviews have found that simple, one off advice from a physician during a routine consultation is associated with at least 2% of smokers quitting smoking and not relapsing for 1 year. Additional encouragement or support may increase the effectiveness of the advice (by a further 3%). Individual advice from a psychologist achieves a similar quit rate (3%), and advice from trained nurse counsellors, or from trained counsellors who are neither doctors nor nurses, increases quit rates compared with minimal intervention. We found limited evidence from one systematic review that telephone counselling may improve quit rates compared to interventions with no personal contact. One systematic review found that self help materials slightly improve smoking cessation compared with no intervention. It found that individually tailored materials were more effective than standard or stage based materials and that telephone counselling increased the effectiveness of postal self help materials.

Benefits: We found four systematic reviews[1–4] and one later RCT.[5] **Physicians:** The first review (search date 2000, 34 RCTs, 28 000 smokers) considered advice given by physicians, most often in the primary care setting, but also in hospitals and other clinics.[1] It found that brief advice improved quit rates compared to no advice (16 trials, 12 with follow up for at least 1 year; 451/7705 [5.9%] with brief advice *v* 241/5870 [4.1%] with no advice; meta-analysis OR 1.69, 95% CI 1.45 to 1.98; ARI 2.5%; NNT 40). Intensive advice slightly improved quit rates compared with minimal advice among smokers not at high risk of disease (10 trials, 7 with follow up for at least 1 year; OR with intensive *v* minimal advice 1.23, 95% CI 1.02 to 1.49). One subsequent RCT tested a brief (10 min) intervention given by general practitioners who had received a 2 hour training.[5] The intervention increased the abstinence rate at 12 months (7.3% with control *v* 13.4% with intervention; NNT 16; $P < 0.05$). **Counsellors:** The second systematic review (search date 1998, 11 RCTs) of interventions by counsellors (other than doctors and nurses) trained in smoking cessation used a broad definition of counselling, which included all contacts with a smoker that lasted at least 10 minutes. Follow up was at least 1 year for six of the RCTs, and was at least 6 months for the rest. The review found that counselling increased the rate of quitting (263/1381 [14%] quit with counselling *v* 194/1899 [10%] with control; OR of quitting 1.55, 95% CI 1.27 to 1.90).[2] **Nurses:** The third review (search date 2001, 22 RCTs, 5 with follow up for < 1 year) considered the effectiveness of smoking interventions delivered by a nurse. It found that advice from a nurse increased the rate of quitting by the end of follow up (meta-analysis of 18 studies: 646/4836 [13.4%] quit with advice *v* 405/3356 [12.1%] with control; OR 1.50, 95% CI 1.29 to 1.73).[3] **Telephone advice:** The final systematic review (search date 2000, 23 RCTs) considered counselling delivered by telephone.[4] Ten of the included trials (9 with follow up for at least 12 months) compared proactive telephone counselling versus minimum intervention (involving no person to person contact). Pooled analysis was not possible because of statistical heterogeneity among trials. However, three trials found that telephone counselling was significantly more effective than minimum intervention; four trials found a non-significant benefit, and none of the trials found significant harms of telephone counselling. **Self help materials:** We found one systematic review (search date 1999, 45 RCTs)[6] and one subsequent RCT[7] that examined effects of providing materials giving advice and information to smokers attempting to give up on their own. It found that self help materials without face to face contact slightly improved smoking cessation compared with no intervention (9 trials, 8 of them with at least 12 months' follow up; OR 1.23, 95% CI 1.02 to 1.49; NNT 100). Individually tailored materials were more effective than standard or stage based materials (8 trials, OR for cessation 1.41, 95% CI 1.14 to 1.75).[6] One subsequent RCT compared postal self help materials alone versus postal self help plus telephone counselling.[7] It found that adding telephone counselling improved quit rates at 12 months compared with self help materials alone (OR 2.2, 95% CI 1.1 to 4.6).[7]

Harms: We found no evidence of harm.

Comment: The effects of advice may appear small, but a year on year reduction of 2% in the number of smokers would represent a significant public health gain (see smoking cessation under primary prevention, p 95). In the systematic review of advice provided by nurses,[3] there was significant heterogeneity of the study results and many studies may not have been adequately randomised (7/18 studies [39%] did not specify the randomisation method and 3 [19%] used an inadequate form of randomisation).

OPTION NICOTINE REPLACEMENT

One systematic review and one subsequent RCT have found that nicotine replacement is an effective component of cessation strategies in smokers who smoke at least 10 cigarettes daily. Fifteen such smokers would have to be treated with nicotine replacement to produce one extra non-smoker at 12 months, but this overestimates effectiveness because relapse will continue after 12 months. Higher dose chewing gum (4 mg) is more effective than lower dose chewing gum (2 mg) in very dependent smokers. We found no clear evidence that any one method of delivery of nicotine is more effective, or evidence of further benefit after 8 weeks' treatment with patches. Long term relapse may occur in people who quit, but the review found that the rate of relapse was not greater in those who quit with the aid of nicotine replacement. Abstinence after 1 week is a strong predictor of 12 month abstinence.

Benefits: **Abstinence at 12 months:** We found one systematic review (search date 2001) that identified 51 trials of nicotine chewing gum, 33 trials of nicotine transdermal patches, four of nicotine intranasal spray, four of inhaled nicotine, and two of sublingual tablets.[8] All forms of nicotine replacement were more effective than placebo. When the abstinence rates for all trials were pooled according to the longest duration of follow up available, nicotine replacement compared with placebo increased the odds of abstinence (1508/7674 [19.7%] with nicotine replacement *v* 1110/9613 [11.5%] with placebo; OR 1.66, 95% CI 1.52 to 1.81). The review found no significant difference in abstinence with different forms of nicotine replacement in indirect comparisons (OR 1.66 for nicotine chewing gum *v* 2.27 for nicotine nasal spray) or direct comparisons (1 RCT, inhaler *v* patch; OR 0.57, 95% CI 0.20 to 1.62). In trials that directly compared 4 mg with 2 mg nicotine chewing gum, the higher dose improved abstinence in highly dependent smokers (OR 2.18, 95% CI 1.49 to 3.17). High dose versus standard dose patches slightly increased abstinence (6 RCTs; OR 1.21, 95% CI 1.03 to 1.42). The review found no evidence of a difference in effectiveness for 16 hour patches versus 24 hour patches, and no difference in effect in trials where the dose was tapered compared with those where the patches were withdrawn abruptly. Use of the patch for 8 weeks was as effective as longer use, and there was very weak evidence in favour of nicotine replacement in relapsed smokers. One included RCT (3585 people) found that abstinence at 1 week was a strong predictor of 12 month abstinence (25% of those abstinent at 1 wk were abstinent at 12 months *v* 2.7% of those not abstinent at 1 wk).[9] One meta-analysis of relapse rates in nicotine replacement trials found that nicotine replacement increased abstinence at 12 months, but that continued nicotine replacement did not significantly affect relapse rates between 6 weeks and 12 months.[10] **Longer term abstinence:** We found three RCTs[11–13] that found nicotine replacement does not affect long term abstinence. In one RCT that compared nicotine spray versus placebo, 47 people abstinent at 1 year were followed for up to a further 2 years and 5 months, after which there was still a significant, although smaller, difference in abstinence (in the longer term 15.4% abstinent with nicotine spray *v* 9.3% with placebo; NNT for 1 extra person to abstain 7 at 1 year *v* 11 at 3.5 years).[11] The second RCT compared 5 months of nicotine patches plus nicotine spray versus the same patches plus a placebo spray. It found no significant difference between treatments after 6 years (16.2% abstinent with nicotine spray *v* 8.5% with placebo spray; P = 0.08).[12] The third trial compared patches delivering different nicotine doses versus placebo patches. The trial followed everyone that quit at 6 weeks for a further 4–5 years and found no significant difference in relapse between the groups. Overall, 73% of people who quit at 6 weeks relapsed.[13]

Harms: Nicotine chewing gum has been associated with hiccups, gastrointestinal disturbances, jaw pain, and orodental problems. Nicotine transdermal patches have been associated with skin sensitivity and irritation. Nicotine inhalers and nasal spray have been associated with local irritation at the site of administration. Nicotine sublingual tablets have been reported to cause hiccups, burning, smarting sensations in the mouth, sore throat, coughing, dry lips, and mouth ulcers.[14]

Comment: Nicotine replacement may not represent an "easy cure" for nicotine addiction, but it does improve the cessation rate. The evidence suggests that the majority of smokers attempting cessation fail at any one attempt or relapse over the next 5 years. Multiple attempts may be needed.

OPTION ACUPUNCTURE

One systematic review has found no evidence that acupuncture increases rates of smoking cessation at 12 months.

Benefits: We found one systematic review (search date 2002, 22 RCTs, 4158 adults, 330 young people aged 12–18 years) comparing acupuncture with sham acupuncture, other treatment, or no treatment.[15] Seven RCTs (2701 people) reported abstinence after at least 12 months. The review found no significant difference in smoking cessation with acupuncture versus control at 12 months (OR 1.08, 95% CI 0.77 to 1.52).

Harms: None were documented.

Comment: None.

OPTION PHYSICAL EXERCISE

One systematic review found limited evidence that exercise might increase smoking cessation.

Benefits: We found one systematic review (search date 1999, 8 RCTs) of exercise versus control interventions.[16] Four small RCTs in the review reported point prevalence of non-smoking at 12 months and found no significant benefit from exercise, but these studies were incufficiently powered to exclude a clinically important effect. One RCT (281 women) found that three exercise sessions a week for 12 weeks plus a cognitive behavioural programme (see glossary, p 55) improved continuous abstinence from smoking at 12 months compared with the behavioural programme alone (16/134 [12%] with exercise *v* 8/147 [5%] with control; ARR +6.5%, 95% CI –19 to +0.0; RR 2.2, 95% CI 0.98 to 4.5).[17]

Harms: None were documented.

Comment: None.

OPTION ANTIDEPRESSANT AND ANXIOLYTIC TREATMENT

Systematic reviews have found that quit rates are significantly increased by bupropion, but not by moclobemide or anxiolytics.

Benefits: **Antidepressants:** We found one systematic review of antidepressants (search date 2001, 18 RCTs).[18] Eight of the RCTs (2649 people) reported 12 month cessation rates. It found that bupropion increased quit rates compared with placebo at 6–12 months (calculated by combining results of 4 RCTs with 12 month follow up and 3 RCTs with 6 month follow up; OR of quitting with bupropion *v* placebo 2.54, 95% CI 1.90 to 3.41; NNT 10). The review found no evidence of statistical heterogeneity between the two follow up times.[18] One RCT included in the review compared combined bupropion plus a nicotine patch versus patch alone. It found that combined treatment improved cessation compared with patch alone (OR 2.65, 95% CI 1.58 to 4.45), but was not more effective than bupropion alone. Another included RCT compared different doses of bupropion (100–300 mg/day) and found that cessation rate was linearly related to dose. Three other included RCTs (2 with 6 months' and 1 with 12 months' follow up) found that nortriptyline improved long term (6–12 month) abstinence rates compared with placebo (OR 2.77, 95% CI 1.73 to 4.44). One RCT of moclobemide found no significant difference in abstinence at 12 months. **Anxiolytics:** We found one systematic review of anxiolytics (search date 2000, 6 RCTs).[19] Four of the RCTs (626 people) reporting 12 month cessation rates found no significant increase in abstinence with anxiolytics versus control treatment.[19]

Harms: Headache, insomnia, and dry mouth were reported in people using bupropion.[19] Nortriptyline can cause sedation and urinary retention, and can be dangerous in overdose. One large RCT found that discontinuation rates caused by adverse events were 3.8% with placebo, 6.6% for nicotine replacement treatment, 11.9% for bupropion, and 11.4% for bupropion plus nicotine replacement treatment.[20] Anxiolytics may cause dependence and withdrawal problems, tolerance, paradoxical effects, and impair driving ability. Allergic reactions to bupropion have been reported in about 1 in 1000 people.

Comment: None.

QUESTION **Are smoking cessation interventions more effective in people at high risk of smoking related disease?**

OPTION **IN PREGNANT WOMEN**

Two systematic reviews have found that antismoking interventions in pregnant women increase abstinence rates and decrease the risk of giving birth to low birthweight babies. The increase in abstinence with non-nicotine replacement interventions was similar to the increase found in trials of nicotine replacement in men and non-pregnant women. One RCT found no evidence that nicotine patches increased quit rates in pregnant women compared with placebo, although birthweight was greater in babies born to mothers given active patches. One RCT found no evidence that a brief intervention delivered by midwives at the booking visit improved quit rates compared with no intervention.

Benefits: We found two systematic reviews[21,22] and three additional RCTs.[23–25] The most recent review (search date 1998, 44 RCTs) assessed smoking cessation interventions in pregnancy. It found that smoking cessation programmes improved abstinence (OR of continued smoking in late pregnancy with antismoking programmes *v* no programmes 0.53, 95% CI 0.47 to 0.60; NNT 16).[22] The findings were similar if the analysis was restricted to trials in which abstinence was confirmed by means other than self reporting. The review also found that antismoking programmes reduced the risk of low birthweight babies, but found no evidence of an effect on the rates of very low birthweight babies or perinatal mortality, although the power to detect such effects was low (OR for low birthweight babies 0.80, 95% CI 0.69 to 0.99). The review calculated that of 100 smokers attending a first antenatal visit, 10 stopped spontaneously and a further six to seven stopped as the result of a smoking cessation programme. Five included trials examined the effects of interventions to prevent relapse in 800 women who had quit smoking. Collectively, these trials found no evidence that the interventions reduced relapse rate.[22] One earlier systematic review (search date not stated, 10 RCTs, 4815 pregnant women)[21] of antismoking interventions included one trial of physician advice, one trial of advice by a health educator, one trial of group sessions, and seven trials of behavioural therapy based on self help manuals. Cessation rates among trials ranged from 1.9–16.7% in the control groups and from 7.1–36.1% in the intervention groups. The review found that antismoking interventions significantly increased the rate of quitting (ARI with intervention *v* no intervention 7.6%, 95% CI 4.3% to 10.8%).[21] Onc additional RCT found that nicotine patches did not significantly alter quit rates in pregnant women compared with placebo. But active patches were associated with greater birthweight in babies born to treated mothers (mean difference in birthweight with nicotine *v* placebo 186 g, 95% CI 35 g to 336 g).[23] The second RCT (1120 pregnant women) compared a brief (10–15 min) smoking intervention delivered by trained midwives at booking interviews versus usual care.[24] It found no significant difference in smoking behaviour between women receiving intervention versus usual care (abstinence in final 12 wks of pregnancy until birth 17% in each group; abstinence for 6 months after birth 7% with intervention *v* 8% with control). The intervention was difficult to implement (see comment below). The third RCT compared motivational interviewing (see glossary, p 56) with usual care in 269 women in their 28th week of pregnancy who had smoked in the past month.[25] It found no significant differences in cessation rate between intervention and control group at 34th week or at 6 months post partum.

Harms: None documented.

Comment: The recent review found that some women quit smoking before their first antenatal visit, and the majority of these will remain abstinent.[22] Recruitment to the RCT comparing midwife delivered intervention versus usual care was slow. Midwives reported that the intervention was difficult to implement because of a lack of time to deliver the intervention at the booking appointment.[24]

OPTION IN PEOPLE AT HIGH RISK OF DISEASE

Systematic reviews and two subsequent RCTs have found that antismoking advice improves smoking cessation in people at high risk of smoking related disease. One RCT found no added benefit from a single session intervention that included a carbon monoxide reading.

Benefits: We found no trials in which the same intervention was used in high and low risk people. We found one systematic review (search date not stated, 4 RCTs, 13 208 healthy men at high risk of heart disease),[21] one systematic review among people admitted to hospital (search date 2000, 15 RCTs),[26] and two subsequent RCTs.[27,28] The first review found that antismoking advice improved smoking cessation rates compared with control interventions among healthy men at high risk of heart disease (ARI of smoking cessation 21%, 95% CI 10 to 31; NNT 5, 95% CI 4 to 10).[21] One early trial (223 men) that was included in the review used non-random allocation after myocardial infarction. The intervention group was given intensive advice by the therapeutic team while in the coronary care unit. The trial found that the self reported cessation rate at 1 year or more was higher in the intervention group than the control group (63% quit in the intervention group *v* 28% in the control group; ARI of quitting 36%, 95% CI 23 to 48).[29] The second review included seven trials (6 of them with at least 12 months' duration) of high intensity behavioural interventions (defined as contact in hospital plus active follow up for at least 1 month) among smokers admitted to hospital. The review found that active intervention increased quit rates compared to usual care (OR 1.82, 95% CI 1.49 to 2.22; NNT about 10). We found two RCTs not included in the reviews. The first compared postal advice on smoking cessation versus no intervention in men aged 30–45 years with either a history of asbestos exposure, or forced expiratory volume in 1 second in the lowest quartile for their age. Postal advice increased the self reported sustained cessation rate at 1 year compared with no intervention (5.6% with postal advice *v* 3.5%; $P < 0.05$; NNT 48).[27] The second RCT compared brief advice (consultation lasting 20–30 min plus a carbon monoxide reading) versus usual care in 540 smokers following myocardial infarction or cardiac bypass surgery.[29] At 12 months the trial found no significant difference between groups for abstinence rates (41% abstinent with usual care *v* 37% with intervention).[28]

Harms: None were documented.

Comment: There was heterogeneity in the four trials included in the review among healthy men at high risk of heart disease, partly because of a less intense intervention in one trial and the recording of a change from cigarettes to other forms of tobacco as success in another. One of the included trials was weakened by use of self reported smoking cessation as an outcome and non-random allocation to the intervention.[29]

QUESTION Does training of professionals increase the effectiveness of smoking cessation interventions?

One systematic review has found that training professionals increases the frequency of antismoking interventions being offered, but found no good evidence that antismoking interventions are more effective if the health professionals delivering the interventions received training. One RCT found that a structured intervention delivered by trained community pharmacists increased smoking cessation rates compared to usual care delivered by untrained community pharmacists.

Benefits: We found one systematic review[30] and one subsequent RCT.[31] The review (search date 2000, 9 RCTs)[30] included eight RCTs of training medical practitioners and one RCT of training dental practitioners to give antismoking advice. All the trials took place in the USA. The training was provided on a group basis, and variously included lectures, videotapes, role plays, and discussion. The importance of setting quit dates and offering follow up was emphasised in most of the training programmes. The review found no good evidence that training professionals leads to higher quit rates in people receiving antismoking interventions from those professionals, although training increased the frequency with which such interventions were offered. Three of the trials used prompts and reminders to practitioners to deploy smoking cessation techniques, and found that prompts increased the frequency of health professional interventions.[30] The later RCT compared a structured smoking cessation intervention delivered by community pharmacists, who had received 3 hours of training versus no specific training or antismoking intervention.[31] Intervention delivered by trained pharmacists improved abstinence compared to usual care (AR of abstinence at 12 months 14.3% with intervention *v* 2.7% with usual care; RR 5.3; NNT 9; CIs not reported; $P < 0.001$).

Harms: None were documented.

Comment: The results of the systematic review should be interpreted with caution because there were variations in the way the analysis allowed for the unit of randomisation.

QUESTION **Which interventions increase physical activity in sedentary people?**

OPTION **COUNSELLING**

We found weak evidence from systematic reviews and subsequent RCTs that sedentary people can be encouraged to increase their physical activity. Interventions that encourage moderate rather than vigorous exercise, and do not require attendance at a special facility, may be more successful. Increases in walking in previously sedentary women can be sustained over at least 10 years. Brief advice from a physician may lead to short term changes in physical activity, but is probably not effective in increasing physical activity beyond 3 months. We found limited evidence from RCTs that primary care consultation with an exercise specialist may increase physical activity at 1 year compared with no advice. We found limited evidence that in primary care more intensive and prolonged advice programmes are likely to be more effective than brief advice alone, at least among women.

Benefits: We found two systematic reviews[32,33] and ten subsequent RCTs.[34–43] The first review (search date 1996, 11 RCTs based in the USA, 1699 people) assessed single factor physical activity promotion.[32] Seven trials evaluated advice to undertake exercise from home (mainly walking, but including jogging and swimming), and six evaluated advice to undertake facility based exercise (including jogging and walking on sports tracks, endurance exercise, games, swimming, and exercise to music classes). An increase in activity in the intervention groups was seen in trials in which home based moderate exercise was encouraged and regular brief follow up of participants was provided. In most of the trials participants were self selected volunteers, so the effects of the interventions may have been exaggerated. The second systematic review (search date not stated, 3 RCTs, 420 people) compared "lifestyle" physical activity interventions with either standard exercise treatment or a control group.[33] Lifestyle interventions were defined as those concerned with the daily accumulation of moderate or vigorous exercise as part of everyday life. The first RCT (60 adults, 65–85 years old) found significantly more self reported physical activity in the lifestyle group than a standard exercise group. The second RCT (235 people, 35–60 years old) found no significant difference in physical activity between the groups. The third RCT (125 women, 23–54 years old) of encouraging walking found no significant difference in walking levels at 30 months' follow up between people receiving an 8 week behavioural intervention and those receiving a 5 minute telephone call and written information about the benefits of exercise, although both groups increased walking. Nine of the additional trials involved primary care delivered interventions.[34–36,38-43] The two trials in which advice was delivered by an exercise specialist rather than a physician found significant improvement in self reported physical activity at long term (> 6 months) follow up compared with controls.[38,39] Short term improvement was found in two further trials, but not maintained at 9 months or 1 year.[35,36] Two quasi-randomised trials (776 and 1142 people in a primary care setting) tested the effect of brief physician advice plus a postal booklet on physical activity.[37,42] Both found short term improvement in self reported physical activity with the intervention versus control. One of the RCTs continued follow up after 12 months and found that a significant difference was not maintained.[37] One RCT conducted in a primary care setting (874 people) compared behavioural counselling versus behavioural counselling plus telephone support versus physician advice and brief education.[41] At 24 months, interventions including behavioural counselling significantly improved cardiorespiratory fitness compared to the briefer intervention among women, but not men (mean difference in VO_2 max for behavioural counselling plus telephone support *v* advice 80.7 mL/min, 99.2% CI 8.1 mL/min to 153.2 mL/min). The trial found no significant effect from adding telephone support to behavioural counselling on cardiorespiratory fitness among men or women. However, self reported activity was similar among all treatment groups, for women and men, at 24 months. One RCT (229 women) of encouraging women to increase walking found significantly increased walking in the intervention group at 10 years' follow up (86% of women available for follow up, median estimated calorie expenditure from self reported amount of walking 1344 kcal/wk with encouragement *v* 924 kcal/wk with no encouragement; P = 0.01).[44] A further RCT (260 people in a primary care setting) compared the additional offer of community walks (led by lay people) versus fitness tests and advice alone.[43] It found no significant difference in physical activity at 12 months' follow up (ARR for achieving at least 120 min moderate intensity activity per wk 6%, 95% CI –5% to +16.4%).

Harms: In the trial comparing behavioural counselling versus brief advice, 60% of participants experienced a musculoskeletal event during the 2 years of the study. About half of these required a visit to the physician. About 5% of all participants were admitted to hospital for a suspected cardiovascular event. The trial lacked a non-intervention control group.[41] We found no evidence that counselling people to increase activity levels increased adverse events compared to no counselling.

Comment: Self reporting of effects by people in a trial, especially where blinding to interventions is not possible (as is the case with advice or encouragement), is a potential source of bias. Several trials are in progress, including one in the UK, in which people in primary care have been randomised to two different methods of encouragement to increase walking or to a no intervention arm.

QUESTION What are effects of exercise advice in high risk people?

OPTION IN WOMEN AGED OVER 80 YEARS

One RCT found exercise advice increased physical activity in women aged over 80 years and decreased the risk of falling.

Benefits: We found no systematic review. One RCT (233 women > 80 years old, conducted in New Zealand) compared four visits from a physiotherapist who advised a course of 30 minutes of home based exercises three times a week that was appropriate for the individual versus a similar number of social visits.[45] After 1 year, women who had received physiotherapist visits were significantly more active than women in the control group, and 42% were still completing the recommended exercise programme at least three times a week. The mean annual rate of falls in the intervention group was 0.87 compared with 1.34 in the control group, a difference of 0.47 falls a year (95% CI 0.04 to 0.90).

Harms: No additional harms in the intervention group were reported.

Comment: None.

QUESTION What are the effects on blood cholesterol of dietary advice to reduce fat, increase polyunsaturated fats, and decrease saturated fats?

OPTION COUNSELLING

Systematic reviews have found that advice on eating a cholesterol lowering diet (i.e. advice to reduce fat intake or increase the polyunsaturated to saturated fatty acid ratio in the diet) leads to a small reduction in blood cholesterol concentrations in the long term (6 months or more). We found no evidence to support the effectiveness of such advice in primary care.

Benefits: **Effects on blood cholesterol:** We found three systematic reviews[14,46,47] and two subsequent RCTs that reported biochemical rather than clinical end points.[48,49] None of the reviews included evidence after 1996. One review (search date 1993) identified five trials of cholesterol lowering dietary advice (principally advice from nutritionists or specially trained counsellors) with follow up for 9–18 months.[46] It found a reduction in blood cholesterol concentration in the intervention group of 0.22 mmol/L (95% CI 0.05 mmol/L to 0.39 mmol/L) compared with the control group. There was significant heterogeneity ($P < 0.02$), with two outlying studies — one showing no effect and one showing a larger effect. This review excluded trials in people at high risk of heart disease. Another systematic review (search date 1994) identified 13 trials of more than 6 months' duration and included people at high risk of heart disease.[14] It found that dietary advice reduced blood cholesterol (mean reduction in blood cholesterol concentration with advice 4.5%, 95% CI 3.9 to 5.1; given a mean baseline cholesterol of 6.3 mmol/L, mean AR about 0.3 mmol/L). The third systematic review (search date 1996, 1 trial,[50] 76 people) found no significant difference between brief versus intensive advice from a general practitioner and dietician on blood cholesterol at 1 year.[47] The first subsequent RCT (186 men and women at high risk of coronary heart disease) compared advice on healthy eating versus no intervention. At 1 year it found no significant differences between groups in total and low density lipoprotein cholesterol concentrations for either sex, even though the reported percentage of energy from fat consumed by both women and men in the advice group decreased significantly compared with that reported by the women and men in the control group.[48] These results may reflect bias caused by self reporting of dietary intake. The second RCT, in 531 men with hypercholesterolaemia (with and without other hyperlipdaemias) and fat intake of about 35%, compared dietary advice aimed at reducing fat intake to 30% versus 26% versus 22%. All interventions were similarly effective for reducing fat intake (total fat intake after intervention about 26% in all groups).[49] **Effects on clinical outcomes:** We found two systematic reviews that reported on morbidity and mortality.[14,51] The first (search date 1994) compared 13 separate and single dietary interventions.[14] It found no significant effect of dietary interventions on total mortality (OR 0.93, 95% CI 0.84 to 1.03) or coronary heart disease mortality (OR 0.93, 95% CI 0.82 to 1.06), but found a reduction in non-fatal myocardial infarction (OR 0.77, 95% CI 0.67 to 0.90). The second review (search date 1999, 27 studies including 40 intervention arms, 30 901 person years) found dietary advice to reduce or modify dietary fat versus no dietary advice had no significant effect on total mortality (HR 0.98, 95% CI 0.86 to 1.12) or cardiovascular disease mortality (HR 0.98, 95% CI 0.77 to 1.07), but significantly reduced cardiovascular disease events (HR 0.84, 95% CI 0.72 to 0.99).[51] RCTs in which people were followed for more than 2 years showed significant reductions in the rate of cardiovascular disease events. The relative protection from cardiovascular disease events was similar in both high and low risk groups, but was significant only in high risk groups.

Harms: We found no evidence about harms.

Comment: The finding of a 0.2–0.3 mmol/L reduction in blood cholesterol in the two systematic reviews accords with the findings of a meta-analysis of the plasma lipid response to changes in dietary fat and cholesterol.[52] The analysis included data from 244 published studies (trial duration 1 day to 6 years), and concluded that adherence to dietary recommendations (30% energy from fat, < 10% saturated fat, and < 300 mg cholesterol/day) compared with average US dietary intake would reduce blood cholesterol by about 5%.

QUESTION **Does dietary advice to reduce sodium intake lead to a sustained fall in blood pressure?**

Systematic reviews and RCTs have found that salt restriction reduces blood pressure in people with normal blood pressure, and in people with hypertension. The effect was more pronounced in older people. We found no evidence of effects on morbidity and mortality.

Benefits: We found three systematic reviews[46,53,54] and three additional RCTs[55–57] about the effects of advice to restrict salt. The first systematic review (search date 1993, 5 trials with follow up for 9–18 months) compared dietary advice (mainly from nutritionists or specially trained counsellors) with control treatment. It found that the advice slightly reduced systolic blood pressure (change in blood pressure, −1.9 mm Hg systolic, 95% CI −3.0 mm Hg to −0.8 mm Hg), but not diastolic blood pressure (−1.2 mm Hg, 95% CI −2.6 mm Hg to +0.2 mm Hg).[46] The second review (search date 1998, 8 RCTs in adults over 44 years with and without hypertension) found no clearly significant systolic blood pressure changes after at least 6 months' follow up with advice on salt restriction versus no dietary advice either in people with hypertension (−2.9 mm Hg, 95% CI −5.8 mm Hg to +0.0 mm Hg) or in people without hypertension (−1.3 mm Hg, 95% CI −2.7 mm Hg to +0.1 mm Hg). Small but significant changes in mean diastolic blood pressure were found in people with hypertension (−2.1 mm Hg, 95% CI −4.0 mm Hg to −0.1 mm Hg) but not in people without hypertension (−0.8 mm Hg, 95% CI −1.8 mm Hg to +0.2 mm Hg).[53] The definitions of hypertension varied between the trials. The third review (search date 1996, 30 RCTs) found that, in people aged over 44 years defined as having hypertension, a reduction in sodium intake of 100 mmol daily resulted in a decrease of 6.3 mm Hg in systolic blood pressure and 2.2 mm Hg in diastolic pressure.[54] For younger people with hypertension, the systolic fall was 2.4 mm Hg and the diastolic fall was negligible. We found three additional RCTs that found similar results.[55–57] The first RCT (975 people) found that advice to restrict salt intake was more effective compared to usual care at 30 months (HR for hypertension, prescription of an antihypertensive drug or a cardiovascular event with advice *v* usual care 0.69, 95% CI 0.59 to 0.81).[55] Subgroup analysis (585 people) found no evidence that advice to reduce salt intake was more effective than advice to reduce weight among people who were overweight at baseline. The second RCT (208 people, analysis performed on 181 participants) compared weight reduction advice versus salt restriction advice versus no intervention. The weight advice group excluded people who were not overweight, whereas salt restriction and control groups included people regardless of weight. Among people of all weights, salt restriction did not significantly reduce the risk of hypertension at 7 years compared to all controls (AR for hypertension at 7 years 22.4% with advice *v* 32.9% with control; CI not provided; P = 0.19).

But in overweight people, weight reduction advice significantly reduced hypertension at 7 years compared to overweight control participants (AR for hypertension at 7 years 18.9% with advice *v* 40.5% in overweight controls; CI not provided; P = 0.02).[56] The third RCT (2382 overweight non-hypertensive people) compared advice to reduce salt versus advice to reduce weight versus both versus usual care. Compared to usual care, advice reduced blood pressure (at 6 months blood pressure decreased by 3.7/2.7 mm Hg with weight loss advice *v* 2.9/1.6 mm Hg with salt reduction advice *v* 4.0/2.8 mm Hg with both; P < 0.001 for all comparisons).[57]

Harms: None reported.

Comment: None.

QUESTION What are the effects of lifestyle interventions to achieve sustained weight loss?

Systematic reviews and subsequent RCTs have found that a combination of advice on diet and exercise, supported by behavioural therapy, is probably more effective in achieving weight loss than either diet or exercise advice alone. A low energy, low fat diet is the most effective lifestyle intervention for weight loss. Combined personal and computerised tailoring of weight loss programmes may improve maintenance of weight loss. RCTs have found no significant differences in weight loss between interventions to promote physical activity. Weight regain is likely, but weight loss of 2–6 kg may be sustained over at least 2 years.

Benefits: We found three systematic reviews[58–60] and 17 additional RCTs.[55,61–76] One systematic review (search date 1995) identified 99 studies, including some that tested either dietary or physical activity interventions with or without a behavioural intervention component. The combination of diet and exercise in conjunction with behavioural therapy produced greater weight loss than diet alone. However, this finding was based on the results of one RCT, in which a mean weight loss of 3.8 kg at 1 year was observed in a group receiving diet guidelines and behavioural intervention compared with a significantly different mean loss of 7.9 kg in a group receiving the same intervention plus a programme of walking.[58] The second systematic review of the detection, prevention, and treatment of obesity (search date 1999, 11 RCTs and additional prospective cohort studies) included eight RCTs comparing dietary prescriptions with exercise, counselling, or behavioural therapy for the treatment of obesity, and three RCTs comparing dietary counselling alone with no intervention. In both comparisons, initial weight loss was followed by gradual weight regain once treatment had stopped (mean difference in weight change at least 2 years after baseline, 2–6 kg for dietary prescription trials, and 2–4 kg for dietary counselling trials).[59] The third systematic review (search date 1997) of RCTs and observational studies similarly found that a combination of diet and exercise, supported by behavioural therapy, was more effective than any one or two of these individual interventions.[60] One additional RCT compared advice on an energy restricted diet to advice on a fat restricted diet.[65] Weight loss was greater on an energy restricted diet than on the fat restricted diet at 6 months (–11.2 kg *v* –6.1 kg; P < 0.001) and at 18 months (–7.5 kg v –1.8 kg; $P < 0.001$). Seven RCTs focused on physical activity.[61–63,67-69,72] The heterogeneity of interventions makes pooling of data inappropriate, but no major differences were found between the various behavioural therapies and exercise regimes. One RCT[64] found behavioural choice therapy versus standard behavioural therapy resulted in greater weight loss at 12 months (–10.1 kg v –4.3 kg; $P < 0.01$). One RCT (166 people) compared standard behavioural therapy plus support from friends with standard behavioural therapy without support. It found no additional weight loss at 16 months with social support from friends (–4.7 kg v –3.0 kg, $P < 0.3$).[66] A further RCT (62 women) found that 1 year weight loss was greater in women following a standard versus a modified cognitive behavioural programme (–3.6 kg v 2.0 kg; $P = 0.02$).[71] One RCT has found that adding meal replacements to a dietician led group intervention improved weight loss at 1 year (9.1% weight loss with replacements v 4.1% without),[73] although another found that adding body image treatment did not significantly improve weight loss compared to dietician led treatment alone.[74] We found two RCTs examining effects of advice to lose weight among people who were overweight and hypertensive. The first (1191 people) found that advice reduced weight and hypertension more than no weight loss advice at 3 years (weight loss at 3 years, 1.8 kg with advice v 0.2 kg with control; RR for hypertension with advice v control 0.81, 95% CI 0.70 to 0.95). Subgroup analysis of the second RCT (585 overweight elderly people with hypertension) found that weight advice reduced body weight more than no weight advice (weight loss at 30 months 4.7 kg v 0.9 kg).[55] One large RCT (588 overweight people) compared three different cognitive behavioural approaches for tailoring lifestyle modification goals: workbook alone (no tailoring of goals); adding computerised computer kiosks with touch screen monitors to help participants tailor goals; and adding both computers and staff consultation to tailor goals. After 12 months, it found that all groups achieved a statistically significant mean weight loss from baseline. It found that combined personal and computerised tailoring improved weight loss compared with workbook alone (mean weight loss 1 kg with workbook v 2.1 kg with computerised tailoring v 3.3 kg with combined personal and computerised tailoring, $P = 0.02$ for workbook v combined group).[76]

Harms: The systematic reviews and RCTs provided no evidence about harms resulting from diet or exercise for weight loss.

Comment: None.

QUESTION **What are the effects of lifestyle interventions to maintain weight loss?**

One systematic review and additional RCTs have found that most types of maintenance strategy result in smaller weight gains or greater weight losses compared with no contact. Strategies that involve personal contact with a therapist, family support, walking training programmes, or multiple interventions, or are weight focused, appear most effective.

Benefits: We found one systematic review[58] and seven additional RCTs.[77–83] The systematic review (search date 1995, 21 studies) compared different types and combinations of interventions. It found that increased contact with a therapist in the long term produced smaller weight gain or greater weight loss, and that additional self help peer groups, self management techniques, or involvement of the family or spouse may increase weight loss. The largest weight loss was seen in programmes using multiple strategies. Two additional small RCTs (102 people[77] and 100 people in two trials[81]) assessed simple strategies without face to face contact with a therapist. Frequent telephone contacts, optional food provision, continued self monitoring, urge control, or relapse prevention did not reduce the rate of weight regain. One small RCT (117 people) found that telephone contacts plus house visits did reduce the rate of weight regain compared with no intervention (3.65 kg *v* 6.42 kg; $P = 0.048$).[78] One further small RCT (80 obese women) found no difference in weight change at 1 year between participants offered relapse prevention training or problem solving compared with no further contact.[83] One RCT (82 women) compared two walking programmes (4.2 MJ/wk or 8.4 MJ/wk) plus diet counselling versus diet counselling alone following a 12 week intensive weight reduction programme.[82] Both walking programmes reduced weight regain at 1 year (reduction in weight gain compared with dietary counselling alone 2.7 kg, 95% CI 0.2 kg to 5.2 kg with low intensity programme and 2.6 kg, 95% CI 0.0 kg to 5.1 kg with high intensity programme). At 2 years, weight regain was not significantly different between high intensity programme and control, but was reduced in the low intensity group (reduction in weight gain 3.5 kg, 95% CI 0.2 kg to 6.8 kg with low intensity programme and 0.2 kg, 95% CI –3.1 kg to +3.6 kg with high intensity programme). One additional small RCT (67 people) found that people on a weight focused programme maintained weight loss better than those on an exercise focused programme (0.8 kg *v* 4.4 kg; $P < 0.01$).[79] One 5 year RCT (489 menopausal women) compared behavioural intervention in two phases aimed at lifestyle changes in diet and physical activity with lifestyle assessment. People in the intervention group were encouraged to lose weight during the first 6 months (phase I), and thereafter maintain this weight loss for a further 12 months (phase II). The intervention resulted in weight loss compared to control during the first 6 months (–8.9 lb *v* –0.8 lb; $P < 0.05$), most of which was sustained over phase II (–6.7 lb *v* +0.6 lb; $P < 0.05$).[80]

Harms: We found no direct evidence that interventions designed to maintain weight loss are harmful.

Comment: Weight regain is common. The resource implication of providing long term maintenance of any weight loss may be a barrier to the routine implementation of maintenance programmes.

QUESTION **What are the effects of lifestyle advice to prevent weight gain?**

One small RCT found that low intensity education increased weight loss. A second RCT found no significant effect on weight gain from a postal newsletter with or without a linked financial incentive. One RCT found that lifestyle advice prevented weight gain in perimenopausal women compared to assessment alone.

Benefits: We found three systematic reviews (search dates 1995,[58] 1999,[59] and not stated[84]) that included the same two RCTs[85,86] and one subsequent RCT.[87] The first RCT (219 people) compared low intensity education with a financial incentive to maintain weight versus an untreated control group. It found significantly greater average weight loss in the intervention group than in the control group (–0.95 kg with intervention *v* –0.14 kg with control; P = 0.03).[85] The second RCT (228 men and 998 women) compared a monthly newsletter versus the newsletter plus a lottery incentive versus no contact. There was no significant difference in weight gain after 3 years between the groups (1.6 kg *v* 1.5 kg *v* 1.8 kg).[86] The later RCT, which was not included in the reviews, compared lifestyle advice versus assessment alone among 535 perimenopausal women. It found that advice reduced weight gain over 2 years (weight gain 0.5 kg with advice *v* 11.5 kg with assessment alone).[87]

Harms: None reported.

Comment: None.

QUESTION What are the effects of training professionals in promoting reduction of body weight?

One systematic review of poor quality RCTs found little evidence on the sustained effect of interventions to improve health professionals' management of obesity. One subsequent small RCT found limited evidence that training for primary care doctors in nutrition counselling plus a support programme reduced body weight of the people in their care over 1 year.

Benefits: We found one systematic review (search date 2000, 18 RCTs, 8 with follow up > 1 year)[88] and one subsequent RCT.[89] The studies in the review were heterogeneous and poor quality. The subsequent RCT (45 people) compared nutrition counselling training plus a support programme for primary care doctors versus usual care.[89] The nutrition supported intervention compared with usual care increased weight loss at 1 year (additional weight loss 2.3 kg; $P < 0.001$).

Harms: None reported.

Comment: The doctors were randomly allocated to treatment but the analysis of results was based on the people in the care of those doctors. No allowance was made for cluster bias. This increases the likelihood that the additional weight loss could have occurred by chance.

GLOSSARY

Behavioural choice therapy A cognitive behavioural intervention based on a decision making model of women's food choice. This relates situation specific eating behaviour to outcomes and goals using decision theory. The outcomes and goals governing food choice extend beyond food related factors to include self esteem and social acceptance.

Cognitive behavioural programme Traditional cognitive behavioural topics (e.g. self monitoring, stimulus control, coping with cravings and high risk situations, stress management, and relaxation techniques) along with topics of particular importance to women (e.g. healthy eating, weight management, mood management, and managing work and family).

Motivational interviewing A goal directed counselling style that helps participants to understand and resolve areas of ambivalence that impede behavioural change.

Standard behavioural therapy A behavioural weight management programme that incorporates moderate calorie restriction to promote weight loss.

Substantive changes

Acupuncture for smoking cessation Update of systematic review, four new RCTs;[15] conclusion unchanged.

Antidepressants and anxiolytics for smoking cessation Update of systematic review.[18] Six new RCTs; conclusion unchanged.

Smoking cessation in pregnant women New RCT comparing motivational interviewing versus usual care;[25] conclusion unchanged.

Smoking cessation in people at high risk of smoking related disease New RCT;[28] conclusion unchanged.

Exercise for the sedentary One additional RCT;[42] conclusions unchanged.

Maintaining weight loss New RCT;[76] found that combined personal and computerised tailoring of weight loss programmes may improve maintenance of weight loss.

Lifestyle interventions to maintain weight loss New RCT;[25] conclusions unchanged.

REFERENCES

1. Silagy C, Stead LF. Physician advice for smoking cessation. In: The Cochrane Library, Issue 2, 2002. Oxford: Update Software. Search date 2000; primary sources Cochrane Tobacco Addiction Group Trials Register and the Cochrane Controlled Trials Register.
2. Lancaster T, Stead LF. Individual behavioural counselling for smoking cessation. In: The Cochrane Library, Issue 2, 2002. Oxford: Update Software. Search date 1998; primary sources Cochrane Tobacco Addiction Group Trials Register.
3. Rice VH, Stead LF. Nursing interventions for smoking cessation. In: The Cochrane Library, Issue 2, 2002. Oxford: Update Software. Search date 2001; primary sources Cochrane Tobacco Addiction Group Trials Register and Cinahl.
4. Stead LF, Lancaster T. Telephone counselling for smoking cessation. In: The Cochrane Library Issue 2, 2002. Oxford: Update Software. Search date 2000; primary source Cochrane Tobacco Addiction Group Trials Register.
5. Pieterse ME, Seydel ER, de Vries H, et al. Effectiveness of a minimal contact smoking cessation program for Dutch general practitioners: a randomized controlled trial. *Prev Med* 2001;32:182–190.
6. Lancaster T, Stead LF. Self-help interventions for smoking cessation (Cochrane review). In: The Cochrane Library Issue 2, 2002. Oxford: Update Software. Search date 1999; primary sources previous reviews and meta-analyses, the Tobacco Addiction Review Group register of controlled trials identified from Medline Express (Silverplatter) to 1999/8 and the Science Citation Index to 9/1999.
7. Miguez MC, Vasquez FL, Becona E. Effectiveness of telephone contact as an adjunct to a self-help program for smoking cessation. A randomized controlled trial in Spanish smokers. *Addict Behav* 2002;27:139–144.
8. Silagy C, Mant D, Fowler G, et al. Nicotine replacement therapy for smoking cessation. In: The Cochrane Library, Issue 2, 2002. Oxford: Update Software. Search date 2001; primary source Cochrane Tobacco Addiction Group Trials Register.
9. Tonneson P, Paoletti P, Gustavsson G, et al. Higher dose nicotine patches increase one year smoking cessation rates: results from the European CEASE trial. *Eur Respir J* 1999;13:238–246.
10. Stapleton J. Cigarette smoking prevalence, cessation and relapse. *Stat Methods Med Res* 1998;7:187–203.
11. Stapleton JA, Sutherland G, Russell MA. How much does relapse after one year erode effectiveness of smoking cessation treatments? Long term follow up of a randomised trial of nicotine nasal spray. *BMJ* 1998;316:830–831.
12. Blondal T, Gudmundsson J, Olafsdottir I, et al. Nicotine nasal spray with nicotine patch for smoking cessation: randomised trial with six years follow up. *BMJ* 1999;318:285–289.
13. Daughton DM, Fortmann SP, Glover ED, et al. The smoking cessation efficacy of varying doses of nicotine patch delivery systems 4 to 5 years post-quit day. *Prev Med* 1999;28:113–118.
14. Ebrahim S, Davey Smith G. Health promotion in older people for the prevention of coronary heart disease and stroke. *Health promotion effectiveness reviews reries*, No 1. London: Health Education Authority, 1996. Search date 1994; primary sources Medline, hand searched reference lists, and citation search on BIDS for Eastern European trials.
15. White AR, Rampes H, Ernst E. Acupuncture for smoking cessation (Cochrane review) In: The Cochrane Library Issue 2, 2002. Oxford: Update Software. Search date 2002; primary sources Cochrane Tobacco Addiction Group Register, Medline, Psychlit, Dissertation Abstracts, Health Planning and Administration, SocialSciSearch, Smoking and Health, Embase, Biological Abstracts, and Drug.
16. Ussher MH, Taylor AH, West R, et al. Does exercise aid smoking cessation? *Addiction* 2000;95:199–208. Search date 1999; primary

sources Medline, Psychlit, Dissertation Abstracts, Sports Discus, hand searched reference lists, and personal contact with research colleagues.

17. Marcus BH, Albrecht AE, King TK, et al. The efficacy of exercise as an aid for smoking cessation in women. *Arch Intern Med* 1999;159:1229–1234.
18. Hughes JR, Stead LF, Lancaster T. Antidepressants for smoking cessation. In: The Cochrane Library, Issue 2, 2002. Oxford: Update Software. Search date 2001; primary source Cochrane Tobacco Addiction Group Trials Register.
19. Hughes JR, Stead LF, Lancaster T. Anxiolytics for smoking cessation. In: The Cochrane Library, Issue 2, 2002. Oxford: Update Software. Search date 2000; primary source Cochrane Tobacco Addiction Group Trials Register.
20. Jorenby DE, Leischow SJ, Nides MA, et al. A controlled trial of sustained-release bupropion, a nicotine patch, or both for smoking cessation. *N Engl J Med* 1999;340:685–691.
21. Law M, Tang JL. An analysis of the effectiveness of interventions intended to help people stop smoking. *Arch Intern Med* 1995;155:1933–1941. Search date not stated; primary sources Medline and Index Medicus.
22. Lumley J, Oliver S, Waters E. Interventions for promoting smoking cessation during pregnancy. In: The Cochrane Library, Issue 2, 2002. Oxford: Update Software. Search date 1998; primary source Cochrane Tobacco Addiction Group Trials Register.
23. Wisborg K, Henriksen TB, Jespersen LB, et al. Nicotine patches for pregnant smokers: a randomized controlled study. *Obstet Gynecol* 2000,96:967–971.
24. Hajek P, West R, Lee A, et al. Randomized trial of a midwife-delivered brief smoking cessation intervention in pregnancy. *Addiction* 2001;96:485–494.
25. Stotts A, DiClememte CC, Dolan-Mullen P. One-to-one. A motivational intervention for resistant pregnant smokers *Addict Behav* 2002;27:275–292.
26. Rigotti NA, Munafro MR, Murphy MFG, et al. Interventions for smoking cessation in hospitalised patients. In: The Cochrane Library, Issue 2, 2002. Oxford: Update Software. Search date 2000; primary sources Cochrane Controlled Trials Register, Centre for Disease Control Smoking and Health database, Cinahl, and experts.
27. Humerfelt S, Eide GE, Kvale G, et al. Effectiveness of postal smoking cessation advice: a randomized controlled trial in young men with reduced FEV_1 and asbestos exposure. *Eur Respir J* 1998;11:284–290.
28. Hajek P, Taylor TZ, Mills P. Brief intervention during hospital admission to help patients to give up smoking after myocardial infarction and bypass surgery: randomized controlled trial. *BMJ* 2002;324:1–6.
29. Burt A, Thornley P, Illingworth D, et al. Stopping smoking after myocardial infarction. *Lancet* 1974;1:304–306.
30. Lancaster T, Silagy C, Fowler G. Training health professionals in smoking cessation. In: The Cochrane Library, Issue 2, 2002. Oxford: Update Software. Search date 2000; primary source Cochrane Tobacco Addiction Group Trials Register.
31. Maguire TA, McElnay JC, Drummond A. A randomized controlled trial of a smoking cessation intervention based in community pharmacies. *Addiction* 2001;96:325–331.
32. Hillsdon M, Thorogood M. A systematic review of physical activity promotion strategies. *Br J Sports Med* 1996;30:84–89. Search date 1996; primary sources Medline, Excerpta Medica, Sport SCISearch, and hand searched reference lists.
33. Dunn AL, Anderson RE, Jakicic JM. Lifestyle physical activity interventions. History, short- and long-term effects and recommendations. *Am J Prev Med* 1998;15:398–412. Search date not stated; primary sources Medline, Current Contents, Biological Abstracts, The Johns Hopkins Medical Institutions Catalog, Sport Discus, and Grateful Med.
34. Goldstein MG, Pinto BM, Marcus BH, et al. Physician-based physical activity counseling for middle-aged and older adults: a randomised trial. *Ann Behav Med* 1999;1:40–47.
35. Harland J, White M, Drinkwater C, et al. The Newcastle exercise project: a randomised controlled trial of methods to promote physical activity in primary care. *BMJ* 1999;319:828–832.
36. Taylor, A, Doust, J, Webborn, N. Randomised controlled trial to examine the effects of a GP exercise referral programme in Hailsham, East Sussex, on modifiable coronary heart disease risk factors. *J Epidemiol Community Health* 1998;52:595–601.
37. Bull F, Jamorozik K. Advice on exercise from a family physician can help sedentary patients to become active. *Am J Prev Med* 1998;15:85–94.
38. Stevens W, Hillsdon M, Thorogood M, et al. Cost-effectiveness of a primary care based physical activity intervention in 45–74 year old men and women; a randomised controlled trial. *Br J Sports Med* 1998;32:236–241.
39. Halbert JA, Silagy CA, Finucane PM, et al. Physical activity and cardiovascular risk factors: effect of advice from an exercise specialist in Australian general practice. *Med J Aust* 2000;173:84–87.
40. Norris SL, Grothaus LC, Buchner DM, et al. Effectiveness of physician-based assessment and counseling for exercise in a staff model HMO. *Prev Med* 2000;30:513–523.
41. The Writing Group for the Activity Counseling Trial Research Group. Effects of physical activity counseling in primary care: the Activity Counseling Trial: a randomised controlled trial. *JAMA* 2001;286:677–687.
42. Smith BJ, Bauman AE, Bull FC, et al. Promoting physical activity in general practice: a controlled trial of written advice and information maeterials. *Br J Sports Med* 2000;34:262–267.
43. Lamb SE, Bartlett HP, Ashley A, et al. Can lay-led walking programmes increase physical activity in middle aged adults? A randomised controlled trial. *J Epidemiol Community Health* 2002;56:246–252.
44. Pereira MA, Kriska AN, Day RD, et al. A randomized walking trial in postmenopausal women. *Arch Intern Med* 1998;158:1695–1701.
45. Campbell AJ, Robertson MC, Gardner MM, et al. Randomised controlled trial of a general practice programme of home based exercise to prevent falls in elderly women. *BMJ* 1997;315:1065–1069.
46. Brunner E, White I, Thorogood M, et al. Can dietary interventions change diet and cardiovascular risk factors? A meta-analysis of randomised controlled trials. *Am J Public Health* 1997;87:1415–1422. Search date 1993; primary sources computer and manual searched databases and journals.
47. Tang JL, Armitage JM, Lancaster T, et al. Systematic review of dietary intervention trials to lower blood total cholesterol in free living subjects. *BMJ* 1998;316:1213–1220. Search date 1996; primary sources Medline, Human Nutrition, Embase, Allied and Alternative Health, hand search of *Am J Clin Nutr*, and reference list checks.

48. Stefanick ML, Mackey S, Sheehan M, et al. Effects of diet and exercise in men and postmenopausal women with low levels of HDL cholesterol and high levels of LDL cholesterol. *N Engl J Med* 1998;339:12–20.
49. Knopp RH, Retzlaff B, Walden C, et al. One year effects of increasingly fat-restricted, carbohydrate-enriched diets in lipoprotein levels in free living subjects. *Proc Soc Exp Biol Med* 2000;225:191–199.
50. Tomson Y, Johannesson M, Aberg H. The costs and effects of two different lipid intervention programmes in primary health care. *J Intern Med* 1995;237:13–17.
51. Hooper L, Summerbell CD, Higgins JPT, et al. Reduced or modified dietary fat for preventing cardiovascular disease. In: The Cochrane Library, Issue 2, 2002. Oxford: Update Software. Search date 1999; primary sources Cochrane Library, Medline, Embase, CAB Abstracts, CVRCT registry, related Cochrane Groups' Trial Registers, trials known to experts in the field, and biographies.
52. Howell WH, McNamara DJ, Tosca MA, et al. Plasma lipid and lipoprotein responses to dietary fat and cholesterol: a meta-analysis. *Am J Clin Nutr* 1997;65:1747–1764. Search date 1994; primary sources Medline, hand search of selected review publications, and bibliographies.
53. Ebrahim S, Davey Smith G. Lowering blood pressure: a systematic review of sustained effects of non-pharmacological interventions. *J Public Health* 1998;2:441–448. Search date 1998; primary sources Medline and hand searches of reference lists.
54. Fodor JG, Whitmore B, Leenen F, et al. Recommendations on dietary salt. *Can Med Assoc J* 1999;160(Suppl 9):29–34. Search date 1996; primary sources Medline, hand searches of reference lists, personal files, and contact with experts.
55. Whelton PK, Appel LJ, Espeland MA, et al. Sodium reduction and weight loss in the treatment of hypertension in older persons. A randomized controlled Trial of Nonpharmacologic Interventions in the Elderly (TONE). *JAMA* 1998;279:839–846.
56. He J, Whelton PK, Appel LJ, et al. Long-term effects of weight loss and dietary sodium reduction on incidence of hypertension. *Hypertension* 2000;35:544–549.
57. The Trials of Hypertension Prevention, Phase II. Effects of weight loss and sodium reduction intervention on blood pressure and hypertension incidence in overweight people with high-normal blood pressure. *Arch Intern Med* 1997;157:657–667.
58. Glenny A-M, O'Meara S, Melville A, et al. The treatment and prevention of obesity: a systematic review of the literature. *Int J Obesity* 887:21;715–737. Published in full as NHS CRD report 1997, No 10. A systematic review of interventions in the treatment and prevention of obesity. http://www.york.ac.uk/inst/crd/obesity.htm (last accessed 03/09/2002). Search date 1995; primary sources Medline, Embase, DHSS data, Current Research in UK, Science citation index, Social science citation index, Conference Proceedings index, Sigle, Dissertation Abstracts, Sport, Drug Info, AMED (Allied and alternative medicine), ASSI (abstracts and indexes), CAB, NTIS (national technical information dB), Directory of Published Proceedings (Interdoc), Purchasing Innovations database, Health promotion database, S.S.R.U., DARE (CRD, database of systematic reviews, NEED, CRD, database of health economic reviews), and all databases searched from starting date to the end of 1995.
59. Douketis JD, Feightner JW, Attia J, et al. Periodic health examination, 1999 update. Detection, prevention and treatment of obesity. Canadian Task Force on Preventive Health Care. *Can Med Assoc J* 1999;160:513–525. Search date 1999; primary sources Medline, Current Contents, and hand searched references.
60. The National Heart, Lung, and Blood Institute. Clinical guidelines on the identification, evaluation, and treatment of overweight and obesity in adults. Bethesda, Maryland: National Institutes of Health, 1998; http://www.nhlbi.nih.gov/guidelines/obesity/ob_home.htm (last accessed 3 Sept 2002) Search date 1997; primary sources Medline, and hand searched reference lists.
61. Wing RR, Polley BA, Venditti E, et al. Lifestyle intervention in overweight individuals with a family history of diabetes. *Diabetes Care* 1998;21:350–359.
62. Anderson RE, Wadden TA, Barlett SJ, et al. Effects of lifestyle activity v structured aerobic exercise in obese women. *JAMA* 1999;281:335–340.
63. Jakicic JM, Winters C, Lang W, et al. Effects of intermittent exercise and use of home exercise equipment on adherence, weight loss, and fitness in overweight women. *JAMA* 1999;282:1554–1560.
64. Sbrocco T, Nedegaard RC, Stone JM, et al. Behavioural choice treatment promotes continuing weight loss. *J Consult Clin Psychol* 1999;67:260–266.
65. Harvey-Berino J. Calorie restriction is more effective for obesity treatment than dietary fat restriction. *Ann Behav Med* 1999;21:35–39.
66. Wing RR, Jeffery RW. Benefits of recruiting participants with friends and increasing social support for weight loss and maintenance. *J Consult Clin Psychol* 1999;67:132–138.
67. Jeffery RW, Wing RR, Thorson C, et al. Use of personal trainers and financial incentives to increase exercise in a behavioural weight loss program. *J Consult Clin Psychol* 1998;66:777–783.
68. Craighead LW, Blum MD. Supervised exercise in behavioural treatment for moderate obesity. *Behav Ther* 1989;20:49–59.
69. Donnelly JE, Jacobsen DJ, Heelan KS, et al. The effects of 18 months of intermittent vs. continuous exercise on aerobic capacity, body weight and composition, and metabolic fitness in previously sedentary, moderately obese females. *Int J Obesity* 2000;24:566–572.
70. Kunz K, Kreimel K, Gurdet C, et al. Comparison of behaviour modification and conventional dietary advice in a long-term weight reduction programme for obese women [abstract]. *Diabetologia* 1982;23:181.
71. Rapoport L, Clark M, Wardle J. Evaluation of a modified cognitive-behavioural programme for weight management. *Int J Obesity* 2000;24:1726–1737.
72. Wing R, Epstein LH, Paternostro-Bayles M, et al. Exercise in a behavioural weight control program for obese patients with type 2 (non insulin dependent) diabetes. *Diabetologica* 1988;31:902–909.
73. Ashley LM, St Jeor ST, Schrage JP, et al. Weight control in the physicians office. *Arch Intern Med* 2001;161:1599–1604.
74. Ramirez EM, Rosen JC. A comparison of weight control and weight control plus body image therapy for obese men and women. *J Consult Clin Psychol* 2001;69:444–446.
75. Stevens VJ, Obarzanek E, Cook NR, et al. for the Trials of Hypertension Prevention Research Group. Long term weight loss and changes in blood

pressure: Results of the Trials of Hypertension Prevention, Phase II. *Ann Intern Med* 2001;134:1–11.
76. Wylie-Rosett J, Swencionis C, Ginsberg M, et al. Computerized weight loss intervention optimises staff time: the clinical and cost results of a controlled clinical trail conducted in a managed care setting. *J Am Dietetic Assoc* 2001;101:1155–1162.
77. Bonato DP, Boland FJ. A comparison of specific strategies for long-term maintenance following a behavioural treatment program for obese women. *Int J Eat Disord* 1986;5:949–958.
78. Hillebrand TH, Wirth A. Evaluation of an outpatient care program for obese patients after an inpatient treatment. *Prav Rehab* 1996;8:83–87.
79. Leermakers EA, Perri MG, Shigaki CL, et al. Effects of exercise-focused versus weight-focused maintenance programs on the management of obesity. *Addict Behav* 1999;24:219–227.
80. Simkin-Silverman LR, Wing RR, Boraz MA, et al. Maintenance of cardiovascular risk factor changes among middle-aged women in a lifestyle intervention trial. *Women's Health: Research on Gender, Behaviour, and Policy* 1998;4:255–271.
81. Wing RR, Jeffery RW, Hellerstedt WL, et al. Effect of frequent phone contacts and optional food provision on maintenance of weight loss. *Ann Behav Med* 1996;18:172–176.
82. Fogelholm M, Kukkonen-Harjula K, Nenonen A, et al. Effects of walking training on weight maintenance after a very-low-energy diet in premenopausal obese women: a randomized controlled trial. *Arch Intern Med* 2000;160:2177–2184.
83. Perri MG, Nezu AM, McKelvey WF, et al. Relapse prevention training and problem-solving therapy in the long-term management of obesity. *J Consult & Clin Psychol* 2001;69:722–726.
84. Hardeman W, Griffin S, Johnston M, et al. Interventions to prevent weight gain: a systematic review of psychological models and behaviour change methods. *Int J Obesity* 2000;4:131–143. Search date not stated; primary sources Medline, Embase, Psychlit, The Cochrane Library, Current Contents, ERIC, HealthStar, Social Science Citation Index, and hand searched reference lists.
85. Forster JL, Jeffery RW, Schmid TL, et al. Preventing weight gain in adults: a pound of prevention. *Health Psychol* 1988;7:515–525.
86. Jeffery RW, French SA. Preventing weight gain in adults: the pound of prevention study. *Am J Public Health* 1999;89:747–751.
87. Kuller LH, Simkin-Silverman LR, Wing RR, et al. Women's health lifestyle project: a randomized clinical trial. *Circulation* 2001;103:32–37.
88. Harvey EL, Glenny A, Kirk SFL, et al. Improving health professionals' management and the organisation of care for overweight and obese people. In: The Cochrane Library, Issue 2, 2002. Oxford: Update Software. Search date 2000; primary sources Specialised Registers of the Cochrane Effective Practice and Organisation of Care Group, the Cochrane Depression, Anxiety and Neurosis Group, the Cochrane Diabetes Group, the Cochrane Controlled Trials Register, Medline, Embase, Cinahl, PsycLit, Sigle, Sociofile, Dissertation Abstracts, Resource Database in Continuing Medical Education, and Conference Papers Index.
89. Ockene IS, Hebert JR, Ockene JK, et al. Effect of physician-delivered nutrition counseling training and an office-support program on saturated fat intake, weight, and serum lipid measurements in a hyperlipidemic population: Worcester area trial for counseling in hyperlipidemia (WATCH). *Arch Intern Med* 1999;159:725–731.

Margaret Thorogood
Reader in Public Health and Preventative Medicine

Melvyn Hillsdon
Lecturer in Health Promotion

London School of Hygiene and Tropical Medicine
University of London
London
UK

Carolyn Summerbell
Reader in Human Nutrition
School of Health
University of Teesside
Middlesborough
UK

Competing interests: None declared.

Heart failure

Search date February 2002

Robert McKelvie

QUESTIONS

INTERVENTIONS

To be covered in future updates
Vasodilators
Coronary revascularisation
Atheroma risk factor modification

See glossary, p 79

Key Messages

Non-drug treatments

- **Exercise** Systematic reviews have found that prescribed exercise training improves functional capacity and quality of life. One subsequent RCT has found that exercise training versus no exercise training significantly reduces fatal or non-fatal cardiac events (NNT 2, 95% CI 2 to 5), hospital readmission for heart failure (NNT 5, 95% CI 4 to 30), and mortality at 12 months (NNT 4, 95% CI 3 to 19).
- **Multidisciplinary interventions** One systematic review has found that multidisciplinary approaches to nutrition, patient counselling, and education versus usual care significantly reduce admissions to hospital, but do not significantly reduce mortality. Analysis by each intervention found that only follow up by a multidisciplinary team reduced admissions to hospital, whereas telephone contact plus improved coordination of primary care had no significant effect.

Clin Evid 2002;8:60–81.

Drug and invasive treatments

- **Amiodarone** Systematic reviews have found weak evidence suggesting that amiodarone versus placebo may reduce mortality.
- **Angiotensin converting enzyme inhibitors** Systematic reviews and RCTs have found that angiotensin converting enzyme inhibitors versus placebo significantly reduce mortality, hospital admission for heart failure, and ischaemic events. Relative benefits are similar in different groups of people, but absolute benefits are greater in people with severe heart failure. RCTs in people with asymptomatic left ventricular systolic dysfunction have found that angiotensin converting enzyme inhibitors versus placebo significantly delay the onset of symptomatic heart failure and reduce cardiovascular events over 40 months.
- **Angiotensin II receptor blockers** One systematic review has found that angiotensin receptor blockers versus placebo reduced all cause mortality and hospital admission in people with New York Heart Association class II–IV heart failure, although the difference was not significant. This may be explained by the small numbers of deaths and admissions reported. It found no significant difference in all cause mortality or hospital admission with angiotensin receptor blockers versus angiotensin converting enzyme inhibitors. It found that angiotensin receptor blockers plus angiotensin converting enzyme inhibitors versus angiotensin converting enzyme inhibitors alone reduced admission for heart failure but did not significantly reduce all cause mortality.
- **Anticoagulation** We found no RCTs of anticoagulation in people with heart failure. We found conflicting evidence from two large retrospective cohort studies.
- **Antiplatelet agents** We found no RCTs of antiplatelet agents in people with heart failure. Retrospective analyses have included too few events to establish or exclude a clinically important effect of antiplatelet agents.
- **β Blockers** Systematic reviews have found strong evidence that adding a β blocker to an angiotensin converting enzyme inhibitor significantly decreases mortality and hospital admission. Limited evidence from a subgroup analysis of one RCT found no significant effect on mortality in black people.
- **Calcium channel blockers** One systematic review has found no significant difference in mortality with second generation dihydropyridine calcium channel blockers versus placebo. RCTs comparing other calcium channel blockers versus placebo found no evidence of benefit.
- **Digoxin (improves morbidity in people already receiving diuretics and angiotensin converting enzyme inhibitors)** One large RCT in people already receiving diuretics and angiotensin converting enzyme inhibitors found that digoxin versus placebo significantly reduces the number of people admitted to hospital for worsening heart failure at 37 months (NNT 13, 95% CI 10 to 17), but did not significantly reduce mortality.
- **Implantable cardiac defibrillators (in people with heart failure and cardiac arrest)** One RCT has found good evidence that an implantable cardiac defibrillator reduces mortality in people with heart failure who have experienced a cardiac arrest.
- **Non-amiodarone antiarrhythmic drugs** Evidence extrapolated from one systematic review in people treated after a myocardial infarction suggests that other antiarrhythmic drugs (apart from β blockers) may increase mortality.
- **Positive inotropes (ibopamine, milrinone, and vesnarinone)** RCTs found that positive inotropic drugs (other than digoxin) versus placebo significantly increased mortality over 6–11 months.

- **Prophylactic use of implantable cardiac defibrillators in people at high risk of arrhythmia** Two RCTs have found that implantable cardiac defibrillators versus medical treatment reduce mortality in people with heart failure and at high risk of arrythmia, whereas one RCT found no significant difference in mortality.
- **Spironolactone in severe heart failure** One RCT in people with severe heart failure taking diuretics, angiotensin converting enzyme inhibitors, and digoxin has found that adding spironolactone versus placebo significantly reduces mortality after 2 years (NNT 9, 95% CI 6 to 15).
- **Treatments for diastolic heart failure** We found no RCTs in people with diastolic heart failure.

DEFINITION Heart failure occurs when abnormality of cardiac function causes failure of the heart to pump blood at a rate sufficient for metabolic requirements, or maintains cardiac output only with a raised filling pressure. It is characterised clinically by breathlessness, effort intolerance, fluid retention, and poor survival. It can be caused by systolic or diastolic dysfunction and is associated with neurohormonal changes.[1] Left ventricular systolic dysfunction (LVSD) is defined as a left ventricular ejection fraction below 0.40. It can be symptomatic or asymptomatic. Defining and diagnosing diastolic heart failure can be difficult. Recently proposed criteria include: (1) clinical evidence of heart failure; (2) normal or mildly abnormal left ventricular systolic function; and (3) evidence of abnormal left ventricular relaxation, filling, diastolic distensibility, or diastolic stiffness.[2] The clinical utility of these criteria is limited by difficulty in standardising assessment of the last criterion.

INCIDENCE/ PREVALENCE Both the incidence and prevalence of heart failure increase with age. Studies of heart failure in the USA and Europe found that under 65 years of age the incidence is 1/1000 men a year and 0.4/1000 women a year. Over 65 years, incidence is 11/1000 men a year and 5/1000 women a year. Under 65 years the prevalence of heart failure is 1/1000 men and 1/1000 women; over 65 years the prevalence is 40/1000 men and 30/1000 women.[3] The prevalence of asymptomatic LVSD is 3% in the general population.[4–6] The mean age of people with asymptomatic LVSD is lower than that for symptomatic individuals. Both heart failure and asymptomatic LVSD are more common in men.[4–6] The prevalence of diastolic heart failure in the community is unknown. The prevalence of heart failure with preserved systolic function in people in hospital with clinical heart failure varies from 13–74%.[7,8] Less than 15% of people with heart failure under 65 years have normal systolic function, whereas the prevalence is about 40% in people over 65 years.[7]

AETIOLOGY/ RISK FACTORS Coronary artery disease is the most common cause of heart failure.[3] Other common causes include hypertension and idiopathic dilated congestive cardiomyopathy. After adjustment for hypertension, the presence of left ventricular hypertrophy remains a risk factor for the development of heart failure. Other risk factors include cigarette smoking, hyperlipidaemia, and diabetes mellitus.[4] The common causes of left ventricular diastolic dysfunction are coronary artery disease and systemic hypertension. Other causes are hypertrophic cardiomyopathy, restrictive or infiltrative cardiomyopathies, and valvular heart disease.[8]

PROGNOSIS The prognosis of heart failure is poor, with 5 year mortality ranging from 26–75%.[3] Up to 16% of people are readmitted with heart failure within 6 months of first admission. In the USA it is the leading cause of hospital admission among people over 65 years old.[3] In people with heart failure, a new myocardial infarction increases the risk of death (RR 7.8, 95% CI 6.9 to 8.8); 34% of all deaths in people with heart failure are preceded by a major ischaemic event.[9] Sudden death, mainly caused by ventricular arrhythmia, is responsible for 25–50% of all deaths, and is the most common cause of death in people with heart failure.[10] The presence of asymptomatic LVSD increases an individual's risk of having a cardiovascular event. One large prevention trial found that for a 5% reduction in ejection fraction the risk ratio for mortality was 1.20 (95% CI 1.13 to 1.29), for hospital admission for heart failure it was 1.28 (95% CI 1.18 to 1.38), and for development of heart failure it was 1.20 (95% CI 1.13 to 1.26).[4] The annual mortality for patients with diastolic heart failure varies in observational studies (1.3–17.5%).[7] Reasons for this variation include age, the presence of coronary artery disease, and variation in the partition value used to define abnormal ventricular systolic function. The annual mortality for left ventricular diastolic dysfunction is lower than that found in patients with systolic dysfunction.[11]

AIMS To relieve symptoms; to improve quality of life; to reduce morbidity and mortality, with minimum adverse effects.

OUTCOMES Functional capacity (assessed by the New York Heart Association [see glossary, p 79] functional classification or more objectively by using standardised exercise testing or the 6 min walk test);[12] quality of life (assessed with questionnaires);[13] mortality; adverse effects of treatment. Proxy measures of clinical outcome (e.g. left ventricular ejection fraction and hospital readmission rates) are used only when clinical outcomes are unavailable.

METHODS *Clinical Evidence* update search and appraisal February 2002. Generally, RCTs with less than 500 people have been excluded because of the number of large RCTs available. If for any comparison very large RCTs exist then much smaller RCTs have been excluded, even if they have more than 500 people.

QUESTION What are the effects of non-drug treatments?

OPTION MULTIDISCIPLINARY

One systematic review has found that multidisciplinary programmes significantly reduce admissions to hospital but did not significantly reduce mortality; analysis by intervention has found that only follow up by a multidisciplinary team reduces admissions to hospital, whereas telephone contact plus improved coordination of primary care has no significant effect.

Benefits: We found one systematic review (search date 1999, 11 RCTs, 2067 people with heart failure) that compared a multidisciplinary programme versus conventional care alone.[14] Multidisciplinary programmes included non-drug treatments such as nutrition advice, counselling, patient education, and exercise training. The review found that multidisciplinary interventions significantly reduced hospital admission (406/1001 [40.6%] with multidisciplinary programme *v* with conventional care 474/1011 [46.9%]; RR 0.87, 95% CI 0.79 to 0.96; 11 RCTs), but did not significantly reduce mortality (104/534 [19.5%] with multidisciplinary programme *v* 121/572 [21.2%] with conventional care; RR 0.94, 95% CI 0.75 to 1.19; 7 RCTs). However, the hospital admission results were heterogeneous by intervention. Specialised follow up by a multidisciplinary team substantially reduced admissions to hospital (RR 0.77, 95% CI 0.68 to 0.86; 1366 people with heart failure; 9 RCTs), but there was no benefit from telephone contact plus improved coordination of primary care services (RR 1.15, 95% CI 0.96 to 1.37; 646 people with heart failure; 2 RCTs).

Harms: The review suggested that disease management programmes may fragment care such that peoples other conditions are overlooked.[14] However, it did not provide evidence to support this.

Comment: Studies were small, involved highly selected patient populations, and were usually performed in academic centres, so results may not generalise to smaller community centres. Studies lasted less than 6 months and it is not known how well people adhere to treatment over the longer term. Larger studies are needed to define the effects on morbidity and mortality of longer term multidisciplinary interventions.

OPTION EXERCISE

Systematic reviews found that prescribed exercise training improved functional capacity and quality of life. One recent RCT also found that exercise significantly reduced adverse cardiac events.

Benefits: We found two systematic reviews (search dates 1993 and not stated),[15,16] two subsequent non-systematic reviews,[17,18] and one subsequent RCT[19] of exercise training in people with heart failure. The reviews identified 20 small RCTs that reported only proxy outcomes (maximum exercise time [see glossary, p 79] oxygen uptake, various biochemical measures, and unvalidated symptom scores) in a small number of people over a few weeks. The subsequent RCT (99 people with heart failure, 88 men) compared 12 months of exercise training versus a group with no exercise training.[19] After 12 months, exercise compared with control improved quality of life ($P < 0.001$), reduced fatal or non-fatal cardiac events (17/50 [34%] with training *v* 37/49 [76%] without exercise; ARR 42%, 95% CI 20% to 58%; RR 0.45, 95% CI 0.23 to 0.73; NNT 2, 95% CI 2 to 5), mortality (9/50 [18%] with training *v* 20/49 [41%] without exercise; RR 0.44, 95% CI 0.20 to 0.87; NNT 4, 95% CI 3 to 19), and reduced hospital readmission for heart failure (5/50 [10%] with training *v* 14/49 [29%] without exercise; ARR 19%, 95% CI 3% to 25%; RR 0.35, 95% CI 0.12 to 0.88; NNT 5, 95% CI 4 to 30).[19]

Harms: The reviews and trial reported no important adverse effects associated with prescribed exercise training.[15,17–19]

Comment: The studies were small, involved highly selected patient populations, and were performed in well resourced academic centres. The results may not generalise to smaller community centres. The specific form of exercise training varied among studies and the relative merits of each strategy are unknown. The studies generally lasted less than 1 year and long term effects are unknown. Larger studies over a longer period are needed.

QUESTION What are the effects of drug treatments in heart failure?

OPTION ANGIOTENSIN CONVERTING ENZYME INHIBITORS

Two systematic reviews and recent RCTs have found that angiotensin converting enzyme inhibitors reduce mortality, hospital admission for heart failure, and ischaemic events in people with heart failure. Relative benefits are similar in different groups of people, but absolute benefits are greater in people with severe heart failure.

Benefits: We found two systematic reviews (search dates 1994 and not stated) of angiotensin converting enzyme (ACE) inhibitors versus placebo in heart failure.[20,21] The first systematic review (search date 1994, 32 RCTs, duration 3–42 months, 7105 people, New York Heart Association [see glossary, p 79] class III or IV) found that ACE inhibitors versus placebo reduced mortality (611/3870 [16%] with ACE inhibitors *v* 709/3235 [22%] with placebo; ARR 6%, 95% CI 4% to 8%; OR 0.77, 95% CI 0.67 to 0.88; NNT 16).[20] Relative reductions in mortality were similar in different subgroups (stratified by age, sex, cause of heart failure, and New York Heart Association class). The second systematic review (search date not stated, 5 RCTs, 12 763 people with left ventricular dysfunction or heart failure of mean duration 35 months) analysed results from individuals in long term and large RCTs that compared ACE inhibitors versus placebo.[21] Three RCTs were in people for 1 year after myocardial infarction. In these three postinfarction trials (5966 people) ACE inhibitor versus placebo significantly reduced mortality (702/2995 [23.4%] with ACE inhibitor *v* 866/2971 [29.1%] with placebo; OR 0.74, 95% CI 0.66 to 0.83), readmission for heart failure (355/2995 [11.9%] with ACE inhibitor *v* 460/2971 [15.5%] with placebo; OR 0.73, 95% CI 0.63 to 0.85), and reinfarction (324/2995 [10.8%] with ACE inhibitor *v* 391/2971 [13.2%] with placebo; OR 0.80, 95% CI 0.69 to 0.94). For all five trials, ACE inhibitors versus placebo reduced mortality (1467/6391 [23.0%] with ACE inhibitor *v* 1710/6372 [26.8%] with placebo; OR 0.80, 95% CI 0.74 to 0.87), reinfarction (571/6391 [8.9%] with ACE inhibitor *v* 703/6372 [11.0%] with placebo; OR 0.79, 95% CI 0.70 to 0.89), and readmission for heart failure (876/6391 [13.7%] with ACE inhibitor *v* 1202/6372 [18.9%] with placebo; OR 0.67, 95% CI 0.61 to 0.74). The relative benefits began soon after the start of treatment, persisted long term, and were independent of age, sex, and baseline use of diuretics, aspirin, and β blockers. Although there was a trend towards greater relative reduction in mortality or readmission for heart failure in people with lower ejection fractions, benefit was apparent over the range examined. **Other ischaemic**

events: Individual RCTs that studied high risk groups found that ACE inhibitors significantly reduced some ischaemic event rates. One RCT in people with left ventricular dysfunction found that ACE inhibitors reduced myocardial infarction (combined fatal or non-fatal myocardial infarction: 9.9% with ACE inhibitor *v* 12.3% with placebo; RR 0.77, 95% CI 0.61 to 0.98), hospital admission for angina (15% with ACE inhibitor *v* 19% with placebo; RR 0.73, 95% CI 0.60 to 0.88), and the combined end point of cardiac death, non-fatal myocardial infarction, or hospital admission for angina (43% with ACE inhibitor *v* 51% with placebo; RR 0.77, 95% CI 0.68 to 0.86).[9] Effects on hospital readmissions were observed shortly after starting ACE inhibitor treatment, although effects on ischaemic events were not apparent for at least 6 months and peaked at 36 months. **Dosage:** We found one large RCT (3164 people with New York Heart Association class II–IV heart failure) that compared low dose lisinopril (2.5 or 5.0 mg/day) versus high dose lisinopril (32.5 or 35 mg/day).[22] It found no significant difference in mortality (717/1596 [44.9%] with low dose *v* 666/1568 [42.5%] with high dose; ARR 2.4%, CI not provided; HR 0.92, 95% CI 0.80 to 1.03; P = 0.128), but found that high dose lisinopril reduced the combined outcome of death or hospital admission for any reason (1338/1596 [83.8%] events with low dose *v* 1250/1568 [79.7%] events with high dose; ARR 4.1%, CI not provided; HR 0.88, 95% CI 0.82 to 0.96; P = 0.002), and reduced admissions for heart failure (1576/1596 [98.7%] admissions with low dose *v* 1199/1568 [76.5%] admissions with high dose; ARR 22.2%; CI not provided; P = 0.002). **Comparison of different angiotensin converting enzyme inhibitors:** The first systematic review found similar benefits with different ACE inhibitors.[20]

Harms: We found no systematic review. The main adverse effects documented in large trials were cough, hypotension, hyperkalaemia, and renal dysfunction. Compared with placebo, ACE inhibitors increased the incidence of cough (37% with ACE inhibitor *v* 31% with placebo; ARI 7%, 95% CI 3% to 11%; RR 1.23, 95% CI 1.11 to 1.35; NNH 14), dizziness or fainting (57% with ACE inhibitor *v* 50% with placebo; ARI 7%, 95% CI 3% to 11%; RR 1.14, 95% CI 1.06 to 1.21; NNH 14), increased creatinine concentrations above 177 μmol/L (10.7% with ACE inhibitor *v* 7.7% placebo; ARI 3.0%, 95% CI 0.6% to 6.0%; RR 1.38, 95% CI 1.09 to 1.67; NNH 34), and increased potassium concentrations above 5.5 mmol/L (AR 6.4% with ACE inhibitor *v* 2.5% with placebo; ARI 4%, 95% CI 2% to 7%; RR 2.56, 95% CI 1.92 to 3.20; NNH 26).[23] Angioedema was not found to be more common with ACE inhibitors than placebo (3.8% taking enalapril *v* 4.1% taking placebo; ARI +0.3%, 95% CI –1.4% to +1.5%).[23] The trial comparing low and high doses of lisinopril found that most adverse effects were more common with high dose (no P value provided; dizziness: 12% with low dose *v* 19% with high dose; hypotension: 7% with low dose *v* 11% with high dose; worsening renal function: 7% with low dose *v* 10% with high dose; significant change in serum potassium concentration: 7% with low dose *v* 7% with high dose), although there was no difference in withdrawal rates between groups (17% discontinued with high dose *v* 18% with low dose). The trial found that cough was less commonly experienced with high dose compared with low dose lisinopril (cough: 13% with low dose *v* 11% with high dose).

Comment: The relative beneficial effects of ACE inhibitors were similar in different subgroups of people with heart failure. Most RCTs evaluated left ventricular function by assessing left ventricular ejection fraction, but some studies defined heart failure clinically, without measurement of left ventricular function in people at high risk of developing heart failure (soon after myocardial infarction). It is unclear whether there are additional benefits from adding ACE inhibitor treatment in people with heart failure who are already taking antiplatelet treatment, and of adding antiplatelet treatment in people with heart failure who are already taking an ACE inhibitor (see antiplatelet agents, p 76).

OPTION ANGIOTENSIN II RECEPTOR BLOCKERS

One systematic review has found that angiotensin receptor blockers versus placebo reduced all cause mortality and hospital admission in people with New York Heart Association class II–IV heart failure, although the difference was not significant. This may be explained by the small numbers of deaths and admissions reported. It found no significant difference in all cause mortality or hospital admission with angiotensin receptor blockers versus angiotensin converting enzyme inhibitors. It found that angiotensin receptor blockers plus angiotensin converting enzyme inhibitors versus angiotensin converting enzyme inhibitors alone reduced admission for heart failure but did not significantly reduce all cause mortality.

Benefits: **Versus placebo:** We found one systematic review (search date 2001, 11 RCTs, 2259 people with New York Heart Association [see glossary, p 79] class II–IV, follow up 4 wks to 2 years).[24] It found that angiotensin receptor blockers versus placebo reduced all cause mortality and admission for heart failure, although the differences were not significant (all cause mortality: 7 RCTs; AR 2% with angiotensin receptor blockers *v* 3% with placebo; OR 0.68, 95% CI 0.38 to 1.22; admission for heart failure: 1 RCT; 8% with angiotensin receptor blockers *v* 12% with placebo; OR 0.67, 95% CI 0.29 to 1.51). The numbers of deaths and admissions were small, which may explain why the difference did not reach significance. **Versus angiotensin converting enzyme inhibitors:** The systematic review identified six RCTs (4682 people with New York Heart Association class II–IV, follow up 4 wks to 1.5 years) comparing angiotensin receptor blockers versus angiotensin converting enzyme (ACE) inhibitors.[24] It found no significant difference between treatments for all cause mortality or rate of admission for heart failure (all cause mortality: 6 RCTs; OR 1.09, 95% CI 0.92 to 1.29; admission for heart failure: 3 RCTs; OR 0.95, 95% CI 0.8 to 1.13). **Plus angiotensin converting enzyme inhibitors versus angiotensin converting enzyme inhibitors alone:** The systematic review identified six RCTs (5712 people with New York Heart Association class II–IV heart failure) comparing angiotensin receptor blockers plus ACE inhibitors versus ACE inhibitors alone.[24] It found that combined treatment significantly reduced hospital admission for heart failure (3 RCTs; OR 0.74, 95% CI 0.64 to 0.86). However, it found no significant difference between treatments for all cause mortality (6 RCTs; OR 1.04, 95% CI 0.91 to 1.20).

Harms: The systematic review did not report on harms.[24]

Comment: In people who are truly intolerant of ACE inhibitors the evidence supports the use of angiotensin II receptor blockers, with the expectation of at least symptomatic improvement of the heart failure.

OPTION POSITIVE INOTROPIC AGENTS

One well designed RCT found that digoxin decreased the rate of hospital admissions for worsening heart failure in people already receiving diuretics and angiotensin converting enzyme inhibitors, although it found no evidence of an effect on mortality. RCTs found evidence that positive inotropic drugs other than digoxin increased mortality in people with heart failure; evidence on morbidity was less clear.

Benefits: **Digoxin:** We found one systematic review (search date 1992, 13 RCTs, duration 3–24 wks, 1138 people with heart failure and sinus rhythm)[25] and one subsequent large RCT.[26] The systematic review found that six of the 13 RCTs enrolled people without assessment of ventricular function and may have included some people with mild or no heart failure. Other limitations of the older trials included crossover designs and small sample sizes. In people who were in sinus rhythm with heart failure, the systematic review found fewer people with clinical worsening of heart failure (52/628 [8.3%] with digoxin *v* 131/631 [20.8%] with placebo; ARR 12.5%, 95% CI 9.5% to 14.7%; RR 0.40, 95% CI 0.29 to 0.54) but did not find a definite effect on mortality (16/628 [2.5%] with digoxin *v* 15/631 [2.4%] with placebo; ARR −0.2%, 95% CI −2.6% to +1.1%; RR 1.07, 95% CI 0.53 to 2.23). The subsequent large RCT (6800 people, 88% male, mean age 64 years, New York Heart Association class I–III [see glossary, p 79], 94% already taking angiotensin converting enzyme inhibitors, 82% taking diuretics) compared blinded additional treatment with either digoxin or placebo for a mean of 37 months.[26] Digoxin did not reduce all cause mortality compared with placebo (1181/3397 [34.8%] with digoxin *v* 1194/3403 [35.1%] with placebo; ARR +0.3%, 95% CI −2.0% to +2.6%; RR 0.99, 95% CI 0.93 to 1.06). The number of people admitted to hospital for worsening heart failure was substantially less with digoxin over 37 months (910/3397 [27%] with digoxin *v* 1180/3403 [35%] with placebo; ARR 8%, 95% CI 6% to 10%; RR 0.77, 95% CI 0.72 to 0.83; NNT 13, 95% CI 10 to 17), as was the combined outcome of death or hospital admission caused by worsening heart failure (1041/3397 [31%] with digoxin *v* 1291/3403 [38%] for placebo; ARR 7.3%, 95% CI 5.1% to 9.4%; RR 0.81, 95% CI 0.75 to 0.87; NNT 14). **Other inotropic agents:** One non-systematic review (6 RCTs, 8006 people) of RCTs found that non-digitalis positive inotropic agents increased mortality compared with placebo.[10] The largest RCT in the review (3833 people with heart failure) found increased mortality with vesnarinone 60 mg daily versus placebo over 9 months (292/1275 [23%] with vesnarinone *v* 242/1280 [19%] with placebo; ARI 4%, 95% CI 1% to 8%; RR 1.21, 95% CI 1.04 to 1.40; NNH 25).[10,27] Another large RCT (1088 people with heart failure) found milrinone versus placebo increased mortality over 6 months (168/561 [30%] with milrinone *v* 127/527 [24%] with placebo; ARI 6.0%, 95% CI 0.5% to 12.0%; RR 1.24, 95% CI 1.02 to 1.49; NNH 17).[28] A third large RCT (1906 people with heart failure) compared ibopamine versus placebo over 11 months.[29] It found that ibopamine increased mortality (232/953 [25%] with ibopamine *v* 193/953 [20%] with placebo; RR 1.26, 95% CI 1.04 to 1.53). The review found that some studies reported improved functional capacity and quality of life, but this was not consistent across all studies.

Harms: We found no systematic review. **Digoxin:** The RCT (6800 people) found that more people had suspected digoxin toxicity in the digoxin group versus placebo (11.9% with digoxin *v* 7.9% with placebo; ARI 4.0%, 95% CI 2.4% to 5.8%; RR 1.5, 95% CI 1.30 to 1.73; NNH 25).[26] The RCT found no evidence that digoxin increased the risk of ventricular fibrillation or tachycardia compared with placebo (37/3397 [1.1%] with digoxin *v* 27/3403 [0.8%] with placebo; ARI +0.3%, 95% CI –0.1% to +1.0%; RR 1.37, 95% CI 0.84 to 2.24). Digoxin compared with placebo increased rates of supraventricular arrhythmia (2.5% with digoxin *v* 1.2% with placebo; ARI 1.3%, 95% CI 0.5% to 2.4%; RR 2.08, 95% CI 1.44 to 2.99; NNH 77) and second or third degree atrioventricular block (1.2% with digoxin *v* 0.4% with placebo; ARI 0.8%, 95% CI 0.2% to 1.8%; RR 2.93, 95% CI 1.61 to 5.34; NNH 126). **Other inotropic agents:** Most RCTs found that inotropic agents other than digoxin increased risk of death (see benefits above).

Comment: None.

OPTION β BLOCKERS

We found strong evidence from systematic reviews that adding β blockers to standard treatment with angiotensin converting enzymes inhibitors in people with moderate and severe heart failure reduces the rate of hospital admission or death. Subgroup analysis in black people found no significant effect on mortality.

Benefits: We found two systematic reviews (search dates 2000 and not stated)[30,31] and two subsequent RCTs of the effects of β blockers in heart failure.[32,33] **In people with any severity of heart failure:** The first systematic review (search date 2000, 22 RCTs, 10 315 people with heart failure) found that β blockers versus placebo significantly reduced the risk of death (444/5273 [8.4%] with β blockers *v* 624/4862 [12.8%] with placebo; OR 0.65, 95% CI 0.53 to 0.80) and hospital admissions (540/5244 [10.3%] with β blockers *v* 754/4832 [15.6%] with placebo; OR 0.64, 95% CI 0.53 to 0.79).[30] This is equivalent to three fewer deaths and four fewer hospital admissions per 100 people treated for 1 year. The results were consistent for selective and non-selective β blockers. Sensitivity analysis and funnel plots found that the results were robust to any reasonable publication bias. **In people with severe**

heart failure: The second systematic review (search date not stated, 4 RCTs, 635 people with class IV heart failure) found that β blockers versus placebo significantly reduced the risk of death (56/313 [17.9%] with β blockers *v* 81/322 [25.1%] with placebo; RR 0.71, 95% CI 0.52 to 0.96). Two subsequent RCTs compared β blockers versus placebo in people with class III or IV heart failure.[32,33] The first RCT (2289 people with class IV heart failure, who were euvolemic [defined as the absence of rales and ascites and the presence of no more than minimal peripheral oedema] and who had an ejection fraction of less than 25%, but were not receiving intensive care, intravenous vasodilators, or positive inotropic drugs) compared carvedilol versus placebo over 10.4 months. It was stopped early because of a significant beneficial effect on survival that exceeded the pre-specified interim monitoring boundaries.[32] It found that β blockers significantly reduced mortality (130/1156 [11.2%] with β blockers *v* 190/1133 [16.8%] with placebo; RR 0.65, 95% CI 0.52 to 0.81) and the combined outcome of death or hospital admission (425/1156 [36.8%] with β blockers *v* 507/1133 [44.7%] with placebo; RR 0.76, 95% CI 0.67 to 0.87). The second RCT compared bucindolol versus placebo in people with severe heart failure (2708 people class III or IV heart failure and ejection fraction ≤ 35%; about 70% of the people were white and 24% were black).[33] The RCT was stopped early because of accumulated evidence from other studies of β blockers. It found that more people died with placebo but the difference did not reach significance (411/1354 [30.4%] with bucindolol *v* 449/1354 [33.1%] with placebo; HR 0.90, 95% CI 0.78 to 1.02). The RCT found a significant interaction of treatment effect with race (black *v* non-black). There was no evidence of benefit in black people (HR 1.17, 95% CI 0.89 to 1.53), although there was a significant effect for non-black people (HR 0.82, 95% CI 0.70 to 0.96).

Harms: Fears that β blockers may cause excessive problems with worsening heart failure, bradyarrhythmia, or hypotension have not been confirmed. One subsequent RCT found that fewer people with carvedilol versus placebo required permanent discontinuation of treatment because of adverse events other than death (P = 0.02).[32] Cumulative withdrawals at 1 year were 14.8% with carvedilol versus 18.5% with placebo. For the subgroup of people with recent or recurrent cardiac decompensation or severely depressed cardiac function the difference in withdrawal rates was greater (17.5% with carvedilol *v* 24.2% with placebo). The subsequent RCT comparing bucindolol versus placebo found that 23% in the bucindolol group and 25% of people in the placebo group permanently discontinued the medication.[33]

Comment: Good evidence was found for the use of β blockers in people with moderate symptoms (New York Heart Association class II or III [see glossary, p 79]) receiving standard treatment, including angiotensin converting enzyme inhibitors. The value of β blockers needs clarification in heart failure with preserved ejection fraction and in asymptomatic left ventricular systolic dysfunction. One recent RCT has shown that carvedilol reduced all cause mortality compared with placebo (AR for death: 12% with carvedilol *v* 15% with placebo; HR 0.77, 95% CI 0.60 to 0.98; P = 0.03) in 1959 people with acute myocardial infarction and left ventricular ejection fraction less than or equal to 40%.[34] The RCTs of β blockers have consistently found a mortality benefit, but it is not clear whether or not the benefit is a class effect. One recent small RCT (150 people) of metoprolol versus carvedilol found some differences in surrogate outcomes, but both drugs produced similar improvements in symptoms, submaximal exercise tolerance, and quality of life.[35] The results for non-black people were consistent between bucindolol and carvedilol. The lack of observed benefit for black people in one RCT[33] raises the possibility that there may be race specific responses to pharmacological treatment for cardiovascular disease.

OPTION CALCIUM CHANNEL BLOCKERS

One systematic review of second generation dihydropyridine calcium channel blockers found no evidence of benefit. RCTs of other calcium channel blockers found no evidence of benefit.

Benefits: **After myocardial infarction:** See calcium channel blockers under acute myocardial infarction, p 011. **Other heart failure:** We found one systematic review (search date not stated) of second generation dihydropyridine calcium channel blockers,[36] one non-systematic review of all calcium channel blockers (3 RCTs, 1790 people with heart failure),[10] and one subsequent RCT.[37] The systematic review (18 RCTs) found two RCTs large enough to assess mortality.[36] Meta-analysis found no significant difference in mortality (1603 people; OR 0.94, 95% CI 0.79 to 1.12).[36] The largest RCT in the non-systematic review (1153 people, [New York Heart Association class III or IV — see glossary, p 79], left ventricular ejection fraction < 0.30, using diuretics, digoxin, and angiotensin converting enzyme inhibitors) found that amlodipine versus placebo had no significant effect on the primary combined end point of all cause mortality and hospital admission for cardiovascular events over 14 months (222/571 [39%] with amlodipine *v* 246/582 [42%] with placebo; ARR +3.4%, 95% CI –2.3% to +8.8%; RR 0.92, 95% CI 0.79 to 1.06).[10,38] Subgroup analysis of people with primary cardiomyopathy found a reduction in mortality (45/209 [22%] with amlodipine *v* 74/212 [35%] with placebo; ARR 13%, 95% CI 5% to 20%; RR 0.62, 95% CI 0.43 to 0.85; NNT 7). There was no significant difference in the group with heart failure caused by coronary artery disease. The second RCT (186 people, idiopathic dilated cardiomyopathy, NYHA class I–III) compared diltiazem versus placebo.[10] It found no evidence of a difference in survival with diltiazem versus placebo in those who did not have a heart transplant, although people on diltiazem had improved cardiac function, exercise capacity, and subjective quality of life. The third RCT (451 people with mild heart failure, NYHA class II or III) compared felodipine versus placebo.[10] No significant beneficial or adverse effect was found. The subsequent RCT (2590 NYHA people with class II–IV heart failure, mean follow up of 1.6 years with placebo and 1.5 with mibefradil) found that more people died with mibefradil but the difference was not significant (350/1295 [27.0%] with mibefradil *v* 319/1295 [24.6%] with placebo; RR 1.10, 95% CI 0.96 to 1.25).[37]

Harms: Calcium channel blockers have been found to exacerbate symptoms of heart failure or increase mortality in people with pulmonary congestion after myocardial infarction or ejection fraction less than 0.40 (see calcium channel blockers under acute myocardial infarction, p 11).[10] The mibefradil RCT found that in people taking digoxin, class I or II antiarrhythmics, amiodarone, or drugs associated with torsade de pointes, mibefradil increased risk of death versus placebo.[37] The review found that second generation dihydropyridine calcium channel blockers did not cause significant adverse effects.[36]

Comment: Many of the RCTs were underpowered and had wide confidence intervals. An RCT of amlodipine in people with primary dilated cardiomyopathy is in progress.

OPTION ALDOSTERONE RECEPTOR ANTAGONISTS

One large RCT of people with severe heart failure (on usual treatment including angiotensin converting enzyme inhibitors) has found that adding an aldosterone receptor antagonist (spironolactone) further reduces mortality.

Benefits: We found no systematic review. We found one RCT of spironolactone (25 mg/day) versus placebo (1663 people with heart failure, New York Heart Association class III or IV [see glossary, p 79], left ventricular ejection fraction < 0.35, all taking angiotensin converting enzyme inhibitors and loop diuretics, and most taking digoxin).[39] The trial was stopped early because of a significant reduction in the primary end point of all cause mortality with spironolactone after 2 years (mortality: 284/822 [35%] with spironolactone *v* 386/841 [46%] with placebo; ARR 11%, 95% CI 7% to 16%; RR 0.75, 95% CI 0.66 to 0.85; NNT 9, 95% CI 6 to 15).[39]

Harms: The RCT found no evidence that spironolactone in combination with an angiotensin converting enzyme inhibitor may result in an increased incidence of clinically significant hyperkalaemia. Gynaecomastia or breast pain were reported in 10% of men given spironolactone and 1% of men given placebo.[39]

Comment: The RCT was large and well designed. As only people with New York Heart Association functional class III or IV were included, these results cannot necessarily be generalised to people with milder heart failure.

OPTION ANTIARRHYTHMIC DRUG TREATMENT

Systematic reviews found weak evidence that amiodarone reduced total mortality in people with heart failure. Extrapolation from one systematic review in people treated after a myocardial infarction suggests that other antiarrhythmic agents may increase mortality in people with heart failure.

Benefits: **Amiodarone:** We found two systematic reviews of the effects of amiodarone versus placebo in heart failure.[40,41] The most recent review (search date 1997, 10 RCTs, 4766 people) included people with a wide range of conditions (symptomatic and asymptomatic heart failure, ventricular arrhythmia, recent myocardial infarction, and recent cardiac arrest).[40] Eight of these RCTs reported the number of deaths. The review found that treatment with amiodarone over 3–24 months reduced the risk of death from any cause compared with placebo or conventional treatment (436/2262 [19%] with amiodarone *v* 507/2263 [22%] with control; ARR 3%, 95% CI 0.8% to 5.3%; RR 0.86, 95% CI 0.76 to 0.96; NNT 32). This review did not perform any subgroup analyses on people with heart failure. The earlier systematic review (search date not stated) found eight RCTs (5101 people after myocardial infarction) of prophylactic amiodarone versus placebo or usual care and five RCTs (1452 people with heart failure).[41] Mean follow up was 16 months. Analysis of results from all 13 RCTs found a lower total mortality with amiodarone than control (annual mortality: 10.9% with amiodarone *v* 12.3% with control). The effect was significant with some methods of calculation (fixed effects model: OR 0.87, 95% CI 0.78 to 0.99) but not with others (random effects model: OR 0.85, 95% CI 0.71 to 1.02). The effect of amiodarone was significantly greater in RCTs that compared amiodarone versus usual care than in placebo controlled RCTs. Deaths classified as arrhythmic death or sudden death were significantly reduced by amiodarone compared with placebo (OR 0.71, 95% CI 0.59 to 0.85). Subgroup analysis found a significant effect of amiodarone in the five heart failure RCTs (annual mortality: 19.9% with amiodarone *v* 24.3% with placebo; OR 0.83, 95% CI 0.70 to 0.99). **Other antiarrhythmics:** Apart from β blockers, other antiarrhythmic drugs seem to increase mortality in people at high risk (see class I antiarrhythmic agents under secondary prevention of ischaemic cardiac events, p 129).

Harms: **Amiodarone:** Amiodarone was not found to increase the non-arrhythmic death rate (OR 1.02, 95% CI 0.87 to 1.19).[41] In placebo controlled RCTs, after 2 years 41% of people in the amiodarone group and 27% in the placebo group had permanently discontinued study medication.[41] In 10 RCTs of amiodarone versus placebo, amiodarone increased the odds of reporting adverse drug reactions compared with placebo (OR 2.22, 95% CI 1.83 to 2.68). Nausea was the most common adverse effect. Hypothyroidism was the most common serious adverse effect (7.0% with amiodarone *v* 1.1% with control). Hyperthyroidism (1.4% with amiodarone *v* 0.5% with control), peripheral neuropathy (0.5% with amiodarone *v* 0.2% with control), lung infiltrates (1.6% with amiodarone *v* 0.5% with control), bradycardia (2.4% with amiodarone *v* 0.8% with control), and liver dysfunction (1.0% with amiodarone *v* 0.4% with control) were all more common in the amiodarone group.[41] **Other antiarrhythmics:** These agents (particularly class I antiarrhythmics) may increase mortality (see class I antiarrhythmic agents under secondary prevention of ischaemic cardiac events, p 129).

Comment: **Amiodarone:** RCTs of amiodarone versus usual treatment found larger effects than placebo controlled trials.[41] These findings suggest bias; unblinded follow up may be associated with reduced usual care or improved adherence with amiodarone. Further studies are required to assess the effects of amiodarone treatment on mortality and morbidity in people with heart failure.

OPTION IMPLANTABLE CARDIAC DEFIBRILLATORS

One RCT has found good evidence that implantable cardiac defibrillator reduces mortality in people with heart failure who have experienced a cardiac arrest. Two RCTs have found that implantable cardiac defibrillators reduce mortality compared with medical treatment in people with heart failure and at high risk of arrhythmia, whereas one RCT found no significant difference in mortality.

Benefits: We found no systematic review. We found four RCTs examining the effects of implantable cardiac defibrillators (ICDs) in people with left ventricular dysfunction.[42–45] The first RCT (1016 people resuscitated after ventricular arrhythmia plus either syncope or other serious cardiac symptom plus left ventricular ejection fraction ≤ 0.40) compared an ICD versus an antiarrhythmic drug (mainly amiodarone).[42] ICDs improved survival at 1, 2, and 3 years (1 year survival: 89.3% with ICD *v* 82.3% with antiarrhythmic; 2 year survival: 81.6% with ICD *v* 73.7% with antiarrhythmic; 3 year survival: 75.4% with ICD *v* 64.1% with antiarrhythmic). The second RCT included 196 people with New York Heart Association class I–III (see glossary, p 79) heart failure and previous myocardial infarction, a left ventricular ejection fraction 0.35 or less, a documented episode of asymptomatic unsustained ventricular tachycardia, and inducible non-suppressible ventricular tachyarrhythmia on electrophysiological study.[43] Ninety five people received an ICD and 101 received conventional medical treatment. The trial found that ICDs reduced mortality over a mean of 27 months (deaths: 15/95 [16%] with ICD [11 from cardiac cause] *v* 39/101 [39%] with conventional treatment [27 from cardiac cause]; HR 0.46, 95% CI 0.26 to 0.82). The third RCT included 1055 people aged under 80 years who were scheduled for coronary artery bypass surgery, had a left ventricular ejection fraction less than 0.36, and had electrocardiographic abnormalities. It found that ICD (446 people) at the time of bypass surgery versus no ICD (454 people) produced no significant difference in mortality over a mean of 32 months (deaths: 101/446 [23%] with ICD [71 from cardiac causes] *v* 95/454 [21%] with control [72 from cardiac causes]; HR 1.07, 95% CI 0.81 to 1.42).[44] The fourth RCT (1232 people with prior myocardial infarction and left ventricular ejection fraction < 0.30) compared an ICD (742 people) versus conventional medical treatment (490 people).[45] It found that ICD reduced all cause mortality after 20 months mean follow up (AR 14.2% with ICD *v* 19.8% with conventional treatment; HR 0.69, 95% CI 0.51 to 0.93, P = 0.016).

Harms: The RCTs found that the main adverse effects of ICDs were infection (about 5%), pneumothorax (about 2%), bleeding requiring further operation (about 1%), serious haematomas (about 3%), cardiac perforation (about 0.2%), problems with defibrillator lead (about 7%), and malfunction of defibrillator generator (about 3%).[42–45]

Comment: The RCTs were in people with reduced left ventricular function and included people with and without previous cardiac arrest or inducible arrhythmia. It is uncertain whether asymptomatic ventricular arrhythmia is in itself a predictor of sudden death in people with moderate or severe heart failure.[46] Several RCTs of prophylactic ICD treatment in people with heart failure and in survivors of acute myocardial infarction are ongoing.[47]

OPTION ANTICOAGULATION

We found no RCTs of anticoagulation in people with heart failure. We found conflicting evidence from two large retrospective cohort studies.

Benefits: We found no systematic review and no RCTs of anticoagulation in people with heart failure. We found conflicting evidence from two large retrospective cohort studies (see comment below).[48,49]

Harms: Neither cohort study reported harms of anticoagulation.

Comment: The first retrospective analysis assessed the effect of anticoagulants used at the discretion of individual investigators in RCTs on the incidence of stroke, peripheral arterial embolism, and pulmonary embolism.[48] The first cohort was from one RCT (642 men with chronic heart failure) comparing hydralazine plus isosorbide dinitrate versus prazosin versus placebo. The second cohort was from another RCT (804 men with chronic heart failure) comparing enalapril versus hydralazine plus isosorbide dinitrate. All people were given digoxin and diuretics. The retrospective analysis found that without treatment the incidence of all thromboembolic events was low (2.7/100 people years in the first RCT; 2.1/100 people years in the second RCT) and that anticoagulation did not reduce the incidence of thromboembolic events (2.9/100 people years in the first RCT; 4.8/100 people years in the second RCT). In this group of people, atrial fibrillation was not found to be associated with a higher risk of thromboembolic events. The second retrospective analysis was from two large RCTs (2569 people with symptomatic and asymptomatic left ventricular dysfunction) that compared enalapril versus placebo.[49] The analysis found that people treated with warfarin at baseline had significantly lower risk of death during follow up (HR adjusted for baseline differences 0.76, 95% CI 0.65 to 0.89). Warfarin use was associated with a reduction in the combined outcome of death plus hospital admission for heart failure (adjusted HR 0.82, 95% CI 0.72 to 0.93). The benefit with warfarin use was not significantly influenced by the presence of symptoms, randomisation to enalapril or placebo, sex, presence of atrial fibrillation, age, ejection fraction, New York Heart Association classification (see glossary, p 79), or cause of heart failure. Warfarin reduced cardiac mortality, specifically deaths that were sudden, or associated with either heart failure or myocardial infarction. Neither of the retrospective studies was designed to determine the incidence of thromboembolic events in heart failure or the effects of treatment. Neither study included information about the intensity of anticoagulation or warfarin use. We found several additional cohort studies that showed a reduction in thromboembolic events with anticoagulation, but they all reported results for too few people to provide useful results. An RCT is needed to compare anticoagulation versus no anticoagulation in people with heart failure.

OPTION ANTIPLATELET AGENTS

We found no RCTs. Retrospective analyses have included too few events to establish or exclude a clinically important effect of antiplatelet agents in people with heart failure. In people not taking angiotensin converting enzyme inhibitors, we found limited evidence from one retrospective cohort analysis that the incidence of thromboembolic events in people with heart failure was low and not significantly improved with antiplatelet treatment. It is unclear from two retrospective cohort analyses, whether there are additional reductions in the incidence of thromboembolic events from adding angiotensin converting enzyme inhibitor treatment to antiplatelet treatment in people with heart failure. It is unclear from one retrospective cohort analysis, whether adding antiplatelet treatment to angiotensin converting enzyme inhibitor treatment in people with heart failure is beneficial.

Benefits: We found no systematic review and no RCTs examining effects of antiplatelet agents in people with heart failure. We found two cohort studies (see comment below).[48,50]

Harms: Neither study reported harms of treatment.

Comment: **In people not taking angiotensin converting enzyme inhibitors:** We found no systematic review and no RCTs. We found one retrospective cohort analysis within one RCT in 642 men with heart failure.[48] The RCT compared hydralazine plus isosorbide dinitrate versus prazosin versus placebo in men receiving digoxin and diuretics. Aspirin, dipyridamole, or both were used at the discretion of the investigators. The number of thromboembolic events was low in both groups (only 1 stroke and no pulmonary or peripheral emboli in 184 people years of treatment with antiplatelet drugs *v* 21 strokes, 4 peripheral, and 4 pulmonary emboli in 1068 people years of treatment without antiplatelet drugs; 0.5 events/100 people years with antiplatelet agents *v* 2.0 events/100 people years without antiplatelet agents; P = 0.07). **In people taking angiotensin converting enzyme inhibitors:** We found no RCTs. We found two large retrospective cohort studies.[48,50] The first retrospective analysis assessed the effect of antiplatelet agents used at the discretion of individual investigators on the incidence of stroke, peripheral arterial embolism, and pulmonary embolism within one RCT.[48] The RCT (804 men with chronic heart failure) compared enalapril versus hydralazine plus isosorbide dinitrate. It found that the incidence of all thromboembolic events was low without antiplatelet treatment and, although antiplatelet agents reduced the thromboembolic rate, the difference was not significant (1.6 events/100 people years with antiplatelet agents *v* 2.1 events/100 people years with no antiplatelet agent; P = 0.48). The second cohort analysis was from two large RCTs that compared enalapril versus placebo (2569 people with symptomatic and asymptomatic left ventricular dysfunction). It found that people treated with antiplatelet agents at baseline had a significantly lower risk of death (HR adjusted for baseline differences 0.82, 95% CI 0.73 to 0.92).[50] Subgroup analysis suggested that an effect of antiplatelet agents might be present in people who were randomised to placebo (mortality HR for antiplatelet treatment at baseline *v* no antiplatelet treatment at baseline 0.68, 95% CI 0.58 to 0.80), but not in people randomised to enalapril (mortality HR for antiplatelet treatment *v* no antiplatelet treatment 1.00, 95% CI 0.85 to 1.17). Both retrospective studies have limitations common to studies with a retrospective cohort design. One study did not report on the proportions of people taking aspirin and other antiplatelet agents.[48] The other study noted that more than 95% of people took aspirin, but the dosage and consistency of antiplatelet use was not recorded.[50] One retrospective non-systematic review (4 RCTs, 96 712 people) provided additional evidence about the effect of aspirin on the benefits of early angiotensin converting enzyme inhibitors in heart failure.[51] It found a similar reduction in 30 day mortality with angiotensin converting enzyme inhibitor versus control for those people not taking aspirin compared to those taking aspirin (aspirin: OR 0.94, 95% CI 0.89 to 0.99; no aspirin: OR 0.90, 95% CI 0.81 to 1.01). However, the analysis may not be valid because the people who did not receive aspirin were older and had a worse baseline prognosis than those taking aspirin. The effects of antiplatelet treatment in combination with ACE inhibitors in people with heart failure requires further research.

QUESTION What are the effects of angiotensin converting enzyme inhibitors in people at high risk of heart failure?

RCTs have found good evidence that angiotensin converting enzyme inhibitors can delay development of symptomatic heart failure and reduce the frequency of cardiovascular events in people with asymptomatic left ventricular systolic dysfunction, and in people with other cardiovascular risk factors for heart failure.

Benefits: **In people with asymptomatic left ventricular systolic dysfunction:** We found no systematic review but found two RCTs. One large RCT examined an angiotensin converting enzyme (ACE) inhibitor (enalapril) versus placebo over 40 months in people with asymptomatic left ventricular systolic dysfunction (LVEF; < 0.35).[52] It found no evidence that enalapril significantly decreased total mortality and cardiovascular mortality compared with placebo (all cause mortality: 313/2111 [14.8%] with ACE inhibitor *v* 334/2117 [15.8%] with placebo; ARR +0.9%, 95% CI –1.3% to +2.9%; RR 0.94, 95% CI 0.81 to 1.08; cardiovascular mortality: 265/2111 [12.6%] with ACE inhibitor *v* 298/2117 [14.1%] with placebo; ARR +1.5%, 95% CI –0.6% to +3.3%; RR 0.89, 95% CI 0.76 to 1.04). During the study more people assigned to the placebo received digoxin, diuretics, or ACE inhibitors that were not part of the study protocol, which may have contributed to the lack of significant difference in mortality between the two groups. Compared with placebo, enalapril reduced symptomatic heart failure, hospital admission for heart failure, and fatal or non-fatal myocardial infarction (symptomatic heart failure: 438/2111 [21%] with ACE inhibitor *v* 640/2117 [30%] with placebo; ARR 9.5%, 95% CI 7% to 12%;

RR 0.69, 95% CI 0.61 to 0.77; NNT 11; admission for heart failure: 306/2111 [15%] with ACE inhibitor *v* 454/2117 [21%] with placebo; ARR 7%, 95% CI 5% to 9%; RR 0.68, 95% CI 0.59 to 0.77; NNT 14; fatal or non-fatal myocardial infarction: 7.6% with ACE inhibitor *v* 9.6% with placebo; ARR 2%, 95% CI 0.4% to 3.4%; RR 0.79, 95% CI 0.65 to 0.96).[9,52] A second RCT in asymptomatic people after myocardial infarction with documented LVSD found that an ACE inhibitor (captopril) reduced mortality and reduced the risk of ischaemic events compared with placebo.[53] **In people with other risk factors:** We found one large RCT comparing ramipril 10 mg daily versus placebo, for a mean of 5 years, in 9297 high risk people (people with vascular disease or diabetes plus one other cardiovascular risk factor) who were not known to have LVSD or heart failure.[54] It found that ramipril reduced the risk of heart failure (9.0% with ramipril *v* 11.5% with placebo; RR 0.77, 95% CI 0.67 to 0.87; $P < 0.001$). Ramipril also reduced the combined risk of myocardial infarction or stroke or cardiovascular death, the risk of these outcomes separately, and all cause mortality (see angiotensin converting enzyme inhibitors under secondary prevention of ischaemic cardiac events, p 129). During the trial, 496 people underwent echocardiography; 2.6% of these people were found to have ejection fraction less than 0.4. Retrospective review of charts found that left ventricular function had been documented in 5193 people; 8.1% had a reduced ejection fraction.

Harms: We found no systematic review. The first RCT over 40 months found that a high proportion of people in both groups reported adverse effects (76% with enalapril *v* 72% with placebo).[52] Dizziness or fainting (46% with enalapril *v* 33% with placebo) and cough (34% with enalapril *v* 27% with placebo) were reported more often in the enalapril group (P value not stated). The incidence of angioedema was the same in both groups (1.4%). Study medication was permanently discontinued by 8% of the people in the enalapril group versus 5% in the placebo group (P value not stated).

Comment: Asymptomatic LVSD is prognostically important, but we found no prospective studies that have assessed the usefulness of screening to detect its presence.

QUESTION What are the effects of treatments for diastolic heart failure?

We found no RCTs in people with diastolic heart failure.

Benefits: We found no systematic review or RCTs in people with diastolic heart failure.

Harms: We found no evidence on the harms of treatments for diastolic heart failure.

Comment: The causes of diastolic dysfunction vary among people with diastolic heart failure. Current treatment is empirical, based on the results of small clinical studies and consists of treating the underlying cause and coexistent conditions with interventions optimised for individuals.[6,55,56] RCTs with clinically relevant outcome measures are needed to determine the benefits and harms of treatment in diastolic heart failure.

GLOSSARY

Exercise time This is the total time in seconds that a person is able to pedal in a standardised symptom limited bicycle ergonometry exercise test.

New York Heart Association classification Classification of severity by symptoms. Class I: no limitation of physical activity; ordinary physical activity does not cause undue fatigue or dyspnoea. Class II: slight limitation of physical activity; comfortable at rest, but ordinary physical activity results in fatigue or dyspnoea. Class III: limitation of physical activity; comfortable at rest, but less than ordinary activity causes fatigue or dyspnoea. Class IV: unable to carry on any physical activity without symptoms; symptoms are present even at rest; if any physical activity is undertaken, symptoms are increased.

Substantive changes

Angiotensin receptor blockers New systematic review;[24] found no significant difference between angiotensin receptor blockers versus placebo or angiotensin converting enzyme inhibitors for all cause mortality or admission for heart failure. Adding angiotensin converting enzyme inhibitors to angiotensin receptor blockers reduced hospital admission for heart failure but did not significantly affect all cause mortality compared with angiotensin converting enzyme inhibitors alone. Categorisation moved from "beneficial" to "likely to be beneficial".

Implantable cardiac defibrillators New RCT;[45] found that implantable defibrillators reduced mortality versus medical treatment in people with reduced systolic function.

REFERENCES

1. Poole-Wilson PA. History, definition, and classification of heart failure. In: Poole-Wilson PA, Colucci WS, Massie BM, et al, eds. *Heart failure. Scientific principles and clinical practice.* London: Churchill Livingston, 1997:269–277.
2. Working Group Report. How to diagnose diastolic heart failure: European Study Group on Diastolic Heart Failure. *Eur Heart J* 1998;19:990–1003.
3. Cowie MR, Mosterd A, Wood DA, et al. The epidemiology of heart failure. *Eur Heart J* 1997;18:208–225.
4. McKelvie RS, Benedict CR, Yusuf S. Prevention of congestive heart failure and management of asymptomatic left ventricular dysfunction. *BMJ* 1999;318:1400–1402.
5. Bröckel U, Hense HW, Museholl M. Prevalence of left ventricular dysfunction in the general population [abstract]. *J Am Coll Cardiol* 1996;27(suppl A):25.
6. Mosterd A, deBruijne MC, Hoes A. Usefulness of echocardiography in detecting left ventricular dysfunction in population-based studies (the Rotterdam study). *Am J Cardiol* 1997;79;103–104.
7. Vasan RS, Benjamin EJ, Levy D. Congestive heart failure with normal left ventricular systolic function. *Arch Intern Med* 1996;156:146–157.
8. Davie AP, Francis CM, Caruana L, et al. The prevalence of left ventricular diastolic filling abnormalities in patients with suspected heart failure. *Eur Heart J* 1997;18:981–984.
9. Yusuf S, Pepine CJ, Garces C, et al. Effect of enalapril on myocardial infarction and unstable angina in patients with low ejection fractions. *Lancet* 1992;340:1173–1178.
10. Gheorghiade M, Benatar D, Konstam MA, et al. Pharmacotherapy for systolic dysfunction: a review of randomized clinical trials. *Am J Cardiol* 1997;80(8B):14H–27H.
11. Gaasch WH. Diagnosis and treatment of heart failure based on LV systolic or diastolic dysfunction. *JAMA* 1994;271:1276–1280.
12. Bittner V, Weiner DH, Yusuf S, et al, for the SOLVD Investigators. Prediction of mortality and morbidity with a 6-minute walk test in patients with left ventricular dysfunction. *JAMA* 1993;270:1702–1707.
13. Rogers WJ, Johnstone DE, Yusuf S, et al, for the SOLVD Investigators. Quality of life among 5 025 patients with left ventricular dysfunction randomized between placebo and enalapril. The studies of left ventricular dysfunction. *J Am Coll Cardiol* 1994;23:393 400.
14. McAlister FA, Lawson FME, Teo KK, et al. A systematic review of randomized trials of disease management programs in heart failure. *Am J Med* 2001;110:378–384. Search date 1999; primary sources Medline, Embase, Cinahl, Sigle, Cochrane Controlled Trials Register, the Cochrane Effective Practice and Organization of Care Study Register, hand searches of bibliographies of identified studies, and personal contact with content experts.
15. Dracup K, Baker DW, Dunbar SB, et al. Management of heart failure. II. Counseling, education and lifestyle modifications. *JAMA* 1994;272:1442–1446. Search date 1993; primary sources Medline and Embase.
16. Piepoli MF, Flater M, Coats AJS. Overview of studies of exercise training in chronic heart failure: the need for a prospective randomized multi-centre European trial. *Eur Heart J* 1998;19:830–841. Search date and primary sources not stated; computer aided search performed.
17. Miller TD, Balady GJ, Fletcher GF. Exercise and its role in the prevention and rehabilitation of cardiovascular disease. *Ann Behav Med* 1997;19:220–229.
18. European Heart Failure Training Group. Experience from controlled trials of physical training in chronic heart failure. Protocol and patient factors in effectiveness in the improvement in exercise tolerance. *Eur Heart J* 1998;19:466–475.

19. Belardinelli R, Georgiou D, Cianci G, et al. Randomized, controlled trial of long-term moderate exercise training in chronic heart failure. Effects on functional capacity, quality of life, and clinical outcomes. *Circulation* 1999;99:1173–1182.
20. Garg R, Yusuf S, for the Collaborative Group on ACE Inhibitor Trials. Overview of randomized trials of angiotensin-converting enzyme inhibitors on mortality and morbidity in patients with heart failure. *JAMA* 1995;273:1450–1456. Search date 1994; primary sources Medline and correspondence with investigators and pharmaceutical companies.
21. Flather M, Yusuf S, Kober L, et al, for the ACE-Inhibitor Myocardial Infarction Collaborative Group. Long-term ACE-inhibitor therapy in patients with heart failure or left-ventricular dysfunction: a systematic overview of data from individual patients. *Lancet* 2000;355:1575–1581. Search date not stated; primary sources Medline, Ovid, hand searches of reference lists, and personal contact with researchers, colleagues, and principal investigators of the trials identified.
22. Packer M, Poole-Wilson PA, Armstrong PW, et al, on behalf of the ATLAS Study Group. Comparative effects of low and high doses of the angiotensin-converting enzyme inhibitor, lisinopril, on morbidity and mortality in chronic heart failure. *Circulation* 1999;100:2312–2318.
23. SOLVD Investigators. Effect of enalapril on survival in patients with reduced left ventricular ejection fractions and congestive heart failure. *N Engl J Med* 1991;325:293–302.
24. Jong P, Demers C, McKelvie RS, et al. Angiotensin receptor blockers in heart failure: meta-analysis of randomized controlled trials. *J Am Coll Cardiol* 2002;39:463–470. Search date 2001; primary sources Medline, Embase, Biological Abstracts, International Pharmaceutical Abstracts, Cochrane Controlled Trials Database, McMaster Cardiovascular Randomized Clinical Trial Registry, and Science Citation Index.
25. Kraus F, Rudolph C, Rudolph W. Wirksamkeit von Digitalis bei Patienten mit chronischer Herzinsuffizienz und Sinusrhythmus. *Herz* 1993;18:95–117. Search date 1992; primary source Medline.
26. Digitalis Investigation Group. The effect of digoxin on mortality and morbidity in patients with heart failure. *N Engl J Med* 1997;336:525–533.
27. Cohn J, Goldstein S, Greenberg B, et al. A dose-dependent increase in mortality with vesnarinone among patients with severe heart failure. *N Engl J Med* 1998;339:1810–1816.
28. Packer M, Carver JR, Rodeheffer RJ, et al, for the PROMISE Study Research Group. Effect of oral milrinone on mortality in severe chronic heart failure. *N Engl J Med* 1991;325:1468–1475.
29. Hampton JR, van Veldhuisen DJ, Kleber FX, et al. Randomised study of effect of ibopamine on survival in patients with advanced severe heart failure. *Lancet* 1997;349:971–977.
30. Brophy JM, Joseph L, Rouleau JL. β-blockers in congestive heart failure: a Bayesian meta-analysis. *Ann Intern Med* 2001;134:550–560. Search date 2000; primary sources Medline, Cochrane Library, Web of Science, and hand searches of reference lists from relevant articles.
31. Whorlow SL, Krum H. Meta-analysis of effect of β-blocker therapy on mortality in patients with New York Heart Association class IV chronic congestive heart failure. *Am J Cardiol* 2000;86:886–889. Search date not stated; primary sources Medline and hand searches of reference lists from relevant reviews.
32. Packer M, Coats A, Fowler MB. Effect of carvedilol on survival in severe chronic heart failure. Engl J Med 2001;344:1651–1658.
33. The Beta-Blocker Evaluation of Survival Trial Investigators. A trial of the β-blocker bucindolol in patients with advanced chronic heart failure. *N Engl J Med* 2001;344:1659–1667.
34. The CAPRICORN Investigators. Effect of carvedilol on outcome after myocardial infarction in patients with left ventricular dysfunction: the CAPRICORN randomized trial. *Lancet* 2001;357:1385–1390.
35. Metra M, Giubbini R, Nodari S, et al. Differential effects of β-blockers in patients with heart failure: a prospective, randomized, double-blind comparison of the long-term effects of metoprolol versus carvedilol. *Circulation* 2000;102:546–551.
36. Cleophas T, van Marum R. Meta-analysis of efficacy and safety of second-generation dihydropyridine calcium channel blockers in heart failure. *Am J Card* 2001;87:487–490. Search date not stated; primary source Medline.
37. Levine TB, Bernink P, Caspi A, et al. Effect of mibefradil, a T-type calcium channel blocker, on morbidity and mortality in moderate to severe congestive heart failure. The MACH-1 study. *Circulation* 2000;101:758–764.
38. Packer M, O'Connor CM, Ghali JK, et al, for the Prospective Randomized Amlodipine Survival Evaluation Study Group. Effect of amlodipine on morbidity and mortality in severe chronic heart failure. *N Engl J Med* 1996;335:1107–1114.
39. Pitt B, Zannad F, Remme WJ, et al, for the Randomized Aldactone Evaluation Study Investigators. The effects of spironolactone on morbidity and mortality in patients with severe heart failure. *N Engl J Med* 1999;341:709–717.
40. Piepoli M, Villani GQ, Ponikowski P, et al. Overview and meta-analysis of randomised trials of amiodarone in chronic heart failure. *Int J Cardiol* 1998;66:1–10. Search date 1997; primary source unspecified computerised literature database.
41. Amiodarone Trials Meta-Analysis Investigators. Effect of prophylactic amiodarone on mortality after acute myocardial infarction and in congestive heart failure: meta-analysis of individual data from 6500 patients in randomised trials. *Lancet* 1997;350:1417–1424. Search date not stated; primary sources literature reviews, computerised literature reviews, and discussion with colleagues.
42. The Antiarrhythmic versus Implantable Defibrillators (AVID) Investigators. A comparison of antiarrhythmic-drug therapy with implantable defibrillators I patients resuscitated from near-fatal ventricular arrhythmias. *N Engl J Med* 1997;337:1576–1583.
43. Moss AJ, Hall WJ, Cannom DS, et al. Improved survival with an implanted defibrillator in patients with coronary disease at high risk for ventricular arrhythmia. *N Engl J Med* 1996;335:1933–1940.
44. Bigger JT for The Coronary Artery Bypass Graft (CABG) Patch Trial Investigators. Prophylactic use of implanted cardiac defibrillators in patients at high risk for ventricular arrhythmias after coronary-artery bypass graft surgery. *N Engl J Med* 1997;337:1569–1575.
45. Moss AJ, Zoreba W, Hall J, et al, for the Multicenter Automatic Defibrillator Implantation Trial II Investigators. Prophylactic implantation of a defibrillator in patients with myocardial infarction and reduced ejection fraction. *N Engl J Med* 2002;346:877–883.
46. Teerlink JR, Jalaluddin M, Anderson S, et al. Ambulatory ventricular arrhythmias in patients with heart failure do not specifically predict an increased risk of sudden death. *Circulation* 2000;101:40–46.

47. Connolly SJ. Prophylactic antiarrhythmic therapy for the prevention of sudden death in high-risk patients: drugs and devices. *Eur Heart J* 1999;(suppl C):31–35.
48. Dunkman WB, Johnson GR, Carson PE, et al, for the V-HeFT Cooperative Studies Group. Incidence of thromboembolic events in congestive heart failure. *Circulation* 1993;87:94–101.
49. Al-Khadra AS, Salem DN, Rand WM, et al. Warfarin anticoagulation and survival: a cohort analysis from the studies of left ventricular dysfunction. *J Am Coll Cardiol* 1998;31:749–753.
50. Al-Khadra AS, Salem DN, Rand WM, et al. Antiplatelet agents and survival: a cohort analysis from the Studies of Left Ventricular Dysfunction (SOLVD) Trial. *J Am Coll Cardiol* 1998;31:419–425.
51. Latini R, Tognoni G, Maggioni AP, et al, on behalf of the Angiotensin-converting Enzyme Inhibitor Myocardial Infarction Collaborative Group. Clinical effects of early angiotensin-converting enzyme inhibitor treatment for acute myocardial infarction are similar in the presence and absence of aspirin. Systematic overview of individual data from 96 712 randomized patients. *J Am Coll Cardiol* 2000;35:1801–1807.
52. SOLVD Investigators. Effect of enalapril on mortality and the development of heart failure in asymptomatic patients with reduced left ventricular ejection fractions. *N Engl J Med* 1992;327:685–691.
53. Rutherford JD, Pfeffer MA, Moyé LA, et al. Effects of captopril on ischaemic events after myocardial infarction. *Circulation* 1994;90:1731–1738.
54. The Heart Outcome Prevention Evaluation Study Investigators. Effects of an angiotensin-converting-enzyme inhibitor, ramipril, on cardiovascular events in high-risk patients. *N Engl J Med* 2000;342:145–153.
55. The Task Force of the Working Group on Heart Failure of the European Society of Cardiology. The treatment of heart failure. *Eur Heart J* 1997;18:736–753.
56. Tendera M. Ageing and heart failure: the place of ACE inhibitors in heart failure with preserved systolic function. *Eur Heart J* 2000;2(suppl I):I8–I14.

Robert McKelvie
Associate Professor of Medicine
McMaster University
Hamilton, ON
Canada

Competing interests: RM has been paid by AstraZeneca and Bristol-Myers Squibb to serve on steering committees and has been paid by AstraZeneca and Merck Frosst to give presentations.

Peripheral arterial disease

Search date December 2001

Sonia Anand and Mark Creager

QUESTIONS

INTERVENTIONS

*Despite the absence of strong evidence from RCTs, there is a consensus belief that bypass surgery is effective for people with severe peripheral vascular disease.

See glossary, p 92.

Key Messages

- **Antiplatelet treatment** Systematic reviews have found that antiplatelet agents versus control treatments significantly reduce the rate of major cardiovascular events over an average of about 2 years. Systematic reviews have found that antiplatelet agents versus placebo or no treatments significantly reduce the risk of arterial occlusion and reduce the risk of revascularisation procedures. The balance of benefits and harms is in favour of treatment for most people with symptomatic peripheral arterial disease, because as a group they are at much greater risk of cardiovascular events.
- **Bypass surgery** One systematic review found that surgery versus percutaneous transluminal angioplasty significantly improved primary patency after 12–24 months, but found no significant difference after 4 years. The review found no significant difference in mortality after 12–24 months. One systematic review found that surgery versus thrombolysis significantly reduced the number of amputations and the number of people reporting ongoing ischaemic pain, but found no significant difference in mortality after 1 year. Although the consensus view is that bypass surgery is the most effective treatment for people with debilitating symptomatic peripheral arterial disease, we found inadequate evidence from RCTs reporting long term clinical outcomes to confirm this view.

- **Cilostazol** Four RCTs in people with intermittent claudication have found that cilostazol versus placebo significantly improves initial claudication distance and absolute claudication distance measured on a treadmill and significantly reduces the proportion of people with symptoms that do not improve. One RCT with a high withdrawal rate found that pentoxifylline versus cilostazol significantly increased the number of people who had no change or deterioration in the initial claudication distance and the absolute claudication distance.
- **Exercise** Systematic reviews in people with chronic stable claudication have found that regular exercise at least three times weekly versus no exercise significantly improves total walking distance and maximal exercise time after 3–12 months.
- **Pentoxifylline** Systematic reviews of small RCTs of variable quality in people with intermittent claudication have found that pentoxifylline versus placebo increases the walking distance by a small amount. One subsequent RCT with a high withdrawal rate found no significant difference in walking distance between pentoxifylline versus placebo, but found that pentoxifylline versus placebo significantly increased the number of people who had no change or deterioration in the initial claudication distance and the absolute claudication distance.
- **Percutaneous transluminal angioplasty (transient benefit only)** Two small RCTs in people with mild to moderate intermittent claudication found limited evidence that angioplasty versus no angioplasty significantly improved walking distance after 6 months but found no significant difference after 2 or 6 years. Four RCTs in people with femoral to popliteal artery stenoses have found no significant difference with angioplasty alone versus angioplasty plus stent placement in patency rates, occlusion rates or clinical improvement.
- **Smoking cessation (based on consensus of opinion)** RCTs of advice to stop smoking are unlikely to be conducted. The consensus view is that smoking cessation improves symptoms in people with intermittent claudication. One systematic review has found observational evidence that continued cigarette smoking by people with intermittent claudication is associated with progression of symptoms, poor prognosis after bypass surgery, amputation, and need for reconstructive surgery. Another systematic review found no good evidence from controlled studies about the effects of advice to stop smoking.

DEFINITION Peripheral arterial disease arises when there is significant narrowing of arteries distal to the arch of the aorta. Narrowing can arise from atheroma, arteritis, local thrombus formation, or embolisation from the heart or more central arteries. This topic includes treatment options for people with symptoms of reduced blood flow to the leg that are likely to arise from atheroma. These symptoms range from calf pain on exercise (intermittent claudication), to rest pain, skin ulceration, or ischaemic necrosis (gangrene) in people with critical ischaemia (see glossary, p 92).

INCIDENCE/ PREVALENCE Peripheral arterial disease is more common in people aged over 50 years than in younger people, and is more common in men than women. The prevalence of peripheral arterial disease of the legs (assessed by non-invasive tests) is about 3% in people under the age of 60 years, but rises to over 20% in people over 75 years.[1] The overall annual incidence of intermittent claudication is 1.5–2.6/1000 men a year and 1.2–3.6/1000 women a year.[2]

AETIOLOGY/ RISK FACTORS Factors associated with the development of peripheral arterial disease include age, gender, cigarette smoking, diabetes mellitus, hypertension, hyperlipidaemia, obesity, and physical inactivity. The strongest association is with smoking (RR 2.0–4.0) and diabetes (RR 2.0–3.0).[3] Acute limb ischaemia (see glossary, p 92) may result from thrombosis arising within a peripheral artery or from embolic occlusion.

PROGNOSIS The symptoms of intermittent claudication can resolve spontaneously, remain stable over many years, or progress rapidly to critical limb ischaemia. About 15% of people with intermittent claudication eventually develop critical leg ischaemia, which endangers the viability of the limb. The incidence of critical limb ischaemia in Denmark and Italy in 1990 was 0.25–0.45/1000 people a year.[4,5] Coronary heart disease is the major cause of death in people with peripheral arterial disease of the legs. Over 5 years, about 20% of people with intermittent claudication have a non-fatal cardiovascular event (myocardial infarction [MI], or stroke).[6] The mortality rate of people with peripheral arterial disease is two to three times higher than that of age and sex matched controls. Overall mortality after the diagnosis of peripheral arterial disease is about 30% after 5 years and 70% after 15 years.[6]

AIMS To reduce symptoms (intermittent claudication), local complications (arterial leg ulcers, critical leg ischaemia), and general complications (MI and stroke).

OUTCOMES **Local outcomes:** Proportion of people with adverse outcomes including a decline in claudication distance, amputation, or adverse effects of treatment, the mean improvement in claudication distance measured on a treadmill or by some other specified means. **General outcomes:** Rates of MI, stroke, and other major cardiovascular events.

METHODS *Clinical Evidence* search and appraisal December 2001.

QUESTION **What are the effects of treatments for people with chronic peripheral arterial disease?**

OPTION **ANTIPLATELET AGENTS**

Systematic reviews have found strong evidence that antiplatelet agents versus control treatments significantly reduce the rate of major cardiovascular events over an average of about 2 years. Systematic reviews have found that antiplatelet agents versus placebo or no treatments significantly reduce the risk of arterial occlusion and the risk of revascularisation procedures. The balance of benefits and harms is in favour of treatment for most people with symptomatic peripheral arterial disease, because as a group they are at much greater risk of cardiovascular events.

Benefits: **Peripheral arterial disease complications:** We found two systematic reviews,[7,8] one of which has subsequently been updated.[9] The first systematic review (search date 1997, 42 RCTs; 9214 people with intermittent claudication [see glossary, p 92], bypass surgery of the leg, or peripheral artery angioplasty) found that antiplatelet treatment compared with no additional treatment significantly reduced the risk of arterial occlusion over 19 months (RRR 0.30; P < 0.00001).[9] The second systematic review (search date 1998, 54 RCTs) found that aspirin versus placebo reduced the number of arterial occlusions and that ticlopidine reduced the risk of revascularisation procedures.[8] **Cardiovascular events:** We found two systematic reviews.[9,10] The first review (search date 1997, 42 RCTs; 9214 people) found that antiplatelet treatment versus control treatment significantly reduced the combined outcome of vascular death, myocardial infarction, or stroke over an average of 2 years (280/4844 [6.0%] with antiplatelet treatment *v* 347/4662 [7%] with control; RR 0.78, 95% CI 0.67 to 0.90; NNT 61, 95% CI 38 to 153).[9] The second systematic review (search date 1999, 39 RCTs) found that antiplatelet treatment versus control significantly reduced the absolute event rate for the combined end point of myocardial infarction, stroke, or vascular death (6.5% with antiplatelet treatment *v* 8.1% with control; OR 0.78, 95% CI 0.63 to 0.96).[10]

Harms: The first review (search date 1990; 35 RCTs; 8098 people with peripheral arterial disease) found no significant difference with antiplatelet treatment versus control treatment in the risk of non-fatal major bleeds (14/2545 [0.55%] *v* 9/2243 [0.40%]; RR 1.37, 95% CI 0.60 to 3.16).[7] The second review (search date 1999, 36 RCTs, 8449 people with peripheral disease) found no significant difference with antiplatelet treatment versus placebo in major bleeding (47/4349 [1%] with antiplatelet treatment *v* 33/4100 [< 1%] with placebo; OR 1.40, 95% CI 0.90 to 2.20), and found no significant difference with aspirin versus other antiplatelet agents in major bleeding (68/3467 [2%] with aspirin *v* 59/3561 [2%] with other antiplatelet agents; RR 1.18, 95% CI 0.84 to 1.67).[10] The number of events was too low to exclude a clinically important increase in major bleeding.[7,10] Across a wide range of people, antiplatelet agents have been found to increase significantly the risk of major haemorrhage (see harms of antiplatelet agents under primary prevention, p 116).

Comment: We found no evidence about the effects of combined clopidogrel and aspirin versus a single antiplatelet agent in people with peripheral arterial disease. Peripheral arterial disease increases the risk of cardiovascular events, so for most people the risk of bleeding is outweighed by the benefits of regular antiplatelet use.

OPTION EXERCISE

Systematic reviews in people with chronic stable claudication have found that regular exercise at least three times weekly versus no exercise significantly improves total walking distance and maximal exercise time after 3–12 months.

Benefits: **Walking exercise versus no exercise:** We found two systematic reviews of exercise versus no exercise in people with chronic stable intermittent claudication (see glossary, p 92) (search dates 1996,[11] and not stated;[12] see comment below). The first review found that exercise programmes (at least 30 min walking as far as claudication permits, at least 3 times weekly, for 3–6 months in people also being treated with surgery, aspirin, or dipyridamole) versus no exercise significantly increased both the initial claudication distance (see glossary, p 92) (4 RCTs; 94 people; difference of means 139 m, 95% CI 31 m to 247 m) and the absolute claudication distance (see glossary, p 92) (5 RCTs; 115 people; difference of means 179 m, 95% CI 60 m to 298 m) after 3–12 months.[13] Control treatments were placebo tablets (2 RCTs) or "instructed to continue with normal lifestyle". The second review (10 RCTs, including all those in the first review) found that exercise versus no exercise increased maximal exercise time (3 RCTs; 53 people; WMD 6.5 min, 95% CI 4.4 to 8.7 min).[12] **Different types of exercise:** All the RCTs included in the systematic reviews involved walking exercise. We found one RCT (67 people with moderate to severe intermittent claudication), which compared arm versus leg exercise of similar intensity.[13] A third group of 15 people was given no exercise, but this group was not created by random allocation. The RCT found no significant difference with arm versus leg exercises in initial claudication distance (122% with arm exercise *v* 93% with leg exercise) and absolute claudication distance (47% with arm exercise *v* 50% with leg exercise) although both groups improved after 6 weeks.

Harms: Neither review gave details of any observed harms of the exercise programmes.[11,14]

Comment: The RCTs in the systematic reviews had low drop out rates.[11,12] Blinding of participants was not possible. Blinding of assessors is not clear from the reviews. Most (5/6) exercise programmes in the second review occurred under supervision.[12] We found one further systematic review of 21 observational studies or RCTs of exercise in 564 people with peripheral arterial disease.[14] This review calculated effects based on the differences in claudication difference after and before exercise treatment, but it made no allowance for any spontaneous improvement that might have occurred in the participants. It reported large increases with exercise in the initial claudication distance (126–351 m) and in the absolute claudication distance (325–723 m), but these estimates were based on observational data. An ongoing Australian RCT is examining the effect of exercise treatment in 1400 men.[12] The benefit from arm exercise remains unconfirmed, but suggests that improved walking may be caused by generally improved cardiovascular function rather than local changes of the peripheral circulation.

OPTION SMOKING CESSATION

RCTs of advice to stop smoking are unlikely to be conducted. The consensus view is that smoking cessation improves symptoms in people with intermittent claudication. One systematic review has found observational evidence that continued cigarette smoking by people with intermittent claudication is associated with progression of symptoms, poor prognosis after bypass surgery, amputation, and need for reconstructive surgery. Another systematic review found no good evidence from controlled studies about the effects of advice to stop smoking.

Benefits: We found no RCTs.

Harms: The reviews did not report on harms (see comment below).[11,15]

Comment: RCTs of advice to stop smoking are unlikely to be conducted, although the consensus view is that smoking cessation improves symptoms in people with intermittent claudication (see glossary, p 92). We found one systematic review (search date 1996; 4 observational studies; 866 people) of advice to quit cigarette smoking versus no advice.[11] The intervention in all the studies was advice to stop smoking. One large observational study in the systematic review found no significant increase in absolute claudication distance (see glossary, p 92) after cessation of smoking.[11] Two other studies found conflicting results about the risk of deteriorating from moderate to severe claudication in people who successfully quit smoking compared with current smokers. The fourth study provided no numerical results. Overall, the review found no good evidence to confirm or refute the consensus view that advice to stop smoking improves symptoms in people with intermittent claudication. An older systematic review (search date 1989) concluded that most of the evidence on the effects of smoking cessation derives from observational studies that have found among cigarette smokers increased risk of onset of intermittent claudication, progression of symptoms, poor progress after bypass surgery, amputation, and the need for reconstructive surgery.[15]

OPTION CILOSTAZOL

Four RCTs in people with intermittent claudication have found that cilostazol versus placebo significantly improves initial claudication distance and absolute claudication distance measured on a treadmill and significantly reduces the proportion of people with symptoms that do not improve. One RCT with a high withdrawal rate found that pentoxifylline versus cilostazol significantly increased the number of people who had no change or deterioration in the claudication distance, the initial claudication distance, and the absolute claudication distance.

Benefits: We found no systematic review. **Versus placebo:** We found four RCTs comparing cilostazol versus placebo (see comment below) (see table 1, p 94).[16–19] The RCTs found that cilostazol versus placebo significantly reduced the risk of claudication being rated as unchanged, worsened, or unsure at the end of each trial (4 RCTs; 1091 people; no heterogeneity; combined RR using fixed effects model 0.71, 95% CI 0.63 to 0.81), and significantly improved the initial claudication distance (see glossary, p 92) (by 38–80 m) and the absolute claudication distance (see glossary, p 92) (by 28–84 m). **Versus pentoxifylline:** See benefits of pentoxifylline, p 88.

Harms: The most recent RCT reported that cilostazol versus placebo significantly increased the number of people who withdrew from the trial because of adverse effects or concerns about safety (39/227 [17%] with cilostazol *v* 24/239 [10%] with placebo; RR 1.71, 95% CI 1.06 to 2.75; ARI 7.1%, 95% CI 0.9% to 13.3%; NNH 14, 95% CI 8 to 111).[16] Side effects of cilostazol included headache (28% *v* 12% with placebo), diarrhoea (19% *v* 8%), abnormal stools (15% *v* 5%), palpitations (17% *v* 2%), and dizziness.[16–19] Cilostazol is a phosphodiesterase inhibitor; RCTs have found that other phosphodiesterase inhibitors (milrinone, vesnarinone) are associated with increased mortality in people with heart failure. However, results aggregated from other studies have not found an excess of cardiovascular events with cilostazol.[20]

Comment: Although the overall results of cilostazol versus placebo indicate a significant effect of cilostazol on increasing walking distance, the RCTs have some weakness of their methods, which may limit the applicability of the results.[16–19] Firstly, none of the RCTs evaluated cilostazol beyond 24 weeks. In addition, the RCTs all had moderate withdrawal rates after randomisation (up to 28.9%).[17] All four RCTs found that withdrawals were more common with cilostazol than placebo (61/227 [27%] *v* 38/239 [16%] with placebo; RR 1.69, 95% CI 1.18 to 2.43; ARI 11%, 95% CI 4% to 18%).[16–19] To allow for these problems, the authors performed an intention to treat analysis using "last available observation carried forward". However, the analysis did not include the 35 people with no observations to carry forward, and the effects of the difference in withdrawals between the groups was not explored adequately (e.g. if people with worsening claudication were more likely to withdraw, then the observed differences may be artefactual). Although cilostazol appears promising, the exact balance of its benefits and harms remains unclear.

OPTION PENTOXIFYLLINE

Systematic reviews of small RCTs of variable quality in people with intermittent claudication have found that pentoxifylline versus placebo increases the walking distance by a small amount. One subsequent RCT with a high withdrawal rate found no significant difference in walking distance between pentoxifylline versus placebo, but found that pentoxifylline versus cilostazol significantly increased the number of people who had no change or deterioration in the initial claudication distance and the absolute claudication distance.

Benefits: We found two systematic reviews,[11,21] and one subsequent RCT.[16] The first review (search date 1994, 29 RCTs of people with Fontaine's classification stage II or III intermittent claudication [see glossary, p 92] for at least 3 months) included RCTs only if they were placebo controlled and double blinded, and used pentoxifylline 600–1800 mg daily for 2–26 weeks.[21] The review found that pentoxifylline versus placebo significantly increased both the initial claudication distance (see glossary, p 92) and the absolute claudication distance (see glossary, p 92) (see table 2, p 94). The second systematic review found similar results (see table 2, p 94).[11] The subsequent RCT (438 people; see comment below) found no significant difference with pentoxifylline versus placebo in the number of people who had no change or deterioration in the claudication distance (72/212 [34%] with pentoxifylline *v* 68/226 [30%] with placebo; RR 1.13, 95% CI 0.86 to 1.48), the initial claudication distance (202 m with pentoxifylline *v* 180 m with placebo; mean difference 22 m; P for change from baseline = 0.07), or the absolute claudication distance (308 m with pentoxifylline *v* 300 m with placebo; mean difference 8 m; P for change from baseline = 0.82) after 24 weeks (see table 2, p 94).[16] **Versus cilostazol:** The subsequent RCT (see comment below) found that pentoxifylline versus cilostazol significantly increased the number of people who had no change or deterioration in the claudication distance (72/212 [34%] with pentoxifylline *v* 47/205 [23%] with cilostazol; RR 1.48, 95% CI 1.08 to 2.03; ARR 11%, 95% CI 2.4% to 20%; NNT 9, 95% CI 5 to 42), the initial claudication distance (202 m with pentoxifylline *v* 218 m with cilostazol; mean difference –16 m; P = 0.0001), and the absolute claudication distance (308 m with pentoxifylline *v* 350 m with cilostazol; mean difference –42 m; P = 0.0005) after 24 weeks.[16]

Harms: The subsequent RCT found that pentoxifylline versus placebo significantly increased the number of people who withdrew from the RCT because of adverse effects or concerns about safety (44/232 [19%] with pentoxifylline *v* 24/239 [10%] with placebo; RR 1.89, 95% CI 1.19 to 3.00; ARI 8.9%, 95% CI 2.6% to 15.3%; NNH 12, 95% CI 7 to 39).[16] Side effects of pentoxifylline included sore throat (14% *v* 7%), dyspepsia, nausea, diarrhoea (8% *v* 5% with placebo; P = 0.31), and vomiting.[16] No life threatening side effects of pentoxifylline have been reported, although RCTs have been too small to date to assess this reliably.

Comment: The systematic reviews contained many RCTs in common.[11,21] Results from the subsequent RCT,[16] have been published in numerous articles without stating clearly whether any contain additional results.[17–19] The subsequent RCT had a high withdrawal rate after randomisation, which could act as a potential source of bias (60/232 [26%] with pentoxifylline *v* 61/237 [26%] with cilostazol). In all RCTs, withdrawals were more common with pentoxifylline (60/232 [26%] *v* 38/239 [16%] with placebo; RR 1.63, 95% CI 1.13 to 2.34; ARI 10%, 95% CI 3% to 17%). To allow for these problems, the published analysis performed an intention to treat analysis using "last available observation carried forward". However, the analysis did not include the 33 people with no observations to carry forward, and the effects of the difference in withdrawals between the groups was not explored adequately (e.g. if people with worsening claudication were more likely to withdraw, then the observed differences may be artefactual). The available evidence is not good enough to define clearly the effects of pentoxifylline.

OPTION PERCUTANEOUS TRANSLUMINAL ANGIOPLASTY

Two small RCTs in people with mild to moderate intermittent claudication found limited evidence that angioplasty versus no angioplasty significantly improved walking distance after 6 months but found no significant difference after 2 or 6 years. Four RCTs in people with femoral to popliteal artery stenoses have found no significant difference with angioplasty alone versus angioplasty plus stent placement in patency rates, occlusion rates, or clinical improvement.

Benefits: **Percutaneous transluminal agioplasty (PTA) versus no PTA:** We found one systematic review (search date not stated; 2 RCTs; 78 men and 20 women with mild to moderate intermittent claudication [see glossary, p 92]) of PTA of the aortoiliac or femoral-popliteal arteries versus no angioplasty.[22] The first RCT identified by the review found that PTA versus no PTA significantly increased the median claudication distance after 6 months (667 m *v* 172 m; P < 0.05), but found no significant difference in median claudication distance or quality of life after 2 years.[23] The second RCT found that PTA versus an exercise programme significantly increased the absolute claudication distance (see glossary, p 92) at 6 months (130 m *v* 50 m; WMD 80 m), but found no significant difference in absolute claudication distance after 6 years (180 m *v* 130 m; WMD 50 m; P > 0.05).[24,25] **PTA versus PTA plus stents:** We found no systematic review, but found five RCTs.[26–30] One RCT (279 people with intermittent claudication and iliac artery stenosis) compared PTA plus routine stent placement versus PTA plus selective stent placement.[26] It found no significant difference in short or long term patency rates. The other four RCTs included people with femoral to popliteal artery stenoses and compared PTA alone versus PTA plus stent placement.[27–30] The first of these four RCTs (51 people) found no significant differences in primary patency assessed by colour flow duplex ultrasound (62% with PTA plus stent *v* 74% with PTA alone; P = 0.22) or in the occlusion rate (5/24 [21%] with PTA plus stent *v* 7% [2/27] with PTA alone; P = 0.16).[27] The second RCT (53 people) found no significant difference in primary patency after 34 months' follow up (68.4% with PTA *v* 62% with PTA plus stent placement). The third RCT (32 people) found no significant difference in "clinical improvement" after 1 year (71% with PTA *v* 60% with PTA plus stent placement; P = 0.17).[30] The fourth RCT (141 people, 154 limbs) found no significant difference in primary patency as determined by angiography after 1 year (63% with PTA *v* 63% with PTA plus stent placement).[28]

Harms: Prospective cohort studies have found that PTA complications include puncture site major bleeding (3.4%), pseudoaneurysms (0.5%), limb loss (0.2%), renal failure secondary to intravenous contrast (0.2%), cardiac complications such as myocardial infarction (0.2%), and death (0.2%).[31,32]

Comment: This limited evidence suggests transient benefit from angioplasty versus no angioplasty. The longer term effects of angioplasty or stent placement on symptoms, bypass surgery, and amputation remain unclear. Angioplasty and selective stent placement appear to be an appropriate strategy for selected iliac stenoses.[21] The long term patency of femoral-popliteal angioplasties is poor, and there is no evidence that the addition of stents confers any additional benefit.[28–30]

OPTION BYPASS SURGERY

One systematic review found that surgery versus percutaneous transluminal angioplasty significantly improved primary patency after 12–24 months, but found no significant difference after 4 years. The review found no significant difference in mortality after 12–24 months. One systematic review found that surgery versus thrombolysis significantly reduced the number of amputations and the number of people reporting ongoing ischaemic pain, but found no significant

difference in mortality after 1 year. Although the consensus view is that bypass surgery is the most effective treatment for people with debilitating symptomatic peripheral arterial disease, we found inadequate evidence from RCTs reporting long term clinical outcomes to confirm this view.

Benefits: **Surgery versus exercise:** We found no RCTs (see comment below). **Surgery versus percutaneous transluminal angioplasty (PTA):** We found one systematic review (search date not stated, 2 RCTs, 365 people with chronic progressive peripheral arterial disease), which found no significant difference with surgery versus PTA in mortality after 12–24 months (OR 1.08, 95% CI 0.61 to 1.89).[33] The review found that surgery versus PTA significantly improved primary patency after 12–24 months (OR 0.62, 95% CI 0.39 to 0.99), but found no significant difference in primary patency after 4 years (P = 0.14). The review found no significant difference in mortality or amputation rates. **Surgery versus thrombolysis:** We found one systematic review (search date not stated, 1 RCT, with acute limb ischaemia), which compared surgery versus thrombolysis using tissue plasminogen activator or urokinase.[33] The review found no significant difference in mortality after 1 year (OR 1.59, 95% CI 0.70 to 3.59). The review found that surgery versus thrombolysis significantly reduced the number of amputations (OR 0.19, 95% CI 0.06 to 0.59) and significantly reduced the number of people reporting ongoing ischaemic pain (OR 0.30, 95% CI 0.17 to 0.50) after 1 year. **Surgery versus PTA plus stent placement:** We found no RCTs of surgery versus PTA plus stent placement that reported long term outcomes.

Harms: Surgery versus PTA increased early procedural complications. Among people having aortoiliac surgery, perioperative mortality (within 30 days of the procedure) was 3.3%, and complications having a major health impact occurred in 8.3%.[34] Among people having infrainguinal bypass surgery, perioperative mortality was about 2% and serious complications occurred in 8%.[35] Among people having PTA with or without stent placement, perioperative mortality was about 1% and serious complications occurred in about 5%.[36]

Comment: The RCTs are small, have different follow up periods, and assessed different outcomes. Indirect comparisons from observational studies of proxy outcomes (primary patency rates) suggest that for aortoiliac stenosis or occlusion, greater patency rates 5 years after intervention are achieved with surgery (6250 [89%] people) compared with PTA (1300 [34–85%] people) or compared with combined PTA and stent placement (816 [54–74%] people).[30–32] Too few people with infrainguinal lesions were included in the RCTs to provide good evidence about surgical management. Indirect comparisons of proxy outcomes in people with infrainguinal lesions suggest worse results after PTA (after 5 years patency 38%, range 34–42%) compared with surgery (patency 80%).[37] Although the consensus view is that bypass surgery is the most effective treatment for people with debilitating symptomatic peripheral arterial disease, we found inadequate evidence from RCTs reporting long term clinical outcomes to confirm this view.

Peripheral arterial disease

GLOSSARY

Absolute claudication distance Also known as the total walking distance; the maximum distance a person can walk before stopping.

Acute limb ischemia An ischemic process which threatens the viability of the limb, and is associated with pain, neurologic deficit, inadequate skin capillary circulation, and/or inaudible arterial flow signals by Doppler examination. This acute process often leads to hospitalisation.

Ankle–brachial index The ratio of the systolic blood pressure in the leg over the systolic blood pressure in the arm.

Critical limb ischemia results in a breakdown of the skin (ulceration or gangrene) or pain in the foot at rest. Critical limb ischemia corresponds to the Fontaine classification III and IV.

Fontaine's classification I: asymptomatic; II: intermittent claudication (see below); II-a: pain free, claudication walking > 200 metres; II-b: pain free, claudication walking < 200 metres; III: rest/nocturnal pain; IV: necrosis/gangrene.

Initial claudication distance The distance a person can walk before the onset of claudication symptoms.

Intermittent claudication Pain, stiffness, or weakness in the leg that develops on walking, intensifies with continued walking until further walking is impossible, and is relieved by rest.

Substantive changes

Antiplatelet agents One new systematic review;[10] conclusions unchanged.

Percutaneous transluminal angioplasty Three new RCTs;[28–30] conclusions unchanged.

Bypass surgery One new systematic review;[33] conclusions unchanged.

REFERENCES

1. Fowkes FGR, Housely E, Cawood EH, et al. Edinburgh Artery Study: prevalence of asymptomatic and symptomatic peripheral arterial disease in the general population. *Int J Epidemiol* 1991;20:384–392.
2. Kannel WB, McGee DL. Update on some epidemiological features of intermittent claudication. *J Am Geriatr Soc* 1985;33:13–18.
3. Maurabito JM, D'Agostino RB, Sibersschatz, et al. Intermittent claudication: a risk profile from the Framingham Heart Study. *Circulation* 1997;96:44–49.
4. Catalano M. Epidemiology of critical limb ischemia: north Italian data. *Eur J Med* 1993;2:11–14.
5. Ebskov L, Schroeder T, Holstein P. Epidemiology of leg amputation: the influence of vascular surgery. *Br J Surg* 1994:81:1600–1603.
6. Leng GC, Lee AJ, Fowkes FG, et al. Incidence, natural history and cardiovascular events in symptomatic and asymptomatic peripheral arterial disease in the general population. *Int J Epidemiol* 1996;25:1172–1181.
7. Antiplatelet Trialists' Collaborative overview of randomized trials of antiplatelet therapy. I: prevention of death, myocardial infarction, and stroke by prolonged antiplatelet therapy in various categories of patients. *BMJ* 1994;308:81–106. Search date 1990; primary sources Medline, Current Contents, hand searches of reference lists of trials and review articles, journal abstracts and meeting proceedings, trial register of the International Committee on Thrombosis and Haemostasis, and personal contacts with colleagues and antiplatelet manufacturers.
8. Girolami B, Bernardi E, Prins MH, et al. Antithrombotic drugs in the primary medical management of intermittent claudication: a meta-analysis. *Thromb Haemost* 1999;81:715–722. Search date 1998; primary sources Medline and hand searches.
9. Antithrombotic, Trialists' Collaboration Collaborative meta-analysis of randomised trials of antiplatelet therapy for prevention of death, myocardial infarction, and stroke in high risk patients. BMJ 2002; 324:71–86. Search date: 1997 Primary sources: Medline, Embase, Derwent, Scisearch, Biosis, the Cochrane Stroke and Peripheral Vascular Disease Group Registers, handsearching of journals, abstracts, and proceedings of meetings, reference lists of trials and review articles and personal contact with colleagues, including representatives of pharmaceutical companies.
10. Robless P, Mikhailidis D, Stansby G. Systematic review of antiplatelt therapy for the prevention of myocaridla infarction, stroke, or vascular death in patients with peripheral vascular disease. *British Journal of Surgery* 2001;88:787–800.
11. Girolami B, Bernardi E, Prins M, et al. Treatment of intermittent claudication with physical training, smoking cessation, pentoxifylline, or nafronyl: a meta-analysis. *Arch Intern Med* 1999;159:337–345. Search date 1996; primary sources Medline and hand searches of reference lists.
12. Leng GC, Fowler B, Ernst E. Exercise for intermittent claudication In: The Cochrane Library, Issue 3, 2000. Oxford: Update Software. Search date not stated; primary sources Cochrane Peripheral Vascular Diseases Group trials register, Embase, reference lists of relevant articles, and personal contact with principal investigators of trials.

13. Walker RD, Nawaz S, Wilkinson CH, et al. Influence of upper- and lower-limb exercise training on cardiovascular function and walking distances in patients with intermittent claudication. *J Vasc Surg* 2000;31:662–669.
14. Gardner A, Poehlman E. Exercise rehabilitation programs for the treatment of claudication pain. *JAMA* 1995;274:975–980. Search date 1993; primary sources Medline and hand searches of bibliographies of reviews, textbooks, and studies located through the computer search.
15. Radack K, Wyderski RJ. Conservative management in intermittent claudication. *Ann Intern Med* 1990;113:135–146. Search date 1989; primary sources Index Medicus, Medline, textbooks, and experts.
16. Dawson DL, Cutler BS, Hiatt WR, et al. A comparison of cilostazol and pentoxifylline for treating intermittent claudication. *Am J Med* 2000;109:523–530.
17. Money SR, Herd A, Isaacsohn JL, et al. Effect of cilostazol on walking distances in patients with intermittent claudication cause by peripheral vascular disease. *J Vasc Surg* 1998;27:267–275.
18. Beebe HG, Dawson D, Cutler B, et al. A new pharmacological treatment for intermittent claudication. *Arch Intern Med* 1999;159:2041–2050.
19. Dawson D, Cutler B, Meeisner M, et al. Cilostazol has beneficial effects in treatment of intermittent claudication. *Circulation* 1998;98.678–686.
20. Hiatt WR. Medical treatment of peripheral arterial disease and claudication. *N Engl J Med* 2001;344:1608–1621.
21. Hood S, Moher D, Barber G. Management of intermittent claudication with pentoxifylline: a meta-analysis of randomized controlled trials. *Can Med Assoc J* 1996;155:1053–1059. Search date 1994; primary sources Medline and hand searches of references lists.
22. Fowkes FG, Gillespie IN. Angioplasty (versus non surgical management) for intermittent claudication. In: The Cochrane Library, Issue 3, 2000. Oxford: Update Software. Search date not stated; primary sources Cochrane Peripheral Vascular Diseases Group Trials Register, Embase, reference lists of relevant articles and conference proceedings, and personal contact with principal investigators of trials.
23. Whyman MR, Fowkes FGR, Kerracher EMG, et al. Randomized controlled trial of percutaneous transluminal angioplasty for intermittent claudication. *Eur J Vasc Endovasc Surg* 1996;12:167–172.
24. Creasy TS, McMillan PJ, Fletcher EWL, et al. Is percutaneous transluminal angioplasty better than exercise for claudication? Preliminary results of a prospective randomized trial. *Eur J Vasc Surg* 1990;4:135–140.
25. Perkins JMT, Collin J, Creasy TS, et al. Exercise training versus angioplasty for stable claudication. Long and medium term results of a prospective, randomized trial. *Eur J Vasc Endovasc Surg* 1996;11:409–413.
26. Teteroo E, van der Graef Y, Bosch J, et al. Randomized comparison of primary stent placement versus primary angioplasty followed by selective stent placement in patients with iliac artery occlusive disease. *Lancet* 1998;351:1153–1159.
27. Vroegindeweij D, Vos L, Tielbeek A, et al. Balloon angioplasty combined with primary stenting versus balloon angioplasty alone in femoropopliteal obstructions: a comparative randomized study. *Cardiovasc Intervent Radiol* 1997;20:420–425.
28. Cejna M, Thurnher S, Illiasch H, et al. PTA versus palmaz stent placement in femeropopliteal artery obstructions: a multicenter prospective randomised study. *Journal of Vascular and interventional radiology* 2001;12:23–31.
29. Grimm J, Muller-Hulsbeck S, Jahnke T, et al. Randomized study to compare PTA alone versus PTA with Palmaz stent placement for femoropopliteal lesions. *J Vasc Interv Radiol* 200;12:935–42.
30. Zdanowski Z, Albrechtsson U, Lundin A, et al. Percutaneous transluminal angioplasty with or without stenting for femoropopliteal occlusions? A randomized controlled study. *Int Angiol* 1999;18:251–5.
31. Becker GJ, Katzen BT, Dake MD. Noncoronary angioplasty. *Radiology* 1989;170:921–940.
32. Matsi PJ, Manninen HI. Complications of lower-limb percutaneous transluminal angioplasty: a prospective analysis of 410 procedures on 295 consecutive patients. *Cardiovasc Intervent Radiol* 1998;21:361–366.
33. Leng GC, Davis M, Baker D. Bypass surgery for chronic lower limb ischemia. Cochrane Library Issue 2, 2002. Oxford: Update Software. Search date 2001; primary sources: Cochrane peripheral vascular diseases group trials register, medline, EMBASE, reference lists of various articles and contact with trial investigators.
34. De Vries SO, Hunink MG. Results of aortic bifurcation grafts for aortoiliac occlusive disease: a meta-analysis. *J Vasc Surg* 1997;26:558–569. Search date 1996; primary sources Medline and hand searches of review articles, original studies, and a vascular surgery textbook.
35. Johnston KW, Rae M, Hogg-Johnston SA, et al. Five-year results of a prospective study of percutaneous transluminal angioplasty. *Ann Surg* 1987;206:403–413.
36. Bosch J, Hunink M. Meta-analysis of the results of percutaneous transluminal angioplasty and stent placement for aortoiliac occlusive disease. *Radiology* 1997;204:87–96. Search date not stated; primary sources Medline and hand searches of reference lists.
37. Johnson KW. Femoral and popliteal arteries: reanalysis of results of balloon angioplasty. *Radiology* 1992;183:767–771.

Sonia Anand
Assistant Professor of Medicine
McMaster University
Hamilton
Canada

Mark Creager
Associate Professor of Medicine
Harvard Medical School
Boston
USA

Competing interests: None declared.

TABLE 1 Cilostazol 200 mg daily versus placebo (see text pp 87, 88).

Ref	Duration (wks)	Number of people: Randomised	Protocol violation	Withdrawn	People self rated as worsened, unchanged, or unsure	Absolute claudication distance (m)	Initial claudication distance (m)
16	24	466	35	64	47/205 (23%) *v* 68/226 (30%); RR 0.76 (95% CI 0.55 to 1.05)	350 *v* 300 (P < 0.001)	218 *v* 180 (P = 0.02)
17	16	298	59	27	53/119 (45%) *v* 78/120 (65%); RR 0.68 (95% CI 0.54 to 0.87)	333 *v* 281	NA
18	24	516	23	75	80/171 (47%) *v* 106/169 (63%); RR 0.75 (95% CI 0.61 to 0.91)	259 *v* 175 (P < 0.001)	138 *v* 96 (P < 0.001)
19	12	81	4	15	27/54 (50%) *v* 22/27 (81%); RR 0.61 (95% CI 0.45 to 0.85)	113 *v* 85 (P = 0.007)	232 *v* 152 (P = 0.002)

m, metres; NA, not available; ref, reference.

TABLE 2 Systematic reviews and a subsequent RCT of pentoxifylline versus placebo (see text, p 88).

Ref	Number of RCTs (people)	Initial claudication distance (m)	Absolute claudication distance (m)
11	13 (600)	21 (95% CI 0.7 to 41)	44 (95% CI 14 to 74)
16	1 (471)	22 (95% CI NA)	8 (95% CI NA)
21	11 (612)	29 (95% CI 13 to 46)	48 (95% CI 18 to 79)

NA, not available; ref, reference.

Primary prevention

Search date March 2002

Clinical Evidence writers on primary prevention

QUESTIONS

INTERVENTIONS

Covered elsewhere in *Clinical Evidence*

See cardiovascular disease in diabetes, p 541

Clin Evid 2002;8:95–128.

Key Messages

Exercise

- **Physical activity** Observational studies have found that moderate to high physical activity significantly reduces coronary heart disease and stroke. They also found that sudden death soon after strenuous exercise was rare, more common in sedentary people, and did not outweigh the benefits.

Diet

- **Antioxidants (other than betacarotene)** Observational studies found insufficient evidence on the effects of vitamin C, vitamin E, copper, zinc, manganese, or flavonoids. Two RCTs found no significant difference in mortality after about 6 years with vitamin E supplements versus placebo.
- **Betacarotene** RCTs found no evidence that betacarotene supplements are effective, and have found that they may be harmful.
- **Eating more fruit and vegetables** Observational studies have found that consumption of fruit and vegetables reduces ischaemic heart disease and stroke. The size and nature of any real effect is uncertain.

Smoking

- **Smoking cessation** Observational studies have found a strong association between smoking and overall mortality and ischaemic vascular disease. Several large cohort studies have found that the increased risk associated with smoking falls after stopping smoking. The risk can take many years to approach that of non-smokers, particularly in those with a history of heavy smoking.

Antithrombotic drugs

- **Anticoagulant treatment (warfarin)** One RCT found that the benefits and harms of oral anticoagulation among individuals without symptoms of cardiovascular disease were finely balanced, and that net effects were uncertain.
- **Aspirin in low risk people** We found insufficient evidence to identify which asymptomatic individuals would benefit overall and which would be harmed by regular treatment with aspirin. Benefits are likely to outweigh risks in people at higher risk.

Interventions aimed at lowing blood pressure

- **Antihypertensive drug treatments in people with hypertension** Systematic reviews have found that initial treatment with diuretics, angiotensin converting enzyme inhibitors, or β blockers reduce morbidity and mortality, with minimal adverse effects. The biggest benefit was seen in those with the highest baseline risk. We found limited evidence from two systematic reviews that diuretics, β blockers, and angiotensin converting enzyme inhibitors reduced coronary heart disease and heart failure more than calcium channel antagonists. However, calcium channel antagonists reduced risk of stroke more than the other agents. One RCT found no significant difference in coronary heart disease outcomes with α blockers versus diuretics, but found that α blockers significantly increased cardiovascular events, particularly congestive cardiac failure at 4 years.
- **Calcium supplementation** We found no RCTs examining the effects of calcium supplementation on morbidity or mortality. We found insufficient evidence on the effects of calcium supplementation specifically in people with hypertension. One systematic review in people with and without hypertension found that calcium supplementation may reduce systolic blood pressure by small amounts.

- **Dietary salt restriction** We found no RCTs of the effects of salt restriction on morbidity or mortality. One systematic review has found that a low salt diet versus a usual diet may lead to modest reductions in blood pressure, with more benefit in people older than 45 years than in younger people (see table 1, p 125).
- **Diuretics in high risk people** Systematic reviews have found that diuretics versus placebo significantly decrease the risk of fatal and non-fatal stroke, cardiac events, and total mortality. The biggest benefit is seen in people with the highest baseline risk. Systematic reviews have found no significant difference in mortality or morbidity with diuretics versus β blockers.
- **Fish oil supplementation** We found no RCTs examining the effects of fish oil supplementation on morbidity or mortality. One systematic review has found that fish oil supplementation in large doses of 3 g daily modestly lowers blood pressure.
- **Low fat, high fruit and vegetable diet** We found no systematic review and no RCTs examining the effects of low fat, high fruit and vegetable diet on morbidity or mortality of people with raised blood pressure. One RCT found that a low fat, high fruit and vegetable diet versus control diet modestly reduced blood pressure.
- **Magnesium supplementation** We found no RCTs examining the effects of magnesium supplementation on morbidity or mortality. We found limited and conflicting evidence on the effect of magnesium supplementation on blood pressure in people with hypertension and normal magnesium concentrations.
- **Physical activity** We found no RCTs examining the effects of exercise on morbidity or mortality. One systematic review has found that aerobic exercise versus no exercise reduces blood pressure.
- **Potassium supplementation** We found no RCTs examining the effects of potassium supplementation on morbidity or mortality. One systematic review has found that a daily potassium supplementation of about 60 mmol (2 g, which is about the amount contained in 5 bananas) reduces blood pressure by small amounts.
- **Reduced alcohol consumption** We found no RCTs examining the effects of reducing alcohol consumption on morbidity or mortality. One systematic review in moderate drinkers (25–50 drinks/wk) found inconclusive evidence regarding effects of alcohol reduction on blood pressure.
- **Smoking cessation** Observational studies have found that smoking is a significant risk factor for cardiovascular disease. We found no direct evidence specifically in people with hypertension that stopping smoking decreases blood pressure.
- **Weight loss** We found no RCTs examining the effects of weight loss on morbidity and mortality. One systematic review and additional RCTs have found that modest weight reduction in obese people with hypertension may lead to modest reductions in blood pressure.

Interventions aimed at lowering cholesterol

- **Cholesterol reduction in high risk people** Systematic reviews have found that reducing cholesterol concentration in asymptomatic people lowers the rate of cardiovascular events. RCTs have found that the magnitude of the benefit is related to an individual's baseline risk of cardiovascular events, and to the degree of cholesterol lowering, rather than to the individual's cholesterol concentration.

Primary prevention

- **Low fat diet** Systematic reviews and RCTs have found that combined use of cholesterol lowering diet and lipid lowering drugs reduces cholesterol concentration more than lifestyle interventions alone.

DEFINITION Primary prevention in this context is the long term management of people at increased risk but with no evidence of cardiovascular disease. Clinically overt ischaemic vascular disease includes acute myocardial infarction, angina, stroke, and peripheral vascular disease. Many adults have no symptoms or obvious signs of vascular disease, even though they have atheroma and are at increased risk of ischaemic vascular events because of one or more risk factors (see aetiology below).

INCIDENCE/ PREVALENCE According to the World Health Report 1999, ischaemic heart disease was the leading single cause for death in the world, the leading single cause for death in high income countries and second to lower respiratory tract infections in low and middle income countries. In 1998 it was still the leading cause for death, with nearly 7.4 million estimated deaths a year in member states of the World Health Organization. This condition had the eighth highest burden of disease in the low and middle income countries (30.7 million disability adjusted life years).[1]

AETIOLOGY/ RISK FACTORS Identified major risk factors for ischaemic vascular disease include increasing age, male sex, raised low density lipoprotein cholesterol, reduced high density lipoprotein cholesterol, raised blood pressure, smoking, diabetes, family history of cardiovascular disease, obesity, and sedentary lifestyle. For many of these risk factors, observational studies show a continuous gradient of increasing risk of cardiovascular disease with increasing levels of the risk factor, with no obvious threshold level. Although by definition event rates are higher in high risk people, of all ischaemic vascular events that occur in the population, most occur in people with intermediate levels of absolute risk because there are many more of them than there are people at high risk; see Appendix 1.[2]

PROGNOSIS A study carried out in Scotland found that about half of people who suffer an acute myocardial infarction die within 28 days, and two thirds of acute myocardial infarctions occur before the person reaches hospital.[3] The benefits of intervention in unselected people with no evidence of cardiovascular disease (primary prevention) are small because in such people the baseline risk is small. However, absolute risk of ischaemic vascular events varies dramatically, even among people with similar levels of blood pressure or cholesterol. Estimates of absolute risk can be based on simple risk equations or tables; see Appendix 1.[4,5]

AIMS To reduce morbidity and mortality from cardiovascular disease, with minimum adverse effects.

OUTCOMES Incidence of fatal and non-fatal cardiovascular events (including coronary, cerebrovascular, renal, and eye disease, and heart failure). Surrogate outcomes include changes in levels of individual risk factors, such as blood pressure.

METHODS *Clinical Evidence* update search and appraisal March 2002.

QUESTION Does physical activity reduce the risk of vascular events in asymptomatic people?

Charles Foster and Michael Murphy

We found strong observational evidence that moderate to high levels of physical activity reduce the risk of non-fatal and fatal coronary heart disease and stroke. People who are physically active (those who undertake moderate levels of activity daily or almost daily, e.g. walking) typically experience 30–50% reductions in relative risk of coronary heart disease compared with people who are sedentary after adjustment for other risk factors. The absolute risk of sudden death after strenuous activity is small (although greatest in people who are habitually sedentary) and does not outweigh observed benefits.

Benefits: **Effects of physical activity on coronary heart disease:** We found no RCTs. Three systematic reviews (search dates 1995[6] and not stated[7,8]) evaluated observational studies and found increased risk of coronary heart disease (CHD) in sedentary compared with active people. Since 1992, 17 large, well conducted prospective, non-randomised studies, with follow up periods ranging from 18 months to 29 years, have specifically examined the association between physical activity and risk of non-fatal or fatal CHD.[9–25] The studies found that risk declined with increasing levels of physical activity (for examples of activity levels see table 1, p 125) (AR for CHD death in people with sedentary lives [rare or no physical activity] 70/10 000 person-years *v* 40/10 000 person-years in people with the highest level of activity [> 3500 kcal/wk]; absolute benefit of high levels of physical activity 30 lives saved/10 000 person-years). A new observational study of women found that at least 1 hour of walking a week predicted lower risk compared to no walking a week (OR 0.49, 95% CI 0.28 to 0.86).[26] **Effects of physical fitness on coronary heart disease:** We found no RCTs. One systematic review (search date not stated) identified seven large, well designed prospective, non-randomised studies of the effects of physical fitness on CHD.[27] All used reproducible measures of physical fitness. Five studies adjusted for other CHD risk factors. These found an increased risk of death from CHD in people with low levels of physical fitness compared with those with high levels (RR of death lowest quartile *v* highest quartile ranged from 1.2–4.0). Most studies reported only baseline measures of physical fitness; thus, not accounting for changes in fitness. One recent large follow up study found lower risk among people who increased their fitness level (RR for cardiovascular disease death compared with those whose level of fitness did not change 0.48, 95% CI 0.31 to 0.74).[28] One recent study showed that high fitness levels seem to slow down the development of atherosclerosis compared to those with lower levels of fitness.[29] A new meta-analysis examining fitness and activity as separate risk factors for CHD concluded that being unfit warrants consideration as a risk factor.[30] **Effects of physical activity on stroke:** We found no RCTs and no systematic review of observational studies. We found 12 observational studies (published between 1990 and 1999), based on 3680 strokes among North American, Japanese, and European populations.[31–44] Most of these found that moderate activity was associated with reduced risk of stroke compared with inactivity (RR of stroke, moderate activity *v* inactivity about 0.5). One cohort study from Japan found that "heavy" physical activity reduced the risk of stroke compared with "moderate" activity (RR of stroke, "heavy" *v* "moderate" activity about 0.3; $P < 0.05$).[42] In most studies, the benefits were greater in older people and in men. Most studies were conducted in white men in late middle age, which potentially limits their applicability to other groups of people. The results usually persisted after adjustment for other known risk factors for stroke (blood pressure, blood lipids, body mass index, and smoking) and after exclusion of people with pre-existing diseases that might limit physical activity and increase risk of stroke. The more recent studies found maximum reduction in the risk of stroke with moderate as opposed to high levels of physical exercise levels.

Harms: No direct evidence of harm was reported in the studies described. We found two studies in people who had experienced non-fatal myocardial infarction, conducted in the USA and Germany. Each involved more than 1000 events and found that 4–7% of these events occurred within 1 hour of strenuous physical activity.[45–47] Strenuous activity was estimated to have raised the relative risk of acute myocardial infarction between two- and sixfold in the hour after activity, with risks returning to baseline after that. However, the absolute risk remained low, variously estimated at six deaths per 100 000 middle aged men a year[48] or 0.3–2.7 events per 10 000 person hours of exercise.[49] Both studies found that the relative risk of acute myocardial infarction after strenuous activity was much higher in people who were habitually sedentary (RR 107, 95% CI 67 to 171) compared with the relative risk in those who engaged in heavy physical exertion on five or more occasions a week (RR 2.4, 95% CI 1.5 to 3.7).[46] Injury is likely to be the most common adverse event, but we found too few population data to measure its risk.

Comment: Findings from these observational studies should be interpreted with caution. The studies varied in definitions of levels of activity and fitness. The level of activity or fitness experienced by each person was not experimentally assigned by an investigator (as in an RCT) but resulted from self selection. Active (or fit) people are likely to differ from inactive (or unfit) people in other ways that also influence their risk of cardiovascular disease. Confounding of this type can be partially controlled by adjustment for other known risk factors (such as age, smoking status, and body mass index), but it is likely that some residual confounding will remain, which could overestimate the effect of exercise. The studies have found that the absolute risk of sudden death during or immediately after physical activity is small and does not outweigh the observed benefits.

QUESTION What intensity and frequency of physical activity improves fitness?

Charles Foster and Michael Murphy

Small RCTs found that at least moderate intensity exercise (equivalent to brisk walking) is necessary to improve fitness. We found insufficient evidence on the effects of short bouts of exercise several times daily compared with longer daily bouts.

Benefits: **Intensity:** We found no systematic review. Numerous small RCTs of varying quality have been conducted in different subpopulations. In general, these found that over a period of 6–12 months low intensity activity programmes produced no measurable changes in maximum oxygen consumption (Vo_2max), whereas moderate intensity activity programmes (equivalent to brisk walking) typically produced improvements of 20% in oxygen consumption in sedentary people. Table 1, p 125 gives the intensity of effort required for a range of physical activities. Two recent RCTs compared structured aerobic exercise (such as step classes and aerobics classes) with lifestyle activity programmes (such as regular walking and using stairs instead of lifts) among obese women[50] and sedentary men and women.[51] Both studies reported similar, significant changes in measures of cardiovascular fitness and blood pressure with each intervention, and these changes were sustained for at least 2 years after intervention. One prospective follow up study of women previously involved in a randomised trial of physical activity found that women who start a programme of regular walking maintain higher levels of physical activity 10 years after the intervention.[52]
Frequency: We found no systematic review. One RCT (36 men) compared 8 weeks of a single daily session of 30 minutes of exercise versus three daily sessions of 10 minutes each.[53] It found no significant difference in fitness benefit between groups.

Harms: None reported.

Comment: None.

QUESTION What are the effects of dietary interventions on the risk of myocardial infarction and stroke in asymptomatic people?

Andy Ness

OPTION EATING MORE FRUIT AND VEGETABLES

Cohort studies have found that eating more fruit and vegetables reduces the risk of myocardial infarction and stroke. The size and nature of any real protective effect is uncertain.

Benefits: **Ischaemic heart disease:** We found no RCTs. We found three systematic reviews of observational studies.[54–57] With addition of recently published studies[58–66] to those reported in the first review (search date 1995),[54] a protective association was observed for ischaemic heart disease in 14/25 (56%) cohort studies. In the second review (search date not stated),[55] the authors calculated a summary measure of the protective association of 15% between those above the 90th centile and those below the 10th centile for fruit and vegetable consumption. In the third review (search date 1998),[56,57] the authors estimated that increased intake of fruit and vegetables of about 150 g daily was associated with a reduced risk of coronary heart disease of 20–40%. The validity of these estimates has been questioned. One large, high quality cohort study found that eating more vegetables was associated with decreased coronary mortality (≥ 117 g vegetables/day *v* < 61 g vegetables/day: RR 0.66, 95% CI 0.46 to 0.96; for fruit, the association was more modest and not significant (≥ 159 g fruit/day *v* < 75 g fruit/day: RR 0.77, 95% CI 0.54 to 1.12).[67] **Stroke:** We found no RCTs but we found two systematic reviews examining the evidence from observational studies for stroke.[54,56,57] With addition of recently published studies[58–65,67] to those reported in the first review (search date 1995),[54] a protective association was observed in 10/16 (63%) cohort studies for stroke. In the second review (search date not stated),[56,57] the authors estimated that increased intake of fruit and vegetables of about 150 g daily was associated with a reduced risk of stroke of 0–25%. The basis for this estimate is not clear. One large, high quality cohort study in US health professionals found that increased fruit and vegetable intake was associated with a decreased risk of ischaemic stroke (RR per daily serving of fruit and vegetables 0.94, 95% CI 0.90 to 0.99; RR in the fifth of the population eating the most fruit and vegetables *v* the fifth eating the least 0.69, 95% CI 0.52 to 0.92).[68]

Harms: None were identified.

Comment: Lack of RCT evidence and deficiencies in the data available from observational studies mean that the size and nature of any real protective effect is uncertain.[69,70] The observed associations could be the result of confounding as people who eat more fruit and vegetables often come from higher socioeconomic groups and have other healthy lifestyles.[71]

OPTION ANTIOXIDANTS

We found no evidence of benefit from betacarotene supplements, and RCTs suggest that they may be harmful. Other antioxidant supplements may be beneficial, but we found insufficient RCT evidence to support their use.

Benefits: **Betacarotene:** We found one systematic review of prospective studies and RCTs (search date not stated, published in 1997), which did not pool data because of heterogeneity among studies.[72] Most prospective cohort studies of betacarotene found a modest protective association with increased intake,[72–75] although several large RCTs of betacarotene supplementation found no evidence of benefit.[75,76] **Vitamin C (ascorbic acid):** We found two systematic reviews (search dates not stated[72] and 1996[77]), which mostly included the same studies, and seven subsequent prospective studies.[62,72,78–82] Three of 14 cohort studies found a significant protective association between vitamin C and coronary heart disease, and 2/11 (18%) studies found a protective association between vitamin C and stroke. We found no large RCTs of vitamin C supplementation alone. Two large RCTs of multivitamin supplements have been carried out in Linxian, China.[72,83–85] One RCT (that was included in the reviews) was carried out in 29 584 people drawn from the general population who were randomised by using a factorial design to one of four arms: arm A — retinol (10 000 IU) and zinc (22.5 mg); arm B — riboflavin (riboflavine) (5.2 mg) and niacin (40 mg); arm C — ascorbic acid (120 mg) and molybdenum (30 μg); and arm D — betacarotene (15 mg), selenium (50 μg), and vitamin E (30 mg). After 6 years the RCT found that people allocated to arm D (betacarotene, selenium, and vitamin E) reduced all cause mortality and death because of stroke (RR for death from any cause arm D *v* other arms 0.91, 95% CI 0.84 to 0.99). It found no reduction in stroke or all cause mortality among the other arms.[72] The other RCT (subsequent to the reviews) included 3318 people with oesophageal dysplasia who were randomised to placebo or a multivitamin supplement that contained 14 vitamins and 12 minerals, including vitamin C (180 mg), vitamin E (60 IU [1 IU = 0.67 mg]), betacarotene (15 mg), and selenium (50 μg). After 6 years it found that the supplement did not significantly reduce stroke or death from all causes (RR for all cause mortality 0.93, 95% CI 0.75 to 1.16; RR for stroke 0.67, 95% CI 0.37 to 1.07).[83,84] **Vitamin E:** We found one systematic review and additional prospective studies.[71] Eight large cohort studies (5 of which were included in the review) have examined the association between vitamin E intake and ischaemic heart disease. Six found a significant protective association,[72,80,86] whereas two found no significant association.[62,87] In three studies the protective association was with dietary vitamin E.[72,84] In the others it was either wholly or mainly with vitamin E supplements.[72,87] In the review, the largest RCT of vitamin E alone versus placebo (in 29 133 Finnish smokers) found that vitamin E did not significantly reduce mortality compared with placebo (RR for death 0.98, 95% CI 0.91 to 1.05) after 5–8 years. (See vitamin C above for the results of the Linxian RCTs.)[72,83–85] Since the review was published the Primary Prevention project (4495 people at high risk of cardiovascular disease in a factorial design to vitamin E [300 mg/day] and aspirin) followed them up for 3.6 years. The trial was stopped early because of the results in the aspirin arm. There was no significant reduction in the risk of cardiovascular events or all cause mortality with vitamin E (RR for all cardiovascular events with vitamin E 0.94, 95% CI 0.77 to 1.16; RR for death from all causes 0.93, 95% CI 0.51 to 1.23).[88] Four cohort studies found no association between vitamin E intake and stroke.[79,81,82,89] In the α-tocopherol and betacarotene supplement RCT (28 519 male Finnish smokers) no significant reduction in overall stroke incidence or stroke mortality was found in those receiving vitamin E (RR of stroke incidence 0.93, 95% CI 0.83 to 1.05; RR of stroke death 1.29, 95% CI 0.94 to 1.76) after 6 years. There was a reduction in incidence from cerebral infarction, but no significant reduction in mortality due to cerebral infarction (RR for cerebral infarction 0.86, 95% CI 0.75 to 0.99; RR for death due to cerebral infarction 0.81, 95% CI 0.49 to 1.32) and an increase in mortality from subarachnoid haemorrhage (RR for subarachnoid haemorrhage 1.50, 95% CI 0.97 to 2.32; RR death 2.81, 95% CI 1.37 to 5.79) and non significant increase in mortality from haemorrhagic stroke (RR 1.64, 95% CI 0.93 to 2.90).[90] **Antioxidant minerals:** We found little epidemiological evidence about the cardioprotective effect of copper, zinc, or manganese on the heart.[91] Cohort studies reported an increased risk of ischaemic heart disease in people with low blood selenium concentrations.[92] Most of these were carried out in Finland, a country with low intakes of antioxidants.[93] (See vitamin C above for the results of the Linxian RCTs.)[72,83–85] **Flavonoids:** We found no systematic review. We found five cohort studies,[93–97] three of which reported a reduced risk of ischaemic heart disease with increased flavonoid intake.[93–95] One of four observational studies reported a reduced risk of stroke with increased flavonoid intake.[57,79,89,94]

Harms: Several large RCTs found that betacarotene supplements may increase cardiovascular mortality (pooled data from 4 RCTs, RR for cardiovascular death 1.12, 95% CI 1.04 to 1.22).[75] Explanations for these results include use of the wrong isomer, the wrong dose, or a detrimental effect on other carotenoid levels.[98,99]

Comment: RCTs of antioxidants such as betacarotene and vitamin E have not produced any evidence of benefit. Routine use of antioxidant supplements is not justified by the currently available evidence. More RCTs of antioxidant supplementation are underway.[100]

QUESTION By how much does smoking cessation, or avoiding starting smoking, reduce risk?

Julian J Nicholas

Observational studies have found that cigarette smoking is strongly related to overall mortality. We found evidence from both observational and randomised studies that cigarette smoking increases the risk of coronary heart disease and stroke. The evidence is strongest for stroke.

Benefits: Several large cohort studies examining the effects of smoking have been reviewed extensively by the US Surgeon General[101] and the UK Royal College of Physicians.[102] The reviews concluded that cigarette smoking was causally related to disease and that smoking cessation substantially reduced the risk of cancer, respiratory disease, coronary heart disease (CHD), and stroke. **Death from all causes:** The longest prospective cohort study, in 34 439 male British doctors whose smoking habits were periodically assessed over 40 years (1951–1991), found a strong association between smoking and increased mortality. It found that smokers were about three times more likely to die in middle age (45–64 years) and twice as likely to die in older age (65–84 years) compared with lifelong non-smokers (CI not provided).[103] The prospective nurses' health study followed 117 001 middle aged female nurses for 12 years. It found that the total mortality in current smokers was nearly twice that in lifelong non-smokers (RR of death 1.87, 95% CI 1.65 to 2.13).[104] **Coronary heart disease:** One review (published in 1990) identified 10 cohort studies, involving 20 million person-years of observation.[101] All studies found a higher incidence of CHD among smokers (pooled RR of death from CHD compared with non-smokers 1.7, CI not provided).[101] People smoking more than 20 cigarettes daily were more likely to have a coronary event (RR 2.5, CI not provided).[102] Middle aged smokers were more likely to experience a first non-fatal acute myocardial infarction compared with people who had never smoked (RR in men 2.9, 95% CI 2.4 to 3.4; RR in women 3.6, 95% CI 3.0 to 4.4).[105,106] One RCT of advice encouraging smoking cessation in 1445 men aged 40–59 years found that more men given advice to stop smoking gave up cigarettes (mean absolute reduction in men continuing to smoke after advice *v* control 53%). The RCT found no evidence that men given advice to stop smoking had a significantly lower mortality from CHD (RR 0.82, 95% CI 0.57 to 1.18).[107] The wide confidence intervals mean that there could have been anything from a 43% decrease to an 18% increase in rates of CHD death in men given advice to quit, regardless of whether they actually gave up smoking. **Stroke:** One systematic review (search date 1998) found 32 studies (17 cohort studies with concurrent or historical controls, 14 case control studies, and one hypertension intervention RCT).[108] It found good evidence that smoking was associated with an increased risk of stroke (RR of stroke in cigarette smokers *v* non-smokers 1.5, 95% CI 1.4 to 1.6).[108] Smoking was associated with an increased risk of cerebral infarction (RR 1.92, 95% CI 1.71 to 2.16) and subarachnoid haemorrhage (RR 2.93, 95% CI 2.48 to 3.46), and a reduced risk of intracerebral haemorrhage (RR 0.74, 95% CI 0.56 to 0.98). The relative risk of stroke in smokers versus non-smokers was highest in those aged under 55 years (RR 2.90, 95% CI 2.40 to 3.59) and lowest in those aged over 74 years (RR 1.11, 95% CI 0.96 to 1.28).

Harms: We found no evidence that stopping smoking increases mortality in any subgroup of smokers.

Comment: We found no evidence of publication or other overt bias that may explain the observed association between smoking and stroke. There was a dose related effect the number of cigarettes smoked and the relative risk for stroke, consistent with a causal relation. The absolute risk reduction from stopping smoking will be highest for those with the highest absolute risk of vascular events.

QUESTION How quickly do risks diminish when smokers stop smoking?

Julian J Nicholas

Observational studies have found that the risk of death and cardiovascular events falls when people stop smoking. The risk can take many years to approach that of non-smokers, particularly in those with a history of heavy smoking.

Benefits: **Death from all causes:** In people who stopped smoking, observational studies found that death rates fell gradually to lie between those of lifelong smokers and people who had never smoked. Estimates for the time required for former smokers to bring their risk of death in line with people who had never smoked varied among studies but may be longer than 15 years.[109] Actuarial projections from one study among British doctors predicted that life expectancy would improve even among people who stopped smoking in later life (≥ 65 years).[103] **Coronary heart disease:** Observational studies found that, in both male and female ex-smokers, the risk of coronary events rapidly declined to a level comparable with that of people who had never smoked after 2–3 years and was independent of the number of cigarettes smoked before quitting.[101] **Stroke:** The US Surgeon General's review of observational studies found that the risk of stroke decreased in ex-smokers compared with smokers (RR of stroke, smokers *v* ex-smokers 1.2, CI not provided) but remained raised for 5–10 years after cessation compared with those who had never smoked (RR of stroke ex-smokers *v* never smokers 1.5, CI not provided).[101] One recent study in 7735 middle aged British men found that 5 years after smoking cessation the risk of stroke in previously light smokers (< 20 cigarettes/day) was identical to that of lifelong non-smokers, but the risk in previously heavy smokers (> 21 cigarettes/day) was still raised compared with lifelong non-smokers (RR of stroke, previously heavy smokers *v* never smokers 2.2, 95% CI 1.1 to 4.3).[110] One observational study in 117 001 middle aged female nurses also found a fall in risk on stopping smoking and found no difference between previously light and previously heavy smokers (RR in all former smokers 2–4 years after stopping smoking 1.17, 95% CI 0.49 to 2.23).[104]

Harms: We found no evidence that stopping smoking increases mortality in any subgroup of smokers.

Comment: For a review of the evidence on methods of changing smoking behaviour, see secondary prevention of ischaemic cardiac events, p 129.

QUESTION **What are the effects of lifestyle changes in asymptomatic people with primary hypertension?**

Cindy Mulrow and Mike Pignone

OPTION **PHYSICAL ACTIVITY**

One systematic review has found that aerobic exercise reduces blood pressure.

Benefits: We found no RCTs examining the effects of exercise on morbidity, mortality, or quality of life. One systematic review (search date 2001, 54 RCTs, 2419 sedentary adults aged > 18 years) examined the effects on blood pressure of at least 2 weeks of regular exercise versus no exercise.[111] Compared with non-exercising control groups, groups randomised to aerobic exercise reduced their systolic blood pressure by 3.8 mm Hg (95% CI 2.7 mm Hg to 5.0 mm Hg) and diastolic blood pressure by 2.6 mm Hg (95% CI 1.8 mm Hg to 3.4 mm Hg). Reductions in blood pressure were seen in hypertensive and non-hypertensive people, and in overweight and normal weight people. RCTs with interventions lasting longer than 6 months in adults aged 45 years or over with hypertension found non-significant mean reductions in blood pressure, with wide confidence intervals (systolic reduction 0.8 mm Hg, 95% CI 5.9 mm Hg reduction to 4.2 mm Hg increase).[112]

Harms: Musculoskeletal injuries can occur, but their frequency was not documented.

Comment: Many adults find aerobic exercise programmes difficult to sustain. The clinical significance of the observed reductions in blood pressure is uncertain. The type and amount of exercise most likely to result in benefits are unclear, with some recent studies showing some benefits with simple increases in lifestyle activity. One cohort study (173 men with hypertension) found that "regular heavy activity several times weekly" compared with no or limited spare time physical activity reduced all cause and cardiovascular mortality (all cause mortality RR 0.43, 95% CI 0.22 to 0.82; cardiovascular mortality RR 0.33, 95% CI 0.11 to 0.94).[113]

OPTION LOW FAT, HIGH FRUIT AND VEGETABLE DIET

We found no systematic review and no RCTs examining the effects of low fat, high fruit and vegetable diet on morbidity or mortality in people with primary hypertension. One RCT found that a low fat, high fruit and vegetable diet modestly reduced blood pressure.

Benefits: We found no systematic review and no RCTs examining the effects of low fat, high fruit and vegetable diet on morbidity or mortality in people with primary hypertension. For evidence from cohort studies in asymptomatic people in general see question on effects of dietary interventions, p 101. One RCT (459 adults with systolic blood pressures of < 160 mm Hg and diastolic blood pressures of 80–90 mm Hg) compared effects on blood pressure of three diets (control diet low in both magnesium and potassium *v* fruit and vegetable diet high in both potassium and magnesium *v* combination of the fruit and vegetable diet with a low fat diet high in both calcium and protein).[114] After 8 weeks the fruit and vegetable diet reduced systolic and diastolic blood pressure compared with the control diet (mean change in systolic blood pressure −2.8 mm Hg, 97.5% CI −4.7 mm Hg to −0.9 mm Hg; mean change in diastolic blood pressure −1.1 mm Hg, 97.5% CI −2.4 mm Hg to +0.3 mm Hg). The combination diet also reduced systolic and diastolic blood pressure compared with the control diet (mean change in systolic blood pressure −5.5 mm Hg, 97.5% CI −7.4 mm Hg to −3.7 mm Hg; mean change in diastolic blood pressure −3.0 mm Hg, 97.5% CI −4.3 to −1.6 mm Hg).

Harms: We found no direct evidence that a low fat, high fruit and vegetable diet is harmful.

Comment: The RCT was of short duration and people were supplied with food during the intervention period.[114] Other studies have found that long term maintenance of particular diets is difficult for many people, although low fat, high fruit and vegetable diets may have multiple benefits (see changing behaviour, p 37).

OPTION REDUCED ALCOHOL CONSUMPTION

One systematic review found inconclusive evidence regarding effects of alcohol reduction on blood pressure.

Benefits: We found no RCTs examining the effects of reducing alcohol consumption on morbidity or mortality. Over 60 population studies have reported associations between alcohol consumption and blood pressure; the relation was found to be generally linear, although several studies reported a threshold effect at about two to three standard drinks daily.[115] Any adverse effect of up to two drinks daily on blood pressure was found to be either small or non-existent. One systematic review (search date 1999, 7 RCTs, 751 people with hypertension; mainly men) found that data were inconclusive on the benefits of reducing alcohol among moderate to heavy drinkers (25–50 drinks/wk).[116]

Harms: We found no direct evidence that reducing alcohol intake to as few as two drinks daily was harmful.

Comment: Most data were from observational studies. RCTs were small and lacked reliable information about adherence. Substantial reductions in alcohol use in both control and intervention groups were observed, with limited ability to detect differences between groups.

OPTION SALT RESTRICTION

One systematic review has found that salt restriction may lead to modest reductions in blood pressure, with more benefit in people older than 45 years than in younger people.

Benefits: We found no RCT examining the effects of salt restriction on morbidity or mortality. We found one systematic review (search date 1997, 58 RCTs, 2161 people with hypertension, age 23–73 years)[117] and two subsequent RCTs,[118,119] which examined the effects of salt restriction on blood pressure. Interventions were low salt diets with or without weight reduction. People in the control groups took their usual diet. Changes in salt intake varied among RCTs in the systematic review; a mean reduction in sodium intake of 118 mmol (6.7 g) daily for 28 days led to reductions of 3.9 mm Hg (95% CI 3.0 mm Hg to 4.8 mm Hg) in systolic blood pressure and 1.9 mm Hg (95% CI 1.3 mm Hg to 2.5 mm Hg) in diastolic blood pressure.[117] One RCT (875 people with hypertension, age 60–80 years, duration 30 months) found that a mean decrease in salt intake of about 40 mmol (2.4 g) daily reduced systolic blood pressure by 2.6 mm Hg (95% CI 0.4 mm Hg to 4.8 mm Hg) and diastolic blood pressure by 1.1 mm Hg (95% CI 0.3 mm Hg rise in diastolic to 2.5 mm Hg fall).[118] Another RCT (412 people with systolic/diastolic blood pressure > 120/80 mm Hg, mean age 48 years, duration 30 days) that tested three different target levels of sodium intake (150, 100, and 50 mmol/day) found significantly lower systolic blood pressure levels with lower sodium intakes.[119] An earlier systematic review (search date 1994) identified 28 RCTs in 1131 people with hypertension. It found that lesser reductions of 60 mmol/day led to smaller reductions in systolic/diastolic blood pressure of 2.2/0.5 mm Hg and found greater effects in RCTs in which mean age was over 45 years (6.3/2.2 mm Hg).[120]

Harms: We found no direct evidence that low salt diets may increase morbidity or mortality.

Comment: Small RCTs tended to report larger reductions in systolic and diastolic blood pressure than larger RCTs. This may be explained by publication bias or less rigorous methodology in small RCTs.[120]

OPTION **SMOKING CESSATION**

Epidemiological data clearly identify that smoking is a significant risk factor for cardiovascular disease. We found no direct evidence that stopping smoking decreases blood pressure in people with hypertension.

Benefits: We found no direct evidence that stopping smoking reduces blood pressure in people with hypertension, although we found good evidence that, in general, smoking cessation reduces risk of cardiovascular disease (see question on how much does smoking cessation, or avoiding starting smoking, reduce risk, p 104).

Harms: We found insufficient evidence in this context.

Comment: None.

OPTION **WEIGHT LOSS**

One systematic review and additional RCTs have found that modest weight reductions of 3–9% of body weight are achievable in motivated middle aged and older adults, and may lead to modest reductions in blood pressure in obese people with hypertension. Many adults find it difficult to maintain weight loss.

Benefits: We found no RCTs examining the effects of weight loss on morbidity and mortality. We found one systematic review (search date 1998, 18 RCTs, 2611 middle aged people, mean age 50 years, mean weight 85 kg, mean systolic/diastolic blood pressure 152/98 mm Hg, 55% men)[121] and two subsequent RCTs[122,123] that examined the effects of weight loss on blood pressure. In the systematic review, caloric intakes ranged from 450–1500 kcal daily; most diets led to weight reductions of 3–9% of body weight. Combined data from the six RCTs that did not vary antihypertensive regimens during the intervention period found that reducing weight reduced systolic and diastolic blood pressures (mean reduction in systolic pressure, weight loss *v* no weight loss 3.0 mm Hg, 95% CI 0.7 mm Hg to 6.8 mm Hg; mean reduction in diastolic blood pressure, weight loss *v* no weight loss 2.9 mm Hg, 95% CI 0.1 mm Hg to 5.7 mm Hg). RCTs that allowed adjustment of antihypertensive regimens found that lower doses and fewer antihypertensive drugs were needed in the weight reduction groups compared with control groups. The two subsequent RCTs found that sustained weight reduction of 2–4 kg significantly reduced systolic blood pressure at 1–3 years by about 1 mm Hg.[122,123]

Harms: We found no direct evidence that intentional gradual weight loss of less than 10% of body weight is harmful in obese adults with hypertension.

Comment: None.

OPTION POTASSIUM SUPPLEMENTATION

One systematic review has found that a daily potassium supplementation of about 60 mmol (2 g, which is about the amount contained in 5 bananas) is feasible for many adults and reduces blood pressure by small amounts.

Benefits: We found no RCTs examining the effects of potassium supplementation on morbidity or mortality. One systematic review (search date 1995, 21 RCTs, 1560 adults with hypertension, age 19–79 years) compared the effects on blood pressure of potassium supplements (60–100 mmol potassium chloride daily) versus placebo or no supplement.[124] It found that, compared with the control interventions, potassium supplements reduced systolic and diastolic blood pressures (mean decrease in systolic blood pressure with potassium supplements 4.4 mm Hg, 95% CI 2.2 mm Hg to 6.6 mm Hg; mean decrease in diastolic blood pressure 2.5 mm Hg, 95% CI 0.1 mm Hg to 4.9 mm Hg).

Harms: We found no direct evidence of harm in people without kidney failure and in people not taking drugs that increase serum potassium concentration. Gastrointestinal adverse effects such as belching, flatulence, diarrhoea, or abdominal discomfort occurred in 2–10% of people.[124]

Comment: None.

OPTION FISH OIL SUPPLEMENTATION

One systematic review has found that fish oil supplementation in large doses of 3 g daily modestly lowers blood pressure.

Benefits: We found no RCTs examining the effects of fish oil supplementation on morbidity or mortality. One systematic review (search date not stated, 7 brief RCTs, 339 people with hypertension, mainly middle aged white men, mean age 50 years) compared effects on blood pressure of fish oil (usually 3 g daily as capsules) versus no supplements or "placebo".[125] The contents of placebo capsules varied among RCTs. Some used oil mixtures containing omega-3 polyunsaturated fatty acids, some without. The review found that fish oil supplements reduced blood pressure compared with control interventions (mean decrease in systolic blood pressure in treatment *v* control 4.5 mm Hg, 95% CI 1.2 mm Hg to 7.8 mm Hg, and mean decrease in diastolic blood pressure in treatment *v* control 2.5 mm Hg, 95% CI 0.6 mm Hg to 4.4 mm Hg).

Harms: Belching, bad breath, fishy taste, and abdominal pain occurred in about a third of people taking high doses of fish oil.[125]

Comment: The RCTs were of short duration and used high doses of fish oil. Such high intake may be difficult to maintain. We found no evidence of beneficial effect on blood pressure at lower intakes.

OPTION CALCIUM SUPPLEMENTATION

We found insufficient evidence on the effects of calcium supplementation specifically in people with hypertension. One systematic review in people both with and without hypertension found that calcium supplementation may reduce systolic blood pressure by small amounts.

Benefits: We found no RCTs examining the effects of calcium supplementation on morbidity or mortality. One systematic review (search date 1994, 42 RCTs, 4560 middle aged people) compared the effects on blood pressure of calcium supplementation (500–2000 mg/day) versus placebo or no supplements.[126] It found that calcium supplements reduced blood pressure by a small amount (mean systolic blood pressure reduction, supplement *v* control 1.4 mm Hg, 95% CI 0.7 mm Hg to 2.2 mm Hg; mean diastolic reduction 0.8 mm Hg, 95% CI 0.2 mm Hg to 1.4 mm Hg).

Harms: Adverse gastrointestinal effects, such as abdominal pain, were generally mild and varied among particular preparations.

Comment: Data relating specifically to people with hypertension are limited by few studies with small sample sizes and short durations.

OPTION MAGNESIUM SUPPLEMENTATION

We found no RCTs examining the effects of magnesium supplementation on morbidity or mortality. We found limited and conflicting evidence on the effect of magnesium supplementation on blood pressure in people with hypertension and normal magnesium concentrations.

Benefits: We found no RCTs examining the effects of magnesium supplementation on morbidity or mortality. A few small, short term RCTs found mixed results on effects on blood pressure reduction.

Harms: We found insufficient evidence.

Comment: None.

QUESTION What are the effects of drug treatment in primary hypertension?

Cindy Mulrow and Mike Pignone

OPTION ANTIHYPERTENSIVE DRUGS VERSUS PLACEBO

Many systematic reviews have found that drug treatment decreases the risk of fatal and non-fatal stroke, cardiac events, and total mortality in specific populations of people. The biggest benefit is seen in people with highest baseline risk of cardiovascular disease.

Benefits: We found many systematic reviews. One review (search date 1997, 17 RCTs with morbidity and mortality outcomes, duration > 1 year, 37 000 people) found that antihypertensive drugs versus placebo produced variable reductions of systolic/diastolic blood pressure that averaged about 12–16/5–10 mm Hg.[127] It found evidence of benefit in total death rate, cardiovascular death rate, stroke, major coronary events, and congestive cardiac failure, but the absolute results depended on age and the severity of the hypertension (see target diastolic blood pressure below). The biggest benefit was seen in those with the highest baseline risk. The RCTs mainly compared placebo versus diuretics (usually thiazides with the addition of amiloride or triamterene) and versus β blockers (usually atenolol or metoprolol) in a stepped care approach. One systematic review (search date 1999, 8 RCTs, 15 693 people) found that, in people aged over 60 years with systolic hypertension, treatment of systolic pressures greater than 160 mm Hg decreased total mortality and fatal and non-fatal cardiovascular events.[128] Absolute benefits were greater in men than women, in people aged over 70 years, and in those with prior cardiovascular events or wider pulse pressure. The relative hazard rates associated with a 10 mm Hg higher initial systolic blood pressure were 1.26 (P = 0.0001) for total mortality, 1.22 (P = 0.02) for stroke, but only 1.07 (P = 0.37) for coronary events. Active treatment reduced total mortality (RR 0.87, 95% CI 0.78 to 0.98; P = 0.02).[128] **Target diastolic blood pressure:** We found one RCT (18 790 people, mean age 62 years, diastolic blood pressures 100–115 mm Hg), which aimed to evaluate the effects on cardiovascular risk of target diastolic blood pressures of 90, 85, and 80 mm Hg.[129] However, mean achieved diastolic blood pressures were 85, 83, and 81 mm Hg, which limited power to detect differences among groups. There were no significant differences in major cardiovascular events among the three groups.

Harms: **Mortality and major morbidity:** One systematic review (search date 1997) comparing diuretics and β blockers versus placebo found no increase in non-cardiovascular mortality in treated people.[127] **Quality of life and tolerability:** One systematic review (search date 1990)[130] and several recent RCTs found that quality of life was not adversely affected and may be improved in those who remain on treatment.[131]

Comment: RCTs included people who were healthier than the general population, with lower rates of cardiovascular risk factors, cardiovascular disease, and comorbidity. People with higher cardiovascular risk can expect greater short term absolute risk reduction than seen in the RCTs, whereas people with major competing risks such as terminal cancer or end stage Alzheimer's disease can expect smaller risk reduction. In the systematic review,[127] five of the RCTs were in middle aged people with mild to moderate hypertension. Seven of the RCTs were in people older than 60 years. On average, every 1000 person-years of treatment in older adults prevented five strokes (95% CI 2 to 8), three coronary events (95% CI 1 to 4), and four cardiovascular deaths (95% CI 1 to 8). Drug treatment in middle aged people prevented one stroke (95% CI 0 to 2) for every 1000 person-years of treatment and did not significantly affect coronary events or mortality. One meta-analysis (7 RCTs, 40 233 people with hypertension) found an increased risk of total and cardiovascular mortality with diastolic blood pressure levels below 85 mm Hg that was not related to antihypertensive treatment.[132]

OPTION COMPARING ANTIHYPERTENSIVE DRUG TREATMENTS

Systematic reviews have found that initial treatment with diuretics, angiotensin converting enzyme inhibitors, or β blockers reduce morbidity and mortality, with minimal adverse effects. RCTs found no significant morbidity or mortality differences among these agents. We found limited evidence from two systematic reviews that diuretics, β blockers, and angiotensin converting enzyme inhibitors reduced coronary heart disease and heart failure more than calcium channel antagonists. However, calcium channel antagonists reduced risk of stroke more than the other agents. One RCT found that a thiazide diuretic is superior to an α blocker in reducing cardiovascular events, particularly congestive heart failure.

Benefits: **β Blockers versus diuretics:** One systematic review (search date 1995, > 48 000 people) identified RCTs comparing effects of high and low dose diuretics versus β blockers.[133] A second systematic review (search date 1998) was limited to 10 RCTs in 16 164 elderly people.[134] These reviews did not summarise direct comparisons of diuretics versus β blockers but compared results of RCTs that used diuretics as preferred treatment versus results of RCTs that used β blockers as preferred treatment. The reviews found no significant difference between diuretics and β blockers for lowering blood pressure. They found that diuretics reduced coronary events, but found no evidence that β blockers reduced coronary events. **Comparison of β blockers, diuretics, angiotensin converting enzyme inhibitors, and calcium channel antagonists:** One systematic review (search date 2000, 8 RCTs) compared different antihypertensive regimens, and found no significant differences in outcome among people initially treated with β blockers, diuretics, or angiotensin converting enzyme (ACE) inhibitors.[135] However, it found that β blockers or diuretics decreased coronary events compared with calcium channel antagonists and increased stroke rate, although there was no significant difference for all cause mortality (OR for mortality, β blockers or diuretics *v* calcium channel antagonists 1.01, 95% CI 0.92 to 1.11). ACE inhibitors did not significantly alter all cause mortality or stroke rate compared with calcium channel antagonists, but decreased coronary events (OR for ACE inhibitors *v* calcium channel antagonist 1.03, 95% CI 0.91 to 1.18 for all cause mortality; 1.02, 95% CI 0.85 to 1.21 for stroke; 0.81, 95% CI 0.68 to 0.97 for coronary events).[135] A second review of similar trials (search date 2001, 9 RCTs, 62 605 hypertensive people) found that diuretics, β blockers, ACE inhibitors, and calcium channel antagonists were all associated with similar reductions in cardiovascular risk.[136] However, calcium channel antagonists reduced risk of stroke and increased risk of myocardial infarction compared with other agents (RR for stroke 0.87, 95% CI 0.76 to 0.99; RR for myocardial infarction 1.19, 1.04 to 1.37).[136] **Comparison of α blockers and diuretics:** A double blind RCT (24 335 high risk people with hypertension), which was included in the systematic review[136], found no significant differences in coronary heart disease outcomes between doxazosin, an α blocker, compared with chlortalidone (chlorthalidone). However, doxazosin versus chlortalidone increased the total number of cardiovascular events after 4 years (25% with doxazosin *v* 22% with chlortalidone; HR 1.25, 95% CI 1.17 to 1.33) and, in particular, increased congestive heart failure (8% with doxazosin *v* 4% with chlortalidone; HR 2.04, 95% CI 1.79 to 2.32).[137] **Drug treatment in people with diabetes:** See cardiovascular disease in diabetes, p 541.

Harms: **Quality of life and tolerability:** In the three long term, double blind comparisons of low dose diuretics, β blockers, ACE inhibitors, and calcium channel blockers, tolerability and overall quality of life indicators tended to be more favourable for diuretics and β blockers than for newer drugs.[138–140] One systematic review (search date 1998) of RCTs comparing thiazides versus β blockers found that thiazides were associated with fewer withdrawals because of adverse effects (RR 0.69, 95% CI 0.63 to 0.76).[141] Adverse effects are agent specific. The recent unblinded RCT comparing diuretics, β blockers, calcium channel antagonists, and ACE inhibitors found that after 5 years' follow up, 26% of people receiving felodipine or isradipine (calcium channel antagonists) reported ankle oedema, 30% receiving enalapril or lisinopril (ACE inhibitors) reported cough, and 9% receiving diuretics, β blockers, or both reported cold hands and feet.[142] **Major harm controversies:** Case control, cohort, and randomised studies suggest that short and intermediate acting dihydropyridine calcium channel blockers, such as nifedipine and isradipine, may increase cardiovascular morbidity and mortality.[143]

Comment: None.

QUESTION What are the effects of lowering cholesterol concentration in asymptomatic people?

Michael Pignone

Systematic reviews have found that in people with an annual risk of coronary heart disease events 0.6–1.5% a year, cholesterol reduction reduces non-fatal myocardial infarction (see cholesterol reduction under secondary prevention of ischaemic cardiac events for additional information, p 129). RCTs have found that absolute benefit is related to an individual's baseline risk of cardiovascular events and to the degree of cholesterol lowering rather than to the individual's cholesterol concentration.

Benefits: **Cholesterol lowering drug treatment:** We found two systematic reviews of any type of cholesterol lowering drug treatment versus placebo or no treatment in people without a diagnosis of coronary heart disease (CHD).[144,145] Both systematic reviews found similar results. The most recent systematic review (search date 1999) found four RCTs (2 with statins, 1 with fibrates, and 1 with cholestyramine, 21 087 people).[144] It found that cholesterol reduction treatment versus placebo significantly reduced CHD events and CHD mortality, but found no significant effect on overall mortality (OR for treatment *v* placebo; 0.70, 95% CI 0.62 to 0.79 for CHD events; 0.71, 95% CI 0.56 to 0.91 for CHD mortality; 0.94, 95% CI 0.81 to 1.09 for overall mortality). **Statins:** We found five systematic reviews (search dates 1995,[146] 1997,[147] 1998,[148] 1999,[144] and not stated[145]) and two subsequent RCTs[149,150] that considered the effect of 3-hydroxy-3-methylglutaryl coenzyme A reductase inhibitors (statins) versus placebo on clinical outcomes in people given long term (≥6 months) treatment. All the systematic reviews included the same two RCTs of statins in primary prevention (13 200 people).[151,152] All the systematic reviews found similar results. After 4–6 years of treatment for primary prevention, statins compared with placebo did not significantly reduce all cause mortality or CHD mortality, but did reduce major coronary events and cardiovascular mortality (all cause mortality: OR 0.87, 95% CI 0.71 to 1.06; CHD mortality OR 0.73, 95% CI 0.51 to 1.05; major coronary events: OR 0.66, 95% CI 0.57 to 0.76; cardiovascular mortality: OR 0.68, 95% CI 0.50 to 0.93).[148] The absolute risk reduction for CHD events, CHD mortality, and total mortality varied with the baseline risk (see figure 1, p 128). The first subsequent RCT (15 454 men and 5082 women) included 7150 people with no diagnosis of CHD but at high risk (1820 had cerebrovascular disease, 2701 had peripheral arterial disease, and 3982 had diabetes).[149] In people with no diagnosis of CHD, simvastatin versus placebo reduced the risk of a major vascular event (major coronary event, stroke, or revascularisation) after 5 years (risk of major vascular event: event rate ratio 0.75, 95% CI 0.67 to 0.84). The second subsequent RCT (246 men with hyperlipidaemia) compared three treatments: diet alone; diet with pravastatin, and diet and probucol. It found that pravastatin reduced cardiovascular events compared with diet alone after 2 years (AR for any cardiovascular event 4.8% with pravastatin *v* 13.6% with diet alone, P value and CI not provided).[150] **Low fat diet:** See changing behaviour, p 037.

Harms: Specific harms of statins are discussed under secondary prevention of ischaemic cardiac events, p 129.

Comment: The CHD event rate in the placebo group of the two large primary prevention RCTs using statins was 0.6%[151] and 1.5%[152] a year. If the 17% relative reduction in total mortality observed in the higher risk west of Scotland RCT is real, then about 110 high risk people without known CHD would need to be treated for 5 years to save one life. One regression analysis of all the major statin trials found that mortality benefits of statins outweigh risks in people with a 10 year CHD risk of more than 13%.[156] **Cholesterol lowering treatment in older people:** We found no RCTs specifically evaluating the effect of cholesterol lowering treatment in asymptomatic people aged over 75 years. One large RCT comparing statin with placebo included more than 5000 people over the age of 70 years. It found major vascular events were reduced to a similar extent in people above and below the age of 70 years.[149] **Cholesterol lowering treatment in women:** Subgroup analyses of two RCTs have found conflicting results. One RCT (5608 men, 997 women) compared statins with placebo for primary prevention in women.[151] It found that lovastatin reduced the risk of CHD events in women but this was not statistically significant (RR 0.54, 95% CI 0.22, 1.35). In the second RCT, the reduction in major event rate was similar in men and women (quantitative results not reported).[149] Other treatments are discussed under changing behaviour, p 37, or were performed in people with known CHD (see secondary prevention of ischaemic cardiac events, p 129). We found one systematic review (search date 1996, 59 RCTs, 173 160 people receiving drug treatments, dietary intervention, or ileal bypass), which did not differentiate primary and secondary prevention and included RCTs of any cholesterol lowering intervention, irrespective of duration, as long as mortality data were reported.[157] Overall, baseline risk was similar in people allocated to all interventions. Among non-surgical treatments, the review found that only statins reduced CHD mortality (RR *v* control: 0.69, 95% CI 0.59 to 0.80 for statins; 0.44, 95% CI 0.18 to 1.07 for n–3 fatty acids; 0.98, 95% CI 0.78 to 1.24 for fibrates; 0.71, 95% CI 0.51 to 0.99 for resins; 1.04, 95% CI 0.93 to 1.17 for hormones; 0.95, 95% CI 0.83 to 1.10 for niacin; 0.91, 95% CI 0.82 to 1.01 for diet), and that only statins and n–3 fatty acids reduced all cause mortality (RR *v* control: 0.79, 95% CI 0.71 to 0.89 for statins; 0.68, 95% CI 0.53 to 0.88 for n–3 fatty acids; 1.06, 95% CI 0.78 to 1.46 for fibrates; 0.85, 95% CI 0.66 to 1.08 for resins; 1.09, 95% CI 1.00 to 1.20 for hormones; 0.96, 95% CI 0.86 to 1.08 for niacin; 0.97, 95% CI 0.81 to 1.15 for diet).[157]

QUESTION What is the role of antithrombotic treatment in asymptomatic people?

Cathie Sudlow

OPTION ASPIRIN

We found the role of antiplatelet treatment in individuals without symptoms of cardiovascular disease to be uncertain. We found insufficient evidence from RCTs to identify which individuals would benefit overall and which would be harmed by regular treatment with aspirin, although those at high and intermediate rather than low risk, would be more likely to gain benefit (see table 2, p 126 and table 3, p 127).

Benefits: We found four recent systematic reviews[158–161], which between them included five large RCTs of aspirin versus control among individuals with no prior history of vascular disease, with or without vascular risk factors.[88,129,162–164] The earliest two trials recruited a total of about 30 000 healthy, mainly middle aged, male doctors (5139 in the UK, randomised between aspirin 500 mg/day and control, and 22 071 in the USA, randomised between aspirin 325 mg every other day and placebo).[162,163] Three subsequent RCTs included asymptomatic people with identifiable risk factors for vascular events. All three had a factorial design. The first compared aspirin 75 mg daily versus placebo and low intensity warfarin versus placebo in 5000 middle aged men with coronary heart disease risk score in the top 20–25% of the population distribution.[165] The second compared aspirin 75 mg daily versus placebo in three groups with different intensities of blood pressure reduction in a total of about 19 000 people with hypertension, most of whom had no history of vascular disease.[129] The third compared aspirin 100 mg daily versus placebo and vitamin E versus placebo in about 4500 people aged more than 50 years, with at least one major cardiovascular risk factor (hypertension, hypercholesterolaemia, diabetes, obesity, family history of premature myocardial infarction, or age ≥65 years).[92] The average control group risk of a serious vascular event (myocardial infarction, stroke, or death from a vascular cause) in each of these trials was low (about 1% a year). Data from these five RCTs were pooled in our own meta-analysis (which is updated for each issue of *Clinical Evidence*, and currently includes about 55 000 people low risk individuals). Results are summarised in table 2, p 126 and table 3, p 127. We found that, overall, aspirin slightly reduced the risk of a serious vascular event (OR 0.86, 95% CI 0.80 to 0.90; ARR 1/1000 people/year), reduced the relative risk of myocardial infarction by about a third (OR 0.71, 95% CI 0.60 to 0.80), but had an uncertain effect on stroke (OR 1.05, 95% CI 0.90 to 1.20). The systematic reviews found similar results.[158–161]. One of these systematic reviews[158] also included an RCT in about 3000 people with diabetes[164] who were at substantially higher average risk of vascular events (about 4% a year) than the low risk individuals in the primary prevention RCTs included in our meta-analysis.

Harms: Serious, potentially life threatening bleeding is the most important adverse effect of aspirin. **Intracranial haemorrhage:** These are uncommon, but they are often fatal and usually cause substantial disability in survivors. We found one relevant systematic review (search date 1997) in which people were randomised to aspirin or control treatment for at least 1 month. It found that aspirin produced a small increased risk of intracranial haemorrhage of about 1/1000 (0.1%) people treated for 3 years.[167] Our meta-analysis of the primary prevention RCTs found a somewhat smaller absolute overall excess of about 0.1/1000 (0.01%) people treated with aspirin per year (see table 3, p 127). **Extracranial haemorrhage:** Major extracranial bleeds occur mainly in the gastrointestinal tract and may require hospital admission or blood transfusion, but do not generally result in permanent disability and are rarely fatal. We found one relevant systematic review of aspirin versus control with a scheduled treatment duration of at least 1 year. It found the relative excess risk of gastrointestinal bleeding with aspirin to be about 70% (OR 1.7, 95% CI 1.5 to 1.9).[168] A recent overview of 15 observational studies, including over 10 000 cases of upper gastrointestinal bleeding or perforation requiring hospitalisation, found the relative risk with aspirin to be 2.5 (95% CI 2.4 to 2.7). If only those studies that had a prospective (and so methodologically more rigorous) design were considered, the relative risk fell to 1.9 (95% CI 1.7 to 2.1), similar to that found in the RCTs.[169] Meta-analysis of primary prevention RCTs found a similar relative excess risk of major extracranial (mainly gastrointestinal) haemorrhage and an absolute excess of about 0.7 major extracranial haemorrhages per 1000 people treated with aspirin a year (see table 3, p 127).

Comment: Since the average risk of a serious vascular event in the primary prevention RCTs (about 1% a year in the control group) was low, the absolute benefit of aspirin was small and was of similar magnitude to the risks of major haemorrhage. Although there was a small reduction in serious vascular events overall, it therefore seems likely that some asymptomatic individuals would gain net benefit whereas others would experience net harm with regular aspirin treatment. The size and direction of the effects of aspirin in particular individuals may well depend on specific factors, such as age, blood pressure, and smoking status. People without symptoms at intermediate rather than low risk of vascular disease may benefit overall, but we found insufficient evidence to be certain.[160,161] However, one large overview of randomised trials of antiplatelet treatment among people at high risk of vascular events (> 3% a year), including people with diabetes, found clear evidence of net benefit (see stroke prevention, p 184, secondary prevention of ischaemic cardiac events, p 129, and cardiovascular disease in diabetes, p 541).[170] Further information will soon be available from a detailed overview of individual participant data from the completed primary prevention RCTs (Baigent C, personal communication, 2001); from the Women's Health Study, comparing aspirin 100 mg daily versus placebo among 40 000 healthy postmenopausal women;[171] and from the Aspirin in Asymptomatic Atherosclerosis RCT, comparing low dose aspirin versus placebo in 3300 middle aged people with asymptomatic atherosclerosis, identified by an ankle brachial pressure index ≥ 0.9 (Fowkes G, personal communication, 2000).

OPTION ANTICOAGULANT TREATMENT

We found evidence from one RCT that the benefits and risks of low intensity oral anticoagulation among individuals without evidence of cardiovascular disease are finely balanced, and the net effects are uncertain.

Benefits: We found no systematic review. We found one RCT assessing anticoagulation (with a low target international normalised ratio of 1.5) among people without evidence of cardiovascular disease.[165] It found that the proportional effects of warfarin were similar among people allocated aspirin or placebo, and overall warfarin non-significantly reduced the odds of a vascular event over about 6.5 years compared with placebo (253 events in 2762 people allocated to warfarin, AR 9.2% *v* 288 events in 2737 people allocated to placebo, AR 10.5%; mean ARR warfarin *v* placebo about 2 events/1000 individuals/year; reduction in odds of vascular event warfarin *v* placebo +14%, 95% CI –2% to +28%). Compared with placebo, warfarin produced a relative reduction in the rate of all ischaemic heart disease (RRR 21%, 95% CI 4% to 35%), but had no significant effect on the rate of stroke (increase in RR +15%, 95% CI –22% to +68%) or other causes of vascular death.[165]

Harms: Allocation to warfarin was associated with a non-significant excess of about 0.4 intracranial bleeds per 1000 individuals a year (14/2762 [0.5%] with warfarin *v* 7/2737 [0.3%] with placebo) and a non-significant excess of extracranial bleeds of about 0.5/1000 individuals a year (21/2545 [0.8%] with warfarin *v* 12/2540 [0.5%] with placebo; RR 1.75, 95% CI 0.86 to 3.5).[165]

Comment: As is the case for aspirin, the benefits and risks of low intensity oral anticoagulation among people without evidence of cardiovascular disease are finely balanced. The number of individuals randomised to date is only about 10% of the number included in primary prevention RCTs of aspirin (see aspirin, p 116), and so the reliable identification of those who may benefit from such treatment will require further large scale randomised evidence.

Substantive changes

Effect of physical activity on blood pressure New systematic review;[111] conclusion unchanged.

Comparing antihypertensive drug treatments New systematic review;[136] conclusion unchanged.

Aspirin New systematic review;[161] conclusion unchanged.

Cholesterol reduction Two new RCTs;[149,150] conclusions unchanged

REFERENCES

1. http://www.who.int/whr/1999/en/report.htm (last accessed 19 Sept 2002).
2. Heller RF, Chinn S, Pedoe HD, et al. How well can we predict coronary heart disease? Findings of the United Kingdom heart disease prevention project. *BMJ* 1984;288:1409–1411.
3. Tunstall-Pedoe H, Morrison C, Woodward M, et al. Sex differences in myocardial infarction and coronary deaths in the Scottish MONICA population of Glasgow 1985 to 1991: presentation, diagnosis, treatment, and 28-day case fatality of 3991 events in men and 1551 events in women. *Circulation* 1996;93:1981–1992.
4. Anderson KV, Odell PM, Wilson PWF, et al. Cardiovascular disease risk profiles. *Am Heart J* 1991;121:293–298.
5. National Health Committee. Guidelines for the management of mildly raised blood pressure in New Zealand. Wellington Ministry of Health, 1993. http://www.nzgg.org.nz/library/gl_complete/bloodpressure/table1.cfm (last accessed 19 Sept 2002).
6. Powell KE, Thompson PD, Caspersen CJ, et al. Physical activity and the incidence of coronary heart disease. *Ann Rev Public Health* 1987;8:253–287. Search date 1995; primary sources computerised searches of personal files, *J Chronic Dis* 1983–1985, and *Am J Epidemiol* 1984–1985.
7. Berlin JA, Colditz GA. A meta-analysis of physical activity in the prevention of coronary heart disease. *Am J Epidemiol* 1990;132:612–628. Search date not stated; primary sources review articles and Medline.
8. Eaton CB. Relation of physical activity and cardiovascular fitness to coronary heart disease. Part I: a meta-analysis of the independent relation of physical activity and coronary heart disease. *J Am Board Fam Pract* 1992;5:31–42. Search date not stated; primary source Medline.
9. Fraser GE, Strahan TM, Sabate J, et al. Effects of traditional coronary risk factors on rates of incident coronary events in a low-risk population: the Adventist health study. *Circulation* 1992;86:406–413.
10. Lindsted KD, Tonstad S, Kuzma JW. Self-report of physical activity and patterns of mortality in Seventh-Day Adventist men. *J Clin Epidemiol* 1991;44:355–364.
11. Folsom AR, Arnett DK, Hutchinson RG, et al. Physical activity and incidence of coronary heart disease in middle-aged women and men. *Med Sci Sports Exerc* 1997;29:901–909.
12. Jensen G, Nyboe J, Appleyard M, et al. Risk factors for acute myocardial infarction in Copenhagen, II: smoking, alcohol intake, physical activity, obesity, oral contraception, diabetes, lipids, and blood pressure. *Eur Heart J* 1991;12:298–308.
13. Simonsick EM, Lafferty ME, Phillips CL, et al. Risk due to inactivity in physically capable older adults. *Am J Public Health* 1993;83:1443–1450.
14. Haapanen N, Miilunpalo S, Vuori I, et al. Association of leisure time physical activity with the risk of coronary heart disease, hypertension and diabetes in middle-aged men and women. *Int J Epidemiol* 1997;26:739–747.
15. Sherman SE, D'Agostino RB, Cobb JL, et al. Does exercise reduce mortality rates in the elderly? Experience from the Framingham heart study. *Am Heart J* 1994;128:965–672.
16. Rodriguez BL, Curb JD, Burchfiel CM, et al. Physical activity and 23-year incidence of coronary heart disease morbidity and mortality among middle-aged men: the Honolulu heart program. *Circulation* 1994;89:2540–2544.
17. Eaton CB, Medalie JH, Flocke SA, et al. Self-reported physical activity predicts long-term coronary heart disease and all-cause mortalities: 21-year follow-up of the Israeli Ischemic heart disease study. *Arch Fam Med* 1995;4:323–329.
18. Stender M, Hense HW, Doring A, et al. Physical activity at work and cardiovascular disease risk: results from the MONICA Augsburg study. *Int J Epidemiol* 1993;22:644–650.
19. Leon AS, Myers MJ, Connett J. Leisure time physical activity and the 16-year risks of mortality from coronary heart disease and all-causes in the multiple risk factor intervention trial (MRFIT). *Int J Sports Med* 1997;18(suppl 3):208–315.
20. Rosolova H, Simon J, Sefrna F. Impact of cardiovascular risk factors on morbidity and mortality in Czech middle-aged men: Pilsen longitudinal study. *Cardiology* 1994;85:61–68.
21. Luoto R, Prattala R, Uutela A, et al. Impact of unhealthy behaviors on cardiovascular mortality in Finland, 1978–1993. *Prev Med* 1998;27:93–100.
22. Woo J, Ho SC, Yuen YK, et al. Cardiovascular risk factors and 18-month mortality and morbidity in an elderly Chinese population aged 70 years and over. *Gerontology* 1998;44:51–55.
23. Gartside PS, Wang P, Glueck CJ. Prospective assessment of coronary heart disease risk factors: the NHANES I epidemiologic follow-up study (NHEFS) 16-year follow-up. *J Am Coll Nutr* 1998;17:263–269.
24. Dorn JP, Cerny FJ, Epstein LH, et al. Work and leisure time physical activity and mortality in men and women from a general population sample. *Ann Epidemiol* 1999;9:366–373.
25. Hakim AA, Curb JD, Petrovitch H, et al. Effects of walking on coronary heart disease in elderly men: the Honolulu heart program. *Circulation* 1999;100:9–13.
26. Pate RR, Pratt M, Blair SN, et al. Physical activity and public health. A recommendation from the Centers for Disease Control and Prevention and the American College of Sports Medicine. *JAMA* 1995;273:402–407.
27. Lee IM, Rexrode KM, Cook NR, et al. Physical activity and coronary heart disease in women: is "no pain, no gain" passe? *JAMA* 2001;285:1447–1454.
28. Eaton CB. Relation of physical activity and cardiovascular fitness to coronary heart disease,

part II: cardiovascular fitness and the safety and efficacy of physical activity prescription. *J Am Board Fam Pract* 1992;5:157–165. Search date not stated; primary sources Medline and hand searches.

29. Blair SN, Kohl HW 3rd, Barlow CE, et al. Changes in physical fitness and all-cause mortality: a prospective study of healthy and unhealthy men. *JAMA* 1995;273:1093–1098.
30. Lakka TA, Laukkanen JA, Rauramaa R, et al. Cardiorespiratory fitness and the progression of carotid atherosclerosis in middle-aged men. *Ann Intern Med* 2001;134:12–20.
31. Williams PT. Physical fitness and activity as separate heart disease risk factors: a meta-analysis. *Med Sci Sports Exerc* 2001;33:754–761.
32. Sacco RL, Gan R, Boden-Albala B, et al. Leisure-time physical activity and ischemic stroke risk: the Northern Manhattan stroke study. *Stroke* 1998;29:380–387.
33. Shinton R. Lifelong exposures and the potential for stroke prevention: the contribution of cigarette smoking, exercise, and body fat. *J Epidemiol Community Health* 1997;51:138–143.
34. Gillum RF, Mussolino ME, Ingram DD. Physical activity and stroke incidence in women and men. The NHANES I epidemiologic follow-up study. *Am J Epidemiol* 1996;143:860–869.
35. Kiely DK, Wolf PA, Cupples LA, et al. Physical activity and stroke risk: the Framingham study [correction appears in *Am J Epidemiol* 1995;141:178]. *Am J Epidemiol* 1994;140:608–620.
36. Abbott RD, Rodriguez BL, Burchfiel CM, et al. Physical activity in older middle-aged men and reduced risk of stroke: the Honolulu heart program. *Am J Epidemiol* 1994;139:881–893.
37. Haheim LL, Holme I, Hjermann I, et al. Risk factors of stroke incidence and mortality: a 12-year follow-up of the Oslo study. *Stroke* 1993;24:1484–1489.
38. Wannamethee G, Shaper AG. Physical activity and stroke in British middle aged men. *BMJ* 1992;304:597–601.
39. Menotti A, Keys A, Blackburn H, et al. Twenty-year stroke mortality and prediction in twelve cohorts of the seven countries study. *Int J Epidemiol* 1990;19:309–315.
40. Lindenstrom E, Boysen G, Nyboe J. Risk factors for stroke in Copenhagen, Denmark. II. Lifestyle factors. *Neuroepidemiology* 1993;12:43–50.
41. Lindenstrom E, Boysen G, Nyboe J. Lifestyle factors and risk of cerebrovascular disease in women: the Copenhagen City heart study. *Stroke* 1993;24:1468–1472.
42. Folsom AR, Prineas RJ, Kaye SA, et al. Incidence of hypertension and stroke in relation to body fat distribution and other risk factors in older women. *Stroke* 1990;21:701–706.
43. Nakayama T, Date C, Yokoyama T, et al. A 15.5-year follow-up study of stroke in a Japanese provincial city: the Shibata study. *Stroke* 1997;28:45–52.
44. Lee IM, Hennekens CH, Berger K, et al. Exercise and risk of stroke in male physicians. *Stroke* 1999;30:1–6.
45. Evenson KR, Rosamond WD, Cai J, et al. Physical activity and ischemic stroke risk: the atherosclerosis in communities study. *Stroke* 1999;30:1333–1339.
46. Mittleman MA, Maclure M, Tofler GH, et al. Triggering of acute myocardial infarction by heavy physical exertion. Protection against triggering by regular exertion: determinants of myocardial infarction onset study investigators. *N Engl J Med* 1993;329:1677–1683.
47. Willich SN, Lewis M, Lowel H, et al. Physical exertion as a trigger of acute myocardial infarction: triggers and mechanisms of myocardial infarction study group. *N Engl J Med* 1993;329:1684–1690.
48. Thompson PD. The cardiovascular complications of vigorous physical activity. *Arch Intern Med* 1996;156:2297–2302.
49. Oberman A. Exercise and the primary prevention of cardiovascular disease. *Am J Cardiol* 1985;55:10–20.
50. Andersen RE, Wadden TA, Bartlett SJ, et al. Effects of lifestyle activity vs structured aerobic exercise in obese women: a randomized trial. *JAMA* 1999;281:335–340.
51. Dunn AL, Marcus BH, Kampert JB, et al. Comparison of lifestyle and structured interventions to increase physical activity and cardiorespiratory fitness: a randomized trial. *JAMA* 1999;281:327–434.
52. Pereira MA, Kriska AM, Day RD, et al. A randomized walking trial in postmenopausal women: effects on physical activity and health 10 years later. *Arch Intern Med* 1998;158:1695–1701.
53. DeBusk RF, Stenestrand U, Sheehan M, et al. Training effects of long versus short bouts of exercise in healthy subjects. *Am J Cardiol* 1990;65:1010–1013.
54. Ness AR, Powles JW. Fruit and vegetables and cardiovascular disease: a review. *Int J Epidemiol* 1997;26:1–13. Search date 1995; primary sources Medline, Embase, and hand searches of personal bibliographies, books, reviews, and citations in located reports.
55. Law MR, Morris JK. By how much does fruit and vegetable consumption reduce the risk of ischaemic heart disease? *Eur J Clin Nutr* 1998;52:549–556. Search date not stated; primary sources Medline, Science Citation Index, and hand searches of review articles.
56. Klerk M, Jansen MCJF, van't Veer P, et al. Fruits and vegetables in chronic disease prevention. Wageningen: Grafisch Bedrijf Ponsen and Looijen, 1998. Search date 1998; primary sources Medline, Current Contents, and Toxline.
57. Knekt P, Isotupa S, Rissanen H, et al. Quercetin intake and the incidence of cerebrovascular disease. *Eur J Clin Nutr* 2000;54:415–417.
58. Key TJA, Thorogood M, Appleby PN, et al. Dietary habits and mortality in 11 000 vegetarians and health conscious people: results of a 17 year follow up. *BMJ* 1996;313:775–779.
59. Pietinen P, Rimm EB, Korhonen P, et al. Intake of dietary fibre and risk of coronary heart disease in a cohort of Finnish men. *Circulation* 1996;94:2720–2727.
60. Mann JI, Appleby PN, Key TJA, et al. Dietary determinants of ischaemic heart disease in health conscious individuals. *Heart* 1997;78:450–455.
61. Geleijnse M. Consumptie van groente en fruit en het risico op myocardinfarct 1997. Basisrapportage. Rotterdam: Erasmus Universiteit (cited in appendix XIII of review by Klerk).
62. Todd S, Woodward M, Tunstall-Pedoe H, et al. Dietary antioxidant vitamins and fiber in the etiology of cardiovascular disease and all-cause mortality: results from the Scottish heart health study. *Am J Epidemiol* 1999;150:1073–1080.
63. Bazzano L, Ogden LG, Vupputuri S, et al. Fruit and vegetable intake reduces cardiovascular mortality: results from the NHANES I epidemiologic follow-up study (NHEFS). Abstract presented at the 40th Annual conference on Cardiovascular Epidemiology and Prevention, San Diego California March 1–4, 2000.

64. Liu S, Lee I-M, Ajani U, et al. Intake of vegetables rich in carotenoids and risk of coronary heart disease in men: the Physicians' Health Study. *Int J Epidemiol* 2001;30:130–135.
65. Lui S, Manson JE, Lee I-M, et al. Fruit and vegetable intake and risk of cardiovascular disease: the Women's Health Study. *Am J Clin Nutr* 2000;72:922–928.
66. Cox BD, Whichelow MJ, Prevost AT. Seasonal consumption of salad vegetables and fresh fruit in relation to the development of cardiovascular disease and cancer. *Public Health Nutr* 2000;3:19–29.
67. van't Veer P, Jansen MCJF, Klerk M, et al. Fruits and vegetables in the prevention of cancer and cardiovascular disease. *Public Health Nutr* 2000;3:103–107.
68. Joshipura KJ, Ascherio A, Manson JE, et al. Fruit and vegetable intake in relation to risk of ischemic stroke. *JAMA* 1999;282:1233–1239.
69. Ness AR, Powles JW. Does eating fruit and vegetables protect against heart attack and stroke? *Chem Indus* 1996;792–794.
70. Ness AR, Powles JW. Dietary habits and mortality in vegetarians and health conscious people: several uncertainties exist. *BMJ* 1997;314:148.
71. Serdula MK, Byers T, Mokhad AH, et al. The association between fruit and vegetable intake and chronic disease risk factors. *Epidemiology* 1996;7:161–165.
72. Lonn EM, Yusuf S. Is there a role for antioxidant vitamins in the prevention of cardiovascular disease? An update on epidemiological and clinical trials data. *Can J Cardiol* 1997;13:957–965. Search date not stated; primary sources Medline, Science Citation Index, and hand searching.
73. Jha P, Flather M, Lonn E, et al. The antioxidant vitamins and cardiovascular disease: a critical review of epidemiologic and clinical trial data. *Ann Intern Med* 1995;123:860–872.
74. Roxrode KM, Manson JE. Antioxidants and coronary heart disease: observational studies. *J Cardiovasc Risk* 1996;3:363–367.
75. Egger M, Schneider M, Davey Smith G. Spurious precision? Meta-analysis of observational studies. *BMJ* 1998;316:140–144.
76. Gaziano JM. Randomized trials of dietary antioxidants in cardiovascular disease prevention and treatment. *J Cardiovasc Risk* 1996;3:368–371.
77. Ness AR, Powles JW, Khaw KT. Vitamin C and cardiovascular disease — a systematic review. *J Cardiovasc Risk* 1997;3:513–521. Search date 1996; primary sources Medline, Embase, and hand searches of personal bibliographies, books, reviews, and citations in located reports.
78. Daviglus ML, Orencia AJ, Dyer AR, et al. Dietary vitamin C, beta-carotene and 30-year risk of stroke: results from the Western Electric study. *Neuroepidemiology* 1997;16:69–77.
79. Hirvonen T, Virtamo J, Korhonen P, et al. Intake of flavonoids, carotenoids, vitamin C and E, and risk of stroke in male smokers. *Stroke* 2000;31:2301–2306.
80. Klipstein-Grobusch K, Geleijnse JM, den Breeijen JH, et al. Dietary antioxidants and risk of myocardial infarction in the elderly: the Rotterdam study. *Am J Clin Nutr* 1999;69:261–266.
81. Ascherio A, Rimm EB, Hernan MA, et al. Relation of consumption of vitamin E, vitamin C, and carotenoids to risk for stroke among men in the United States. *Ann Intern Med* 1999;130:963–970.
82. Yochum L, Folsom AR, Kushi LH. Intake of antioxidant vitamins and risk of death from stroke in postmenopausal women. *Am J Clin Nutr* 2000;72:476–483.
83. Li J, Taylor PR, Li B, et al. Nutrition intervention trials in Linxian, China: multiple vitamin/mineral supplementation, cancer incidence, and disease-specific mortality among adults with esophageal dysplasia. *J Natl Cancer Inst* 1993;85:1492–1498.
84. Mark SD, Wang W, Fraumeni JF, et al. Lowered risks of hypertension and cerebrovascular disease after vitamin/mineral supplementation. *Am J Epidemiol* 1996;143:658–664.
85. Mark SD, Wang W, Fraumeni JFJ, et al. Do nutritional supplements lower the risk of stroke or hypertension? *Epidemiology* 1998;9:9–15.
86. Losonczy KG, Harris TB, Havlik RJ. Vitamin E and vitamin C supplement use and risk of all-cause and coronary mortality in older persons: the established populations for epidemiologic studies of the elderly. *Am J Clin Nutr* 1996;64:190–196.
87. Sahyoun NR, Jacques PF, Russell RM. Carotenoids, vitamin C and E, and mortality in an elderly population. *Am J Epidemiol* 1996;144:501–511.
88. Collaborative group of the Primary Prevention Project (PPP). Low-dose aspirin and vitamin E in people at cardiovascular risk: a randomised trial in general practice. *Lancet* 2001;357:89–95.
89. Keli SO, Hertog MGL, Feskens EJM, et al. Dietary flavonoids, antioxidant vitamins, and incidence of stroke. *Arch Intern Med* 1996;156:637–642.
90. Leppälä JM, Virtamo J, Fogelholm R, et al. Controlled trial of α-tocopherol and β-carotene supplements on stroke incidence and mortality in male smokers *Arterioscler Thromb Vasc Biol* 2000;20:230–235
91. Houtman JP. Trace elements and cardiovascular disease. *J Cardiovasc Risk* 1996;3:18–25.
92. Nève J. Selenium as a risk factor for cardiovascular disease. *J Cardiovasc Risk* 1996;3:42–47.
93. Hertog MGL, Feskens EJM, Holliman PCH, et al. Dietary antioxidant flavonoids and risk of coronary heart disease: the Zutphen elderly study. *Lancet* 1993;342:1007–1011.
94. Yochum L, Kushi LH, Meyer K, et al. Dietary flavonoid intake and risk of cardiovascular disease in postmenopausal women. *Am J Epidemiol* 1999;149:943–949.
95. Knekt P, Jarvinen R, Reunanen A, et al. Flavonoid intake and coronary mortality in Finland: a cohort study. *BMJ* 1996;312:478–481.
96. Rimm EB, Katan MB, Ascherio A, et al. Relation between intake of flavonoids and risk for coronary heart disease in male health professionals. *Ann Intern Med* 1996;125:384–389.
97. Hertog MGL, Sweetnam PM, Fehily AM. Antioxidant flavonols and ischemic heart disease in a Welsh population of men: the Caerphilly study. *Am J Clin Nutr* 1997;65:1489–1494.
98. Doering WV. Antioxidant vitamins, cancer, and cardiovascular disease. *N Engl J Med* 1996;335:1065.
99. Pietrzik K. Antioxidant vitamins, cancer, and cardiovascular disease. *N Engl J Med* 1996;335:1065–1066.
100. Hennekens CH, Gaziano JM, Manson JE, et al. Antioxidant vitamin cardiovascular disease hypothesis is still promising, but still unproven: the need for randomised trials. *Am J Clin Nutr* 1995;62(suppl):1377–1380.
101. US Department of Health and Human Services. The health benefits of smoking cessation: a report of the Surgeon General. Rockville, Maryland: US Department of Health and Human

Services, Public Health Service, Centers for Disease Control, 1990. DHHS Publication (CDC) 90-8416.
102. Royal College of Physicians. *Smoking and health now*. London: Pitman Medical and Scientific Publishing, 1971.
103. Doll R, Peto R, Wheatley K, et al. Mortality in relation to smoking: 40 years' observations on male British doctors. *BMJ* 1994;309:901–911.
104. Kawachi I, Colditz GA, Stampfer MJ, et al. Smoking cessation in relation to total mortality rates in women: a prospective cohort study. *Ann Intern Med* 1993;119:992–1000.
105. Rosenberg L, Kaufman DW, Helmrich SP, et al. The risk of myocardial infarction after quitting smoking in men under 55 years of age. *N Engl J Med* 1985;313:1511–1514.
106. Rosenberg L, Palmer JR, Shapiro S. Decline in the risk of myocardial infarction among women who stop smoking. *N Engl J Med* 1990;322:213–217.
107. Rose G, Hamilton PJ, Colwell L, et al. A randomised controlled trial of anti-smoking advice: 10-year results. *J Epidemiol Community Health* 1982;36:102–108.
108. Shinton R, Beevers G. Meta-analysis of relation between cigarette smoking and stroke. *BMJ* 1989;298:789–794. Search date 1988; primary source index references from three studies on cigarette smoking and stroke on medicine.
109. Rogot E, Murray JL. Smoking and causes of death among US veterans: 16 years of observation. *Public Health Rep* 1980;95:213–222.
110. Wannamethee SG, Shaper AG, Ebrahim S. History of parental death from stroke or heart trouble and the risk of stroke in middle-aged men. *Stroke* 1996;27:1492–1498.
111. Whelton SP, Chin A, Xin X, et al. Effect of aerobic exercise on blood pressure: a meta-analysis of randomized, controlled trials. *Ann Intern Med* 2002;136:493–503.
112. Ebrahim S, Davey Smith G. Lowering blood pressure: a systematic review of sustained non-pharmacological interventions. *J Public Health Med* 1998;20:441–448. Search date 1995; primary source Medline.
113. Engstom G, Hedblad B, Janzon L. Hypertensive men who exercise regularly have lower rate of cardiovascular mortality. *J Hypertens* 1999;17:737–742.
114. Appel LJ, Moore TJ, Obarzanek E, et al. A clinical trial of the effects of dietary patterns on blood pressure. *N Engl J Med* 1997;336:1117–1124.
115. Beilin LJ, Puddey IB, Burke V. Alcohol and hypertension: kill or cure? *J Hum Hypertens* 1996;10(suppl 2):1–5.
116. Xin X, HE J, Frontini MG, et al. Effects of alcohol reduction on blood pressure: a meta-analysis of randomized controlled trials. *Hypertension*. 2001;38:1112–1117. Search date 1999; primary sources Medline and reference lists of retrieved articles.
117. Graudal NA, Galloe AM, Garred P. Effects of sodium restriction on blood pressure, renin, aldosterone, catecholamines, cholesterols, and triglyceride. *JAMA* 1998;279:1383–1391. Search date 1997; primary source Medline.
118. Whelton PK, Appel LJ, Espelland MA, et al. Sodium reduction and weight loss in the treatment of hypertension in older persons: a randomized controlled trial of non pharmacologic interventions in the elderly (TONE). *JAMA* 1998;279:839–846.
119. Sacks FM, Svetkey LP, Vollmer WM, et al. Effects on blood pressure of reduced dietary sodium and the dietary approaches to stop hypertension (DASH) diet. *N Engl J Med* 2001;344:3–10
120. Midgley JP, Matthew AG, Greenwood CMT, et al. Effect of reduced dietary sodium on blood pressure. *JAMA* 1996;275:1590–1597. Search date 1994; primary sources Medline and Current Contents.
121. Mulrow CD, Chiquette E, Angel L, et al. Dieting to reduce body weight for controlling hypertension in adults. In: The Cochrane Library, Issue 2, 2002. Oxford: Update Software. Search date 1998; primary source Cochrane Library, Medline, and contact with experts in the field.
122. Metz JA, Stern JS, Kris-Etherton P, et al. A randomized trial of improved weight loss with a prepared meal plan in overweight and obese patients. *Arch Intern Med* 2000;160:2150–2158.
123. Stevens VJ, Obarzanek E, Cook NR, et al. Long-term weight loss and changes in blood pressure: results of the Trials of Hypertension Prevention, phase II. *Ann Intern Med* 2001;134:1–11.
124. Whelton PK, He J, Cutler JA, et al. Effects of oral potassium on blood pressure: meta-analysis of randomized controlled clinical trials. *JAMA* 1997;277:1624–1632. Search date 1995; primary source Medline.
125. Morris MC, Sacks F, Rosner B. Does fish oil lower blood pressure? A meta-analysis of controlled clinical trials. *Circulation* 1993;88:523–533. Search date not stated; primary source Index Medicus.
126. Griffith LE, Guyatt GH, Cook RJ, et al. The influence of dietary and nondietary calcium supplementation on blood pressure. *Am J Hypertens* 1999;12:84–92. Search date 1994; primary sources Medline and Embase.
127. Gueyffier F, Froment A, Gouton M. New meta-analysis of treatment trials of hypertension: improving the estimate of therapeutic benefit. *J Hum Hypertens* 1996;10:1–8. Search date 1997; primary source Medline.
128. Staessen JA, Gasowski J, Wang JG, et al. Risks of untreated and treated isolated systolic hypertension in the elderly: meta-analysis of outcome trials. *Lancet* 2000;355:865–872. Search date 1999; primary sources other systematic reviews and reports from collaborative trialists.
129. Hansson L, Zanchetti AZ, Carruthers SG, et al. Effects of intensive blood pressure lowering and low-dose aspirin in patients with hypertension: principal results of the hypertension optimal treatment (HOT) trial. *Lancet* 1998;351:1755–1762.
130. Beto JA, Bansal VK. Quality of life in treatment of hypertension: a meta-analysis of clinical trials. *Am J Hypertens* 1992;5:125–133. Search date 1990; primary sources Medline and ERIC.
131. Croog SH, Levine S, Testa MA. The effects of antihypertensive therapy on quality of life. *N Engl J Med* 1986;314:1657–1664.
132. Boutitie F, Gueyffier F, Pocock S, et al. J-Shaped relationship between blood pressure and mortality in hypertensive patients: new insights from a meta-analysis of individual-patient data. *Ann Intern Med* 2002;136:438–448.
133. Psaty BM, Smith NS, Siscovick DS, et al. Health outcomes associated with antihypertensive therapies used as first line agents: a systematic review and meta-analysis. *JAMA* 1997;277:739–745. Search date 1995; primary source Medline.
134. Messerli FH, Grossman E, Goldbourt U. Are beta blockers efficacious as first-line therapy for

hypertension in the elderly? A systematic review. *JAMA* 1998;279:1903–1907. Search date 1998; primary source Medline.

135. Blood Pressure Lowering Treatment Trialists' Collaboration. Effects of ACE inhibitors, calcium antagonists, and other blood-pressure-lowering drugs: results of prospectively designed overviews of trials. *Lancet* 2000;356:1955–1964. Search date 2000; primary sources WHO-International Society of Hypertension registry of randomised trials; trials were sought that had not published or presented their results before July 1995.
136. Staessen JA, Wang JG, Thijs L. Cardiovascular protection and blood pressure reduction: a meta-analysis. *Lancet* 2001;358:1305–1315.
137. The ALLHAT Officers and Coordinators for the ALLHAT Collaborative Research Group. Major cardiovascular events in hypertensive patients randomized to doxazosin vs chlorthalidone: the antihypertensive and lipid-lowering treatment to prevent heart attack trial (ALLHAT). *JAMA* 2000;283:1967–1975.
138. Neaton JD, Grimm RH, Prineas RJ, et al. Treatment of mild hypertension study: final results. *JAMA* 1993;270:713–724.
139. Materson BJ, Reda DJ, Cushman WC, et al. Single drug therapy for hypertension in men. *N Engl J Med* 1993;328:914–921.
140. Philipp T, Anlauf M, Distler A, et al. Randomised, double blind, multicentre comparison of hydrochlorothiazide, atenolol, nitrendipine, and enalapril in antihypertensive treatment: results of the HANE study. *BMJ* 1997;315:154–159.
141. Wright JM, Lee CH, Chambers CK. Systematic review of antihypertensive therapies: does the evidence assist in choosing a first line drug? *Can Med Assoc J* 1999;161:25–32. Search date 1998; primary sources Medline and Cochrane Library.
142. Hansson L, Zanchetti AZ, Carruthers SG, et al. Effects of intensive blood pressure lowering and low-dose aspirin in patients with hypertension: principal results of the hypertension optimal treatment (HOT) trial. *Lancet* 1998;351:1755–1762.
143. Cutler JA. Calcium channel blockers for hypertension — uncertainty continues. *N Engl J Med* 1998;338:679–680.
144. Pignone M, Phillips C, Mulrow C. Use of lipid lowering drugs for primary prevention of coronary heart disease: meta-analysis of randomised trials. *BMJ* 2000;321:983–986. Search date 1999; primary sources Medline, Cochrane Library, and hand searches of bibliographies of systematic reviews and clinical practice guidelines.
145. Cucherat M, Lievre M, Gueyffier F. Clinical benefits of cholesterol lowering treatments. Meta-analysis of randomized therapeutic trials. *Presse Med* 2000 May 13;29:965–976. Search date and primary sources not stated.
146. Katerndahl DA, Lawler WR. Variability in meta-analytic results concerning the value of cholesterol reduction in coronary heart disease: a meta-meta-analysis. *Am J Epidemiol* 1999;149:429–441. Search date 1995; primary sources Medline and meta-analysis bibliographies.
147. Ebrahim S, Davey Smith G, McCabe CCC, et al. What role for statins? A review and economic model. *Health Technol Assess* 1999;3(10):i–iv, 1–91. Search dates 1997; primary sources Medline, Cochrane Controlled Trials Register, and personal contact with investigators working in the field of cholesterol lowering.
148. LaRosa JC, He J, Vupputuri S. Effect of statins on risk of coronary disease: a meta-analysis of randomized controlled trials. *JAMA* 1999;282:2340–2346. Search date 1998; primary sources Medline, bibliographies, and authors' reference files.
149. Heart Protection Study Collaborative Group MRC/BHF Heart Protection Study of cholesterol lowering with simvastatin in 20536 high-risk individuals: a randomised placebo-controlled trial. *Lancet* 2002;360:7–22.
150. Sawayama Y, Shimuzu C, Maeda N, et al. Effects of probucol and pravastatin on common carotid atherosclerosis in patients with asymptomatic hypercholesterolemia. Fukuoka Atherosclerosis Trial (FAST). *J Am Coll Cardiol* 2002;39:610–616.
151. Downs JR, Clearfield M, Weis S, et al. Primary prevention of acute coronary events with lovastatin in men and women with average cholesterol levels: results of the AFCAPS/TexCAPS. *JAMA* 1998;279:1615–1622.
152. Shepherd J, Cobbe SM, Ford I, et al. Prevention of coronary heart disease with pravastatin in men with hypercholesterolemia. *N Engl J Med* 1995;333:1301–1307.
153. Scandinavian Simvastatin Survival Study Group. Randomized trial of cholesterol lowering in 4444 patients with coronary heart disease: the Scandinavian simvastatin survival study (4S). *Lancet* 1995;344:1383–1389.
154. Long-term Intervention with Pravastatin in Ischemic Disease (LIPID) Study Program. Prevention of cardiovascular events and death with pravastatin in patients with coronary heart disease and a broad range of initial cholesterol levels. *N Engl J Med* 1998;339:1349–1357.
155. Sacks FM, Pfeffer MA, Moye LA, et al. Effect of pravastatin on coronary events after myocardial infarction in patients with average cholesterol levels. *N Engl J Med* 1996;335:1001–1009.
156. Jackson PR, Wallis EJ, Haq IU, et al. Statins for primary prevention: at what coronary risk is safety assured? *Br J Clin Pharmacol* 2001;52:439–446.
157. Bucher HC, Griffith LE, Guyatt G. Systematic review on the risk and benefit of different cholesterol-lowering interventions. *Arterioscler Thromb Vasc Biol* 1999:19;187–195. Search date 1996; primary sources Medline, Embase, and hand searches of bibliographies.
158. Hart RG, Halperin JL, McBride R, et al. Aspirin for the primary prevention of stroke and other major vascular events. Meta-analysis and hypotheses. *Arch Neurol* 2000;57:326–332. Search date 1998; primary sources unspecified computerised medical databases, Cochrane Collaboration Registry, and hand searched references of Antiplatelet Trialists' Collaboration publications.
159. Hebert PR, Hennekens CH. An overview of the 4 randomized trials of aspirin therapy in the primary prevention of vascular disease. *Arch Int Med* 2000;160:3123–3127. Search date and primary sources not stated.
160. Sanmuganathan PS, Ghahramani P, Jackson PR, et al. Aspirin for primary prevention of coronary heart disease: safety and absolute benefit related to coronary risk derived from a meta-analysis of randomised trials. *Heart* 2001;85:265–271. Search date not stated; primary sources Medline and previous meta-analyses and review articles.
161. Hayden M, Pignone M, Phillips C, et al. Aspirin for the primary prevention of cardiovascular events: a summary of the evidence for the US preventive services task force. *Ann Intern Med* 2002;136:161–172.

162. Peto R, Gray R, Collins R, et al. Randomised trial of prophylactic daily aspirin in British male doctors. *BMJ* 1988;296:313–316.
163. Steering Committee of the Physicians' Health Study Research Group. Final report on the aspirin component of the ongoing physicians' health study. *N Engl J Med* 1989;321:129–135.
164. ETDRS Investigators. Aspirin effects on mortality and morbidity in patients with diabetes mellitus. Early treatment diabetic retinopathy study report 14. *JAMA* 1992;268:1292–1300.
165. Medical Research Council's General Practice Research Framework. Thrombosis prevention trial: randomised trial of low-intensity anticoagulation with warfarin and low dose aspirin in the primary prevention of ischaemic heart disease in men at increased risk. *Lancet* 1998;351:233–241.
166. Antiplatelet Trialists' Collaboration. Collaborative overview of randomised trials of antiplatelet therapy — I: prevention of death, myocardial infarction, and stroke by prolonged antiplatelet therapy in various categories of patients. *BMJ* 1994;308:81–106. Search date 1990; primary sources Medline, Current Contents, hand searches of reference list of trials and review articles, journal abstracts and meeting proceedings, trial register of the International Committee on Thrombosis and Haemostasis, and personal contacts with colleagues and antiplatelet manufacuters.
167. He J, Whelton PK, Vu B, et al. Aspirin and risk of hemorrhagic stroke: a meta-analysis of randomized controlled trials. *JAMA* 1998;280:1930–1935. Search date 1997; primary sources Medline, the authors' reference files, and reference lists from original communications and review articles.
168. Derry S, Loke YK. Risk of gastrointestinal haemorrhage with long term use of aspirin: meta-analysis. *BMJ* 2000;321:1183–1187. Search date not stated; primary sources Medline, Embase, and reference lists from previous review papers and retrieved trials.
169. García Rodríguez LA, Hernández-Díaz S, De Abajo FJ. Association between aspirin and upper gastrointestinal complications: a systematic review of epidemiologic studies. *Br J Clin Pharmacol Zool* 2001;52:563–571.
170. Antithrombotic Trialists' Collaboration. Collaborative meta-analysis of randomised trials of antiplatelet therapy for prevention of death, myocardial infarction, and stroke in high risk patients. *BMJ* 2002;324:71–86.
171. Buring JE, Hennekens CH. Women's health study: summary of the study design. *J Myocard Ischemia* 1992;4:27–29.

Michael Murphy
Director, ICRF General Practice Research Group

Charles Foster
British Heart Foundation Scientist

University of Oxford
Oxford
UK

Cathie Sudlow
Wellcome Clinician Scientist
Department of Clinical Neurosciences
University of Edinburgh
Edinburgh
UK

Julian Nicholas
Resident Physician
Mayo Clinic
Rochester
USA

Cindy Mulrow
Professor of Medicine
University of Texas Health Science Center
San Antonio
USA

Andy Ness
Senior Lecturer in Epidemiology
University of Bristol
Bristol
UK

Michael Pignone
Assistant Professor of Medicine
Division of General Internal Medicine
University of North Carolina
Chapel Hill
USA

Competing interests: CM has participated in multicentre research trials evaluating antihypertensive agents that were funded by industry; other authors, none declared.

TABLE 1 **Examples of common physical activities by intensity of effort required in multiples of the resting rate of oxygen consumption during physical activity (see text, p 99). Published in *JAMA* 1995;273:402–407.[26]**

Activity type	Light activity (< 3.0 METs)	Moderate activity (3.0–6.0 METs)	Vigorous activity (> 6.0 METs)
Walking	Slowly (1–2 mph)	Briskly (3–4 mph)	Briskly uphill or with a load
Swimming	Treading slowly	Moderate effort	Fast treading or swimming
Cycling	NA	For pleasure or transport (≤ 10 mph)	Fast or racing (> 10 mph)
Golf	Power cart	Pulling cart or carrying clubs	NA
Boating	Power boat	Canoeing leisurely	Canoeing rapidly (> 4 mph)
Home care	Carpet sweeping	General cleaning	Moving furniture
Mowing lawn	Riding mower	Power mower	Hand mower
Home repair	Carpentry	Painting	NA

METs, work metabolic rate/resting metabolic rate; 1 MET represents the rate of oxygen consumption of a seated adult at rest; mph, miles per hour; NA, not applicable.

TABLE 2 Effects of aspirin on vascular events (myocardial infarction, stroke, or vascular death) in RCTs among individuals without evidence of cardiovascular disease (see text, p 116).

Trials (duration)	Annual risk of vascular event (control)	Vascular events: Antiplatelet, control, and odds ratio* (CI†)	Events avoided per 1000 person-years	Myocardial infarction: Antiplatelet, control, and odds ratio* (CI†)	Stroke: Antiplatelet, control, and odds ratio* (CI†)
UK doctors[162] (70 months)	1.5%	288/3429, 280/3420‡, 1.03 (0.6 to 2.3)	–0.4	169/3429, 176/3420‡, 0.96 (0.7 to 1.4)	91/3429, 78/3420‡, 1.16 (0.7 to 1.9)
US physicians[163] (60 months)	0.7%	321/11037, 387/11034, 0.82 (0.7 to 1.0)	1.2	139/11037, 239/11034, 0.58 (0.5 to 0.8)	119/11 037, 98/11 034, 1.22 (0.9 to 1.7)
TPT[165] (76 months)	1.8%	239/2545, 270/2540, 0.87 (0.7 to 1.1)	2.0	154/2545, 190/2540, 0.80 (0.7 to 1.1)	47/2545, 48/2540, 0.98 (0.6 to 1.7)
HOT[142] (46 months)	1.0%	315/9399, 368/9391, 0.85 (0.7 to 1.0)	1.5	82/9399, 127/9391, 0.65 (0.5 to 0.9)	146/9399, 148/9391, 0.99 (0.7 to 1.3)
PPP[88] (44 months)	0.8%	45/2226, 64/2269, 0.71 (0.4 to 1.2)	2.2	19/2226, 28/2269, 0.69 (0.3 to 1.5)	16/2226, 24/2269, 0.68 (0.3 to 1.6)
All trials (56 months)	1.0%	1208/28 636 (4.2%), 1369/28 654 (4.8%), 0.86§ (0.8 to 0.9)	1.2	563/28 636 (2.0%), 760/28 654 (2.4%), 0.71§ (0.6 to 0.8)	419/28 636 (1.5%), 396/28 654 (1.4%), 1.05§ (0.9 to 1.2)

Data from individual trial publications and from the APT overview (1994).[166] The effects of aspirin were similar in the absence or presence of warfarin, so the data presented are not stratified by warfarin allocation. * Odds ratios calculated using the "observed minus expected" method;[166] † 99% CI for individual trials 95% CI for "All trials"; ‡ Number of patients in control group was 1710 (randomisation ratio 2 : 1); numerator and denominator multiplied by 2 to calculate totals for absolute differences between antiplatelet and control group event rates; actual numbers of events used to calculate odds ratios and confidence intervals; ¶ Weighted by study size; § Heterogeneity of odds ratios between five trials not significant ($P > 0.05$).

TABLE 3 **Effects of aspirin on intracranial and major extracranial haemorrhages in RCTs among individuals without evidence of cardiovascular disease (see text, p 116).**

Trials	Antiplatelet	Control	Summary odds ratio* (95% CI)	Excess bleeds per 1000 patients treated per year
Intracranial bleeds				
UK doctors[160]	13/3429	12/3420†		
US physicians[161]	23/11037	12/11034		
TPT[164]	12/2545	6/2540		
HOT[132]	14/9399	15/9391		
PPP[96]	2/2226	3/2269		
All trials	**64/28 636 (0.22%)**	**48/28654 (0.17%)**	**1.4(0.9 to 2.0)**	**0.1 (P = 0.1)**
Major extracranial bleeds				
UK Doctors[160]	21/3429	20/3420†		
US Physicians[161]	48/1 037	28/11 034		
TPT[164]	20/2545	13/2540		
HOT[132]	122/9399	63/9391		
All trials	**211/26 410 (0.8%)**	**134/28 095 (0.5%)**	**1.7(1.4 to 2.1)**	**0.7 (P < 0.00001)**

Data from individual trial publications. *Odds ratios calculated using the "observed minus expected" method.[166]
†Number of patients in control group was 1710 (randomisation ratio 2 : 1); numerator and denominator multiplied by 2 to calculate totals for absolute differences between antiplatelet and control group event rates; actual numbers of events used to calculate odds ratios and confidence intervals.

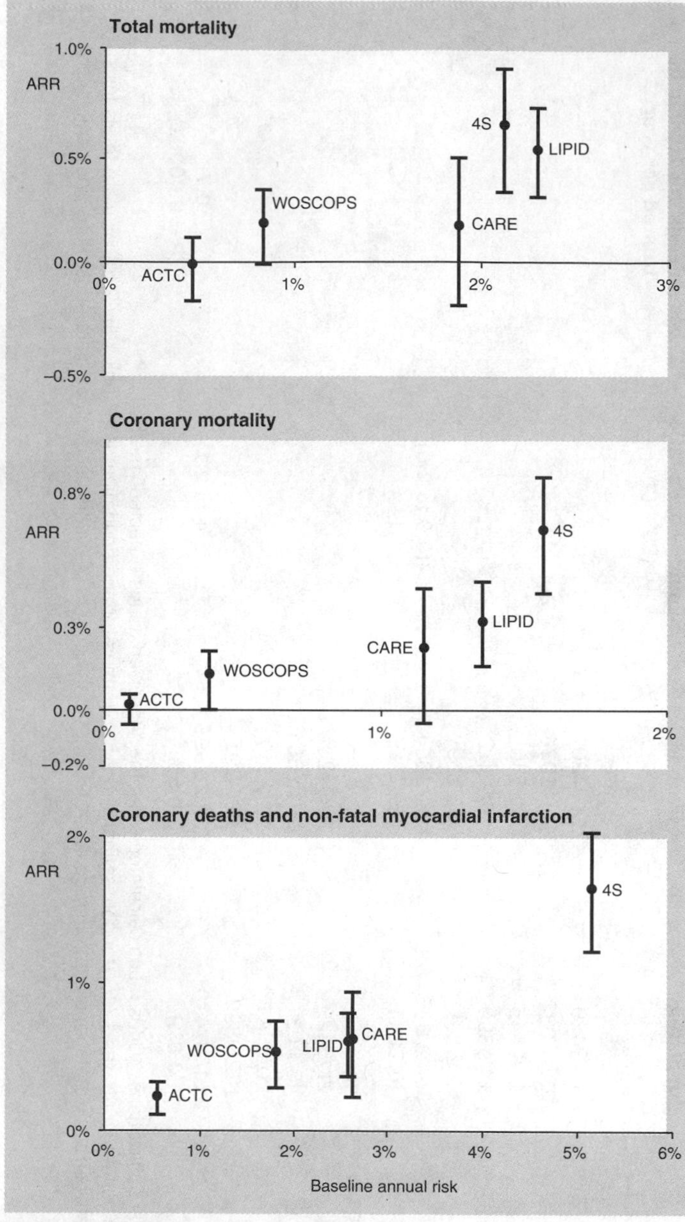

FIGURE 1 **Effects of cholesterol lowering: relation between the ARR (for annual total mortality, coronary heart disease mortality, coronary deaths, and non-fatal myocardial infarction) and the baseline risk of those events in the placebo group for five large statin trials (ACTC = AFCAPS/TexCAPS,[151] 4S,[153] LIPID,[154] CARE,[155] WOSCOPS[152]) (see text, p 114).**

Secondary prevention of ischaemic cardiac events

Search date March 2002

Clinical Evidence writers on secondary prevention of ischaemic cardiac events

QUESTIONS

INTERVENTIONS

See glossary, p 161

Clin Evid 2002;8:129–168.

Secondary prevention of ischaemic cardiac events

Key Messages

Antithrombotic treatment

- **Adding anticoagulants to antiplatelet treatment** One systematic review and one subsequent RCT found no evidence that addition of oral anticoagulation at low (INR < 1.5) or moderate (INR 1.5–3) intensity to aspirin reduced risk of death or recurrent cardiac events, but found an increased risk of major haemorrhage.
- **Anticoagulants in the absence of antiplatelet treatment** One systematic review has found that high or moderate intensity oral anticoagulants given alone significantly reduce the risk of serious vascular events in people with coronary artery disease, but are associated with substantial risk of haemorrhage.
- **Any oral antiplatelet treatment** One systematic review has found that prolonged antiplatelet treatment versus placebo or no antiplatelet treatment reduces the risk of serious vascular events in people at high risk of ischaemic cardiac events.
- **Aspirin** One systematic review has found that, for prolonged use, aspirin 75–150 mg daily is as effective as higher doses, but found insufficient evidence that doses below 75 mg daily are as effective.
- **Oral glycoprotein IIb/IIIa receptor inhibitors** One systematic review in people with acute coronary syndromes or undergoing percutaneous coronary interventions has found that oral glycoprotein IIb/IIIa receptor inhibitors versus placebo increase risk of mortality and bleeding.
- **Thienopyridines** One systematic review has found that clopidogrel is at least as safe and effective as aspirin in people at high risk of vascular events.

Other drug treatments

- **Angiotensin converting enzyme inhibitors in high risk people without left ventricular dysfunction** One large RCT in people without left ventricular dysfunction found that ramipril versus placebo significantly reduced the combined outcome of cardiovascular death, stroke, and myocardial infarction after about 5 years (NNT 27, 95% CI 20 to 45).
- **Angiotensin converting enzyme inhibitors in people with left ventricular dysfunction** One systematic review has found that in people who have had a myocardial infarction and have left ventricular dysfunction, angiotensin converting enzyme inhibitors versus placebo significantly reduce mortality (NNT 17, CI not available), admission to hospital for congestive heart failure (NNT 28, CI not available), and recurrent non-fatal myocardial infarction (NNT 43, CI not available) after 2 years' treatment.
- **Amiodarone in selected high risk people** Two systematic reviews have found that amiodarone versus placebo significantly reduces the risk of sudden cardiac death, and reduces mortality at 1 year in people at high risk of death after myocardial infarction.
- **β Blockers** Systematic reviews in people after myocardial infarction have found that long term β blockers reduce all cause mortality, coronary mortality, recurrent non-fatal myocardial infarction, and sudden death. One RCT found that about 25% of people suffer adverse effects.
- **Calcium channel blockers (dihydropyridines)** One systematic review found non-significantly higher mortality with dihydropyridines compared with placebo.

- **Calcium channel blockers (diltiazem and verapamil)** One systematic review found no benefit from calcium channel blockers in people after myocardial infarction or with chronic coronary heart disease. Diltiazem and verapamil may reduce rates of reinfarction and refractory angina in people after myocardial infarction who do not have heart failure.
- **Class I antiarrhythmic agents** One systematic review has found that class I antiarrhythmic agents versus placebo given after myocardial infarction significantly increase the risk of cardiovascular mortality and sudden death.
- **Hormone replacement therapy** One large RCT found no evidence that hormone replacement therapy versus placebo reduces major cardiovascular events in postmenopausal women with established coronary artery disease.
- **Sotalol** One RCT found limited evidence that sotalol versus placebo significantly increased mortality within 1 year.

Cholesterol reduction

- **Cholesterol lowering drugs** Systematic reviews and large subsequent RCTs have found that lowering cholesterol in people at high risk of ischaemic coronary events substantially reduces the risk of overall mortality, cardiovascular mortality, and non-fatal cardiovascular events. One systematic review of primary and secondary prevention trials found that statins, in people also given dietary advice, were the only non-surgical treatment for cholesterol reduction to significantly reduce mortality. One systematic review found that the absolute benefits increase as baseline risk increases, but are not additionally influenced by the person's absolute cholesterol concentration.

Blood pressure reduction

- **Blood pressure lowering in people at high risk of ischaemic coronary events** We found no direct evidence of the effects of blood pressure lowering in people with established coronary heart disease. Observational studies, and extrapolation of primary prevention trials of blood pressure reduction, support the lowering of blood pressure in those at high risk of ischaemic coronary events. The evidence for benefit is strongest for β blockers, although not specifically in people with hypertension. The target blood pressure in these people is not clear. Angiotensin converting enzyme inhibitors, calcium channel blockers, and β blockers are discussed separately.

Non-drug treatments

- **Advice to eat less fat** RCTs found no strong evidence that low fat diets reduced mortality at 2 years.
- **β Carotene** Large RCTs found no evidence of benefit with β carotene, and one RCT found evidence of a significant increase in mortality. Four large RCTs of β carotene supplementation in primary prevention found no cardiovascular benefits, and two of the RCTs raised concerns about increased mortality.
- **Cardiac rehabilitation** One systematic review has found that cardiac rehabilitation including exercise reduces the risk of major cardiac events.
- **Eating more fish (particularly oily fish)** One RCT has found that advising people with coronary heart disease to eat more fish (particularly oily fish) significantly reduces mortality at 2 years (NNT 29, 95% CI 17 to 129). A second RCT found that fish oil capsules significantly reduced mortality at 3.5 years.
- **Exercise without cardiac rehabilitation** One systematic review has found that exercise alone versus usual care significantly reduces mortality.

Secondary prevention of ischaemic cardiac events

- **Mediterranean diet** One RCT has found that advising people with coronary artery disease to eat more bread, fruit, vegetables, and fish, and less meat, and to replace butter and cream with rapeseed margarine significantly reduces mortality at 27 months (NNT 26, 95% CI 14 to 299).
- **Psychosocial treatment** One systematic review of mainly poor quality RCTs found that psychological treatments versus usual treatment may decrease rates of myocardial infarction or cardiac death in people with coronary heart disease.
- **Smoking cessation** We found no RCTs of the effects of smoking cessation on cardiovascular events in people with coronary heart disease. Moderate evidence from epidemiological studies indicates that people with coronary heart disease who stop smoking, rapidly reduce their risk of recurrent coronary events or death. Treatment with nicotine patches seems safe in people with coronary heart disease.
- **Stress management** One systematic review of mainly poor quality RCTs found that stress management may decrease rates of myocardial infarction or cardiac death in people with coronary heart disease.
- **Vitamin C** Pooled analysis of three small RCTs found no evidence that vitamin C versus placebo provided any substantial benefit.
- **Vitamin E** Pooled analysis of four large RCTs found no evidence that vitamin E versus placebo given for 1.3–4.5 years altered cardiovascular events and all cause mortality.

Surgical treatments

- **Coronary artery bypass grafting versus coronary percutaneous transluminal angioplasty for multi vessel disease** One systematic review has found that coronary artery bypass grafting versus percutaneous transluminal angioplasty has no significant effect on death, myocardial infarction, or quality of life. Percutaneous transluminal angioplasty is less invasive but increased the number of repeat procedures.
- **Coronary artery bypass grafting versus medical treatment alone** One systematic review found that coronary artery bypass grafting reduced the risk of death from coronary artery disease at 5 and 10 years compared with medical treatment alone. Greater benefit occurred in people with poor left ventricular function. One subsequent RCT in people with asymptomatic disease found that revascularisation with coronary artery bypass grafting or coronary percutaneous transluminal angioplasty versus medical treatment alone reduced mortality at 2 years.
- **Coronary percutaneous transluminal angioplasty versus medical treatment alone** One systematic review found that coronary percutaneous transluminal angioplasty versus medical treatment alone improved angina, but was associated with a higher rate of coronary artery bypass grafting. The review found higher mortality and rates of myocardial infarction with percutaneous transluminal angioplasty versus medical treatment but the difference was not significant. RCTs have found that percutaneous transluminal angioplasty is associated with increased risk of emergency coronary artery bypass grafting and myocardial infarction during and soon after the procedure. One RCT found that percutaneous transluminal angioplasty reduced cardiac events and improved angina severity compared with medical treatment alone in people over the age of 75 years.

- **Intracoronary stents versus coronary percutaneous transluminal angioplasty alone** One systematic review found that intracoronary stents versus coronary percutaneous transluminal angioplasty alone significantly reduce the need for repeat vascularisation. It found no significant difference in mortality or myocardial infarction, but crossover rates from percutaneous transluminal angioplasty alone to stent were high. RCTs found that intracoronary stents improved outcomes after 4–9 months compared with percutaneous transluminal angioplasty alone in people with previous coronary artery bypass grafting, chronic total occlusions, and for treatment of restenosis after initial percutaneous transluminal angioplasty.

DEFINITION Secondary prevention in this context is the long term management of people with a prior acute myocardial infarction, and of people at high risk of ischaemic cardiac events for other reasons, such as a history of angina or coronary surgical procedures.

INCIDENCE/ PREVALENCE Coronary artery disease is the leading cause of mortality in developed countries and is becoming a major cause of morbidity and mortality in developing countries. There are pronounced international, regional, and temporal differences in death rates. In the USA, the prevalence of overt coronary artery disease approaches 4%.[1]

AETIOLOGY/ RISK FACTORS Most ischaemic cardiac events are associated with atheromatous plaques that can cause acute obstruction of coronary vessels. Atheroma is more likely in elderly people, in those with established coronary artery disease, and in those with risk factors (such as smoking, hypertension, high cholesterol, and diabetes mellitus).

PROGNOSIS Almost 50% of those who suffer an acute myocardial infarction die before they reach hospital. Of those admitted to hospital, 7–15% die in hospital and another 7–15% die during the following year. People who survive the acute stage of myocardial infarction fall into three prognostic groups, based on their baseline risk (see table 1, p 166);[2–4] high (20% of all survivors), moderate (55%), and low (25%) risk. Long term prognosis depends on the degree of left ventricular dysfunction, the presence of residual ischaemia, and the extent of any electrical instability. Further risk stratification procedures include assessment of left ventricular function (by echocardiography or nuclear ventriculography) and of myocardial ischaemia (by non-invasive stress testing).[4–8] Those with low left ventricular ejection fraction, ischaemia, or poor functional status can be assessed further by cardiac catheterisation.[9]

AIMS To improve long term survival and quality of life; to prevent (recurrent) myocardial infarction, unstable angina, left ventricular dysfunction, heart failure, and sudden cardiac death; and to restore and maintain normal activities.

OUTCOMES Mortality (total, cardiovascular, coronary, sudden death, non-cardiovascular); morbidity (myocardial infarction, severe angina, stroke); quality of life.

METHODS *Clinical Evidence* update search and appraisal March 2002.

QUESTION What are the effects of antithrombotic treatment?

Cathie Sudlow

OPTION ANY ORAL ANTIPLATELET TREATMENT

One systematic review has found that prolonged antiplatelet treatment reduces the risk of serious vascular events in people at high risk of ischaemic cardiac events.

Benefits: **Oral antiplatelet treatment versus no antiplatelet treatment:** We found one systematic review (search date 1997, 195 RCTs, > 140 000 high risk people) comparing an antiplatelet regimen (mostly aspirin) versus no antiplatelet treatment (including placebo).[10] It found that antiplatelet treatment reduced the odds of a serious vascular event (myocardial infarction, stroke, or vascular death) by 25% among all types of high risk people (OR 0.75, 95% CI 0.72 to 0.78), excluding those with acute ischaemic stroke (among whom the proportional benefits were smaller).[10] The proportional effects of antiplatelet treatment were similar regardless of whether the people were included on the basis of a prior or acute myocardial infarction, prior stroke or transient ischaemic attack, stable or unstable angina, peripheral arterial disease, atrial fibrillation, or other high risk condition. Most of these people were at high risk of ischaemic cardiac events, and some (including those with a history of myocardial infarction, those with stable angina, and those who had undergone coronary revascularisation procedures) were at particularly high risk. Among the 20 000 people with a prior myocardial infarction it was estimated that antiplatelet treatment prevented 18 non-fatal recurrent myocardial infarctions, five non-fatal strokes, and 14 vascular deaths per 1000 people treated for about 2 years. The review also found that antiplatelet treatment reduced the risk of all cause mortality (see figure 1, p 167).

Harms: **Oral antiplatelet treatment:** The most important adverse effect of antiplatelet treatment is haemorrhage, particularly intracranial haemorrhage because it is frequently fatal or disabling. The systematic review (search date 1997) found a proportional increase in the risk of intracranial haemorrhage of about a quarter (OR 1.22, 95% CI 1.03 to 1.44). However, the absolute excess risk was no more than one or two events per 1000 people a year.[10] Antiplatelet treatment was associated with about a 60% increased odds of extracranial haemorrhage (mainly from the gastrointestinal tract) (OR 1.6, 95% CI 1.4 to 1.8) corresponding to an absolute excess risk of about 1–2/1000 people treated a year with a prior myocardial infarction. Most of the extracranial haemorrhages were non-fatal.[10]

Comment: Among people at high risk of cardiac events, the large absolute reductions in serious vascular events associated with antiplatelet treatment far outweigh any absolute risks.

OPTION ASPIRIN

One systematic review has found that for prolonged use, aspirin 75–150 mg daily is as effective as higher doses, but found insufficient evidence that doses below 75 mg daily are as effective. It found no clear evidence that any alternative antiplatelet regimen is superior to aspirin in the long term secondary prevention of vascular events, but found that clopidogrel is at least as effective and as safe as aspirin.

Benefits: **Versus no aspirin:** We found one systematic review (search date 1997, 195 RCTs, > 140 000 high risk people) comparing an antiplatelet regimen versus no antiplatelet treatment (including placebo).[10] Aspirin was by far the most widely studied antiplatelet drug in the systematic review. Among almost 60 000 people, excluding those with acute ischaemic stroke, aspirin reduced the odds of a serious vascular event by about a quarter compared with control (OR 0.77, 95% CI 0.73 to 0.81).[10] **Different daily doses:** Direct comparisons (3197 high risk people) between daily doses of 500–1500 mg versus 75–325 mg found no significant difference in effect (OR higher versus lower dose 0.97, 95% CI 0.79 to 1.19).[10] A subsequent RCT (2849 high risk people) compared four doses of aspirin, two lower doses (81 or 325 mg/day), and two higher doses (650 or 1300 mg/day). It found that the combined rate of myocardial infarction, stroke, or death was slightly lower in the lower dose than in the higher dose groups at 3 months (AR 6.2% with lower doses *v* 8.4% with higher doses; P = 0.03).[11] Direct comparisons (3570 people in the review) between daily doses greater than or equal to 75 mg and less than 75 mg daily found no significant difference, but the confidence intervals included a potentially clinically important difference (OR higher *v* lower doses 1.08, 95% CI 0.90 to 1.31).[10] Indirect comparisons of trials in the review comparing different daily aspirin doses versus control among people at high risk (excluding those with acute ischaemic stroke) found similar reductions in serious vascular events for the higher daily doses 500–1500 mg daily (OR 0.81, 95% CI 0.75 to 0.87), 160–325 mg daily (OR 0.74, 95% CI 0.69 to 0.80), 75–150 mg daily (OR 0.68, 95% CI 0.59 to 0.79), but somewhat smaller effect with less than 75 mg daily (OR 0.87, 95% CI 0.74 to 1.03)(see figure 2, p 168).[10] **Versus or with thienopyridines:** See benefits of thienopyridines, p 136. **Versus or with anticoagulants:** See benefits of oral anticoagulants in absence of antiplatelet treatment, p 138. See benefits of oral anticoagulants in addition to antiplatelet treatment, p 138.

Harms: **Intracranial haemorrhage:** A systematic review of aspirin versus control for at least 1 month found that aspirin produced a small increased risk of intracranial haemorrhage of about 1/1000 (0.1%) people treated for 3 years.[12] There was no clear variation in risk with the dose of aspirin used. In RCTs directly comparing different daily doses there was no significant difference in the risk of intracranial haemorrhage, but the number of events was small and the confidence intervals wide.[11,13,14] Two observational studies (1 case control and 1 cohort study) found a dose dependent association between aspirin and intracranial haemorrhage, but the methods of these studies prevent firm conclusions being drawn.[15,16] **Extracranial haemorrhage:** The systematic review (search date 1997) found that aspirin slightly increased the risk of major extracranial haemorrhage, similar to the risk for antiplatelet treatment in general (see harms of antiplatelet treatment, p 134). It found that the risk of major extracranial haemorrhage was similar with different daily doses (numerical results not presented).[10] **Gastrointestinal haemorrhage:** A systematic review (search date 1999) of aspirin versus control found an increased risk of gastrointestinal haemorrhage with aspirin (OR 1.68, 95% CI 1.51 to 1.88), with no definite variation in risk between doses or different formulations.[17] RCTs directly comparing different doses of aspirin found a trend towards more gastrointestinal haemorrhages with high (500–1500 mg/day) versus medium (75–325 mg/day) doses (OR 1.7, 95% CI 0.9 to 2.1), but no difference between medium (283 mg/day) and low (30 mg/day) doses (OR 1.2, 95% CI 0.7 to 2.0).[11,13,14] A recent overview of 15 observational studies including over 10 000 cases of upper gastrointestinal haemorrhage or perforation requiring admission to hospital, found a more than doubled increased risk with aspirin (RR 2.5, 95% CI 2.4 to 2.7).[18] Restricting the analysis to prospective studies gave a lower risk (RR 1.9, 95% CI 1.7 to 2.1), similar to that found in the RCTs.[17,18] **Upper gastrointestinal symptoms:** RCTs directly comparing different doses of aspirin found that high dose (500–1500 mg/day) significantly increased the odds of upper gastrointestinal symptoms compared with medium dose (75–325 mg/day; OR 1.3, 95% CI 1.1 to 1.5),[11,13] and that medium dose (283 mg/day) aspirin was associated with non-significantly higher odds of upper gastrointestinal upset compared with low dose (30 mg/day) (OR 1.1, 95% CI 0.9 to 1.4).[14]

Comment: Among people at high risk of cardiac events, the large absolute reductions in serious vascular events associated with aspirin far outweigh any absolute risks.

OPTION THIENOPYRIDINES (CLOPIDOGREL OR TICLOPIDINE)

One RCT has found that clopidogrel is at least as effective at preventing vascular events and is at least as safe as aspirin in people with a history of cardiovascular disease.

Benefits: **Versus aspirin:** One RCT (19 185 people with a history of myocardial infarction, stroke, or peripheral arterial disease) compared clopidogrel (75 mg/day) versus aspirin (325 mg/day).[19] It found that clopidogrel reduced the odds of a serious vascular event by 10% (OR 0.9, 95% CI 0.82 to 0.99). One systematic review found similar, but non-significant results for ticlopidine (a thienopyridine similar to clopidogrel) versus aspirin (4 RCTs, 3791 high risk people, RR 0.88, 95% CI 0.75 to 1.03).[10] We found one subsequent RCT comparing ticlopidine versus aspirin.[20] It found a non-significant lower risk of a vascular event (OR 0.69, 95% 0.31 to 1.48). A separate systematic review comparing ticlopidine or clopidogrel versus aspirin (search date 1999, 4 RCTs, 22 656 people at high risk of vascular disease, most of whom were included in the trial comparing clopidogrel with aspirin[20]) found that ticlopidine or clopidogrel reduced the odds of a vascular event compared with aspirin (OR 0.91, 95% CI 0.84 to 0.98).[21] However, there was substantial uncertainty about the absolute size of any additional benefit (average 11 events prevented/1000 people treated for 2 years, 95% CI 2 to 19). **Thienopyridines plus aspirin versus aspirin alone:** We found no completed long term trials of the effects of adding clopidogrel to aspirin among people at high risk of occlusive arterial disease but without an acute cardiovascular event. We found one RCT in people with acute coronary syndromes (see comment below).

Harms: One systematic review of randomised trials of the thienopyridine derivatives versus aspirin found that the thienopyridines produced significantly less gastrointestinal haemorrhage and upper gastrointestinal upset than aspirin.[21] However, the odds of skin rash and diarrhoea were doubled with ticlopidine and increased by about a third with clopidogrel. Ticlopidine (but not clopidogrel) increased the odds of neutropenia. Observational studies have also found that ticlopidine is associated with thrombocytopenia and thrombotic thrombocytopenic purpura.[22,23] However, we found no clear evidence of an excess of haematological adverse effects with clopidogrel.[24,25] Three RCTs (about 2700 people undergoing coronary artery stenting) of clopidogrel plus aspirin versus ticlopidine plus aspirin suggested better safety and tolerability with clopidogrel versus ticlopidine.[26–28]

Comment: One RCT (about 12 500 people within 24 h of onset of an acute coronary syndrome without ST segment elevation) compared clopidogrel plus aspirin versus placebo plus aspirin.[29] After 3–12 months' treatment, it found that adding clopidogrel to aspirin significantly reduced the risk of a major vascular event (RR 0.88, 95% CI 0.72 to 0.90).[29] See antiplatelets under unstable angina, p 225. The trial found that combined treatment increased risk of major haemorrhages (mainly gastrointestinal) and bleeding at sites of arterial punctures (RR 1.38, 95% CI 1.13 to 1.67), but did not increase intracranial, life-threatening, or fatal haemorrhages compared with aspirin alone.[29] An RCT of the effects of adding clopidogrel to aspirin in people with acute myocardial infarction is under way.[30]

OPTION ORAL GLYCOPROTEIN IIB/IIIA RECEPTOR INHIBITORS New

One systematic review in people with acute coronary syndromes or undergoing percutaneous coronary interventions has found that oral glycoprotein IIb/IIIa receptor inhibitors versus placebo increase risk of mortality and bleeding.

Benefits: One systematic review in people with acute coronary syndrome or undergoing percutaneous coronary intervention (search date 2000, 4 RCTs, 33 326 people) found that oral glycoprotein IIb/IIIa receptor inhibitors versus placebo increased mortality but did not significantly affect the risk of myocardial infarction after 3–10 months (mortality: pooled OR 1.37, 95% CI 1.13 to 1.66; myocardial infarction: pooled OR 1.04, 95% CI 0.93 to 1.16).[31]

Harms: The review found that oral glycoprotein IIb/IIIa receptor inhibitors increased all cause mortality and major bleeding compared with placebo. One subsequent RCT (9200 people with a recent myocardial infarction, unstable angina, ischaemic stroke/transient ischaemic attack, or peripheral arterial disease) assessing the effects of adding an oral glycoprotein IIb/IIIa receptor inhibitor to aspirin was stopped early because of safety concerns.[32]

Comment: None.

OPTION ORAL ANTICOAGULANTS IN THE ABSENCE OF ANTIPLATELET TREATMENT

One systematic review has found that high or moderate intensity oral anticoagulants given alone reduce the risk of serious vascular events in people with coronary artery disease, but are associated with substantial risks of haemorrhage. Oral anticoagulants require regular monitoring for intensity of anticoagulant effect.

Benefits: We found one systematic review (search date 1999) of the effects of oral anticoagulation in people with coronary artery disease.[33] It identified 16 RCTs of high intensity anticoagulation (international normalised ratio [see glossary, p 161] > 2.8) versus control (either no anticoagulation or placebo) in 10 056 people, and four RCTs of moderate intensity anticoagulation (INR 2–3) versus control in 1365 people. Antiplatelet treatment was not routinely given in any of these 20 trials. The review found that high intensity anticoagulation reduced the odds of the combined outcome of mortality, myocardial infarction, or stroke compared with control (OR 0.57, 95% CI 0.51 to 0.63; about 98 events avoided/1000 people treated). Compared with control, moderate intensity anticoagulation was associated with a smaller non-significant reduction.[33] In direct comparisons of high or moderate intensity oral anticoagulation with aspirin, the effects on mortality, myocardial infarction, or stroke were similar (OR 1.04, 95% CI 0.80 to 1.34).[33]

Harms: Compared with control, high intensity anticoagulation increased the odds of major (mainly extracranial) haemorrhage by about sixfold (OR 6.0, 95% CI 4.4 to 8.2; absolute increase of 39 events/1000 people treated), and moderate intensity anticoagulation also increased the odds of major haemorrhage by about eightfold (OR 7.7, 95% CI 3.3 to 17.6).[33] Compared with aspirin, high or moderate intensity oral anticoagulation increased the odds of major haemorrhage more than twofold (OR 2.4, 95% CI 1.6 to 3.6).[33]

Comment: Oral anticoagulants provide substantial protection against vascular events in the absence of antiplatelet treatment, but the risks of serious haemorrhage are higher than for antiplatelet treatment and regular monitoring is required. Aspirin provides similar protection, but is safer and easier to use (see harms under antiplatelet treatment, p 134).

OPTION ORAL ANTICOAGULANTS IN ADDITION TO ANTIPLATELET TREATMENT

One systematic review found no evidence that the addition of low intensity oral anticoagulation (target international normalised ratio < 1.5) to aspirin reduced mortality, myocardial infarction, and stroke. One

systematic review and subsequent RCTs found that adding moderate intensity oral anticoagulation (target international normalised ratio 1.5–3.0) to aspirin did not reduce the risk of recurrent cardiovascular events or mortality compared with aspirin alone, although it increased the risk of major haemorrhage.

Benefits: We found one systematic review (search date 1999, 6 RCTs, 8915 people with coronary artery disease) of adding an oral anticoagulant regimen to aspirin.[33] Three of these RCTs assessed the addition of a low intensity (target international normalised ratio [see glossary, p 161] < 1.5) regimen to aspirin in a total of 8435 people, and found no significant reduction in the odds of mortality, myocardial infarction, or stroke (OR 0.91, 95% CI 0.79 to 1.06).[33] Trials assessing the addition of a moderate intensity (INR 2–3) oral anticoagulant regimen to aspirin were too small (480 people) to produce reliable estimates of efficacy and safety.[33] We found one subsequent RCT (3712 people with unstable angina) of 5 months' oral anticoagulant treatment (target INR 2.0–2.5) plus standard treatment (usually including aspirin) versus standard treatment alone.[34] When this trial was included in a meta-analysis with the previous trials assessing the addition of moderate intensity oral anticoagulation to aspirin, oral anticoagulation was associated with a non-significant reduction in mortality, myocardial infarction, or stroke (OR 0.83; 95% CI 0.66 to 1.03).[33] We found one subsequent unblinded RCT (5059 people with myocardial infarction in the previous 14 days), that compared warfarin (target INR 1.5–2.5) plus aspirin (81 mg/day) versus aspirin alone (162 mg/day).[35] It found no significant differences between treatments in mortality, recurrent myocardial infarction, or stroke after a median of 2.7 years (mortality 17.6% with warfarin plus aspirin *v* 17.3% with aspirin alone, P = 0.8; AR for recurrent myocardial infarction 13.3% with warfarin plus aspirin *v* 13.1% with aspirin alone, P = 0.8; AR for stroke 3.1% with warfarin plus aspirin *v* 3.5% with aspirin alone, P = 0.5).

Harms: The systematic review found a non-significant excess of major haemorrhage with the addition of low intensity oral anticoagulation to aspirin (OR 1.29, 95% CI 0.96 to 1.75).[33] An updated meta-analysis assessing the addition of moderate intensity oral anticoagulation to aspirin included the RCTs from the systematic review[33] and one subsequent trial[34] (total of 4192 people with coronary artery disease). It found a clear excess of major haemorrhage in people allocated oral anticoagulation (OR 1.95, 95% CI 1.27 to 2.98).[34] One of the more recent RCTs (5059 people) examining the addition to aspirin of moderate intensity anticoagulation also found that combined treatment increased risk of major haemorrhage (RR 1.78, 95% CI 1.27 to 2.72).[35]

Comment: The issue of whether adding a moderately intense oral anticoagulant regimen to aspirin provides additional net benefit to people at high risk of ischaemic cardiac events is being assessed in several ongoing RCTs. One RCT (135 people with unstable angina or non-ST segment myocardial infarction, with prior coronary artery bypass grafting) compared three treatments: aspirin alone (80 mg/day) plus placebo; warfarin (target INR 2.0–2.5) plus placebo, and aspirin plus warfarin.[36] It found no significant difference among treatments for rates of primary end point (death or myocardial infarction or unstable angina requiring admission to hospital at 1 year; AR 14.6% with warfarin alone *v* 11.5% with aspirin alone *v* 11.3% with combination, P = 0.76).[36] However, it found no significant difference for major haemorrhage among people taking warfarin compared with those who were not. Event rates were low and the study may have lacked power to detect a clinically important difference for adverse effects.[36]

QUESTION What are the effects of other drug treatments?

Eva Lonn

OPTION β BLOCKERS

Systematic reviews have found strong evidence that β blockers reduce the risk of all cause mortality, coronary mortality, recurrent non-fatal myocardial infarction, and sudden death in people after myocardial infarction. Most benefit was seen in those at highest risk of mortality after a myocardial infarction (> 50 years old; previous myocardial infarction, angina pectoris, hypertension, or treatment with digitalis; transient mechanical or electrical failure; higher heart rate at study entry). About 25% of people suffered adverse effects.

Benefits: **Survival and reinfarction:** One systematic review (search date 1993, 26 RCTs, > 24 000 people) compared oral β blockers versus placebo within days or weeks of an acute myocardial infarction (late intervention trials) and continued for between 6 weeks to 3 years.[37] Most RCTs followed people for 1 year. The review found improved survival in people given β blockers (RR 0.77, 95% CI 0.70 to 0.86).[37] One prior systematic review (search date not stated, 24 RCTs) found that long term use of β blockers versus placebo after myocardial infarction reduced total mortality (RR about 0.80; NNT 48), sudden death (RR about 0.70; NNT 63), and non-fatal reinfarction (RR about 0.75; NNT 56).[38] **Anginal symptoms:** We found no good RCTs assessing the antianginal effects of β blockers in people after myocardial infarction. One trial found atenolol more effective than placebo in people with chronic stable effort angina or silent ischaemia.[39] **Different types of β blockers:** The earlier review found no differences between β blockers with and without cardioselectivity or membrane stabilising properties, but it raised concerns about the lack of efficacy of β blockers with intrinsic sympathomimetic activity in long term management after myocardial infarction.[38] One RCT (607 people after myocardial infarction) found that acebutolol, a β blocker with moderate partial agonist activity, decreased 1 year mortality compared with placebo (AR of death: 11% with placebo *v* 6% with acebutolol; RR 0.52, 95% CI 0.29 to 0.91).[40] **Effects in different subgroups:** One systematic review (search date 1983, 9 RCTs) compared β blockers versus placebo started more than 24 hours after onset of symptoms of acute myocardial infarction and continued for 9–24 months.[41] Pooled analysis of individual data (13 679 people) found that the benefits of β blockers versus placebo on mortality seemed comparable in men and women. The highest absolute benefit from β blockers was found in subgroups with the highest baseline risks (i.e. those with the highest mortality on placebo), those over 50 years of age; those with a history of previous myocardial infarction, angina pectoris, hypertension, or treatment with digitalis; those with transient signs or symptoms of mechanical or electrical failure in the early phases of myocardial infarction; and those with a higher heart rate at study entry. Low risk subgroups had smaller mean absolute benefit.

Harms: Adverse effects include shortness of breath, bronchospasm, bradycardia, hypotension, heart block, cold hands and feet, diarrhoea, fatigue, reduced sexual activity, depression, nightmares, faintness, insomnia, syncope, and hallucinations. Rates vary in different studies. One RCT reported an absolute risk increase for any adverse effect on propranolol compared with placebo of 24% (no CI available; NNH 4). Serious adverse effects were uncommon and only a small proportion of people withdrew from the study as a result.[42]

Comment: Continued benefit from β blockers has been reported up to 6 years after myocardial infarction (ARR for mortality: 5.9%, P = 0.003; RR 0.82, no CI available). However, the study was not blinded after 33 months.

OPTION ANGIOTENSIN CONVERTING ENZYME INHIBITORS

One systematic review has found that in people who have had a myocardial infarction and have left ventricular dysfunction, angiotensin converting enzyme inhibitors versus placebo reduce mortality, admission to hospital for congestive heart failure, and recurrent non-fatal myocardial infarction. One large RCT in people without left ventricular dysfunction found that ramipril versus placebo reduced cardiovascular death, stroke, and myocardial infarction.

Benefits: **In people with left ventricular dysfunction:** One systematic review (search date not stated, 3 RCTs, 5966 people)[43] compared angiotensin converting enzyme (ACE) inhibitors (captopril, ramipril, or trandolapril) versus placebo started 3–16 days after acute myocardial infarction and continued for 15–42 months. It analysed individual data from 5966 people with a recent myocardial infarction and with clinical manifestations of congestive heart failure or moderate left ventricular dysfunction (left ventricular ejection fraction ≥ 35–40%). ACE inhibitors versus placebo significantly reduced mortality (702/2995 [23.4%] with ACE *v* 866/2971 [29.1%] with control; OR 0.74, 95% CI 0.66 to 0.83; NNT 17 people treated for about 2 years to prevent 1 death, CI not provided), admission to hospital for congestive heart failure (355/2995 [11.9%] with ACE *v* 460/2971 [15.5%] with control; OR 0.73, 95% CI 0.63 to 0.85; NNT 28, CI not available), and recurrent non-fatal myocardial infarction (324/2995 [10.8%] with ACE *v* 391/2971 [13.1%] with control; OR 0.80, 95% CI 0.69 to 0.94; NNT 43, CI not available). **In people without impaired ventricular function or evidence of congestive heart failure:** We found no systematic review but found one large RCT (9297 people at high risk of cardiovascular events).[44] It found that ramipril (10 mg/day) versus placebo reduced the composite primary outcome of cardiovascular death, myocardial infarction, or stroke over an average of 4.7 years (RR for composite outcome: 0.78, 95% CI 0.70 to 0.86, NNT 27, 95% CI 20 to 45; RR for cardiovascular death: 0.74, 95% CI 0.64 to 0.87, NNT 50, CI not available; RR for myocardial infarction: 0.80, 95% CI 0.70 to 0.90, NNT 42, CI not available; RR for stroke: 0.68, 95% CI 0.56 to 0.84, NNT 67, CI not available; RR for death from all causes: 0.84, 95% CI 0.75 to 0.95, NNT 56, CI not available). The RCT found that ramipril reduced the need for revascularisation procedures and reduced heart failure related outcomes (need for revascularisation: RR 0.85, no CI available; heart failure related outcomes: RR 0.77, no CI available). Ramipril versus placebo produced benefit in all subgroups examined, including women and men; people aged over and under 65 years; those with and without a history of coronary artery disease, hypertension, diabetes, peripheral vascular disease, cerebrovascular disease, and those with and without microalbuminuria at study entry.[44] **In people with diabetes:** See antihypertensive treatment under cardiovascular disease in diabetes, p 541.[45]

Harms: The major adverse effects reported in these trials were cough (ARI 5–10% with ACE inhibitors *v* placebo), dizziness, hypotension (ARI with 5–10% ACE inhibitors *v* placebo), renal failure (ARI < 3% with ACE inhibitors *v* placebo), hyperkalaemia (ARI < 3% with ACE inhibitors *v* placebo), angina, syncope, diarrhoea (ARI 2% with ACE inhibitors *v* placebo), and, for captopril, alteration in taste (2% of captopril users).[43]

Comment: There are several other ongoing large RCTs assessing ACE inhibitors in people without clinical manifestations of heart failure and with no or with mild impairment in left ventricular systolic function. These include one trial of trandolapril in 8000 people with coronary artery disease, and one trial of perindopril in 10 500 people with stable coronary artery disease.[46]

OPTION **CLASS I ANTIARRHYTHMIC AGENTS (QUINIDINE, PROCAINAMIDE, DISOPYRIMIDE, ENCAINIDE, FLECAINIDE, AND MORACIZINE)**

One systematic review has found that class I antiarrhythmic agents after myocardial infarction increase the risk of cardiovascular mortality and sudden death.

Benefits: None (see harms below).

Harms: One systematic review (search date 1993, 51 RCTs, 23 229 people) compared class I antiarrhythmic drugs versus placebo given acutely and later in the management of myocardial infarction.[37] The review found that the antiarrhythmic agents increased mortality (AR of death 5.6% with class I antiarrhythmic *v* 5.0% with placebo; OR 1.14, 95% CI 1.01 to 1.28). One RCT (1498 people with myocardial infarction and asymptomatic or mildly symptomatic ventricular arrhythmia) found that encainide or flecainide versus placebo increased the risk of death or cardiac arrest after 10 months (RR 2.38, 95% CI 1.59 to 3.57; NNH 17).[47]

Comment: The evidence implies that class I antiarrhythmic drugs should not be used in people after myocardial infarction or with significant coronary artery disease.

OPTION CLASS III ANTIARRHYTHMIC AGENTS (AMIODARONE, SOTALOL)

Systematic reviews have found that amiodarone versus placebo reduces the risk of sudden death and marginally reduces mortality in people at high risk of death after myocardial infarction. One RCT found limited evidence that sotalol versus placebo significantly increased mortality within 1 year.

Benefits: **Amiodarone:** We found two systematic reviews.[48,49] The first systematic review (search date not stated, individual data from 6553 high risk people in 13 RCTs) compared amiodarone versus control treatments.[48] People were selected with a recent myocardial infarction and a high risk of death from cardiac arrhythmia (based on low left ventricular ejection fraction, frequent ventricular premature depolarisation, or non-sustained ventricular tachycardia, but no history of sustained symptomatic ventricular tachycardia or ventricular fibrillation); 78% of people from eight RCTs had a recent myocardial infarction, and 22% of people from five RCTs had congestive heart failure.[48] Most trials were placebo controlled with a mean follow up of about 1.5 years. The people with congestive heart failure were symptomatic but stable and did not have a recent myocardial infarction, although in most cases the heart failure was ischaemic in origin. All RCTs used a loading dose of amiodarone (400 mg/day for 28 days or 800 mg/day for 14 days) followed by a maintenance dose (200–400 mg/day). Amiodarone versus placebo significantly reduced total mortality (AR for total mortality: 10.9% a year with amiodarone *v* 12.3% a year with placebo; RR 0.87, 95% CI 0.78 to 0.99; NNT 71 a year to avoid 1 additional death) and rates of sudden cardiac death (RR 0.71, 95% CI 0.59 to 0.85; NNT 59). Amiodarone had similar effects in the studies after myocardial infarction and congestive heart failure. The second systematic review (search date 1997, 5864 people with myocardial infarction, congestive heart failure, left ventricular dysfunction, or cardiac arrest) found similar results.[49] **Sotalol:** We found one RCT (3121 people with myocardial infarction and left ventricular dysfunction), which found increased mortality with the class III antiarrhythmic agent sotalol versus placebo (AR for death: 5.0% with sotalol *v* 3.1% with placebo; RR 1.65, 95% CI 1.15 to 2.36). The trial was terminated prematurely after less than 1 year.[50]

Harms: Adverse events leading to discontinuation of amiodarone were hypothyroidism (expressed as events per 100 person-years: 7.0 with amiodarone *v* 1.1 with placebo; OR 7.3), hyperthyroidism (1.4 with amiodarone *v* 0.5 with placebo; OR 2.5), peripheral neuropathy (0.5 with amiodarone *v* 0.2 with placebo; OR 2.8), lung infiltrates (1.6 with amiodarone *v* 0.5 with placebo; OR 3.1), bradycardia (2.4 with amiodarone *v* 0.8 with placebo; OR 2.6), and liver dysfunction (1.0 with amiodarone *v* 0.4 with placebo; OR 2.7).[48]

Comment: The conclusions of the review are probably specific to amiodarone.[48,49] The two largest RCTs of amiodarone after myocardial infarction found a favourable interaction between β blockers and amiodarone, with additional reduction in cardiac mortality.[51,52]

OPTION CALCIUM CHANNEL BLOCKERS

One systematic review found no benefit from calcium channel blockers in people after myocardial infarction or with chronic coronary heart disease. Diltiazem and verapamil may reduce rates of reinfarction and refractory angina in people after myocardial infarction who do not have heart failure. The review found non-significantly higher mortality with dihydropyridines compared with placebo.

Benefits: One systematic review (search date 1993, 24 RCTs) compared calcium channel blockers (including dihydropyridines, diltiazem, and verapamil) versus placebo given early or late during the course of acute myocardial infarction or unstable angina and continued in the intermediate or long term.[37] Two of the RCTs used angiographic regression of coronary stenosis as an outcome in people with stable coronary heart disease treated with calcium channel blockers. The review found no significant difference in the absolute risk of death compared with placebo (AR 9.7% with calcium channel blockers *v* 9.3% with placebo; ARI with calcium channel blockers versus placebo +0.4%, 95% CI –0.4% to +1.2%; OR 1.04, 95% CI 0.95 to 1.14). **Diltiazem and verapamil:** The review found no significant effect compared with placebo (OR 0.95, 95% CI 0.82 to 1.09).[37] Three RCTs comparing diltiazem or verapamil versus placebo found decreased rates of recurrent infarction and refractory angina with active treatment but only for those people without signs or symptoms of heart failure. For those with clinical manifestations of heart failure, the trends were towards harm.[53–55] **Dihydropyridines:** The review found non-significantly higher mortality with dihydropyridines compared with placebo (OR 1.16, 95% CI 0.99 to 1.35). Several individual RCTs of dihydropyridines found increased mortality, particularly when these agents were started early in the course of acute myocardial infarction and in the absence of β blockers.

Harms: Adverse effects reported of verapamil and diltiazem include atrioventricular block, atrial bradycardia, new onset heart failure, hypotension, dizziness, oedema, rash, constipation, and pruritus.

Comment: We found little good evidence on newer generation dihydropyridines, such as amlodipine and felodipine, in people after myocardial infarction but these have been found to be safe in people with heart failure, including heart failure of ischaemic origin.

OPTION HORMONE REPLACEMENT THERAPY

One large, well designed RCT of hormone replacement therapy versus placebo found no reduction of major cardiovascular events in postmenopausal women with established coronary artery disease, despite evidence from RCTs that hormone replacement therapy improves some cardiovascular risk factors.

Benefits: **Combined oestrogen and progestins:** We found no systematic review. One large RCT (2763 postmenopausal women with coronary heart disease) found that conjugated equine oestrogen (0.625 mg/day) plus medroxyprogesterone acetate (2.5 mg/day) versus placebo for an average of 4.1 years produced no significant difference in the risk of non-fatal myocardial infarction or deaths caused by coronary heart disease (172/1380 [12.5%] with hormone replacement therapy *v* 176/1383 [12.7%] with placebo; ARR +0.3%, 95% CI −2.2% to +2.7%; RR 0.98, 95% CI 0.80 to 1.19).[56] It also found no significant difference in secondary cardiovascular outcomes (coronary revascularisation, unstable angina, congestive heart failure, resuscitated cardiac arrest, stroke or transient ischaemic attack, and peripheral arterial disease) or in all cause mortality. **Oestrogen alone:** We found no good RCTs of oestrogen alone in the secondary prevention of coronary heart disease in postmenopausal women. One RCT found that high dose oestrogen (5 mg/day conjugated equine oestrogen) increased the risk of myocardial infarction and thromboembolic events in men with pre-existing coronary heart disease.[57]

Harms: Pooled estimates from observational studies found an increased risk of endometrial cancer (RR > 8) and of breast cancer (RR 1.25–1.46) when oestrogen was used for more than 8 years. In most observational studies, the addition of progestins prevented endometrial cancer but not breast cancer. The risk of venous thromboembolism, including pulmonary embolism and deep vein thrombosis, was three to four times higher with hormone replacement therapy than without. However, because the incidence of venous thromboembolism is low in postmenopausal women, the absolute increase in risk was only about one to two additional cases of venous thromboembolism in 5000 users a year.[58] In one RCT,[56] more women in the HRT group than in the placebo group experienced venous thromboembolism (34/1380 [2.5%] with HRT *v* 12/1383 [0.9%] with placebo; OR 2.65, 95% CI 1.48 to 4.75) and gall bladder disease (84/1380 [6.1%] with HRT *v* 62/1383 [4.5%] with placebo; OR 1.38, 95% CI 0.99 to 1.92).

Comment: Many observational studies have found reduced rates of clinical events caused by coronary heart disease in postmenopausal women using HRT, especially in women with pre-existing coronary heart disease. Hormone users experienced 35–80% fewer recurrent events than non-users.[59,60] Several RCTs have found that HRT improves cardiovascular risk factors.[61] It is not known whether studies longer than 4 years would show a benefit.

QUESTION What are the effects of cholesterol reduction?

Michael Pignone

Systematic reviews and large subsequent RCTs have found that lowering cholesterol in people at high risk of ischaemic coronary events substantially reduces overall mortality, cardiovascular mortality, and non-fatal cardiovascular events. One systematic review of primary and secondary prevention trials found that statins, in people also given dietary advice, were the only non-surgical treatment for cholesterol reduction to significantly reduce mortality. One systematic review found that the absolute benefits increase as baseline risk increases, but are not additionally influenced by the person's absolute cholesterol concentration.

Benefits: **All cholesterol treatments:** We found one systematic review (search date 1996, 59 RCTs, 173 160 people), which did not differentiate primary and secondary prevention, and included RCTs of any cholesterol lowering intervention, irrespective of duration, as long as mortality data were reported.[62] It included drug treatments (statins, n–3 fatty acids, fibrates, resins, hormones, or niacin), dietary intervention alone, or surgery (ileal bypass) alone. Overall, baseline risk was similar among all intervention groups. Among non-surgical treatments, the review found that only statins reduced coronary heart disease mortality, and that only statins and n–3 fatty acids significantly reduced all cause mortality (RR of coronary heart disease mortality: statins *v* control 0.69, 95% CI 0.59 to 0.80; n–3 fatty acids *v* control 0.44, 95% CI 0.18 to 1.07; fibrates *v* control 0.98, 95% CI 0.78 to 1.24; resins *v* control 0.71, 95% CI 0.51 to 0.99; hormones *v* control 1.04, 95% CI 0.93 to 1.17; niacin *v* control 0.95, 95% CI 0.83 to 1.10; diet *v* control 0.91, 95% CI 0.82 to 1.01. RR of all cause mortality: statins *v* control 0.79, 95% CI 0.71 to 0.89; n–3 fatty acids *v* control 0.68, 95% CI 0.53 to 0.88; fibrates *v* control 1.06, 95% CI 0.78 to 1.46; resins *v* control 0.85, 95% CI 0.66 to 1.08; hormone *v* control 1.09, 95% CI 1.00 to 1.20; niacin *v* control 0.96, 95% CI 0.86 to 1.08; diet *v* control 0.97, 95% CI 0.81 to 1.15).[62] **Statins:** We found one systematic review (search date 1998, 5 RCTs, 30 817 people) that compared long term (≥ 4 years) treatment with statins versus placebo.[63] Combining the three secondary prevention trials, the review found that statins reduced coronary heart disease mortality, cardiovascular mortality, and all cause mortality compared with placebo over a mean of 5.4 years (coronary heart disease mortality: OR 0.71, 95% CI 0.63 to 0.80; cardiovascular mortality: OR 0.73, 95% CI 0.66 to 0.82; all cause mortality: OR 0.77, 95% CI 0.70 to 0.85). One subsequent RCT (20 536 adults with total cholesterol > 3.5 mmol/L [an inclusion threshold lower than previous statin trials], including > 5000 women and > 5000 people over 70 years of age) compared simvastatin (40 mg) versus placebo. The study included both primary and secondary prevention populations.[64] After a mean of 5.5 years follow up, simvastatin reduced total mortality and major vascular events compared with placebo (all cause mortality: 12.9% with simvastatin *v* 14.7% with placebo, RR 0.87, 95% CI 0.81 to 0.94; major vascular events 19.8% with simvastatin *v* 25.2% with placebo, RR 0.76, 95% CI 0.72 to 0.81). **Effects of statins in different groups of people:** Combining results from primary and secondary prevention trials, the review found that, compared with placebo, statins reduced coronary events by a similar proportion in men (OR 0.69, 95% CI 0.65 to 0.74; ARR 3.7%, 95% CI 2.9% to 4.4%), in women (OR 0.71, 95% CI 0.64 to 0.76; ARR 3.3%, 95% CI 1.3% to 5.2%), in people under 65 years (OR 0.69, 95% CI 0.64 to 0.76; ARR 3.2%, 95% CI 2.4% to 4.0%), and in people over 65 years (OR 0.68, 95% CI 0.61 to 0.77; ARR 4.4%, 95% CI 3.0% to 5.8%). The reduction of coronary heart disease events in women involved more non-fatal and fewer fatal events than in men. One large RCT found no significant difference in mortality with statins versus placebo for the subgroup of women, but the confidence interval was wide (28/407 [6.9%] with simvastatin *v* 25/420 [6.0%], RR 1.16, 95% CI 0.68 to 1.99).[65] One recent RCT that was not included in the review found that relative risk reductions were similar for people with initial total cholesterol levels of under 5.0 mmol/L compared with people with levels over 5.0 mmol/L and for women and the elderly compared with younger men.[64] One RCT compared early initiation of atorvastatin (80 mg/day started 1–4 days after admission) versus placebo in people with unstable angina or non-Q wave myocardial infarction.[66] After 3 months, it found no significant difference between treatments for coronary event rates, although atorvastatin reduced readmission rate for recurrent ischaemia compared with placebo (AR for readmission for ischaemia: 6.2% with atorvastatin *v* 8.4% with placebo, RR 0.74, 95% CI 0.57 to 0.95). **Intensity of statin treatment:** We found one RCT (1351 people with a history of saphenous vein coronary artery bypass grafting) that compared aggressive reduction of cholesterol with lovastatin and, if necessary, colestyramone (cholestyramine) (aiming for target low density lipoprotein cholesterol 1.6–2.2 mmol/L [60–85 mg/dL]) with more moderate reduction (target low density lipoprotein cholesterol 3.4–3.7 mmol/L [130–140 mg/dL]) with the same drugs.[67] The trial found that aggressive treatment reduced the risk of needing repeat revascularisation at 4 years (6.5% with aggressive treatment *v* 9.2% with moderate treatment, $P = 0.03$). After an additional 3 years, aggressive treatment reduced the risk of revascularisation and cardiovascular death compared with moderate treatment (AR of revascularisation 19% with aggressive treatment *v* 27% with moderate treatment, $P = 0.0006$; AR for cardiovascular death, 7.4% with aggressive treatment *v* 11.3% with moderate treatment, $P = 0.03$).[67] **Fibrates:** We found one systematic review (search date not stated, 4 RCTs)[68] and two additional RCTs.[69,70] The systematic review compared fibrates versus placebo in people with known coronary heart disease. The review identified one RCT (2531 men with coronary heart disease and a level of high density lipoprotein cholesterol > 1 mmol/L) that found gemfibrozil versus placebo reduced the composite outcome of non-fatal myocardial infarction plus death from coronary heart disease after a median of 5.1 years (AR 219/1264 [17%] for gemfibrozil *v* 275/1267 [22%] for placebo; ARR 4.4%, 95% CI 1.4% to 7.0%; RR 0.80, 95% CI 0.68 to 0.94; NNT 23, 95% CI 14 to 73). The review identified three trials comparing clofibrate versus placebo, which found no consistent difference between groups. The two additional RCTs[69,70] both compared bezafibrate versus placebo. The larger RCT (3090 people selected with previous myocardial infarction or stable angina, high density lipoprotein cholesterol < 45 mg/dL, and low density lipoprotein cholesterol < 180 mg/dL) found that bezafibrate versus placebo did not significantly reduce all cause mortality or the composite end point of myocardial infarction plus sudden death (AR for myocardial infarction or sudden death: 13.6% with bezafibrate *v* 15.0% with placebo; cumulative RR 0.91; $P = 0.26$).[69] The smaller RCT (92 young male survivors of myocardial infarction) found that bezafibrate versus placebo significantly reduced the combined outcome of death, reinfarction, plus revascularisation (3/47 [6%] with bezafibrate *v* 11/45 [24%], RR 0.26, 95% CI 0.08 to 0.88).[70] **Cholesterol lowering versus angioplasty:** We found no systematic review. One RCT found that aggressive lipid lowering treatment was as effective as percutaneous transluminal angioplasty for reducing ischaemic events, although anginal symptoms were reduced more by percutaneous transluminal angioplasty (see percutaneous transluminal angioplasty versus medical treatment, p 156).

Harms: Total non-cardiovascular events, total and tissue specific cancers, and accident and violent deaths have been reported in statin trials. However, the systematic review of long term statin trials found no significant difference between statins and placebo in terms of non-cardiovascular mortality, cancer incidence, asymptomatic elevation of creatine kinase (> 10 times upper reference limit), or elevation of transaminases (> 3 times upper reference limit) during a mean of 5.4 years of treatment (OR of event, statin *v* placebo for non-cardiovascular mortality 0.93, 95% CI 0.81 to 1.07; for cancer 0.99, 95% CI 0.90 to 1.08; for creatine kinase increase 1.25, 95% CI 0.83 to 1.89; for transaminase increase 1.13, 95% CI 0.95 to 1.33).[65] We found no evidence of additional harm associated with cholesterol lowering in elderly people, or in people after acute myocardial infarction.

Comment: Multivariate analysis in one systematic review (search date 1996) indicates that in a wide range of clinical contexts the relative risk reduction depends on the percent reduction in total or low density lipoprotein cholesterol and is not otherwise dependent on the method by which cholesterol is lowered. The absolute benefit over several years of lowering cholesterol will therefore be greatest in people with the highest baseline risk of an ischaemic cardiac event. Even if the relative risk reduction attenuates at older age, the absolute risk reduction for ischaemic cardiac events may be higher in elderly people than in younger people. The Women's Health Initiative (48 000 people, completion 2007, diet, up to age 79 years),[71] and the Antihypertensive and Lipid Lowering Treatment to Prevent Heart Disease Trial (10 000 people, completion 2002, pravastatin, no upper age limit) are ongoing.[72] We found no large direct comparisons of cholesterol modifying drugs; it remains unclear whether any one drug has advantages over others in subgroups of high risk people with particular lipid abnormalities. Because the main aim of treatment is to reduce absolute risk (rather than to reduce the cholesterol to any particular concentration), treatments aimed at lowering cholesterol need assessing for effectiveness in comparison and in combination with other possible risk factor interventions in each individual. People in the large statin trials in both treatment and placebo groups were given dietary advice aimed at lowering cholesterol.

QUESTION What are the effects of blood pressure reduction?

Eva Lonn

We found no direct evidence of the effects of blood pressure lowering in people with established coronary heart disease. Observational studies, and extrapolation of primary prevention trials of blood pressure reduction, support the lowering of blood pressure in those at high risk of ischaemic coronary events. The evidence for benefit is strongest for β blockers, although not specifically in people with hypertension. The target blood pressure in these people is not clear.

Benefits: We found no systematic review and no RCTs designed specifically to examine blood pressure reduction in those with established coronary heart disease. Prospective epidemiological studies have established that blood pressure continues to be a risk factor for cardiovascular events in people who have already experienced myocardial infarction. Prospective follow up of 5362 men who reported prior myocardial infarction during screening for one large RCT found no detectable association between systolic blood pressure and coronary heart disease mortality, and increased coronary heart disease mortality for those with lowest diastolic blood pressure in the first 2 years.[73] After 15 years there were highly significant linear associations between both systolic and diastolic blood pressure and increased risk of coronary heart disease mortality (stronger relation for systolic blood pressure), with apparent benefit for men with blood pressure maintained at levels lower than the arbitrarily defined "normal" levels. Experimental evidence of benefit from lowering of blood pressure in those with coronary heart disease requires extrapolation from primary prevention trials, because trials of antihypertensive treatment in elderly people[74–76] are likely to have included those with preclinical coronary heart disease. Mortality benefit has been established for β blockers after myocardial infarction (see beta blockers, p 140), for verapamil and diltiazem after myocardial infarction in those without heart failure (see calcium channel blockers, p 144), and for angiotensin converting enzyme inhibitors after myocardial infarction, especially in those with heart failure (see angiotensin converting enzyme inhibitors, p 141).

Harms: Some observational studies have found increased mortality among those with low diastolic blood pressure.[77] Trials in elderly people of blood pressure lowering for hypertension or while treating heart failure[78] found no evidence of a J-shaped relation between blood pressure and death.

Comment: Without specific studies comparing different antihypertensive treatments, the available evidence is strongest for a beneficial effect of β blockers when treating survivors of a myocardial infarction who have hypertension. We found no specific evidence about the target level of blood pressure.

QUESTION What are the effects of non-drug treatments?

Andy Ness and Eva Lonn

OPTION DIETARY INTERVENTIONS

One RCT found that advising people with coronary heart disease to eat more fruit and vegetables, bread, pasta, potatoes, olive oil, and rapeseed margarine (i.e. a Mediterranean diet) may result in a substantial survival benefit. We found no strong evidence from RCTs for a beneficial effect of low fat or high fibre diets on major non-fatal coronary heart disease events or coronary heart disease mortality. One RCT has found that advising people with coronary heart disease to eat more fish (particularly oily fish) significantly reduces mortality at 2 years. A second RCT found that fish oil capsules significantly reduced mortality at 3.5 years.

Benefits: **Low fat diets:** One systematic review (search date not stated) found no evidence that allocation to a low fat diet reduced mortality from coronary heart disease in people after myocardial infarction (RR 0.94, 95% CI 0.84 to 1.06).[79] One large RCT included in the review (2033 middle aged men with a recent myocardial infarction) compared three dietary options: fat advice (to eat less fat), fibre advice (to eat more cereal fibre), and fish advice (to eat at least 2 portions of oily fish a week).[80] Advice to reduce fat was complicated and, though fat intake reduced only slightly in the fat advice group, fruit and vegetable intake increased by about 40 g daily.[81] However, there was no significant reduction in mortality (unadjusted RR at 2 years for death from any cause 0.97, 95% CI 0.75 to 1.27). **High fibre diets:** In the RCT, people advised to eat more fibre doubled their intake, but survival was non-significantly worse (unadjusted RR at 2 years for death from any cause 1.23, 95% CI 0.95 to 1.60).[80] **High fish diets:** In the RCT, those advised to eat more fish ate three times as much fish, although about 14% could not tolerate the fish and were given fish oil capsules. Those given fish advice were significantly less likely to die within 2 years (94/1015 [9.3%] with fish advice *v* 130/1018 [12.8%] with no fish advice, NNT 29, 95% CI 17 to 129, RR 0.71, 95% CI 0.54 to 0.93).[80] In a second trial, 11 324 people who had survived a recent myocardial infarction were randomised to receive 1 g daily of n–3 polyunsaturated fatty acids (fish oil) or no fish oil. Those given fish oil were less likely to die within 3.5 years (RR 0.86, 95% CI 0.76 to 0.97).[82] **Mediterranean diet:** One RCT (605 middle aged people with a recent myocardial infarction) compared advice to eat a Mediterranean diet (more bread, fruit and vegetables, fish, and less meat, and to replace butter and cream with rapeseed margarine) versus usual dietary advice.[83] There were several dietary differences between the groups. Fruit intake, for example, was about 50 g daily higher in the intervention group than the control group. After 27 months, the trial was stopped prematurely because of significantly better outcomes in the intervention group (mortality: 8/302 [2.6%] with intervention *v* 20/303 [6.6%] with usual dietary advice, adjusted RR of death 0.24, 97% CI 0.15 to 0.91 [97% CI to allow for early stopping]; NNT 25, 95% CI 14 to 299 over 27 months).[83]

Harms: No major adverse effects have been reported.

Comment: Diets low in saturated fat and cholesterol can lead to 10–15% reductions in cholesterol concentrations in highly controlled settings, such as in metabolic wards.[84] In people in the community the effects are smaller: 3–5% reductions in cholesterol concentrations in general population studies and 9% reductions in people after myocardial infarction.[79,85–87] Several RCTs of intensive dietary intervention in conjunction with multifactorial risk reduction treatment found decreased progression of anatomic extent of coronary heart disease on angiography.[88] A trial of advice to eat more fruit and vegetables in men with angina is underway (Burr M, personal communication, 2001) **Effect on cardiovascular risk factors:** Other studies have investigated the effects of dietary interventions on cardiovascular risk factors rather than the effect on cardiovascular morbidity and mortality. One systematic review (search date 1992) suggested that garlic may reduce cholesterol by about

10%.[89] Some trials in this review had problems with their methods. More recent reports (published in 1998) found no effects of garlic powder or garlic oil on cholesterol concentrations.[90,91] One systematic review (search date 1991) reported modest reductions in cholesterol levels of 2–5% from oats and psyllium enriched cereals (high fibre diets), although we found no evidence that high fibre diets reduce mortality in people with coronary heart disease.[92] One systematic review (search date 1991) of soy protein also reported modest reductions in cholesterol concentrations.[92]

OPTION ANTIOXIDANT VITAMINS (VITAMIN E, β CAROTENE, VITAMIN C)

Pooled analysis from four large RCTs found no evidence that vitamin E altered cardiovascular events and all cause mortality compared with placebo when given for 1.3–4.5 years. Pooled analysis from three small RCTs found no evidence that vitamin C provided any substantial benefit. Large RCTs found no evidence of benefit with β carotene, and one RCT found evidence of a significant increase in mortality. Four large RCTs of β carotene supplementation in primary prevention found no cardiovascular benefits, and two of the RCTs raised concerns about increased mortality.

Benefits: We found no systematic review. **Vitamin E and β carotene:** We found four large RCTs of vitamin E in people with coronary artery disease.[82,93–95] The first RCT (2002 people with angiographically proved ischaemic heart disease)[93] used a high dose of vitamin E (400 or 800 IU) and follow up was brief (median 510 days). The RCT found that vitamin E reduced non-fatal coronary events (RR 0.23, 95% CI 0.11 to 0.47), but also found a non-significant increase in coronary death (RR 1.18, 95% CI 0.62 to 2.27) and all cause mortality. The second RCT (29 133 male Finnish smokers) compared β carotene supplements versus vitamin E supplements versus both versus placebo.[94] The dose of vitamin E (50 mg/day) was smaller than that used in the first trial. In the subgroup analysis of data from the 1862 men with prior myocardial infarction, the trial found that vitamin E reduced non-fatal myocardial infarction (RR 0.62, 95% CI 0.41 to 0.96) but non-significantly increased coronary death (RR 1.33, 95% CI 0.86 to 2.05).[94] There were significantly more deaths from coronary heart disease on β carotene and β carotene plus vitamin E than placebo. There was no significant difference between vitamin E alone and placebo. The third RCT (11 324 people ≤ 3 months after myocardial infarction)[82] used a factorial design to compare vitamin E (300 mg/day) versus no vitamin E (as well as fish oil *v* no fish oil). After 3.5 years there was a small and non-significant reduction in the risk of cardiovascular death and deaths from all causes in those who received vitamin E compared with those who did not (all cause mortality: RR 0.92, 95% CI 0.82 to 1.04). There was no significant change in the rate of non-fatal coronary events in those who received vitamin E (RR 1.04, 95% CI 0.88 to 1.22).[82] The fourth RCT (9541 people at high cardiovascular risk, 80% with prior clinical coronary artery disease, remainder with other atherosclerotic disease or diabetes with ≥ 1 additional cardiovascular risk factor) compared natural source vitamin E (D-α tocopherol acetate, 400 IU/day) versus placebo and followed people for an average of 4.7 years.[95] It found no significant differences in any cardiovascular outcomes between vitamin E and placebo (AR for major fatal or non-fatal cardiovascular event 16.2% with vitamin E *v* 15.5% with placebo, $P > 0.05$; AR for cardiovascular death 7.2% with vitamin E *v* 6.9% with placebo, $P > 0.05$; AR for non-fatal myocardial infarction 11.2% *v* 11.0% with placebo, $P > 0.05$; AR for stroke 4.4% with vitamin E *v* 3.8% with placebo, $P > 0.05$; AR for death from any cause 11.2% with vitamin E *v* 11.2% with placebo, $P > 0.05$). Pooled analysis from all four of these major RCTs found no evidence that vitamin E altered cardiovascular events and all cause mortality compared with placebo when given for 1.3–4.5 years. One additional smaller RCT (196 people on haemodialysis, aged 40–75 years) compared high dose vitamin E (800 IU/day) versus placebo.[96] After a median of 519 days, it found that vitamin E reduced the rate of combined cardiovascular end points but found no significant effect for all cause mortality (cardiovascular end points: vitamin E *v* placebo RR 0.54, 95% CI 0.23 to 0.89; mortality: vitamin E *v* placebo RR 1.09, 95% CI 0.70 to 1.70).[96] **Vitamin C:** We found four small RCTs comparing vitamin C with placebo.[97–100] The first RCT (538 people admitted to an acute geriatric unit) compared vitamin C (200 mg/day) versus placebo for 6 months.[97] The second RCT (297 elderly people with low vitamin C levels) compared vitamin C (150 mg/day for 12 wks, then 50 mg/day) versus placebo for 2 years.[98] The third RCT (199 elderly people) compared vitamin C (200 mg/day) versus placebo for 6 months.[99] The three RCTs were small and brief, and their combined results provide no evidence of any substantial early benefit of vitamin C supplementation (mortality: vitamin *v* placebo RR 1.08, 95% CI 0.93 to 1.26). The fourth small RCT (160 people) found no significant difference in the rate of cardiovascular events between antioxidants vitamins (vitamin E, vitamin C, β carotene, and selenium) versus placebo.[100]

Harms: Two of the trials of vitamin E found non-significant increases in the risk of coronary death (see benefits above).[93,97] Four large RCTs of β carotene supplementation in primary prevention found no cardiovascular benefits, and two of the trials raised concerns about increased mortality (cardiovascular death: β carotene *v* placebo RR 1.12, 95% CI 1.04 to 1.22) and cancer rates.[101]

Comment: One systematic review (search date 1996) of epidemiological studies found consistent associations between increased dietary intake, supplemental intake of vitamin E, or both, and lower cardiovascular risk and less consistent associations for β carotene and vitamin C.[101] Most observational studies of antioxidants have excluded people with pre-existing disease.[102,103] The results of the trial in people on haemodialysis raises the possibility that high dose vitamin E supplementation may be beneficial in those at high absolute risk of coronary events.[96] Further trials in such groups are required to confirm or refute this finding. The Heart Protection Study (results not fully published at time of search, 20 536 people aged 40–80 years with prior cardiovascular events or at high risk for vascular disease) compared a combination of antioxidant vitamins (vitamin C 250 mg, vitamin E 600 mg, and β carotene 20 mg) versus placebo. After 5.5 years, the antioxidant treatment had no significant effect on total mortality and major cardiovascular events.[104]

OPTION CARDIAC REHABILITATION INCLUDING EXERCISE

One systematic review has found that cardiac rehabilitation including exercise reduces the risk of major cardiac events in people after myocardial infarction. It found that exercise alone reduced the risk of a major cardiac event, and probably reduced mortality.

Benefits: We found one systematic review (search date 1998).[105] **Cardiac rehabilitation:** The review identified 42 RCTs of cardiac rehabilitation including exercise versus usual care (7683 people, who have had myocardial infarction, coronary artery bypass grafting [CABG], or percutaneous transluminal coronary angioplasty, or who have angina pectoris or coronary artery disease defined by angiography). It found that cardiac rehabilitation including exercise reduced the composite end point of mortality, non-fatal myocardial infarction, CABG, percutaneous transluminal angioplasty (636/3863 [16.5%] with cardiac rehabilitation *v* 734/3820 [19.2%] with usual care, RR 0.85, 95% CI 0.77 to 0.93). It found limited evidence of a reduction in mortality but significance was sensitive to the quality of the trials.[105] **Exercise alone:** The review identified 12 RCTs of exercise alone versus usual care (2582 people, who have had myocardial infarction, CABG, or percutaneous transluminal angioplasty, or who have angina pectoris or coronary artery disease defined by angiography). It found that exercise significantly reduced mortality (93/1297 [7.2%] with exercise *v* 122/1285 [9.5%] with usual care, RR 0.76, 95% CI 0.59 to 0.98). It was associated with a reduction in the composite end point of mortality, non-fatal myocardial infarction, CABG, and percutaneous transluminal angioplasty, but the difference was not significant (183/1297 [14.1%] with exercise *v* 216/1285 [16.8%] with usual care, RR 0.85, 95% CI 0.71 to 1.01).[105]

Harms: Rates of adverse cardiovascular outcomes (syncope, arrhythmia, myocardial infarction, or sudden death) were low (2–3/100 000 person h) in supervised rehabilitation programmes, and rates of fatal cardiac events during or immediately after exercise training, were reported in two older surveys as ranging from 1/116 400 to 1/784 000 person hours.[106]

Comment: The review included some RCTs performed before the widespread use of thrombolytic agents and β blockers after myocardial infarction.[105] Most people were white men, without comorbidity, and under 70 years of age. Other interventions aimed at risk factor modification were often provided in the intervention groups (including nutritional education, counselling in behavioural modification, and, in some trials, lipid lowering medications). We found no strong evidence that exercise training and cardiac rehabilitation programmes increased the proportion of people returning to work after myocardial infarction.

OPTION SMOKING CESSATION

We found no RCTs of the effects of smoking cessation on cardiovascular events in people with coronary heart disease. Moderate quality evidence from epidemiological studies indicates that people with coronary heart disease who stop smoking, rapidly reduce their risk of recurrent coronary events or death. Treatment with nicotine patches seems safe in people with coronary heart disease.

Benefits: We found no RCTs assessing the effects of smoking cessation on coronary morbidity and mortality. Many observational studies have found that people with coronary heart disease who stop smoking, rapidly reduce their risk of cardiac death and myocardial infarction (recurrent coronary events or premature death compared with continuing smokers: RR about 0.50).[107] See smoking cessation under primary prevention for more details, p 95. The studies found that about 50% of the benefits occur in the first year of stopping smoking, followed by a more gradual decrease in risk, reaching the risk of never smokers after several years of abstinence.[107] Among people with peripheral arterial disease and stroke, smoking cessation has been shown in observational studies to be associated with improved exercise tolerance, decreased risk of amputation, improved survival, and reduced risk of recurrent stroke.

Harms: Two recent RCTs found no evidence that nicotine replacement using transdermal patches in people with stable coronary heart disease increased cardiovascular events.[108,109]

Comment: One RCT compared the impact of firm and detailed advice to stop smoking (125 survivors of acute myocardial infarction) versus conventional advice (85 people).[110] Allocation to the intervention or control group was determined by day of admission. At over 1 year after admission, 62% of the intervention group and 28% of the control group were non-smokers. Morbidity and mortality were not reported.

OPTION PSYCHOLOGICAL AND STRESS MANAGEMENT

One systematic review of mainly poor quality RCTs found that psychosocial treatments may decrease rates of myocardial infarction or cardiac death in people with coronary heart disease.

Benefits: One systematic review (search date not stated, 23 RCTs, 3180 people with coronary artery disease) compared a diverse range of psychosocial treatments (2024 people) versus usual treatment (1156 people).[111] Mortality results were available in only 12 RCTs. Psychosocial interventions versus control interventions significantly reduced mortality (OR survival 1.70, 95% CI 1.09 to 2.64) and non-fatal events in the first 2 years after myocardial infarction (OR for no event 1.84, 95% CI 1.12 to 2.99).[111]

Harms: No specific harms were reported.

Comment: These results should be interpreted with caution because of limits of the methods of the individual RCTs and the diversity of interventions (relaxation, stress management, counselling). The RCTs were generally small, with short follow up, and used non-uniform outcome measures. Methods of concealment allocation were not assessed. The authors of the review acknowledged the strong possibility of publication bias but made no attempt to measure it. The results were inconsistent across trials.[112] Several observational studies have found that depression and social isolation (lack of social and emotional support) are independent predictors of mortality and non-fatal coronary heart disease events in people after myocardial infarction.[113]

QUESTION What are the effects of surgical treatments?

Charanjit Rihal

OPTION CORONARY ARTERY BYPASS GRAFTING VERSUS MEDICAL TREATMENT ALONE

One systematic review found that coronary artery bypass grafts reduced the risk of death from coronary artery disease at 5 and 10 years compared with medical treatment alone. Greater benefit occurred in people with poor left ventricular function. One subsequent RCT in people with asymptomatic disease found that revascularisation with coronary artery bypass grafting or coronary percutaneous transluminal angioplasty versus medical treatment alone reduced mortality at 2 years.

Benefits: We found one systematic review comparing coronary artery bypass grafting (CABG) with medical treatment alone[114] and one subsequent RCT in asymptomatic people of revascularisation with CABG or coronary percutaneous transluminal angioplasty versus medical treatment alone.[115] In the systematic review (search date not stated, 7 RCTs, individual results from 2649 people with coronary heart disease) most people were middle aged men with multivessel disease but good left ventricular function who were enrolled from 1972–1984 (97% were male; 82% 41–60 years old; 80% with ejection fraction > 50%; 60% with prior myocardial infarction; and 83% with 2 or 3 vessel disease).[114] People assigned to CABG also received medical treatment, and 40% initially assigned to medical treatment underwent CABG in the following 10 years. The systematic review found that CABG versus medical treatment reduced deaths at 5 and 10 years (death at 5 years: RR 0.61 95% CI 0.48 to 0.77; death at 10 years: RR 0.83, 95% CI 0.70 to 0.98).[114] Most trials did not collect data on recurrent angina or quality of life. **Effects in people with reduced versus normal left ventricular function:** The systematic review found that the relative benefits were similar in people with normal versus reduced left ventricular function (death: OR 0.61, 95% CI 0.46 to 0.81 if left ventricular function was normal; OR 0.59. 95% CI 0.39 to 0.91 if left ventricular function was reduced).[114] The absolute benefit of CABG was greater in people with a reduced left ventricular function because the baseline risk of death was higher. **Effects in people with different numbers of diseased vessels:** The systematic review found lower mortality with CABG versus medical treatment in people with single vessel, two vessel, three vessel, and left main stem disease, but for single vessel and two vessel disease the difference was not statistically significant, possibly because the number of deaths was small (RR with single vessel disease 0.54, 95% CI 0.22

to 1.33; with two vessel disease 0.84, 95% CI 0.54 to 1.32; with three vessel disease 0.58, 95% CI 0.42 to 0.80; with left main stem disease 0.32, 95% CI 0.15 to 0.70).[114] **Effects in asymptomatic people:** We found one RCT (558 people) of revascularisation with CABG or percutaneous transluminal angioplasty versus symptom guided treatment versus electrocardiogram and symptom guided treatment in people with asymptomatic ischaemia identified by exercise test or ambulatory electrocardiogram.[115] It found that revascularisation versus medical treatment alone reduced death or myocardial infarction at 2 years (death or myocardial infarction: AR 4.7% with revascularisation *v* 8.8% with symptom guided treatment *v* 12.1% with symptom plus electrocardiogram guided treatment; $P < 0.04$).

Harms: In the systematic review, of the 1240 people who underwent CABG, 40 (3.2%) died and 88 (7.1%) had documented non-fatal myocardial infarction within 30 days of the procedure. At 1 year, the estimated incidence of death or myocardial infarction was significantly higher with CABG versus medical treatment (11.6% with CABG *v* 8% with medical treatment, RR 1.45, 95% CI 1.18 to 2.03).[114] The diagnosis of myocardial infarction after CABG is difficult, and true incidence may be higher.

Comment: The results of the systematic review may not be easily generalised to current practice. People were 65 years or younger, but more than 50% of CABG procedures are now performed on people over 65 years of age. Almost all people were male. High risk people, such as those with severe angina and left main coronary artery stenosis, were under-represented. Internal thoracic artery grafts were used in fewer than 5% of people. Lipid lowering agents (particularly statins) and aspirin were used infrequently (aspirin used in 3% of people at enrolment). Only about 50% of people were taking β blockers. The systematic review may underestimate the real benefits of CABG in comparison with medical treatment alone because medical and surgical treatment for coronary artery disease were not mutually exclusive; by 5 years, 25% of people receiving medical treatment had undergone CABG surgery and by 10 years, 41% had undergone CABG surgery. The underestimate of effect would be greatest among people at high risk. People with previous CABG have not been studied in RCTs, although they now represent a growing proportion of those undergoing CABG.

OPTION CORONARY PERCUTANEOUS TRANSLUMINAL ANGIOPLASTY VERSUS MEDICAL TREATMENT ALONE

One systematic review found that coronary percutaneous transluminal angioplasty versus medical treatment alone improved angina, but was associated with a higher rate of coronary artery bypass grafting. The review found higher mortality and rates of myocardial infarction with percutaneous transluminal angioplasty versus medical treatment but the difference was not significant. RCTs have found that percutaneous transluminal angioplasty was associated with increased risk of emergency coronary artery bypass grafting and myocardial infarction

during and soon after the procedure. One RCT found that percutaneous transluminal angioplasty reduced cardiac events and improved angina severity compared with medical treatment alone in people over the age of 75 years.

Benefits: We found one systematic review (search date 1998, 6 RCTs, 1904 people with stable coronary artery disease) comparing coronary percutaneous transluminal angioplasty (PTA) versus medical treatment alone.[116] Follow up varied from 6–57 months. It found that PTA versus medical treatment alone reduced angina, but increased subsequent coronary artery bypass grafting (CABG) (angina: RR 0.70, 95% CI 0.50 to 0.98; CABG: RR 1.59, 95% CI 1.09 to 2.32). It found higher mortality and myocardial infarction with PTA versus medical treatment alone but the difference was not significant (death: RR 1.32, 95% CI 0.65 to 2.70; myocardial infarction: RR 1.42, 95% CI 0.90 to 2.25). The review found significant heterogeneity between trials. The largest RCT identified by the review (1018 people) found that PTA versus medical treatment improved physical functioning, vitality, and general health at 1 year (proportion of people rating their health "much improved": 33% of people treated with PTA *v* 22% with medical treatment alone; P = 0.008), but found no significant difference at 3 years.[117] The improvements were related to breathlessness, angina, and treadmill tolerance. High transfer (27%) from the medical to PTA group may partly explain the lack of difference between groups at 3 years. **Effects in elderly people:** One RCT (305 people aged > 75 years with chronic refractory angina) compared PTA versus medical treatment alone.[118] It found that PTA reduced all adverse cardiac events and decreased anginal severity compared with medical treatment, but had no significant effect on deaths or non-fatal myocardial infarctions after 6 months (adverse cardiac events: AR 19% with PTA *v* 49% with medical treatment alone, P < 0.0001; change in angina class: –2.0 with PTA *v* –1.6 with medical treatment alone, P < 0.0001; deaths: AR 8.5% with PTA *v* 4.1% with medical treatment alone, P = 0.15; non-fatal infarctions: AR 7.8% with PTA *v* 11.5% with medical treatment alone, P = 0.46). **Effects in people with different angina severity:** One of the RCTs in the systematic review found that antianginal benefit from PTA was limited to people with moderate to severe (grade 2 or worse) angina (20% lower incidence of angina and 1 min longer treadmill exercise times compared with medical treatment).[119] People with mild symptoms at enrolment derived no significant improvement in symptoms. **Effects in asymptomatic people:** We found one RCT (558 people) of revascularisation with CABG or PTA versus symptom guided treatment versus electrocardiogram and symptom guided treatment in people with asymptomatic ischaemia identified by exercise test or ambulatory electrocardiogram[115] (see benefits of coronary artery bypass grafting versus medical treatment alone, p 155).

Harms: Procedural death and myocardial infarction, as well as repeat procedures for restenosis, are the main hazards of PTA. Four RCTs included in the review reported complications of PTA. In the first RCT, two (1.9%) emergency CABG operations and five (4.8%) myocardial infarctions occurred at the time of the procedure. By 6 months, the PTA group had higher rates of CABG surgery (7% with PTA *v* 0% with medical treatment alone) and non-protocol PTA (15.2% with PTA *v* 10.3% with medical treatment alone).[119,120] In the second RCT, the higher mortality or rate of myocardial infarction with PTA was attributable to one death and seven procedure related myocardial infarctions.[118] The third RCT found a procedure related CABG rate and myocardial infarction rate of 2.8% each, and the fourth found rates of 2.0% for CABG and 3.0% for myocardial infarction.[115]

Comment: We found good evidence that PTA treats the symptoms of angina, but we found no evidence that it reduces the overall incidence of death or myocardial infarction in people with stable angina. This could be because of the risk of complications during and soon after the procedure, and because most PTAs are performed for single vessel disease.

OPTION CORONARY PERCUTANEOUS TRANSLUMINAL ANGIOPLASTY VERSUS CORONARY ARTERY BYPASS GRAFTING

One systematic review has found that percutaneous transluminal angioplasty versus coronary artery bypass grafting has no significant effect on mortality, the risk of myocardial infarction, or quality of life. Percutaneous transluminal angioplasty is less invasive but increased the number of repeat procedures. The relevant RCTs were too small to exclude a 20–30% relative difference in mortality.

Benefits: We found one systematic review (search date not stated, 8 RCTs, 3371 people)[122], one subsequent RCT[123], one subsequent non-systematic review, (including the subsequent RCT),[124] which compared percutaneous transluminal angioplasty (PTA) versus coronary artery bypass grafting (CABG). **Angina:** The systematic review found that the prevalence of moderate to severe angina (grade 2 or worse) was significantly higher after PTA than after CABG at 1 year (RR 1.6, 95% CI 1.3 to 1.9).[122] After 3 years this difference had decreased (RR 1.2, 95% CI 1.0 to 1.5). **Mortality:** The systematic review found that PTA did not reduce deaths compared with CABG after 1 year (RR 1.08, 95% CI 0.79 to 1.50),[122] the subsequent RCT (392 people) found no significant difference in deaths between CABG versus PTA after 8 years, although the trial was too small to exclude a clinically important difference (AR for survival 83% with CABG *v* 79% with PTA; P = 0.40).[124] The subsequent non-systematic review found that mortality was not significantly different between PTA versus CABG (OR 1.09, 95% CI 0.88 to 1.35).[123] **Repeat procedures:** The systematic review found that PTA increased subsequent procedures compared with CABG (subsequent CABG: RR 1.59, 95% CI 1.09 to 2.32; subsequent PTA: RR 1.29, 95% CI 0.71 to 3.36).[122] **Quality of life:** Two of the RCTs included in the systematic review found no difference in quality of life between people who had PTA and people who had CABG over 3–5 years.[125,126]

Harms: See harms under percutaneous transluminal angioplasty versus medical treatment, p 157. CABG is more invasive than PTA, but PTA is associated with a greater need for repeat procedures.

Comment: Although no major differences in death or myocardial infarction were observed in the systematic review[122] these trials enrolled people at relatively low risk of cardiac events, so it is premature to conclude that PTA and CABG are equivalent for people with multivessel disease. Fewer than 20% of people had left ventricular dysfunction, almost 70% had one or two vessel disease, and observed mortality was only 2.6% for the first year and 1.1% for the second year. People enrolled in the largest trial more closely approximated to moderate risk people, but this was caused primarily by the higher proportion of people with diabetes mellitus.[127] Even in that trial nearly 60% of people had two vessel coronary artery disease. The total number of people enrolled in the nine trials so far is not adequate to show anything less than a 20–30% difference in mortality between PTA and CABG. Subgroup analysis of one RCT (1829 people) found that in people with diabetes (353 people) CABG reduced deaths compared with PTA after 7 years[127] (see coronary artery bypass grafting v percutaneous transluminal angioplasty in cardiovascular disease in diabetes, p 541). This difference was not found in people without diabetes or any other subgroup (deaths in people without diabetes: AR 13.6% with CABG *v* 13.2% with PTA; P = 0.72).[127]

OPTION INTRACORONARY STENTS VERSUS CORONARY PERCUTANEOUS TRANSLUMINAL ANGIOPLASTY ALONE

One systematic review has found that intracoronary stents versus coronary percutaneous transluminal angioplasty alone significantly reduce the need for repeat vascularisation. It found no significant difference in mortality or myocardial infarction, but crossover rates from percutaneous transluminal angioplasty alone to stent were high. RCTs found that intracoronary stents improved outcomes after 4–9 months compared with percutaneous transluminal angioplasty alone in people with previous coronary artery bypass grafting, chronic total occlusions, and for treatment of restenosis after initial percutaneous transluminal angioplasty.

Benefits: We found one systematic review (search date 1999, 11 RCTs with 4–11 months' follow up, 4815 people) of stents versus percutaneous transluminal angioplasty (PTA) alone.[129] It found a significant reduction in cardiac event rates after 4–11 months with stents compared with PTA alone (composite of death, myocardial infarction, or repeat vascularisation; 17.9% with stent *v* 24.1% with PTA; OR 0.68, 95% CI 0.59 to 0.78). Stents reduced repeat vascularisation compared with PTA alone (12.4% with stent *v* 20.6% with PTA alone; OR 0.54, 95% CI 0.45 to 0.65), whereas there was no significant difference in deaths (0.9% with stent *v* 1.3% with PTA alone; OR 0.68, 95% CI 0.40 to 1.14) or myocardial infarctions (4.4% with stent *v* 3.6% with PTA alone; OR 1.23, 95% CI 0.88 to 1.72). Seven RCTs with follow up over 1 year found a significant reduction in cardiac events with stents compared with PTA alone (19.5% with stent *v* 28.1% with PTA alone, OR 0.62, 95% CI 0.52 to 0.74). **In saphenous vein graft lesions in people with prior coronary artery bypass grafting:** We found one RCT (220 people) comparing stents with PTA alone for stenosed saphenous vein grafts.[130] There was no significant difference in rates of restenosis

(37% with stent *v* 46% with PTA alone; P = 0.24) after 6 months, but stents compared with PTA alone reduced death, myocardial infarction, coronary artery bypass grafting, or repeat PTA (27% with stent *v* 42% with PTA alone; P = 0.03). **In people with total occlusions:** We found three RCTs comparing stents with PTA alone in people with chronic totally occluded coronary arteries.[131–133] The first RCT (119 people) found that stent compared with PTA alone reduced angina, angiographic restenosis, and repeat procedures (angina free at 6 months: 57% with stent *v* 24% with PTA alone; P < 0.001; > 50% stenosis on follow up angiography: 32% with stent *v* 74% with PTA alone; P < 0.001; repeat procedures: 22% with stent *v* 42% with PTA alone; P = 0.03).[131] The second RCT (110 people) found that stents compared with PTA alone reduced restenosis and repeat procedures after 9 months (restenosis: 32% with stent *v* 68%; with PTA alone; P < 0.001; repeat procedures: 5% with stent *v* 22% with PTA alone; P = 0.04).[132] The third RCT (110 people) found that stents versus PTA alone reduced restenosis and repeat PTA after 4 months (restenosis: 26% with stent *v* 62% with PTA alone; P = 0.01; repeat PTA: 24% with stent *v* 55% with PTA alone; P = 0.05). No deaths or coronary artery bypass grafting operations occurred in either group. The incidence of myocardial infarction was low in both groups (0% with stent *v* 2% with PTA alone, P > 0.05).[133] **For treatment of restenosis after initial percutaneous transluminal angioplasty:** We found one RCT (383 people) of coronary stent versus PTA alone for treatment of restenosis. It found that stents versus PTA alone reduced restenosis and repeat procedures, and increased survival free of myocardial infarction and repeat revascularisation after 6 months (restenosis: 18% with stent *v* 32% with PTA alone; P = 0.03; repeat procedures: 10% with stent *v* 27% with PTA alone; P = 0.001; survival free of myocardial infarction or repeat revascularisation: 84% with stent *v* 72% with PTA alone; P = 0.04).[134]

Harms: Initially, aggressive combination antithrombotic and anticoagulant regimens were used after stenting because of a high incidence of stent thrombosis and myocardial infarction. These regimens led to a high incidence of arterial access site haemorrhage.[124] More recently, improved stent techniques and use of aspirin and ticlopidine have reduced both stent thrombosis and arterial access site haemorrhage.[130,134] Currently, the risk of stent thrombosis is less than 1%.[135–137] Haemorrhage (particularly femoral artery haemorrhage) was more frequent after stenting than PTA alone,[138] but occurred in less than 3% after stenting when antiplatelet drugs were used without long term anticoagulants.

Comment: It is unclear whether stenting influences the relative benefits and harms of percutaneous procedures compared with coronary artery bypass grafting. Coronary stents are associated with fewer repeat revascularisation procedures and less angiographic restenosis than PTA. Rates of death and myocardial infarction are low in the RCTs and are not significantly different between stents and PTA. However, any potential differences may be masked by the crossover to stents after poor results (such as dissection) immediately after PTA.

GLOSSARY

International normalised ratio (INR) A value derived from a standardised laboratory test that measures the effect of an anticoagulant. The laboratory materials used in the test are calibrated against internationally accepted standard reference preparations, so that variability between laboratories and different reagents is minimised. Normal blood has an INR of 1. Therapeutic anticoagulation often aims to achieve an INR value of 2.0–3.5.

Substantive changes

Oral anticoagulants in addition to antiplatelet treatment One new RCT;[35] found no evidence of benefit from addition of moderate intensity oral anticoagulation to aspirin, compared to aspirin alone.

Cholesterol reduction New RCT;[64] conclusions unchanged.

Cholesterol reduction New RCT;[66] found that atorvastatin reduces the number of emergency re-admissions for recurrent ischaemia in people admitted with unstable angina or non-Q wave myocardial infarction.

Coronary percutaneous transluminal angioplasty versus medical treatment New RCT;[118] found that in elderly people, PTA reduced the risk of adverse cardiac events, as well as improved the severity of angina and improved quality of life when compared to medical treatment.

REFERENCES

1. Greaves EJ, Gillum BS. 1994 Summary: national hospital discharge survey. Advance data from Vital and Health Statistics, no. 278. Hyattsville, Maryland, USA: National Center for Health Statistics, 1996.
2. Shaw LJ, Peterson ED, Kesler K, et al. A meta-analysis of predischarge risk stratification after acute myocardial infarction with stress electrocardiographic, myocardial perfusion, and ventricular function imaging. *Am J Cardiol* 1996;78:1327–1337. Search date 1995; primary sources Medline and hand searches of bibliographies of review articles.
3. Kudenchuk PJ, Maynard C, Martin JS, et al. Comparison, presentation, treatment and outcome of acute myocardial infarction in men versus women (the myocardial infarction triage and intervention registry). *Am J Cardiol* 1996;78:9–14.
4. The Task Force on the Management of Acute Myocardial Infarction of the European Society of Cardiology. Acute myocardial infarction: pre-hospital and in-hospital management. *Eur Heart J* 1996;17:43–63.
5. Peterson ED, Shaw LJ, Califf RM. Clinical guideline: part II. Risk stratification after myocardial infarction. *Ann Intern Med* 1997;126:561–582.
6. The Multicenter Postinfarction Research Group. Risk stratification and survival after myocardial infarction. *N Engl J Med* 1983;309;331–336.
7. American College of Cardiology/American Heart Association Task Force on Practice Guidelines (Committee on Exercise Testing). ACC/AHA guidelines for exercise testing. *J Am Coll Cardiol* 1997;30:260–315.
8. Fallen E, Cairns J, Dafoe W, et al. Management of the postmyocardial infarction patient: a consensus report — revision of the 1991 CCS guidelines. *Can J Cardiol* 1995;11:477–486.
9. Madsen JK, Grande P, Saunamaki, et al. Danish multicenter randomized study of invasive versus conservative treatment in patients with inducible ischemia after thrombolysis in acute myocardial infarction (DANAMI). DANish trial in Acute Myocardial Infarction. *Circulation* 1997;96:748–755.
10. Antithrombotic Trialists' Collaboration. Collaborative meta-analysis of randomised trials of antiplatelet therapy for prevention of death, myocardial infarction and stroke in high risk patients. *BMJ* 2002;324:71–86. Search date 1997; primary sources Medline, Embase, Derwent, Scisearch, and Biosis, in additional trials registers of Cochrane Stroke and Peripheral Vascular Diseases Group, hand searches of journals, abstracts, and conference proceedings, and contact with experts.
11. Taylor DW, Barnett HJM, Haynes RB, et al. Low-dose and high-dose acetylsalicylic acid for patients undergoing carotid endarterectomy: a randomised controlled trial. *Lancet* 1999;353:2179–2184.
12. He J, Whelton PK, Vu B, et al. Aspirin and risk of hemorrhagic stroke. A meta-analysis of randomised controlled trials. *JAMA* 1998;280:1930–1935.
13. Farrell B, Godwin J, Richards S, et al. The United Kingdom transient ischaemic attack (UK-TIA) aspirin trial: final results. *J Neurol Neurosurg Psychiatry* 1991;54:1044–1054.
14. Dutch TIA Trial Study Group. A comparison of two doses of aspirin (30 mg vs 283 mg a day) in patients after a transient ischemic attack or minor ischemic stroke. *N Engl J Med* 1991;325:1261–1266.
15. Thrift AG, McNeil JJ, Forbes A, et al. Risk factors for cerebral hemorrhage in the era of well-controlled hypertension. Melbourne Risk Factor Study (MERFS) Group. *Stroke* 1996;27:2020–2025.
16. Iso H, Hennekens CH, Stampfer MJ, et al. Prospective study of aspirin use and risk of stroke in women. *Stroke* 1999;30:1764–1771.
17. Derry S, Loke YK. Risk of gastrointestinal haemorrhage with long term use of aspirin: meta-analysis. *BMJ* 2000;321:1183–1187. Search date 1999; primary sources Medline, Embase, and reference lists of existing systematic reviews.

18. García Rodríguez LA, Hernández-Díaz S, de Abajo FJ. Association between aspirin and upper gastrointestinal complications. Systematic review of epidemiologic studies. *Br J Clin Pharmacol* 2001;52:563–571.
19. CAPRIE Steering Committee. A randomised, blinded, trial of clopidogrel versus aspirin in patients at risk of ischaemic events. *Lancet* 1996;348:1329–1339.
20. Scrutinio D, Cimminiello C, Marubini E, et al. Ticlopidine versus aspirin after myocardial infarction (STAMI) trial. *J Am Coll Cardiol* 2001;37:1259–1265.
21. Hankey GJ, Sudlow CLM, Dunbabin DW. Thienopyridine derivatives (ticlopidine, clopidogrel) versus aspirin for preventing stroke and other serious vascular events in high vascular risk patients. In: The Cochrane Library, Issue 2, 2002. Oxford: Update Software. Search date 1999; primary sources Medline, Embase, Cochrane Stroke Group Register, Antithrombotics Trialists' database, authors of trials, and drug manufacturers.
22. Moloney BA. An analysis of the side effects of ticlopidine. In: Hass WK, Easton JD, eds. *Ticlopidine, platelets and vascular disease*. New York: Springer, 1993:117–139.
23. Bennett CL, Davidson CJ, Raisch DW, et al. Thrombotic thrombocytopenic purpura associated with ticlopidine in the setting of coronary artery stents and stroke prevention. *Arch Int Med* 1999;159:2524–2528.
24. Bennett CL, Connors JM, Carwile JM, et al. Thrombotic thrombocytopenic purpura associated with clopidogrel. *N Engl J Med* 2000;342:1773–1777.
25. Hankey GJ. Clopidogrel and thrombotic thrombocytopenic purpura. *Lancet* 2000;356:269–270.
26. Müller C, Büttner HJ, Petersen J, et al. A randomized comparison of clopidogrel and aspirin versus ticlopidine and aspirin after the placement of coronary-artery stents. *Circulation* 2000;101:590–593.
27. Bertrand ME, Rupprecht H-J, Urban P, et al, for the CLASSICS Investigators. Double-blind study of the safety of clopidogrel with and without a loading dose in combination with aspirin compared with ticlopidine in combination with aspirin after coronary stenting. The Clopidogrel Aspirin Stent International Cooperative Study (CLASSICS). *Circulation* 2000;102:624–629.
28. Taniuchi M, Kurz HI, Lasala JM. Randomized comparison of ticlopidine and clopidogrel after intracoronary stent implantation in a broad patient population. *Circulation* 2001;104:539–543.
29. The Clopidogrel in Unstable Angina to Prevent Recurrent Events (CURE) Trial Investigators. Effects of clopidogrel in addition to aspirin in patients with acute coronary syndromes without ST-segment elevation. *N Engl J Med* 2001;345:494–502.
30. Second Chinese Cardiac Study (CCS-2) Collaborative Group. Rationale, design and organisation of the Second Chinese Cardiac Study (CCS-2): a randomised trial of clopidogrel plus aspirin, and of metoprolol, among patients with suspected acute myocardial infarction. *J Cardiovasc Risk* 2000;7:435–441.
31. Chew DP, Bhatt DL, Sapp S, et al. Increased mortality with oral platelet glycoprotein IIb/IIIa antagonists. *Circulation* 2001;103:201–206. Search date 2000; primary source Medline.
32. SoRelle R. SmithKline Beecham halts tests of lotrafiban, an oral glycoprotein IIb/IIIa inhibitor. *Circulation* 2001;103:E9001–9002.
33. Anand SS, Yusuf S. Oral anticoagulant therapy in patients with coronary artery disease: a meta-analysis. *JAMA* 1999;282:2058–2067. Search date 1999; primary sources Medline, Embase, Current Contents, hand searches of reference lists, experts, and pharmaceutical companies.
34. The Organization to Assess Strategies for Ischemic Syndromes (OASIS) Investigators. Effects of long-term, moderate intensity oral anticoagulation in addition to aspirin in unstable angina. *J Am Coll Cardiol* 2001;37:475–484.
35. Fiore LD, Ezekowitz MD, Brophy MT, et al, for the Combination Hemotherapy and Mortality Prevention (CHAMP) Study Group. Department of Veterans Affairs Cooperative Studies Program clinical trial comparing combined warfarin and aspirin with aspirin alone in survivors of acute myocardial infarction. Primary results of the CHAMP study. *Circulation* 2002;105:557–563.
36. Huynh T, Theroux P, Bogaty P, et al. Aspirin, warfarin, or the combination for secondary prevention of coronary events in patients with acute coronary syndromes and prior coronary artery bypass surgery. *Circulation* 2001;103:3069–3074.
37. Teo KK, Yusuf S, Furberg CD. Effects of prophylactic antiarrhythmic drug therapy in acute myocardial infarction. *JAMA* 1993;270:1589–1595. Search date 1993; primary sources Medline, hand searches of reference lists, and details of unpublished trials sought from pharmaceutical industry/other investigators.
38. Yusuf S, Peto R, Lewis J, et al. Beta blockade during and after myocardial infarction: an overview of the randomized trials. *Prog Cardiovasc Dis* 1985;27:335–371. Search date and primary sources not stated.
39. Pepine CJ, Cohn PF, Deedwania PC, et al. Effects of treatment on outcome in mildly symptomatic patients with ischemia during daily life: the atenolol silent ischemia study (ASIST). *Circulation* 1994;90:762–768.
40. Boissel J-P, Leizerovicz A, Picolet H, et al. Secondary prevention after high-risk acute myocardial infarction with low-dose acebutolol. *Am J Cardiol* 1990;66:251–260.
41. The Beta-Blocker Pooling Project Research Group. The Beta-Blocker Pooling Project (BBPP): subgroup findings from randomized trials in post infarction patients. *Eur Heart J* 1988;9:8–16. Search date 1983; primary sources not stated.
42. Beta-blocker Heart Attack Trial Research Group. A randomized trial of propranolol in patients with acute myocardial infarction: I. mortality results. *JAMA* 1982;247:1707–1714.
43. Flather MD, Yusuf S, Kober L, et al. Long-term ACE-inhibitor therapy in patients with heart failure or left-ventricular dysfunction: a systematic overview of data from individual patients. ACE-Inhibitor Myocardial Infarction Collaborative Group. *Lancet* 2000 6;355:1575–81. Search date not stated; primary sources Medline, hand searches of reference lists, and contact with experts.
44. The Heart Outcomes Prevention Evaluation (HOPE) Investigators. Effects of an angiotensin-converting enzyme inhibitor, ramipril, on cardiovascular events in high-risk patients. *N Engl J Med* 2000;342;145–153.
45. Heart Outcomes Prevention Evaluation (HOPE) Investigators. Effects of ramipril on cardiovascular and microvascular outcomes on people with diabetes mellitus: results of the hope study and MICRO-HOPE substudy. *Lancet* 2000;355:253–259.

46. Yusuf S, Lonn E. Anti-ischaemic effects of ACE inhibitors: review of current clinical evidence and ongoing clinical trials. *Eur Heart J* 1998;19:J36–J44.
47. Echt DS, Liebson PR, Mitchell LB, et al. Mortality and morbidity in patients receiving encainide, flecainide, or placebo. The Cardiac Arrhythmia Suppression Trial. *N Engl J Med* 1991;324:781–788.
48. Amiodarone Trials Meta-Analysis Investigators. Effect of prophylactic amiodarone on mortality after acute myocardial infarction and in congestive heart failure: meta-analysis of individual data from 6500 patients in randomised trials. *Lancet* 1997;350:1417–1424. Search date and primary sources not stated.
49. Sim I, McDonald KM, Lavori PW, et al. Quantitative overview of randomized trials of amiodarone to prevent sudden cardiac death. *Circulation* 1997;96:2823–2829. Search date 1997; primary sources Medline and Biosis.
50. Waldo AL, Camm AJ, de Ruyter H, et al, for the SWORD Investigators. Effect of d-sotalol on mortality in patients with left ventricular dysfunction after recent and remote myocardial infarction. *Lancet* 1996;348:7–12.
51. Cairns JA, Connolly SJ, Roberts R, et al, for the Canadian Amiodarone Myocardial Infarction Arrhythmia Trial Investigators. Randomized trial of outcome after myocardial infarction in patients with frequent or repetitive ventricular premature depolarisations: CAMIAT. *Lancet* 1997;349:675–682.
52. Julian DG, Camm AJ, Janse MJ, et al, for the European Myocardial Infarct Amiodarone Trial Investigators. Randomised trial of effect of amiodarone on mortality in patients with left-ventricular dysfunction after recent myocardial infarction: EMIAT. *Lancet* 1997;349:667–674.
53. Gibson R, Boden WE, Theroux P, et al. Diltiazem and reinfarction in patients with non-Q-wave myocardial infarction. Results of a double-blind, randomized, multicenter trial. *N Engl J Med* 1986;315:423–429.
54. The Multicenter Diltiazem Postinfarction Trial Research Group. The effect of diltiazem on mortality and reinfarction after myocardial infarction. *N Engl J Med* 1988;319:385–392.
55. The Danish Study Group on Verapamil in Myocardial Infarction. Effect of verapamil on mortality and major events after acute myocardial infarction: the Danish verapamil infarction trial II (DAVIT II). *Am J Cardiol* 1990;66:779–785.
56. Hulley S, Grady D, Bush T, et al. Randomized trial of estrogen plus progestin for secondary prevention of coronary heart disease in postmenopausal women. *JAMA* 1998;280:605–613.
57. Coronary Drug Research Project Research Group. The coronary drug project: initial findings leading to modifications of its research protocol. *JAMA* 1970;214:1303–1313.
58. Daly E, Vessey MP, Hawkins MM, et al. Risk of venous thromboembolism in users of hormone replacement therapy. *Lancet* 1996;348:977–980.
59. Newton KM, LaCroix AZ, McKnight B, et al. Estrogen replacement therapy and prognosis after first myocardial infarction. *Am J Epidemiol* 1997;145:269–277.
60. Sullivan JM, El-Zeky F, Vander Zwaag R, et al. Effect on survival of estrogen replacement therapy after coronary artery bypass grafting. *Am J Cardiol* 1997;79:847–850.
61. The Writing Group for the PEPI Trial. Effects of estrogen or estrogen/progestin regimens on heart disease risk factors in postmenopausal women. *JAMA* 1995;273:199–208.
62. Bucher HC, Griffith LE, Guyatt G. Systematic review on the risk and benefit of different cholesterol-lowering interventions. *Arterioscler Thromb Vasc Biol* 1999;19:187–195. Search date 1996; primary sources Medline, Embase, and bibliographic searches.
63. Miettinen TA, Pyorala K, Olsson AG, et al. Cholesterol-lowering therapy in women and elderly patients with myocardial infarction or angina pectoris: findings from the Scandinavian Simvastatin Survival Study (4S). *Circulation* 1997;96:4211–4218.
64. Heart Protection Study Collaborative Group. MRC/BHF Heart Protection Study of cholesterol lowering with simvastatin in 20 536 high-risk individuals: a randomised placebo-controlled trial. *Lancet* 2002;360:7M–22M.
65. LaRosa JC, He J, Vupputuri S. Effect of statins on risk of coronary disease: a meta-analysis of randomized controlled trials. *JAMA* 1999;282:2340–2346. Search date 1998; primary sources Medline, bibliographies, and authors' reference files.
66. Schwartz GG, Olsson AG, Ezekowitz MD, et al. Effects of atorvastatin on early recurrent ischemic events in acute coronary syndromes: the MIRACL study: a randomized controlled trial. *JAMA* 2001;285:1711–1718.
67. Knatterud GL, Rosenberg Y, Campeau L, et al. Long-term effects on clinical outcomes of aggressive lowering of low-density lipoprotein cholesterol levels and low-dose anticoagulation in the post coronary artery bypass graft trial. Post CABG Investigators. *Circulation* 2000;102:157–165.
68. Montagne O, Vedel I, Durand-Zaleski I. Assessment of the impact of fibrates and diet on survival and their cost-effectiveness: evidence from randomized, controlled trials in coronary heart disease and health economic evaluations. *Clin Ther* 1999;21:2027–2035. Search date not stated; primary sources Medline, hand searches of reference lists, and systematic reviews.
69. Schlesinger Z, Vered Z, Friedenson A, et al. Secondary prevention by raising HDL cholesterol and reducing triglycerides in patients with coronary artery disease: the Bezafibrate Infarction Prevention (BIP) study. *Circulation* 2000;102:21–27.
70. Ericsson CG, Hamsten A, Nilsson J, et al. Angiographic assessment of effects of bezafibrate on progression of coronary artery disease in young male postinfarction patients. *Lancet* 1996;347:849–853.
71. The Women's Health Initiative Study Group. Design of the women's health initiative clinical trial and observational study. *Control Clin Trials* 1998;19:61–109.
72. Davis BR, Cutler JA Gordon DJ, et al, for the ALLHAT Research Group. Rationale and design for the antihypertensive and lipid lowering treatment to prevent heart attack trial (ALLHAT). *Am J Hypertens* 1996;9:342–360.
73. Flack JM, Neaton J, Grimm R, et al. Blood pressure and mortality among men with prior myocardial infarction. *Circulation* 1995;92;2437–2445.
74. Dahlof B, Lindholm LH, Hansson L, et al. Morbidity and mortality in the Swedish trial in old patients with hypertension (STOP-hypertension). *Lancet* 1991;338:1281–1285.
75. Medical Research Council Working Party. MRC trial on treatment of hypertension in older adults: principal results. *BMJ* 1992;304:405–412.
76. Systolic Hypertension in Elderly Patients (SHEP) Cooperative Research Group. Prevention of stroke

by antihypertensive treatment in older persons with isolated systolic hypertension. *JAMA* 1991;265:3255–3264.
77. D'Agostini RB, Belanger AJ, Kannel WB, et al. Relationship of low diastolic blood pressure to coronary heart disease death in presence of myocardial infarction: the Framingham study. *BMJ* 1991;303:385–389.
78. Pfeffer MA, Braunwald E, Moye LA, et al. Effect of captopril on mortality and morbidity in patients with left ventricular dysfunction after myocardial infarction: results of the survival and ventricular enlargement trial. *N Engl J Med* 1992;327:669–677.
79. NHS Centre for Reviews and Dissemination, University of York. Cholesterol and coronary heart disease: screening and treatment. *Eff Health Care* 1998;4:1. Search date and primary sources not stated.
80. Burr ML, Fehily AM, Gilbert JF, et al. Effects of changes in fat, fish, and fibre intakes on death and myocardial reinfarction: Diet And Reinfarction Trial (DART). *Lancet* 1989;2:757–761.
81. Fehily AM, Vaughan-Williams E, Shiels K, et al. The effect of dietary advice on nutrient intakes: evidence from the Diet And Reinfarction Trial (DART). *J Hum Nutr Diet* 1989;2:225–235.
82. GISSI-Prevenzione Investigators. Dietary supplementation with n–3 polyunsaturated fatty acids and vitamin E after myocardial infarction: results of the GISSI-Prevenzione. *Lancet* 1999;354:447–455.
83. De Lorgeril M, Renaud S, Mamelle N, et al. Mediterranean alpha-linolenic acid-rich diet in secondary prevention of coronary heart disease. *Lancet* 1994;343:1454–1459.
84. Clarke R, Frost C, Collins R, et al. Dietary lipids and blood cholesterol: quantitative meta-analysis of metabolic ward studies. *BMJ* 1997;314:112–117. Search date 1995; primary sources Medline, and hand searches of reference lists and nutrition journals.
85. Tang JL, Armitage JM, Lancaster T, et al. Systematic review of dietary intervention trials to lower blood total cholesterol in free-living subjects. *BMJ* 1998;316:1213–1220. Search date 1997; primary sources Medline, Human Nutrition, Embase, and Allied and Alternative Medicine, hand searches the *Am J Clin Nutr*, and references of review articles.
86. Brunner E, White I, Thorogood M, et al. Can dietary interventions change diet and cardiovascular risk factors? A meta-analysis of randomized controlled trials. *Am J Public Health* 1997;87:1415–1422. Search date 1993; primary sources Medline and hand searches of selected journals.
87. Ebrahim S, Davey SG. *Health promotion in older people for the prevention of coronary heart disease and stroke*. London: Health Education Authority, 1996.
88. Waters D. Lessons from coronary atherosclerosis "regression" trials. *Cardiol Clin* 1996;14:31–50.
89. Silagy C, Neil A. Garlic as a lipid lowering agent: a meta-analysis. *J R Coll Physicians Lond* 1994;28:39–45. Search date 1992; primary sources Medline, Alternative Medicine database, contact with authors of published studies, manufacturers, and hand searches of references.
90. Isaacson JL, Moser M, Stein EA, et al. Garlic powder and plasma lipids and lipoproteins. *Arch Intern Med* 1998;158:1189–119.
91. Berthold HK, Sudhop T, von Bergmann K. Effect of a garlic oil preparation on serum lipoproteins and cholesterol metabolism. *JAMA* 1998;279:1900–1902.
92. Ripsin CM, Keenan JM, Jacobs DR Jr, et al. Oat products and lipid lowering: a meta-analysis. *JAMA* 1992;267:3317–3325. Search date 1991; primary sources Medline and unpublished trials solicited from all known investigators of lipid–oats association.
93. Stephens NG, Parsons A, Schofield PM, et al. Randomised controlled trial of vitamin E in patients with coronary disease: Cambridge Heart Antioxidant Study (CHAOS). *Lancet* 1996;347:781–786.
94. Rapola JM, Virtamo J, Ripatti S, et al. Randomised trial of alpha-tocopherol and beta-carotene supplements on incidence of major coronary events in men with previous myocardial infarction. *Lancet* 1997;349:1715–1720.
95. The Heart Outcomes Prevention Evaluation Study Investigators. Vitamin E supplementation and cardiovascular events in high-risk patients. The Heart Outcomes Prevention Evaluation Study Investigators. *N Engl J Med* 2000;342:154–160.
96. Boaz M, Smetana S, Weinstein T, et al. Secondary prevention with antioxidants of cardiovascular disease in endstage renal disease (SPACE): randomised placebo-controlled trial. *Lancet* 2000;356:1213–1218.
97. Wilson TS, Datta SB, Murrell JS, et al. Relation of vitamin C levels to mortality in a geriatric hospital: a study of the effect of vitamin C administration. *Age Aging* 1973;2:163–170.
98. Burr ML, Hurley RJ, Sweetnam PM. Vitamin C supplementation of old people with low blood levels. *Gerontol Clin* 1975;17:236–243.
99. Hunt C, Chakkravorty NK, Annan G. The clinical and biochemical effects of vitamin C supplementation in short-stay hospitalized geriatric patients. *Int J Vitam Nutr Res* 1984;54:65–74.
100. Brown BG, Zhao X-Q, Chait A, et al. Simvastatin and niacin, antioxidant vitamins, or the combination for the prevention of coronary disease. *N Engl J Med* 2001;345:1583–1592.
101. Lonn EM, Yusuf S. Is there a role for antioxidant vitamins in the prevention of cardiovascular diseases? An update on epidemiological and clinical trials data. *Can J Cardiol* 1997;13:957–965. Search date 1996; primary sources Medline and one reference from 1997.
102. Jha P, Flather M, Lonn E, et al. The antioxidant vitamins and cardiovascular disease: a critical review of epidemiologic and clinical trial data. *Ann Intern Med* 1995;123:860–872.
103. Ness AR, Powles JW, Khaw KT. Vitamin C and cardiovascular disease: a systematic review. *J Cardiovasc Risk* 1997;3:513–521. Search date not stated; primary sources Medline, experts, and hand searches of references.
104. Collins R, Peto R, Armitage J. The MRC/BHF heart protection study: preliminary results. *Int J Clin Pract* 2002;56:53.
105. Jolliffe JA, Rees K, Taylor RS, et al. Exercise-based rehabilitation for coronary heart disease. In: The Cochrane Library, Issue 2, 2002. Oxford: Update Software. Search date 1998; primary sources Cardiovascular RCT register at McMaster University, Cochrane Controlled Trials Register, Medline, Embase, Cinahl, Amed, Bids, ISI, and Sportsdiscus, hand searches of reference lists, conference proceedings, and contact with experts.
106. Wenger NK, Froelicher NS, Smith LK, et al. *Cardiac rehabilitation and secondary prevention*. Rockville, Maryland: Agency for Health Care Policy and Research and National Heart, Lung and Blood Institute, 1995. Search date and primary source not stated.

107. US Department of Health and Human Services. *The health benefits of smoking cessation: a report of the surgeon general*. Bethesda, Maryland: US DHSS, 1990.
108. Working Group for the Study of Transdermal Nicotine in Patients with Coronary Artery Disease. Nicotine replacement therapy for patients with coronary artery disease. *Arch Intern Med* 1994;154:989–995.
109. Joseph AM, Norman SM, Ferry LH, et al. The safety of transdermal nicotine as an aid to smoking cessation in patients with cardiac disease. *N Engl J Med* 1996;335:1792–1798.
110. Burt A, Thornley P, Illingworth D, et al. Stopping smoking after myocardial infarction. *Lancet* 1974;1:304–306.
111. Linden W, Stossel C, Maurice J. Psychosocial interventions in patients with coronary artery disease: a meta-analysis. *Arch Intern Med* 1996;156:745–752. Search date and primary sources not stated.
112. US Department of Health and Human Services. Cardiac rehabilitation. AHCPR Publication No 96–0672, 1995;121–128.
113. Hemingway H, Marmot M. Psychosocial factors in the primary and secondary prevention of coronary heart disease: a systematic review. In: Yusuf S, Cairns JA, Camm AJ, et al, eds. *Evidence based cardiology*. London: BMJ Books, 1998. Search date 1996; primary sources Medline, and manual searches of bibliographics of retrieved articles and review articles.
114. Yusuf S, Zucker D, Peduzzi P, et al. Effect of coronary artery bypass graft surgery on survival: overview of 10-year results from randomized trials by the Coronary Artery Bypass Graft Surgery Trialists Collaboration. *Lancet* 1994;344:563–570. Search date and primary sources not stated.
115. Davies RF, Goldberg AD, Forman S, et al. Asymptomatic Cardiac Ischemia Pilot (ACIP) study two-year follow-up: outcomes of patients randomized to initial strategies of medical therapy versus revascularization. *Circulation* 1997;95:2037–2043.
116. Bucher HC, Hengstler P, Schindler C, et al. Percutaneous transluminal coronary angioplasty versus medical treatment for non-acute coronary heart disease: meta-analysis of randomised controlled trials. *BMJ* 2000;321:73–77. Search date 1998; primary sources Medline, Embase, Cochrane Library, Biological Abstracts, Health Periodicals Database, Pascal, and hand searches of references.
117. Pocock SJ, Henderson RA, Clayton T, et al. Quality of life after coronary angioplasty or continued medical treatment for angina: three-year follow-up in the RITA-2 trial. Randomized Intervention Treatment of Angina. *J Am Coll Cardiol* 2000;35:907–914.
118. TIME investigators. Trial of invasive versus medical therapy in elderly patients with chronic symptomatic coronary-artery disease (TIME): a randomised trial. *Lancet* 2001;358:951–957.
119. RITA-2 Trial Participants. Coronary angioplasty versus medical therapy for angina: the second randomized intervention treatment of angina (RITA-2) trial. *Lancet* 1997;350:461–468.
120. Parisi AF, Folland ED, Hartigan P. A comparison of angioplasty with medical therapy in the treatment of single-vessel coronary artery disease. *N Engl J Med* 1992;326:10–16.
121. Morris KG, Folland ED, Hartigan PM, et al. Unstable angina in late follow-up of the ACME trial. *Circulation* 1995;92(suppl S):3484.
122. Pocock SJ, Henderson RA, Rickards AF, et al. Meta-analysis of randomized trials comparing coronary angioplasty with bypass surgery. *Lancet* 1995;346:1184–1189. Search date and primary sources not stated.
123. Rihal CS, Gersh BJ, Yusuf S. Chronic coronary artery disease: coronary artery bypass surgery vs percutaneous transluminal coronary angioplasty vs medical therapy. In: Yusuf S, Cairns JA, Camm JA, et al, eds. *Evidence based cardiology*. London: BMJ Books, 1998.
124. King SB, Kosinski AS, Guyton RA, et al. Eight-year mortality in the Emory Angioplasty versus Surgery Trial (EAST). *J Am Coll Cardiol* 2000;35:1116–1121.
125. Hlatky MA, Rogers WJ, Johnstone I, et al. Medical care costs and quality of life after randomization to coronary angioplasty or coronary bypass surgery. *N Engl J Med* 1997;336:92–99.
126. Währborg P. Quality of life after coronary angioplasty or bypass surgery. *Eur Heart J* 1999;20:653–658.
127. Bypass Angioplasty Revascularization Investigation (BARI) Investigators. Comparison of coronary bypass surgery with angioplasty in patients with multivessel disease. *N Engl J Med* 1996;335:217–225.
128. The BARI Investigators. Seven-year outcome in the Bypass Angioplasty Revascularization Investigation (BARI) by treatment and diabetic status. *J Am Coll Cardiol* 2000;35:1122–1129.
129. National Institute of Clinical Excellence http://www.nice.org.uk/pdf/HTAReport-Stents.pdf (last accessed 19 September 2002). Search date 1999; primary sources Medline, Embase, Bids, Cochrane Library, and York HTA.
130. Savage MP, Douglas JS Jr, Fischman DL, et al. Stent placement compared with balloon angioplasty for obstructed coronary bypass grafts. *N Engl J Med* 1997;337:740–747.
131. Sirnes P, Golf S, Yngvar M, et al. Stenting In Chronic Coronary Occlusion (SICCO): a randomized controlled trial of adding stent implantation after successful angioplasty. *J Am Coll Cardiol* 1996;28:1444–1451.
132. Rubartelli P, Niccoli L, Verna E, et al. Stent implantation versus balloon angioplasty in chronic coronary occlusions: results from the GISSOC trial. Gruppo Italiano di Studio sullo Stent nelle Occlusioni Coronariche. *J Am Coll Cardiol* 1998;32:90–96.
133. Sievert H, Rohde S, Utech A, et al. Stent or Angioplasty after Recanalization of Chronic Coronary Occlusions? (The SARECCO trial). *Am J Cardiol* 1999;84:386–390.
134. Erbel R, Haude M, Hopp HW, et al. Coronary artery stenting compared with balloon angioplasty for restenosis after initial balloon angioplasty. *N Engl J Med* 1998;23:1672–1688.
135. Versaci F, Gaspardone A, Tomai F, et al. A comparison of coronary-artery stenting with angioplasty for isolated stenosis of the proximal left anterior descending coronary artery. *N Engl J Med* 1997;336:817–822.
136. Schomig A, Neumann FJ, Kastrati A, et al. A randomized comparison of antiplatelet and anticoagulation therapy after the placement of intracoronary stents. *N Engl J Med* 1996;334:1084–1089.
137. Leon MB, Baim DS, Gordon P, et al. Clinical and angiographic results from the Stent Anticoagulation Regimen Study (STARS). *Circulation* 1996;94(suppl S):4002.
138. Witkowski A, Ruzyllo W, Gil R, et al. A randomized comparison of elective high-pressure stenting with balloon angioplasty: six-month angiographic and two-year clinical follow-up. *Am Heart J* 2000;140:264–271.

Secondary prevention of ischaemic cardiac events

Cathie Sudlow
Wellcome Clinician Scientist
Western General Hospital
University of Edinburgh
Edinburgh, UK

Eva Lonn
Associate Professor of Medicine
Hamilton General Hospital
Hamilton, Canada

Michael Pignone
Division of General Internal Medicine
University of North Carolina
Chapel Hill, USA

Andrew Ness
Senior Lecturer in Epidemiology
University of Bristol
Bristol, UK

Charanjit Rihal
Consultant Cardiologist
Mayo Clinic and Mayo Foundation
Rochester, USA

Competing interests: CR none declared. AN none declared. EL has reveived reimbursement for participating at symposiums, presentations of lectures and organising education activities for different pharmaceutical companies. CR none declared. CS on one occasion received fee from Sanofi-Synthelabo for giving a talk at a GP meeting.

TABLE 1 **Prognostic groups for people who survive the acute stage of myocardial infarction (see text, p 133).**

Baseline risk	1 year mortality	Clinical markers[2–4]
High	10–50%	Older age; history or previous myocardial infarction; reduced exercise tolerance (New York Heart Association functional classes II–IV) before admission; clinical signs of heart failure in the first 2 days (Killip classes IIb, III, and IV) or persistent heart failure on days 3–5 after infarction; early increased heart rate; persistent or early appearance of angina at rest or with minimal exertion; and multiple or complex ventricular arrhythmias during monitoring in hospital.
Moderate	10%	ND
Low	2–5%	Younger age (< 55 years), no previous myocardial infarction, an event free course during the first 5 days after myocardial infarction.[2]

ND, no data.

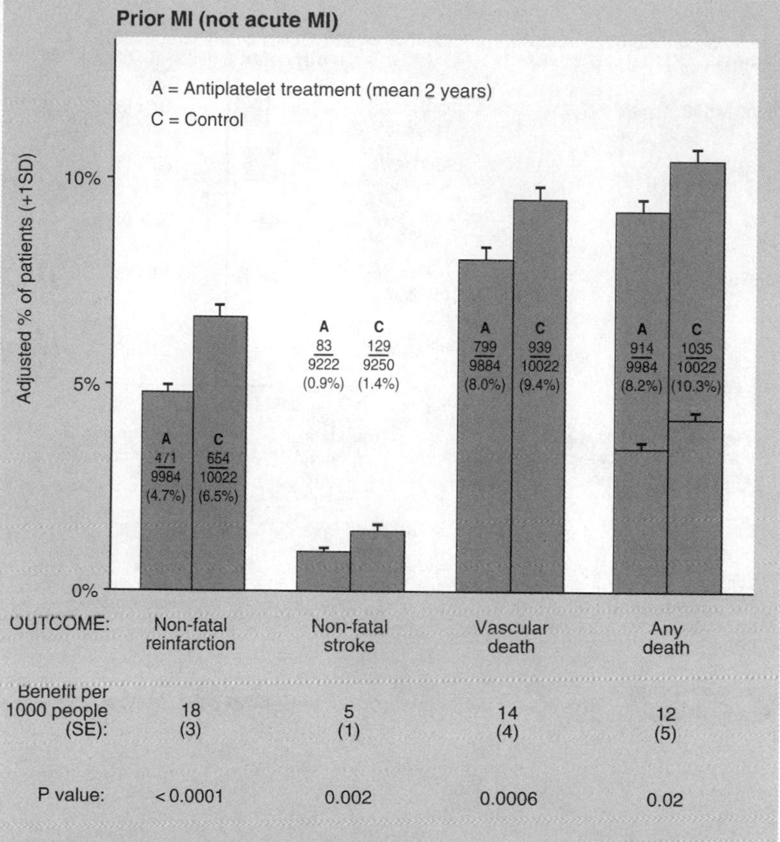

FIGURE 1 **The absolute effects of antiplatelet treatment on various outcomes in people with prior myocardial infarction: results of a systematic review.[10] The columns show the absolute risks over 2 years for each outcome. The error bars represent standard deviations. In the "any death" column, non-vascular deaths are represented by lower horizontal lines (see text, p 134).**

Aspirin daily dose (mg)	No of trials†	Events/patients Aspirin (%)	Control (%)	Odds ratio (95% CI Random) Aspirin:control	Odds reduction (SD)	2P
500–1500	34	1621/11215 (14.5%)	1930/11236 (17.2%)		19% (3)	< 0.00001
160–325	19	1526/13240 (11.5%)	1963/13273 (14.8%)		25% (3)	< 0.00001
75–150	12	370/3370 (11.0%)	519/3406 (15.2%)		32% (6)	< 0.00001
< 75	3	316/1827 (17.3%)	354/1828 (19.4%)		13% (8)	NS
Total	65	3833/29652 (12.9%)	4766/29743 (16.0%)		23% (2)	< 0.00001

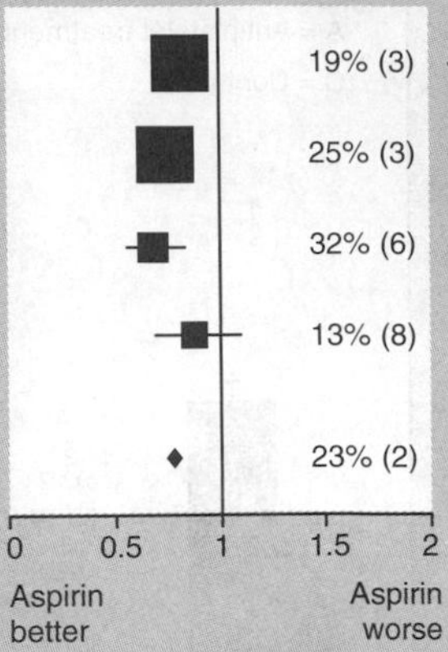

Heterogeneity between 4 dose categories:
χ^2 3df = 7.7: P = 0.06

† Some trials contributed to more than one daily dose category.

Typical odds ratio for each category shown as square (with area proportional to the variance of observed - expected) together with its 99% confidence interval (horizontal line). Typical odds ratio for the total shown as diamond with its 95% confidence interval (horizontal line = width of diamond). Vertical dotted line passes through point estimate of typical odds ratio for total.

FIGURE 2 **Effects of different doses of aspirin (see text, p 134).**

Stroke management

Search date January 2002

Gord Gubitz and Peter Sandercock

QUESTIONS

INTERVENTIONS

See glossary, p 180

Key Messages

Acute ischaemic stroke

- **Acute reduction in blood pressure** One systematic review found insufficient evidence about the effects of antihypertensives versus placebo, but RCTs have suggested that people treated with antihypertensive agents may have a worse clinical outcome and increased mortality.
- **Aspirin** One systematic review in people with ischaemic stroke confirmed by computerised tomography scan has found that aspirin versus placebo within 48 hours of stroke onset significantly reduces death or dependency at 6 months (NNT 77, 95% CI 43 to 333) and significantly increases the number of people making a complete recovery (NNT 91, 95% CI 50 to 500). We found indirect evidence that aspirin should not be delayed if a computerised tomography scan is not available within 48 hours: results from two large RCTs found no significant difference in further stroke or death with aspirin versus placebo in people who were subsequently found to have haemorrhagic rather than ischaemic stroke.

Stroke management

- **Immediate systemic anticoagulation** One systematic review comparing systemic anticoagulants (unfractionated heparin, low molecular weight heparin, heparinoids, oral anticoagulants, or specific thrombin inhibitors) versus usual care without systemic anticoagulants found no significant difference in death or dependence after 3–6 months. One systematic review has found that immediate systemic anticoagulation significantly reduces the risk of deep venous thrombosis (NNT 3, 95% CI 2 to 4) and symptomatic pulmonary embolus (NNT 333, 95% CI 167 to 1000), but increases the risk of intracranial haemorrhage (NNH 108, 95% CI 85 to 147) or extracranial haemorrhage (NNH 109, 95% CI 87 to 149). One RCT in people with acute ischaemic stroke and atrial fibrillation found no significant difference with low molecular weight heparin versus aspirin in recurrent ischaemic stroke within 14 days. One RCT in people within 48 hours of stroke onset found no significant difference with high or low dose tinzaparin versus aspirin in people achieving functional independence at 6 months.
- **Neuroprotective agents (calcium channel antagonists, γ-aminobutyric acid agonists, lubeluzole, glycine antagonists, tirilazad, N-methyl-D-aspartate antagonists)** RCTs found no evidence that, compared with placebo, calcium channel antagonists, tirilazad, lubeluzole, γ-aminobutyric acid agonists, glycine antagonists, or N-methyl-D-aspartate antagonists significantly improve clinical outcomes. One systematic review found that lubeluzole versus placebo was associated with a significant increase in the risk of having Q-T prolongation to more than 450 ms on electrocardiography (NNH 45, 95% CI 23 to 1000).
- **Specialised care** One systematic review has found that specialist stroke rehabilitation units versus alternate (less organised) care significantly reduce death or dependency after 1 year (NNT 21, 95% CI 13 to 63).
- **Thrombolysis** One systematic review has found that thrombolysis versus placebo significantly reduces the risk of death or dependency in the long term (NNT 24, 95% CI 14 to 83), but significantly increases the risk of death from intracranial haemorrhage measured in the first 7–10 days (NNH 23, 95% CI 19 to 29).

Intracerebral haematomas

- **Evacuation** We found that the balance between benefits and harms has not been clearly established for the evacuation of supratentorial haematomas. We found no evidence from RCTs on the role of evacuation or ventricular shunting in people with infratentorial haematoma whose consciousness level is declining.

DEFINITION Stroke is characterised by rapidly developing clinical symptoms and signs of focal, and at times global, loss of cerebral function lasting more than 24 hours or leading to death, with no apparent cause other than that of vascular origin.[1] Ischaemic stroke is stroke caused by vascular insufficiency (such as cerebrovascular thromboembolism) rather than haemorrhage.

INCIDENCE/ PREVALENCE Stroke is the third most common cause of death in most developed countries.[2] It is a worldwide problem; about 4.5 million people die from stroke a year. Stroke can occur at any age, but half of all strokes occur in people over 70 years old.[3]

AETIOLOGY/ RISK FACTORS About 80% of all acute strokes are caused by cerebral infarction, usually resulting from thrombotic or embolic occlusion of a cerebral artery.[4] The remainder are caused either by intracerebral or subarachnoid haemorrhage.

PROGNOSIS About 10% of all people with acute ischaemic strokes will die within 30 days of stroke onset.[5] Of those who survive the acute event, about 50% will experience some level of disability after 6 months.[6]

AIMS To minimise impairment, disability, secondary complications, and adverse effects from treatment.

OUTCOMES Risk of death or dependency (generally assessed as the proportion of people dead or requiring physical assistance for transfers, mobility, dressing, feeding, or toileting 3–6 months after stroke onset);[6] quality of life.

METHODS *Clinical Evidence* search and appraisal January 2002.

QUESTION What are the effects of specialised care in people with stroke?

One systematic review has found that specialist stroke rehabilitation units versus alternate (less organised) care significantly reduces death or dependency after 1 year. Prospective observational data suggest these findings may be reproducible in routine clinical settings.

Benefits: We found one systematic review (search date 2001, 23 RCTs, 4911 people with stroke) comparing specialised stroke rehabilitation versus conventional care.[7] In most trials, the specialised stroke rehabilitation unit consisted of a designated area or ward, although some trials used a mobile "stroke team". People in these trials were usually transferred to stroke unit care within the first or second week after stroke onset. It found people cared for in a stroke rehabilitation unit had lower rates of death or dependency after a median follow up of 1 year (AR 60.5% without stroke unit *v* 55.8% with stroke unit, ARR 4.7%, 95% CI 1.6% to 7.8%; NNT 21, 95% CI 13 to 63; OR 0.78, 95% CI 0.68 to 0.89) (see figure 1, p 183).[7] The duration of stay was calculated differently for many of the trials, so the consequent heterogeneity between results limits generalisability. However, overall, duration of stay in the stroke unit was about 6 days (95% CI 2 to 10 days) shorter than duration of stay in a non-stroke unit setting. The review found that organised stroke unit care versus alternate service significantly reduced death or dependency at 5 years' follow up (223/286 [78%] with organised stroke unit care *v* 214/249 [86%] with alternate care; RR 0.91, 95% CI 0.84 to 0.99).[7] One RCT (220 people) included in the review found that care in a combined acute and rehabilitation unit compared with care in general wards increased the proportion of people able to live at home 10 years after their stroke (ARI 11%, 95% CI 1.9% to 20%; NNT 9, 95% CI 5 to 52).[11] We found one additional RCT, which randomised 76 people 2–10 days after their stroke to either an integrated care pathway (see glossary, p 180) or to conventional multidisciplinary care on a stroke rehabilitation unit in the UK.[12] All received similar occupational and physical therapy. Conventional treatment versus the integrated care pathway produced more improvement in the Barthel Index from 4–12 weeks

(CI not provided; $P < 0.01$), and higher scores on the Euroquol (Quality of Life Scale) after 6 months ($P < 0.05$). It found no significant difference between the two treatments in mortality, duration of hospital stay, or the proportion of people requiring long term institutional care.

Harms: No detrimental effects attributable to stroke units were reported.[7]

Comment: Although the proportional reduction in death or dependency seems larger with thrombolysis (see thrombolysis option, p 172), stroke unit care is applicable to most people with stroke whereas thrombolysis is applicable only to a small proportion. The systematic review did not provide evidence about which aspects of the multidisciplinary approach led to improved outcome,[7] although one limited retrospective analysis of one of the RCTs found that several factors, including early mobilisation, increased use of oxygen, intravenous saline solutions, and antipyretics, might have been responsible.[13] Most of the trials excluded the most mild and severe strokes. After publication of the systematic review,[7] prospective observational data have been collected in one large series of over 14 000 people in 80 Swedish hospitals.[14] In this series, people admitted to stroke units had reduced dependence at 3 months (RRR 6%, 95% CI 1% to 11%). Although biases are inherent in such observational data, the findings suggest that the results of the meta-analysis may be reproducible in routine clinical settings.

QUESTION What are the effects of medical treatment in acute ischaemic stroke?

OPTION THROMBOLYSIS

One systematic review has found that thrombolysis versus placebo significantly reduces the risk of death or dependency in the long term, but significantly increases the risk of death from intracranial haemorrhage measured in the first 7–10 days.

Benefits: We found one systematic review (search date 1999, 17 RCTs, 5216 highly selected people) comparing thrombolysis with placebo given soon after the onset of stroke.[8] All trials used computerised tomography or magnetic resonance scanning before randomisation to exclude intracranial haemorrhage or other non-stroke disorders. Results for three different thrombolytic agents (streptokinase, urokinase, and recombinant tissue plasminogen activator) were included, but direct comparison of different thrombolytic drugs was not possible. Two trials used intra-arterial administration and the rest used the intravenous route. Thrombolysis significantly reduced the risk of death or dependency at the end of the studies (ARR 4.2%, 95% CI 1.2% to 7.2%; RRR 7%, 95% CI 3% to 12%; NNT 24, 95% CI 14 to 83) (see figure 1, p 183 and figure 2, p 183).[8] In the subset of trials that assessed intravenous recombinant tissue plasminogen activator, the findings were similar (ARR 5.7%, 95% CI 2.0% to 9.4%; RRR 10%, 95% CI 4% to 16%; NNT 18, 95% CI 11 to 50). One meta-analysis (4 RCTs, individual results of 1292 people with acute ischaemic stroke treated with streptokinase or placebo) found that streptokinase versus placebo had no clear effect on the proportion of people dead or dependent at 3 months, and included the possibility of both substantial benefit or substantial harm (RRR +1%, 95% CI –6% to +8%).[15] People allocated to streptokinase were more likely to be dead after 3 months (RRI 46%, 95% CI 24% to 73%). The combination of aspirin plus streptokinase significantly increased mortality at 3 months (P = 0.005), but this did not affect the combined risk of death or severe disability (CI not provided; P = 0.28).

Harms: **Fatal intracranial haemorrhage:** In the systematic review, thrombolysis increased fatal intracranial haemorrhage compared with placebo measured in the first 7–10 days (ARI 4.4%, 95% CI 3.4% to 5.4%; RRI 396%, 95% CI 220% to 668%; NNH 23, 95% CI 19 to 29).[8] In the subset of trials that assessed intravenous recombinant tissue plasminogen activator, the findings were similar (ARI 2.9%, 95% CI 1.7% to 4.1%; RRI 259%, 95% CI 102% to 536%; NNH 34, 95% CI 24 to 59). **Death:** In the systematic review, thrombolysis compared with placebo increased the risk of death by the end of the follow up (ARI 3.3%, 95% CI 1.2% to 5.4%; RRI 23%, 95% CI 10% to 38%; NNH 30, 95% CI 19 to 83).[8] This excess of deaths was offset by fewer people being alive but dependent 6 months after stroke onset. The net effect was a reduction in the number of people who were dead or dependent.

Comment: There was no significant heterogeneity of treatment effect overall, but heterogeneity of results was noted for the outcomes of death, and death or dependency at final follow up among the eight trials of intravenous recombinant tissue plasminogen activator.[8] Explanations may include the combined use of antithrombotic agents (aspirin or heparin within the first 24 h of thrombolysis), stroke severity, the presence of early ischaemic changes on computerised tomography scan, and the time from stroke onset to randomisation. A subgroup analysis suggested that thrombolysis may be more beneficial if given within 3 hours of symptom onset, but the duration of the "therapeutic time window" could not be determined reliably. Most of the trial results were of outcome at 3 months; only one trial reported 1 year outcome data.[16] We found little evidence about which people are most and least likely to benefit from thrombolysis. A number of trials of different thrombolytic regimens are underway.[17] In addition, preliminary information from a meta-analysis of individual patient data from the recombinant tissue plasminogen activator trials by the ECASS, NINDS, and ATLANTIS investigators was recently reported at a platform session of the 27th International Stroke Conference; full publication is awaited, and will be presented in future *Clinical Evidence* updates (B Thomas, personal communication, 2002).

OPTION ASPIRIN

One systematic review in people with ischaemic stroke confirmed by computerised tomography scan has found that aspirin versus placebo within 48 hours of stroke onset significantly reduces death or dependency at 6 months and significantly increases the number of people making a

complete recovery. We found indirect evidence that aspirin should not be delayed if a computerised tomography scan is not available within 48 hours; results from two large RCTs found no significant difference in further stroke or death with aspirin versus placebo in people who were subsequently found to have haemorrhagic rather than ischaemic stroke.

Benefits: **Early use of aspirin:** We found one systematic review (search date 1999, 8 RCTs, 41 325 people with definite or presumed ischaemic stroke), which compared antiplatelet treatment started within 14 days of the stroke versus placebo.[18] Of the data in the systematic review, 98% came from two large RCTs of aspirin (160–300 mg daily) started within 48 hours of stroke onset.[9,10] Most people had an ischaemic stroke confirmed by computerised tomography scan before randomisation, but people who were conscious could be randomised before computerised tomography scan if the stroke was very likely to be ischaemic on clinical grounds. Treatment duration varied from 10–28 days. Aspirin started within the first 48 hours of acute ischaemic stroke reduced death or dependency at 6 months' follow up (RRR 3%, 95% CI 1% to 5%; NNT 77, 95% CI 43 to 333) (see figure 1, p 183) and increased the number of people making a complete recovery (NNT 91, 95% CI 50 to 500). A prospective combined analysis[19] of the two large RCTs[9,10] found a significant reduction in the outcome of further stroke or death with aspirin versus placebo (ARR 0.9%, 95% CI 0.75% to 1.85%; NNT 111, 95% CI 54 to 133). The effect was similar across subgroups (older *v* younger; male *v* female; impaired consciousness or not; atrial fibrillation or not; blood pressure; stroke subtype; timing of computerised tomography scanning). For the 773 people subsequently found to have had a haemorrhagic stroke rather than an ischaemic stroke, the subgroup analysis found no difference in the outcome of further stroke or death between those who were randomised to aspirin versus placebo (16% *v* 18%; ARR +2.0%, 95% CI –4.0% to +6.6%).[19] **Long term treatment:** See aspirin under stroke prevention, p 184.

Harms: Aspirin caused an excess of about two intracranial and four extracranial haemorrhages per 1000 people treated, but these small risks were more than offset by the reductions in death and disability from other causes both in the short term[18] and in the long term.[20] Common adverse effects of aspirin (such as dyspepsia and constipation) were dose related.[21]

Comment: We found no clear evidence that any one dose of aspirin is more effective than any other in the treatment of acute ischaemic stroke. One recent meta-regression analysis of the dose–response effect of aspirin on stroke found a uniform effect of aspirin in a range of doses from 50–1500 mg daily.[22] People unable to swallow safely after a stroke may be given aspirin as a suppository.

OPTION **IMMEDIATE SYSTEMIC ANTICOAGULATION**

One systematic review comparing systemic anticoagulants (unfractionated heparin, low molecular weight heparin, heparinoids, oral anticoagulants, or specific thrombin inhibitors) versus usual care without systemic anticoagulants has found no significant difference in death or

dependence after 3–6 months. One systematic review has found that immediate systemic anticoagulation significantly reduces the risk of deep venous thrombosis and symptomatic pulmonary embolus, but increases the risk of intracranial haemorrhage or extracranial haemorrhage. One RCT in people with acute ischaemic stroke and atrial fibrillation found no significant difference with low molecular weight heparin versus aspirin in recurrent ischaemic stroke within 14 days. One RCT in people within 48 hours of stroke onset found no significant difference with high or low dose tinzaparin versus aspirin in people achieving functional independence at 6 months.

Benefits: **Death or dependency:** We found one systematic review (search date 1999, 21 RCTs, 23 427 people)[23] and three subsequent RCTs.[24–26] The systematic review compared unfractionated heparin, low molecular weight heparin, heparinoids, oral anticoagulants, or specific thrombin inhibitors versus usual care without systemic anticoagulants.[23] Over 80% of the data came from one trial, which randomised people with any severity of stroke to either subcutaneous heparin or placebo, usually after exclusion of haemorrhage by computerised tomography scan.[10] The systematic review found no significant difference in the proportion of people dead or dependent in the treatment and control groups at the end of follow up (3–6 months after the stroke: ARR +0.4%, 95% CI –0.9% to +1.7%; RRR 0%, 95% CI –2% to +3%).[23] There was no clear short or long term benefit of anticoagulants in any prespecified subgroups (stroke of presumed cardioembolic origin *v* others; different anticoagulants). The first subsequent RCT (449 people with acute stroke and atrial fibrillation) found no significant difference between dalteparin (a low molecular weight heparin) versus aspirin for the primary outcome of recurrent ischaemic stroke during the first 14 days (ARI +1.0%, 95% CI –3.6% to +6.2%) or for secondary outcomes, including functional outcome at 3 months.[24] The second RCT randomised 404 people to one of four different doses of certoparin (a low molecular weight heparin) within 12 hours of stroke onset.[25] There was no difference in neurological outcome between the four groups 3 months after treatment. The third RCT (1486 people) compared aspirin versus two different doses of tinzaparin (a low molecular weight heparin) within 48 hours of stroke onset.[26] It found no significant difference among the three groups for achieving functional independence at 6 months (AR for independence 41.5% with tinzaparin 175 anti-Xa IU/kg/daily *v* 42.4% with tinzaparin 100 anti-Xa IU/kg/daily *v* 42.5% with aspirin 300 mg/daily). **Deep venous thrombosis and pulmonary embolism:** We found three systematic reviews.[23,27,28] The first systematic review (search date 1999) included 10 small heterogeneous RCTs (22 000 people), which assessed anticoagulants in 916 people at high risk of deep venous thrombosis after their stroke.[23] Anticoagulation compared with control reduced the risk of deep vein thrombosis (ARR 29%, 95% CI 24% to 35%; RRR 64%, 95% CI 54% to 71%; NNT 3, 95% CI 2 to 4) and reduced symptomatic pulmonary embolism (ARR 0.3%, 95% CI 0.1% to 0.6%; RRR 38%, 95% CI 16% to 54%; NNT 333, 95% CI 167 to 1000). No RCT performed investigations in all people to rule out silent events. The frequency of reported pulmonary emboli was low and varied among RCTs, so there may have been under ascertainment.

Two other systematic reviews (search dates 1999[28] and 2001,[27] same 5 RCTs in each review, 705 people with acute ischaemic stroke) found that low molecular weight heparins or heparinoids versus unfractionated heparin significantly reduced deep venous thrombosis (AR 13% with low molecular weight heparins or heparinoids *v* 22% with unfractionated heparin; ARR 9%, 95% CI 4.5% to 16%). The number of events was too small to estimate the effects of low molecular weight heparins or heparinoids versus unfractionated heparin on death, intracranial haemorrhage, or functional outcome in survivors.

Harms: One systematic review found that anticoagulation slightly increased symptomatic intracranial haemorrhages within 14 days of starting treatment compared with control (ARI 0.93%, 95% CI 0.68% to 1.18%; RRI 163%, 95% CI 95% to 255%; NNH 108, 95% CI 85 to 147).[23] The large trial of subcutaneous heparin found that this effect was dose dependent (symptomatic intracranial haemorrhage by using medium dose compared with low dose heparin for 14 days; RRI 143%, 95% CI 82% to 204%; NNH 97, 95% CI 68 to 169).[10] The review also found a dose dependent increase in major extracranial haemorrhages after 14 days of treatment with anticoagulants (ARI 0.91%, 95% CI 0.67% to 1.15%; RRI 231%, 95% CI 136% to 365%; NNH 109, 95% CI 87 to 149).[23] The subsequent RCT of dalteparin versus aspirin for people with acute stroke and atrial fibrillation found no difference in adverse events, including symptomatic or asymptomatic intracerebral haemorrhage, progression of symptoms, or early or late death.[24] As in the systematic review,[23] the RCT comparing different doses of certoparin found that intracranial haemorrhage occurred more often in those receiving a higher dose of anticoagulant.[25] However, the overall number of people experiencing haemorrhagic complications in the RCT may have been artificially lowered because the study protocol was changed during the trial period so as to exclude people with early ischaemic changes on computerised tomography scan. The RCT comparing different doses of tinzaparin found that high dose tinzaprin versus aspirin significantly increased symptomatic intracranial haemorrhage (AR 1.5% with high dose tinzaparin *v* 0.2% with aspirin; OR 7.2, 95% CI 1.1 to 163).[26]

Comment: Alternative treatments to prevent deep venous thrombosis and pulmonary embolism after acute ischaemic stroke include aspirin and compression stockings. The evidence relating to these will be reviewed in future *Clinical Evidence* updates.

OPTION **BLOOD PRESSURE REDUCTION**

One systematic review found insufficient evidence about the effects of antihypertensives versus placebo, but RCTs have suggested that people treated with antihypertensive agents may have a worse clinical outcome and increased mortality.

Benefits: We found one systematic review (search date 2000, 5 RCTs, 281 people with acute stroke) comparing blood pressure lowering treatment with placebo.[29] Several different antihypertensive agents were used. The trials collected insufficient clinical data to allow an analysis of the relation between changes in blood pressure and clinical outcome.

Harms: Two placebo controlled RCTs have suggested that people treated with antihypertensive agents may have a worse clinical outcome and increased mortality.[30,31] The first RCT (295 people with acute ischaemic stroke) compared nimodipine (a calcium channel antagonist) with placebo.[30] The trial was stopped prematurely because of an excess of unfavourable neurological outcomes in the nimodipine treated group. Exploratory analyses confirmed that this negative correlation was related to reductions in mean arterial blood pressure (CI not provided; $P = 0.02$) and diastolic blood pressure ($P = 0.0005$). The second RCT (302 people with acute ischaemic stroke) assessed β blockers (atenolol or propranolol).[31] There was a non-significant increase in death for people taking β blockers, and no difference in the proportion of people achieving a good outcome. One systematic review (search date 1994, 9 RCTs, 3719 people with acute stroke) compared nimodipine versus placebo; no net benefit was found.[32] A second review (24 RCTs, 6894 people) found a non-significant increase in the risk of death with calcium channel antagonists versus placebo (RRI 8%, 95% CI 1% reduction to 18% increase).[33] Although treatment with calcium channel antagonists in these trials was intended for neuroprotection, blood pressure was lower in the treatment group in several trials.

Comment: Population based studies suggest a direct and continuous association between blood pressure and the risk of recurrent stroke.[34] However, acute blood pressure lowering in acute ischaemic stroke may lead to increased cerebral ischaemia. The systematic review[29] identified several ongoing RCTs. We identified one additional ongoing RCT not included in the review.[35]

OPTION NEUROPROTECTIVE AGENTS

RCTs found no evidence that compared with placebo, calcium channel antagonists, lubeluzole, γ-aminobutyric acid agonists, tirilazad, glycine antagonists, or N-methyl-D-aspartate antagonists significantly improved clinical outcomes. One systematic review found that lubeluzole versus placebo was associated with a significant increase in the risk of having Q-T prolongation to more than 450 ms on electrocardiography.

Benefits: We found no systematic reviews assessing the general effectiveness of neuroprotective agents in acute ischaemic stroke. **Calcium channel antagonists:** We found two systematic reviews comparing calcium channel antagonists with placebo.[36,37] The first review (search date 1999, 28 RCTs, 7521 people with acute ischaemic stroke) found that calcium channel antagonists did not significantly reduce the risk of poor outcome (including death) at the end of the follow up period compared with placebo (ARI of poor outcome +4.9%, 95% CI –2.5% to +7.3%; RRI +4%, 95% CI –2% to +9%).[36] The second review (search date 1999)[37] includes one additional RCT (454 people)[38] that was stopped prematurely because of publication of the first review.[36] Inclusion of its data does not change the results of the first review. **γ-Aminobutyric acid agonists:** We found one systematic review (search date not stated, 3 RCTs, 1002 people with acute ischaemic stroke), which found no significant difference between piracetam (a γ-aminobutyric acid agonist) and control groups for the number of people dead or dependent at the end of follow up (ARI +0.2%, 95% CI –6.0% to +6.4%; RRI 0%, 95% CI –11% to +9%).[39] We found one RCT (1360 people with acute stroke), which identified no significant effect of clomethiazole (chlormethiazole; a γ-aminobutyric acid agonist) versus placebo on achievement of functional independence (ARR +1.5%, 95% CI –4.0% to +6.6%; RRR +3.0%, 95% CI –7% to +13%).[40] **Lubeluzole:** We found one systematic review (search date 2001, 5 RCTs, 3510 people) that compared lubeluzole (5, 10, or 20 mg daily for 5 days) versus placebo.[41] It found no significant difference with any dose of lubeluzole versus placebo in death or dependency at the end of follow up (after 4–12 wks' follow up, AR 54.6% with lubeluzole *v* 53.4% with placebo; ARI +1.2%, 95% CI –2.5% to +6.2%). **Glycine antagonists:** We found two RCTs.[42,43] One RCT (1804 conscious people with limb weakness assessed within 6 h of stroke onset) found no significant difference between gavestinel (a glycine antagonist) versus placebo in survival and outcome at 3 months as measured using the Barthel Index (ARR +1.0%, 95% CI –3.5% to +6.0%).[42] The second RCT (1367 people with predefined level of limb weakness and functional independence before stroke) also found no significant difference in survival and outcome at 3 months, measured using the Barthel Index (ARI +1.9%, 95% CI –3.8% to +6.4%).[43] **N-methyl-D-aspartate antagonists:** Two recent RCTs assessing the N-methyl-D-aspartate antagonist (see glossary, p 180) selfotel found no significant difference in the proportion of people with a Barthel Index over 60, but data were limited as the trials were terminated because of adverse outcomes after only 31% of the total planned patient enrolment.[44] **Tirilazad:** We found one systematic review (search date 2001, 6 RCTs, 1757 people) comparing tirilazad (a steroid derivative) versus placebo in people with acute ischaemic stroke.[45] Tirilazad increased death and disability at 3 months' follow up when measured using the expanded Barthel Index (ARI +3.9%, 95% CI –0.8% to +8.6%).[45]

Harms: In the systematic review of calcium channel antagonists, indirect and limited comparisons of intravenous versus oral administration found no significant difference in adverse events (ARI of adverse events, iv *v* oral, +2.3%, 95% CI –0.9% to +3.7%; RRI +17%, 95% CI –3% to +41%).[36] In the systematic review of piracetam, there was a non-significant increase in death with piracetam versus placebo, which was no longer apparent after correction for imbalance in stroke severity.[39] The systematic review of lubeluzole found that at any dose, lubeluzole was associated with a significant increase in the risk of having a heart conduction disorder (Q-T prolongation to more than 450 ms on electrocardiography) at the end of follow up (AR with lubeluzole 11.9% *v* 9.74% with control; ARI 2.2%, 95% CI 0.1% to 4.2%; NNH 45, 95% CI 23 to 1000).[41] Lubeluzole did not significantly increase heart rhythm disorders (atrial fibrillation, ventricular tachycardia or fibrillation, torsade de pointes) at the end of the scheduled follow up (OR 1.28, 95% CI 0.97 to 1.69) The trials of selfotel were terminated after enrolling 567 people because of greater early mortality in the selfotel groups.[44] The systematic review of tirilazad found an increased risk of injection site phlebitis compared with placebo (ARI 12.2%, 95% CI 8.7% to 15.7%).[45]

Comment: The effects of the cell membrane precursor citicholine have been assessed in small trials, and a systematic review is in progress.[46] Systematic reviews are being developed for antioxidants and for excitatory amino acid modulators.[47] Several RCTs are ongoing, including one of intravenous magnesium sulphate[48] and another of diazepam (a γ-aminobutyric acid agonist).[49]

QUESTION What are the effects of surgical treatment for intracerebral haematomas?

OPTION EVACUATION

We found that the balance between benefits and harms has not been clearly established for the evacuation of supratentorial haematomas. We found no evidence from RCTs on the role of evacuation or ventricular shunting in people with infratentorial haematoma whose consciousness level is declining.

Benefits: **For supratentorial haematomas:** We found three systematic reviews.[50–52] The first review (search date 1998)[50] and second review (search date 1997)[51] both assessed the same four RCTs comparing surgery (craniotomy in 3 trials and endoscopy in 1 trial) versus best medical treatment in 354 people with primary supratentorial intracerebral haemorrhage. The second review also assessed information from case series.[51] Overall, neither review found significant short or long term differences between surgical and medical treatment for death or disability (ARI +3.3%, 95% CI –5.9% to +12.5%; RRI +5%, 95% CI –7% to +19%). The third review (search date 1999)[52] includes several analyses. The first analysis includes results from seven RCTs (530 people), including two RCTs not included in either of the first two systematic reviews. The overall results are similar to those of the first two systematic reviews, with no significant difference in death or disability for surgically treated people (ARI +3.5%, 95% CI –4.4% to +11.4%). A further analysis of results from only recent, post-computerised tomography, well constructed, balanced trials (5 trials, 224 people in total) did not find a significant difference between the two groups (ARR +9.3%, 95% CI –2.6% to +21.2%). **For infratentorial haematomas:** We found no evidence from systematic reviews or RCTs on the role of surgical evacuation or ventricular shunting.[53]

Harms: The two earlier reviews undertook subgroup analyses separating results for craniotomy and endoscopy. They found that for the 254 people randomised to craniotomy rather than best medical treatment, there was increased death and disability (ARI 12%, 95%

CI 1.8% to 22%; RRI 17%, 95% CI 2% to 34%; NNH 8, 95% CI 5 to 56).[50,51] For the 100 people randomised to endoscopy rather than best medical practice, there was no significant effect on death and disability (RRR 24%, 95% CI –2% to +44%). The third systematic review did not evaluate these adverse outcomes.[52]

Comment: Current practice is based on the consensus that people with infratentorial (cerebellar) haematomas whose consciousness level is declining probably benefit from evacuation of the haematoma. We identified one ongoing multicentre trial comparing a policy of "early surgical evacuation" of haematoma versus "initial conservative treatment" in people with spontaneous intracerebral haemorrhage.[54]

GLOSSARY

Integrated care pathway A model of care that includes definition of therapeutic goals and specification of a timed plan designed to promote multidisciplinary care, improve discharge planning, and reduce the duration of hospital stay.

N-methyl-D-aspartate antagonist Glutamate can bind to N-methyl-D-aspartate receptors on cell surfaces. One hypothesis proposed that glutamate released during a stroke can cause further harm to neurones by stimulating the N-methyl-D-aspartate receptors. N-Methyl-D-aspartate antagonists block these receptors.

Substantive changes

Specialised care in people with stroke Updated systematic review;[7] conclusion unchanged.

Immediate systemic anticoagulation New RCT;[26] conclusion unchanged.

Neuroprotective agents New systematic review;[41] no new evidence of benefit of lubeluzole but more evidence of harm.

Neuroprotective agents Updated systematic review assessing tirilazad;[45] conclusion unchanged.

REFERENCES

1. Hatano S. Experience from a multicentre stroke register: a preliminary report. *Bull World Health Organ* 1976;54:541–553.
2. Bonita R. Epidemiology of stroke. *Lancet* 1992;339:342–344.
3. Bamford J, Sandercock P, Dennis M, et al. A prospective study of acute cerebrovascular disease in the community: the Oxfordshire community stroke project, 1981–1986. 1. Methodology, demography and incident cases of first ever stroke. *J Neurol Neurosurg Psychiatry* 1988;51:1373–1380.
4. Bamford J, Dennis M, Sandercock P, et al. A prospective study of acute cerebrovascular disease in the community: the Oxfordshire community stroke project, 1981–1986. 2. Incidence, case fatality rates and overall outcome at one year of cerebral infarction, primary intracerebral and subarachnoid haemorrhage. *J Neurol Neurosurg Psychiatry* 1990;53:16–22.
5. Bamford J, Dennis M, Sandercock P, et al. The frequency, causes and timing of death within 30 days of a first stroke: the Oxfordshire community stroke project. *J Neurol Neurosurg Psychiatry* 1990;53:824–829.
6. Wade DT. Functional abilities after stroke: measurement, natural history and prognosis. *J Neurol Neurosurg Psychiatry* 1987;50:177–182.
7. Stroke Unit Trialists' Collaboration. Organised inpatient (stroke unit) care for stroke. In: The Cochrane Library, Issue 1, 2002. Oxford: Update Software. Search date 2001; primary sources Cochrane Stroke Group Specialised Trials Register and hand searches of reference lists of relevant articles and personal contact with colleagues.
8. Wardlaw JM, del Zoppo G, Yamaguchi T. Thrombolysis for acute ischaemic stroke. In: The Cochrane Library, Issue 1, 2002. Oxford: Update Software. Search date 1999; primary sources Cochrane Stroke Group Specialised Register of Controlled Trials, Embase, hand searches of relevant journals and references listed in relevant papers, and personal contact with pharmaceutical companies and principal investigators of trials.
9. CAST (Chinese Acute Stroke Trial) Collaborative Group. Randomised placebo-controlled trial of early aspirin use in 20 000 patients with acute ischaemic stroke. *Lancet* 1997;349:1641–1649.
10. International Stroke Trial Collaborative Group. The international stroke trial (IST): a randomised trial of aspirin, heparin, both or neither among 19 435 patients with acute ischaemic stroke. *Lancet* 1997;349:1569–1581.
11. Indredavik B, Bakke RPT, Slordahl SA, et al. Stroke unit treatment. 10-year follow-up. *Stroke* 1999;30:1524–1527.
12. Sulch D, Perez I, Melbourn A, Kalra L. Randomized controlled trial of integrated (managed) care pathway for stroke rehabilitation. *Stroke* 2000;31:1929–1934.

13. Indredavik B, Bakke RPT, Slordahl SA, et al. Treatment in a combined acute and rehabilitation stroke unit. Which aspects are most important. *Stroke* 1999;30:917–923.
14. Stegmayr B, Asplund K, Hulter-Asberg K, et al. Stroke units in their natural habitat: can results of randomized trials be reproduced in routine clinical practice? For the risk-stroke collaboration. *Stroke* 1999;30:709–714.
15. Cornu C, Boutitie F, Candelise L, et al. Streptokinase in acute ischemic stroke: an individual patient data meta-analysis: the thrombolysis in acute stroke pooling project. *Stroke* 2000;31:1555–1560.
16. Kwiatkowski T, Libman R, Frankel M, et al. Effects of tissue plasminogen activator for acute ischemic stroke at one year. National Institute of Neurological Disorders and stroke recombinant tissue plasminogen activator stroke study group. *N Engl J Med* 1999;340:1781–1787.
17. Internet Stroke Center: http://www.strokecenter.org/trials (last accessed 5 Sept 2002).
18. Gubitz G, Sandercock P, Counsell C. Antiplatelet therapy for acute ischaemic stroke. In: The Cochrane Library, Issue 1, 2002. Oxford: Update Software. Search date 1999; primary sources Cochrane Stroke Group Specialised Register of Controlled Trials, the Register of the Antiplatelet Trialists' Collaboration, MedStrategy, and personal contact with pharmaceutical companies.
19. Chen Z, Sandercock P, Pan H, et al. Indications for early aspirin use in acute ischemic stroke: a combined analysis of 40 000 randomized patients from the Chinese Acute Stroke Trial and the International Stroke Trial. *Stroke* 2000;31:1240–1249.
20. Antithrombotic Trialists' Collaboration. Collaborative meta-analysis of randomised trials of antiplatelet therapy for prevention of death, myocardial infarction, and stroke in high risk patients. *BMJ* 2002;324:71– 86. Search date 1997; primary sources Medline, Embase, Derwent, Scisearch, Biosis, Cochrane Stroke Group Controlled Trials Register, Cochrane Peripheral Vascular Disease Group Controlled Trials Register, hand searches of journals, abstracts and proceedings of meetings, reference lists from relevant articles, and personal contact with colleagues and pharmaceutical companies.
21. Slattery J, Warlow CP, Shorrock CJ, Langman MJS. Risks of gastrointestinal bleeding during secondary prevention of vascular events with aspirin analysis of gastrointestinal bleeding during the UK-TIA trial. *Gut* 1995;37:509–511.
22. Johnson ES, Lanes SF, Wentworth CE, et al. A metaregression analysis of the dose–response effect of aspirin on stroke. *Arch Intern Med* 1999;159:1248–1253.
23. Gubitz G, Counsell C, Sandercock P, et al. Anticoagulants for acute ischaemic stroke. In: The Cochrane Library, Issue 1, 2002. Oxford: Update Software. Search date 1999; primary sources Cochrane Stroke Group Specialised Register of Controlled Trials, trials register held by the Antithrombotic Therapy Trialist's Collaboration, MedStrategy, and personal contact with pharmaceutical companies.
24. Berge E, Abdelnoor M, Nakstad P, et al. Low-molecular-weight heparin versus aspirin in people with acute ischaemic stroke and atrial fibrillation: a double-blind randomised study. HAEST Study Group. Heparin in Acute Embolic Stroke Trial. *Lancet* 2000;355:1205–1210.
25. Diener H, Ringelstein E, von Kummer R, et al. Treatment of acute ischemic stroke with the low-molecular-weight heparin certoparin: results of the TOPAS Trial. *Stroke* 2001;32:22–29.
26. Bath P, Lindenstrome E, Bioysen G, et al. Tinzaparin in acute ischaemic stroke (TAIST): a randomised aspirin-controlled trial. *Lancet* 2001;358:702–710.
27. Counsell C, Sandercock P. Low-molecular-weight heparins or heparinoids versus standard unfractionated heparin for acute ischaemic stroke (Cochrane Review). In: The Cochrane Library, Issue 1, 2002. Oxford: Update Software. Search date 2001; primary sources Cochrane Stroke Group Specialised Trials Register, MedStrategy, and personal contact with pharmaceutical companies.
28. Bath P, Iddenden R, Bath F. Low-molecular-weight heparins and heparinoids in acute ischemic stroke: a meta-analysis of randomized controlled trials. *Stroke* 2000;31:1770–1778. Search date 1999; primary sources Cochrane Stroke Group Database of Trials in Acute Stroke, Cochrane Library, and hand searches of reference lists of identified publications.
29. Blood pressure in Acute Stroke Collaboration (BASC). Interventions for deliberately altering blood pressure in acute stroke. In: The Cochrane Library, Issue 1, 2002. Oxford: Update Software. Search date 2000; primary sources Cochrane Stroke Group Specialised Register of Controlled Trials, Cochrane Library (CDSR, CCTR), Medline, Embase, Bids, ISI-Science Citation Index, hand searches of reference lists of existing reviews and the ongoing trials section of the journal *Stroke*, and personal contact with research workers in the field and pharmaceutical companies.
30. Wahlgren NG, MacMahon DG, DeKeyser J, et al. Intravenous nimodipine west European stroke trial (INWEST) of nimodipine in the treatment of acute ischaemic stroke. *Cerebrovasc Dis* 1994;4:204–210.
31. Barer DH, Cruickshank JM, Ebrahim SB, et al. Low dose beta blockade in acute stroke (BEST trial): an evaluation. *BMJ* 1988;296:737–741.
32. Mohr JP, Orgogozo JM, Harrison MJG, et al. Meta-analysis of oral nimodipine trials in acute ischaemic stroke. *Cerebrovasc Dis* 1994;4:197–203. Search date 1994; primary source Bayer database.
33. Horn J, Orgogozo JM, Limburg M. Review on calcium antagonists in ischaemic stroke: mortality data. *Cerebrovasc Dis* 1998;8(suppl 4):27.
34. Rodgers A, MacMahon S, Gamble G. Blood pressure and risk of stroke patients with cerebrovascular disease. *BMJ* 1996;313:147.
35. Schrader J, Rothemeyer M, Luders S, et al. Hypertension and stroke – rationale behind the ACCESS trial. *Basic Res Cardiol* 1998;93(suppl 2):69–78.
36. Horn J, Limburg M. Calcium antagonists for acute ischemic stroke. In: The Cochrane Library, Issue 1, 2002. Oxford: Update Software. Search date 1999; primary sources Cochrane Stroke Group Specialised Register of Controlled Trials and personal contact with trialists.
37. Horn J, Limburg M. Calcium antagonists for ischemic stroke: a systematic review. *Stroke* 2001;32:570–576. Search date 1999; primary sources Cochrane Collaboration Stroke Group Specialized Register of Controlled Trials, and personal contact with principal investigators and company representatives.
38. Horn J, de Haan R, Vermeulen M, et al. Very Early Nimodipine Use in Stroke (VENUS). A randomized, double-blind, placebo-controlled trail. *Stroke* 2001;32:461–465.
39. Ricci S, Celani MG, Cantisani AT, et al. Piracetam for acute ischaemic stroke (Cochrane Review). In: The Cochrane Library, Issue 1, 2002. Oxford:

Update Software. Search date not stated; primary sources Cochrane Stroke Review Group trials register, Medline, Embase, BIDIS ISI, hand searches of relevant journals, and personal contact with the manufacturer.
40. Wahlgren NG, Ranasinha KW, Rosolacci T, et al. Clomethiazole acute stroke study (CLASS): results of a randomised, controlled trial of clomethiazole versus placebo in 1360 acute stroke patients. *Stroke* 1999;30:21–28.
41. Gandolfo C, Sandercock P, Conti M. Lubeluzole for acute ischaemic stroke. In: The Cochrane Library, Issue 1, 2002. Oxford: Update Software. Search date 2001; primary sources Cochrane Stroke Group Specialised Register of Controlled Trials, Cochrane Controlled Trials Register (CENTRAL/CCTR), Medline, Embase, Pascal BioMed, Current Contents, hand searches of all references in relevant papers, and personal contact with Janssen Research Foundation.
42. Lees K, Asplund K, Carolei A, et al. Glycine antogonist (gavestinel) in neuroprotection (GAIN International) in people with acute stroke: a randomised controlled trial. *Lancet* 2000;355:1949–1954.
43. Sacco R, DeRosa J, Haley E Jr, et al. for the GAIN Americas Investigators. Glycine Antagonist in Neuroprotection for Patients with Acute Stroke. GAIN Americas: a randomized controlled trial. *JAMA* 2001;285:1719–1728.
44. Davis S, Lees K, Albers G, et al. for the ASSIST Investigators. Selfotel in acute ischemic stroke. Possible neurotoxic effects of an NMDA antagonist. *Stroke* 2000;31:347–354.
45. The Tirilazad International Steering Committee. Tirilazad for acute ischaemic stroke. In: The Cochrane Library, Issue 1, 2002. Oxford: Update Software. Search date 2001; primary sources Cochrane Stroke Group Specialised Trials Register, Cochrane Controlled Trials Register (CENTRAL/CCTR), the Cochrane Library, hand searches of a publication on the quality of acute stroke RCTs, and personal contact with Pharmacia & Upjohn.
46. Saver JL, Wilterdink J. Choline precursors for acute and subacute ischemic and hemorrhagic stroke (Protocol for a Cochrane Review). In: The Cochrane Library, Issue 1, 2002. Oxford: Update Software.
47. Cochrane Stroke Review Group. Department of Clinical Neurosciences, Western General Hospital, Crewe Road, Edinburgh, UK EH4 2XU. http://www.dcn.ed.ac.uk/csrg (last accessed 5 Sept 2002).
48. Muir KW, Lees KR. IMAGES. Intravenous magnesium efficacy in stroke trial [abstract]. *Cerebrovasc Dis* 1996;6:75P383.
49. Lodder J, van Raak L, Kessels F, Hilton A. Early GABA-ergic activation study in stroke (EGASIS). *Cerebrovasc Dis* 2000;10(suppl 2):80.
50. Prasad K , Shrivastava A. Surgery for primary supratentorial intracerebral haemorrhage. In: The Cochrane Library, Issue 1, 2002. Oxford: Update Software. Search date 1998; primary sources Cochrane Stroke Group Trials Register and hand searches of reference lists of articles identified, three relevant monographs and issues of *Curr Opin Neurol Neurosurg* and *Neurosurg Clin N Am*.
51. Hankey G, Hon C. Surgery for primary intracerebral hemorrhage: is it safe and effective? A systematic review of case series and randomised trials. *Stroke* 1997;28:2126–2132. Search date 1997; primary sources Medline, and hand searches of reference lists of identified articles, published epidemiological studies, and reviews.
52. Fernandes HM, Gregson B, Siddique S, et al. Surgery in intracerebral hemorrhage: the uncertainty continues. *Stroke* 2000;31:2511–2516. Search date 1999; primary sources Ovid databases (unspecified), Medline, and hand searches of the reference lists of identified articles and relevant cited references.
53. Warlow CP, Dennis MS, van Gijn J, et al, eds. Treatment of primary intracerebral haemorrhage. In: *Stroke: a practical guide to management*. Oxford: Blackwell Science, 1996:430–437.
54. Mendelow A. International Surgical Trial in Intracerebral Haemorrhage (ISTICH). *Stroke* 2000;31:2539.

Gord Gubitz
Assistant Professor
Division of Neurology
Dalhousie University
Halifax
Canada

Peter Sandercock
Professor of Neurology
Neurosciences Trials Unit
University of Edinburgh
Edinburgh
UK

Competing interests: GG none declared. PS was the Principal Investigator of the second International Stroke Trial (IST-2). The trial was partly funded by Glaxo-Wellcome. He is also Chairman of the Steering Committee for the third International Stroke Trial (IST3) of thrombolysis in acute stroke. The start-up phase of trial is currently funded by a grant from the Stroke Association. Boehringer Ingelheim have donated trial drug and placebo for the 300 patients to be included in the start-up phase. PS has received honoraria for lectures, single consultations and travel expenses from a variety of pharmaceutical companies including: Boehringer Ingelheim, Sanofi, BNS, MSD, Servier, Glaxo-Wellcome, Lilly, Centocor.

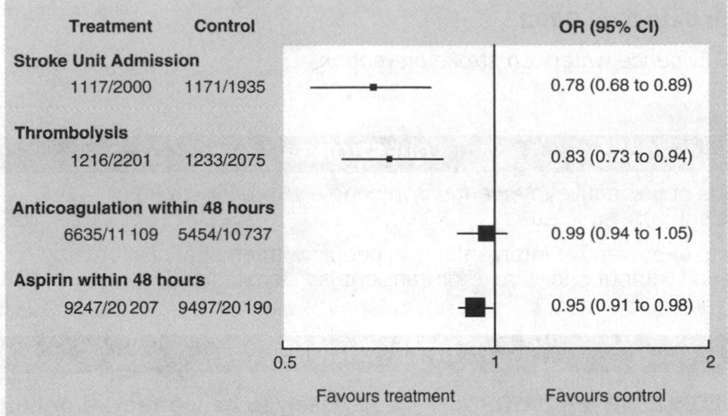

FIGURE 1 **Proportional effects on "death or dependency" at the end of scheduled follow up: results of systematic reviews.[7–10] Data refer only to benefits and not to harms (see text, p 174).**

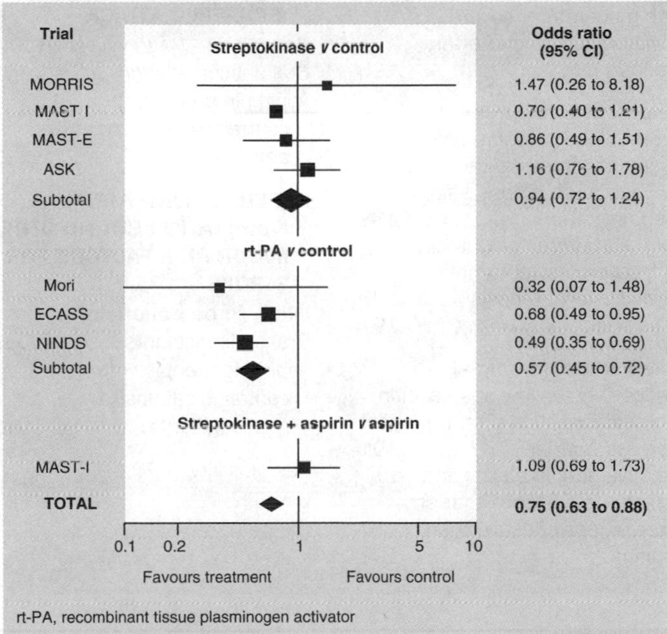

FIGURE 2 **Effect of thrombolysis on death and dependency at end of trial: results of review (see text, p 172). Figure reproduced with permission. Wardlaw JM, Warlow CP, Counsell C. Systematic review of evidence on thrombolytic therapy for acute ischaemic stroke. *Lancet* 1997;350:607–614. © by The Lancet Ltd, 1997.**

Stroke prevention

Search date May 2002

Clinical Evidence writers on stroke prevention

QUESTIONS

INTERVENTIONS

See glossary, p 202

Key Messages

In people with a prior stroke or transient ischaemic attack

- **Alternative antiplatelet agents to aspirin** Systematic reviews have found no good evidence that any antiplatelet treatment is superior to aspirin for long term secondary prevention of serious vascular events.
- **Antiplatelet treatment** One systematic review found that antiplatelet treatment reduces the risk of serious vascular events in people with prior stroke or transient ischaemic attack compared with placebo or no antiplatelet treatment.

Clin Evid 2002;8:184–208.

- **Blood pressure reduction** One systematic review and one subsequent RCT found that antihypertensive treatment reduced stroke among people with a prior stroke or transient ischaemic attack, whether they were hypertensive or not.
- **Carotid angioplasty** RCTs found insufficient evidence about the effects of carotid angioplasty versus best "medical treatment".
- **Carotid endarterectomy in people with severe asymptomatic carotid artery stenosis** Systematic reviews in people with no carotid territory transient ischaemic event or minor stroke within the past few months found limited evidence suggesting that carotid endarterectomy versus medical treatment may significantly reduce the risk of perioperative stroke or death or subsequent ipsilateral stroke over 3 years. However, as the risk of death without surgery in asymptomatic people is relatively low, the balance of benefits and harms from surgery remains unclear.
- **Carotid endarterectomy in people with moderate or severe symptomatic carotid artery stenosis** One systematic review in people with a recent carotid territory transient ischaemic event or non-disabling ischaemic stroke has found that carotid endarterectomy versus control treatment significantly reduces the risk of major stroke or death (NNT 15, 95% CI 10 to 31).
- **Cholesterol reduction** One large RCT has found that simvastatin versus placebo reduced major vascular events, including stroke, in people with prior stroke or transient ischaemic attack over about 5 years. RCTs have found no evidence that non-statin treatments versus placebo or no treatment reduced stroke.
- **Different blood pressure lowering regimens** Systematic reviews found no clear evidence of a difference in effectiveness between different antihypertensive drugs. One systematic review found that more intensive treatment reduced stroke and major cardiovascular events, but not mortality, compared with less intensive treatment.
- **High dose versus low dose aspirin (no additional benefit but may increase harms)** One systematic review and one subsequent RCT have found that low dose aspirin (75–150 mg) daily is as effective as higher doses in the prevention of serious vascular events. There was insufficient evidence that doses lower than 75 mg daily are as effective. One systematic review found no association between the dose of aspirin and risk of major extracranial haemorrhage in either direct or indirect comparisons. Another systematic review found no association between the dose of aspirin and risk of gastrointestinal bleeding in an indirect comparison. RCTs directly comparing different doses of aspirin found an increased risk of upper gastrointestinal upset with high (500–1500 mg daily) versus medium (75–325 mg daily) doses. One systematic review of observational studies found an increased risk of gastrointestinal complications with doses of aspirin greater than 300 mg daily. One systematic review found no association between dose of aspirin and risk of intracranial haemorrhage.
- **Oral anticoagulation in people with prior cerebrovascular ischaemia and sinus rhythm** One systematic review in people with prior cerebral ischaemia and in normal sinus rhythm found no significant difference with anticoagulation versus placebo for death or dependency, mortality, or recurrent stroke at about 2 years, but found a significantly increased risk of fatal intracranial haemorrhage (NNH 49, 95% CI 27 to 240). One systematic review has found no

significant difference between high intensity (international normalised ratio 3.0–4.5) or low intensity (international normalised ratio 2.5–3.5) anticoagulation versus antiplatelet treatment for preventing recurrent stroke in people with recent cerebral ischaemia of presumed arterial (non-cardiac) origin. High intensity anticoagulation increased the risk of major bleeding compared with antiplatelet treatment.

In people with atrial fibrillation and a prior stroke or transient ischaemic attack

- **Aspirin in people with contraindications to anticoagulants** Systematic reviews have found that aspirin versus placebo reduces the risk of stroke, but found that aspirin is less effective than anticoagulants. These findings support the use of aspirin in people with atrial fibrillation and contraindications to anticoagulants.
- **Oral anticoagulation** Systematic reviews have found that adjusted dose warfarin versus placebo significantly reduces the risk of stroke. Systematic reviews have also found that warfarin versus aspirin significantly reduces the risk of stroke in people with previous stroke or transient ischaemic attack.

In people with atrial fibrillation but no other major risk factors for stroke

- **Aspirin in people with contraindications to anticoagulants** One systematic review has found that aspirin versus placebo significantly reduces the risk of stroke (NNT 45, 95% CI 24 to 333), but another review found no significant difference. These findings support the use of aspirin in people with atrial fibrillation and contraindications to anticoagulants.
- **Oral anticoagulation** One systematic review has found that warfarin versus placebo significantly reduces fatal and non-fatal ischaemic stroke (NNT 25, 95% CI 18 to 42), provided there is a low risk of bleeding and careful monitoring. The people in the review had a mean age of 69 years. One overview in people less than 65 years old has found no significant difference in the annual stroke rate with warfarin versus placebo.

DEFINITION Prevention in this context is the long term management of people with a prior stroke or transient ischaemic attack, and of people at high risk of stroke (see glossary, p 202) for other reasons such as atrial fibrillation. **Stroke:** See definition under stroke management, p 169. **Transient ischaemic attack:** Similar to a mild ischaemic stroke except that symptoms last for less than 24 hours.[1]

INCIDENCE/ PREVALENCE See incidence/prevalence under stroke management, p 169.

AETIOLOGY/ RISK FACTORS See aetiology under stroke management, p 169. Risk factors for stroke include prior stroke or transient ischaemic attack, increasing age, hypertension, diabetes, cigarette smoking, and emboli associated with atrial fibrillation, artificial heart valves, or myocardial infarction. The relation with cholesterol is less clear; an overview of prospective studies among healthy middle aged individuals found no association between total cholesterol and overall stroke risk.[2] However, one review of prospective observational studies in eastern Asian people found that cholesterol was positively associated with ischaemic stroke but negatively associated with haemorrhagic stroke.[3]

PROGNOSIS People with a history of stroke or transient ischaemic attack are at high risk of all vascular events, such as myocardial infarction, but are at particular risk of subsequent stroke (about 10% in the first year and about 5% each year thereafter); see figure 1, p 208, and figure 1 in secondary prevention of ischaemic cardiac events, p 129.[5,6] People with intermittent atrial fibrillation treated with aspirin should be considered at similar risk of stroke, compared to people with sustained atrial fibrillation treated with aspirin (rate of ischaemic stroke/year: 3.2% with intermittent *v* 3.3% with sustained).[7]

AIMS To prevent death or disabling stroke, as well as other serious non-fatal outcomes, especially myocardial infarction, with minimal adverse effects from treatment.

OUTCOMES Dependency; myocardial infarction; stroke; and mortality.

METHODS *Clinical Evidence* update search and appraisal May 2002, plus handsearches of vascular, neurology, and general medical journals for options authored by Cathie Sudlow.

QUESTION What are the effects of interventions in people with prior stroke or transient ischaemic attack?

OPTION BLOOD PRESSURE REDUCTION VERSUS NO BLOOD PRESSURE REDUCTION

Cathie Sudlow

One systematic review and one subsequent RCT found that antihypertensive treatment reduced stroke in people with a prior stroke or transient ischaemic attack, whether they were hypertensive or not.

Benefits: We found one systematic review[8] and one subsequent RCT[9] of antihypertensive treatment versus placebo, no treatment, or usual care in people with a prior stroke or transient ischaemic attack. The systematic review (9 RCTs, search date not stated, 6753 people with a prior stroke or transient ischaemic attack) found that antihypertensive treatment significantly reduced stroke and major cardiovascular events compared with placebo, no treatment, or usual care over 2–7 years (stroke: RR 0.72, 95% CI 0.61 to 0.85; major cardiovascular events: RR 0.79, 95% CI 0.68 to 0.91).[8] Over 80% of people in the review were included in a single large RCT, the results of which have only been published in preliminary form.[10] The subsequent RCT (6105 people with a prior stroke or transient ischaemic attack with and without hypertension) compared the angiotensin converting enzyme inhibitor perindopril plus indapamide (added at the discretion of the physician) versus placebo.[9] It found that active treatment versus placebo reduced stroke but not deaths after about 4 years (stroke: AR 10% with treatment *v* 14% with placebo; RR 0.72, 95% CI 0.62 to 0.83; deaths: AR with treatment 10% *v* 10% with placebo; RR 0.96, 95% CI 0.82 to 1.12). Relative risks were similar in people with and without hypertension.

Harms: In people with a history of stroke, reports of an apparently J-shaped relationship between blood pressure and subsequent stroke have led to concerns that blood pressure reduction may increase the risk of recurrent stroke, perhaps because of reduced cerebral perfusion, particularly among people with extracranial carotid or vertebral artery stenosis.[11] However, observational studies found no evidence of a threshold of diastolic blood pressure below which there was no reduction in stroke.[11,12]

Comment: The systematic review found that the effects of blood pressure lowering were similar in people with and without a history of stroke or transient ischaemic attack.[8]

OPTION DIFFERENT BLOOD PRESSURE LOWERING REGIMENS

Cathie Sudlow

Systematic reviews found no clear evidence of a difference in effectiveness between different antihypertensive drugs. One systematic review found that more intensive treatment reduced stroke and major cardiovascular events, but not mortality, compared with less intensive treatment.

Benefits: We found no RCTs comparing different antihypertensive regimens specifically among people with a prior stroke or transient ischaemic attack. We found three systematic reviews[13–15] and one subsequent RCT[16] that compared effects of different antihypertensive treatments on stroke and other vascular outcomes in people with hypertension. One systematic review (search date 1997, 5 RCTs, about 18 000 people) found no significant difference between diuretics versus β blockers in death, stroke, or coronary artery disease.[13] The second systematic review (search date not stated, 15 RCTs)[14] compared more intensive versus less intensive treatment (3 RCTs, about 20 000 people); angiotensin converting enzyme inhibitors versus diuretics or β blockers (3 RCTs, about 16 000 people); calcium channel antagonists versus diuretics or β blockers (5 RCTs, about 23 000 people); and angiotensin converting enzyme inhibitors versus calcium channel antagonists (2 RCTs, about 5000 people). It found that more intensive treatment (target diastolic blood pressure 75–85 mm Hg) versus less intensive treatment (target diastolic blood pressure 85–105 mm Hg) significantly reduced stroke and major cardiovascular events, but not death (stroke: RR 0.80, 95% CI 0.65 to 0.98; major cardiovascular events: RR 0.85, 95% CI 0.76 to 0.96; death: RR 0.97, 95% CI 0.85 to 1.11). It found no significant difference with angiotensin converting enzyme inhibitors versus diuretics or β blockers in stroke, other vascular outcomes, or death (stroke: RR 1.05, 95% CI 0.92 to 1.19; death: RR 1.03, 95% CI 0.93 to 1.14). Calcium channel antagonists versus diuretics or β blockers reduced stroke (stroke: RR 0.87, 95% CI 0.77 to 0.98), but slightly increased coronary heart disease (RR 0.81, 95% CI 0.68 to 0.97), and had no significant effect on death or other vascular outcomes (death: RR 1.01, 95% CI 0.92 to 1.11). Angiotensin converting enzyme inhibitors versus calcium channel antagonists reduced coronary heart disease, but had no significant effect on stroke or death (coronary heart disease: RR 0.81, 95% CI 0.68 to 0.97; stroke: RR 1.02,

95% CI 0.85 to 1.21; death: RR 1.03, 95% CI 0.91 to 1.18). However, the RCTs included in this comparison were statistically heterogeneous so the results of the analysis should be treated with caution. The third systematic review (search date not stated) found similar results to the second review.[15] It suggested that results for different antihypertensive drugs could be explained by the blood pressure differences between randomised groups. The subsequent RCT (9193 people with hypertension, 728 of whom had a history of cerebrovascular disease) compared an angiotensin II receptor blocker (losartan) with a β blocker (atenolol).[16] It found that losartan versus atenolol significantly reduced the combined outcome of cardiovascular death, myocardial infarction, and stroke after 5 years (AR 14% with atenolol *v* 12% with losartan; HR 0.85, 95% CI 0.76 to 0.96). Blood pressure reduction was similar in both treatment groups (systolic/diastolic: about 30/17 mm Hg).

Harms: See harms under blood pressure reduction, p 188.

Comment: It has been suggested that both angiotensin converting enzyme inhibitors and angiotensin II receptor blockers produce reductions in vascular outcomes beyond what might be expected from their effects on blood pressure.[16,17]

OPTION CHOLESTEROL REDUCTION

Cathie Sudlow

One large RCT has found that simvastatin versus placebo reduced major vascular events, including stroke, in people with prior stroke or transient ischaemic attack. RCTs have found no evidence that non-statin treatments versus placebo or no treatment reduced stroke.

Benefits: **Statins:** We found several systematic reviews (about 38 000 people with and without a history of coronary heart disease) that assessed the effects of reducing cholesterol with a statin on coronary heart disease and also reported on stroke as an outcome. The RCTs included did not specifically aim to include people with a prior stroke or transient ischaemic attack (TIA). One systematic review (search date 1995, 14 RCTs)[18] and one additional RCT[19] included all of the relevant results, which are summarised in table 1 (see table 1, p 207). The review found that reducing mean total cholesterol with a statin by 21% over an average of 4 years reduced the relative odds of stroke by 24% (see table 1, p 207). We found one subsequent RCT (20 536 people with coronary heart disease, other occlusive vascular disease, or diabetes, 3280 of whom had a history of cerebrovascular disease and over 4000 of whom had a pretreatment cholesterol of < 5.0 mmol/L) that compared simvastatin 40 mg daily versus placebo[20] (see table 1, p 207). It found that simvastatin versus placebo reduced mean total cholesterol by 24%, reduced stroke, major vascular events (major coronary events, strokes, and coronary or non-coronary revascularisations), and deaths over 5 years (stroke: AR 4% with simvastatin *v* 6% with placebo; RR 0.75, 95% CI 0.66 to 0.85; major vascular events: AR 20% with simvastatin *v* 25% with placebo; RR 0.76, 95% CI 0.72 to 0.81; deaths: AR 13% with simvastatin *v* 15% with placebo; RR 0.87, 95% CI 0.81 to 0.94). The relative risk of major vascular events was similar and separately significant in people with and without a history of coronary artery disease, among those with a history of ischaemic stroke or TIA, peripheral vascular disease, and diabetes, and among those with different pretreatment concentrations of cholesterol and triglycerides. **Non-statin treatments:** We found one overview,[21] one subsequent RCT,[22] and one additional RCT[23] that assessed the outcome of stroke. The overview (11 RCTs) compared reducing cholesterol with a non-statin treatment (fibrate, resin, or diet) versus placebo or no treatment.[21] It found no significant difference with a non-statin treatment versus placebo in the risk of stroke (OR 0.99, 95% CI 0.82 to 1.21). Results for people with previous stroke or TIA were not provided separately. The subsequent RCT (2531 men with coronary heart disease)[22] found no significant difference with gemfibrozil versus placebo in the risk of stroke (AR 5% with gemfibrozil *v* 6% with placebo; RRR +25%, 95% CI –6% to +47%). Results on people with previous stroke or TIA were not provided separately. The additional RCT (532 men who had a previous stroke or TIA)[23] found no significant difference between clofibrate versus placebo in death after 3.5 years (AR 13% with clofibrate *v* 19% with placebo; P value not provided).

Harms: It had been suggested that statins may increase haemorrhagic stroke.[3,18] However, the subsequent RCT found that simvastatin did not increase haemorrhagic stroke.[20]

Comment: An RCT comparing atorvastatin versus placebo in 4200 people with minor stroke or TIA is in progress.[24] A planned overview of individual participant data from all RCTs of cholesterol reduction aims to summarise the effects of reducing cholesterol in different groups of people, including those with a prior stroke or TIA.[25]

OPTION ANTIPLATELET TREATMENT VERSUS NO ANTIPLATELET TREATMENT

Cathie Sudlow

One systematic review found that prolonged antiplatelet treatment versus placebo or no antiplatelet treatment reduces the risk of serious vascular events in people with prior stroke or transient ischaemic attack.

Benefits: We found one systematic review (search date 1997, 195 RCTs, about 135 640 people at high risk of vascular disease: previous stroke or transient ischaemic attack [TIA], acute stroke, ischaemic heart disease, heart failure, cardiac valve disease, atrial fibrillation, peripheral arterial disease, diabetes, and haemodialysis) comparing antiplatelet treatment (mostly aspirin) versus placebo or no antiplatelet treatment.[4] It found that in people with prior stroke or TIA (21 RCTs, 18 270 people), antiplatelet treatment reduced serious vascular events (stroke, myocardial infarction, or vascular death) compared with placebo or no antiplatelet treatment after

3 years (AR 18% with antiplatelet *v* 21% with placebo or no antiplatelet treatment; OR 0.78, 95% CI 0.73 to 0.85). Antiplatelet treatment also reduced the separate outcomes of stroke, myocardial infarction, vascular death, and death (see figure 1, p 208). For every 1000 people with a prior stroke or TIA treated for about 3 years, antiplatelet treatment prevented 25 non-fatal strokes, six non-fatal myocardial infarctions, and 15 deaths.[4]

Harms: The systematic review found that antiplatelet treatment versus no antiplatelet treatment in people with prior stroke or TIA increased major extracranial haemorrhage (haemorrhages requiring hospital admission or blood transfusion), and intracranial haemorrhage (intracranial haemorrhage: AR 0.64% with antiplatelet *v* 0.56% with no antiplatelet; OR 1.2; CI not provided; major extracranial haemorrhage: AR 0.97% with antiplatelet *v* 0.47% with no antiplatelet; OR 2.0; CI not provided).[4] We found one systematic review (search date 1999, 24 RCTs) assessing the effects of aspirin on gastrointestinal bleeding.[26] It found that aspirin versus placebo or no aspirin increased gastrointestinal bleeding (OR 1.68, 95% CI 1.51 to 1.88). Another systematic review (search date 1997, 16 RCTs, 55 462 people)[27] found that aspirin increased intracranial haemorrhage by about one event per 1000 people treated for 3 years.

Comment: In people at high risk of vascular disease, including those with a prior ischaemic stroke or TIA, the large absolute reductions in serious vascular events produced by antiplatelet treatment far outweighed any absolute hazards.

OPTION HIGH DOSE VERSUS LOW DOSE ASPIRIN New

Cathie Sudlow

One systematic review and one subsequent RCT have found that low dose aspirin (75–150 mg daily) is as effective as higher doses in the prevention of serious vascular events. There was insufficient evidence that doses lower than 75 mg daily are as effective. One systematic review found no association between the dose of aspirin and risk of major extracranial haemorrhage in either direct or indirect comparisons. Another systematic review found no association between the dose of aspirin and risk of gastrointestinal bleeding in an indirect comparison. RCTs directly comparing different doses of aspirin found an increased risk of upper gastrointestinal upset with high (500–1500 mg daily) versus medium (75–325 mg daily) daily doses. One systematic review of observational studies found an increase in risk of gastrointestinal complications with doses of aspirin greater than 300 mg daily. One systematic review found no association between dose of aspirin and risk of intracranial haemorrhage.

Benefits: We found one systematic review (search date 1997, 7225 people at high risk of vascular disease in RCTs comparing different doses of aspirin; and about 60 000 people at high risk of vascular disease, excluding those with acute stroke, in RCTs comparing different doses of aspirin versus placebo or no aspirin)[4] and one subsequent RCT[28] that compared the effects of higher versus lower dose aspirin on stroke. The systematic review found no significant difference between aspirin 500–1500 mg daily versus 75–325 mg daily in serious vascular events (stroke, myocardial infarction, or vascular death; OR 0.97, 95% CI 0.79 to 1.19).[4] It also found that doses of 75 mg or more did not reduce serious vascular events compared with doses lower than 75 mg (OR 1.08, 95% CI 0.90 to 1.31). However, the comparison lacked power to exclude a clinically important difference. The results in people with prior stroke or transient ischaemic attack were not presented separately. The systematic review also found that different aspirin doses versus placebo or no antiplatelet treatment reduced serious vascular events by similar amounts for the higher daily doses (500–1500 mg daily *v* placebo or no antiplatelet treatment: OR 0.81, 95% CI 0.75 to 0.87; 160–325 mg daily *v* placebo or no antiplatelet treatment: OR 0.74, 95% CI 0.69 to 0.80; 75–150 mg daily *v* placebo or no antiplatelet treatment: OR 0.68, 95% CI 0.59 to 0.79) but by a smaller amount for lower doses (< 75 mg daily *v* placebo or no antiplatelet treatment: OR 0.87, 95% CI 0.74 to 1.03). See figure 2 in secondary prevention of ischaemic cardiac events, p 129. People with acute stroke were excluded from these analyses. The results in people with prior stroke or transient ischaemic attack were not presented separately. The subsequent RCT (2849 people scheduled for carotid endarterectomy, most of whom had prior stroke or transient ischaemic attack) compared low dose aspirin (81 and 325 mg daily) versus high dose aspirin (650 and 1300 mg daily).[28] It found that high dose versus low dose aspirin increased the combined outcome of stroke, myocardial infarction, and death after 3 months (AR 8.4% with high dose *v* 6.2% with low dose; RR 1.34, 95% CI 1.03 to 1.75).

Harms: **Extracranial haemorrhage:** The systematic review found that the proportional increase in risk of major extracranial haemorrhage was similar with all daily aspirin doses. In direct comparisons, 75–325 mg aspirin did not increase major extracranial haemorrhage compared with doses lower than 75 mg (AR 2.5% with 75–325 mg daily *v* 1.8% with < 75 mg daily; $P > 0.05$).[6] We found one systematic review (search date 1999, 24 RCTs) of the effects of aspirin on gastrointestinal bleeding.[26] Indirect comparisons in a metaregression analysis found no association between dose of aspirin and risk of gastrointestinal bleeds. RCTs directly comparing different daily doses of aspirin have found a trend towards more gastrointestinal haemorrhage and a significant increase in upper gastrointestinal symptoms with high (500–1500 mg) versus medium (75–325 mg) doses (upper gastrointestinal symptoms, OR 1.3, 95% CI 1.1 to 1.5), but no significant difference in these outcomes between 283 mg and 30 mg daily.[28–30] We found one systematic review of observational studies (search date 2001, 5 studies) of the effects of different doses of aspirin on the risk of upper gastrointestinal complications (bleeding, perforation, or upper gastrointestinal event leading to hospital admission or visit to specialist).[31] It found greater risks of upper gastrointestinal complications with doses of aspirin greater than 300 mg daily. **Intracranial haemorrhage:** We found one systematic review (search date 1997, 16 RCTs, 55 462 people) of the effects of aspirin on intracranial haemorrhage.[27] It found no clear variation in risk with the dose of aspirin used. Three RCTs directly compared different daily doses of aspirin and found no significant differences in the risk of intracranial haemorrhage, but lacked power to detect clinically important differences.[28–30]

Comment: None.

OPTION ALTERNATIVE ANTIPLATELET AGENTS TO ASPIRIN New

Cathie Sudlow

Systematic reviews have found no good evidence that any antiplatelet regimen is superior to aspirin for long term secondary prevention of serious vascular events.

Benefits: **Thienopyridines (clopidogrel and ticlopidine) versus aspirin:** We found two systematic reviews (search dates 1997[4] and 1999[32]) that compared thienopyridines versus aspirin. The first systematic review (4 RCTs, 3791 people at high risk of vascular disease) found no significant difference with ticlopidine versus aspirin in serious vascular events (stroke, myocardial infarction, or vascular death) (AR 21% with ticlopidine *v* 23% with aspirin; OR presented graphically; P value not provided).[4] It also found that the risk of serious vascular events was similar with clopidogrel versus aspirin (1 RCT; 19 185 people; AR 10% with clopidogrel *v* 11% with aspirin; OR 0.90, 95% CI 0.82 to 0.99). The second systematic review (4 RCTs)[32] found that ticlopidine or clopidogrel versus aspirin marginally reduced vascular events after about 2 years (OR 0.91, 95% CI 0.84 to 0.98; ARR 1.1%, 95% CI 0.2% to 1.9%). **Dipyridamole plus aspirin:** We found one systematic review (search date 1997, 25 relevant RCTs, 10 404 people comparing dipyridamole plus aspirin versus aspirin alone).[4] It found no significant difference with adding dipyridamole to aspirin in serious vascular events (stroke, myocardial infarction, or vascular death) (AR 11.8% with combination treatment *v* 12.4% with aspirin alone; OR 0.94, 95% CI 0.83 to 1.06).

Harms: **Thienopyridines (clopidogrel and ticlopidine):** The second systematic review[32] of thienopyridines versus aspirin found that the thienopyridines reduced gastrointestinal haemorrhage and upper gastrointestinal symptoms compared with aspirin (gastrointestinal haemorrhage: OR 0.71, 95% CI: 0.59 to 0.86; indigestion, nausea, or vomiting: OR 0.84, 95% CI: 0.78 to 0.90). However, thienopyridines increased the incidence of skin rash and diarrhoea compared with aspirin (skin rash: clopidogrel *v* aspirin, OR 1.3, 95% CI 1.2 to 1.5; ticlopidine *v* aspirin, OR 2.2, 95% CI 1.7 to 2.9; diarrhoea: clopidogrel *v* aspirin, OR 1.3, 95% CI 1.2 to 1.6; ticlopidine *v* aspirin, OR 2.3, 95% CI 1.9 to 2.8). Ticlopidine (but not clopidogrel) increased neutropenia compared with aspirin (OR 2.7, 95% CI 1.5 to 4.8). Observational studies have found that ticlopidine is associated with thrombocytopenia and thrombotic thrombocytopenic purpura.[33,34] **Dipyridamole:** One RCT found that combination treatment with dipyridamole plus aspirin was discontinued more frequently for adverse effects than aspirin alone.[35]

Comment: One large RCT has assessed effects of adding clopidogrel to aspirin among people with unstable angina (see benefits of antiplatelet treatments in unstable angina, p 225).[36] A further large RCT is currently assessing the effects of alternative antiplatelet regimens among people with acute myocardial infarction.[37] One ongoing RCT is comparing effects of oral anticoagulation, aspirin plus dipyridamole, and aspirin alone among 4500 people with a prior transient ischaemic attack or minor ischaemic stroke.[38]

OPTION LONG TERM ORAL ANTICOAGULATION IN PEOPLE WITH RECENT CEREBRAL ISCHAEMIA AND IN SINUS RHYTHM

Gord Gubitz and Peter Sandercock

One systematic review has found no significant difference between anticoagulation versus placebo for preventing recurrent stroke after presumed ischaemic stroke in people in normal sinus rhythm. Anticoagulants increased the risk of fatal intracranial and extracranial haemorrhage compared with placebo. One systematic review has found no significant difference between high or low intensity anticoagulation versus antiplatelet treatment for preventing recurrent stroke in people with recent cerebral ischaemia of presumed arterial (non-cardiac) origin. High intensity anticoagulation increased the risk of major bleeding compared with antiplatelet treatment.

Benefits: **Versus placebo:** We found one systematic review (search date not stated, 9 small RCTs, 1214 people in sinus rhythm with previous non-embolic presumed ischaemic stroke or transient ischaemic attack, mean duration 1.8 years).[39] It found no clear benefit of oral anticoagulants (warfarin, dicoumarol, or phenindione) versus placebo on death or dependency (ARR +4%, 95% CI –6% to +14%; RRR +5%, 95% CI –9% to +18%), or on mortality or recurrent stroke. **Versus antiplatelet treatment:** We found one systematic review (search date 1999, 4 RCTs, 1870 people) comparing long term (> 6 months) treatment with oral anticoagulants (warfarin, phenprocoumarin, or acenocoumarol [nicoumalone]) versus antiplatelet treatment in people with a history of transient ischaemic attack or minor stroke of presumed arterial (non-cardiac) origin in the past 6 months.[40] It found no significant difference between high intensity (INR [see glossary, p 202] 3.0–4.5) or low intensity (INR 2.1–3.5) anticoagulation versus antiplatelet treatment for preventing recurrent stroke (low intensity anticoagulation *v* antiplatelet treatment: ARR +0.2%, 95% CI –4.0% to +4.3%; RR 0.96, 95% CI 0.38 to 2.42; high intensity anticoagulation *v* antiplatelet treatment: ARR –0.1%, 95% CI –1.7% to +1.5%; RR 1.02, 95% CI 0.49 to 2.13).

Harms: **Versus placebo:** The first review found that anticoagulants increased the risk of fatal intracranial haemorrhage (ARI 2.0%, 95% CI 0.4% to 3.6%; RR 2.51, 95% CI 1.12 to 5.60; NNH 49 people treated with anticoagulants over 1.8 years for 1 additional non-fatal extracranial haemorrhage, 95% CI 27 to 240).[39] The risk of fatal and non-fatal extracranial haemorrhage was also increased by anticoagulants compared with placebo (ARI 5.1%, 95% CI 3.0% to 7.2%; RR 5.86, 95% CI 2.39 to 14.3; NNH 20, 95% CI 14 to 33).

Versus antiplatelet treatment: The review comparing anticoagulants versus antiplatelet treatment found no significant difference in risk of major intracranial or extracranial bleeding with low intensity anticoagulation (INR 2.1–3.6) versus antiplatelet treatment (RR 1.19, 95% CI 0.59 to 2.41).[40] However, high intensity anticoagulation (INR 3.0–4.5) significantly increased the risk of major intracranial or extracranial bleeding (RR 1.08, 95% CI 1.03 to 1.20).

Comment: **Versus placebo:** The trials in the systematic review all had major problems with their methods, including poor monitoring of anticoagulation.[39] All were completed before introducing routine computerised tomography scanning, which means that people with primary haemorrhagic strokes could have been included. The systematic review could not, therefore, provide a reliable and precise overall estimate of the balance of risk and benefit regarding death or dependency. Most people in the trial comparing warfarin and aspirin did have a computerised tomography scan, but an adverse outcome was still seen with anticoagulants. Two further RCTs are in progress: one compares a lower intensity of adjusted dose warfarin (to maintain an INR of 1.4–2.8) with aspirin 325 mg four times daily within 30 days after stroke and treated for at least 2 years,[41] whereas the other assesses warfarin (to maintain an INR of 2.0–3.0) versus aspirin (any dose between 30–325 mg daily) versus aspirin plus dipyridamole (400 mg daily).[42]

OPTION CAROTID ENDARTERECTOMY FOR PEOPLE WITH RECENT CAROTID TERRITORY ISCHAEMIA

Gord Gubitz and Peter Sandercock

One systematic review has found that carotid endarterectomy reduces the risk of major stroke and death in people with a recent carotid territory transient ischaemic attack or non-disabling ischaemic stroke who have moderate or severe symptomatic stenosis of the ipsilateral carotid artery. Evidence from two other systematic reviews suggest a possible benefit in people with asymptomatic but severe stenosis, but the results of a new large scale trial are awaited. One systematic review found no evidence that eversion carotid endarterectomy is more beneficial than conventional carotid endarterectomy.

Benefits: **People with symptomatic stenosis:** We found one systematic review (search date 1999, 3 RCTs, 6143 people with a recent neurological event in the territory of a stenosed ipsilateral carotid artery) comparing carotid surgery versus control treatment;[43] 96% of these data came from two large RCTs.[44,45] People were randomised within 4 and 6 months of the onset of vascular symptoms. The trials used different methods to measure degree of stenosis. The trials included 1247 people with severe stenosis (80–99%[44] and 70–99%[45]), 1259 people with moderate stenosis (70–79%[44] and 50–69%[45]), and 3397 people with mild stenosis (< 70%[44] and < 50%[45]). The degree of benefit from surgery was related to the degree of stenosis. For people with severe stenosis, there was a significant decrease in the subsequent risk of major stroke or death (ARR 6.7%, 95% CI 3.2% to 10.0%; RR 0.52, 95% CI 0.37 to 0.73; NNT 15, 95% CI 10 to 31). People with moderate stenosis also benefited (ARR 4.7%, 95% CI 0.8% to 8.7%; RR 0.73, 95% CI 0.56 to 0.95; NNT 21, 95% CI 11 to 125). People with mild stenosis did not have a significantly reduced risk of stroke (RR 0.80, 95% CI 0.56 to 1.0). In the trial with longer follow up, the annual risk of stroke after 3 years was not significantly different between people who had had surgery and those who had not.[44] In the other trial, people with severe stenosis had a benefit from endarterectomy at 8 years' follow up.[46] **People with asymptomatic stenosis:** We found two systematic reviews (search dates 1998) assessing carotid endarterectomy for asymptomatic carotid stenosis (no carotid territory transient ischaemic attack or minor stroke within the past few months).[47,48] One review included results from five RCTs (2440 people).[47] The other review included results from 2203 people from four of these five RCTs, after excluding the fifth RCT because of weak methods.[48] Both reviews found similar results. Carotid endarterectomy reduced the risk of perioperative stroke, death, or subsequent ipsilateral stroke (for the review of 4 RCTs:[48] AR 4.9% over 3 years in the surgical group *v* 6.8% in the medical group; ARR 1.9%, 95% CI 0.1% to 3.9%; NNT 52, 95% CI 26 to 1000; for the review of 5 RCTs:[47] 4.7% over 3 years in the surgical group *v* 7.4% in the medical group; ARR 2.7%, 95% CI 0.8% to 4.6%; NNT 37, 95% CI 22 to 125). Although the risk of perioperative stroke or death from carotid surgery for people with asymptomatic stenosis seems to be lower than in people with symptomatic stenosis, the risk of stroke or death without surgery in asymptomatic people is relatively low and so, for most people, the balance of risk and benefit from surgery remains unclear.[47,48] **Eversion carotid endarterectomy versus conventional carotid endarterectomy:** We found one systematic review (search date 1999, 5 RCTs, 2645 people, 2590 carotid arteries) that compared eversion carotid endarterectomy versus conventional carotid endarterectomy (see glossary, p 202) performed either with primary closure or patch angioplasty.[49] Overall, the review found no significant differences in the rate of perioperative stroke, stroke or death, local complication rate, and rate of neurological events (for stroke or death: AR 1.7% with eversion *v* 2.6% with conventional, ARR +0.9%, 95% CI –0.3% to +2.1%; for stroke: AR 1.4% with eversion *v* 1.7% with conventional, ARR +0.3%, 95% CI –0.7% to +1.3%).

Harms: **People with symptomatic stenosis:** The systematic review of endarterectomy for symptomatic stenosis found that carotid surgery was associated with a definite risk of recurrent stroke or death.[43] The relative risk of disabling stroke or death within 30 days of randomisation was 2.5 (95% CI 1.6 to 3.8). A second systematic review (search date 1996, 36 studies) identified several risk factors for operative stroke and death from carotid endarterectomy, including female sex, occlusion of the contralateral internal carotid artery, stenosis of the ipsilateral external carotid artery, and systolic blood pressure greater than 180 mm Hg.[50] Endarterectomy is also associated with other postoperative complications, including wound infection (3%), wound haematoma (5%), and lower cranial nerve injury (5–7%). **People with asymptomatic stenosis:** Given the low prevalence of severe carotid stenosis in the general population, there is concern that screening and surgical intervention in asymptomatic people may result in more strokes than it prevents.[51]

Comment: **People with symptomatic stenosis:** The two RCTs contributing most of the data to the systematic review[44,45] used different techniques to measure the degree of carotid stenosis, but conversion charts are available and were used in the systematic review.[43] The trials, as well as observational studies,[5] found that risk of recurrent stroke was highest about the time of the symptomatic event. Subgroup analysis of one RCT included in the review found that, compared to medical treatment, endarterectomy for greater than 70% symptomatic stenosis reduced ipsilateral stroke to a greater extent in older people than younger people (at 2 years, for people > 75 years: ARR of stroke with endarterectomy *v* medical treatment 28.9%, 95% CI 12.9% to 44.9%; NNT 3, 95% CI 2 to 8; for people aged 65–74 years: ARR 15.1%, 95% CI 7.2% to 23.0%; NNT 7, 95% CI 4 to 14; for people aged < 65 years: ARR 9.7%, 95% CI 1.5% to 17.9%; NNT 10, 95% CI 6 to 67).[52] Among people with 50–69% stenosis, only the older (> 75 years) age group significantly benefited from endarterectomy (ARR for ipsilateral stroke at 2 years 17.3%, 95% CI 6.6% to 28.0%; NNT 6, 95% CI 4 to 15). Participating surgeons were experienced and people with other life threatening comorbidity were excluded. **People with asymptomatic stenosis:** A large scale trial is ongoing.[53]

OPTION CAROTID AND VERTEBRAL PERCUTANEOUS TRANSLUMINAL ANGIOPLASTY

Gord Gubitz and Peter Sandercock

We found that carotid or vertebral percutaneous transluminal angioplasty has not been adequately assessed in people with a recent carotid or vertebral territory transient ischaemic attack or non-disabling ischaemic stroke who have severe stenosis of the ipsilateral carotid or vertebral artery.

Benefits: We found no systematic review. **Carotid percutaneous transluminal angioplasty:** One RCT (504 people with a recent carotid territory transient ischaemic attack or non-disabling ischaemic stroke with stenosis of the ipsilateral carotid artery) compared "best medical treatment" plus carotid percutaneous transluminal angioplasty (PTA) versus "best medical treatment" plus carotid endarterectomy.[54] The rates of major outcome events within 30 days of first treatment did not differ significantly between endovascular treatment and surgery (AR for disabling stroke or death 6.4% with PTA *v* 5.9% with surgery; AR for stroke lasting more than 7 days or death 10.0% with PTA *v* 9.9% with surgery). The trial found no significant difference between treatments for ipsilateral stroke rate up to 3 years after randomisation (adjusted HR 1.04, 95% CI 0.63 to 1.70, P = 0.9). **Vertebral artery; PTA:** The RCT also compared vertebral PTA versus "best medical treatment" in 16 people, but did not provide enough data for reliable estimates of efficacy.[54]

Harms: The RCT found that cranial neuropathy was more common with surgery (22 people [8.7%] undergoing surgery *v* 0 people after endovascular treatment; P < 0.0001). Major groin or neck haematoma occurred less often after endovascular treatment than after surgery (3 people with endovascular treatment [1.2%] *v* 17 people with surgery [6.7%]; P < 0.0015).[54]

Comment: The RCT comparing endovascular treatment versus surgery had low power, and results lacked precision.[54] Two ongoing RCTs are comparing carotid endarterectomy versus primary stenting in people with recently symptomatic severe carotid stenosis.[55,56]

QUESTION What are the effects of anticoagulant and antiplatelet treatment in people with atrial fibrillation?

Gord Gubitz, Peter Sandercock, and Gregory YH Lip

Systematic reviews have found that people with atrial fibrillation at high risk of stroke and with no contraindications are likely to benefit from anticoagulation. However, one recent systematic review has questioned the quality of existing RCTs and reviews and suggested that more trials are needed to establish effects of anticoagulation. Antiplatelet agents are less effective than warfarin and are associated with a lower bleeding risk, but are a reasonable alternative if warfarin is contraindicated or if risk of ischaemic stroke is low. The best time to begin anticoagulation after an ischaemic stroke is unclear.

Benefits: Three risk strata have been identified based on evidence derived from one overview of five RCTs[57] and one subsequent RCT.[58] Most reviews have stratified effects of treatment in terms of these risk categories. However, one recent systematic review (search date 1999), which did not stratify for perceived risk, has suggested that RCTs may be too heterogeneous to determine effects of long term oral anticoagulation versus placebo among people with non-rheumatic atrial fibrillation (see comment below).[59] **People with atrial fibrillation at high risk of stroke, adjusted dose warfarin versus placebo:** We found one overview[57] and three systematic reviews[60–62] examining the effect of warfarin in different groups of people with atrial fibrillation at high risk of stroke (see glossary, p 202). The overview (5 RCTs, 2461 elderly people with atrial fibrillation and a variety of stroke risks) compared warfarin versus placebo.[57] It found that anticoagulation reduced the risk of stroke (ARR after a mean of 5 years 4.4%, 95% CI 2.8% to 6.0%; RR 0.32, 95% CI 0.21 to 0.50; NNT 23 over 1 year, 95% CI 17 to 36). The first systematic review (search date not stated) identified two RCTs comparing warfarin with placebo in 1053 people with chronic non-rheumatic atrial fibrillation and a history of prior stroke or transient ischaemic attack (TIA).[60] Most people (98%) came from one double blind RCT (669 people within 3 months of a minor stroke or TIA,[63] which compared anticoagulant (target INR [see glossary, p 202] 2.5–4.0) versus aspirin versus placebo. It found that anticoagulants reduced the risk of recurrent stroke over about 2 years (ARR 13.7%, 95% CI 7.3% to 20.1%; RR 0.39, 95% CI 0.25 to 0.63; NNT 7 over 1 year, 95% CI 5 to 14). The second systematic review (search date 1999, 16 RCTs, 9874 people) included six RCTs (2900 people) of adjusted dose warfarin versus placebo (5 RCTs) or versus control (1 RCT) in high risk people (45% had hypertension, 20% had experienced a previous stroke or TIA).[61] These six RCTs included five trials in people without prior cerebral ischaemia (primary prevention trials) and one RCT in people with prior cerebral ischaemia (secondary prevention trial).[64] Target INR varied among RCTs (2.0–2.6 in primary prevention RCTs and 2.9 in the secondary prevention RCT). The results of this systematic review were similar to the others. The meta-analysis found that adjusted dose warfarin reduced the risk of stroke (5 primary prevention RCTs: ARR 4.0%, 95% CI 2.3% to 5.7%; NNT 25, 95% CI 18 to 43; 1 secondary prevention RCT: ARR 14.5%, 95% CI 7.7% to 21.3%; NNT 7, 95% CI 5 to 13; combined primary and secondary prevention RCTs: ARR 5.5%, 95% CI 3.7% to 7.3%; NNT 18, 95% CI 14 to 27). The third systematic review (search date 1999, 14 RCTs) identified the same warfarin versus placebo trials and found similar results.[62] **Adjusted dose warfarin versus minidose warfarin in people with atrial fibrillation and high risk of stroke:** We found no systematic review or RCTs of low dose warfarin regimens in people with atrial fibrillation and a recent TIA or acute stroke. We found one RCT (1044 people with atrial fibrillation at high risk of stroke), which compared low, fixed dose warfarin (target INR 1.2–1.5) plus aspirin (325 mg daily) with standard adjusted dose warfarin treatment (target INR 2.0–3.0).[58] Adjusted dose warfarin significantly reduced the combined rate of ischaemic stroke or systemic embolism (ARR 6.0%, 95% CI 3.4% to 8.6%; NNT 17, 95% CI 12 to 29), and of disabling or fatal stroke (ARR 3.9%, 95% CI 1.6% to 6.1%; NNT 26, 95% CI 16 to 63). We found three additional RCTs,[65–67] which aimed to assess adjusted dose warfarin versus low dose warfarin and aspirin, but were stopped prematurely when the results of the earlier trial[58] were published. Analyses of the optimal anticoagulation intensity for stroke prevention in atrial fibrillation found that stroke risk was substantially increased at INR levels below 2.[64,68] **Adjusted dose warfarin versus aspirin in people with atrial fibrillation and high risk of stroke:** We found two systematic reviews of warfarin versus different antiplatelet regimens in people at high risk of stroke.[61,69] The first systematic review (search date not stated, 1 RCT)[69] found that in elderly people with atrial fibrillation and a prior history of stroke or TIA, warfarin (target INR 2.5–4.0) reduced the risk of stroke compared to aspirin 300 mg daily (22.6% with aspirin *v* 8.9% with warfarin; ARR 14%, 95% CI 7% to 20%; RR 0.39, 95% CI 0.24 to 0.64; NNT 7, 95% CI 5 to 14).[69] The second systematic review (search date 1999, 16 RCTs, 9874 people) included five RCTs (4 primary prevention and 1 secondary prevention RCTs; 2837 people) of adjusted dose warfarin versus aspirin in high risk people (45% had hypertension, 20% had experienced a previous stroke or TIA).[61] Target INR varied among RCTs (2.0–4.5 in primary prevention RCTs, 2.5–4.0 in the secondary prevention RCT). Adjusted dose warfarin versus aspirin reduced the overall risk of stroke (ARR 2.9%, 95% CI 0.9% to 4.8%; NNT 34, 95% CI 21 to 111). The effect varied widely among the five RCTs, none of which were blinded. **Adjusted dose warfarin versus other antiplatelet treatment in people with atrial fibrillation and high risk of stroke:** One systematic review (search date 1999) compared adjusted dose warfarin versus other antiplatelet agents such as indobufen.[61] One RCT included in the review (916 people within 15 days of stroke onset) compared warfarin (INR 2.0–3.5) with indobufen.[70] It found no significant difference in the rate of recurrent stroke between the two groups (5% for indobufen *v* 4% for warfarin; ARR +1.0%, 95% CI −1.7% to +3.7%). **Adjusted warfarin versus any antiplatelet agents in people with atrial**

fibrillation and high risk of stroke: We found one systematic review (search date 1999, 6 RCTs, 3298 people) of aspirin or indobufen versus warfarin.[59] It found that warfarin reduced stroke more than antiplatelet agents (ARR 1.8%, 95% CI 0.4% to 3.2%; NNT 56, 95% CI 31 to 250). **Aspirin versus placebo in people with atrial fibrillation and high risk of stroke:** We found one systematic review (search date 1999, 5 RCTs, 2769 people with atrial fibrillation and prior stroke or TIA).[62] Aspirin reduced the risk of stroke, although the confidence interval included the possibility of no benefit (ARR +1.8%, 95% CI –0.4% to +4.0%). **In people with atrial fibrillation at moderate risk of stroke:** See glossary, p 203. We found no RCT that considered this group specifically. **Anticoagulants in people with atrial fibrillation at low risk of stroke:** See glossary, p 203. We found one systematic review[71] and one overview[57] comparing warfarin versus placebo in people with atrial fibrillation and a variety of stroke risks. Both reviews included the same five RCTs. The overview (2461 people) found that, for people younger than 65 years with atrial fibrillation (but no history of hypertension, stroke, TIA, or diabetes), the annual stroke rate was the same with warfarin or placebo (1% a year).[57] The systematic review (search date 1999, 2313 people, mean age 69 years, 20% aged > 75 years; 45% had hypertension, 15% diabetes, and 15% a prior history of myocardial infarction) found that warfarin (INR 2.0–2.6) versus placebo reduced fatal and non-fatal ischaemic stroke (ARR 4.0%, 95% CI 2.4% to 5.6%; NNT 25, 95% CI 18 to 42), reduced all ischaemic strokes or intracranial haemorrhage (ARR 4.5%, 95% CI 2.8% to 6.2%; NNT 22, 95% CI 16 to 36), and reduced the combined outcome of disabling or fatal ischaemic stroke or intracranial haemorrhage (ARR 1.8%, 95% CI 0.5% to 3.1%; NNT 56, 95% CI 32 to 200).[71] **Antiplatelet treatment in people with atrial fibrillation and low risk of stroke:** We found two systematic reviews.[61,72] The first (search date 1999, 2 RCTs, 1680 people with either paroxysmal or sustained non-valvular atrial fibrillation confirmed by electrocardiogram but without previous stroke or TIA, 30% aged > 75 years) compared aspirin with placebo.[72] In primary prevention, aspirin did not significantly reduce ischaemic stroke (OR 0.71, 95% CI 0.46 to 1.10; ARR +1.6%, 95% CI –0.5% to +3.7%), all stroke (OR 0.70, 95% CI 0.45 to 1.08; ARR +1.8%; 95% CI –0.5% to +3.9%), all disabling or fatal stroke (OR 0.88, 95% CI 0.48 to 1.58; ARR +0.4%, 95% CI –1.2% to +2.0%), or the composite end point of stroke, myocardial infarction, or vascular death (OR 0.76, 95% CI 0.54 to 1.05; ARR +2.3%, 95% CI –0.4% to +5.0%). The second systematic review (search date 1999)[61] included three RCTs of primary prevention. The average rate of stroke among people taking placebo was 5.2%. Meta-analysis of the three RCTs found that antiplatelet treatment versus placebo reduced the risk of stroke (ARR 2.2%, 95% CI 0.3% to 4.1%; NNT 45, 95% CI 24 to 333).

Harms: The major risk of anticoagulants and antiplatelet agents was haemorrhage. In the overview assessing elderly people with variable risk factors for stroke, the absolute risk of major bleeding was 1% for placebo, 1% for aspirin, and 1.3% for warfarin.[57] Another systematic review[61] found the absolute risk of intracranial haemorrhage increased from 0.1% a year with control to 0.3% a year with warfarin, but the difference was not significant. The absolute risks were three times higher in people who had bled previously. Both bleeding and haemorrhagic stroke were more common in people aged over 75 years. The risk of death after a major bleed was 13–33%, and risk of subsequent morbidity in those who survived a major bleed was 15%. The risk of bleeding was associated with an INR greater than 3, fluctuating INRs, and uncontrolled hypertension. In a systematic review (search date not stated, 2 RCTs) major extracranial bleeding was more frequent with anticoagulation treatment than placebo (ARI 4.9%, 95% CI 1.6% to 8.2%; RR 6.2, 95% CI 1.4 to 27.1; NNH 20, 95% CI 12 to 63).[60] The studies were too small to define the rate of intracranial haemorrhage (none occurred). In a systematic review (search date not stated) comparing anticoagulants and antiplatelet treatment, major extracranial bleeding was more frequent with anticoagulation (ARI 4.9%, 95% CI 1.6% to 8.2%; RR 6.4, 95% CI 1.5 to 28.1; NNH 20, 95% CI 12 to 63).[69] The studies were too small to define the rate of intracranial haemorrhage (in 1 RCT, none of the people on anticoagulant and 1 person on aspirin had an intracranial bleed). In the systematic review of oral anticoagulants versus placebo in low risk people,[71] the number of intracranial haemorrhages was small with a non-significant increase in the treatment group (5 in the treatment group and 2 in the control group). Likewise, in the systematic review assessing antiplatelet treatment in low risk people with atrial fibrillation,[72] too few haemorrhages occurred to characterise the effects of aspirin. One more recent systematic review found no evidence that warfarin significantly increased the risk of major haemorrhage compared with placebo among people with no prior TIA or stroke (5 RCTs, 2415 people; ARI for major haemorrhage warfarin *v* placebo +0.8%, 95% CI −1.3% to +2.9%).[62] However, if people with prior stroke or TIA were included, warfarin significantly increased major haemorrhage (6 RCTs, ARI warfarin *v* placebo 1.3%, 95% CI 0.4% to 2.2%; NNH 77, 95% CI 45 to 250). The systematic review found no evidence of a difference in major haemorrhage between warfarin and aspirin; warfarin and any antiplatelet agent; warfarin and low dose warfarin plus aspirin; and low molecular weight heparin and placebo; however, the review may have lacked power to detect a clinically important difference.[62]

Comment: One recent systematic review (search date 1999, 5 RCTs, 3298 people) has found results that conflict with those of previous reviews.[59] The review questions the methods and highlights the heterogeneity of RCTs of oral anticoagulation in people with non-rheumatic atrial fibrillation. People in the RCTs were highly selected (< 10%, range 3–40% of eligible people were randomised); many were excluded after assessments for the absence of contraindications and physicians' refusal to enter them into the study. Many of the studies were not double blinded and in some studies there was poor agreement between raters for "soft" neurological end points. The frequent monitoring of warfarin treatment under trial conditions and motivation of people/investigators was probably more than that seen in usual clinical practice. The review has suggested that considerable uncertainty remains about benefits of long term anticoagulation in people with non-rheumatic atrial fibrillation. The review has different inclusion and exclusion criteria than previously published reviews and includes a trial not included in previous reviews.[58] Unlike previous reviews, the recent systematic review did not stratify people for perceived stroke risk and identified no significant difference between anticoagulant versus placebo with either a fixed effects model or a random effects model, which was employed to account for heterogeneity of underlying trials (fixed effects: OR 0.74, 95% CI 0.39 to 1.40 for stroke deaths; OR 0.86, 95% CI 0.16 to 1.17 for vascular deaths; random effects: OR 0.79, 95% CI 0.61 to 1.02 for combined fatal and non-fatal events).[59] The publication of this review has led to debate and uncertainty about clinical effectiveness of long term anticoagulation in people with non-rheumatic atrial fibrillation. Decisions to treat should be informed by considering trade-offs between benefits and harms, and each person's treatment preferences.[73–78] We found net benefit of anticoagulation for people in atrial fibrillation who have had a TIA or stroke, or who are over 75 years of age and at a high risk of stroke. We found less clear cut evidence for those aged 65–75 years at high risk, and for those with moderate risk (i.e. > 65 years and not in a high risk group or < 65 years with clinical risk factors), or for those at low risk (< 65 years with no other risk factors). The benefits of warfarin in the RCTs may not translate into effectiveness in clinical practice.[59,79,80] In the RCTs, most strokes in people randomised to warfarin occurred while they were not in fact taking warfarin, or were significantly underanticoagulated at the time of the event. A recent systematic review[81] (search date not stated, 410 people) identified three trials comparing the outcomes of people treated with anticoagulants in the community to the pooled results of the RCTs. The authors confirmed that people who undergo anticoagulation for atrial fibrillation in actual clinical practice are generally older and have more comorbid conditions than people enrolled in RCTs. However, both groups had similar rates of stroke and major bleeding. This risk of minor bleeding was higher in the community group, and it was suggested that these people may require more intensive monitoring in routine practice. **Timing of anticoagulation:** The best time to start anticoagulation after an ischaemic stroke is unclear, but aspirin reduces the risk of recurrent stroke in such people with or without atrial fibrillation, suggesting that it is reasonable to use aspirin until it is considered safe to start oral anticoagulants.[82]

GLOSSARY

Conventional carotid endarterectomy This is more commonly employed and involves a longitudinal arteriotomy of the carotid artery.

Eversion carotid endarterectomy This involves a transverse arteriotomy and reimplantation of the carotid artery.

International normalised ratio (INR) A value derived from a standardised laboratory test that measures the effect of an anticoagulant like warfarin. The laboratory materials used in the test are calibrated against internationally accepted standard reference preparations, so that variability between laboratories and different reagents is minimised. Normal blood has an INR of 1. Therapeutic anticoagulation often aims to achieve an INR value of 2.0–3.5.

People at high risk of stroke People of any age with a previous transient ischaemic attack or stroke or a history of rheumatic vascular disease, coronary artery disease, congestive heart failure, and impaired left ventricular function or echocardiography; and people aged 75 years and over with hypertension, diabetes, or both.

People at moderate risk of stroke People aged over 65 years who are not in the high risk group; and people aged under 65 years with clinical risk factors, including diabetes, hypertension, peripheral arterial disease, and ischaemic heart disease.

People at low risk of stroke All other people aged less than 65 years with no history of stroke, transient ischaemic attack, embolism, hypertension, diabetes, or other clinical risk factors.

Substantive changes

Blood pressure reduction versus no blood pressure reduction New systematic review;[8] conclusions unchanged.

Cholesterol reduction New RCT;[20] found that simvastatin versus placebo reduced major vascular events, including stroke, in people with prior stroke or transient ischaemic attack.

Long term oral anticoagulation for people in normal sinus rhythm New systematic review;[37] found no significant difference between long term oral anticoagulation and antiplatelet treatment for preventing recurrent stroke, and no significant difference in major bleeding between low intensity anticoagulation versus antiplatelet treatment. High intensity anticoagulation increased major bleeding risks compared with antiplatelet treatment.

REFERENCES

1. Hankey GJ, Warlow CP. *Transient ischaemic attacks of the brain and eye*. London: WB Saunders, 1994.
2. Prospective Studies Collaboration. Cholesterol, diastolic blood pressure, and stroke: 13 000 strokes in 450 000 people in 45 prospective cohorts. *Lancet* 1995;346:1647–1653.
3. Eastern Stroke and Coronary Heart Disease Collaborative Research Group. Blood pressure, cholesterol, and stroke in eastern Asia. *Lancet* 1998;352:1801–1807.
4. Antithrombotic Trialists' Collaboration Collaborative meta-analysis of randomised trials of antiplatelet therapy for prevention of death, myocardial infarction, and stroke in high risk patients. *BMJ* 2002;324:71–86. Corrections: *BMJ* 2002;324:141. Search date 1997; primary sources Medline, Embase, Derwent, SciSearch, Biosis, searching the trials registers of the Cochrane Stroke and Peripheral Vascular Disease Groups trials registers, and hand searches of selected journals, proceedings of meetings, reference lists of trials and review articles, and personal contact with colleagues and representatives of pharmaceutical companies.
5. Warlow CP, Dennis MS, Van Gijn J, et al. Predicting recurrent stroke and other serious vascular events. In: *Stroke. A practical guide to management*. Oxford: Blackwell Science, 1996:545–552.
6. Antiplatelet Trialists' Collaboration. Collaborative overview of randomised trials of antiplatelet therapy — I: prevention of death, myocardial infarction, and stroke by prolonged antiplatelet therapy in various categories of patients. *BMJ* 1994;308:81–106. Search date 1990; primary sources Medline, Current Contents, hand searches of journals, reference lists, and conference proceedings, and contact with authors of trials and manufacturers.
7. Hart RG, Pearce LA, Rothbart RM, et al. Stroke with intermittent atrial fibrillation: incidence and predictors during aspirin therapy. Stroke Prevention in Atrial fibrillation Investigators. *J Am Coll Cardiol* 2000;35:183–187.
8. The INDANA Project Collaborators. Effect of antihypertensive treatment in patients having already suffered from stroke. *Stroke* 1997;28:2557–2562. Search date not stated; primary sources electronic medical databases; survey of specialised and general medical journals and congress proceedings and consultanting experts.
9. PROGRESS Collaborative Group. Randomised trial of a perindopril-based blood-pressure-lowering regimen among 6105 individuals with previous stroke or transient ischaemic attack. *Lancet* 2001;358:1033–1041.
10. PATS Collaborating Group. Post-stroke antihypertensive treatment study: a preliminary result. *Chinese Med J* 1995;108:710–717.
11. Rodgers A, MacMahon S, Gamble G, et al, for the United Kingdom Transient Ischaemic Attack Collaborative Group. Blood pressure and risk of stroke in patients with cerebrovascular disease. *BMJ* 1996;313:147.
12. Neal B, Clark T, MacMahon S, et al, on behalf of the Antithrombotic Trialists' Collaboration. Blood pressure and the risk of recurrent vascular disease. *Am J Hypertension* 1998;11:25A–26A.
13. Wright JM, Lee C-H, Chambers GK. Systematic review of antihypertensive therapies: does the evidence assist in choosing a first-line drug? *Can Med Assoc J* 1999;161:25–32. Search date 1997; primary sources Medline, Cochrane Library (Issue 2, 1998), and references from previous meta-analyses published between 1980 and 1997.
14. Blood Pressure Lowering Treatment Trialists' Collaboration. Effects of ACE inhibitors, calcium antagonists, and other blood-pressure-lowering drugs: results of prospectively designed overviews of randomised trials. *Lancet* 2000;356:1955–1964. Search date not stated; primary sources result from a collaboration of trialists providing a limited data set for inclusion in the overview analyses.
15. Staessen JA, Wang J-G, Thijs L. Cardiovascular protection and blood pressure reduction: a meta-analysis. *Lancet* 2001;358:1305–1315.

Search date not stated; primary sources Medline and hand searches of reference lists of previous overviews.

16. Dahlöf B, Devereux RB, Kjeldsen SE, et al, for the LIFE study group. Cardiovascular morbidity and mortality in the Losartan Intervention for Endpoint reduction in hypertension study (LIFE): a randomised trial against atenolol. *Lancet* 2002;359:995–1003.
17. Sleight P, Yusuf S, Pogue J, et al, for the Heart Outcomes Prevention Evaluation (HOPE) study investigators. Blood-pressure reduction and cardiovascular risk in HOPE study. *Lancet* 2001;358:2130–2131.
18. Hebert PR, Gaziano JM, Chan KS, et al. Cholesterol lowering with statin drugs, risk of stroke, and total mortality: an overview of randomized trials. *JAMA* 1997;278:313–321. Search date 1995; primary sources electronic databases, reference lists, authors of trials and funding agencies. Cholesterol and Current Events (CARE) data added in 1996.
19. The Long-term Intervention with Pravastatin in Ischaemic Disease (LIPID) study group. Prevention of cardiovascular events and death with pravastatin in patients with coronary heart disease and a broad range of initial cholesterol levels. *N Engl J Med* 1998;339:1349–1357.
20. Heart Protection Study Collaborative Group. MRC/BHF Heart Protection Study of cholesterol lowering with simvastatin in 20 536 high-risk individuals: a randomised placebo-controlled trial. *Lancet* 2002;360:7–22.
21. Hebert PR, Gaziano M, Hennekens CH. An overview of trials of cholesterol lowering and risk of stroke. *Arch Intern Med* 1995;155:50–55.
22. Rubins HB, Robins SJ, Collins D, et al. Gemfibrozil for the secondary prevention of coronary heart disease in men with low levels of high-density lipoprotein cholesterol. *N Engl J Med* 1999;341:410–418.
23. Anonymous. The treatment of cerebrovascular disease with clofibrate. Final report of the Veterans' Administration Cooperative Study of Atherosclerosis, neurology section. *Stroke* 1973;4:684–693.
24. Welch KMA. Stroke Prevention by Aggressive Reduction in Cholesterol Levels (SPARCL). *Stroke* 2000;31:2541.
25. Cholesterol Treatment Trialists' Collaboration. Protocol for a prospective collaborative overview of all current and planned randomized trials of cholesterol treatment regimens. *Am J Cardiol* 1995;75:1130–1134.
26. Derry S, Loke YK. Risk of gastrointestinal haemorrhage with long term use of aspirin: meta-analysis. *BMJ* 2000;321:1183–1187. Search date 1999; primary sources Medline, Embase, and hand searches of reference lists from previous review papers and retrieved trials.
27. He J, Whelton PK, Vu B, et al. Aspirin and risk of hemorrhagic stroke. A meta-analysis of randomised controlled trials. *JAMA* 1998;280:1930–1935. Search date 1997; primary sources Medline and hand searches of reference lists of relevant articles.
28. The Dutch TIA Study Group. A comparison of two doses of aspirin (30 mg vs 283 mg a day) in patients after a transient ischaemic attack or minor ischaemic stroke. *N Engl J Med* 1991;325:1261–1266.
29. Farrell B, Godwin J, Richards S, et al. The United Kingdom transient ischaemic attack (UK-TIA) aspirin trial: final results. *J Neurol Neurosurg Psychiatry* 1991;54:1044–1054.
30. Taylor DW, Barnett HJM, Haynes RB, et al, for the ASA and Carotid Endarterectomy (ACE) Trial Collaborators. Low-dose and high-dose acetylsalicylic acid for patients undergoing carotid endarterectomy: a randomised controlled trial. *Lancet* 1999;353:2179–2184.
31. Garc a Rodr guez LA, Hernández-D az S, de Abajo FJ. Association between aspirin and upper gastrointestinal complications. Systematic review of epidemioligic studies. *Br J Clin Pharmacol* 2001;52;563–571. Search date 2001; primary sources Medline and hand searches of reference lists of reviews.
32. Hankey GJ, Sudlow CLM, Dunbabin DW. Thienopyridine derivatives (ticlopidine, clopidogrel) versus aspirin for preventing stroke and other serious vascular events in high vascular risk patients. In: The Cochrane Library, Issue 3, 2001. Oxford: Update Software. Search date 1999; primary sources Cochrane Stroke Group Trials Register, Antithrombotic Trialists' Collaboration database, and personal contact with the Sanofi pharmaceutical company.
33. Moloney BA. An analysis of the side effects of ticlopidine. In: Hass WK, Easton JD, eds. *Ticlopidine, platelets and vascular disease*. New York: Springer, 1993:117–139.
34. Bennett CL, Davidson CJ, Raisch DW, et al. Thrombotic thrombocytopenic purpura associated with ticlopidine in the setting of coronary artery stents and stroke prevention. *Arch Int Med* 1999;159:2524–2528.
35. Diener HC, Cunha L, Forbes C, et al. European secondary prevention study 2: dipyridamole and acetylsalicylic acid in the secondary prevention of stroke. *J Neurol Sci* 1996;143:1–13.
36. The Clopidogrel in Unstable Angina to Prevent Recurrent Events (CURE) Trial Investigators. Effects of clopidogrel in addition to aspirin in patients with acute coronary syndromes without ST-segment elevation. *N Engl J Med* 2001;345:494–502.
37. Second Chinese Cardiac Study (CCS-2) Collaborative Group. Rationale, design and organisation of the Second Chinese Cardiac Study (CCS-2): a randomised trial of clopidogrel plus aspirin, and of metoprolol, among patients with suspected acute myocardial infarction. *J Cardiovasc Risk* 2000;7:435–441.
38. De Schryver ELLM, on behalf of the European/Australian Stroke Prevention in Reversible Ischaemia Trial (ESPRIT) Group. Design of ESPRIT: an international randomized trial for secondary prevention after non-disabling cerebral ischaemia of arterial origin. *Cerebrovasc Dis* 2000;10:147–150.
39. Liu M, Counsell C, Sandercock P. Anticoagulants for preventing recurrence following ischaemic stroke or transient ischaemic attack. In: The Cochrane Library, Issue 3, 2001. Oxford: Update Software. Search date not stated; primary sources Cochrane Stroke Group Trials Register, and contact with companies marketing anticoagulant agents.
40. Algra A, De Schryver ELLM, van Gijn J, et al. Oral anticoagulants versus antiplatelet therapy for preventing further vascular events after transient ischaemic attack or minor stroke of presumed arterial origin (Cochrane Review). In: The Cochrane Library, Issue 2, 2002. Oxford: Update Software.
41. Mohr J, for the WARSS Group. Design considerations for the warfarin-antiplatelet recurrent stroke study. *Cerebrovasc Dis* 1995;5:156–157.
42. De Schryvfer E, for the ESPRIT Study Group. ESPRIT: mild anticoagulation, acetylsalicylic acid plus dipyridamole or acetylsalicylic acid alone after cerebral ischaemia of arterial origin [abstract]. *Cerebrovasc Dis* 1998;8(suppl 4):83.

43. Cina C, Clase C, Haynes R. Carotid endarterectomy for symptomatic stenosis. In: The Cochrane Library, Issue 3, 2001. Oxford: Update Software. Search date 1999; primary sources Cochrane Stroke Group Specialised Register of Trials, Medline, Embase, Healthstar, Serline, Cochrane Controlled Trials Register, DARE, and Best Evidence.
44. European Carotid Surgery Trialists' Collaborative Group. Randomised trial of endarterectomy for recently symptomatic carotid stenosis: final results of the MRC European carotid surgery trial. *Lancet* 1998;351:1379–1387.
45. North American Symptomatic Carotid Endarterectomy Trial Collaborators. Beneficial effect of carotid endarterectomy in symptomatic patients with high-grade carotid stenosis. *N Engl J Med* 1991;325:445–453.
46. Barnett HJ, Taylor DW, Eliasziw M, et al. Benefit of carotid endarterectomy in patients with symptomatic moderate or severe stenosis. North American symptomatic carotid endarterectomy trial collaborators. *N Engl J Med* 1998;339:1415–1425.
47. Benavente O, Moher D, Pham B. Carotid endarterectomy for asymptomatic carotid stenosis: a meta-analysis. *BMJ* 1998;317:1477–1480. Search date 1998; primary sources Medline, Cochrane Controlled Trials Register, Ottawa Stroke Trials Register, Current Contents, and hand searches.
48. Chambers BR, You RX, Donnan GA. Carotid endarterectomy for asymptomatic carotid stenosis. In: The Cochrane Library, Issue 3, 2001. Oxford: Update Software. Search date 1998; primary sources Cochrane Stroke Group Trials Register, Medline, Current Contents, hand searches of reference lists, and contact with researchers in the field.
49. Cao PG, De Rango P, Zannetti S, et al. Eversion versus conventional carotid endarterectomy for preventing stroke. In: The Cochrane Library, Issue 4, 2001. Oxford: Update Software. Search date 1999; primary sources Medline, Cochrane Stroke Group Trials Register, hand searches of surgical journals and conference proceedings, and contact with experts.
50. Rothwell P, Slattery J, Warlow C. Clinical and angiographic predictors of stroke and death from carotid endarterectomy: systematic review. *BMJ* 1997;315:1571–1577. Search date 1996; primary sources Medline, Cochrane Collaboration Stroke database, and hand searches of reference lists.
51. Whitty C, Sudlow C, Warlow C. Investigating individual subjects and screening populations for asymptomatic carotid stenosis can be harmful. *J Neurol Neurosurg Psychiatry* 1998;64:619–623.
52. Alamowitch S, Eliasziw, M, Algra A, et al, for the North American Symptomatic Carotid Endarterectomy Trial (NASCET) Group. Risk, causes, and prevention of ischaemic stroke in elderly patients with symptomatic internal-carotid-artery stenosis. *Lancet* 2001;357:1154–1160.
53. Halliday A, Thomas D, Manssfield A. The asymptomatic carotid surgery trial (ACST). Rationale and design. *Eur J Vascular Surg* 1994;8:703–710.
54. CAVATAS Investigators. Endovascular versus surgical treatment in patents with carotid stenosis in the Carotid and Vertebral Artery Transluminal Angioplasty Study (CAVATAS): a randomised trial. *Lancet* 2001;357;1729–1737.
55. Brown M. The International Carotid Stenting Study [abstract]. *Stroke* 2000;31:2812.
56. Al-Mubarek N, Roubin G, Hobson R, et al. Credentialing of Stent Operators for the Carotid Revascularization Endarterectomy vs Stenting Trial (CREST) [abstract]. *Stroke* 2000;31:292.
57. Atrial Fibrillation Investigators. Risk factors for stroke and efficacy of antithrombotic therapy in atrial fibrillation. *Arch Intern Med* 1994;154:1449–1457.
58. Stroke Prevention in Atrial Fibrillation Investigators. Adjusted-dose warfarin versus low-intensity, fixed-dose warfarin plus aspirin for high-risk patients with atrial fibrillation: stroke prevention in atrial fibrillation III randomised clinical trial. *Lancet* 1996;348:633–638.
59. Taylor F, Cohen H, Ebrahim S. Systematic review of long term anticoagulation or antiplatelet treatment in patients with non-rheumatic atrial fibrillation. *BMJ* 2001;322:321–326. Search date 1999; primary sources Cochrane Central database, Embase, Medline, Cinahl, Sigle, hand searches of reference lists, and personal contact with experts.
60. Koudstaal P. Anticoagulants for preventing stroke in patients with non-rheumatic atrial fibrillation and a history of stroke or transient ischemic attacks. In: The Cochrane Library, Issue 2, 2002. Oxford: Update Software. Search date not stated; primary source Cochrane Stroke Group Trials Register and contact with trialists.
61. Hart R, Benavente O, McBride R, et al. Antithrombotic therapy to prevent stroke in patients with atrial fibrillation: a meta-analysis. Ann Intern Med 1999;131:492–501. Search date 1999; primary sources Medline, Cochrane Database, and Antithrombotic Trialists' Collaboration database.
62. Segal JB, McNamara RL, Miller MR, et al. Anticoagulants or antiplatelet therapy for non-rheumatic atrial fibrillation and flutter. In: The Cochrane Library, Issue 2, 2002. Oxford: Update Software. Search date 1999; primary sources Medline, Embase, Cochrane Heart Group Trials Register, hand searches of selected journals and conference proceedings, and contact with experts.
63. European Atrial Fibrillation Trial Study Group. Secondary prevention in non-rheumatic atrial fibrillation after transient ischaemic attack or minor stroke. *Lancet* 1993;342:1255.
64. The European Atrial Fibrillation Trial Study Group. Optimal oral anticoagulant therapy in patients with non-rheumatic atrial fibrillation and recent cerebral ischemia. *N Engl J Med* 1995;333:5–10.
65. Pengo V, Zasso Z, Barbero F, et al. Effectiveness of fixed minidose warfarin in the prevention of thromboembolism and vascular death in nonrheumatic atrial fibrillation. *Am J Cardiol* 1998;82:433–437.
66. Gullov A, Koefoed B, Petersen P, et al. Fixed minidose warfarin and aspirin alone and in combination vs adjusted-dose warfarin for stroke prevention in atrial fibrillation. Second Copenhagen Atrial Fibrillation, Aspirin, and Anticoagulation Study. *Arch Intern Med* 1998;158:1513–1521.
67. Hellemons B, Langenberg M, Lodder J, et al. Primary prevention of arterial thrombo-embolism in non-rheumatic atrial fibrillation in primary care: randomised controlled trial comparing two intensities of coumarin with aspirin. *BMJ* 1999;319:958–964.
68. Hylek EM, Skates SJ, Sheehan MA, et al. An analysis of the lowest effective intensity of prophylactic anticoagulation for patients with non-rheumatic atrial fibrillation. *N Engl J Med* 1996;335:540–546.
69. Koudstaal P. Anticoagulants versus antiplatelet therapy for preventing stroke in patients with non-rheumatic atrial fibrillation and a history of

stroke or transient ischemic attacks. In: The Cochrane Library, Issue 2, 2002. Oxford: Update Software. Search date not stated; primary sources Cochrane Stroke Group Trials Register and contact with trialists.
70. Morocutti C, Amabile G, Fattapposta F, et al, for the SIFA Investigators. Indobufen versus warfarin in the secondary prevention of major vascular events in non-rheumatic atrial fibrillation. *Stroke* 1997;28:1015–1021.
71. Benavente O, Hart R, Koudstaal P, et al. Oral anticoagulants for preventing stroke in patients with non-valvular atrial fibrillation and no previous history of stroke or transient ischemic attacks. In: The Cochrane Library, Issue 2, 2002. Oxford: Update Software. Search date 1999; primary sources Cochrane Stroke Group Specialised Register of Trials, Medline, Antithrombotic Trialists' Collaboration database, and hand searches of reference lists of relevant articles.
72. Benavente O, Hart R, Koudstaal P, et al. Antiplatelet therapy for preventing stroke in patients with non-valvular atrial fibrillation and no previous history of stroke or transient ischemic attacks. In: The Cochrane Library, Issue 2, 2002. Oxford: Update Software. Search date 1999; primary sources Medline, Cochrane Specialised Register of Trials, and hand searches of reference lists of relevant articles.
73. Lip G. Thromboprophylaxis for atrial fibrillation. *Lancet* 1999;353:4–6.
74. Ezekowitz M, Levine J. Preventing stroke in patients with atrial fibrillation. *JAMA* 1999;281:1830–1835.
75. Hart R, Sherman D, Easton D, et al. Prevention of stroke in patients with non-valvular atrial fibrillation. *Neurology* 1998;51:674–681.
76. Feinberg W. Anticoagulation for prevention of stroke. *Neurology* 1998;51(suppl 3):20–22.
77. Albers G. Choice of antithrombotic therapy for stroke prevention in atrial fibrillation. Warfarin, aspirin, or both? *Arch Intern Med* 1998;158:1487–1491.
78. Nademanee K, Kosar E. Long-term antithrombotic treatment for atrial fibrillation. *Am J Cardiol* 1998;82:37N–42N.
79. Green CJ, Hadorn DC, Bassett K, et al. Anticoagulation in chronic non-valvular atrial fibrillation: a critical appraisal and meta-analysis. *Can J Cardiol* 1997;13:811–815.
80. Blakely J. Anticoagulation in chronic non-valvular atrial fibrillation: appraisal of two meta-analyses. *Can J Cardiol* 1998;14:945–948.
81. Evans A, Kalra L. Are the results of randomized controlled trials on anticoagulation in patients with atrial fibrillation generalizable to clinical practice? *Arch Intern Med* 2001;161:1443–1447. Search date not stated; primary sources Medline, Cochrane Library, and hand searches of reference lists of relevant retrieved articles.
82. Chen ZM, Sandercock P, Pan HC, et al. Indications for early aspirin use in acute ischemic stroke: a combined analysis of 40 000 randomized patients from the Chinese acute stroke trial and the international stroke trial. On behalf of the CAST and IST collaborative groups. *Stroke* 2000;31:1240–1249.

Cathie Sudlow
Wellcome Clinician Scientist
Department of Clinical Neurosciences
University of Edinburgh
Edinburgh, UK

Gord Gubitz
Assistant Professor
Division of Neurology
Dalhousie University
Halifax, Canada

Peter Sandercock
Professor in Neurology
Neurosciences Trials Unit
University of Edinburgh
Edinburgh, UK

Gregory Lip
Consultant Cardiologist and Professor of Cardiovascular Medicine
City Hospital
Birmingham, UK

Competing interests: PS was the Principal Investigator of the second International Stroke Trial (IST-2). The trial was partly funded by Glaxo-Wellcome. He is also Chairman of the Steering Committee for the third International Stroke Trial (IST3) of thrombolysis in acute stroke. The start-up phase of trial is currently funded by a grant from the Stroke Association. Boehringer Ingelheim have donated trial drug and placebo for the 300 patients to be included in the start-up phase. PS has received honoraria for lectures, single consultations and travel expenses from a variety of pharmaceutical companies including: Boehringer Ingelheim, Sanofi, BNS, MSD, Servier, Glaxo-Wellcome, Lilly, Centocor. GG and GL none declared. CS on one occasion received fee from Sanofi-Synthelabo for giving a talk at a GP meeting.

TABLE 1 **Effects of cholesterol reduction with a statin on risk of stroke: results of systematic review[18] and RCTs (see text, p 191).[19,20]**

	Number of		Mean pretreatment cholesterol (mmol/L)	Average follow up duration (years)	Mean reduction in cholesterol* (%)	Summary OR (95% CI) for active treatment *v* control	
	People	Strokes				Fatal or non-fatal stroke	Fatal stroke
1997 overview (14 RCTs)[18] + LIPID trial[19]	38 000	827	6.3	4	21	0.76† (0.66 to 0.87)	0.99† (0.67 to 1.45)
Heart Protection Study[20]	20 000	1029	5.9	5	24	0.75 (0.66 to 0.85)	0.81 (0.62 to 1.1)
All trials	58 000	1856	6.2	4.4	23	0.75 (0.67 to 0.83)	0.86 (0.69 to 1.1)

*Weighted by trial size; †the findings of other published overviews were consistent with the results shown here.

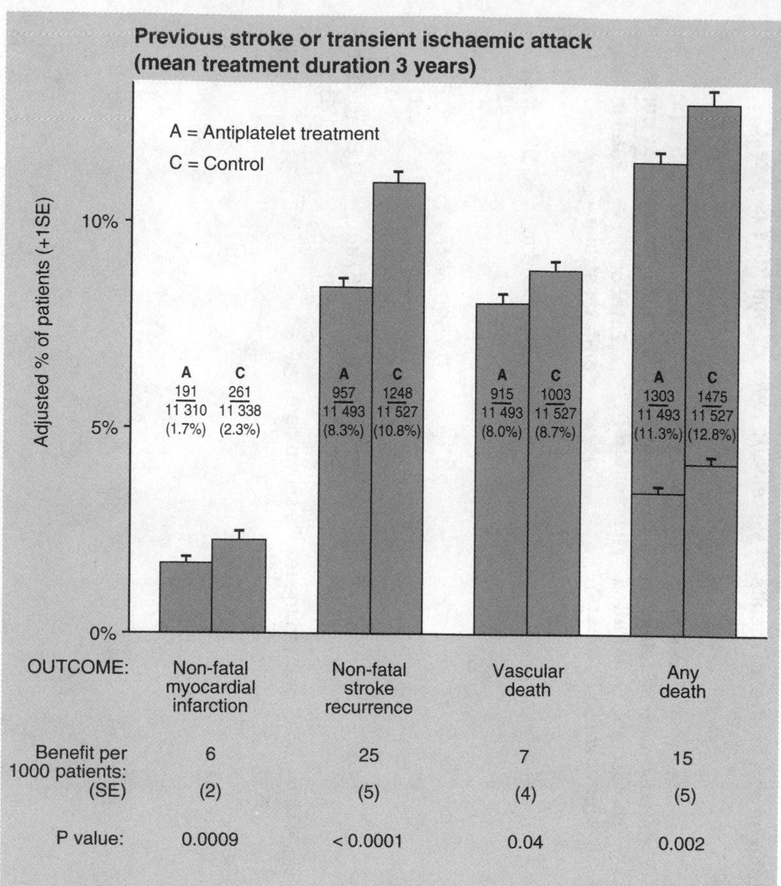

FIGURE 1 **Absolute effects of antiplatelet treatment on various outcomes in 21 trials in people with a prior (presumed ischaemic) stroke or transient ischaemic attack. The columns show the absolute risks over 3 years for each outcome. The error bars represent standard deviations. In the "any death" column, non-vascular deaths are represented by lower horizontal lines (see text, p 190). Adapted with permission.[4]**

Thromboembolism

Search date March 2002

David Fitzmaurice, FD Richard Hobbs, and Richard McManus

QUESTIONS

INTERVENTIONS

To be covered in future updates
Compression stockings for deep vein thrombosis
Oral antithrombotic agents (such as glycoprotein IIb/IIIa antagonists)
Inferior vena cava filters
Aspirin
Thromboembolism in pregnancy

See glossary, p 222

Key Messages

Proximal deep vein thrombosis

- **Oral anticoagulants** One RCT found that combined acenocoumarol plus intravenous unfractionated heparin versus acenocoumarol alone for initial treatment reduced recurrence of proximal deep vein thrombosis within 6 months. Systematic reviews have found that longer versus shorter duration of anticoagulation is associated with significantly fewer deep vein thrombosis recurrences or thromboembolic complications. One non-systematic review found limited evidence that longer versus shorter duration of warfarin treatment was associated with a significantly increased risk of major haemorrhage, but another non-systematic review found no significantly increased risk. The absolute risk of recurrent venous thromboembolism decreases with time, but the relative risk reduction with treatment remains constant. Harms of treatment, including major haemorrhage, continue during prolonged treatment. Individual people have different risk profiles. It is likely that the optimal duration of anticoagulation will vary between people.

- **Unfractionated and low molecular weight heparin** One systematic review has found no significant difference with long term low molecular weight heparin versus oral anticoagulation in recurrent thromboembolism, major haemorrhage, or mortality. Systematic reviews have found that low molecular weight heparin is at least as effective as unfractionated heparin in reducing the incidence of recurrent thromboembolic disease, and have found that short term low molecular weight heparin versus unfractionated heparin is associated with a significantly decreased risk of major haemorrhage.

Isolated calf vein thrombosis

- **Warfarin plus heparin** One RCT found that warfarin plus intravenous unfractionated heparin versus heparin alone (international normalised ratio 2.5–4.2) reduced the rate of proximal extension. One unblinded RCT found no significant difference in recurrent thromboembolism with 6 versus 12 weeks of anticoagulation.

Pulmonary embolism

- **Oral anticoagulants** We found no direct evidence about the optimum intensity and duration of anticoagulation in people with pulmonary embolism. The best available evidence requires extrapolation of results from studies of people with proximal deep vein thrombosis.
- **Thrombolysis** One systematic review in people with pulmonary embolism has found no significant difference in mortality with thrombolysis plus heparin versus heparin alone, and has found that thrombolysis may increase the incidence of intracranial haemorrhage. One small RCT identified by the review found limited evidence that thrombolysis may reduce mortality in people with shock due to massive pulmonary embolism.
- **Unfractionated and low molecular weight heparin** One small RCT found that heparin plus warfarin versus no anticoagulation significantly reduced mortality at 1 year in people with pulmonary embolism (NNT 4, 95% CI 2 to 16). One RCT in people with symptomatic pulmonary embolism who did not receive thrombolysis or embolectomy found no significant difference with low molecular weight heparin versus unfractionated heparin in mortality or new episodes of thromboembolism. Another RCT in people with proximal deep vein thrombosis without clinical signs or symptoms of pulmonary embolism but with high probability lung scan findings found that fixed dose low molecular weight heparin versus intravenous heparin significantly reduced the proportion of people with new episodes of venous thromboembolism.

Computerised decision support of oral anticoagulation

- We found no RCTs of computerised decision support versus usual management of oral anticoagulation that used clinically important outcomes (major haemorrhage or death).
- One systematic review and three subsequent RCTs have found that computerised decision support in oral anticoagulation significantly increases time spent in the target international normalised ratio range. Another subsequent RCT found no significant difference with computerised decision support versus standard manual support in the time spent in the target international normalised ratio range. A subsequent RCT of initiation of warfarin found no significant difference with computerised decision support versus usual care in the time taken to reach therapeutic levels of anticoagulation.

DEFINITION **Venous thromboembolism** is any thromboembolic event occurring within the venous system, including deep vein thrombosis and pulmonary embolism. **Deep vein thrombosis** is a radiologically confirmed partial or total thrombotic occlusion of the deep venous system of the legs sufficient to produce symptoms of pain or swelling. **Proximal deep vein thrombosis** affects the veins above the knee (popliteal, superficial femoral, common femoral, and iliac veins). **Isolated calf vein thrombosis** is confined to the deep veins of the calf and does not affect the veins above the knee. **Pulmonary embolism** is radiologically confirmed partial or total thromboembolic occlusion of pulmonary arteries, sufficient to cause symptoms of breathlessness, chest pain, or both. **Post-thrombotic syndrome** is oedema, ulceration, and impaired viability of the subcutaneous tissues of the leg occurring after deep vein thrombosis. **Recurrence** refers to symptomatic deterioration due to a further (radiologically confirmed) thrombosis, after a previously confirmed thromboembolic event, where there had been an initial partial or total symptomatic improvement. **Extension** refers to a radiologically confirmed new, constant, symptomatic intraluminal filling defect extending from an existing thrombosis.

INCIDENCE/ PREVALENCE We found no reliable study of the incidence/prevalence of deep vein thrombosis or pulmonary embolism in the UK. A prospective Scandinavian study found an annual incidence of 1.6–1.8/1000 people in the general population.[1,2] One postmortem study estimated that 600 000 people develop pulmonary embolism each year in the USA, of whom 60 000 die as a result.[3]

AETIOLOGY/ RISK FACTORS Risk factors for deep vein thrombosis include immobility, surgery (particularly orthopaedic), malignancy, smoking, pregnancy, older age, and inherited or acquired prothrombotic clotting disorders.[4] Evidence for these factors is mainly observational. The oral contraceptive pill is associated with increased risk of death due to venous thromboembolism (ARI with any combined oral contraception: 1–3/million women a year).[5] The principal cause of pulmonary embolism is a deep vein thrombosis.[4]

PROGNOSIS The annual recurrence rate of symptomatic calf vein thrombosis in people without recent surgery is over 25%.[6,7] Proximal extension develops in 40–50% of people with symptomatic calf vein thrombosis.[8] Proximal deep vein thrombosis may cause fatal or non-fatal pulmonary embolism, recurrent venous thrombosis, and the post-thrombotic syndrome. One observational study published in 1946 found 20% mortality from pulmonary emboli in people in hospital with untreated deep vein thrombosis.[9] One non-systematic review of observational studies found that, in people after recent surgery who have an asymptomatic calf vein deep vein thrombosis, the rate of fatal pulmonary embolism was 13–15%.[10] The incidence of other complications without treatment is not known. The risk of recurrent venous thrombosis and complications is increased by thrombotic risk factors.[11]

AIMS To reduce acute symptoms of deep vein thrombosis and to prevent morbidity and mortality associated with thrombus extension, the post-thrombotic syndrome, and pulmonary embolisation; to reduce recurrence; to minimise any adverse effects of treatment.

OUTCOMES Rates of symptomatic recurrence, post-thrombotic syndrome, symptomatic pulmonary embolism, and death. Proxy outcomes include radiological evidence of clot extension or pulmonary embolism.

METHODS *Clinical Evidence* update search and appraisal March 2002. Observational studies were used for estimating incidence, prevalence, and adverse event rates. RCTs were included only if participants and outcomes were objectively defined, and if the trial provided dose ranges (with adjusted dosing schedules for oral anticoagulation and unfractionated heparin) and independent, blinded outcome assessment.

QUESTION What are the effects of treatments for proximal deep vein thrombosis?

OPTION ANTICOAGULATION

Warfarin versus placebo: we found no RCTs. Acenocoumarol plus intravenous unfractionated heparin versus acenocoumarol alone for initial treatment: one RCT found reduced recurrence of proximal deep vein thrombosis. Longer versus shorter duration of anticoagulation: systematic reviews have found significantly fewer deep vein thrombosis recurrences with longer anticoagulation. One non-systematic review found limited evidence of significantly increased major haemorrhage, but another non-systematic review found no significant increase. Low molecular weight heparin versus unfractionated heparin: systematic reviews have found that low molecular weight heparin is at least as effective as unfractionated heparin in reducing the incidence of recurrent thromboembolic disease, and have found that short term low molecular weight heparin versus unfractionated heparin is associated with a significantly decreased risk of major haemorrhage. Long term low molecular weight heparin versus oral anticoagulation: one systematic review has found no significant difference with long term low molecular weight heparin versus oral anticoagulation in recurrent thromboembolism, major haemorrhage, or mortality. Heparin treatment at home versus in hospital: one systematic review has found limited evidence of no significant difference in recurrence of thromboembolism.

Benefits: **Warfarin versus placebo:** We found no systematic review and no RCTs. **Acenocoumarol plus intravenous unfractionated heparin versus acenocoumarol alone for initial treatment:** We found no systematic review. One RCT (120 people with proximal deep vein thrombosis) found that combined intravenous unfractionated heparin plus acenocoumarol versus acenocoumarol alone reduced recurrence at interim analysis at 6 months; although the difference did not quite reach significance and, as a result, the trial was stopped (12/60 [20%] with warfarin alone *v* 4/60 [7%] with combined treatment; P = 0.058).[12] **Longer versus shorter duration of anticoagulation:** We found two systematic reviews[13,14] and two subsequent open label RCTs.[15,16] The first systematic review (search date 2000, 4 RCTs, 1500 people) included two RCTs of people with a first episode of venous thromboembolism, one RCT in people with a second episode of venous thromboembolism, and one RCT in people with acute proximal deep vein thrombosis.[13] The periods of treatment compared were different in all four RCTs: 4 weeks versus 3 months, 6 weeks versus 6 months, 3 months versus 27 months, and 6 months versus 4 years. In all RCTs, anticoagulant doses were adjusted to achieve an international normalised ratio (see glossary, p 222) of 2.0–3.0. The review found that prolonged versus shorter treatment significantly reduced thromboembolic complications (AR 7/758 [0.9%] in the long arm *v* 91/742 [12.3%] in the short arm; RR 0.08, 95% CI 0.04 to 0.16; NNT 9, 95% CI 8 to 12). However, it found no significant reduction in mortality with prolonged versus shorter treatment (AR 37/758 [4.9%] in the long arm *v* 50/742 [6.7%] in the short arm; RR 0.72, 95% CI 0.48 to 1.08).[13] The second systematic review (search date not stated, 7 RCTs, 2304 people) included three of the same RCTs as the first systematic review plus four RCTs that had been excluded from the first systematic review on methodological grounds (either because of problems with blinding of outcomes or lack of an objective test to confirm thromboembolism).[14] There was wide variation in the duration of short term (3–12 wks) and longer term (12 wks to 2 years) RCTs. This review also found that longer versus shorter duration of anticoagulation reduced the risk of recurrent thromboembolism (74/1156 [6.4%] events per person with longer duration *v* 127/1148 [11.1%] with shorter duration; RR 0.60, 95% CI 0.45 to 0.79; NNT 22, 95% CI 15 to 43). The first subsequent RCT (736 people, including 539 with proximal deep vein thrombosis and/or pulmonary embolism; open label) comparing fluindione for 3 months versus 6 months found no significant difference in the risk of recurrent thromboembolism, although the confidence interval was wide (AR 21/270 [7.8%] with 3 months treatment *v* 23/269 [8.6%] with 6 months; ARR +0.8%, 95% CI −3.9% to +5.4%; RR 0.93, 95% CI 0.53 to 1.65).[15] The second subsequent RCT (267 people with a first episode of symptomatic proximal deep vein thrombosis; open label) compared warfarin or acenocoumarol treatment for 3 months versus 12 months.[16] It found no significant difference in recurrence of venous thromboembolism over a mean of 3 years (21/134 [15.7%] with 12 months *v* 21/133 [15.8%] with 3 months treatment; RR 0.99, 95% CI 0.57 to 1.73). Mean time to recurrence was shorter with 3 months versus 12 months treatment (11.2 months with 3 months *v* 16 months with 12 months; no further data provided).[16] **Intensity of anticoagulation:** We found one RCT (96 people with a first episode of idiopathic venous thromboembolism) comparing international normalised ratio targets of 2.0–3.0 versus 3.0–4.5 for 12 weeks' treatment with warfarin after an initial course of intravenous heparin. It found similar recurrence rates at 10 months for both international normalised ratio target ranges (1/47 [2.1%] with lower range *v* 1/49 [2.0%] with higher range; $P > 0.05$), but found significantly fewer haemorrhagic events with the lower target range (2/47 [4.3%] *v* 11/49 [22.4%]; ARR 18%, 95% CI 5% to 32%; RR 0.19, 95% CI 0.04 to 0.81; NNT 6, 95% CI 4 to 23).[17] **Abrupt versus gradual discontinuation of warfarin:** One RCT (41 people with deep vein thrombosis who had received intravenous heparin for 3–5 days followed by warfarin for 3–6 months) compared abrupt withdrawal of warfarin versus an additional month of warfarin at a fixed low dose of 1.25 mg daily.[18]

It found no difference in recurrence (3 people with abrupt withdrawal *v* 1 person with gradual withdrawal). **Low molecular weight heparin (LMWH) versus unfractionated heparin in people with proximal deep vein thrombosis:** We found two systematic reviews[19,20] and one subsequent unblinded RCT[21] in people with symptomatic proximal deep vein thrombosis. The first systematic review (search date 1993, 16 RCTs, 2045 people) found that LMWH (see glossary, p 222) versus unfractionated heparin significantly reduced thrombus extension (ARs not provided; OR 0.45, 95% CI 0.25 to 0.81).[19] The second systematic review (search date 1994, 10 RCTs, 1424 people) found that LMWH versus unfractionated heparin significantly reduced symptomatic thromboembolic complications (ARs not provided; RR 0.47, 95% CI 0.27 to 0.82) and mortality (RR 0.53, 95% CI 0.31 to 0.90).[20] The subsequent unblinded RCT (961 people) compared LMWH twice daily for 1 week versus LMWH once daily for 4 weeks versus intravenous unfractionated heparin.[21] It found that both LMWH regimens versus unfractionated heparin significantly increased thrombus regression at 21 days (167/312 [53.5%] with once daily LMWH *v* 129/321 [40.2%] with unfractionated heparin; RR 1.29, 97.5% CI 1.08 to 1.53; 175/328 [53.4%] with twice daily LMWH *v* 129/321 [40.2%] with unfractionated heparin; RR 1.28, 97.5% CI 1.08 to 1.52). It found that twice daily LMWH versus unfractionated heparin significantly reduced recurrent thromboembolism at 90 days (7/388 [1.8%] with twice daily LMWH *v* 24/375 [6.4%] with unfractionated heparin; RR 0.28, 97.5% CI 0.11 to 0.74), but found no significant difference with once daily LMWH versus unfractionated heparin in recurrent thromboembolism (13/374 [3.5%] with once daily LMWH *v* 24/375 [6.4%] with unfractionated heparin; RR 0.55, 97.5% CI 0.24 to 1.16). **LMWH versus unfractionated heparin in people with symptomatic venous thromboembolism:** We found six systematic reviews[22–27] and two subsequent RCTs[28,29] of LMWH versus unfractionated heparin in people with symptomatic venous thromboembolism located at sites other than just the proximal calf. The first systematic review (search date 1999, 14 RCTs, 4754 people) included five RCTs (blinded and unblinded, 1636 people) of proximal deep vein thrombosis.[22] It found that LMWH versus unfractionated heparin significantly reduced thrombotic complications (AR 39/814 [4.8%] with LMWH *v* 64/822 [7.8%] with unfractionated heparin; OR 0.60, 95% CI 0.40 to 0.89). Overall mortality was also reduced (AR 44/814 [5.4%] with LMWH *v* 68/822 [8.3%] with unfractionated heparin; OR 0.64, 95% CI 0.43 to 0.93). Eight of the 14 RCTs in the systematic review included people with symptomatic deep vein thrombosis of the leg without symptoms of pulmonary embolism, and these accounted for about 75% of all participants. Analysis of the seven RCTs that concealed treatment allocation found no difference in recurrent venous thromboembolism during initial treatment (AR 34/1569 [2.2%] with LMWH *v* 43/1595 [2.7%] with unfractionated heparin; OR 0.80, 95% CI 0.51 to 1.26), in recurrent venous thromboembolism at the end of 1–6 months' follow up (AR 75/1671 [4.5%] with LMWH *v* 92/1693 [5.4%] with unfractionated heparin; OR 0.82, 95% CI 0.60 to 1.12), in overall mortality (AR 123/1671 [7.4%] with LMWH *v* 150/1694 [8.9%] with unfractionated heparin; OR 0.82,

95% CI 0.64 to 1.05), or in major haemorrhage (see glossary, p 222).[22] The second systematic review (search date 1999, 21 blinded and unblinded RCTs, 4472 people) included nine RCTs excluded from the first systematic review on methodological grounds (dose of unfractionated heparin not adjusted, adjustment of dose of LMWH, and intravenous administration of LMWH).[26] Results for people with proximal deep vein thrombosis alone were not analysed separately. It found that LMWH versus unfractionated heparin significantly improved clot regression (OR 0.73, 95% CI 0.59 to 0.90), reduced the incidence of haemorrhage (OR 0.65, 95% CI 0.43 to 0.98; P = 0.047), and reduced mortality (OR 0.68, 95% CI 0.50 to 0.91; P = 0.01). It found no significant difference in recurrent thromboembolism (OR 0.78, 95% CI 0.59 to 1.04; P = 0.10). The third systematic review (search date not stated, 16 unblinded and blinded RCTs, 6042 people) included 14 RCTs from the first systematic review and two RCTs published after the search date of the first review.[27] It found that LMWH versus unfractionated heparin significantly reduced recurrent venous thromboembolism (ARs not provided; OR 0.66, 95% CI 0.51 to 0.86). The other three systematic reviews (search dates 1996,[23] 1999,[24] and not stated[25]), which included many of the same trials, found no significant difference in recurrent venous thromboembolism or pulmonary embolism with unfractionated heparin versus LMWH, and found a significant difference in favour of LMWH for total mortality over 3 months. The first subsequent RCT (294 people with acute proximal deep vein thrombosis, unblinded) compared intravenous unfractionated heparin in hospital versus LMWH twice daily given mainly at home (outpatients) or alternatively in hospital versus subcutaneous heparin calcium given at home. It found no significant difference in recurrent deep vein thrombosis (6/98 [6%] with unfractionated heparin *v* 6/97 [6%] with LMWH *v* 7/99 [7%] with subcutaneous heparin calcium).[28] See systematic anticoagulation under stroke management, p 169. The second subsequent RCT (900 people with symptomatic lower extremity deep vein thrombosis, including 287 with pulmonary embolism) compared unfractionated heparin versus enoxaparin once or twice daily. It found no significant difference in recurrent thromboembolism at 3 months (12/290 [4.1%] with unfractionated heparin *v* 22/610 [3.6%] with enoxaparin; ARR +0.5%, 95% CI −2% to +3%).[29] **Once daily versus twice daily LMWH:** We found one systematic review (search date 1999, 5 RCTs, 1522 people with symptomatic proximal deep vein thrombosis) comparing once versus twice daily LMWH for 5–10 days.[30] It found that once versus twice daily LMWH reduced the proportion of people with symptomatic or asymptomatic venous thromboembolism at 10 days or 3 months, but the difference was not significant (symptomatic venous thromboembolism at 10 days: 5 RCTs, OR 0.82, 95% CI 0.26 to 2.49; at 3 months: 3 RCTs, OR 0.85, 95% CI 0.48 to 1.49). **Long term LMWH versus oral anticoagulation:** We found one systematic review (search date 2001, 7 RCTs, 1137 people with proximal deep vein thrombosis treated initially with LMWH or unfractionated heparin for 5–10 days) comparing long term oral anticoagulation versus long term LMWH.[31] It found no significant difference with

LMWH versus oral anticoagulation in recurrent symptomatic thromboembolism (27/568 [4.8%] *v* 38/569 [6.7%]; OR 0.70, 95% CI 0.42 to 1.16) or mortality (21/568 [4.0%] *v* 14/569 [2.5%]; OR 1.51, 95% CI 0.77 to 2.97).[31] **Home versus hospital treatment with short term heparin:** We found one systematic review (search date 2000, 3 RCTs, 1104 people).[32] Two of the RCTs in the systematic review compared LMWH at home versus unfractionated heparin in hospital, the other RCT compared LMWH both at home and in hospital. The RCTs had methodological problems, including high exclusion rates and partial hospital treatment in the home treatment arms. The systematic review found no significant difference between treatments in recurrence of thromboembolism, minor bleeding, major haemorrhage, or mortality.[32]

Harms: **Warfarin:** Two non-systematic reviews of RCTs and cohort studies found annual bleeding rates of 0–5% (fatal bleeding) and 2–8% (major bleeds).[33,34] Rates depended on how bleeding was defined and the intensity of anticoagulation. **Acenocoumarol plus intravenous unfractionated heparin versus acenocoumarol alone for initial treatment:** In the RCT comparing acenocoumarol plus heparin versus acenocoumarol alone: one person in the combined treatment group committed suicide at 6 months. There were two cancer related deaths, confirmed by postmortem examination, in the group treated with warfarin alone; one in week 11 and the other in week 12.[12] **Longer versus shorter duration of anticoagulation:** No individual study in either review comparing length of anticoagulation found a significant increase in bleeding complications during prolonged versus shorter treatment for venous thromboembolism.[13,14] Both reviews included studies with different periods of treatment and the populations studied had different types of venous thromboembolism (see benefits above). The first review found that prolonged versus shorter anticoagulation significantly increased the risk of major haemorrhage (19/758 [2.5%] with prolonged anticoagulation *v* 4/742 [0.5%] with shorter anticoagulation; OR 3.75, 95% CI 1.63 to 8.62).[13] The second review found a greater risk of major haemorrhage with prolonged versus shorter anticoagulation, but the difference was not significant (10/917 [1.1%] with prolonged treatment *v* 6/906 [0.7%] with shorter treatment; RR 1.43, 95% CI 0.51 to 4.01).[14] **LMWH versus unfractionated heparin:** One systematic review (3306 people treated for at least 5 days) found no significant difference with LMWH versus unfractionated heparin in the risk of thrombocytopenia (RR 0.85, 95% CI 0.45 to 1.62).[23] Another systematic review in people with venous thromboembolism found no significant difference with LMWH versus unfractionated heparin in the risk of major haemorrhage (AR 27/1791 [1.5%] *v* 39/1827 [2.1%]; OR 0.71, 95% CI 0.43 to 1.15).[22] In this systematic review, pooling of blinded and unblinded RCTs found that the risk of major haemorrhage was 1–2% for up to 10 days' treatment with either LMWH or unfractionated heparin. Analysis of the five RCTs in the review of people with proximal thrombosis (blinded and unblinded, 1636 people) found that short term LMWH versus unfractionated heparin significantly reduced major haemorrhage (8/814 [1.0%] *v* 19/822 [2.3%]; OR 0.44, 95% CI 0.21 to 0.95).[22] Three other systematic reviews, covering many of the same trials, found similar significant reductions in major haemorrhage.[23–25] A fifth systematic review (4472 people) found no significant difference with twice daily LMWH versus unfractionated heparin in major haemorrhage (OR 0.79, 95% CI 0.47 to 1.32), but found that once daily LMWH versus unfractionated heparin significantly reduced major haemorrhage (OR 0.07, 95% CI 0.01 to 0.54).[26] A sixth systematic review (6055 people) found that LMWH versus unfractionated heparin significantly reduced the frequency of major haemorrhage (OR 0.56, 95% CI 0.38 to 0.83).[27] One of the systematic reviews in people with deep vein thrombosis found that unfractionated heparin versus LMWH was associated with higher rates of clinically important bleeding (ARs not provided; unfractionated heparin *v* LMWH RR 2.48, 95% CI 1.27 to 6.67) and death.[20] **Long term LMWH versus anticoagulation:** One systematic review found that long term anticoagulation versus long term LMWH significantly reduced major haemorrhage (7 RCTs; 5/568 [0.9%] *v* 14/569 [2.5%]; OR 0.38, 95% CI 0.15 to 0.94) but, when only high quality RCTs were included, it found no significant difference in major haemorrhage with long term LMWH versus anticoagulation (3 RCTs; 4/236 [1.7%] *v* 5/241 [2.1%]; OR 0.80, 95% CI 0.21 to 3.00).[31]

Comment: **Studies assessing harm:** These varied in regard to diagnostic criteria, definitions of adverse events, and intensity of anticoagulation, making interpretation difficult. **Duration of warfarin treatment:** The absolute risk of recurrent venous thromboembolism decreases with time, whereas the relative risk reduction with treatment remains constant. Observed recurrence of venous thromboembolism is therefore dependent on length of follow up. Harms of treatment, including major haemorrhage, continue during prolonged treatment. Individual people have different risk profiles and it is likely that the optimal duration of anticoagulation will vary between people.

QUESTION What are the effects of treatment for isolated calf vein thrombosis?

OPTION ANTICOAGULATION

One RCT found that warfarin plus intravenous unfractionated heparin versus heparin alone (international normalised ratio 2.5–4.2) reduced rates of proximal extension. One unblinded RCT found no significant difference in recurrent thromboembolism with 6 versus 12 weeks of anticoagulation.

Benefits: **Warfarin versus placebo:** We found no systematic review and no RCTs. **Warfarin plus heparin versus warfarin alone:** We found no systematic review. We found one RCT that compared intravenous unfractionated heparin (international normalised ratio [see glossary, p 222] 2.5–4.2) for at least 5 days with or without 3 months of warfarin. It found that heparin plus warfarin reduced proximal extension of clot at 1 year compared with heparin alone (1/23 [4%] people with heparin plus warfarin *v* 9/28 [32%] people with heparin alone; ARR 28%, 95% CI 9% to 47%).[6] **Duration of anticoagulation:** We found one unblinded RCT (736 people, including 197 with isolated calf vein thrombosis) comparing 6 weeks versus 12 weeks of anticoagulation, which found no significant difference in recurrence of venous thromboembolism (AR 2/105 [1.9%] with 6 wks treatment *v* 3/92 [3.3%] with 12 wks; RR 0.58, 95% CI 0.10 to 3.36).[15]

Harms: See harms of anticoagulation under treatments for proximal deep vein thrombosis, p 216. **Duration of anticoagulation:** One RCT (197 people) found no significant difference in rate of haemorrhage with 6 weeks versus 12 weeks of anticoagulation (AR 13/105 [12.4%] with 6 wks treatment *v* 19/92 [20.6%] with 12 wks; RR 0.59, 95% CI 0.31 to 1.26).[15]

Comment: Many reported cases of isolated calf vein thrombosis are asymptomatic but detected radiologically for research purposes. We found limited evidence on the clinical significance of asymptomatic calf vein thrombosis. Similarly, studies into the incidence of pulmonary embolism associated with isolated calf vein thrombosis detected asymptomatic embolism by ventilation–perfusion scanning, and it is not clear what the clinical significance of these findings are.

QUESTION **What are the effects of treatments for pulmonary embolism?**

OPTION **ANTICOAGULATION**

We found no direct evidence in people with pulmonary embolism about the optimum intensity and duration of anticoagulation. Evidence for intensity and duration of treatment has been extrapolated from studies in people with proximal deep vein thrombosis and any venous thromboembolism. One small RCT found that heparin plus warfarin versus no anticoagulation significantly reduced mortality in people with pulmonary embolism. One RCT in people with symptomatic pulmonary embolism who did not receive thrombolysis or embolectomy found no significant difference with low molecular weight heparin versus unfractionated heparin in mortality or new episodes of thromboembolism. Another RCT in people with proximal deep vein thrombosis without clinical signs or symptoms of pulmonary embolism but with high probability lung scan findings found that low molecular weight heparin versus intravenous heparin significantly reduced the proportion of people with new episodes of venous thromboembolism.

Benefits: We found no RCTs of heparin versus placebo, warfarin versus placebo, or heparin plus warfarin versus heparin alone or versus warfarin alone. **Heparin plus warfarin versus no anticoagulation:** We found no systematic review. We found one RCT (published 1960; 35 people with pulmonary embolism) comparing heparin plus warfarin versus no anticoagulation.[35] It found that anticoagulation significantly reduced mortality at 1 year (0/16 deaths [0%] with anticoagulation *v* 5/19 deaths [26%] with no anticoagulation; NNT 4, 95% CI 2 to 16). **Duration and intensity of anticoagulation:** We found no direct evidence in people with pulmonary embolism. Evidence for intensity and duration of treatment has been extrapolated from studies in people with proximal deep vein thrombosis and any venous thromboembolism. These trials found that bleeding rates were increased by higher international normalised ratio (see glossary, p 222) target ranges (international normalised ratio 3.0–4.5), but recurrence rates were not significantly different compared with a lower range (international normalised ratio 2.0–3.0), and that longer courses of anticoagulation reduced recurrence compared with shorter courses (see benefits of anticoagulation under treatments for proximal deep vein thrombosis, p 212). **Low molecular weight heparin (LMWH) versus**

unfractionated heparin: We found no systematic review. We found two RCTs.[36,37] The first RCT (612 people with symptomatic pulmonary embolism who did not receive thrombolysis or embolectomy) found no significant difference with LMWH (see glossary, p 222) (tinzaparin) versus intravenous heparin in mortality (AR 12/304 [3.9%] with tinzaparin *v* 14/308 [4.5%] with heparin; P = 0.7) or recurrent thromboembolism (5/304 [1.6%] with tinzaparin *v* 6/308 [1.9%] with heparin; P = 0.8).[36] The second RCT (200 people with proximal deep vein thrombosis without clinical signs or symptoms of pulmonary embolism but with high probability lung scan findings) found that fixed dose LMWH given once daily versus dose adjusted intravenous heparin significantly reduced the proportion of people with new episodes of venous thromboembolism (AR 0/97 [0%] with LMWH *v* 7/103 [6.8%] with iv heparin; P = 0.01).[37]

Harms: The first RCT comparing LMWH versus unfractionated heparin found no significant difference in the rate of major haemorrhage (see glossary, p 222) (3/304 [1.0%] with LMWH *v* 5/308 [1.6%] with unfractionated heparin; P = 0.5).[36] The second RCT also found no significant difference in the risk of major haemorrhage (1/97 [1%] with LMWH *v* 2/103 [2%] with iv heparin; P = 0.6).[37] See harms of anticoagulation under treatments for proximal deep vein thrombosis, p 216.

Comment: In the two RCTs,[36,37] the incidence of major haemorrhage was low and the number of people was too small to detect a clinically important difference.

OPTION THROMBOLYSIS New

One systematic review in people with pulmonary embolism has found no significant difference in mortality with thrombolysis plus heparin versus heparin alone, and has found that thrombolysis may increase the incidence of intracranial haemorrhage. One small RCT identified by the review found limited evidence that thrombolysis may reduce mortality in people with shock due to massive pulmonary embolism.

Benefits: We found one systematic review,[38] and one large non-randomised trial (see comment below).[39] **Versus heparin:** The systematic review (search date 1998) identified nine RCTs comparing various thrombolytic agents versus heparin.[38] The review did not perform a meta-analysis. The largest RCT (160 people with angiographically documented pulmonary embolism) identified by the review compared a 12 hour infusion of urokinase followed by heparin versus heparin alone. It found no significant difference between treatments in mortality (7/78 [9%] *v* 6/82 [7%]; RR 1.23, 95% CI 0.43 to 3.49) or recurrent pulmonary embolism at 12 months (15/78 [19%] *v* 12/82 [15%]; RR 1.31, 95% CI 0.66 to 2.63). Seven short term RCTs identified by the review compared urokinase, streptokinase, or recombinant tissue-type plasminogen activator followed by heparin versus heparin alone, where heparin was adjusted to maintain a therapeutic partial thromboplastin time. They found no significant difference in mortality or recurrent embolism at 24 hours to 30 days. One small RCT identified by the review (8 people with shock related to pulmonary embolism) comparing bolus streptokinase versus heparin found limited evidence that streptokinase reduced mortality (0/4 [0%] with streptokinase *v* 4/4 [100%] with heparin). However, these results should be interpreted with caution as people receiving heparin alone had a much longer delay between onset of symptoms and initiation of treatment than people receiving streptokinase.[38] **Versus each other:** The systematic review identified six RCTs (491 people) comparing different thrombolytic agents versus each other.[38] It found no significant difference in mortality or recurrent pulmonary embolism with different thrombolytics.

Harms: One systematic review (search date not stated) assessing haemorrhagic complications of anticoagulation identified the same 16 RCTs.[40] It found no difference in the proportion of people who had major bleeding events with thrombolysis versus thrombolytics plus heparin or versus heparin alone (thrombolytics 0–48% *v* thrombolytics plus heparin 0–45% *v* heparin alone 0–27%).[40] It also found no difference between different thrombolytic agents in the proportion of people who had major bleeding events (9–14%). It found that intravenous thrombolytics versus heparin increased the proportion of people who had an intracranial haemorrhage (896 people; 1.2% with thrombolytics [half of which were fatal] *v* 0% with heparin alone).[40]

Comment: **Versus heparin:** One additional, non-randomised trial (719 people), which excluded people with shock, found limited evidence that thrombolytics versus heparin reduced overall mortality (8/169 [5%] *v* 61/550 [11%]; RR 0.43, 95% CI 0.21 to 0.87) and recurrent pulmonary embolism over 30 days (13/169 [8%] *v* 103/550 [19%]; RR 0.25, 95% CI 0.13 to 0.51).[39] However, these results should be interpreted with caution as people receiving heparin were older and more likely to have underlying cardiac or pulmonary disease than those receiving thrombolytics.

QUESTION What are the effects of computerised decision support on oral anticoagulation management?

We found no RCTs of computerised decision support versus usual management of oral anticoagulation that used clinically important outcomes (major haemorrhage or death). One systematic review and three subsequent RCTs have found that computerised decision support in oral anticoagulation significantly increases time spent in the target international normalised ratio range. Another subsequent RCT found no significant difference with computerised decision support versus standard manual support in the time spent in the target international normalised ratio range. A subsequent RCT of initiation of warfarin found no significant difference with computerised decision support versus usual care in the time taken to reach therapeutic levels of anticoagulation. Most RCTs were small and brief.

Benefits: **Clinical outcomes:** We found no systematic review and no RCTs. **Laboratory outcomes:** We found three systematic reviews[41–43] and five subsequent RCTs.[44–48] The first review (search date 1997, 9 RCTs, 1336 people) included eight RCTs using warfarin and one using heparin.[41] The computer systems advised the doses for initiation of anticoagulation (2 RCTs) and for maintenance of anticoagulation (6 RCTs). Follow up was short (15 days to 12 months). Indications for treatment included cardiac diseases and venous thrombosis. The outcome reported by 7/9 RCTs (693 people) in the systematic review was the proportion of days within the target range of anticoagulation. The review found that computerised decision support (see glossary, p 222) versus usual care increased the time that the international normalised ratio (see glossary, p 222) was in the target range (OR 1.29, 95% CI 1.12 to 1.49). One included trial (small and with the largest effect) introduced significant heterogeneity between the trials and therefore was excluded (OR for remaining RCTs 1.25, 95% CI 1.08 to 1.45). The other two systematic reviews (search dates 1998[42] and 1996[43]) included computer support for determining the dose for a wider range of drugs and included seven[42] and four[43] RCTs of the nine found by the first systematic review.[41] These reviews did not provide a discrete analysis of the RCTs of computer support of oral anticoagulation. The first subsequent RCT (122 people on warfarin after hip replacement) compared usual care versus computerised decision support.[44] Only initiation of warfarin was studied. It found no significant difference in the time taken to reach therapeutic levels of anticoagulation (4.7 days with usual care *v* 2.8 days with computerised decision support). The second subsequent RCT compared a computerised decision support dosing system versus physician adjusted dosing in five hospitals.[45] People who were taking warfarin for at least 6 days were selected (285 people) and followed for at least 3 months (results from 254 people [89%] were analysed). People managed by computerised decision support spent significantly more time with their international normalised ratio in the target range than people managed conventionally (63% with computerised decision support *v* 53% with conventional management; $P < 0.05$). The third subsequent RCT (244 people) compared a package of care that included computerised decision support versus traditional hospital outpatient management. The intervention was based in primary care: a practice nurse clinic that included near patient international normalised ratio testing and computerised decision support. It found significantly more time spent in the target range after 12 months with packaged care versus traditional outpatient management (69% *v* 57%; $P < 0.001$), but no difference in the proportion of tests in range (61% with intervention *v* 51% with control) or in the point prevalence of tests in range (71% *v* 62%).[46] The fourth subsequent RCT (101 people receiving oral anticoagulation after heart valve replacement) compared a computerised decision support system versus standard manual monitoring of international normalised ratio over 315 days.[47] It found no significant difference in the proportion of international normalised ratios in the target range or time spent in the target range (no further data and no mean follow up time provided). It found that people had significantly fewer dose changes with computerised versus standard manual monitoring (31% with computerised *v* 47% with manual; $P = 0.02$). The fifth subsequent RCT (335 people receiving initiation, 916 people receiving maintenance anticoagulation treatment for a variety of indications) compared a computerised decision support system for both dosing and appointment scheduling versus standard manual monitoring by "expert physicians".[48] It found that significantly more people managed by computerised decision support versus standard monitoring achieved a stable international normalised ratio in the first month (39% with computerised decision support *v* 27% with standard monitoring; $P < 0.01$) and spent more time with their international normalised ratio in the target range (71% with computerised decision support *v* 68% with standard monitoring; $P < 0.001$).

Harms: **Major haemorrhage:** See glossary, p 222. One systematic review (search date 1997, 9 RCTs, 1336 people) found major haemorrhages in 14/700 (2%) people with computerised decision support versus 25/636 (4%) in the control group.[41] Most of the events occurred in one study making meta-analysis inappropriate. One RCT found no significant difference in overall mortality or serious adverse events with computerised decision support versus usual care.[46]

Comment: We found only limited evidence (from small trials with short follow up of proxy outcomes) on the use of computerised decision support in oral anticoagulation management. Computerised decision support for oral anticoagulation seems to be at least as effective as human performance in terms of time spent in the target international normalised ratio range. It is not clear if this will translate to improved clinical outcomes. Larger and longer trials that measure clinical outcomes (particularly harms) are needed.

GLOSSARY

Computerised decision support system A computer program that provides advice on the significance and implications of clinical findings or laboratory results.
International normalised ratio (INR) A value derived from a standardised laboratory test that measures the effect of an anticoagulant. The laboratory materials used in the test are calibrated against internationally accepted standard reference preparations, so that variability between laboratories and different reagents is minimised. Normal blood has an international normalised ratio of 1. Therapeutic anticoagulation often aims to achieve an international normalised ratio value of 2.0–3.5.
Low molecular weight heparins (LMWH) are made from heparin using chemical or enzymatic methods. The various formulations of LMWH differ in mean molecular weight, composition, and anticoagulant activity. As a group, LMWHs have distinct properties and it is not yet clear that one LMWH will behave exactly like another. Some subcutaneously administered LMWHs do not require monitoring.
Major haemorrhage Exact definitions vary between studies but usually a major haemorrhage is one involving intracranial, retroperitoneal, joint, or muscle bleeding leading directly to death or requiring admission to hospital to stop the bleeding or provide a blood transfusion. All other haemorrhages are classified as minor.

Substantive changes

Anticoagulation; duration of anticoagulation One new RCT;[16] conclusions unchanged.
Anticoagulation; once daily versus twice daily low molecular weight heparin One new systematic review found that once versus twice daily low molecular weight heparin reduced the proportion of people with symptomatic or asymptomatic venous thromboembolism at 10 days or 3 months, but the difference was not significant.[30]
Computerised decision support One new RCT;[48] conclusions unchanged.

REFERENCES

1. Nordstrom M, Linblad B, Bergqvist D, et al. A prospective study of the incidence of deep-vein thrombosis within a defined urban population. *Arch Intern Med* 1992;326:155–160.
2. Hansson PO, Werlin L, Tibblin G, et al. Deep vein thrombosis and pulmonary embolism in the general population. *Arch Intern Med* 1997;157:1665–1670.

3. Rubinstein I, Murray D, Hoffstein V. Fatal pulmonary emboli in hospitalised patients: an autopsy study. *Arch Intern Med* 1988;148:1425–1426.
4. Hirsh J, Hoak J. Management of deep vein thrombosis and pulmonary embolism. *Circulation* 1996;93:2212–2245.
5. Farley TMM, Meirik O, Chang CL, et al. Effects of different progestogens in low oestrogen oral contraceptives on venous thromboembolic disease. *Lancet* 1995;346:1582–1588.
6. Lagerstedt C, Olsson C, Fagher B, et al. Need for long term anticoagulant treatment in symptomatic calf vein thrombosis. *Lancet* 1985;334:515–518.
7. Lohr J, Kerr T, Lutter K, et al. Lower extremity calf thrombosis: to treat or not to treat? *J Vasc Surg* 1991;14:618–623.
8. Kakkar VV, Howe CT, Flanc C, et al. Natural history of postoperative deep vein thrombosis. *Lancet* 1969;ii:230–232.
9. Zilliacus H. On the specific treatment of thrombosis and pulmonary embolism with anticoagulants, with a particular reference to the post thrombotic sequelae. *Acta Med Scand* 1946;170:1–221.
10. Giannoukas AD, Labropoulos N, Burke P, et al. Calf deep vein thrombosis: a review of the literature. *Eur J Vasc Endovasc Surg* 1995;10:398–404.
11. Lensing AWA, Prandoni P, Prins MH, et al. Deep-vein thrombosis. *Lancet* 1999;353:479–485.
12. Brandjes DPM, Heijboer H, Buller HR, et al. Acenocoumarol and heparin compared with acenocoumarol alone in the initial treatment of proximal-vein thrombosis. *N Engl J Med* 1992;327:1485–1489.
13. Hutten BA, Prins MH. Duration of treatment with vitamin K antagonists in symptomatic venous thromboembolism. In: The Cochrane Library, Issue 1, 2002. Oxford: Update Software. Search date 2000; primary sources Medline, Embase, hand searching relevant journals, and personal contacts.
14. Pinede L, Duhaut P, Cucherat M, et al. Comparison of long versus short duration of anticoagulant therapy after a first episode of venous thromboembolism: a meta-analysis of randomized, controlled trials. *J Intern Med* 2000;247:553–562. Search date not stated; primary sources Medline, Embase, Cochrane Controlled Trials Register, and hand searched reference lists.
15. Pinede L, Ninet J, Duhaut P, et al. Comparison of 3 and 6 months of oral anticoagulant therapy after a first episode of proximal deep vein thrombosis or pulmonary embolism and comparison of 6 and 12 weeks of therapy after isolated calf deep vein thrombosis. *Circulation* 2001;103:2453–2460.
16. Agnelli G, Prandoni P, Santamaria MG, et al. Three months versus one year of oral anticoagulant therapy for idiopathic deep venous thrombosis. Warfarin Optimal Duration Italian Trial Investigators. *N Engl J Med* 2001;345:165–169.
17. Hull R, Hirsh J, Jay RM, et al. Different intensities of oral anticoagulant therapy in the treatment of proximal vein thrombosis. *N Engl J Med* 1982;307:1676–1681.
18. Ascani A, Iorio A, Agnelli G. Withdrawal of warfarin after deep vein thrombosis: effects of a low fixed dose on rebound thrombin generation. *Blood Coagul Fibrinolysis* 1999;10:291–295.
19. Leisorovicz A, Simonneau G, Decousous H, et al. Comparison of efficacy and safety of low molecular weight heparins and unfractionated heparin in initial treatment of deep venous thrombosis: a meta-analysis. *BMJ* 1994;309:299–304. Search date 1993; primary sources Medline and hand searched references.
20. Lensing AWA, Prins MH, Davidson BL, et al. Treatment of deep venous thrombosis with low-molecular weight heparins. *Arch Intern Med* 1995;155:601–607. Search date 1994; primary sources Medline, manual search, and hand searched references.
21. Breddin HK, Hach-Wunderle V, Nakov R, et al. Effects of a low-molecular-weight heparin on thrombus regression and recurrent thromboembolism in patients with deep-vein thrombosis. *N Engl J Med* 2001;344:626–631.
22. Van den Belt AGM, Prins MH, Lensing AWA, et al. Fixed dose subcutaneous low molecular weight heparins versus adjusted dose unfractionated heparin for venous thromboembolism. In: The Cochrane Library, Issue 1, 2002. Oxford: Update Software. Search date 1999; primary sources Medline, Embase, LILACS, contact with researchers and pharmaceutical companies, and hand searched references.
23. Dolovich LR, Ginsberg JS, Douketis JD, et al. A meta-analysis comparing low-molecular-weight heparins with unfractionated heparin in the treatment of venous thromboembolism. *Arch Intern Med* 2000;160:181–188. Search date 1996; primary sources Medline, HEALTH, The Cochrane Library, and hand searched references.
24. Bijsterveld NR, Hettiarachchi R, Peters R, et al. Low-molecular weight heparins in venous and arterial thrombotic disease. *Thromb Haemost* 1999;82(suppl 1):139–147. Search date 1999; primary sources Medline, Embase, principal study investigators, and hand searched references.
25. Rohan JK, Hettiarachchi RJ, Prins MH, et al. Low molecular weight heparin versus unfractionated heparin in the initial treatment of venous thromboembolism. *Curr Opin Pulmon Med* 1998;4:220–225. Search date not stated; primary sources Medline, Current Contents, and Embase.
26. Rocha E, Martinez-Gonzalez MA, Montes R, et al. Do the low molecular weight heparins improve efficacy and safety of the treatment of deep venous thrombosis? A meta-analysis. *Haematologica* 2000;85:935–942. Search date 1999; primary sources Medline, Excerpta Medica, and conference abstracts.
27. Van der Heijden JF, Prins MH, Buller HR. For the initial treatment of venous thromboembolism: are all low-molecular-weight heparin compounds the same? *Thromb Res* 2000;10:V121–V130. Search date not stated; primary sources Medline, Embase, and Current Contents.
28. Belcaro G, Nicolaides AN, Cesarone MR, et al. Comparison of low-molecular-weight heparin, administered primarily at home, with unfractionated heparin, administered in hospital, and subcutaneous heparin, administered at home for deep-vein thrombosis. *Angiology* 1999;50:781–787.
29. Merli G, Spiro TF, Olsson CG, et al. Subcutaneous enoxaparin once or twice daily compared with intravenous unfractionated heparin for treatment of venous thromboembolic disease. *Ann Intern Med* 2001;134:191–202.
30. Couturaud F, Julian JA, Kearon C. Low molecular weight heparin administered once versus twice daily in patients with venous thromboembolism: a meta-analysis. *Thromb Haemost* 2001;86:980–984. Search date 1999; primary sources Medline, the Cochrane Library, hand searches of reference lists, and personal files of local experts.
31. Van Der Heijden JF, Hutten BA, Buller HR, et al. Vitamin K antagonists or low-molecular-weight

heparin for the long term treatment of symptomatic venous thromboembolism. In: The Cochrane Library, Issue 1, 2002. Oxford: Update Software. Search date 2001; primary sources Medline, Embase, Current Contents, hand searching relevant journals, and personal contacts.

32. Schraibman IG, Milne AA, Royle EM. Home versus in-patient treatment for deep vein thrombosis. In: The Cochrane Library, Issue 1, 2002. Oxford: Update Software. Search date 2000; primary sources Medline, Embase, Cochrane Controlled Trials Register, and hand searching of relevant journals.
33. Landefeld CS, Beyth RJ. Anticoagulant related bleeding: clinical epidemiology, prediction, and prevention. *Am J Med* 1993;95:315–328.
34. Levine MN, Hirsh J, Landefeld CS, Raskob G. Haemorrhagic complications of anticoagulant treatment. *Chest* 1992;102(suppl):352–363.
35. Barrit DW, Jordan SC. Anticoagulant drugs in the treatment of pulmonary embolism: a controlled trial. *Lancet* 1960;i:1309–1312.
36. Simonneau G, Sors H, Charbonnier B, et al. A comparison of low-molecular weight heparin with unfractionated heparin for acute pulmonary embolism. *N Engl J Med* 1997;337:663–669.
37. Hull RD, Raskob GE, Brant RF, et al. Low-molecular-weight heparin vs heparin in the treatment of patients with pulmonary embolism. American–Canadian Thrombosis Study Group. *Arch Intern Med* 2000;160:229–236.
38. Arcasoy SM, Kreit JW. Thrombolytic therapy for pulmonary embolism. A comprehensive review of current evidence. *Chest* 1999;115:1695–1707. Search date 1998; primary sources Medline and hand searches of reference lists of retrieved articles.
39. Konstantinides S, Geibel A, Olschewski M, et al. Association between thrombolytic treatment and the prognosis of haemodynamically stable patients with major pulmonary embolism: results of a multicentre registry. *Circulation* 1997;96:882–888.
40. Levine MN, Goldhaber SZ, Gore JM, et al. Haemorrhagic complications of thrombolytic therapy in the treatment of myocardial infarction and venous thromboembolism. *Chest* 1995;108:291S–301S. Search date not stated; primary sources not stated.
41. Chatellier G, Colombet I, Degoulet P. An overview of the effect of computer-assisted management of anticoagulant therapy on the quality of anticoagulation. *Int J Med Informatics* 1998;49:311–320. Search date 1997; primary source Medline.
42. Hunt DL, Haynes RB, Hanna SE, et al. Effects of computer-based clinical decision support systems on physician performance and patient outcomes: a systematic review. *JAMA* 1998;280:1339–1346. Search date 1998; primary sources Medline, Embase, Inspec, SciSearch, Cochrane Library, hand searching of reference lists, and personal contact with authors.
43. Walton RT, Dovey S, Harvey E, et al. Computerised advice on drug dosage to improve prescribing practice. Search date 1996; primary sources The Cochrane Effective Practice and Organisation of Care Group specialised register, Medline, Embase, and hand searches of the journal *Therapeutic Drug Monitoring*, reference lists of articles, and contact with experts in the field.
44. Motykie GD, Mokhtee D, Zebala LP, et al. The use of a Bayseian Forecasting Model in the management of warfarin therapy after total hip arthroplasty. *J Arthroplasty* 1999;14:988–993.
45. Poller L, Shiach CR, MacCallum PK, et al. Multicentre randomised study of computerised anticoagulant dosage. European Concerted Action on Anticoagulation. *Lancet* 1998;352:1505–1509.
46. Fitzmaurice DA, Hobbs FDR, Murray ET, et al. Oral anticoagulation management in primary care with the use of computerized decision support and near-patient testing. Randomized Controlled Trial. *Arch Intern Med* 2000;160:2343–2348.
47. Ageno W, Turpie AG. A randomized comparison of a computer-based dosing program with a manual system to monitor oral anticoagulant therapy. *Thromb Res* 1998;91:237–240.
48. Manotti C, Moia M, Palareti G, et al. Effect of computer-aided management on the quality of treatment in anticoagulated patients: a prospective, randomized, multicenter trial of APROAT (Automated PRogram for Oral Anticoagulant Treatment). *Haematologica* 2001;86:1060–1070.

David Fitzmaurice
Senior Lecturer

FD Richard Hobbs
Professor

Richard McManus
Clinical Research Fellow

Department of Primary Care and General Practice
The Medical School University of Birmingham, Birmingham, UK

Competing interests: RM none declared. FDRH is a member of the European Society of Cardiology (ESC) Working Party on Heart Failure, Treasurer of the British Society for Heart Failure, and Chair of the British Primary Care Cardiovascular Society (PCCS). He has received travel sponsorship and honoraria from several multinational biotechnology and pharmaceutical companies with cardiovascular products for plenary talks and attendance at major cardiology scientific congresses and conferences. DF has received reimbursement for attendance at scientific meetings from Leo Laboratories who make tinzaparin, a low molecular weight heparin. The Department of Primary Care and General Practice at the University of Birmingham, where the authors work, has a computerised decision support programme that is commercially available.

Unstable angina

Search date April 2002

Madhu Natarajan

QUESTIONS

INTERVENTIONS

Key Messages

- **Adenosine diphosphate inhibitors** One RCT found that clopidogrel versus placebo reduced death, myocardial infarction, and stroke after 9 months. Clopidogrel increased the risk of major bleeding, but not haemorrhagic strokes. Another RCT found that ticlopidine versus conventional treatment reduced vascular deaths and non-fatal myocardial infarction after 6 months (NNT 16, 95% CI 9 to 62), but was associated with neutropenia.
- **Aspirin** One systematic review has found that aspirin versus placebo significantly reduces the risk of death, myocardial infarction, and stroke at 6 months (NNT 20, 95% CI 15 to 34).
- **Calcium channel blockers** One systematic review has found that calcium channel blockers versus placebo or versus standard treatment did not reduce death or myocardial infarction.
- **Direct thrombin inhibitors** One systematic review has found that direct thrombin inhibitors versus heparin reduces death and myocardial infarction after 30 days.
- **Intravenous glycoprotein IIb/IIIa inhibitors** One systematic review has found that intravenous glycoprotein IIb/IIIa inhibitors reduce death or myocardial infarction compared with placebo, but increase the risk of major bleeding complications.

Unstable angina

- **Low molecular weight heparins** One systematic review has found that low molecular weight heparin reduced death or myocardial infarction in people taking aspirin, and did not increase bleeding complications in the first 7 days after onset of symptoms. It also found that longer term treatment with low molecular weight heparin versus placebo did not reduce death or myocardial infarction, and increased major bleeding. One systematic review found that low molecular weight heparin versus unfrationated heparin did not reduce death or myocardial infarction.
- **Oral glycoprotein IIb/IIIa inhibitors** One systematic review found that oral glycoprotein IIb/IIIa inhibitors did not reduce mortality, myocardial infarction, or recurrent ischaemia but increased bleeding events.
- **Routine early invasive treatment** Two RCTs found that that early invasive treatment reduced death and myocardial infarction, but two RCTs found that early invasive treatment did not reduce death and myocardial infarction.
- **Unfractionated heparin added to aspirin** Two systematic reviews have found that adding unfractionated heparin to aspirin in people with unstable angina reduces death or myocardial infarction with no significant increase in major bleeding after 1 week of treatment. One systematic review found that adding unfractionated heparin to aspirin does not reduce death or myocardial infarction after 12 weeks.
- **Warfarin** Five RCTs found no significant difference in myocardial infarction or death with the addition of warfarin to standard treatment. One RCT found that warfarin was associated with an increase in major bleeding.
- **β Blockers; nitrates** We found insufficient evidence of the effects of these interventions.

DEFINITION Unstable angina is distinguished from stable angina, acute myocardial infarction, and non-cardiac pain by the pattern of symptoms (characteristic pain present at rest or on lower levels of activity), the severity of symptoms (recently increasing intensity, frequency, or duration), and the absence of persistent ST segment elevation on a resting electrocardiogram. Unstable angina includes a variety of different clinical patterns: angina at rest of up to 1 week's duration; angina increasing in severity to moderate or severe pain; non-Q wave myocardial infarction; and post-myocardial infarction angina continuing for longer than 24 hours.

INCIDENCE/ PREVALENCE In industrialised countries, the annual incidence of unstable angina is about 6/10 000 people in the general population.

AETIOLOGY/ RISK FACTORS Risk factors are the same as for other manifestations of ischaemic heart disease: older age, previous atheromatous cardiovascular disease, diabetes mellitus, smoking cigarettes, hypertension, hypercholesterolaemia, male sex, and a family history of ischaemic heart disease. Unstable angina can also occur in association with other disorders of the circulation, including heart valve disease, arrhythmia, and cardiomyopathy.

PROGNOSIS In people taking aspirin, the incidence of serious adverse outcomes (such as death, acute myocardial infarction, or refractory angina requiring emergency revascularisation) is 5–10% within the first 7 days and about 15% at 30 days. Between 5% and 14% of people with unstable angina die in the year after diagnosis, with about half of these deaths occurring within 4 weeks of diagnosis. No single factor identifies people at higher risk of an adverse event. Risk factors include severity of presentation (e.g. duration of pain, rapidity of progression, evidence of heart failure), medical history (e.g. previous unstable angina, acute myocardial infarction, left ventricular dysfunction), other clinical parameters (e.g. age, diabetes), electrocardiogram changes (e.g. severity of ST segment depression, deep T wave inversion, transient ST segment elevation), biochemical parameters (e.g. troponin concentration), and change in clinical status (e.g. recurrent chest pain, silent ischaemia, haemodynamic instability).

AIMS To relieve pain and ischaemia; to prevent death and myocardial infarction; to identify people at high risk who require revascularisation; to facilitate early hospital discharge in people at low and medium risk; to modify risk factors; to prevent death, myocardial infarction, and recurrent ischaemia after discharge from hospital, with minimum adverse effects.

OUTCOMES Rate of death or myocardial infarction (often measured at 2, 7, and 30 days, and 6 months after randomisation); and adverse effects of treatment. Some RCTs include rates of refractory ischaemia or readmission for unstable angina.

METHODS *Clinical Evidence* update search and appraisal April 2002.

QUESTION What are the effects of antiplatelet treatments?

OPTION ASPIRIN

One systematic review has found that aspirin alone versus placebo reduces the risk of death, myocardial infarction, and stroke in people with unstable angina. The evidence suggests no added cardiovascular benefit, and possible added harm, from doses of aspirin over 325 mg daily.

Benefits: One systematic review (search date 1990, 145 RCTs, 100 000 people) compared antiplatelet treatment versus placebo.[1] Seven of these trials included a total of 4000 people with unstable angina. The review found that antiplatelet treatment (mostly medium dose aspirin, 75–325 mg daily) reduced the combined outcome of vascular death, myocardial infarction, or stroke at 6 months (AR 14% with placebo *v* 9% with antiplatelet treatment; RR 0.65, 95% CI 0.51 to 0.79; NNT 20, 95% CI 15 to 34). This means that 20 people would need to be treated with aspirin rather than placebo to prevent one additional event in 6 months. Individual trials within the systematic review showed consistent benefit from daily aspirin in terms of reduced deaths and myocardial infarction.

Harms: The review found that people taking doses of aspirin of 75–1200 mg daily had no significant adverse events, including gastrointestinal intolerance or bleeding.[1] However, the sum of the evidence suggests no added cardiovascular benefit, and greater incidence of gastrointestinal effects, for aspirin doses greater than 325 mg daily. Some people are allergic to aspirin.

Comment: The systematic review covered a wide range of people with different morbidities and levels of risk. Its results should be generalisable to routine practice.[1] People with unstable angina who are allergic or who do not respond to aspirin will need alternative antiplatelet treatment.

OPTION ADENOSINE DIPHOSPHATE INHIBITORS New

Two RCTs found that clopidogrel or ticlopidine reduced death and myocardial infarction compared with placebo or conventional treatment alone. One RCT found that clopidogrel increased major bleeding, but not haemorrhagic strokes after 6–9 months. The other RCT found that ticlopidine was associated with neutropenia. These drugs may be an alternative in people who are intolerant of or allergic to aspirin.

Benefits: We found no systematic review. We found two RCTs comparing adenosine diphosphate inhibitors versus placebo or conventional treatment.[2,3] The first RCT (12 562 people) compared clopidogrel (300 mg orally within 24 h of onset of symptoms followed by 75 mg daily) versus placebo.[2] It found that clopidogrel significantly reduced the combined outcome of death, myocardial infarction, and stroke after 9 months (AR 9% with clopidogrel *v* 11% with placebo; OR 0.8, 95% CI 0.7 to 0.9; NNT 50; CI not provided). The second RCT (652 people)[3] found that ticlopidine versus conventional treatment significantly reduced the combined outcome of vascular deaths and myocardial infarction after 6 months (RR 0.5, 95% CI 0.2 to 0.9; NNT 16, 95% CI 9 to 62).

Harms: In the first RCT, clopidogrel versus placebo increased major bleeding complications, but not haemorrhagic strokes (major bleeding 3.7% with clopidogrel *v* 2.7% with placebo, OR 1.4, 95% CI 1.1 to 1.7; haemorrhagic stroke 0.1% with clopidogrel *v* 0.1% with placebo, P value and OR not provided).[2] Reversible neutropenia has been reported in 1–2% of people taking ticlopidine.

Comment: Clopidogrel and ticlopidine are also associated with other adverse effects including diarrhoea and rash.

OPTION INTRAVENOUS GLYCOPROTEIN IIB/IIIA PLATELET RECEPTOR INHIBITORS

One systematic review found that intravenous glycoprotein IIb/IIIa inhibitors versus placebo reduced death or myocardial infarction, but increased the risk of major bleeding complications.

Benefits: We found one systematic review (search date 2001, 8 RCTs, 30 006 people) comparing intravenous glycoprotein IIb/IIIa inhibitors with placebo.[4] It found that intravenous glycoprotein IIb/IIIa inhibitors significantly reduced the combined outcome of death and myocardial infarction at 30 days and 6 months (at 30 days: 8 RCTs; AR 10.8% with inhibitors *v* 11.8% with placebo; OR 0.91, 95% CI 0.85 to 0.98; at 6 months: 4 RCTs, AR 13.3% with inhibitors *v* 14.6% with placebo; OR 0.88, 95% CI 0.81 to 0.95).[4]

Harms: The systematic review found that intravenous glycoprotein IIb/IIIa inhibitors versus placebo increased major bleeding complications at 30 days (AR 3.7% with inhibitors *v* 3.6% with placebo; OR 1.27, 95% CI 1.22 to 1.44).[4]

Comment: A small trial of adding a glycoprotein IIb/IIIa inhibitor to standard treatment suggests that a "dose ceiling" may exist beyond which escalation of dose results in higher bleeding complications with no increase in efficacy.[5]

OPTION ORAL GLYCOPROTEIN IIB/IIIA PLATELET RECEPTOR INHIBITORS

One systematic review found that oral glycoprotein IIb/IIIa inhibitors did not reduce the combined outcome of death, myocardial infarction, and recurrent ischaemia, but increased bleeding events.

Benefits: We found one systematic review (search date not stated, 4 RCTs, 26 462 people) comparing combinations of oral glycoprotein IIb/IIIa inhibitors, aspirin, and placebo.[5] Three of the RCTs were reported as abstracts only. The systematic review found that oral glycoprotein IIb/IIIa inhibitors versus aspirin did not reduce the combined outcome of death, myocardial infarction, and severe ischaemia after 90 days (results from fully reported RCT: AR 10.1% with sibrafiban *v* 9.8% with aspirin; difference not statistically significant; OR and P value not provided).

Harms: The fully reported RCT in the systematic review found that sibrafiban increased major bleeding versus aspirin (AR 27% with low dose sibrafiban *v* 19% with aspirin; OR and P value not provided). One RCT in the systematic review comparing sibrafiban plus aspirin versus placebo plus aspirin was stopped early because of the findings of the fully reported RCT. A further RCT in the systematic review comparing orbofiban plus aspirin versus placebo plus aspirin was stopped early because orbofiban plus aspirin increased mortality compared with placebo plus aspirin at 30 days (quantitative data not provided). One RCT in the systematic review comparing different doses of lefradafiban plus aspirin versus placebo plus aspirin stopped recruiting to the high dose lefradafiban plus aspirin group because of increased bleeding (AR 11% with high dose lefradafiban *v* 3% with low and medium dose lefradafiban *v* 1% with placebo; P value not provided).

Comment: None.

QUESTION What are the effects of antithrombin treatments?

OPTION UNFRACTIONATED HEPARIN

Two systematic reviews found that adding unfractionated heparin to aspirin in people with unstable angina reduced death or myocardial infarction after 1 week. One systematic review found that adding unfractionated heparin to aspirin did not reduce death or myocardial infarction after 12 weeks.

Benefits: **Added to aspirin:** We found two systematic reviews (search dates 1995[6] and not stated[7]). Both included the same six RCTs in 1353 people with unstable angina who were treated with either unfractionated heparin plus aspirin or aspirin alone for 2–7 days. The most recent review found that unfractionated heparin plus aspirin versus aspirin alone reduced the risk of death or myocardial infarction after

7 days (AR 8% with unfractionated heparin plus aspirin *v* 10% with aspirin alone; OR 0.67, 95% CI 0.45 to 0.99).[7] The older systematic review found that heparin plus aspirin versus aspirin did not reduce death or myocardial infarction after 12 weeks (AR 12% with unfractionated heparin plus aspirin *v* 14% with aspirin; RR 0.82, 95% CI 0.56 to 1.20).[6] **Versus low molecular weight heparin:** See benefits of low molecular weight heparin, p 230.

Harms: The older systematic review found that heparin plus aspirin did not significantly increase major bleeding compared with aspirin alone (AR 1.5% with unfractionated heparin plus aspirin *v* 0.4% with aspirin; RR 1.89, 95% CI 0.66 to 5.38).[6]

Comment: None.

OPTION LOW MOLECULAR WEIGHT HEPARINS

One systematic review has found that low molecular weight heparin versus placebo or no treatment reduced death or myocardial infarction in people taking aspirin and did not increase bleeding complications in the first 7 days after an episode of unstable angina. It also found that longer term treatment with low molecular weight heparin versus placebo did not reduce death or myocardial infarction. One systematic review found no significant difference between low molecular weight heparin versus unfractionated heparin in death or myocardial infarction. Long term low molecular weight heparin increased major bleeding compared with placebo, but not compared with unfractionated heparin.

Benefits: **Versus placebo or no heparin treatment:** We found one systematic review (search date not stated, 7 RCTs) comparing low molecular weight heparin (LMWH) versus placebo or no heparin treatment.[7] The systematic review found two RCTs (1639 people already taking aspirin) comparing LMWH versus no heparin or placebo for up to 7 days. It found that LMWH reduced death or myocardial infarction compared with no heparin or placebo during treatment (OR 0.34, 95% CI 0.20 to 0.58). The systematic review found five RCTs (12 099 people) comparing longer term LMWH (up to 90 days) versus placebo. It found that LMWH did not reduce death or myocardial infarction after 90 days compared with placebo (OR 0.98, 95% CI 0.81 to 1.17). **Versus unfractionated heparin:** We found one systematic review (search date not stated, 5 RCTs, 12 171 people) comparing an equal duration (maximum 8 days) of LMWH versus unfractionated heparin.[7] It found that LMWH did not significantly reduce the combined outcome of death or myocardial infarction compared with unfractionated heparin (OR 0.88, 95% CI 0.69 to 1.12).

Harms: The systematic review found no significant difference between LMWH versus unfractionated heparin in the frequency of major bleeds (OR 1.00, 95% CI 0.64 to 1.57)[7] (see harms of unfractionated heparin, p 230). Long term LMWH versus placebo significantly increased the risk of major bleeding (OR 2.26, 95% CI 1.63 to 3.14): equivalent to an excess of 12 bleeds for every 1000 people treated.[7]

Comment: LMWH may be more attractive than unfractionated heparin for routine short term use because coagulation monitoring is not required and it can be self administered after discharge.

OPTION DIRECT THROMBIN INHIBITORS *New*

One systematic review has found that direct thrombin inhibitors versus heparin reduce death and myocardial infarction.

Benefits: We found one systematic review (search date not stated, 11 RCTs, 35 070 people) comparing 7 days' treatment with direct thrombin inhibitors (hirudin, argatroban, bivalirudin, efegatran, inogatran) versus heparin.[8] It found that direct thrombin inhibitors reduced death or myocardial infarction compared with heparin after 30 days (AR 7.4% with direct thrombin inhibitors *v* 8.2% with heparin; RR 0.91, 95% CI 0.84 to 0.99).[8]

Harms: The systematic review found that, compared with heparin, direct thrombin inhibitors reduced the risk of major bleeding during treatment (major bleeding; AR 1.9% with direct thrombin inhibitors *v* 2.3% with heparin; OR 0.75, 95% CI 0.65 to 0.87), and found no significant difference between the risk of stroke at 30 days (stroke; AR 0.6% with direct thrombin inhibitors *v* 0.6% with heparin; OR 1.01, 95% CI 0.78 to 1.31).[8]

Comment: None.

OPTION WARFARIN *New*

Five RCTs found no significant difference in myocardial infarction or death with the addition of warfarin to standard treatment. One RCT found that warfarin was associated with an increase in major bleeding.

Benefits: We found no systematic review. We found five RCTs comparing warfarin versus no warfarin in addition to usual treatment.[9–12] Two of the RCTs were reported in the same journal article.[10] The first RCT (214 people) compared warfarin plus aspirin versus aspirin alone.[9] It found that warfarin (target international normalised ratio [see glossary, p 234] 2.0–2.5) plus aspirin reduced the combined outcome of recurrent angina, myocardial infarction, or death after 12 weeks (AR 13% with warfarin plus aspirin *v* 25% with aspirin; P = 0.06). The second RCT (309 people) compared warfarin (fixed dose 3 mg daily) plus aspirin versus aspirin alone.[10] It found no significant difference between warfarin plus aspirin versus aspirin alone in the combined outcome of refractory angina, myocardial infarction, and death after 6 months (AR 7% with warfarin plus aspirin *v* 4% with aspirin alone; RR 1.66, 95% CI 0.62 to 4.44). The third RCT (197 people) compared warfarin (target international normalised ratio 2.0–2.5) plus aspirin versus aspirin alone.[10] It found no significant difference with adding warfarin to aspirin in the combined outcome of refractory angina, myocardial infarction, and death after 6 months (AR 5% with warfarin plus aspirin *v* 12% with aspirin alone; RR 0.42, 95% CI 0.15 to 1.15). The fourth RCT (3712 people) compared adding warfarin (target international normalised ratio 2.0–2.5) to standard treatment versus no warfarin.[11] It found no significant difference with adding warfarin in the combined outcome of death, myocardial infarction, and stroke after 5 months (8% with warfarin *v* 8% with no warfarin; RR 0.90, 95% CI 0.72 to 1.14). The fifth RCT (135 people with prior coronary artery bypass grafts) compared warfarin plus aspirin, warfarin plus placebo, and aspirin plus placebo.[12] It found no significant difference between treatments in the combined outcome of death, myocardial infarction, and hospital admission for unstable angina after 1 year (AR 11% with warfarin plus aspirin *v* 14% with warfarin plus placebo *v* 12% with aspirin plus placebo; P = 0.76).

Harms: In the fourth RCT, warfarin versus standard treatment alone increased major bleeding (AR 2.7% *v* 1.3%; RR 1.99, 95% CI 1.23 to 3.22; NNH 71; CI not provided).[11]

Comment: None.

QUESTION What are the effects of anti-ischaemic treatments?

OPTION NITRATES, β BLOCKERS, AND CALCIUM CHANNEL BLOCKERS

We found insufficient evidence on the effects of nitrates and β blockers on mortality or myocardial infarction. One systematic review found no significant difference between calcium channel blockers versus placebo or standard treatment on mortality or myocardial infarction. Short acting dihydropyridine calcium channel blockers may increase mortality.

Benefits: We found no systematic review. **Nitrates:** We found one RCT (162 people) comparing intravenous glyceryl trinitrate versus placebo for 48 hours.[13] It found that glyceryl trinitrate significantly reduced the proportion of people with more than two episodes of chest pain and one new episode lasting more than 20 minutes (18% with glyceryl trinitrate *v* 36% with placebo; RR 0.50, 95% CI 0.25 to 0.90) and the proportion of people needing more than two additional sublingual glyceryl trinitrate tablets (16% with glyceryl trinitrate *v* 31% with placebo; RR 0.52, 95% CI 0.26 to 0.97). We found one RCT (200 people within 6 months of percutaneous transluminal coronary angioplasty) comparing intravenous glyceryl trinitrate alone, heparin alone, glyceryl trinitrate plus heparin, and placebo.[14] It found that recurrent angina occurred significantly less frequently in people treated with glyceryl trinitrate alone and glyceryl trinitrate plus heparin compared with placebo, but there was no benefit from heparin alone or additional benefit from combination treatment ($P < 0.003$ for glyceryl trinitrate alone and for glyceryl trinitrate plus heparin *v* placebo; CI not provided). **β Blockers:** We found two RCTs.[15,16] The first RCT (338 people with rest angina not receiving a β blocker) compared nifedipine, metoprolol, both, or neither versus placebo.[15] It found that metoprolol versus nifedipine significantly reduced the combined outcome of recurrent angina and myocardial infarction within 48 hours (28% with metoprolol *v* 47% with nifedipine; RR 0.66, 95% CI 0.43 to 0.98). The second RCT (81 people with unstable angina on "optimal doses" of nitrates and nifedipine) compared propranolol (≥ 160 mg daily) versus placebo.[16] It found no significant difference in death, myocardial infarction, and requirement for coronary artery bypass grafting or percutaneous coronary interventions at 30 days (38% with propranolol v 46% with placebo; RR 0.83, 95% CI 0.44 to 1.30). People taking propranolol had a lower cumulative probability of experiencing recurrent rest angina over the first 4 days of the trial. The mean number of clinical episodes of angina, duration of angina, glyceryl trinitrate requirement, and ischaemic ST changes by continuous electrocardiogram monitoring was also lower. **Calcium channel blockers:** We found one systematic review (search date not stated, 6 RCTs, 1109 people) comparing calcium channel blockers versus control treatment (3 RCTs used propranolol as a control and 3 used placebo).[17] The duration of the RCTs ranged from 48 hours (4 RCTs) to 4 months (2 RCTs). The review found no significant difference between calcium channel blockers versus control in rates of myocardial infarction or death.

Harms: Hypotension is a potential adverse effect of nitrates. Both older and more recent large RCTs in people with other ischaemic conditions showed that nitrates were safe and well tolerated when used judiciously in clinically appropriate doses. Potential adverse effects of β blockers include bradycardia, exacerbation of reactive airways disease, and hypoglycaemia in diabetics. Observational studies have reported increased mortality with short acting calcium channel blockers (such as nifedipine) in people with coronary heart disease.[18,19]

Comment: We found no good evidence that anti-ischaemic drugs (nitrates, β blockers, calcium channel blockers) prevent death or myocardial infarction. Consensus suggests that until further data are available, intravenous nitrates remain the preferred treatment together with heparin and aspirin in unstable angina.

QUESTION What are the effects of invasive treatments?

OPTION EARLY ROUTINE CARDIAC CATHETERISATION AND REVASCULARISATION

Four RCTs found conflicting evidence on the effects of early invasive treatment versus conservative treatment.

Benefits: We found no systematic review. We found four RCTs comparing early routine angiography and revascularisation if appropriate versus medical treatment alone.[20–23] The first RCT (2457 people) compared invasive treatment within the first 7 days versus non-invasive treatment plus planned coronary angiography.[20] Invasive treatment significantly reduced the combined outcome of death and myocardial infarction compared with non-invasive treatment after 6 months (AR 9% with invasive treatment v 12% with non-invasive treatment; RR 0.78, 95% CI 0.62 to 0.98; NNT 38; CI not provided). The second RCT (2220 people) compared cardiac catheterisation at 4–48 hours and revascularisation (if appropriate) after a cardiovascular event versus standard treatment.[21] It found that cardiac catheterisation reduced the combined outcome of death, myocardial infarction, and readmission for unstable angina after 6 months (AR 16% with catheterisation v 19% with standard treatment; OR 0.78, 95% CI 0.62 to 0.97; NNT 34; CI not provided). The third RCT (1473 people) compared early cardiac catheterisation at 18–48 hours versus standard treatment.[22] Early cardiac catheterisation did not reduce death or myocardial infarction but did reduce hospital admissions after 1 year (death or myocardial infarction: 11% with cardiac catheterisation *v* 12% with standard treatment, P = 0.42; hospital admissions: 26% with cardiac catheterisation *v* 33% with standard treatment; P < 0.005; NNT 14; CI not provided). The fourth RCT (920 people) compared invasive with conservative treatment.[23] Invasive treatment did not reduce the combined outcome of death or myocardial infarction compared with conservative treatment after 12–44 months (RR 0.87, 95% CI 0.68 to 1.10).

Harms: The first RCT found that early invasive treatment increased major bleeding but not stroke compared with non-invasive treatment (major bleeds: AR 1.6% with invasive treatment *v* 0.7% with non-invasive treatment; NNH 111; CI not provided).[22] The second RCT found that cardiac catheterisation increased bleeding compared with standard treatment (6% with cardiac catheterisation *v* 3% with standard treatment; P < 0.01: NNH 34; CI not provided).[23] The third RCT found that early cardiac catheterisation did not increase complication rates (death, myocardial infarction, emergency coronary artery bypass grafting, abrupt vessel closure, haemorrhage, serious hypotension) compared with conservative treatment (AR 14% with cardiac catheterisation *v* 13% with conservative treatment; P = 0.38; NNH 100; CI not provided).[24]

Comment: All trials have reported only short term and medium term follow up, so we cannot exclude a long term difference in effect between early invasive and early non-invasive strategies. There may be subgroups of people who benefit particularly from either invasive or conservative treatment. Advances in catheterisation and revascularisation technology and periprocedural management may reduce the early risks of invasive treatment in the future.

GLOSSARY

International normalised ratio (INR) A value derived from a standardised laboratory test that measures the effect of an anticoagulant. The laboratory materials used in the test are calibrated against internationally accepted standard reference preparations, so that variability between laboratories and different reagents is minimised. Normal blood has an international normalised ratio of 1. Therapeutic anticoagulation often aims to achieve an international normalised ratio value of 2.0–3.5.

Substantive changes

Intravenous glycoprotein IIb/IIIa platelet receptor inhibitors New systematic review;[4] conclusions unchanged.

Early routine cardiac catheterisation and revascularisation New RCT;[23] conclusions unchanged.

REFERENCES

1. Antiplatelet Trialists' Collaboration. Collaborative overview of randomised trials of antiplatelet therapy. I: Prevention of death, myocardial infarction, and stroke by prolonged antiplatelet therapy in various categories of patients. *BMJ* 1994;308:81–106. Search date 1990; primary sources Medline and Current Contents.
2. Yusuf S, Zhao F, Mehta S, et al. The Clopidogrel in Unstable Angina to Prevent Recurrent Events (CURE) trial. *N Engl J Med* 2001;345:494–502.
3. Balsano F, Rizzon P, Violi F, et al, and the Studio della Ticlopidina nell'Angina Instabile Group. Antiplatelet treatment with ticlopidine in unstable angina: a controlled multicentre clinical trial. *Circulation* 1990;82:17–26.
4. Bosch X, Marrugat J. Platelet glycoprotein IIb/IIIa blockers for percutaneous coronary revascularization, and unstable angina and non-ST-segment elevation myocardial infarction (Cochrane Review). In: The Cochrane Library, Issue 2, 2002. Oxford: Update Software. Search date

2001; primary sources Cochrane Library, Medline, Embase, reference lists of articles, medical internet sites, and hand searches of abstracts from cardiology congresses.

5. McDonagh MS, Bachmann LM, Golder S, et al. A rapid and systematic review of the clinical effectiveness and cost-effectiveness of glycoprotein IIb/IIIa antagonists in the medical management of unstable angina. *Health Technol Assess* 2000;4:1–95. Search date not stated; primary sources Cochrane Library, Embase, Medline, National Research Register, and various Internet and online resources.
6. Oler A, Whooley MA, Oler J, et al. Adding heparin to aspirin reduces the incidence of myocardial infarction and death in patients with unstable angina: a meta-analysis. *JAMA* 1996;276:811–815. Search date 1995; primary sources Medline, hand search of reference lists, and consultation with experts.
7. Eikelboom JW, Anand SS, Malmberg K, et al. Unfractionated heparin and low molecular weight heparin in acute coronary syndrome without ST elevation: a meta-analysis. *Lancet* 2000;355:1936–1942. Search date not stated; primary sources Medline and Embase, reference lists of published papers, and experts canvassed for unpublished trials, and personal data.
8. The Direct Thrombin Inhibitor Trialists' Collaborative Group. Direct thrombin inhibitors in acute coronary syndromes: principal results of a meta-analysis based on individual patients' data. *Lancet* 2002;359:294–302. Search date not stated; primary sources Medline, Embase, Cochrane Library, and conference abstracts and proceedings.
9. Cohen M, Adams PC, Parry G, et al. Combination antithrombotic therapy in unstable rest angina and non-Q-wave infarction in nonprior aspirin users. Primary endpoints analysis from the ATACS trial. Antithrombotic Therapy in Acute Coronary Syndromes Research Group. *Circulation* 1994;89:81–88.
10. Anand SS, Yusuf S, Pogue J, et al. Long-term oral anticoagulant therapy in patients with unstable angina or suspected non-Q-wave myocardial infarction: organization to assess strategies for ischaemic syndromes (OASIS) pilot study results. *Circulation* 1998;98:1064–1070.
11. OASIS Investigators. Effects of long-term, moderate-intensity oral anticoagulation in addition to aspirin in unstable angina. *J Am Coll Cardiol* 2001;37:475–484.
12. Hunyh T, Theroux P, Bogaty P, et al. Aspirin, warfarin, or the combination for secondary prevention of coronary events in patients with acute coronary syndromes and prior coronary artery bypass surgery. *Circulation* 2001;103:3069–3074.
13. Karlberg KE, Saldeen T, Wallin R, et al. Intravenous nitroglycerine reduces ischaemia in unstable angina pectoris: a double-blind placebo-controlled study. *J Intern Med* 1998;243:25–31.
14. Douchet S, Malekianpour M, Theroux P, et al. Randomized trial comparing intravenous nitroglycerin and heparin for treatment of unstable angina secondary or restenosis after coronary artery angioplasty. *Circulation* 2000;101:955–961.
15. HINT Research Group. Early treatment of unstable angina in the coronary care unit: a randomized, double blind, placebo controlled comparison of recurrent ischaemia in patients treated with nifedipine or metoprolol or both. *Br Heart J* 1986;56:400–413.
16. Gottlieb SO, Weisfeldt ML, Ouyang P, et al. Effect of the addition of propranolol to therapy with nifedipine for unstable angina pectoris: a randomized, double-blind, placebo-controlled trial. *Circulation* 1986;73:331–337.
17. Held PH, Yusuf S, Furberg CD. Calcium channel blockers in acute myocardial infarction and unstable angina: an overview. *BMJ* 1989;299:1187–1192. Search date not stated; primary sources not specified in detail.
18. Furberg CD, Psaty BM, Meyer JV. Nifedipine: dose-related increase in mortality in patients with coronary heart disease. *Circulation* 1995;92:1326–1331. Search date and primary sources not stated.
19. WHO-ISH Study. Ad hoc subcommittee of the liaison committee of the World Health Organization and the International Society of Hypertension: effects of calcium antagonists on the risks of coronary heart disease, cancer and bleeding. *J Hypertens* 1997:15:105–115.
20. FRISC II Investigators. Invasive compared with non-invasive treatment in unstable coronary-artery disease: FRISC II prospective randomised multicentre study. Fragmin and Fast Revascularisation during Instability in Coronary artery disease Investigators. *Lancet* 1999;354(9180):694–695.
21. Cannon CP, Weintraub WS, Demopoulos LA, et al. Treat Angina with Aggrastat and Determine Cost of Therapy with an Invasive or Conservative Strategy (TACTICS). *New Engl J Med* 2001;344:1879–1887.
22. The TIMI IIIB Investigators. Effects of tissue plasminogen activator and a comparison of early invasive and conservative strategies in unstable angina and non-Q-wave myocardial infarction. Results of the TIMI IIIB trial. *Circulation* 1994;89:1545–1556.
23. Anderson V, Cannon CP, Stone PH, et al, for the TIMI IIIB Investigators. One-year results of the thrombolysis in myocardial infarction (TIMI) IIIB clinical trial: a randomized comparison of tissue-type plasminogen activator versus placebo and early invasive versus early conservative strategies in unstable angina and non-Q wave myocardial infarction. *J Am Coll Cardiol* 1995;26:1643–1650.
24. Boden WE, O'Rourke RA, Crawford MH, et al, for the VANQWISH Trial Investigators. Outcomes in patients with acute non-Q-wave myocardial infarction randomly assigned to an invasive as compared with a conservative management strategy. *N Engl J Med* 1998;338:1785–1792.

Madhu Natarajan
Division of Cardiology
McMaster University
Hamilton
Canada

Competing interests: None declared.

Absence seizures in children

Search date May 2002

Ewa Posner

QUESTIONS

INTERVENTIONS

* We found no RCT evidence for valproate or ethosuximide versus placebo but there is consensus belief that valproate and ethosuximide have beneficial effect in typical absence seizures.

See glossary, p 241

Key Messages

- **Ethosuximide** We found no systematic review or RCTs comparing ethosuximide versus placebo. There is consensus that ethosuximide is beneficial. Ethosuximide is associated with rare but serious adverse effects, including aplastic anaemia, skin reactions, and renal and hepatic impairment. We found no RCTs comparing ethosuximide versus other anticonvulsants (except valproate) in children with typical absence seizures.
- **Gabapentin** One brief RCT found no significant difference between gabapentin versus placebo in frequency of typical absence seizures.
- **Lamotrigine** One RCT found that lamotrigine versus placebo significantly increased the number of children who remained seizure free, but lamotrigine is associated with serious skin reactions. We found no RCTs comparing lamotrigine versus other anticonvulsants in children with typical absence seizures.
- **Valproate** We found no RCTs comparing valproate versus placebo. There is consensus that valproate is beneficial. Valproate is associated with rare but serious adverse effects, including behavioural and cognitive abnormalities, liver necrosis, and pancreatitis. Three small RCTs found no significant difference between valproate and ethosuximide. We found no RCTs comparing valproate versus other anticonvulsants (except ethosuximide) in children with typical absence seizures.

DEFINITION Absence seizures are sudden, short (seconds) episodes of unconsciousness. Depending on electroencephalogram findings they are divided into typical and atypical seizures. Typical absence seizures are associated with an electroencephalogram showing regular symmetrical three cycles a second generalised spike and wave complexes. Absence seizures may be the only type of seizures experienced by a child and this then constitutes an epileptic syndrome (see glossary, p 241) called childhood absence epilepsy. In many children, typical absence seizures coexist with other types of seizures. Atypical absence seizures do not show the characteristic (for typical absence seizures) electroencephalogram pattern; are usually one of many types of seizures in a child with a background of learning disability and severe epilepsy; and tend to be less defined in time.[1] This differentiation into typical versus atypical seizures is important as the natural history and response to treatment varies in the two groups. Interventions for atypical absence seizures are not included in this topic.

INCIDENCE/ PREVALENCE About 10% of seizures in children with epilepsy are typical absence seizures.[1]

AETIOLOGY/ RISK FACTORS The cause is presumed to be genetic.

PROGNOSIS In childhood absence epilepsy, where typical absence seizures are the only type of seizures suffered by the child, the prognosis is excellent, the seizures cease spontaneously after a few years. In other epileptic syndromes (where absence seizures may coexist with other types of seizures) prognosis is varied, depending on the syndrome. Absence seizures have significant impact on quality of life. The episode of unconsciousness may occur at any time. Absence seizures usually occur without warning. Affected children need to take precaution to prevent injury during absences. Often school staff are the first to notice the recurrent episodes of absence seizures and the treatment is necessitated by the impact on learning.

AIMS Cessation or decrease in the frequency of seizures, with minimum adverse effects of treatment.

OUTCOMES Seizure frequency measured as normalisation of the electroencephalogram; adverse effects of treatment with anticonvulsants. We found no studies assessing quality of life.

METHODS *Clinical Evidence* search and appraisal May 2002. The author also searched the Cochrane Epilepsy Group trials register in March 2001.

QUESTION What are the effects of treatments for typical absence seizures in children? New

OPTION VALPROATE

We found no RCTs comparing valproate versus placebo. There is consensus that valproate is beneficial. Valproate is associated with rare but serious adverse effects, including behavioural and cognitive abnormalities, liver necrosis, and pancreatitits. Three small RCTs found no significant difference between valproate and ethosuximide. We found no RCTs comparing valproate versus other anticonvulsants (except ethosuximide) in children with typical absence seizures.

Benefits: We found no systematic review. **Versus placebo:** We found no RCTs comparing sodium valproate or valproic acid versus placebo. **Versus ethosuximide:** We found three RCTs.[2–4] The first RCT (45 children and adolescents aged 4–18 years with absence seizures, including children with other seizure types, children refractory to anticonvulsant treatment, and naïve children who had not previously received any anticonvulsant treatment) compared valproic acid versus ethosuximide followed by a crossover after 6 weeks.[3] Response to treatment was defined as no generalised spike-wave discharges on 12 hour telemetered electroencephalogram. The RCT found no significant difference in response with valproic acid versus ethosuximide at 6 weeks (naïve: 6/7 [85.7%] with valproic acid *v* 4/9 [44.4%] with ethosuximide; RR 1.93, 95% CI 0.88 to 4.25; refractory: 3/15 [20%] with valproic acid *v* 4/14 [28.6%] with ethosuximide; RR 0.70, 95% CI 0.19 to 2.59).[3] The second RCT (28 naïve children and adolescents aged 4–15 years with typical absence seizures) compared sodium valproate versus ethosuximide for up to 4 years. Response was measured by 6 hour telemetry at two intervals of 6 months and parent and teacher reports of seizure frequency. The RCT found no significant difference with sodium valproate versus ethosuximide in overall improvement (> 50% decrease in the seizure frequency over 6 months, 12/14 [85.7%] with sodium valproate *v* 11/13 [84.6 %] with ethosuximide; RR 1.01, 95% CI 0.74 to 1.39).[2] The third RCT (20 children aged 5–8 years) compared sodium valproate versus ethosuximide for up to 2 years in children with recent (< 6 months) onset of absence seizures.[4] Seizure frequency was assessed using parent completed record cards and electroencephalogram recordings. The RCT found no significant difference in complete remission of seizures with sodium valproate versus ethosuximide (7/10 [70%] with sodium valproate *v* 8/10 [80%] with ethosuximide; RR 0.88, 95% CI 0.53 to 1.46).[4] **Versus other anticonvulsants:** We found no RCTs.

Harms: **Versus placebo:** We found no RCTs comparing valproate versus placebo. Common adverse effects associated with valproic acid include dyspepsia, weight gain, tremor, transient hair loss, and haematological abnormalities. Rare adverse effects include behavioural and cognitive abnormalities, potentially fatal liver necrosis, and pancreatitis.[1] **Versus ethosuximide:** One RCT reported adverse effects in children who had not previously received any anticonvulsant treatment. The adverse effects with valproic acid and ethosuximide included nausea, vomiting, poor appetite, drowsiness, dizziness, headache, and leukopenia. Transient thrombocytopenia occurred in two children with valproic acid. No child withdrew from the trial because of these effects.[3] Another RCT reported acute pancreatitis (1 child) and weight gain not responding to dietary restriction (1 child) with sodium valproate, and drowsiness (1 child receiving a high dose of ethosuximide).[2] A third RCT reported infrequent adverse effects with both sodium valproate (transient nausea and vomiting, decreased number of platelets without thrombocytopenia) and ethosuximide (tiredness).[4]

Comment: The RCTs comparing sodium valproate versus ethosuximide suggest a beneficial effect with sodium valproate and ethosuximide.[2–4] We found a mention of one study (crossover, 35 children with typical absence seizures) comparing sodium valproate versus ethosuximide or placebo for 4 weeks;[5] this is an old study reported in Japanese. A summary of the results in English reported together with another RCT [2] suggests that it found no significant difference between sodium valproate versus ethosuximide.[5]

OPTION ETHOSUXIMIDE

We found no systematic review or RCTs comparing ethosuximide versus placebo. There is consensus that ethosuximide is beneficial. Ethosuximide is associated with rare but serious adverse effects, including aplastic anaemia, skin reactions, and renal and hepatic impairment. We found no RCTs comparing ethosuximide versus other anticonvulsants (except valproate) in children with typical absence seizures.

Benefits: We found no systematic review. **Versus placebo:** We found no systematic review or RCTs comparing ethosuximide versus placebo. **Versus valproate:** See benefits of valproate, p 238. **Versus other anticonvulsants:** We found no RCTs.

Harms: **Versus placebo:** We found no RCTs comparing ethosuximide versus placebo. Common adverse effects associated with ethosuximide include gastrointestinal disturbances, anorexia, weight loss, drowsiness, photophobia, headache, and behaviour disturbances and psychotic disturbances. Rare adverse effects include aplastic anaemia, serious skin reactions, and renal and hepatic impairment.[1] **Versus valproate:** See harms of valproate, p 238.

Comment: None.

OPTION LAMOTRIGINE

One RCT found that lamotrigine versus placebo significantly increased the number of children who remained seizure free, but lamotrigine is associated with serious skin reactions. We found no RCTs comparing lamotrigine versus other anticonvulsants.

Benefits: We found no systematic review. **Versus placebo:** We found one RCT (45 children and adolescents aged 3–15 years with newly diagnosed typical absence seizures) comparing lamotrigine versus placebo for 4 weeks.[6] Response was measured with 24 hour ambulatory electroencephalogram and a hyperventilation test during the electroencephalogram. The RCT found that lamotrigine versus placebo significantly increased the number of children who remained seizure free for 4 weeks (64% with lamotrigine v 21% with placebo; P = 0.03).[6] **Versus other anticonvulsants:** We found no RCTs.

Harms: The RCT reported abdominal pain, headache, nausea, anorexia, dizziness, and hyperkinesia with lamotrigine.[6] Skin rash was reported in 10/29 (35%) children, but only in one did the investigator consider it to be causally related to lamotrigine.[6] We found two open label add-on studies reporting on adverse effects of lamotrigine.[7,8] One add-on study (117 children aged 0–17 years with various drug resistant epilepsies) reported adverse effects in 25/117 (21%) children during treatment with lamotrigine, including skin rash (mainly in children also receiving sodium valproate), ataxia, drowsiness, headache, and vomiting. Skin rash was reported as the main adverse effect, occurring in 12 children (10 children were receiving valproic acid), 1–18 days after initiation of lamotrigine. The rash was maculopapular, beginning on the face and spreading to the trunk and limbs in 2–3 days. No correlation was found with lamotrigine blood levels.[8] Another add-on study (285 children aged < 13 years with refractory epilepsies and ≥ 2 seizure types) found that rash was the most common adverse event leading to discontinuation of lamotrigine (withdrawal of 21/285 [7.4%] from the study).[7] A higher rate of withdrawal was reported from the group receiving concomitant sodium valproate (occurrence of rash according to concomitant medication, sodium valproate 22.8%, carbamazepine 11.7%, and phenytoin 10.8%). Other adverse events leading to withdrawal of two or more children treated with lamotrigine were increased seizure frequency (1.8%), somnolence (1.1%), agitation (0.7%), ataxia (0.7%), fever (0.7%), and vomiting (0.75%).[7] Serious skin rash leading to admission to hospital has been found in 1% of children.[1]

Comment: The RCT[6] randomised a group of children who responded to treatment with lamotrigine in an open label trial (potentially introducing selection bias).[6]

OPTION GABAPENTIN

One brief RCT found no significant difference between gabapentin versus placebo in frequency of typical absence seizures.

Benefits: We found no systematic review. **Versus placebo:** We found one RCT (33 children aged 4–16 years with absence seizures) comparing gabapentin (15–20 mg/kg daily) versus placebo.[9] The study consisted of a 2 week double blind treatment phase followed by a 6 week open label phase. Response was assessed as the change from baseline in seizure frequency (measured with quantified electroencephalogram) after 2 weeks. The RCT found no significant difference between gabapentin versus placebo in frequency of typical absence seizures after 2 weeks.[9] **Versus other anticonvulsants:** We found no RCTs.

Harms: The RCT found that somnolence and dizziness were the most frequent adverse events. All reported adverse events were mild to moderate and no children withdrew from the study because of adverse effects of treatment.[9] This is consistent with the adverse effect profile of gabapentin reported by one other study.[10]

Comment: The RCT[9] was of short duration and used relatively small doses of gabapentin. The target dosage range was 15–20 mg/kg daily, although the current maintenance dose used in children with other epilepsies is 30 mg/kg daily.

GLOSSARY

Epileptic syndrome The term used in the classification of childhood seizure disorders. It relates to a recognisable clinical and electroencephalogram pattern.

REFERENCES

1. Panayiotopoulos CP. Treatment of typical absence seizures and related epileptic syndromes. *Paediatr Drugs* 2001;3:379–403.
2. Callaghan N, O'Hare J, O'Driscoll D, et al. Comparative study of ethosuximide and sodium valproate in the treatment of typical absence seizures (petit mal). *Dev Med Child Neurol* 1982;24:830–836.
3. Sato S, White BG, Penry JK, et al. Valproic acid versus ethosuximide in the treatment of absence seizures. *Neurology* 1982;32:157–163.
4. Martinovic Z. Comparison of ethosuximide with sodium valproate as monotherapies of absence seizures. In: Parsonage M, et al. *Advances in Epileptology: 14th Epilepsy International Symposium.* New York: Raven Press, 1983:301–305.
5. Suzuki M, Maruyama H, Ishibashi Y, et al. The clinical efficacy of sodium dipropylacetate and ethosuximide for infantile epilepsy by double-blind method: especially focusing on pure minor seizure. *Igakunoayum* 1972;82:470–488.
6. Frank LM, Enlow T, Holmes GL, et al. Lamictal (lamotrigine) monotherapy for typical absence seizures in children. *Epilepsia* 1999;40:973–979.
7. Besag FM, Wallace SJ, Dulac O, et al. Lamotrigine for the treatment of epilepsy in childhood. *J Pediatr* 1995;127:991–997.
8. Schlumberger E, Chavez F, Palacios L, et al. Lamotrigine in treatment of 120 children with epilepsy. *Epilepsia* 1994;35:359–367.
9. Trudeau V, Myers S, LaMoreaux L, et al. Gabapentin in naïve childhood absence epilepsy: results from two double-blind, placebo-controlled, multicenter studies. *J Child Neurol* 1996;11:470–475.
10. Anhut H, Ashman P, Feuerstein TJ, et al. Gabapentin (Neurontin) as add-on therapy in patients with partial seizures: a double-blind, placebo-controlled study. *Epilepsia* 1994;35:795–801.

Ewa Posner
Specialist Registrar in Paediatrics
Royal Victoria Infirmary
Newcastle upon Tyne
UK

Competing interests: None declared.

Acute gastroenteritis in children

Search date June 2002

Jacqueline Dalby-Payne and Elizabeth Elliott

QUESTIONS

INTERVENTIONS

To be covered in future updates
Food based oral rehydration solutions
Lactobacillus as an adjuvant to rehydration treatment
Naso–gastric administration of oral rehydration
Anti-emetics

See glossary, p 246

Key Messages

- **Clear fluids (other than oral rehydration solutions)** We found no systematic review or RCTs on "clear fluids" (water, carbonated drinks, and translucent fruit juices) versus oral rehydration solutions for treatment of mild to moderate dehydration caused by acute gastroenteritis.
- **Intravenous fluids (as effective as oral rehydration solutions)** One systematic review in children with mild to moderate dehydration found no significant difference with oral rehydration solutions versus intravenous fluids in duration of diarrhoea, time spent in hospital, or weight gain at discharge. One RCT in children with severe dehydration found that intravenous fluids versus oral rehydration solutions significantly increased the duration of diarrhoea and reduced weight gain at discharge, and were associated with more adverse effects.
- **Lactose-free feeds (for duration of diarrhoea)** One systematic review has found that lactose-free feeds versus lactose-containing feeds reduce the duration of diarrhoea in children with mild to severe dehydration. Subsequent RCTs found conflicting results.
- **Loperamide (reduces duration of diarrhoea, but adverse effects unclear)** Two RCTs found that, in children with mild to moderate dehydration, loperamide versus placebo significantly reduces the duration of diarrhoea. Another RCT found no significant difference with loperamide versus placebo in the duration of diarrhoea. We found insufficient evidence about adverse effects.
- **Oral rehydration solutions (as effective as iv fluids)** See intravenous fluids above.

Clin Evid 2002;8:242–250.

DEFINITION Acute gastroenteritis is characterised by rapid onset of diarrhoea with or without vomiting, nausea, fever, and abdominal pain.[1] In children, the symptoms and signs can be non-specific.[2] Diarrhoea is defined as the frequent passage of unformed liquid stools.[3]

INCIDENCE/ PREVALENCE Worldwide, about 3–5 billion cases of acute gastroenteritis occur in children under 5 years of age each year.[4] In the UK, acute gastroenteritis accounts for 204/1000 general practitioner consultations each year in children under 5 years of age.[5] Gastroenteritis leads to hospital admission in 7/1000 children under 5 years of age per year in the UK[5] and 13/1000 in the USA.[6] In Australia, gastroenteritis accounts for 6% of all hospital admissions in children under 15 years of age.[7]

AETIOLOGY/ RISK FACTORS In developed countries, acute gastroenteritis is predominantly caused by viruses (87%), of which rotavirus is most common;[8–11] bacteria cause most of the remaining cases, predominantly Campylobacter, Salmonella, Shigella, and *Escherichia coli*. In developing countries bacterial pathogens are more frequent, although rotavirus is also a major cause of gastroenteritis.

PROGNOSIS Acute gastroenteritis is usually self limiting but if untreated can result in morbidity and mortality secondary to water and electrolyte losses. Acute diarrhoea causes 4 million deaths per year in children under 5 years of age in Asia (excluding China), Africa, and Latin America, and over 80% of deaths occur in children under 2 years of age.[12] Although death is uncommon in developed countries, dehydration secondary to gastroenteritis is a significant cause of morbidity and need for hospital admission.[6,7,13]

AIMS To reduce the duration of diarrhoea and quantity of stool output, and duration of hospital stay; to prevent and treat dehydration; to promote weight gain following rehydration; to prevent persistent diarrhoea associated with lactose intolerance (see glossary, p 246).

OUTCOMES Total stool volume; duration of diarrhoea (time until permanent cessation); failure rate of oral rehydration treatment (as defined by individual RCTs); weight gain following rehydration; length of hospital stay; mortality.

METHODS *Clinical Evidence* search and appraisal June 2002.

QUESTION What are the effects of treatments for acute gastroenteritis?

OPTION CLEAR FLUIDS

We found no systematic review or RCTs on "clear fluids" (water, carbonated drinks, and translucent fruit juices) versus oral rehydration solutions for treatment of mild to moderate dehydration caused by acute gastroenteritis.

Benefits: We found no systematic review or RCTs of "clear fluids" versus oral rehydration solutions (see comment below).

Harms: We found no RCTs.

Comment: In this review, oral rehydration solutions are defined as glucose plus electrolyte or food (e.g. rice) based electrolyte solutions. Fruit juices and carbonated drinks are low in sodium and potassium, and usually have a high sugar content, which can exacerbate diarrhoea.

OPTION ORAL VERSUS INTRAVENOUS FLUIDS

One systematic review in children with mild to moderate dehydration in developed countries found no significant difference between oral rehydration solutions versus intravenous fluids in duration of diarrhoea, time spent in hospital, or weight gain at discharge. One RCT in children with severe dehydration in a developing country found that oral rehydration solutions versus intravenous fluids significantly reduced the duration of diarrhoea and increased weight gain at discharge, and was associated with fewer adverse effects.

Benefits: **Mild to moderate dehydration:** We found one systematic review (search date 1993, 6 RCTs, 371 children in developed countries with acute gastroenteritis, most with mild to moderate dehydration and in hospital)[14] and two additional RCTs comparing oral rehydration solutions versus intravenous fluids(see table 1, p 248).[21,22] The review and the additional RCTs found no significant difference with oral versus intravenous fluids in the duration of diarrhoea, time spent in hospital, or weight gain at discharge. If children responded poorly to oral fluids they were given intravenous fluids, which was used as a measure of failure of oral fluids. However, the failure rate of intravenous treatment was not recorded. **Severe dehydration:** We found one RCT (470 children in Iran with acute gastroenteritis with severe dehydration) comparing oral rehydration solutions versus intravenous fluids (see table 1, p 248).[23] It found that oral versus intravenous treatment significantly reduced the duration of diarrhoea (4.8 days *v* 5.5 days; difference 0.7 days; P < 0.01), and increased weight gain at discharge (percentage increase in admission weight 9% *v* 7%; P < 0.001). Failure of oral treatment (defined as the need to move to intravenous treatment) occurred in 1/236 children (0.4%; 95% CI not provided). It found no significant difference in mortality rate with oral versus intravenous fluids (2/236 [1%] *v* 5/234 [2%]; RR 0.4, 95% CI 0.08 to 2.02). No cause of death was given.

Harms: **Mild to moderate dehydration:** The systematic review reported no adverse effects.[14] One additional RCT (100 children in Afghanistan) reported fever and rigors in 9/50 children (18%) receiving intravenous fluids versus none receiving oral fluids.[21] **Severe dehydration:** The RCT in children in Iran found that significantly more children receiving intravenous treatment vomited during the first 6 hours of rehydration (70/234 [30%] *v* 47/236 [20%]; RR 0.64, 95% CI 0.46 to 0.89).[23] There was no significant difference in the risk of peri-orbital oedema (RR 0.99, 95% CI 0.25 to 3.92) or abdominal distention (RR 8.9, 95% CI 0.48 to 164). Phlebitis at the injection site requiring antibiotics occurred in 5/234 (2%) of children. In the same RCT, subgroup analysis of 58 children with hypernatraemia found that fewer children taking oral versus intravenous fluids developed seizures during rehydration, although the difference did not quite reach significance (2/34 [6%] *v* 6/24 [25%]; RR 0.23, 95% CI 0.05 to 1.07).

Comment: The quality of the RCTs was difficult to assess because of poor reporting; only one reported the method of allocation concealment[17] and one reported the method of randomisation.[21] Blinding of outcomes was impossible owing to the nature of the intervention. Intention to treat analysis was used in all but one RCT.[17]

OPTION LOPERAMIDE

Two RCTs found that, in children with mild to moderate dehydration, loperamide versus placebo significantly reduced the duration of diarrhoea. Another RCT found no significant difference between loperamide versus placebo in the duration of diarrhoea. We found insufficient evidence to assess the risk of adverse effects.

Benefits: We found no systematic review. We found five RCTs in children with acute diarrhoea (701 children, most with mild to moderate dehydration) (see table 2, p 249).[24–28] Of the three RCTs that assessed the duration of diarrhoea, two[24,26] found that loperamide versus placebo significantly reduced duration of diarrhoea (largest RCT, 315 children; risk of having diarrhoea at 24 h, 36/100 [36%] loperamide *v* 112/203 [55%] with placebo; RR 0.83, 95% CI 0.73 to 0.94).[24] Another RCT found no significant difference.[25] The results of other outcomes are included in table 2, p 249.

Harms: Four RCTs reported no adverse effects from loperamide.[24 26,28] One RCT found significantly more mild abdominal distension, excessive sleep, and lethargy in children taking loperamide versus placebo (3/16 [19%] with loperamide 0.8 mg/kg *v* 1/18 [6%] taking 0.4 mg/kg *v* 0/18 [0%] taking placebo; RR loperamide *v* placebo 4.9, 95% CI 0.28 to 86). Adverse effects caused one child to withdraw from the trial.[27] We found one evidence based guideline that identified case studies reporting lethargy, intestinal ileus, respiratory depression, and coma, especially in infants.[2]

Comment: We found insufficient evidence to estimate accurately the risk of adverse effects of loperamide in children.

OPTION LACTOSE-FREE FEEDS

One systematic review has found that lactose-free feeds versus lactose-containing feeds reduce the duration of diarrhoea in children with mild to severe dehydration. Subsequent RCTs found conflicting results.

Benefits: We found one systematic review (search date not stated, 13 RCTs, 873 children with mild to severe dehydration)[29] and four subsequent RCTs[30–33] comparing lactose-containing versus lactose-free feeds. The review was limited by flaws in its methodology (see comment below). It found that lactose-containing versus lactose-free feeds significantly increased "treatment failure" (89/399 [22%] *v* 56/474 [12%]; RR 2.1, 95% CI 1.6 to 2.7). The definition of treatment failure varied between trials and included increasing severity or persistence of diarrhoea or recurrence of dehydration. It found that lactose-free feeds versus lactose-containing feeds significantly reduced the duration of diarrhoea (9 RCTs; 826 children with mild or no dehydration receiving oral rehydration treatment; 92 h with lactose *v* 88 h with lactose-free; SMD 0.2 h after initiation of the study; P = 0.001). When the three RCTs that included children given additional solid food were excluded, it found that lactose-free versus lactose-containing feeds also significantly reduced the duration of diarrhoea (6 RCTs; 604 children; 95 h with lactose *v* 82 h with lactose-free; SMD 0.3 h; P < 0.001). Children receiving lactose-free versus lactose-containing feeds had significantly reduced stool frequency (4 RCTs; 387 children; 4.0 stool movements/day with lactose *v* 3.5 with lactose-free; SMD 0.3; P < 0.004). Total stool volume was greater in children who received lactose-containing diets (4 RCTs; 209 children; SMD 0.4 g; P = 0.002). Differences in weight gain during treatment could not be assessed because of the use of solid food in two studies and considerable heterogeneity between studies. We found four subsequent RCTs (see table 3, p 250).[30–33] Two found that lactose-free versus lactose-containing feeds significantly reduced the duration of diarrhoea,[30,33] and the other two found no significant difference.[31,32] The results of other outcomes are summarised in table 3, p 250.

Harms: The one RCT assessing adverse effects reported none in the treatment or control groups.[32]

Comment: Although the systematic review stated criteria for inclusion and exclusion of RCTs, only published studies were included and the method of determining RCT quality was not stated.[29] There was considerable heterogeneity between studies. Lactose-free feeds were superior to lactose-containing feeds for the duration of diarrhoea. Differences for other outcomes, although statistically significant, were not clinically important.

GLOSSARY

Lactose intolerance Malabsorption of lactose can occur for a short period after acute gastroenteritis because of mucosal damage and temporary lactase deficiency.

REFERENCES

1. Armon K, Elliott EJ. Acute gastroenteritis. In; Moyer VA, Elliott EJ, Davis RL, eds. *Evidence Based Pediatrics and Child Health*. London: BMJ Books, 2000;273–286.
2. American Academy of Pediatrics (APP). Practice parameter: the management of acute gastroenteritis in young children. American Academy of Pediatrics, Provisional Committee on Quality Improvement, Subcommittee on Acute Gastroenteritis. *Pediatrics* 1996;97:424–435.
3. Critchley M. *Butterworths Medical Dictionary Second Edition.* London: Butterworths & Co, 1986.
4. OPCS. *Mid-1993 population estimates for England and Wales.* London: HMSO, 1994.
5. OPCS. *Morbidity statistics from general practice. Fourth national study, 1991–1992.* London: HMSO, 1993.
6. Glass RI, Lew JF, Gangarosa RE, et al. Estimates of morbidity and mortality rates for diarrheal diseases in American children. *J Pediatr* 1991;118:S27–S33.
7. Elliott EJ, Backhouse JA, Leach JW. Pre-admission management of acute gastroenteritis. *J Paediatr Child Health* 1996;32:18–21.
8. Conway SP, Phillips RR, Panday S. Admission to hospital with gastroenteritis. *Arch Dis Child* 1990;65:579–584.
9. Finkelstein JA, Schwartz JS, Torrey S, et al. Common clinical features as predictors of bacterial diarrhea in infants. *Am J Emerg Med* 1989;7:469–473.
10. DeWitt TG, Humphrey KF, McCarthy P. Clinical predictors of acute bacterial diarrhea in young children. *Pediatrics* 1985;76:551–556.
11. Ferson MJ. Hospitalisations for rotavirus gastroenteritis among children under five years of age in New South Wales. *Med J Aust* 1996;164:273–276.
12. Anonymous. *A manual for the treatment of diarrhoea. Programme for the control of diarrhoeal diseases.* Geneva: WHO, 1990.
13. Conway SP, Phillips RR, Panday S. Admission to hospital with gastroenteritis. *Arch Dis Child* 1990;65:579–584.
14. Gavin N, Merrick N, Davidson B. Efficacy of glucose-based oral rehydration therapy. *Pediatrics* 1996;98:45–51. Search date 1993; primary sources Medline and experts and organisations involved in diarrhoea treatment contacted.
15. Santosham M, Daum RS, Dillman L, et al. Oral rehydration therapy of infantile diarrhea: a controlled study of well-nourished children hospitalized in the United States and Panama. *N Engl J Med* 1982;306:1070–1076.

16. Listernick R, Zieserl E, Davis AT. Outpatient oral rehydration in the United States. *Am J Dis Child* 1986;140:211–215.
17. Mackenzie A, Barnes G. Randomised controlled trial comparing oral and intravenous rehydration therapy in children with diarrhoea. *BMJ* 1991;303:393–396.
18. Tamer AM, Friedman LB, Maxwell SR, et al. Oral rehydration of infants in a large urban US medical center. *J Pediatr* 1985;107:14–19.
19. Vesikari T, Isolauri E, Baer M. A comparative trial of rapid oral and intravenous rehydration in acute diarrhoea. *Acta Paediatr Scand* 1987;76:300–305.
20. Issenman RM, Leung AK. Oral and intravenous rehydration of children. *Can Fam Physician* 1993;39:2129–2136.
21. Singh M, Mahmoodi A, Arya LS, et al. Controlled trial of oral versus intravenous rehydration in the management of acute gastroenteritis. *Indian J Med Res* 1982;75:691–693.
22. Oritiz A. Rehidratacion oral: Experiencia en el manejo de pacientes con gastroenteritis aguda en la sala de emergencia hospital pediatrico. *Bol Asoc Med P R* 1990;82:227–233.
23. Sharifi J, Ghavami F, Nowrouzi Z, et al. Oral versus intravenous rehydration therapy in severe gastroenteritis. *Arch Dis Child* 1985;60:856–860.
24. Diarrhoeal Diseases Study Group (UK). Loperamide in acute diarrhoea in childhood: results of a double blind, placebo controlled multicentre clinical trial. *BMJ Clin Res Ed* 1984;289:1263–1267.
25. Owens JR, Broadhead R, Hendrickse RG, et al. Loperamide in the treatment of acute gastroenteritis in early childhood. Report of a two centre, double-blind, controlled clinical trial. *Ann Trop Paediatr* 1981;1:135–141.
26. Kassem AS, Madkour AA, Massoud BZ, et al. Loperamide in acute childhood diarrhoea: a double blind controlled trial. *J Diarrhoeal Dis Res* 1983;1:10–16.
27. Karrar ZA, Abdulla MA, Moody JB, et al. Loperamide in acute diarrhoea in childhood: results of a double blind, placebo controlled clinical trial. *Ann Trop Paediatr* 1987;7:122–127.
28. Bowie MD, Hill ID, Mann MD. Loperamide for treatment of acute diarrhoea in infants and young children. A double-blind placebo-controlled trial. *S Afr Med J* 1995;85:885–887.
29. Brown KH, Peerson JM, Fontaine O. Use of nonhuman milks in the dietary management of young children with acute diarrhea: a meta-analysis of clinical trials. *Pediatrics* 1994;93:17–27. Search date not stated; primary sources Medline, hand searches of reference lists, and researchers contacted.
30. Allen UD, McLeod K, Wang EE. Cow's milk versus soy-based formula in mild and moderate diarrhea: a randomized, controlled trial. *Acta Paediatrica* 1994;83:183–187.
31. Clemente YF, Tapia CC, Comino AL, et al. Lactose-free formula versus adapted formula in acute infantile diarrhea. *An Esp Pediatr* 1993;39:309–312.
32. Lozano JM, Cespedes JA. Lactose vs. lactose free regimen in children with acute diarrhoea: a randomized controlled trial. *Arch Latinoam Nutr* 1994;44:6–11.
33. Fayad IM, Hashem M, Husseine A, et al. Comparison of soy-based formulas with lactose and with sucrose in the treatment of acute diarrhoea in infants. *Arch Pediatr Adolesc Med* 1999;153:675–680.

Jacqueline Dalby-Payne
Lecturer

Elizabeth Elliott
Staff Specialist General Paediatrician
The Children's Hospital at Westmead
Sydney
Australia

Competing interests: None declared.

TABLE 1 Oral versus intravenous fluids in mild to moderate[15–22] and severe dehydration[23] (see text, p 244).

Intervention (Na^+ concentration)	Participants (age)	Duration of diarrhoea (d)	Stay in hospital (d)	Weight gain (%)	Stool output (mL/kg)	Failure of oral treatment (defined as the need to revert to iv treatment)*
Oral versus intravenous fluids in mild to moderate dehydration						
ORS (90, 50) *v* iv[15]	52 children from US and 94 children in Panama with acute diarrhoea (3–24 months)	NS	NR	NS	US: ORS (90) *v* iv (NS); ORS (50) *v* iv (193 *v* 112; $P < 0.02$). Panama: ORS (90) *v* iv (90 *v* 168; $P < 0.001$); ORS (50) *v* iv (NS)	1/98 (1%)
ORS (60) *v* iv[16]	29 children with acute diarrhoea (3–24 months)	NR	NR	NS	NR	2/15 (13%)
ORS (50) *v* iv[17]	111 children with acute diarrhoea (3–36 months)	NR	NS	NR	NR	2/52 (4%)
ORS (75, 50) *v* iv[18]	100 children with acute diarrhoea (3–33 months)	NR	NS	NS	NR	3/50 (6%)
ORS (60) *v* iv[19]	37 children with acute diarrhoea (< 5 y)	ORS < iv (1.0 ± 0.5 *v* 2.6 ± 1.6; $P < 0.001$)	ORS < iv (2.7 ± 1.0 *v* 3.9 ± 1.7; $P < 0.001$)	ORS > iv ORS + 314 g *v* –16 g; $P < 0.05$	NS	2/20(10%)
ORS (45, 74) *v* iv[20]	42 children with acute diarrhoea (6–31 months)	NR	NR	NS	NR	4/22 (18%)
ORS (3.5 g/L) *v* iv[21]	100 children with acute diarrhoea (mean age 11 y)	NS	NR	NS	NR	NR
ORS (75) *v* iv[22]	31 children with acute diarrhoea (mean age 4–5 y)	NS	NR	NS	NR	NR
Oral versus iv fluids in severe dehydration						
ORS (80, 40) *v* iv[23]	470 children with acute diarrhoea (1–18 months)	ORS < iv (4.8 *v* 5.5; $P < 0.01$)	NR	ORS > iv (8.9% *v* 7.3%; $P < 0.001$)	NR	1/236 (0.4%)

d, days; iv, intravenous; NR, not reported; NS, non-significant; ORS, oral rehydration solution; y, year. *Although this outcome measures treatment failure of oral treatment it is not a comparative outcome as the number of children responding poorly to intravenous treatment was not recorded.

TABLE 2 **Loperamide in mild to moderate dehydration: results of placebo controlled RCTs (see text, p 245).[24–28]**

Intervention (loperamide dose mg/kg/day)	Participants	Duration of diarrhoea	Stay in hospital	Weight gain	Stool output
Loperamide (0.4, 0.8) *v* placebo[24]	315 children with acute diarrhoea and mild to moderate dehydration (3 months to 3 years)	L < P; risk of having ciarrhoea at 24 hours; RR 0.83. 95% CI 0.73 to 0.94.	NS	L > P; children with increased weight at 3 days: loperamide 0.8 mg *v* 0.4 mg *v* placebo: 58% *v* 51% *v* 36%	NR
Loperamide (0.2) *v* placebo[25]	50 children with acute diarrhoea (1–4 years)	NS	NS	NS	NR
Loperamide (0.2) *v* placebo[26]	100 children with acute diarrhoea and mild to moderate dehydration (< 2 years)	L < P; 59.1 hour *v* 81.1 hour; P < 0.05	NR	NS	NS
Loperamide (0.4, 0.8) *v* placebo[27]	53 children with acute diarrhoea (3 months to 3 years)	NR	NR	L > P; children with increased weight at 3 days: loperamide 0.8 mg *v* 0.4 mg *v* placebo: 88% *v* 50% *v* 39%; RR 0.53, 95% CI 0.29 to 0.97	NR
Loperamide (0.8) *v* placebo[28]	185 children with acute gastroenteritis and mild to moderate dehydration (3–18 months).	NR	NS	NR	NR

L, loperamide; NR, not reported; NS, non-significant; P, placebo.

TABLE 3 **Lactose-containing versus lactose-free feeds in children with mild to severe dehydration: results of subsequent RCTs (see text, p 246).[30–33]**

Intervention	Participants	Duration of diarrhoea	Weight gain	Total stool output (mL/kg)	Treatment failure
Cow's milk *v* soy-based formula[30]	76 children with acute diarrhoea and mild to moderate dehydration (2–12 months)	L > LF; 6.6 *v* 4.5 days; $P < 0.01$	NS	NR	NS
Lactose *v* lactose-free formula[31]	60 children with acute diarrhoea (< 1 year)	NS	NS	NR	NR
Lactose *v* lactose-free formula[32]	52 children with acute diarrhoea and mild to moderate dehydration (1–24 months)	NS	NS	NR	NS
Soy-based formula with lactose *v* soy-based formula with sucrose[33]	200 boys with acute diarrhoea (3–18 months)	L > LF; 39 hours *v* 23 hours; $P > 0.001$	NS	L > LF; mean 164 (95% CI 131 to 208) *v* 89 (95% 55 to 87); $P < 0.001$	NS

NR, not recorded; NS, non-significant; L, lactose-containing; LF, lactose-free.

Acute otitis media

Search date February 2002

Paddy O'Neill

QUESTIONS

INTERVENTIONS

Key Messages

Treatment

- **Antibiotics versus placebo** We found four systematic reviews comparing antibiotics versus placebo in acute otitis media (AOM) but using different inclusion criteria and outcome measures. One review in children aged 4 months to 18 years found a significant reduction in symptoms with a range of antibiotics (cephalosporins, erythromycin, penicillins, trimethoprim–sulfamethoxazole [co-trimoxazole]) versus placebo after 7–14 days of treatment (NNT 7, 95% CI 5 to 12). Another review in children aged < 2 years found no significant difference in clinical improvement with antibiotics (penicillins, sulphonamides, co-trimoxazole) versus placebo alone or versus placebo with myringotomy. A third review in children aged 4 months to 18 years found that antibiotics (ampicillin, amoxicillin) versus placebo or observational treatment significantly reduced clinical failure rate within 2–7 days (NNT 8, 95% CI 5 to 36). The final review in children aged 6 months to 15 years found that early use of antibiotics (erythromycin, penicillins) versus placebo significantly reduced the proportion of children still in pain 2–7 days after presentation (NNT 17, 95% CI 11 to 40) and reduced the risk of developing contralateral AOM. This review also found that antibiotics increased the risk of vomiting, diarrhoea, or rashes (NNH 17, 95% CI 9 to 152).

- **Choice of antibiotic regimen** One systematic review in children aged 4 months to 18 years found no significant differences between a range of antibiotics in rate of treatment success at 7–14 days or of middle ear effusion at 30 days. Another systematic review in children aged 4 weeks to 18 years found no significant difference between antibiotics in clinical failure rates within 7–14 days. The second review also found that adverse effects, primarily gastrointestinal, were more common with cefixime versus amoxicillin or ampicillin (NNH 12, 95% CI 8 to 27), and were more common with amoxicillin/clavulanate (original formulation) versus azithromycin (NNH 6, 95% CI 4 to 13).
- **Ibuprofen** One RCT in children aged 1–6 years receiving antibiotic treatment found that ibuprofen versus placebo significantly reduced earache as assessed by parental observation after 2 days (NNT 5, 95% CI 3 to 15).
- **Immediate versus delayed antibiotic treatment** One RCT in children aged 6 months to 10 years found that immediate versus delayed antibiotic treatment significantly reduced the number of days of earache, ear discharge, and amount of daily paracetamol used after the first 24 hours of illness but found no difference in daily pain scores. It also found a significant increase in diarrhoea with immediate versus delayed antibiotic treatment (NNH 11, 95% CI 5 to 125).
- **Paracetamol** One RCT in children aged 1–6 years receiving antibiotic treatment found that paracetamol versus placebo significantly reduced earache as assessed by parental observation after 2 days (NNT 6, 95% CI 3 to 28).
- **Short versus longer courses of antibiotics** One systematic review and two subsequent RCTs have found that 10 day versus 5 day courses of antibiotics significantly reduce treatment failure, relapse, and reinfection at 8–10 days, but found no significant difference at 20–30 days.

Prevention of recurrence

- **Long term antibiotic prophylaxis** One systematic review in children and adults has found that long term antibiotic prophylaxis versus placebo significantly reduces recurrence of AOM after 1 month (NNT 9, 95% CI 5 to 33). However, one subsequent RCT in childrean aged 3 months to 6 years found no significant difference between antibiotic prophylaxis and placebo in preventing recurrence. We found insufficient evidence on which antibiotic to use, for how long, and how many previous episodes of AOM justify starting preventive treatment.
- **Xylitol chewing gum or syrup** One RCT found that xylitol syrup or chewing gum versus control significantly reduced the incidence of AOM over 3 months. It found no significant difference with xylitol lozenges versus control gum. More children taking xylitol versus control withdrew because of abdominal pain or other unspecified reasons.

DEFINITION Otitis media is an inflammation in the middle ear. Subcategories include acute otitis media (AOM), recurrent AOM, and chronic suppurative otitis media. AOM is the presence of middle ear effusion in conjunction with rapid onset of one or more signs or symptoms of inflammation of the middle ear. Uncomplicated AOM is limited to the middle ear cleft.[1] AOM presents with systemic and local signs, and has a rapid onset. The persistence of an effusion beyond 3 months without signs of infection defines otitis media with effusion (also known as "glue ear"). Chronic suppurative otitis media is characterised by continuing inflammation in the middle ear causing discharge (otorrhoea) through a perforated tympanic membrane.

INCIDENCE/ PREVALENCE AOM is common and has a high morbidity and low mortality. In the UK, about 30% of children under 3 years of age visit their general practitioner with AOM each year and 97% receive antimicrobial treatment.[2] By 3 months of age, 10% of children have had an episode of AOM. It is the most common reason for outpatient antimicrobial treatment in the USA.[3]

AETIOLOGY/ RISK FACTORS The most common bacterial causes for AOM in the USA and UK are *Streptococcus pneumoniae*, *Haemophilus influenzae*, and *Moraxella catarrhalis*.[2] Similar pathogens are found in Colombia.[4] The incidence of penicillin resistant *S pneumoniae* has risen, but rates differ between countries. The most important risk factors for AOM are young age and attendance at daycare centres such as nursery schools. Other risk factors include being white; male sex; a history of enlarged adenoids, tonsillitis, or asthma; multiple previous episodes; bottle feeding; a history of ear infections in parents or siblings; and use of a soother or pacifier. The evidence for an effect of environmental tobacco smoke is controversial.[2]

PROGNOSIS In about 80% of children the condition resolves in about 3 days without antibiotic treatment. Serious complications are rare but include hearing loss, mastoiditis, meningitis, and recurrent attacks.[2] The World Health Organization estimates that each year 51 000 children under the age of 5 years die from complications of otitis media in developing countries.[5]

AIMS To reduce the severity and duration of pain and other symptoms, to prevent complications, and to minimise adverse effects of treatment.

OUTCOMES Pain control (in infants this can be assessed by surrogate measures such as parental observation of distress/crying and analgesic use); incidence of complications such as deafness (usually divided into short and long term hearing loss), recurrent attacks of AOM, mastoiditis (see glossary, p 260), and meningitis; resolution of otoscopic appearances; incidence of adverse effects of treatment.

METHODS *Clinical Evidence* update search and appraisal February 2002.

QUESTION **What are the effects of treatments?**

OPTION **ANALGESICS**

One RCT in children receiving antibiotic treatment found that ibuprofen or paracetamol versus placebo significantly reduced earache as assessed by parental observation after 2 days.

Benefits: We found no systematic review but found one RCT (219 children aged 1–6 years with otoscopically diagnosed acute otitis media and receiving antibiotic treatment with cefaclor for 7 days) comparing the effect of three times daily treatment with ibuprofen or paracetamol versus placebo for 48 hours on earache (otalgia) and related outcomes.[6] It found that ibuprofen versus placebo significantly reduced earache after 2 days as assessed by parental observation (AR 5/71 [7%] with ibuprofen *v* 19/75 [25%] with placebo; RR 0.28, 95% CI 0.11 to 0.71; NNT 5, 95% CI 3 to 15) and with paracetamol versus placebo (AR 7/73 [10%] *v* 19/75 [25%] with placebo; RR 0.38, 95% CI 0.17 to 0.85; NNT 6, 95% CI 3 to 28). It found no difference between paracetamol and ibuprofen for reducing earache, and no difference between ibuprofen or paracetamol and placebo for other outcomes (appearance of the tympanic membrane; rectal temperature; and parental assessment of appetite, sleep, and playing activity).

Harms: The RCT found that 11 children experienced mild nausea, vomiting, and abdominal pain (5 [7%] taking ibuprofen, 3 [4%] taking paracetamol, and 3 [4%] taking placebo). None were withdrawn from treatment.[6]

Comment: The evidence from this RCT is limited because the assessment of the child's pain relief was based on parental observation using a scale of 0 or 1.[6] The paracetamol versus placebo result has been recalculated by *Clinical Evidence* from data in the original publication, and corrects the stated conclusions of the RCT.

OPTION ANTIBIOTICS

We found four systematic reviews comparing antibiotics versus placebo in acute otitis media, which used different inclusion criteria and outcome measures. Three reviews found that a range of antibiotics versus placebo significantly reduced symptoms, clinical failure rate, and pain in children aged 4 weeks to 18 years. One of these three reviews also found that antibiotics increased the risk of vomiting, diarrhoea, or rashes. Another review found no significant difference in clinical improvement with antibiotics versus placebo alone or versus placebo with myringotomy in children under 2 years of age.

Benefits: We found four systematic reviews.[1,7–9] **Versus placebo or no treatment:** One systematic review (search date 1992, 33 RCTs, 5400 children aged 4 months to 18 years) identified four RCTs (535 children receiving analgesics or other symptomatic relief).[7] Acute otitis media (AOM) was defined as bulging or opacification of the tympanic membrane with or without erythema, accompanied by at least one of the following signs: fever, otalgia, irritability, otorrhoea, lethargy, anorexia, vomiting, diarrhoea, and mobility of the tympanic membrane absent or markedly decreased. It found a significant reduction in symptoms with a range of antibiotics (cephalosporins, erythromycin, penicillins, trimethoprim–sulfamethoxazole [co-trimoxazole]) versus placebo after 7–14 days of treatment (ARR 13.7%, 95% CI 8.2% to 19.2%; NNT 7, 95% CI 5 to 12).[7] The second systematic review (search date 1997, 741 children aged < 2 years) identified four RCTs comparing antibiotics (penicillins, sulphonamide, amoxicillin/clavulanic acid [co-amoxiclav]) versus placebo alone or versus placebo with myringotomy.[8] Three RCTs used diagnosis of AOM based on otoscopic appearance of the tympanic membrane and clinical signs of acute infection, two RCTs used otoscopy alone, and one RCT did not state diagnostic criteria. The systematic review found no significant difference between antibiotics versus placebo in symptomatic clinical improvement within 7 days (OR 1.31, 95% CI 0.83 to 2.08). Otoscopic appearance, middle ear effusion, and bacteriology were not considered as end points.[8] A third systematic review (search date

1999, 5 RCTs, 1518 children aged 4 wks to 18 years) compared the effects of antibiotics (ampicillin, amoxicillin [amoxycillin]) versus placebo or observational treatment on clinical failure rate.[1] AOM was defined as the presence of middle ear effusion in conjunction with rapid onset of one or more signs or symptoms of inflammation of the middle ear, and was categorised as uncomplicated AOM when limited to the middle ear cleft. Clinical failure was defined as the presence of pain, fever, middle ear effusion, clinical signs of otitis media, or suppurative complications such as mastoiditis (see glossary, p 260). The review found that antibiotics (ampicillin, amoxicillin) versus placebo or observational treatment significantly reduced clinical failure rate within 2–7 days (reduction of 12.3%, 95% CI 21.8 to 2.8; NNT 8, 95% CI 5 to 36).[1] A fourth systematic review (search date 2000, 2288 children aged 6 months to 15 years, 9 RCTs) compared early use of antibiotics (erythromycin, penicillins, sulphonamides) versus placebo.[9] AOM was defined as acute earache with at least one abnormal eardrum, otoscopic middle ear effusion, and general signs and symptoms. Pain was assessed using parental report/score card/diary or clinician assessment at 4 days. The review found that antibiotics versus placebo significantly reduced the proportion of children still in pain 2–7 days after presentation (175/1160 [15.1%] with antibiotics *v* 234/1128 [20.7%] with placebo; ARR 5.6%, 95% CI 2.5% to 8.7%; RR 0.72, 95% CI 0.62 to 0.85; NNT 17, 95% CI 11 to 40). In addition, fewer children experienced contralateral AOM (35/329 [10.6%] with antibiotics *v* 56/337 [16.6%] with placebo; ARR 5.9%, 95% CI 1.0% to 10.8%; RR 0.65 95% CI 0.45 to 0.94). The review found no difference in the rate of subsequent recurrence of AOM (187/864 [21.6%] with antibiotics *v* 175/804 [21.8%] with placebo; RR 0.99, 95% CI 0.83 to 1.19), abnormal tympanometry at 1 month (85/234 [36.3%] with antibiotics *v* 91/238 [38.2%] with placebo; RR 0.94, 95% CI 0.74 to 1.19), or abnormal tympanometry at 3 months (38/182 [20.9%] with antibiotics *v* 49/188 [26.1%] with placebo; RR 0.80, 95% CI 0.55 to 1.16). Four RCTs (717 children) reported pain outcomes (parental report of pain or symptom diary) 24 hours after presentation. All four found no difference in pain outcomes with antibiotics versus placebo (RR 1.02, 95% CI 0.85 to 1.22). Most RCTs did not state the time interval between onset of symptoms and starting treatment; the two RCTs that did stated 1–24 hours and about 30 hours. Only 1/2202 children developed mastoiditis (in a penicillin treated group).[9]

Harms: Two systematic reviews gave no information on adverse events.[7,8] The third systematic review found that adverse effects, primarily gastrointestinal, were more common in children on cefixime than in those on amoxicillin or ampicillin (5 RCTs, rate difference 8.4%, 95% CI 3.8 to 13.1; NNH 12, 95% CI 8 to 27) and were more common in children on amoxicillin/clavulanate (original formulation) than in those on azithromycin (3 RCTs, rate difference −18.0, 95% CI −28.0 to −8.0; NNH 6, 95% CI 4 to 13).[1] The fourth systematic review found that antibiotics increased the risk of vomiting, diarrhoea, or rashes (AR 57/345 [17%] with antibiotics *v* 38/353 [11%] with control; RR 1.55, 95% CI 1.11 to 2.16; NNH 17, 95% CI 9 to 152).[9]

Comment: One systematic review[7] excluded two placebo controlled trials that were included in another review[9] because they included myringotomy as part of the treatment. This may have biased the results in favour of antibiotic treatment and may explain the higher absolute risk reduction quoted in the first review.[7] Another systematic review commented on the difficulty of performing meta-analyses because of the varying criteria between studies for defining AOM and outcome measures.[1] The variation between the systematic reviews that provide numbers needed to treat for the effect of antibiotics versus placebo is because of differences in entry criteria and outcome measures. We found inadequate evidence for the effectiveness of antibiotics in countries where the incidence of complicating mastoiditis is high.

OPTION CHOICE OF ANTIBIOTIC REGIMEN

One systematic review in children aged 4 months to 18 years found no significant difference between a range of antibiotics in rate of treatment success at 7–14 days or of middle ear effusion at 30 days. Another systematic review in children aged 4 weeks to 18 years found no significant difference between antibiotics in clinical failure rates within 7–14 days. The second review also found that adverse effects, primarily gastrointestinal, and were more common in children on cefixime than in those on amoxicillin or ampicillin, were more common in children on amoxicillin/clavulanate (original formulation) than in those on azithromycin.

Benefits: We found two systematic reviews.[1,7] One systematic review (search date 1992, 33 RCTs, 5400 children aged 4 months to 18 years) compared a range of antibiotics (cephalosporins, erythromycin, penicillins, co-trimoxazole).[7] Acute otitis media (AOM) was defined as bulging or opacification of the tympanic membrane with or without erythema, accompanied by at least one sign (fever, otalgia, irritability, otorrhoea, lethargy, anorexia, vomiting, diarrhoea, mobility of the tympanic membrane absent or markedly decreased). Treatment success was defined as the absence of all presenting signs and symptoms of AOM at the evaluation point closest to 7–17 days after start of treatment. The systematic review found no significant differences between different antibiotics in rate of treatment success at 7–14 days or of middle ear effusion at 30 days.[7] A second systematic review (search date 1999) found no significant difference between penicillin versus ampicillin or amoxicillin (amoxycillin) in clinical failure rates within 7–14 days (3 RCTs, 491 children aged 4 wks to 18 years; clinical failure rate difference 4.5%, 95% CI –1.8% to +10.7%).[1] The same review found no significant difference in clinical failure rates within 3–7 days with cefaclor versus ampicillin or amoxicillin (4 RCTs, 56 children aged 4 wks to 18 years; clinical failure rate difference –5.4%, 95% CI –15.2% to +4.4%). Clinical failure was defined as the presence of pain, fever, middle ear effusion, clinical signs of otitis media, or suppurative complications such as mastoiditis (see glossary, p 260).[1]

Harms: See harms of antibiotics, p 255.

Comment: None.

OPTION **IMMEDIATE VERSUS DELAYED ANTIBIOTIC TREATMENT**

One RCT in children aged 6 months to 10 years found that immediate versus delayed antibiotic treatment significantly reduced the number of days of earache, ear discharge, and amount of daily paracetamol used after the first 24 hours of illness, but found no significant difference in daily pain scores. It also found a significant increase in diarrhoea with immediate versus delayed antibiotic treatment.

Benefits: We found one RCT (315 children aged 6 months to 10 years) comparing immediate versus delayed antibiotic (amoxicillin [amoxycillin] or erythromycin) use.[10] Acute otitis media (AOM) was defined as acute otalgia and otoscopic evidence of acute inflammation of the ear drum such as dullness or cloudiness with erythema, bulging, or perforation. Immediate antibiotic treatment was defined as a prescription given to parents at the initial consultation. Delayed antibiotic treatment was defined as parents asked to wait 72 hours after seeing the doctor before using the prescription and only if the child still had substantial otalgia or fever, or was not starting to get better. Earache was assessed from daily diary of symptoms and perceived severity of pain scores (1 = no pain to 10 = extreme pain). The RCT found that, after the first 24 hours of illness, immediate versus delayed antibiotic use reduced the duration of earache (mean difference –1.10 days, 95% CI –0.54 to –1.48 days), duration of ear discharge (mean difference –0.66 days, 95% CI –0.19 to –1.13 days), number of disturbed nights (mean difference –0.72 days, 95% CI –0.30 to –1.13 days), number of days crying (mean difference –0.69 days, 95% CI –0.31 to –1.08 days), and the number of teaspoons of paracetamol used (mean difference –0.52 teaspoons daily, 95% CI –0.26 to –0.79 teaspoons daily). The RCT found no significant difference in mean daily pain score (mean difference –0.16, 95% CI –0.42 to +0.11), number of daily episodes of distress (mean difference –0.12, 95% CI –0.34 to +0.11), or days absence from school (mean difference –0.18 days, 95% CI –0.76 to +0.41 days).

Harms: The RCT found that immediate treatment increased diarrhoea (AR 25/135 [19%] with immediate *v* 14/150 [9%] with delayed; RR 1.9, 95% CI 1.08 to 3.66; NNH 11, 95% CI 5 to 125), but had no significant effect on rash (AR 6/133 [5%] with immediate *v* 8/149 [5%] with delayed; RR 0.84, 95% CI 0.30 to 2.36).[10]

Comment: None.

OPTION **SHORT VERSUS LONGER COURSES OF ANTIBIOTICS**

One systematic review has found that 10 day versus 5 day courses of antibiotics reduce treatment failure, relapse, or reinfection in the short term (at 8–19 days), but found no significant difference in the long term (at 20–30 days). Two subsequent RCTs found similar results.

Benefits: We found one systematic review[11] and two subsequent RCTs.[12,13] The systematic review (search date 1998, 30 RCTs in children aged 4 wks to 18 years with acute otitis media) found that treatment failure, relapse, or reinfection at an early evaluation (8–19 days) was more likely to occur with shorter courses of antibiotics (5 days) than with longer courses (8–10 days; summary OR *v* longer courses 1.52, 95% CI 1.17 to 1.98). However, by 20–30 days there were no differences between treatment groups (summary OR 1.22, 95% CI 0.98 to 1.54).[11] The first subsequent RCT (385 younger children with newly diagnosed acute otitis media, mean age 13.3 months, range 4.0–30.0 months) compared amoxicillin (amoxycillin)/clavulanate in three divided doses for 10 days versus 5 days followed by 5 days of placebo.[12] Clinical success or failure was assessed at 12–14 days and again at 28–42 days after starting treatment. Intention to treat analysis found that the 10 day versus the 5 day regimen increased clinical success on days 12–14 (AR 158/186 [85%] for 10 days *v* 141/192 [73%] for 5 days; RR 1.16, 95% CI 1.04 to 1.28; NNT 8, 95% CI 5 to 30). However, by days 28–42 there was no significant difference in clinical success between the two groups (AR 108/185 [58%] for 10 days *v* 102/190 [54%] for 5 days; RR 1.09, 95% CI 0.91 to 1.30). The second subsequent RCT compared cefpodoxime/proxetil twice daily at 8 mg/kg daily for 10 days versus for 5 days followed by 5 days of placebo. It found that success rates were higher with the 10 day versus the 5 day treatment group after 12–14 days (AR 199/222 [90%] for 10 day treatment *v* 180/226 [80%] for 5 day treatment; RR 1.13, 95% CI 1.04 to 1.22; NNT 10, 95% CI 6 to 30), but no significant difference was found after 28–42 days (AR 149/222 [67%] for 10-day treatment *v* 141/226 [62%] for 5 day treatment; RR 1.08, 95% CI 0.94 to 1.23).[13]

Harms: The systematic review[11] and the two subsequent RCTs[12,13] found no difference with short versus long courses of antibiotics in diarrhoea and/or vomiting and rash.

Comment: None.

QUESTION What are the effects of interventions to prevent recurrence?

OPTION LONG TERM ANTIBIOTIC TREATMENT

One systematic review in children and adults has found that long term antibiotic prophylaxis versus placebo reduces recurrence of acute otitis media. However, one subsequent RCT in children aged 3 months to 6 years found no significant difference between antibiotic prophylaxis and placebo. We found insufficient evidence on which antibiotic to use, for how long, and how many episodes of acute otitis media justify starting preventive treatment.

Benefits: **Versus placebo:** We found one systematic review[14] and one subsequent RCT.[15] The systematic review (search date 1993) identified 33 RCTs comparing antibiotics versus placebo to prevent recurrent acute otitis media (AOM) and otitis media with effusion.[14] Nine of the trials (945 people) looked at recurrent AOM only. It was not clear from the review which of the studies referred only to children; four either included the word "children" in the title or appeared in paediatric journals. Most studies defined recurrent AOM as at least three episodes of AOM in 6 months. The most commonly used antibiotics were amoxicillin (amoxycillin), co-trimoxazole, and sulfamethoxazole (sulphamethoxazole), given for 3 months to 2 years. All nine studies showed a lower rate of recurrence with antibiotic treatment, although in seven of the studies the difference was not significant. Overall, the review found that antibiotics significantly reduced recurrence of AOM (AR of recurrence per person per month 8% with antibiotics *v* 19% with placebo; ARR 11%, 95% CI 3% to 19%; NNT per month to prevent 1 acute episode 9, 95% CI 5 to 33). The subsequent RCT (194 children aged 3 months to 6 years with 3 documented episodes of AOM within the preceding 6 months) compared amoxicillin 20 mg/kg/day either once or twice daily versus placebo.[15] The children were followed up monthly if asymptomatic or within 3–5 days if they had symptoms of upper respiratory tract infection for up to 90 days. The RCT found no significant difference between antibiotics versus placebo in preventing recurrent AOM (RR of remaining AOM free, diagnosed by otoscopy and tympanometry 1.00, 95% CI 0.66 to 1.52 using completer analysis, 36 children lost to follow up). Calculations including those children lost to follow up yielded similar results whether the outcomes were assumed in favour of placebo or in favour of antibiotics. **Choice and duration of antibiotic:** The systematic review found no significant difference in rate of recurrence between antibiotics.[14] Greater treatment effect was seen with treatment lasting less than 6 months, but the confidence intervals overlapped (ARR for recurrence with courses < 6 months 21%, 95% CI 7% to 49%; ARR with courses > 6 months 4%, 95% CI 1% to 9%).

Harms: The studies gave no information on harms.

Comment: None.

OPTION XYLITOL CHEWING GUM OR SYRUP

One RCT found that xylitol syrup or chewing gum versus control reduced the incidence of acute otitis media. It found no significant difference with xylitol lozenges versus control gum. More children taking xylitol versus control withdrew because of abdominal pain or other unspecified reasons.

Benefits: We found no systematic review but found one RCT (857 children, 54% boys) comparing xylitol (either as chewing gum, syrup, or lozenges) versus control (syrup or chewing gum).[16] The RCT randomised children into two groups according to their ability to chew gum. Children who could chew gum received xylitol gum (8.4 g/day, 179 children), xylitol lozenges (10 g/day, 176 children), or control gum (xylitol 0.5 g/day, 178 children). Children who could not chew gum received xylitol syrup (10 g/day, 159 children) or control syrup (0.5 g day, 165 children). Each time the child showed any signs of acute respiratory infection, acute otitis media (AOM) was excluded using tympanometry and otoscopy. Follow up was for 3 months. In the first group, xylitol gum versus control gum significantly reduced the number of children with at least one episode of AOM (AR 29/179 [16%] *v* 49/178 [28%]; RR 0.59, 95% CI 0.39 to 0.89; NNT 8, 95% CI 5 to 36) but no significant difference was found with xylitol lozenges versus control gum (AR 39/176 [22%] *v* 49/178 [28%];

RR 0.81, 95% CI 0.56 to 1.16). In the second group, xylitol syrup versus control syrup significantly reduced the number of children with at least one episode of AOM (AR 46/159 [29%] *v* 68/165 [41%]; RR 0.70, 95% CI 0.52 to 0.95; NNT 8, 95% CI 4 to 53).

Harms: The RCT found that more children taking xylitol lozenges or syrup versus control treatment withdrew from the trial (xylitol lozenges *v* control gum, 26/176 [15%] *v* 8/178 [5%], $P < 0.001$; xylitol syrup *v* control syrup, 30/159 [19%] *v* 17/165 [10%]; CI not provided; $P < 0.03$).[16] Most withdrawals were because of either an unwillingness to take the intervention, having left the area, or because of abdominal discomfort. We found no evidence on the long term effects of xylitol.

Comment: The children in this study received xylitol or the control intervention five times daily, a regimen that might be difficult to maintain long term.[16] The incidence of AOM in those who withdrew from the trial was not described; therefore, the reported effect of xylitol may be underestimated or overestimated.

GLOSSARY

Mastoiditis The presence of infection in mastoid cavity.
Myringotomy The surgical creation of a perforation in tympanic membrane.

Substantive changes

Antibiotics One additional systematic review;[1] evaluation of clinical failure rate as outcome. Conclusion unchanged.
Choice of antibiotic regimen One additional systematic review;[1] conclusion unchanged.

REFERENCES

1. Marcy M, Takata G, Shekelle P, et al. *Management of Acute Otitis Media. Evidence Report/Technology Assessment No.15*. (Prepared by the Southern California Evidence Based Practice Centre under contract No. 290–97–0001.) AHRQ Publication No. 01-E010. Rockville, MD: Agency for Healthcare Research and Quality, May 2001. Search date 1999.
2. Froom J, Culpepper L, Jacobs M, et al. Antimicrobials for acute otitis media? A review from the International Primary Care Network. *BMJ* 1997;315:98–102.
3. Del Mar C, Glasziou P, Hayem M. Are antibiotics indicated as initial treatment for children with acute otitis media? A meta-analysis. *BMJ* 1997;314:1526–1529. Search date 1994; primary sources Medline and Current Contents.
4. Berman S. Otitis media in developing countries. *Pediatrics* 1995;96:126–131.
5. World Health Organization. *World Development Report 1993: Investing in Health*. Oxford: Oxford University Press, 1993:215–222.
6. Bertin L, Pons G, d'Athis P, et al. A randomized double blind multicentre controlled trial of ibuprofen versus acetaminophen and placebo for symptoms of acute otitis media in children. *Fundam Clin Pharmacol* 1996;10:387–392.
7. Rosenfeld RM, Vertrees JE, Carr J, et al. Clinical efficacy of antimicrobial drugs for acute otitis media: meta-analysis of 5400 children from thirty-three randomised trials. *J Pediatr* 1994;124:355–367. Search date 1992; primary sources Medline and Current Contents.
8. Damoiseaux RA, van Balen FAM, Hoes AW, et al. Antibiotic treatment of acute otitis media in children under two years of age: evidence based? *Br J Gen Pract* 1998;48:1861–1864. Search date 1997; primary sources Medline, Embase, and hand searched references.
9. Glasziou PP, Del Mar CB, Sanders SL. Antibiotics for acute otitis media in children (Cochrane Review). In: The Cochrane Library, Issue 1, 2002. Oxford: Update Software. Search date 2000; primary sources Medline, Current Contents, and reference lists.
10. Little P, Gould C, Williamson I, et al J. Pragmatic randomised controlled trial of two prescribing strategies for childhood acute otitis media. *BMJ* 2001;322:336–342.
11. Kozyrskyj AL, Hildes-Ripstein GE, Longstaffe SEA, et al. Short course antibiotics for acute otitis media. In: The Cochrane Library, Issue 1, 2002. Oxford: Update Software. Search date 1998; primary sources Medline, Embase, Science Citation Index, Current Contents, hand searches of reference lists, and personal contacts.
12. Cohen R, Levy C, Boucherat M, et al. A multicenter randomized, double blind trial of 5 versus 10 days of antibiotic therapy for acute otitis media in young children. *J Pediatr* 1998;133:634–639.
13. Cohen R, Levy C, Boucherat M, et al. Five vs. ten days of antibiotic therapy for acute otitis media in young children. *Pediatr Infect Dis J* 2000;19:458–463.
14. Williams RL, Chalmers TC, Stange KC, et al. Use of antibiotics in preventing recurrent acute otitis media and in treating otitis media with effusion: a meta-analytic attempt to resolve the brouhaha. *JAMA* 1993;270:1344–1351. (Published erratum

appears in *JAMA* 1994;27:430.) Search date 1993; primary sources Medline and Current Contents.

15. Roark R, Berman S. Continuous twice daily or once daily amoxycillin prophylaxis compared with placebo for children with recurrent acute otitis media. *Pediatr Infect Dis J* 1997;16:376–378.
16. Uhari M, Kontiokari T, Niemela MA. Novel use of xylitol sugar in preventing acute otitis media. *Pediatrics* 1998;102:879–884.

Paddy O'Neill
General Practitioner
Norton Medical Centre
Stockton on Tees
UK

Competing interests: None declared.

Asthma in children

Search date June 2001

Duncan Keeley

QUESTIONS

INTERVENTIONS

*No RCT, but observational evidence and strong consensus belief that oxygen is beneficial.

See glossary, p 277.

Key Messages

Treating acute asthma in children

- **High dose inhaled corticosteroids** One systematic review in children with acute moderately severe asthma has found no consistent difference in hospital admissions or forced expiratory volume in 1 second between initial treatment with high dose inhaled corticosteroids versus oral corticosteroids. One subsequent RCT found that inhaled versus oral corticosteroids significantly improved lung function. One RCT in children with severe attacks found that oral corticosteroids versus inhaled corticosteroids improved lung function and reduced hospital admissions.
- **Intravenous theophylline** One systematic review found no significant difference with intravenous theophylline versus placebo added to routine treatment, but the trials in the review may have been too small to exclude a clinically important benefit. One subsequent RCT found that intravenous aminophylline versus placebo significantly improved FEV_1 at 6 hours and reduced the liklihood of intubation.
- **Ipratropium bromide added to β_2 agonists** One systematic review has found that in children with mild to severe asthma exacerbations, multiple doses of ipratropium bromide plus a β_2 agonist (fenoterol or salbutamol) versus a β_2 agonist alone significantly reduce hospital admissions (NNT 13, 95% CI 8 to 32) and improve lung function. In children with mild to moderate asthma exacerbations, a single dose of ipratropium bromide plus a β_2 agonist (fenoterol, salbutamol, or terbutaline) versus a β_2 agonist alone significantly improves lung function for up to 2 hours, but does not significantly reduce hospital admissions.
- **Metered dose inhaler plus spacer devices for delivery of β_2 agonists (as effective as nebulisers)** One systematic review in children with acute but not life threatening asthma who were old enough to use a spacer, has found no significant difference in hospital admission rates with a metered dose inhaler plus a spacer versus nebulisation for delivering β_2 agonists (fenoterol, salbutamol, or terbutaline) or β agonist (orciprenaline). Children using metered dose inhaler with spacer may have shorter stays in emergency departments, less hypoxia, and lower pulse rates compared to children receiving β_2 agonist by nebulisation.
- **Oral corticosteroids** One systematic review has found that oral corticosteroids (prednisone or prednisolone) versus placebo within 45 minutes of an acute asthma attack significantly reduces hospital admission.
- **Oxygen** One prospective cohort study and clinical experience support the need for oxygen in acute asthma.

Single agent prophylaxis in childhood asthma

- **Inhaled corticosteroids** One systematic review has found that prophylactic inhaled corticosteroids (betamethasone, beclometasone, budesonide, flunisolide, or fluticasone) versus placebo significantly improve symptoms and lung function. One RCT found no significant difference in symptoms with inhaled beclomethasone versus theophylline. RCTs have found that inhaled corticosteroids (beclometasone, budesonide, or fluticasone) versus inhaled long acting β_2 agonists (salmeterol) or inhaled nedocromil improve symptoms and lung function. Two systematic reviews of studies with long term follow up and a subsequent long term RCT have found no evidence of growth retardation in children with asthma treated with inhaled corticosteroids. Shorter term studies found reduced growth velocity.

Additional treatments in childhood asthma inadequately controlled by standard dose inhaled corticosteroids

- **Addition of increased dose of inhaled corticosteroid** One RCT in children taking beclometasone comparing the addition of a second dose of inhaled corticosteroid (beclometasone) versus placebo found no significant difference in lung function, symptom scores, or exacerbation rates, but found significant reduction of growth velocity at 1 year.
- **Addition of long acting β_2 agonists** One RCT in children taking beclometasone comparing the addition of a second dose of a long acting β_2 agonist (salmeterol) versus placebo found that salmeterol significantly increased peak expiratory flow rates in the first few months of treatment but found no increase after 1 year. A second RCT in children taking inhaled corticosteroids found that the addition of salmeterol versus placebo increased morning peak expiratory flow rates and symptom free days at 3 months.
- **Addition of oral leukotriene receptor antagonists** One crossover RCT in children with persistent asthma who had been taking inhaled corticosteroids (budesonide) for at least 6 weeks found that the addition of a leukotriene receptor antagonist (montelukast) versus placebo significantly improved lung function and decreased the proportion of days with asthma exacerbations over 4 weeks.
- **Addition of oral theophylline** One small RCT found that addition of theophylline versus placebo to previous treatment significantly increased the proportion of symptom free days and significantly reduced the use of additional β agonist (orciprenaline) and additional corticosteroid (beclometasone or prednisolone) over 4 weeks.

Treating acute wheeze in infants

- **β_2 Agonists delivered by nebuliser or metered dose inhaler/spacer** We found conflicting evidence from RCTs. Transient hypoxia may be caused by nebulised bronchodilators, particularly with air driven nebulisers, and seems less likely when using metered dose inhalers/spacers (see bronchiolitis, p 291).
- **Inhaled ipratropium bromide** One systematic review found limited and conflicting evidence on the effects of ipratropium bromide.
- **Oral corticosteroids** One RCT found no evidence that oral corticosteroids versus placebo improved outcomes over 56 episodes of acute wheezing in infants.

Prophylaxis in wheezing infants

- RCTs found insufficient evidence on the effects of prophylaxis with inhaled corticosteroids, continous oral theophylline or sodium cromoglicate (cromoglycate) in wheezing infants.

DEFINITION **Childhood asthma** is characterised by chronic or recurrent cough and wheeze. The diagnosis is confirmed by demonstrating reversible airway obstruction in children old enough to perform peak flow measurements or spirometry. Diagnosing asthma in children requires exclusion of other causes of recurrent respiratory symptoms. **Wheezing in infancy** may be caused by acute viral infection (see bronchiolitis, p 291), episodic viral associated wheeze, or asthma. These are not easy to distinguish clinically.

INCIDENCE/ PREVALENCE Surveys have found increasing prevalence of wheeze and shortness of breath, and diagnosed asthma in children. The increase is more than can be explained by an increased readiness to diagnose asthma. One questionnaire study from Aberdeen, Scotland, surveyed 2510 children aged 8–13 years in 1964 and 3403 children in 1989. Over the 25 years, prevalence of wheeze rose from 10% to 20%; episodes of shortness of breath from 5% to 10%; and diagnosis of asthma from 4% to 10%.[1] One prospective cohort study (826 neonates reviewed at 3 and 6 years of age) found that 34% had experienced at least one wheezing illness before age 3 years, 14% wheezed before age 3 years and were still wheezing at age 6, and 15% had a wheezing illness in the past year at age 6 but had not wheezed before age 3.[2]

AETIOLOGY/ RISK FACTORS Asthma is more common in children with a personal or family history of atopy. Precipitating factors include infection, house dust mites, allergens from pet animals, exposure to tobacco smoke, and anxiety.

PROGNOSIS A historical cohort study of wheezing in the first year of life found that 14% of children with one attack and 23% of children with four or more attacks (recalled at age 5 years) had experienced at least one wheezing illness in the past year at age 10.[3]

AIMS To reduce or abolish cough and wheeze; to attain best possible lung function; to reduce the risk of severe attacks; to minimise sleep disturbance and absence from school; to minimise adverse effects of treatment; and to allow normal growth.

OUTCOMES Wheeze; cough; nights disturbed by asthma; days lost from school or normal activities; hospital admission and duration of stay in hospital (subjective proxy outcome measures for severity of asthma exacerbations); lung function tests (peak expiratory flow rates and forced expiratory volume in 1 second); blood oxygen saturation in acute attacks; and airway hyperresponsiveness (measured using methacholine challenge tests).

METHODS *Clinical Evidence* search and appraisal June 2001.

QUESTION **What are the effects of treatments for acute asthma in children?**

OPTION **OXYGEN**

One prospective cohort study and clinical experience support the need for oxygen in acute asthma.

Benefits: We found no systematic review or RCTs. One double blind, prospective cohort study (280 children) found that decreased oxygen saturation upon entry to an emergency department was correlated with increased treatment with intravenous aminophylline (see glossary, p 277) and corticosteroids, and increased rates of hospital admission or subsequent readmission (arterial oxygen saturation ≤91% *v* arterial oxygen saturation ≥96%: OR 35, 95% CI 11 to 150; for arterial oxygen saturation 92–95% *v* ≥96%: OR 4.2, 95% CI 2.2 to 8.8).[4]

Harms: We found no evidence about harms.

Comment: A RCT of oxygen versus no oxygen treatment in acute severe asthma would be considered unethical. The cohort study does not address directly whether oxygen should be given therapeutically but it does suggest, along with clinical experience, that oxygen should continue to be given promptly to children with acute asthma.[4]

OPTION IPRATROPIUM BROMIDE ADDED TO β_2 AGONISTS

One systematic review has found that multiple doses of ipratropium bromide plus a β_2 agonist (fenoterol or salbutamol) versus the β_2 agonist alone reduce hospital admission rates and improve lung function in children with severe asthma exacerbations. Combination treatment with a single dose of ipratropium bromide plus a β_2 agonist (fenoterol, salbutamol, or terbutaline) versus the β_2 agonist alone improves lung function but does not reduce hospital admission rates in children with mild to moderate asthma exacerbations.

Benefits: We found one systematic review (search date 2000, 13 RCTs, children aged 18 months to 17 years with acute asthma) comparing effects of combined inhaled anticholinergics plus β_2 agonists versus β_2 agonists alone on hospital admission rate.[5] **Single dose:** The systematic review found that in children with mild to moderate exacerbations, adding a single dose of ipratropium bromide to β_2 agonists (fenoterol, salbutamol (see glossary, p 277) or terbutaline) versus the β_2 agonist alone significantly improved forced expiratory volume in 1 second (FEV_1) at 1 hour (3 RCTs: SMD 0.57, 95% CI 0.21 to 0.93) and at 2 hours (3 RCTs: SMD 0.53, 95% CI 0.17 to 0.90), but found no significant reduction in hospital admission (3 RCTs: RR 0.93, 95% CI 0.65 to 1.32).[5] **Multiple doses:** The systematic review found that in children with mild, moderate, or severe exacerbations, adding multiple doses of ipratropium bromide to a β_2 agonist (fenoterol or salbutamol) improved FEV_1 (4 RCTs: WMD 9.7 of predicted FEV_1, 95% CI 5.7 to 13.7, 1 h after last ipratropium bromide inhalation) and reduced hospital admissions (6 RCTs: RR 0.75, 95% CI 0.62 to 0.89; NNT 13, 95% CI 8 to 32). Subgroup analysis found significant reduction only in children with severe exacerbations (baseline FEV_1 < 50% of predicted or change of 7 to 9 in baseline clinical score after last combined inhalation, RR 0.71, 95% CI 0.58 to 0.89; NNT 7, 95% CI 5 to 20).[5]

Harms: The systematic review found no significant increase in risk of nausea (3 RCTs: RR 0.59, 95% CI 0.30 to 1.14), vomiting (3 RCTs: RR 1.03, 95% CI 0.37 to 2.87), or tremor (4 RCTs: RR 1.01, 95% CI 0.63 to 1.63) in children treated with multiple doses of ipratropium bromide.[5]

Comment: None.

OPTION **METERED DOSE INHALER PLUS SPACER DEVICES VERSUS NEBULISERS FOR DELIVERING β_2 AGONISTS**

One systematic review, in children with acute but not life threatening asthma who were old enough to use a spacer, has found no significant difference in hospital admission rates with a metered dose inhaler plus a spacer versus nebulisation for delivery of β_2 agonists (fenoterol, salbutamol or terbutaline) or β agonist (orciprenaline). Children using a metered dose inhaler with a spacer may have shorter stays in emergency departments, less hypoxia, and lower pulse rates compared with children receivingβ_2 agonist by nebulisation.

Benefits: We found one systematic review (search date 1999, 16 RCTs, 686 children with acute asthma but excluding life threatening asthma) comparing spacer/holding chamber attached to a metered dose inhaler versus single or multiple treatment with nebuliser for delivery of β_2 agonists (fenoterol, salbutamol (see glossary, p 277) or terbutaline) or β agonist (orciprenaline [see glossary, p 277]).[6] The review found no significant difference between spacer and multiple treatments with nebulisers in hospital admission rates (OR 0.91, 95% CI 0.4 to 2.1). It found a significant increase in pulse rate with nebulisers (WMD 8.3% from baseline, 95% CI 5.0% to 11.5%). One RCT (152 children ≥2 years) found that the time spent in the emergency department was shorter in children using metered dose inhaler plus spacer (WMD −37 min, 95% CI −50 to −24 min).[7] Two small RCTs included in the review comparing delivery of β_2 agonists (salbutamol or terbutaline) via spacer versus single treatment with nebuliser found less deterioration in blood gases with the spacer.[6]

Harms: The systematic review found no significant deterioration in any of the outcome measures with delivery of β_2 agonists using metered dose inhaler plus a spacer versus nebulisation.[6]

Comment: These findings suggest that, in children old enough to use a spacer, metered dose inhaler with spacer could be substituted for nebulisation in the treatment of acute asthma in emergency departments and hospital wards.

OPTION **ORAL CORTICOSTEROIDS**

One systematic review has found that early oral corticosteroids (prednisone or prednisolone) versus placebo reduce hospital admission in children with acute asthma exacerbations.

Benefits: We found one systematic review (search date 1999, 3 RCTs comparing corticosteroid v placebo within 45 min of arrival at the emergency department).[8] It found that oral corticosteroid (1–2 mg/kg prednisone or prednisolone) versus placebo significantly reduced admission rates in children with acute asthma exacerbations (OR 0.24, 95% CI 0.11 to 0.53).[8]

Harms: The systematic review included RCTs in adults and did not report separately on adverse reactions in children given oral corticosteroids; overall it found no significant difference with oral corticosteroids versus placebo.[8] We found few reports of adverse effects with short courses of systemic corticosteroids. Several case reports have associated systemic corticosteroid treatment with severe varicella infection. One case control study (167 cases, 134 controls) in otherwise immunocompetent children with complicated and uncomplicated varicella infection did not find significant risk attributable to corticosteroid exposure (OR 1.6, 95% CI 0.2 to 17), but it was too small to exclude a clinically important risk.[9]

Comment: None.

OPTION HIGH DOSE INHALED CORTICOSTEROIDS

One systematic review has found no consistent differences in hospital admission rates or increase in flow expiratory volume in 1 second between initial treatment with high dose inhaled corticosteroids versus oral corticosteroids in acute moderately severe asthma. Three RCTs found no significant difference; one RCT in children with severe attacks found that oral corticosteroids reduced hospital admission and improved lung function. One subsequent RCT found that inhaled corticosteroids improved lung function.

Benefits: **High dose inhaled versus oral:** We found one systematic review (search date not stated, 4 RCTs),[10] one subsequent RCT,[11] and one additional RCT.[12] The systematic review compared effects of initial treatment with high dose inhaled corticosteroids versus oral corticosteroids in hospital emergency departments on admission rates.[10] The results from the four RCTs were not pooled because of marked heterogeneity between studies. One RCT (100 children with acute asthma ≥ 5 years, mean initial flow expiratory volume in 1 second [FEV_1] 45%) compared fluticasone (2 mg through metered dose inhaler with spacer) versus prednisone (2 mg/kg orally).[13] It found that prednisone reduced hospital admission (10% prednisone *v* 31% fluticasone; $P = 0.01$) and increased mean FEV_1 at 4 hours (9% fluticasone *v* 19% prednisone; $P \leq 0.001$).[13] The second RCT (111 children aged 1–17 years) compared dexamethasone (1.5 mg/kg via nebuliser) versus prednisone (2 mg orally).[14] It found no significant difference between nebulised dexmethasone versus oral prednisone in hospital admission (12/56 [21%] with dexamethasone *v* 44/55 [31%] with prednisone; ARR 9.5%, 95% CI –8% to 21%; RR 0.69, 95% CI 0.36 to 1.27), but found fewer relapses with nebulised dexamethasone within 48 hours after discharge (0/44 [0%] *v* 6/38 [16%]; ARR –16%, 95% CI –27% to –4.5%); however, all children in the RCT received a 5 day course of prednisone (2 mg/kg daily) on discharge.[14] Two other RCTs compared budesonide (800 μg via nebuliser at 1, 30, and 60 mins; 1600 μg via turbohaler) versus prednisolone (2 mg/kg orally).[15,16] Overall, no significant differences were found between the groups in admission rates (OR for inhaled corticosteroids *v* oral corticosteroids 0.49, 95% CI 0.22 to 1.07).[15,16] The subsequent RCT (321 children aged 4–16 years, peak expiratory flow rate 40–75% predicted) compared nebulised fluticasone (1 mg twice daily for 7 days) versus oral prednisolone (2 mg/kg for 4 days then 1 mg/kg for 3 days). It found that nebulised fluticasone versus oral prednisolone improved mean morning peak expiratory flow rate over 7 days (difference 9.5 L/min, 95% CI 2 L/min to 17 L/min). No significant differences were found in symptom scores, withdrawals, or adverse events.[11] The additional RCT (46 children, aged 15–16 years, admitted to hospital with severe exacerbations of asthma) compared nebulised budesonide 2 mg hourly with oral prednisolone 2 mg/kg at admission and after 24 hours.[12] It found no significant difference between groups in FEV_1 at 24 hours or at 3 and 24 days after admission. All children in this trial were treated with 800 μg budesonide daily following discharge from hospital.

Harms: The systematic review found no significant adverse effects with inhaled corticosteroids.[10]

Comment: These RCTs suggest that high dose inhaled corticosteroids may be substituted for oral corticosteroids in the initial phase of treatment of moderately severe acute asthma. This may be useful for children who vomit oral corticosteroids or for children with frequent exacerbations where there is concern about the cumulative dose of oral steroids. One RCT was funded by the manufacturers of fluticasone.[11]

OPTION INTRAVENOUS THEOPHYLLINE

One systematic review found no significant difference with intravenous theophylline versus placebo added to routine treatment, but the trials in the review may have been too small to exclude a clinically important benefit. One subsequent RCT found that intravenous aminophylline versus placebo significantly improved FEV_1 at 6 hours and reduced the liklihood of intubation, but found that significantly more children receiving aminophylline versus placebo had infusions stopped because of adverse effects (mainly nausea and vomiting).

Benefits: We found one systematic review (search date 1994, 6 small RCTs, 164 children aged 1.5–18 years)[17] and one subsequent RCT.[18] The review found no significant difference with intravenous theophylline versus placebo added to routine treatment (mean difference in forced expiratory volume in 1 second [FEV_1] +39% of predicted; P = 0.25).[17] The subsequent RCT (163 children aged 1–19 years with acute asthma, 43% admitted to intensive care) compared intravenous aminophylline (see glossary, p 277) versus placebo. It found significantly greater improvement in FEV_1 at 6 hours (mean increase in FEV_1 10%, 95% CI 4% to 17%), less additional oxygen needed in the first 30 hours (median 6 h with additional intravenous *v* 18 h with placebo; P = 0.015) and significantly reduced likelihood of intubation (absolute risk 0% with aminophylline *v* 6% with placebo; P = 0.03).[18]

Harms: The systematic review (search date 1994) did not specifically look for information on adverse effects but concluded that theophylline may have slight detrimental effect as children receiving theophylline versus placebo had slightly longer hospital stays (mean difference 0.31 days; P = 0.03) and received more β_2 agonist (salbutamol) treatments (mean difference 2.1; P = 0.02).[17] The subsequent RCT found that significantly more children had their infusions stopped with aminophylline versus placebo because of adverse effects (mainly nausea and vomiting) (32% *v* 5%; OR 8.7, 95% CI 2.9 to 28.4; P < 0.0001).[18] Theophylline can cause serious adverse effects (cardiac arrhythmia or convulsion) if therapeutic blood concentrations are exceeded.

Comment: The trials in the review were too small to exclude a clinically important effect.

QUESTION What are the effects of single agent prophylaxis in childhood asthma?

OPTION INHALED CORTICOSTEROIDS

One systematic review has found that prophylactic inhaled corticosteroids (betamethasone, beclometasone, budesonide, flunisolide, or fluticasone) versus placebo improve symptoms and lung function in children with asthma. RCTs have found that inhaled corticosteroids (beclometasone, budesonide, or fluticasone) versus inhaled long acting β_2 agonists (salmeterol) or inhaled nedocromil improve symptoms and lung function in children with asthma. One RCT found no significant difference in improving symptoms with inhaled beclometasone versus theophylline. Two systematic reviews of studies with long term follow up and a subsequent long term RCT have found no evidence of growth retardation in children with asthma treated with inhaled corticosteroids. Some shorter term studies found reduced growth velocity.

Benefits: **Versus placebo:** We found one systematic review (search date 1996, 24 RCTs, 1087 children, 10/24 RCTs in preschool children, duration 4–88 wks) comparing effects of regular inhaled corticosteroids (betamethasone, beclometasone [beclomethasone], budesonide, flunisolide, or fluticasone) versus placebo on asthma symptoms (see comment below), concomitant drug use, and peak expiratory flow rate (PEFR).[19] It found that corticosteroids significantly improved symptom score (overall weighted relative improvement in symptom score 50%, 95% CI 49% to 51%), reduced β_2 agonist use (RR 0.37, 95% CI 0.36 to 0.38), reduced oral corticosteroid use (RR 0.68, 95% CI 0.66 to 0.70), and improved peak flow rate (weighted mean improvement in PEFR 11% predicted, 95% CI 9.5% to 12.5%). **Versus theophylline:** We found no systematic review. We found one RCT (195 children aged 6–16 years, followed for 12 months) comparing inhaled beclometasone (360 μg daily) versus oral theophylline.[20] It found no significant difference with inhaled beclometasone versus oral theophylline in the mean asthma symptom score (0 = no symptoms, 6 = incapacitating symptoms: mean score 0.5 to 0.8 for beclometasone *v* 0.6 to 0.9 for theophylline) with less use of bronchodilators and oral corticosteroids with inhaled beclometasone. **Versus sodium cromoglicate (cromoglycate):** We found no systematic review. Several small comparative RCTs have found sodium cromoglicate to be less effective than inhaled corticosteroids in improving symptoms and lung function. **Versus nedocromil:** We found one RCT (1041 children aged 5–12 years, forced expiratory volume in 1 second [FEV_1] 94% predicted) that compared inhaled budesonide (200 μg twice daily) and inhaled nedocromil (8 mg twice daily) versus placebo for 4–6 years.[21] It found that budesonide was superior to nedocromil, and that nedocromil was superior to placebo in several measures of asthma symptoms and morbidity (see table 1, p 279). The mean change in post-bronchodilator FEV_1 over the study period was not signficantly different among the three groups. **Versus inhaled long acting β_2 agonists:** We found no systematic review but found two RCTs of beclometasone (200 µg twice daily) versus salmeterol (50 µg twice daily) for 1 year. The first RCT (67 children aged 6–16 years) found that beclometasone was more effective than salmeterol in improving FEV_1 (mean change of FEV_1 −4.5% of predicted with salmeterol, 95% CI −9.0% to +0.1% *v* 10% with beclometasone, 95% CI not provided; mean difference beclometasone *v* salmeterol 14.2%, 95% CI 8.3% to 20%), reducing use of rescue salbutamol (see glossary, p 277) (0.44 uses/day with salmeterol *v* 0.07 uses/day with beclometasone; $P \leq 0.001$).[22] Both treatments improved symptom scores (3% of children asymptomatic before the trial with salmeterol *v* 6% with beclometasone; 36% at 1 year with salmeterol *v* 55% with beclometasone) and PEFR (improvement in morning PEFR 49 L/min with salmeterol *v* 61 L/min with beclometasone), but there was no significant difference between treatments at 1 year. There were two exacerbations in the beclometasone group compared with 17 in the salmeterol group. The second RCT (241 children aged 6–14 years) compared beclometasone (81 children) versus salmeterol (80 children) versus placebo (80 children).[23] It found that beclometasone reduced airway hyperresponsiveness more than salmeterol ($P = 0.003$). Beclometasone versus placebo reduced rescue bronchodilator use ($P \leq 0.001$) and treatment withdrawals because of exacerbations ($P = 0.03$). Salmeterol versus placebo did not significantly reduce the use of a rescue bronchodilator ($P = 0.09$) or treatment withdrawals because of exacerbations ($P = 0.55$). Both salmeterol and beclometasone improved FEV_1 compared with placebo, but the difference between beclometasone and salmeterol was not significant. **Versus oral leukotriene receptor antagonists:** We found one systematic review (search date 1999, 10 RCTs).[24] All studies were brief (6–12 wks), although some had longer unblinded extensions. Only two studies included children. One of these (involving montelukast) remains unpublished. Another study (451 people aged 12 years and older) compared zafirlukast and low dose fluticasone. It found that fluticasone caused greater improvement in lung function (increase in mean morning PEFR 50 L/min *v* 12 L/min) and symptoms (change in percentage of symptom free days 28% *v* 16%).[25] The systematic review, mainly of results for adults, found similar exacerbation rates but inhaled corticosteroids resulted in better improvements in lung function and symptoms when compared with leukotriene receptor antagonists. We found 1 RCT (336 children, 6–14 years; 8 wk duration) comparing oral montelukast versus placebo in children with asthma (FEV_1 50% to 85% of predicted value). It found improvement with montelukast versus placebo (increase from baseline FEV_1 8.23%, 95% CI 6.3% to 10.1% *v* 3.6%, 95% CI 1.3 to 5.9%; $P < 0.001$).[26]

Harms: **Inhaled corticosteroids versus placebo:** One systematic review (search date 1996) found no significant difference with inhaled corticosteroids (betamethasone, budesonide, flunisolide, or fluticasone) versus placebo in adrenal function (12 RCTs) and found clinical cases of oral candidiasis (four RCTs).[19] Observational studies have found little or no biochemical evidence of change in bone metabolism with inhaled corticosteroids.[27,28] Two cross sectional studies using a slit lamp to screen for lenticular changes in children taking long term inhaled corticosteroids (beclometasone, budesonide) found no posterior subcapsular cataracts.[29,30] The systematic review identified eight RCTs reporting growth velocity and found no significant difference with inhaled corticosteroids versus placebo.[19] One systematic review (search date 1993, 21 studies) reported height for age in 810 children with asthma treated with oral or inhaled corticosteroids. It found no evidence of growth impairment with inhaled beclometasone (12 studies, 331 children).[31] A second systematic review (search date 1999, 3 RCTs) identified one RCT (94 children, 7–9 years) comparing effect of inhaled beclometasone 400 μg daily versus placebo on growth as a primary outcome measure in children with recurrent viral induced wheeze.[32] It found a significant decrease in growth with beclometasone versus placebo (mean growth at end of 7 month treatment period, 2.7 cm *v* 3.7 cm; 95% CI –1.4 to –0.6; $P < 0.0001$) and found no significant catch up growth during a follow up 4 month washout period).[33] A large RCT (1041 children with mild to moderate asthma) compared budesonide (400 μg daily) versus nedocromil versus placebo with 4–6 years' follow up.[21] The mean increase in height in the budesonide group was 1.1 cm less than in the placebo group (22.7 cm *v* 23.8 cm; $P = 0.005$); the difference occurred mainly within the first year of treatment.[21] Two RCTs comparing beclometasone with salmeterol found slowing in linear growth with beclometasone (growth over year of treatment 5.4 cm[22] and 6.1 cm in the salmeterol groups, 4.0 cm[22] and 4.7 cm[23] in the beclometasone groups; $P = 0.004$;[22] $P = 0.007$).[23] **Theophylline:** One RCT found that continuous oral theophylline was associated with a higher frequency of headache, gastric irritation, and tremor than beclometasone (360 μg daily).[20] One systematic review (search date not stated, 12 studies, 340 children) of the behavioural and cognitive effects of theophylline found no evidence of significant adverse effects.[34] Another RCT compared inhaled beclometasone (360 μg daily) versus oral theophylline for 1 year.[20] It found a significantly higher rate of growth (more notable in boys) with the theophylline group (mean rate of growth in prepubescent boys 4.3 cm/year *v* 6.2 cm/year). This effect was not sufficient to be noticed by the children or by their parents, and no child was withdrawn from the study on this account.[20] **Sodium cromoglicate (cromoglycate):** Sodium cromoglicate may cause cough, throat irritation, and bronchoconstriction, but no long term adverse effects have been reported. **Versus theophylline or sodium cromoglicate:** One controlled, prospective study compared 216 children treated with budesonide (400–600 μg daily) with 62 children treated with theophylline or sodium cromoglicate over 3–5 years' follow up.[35] No significant changes in growth velocity were found at doses up to 400 μg (5.5 cm/year with budesonide *v* 5.6 cm/year with controls). The adult height of 142 of these budesonide treated children (mean treatment period 9.2 years, mean daily dosage 412 μg) was compared with 18 controls never treated with inhaled corticosteroids and 51 healthy siblings. There were no significant differences. Children in all groups attained their target adult height (mean difference between measured and target adult height: +0.3 cm, 95% CI –0.6 to +1.2 for budesonide treated children; –0.2 cm, 95% CI –2.4 to +2.1 for control children with asthma; +0.9 cm,

95% CI –0.4 to +2.2 for healthy siblings).[36] **Inhaled long acting β_2 agonists:** These agents occasionally cause tremor or tachycardia. Three large RCTs found no evidence of important adverse effects from salmeterol over 1 year.[22,23,37] **Oral leukotriene receptor antagonists:** One placebo controlled RCT found similar incidence of adverse effects with leukotriene receptor antagonists and with placebo.[26] A systematic review (search date 1994) found that leukotriene receptor antagonists compared with corticosteroids were associated with increased risk of withdrawal because of adverse effects (3 RCTs; RR 1.9, 95% CI 1.1 to 3.3).[24] Gastrointestinal symptoms and headaches have been reported with both montelukast and zafirlukast. Allergic granulomatosis (Churg Strauss syndrome) has been reported in people taking either drug, possibly because of reduction in steroid treatment unmasking a pre-existing condition.

Comment: None.

QUESTION What are the effects of additional treatments in childhood asthma inadequately controlled by standard dose inhaled corticosteroids?

OPTION INCREASED DOSE OF INHALED CORTICOSTEROID

One RCT, of the addition of a second dose of inhaled corticosteroid (beclometasone) to previous treatment, found no significant differences in lung function, symptom scores, exacerbation rates, or bronchial reactivity and found an adverse effect on growth velocity at 1 year.

Benefits: We found no systematic review but found one RCT (177 children, age 6–16 years, 1 year of follow up, mean pre-bronchodilator flow expiratory volume in 1 second [FEV_1] 86% predicted) comparing beclometasone (beclomethasone) (200 µg twice daily), salmeterol (50 µg twice daily), and placebo in children already taking beclometasone (200 µg twice daily).[38] No significant differences were found at 1 year in lung function (mean change in FEV_1: 5.8% of predicted, 95% CI 2.9% to 8.7% with double dose beclometasone *v* 4.3%, 95% CI 2.1 to 6.5 with placebo), symptom scores, exacerbation rates, bronchial reactivity, or changes in airway responsiveness (1.30 units of methacholine, 95% CI 0.73 to 1.87 with salmeterol *v* 0.80, 95% CI 0.33 to 1.27 with placebo). No benefit of either adding salmeterol or a second dose of beclometasone was found in this group of children whose compliance with pre-existing medication was good.

Harms: Growth was significantly slower in children receiving higher dose inhaled corticosteroids (3.6 cm, 95% CI 3.0 to 4.2 with double dose beclometasone *v* 5.1 cm, 95% CI 4.5 to 5.7 with salmeterol *v* 4.5 cm, 95% CI 3.8 to 5.2 with placebo).

Comment: Higher dose inhaled corticosteroids are frequently used despite lack of evidence of benefit. In some children, higher prescribed doses may compensate for poor compliance or incorrect inhaler technique.

OPTION ADDITION OF REGULAR LONG ACTING β_2 AGONIST

One RCT found that addition of a long acting β_2 agonist (salmeterol) versus placebo significantly increased peak expiratory flow rates in the first few months of treatment, but found no significant increase after 1 year. A second short term RCT also found increased morning peak expiratory flow rates and more symptom free days at 3 months with addition of a long acting β_2 agonist (salmeterol).

Benefits: We found no systematic review but found two RCTs.[38,39] One RCT (177 children) found that at 1 year the addition of salmeterol did not improve lung function, airway responsiveness, symptom scores, exacerbation rates, or bronchial reactivity.[38] Salmeterol versus placebo increased mean morning peak expiratory flow rates (PEFRs) slightly after 3 months (difference: +12 L/min). There were no significant differences in symptom scores at any time. The second RCT (210 children, 4–16 years, 12 weeks' follow up, mean morning PFER 79% predicted) compared salmeterol (50 μg twice daily) versus placebo in children inadequately controlled on inhaled corticosteroids (average dose 750 μg daily).[39] At 12 weeks, mean morning PEFR (relative to the predicted PEFR) was 4% higher in the salmeterol group. Mean evening PEFR was not significantly different. The median proportion of symptom free days improved more with salmeterol than with placebo (60% *v* 30% for the third month of treatment).

Harms: The RCTs found no significant adverse effects associated with salmeterol.[38,39]

Comment: The second RCT was organised and funded by the manufacturer of salmeterol. Studies of adults with poor control on low dose inhaled corticosteroids have found greater benefit with additional long-acting β_2 agonists than with higher doses of inhaled steroid (see salmeterol v high dose inhaled corticosteroids under adult asthma, p 1506).

OPTION ADDITION OF ORAL THEOPHYLLINE

One small brief RCT found that addition of theophylline versus placebo to previous treatment significantly increased the number of symptom free days and significantly reduced the use of additional β agonist and additional corticosteroid medication. We found insufficient evidence to weigh these short term benefits and possible long term harms.

Benefits: We found no systematic review but found one RCT (double blind crossover trial, 33 children, age 6–19 years, recruited from a hospital asthma clinic, 22 children used inhaled beclometasone [beclomethasone] [mean 533 μg/day], 11 used oral prednisolone [mean 30 mg alternate days]).[40] It found that the addition for 4 weeks of oral theophylline (serum concentration 10–20 μg/mL) versus placebo increased the mean number of symptom free days (63% with theophylline *v* 42% with placebo; $P \leq 0.01$). Inhaled β agonist (orciprenaline (see glossary, p 277)) was needed twice as often with placebo (0.5 doses/day with theophylline *v* 1.0 with placebo; $P \leq 0.01$). Additional daily prednisolone was needed by fewer children while on theophylline than while on placebo (3/32 with theophylline *v* 10/32 with placebo; $P = 0.02$).

Harms: In the RCT, short term adverse effects included mild transient headache and nausea in six children after the crossover from placebo to the theophylline dose that they had previously tolerated.[40]

Comment: One child was excluded from the analysis because of poor compliance. The RCT was too brief to assess long term harms.

OPTION ADDITION OF ORAL LEUKOTRIENE RECEPTOR ANTAGONISTS

One crossover RCT in children with persistent asthma found small improvements in lung function and fewer asthma exacerbation days over 4 weeks with addition of a leukotriene receptor antagonist (montelukast) to inhaled corticosteroid (budesonide).

Benefits: We found no systematic review but found one crossover RCT (279 children aged 6–14 years previously treated with inhaled corticosteroid for at least 6 wks, with mean flow expiratory volume in 1 second (FEV_1) 78% predicted after 1 month run-in with budesonide 200 µg) comparing adding oral montelukast 5 mg versus placebo to inhaled budesonide over 4 weeks.[41] It found a slight increase in FEV_1 with montelukast versus placebo (primary efficacy analysis of 251 children, relative change of FEV_1, relative to baseline: 4.6% v 3.3%, 95% CI –0.1 to 2.7%, P = 0.06; per-protocol analysis of 205 children, 6.0% v 4.1%, 95% CI 0.5 to 3.4%; P = 0.01). It found fewer asthma exacerbation days (decrease from baseline peak flow of > 20%, or increase from baseline of β_2 agonist use of > 70%) with montelukast versus placebo (12.2% v 15.9%; P = 0.001). No significant differences were found in quality of life measurements, global evaluations, or asthma attacks requiring unscheduled medical intervention or treatment with oral corticosteroid.

Harms: The RCT found no significant difference with montelukast versus placebo in asthma exacerbation, upper respiratory tract infection, headache, cough, pharyngitis, and fever.[41]

Comment: The RCT in children was brief (4 wks treatment).[41] We found one large RCT of montelukast added to beclometasone in adults with inadequately controlled asthma that found benefit over a 16 week period.[42] Both RCTs were funded by the manufacturers of montelukast.

QUESTION What are the effects of treatments for acute wheezing in infancy?

OPTION β_2 AGONISTS DELIVERED BY NEBULISER OR METERED DOSE INHALER/SPACER

We found conflicting evidence from RCTs. Transient hypoxia may be caused by nebulised bronchodilators, particularly with air driven nebulisers, and seems less likely with metered dose inhalers plus spacers (see bronchiolitis, p 291).

Benefits: We found no systematic review but found many hospital based RCTs of nebulised β_2 agonists versus normal saline in infants and young children with acute wheezing. Some, but not all, have found short term improvements in clinical respiratory distress scores with β_2

agonists.[43] We found no large RCTs with clinical outcomes. Small RCTs with physiological rather than clinical end points found that giving β_2 agonists by metered dose inhaler with spacer to wheezy infants was effective, with less likelihood than nebulisation to show transient reduction of lung function.[44,45] A large single blind RCT (123 children aged 1–24 months with moderate to severe wheezing, city hospital emergency department in Santiago, Chile) compared nebulised salbutamol (see glossary, p 277) (0.25 mg/kg 3 times in 1 h) with salbutamol by metered dose inhaler plus spacer (2 puffs 5 times in 1 h). In children assessed as non-responders after the first hour, treatment was repeated for a second hour together with intramuscular betamethasone. Withholding of β_2 agonists from a control group was considered unethical. Reduction in clinical severity score (≤ 5) was significantly better with metered dose inhaler plus spacer versus nebulisation after 1 hour (clinical severity score ≤ 5: 56/62 [90%] *v* 43/61 [71%]; OR 3.9, 95% CI 1.5 to 10.4; $P = 0.01$) but not after 2 hours (100% *v* 94%; $P > 0.05$). Only one child (in the nebuliser group) was hospitalised because of treatment failure.[46]

Harms: Some infants have transiently decreased oxygen saturation after nebulisation, especially with air driven nebulisers.[43] Nebulised β_2 agonists are known to cause tachycardia, tremor, and hypokalaemia, but serious adverse effects are rare.

Comment: None.

OPTION INHALED IPRATROPIUM BROMIDE

We found limited and conflicting evidence from one systematic review on the effects of inhaled ipratropium bromide for clinical outcomes in wheezing children.

Benefits: We found one systematic review (search date 1998, 321 children, six RCTs) of ipratropium bromide for wheeze in children under 2 years.[47] One included RCT found that adding ipratropium bromide to β_2 agonists resulted in fewer children receiving further treatment 45 minutes after initial treatment in the emergency room (OR 0.22, 95% CI 0.08 to 0.61), but a second similar study found no additional benefit. A third included RCT (31 hospitalised children) comparing ipratropium bromide versus placebo found no significant difference in the duration of hospitalisation (WMD –0.4 days, 95% CI –1.4 to +0.61). Adding ipratropium bromide to β_2 agonist had no effect on duration of hospitalisation compared with β_2 agonist alone (WMD –0.4 days, 95% CI –1.41 to +0.61). In one home based, 2 month crossover trial, parents preferred regular nebulised ipratropium bromide to nebulised water, but there was no significant reduction in the frequency of reported symptoms during treatment.[47]

Harms: No evidence of harm specific to the use of ipratropium bromide was found in these studies.

Comment: The studies were too small to exclude a clinically important effect of ipratropium bromide.

OPTION ORAL CORTICOSTEROIDS

We found no evidence that oral corticosteroids improve outcomes in acute wheezing infants.

Benefits: We found no systematic review. One outpatient study compared oral prednisolone versus placebo (38 acutely wheezing children aged 3–17 months, including 30 children previously admitted with wheeze). It found no significant differences in outcome between the two groups in the 56 episodes studied.[48]

Harms: No important adverse effects were identified.[48]

Comment: Acute infantile wheezing may be because of bronchiolitis. This is often difficult to separate from other acute wheezing, and is dealt with elsewhere (see bronchiolitis, p 291).

QUESTION What are the effects of prophylaxis in wheezing infants?

We found weak and conflicting evidence on the effects of prophylaxis with inhaled corticosteroids in wheezing infants.

Benefits: We found no systematic review. We found inconsistent results of placebo controlled trials on inhaled corticosteroids in recurrent or persistent infant wheezing. Some found improvements in symptom scores and reduced administration of additional treatments. Other studies did not find beneficial effect. We found a greater tendency for positive findings in studies of older children and in studies involving administration by metered dose inhaler and spacer rather than nebuliser. We found no RCTs of continuous oral theophylline in infants, and the small numbers of trials with inhaled sodium cromoglicate (cromoglycate) were mainly negative.

Harms: We found no good evidence on the long term safety of treatment with continuous inhaled corticosteroids in infancy. Known effects of using nebuliser and facemasks include oral candidiasis and thinning of facial skin.

Comment: Administering inhaled treatments to infants is difficult. RCTs of treatment for infant wheezing used a variety of drugs, dosages, and devices, and were sometimes conducted in populations with differing proportions of children with asthma rather than other types of infant wheeze. These factors may explain the inconsistent results.

GLOSSARY

Aminophylline A stable combination of theophylline and ethylenediamine; the ethylenediamine is added to increase the solubility of theophylline in water.
Orciprenaline is known as metaproterenol in USA; it is a non-selective β agonist.
Salbutamol is known as albuterol in USA; it is a short acting selective β_2 agonist.

REFERENCES

1. Russell G, Ninan TK. Respiratory symptoms and atopy in Aberdeen school children: evidence from two surveys 25 years apart. *BMJ* 1992;304:873–875.
2. Martinez FD, Wright AL, Taussig L, et al. Asthma and wheezing in the first six years of life. *N Engl J Med* 1995;333:132–138.
3. Park ES, Golding J, Carswell F, et al. Pre-school wheezing and prognosis at 10. Arch Dis Child 1986;61:642–646.
4. Geelhoed GC, Landau LI, Le Souef PN. Evaluation of SaO2 as a predictor of outcome in 280 children presenting with acute asthma. *Ann Emerg Med* 1994;23:1236–1241.

5. Plotnick LH, Ducharme FM. Combined inhaled anticholinergics and β_2 agonists in the initial management of acute paediatric asthma. In: The Cochrane Library, Issue 2, 2001. Oxford: Update Software. Search date 2000; primary sources Medline, Embase, Cinahl, hand searches of bibliographies of references, and contact with pharmaceutical companies for details of unpublished trials and personal contacts.
6. Cates CJ. Holding chambers versus nebulisers for β-agonist treatment of acute asthma. In: The Cochrane Library, Issue 2, 2001. Oxford: Update Software. Search date 1999; primary sources Medline and Cochrane Airways Review Group Register.
7. Chou KJ, Cunningham SJ, Crain EF. Metered-dose inhalers with spacers vs nebulizers for pediatric asthma. *Arch Pediatr Adolesc Med* 1995;149:201–205.
8. Rowe BH, Spooner C, Ducharme FM, Bretzlaff JA, Bota GW. Early emergency department treatment of acute asthma with systemic corticosteroids (Cochrane Review) In: The Cochrane Library, Issue 2, 2001 Oxford: Update Software. Last amended November 2000. Search date 1999; primary sources cochrane Airways Review Group Register, Embase, Medline, Cinahl, and hand searches.
9. Patel H, Macarthur C, Johnson D. Recent corticosteroids use and the risk of complicated varicella in otherwise immunocompetent children. *Arch Pediatr Adolesc Med* 1996;150:409–414.
10. Edmonds ML, Camargo CA Jr, Pollack CV Jr, Rowe BH. Early use of inhaled corticosteroids in the emergency department treatment of acute asthma. In: The Cochrane Library, Issue 2, 2002. Oxford: Update Software. Search date not stated; primary sources Cochrane Airways Group Register, and hand searches of bibliographies.
11. Manjra AI, Price J, Lenney W et al. Efficacy of nebulised fluticasone propionate compared with oral prednisolone in children with an acute exacerbation of asthma. *Respir Med* 2000;94:1206–1214
12. Matthews EE, Curtis PD, McLain B, Morris L, Turbitt M. Nebulized budesonide versus oral steroid in severe exacerbations of childhood asthma. *Acta Paediatr* 1999;88:841–843.
13. Schuh S, Resiman J, Alshehri M, et al. A compariosn of inhaled fluticasone and oral prednisone for children with severe acute asthma. *N Engl J Med* 2000;343:689–694.
14. Scarfone RJ, Loiselle JM, Wiley JF II, et al. Nebulized dexamethasone versus oral prednisone in the emergency treatment of asthmatic children. *Ann Emerg Med* 1995;26:480–486.
15. Volowitz B, Bentur L, Finkelstein Y, et al. Effectiveness and safety of inhaled corticosteroids in controlling acute asthma attacks in children who were treated in the emergency department: a controlled comparative study with oral prednisolone. *J Allergy Clin Immunol* 1998;102:1605–1609.
16. Devidayal S, Singhi S, Kumar L, Jayshree M. Efficacy of nebulized budesonide compared to oral prednisolone in acute bronchial asthma. *Acta Paediatr* 1999;88:835–840.
17. Goodman DC, Littenberg B, O'Connor GT, et al. Theophylline in acute childhood asthma: a meta-analysis of its efficacy. Pediatr Pulmonol 1996;21:211–218. Search date 1994; primary source Medline.
18. Yung M, South M. Randomised controlled trial of aminophylline for severe acute asthma. *Arch Dis Child* 1998;79:405–410.
19. Calpin C, Macarthur C, Stephens D, et al. Effectiveness of prophylactic inhaled steroids in childhood asthma: a systematic review of the literature. *J Allergy Clin Immunol* 1997;100:452–457. Search date 1996; primary source Medline.
20. Tinkelman DG, Reed C, Nelson H, et al. Aerosol beclomethasone diproprionate compared with theophylline as primary treatment of chronic, mild to moderately severe asthma in children. *Pediatrics* 1993;92:64–77.
21. The Childhood Asthma Management Program Research Group. Long-term effects of budesonide or nedocromil in children with asthma. *N Engl J Med* 2000;343:1054–1063.
22. Verberne A, Frost C, Roorda R, et al. One year treatment with salmeterol compared with beclomethasone in children with asthma. *Am J Respir Crit Care Med* 1997;156:688–695.
23. Simons FER and the Canadian Beclomethasone Diproprionate – Salmeterol Xinafoate Study Group. A comparison of beclomethasone, salmeterol and placebo in children with asthma. *N Engl J Med* 1997;337:1659–1665.
24. Ducharme FM, Hicks GC. Anti-leukotriene agents compared to inhaled corticosteroids in the management of recurrent and/or acute asthma. In: The Cochrane Library, Issue 3, 2000. Search date 1999; primary sources Medline, Embase, Cinahl, hand searches of reference lists, and personal contact with colleagues and internal headquarters of leukotriene producers.
25. Bleecker ER, Welch MJ, Weinstein SF, et al. Low dose inhaled fluticasone proprionate versus oral zafirlukast in the treatment of persistent asthma. *J Allergy Clin Immunol* 2000;105(6 Pt 1):1123–1129.
26. Knorr B, Matz J, Bernstein JA, et al. Montelukast for chronic asthma in 6–14 year old children. *JAMA* 1998;279:1181–1186.
27. Wolthers OD, Riis BJ, Pedersen S. Bone turnover in asthmatic children treated with oral prednisolone or inhaled budesonide. *Pediatr Pulmonol* 1993;16:341–346.
28. Reilly SM, Hambleton G, Adams JE, Mughaal MZ. Bone density in asthmatic children treated with inhaled corticosteroids. *Arch Dis Child* 2001;84(2):183–184.
29. Simons FE, Persaud MP, Gillespie CA, et al. Absence of posterior subcapsular cataracts in young patients treated with inhaled corticosteroids. *Lancet* 1993;342:776–778.
30. Abuektish F, Kirkpatrick JN, Russell G. Posterior subcapsular cataract and inhaled steroid therapy. *Thorax* 1995;50:674–676.
31. Allen DB, Mullen M, Mullen B. A meta-analysis of the effect of oral and inhaled steroids on growth. *J Allergy Clin Immunol* 1994;93:967–976. Search date 1993; primary sources literature search of leading medical journals 1956–1993.
32. Sharek PJ, Bergman DA. Beclomethasone for asthma in children: effects on linear growth. In: The Cochrane Library, Issue 2, 2001. Oxford: Update Software. Search date 1999; primary source Cochrane Airways Group Asthma Trials Register.
33. Doull 1995, Freezer NJ, Holgate ST. Growth of prepubertal children with mild asthma treated with inhaled beclometasone dipropionate. *Am J Resp Crit Care Med* 1995;151:1715–1719.
34. Stein MA, Krasowski M, Leventhal BL, et al. Behavioural and cognitive effects of theophylline and caffeine. *Arch Pediatr Adolesc Med* 1996;50:284–288. Search date not stated; primary sources Medline, Psychlit, Dissertation Abstracts, and hand searched references.
35. Agertoft L, Pedersen S. Effects of long-term treatment with an inhaled corticosteroid on growth and pulmonary function in asthmatic children. *Respir Med* 1994;88:373–381.

36. Agertoft L, Pedersen S. Effect of long-term treatment with inhaled budesonide on adult height in children with asthma. *N Engl J Med* 2000;343:1064–1069.
37. Lenney W, Pedersen S, Boner AL, Ebbutt A, Jenkins M, on behalf of an international study group. Efficacy and safety of salmeterol in childhood asthma. *Eur J Pediatr* 1995;154:983–990.
38. Verberne A, Frost C, Duiverman E, Grol M, Kerrebijn K. Addition of salmeterol versus doubling the dose of beclomethasone in children with asthma. *Am J Respir Crit Care Med* 1998;158:213–219.
39. Russell G, Williams DAJ, Weller P, Price J. Salmeterol xinafoate in children on high dose inhaled steroids. *Ann Allergy Asthma Immunol* 1995;75:423–428.
40. Nassif EG, Weinberger M, Thompson R, Huntley W. The value of maintenance theophylline in steroid dependent asthma. *N Engl J Med* 1981;304:71–75.
41. Simons FER, Villa JR, Lee BW, et al. Montelukast added to budesonide in children with persistent asthma: a randomized double blind crossover study. *J Pediatr* 2001;138(5):694–698.
42. Laviolette M, Malmstrom K, Lu S, et al. Montelukast added to inhaled beclomethasone in treatment of asthma. *Am J Respir Crit Care Med* 1999;160:1862–1868.
43. Alario AJ, Lewander W, Dennehy P, et al. The efficacy of nebulised metaproterenol in wheezing infants and young children. *Am J Dis Child* 1992;146:412–418.
44. Kraemer R, Frey U, Sommer CW, et al. Short-term effect of albuterol, delivered via a new auxiliary device, in wheezy infants. *Am Rev Respir Dis* 1991;144:347–351.
45. Yuksel B, Greenough A. Comparison of the effects on lung function of different methods of bronchodilator administration. *Respir Med* 1994;88:22.
46. Rubilar L, Castro-Rodrguez JA, Girardi G. Randomized controlled trial of salbutamol via metered-dose inhaler with spacer verus nebuliser for acute wheezing in children less than 2 years of age. *Pediatr Pulmonol* 2000;29:264–269.
47. Everard M, Kurian M. Anticholinergic drugs for wheeze in children under the age of two years. In: The Cochrane Library, Issue 2, 2001. Oxford: Update Software. Search date 1998; primary sources Cochrane Airways Group Register and hand search of respiratory care and paediatric journals.
48. Webb M, Henry R, Milner AD. Oral corticosteroids for wheezing attacks under 18 months. *Arch Dis Child* 1986;61:15–19.

Duncan Keeley
General Practitioner
Thame, Oxfordshire, UK

Competing interests: The author has received occasional consultancy fees or assistance with organisation of, or travel to, meetings from companies including Allen and Hanburys, Astra, MSD, Zeneca, 3M, and Boots.

TABLE 1 **Comparison of inhaled budesonide, nedocromil, and placebo over 4–6 years on several measures of asthma symptoms and morbidity (see text, p 270).[21]**

Intervention	Budesonide (311 children)	Nedocromil (312 children)	Placebo (418 children)
Prednisone courses per 100 person years	70	102	122
Urgent care visits due to asthma per 100 person years	12	16	22
Hospitalisations due to asthma per 100 person years	2.5	4.3	4.4
Beclomethasone or other asthma medications added	6.6%	17.1%	18.7%

Attention deficit hyperactivity disorder in children

Search date April 2002

Paul Ramchandani, Carol Joughin, and Morris Zwi

QUESTIONS

INTERVENTIONS

To be covered in future updates
Antidepressants
Antipsychotics
Caffeine
Lithium
Parent training
Pemoline
Attention deficit hyperactivity disorder in children with Tourette's syndrome

See glossary, p 288

Key Messages

- **Clonidine** Limited evidence from one systematic review suggests that clonidine versus placebo for 4–12 weeks reduces core symptoms, but the clinical importance of these findings is unclear.
- **Dexamfetamine** Limited evidence from two systematic reviews suggests that dexamfetamine versus placebo significantly improves some behavioural outcomes but increases anorexia and appetite disturbance. The second systematic review could not draw firm conclusions about the effects of dexamfetamine versus methylphenidate.
- **Methylphenidate** A systematic review has found that methylphenidate versus placebo significantly reduces core symptoms in children aged 5–18 years, but may disturb sleep and appetite. The review could not draw firm conclusions about the effects of methylphenidate versus dexamfetamine or versus tricyclic antidepressants. The review also found that methylphenidate versus psychological/behavioural treatment improves symptoms in the medium term, but the clinical importance of these findings is unclear.
- **Methylphenidate plus behavioural treatment** One systematic review found inconsistent results for combination treatments (medication plus psychological/behavioural treatment) versus placebo. A second systematic review has found that combination treatments versus psychological/behavioural treatments alone significantly improve attention deficit hyperactivity disorder symptoms.

Clin Evid 2002;8:280–290.

- **Psychological/behavioural treatment** One systematic review of two small RCTs found insufficient evidence about the effects of psychological/behavioural treatment versus standard care. One large subsequent RCT found no significant difference between psychological/behavioural treatment versus standard care in behaviour rating scales.

DEFINITION Attention deficit hyperactivity disorder is "a persistent pattern of inattention and/or hyperactivity and impulsivity that is more frequent and severe than is typically observed in individuals at a comparable level of development" (DSM-IV).[1] Inattention, hyperactivity, and impulsivity are commonly known as the core symptoms (see glossary, p 288) of attention deficit hyperactivity disorder. Symptoms must be present for at least 6 months, observed before the age of 7 years, and "clinically significant impairment in social, academic, or occupational functioning" must be evident in more than one setting. The symptoms must not be better explained by another disorder, such as an anxiety disorder (see glossary, p 288), mood disorder, psychosis, or autistic disorder.[1] The World Health Organization's *International statistical classification of diseases and related health problems* (ICD-10)[2] uses the term "hyperkinetic disorder" for a more restricted diagnosis. It differs from the DSM-IV classification[3] as all three problems of attention, hyperactivity, and impulsiveness must be present, more stringent criteria for "pervasiveness" across situations must be met, and the presence of another disorder is an exclusion criterion.

INCIDENCE/ PREVALENCE Prevalence estimates of attention deficit hyperactivity disorder vary according to the diagnostic criteria used and the population sampled. DSM-IV prevalence estimates among school children range from 3–5%,[1] but other estimates vary from 1.7–16%.[4,5] No objective test exists to confirm the diagnosis of attention deficit hyperactivity disorder, which remains a clinical diagnosis. Other conditions frequently co-exist with attention deficit hyperactivity disorder. Oppositional defiant disorder (see glossary, p 288) is present in 35% (95% CI 27% to 44%) of children with attention deficit hyperactivity disorder, conduct disorder (see glossary, p 288) in 26% (95% CI 13% to 41%), anxiety disorder in 26% (95% CI 18% to 35%), and depressive disorder (see glossary, p 288) in 18% (95% CI 11% to 27%).[6]

AETIOLOGY/ RISK FACTORS The underlying causes of attention deficit hyperactivity disorder are not known.[6] There is limited evidence that it has a genetic component.[7–9] Risk factors also include psychosocial factors.[10] There is increased risk in boys compared to girls, with ratios varying from 3 : 1[6] to 4 : 1.[3]

PROGNOSIS More than 70% of hyperactive children may continue to meet criteria for attention deficit hyperactivity disorder in adolescence, and up to 65% of adolescents may continue to meet criteria for attention deficit hyperactivity disorder in adulthood.[5] Changes in diagnostic criteria cause difficulty with interpretation of the few outcome studies. One cohort of boys followed up for an average of 16 years found a ninefold increase in antisocial personality disorder and a fourfold increase in substance misuse disorder.[7]

AIMS	To reduce inattention, hyperactivity and impulsivity, and to improve psychosocial and educational functioning in affected children and adolescents, with minimal adverse effects of treatment.
OUTCOMES	Children's behaviour, such as Conners Teacher's Rating Scales (see glossary, p 288); school performance, such as School Situations Questionnaire (see glossary, p 288); adverse effects.
METHODS	*Clinical Evidence* update search and appraisal April 2002

QUESTION **What are the effects of treatments for attention deficit hyperactivity disorder in children?**

OPTION **METHYLPHENIDATE**

One systematic review and subsequent RCTs have found that methylphenidate versus placebo reduces core symptoms of attention deficit hyperactivity disorder in the short term but may disturb sleep and appetite. The review could not draw firm conclusions about the effects of methylphenidate versus dexamfetamine or tricyclic antidepressants. The review also found that methylphenidate versus psychological/behavioural treatment improves symptoms in the medium term, but the clinical importance of these findings is unclear.

Benefits: We found one systematic review (search date 2000)[11] and four subsequent RCTs.[12–15] Most studies were conducted in the USA, used a diagnosis of attention deficit disorder (DSM-III) or attention deficit hyperactivity disorder (DSM-IIIR or DSM-IV), and included children aged 5–18 years, mostly recruited from psychiatric and other hospital outpatient clinics. **Versus placebo:** The systematic review included, but did not pool results from, 13 rigorously selected short term RCTs (1177 children aged 5–18 years).[11] Three RCTs (99 children) found no significant difference in core symptoms (see glossary, p 288) between methylphenidate versus placebo. The other 10 RCTs found that methylphenidate (dose range 0.56–0.72 mg/kg/day or 5–35 mg/day for trials reporting in those units) versus placebo significantly improved the scores on Conners Teacher's Rating Scale (see glossary, p 288) hyperactivity index ($P < 0.05$); see comment below. The same systematic review found similar results in 17 other RCTs (643 children), which were less stringent in terms of homogeneity of participants, outcome measures, and methodological quality. The first subsequent RCT (parallel design 276 children aged 6–12 years with attention deficit hyperactivity disorder but excluding children with Tourette's syndrome, ongoing seizure disorder, or psychotic disorder, and girls who had reached menarche) compared conventional (3 times a day dosing) and sustained release (once daily dosing) formulations of methylphenidate versus placebo.[12] The RCT found that methylphenidate versus placebo significantly improved attention and behaviour at school (measured using Teacher IOWA Conners I/O subscale score, $P < 0.001$) throughout the 4 week period of the study. It found no significant difference between conventional and sustained release formulations of methylphenidate. The second subsequent RCT (crossover design, 68 children aged 6–12 years) found similar benefit for slow release methylphenidate compared to placebo, and broad equivalence with conventional methylphenidate.[13] Two other subsequent RCTs (crossover design, one in 45 adolescents mean age 13.8 years and other in 136 boys aged 7–12 years) also favoured methylphenidate over placebo.[14,15] **Versus dexamfetamine (dexamphetamine):** The systematic review[11] identified four poorly reported crossover RCTs (224 children, aged 5–18 years) comparing methylphenidate (dose range 0.6 mg–4.5 mg/kg/day or 20 mg/day for trials reporting in those units) versus dexamfetamine (dose 0.39–2.6 mg/kg/day or 10 mg/day for trials reporting in those units) but, because of heterogeneity, could not pool their results. Three RCTs (99 children, aged 5–12 years) found no significant difference with methylphenidate versus dexamfetamine in the outcomes of interest. The other RCT found improvement with methylphenidate versus dexamfetamine for teacher reported, but not parent reported, outcomes. No firm conclusions can be drawn. **Versus clonidine or combined treatment:** See versus methylphenidate or combined treatment, p 285. **Versus tricyclic antidepressants:** The systematic review[11] identified, but could not pool, the results of two poorly reported crossover RCTs (105 children) comparing methylphenidate (dose 0.4 mg/kg/day or mean 20 mg/day for trials reporting in those units) versus imipramine (dose 1–2 mg/kg/day or mean 65 mg/day for trials reporting in those units). One RCT (75 children) found no significant differences in clinical outcomes after 1 year, and the other RCT (30 children) found that imipramine versus methylphenidate improved some but not all outcomes in the short term. No firm conclusions can be drawn. **Versus psychological/behavioural treatment:** We found one systematic review (search date 2000) that identified four RCTs comparing methylphenidate versus psychological/behavioural treatment (see glossary, p 288).[11] Three of the RCTs (192 children aged 5–12 years) were poorly reported and compared a variety of psychological/behavioural treatments (individual cognitive training [see glossary, p 288] over 12 wks; parent and teacher training; behaviour treatment for 8 wks) versus methylphenidate (5–60 mg/day). Overall, these three RCTs found limited evidence that, in the medium term (12–52 wks), methylphenidate versus psychological/behavioural treatment improved symptoms. The fourth RCT (579 children aged 7–10 years) compared medication treatment (144 children, double blind titration of methylphenidate dose, switched to alternative medication after 28 days if response unsatisfactory, mean initial dose 30.5 mg/day) versus intensive behavioural management versus combined medication and intensive behavioural management versus standard community care.[16] A total of 74% of the children in the medication group were taking methylphenidate at the end of the study. Initial results were not presented as the number of children who improved, but only as P values. Methylphenidate versus psychological/behaviour treatment improved some, but not all, of the symptoms of attention deficit disorder. Subsequent secondary analysis has developed these findings (see comment below).

Harms: The systematic review (search date 2000)[11] did not combine results on harms because of heterogeneity and incomplete data reporting. It presented the number of RCTs that had found significant results (see comment below). **Versus placebo:** The following symptoms were found by at least one RCT included in the systematic review to be significantly more common in children receiving methylphenidate: sleep disorders; anorexia or appetite disturbance; headache; motor tics; irritability; and abdominal pain (see table 1, p 290). Three subsequent RCTs[12–14] reported similar adverse effects (see table 1, p 290). The third subsequent RCT[15] did not report on adverse effects. We found no good evidence of effects of methylphenidate on growth rates in children. **Versus dexamfetamine:** Out of the four RCTs identified by the systematic review, two RCTs reported no significant difference with methylphenidate versus dexamfetamine for anorexia or appetite disturbance and one RCT reported no significant difference in motor tics, abdominal pain, and irritability. **Versus clonidine or combined treatment:** See versus methylphenidate or combined treatment, p 285. **Versus psychological/behavioural treatment:** The one large RCT comparing medication with intensive behavioural treatment (see glossary, p 288)[16] found that, of the children receiving either medication management or combined medication and intensive behavioural treatment, 50% reported mild adverse effects, 11% had moderate adverse effects, and 3% experienced severe adverse effects.

Comment: The fourth RCT comparing medication versus intensive behavioural treatment (see glossary, p 288) is the largest and most rigorous currently available RCT of attention deficit hyperactivity disorder treatments.[16] Subsequent secondary analysis suggests that 56% of the children taking medication improved compared with these in the behavioural treatment group.[17] There is also a suggestion that children with comorbid behaviour problems (oppositional defiant disorder/conduct disorder) demonstrated a stronger response to medication than those without comorbid behaviour problems, and that children with attention deficit hyperactivity disorder and anxiety disorders were likely to respond equally well to behavioural or medication treatments.[18] There are some concerns about the methods used in the RCT and caution should be exercised when using the results of secondary analysis, as they are more susceptible to bias than the primary outcome analyses.[19] It should also be noted that the principal outcome measures were rating scales based on impressions of parents and teachers; they did not include the children's views or direct measures of their response to treatment. Long term effects on psychosocial adjustment, educational success, or behavioural improvement are unclear. We found no evidence about methylphenidate for pre-school children.[20] The abbreviated Conners Teacher's Rating Scale (see glossary, p 288) has been used widely in treatment studies and has been researched, validated, and standardised to measure treatment effects in attention deficit hyperactivity disorder.[21] However, the clinical importance of the effect of methylphenidate versus placebo on the abbreviated Conners Teacher's Rating Scale remains unclear.

OPTION DEXAMFETAMINE SULPHATE

Limited evidence from two systematic reviews and a subsequent RCT suggests that dexamfetamine versus placebo improves some behavioural outcomes.

Benefits: **Versus placebo:** We found two systematic reviews[5,20] and a subsequent RCT.[22] The first systematic review (search date 1997, 4 RCTs, 61 children aged 6–12 years, dexamfetamine [dexamphetamine] 0.46–0.75 mg/kg/day) found that dexamfetamine versus placebo improved the change in the abbreviated Conners Teacher's Rating Scale (see glossary, p 288) (WMD –4.8, 95% CI –6.4 to –2.9).[20] The second later systematic review (search date 1997, 3 RCTs, 150 children aged 6–16 years, dexamfetamine 5–20 mg/day) only evaluated longer term studies (> 12 wks).[5] It found some evidence of positive outcomes (including improved concentration and hyperactivity) with dexamfetamine versus placebo. However, some methodological problems were identified with the studies in this review.[5] The subsequent RCT (crossover design, 35 children aged 6–12 years) found significant improvement with slow release formulation of dexamfetamine versus placebo on two rating scales (including the hyperactivity index of the Conners Teacher Rating Scale, $P < 0.001$).[22] **Versus methylphenidate:** See benefits of methylphenidate, p 282.

Harms: **Versus placebo:** The first systematic review made a non-specific comment about adverse effects, only two RCTs reported people withdrawing from the trial because of adverse events.[20] The second systematic review found that dexamfetamine significantly increased anorexia and appetite disturbance in three RCTs.[5] The subsequent RCT reported decreased appetite, weight loss, and sleep disturbance.[22] **Versus methylphenidate:** See harms of methylphenidate, p 284.

Comment: See comment of methylphenidate for the principal outcome measures, p 284.

OPTION CLONIDINE

Limited evidence from one systematic review suggests that clonidine versus placebo reduces core attention deficit hyperactivity disorder symptoms, but the clinical importance of these findings is unclear.

Benefits: **Versus placebo:** We found one systematic review (search date 1999, 6 RCTs, 143 children, mean age 11 years, dose of clonidine 0.1–0.24 mg/day for 4–12 wks).[23] One of the six RCTs was a comparison of clonidine versus methylphenidate,[24] rather than versus placebo, and the rating scales of the clinical features of attention deficit hyperactivity disorder completed by parents, teachers, and clinicians were combined in the systematic review. A meta-analysis of the six RCTs found that clonidine versus placebo improved this combined rating scale (effect size 0.58, 95% CI 0.27 to 0.89). The clinical importance of this result is unclear (see comment below), and the results should be treated with caution. **Versus methylphenidate or combined treatment:** We found no systematic review but found one small RCT (3 groups of 8 boys aged

6–16 years with attention deficit hyperactivity disorder and either co-morbid oppositional defiant disorder or conduct disorder [see glossary, p 288]) comparing clonidine (mean dose 0.17 mg/day) versus methylphenidate (mean dose 35 mg/day) versus clonidine plus methylphenidate.[24] Most outcomes were not significantly different between the three groups. However, methylphenidate versus clonidine significantly improved the teacher reported School Situations Questionnaire (see glossary, p 288) ($P < 0.009$). The clinical importance of this isolated result from a single small RCT is unclear.

Harms: **Versus placebo:** The systematic review[23] included information from 10 studies of harms. Not all were high quality RCTs, and their results are difficult to interpret. In children taking clonidine, nine of 10 studies found sedation in children; six studies found increased irritability. Electrocardiographs were recorded in two placebo controlled RCTs, which found no abnormalities. **Versus methylphenidate or combined treatment:** One small RCT (24 boys)[24] found that two of eight children on clonidine developed new onset bradycardia. Four of eight children on a combination of clonidine and methylphenidate developed bradycardia.

Comment: The systematic review[23] noted larger effect sizes in smaller and lower quality studies. Inclusion of the RCT of clonidine versus methylphenidate[24] in the systematic review creates difficulties in using that review to indicate the effects of clonidine versus placebo. The RCT[24] had a larger effect size than most other included studies, and it is likely to have inflated the final result of the meta-analysis. The results used by the systematic review for that RCT were not described in the original RCT report, and may have been a less reliable comparison of baseline and end of the study measures rather than a rigorous comparison of randomly allocated groups. Harms were reported as the number of studies that recorded a specific adverse effect or not rather then the number of children experiencing adverse effects.

OPTION PSYCHOLOGICAL/BEHAVIOURAL TREATMENT

One systematic review of two small RCTs found insufficient evidence; one subsequent RCT found no significant difference with psychological/ behavioural treatment versus standard care in behavioural rating scales.

Benefits: **Versus standard care:** We found one systematic review (search date 1997, 2 RCTs, 50 children aged 6–13 years)[20] and a subsequent RCT.[16] The systematic review found no significant difference between psychological/behavioural treatment (see glossary, p 288) versus standard care in teacher rating scales (SMD –0.40, 95% CI –1.28 to +0.48) or parent ratings (1 RCT, 26 children, WMD –3.8, CI –9.6 to +2.0). The RCTs identified by the systematic review were small and the clinical importance of these results is unclear. The subsequent RCT (290 children) found no significant difference between intensive behavioural treatments versus standard community care.[16] In children with comorbid anxiety disorders (see glossary, p 288), the RCT found that intensive behavioural treatment resulted in better clinical outcomes. **Versus methylphenidate:** See benefits of methylphenidate, p 282.

Harms: The systematic review and subsequent RCT did not make any comment about adverse effects.[16,20]

Comment: Children in the trials had different diagnoses, presentations, and clinical needs. Secondary analysis of one RCT[16] suggests small benefit with intensive behavioural treatment versus standard community care (34% of children improved with intensive behavioural treatment v 25% with standard community care).[13] However, caution should be exercised in interpreting the results of secondary analysis as they are more susceptible to bias than the primary outcome analyses.[19]

OPTION MEDICATION PLUS PSYCHOLOGICAL/BEHAVIOURAL TREATMENT

One systematic review found inconsistent results for combination treatments (methylphenidate plus psychological/behavioural treatment) versus placebo in attention deficit hyperactivity disorder. A second systematic review found that combination treatments versus psychological/behavioural treatments (see glossary, p 288) alone significantly improved attention deficit hyperactivity disorder symptoms.

Benefits: **Versus control/placebo:** We found one systematic review (search date 1997, 3 RCTs, 35 children aged 5–13 years).[20] It found that combination of methylphenidate with psychological/behavioural treatments versus control/placebo improved parent ratings of attention deficit hyperactivity disorder (Conners Parent's Rating Scale WMD −7.3, 95% CI −12.3 to −2.4), but not teacher ratings of attention deficit hyperactivity disorder (Conners Teacher's Rating Scale [see glossary, p 288] WMD 3.8, 95% CI −2.0 to +9.6). The clinical importance of these findings is unclear.[20] **Versus stimulant drugs alone:** See benefits of methylphenidate, p 282. **Versus psychological/behavioural treatments alone:** We found one systematic review (search date 2000, 11 RCTs, 428 children aged 5–18 years).[11] It found that methylphenidate plus behavioural treatments versus behavioural treatments alone significantly improved attention deficit hyperactivity disorder behaviours, symptoms, and measures of academic achievement. No significant difference was found in social skills or in measures of the relationship between parents and children.[11] The review separately assessed one RCT,[12] which found that combined drug and intensive behavioural treatment versus intensive behavioural treatment alone significantly improved three of five measures of attention deficit hyperactivity disorder core symptoms (see glossary, p 288), one of three measures of aggression/oppositional behaviour, one of three measures of anxiety depression, and one of three measures of academic achievement.[16]

Harms: The RCTs did not report any adverse effects. See harms of methylphenidate, p 284.

Comment: The RCT[16] is the largest and most methodologically rigorous study of attention deficit hyperactivity disorder treatments, with high standards for reporting and follow up of nearly all children (see comment under methylphenidate, p 284).[19] The results of a secondary analysis of this RCT[12] suggest that children with attention deficit hyperactivity disorder and comorbid anxiety respond equally well to medication management or intensive behavioural treatment (see comment about secondary analysis under methylphenidate, p 284);[18] but secondary analysis indicated that combined medication management plus intensive behavioural treatment was better than medication management alone.[18]

GLOSSARY

Anxiety disorder A range of conditions with features including apprehension, motor tension, and autonomic overactivity.
Behavioural treatment Treatment using insights from learning theory to achieve specific changes in behaviour. It is usually highly structured. It can be used with either children with attention deficit hyperactivity disorder or their parents/carers.
Cognitive training Brief structured treatment aimed at changing dysfunctional beliefs.
Conduct disorder Conduct disorders include a repetitive pattern of antisocial, aggressive, or defiant conduct that violate age appropriate social expectations.[2]
Conners Teacher's Rating Scales Widely used rating scales for assessment of symptoms of attention deficit hyperactivity disorder used extensively in both clinical work and epidemiological studies. There are 10 item parent and teacher questionnaires that can be used for children aged 3–17 years.
Core symptoms Inattention, hyperactivity, and impulsivity are commonly known as the core symptoms of attention deficit hyperactivity disorder.[5]
Depressive disorder Characterised by persistent low mood, loss of interest and enjoyment, and reduced energy.
Oppositional defiant disorder The presence of markedly defiant, disobedient, provocative behaviour, but without the severely dissocial or aggressive acts seen in conduct disorder.[2]
Psychological/behavioural treatments Includes any of the following methods: contingency management methods (e.g. behaviour modification); cognitive–behavioural therapy; individual psychotherapy; parent training or education; teacher training and education; parent and family counselling/therapy; social skills training; and electroencephalogram, biofeedback, or relaxation treatment.
School Situations Questionnaire A teacher completed questionnaire that measures the pervasiveness of child behaviour problems across 12 school situations.[25]

Substantive changes

Methylphenidate versus placebo Four new RCTs;[12–15] conclusions unchanged.
Dexamfetamine (dexamphetamine) versus placebo One new RCT;[22] conclusions unchanged.

REFERENCES

1. American Psychiatric Association. *Diagnostic and statistical manual of mental disorders (DSM-IV), 4th ed.* Washington, DC: American Psychiatric Association, 1994.
2. World Health Organization. *International statistical classification of diseases and related health problems, 10th rev ed.* Geneva: World Health Organization, 1994.
3. Taylor E, Sergeant J, Doepfner M, et al. Clinical guidelines for hyperkinetic disorder. European Society for Child and Adolescent Psychiatry. *Eur Child Adolesc Psychiatry* 1998;7:184–200.
4. Goldman LS, Genel M, Bezman RJ, et al. Diagnosis and treatment of attention-deficit/hyperactivity disorder in children and adolescents. Council on Scientific Affairs, American Medical Association. *JAMA* 1998;279:1100–1107.
5. Jadad AR, Boyle M, Cunningham C, et al. *Treatment of attention-deficit/hyperactivity disorder.* Evidence report/technology assessment No 11. (Prepared by McMaster University under Contract No. 290–97-0017). Rockville MD: Agency for Health Care Policy and Research and Quality, 1999. Search date 1997; primary sources Medline, Cinahl, HealthStar, PsychInfo, Embase, Cochrane Library, hand searched reference lists, and organisations funding research on attention deficit hyperactivity disorder and researchers contacted. http://hstat.nlm.nih.gov/hq/Hquest/screen/DirectAccess/db/3143 (last accessed 10/09/2002).
6. Green M, Wong M, Atkins D, et al. *Diagnosis and treatment of attention-deficit/hyperactivity disorder in children and adolescents.* Council on Scientific Affairs, American Medical Association. Technical

Review No. 3 (Prepared by Technical Resources International, Inc. under Contract No. 290–94-2024.). Rockville MD: Agency for Health Care Policy and Research, AHCPR Publication No. 99–0050, 1999.

7. Finkel MF. The diagnosis and treatment of the adult attention deficit hyperactivity disorders. *Neurologist* 1997;3:31–44.
8. Hertzig MEE, Farber EAE. *Annual progress in child psychiatry and child development, 1996.* New York: Brunner/Mazel Inc, 1997:602.
9. Kaminester DD. Attention deficit hyperactivity disorder and methylphenidate: When society misunderstands medicine. *McGill J Med* 1997;3:105–114.
10. Taylor E, Sandberg S, Thorley G, et al. *The epidemiology of childhood hyperactivity. Maudsley monographs*. London: Institute of Psychiatry, 1991:33.
11. Lord J, Paisley S. *The clinical effectiveness and cost-effectiveness of methylphenidate for hyperactivity in childhood.* London: National Institute for Clinical Excellence, Version 2, August 2000. Search date 2000; primary sources Jadad et al.[5], Medline, Cinahl, Healthstar, PsychInfo, and Embase.
12. Wolraich ML, Greenhill LL, Pelham W, et al. Randomized, controlled trial of oros methylphenidate once a day in children with attention-deficit/hyperactivity disorder. *Pediatrics* 2001;108:883–892.
13. Pelham WE, Gnagy EM, Burrows-MacLean L, et al. Once-a-day Concerta methylphenidate versus three-times-daily methylphenidate in laboratory and natural settings. *Pediatrics* 2001;107:E105
14. Evans SW, Pelham WE, Smith BH, et al. Dose-response effects of methylphenidate on ecologically valid measures of academic performance and classroom behavior in adolescents with ADHD. *Exp Clin Psychopharmacol* 2001;9(2):163–175.
15. Pelham WE, Hoza B, Pillow DR, et al. Effects of methylphenidate and expectancy on children with ADHD: behavior, academic performance, and attributions in a summer treatment program and regular classroom settings. *J Consult Clin Psychol* 2002;70(2):320–335.
16. Jensen PS, Arnold LE, Richters JE, et al. A 14-month randomized clinical trial of treatment strategies for attention-deficit/hyperactivity disorder. The MTA Cooperative Group. Multimodal Treatment Study of Children with ADHD. *Arch Gen Psychiatry* 1999;56:1073–1086.
17. Swanson JM, Kraemer HC, Hinshaw SP, et al. Clinical relevance of the primary findings of the MTA; success rates based on severity of ADHD and ODD symptoms at the end of treatment. *J Am Acad Child Adolesc Psychiatry* 2001;40:168–179.
18. Jensen PS, Hinshaw SP, Kraemer HP, et al. ADHD comorbidity findings from MTA study: comparing comorbid subgroups. *J Am Acad Child Adolesc Psychiatry* 2001;40:147–158.
19. Boyle MH, Jadad AR. Lessons from large trials: the MTA study as a model for evaluating the treatment of childhood psychiatric disorder. *Can J Psychiatry* 1999;44:991–998.
20. Miller A, Lee SK, Raina P, et al. A review of therapies for attention-deficit/hyperactivity disorder. Canadian Coordinating Office for Health Technology Assessment, 1998. Search date 1997; primary sources Medline, Current Contents, hand search of review articles, textbooks, British Columbia Methylphenidate Survey, and Intercontinental Medical Statistics for information on drug prescription and utilization in Canada.
21. Goyette CH, Conners CK, Ulrich RF. Normative data on revised Conners Parent and Teacher Rating scales. *J Abnorm Child Psychol* 1978;6:221–236.
22. James RS, Sharp WS, Bastain TM, et al. Double-blind, placebo-controlled study of single-dose amphetamine formulations in ADHD. *J Am Acad Child Adolesc Psychiatry* 2001;40:1268–1276.
23. Connor DF, Fletcher KE, Swanson JM. A meta-analysis of clonidine for symptoms of attention-deficit hyperactivity disorder. *J Am Acad Child Adolesc Psychiatry* 1999;38:1551–1559. Search date 1999; primary sources Medline, PsychInfo, Current Contents, Social and Behavioral Sciences, Current Contents Clinical Medicine, and hand searches of non-peer reviewed research reports, book chapters, chapter bibliographies, and individual report references.
24. Connor DF, Barkley RA, Davis HT. A pilot study of methylphenidate, clonidine, or the combination in ADHD comorbid with aggressive oppositional defiant or conduct disorder. *Clin Pediatr (Phila)* 2000;39:15–25.
25. Barkley RA. *Attention-deficit hyperactivity disorder: a handbook for diagnosis and treatment*. New York: Guilford Press, 1990.

Paul Ramchandani
MRC Research Training Fellow
University of Oxford
Department of Psychiatry
Warneford Hospital, Oxford, UK

Carol Joughin
Project Manager
FOCUS, Royal College of Psychiatrists' Research Unit, London, UK

Morris Zwi
Consultant Child
and Adolescent Psychiatrist
Child and Family Consultation Centre, Richmond, Surrey, UK

Competing interests: None declared. The opinions expressed are those of the authors and do not necessarily reflect those of the Royal College of Psychiatrists.

TABLE 1 **The number of RCTs reporting significant adverse effects with methylphenidate versus placebo (see text, p 284).[11] Published with permission © NICE 2000.**

Adverse effect	Number of trials
Anorexia or appetite disturbance	7/12 (58%)
Motor tics	1/2 (50%)
Irritability	2/9 (22%)
Sleep disorder	4/20 (20%)
Abdominal pain	2/10 (20%)
Headache	2/10 (20%)

Bronchiolitis

Search date June 2002

Juan Manuel Lozano

QUESTIONS

INTERVENTIONS

See glossary, p 300

Key Messages

Prevention

- **Nursing interventions (cohort segregation, handwashing, gowns, masks, gloves, and goggles) in children admitted to hospital** We found no RCTs about the effects of these interventions.
- **Respiratory syncytial virus immunoglobulins or palivizumab (monoclonal antibody) in children at high risk** One systematic review has found that, in children born prematurely, in children with bronchopulmonary dysplasia, and in children with a combination of risk factors, prophylactic respiratory syncytial virus immunoglobulin or palivizumab (monoclonal antibody) versus placebo or no prophylaxis reduces admission rates to hospital and intensive care units.

Treatment

- **Antibiotics (routine)** We found no evidence on children with bronchiolitis alone. One unblinded RCT in children with bronchiolitis and uncomplicated pneumonia (crackles on auscultation or consolidation on a chest radiograph) found no significant difference in clinical scores with routine use of antibiotics (ampicillin, penicillin, or erythromycin) versus placebo, but may not have been sufficiently powered to exclude a clinically important effect.

Clin Evid 2002;8:291–303.

- **Bronchodilators** Systematic reviews have found that inhaled bronchodilators versus placebo significantly improve overall clinical scores in the short term in children treated in hospital, emergency departments and outpatient clinics, but have found no evidence that bronchodilators reduce admission rates or produce a clinically important improvement in oxygen saturation.
- **Corticosteroids** One systematic review and nine additional RCTs found limited and conflicting evidence on the effects of corticosteroids versus placebo.
- **Respiratory syncytial virus immunoglobulins, pooled immunoglobulins or palivizumab (monoclonal antibody)** RCTs found insufficient evidence on the effects of immunoglobulin treatment.
- **Ribavirin** One systematic review in children admitted to hospital with respiratory syncytial virus bronchiolitis found no significant difference in mortality, risk of respiratory deterioration, or duration of hospital stay with ribavarin versus placebo, but found that ribavirin significantly reduced the duration of ventilation. One small subsequent RCT found no significant difference with ribavarin versus placebo in hospital stay, oxygen needs, recurrence of disease, or admission rates, but it may have been too small to exclude a clinically important difference.

DEFINITION Bronchiolitis is a virally induced acute bronchiolar inflammation that is associated with signs and symptoms of airway obstruction. Diagnosis is based on clinical findings. Clinical manifestations include fever, rhinitis (inflammation of the nasal mucosa), tachypnoea, expiratory wheezing, cough, rales, use of accessory muscles, apnoea (absence of breathing), dyspnoea (difficulty in breathing), alar flaring (flaring of the nostrils), and retractions (indrawing of the intercostal soft tissues on inspiration). Disease severity (see glossary, p 300) of bronchiolitis may be classified clinically as mild, moderate, or severe.

INCIDENCE/ PREVALENCE Bronchiolitis is the most common lower respiratory tract infection in infants, occurring in a seasonal pattern with highest incidence in the winter in temperate climates,[1] and in the rainy season in warmer countries. Each year in the USA, about 21% of infants have lower respiratory tract disease and 6–10/1000 infants are admitted to hospital for bronchiolitis (1–2% of children > 12 months of age).[2] The peak rate of admission occurs in infants aged between 2 and 6 months.[3]

AETIOLOGY/ RISK FACTORS Respiratory syncytial virus is responsible for bronchiolitis in 70% of cases. This figure reaches 80–100% in the winter months. However, in early spring, parainfluenza virus type 3 is often responsible.[1]

PROGNOSIS **Morbidity and mortality:** Disease severity is related to the size of the infant, and to the proximity and frequency of contact with infective infants. Children at increased risk of morbidity and mortality are those with congenital heart disease, chronic lung disease, history of premature birth, hypoxia, and age less than 6 weeks.[4] Other factors associated with a prolonged or complicated hospital stay include a history of apnoea or respiratory arrest, pulmonary consolidation seen on a chest radiograph, and (in North America) native American or Inuit race.[5] The risk of death within 2 weeks is high for children with congenital heart disease (3.4%) or chronic lung disease (3.5%) as compared with other groups combined (0.1%).[4] Rates of admission to intensive care units (range 31–36%)

and need for mechanical ventilation (range 11–19%) are similar among all high risk groups.[4] The percentage of these children needing oxygen supplementation is also high (range 63–80%).[4] In contrast, rates of intensive care unit admission and ventilation in such children are markedly lower (15% and 8%).[6] **Long term prognosis:** Information on long term prognosis varies among studies. One small prospective study of two matched cohorts (25 children with bronchiolitis; 25 children without) found no evidence that bronchiolitis requiring outpatient treatment is associated with an increased risk of asthma in the long term.[7] Possible confounding factors include variation in illness severity, smoke exposure, and being in overcrowded environments.[8] We found one prospective study in 50 randomly selected infants admitted with bronchiolitis, followed up by questionnaire for 5 years and a visit in the fifth year. It found a doubling of asthma incidence compared with the general population, although there was large (30%) loss to follow up and no matched control group.[9]

AIMS To decrease morbidity and mortality, shorten hospital stay, and prevent transmission of infection, with minimum adverse effects.

OUTCOMES Death rate; rates of hospital admission; rate of intubation or admission to intensive care units; clinical score (clinical score is a subjective, unvalidated measure that is based on judgements made by the clinician); rates of clinical and serological infection. Oxygen saturation is a proxy outcome, but the clinical significance and sensitivity of this outcome are unclear.

METHODS *Clinical Evidence* search and appraisal June 2002.

QUESTION What are the effects of prophylactic measures in high risk children?

OPTION IMMUNOGLOBULINS

One systematic review has found that, in children born prematurely or children with bronchopulmonary dysplasia, prophylactic respiratory syncytial virus immunoglobulin (RSV Ig) or palivizumab (monoclonal antibody) versus placebo or no prophylaxis given monthly reduces hospital admission and admission to intensive care.

Benefits: We found one systematic review (search date 1999, 4 RCTs, 2598 children) comparing monthly RSV Ig or palivizumab (monoclonal antibody) versus placebo or no prophylaxis.[10] Three of the RCTs used intravenous RSV Ig and one used intramuscular palivizumab. Two of the RCTs using RSV Ig were unblinded and both of them used no prophylaxis as the control intervention. The review found that RSV Ig or palivizumab versus placebo reduced admission to hospital (95/1535 [6%] for RSV Ig or palivizumab *v* 138/1063 [13%] with placebo; OR 0.48, 95% CI 0.37 to 0.64) and intensive care unit (27/1535 [2%] for RSV Ig or palivizumab *v* 43/1063 [4%] with placebo; OR 0.47, 95% CI 0.29 to 0.77), but did not reduce the incidence of mechanical ventilation (16/1535 [1%] for RSV Ig or palivizumab *v* 14/1063 [1%] with placebo; OR 0.99, 95% CI 0.48 to 2.07).

Harms: See harms of immunoglobulins, p 300.

Comment: Premature infants included in the RCTs were children under 6 months old, with gestational age at birth less than either 32 or 35 weeks. Children with bronchopulmonary dysplasia were under 2 years old and still undergoing treatment for this anomaly. Planned subgroup analysis in the review found that prophylaxis reduced hospital admission in children whose only risk factor was prematurity (OR 0.27, 95% CI 0.15 to 0.49) and in children with bronchopulmonary dysplasia alone (OR 0.54, 95% CI 0.37 to 0.80), but not in children with cardiac comorbidity alone (OR 0.64, 95% CI 0.37 to 1.10).[10] A cost-effectiveness analysis suggests that the clinical effect of palivizumab when used in all children who meet the licensed indication for it is small, and its benefits are likely to be clinically and economically relevant in children at the highest risk.[11]

QUESTION **What are the effects of measures to prevent transmission in hospital?**

OPTION **NURSING INTERVENTIONS (COHORT SEGREGATION, HANDWASHING, GOWNS, MASKS, GLOVES, AND GOGGLES)**

We found no direct evidence from RCTs that cohort segregation, handwashing, use of gowns, masks, gloves, or goggles reduced nosocomial transmission of respiratory syncytial virus to other children.

Benefits: We found no systematic review and no good quality RCTs examining effects of cohort segregation (see glossary, p 300), handwashing, gowns, masks, gloves, or goggles, used either singly or in combination, on nosocomial transmission of bronchiolitis in children.

Harms: **Cohort segregation:** Potential risks associated with cohort segregation include misdiagnosing respiratory syncytial virus infection and putting non-infected patients at risk by subsequent placement into the wrong cohort. **Handwashing:** Dermatitis is a potential adverse effect of repeated handwashing with some products. **Other interventions:** No harms reported.

Comment: Handwashing is a well established technique for reducing cross-infection in other contexts, and so RCTs may not be ethically feasible. **Single nursing interventions:** We found four observational studies comparing nosocomial infection rates in separate series of children before and after introduction of cohort segregation, handwashing, gowns and masks, and goggles.[12–15] No study adjusted results for variations in baseline incidence. Three studies found a lower incidence of transmission after introduction of cohort segregation alone, handwashing alone, and eye–nose goggles alone.[12–14] The fourth study found no significant difference in transmission after introducing gowns and masks.[15] **Combinations of nursing interventions:** We found one RCT (58 medical personnel caring for children admitted with bronchiolitis), which found no significant difference in nosocomial infection rate in staff when they used gowns and masks in addition to handwashing (5/28 [18%] of those using gowns, masks, and handwashing *v* 4/30 [13%] in the control group; RR 1.3, 95% CI 0.4 to 3.6).[16] The RCT did not report transmission rates in the children. One non-randomised prospective trial (233 children at risk of severe nosocomial infection) compared transmission rates in wards adopting different nursing policies.[17] It found that a combination of cohort segregation, gowns, and gloves reduced nosocomial transmission rates compared with all other policies (cohort segregation alone, gown and gloves alone, no special precautions) taken together. However, the control interventions did not remain constant throughout the trial, the results were based on an interim analysis, and the definition of "at risk" children was not clearly stated.

QUESTION **What are the effects of treatment for children with bronchiolitis?**

OPTION **BRONCHODILATORS (INHALED SALBUTAMOL, INHALED ADRENALINE [EPINEPHRINE])**

Two good quality systematic reviews have found that, when compared with placebo, inhaled bronchodilators achieve short term improvement in overall clinical scores in children treated in hospital, emergency departments, and outpatient clinics, although they have found no evidence that bronchodilators reduce admission rates or produce a clinically important improvement in oxygen saturation. One subsequent RCT found no evidence that nebulised adrenaline, as compared with saline placebo, changed short term outcomes during the first 4 days of illness in infants. One small RCT found that nebulised adrenaline reduced the hospitalisation rate when compared with salbutamol. However, these results await confirmation.

Benefits: **Versus placebo:** We found two systematic reviews[18,19] and one subsequent RCT.[20] The first review (search date 1998, 8 RCTs, 485 children) evaluated children in outpatient clinics or the emergency department and after admission to hospital.[18] The second review (search date 1995, 5 RCTs, 251 children) considered children treated in outpatient clinics.[19] Four RCTs were common to both reviews. The first review found that, in the short term, bronchodilators improved clinical scores in children with mild and moderately severe bronchiolitis (lack of improvement in clinical score, bronchodilator *v* placebo, RR 0.76, 95% CI 0.60 to 0.95).[18] Both reviews found evidence that bronchodilators improved oxygen saturation by a clinically unimportant amount (mean difference in oxygen saturation +1.2%, 95% CI +0.8% to +1.6%[19]). Both reviews found no evidence that bronchodilators versus placebo reduced admission rates in children treated in outpatient clinics or the emergency department (RR 0.85, 95% CI 0.47 to 1.53;[18] 23/97 [24%] children treated with bronchodilator admitted *v* 21/90 [23%] with placebo, RR 1.0, 95% CI 0.6 to 1.7[19]). The subsequent RCT (38 infants without previous wheezing episodes) compared a single dose (3 mg in 3 mL) of nebulised levo-adrenaline (epinephrine) versus 0.9% saline placebo during the first 4 days of their respiratory illness.[20] There were no significant differences in respiratory and heart rates, oxygen saturation, and the RDAI (see glossary, p 300) measured during the following 60 minutes. Results were reported graphically. **Versus other treatments:** We found three

RCTs comparing nebulised adrenaline versus salbutamol (see table 1, p 302).[21–23] The first RCT (24 sedated hospitalised infants without previous wheeze) found a significant improvement in clinical scores after administration of racemic epinephrine, as compared with baseline score (mean difference 1.8, 95% CI 0.79 to 2.80), which was not present after salbutamol inhalation (mean difference 0.4, 95% CI –0.61 to +1.40).[21] However, the clinical importance of this finding is not clear, and a comparison between groups was not provided. The second RCT (42 infants aged 6 wks to 1 year seen in the emergency department) compared inhaled adrenaline versus salbutamol.[22] It found a significant improvement in oxygen saturation after 60 minutes of treatment in favour of adrenaline (mean difference 2%, CI not provided; P = 0.02). The clinical importance of this finding is unclear, given that this was one of many statistical comparisons and because the change is below the 3% difference in oxygen saturation that the authors had previously established as clinically important. It also found a significant reduction in admissions (7/20 [35%] with adrenaline *v* 17/21 [81%] with salbutamol; RR 0.43, 95% CI 0.23 to 0.81; NNT 3, 95% CI 2 to 7). The third RCT (100 infants aged 1–24 months, randomised in the emergency department to 4 treatments: nebulised racemic epinephrine followed by saline placebo; nebulised salbutamol followed by saline placebo; saline placebo followed by racemic epinephrine; saline placebo followed by salbutamol) found no significant differences in RDAI scores between the four groups during the study.[23]

Harms: One systematic review reported tachycardia, increased blood pressure, decreased oxygen saturation, flushing, hyperactivity, prolonged cough, and tremor following use of bronchodilators.[18] The review did not report the frequency of adverse events. The second review did not report harms.[19] One RCT reported a higher incidence of pallor in children treated with adrenaline than in those receiving salbutamol (at 30 min: 10/20 [50%] with epinephrine *v* 3/21 [14%] with salbutamol; RR 3.5, 95% CI 1.12 to 10.9; NNH 3, 95% CI 2 to 8).[22] Three RCTs made no mention of harms.[20,21,23]

Comment: None of the RCTs considered respiratory failure as an outcome. One systematic review found significant heterogeneity among RCTs in the effects of bronchodilators on oxygen saturation.[18] Discrepancies in primary studies included differences in study populations such as inclusion of sedated children, short duration of follow up, and validity of clinical scores. Bronchodilators may improve the clinical appearance of a child through a general stimulatory effect rather than by improving respiratory function.[24]

OPTION CORTICOSTEROIDS

One systematic review and nine additional RCTs found limited and conflicting evidence on the effects of corticosteroids versus placebo.

Benefits: We found one systematic review (search date 1999, 6 RCTs, 347 children in hospital)[25] and nine additional RCTs (928 children) of corticosteroids versus placebo in children with bronchiolitis.[26–34] Three of the additional RCTs had been mentioned in the systematic review but excluded because of data inconsistency,[30] treatment outside hospital,[31] or failure to report the outcome markers sought by the systematic review.[32] The systematic review found no significant difference in the mean duration of stay (5 RCTs, 229 children: WMD −0.43 days, 95% CI −1.05 to +0.18 days), in the RCTs with clearly identified randomisation methods (4 RCTs, 253 children: WMD −0.35 days, 95% CI −0.84 to +0.14 days), and after exclusion of RCTs that included children with previous wheezing (4 RCTs, 264 children: WMD −0.29 days, 95% CI −0.71 to +0.13 days).[25] Interpretation of the effect of corticosteroids versus placebo on clinical symptoms found by the systematic review is difficult (see comment below). The RCTs in the systematic review reported different clinical scales at varying times after starting treatment. The scales usually included measurements of oxygen saturation, wheezing, accessory muscle use, and respiratory rate. Results reported 72 hours after starting treatment were too heterogeneous for analysis. Only three RCTs (197 children) provided results for 24 hours after starting treatment. The systematic review pooled the standardised effect size for clinical scores from these three RCTs and found that corticosteroids versus placebo produced a significant improvement. Although statistically significant, the clinical importance of such an improvement is not clear because different scales are combined across studies. Seven of the nine additional RCTs that compared the clinical score found no significant benefit from corticosteroids (see table 2, p 303).[26–29,31-33] One RCT found a significant transient improvement in a "bronchiolitis score" with oral prednisolone for 2 days.[33] This is of doubtful clinical importance. One subsequent RCT (70 children between 8 wks and 23 months old without previous wheezing episodes) compared oral dexamethasone (1 mg/kg) versus placebo in the emergency department, along with nebulised salbutamol. After a 4 hour observation period, children were discharged to their homes and continued to receive either daily oral dexamethasone (0.6 mg/kg/dose) or placebo for 5 days, as well as inhaled salbutamol. A significant reduction in the RACS (see glossary, p 300) measured after 4 hours was found in the dexamethasone group versus placebo (means difference −1.8, 95% CI −0.175 to −3.425), but no significant difference was found at day 7 (difference in means 0.4, 95% CI −2.1 to 2.8). Admission rates measured at the emergency ward were significantly reduced with dexamethasone (7/36 [19%] with dexamethasone *v* 15/34 [44%] with placebo; RR 0.44, 95% CI 0.21 to 0.95).[34] Three small long term follow up RCTs (3 years,[35] 3–5 years,[36] and 2 years[37]) used telephone questionnaires to examine the effect of corticosteroids during the acute episode on subsequent wheezing. Two of the three RCTs did not observe any benefit from corticosteroids. The third was an unblinded RCT in which 117 hospitalised infants (mean age 2.6 months, requiring hospital treatment because of respiratory syncytial virus bronchiolitis) were allocated to be in a control group (41 infants), and received inhaled budesonide for 7 days (40 infants) or inhaled budesonide for 2 months (36 infants).[37] However, this RCT had several problems that compromised its validity (see comment below).

Harms: The acute adverse effects of oral corticosteroids are well documented, and include hyperglycaemia and immunosuppression. The RCTs did not give information on these. See harms of corticosteroids in asthma in children, p 262.

Comment: The evidence presented in the systematic review[25] is difficult to interpret because some of the RCTs did not exclude children with a history of wheezing who may have asthma, a condition likely to respond to corticosteroids. The clinical scales used in the RCTs included oxygen saturation, but the clinical relevance of changes in this parameter are unclear. Even if the results are accepted at face value, the clinical significance of an effect size is unclear. Furthermore, eight RCTs with more than double the number of people were not included in the meta-analysis. All of these RCTs, except one, did not find a benefit of corticosteroids, and the single RCT that did only observed a transient improvement in clinical score at one timepoint. Another systematic review is under way (Wang E, personal communication, 2001). We found inadequate evidence to evaluate the effects of systemic versus inhaled corticosteroids. The unblinded RCT comparing two different regimens of inhaled budesonide in hospitalised children had several problems that further compromised its validity.[37] Diagnosis of asthma was based only on a telephone survey; the children were not assessed to establish whether they had received additional interventions or exposures that could explain the results.

OPTION ANTIBIOTICS (ROUTINE)

One unblinded RCT found no evidence that routine antibiotics (ampicillin, penicillin, or erythromycin) versus no antibiotics are of clinical benefit in children admitted to hospital with bronchiolitis and uncomplicated respiratory syncytial virus pneumonia, although the RCT may have been too small to exclude a clinically important effect.

Benefits: We found no systematic review. We found one unblinded RCT (138 children admitted to hospital with clinically apparent pneumonia, 45% of whom were diagnosed with respiratory syncytial virus infection) comparing the routine use of antibiotics (ampicillin, penicillin, or erythromycin) versus no antibiotics (no placebo see comment below).[38] It found no significant difference between treatment groups in the proportion of children infected with respiratory syncytial virus. It found no evidence that antibiotics reduced duration of hospital stay or respiratory rate, or improved clinical symptoms, clinical signs, or radiographic assessment scores for pulmonary disease.

Harms: The RCT did not report harms, although potential risks include superinfection with resistant bacteria and drug reactions.

Comment: The RCT was unblinded and used block randomisation (children were randomised in groups of 20).[38] This reduces confidence in the results. The RCT may have been too small to exclude a clinically important effect. Two children initially treated without antibiotics were switched to antibiotics because of complicating purulent infections. Analysis was by intention to treat.

OPTION RIBAVIRIN

One systematic review found no good evidence that ribavirin reduced mortality, risk of respiratory deterioration, or duration of hospital stay in children admitted to hospital with respiratory syncytial virus bronchiolitis. It found some evidence that ribavirin reduced the duration of mechanical ventilation. One subsequent RCT found no evidence that ribavirin reduced duration of hospital stay or admission rate due to lower respiratory tract symptoms during the first year after the acute episode.

Benefits: We found one systematic review (search date 1999, 10 small RCTs).[39] The review found that, in children and infants hospitalised with respiratory syncytial virus bronchiolitis, ribavirin (tribavirin) compared with placebo did not significantly reduce mortality (5/86 [6%] with ribavirin *v* 7/72 [10%] with placebo; RR 0.61, 95% CI 0.21 to 1.75), respiratory deterioration (4/56 [7%] with ribavirin *v* 11/60 [18%] with placebo; RR 0.42, 95% CI 0.15 to 1.17), or duration of hospital stay (1.9 days less with ribavirin *v* placebo, 95% CI –0.9 to +4.6 days), but duration of ventilation was significantly reduced (1.2 days, 95% CI 0.2 to 3.4 days).[39] The high mortality in both groups may have been because of severe disease at baseline. One subsequent RCT (40 hospitalised infants who received ribavirin or placebo within 12 h of admission) found no significant differences in outcomes measured during the acute episode, such as the duration of oxygen supplementation need (ribavirin 2.72 days *v* placebo 1.92 days; mean difference 0.80 days, 95% CI –0.73 to +2.32 days) or hospital stay (ribavirin 4.94 days *v* placebo 3.36 days; mean difference 1.58 days, 95% CI –0.18 to +3.35 days).[40] That RCT also followed the infants for 1 year after the initial episode. It found no significant differences in admission rates associated with recurrent lower respiratory illness (2/16 [13%] with ribavirin *v* 3/19 [16%] with placebo; RR 0.79, 95% CI 0.15 to 4.17) or use of bronchodilators (5/16 [31%] with ribavirin *v* 8/19 [42%] with placebo; RR 0.74, 95% CI 0.30 to 1.82). However, the sample size may have been too small to rule out a clinically important difference.

Harms: We found no results from prospective studies. The review did not report harms.[39] We found case reports of headaches and contact lens dysfunction in carers. Ribavirin has been reported to be associated with acute bronchospasm in treated children. The standard aerosol is sticky, and clogging of ventilatory equipment has been reported.[41]

Comment: We found one small prospective study comparing pulmonary function tests in 54 children previously randomised to inpatient treatment with ribavirin or placebo.[42] It found no evidence of long term differences in outcome, although the study was not sufficiently powerful to rule out a clinically important difference.

OPTION IMMUNOGLOBULINS

Small, low powered RCTs found insufficient evidence about the effects of immunoglobulins versus albumin solution or versus saline in children admitted to hospital with bronchiolitis.

Benefits: We found no systematic review but found five RCTs (4 using albumin solution as control, 1 using saline, 335 children in total).[43–47] Two RCTs used pooled immunoglobulins, two RCTs used respiratory syncytial virus immunoglobulin (RSV Ig), and one RCT used palivizumab (synthetic monoclonal antibody). Neither RCT using RSV Ig found evidence that RSV Ig shortened duration of hospital stay compared with albumin (in high risk children [see glossary, p 300]: mean duration of hospital stay 8.41 days with RSV Ig *v* 8.89 days with albumin, P = NS; in non-high risk children: mean stay 4.58 days with RSV Ig *v* 5.52 days with albumin, P = NS; CIs not reported).[43,44] The third RCT (35 children) found no evidence that palivizumab reduced duration of hospital stay (mean 14.5 days, 95% CI 12.4 to 16.6 days with RSV Ig *v* 11.5 days, 95% CI 10.0 to 13.0 with placebo; P = 0.25), duration of ventilation (mean 8.8 days, 95% CI 6.5 to 11.1 days with palivizumab *v* 6.2 days, 95% CI 4.7 to 7.7 days with placebo; P = 0.45), or duration of treatment with supplemental oxygen (mean 12.3 days, 95% CI 10.0 to 14.6 days with palivizumab *v* 9.5 days, 95% CI 7.9 to 11.1 days with placebo; P = 0.47).[47] Neither of the remaining RCTs found any evidence that pooled immunoglobulins improved outcome in children with bronchiolitis.

Harms: The RCTs found that RSV Ig was associated with elevation in liver enzymes and anoxic spells (no frequencies provided).[43] One unblinded RCT (249 children) of prophylactic RSV Ig found that adverse effects occurred in about 3% of treated children.[10] That RCT and a subsequent analysis of the data found that effects included increased respiratory rate, mild fluid overload during the first infusion, urticarial reaction at the infusion site, mild decreases in oxygen saturation, and fever (no frequencies provided).[10,48]

Comment: Four RCTs used albumin as control. The effects of albumin in bronchiolitis are not known.

GLOSSARY

Cohort segregation Children infected with different viral strains are segregated from each other and treated separately, with the aim of preventing cross-infection.
Disease severity Mild: not requiring hospitalisation. Moderate: requiring hospitalisation but not intubation. Severe: requiring intubation or artificial ventilation.
High risk children Premature infants with or without bronchopulmonary dysplasia, or infants and children with congenital heart disease.
RACS Respiratory Assessment Change Score.
RDAI Respiratory Distress Assessment Instrument.

Substantive changes

Bronchodilators One additional RCT versus placebo[20] and three comparing different interventions;[21–23] conclusions unchanged.
Corticosteroids One additional RCT versus placebo;[34] conclusions unchanged.

REFERENCES

1. Phelan P, Olinsky A, Robertson C. *Respiratory illness in children.* 4th ed. London: Blackwell Scientific Publications, 1994.
2. Gruber W. Bronchiolitis. In: Long S, Pickering L, Prober C, eds. *Principles and practice of pediatric infectious diseases.* 1st ed. New York: Churchill Livingstone, 1997:1821.
3. Glezen WP, Taber LH, Frank AL, et al. Risk of primary infection and reinfection with respiratory syncytial virus. *Am J Dis Child* 1986;140:543–546.
4. Navas L, Wang E, de Carvalho V, et al. Improved outcome of respiratory syncytial virus infections in a high-risk hospitalized population of Canadian children. *J Pediatr* 1992;121:348–354.

5. Wang EEL, Law BJ, Stephens D, PICNIC. Pediatric Investigators Collaborative Network on Infections in Canada (PICNIC) study of morbidity and risk factors with RSV disease. *J Pediatr* 1995;126:212–219.
6. Wang EEL, Law BJ, Boucher F, et al. Pediatric Investigators Collaborative Network on Infections in Canada (PICNIC) study of admission and management variation in patients hospitalized with respiratory syncytial viral lower respiratory infection. *J Pediatr* 1996;129:390–395.
7. McConnochie KM, Mark JD, McBride JT, et al. Normal pulmonary function measurements and airway reactivity in childhood after mild bronchiolitis. *J Pediatr* 1985;107:54–58.
8. McConnochie KM, Roghmann KJ. Parental smoking, presence of older siblings and family history of asthma increase risk of bronchiolitis. *Am J Dis Child* 1986;140:806–812.
9. Sly PD, Hibbert ME. Childhood asthma following hospitalization with acute viral bronchiolitis in infancy. *Pediatr Pulmonol* 1989;7:153–158.
10. Wang EEL, Tang NK. Immunoglobulin for preventing respiratory syncytial virus infection. In: The Cochrane Library, Issue 3, 2001. Oxford: Update Software. Search date 1999; primary sources Cochrane Acute Respiratory Infections Trials Register, Medline, abstracts from the Pediatric Academy Meetings and the Intersciences Conference on Antimicrobial Agents and Chemotherapy from 1994–1997.
11. Simpson S, Burls A. *A systematic review of the effectiveness and cost-effectiveness of palivizumab (Synagis®) in the prevention of respiratory syncytial virus (RSV) infection in infants at high risk of infection*. Birmingham: West Midlands Health Technology Assessment Group, University of Birmingham, 2001.
12. Krasinski K, LaCouture R, Holzman R, et al. Screening for respiratory syncytial virus and assignment to a cohort at admission to reduce nosocomial transmission. *J Pediatr* 1990;116:894–898.
13. Isaacs D, Dickson H, O'Callaghan C, et al. Handwashing and cohorting in prevention of hospital acquired infections with respiratory syncytial virus. *Arch Dis Child* 1991;66:227–231.
14. Gala CL, Hall CB, Schnabel KC, et al. The use of eye-nose goggles to control nosocomial respiratory syncytial virus infection. *JAMA* 1986;256:2706–2708.
15. Hall CB, Douglas RG. Nosocomial respiratory syncytial virus infections: should gowns and masks be used? *Am J Dis Child* 1981;135:512–515.
16. Murphy D, Todd JK, Chao RK, et al. The use of gowns and masks to control respiratory illness in pediatric hospital personnel. *J Pediatr* 1981;99:746–750.
17. Madge P, Paton JY, McColl JH, et al. Prospective controlled study of four infection-control procedures to prevent nosocomial infection with respiratory syncytial virus. *Lancet* 1992;340:1079–1083.
18. Kellner JD, Ohlsson A, Gadomski AM, et al. Bronchodilators for bronchiolitis. In: The Cochrane Library, Issue 3, 2001. Oxford: Update Software. Search date 1998; primary sources Medline, Embase, Reference Update, reference lists of articles, and files of the authors.
19. Flores G, Horwitz RI. Efficacy of beta 2-agonists in bronchiolitis: a reappraisal and meta-analysis. *Pediatrics* 1997;100:233–239. Search date 1995; primary sources Medline and hand searched references and selected journals.
20. Abul-Ainine A, Luyt D. Short term effects of adrenaline in bronchiolitis: a randomised controlled trial. *Arch Dis Child* 2002;86:276–279.
21. Sanchez I, De Koster J, Powell RE, et al. Effect of racemic epinephrine and salbutamol on clinical score and pulmonary mechanics in infants with bronchiolitis. *J Pediatr* 1993;122:145–151.
22. Menon K, Sutcliffe T, Klassen TP. A randomized trial comparing the efficacy of epinephrine with salbutamol in the treatment of acute bronchiolitis. *J Pediatr* 1995;126:1004–1007.
23. Reijonen T, Korppi M, Pitkakangas S, et al. The clinical efficacy of nebulized racemic epinephrine and albuterol in acute bronchiolitis. *Arch Pediatr Adolesc Med* 1995;149:686–692.
24. Gadomski AM, Lichenstein R, Horton L, et al. Efficacy of albuterol in the management of bronchiolitis. *Pediatrics* 1994;93:907–912.
25. Garrison MM, Christakis DA, Harvey E, et al. Systemic corticosteroids in infant bronchiolitis: a meta-analysis. *Pediatrics* 2000;105:e44. Search date 1999; primary sources Medline, Embase, and Cochrane Clinical Trials Registry.
26. Richter H, Seddon P. Early nebulized budesonide in the treatment of bronchiolitis and the prevention of postbronchiolitic wheezing. *J Pediatr* 1998;132:849–853.
27. Bulow SM, Nir M, Levin E. Prednisolone treatment for respiratory syncytial virus infection: a randomized controlled trial of 147 infants. *Pediatrics* 1999;104:77.
28. Tal A, Bavilski C, Yohai D, et al. Dexamethasone and salbutamol in the treatment of acute wheezing in infants. *Pediatrics* 1983;71:13–18.
29. Cade A, Brownlee KG, Conway SP. Randomised placebo-controlled trial of nebulised corticosteroids in acute respiratory syncytial viral bronchiolitis. *Arch Dis Child* 2000;82:126–130.
30. Connolly JH, Field CM, Glasgow JF, et al. A double blind trial of prednisolone in epidemic bronchiolitis due to respiratory syncytial virus. *Acta Paediatr Scand* 1969;58:116–120.
31. Berger I, Argaman Z, Schwartz SB. Efficacy of corticosteroids in acute bronchiolitis: short-term and long-term follow-up. *Pediatr Pulmonol* 1998;26:162–166.
32. Leer JA, Green JL, Heimlich EM, et al. Corticosteroid treatment in bronchiolitis. A controlled collaborative study in 297 infants and children. *Am J Dis Child* 1969;117:495–503.
33. Goebel J, Estrada B, Quinonez J, et al. Prednisolone plus albuterol versus albuterol alone in mild to moderate bronchiolitis. *Clin Pediatr* 2000;39:213–220.
34. Schuh S, Coates AL, Binnie R, et al. Efficacy of oral dexamethasone in outpatients with acute bronchiolitis. *J Pediatr* 2002;140:27–32.
35. Reijonen TM, Kotaniemi-Syrjanen A, Korhonen K, et al. Predictors of asthma three years after hospital admission for wheezing in infancy. *Pediatrics* 2000;106:1406–1412.
36. Van Woensel JBM, Kimpen JLL, Sprikkelman AB, et al. Long-term effects of prednisolone in the acute phase of bronchiolitis caused by respiratory syncytial virus. *Pediatr Pulmonol* 2000;30:92–96.
37. Kajosaari M, Syvanen P, Forars M, et al. Inhaled corticosteroids during and after respiratory syncytial virus-bronchiolitis may decrease subsequent asthma. *Pediatr Allergy Immunol* 2000;11:198–202.
38. Fris B, Andersen P, Brenoe E, et al. Antibiotic treatment of pneumonia and bronchiolitis: a prospective randomised study. *Arch Dis Child* 1984;59:1038–1045.
39. Randolph AG, Wang EEL. Ribavirin for respiratory syncytial virus lower respiratory tract infection. In: The Cochrane Library, Issue 3, 2001. Oxford: Update Software. Search date 1999; primary sources Medline, hand searched references, and noted experts contacted.

40. Everard ML, Swarbrick A, Rigby AS, et al. The effect of ribavirin to treat previously healthy infants admitted with acute bronchiolitis on acute and chronic respiratory morbidity. *Respir Med* 2001;95:275–280.
41. Johnson EM. Developmental toxicity and safety evaluations of ribavirin. *Pediatr Infect Dis J* 1997;9(suppl):85–87.
42. Long CE, Voter KZ, Barker WH, et al. Long term follow-up of children hospitalized with respiratory syncytial virus lower respiratory tract infection and randomly treated with ribavirin or placebo. *Pediatr Infect Dis J* 1997;16:1023–1028.
43. Rodriguez WJ, Gruber WC, Welliver RC, et al. Respiratory syncytial virus (RSV) immune globulin intravenous therapy for RSV lower respiratory tract infection in infants and young children at high risk for severe RSV infections. *Pediatrics* 1997;99:454–461.
44. Rodriguez WJ, Gruber WC, Groothuis JR, et al. Respiratory syncytial virus immune globulin treatment of RSV lower respiratory tract infection in previously healthy children. *Pediatrics* 1997;100:937–942.
45. Hemming VG, Rodriguez W, Kim HW, et al. Intravenous immunoglobulin treatment of respiratory syncytial virus infections in infants and young children. *Antimicrob Agents Chemother* 1987;31:1882–1886.
46. Rimensberger PC, Burek-Kozlowska A, Morell A, et al. Aerosolized immunoglobulin treatment of respiratory syncytial virus infection in infants. *Pediatr Infect Dis J* 1996;15:209–216.
47. Malley R, DeVincenzo J, Ramilo O, et al. Reduction of respiratory syncytial virus (RSV) in tracheal aspirates in intubated infants by use of humanized monoclonal antibody to RSV F protein. *J Infect Dis* 1998;178:1555–1561.
48. Groothuis JR, Levin MJ, Rodriguez W, et al. Use of intravenous gamma globulin to passively immunize high-risk children against respiratory syncytial virus: safety and pharmacokinetics. *Antimicrob Agents Chemother* 1991;35:1469–1473.

Juan Manuel Lozano
Associate Professor
Department of Paediatrics and Clinical Epidemiology Unit
School of Medicine Universidad Javeriana
Bogotá DC
Colombia

Competing interests: None declared.

TABLE 1 Studies of adrenaline (epinephrine) versus salbutamol in bronchiolitis: results of RCTs (see text, p 296).

Ref	Allocation/ blinding	Intervention	Number of children	Outcome	Results
21	Random/ blinded, crossover design	Nebulised racemic adrenaline or salbutamol	24 Inpatients	Clinical score at 20–30 min	Improvement with adrenaline
22	Random/ blinded	Nebulised adrenaline or salbutamol	41 emergency room patients	Pulse oximetry; RDAI scores at 30, 60, and 90 min; admission rate	Transient effect at 60 min; fewer admissions
23	Random/ blinded, factorial design	Nebulised racemic adrenaline, salbutamol or saline placebo	100 emergency room patients	RDAI and RACS scores at 15 and 30 min	Unclear differences

RACS, Respiratory Assessment Change Score; RDAI, Respiratory Distress Assessment Instrument.

TABLE 2 Studies of corticosteroids versus placebo in bronchiolitis: results of RCTs (see text, p 297).

Ref	Allocation/blinding	Intervention	Number of children	Outcome	Results
26	Random/blinded	Nebulised budesonide	40	Clinical score and condition at 6 months	No benefit
27	Random/blinded	Prednisolone/ methylprednisolone	147	Hospital stay; supportive measures in hospital; condition at 1 month and 1 year after discharge	No benefit
28	Random/blinded, factorial design	Dexamethasone/placebo salbutamol/placebo	32	Clinical score and hospital stay	No benefit
29	Random/blinded	Budesonide	161	Hospital stay; time taken to be symptom free; readmission rates; GP consultation	No benefit
30	Random/blinded	Prednisolone	95	Duration of illness after hospitalisation	No benefit
31	Random/blinded	All had salbutamol; prednisone	38	Clinical score; oxygen saturation; condition at 7 days and 2 years later	No benefit
32	Random/blinded	Betamethasone	297	Nine respiratory tract signs; fever and complications after admission	No benefit
33	Random/blinded	All children received salbutamol (oral or inhaled) prednisolone	48	Bronchiolitis score at day 2	Transient effect only on day 2
34	Random/blinded	Oral dexamethasone	70	Clinical score and admission rate	Improvement in clinical score and admission rate

Cardiorespiratory arrest

Search date February 2002

Kate Ackerman and David Creery

QUESTIONS

INTERVENTIONS

*Although we found no direct evidence to support their use, widespread consensus holds that these interventions should be universally applied to children who have arrested on the basis of indirect evidence and extrapolation from adult data. Placebo controlled trials would be considered unethical.

See glossary, p 310

Key Messages

- **Bystander cardiopulmonary resuscitation** It is widely accepted that cardiopulmonary resuscitation should be undertaken in children who have arrested. Placebo controlled trials would be considered unethical. One systematic review of observational studies has found that children who received bystander cardiopulmonary resuscitation versus no bystander cardiopulmonary resuscitation were more likely to survive to hospital discharge.
- **Intubation versus bag-mask ventilation** One controlled clinical trial, in children requiring airway management in the community, found no significant difference with endotracheal intubation versus bag-mask ventilation in survival or neurological outcome.
- **Airway management and ventilation; direct current cardiac shock; standard dose intravenous adrenaline (epinephrine)** Although we found no direct evidence to support their use, widespread consensus based on indirect evidence and extrapolation from adult data holds that these interventions should be universally applied to children who have arrested. Placebo controlled trials would be considered unethical.
- **High dose intravenous adrenaline (epinephrine); intravenous bicarbonate; intravenous calcium; training parents to perform cardiopulmonary resuscitation** We found no RCTs or prospective cohort studies on the effects of these interventions in children who have arrested in the community.

DEFINITION Non-submersion out of hospital cardiorespiratory arrest in children is a state of pulselessness and apnoea occurring outside of a medical facility and not caused by submersion in water.[1]

INCIDENCE/ PREVALENCE We found 12 studies (3 prospective, 9 retrospective) reporting the incidence of non-submersion out of hospital cardiorespiratory arrest in children (see table 1, p 311).[2–13] Eleven studies reported the incidence in both adults and children, and eight reported the incidence in children.[2–9,11-13] Incidence of arrests in the general population ranged from 2.2–5.7/100 000 people a year (mean 3.1, 95% CI 2.1 to 4.1). Incidence of arrests in children ranged from 6.9–18.0/100 000 children a year (mean 10.6, 95% CI 7.1 to 14.1).[8] One prospective study (300 children) found that about 50% of out of hospital cardiorespiratory arrests occurred in children under 12 months, and about two thirds occurred in children under 18 months.[11]

AETIOLOGY/ RISK FACTORS We found 26 studies reporting the causes of non-submersion pulseless arrests (see glossary, p 310) in a total of 1574 children. The commonest causes of arrest were undetermined causes as in sudden infant death syndrome (see glossary, p 310) (39%), trauma (18%), chronic disease (7%), and pneumonia (4%) (see table 2, p 312).[1,3-12,14-28]

PROGNOSIS We found no systematic review that investigated non-submersion arrests alone. We found 27 studies (5 prospective, 22 retrospective; total of 1754 children) that reported only on out of hospital arrest.[1–12,14-28] The overall survival rate following out of hospital arrest was 5% (87 children). Nineteen of these studies (1140 children) found that of the 48 surviving children, 12 (25%) had no or mild neurological disability and 36 (75%) had moderate or severe neurological disability. We found one systematic review (search date 1997), which reported outcomes after cardiopulmonary resuscitation for both in hospital and out of hospital arrests of any cause, including submersion in children.[29] Studies were excluded if they did not report survival. The review found evidence from prospective and retrospective observational studies that out of hospital arrest of any cause in children carries a poorer prognosis than arrest within hospital (132/1568 children [8%] survived to hospital discharge after out of hospital arrest *v* 129/544 children [24%] after in hospital arrests). About half of the survivors were involved in studies that reported neurological outcome. Of these, survival with "good neurological outcome" (i.e. normal or mild neurological deficit) was higher in children who arrested in hospital compared with those who arrested elsewhere (60/77 surviving children [78%] in hospital *v* 28/68 [41%] elsewhere).[29]

AIMS To improve survival and minimise neurological sequelae in children suffering non-submersion out of hospital cardiorespiratory arrest.

OUTCOMES Out of hospital death rate; rate of death in hospital without return of spontaneous circulation; return of spontaneous circulation with subsequent death in hospital; and return of spontaneous circulation with successful hospital discharge with mild, moderate, severe, or no neurological sequelae; adverse effects of treatment.

METHODS *Clinical Evidence* search and appraisal February 2002. In addition, we searched citation lists of retrieved articles and relevant review articles. Studies reporting out of hospital arrest in adults that listed "adolescent" as a MeSH heading were also reviewed. Both authors reviewed the retrieved studies independently and differences were resolved by discussion. We selected studies reporting out of hospital cardiorespiratory arrests in children. Studies were excluded if data relating to submersion could not be differentiated from non-submersion data (except where we found no data relating exclusively to non-submersion arrest; in such cases we have included studies that did not differentiate these types of arrest, and have made it clear that such evidence is limited by this fact). Some features of cardiorespiratory arrest in adults appear to be different from arrest in children, so studies were excluded if data for adults could not be differentiated from data for children.

QUESTION What are the effects of treatments for non-submersion out of hospital cardiorespiratory arrest?

OPTION AIRWAY MANAGEMENT AND VENTILATION

It is widely accepted that good airway management and rapid ventilation should be undertaken in a child who has arrested, and it would be considered unethical to test its role in a placebo controlled trial.

Benefits: We found no studies comparing airway management and ventilation versus no intervention.

Harms: We found insufficient information.

Comment: It would be considered unethical to test the role of airway management and ventilation in a placebo controlled trial.

OPTION INTUBATION VERSUS BAG-MASK VENTILATION

One controlled trial found no evidence of a difference in survival or neurological outcome between bag-mask ventilation and endotracheal intubation in children requiring airway management in the community.

Benefits: We found no systematic review. We found one high quality controlled trial (830 children requiring airway management in the community, including 98 children who had arrested after submersion) comparing (using alternate day allocation) bag-mask ventilation versus endotracheal intubation (given by paramedic staff trained in these techniques).[30] Treatments were not randomised; each was allocated on alternate days. Analysis was by intention to treat (see comment below). The trial found no significant difference in rates of survival or good neurological outcome (normal, mild deficit, or no change from baseline function) between the two treatment groups (105/349 [30%] survived after bag-mask ventilation *v* 90/373 [24%] after intubation; OR 1.36, 95% CI 0.97 to 1.89; good neurological outcome achieved in 80/349 [23%] of children after bag-mask ventilation *v* 70/373 [19%] after intubation; OR 1.27, 95% CI 0.89 to 1.83; OR for non-submersion cardiorespiratory arrest calculated by author).

Harms: The trial found that time spent at the scene of the arrest was longer when intubation was intended, and this was the only significant determinant of a longer total time from dispatch of paramedic team to arrival at hospital (mean time at scene 9 min with bag-mask *v* 11 min with intubation; P < 0.001; mean total time 20 min with bag-mask *v* 23 min with intubation; P < 0.001).[30] However, the trial found no significant difference between bag-mask ventilation and intubation for complications common to both treatments (complications in 727 children for whom data were available, bag-mask *v* intubation: gastric distension 31% *v* 7%; P = 0.20; vomiting 14% *v* 14%; P = 0.82; aspiration 14% *v* 15%; P = 0.84; oral or airway trauma 1% *v* 2%; P = 0.24). A total of 186 children across both treatment groups were thought by paramedical staff to be successfully intubated. Of these, oesophageal intubation occurred in three children (2%); the tube became dislodged in 27 children (14%; unrecognised in 12 children, recognised in 15); right main bronchus intubation occurred in 33 children (18%); and an incorrect size of tube was used in 44 children (24%). Death occurred in all but one of the children with oesophageal intubation or unrecognised dislodging of the tube.[30]

Comment: **Population characteristics:** The baseline characteristics of children did not differ significantly between groups in age, sex, ethnicity, or cause of arrest. The trial did not report the frequency of pulseless arrest (see glossary, p 310) versus respiratory arrest (see glossary, p 310). **Intention to treat:** Intubation and bag mask ventilation are not mutually exclusive. The study protocol allowed bag-mask ventilation before intubation and after unsuccessful intubation. Of 420 children allocated to intubation, 115 received bag-mask ventilation before intubation, 128 received bag-mask ventilation after attempted intubation, four were lost to follow up, and the remainder received intubation that was believed to be successful. Of 410 children allocated to bag-mask ventilation, 10 children were intubated successfully (although in violation of study protocol), nine received bag-mask ventilation after attempted intubation, six were lost to follow up, and the remainder received bag-mask ventilation in accordance with study protocol.[30]

OPTION INTRAVENOUS ADRENALINE (EPINEPHRINE)

Intravenous adrenaline (epinephrine) at "standard dose" (0.01 mg/kg) is a widely accepted treatment for establishing return of spontaneous circulation. We found no prospective evidence comparing adrenaline (epinephrine) versus placebo, or comparing standard or single doses versus high or multiple doses of adrenaline (epinephrine), in children who have arrested in the community.

Benefits: We found no systematic review, no RCTs, and no prospective observational studies.

Harms: We found no prospective data in this context.

Comment: **Versus placebo:** Standard dose adrenaline (epinephrine) is a widely accepted treatment for arrests in children. Placebo controlled trials would be considered unethical. **High versus low dose:** Two small retrospective studies (128 people) found no evidence of a difference in survival to hospital discharge between low or single dose and high or multiple dose adrenaline (epinephrine), although the studies were too small to rule out an effect.[8,12]

OPTION INTRAVENOUS BICARBONATE

We found no RCTs on the effects of intravenous bicarbonate in out of hospital cardiorespiratory arrest in children.

Benefits: We found no RCTs.

Harms: We found insufficient evidence.

Comment: Bicarbonate is widely believed to be effective in arrest associated with hyperkalaemic ventricular tachycardia or fibrillation, but we found no prospective evidence supporting this.

OPTION INTRAVENOUS CALCIUM

We found no RCTs on the effects of intravenous calcium in out of hospital cardiorespiratory arrest in children.

Benefits: We found no RCTs.

Harms: We found insufficient evidence.

Comment: Calcium is widely believed to be effective in arrest associated with hyperkalaemic ventricular tachycardia or fibrillation, but we found no prospective evidence supporting this.

OPTION BYSTANDER CARDIOPULMONARY RESUSCITATION

It is widely accepted that cardiopulmonary resuscitation and ventilation should be undertaken in children who have arrested. Placebo controlled trials would be considered unethical. We found no RCTs on the effects of training parents to perform cardiopulmonary resuscitation. One systematic review of observational studies has found that children who were witnessed having an arrest and who received bystander cardiopulmonary resuscitation were more likely to survive to hospital discharge.

Benefits: We found no RCTs. We found one systematic review (search date 1997) of prospective and retrospective studies.[29] This concluded that survival was improved in children who were witnessed to arrest and received cardiopulmonary resuscitation from a bystander. Of 150 witnessed arrests outside hospital, 28/150 (19%) survived to hospital discharge. Of those children who received bystander cardiopulmonary resuscitation, 20/76 (26%) survived to discharge.[29] The review did not report survival rates in children whose arrests were not witnessed, but the overall survival rate for out of hospital cardiac arrest was 8%. **Training parents to perform cardiopulmonary resuscitation:** We found no systematic review and no RCTs examining the effects of training parents to perform cardiopulmonary resuscitation in children who have arrested outside hospital.

Harms: Potential harms include those resulting from unnecessary chest compression after respiratory arrest with intact circulation.

Comment: The review of observational studies found that children who received bystander cardiopulmonary resuscitation had a hospital discharge rate of 20/76 (26%) versus 8/74 (11%) for children who also had their arrests witnessed but had not received cardiopulmonary resuscitation. Cardiopulmonary resuscitation was not randomly allocated and children resuscitated may be systematically different from those who did not receive resuscitation. The apparent survival rates for witnessed arrests and arrests with bystander initiated cardiopulmonary resuscitation may be artificially high because of inappropriate evaluation of true arrest. However, assuming confounding variables were evenly distributed between groups, then the best estimate of the benefit of cardiopulmonary resuscitation is a 15% absolute increase in the probability that children will be discharged alive from hospital.

OPTION DIRECT CURRENT CARDIAC SHOCK

It is widely accepted that children who arrest outside hospital and are found to have ventricular fibrillation or pulseless ventricular tachycardia should receive direct current cardiac shock treatment. Placebo controlled trials would be considered unethical. We found no RCTs on the effects of direct current cardiac shock in children who have arrested in the community, regardless of the heart rhythm.

Benefits: We found no systematic review and no RCTs.

Harms: We found insufficient evidence.

Comment: **In children with ventricular fibrillation:** One retrospective study (29 children with ventricular fibrillation who had arrested out of hospital from a variety of causes, including submersion) found that of 27 children who were defibrillated, 11 survived (5 with no sequelae, 6 with severe disability). The five children with good outcome all received defibrillation within 10 minutes of arrest (time to defibrillation not given for those who died). Data on the two children who were not defibrillated were not presented.[31] **In children with asystole:** One retrospective study in 90 children with asystole (see glossary, p 310) (including those who had arrested after submersion) found that 49 (54%) had received direct current cardiac shock treatment. None of the children survived to hospital discharge, regardless of whether or not direct current cardiac shock was given.[32] We found one systematic review (search date 1997) of observational studies (1420 children who had arrested outside hospital) that recorded electrocardiogram rhythm.[29] Bradyasystole or pulseless electrical activity (see glossary, p 310) were found in 73%, whereas ventricular fibrillation or pulseless ventricular tachycardia (see glossary, p 310) were found in 10%.[29] The review found that survival after ventricular fibrillation or ventricular tachycardia arrest was higher than after asystolic arrest in children. Survival to discharge reported in the systematic review was 39/802 (5%) for children with initial rhythm asystole (see glossary, p 310) and 30% (29/97) with initial rhythm ventricular fibrillation (see glossary, p 310) or ventricular tachycardia.[29]

GLOSSARY

Asystole The absence of cardiac electrical activity
Bradyasystole Bradycardia clinically indistinguishable from asystole
Initial rhythm asystole The absence of cardiac electrical activity at initial determination
Initial rhythm ventricular fibrillation Electrical rhythm is ventricular fibrillation at initial determination
Pulseless arrest Absence of palpable pulse
Pulseless electrical activity The presence of cardiac electrical activity in absence of a palpable pulse
Pulseless ventricular tachycardia Electrical rhythm of ventricular tachycardia in absence of a palpable pulse
Respiratory arrest Absence of respiratory activity
Sudden infant death syndrome The sudden unexpected death of a child, usually between the ages of 1 month and 1 year, for which a thorough postmortem examination does not define an adequate cause of death. Near miss sudden infant death syndrome refers to survival of a child after an unexpected arrest of unknown cause

REFERENCES

1. Schindler MB, Bohn D, Cox PN, et al. Outcome of out of hospital cardiac or respiratory arrest in children. *N Engl J Med* 1996;335:1473–1479.
2. Broides A, Sofer S, Press J. Outcome of out of hospital cardiopulmonary arrest in children admitted to the emergency room. *Isr Med Assoc J* 2000;2:672–674.
3. Eisenberg M, Bergner L, Hallstrom A. Epidemiology of cardiac arrest and resuscitation in children. *Ann Emerg Med* 1983;12:672–674.
4. Applebaum D, Slater PE. Should the Mobile Intensive Care Unit respond to pediatric emergencies? *Clin Pediatr (Phila)* 1986;25:620–623.
5. Tsai A, Kallsen G. Epidemiology of pediatric prehospital care. *Ann Emerg Med* 1987;16:284–292.
6. Thompson JE, Bonner B, Lower GM. Pediatric cardiopulmonary arrests in rural populations. *Pediatrics* 1990;86:302–306.
7. Safranek DJ, Eisenberg MS, Larsen MP. The epidemiology of cardiac arrest in young adults. *Ann Emerg Med* 1992;21:1102–1106.
8. Dieckmann RA, Vardis R. High-dose epinephrine in pediatric out of hospital cardiopulmonary arrest. *Pediatrics* 1995;95:901–913.
9. Kuisma M, Suominen P, Korpela R. Paediatric out of hospital cardiac arrests — epidemiology and outcome. *Resuscitation* 1995;30:141–150.
10. Ronco R, King W, Donley DK, Tilden SJ. Outcome and cost at a children's hospital following resuscitation for out of hospital cardiopulmonary arrest. *Arch Pediatr Adolesc Med* 1995;149:210–214.
11. Sirbaugh PE, Pepe PE, Shook JE, et al. A prospective, population-based study of the demographics, epidemiology, management, and outcome of out of hospital pediatric cardiopulmonary arrest. *Ann Emerg Med* 1999;33:174–184.
12. Friesen RM, Duncan P, Tweed WA, Bristow G. Appraisal of pediatric cardiopulmonary resuscitation. *Can Med Assoc J* 1982;126:1055–1058.
13. Hu SC. Out of hospital cardiac arrest in an Oriental metropolitan city. *Am J Emerg Med* 1994;12:491–494.
14. Barzilay Z, Somekh E, Sagy M, Boichis H. Pediatric cardiopulmonary resuscitation outcome. *J Med* 1988;19:229–241.
15. Bhende MS, Thompson AE. Evaluation of an end-tidal CO_2 detector during pediatric cardiopulmonary resuscitation. *Pediatrics* 1995;95:395–399.
16. Brunette DD, Fischer R. Intravascular access in pediatric cardiac arrest. *Am J Emerg Med* 1988;6:577–579.
17. Clinton JE, McGill J, Irwin G, Peterson G, Lilja GP, Ruiz E. Cardiac arrest under age 40: etiology and prognosis. *Ann Emerg Med* 1984;13:1011–1015.
18. Hazinski MF, Chahine AA, Holcomb GW, Morris JA. Outcome of cardiovascular collapse in pediatric blunt trauma. *Ann Emerg Med* 1994;23:1229–1235.
19. Losek JD, Hennes H, Glaeser P, Hendley G, Nelson DB. Prehospital care of the pulseless, nonbreathing pediatric patient. *Am J Emerg Med* 1987;5:370–374.
20. Ludwig S, Kettrick RG, Parker M. Pediatric cardiopulmonary resuscitation. A review of 130 cases. *Clin Pediatr (Phila)* 1984;23:71–75.
21. Nichols DG, Kettrick RG, Swedlow DB, Lee S, Passman R, Ludwig S. Factors influencing outcome of cardiopulmonary resuscitation in children. *Pediatr Emerg Care* 1986;2:1–5.

22. O'Rourke PP. Outcome of children who are apneic and pulseless in the emergency room. *Crit Care Med* 1986;14:466–468.
23. Rosenberg NM. Pediatric cardiopulmonary arrest in the emergency department. *Am J Emerg Med* 1984;2:497–499.
24. Sheikh A, Brogan T. Outcome and cost of open- and closed-chest cardiopulmonary resuscitation in pediatric cardiac arrests. *Pediatrics* 1994;93:392–398.
25. Suominen P, Rasanen J, Kivioja A. Efficacy of cardiopulmonary resuscitation in pulseless paediatric trauma patients. *Resuscitation* 1998;36:9–13.
26. Suominen P, Korpela R, Kuisma M, Silfvast T, Olkkola KT. Paediatric cardiac arrest and resuscitation provided by physician-staffed emergency care units. *Acta Anaesthesiol Scand* 1997;41:260–265.
27. Torphy DE, Minter MG, Thompson BM. Cardiorespiratory arrest and resuscitation of children. *Am J Dis Child* 1984;138:1099–1102.
28. Walsh R. Outcome of pre-hospital CPR in the pediatric trauma patient [abstract]. *Crit Care Med* 1994;22:A162.
29. Young KD, Seidel JS. Pediatric cardiopulmonary resuscitation: a collective review. *Ann Emerg Med* 1999;33:195–205. Search date 1997; primary sources Medline and bibliographic search.
30. Gausche M, Lewis RJ, Stratton SJ, et al. Effect of out of hospital pediatric endotracheal intubation on survival and neurological outcome. *JAMA* 2000;283:783–790.
31. Mogayzel C, Quan L, Graves JR, Tiedeman D, Fahrenbruch C, Herndon P. Out of hospital ventricular fibrillation in children and adolescents: causes and outcomes. *Ann Emerg Med* 1995;25:484–491.
32. Losek JD, Hennes H, Glaeser PW, Smith DS, Hendley G. Prehospital countershock treatment of pediatric asystole. *Am J Emerg Med* 1989;7:571–575.

Kate Ackerman
The Children's Hospital
Boston
USA

David Creery
Children's Hospital of Eastern Ontario
Ottawa
Canada

Competing interests: None declared.

TABLE 1 **Incidence of non-submersion out of hospital cardiorespiratory arrest in children* (see text, p 305).**

Reference	Location	Year	Incidence per 100 000 people in total population	Incidence per 100 000 children
12	Manitoba, Canada	1982	2.9	ND
3	King County, USA	1983	2.4	9.9
4	Jerusalem, Israel	1986	2.5	6.9
5	Fresno, USA	1987	5.7	ND
6	Midwestern USA	1990	4.7	ND
7	King County, USA	1992	2.4	10.1
13	Taipei, Taiwan	1994	1.3	ND
8	San Francisco, USA	1995	2.2	16.1
9	Helsinki, Finland	1995	1.4	9.1
10	Birmingham, USA	1995	ND	6.9
11	Houston, USA	1999	4.9	18.0
2	Southern Israel	2000	3.5	7.8

* Incidence represents arrests per 100 000 population per year. ND, no data.

TABLE 2 **Causes of non-submersion out of hospital cardiorespiratory arrest in children* (see text, p 305).**

Cause	Number of arrests (%)	Number of survivors (%)
Undetermined	691 (43.9)	1 (0.1)
Trauma	311 (19.8)	10 (3.2)
Chronic disease	126 (8.0)	9 (7.1)
Pneumonia	75 (4.8)	6 (8.0)
Non-accidental injury	23 (1.5)	2 (8.7)
Aspiration	20 (1.3)	0 (0)
Overdose	19 (1.2)	3 (15.8)
Other	309 (19.6)	28 (9.1)
Total	**1574 (100)**	**59 (3.7)**

*Figures represent the numbers of arrests/survivors in children with each diagnosis.

Constipation

Search date April 2002

Gregory Rubin

QUESTIONS

INTERVENTIONS

*Not widely licensed for use in children. Clinical use in adults recently restricted because of heart rhythm abnormalities. See comments on cisapride under gastro-oesophageal reflux in children, p 340.

Key Messages

- **Biofeedback training (short term benefit only)** Three RCTs found that biofeedback plus conventional treatment (laxatives alone or laxatives plus dietary advice and toilet training) versus conventional treatment alone significantly improved defaecation dynamics and reduced rates of soiling after 3–7 months. Two of the RCTs found no significant difference after 1 year.
- **Cisapride** RCTs in an outpatient setting in people aged 2–18 years found that cisapride versus placebo significantly improved stool frequency and symptoms of constipation after 8–12 weeks of treatment. We found no evidence in primary care settings. Cisapride has been withdrawn in several countries because of suspected adverse cardiac effects.
- **Increased dietary fibre** We found no RCTs in children on the effects of increasing dietary fibre.
- **Medical treatment plus toilet training** One small RCT in children with encopresis found short term benefit from the addition of toilet training to medical treatment (enemas and osmotic or stimulant laxatives).
- **Osmotic laxatives** One RCT in children aged 8 months to 16 years found no significant difference with lactitol versus lactulose in stool frequency and consistency of stools, but found that lactulose significantly increased the proportion of children with abdominal pain and flatulence. Another RCT in children aged 11 months to 13 years found that lactitol versus lactulose significantly increased stool frequency and consistency after 15 days' treatment. A third RCT in infants aged 0–6 months found that lactulose significantly improved ease of evacuation and consistency of stools from baseline after 14 days' treatment. However, the benefits shown in these three RCTs are comparisons of outcomes before and after treatment, and were not necessarily because of the treatments.

- **Stimulant laxatives** We found no RCTs in children on the effects of stimulant laxatives versus placebo or alternative treatments. One small RCT in children with encopresis found short term benefit from the addition of toilet training or biofeedback to stimulant or osmotic laxatives.

DEFINITION Constipation is characterised by infrequent bowel evacuations; hard, small faeces; or difficult or painful defaecation. The frequency of bowel evacuation varies from person to person.[1] Encopresis is defined as involuntary bowel movements in inappropriate places at least once a month for 3 months or more, in children aged 4 years and older.[2]

INCIDENCE/ PREVALENCE Constipation with or without encopresis is common in children. It accounts for 3% of consultations to paediatric outpatient clinics and 25% of paediatric gastroenterology consultations in the USA.[3] Encopresis has been reported in 2% of children at school entry. The peak incidence is at 2–4 years of age.

AETIOLOGY/ RISK FACTORS No cause is discovered in 90–95% of children with constipation. Low fibre intake and a family history of constipation may be associated factors.[4] Psychosocial factors are often suspected, although most children with constipation are developmentally normal.[3] Chronic constipation can lead to progressive faecal retention, distension of the rectum, and loss of sensory and motor function. Organic causes for constipation are uncommon, but include Hirschsprung's disease (1/5000 births; male : female 4 : 1; constipation invariably present from birth), cystic fibrosis, anorectal physiological abnormalities, anal fissures, constipating drugs, dehydrating metabolic conditions, and other forms of malabsorption.[3]

PROGNOSIS Childhood constipation can be difficult to treat and often requires prolonged support, explanation, and medical treatment. In one long term follow up study of children presenting under the age of 5 years, 50% recovered within 1 year and 65–70% recovered within 2 years; the remainder required laxatives for daily bowel movements or continued to soil for years.[3] It is not known what proportion continue to have problems into adult life, although adults presenting with megarectum or megacolon often have a history of bowel problems from childhood.

AIMS To remove faecal impaction and to restore a bowel habit in which stools are soft and passed without discomfort.

OUTCOMES Number of defaecations per week; number of episodes of soiling per month; gut transit time as measured by timing the passage of radio-opaque pellets, which may be ingested within a gelatin capsule; use of laxatives.

METHODS *Clinical Evidence* update search and appraisal April 2002. Keywords: constipation, diet therapy, diagnosis, therapy, psychology, stimulant laxatives, dietary fibre, lactulose. The search was limited to infants and children. Trials were selected for inclusion if they focused on the management of constipation or encopresis, or both; if they were relevant to primary health care; and if they included children without an organic cause for constipation.

QUESTION What are the effects of treatments?

OPTION INCREASED DIETARY FIBRE

We found no RCTs on the effects of increasing dietary fibre in children.

Benefits: We found no systematic review or RCTs.

Harms: We found no good evidence.

Comment: None.

OPTION CISAPRIDE

Two RCTs in people aged 2–18 years found that cisapride versus placebo significantly improved stool frequency and symptoms of constipation after 8–12 weeks of treatment in an outpatient setting. We found no evidence from primary care settings. Cisapride has been withdrawn in several countries because of suspected adverse cardiac effects.

Benefits: We found no systematic review but found two RCTs.[5,6] One RCT (69 people, aged 4–18 years, attending hospital with constipation defined as pain, difficulty in defaecation, or ≤3–4 bowel movements/wk for at least 3 months in the absence of a history of bowel disease) compared cisapride (0.3 mg/kg/day as a syrup) versus placebo following clearance of accumulated stool. It found that after 8 weeks, cisapride significantly increased stool frequency (mean stool frequency/wk 6.75 with cisapride *v* 1.31 with placebo) and decreased gut transit time.[5] The second RCT (40 children, aged 2–16 years with a history of chronic constipation referred for evaluation to a paediatric hospital gastroenterology clinic) found significant benefit for cisapride over placebo at 12 weeks, measured by a composite of improved stool frequency, absence of faecal soiling, and no use of other laxatives (improvement in composite index 14/20 [70%] with cisapride *v* 7/20 [35%] with placebo; RR 2.00, CI 1.03 to 3.88; NNT 3, 95% CI 1 to 24).[6]

Harms: The RCTs did not report harms (see comment below).[5,6]

Comment: Cisapride is licensed for use in children in the Republic of Ireland. Its license has been suspended in the UK and Germany, and its marketing stopped in the USA because of its association with heart rhythm abnormalities in adults. See comments on cisapride under gastro-oesophageal reflux in children, p 344. An RCT comparing cisapride plus magnesium oxide versus magnesium oxide alone is being translated.[7]

OPTION OSMOTIC LAXATIVES

One RCT in children aged 8 months to 16 years found no significant difference with lactitol versus lactulose in stool frequency and consistency of stools, but found that lactulose significantly increased the proportion of children with abdominal pain and flatulence. Another RCT in children aged 11 months to 13 years found limited evidence that lactitol versus lactulose significantly increased stool frequency and consistency from baseline after 15 days' treatment. A third RCT in infants aged 0–6

months found that lactulose significantly improved ease of evacuation and consistency of stools from baseline after 14 days' treatment. However, the benefits shown in these three RCTs are comparisons of outcomes before and after treatment, and were not necessarily because of the treatments. One small RCT in children with encopresis found short term benefit from the addition of toilet training or biofeedback to stimulant or osmotic laxatives.

Benefits: We found no systematic review and no placebo controlled trials of osmotic laxatives in children. We found two small RCTs comparing the effects of lactitol versus lactulose on stool frequency and consistency.[8,9] The first RCT (51 children, aged 8 months to 16 years visiting a physician for chronic idiopathic constipation) found no significant difference in stool frequency or consistency of stools with lactitol versus lactulose.[8] It found that both lactitol and lactulose doubled stool frequency at 4 weeks compared with baseline, and significantly increased the proportion of children with normal stool consistency at 2 weeks. The second RCT (39 children, aged 11 months to 13 years) found that lactitol versus lactulose significantly increased stool frequency and consistency of stools after 15 days' treatment (English abstract only; detailed results will be reported following translation).[9] A third RCT (220 non-breastfed, constipated infants aged 0–6 months) compared 2% and 4% lactulose mixed with an artificial milk preparation.[10] At 14 days, over 90% of parents in both groups reported easy passage of normal or thin consistency stools ($P < 0.05$ compared with baseline). **With toilet training or biofeedback:** One RCT (87 children with encopresis) compared medical treatment (enemas and osmotic or stimulant laxatives) with and without toilet training.[11] A third arm of the trial evaluated biofeedback. Children receiving toilet training used significantly fewer laxatives and required fewer treatment sessions than those in the other two groups. Toilet training and biofeedback produced similar reductions in rates of soiling, which were greater than those achieved by medical treatment alone ($P < 0.04$).

Harms: The first RCT found that significantly fewer children taking lactitol versus lactulose had abdominal pain (22% with lactitol *v* 58% with lactulose; $P < 0.005$) or flatulence (30% with lactitol *v* 63% with lactulose; $P < 0.01$).[8]

Comment: The benefits shown in these RCTs are comparisons of outcomes before and after treatment, and were not necessarily because of the treatments.[8–10] Toilet training consisted of reinforcement and scheduling to promote response to the urge to defaecate, and instruction and modelling to promote appropriate straining.[11]

OPTION STIMULANT LAXATIVES

We found no RCTs in children on the effects of stimulant laxatives versus placebo or alternative treatments. One small RCT found short term benefit from the addition of toilet training or biofeedback to stimulant or osmotic laxatives.

Benefits: We found one systematic review (search date not stated), which found no RCTs of adequate methodological rigour comparing stimulant laxatives versus either placebo or alternative treatment in children.[12] We found no placebo controlled RCTs of the effects of stimulant laxatives in children. **With toilet training or biofeedback:** See osmotic laxatives, p 315.

Harms: None identified.

Comment: The studies identified by the review were all comparative, used multiple interventions, and had small sample sizes.[12] One quasi-randomised study (using last hospital number digit to allocate patients) compared senna versus mineral oil concentrate in 37 children (aged 3–12 years) with chronic constipation.[13] The study found that senna versus mineral oil was less effective in reducing involuntary faecal soiling after 6 months (8/18 [44%] with senna *v* 1/19 [5%] with mineral oil; RR 8.44, 95% CI 1.52 to 16.70). No significant differences were found in the number of children with relapses of constipation symptoms during the treatment period (12/19 [63%] with senna *v* 16/18 [89%] with mineral oil; RR 0.71, 95% CI 0.48 to 1.04).[13]

OPTION BIOFEEDBACK TRAINING

Three RCTs found that biofeedback plus conventional treatment (laxatives alone or laxatives plus dietary advice and toilet training) versus conventional treatment alone significantly improved defaecation dynamics and reduced rates of soiling after 3–7 months. Two of the RCTs found no significant difference in soiling, stool frequency, or laxative use after 1 year.

Benefits: We found no systematic review. Four RCTs compared conventional treatment (laxatives alone or laxatives plus dietary advice and toilet training) with or without biofeedback in 87,[11] 192,[14] 129,[15] and 41[16] children with constipation, encopresis, or both. The biofeedback compared 2–6 weeks of training[16] or seminars.[14] Three RCTs found that biofeedback significantly improved defaecation dynamics[14,16] and rates of soiling[11] after 3–7 months, but none of the RCTs found significant improvement in soiling, stool frequency, or laxative use at 1 year or more.

Harms: The RCTs gave no information on adverse effects.[11,14–16]

Comment: None.

REFERENCES

1. Nelson R, Wagget J, Lennard-Jones JE, et al. Constipation and megacolon in children and adults. In: Misiewicz JJ, Pounder RE, Venables CW, eds. *Diseases of the gut and pancreas*. 2nd ed. Oxford: Blackwell Science, 1994; 843–864.
2. American Psychiatric Association. *Diagnostic and statistical manual of mental disorders*. 4th ed. Washington, DC: American Psychiatric Association, 1994.
3. Loening-Baucke V. Chronic constipation in children. *Gastroenterology* 1993;105:557–1563.
4. Roma E, Adamidis D, Nikolara R, Constantopoulos A, Messaritakis J. Diet and chronic constipation in children: the role of fiber. *J Pediatr Gastroenterol Nutr* 1999;28:169–174.
5. Halibi IM. Cisapride in the management of chronic pediatric constipation. *J Pediatr Gastroenterol Nutr* 1999;28:199–202.
6. Nurko MD, Garcia-Aranda JA, Worona LB, et al. Cisapride for the treatment of constipation in children: a double blind study. *J Pediatr* 2000;136:35–40.
7. Ni YH, Lin CC, Chang SH, et al. Use of cisapride with magnesium oxide in chronic pediatric constipation. *Acta Paediatr Taiwan* 2001;42:345–349.
8. Pitzalis G, Mariani P, Chiarini-Testa MR, et al. Lactitol in chronic idiopathic constipation of childhood. *Pediatr Med Chir* 1995;17:223–226.

9. Martino AM, Pesce F, Rosati U. The effects of lactitol in the treatment of intestinal stasis in childhood. *Minerva Pediatr* 1992;44:319–323.
10. Hejlp M, Kamper J, Ebbesen F, et al. Infantile constipation and allomin-lactulose. Treatment of infantile constipation in infants fed with breast milk substitutes: a controlled trial of 2% and 4% allomin-lactulose. *Ugeskr Laeger* 1990;152:1819–1822.
11. Cox DJ, Sutphen J, Borowitz S, et al. Contribution of behaviour therapy and biofeedback to laxative therapy in the treatment of pediatric encopresis. *Ann Behav Med* 1998;20:70–76.
12. Price KJ, Elliott TM. What is the role of stimulant laxatives in the management of childhood constipation and soiling? In: The Cochrane Library, Issue 3, 2001. Oxford: Update Software. Search date not stated.
13. Sondheimer JM, Gervaise EP. Lubricant versus laxative in the treatment of chronic functional constipation of children: a comparative study. *J Pediatr Gastroenterol Nutr* 1982;1:223–226.
14. Van der Plas RN, Benninga MA, Büller HA, et al. Biofeedback training in treatment of childhood constipation: a randomised controlled study. *Lancet* 1996;348:776–780.
15. Loening-Baucke V. Biofeedback treatment for chronic constipation and encopresis in childhood: long term outcome. *Pediatrics* 1995;96:105–111.
16. Loening-Baucke V. Modulation of abnormal defecation dynamics by biofeedback treatment in chronically constipated children with encopresis. *J Pediatr* 1990;116:214–222.

Gregory Rubin
Professor of Primary Care
University of Sunderland
Sunderland
UK

Competing interests: None declared.

Croup

Search date January 2002

Martin Osmond

QUESTIONS

INTERVENTIONS

See glossary, p 328

Key Messages

- None of the RCTs we reviewed, in over 1000 infants with childhood croup, described any deaths related either to croup itself or to any associated treatment.

Primary care settings

- **Treatment in primary care settings** We found no RCTs on interventions for croup.

Primary paediatric assessment units

- **Nebulised adrenaline (epinephrine) versus placebo** One small RCT in children with stridor at rest has found that nebulised adrenaline versus placebo significantly improves symptoms within 30 minutes. Symptoms returned to pre-intervention severity within 2 hours in a third of children. One small RCT found no evidence of a difference between nebulised adrenaline and inhaled helium–oxygen mixture for symptom improvement.

- **Nebulised steroids versus placebo** RCTs conducted in children given humidified oxygen have found that nebulised steroids versus placebo significantly reduce poor responses after 2–5 hours, and reduce admissions to hospital (NNT 4, 95% CI 3 to 8). They found no significant difference in reattendance to any medical practitioner or institution after 1 week.
- **Systemic steroids versus placebo** Three RCTs have found that a single dose of oral or intramuscular dexamethasone versus placebo significantly improves symptoms within 5 hours, reduces admissions to hospital (NNT 2, 95% CI 1 to 3), and reduces reattendance to any medical practitioner or institution within 1 week of discharge (NNT 12, 95% CI 6 to 60).
- **Systemic versus nebulised steroids** RCTs have found no significant difference between systemic dexamethasone versus nebulised budesonide in improvement in symptoms or reattendance after discharge, but found that dexamethasone significantly reduced the number of children admitted to hospital.

Hospital setting

- **High versus low dose systemic steroid regimens** One RCT found limited evidence that a single dose of oral dexamethasone (0.3 mg.kg) is as effective as 0.6 mg/kg in children.
- **Inhalation of humidified air/oxygen** We found insufficient evidence from one RCT on the effects of humidified air or oxygen in children with croup.
- **Nebulised adrenaline versus placebo** One small RCT has found that nebulised adrenaline versus placebo significantly improves symptoms within 30 minutes, but found no significant difference after 2 hours. Two small RCTs found no significant difference between nebulised adrenaline versus placebo, but they may have been too small to exclude a clinically important difference.
- **Nebulised adrenaline versus steroids** We found insufficient evidence from one RCT to compare the effects of nebulised adrenaline versus steroids.
- **Nebulised steroids versus placebo** RCTs have found that nebulised steroids versus placebo significantly improve symptoms after 2 hours (NNT 2, 95% CI 1 to 8), reduce hospital stay, and reduce further medical attendance within 3 days of discharge.
- **Systemic steroids versus placebo** RCTs have found that systemic steroids versus placebo significantly improve symptoms after 12–24 hours (NNT 7, 95% CI 5 to 10) and reduce the length of hospital stay in children with croup.
- **Systemic versus nebulised steroids** We found no RCTs on the effects of systemic versus nebulised steroids in children with croup.

DEFINITION Croup is an acute clinical syndrome that is characterised by a harsh, barking cough, inspiratory stridor, and hoarse voice, caused by laryngeal or tracheal obstruction. Mild fever and rhinorrhoea may also be present. The most important differential diagnoses are acute epiglottitis, inhalation of a foreign body, and bacterial tracheitis.

INCIDENCE/ PREVALENCE Croup occurs in about 3% of children aged under 6 years per year,[1] and causes 2–3% of hospital admissions in young children in the UK.[2] One retrospective Belgian study of 5 to 8 year old children found that 16% of children had suffered from croup, and 5% had experienced recurrent croup (3 or more episodes).[3]

AETIOLOGY/ RISK FACTORS Croup is believed to be mainly viral in origin, but atopy plays a part in some children. The most common virus isolated is parainfluenza types 1, 2, or 3. Other viruses include influenza, adenovirus, respiratory syncytial virus, and rhinovirus.

PROGNOSIS Fewer than 2% of children with croup are admitted to hospital in the UK.[1] Of those admitted, only 1–2% require intubation. Mortality is low; out of 208 children who were given artificial airways over a 10 year period, two died.[4] Symptoms of upper airway obstruction can be extremely distressing to the child and to the family.

AIMS To reduce suffering and distress, need for hospital admission, duration of hospital stay, rates of intubation, and mortality, without undue adverse effects of treatment.

OUTCOMES Severity of symptoms and signs of upper airway obstruction, visits to a medical practitioner or reattendance to an accident and emergency department, intubation rates, mortality, and adverse effects of treatment. For interventions in paediatric assessment units (see glossary, p 328), we sought rates of hospital admission. For in-hospital treatment, we sought duration of admission. A commonly used definition of a clinically significant improvement is 2 points or more of the validated Westley croup score (maximum score, or most severe, 17)[5] within a predefined timescale. The Westley score comprises the sum of five clinical parameters: consciousness level, cyanosis, stridor, air entry, and chest wall retractions. Intubation and death are rare in children with croup, and so trials recruiting large numbers of children would be needed to exclude a difference in rates between interventions.

METHODS *Clinical Evidence* update search and appraisal January 2002. Data were extracted from trials that used randomisation (not quasi-randomisation) and intention to treat analysis. Common exclusion criteria were previous upper airway abnormalities, previous prolonged intubation, severe croup (cyanosis with impaired consciousness), and recent treatment with steroids. The conclusions presented should not be applied to children with these clinical features. Most children in the studies were cared for in institutions with excellent staffing and monitoring facilities. RCTs performed in hospital settings studied children with more severe croup than did those that were performed in paediatric assessment units. The division of interventions by setting also reflects the differing outcomes that may be relevant in each setting.

QUESTION **What are the effects of treatment in primary care settings?**

We found no RCTs on interventions for croup in primary care settings.

Benefits: We found no systematic review or RCTs evaluating interventions versus placebo in acute childhood croup in primary care settings.

Harms: We found no RCTs.

Comment: It is surprising that there is no evidence relating to children with croup in the primary care setting because this is where the great majority of children with croup are treated.

QUESTION What are the effects of treatment in primary paediatric assessment units?

OPTION SYSTEMIC STEROIDS VERSUS PLACEBO IN PAEDIATRIC ASSESSMENT UNITS

Three RCTs have found that a single dose of oral or intramuscular dexamethasone versus placebo significantly improves symptoms within 5 hours, reduces the likelihood of admission to hospital by 75%, and reduces the need for further treatment after discharge by 70%.

Benefits: We found two systematic reviews (both search dates 1997), which included three relevant trials of systemic steroids versus placebo for children with croup in paediatric assessment units (PAUs) — see glossary, p 328.[6,7] However, they did not analyse these three trials[8–10] separately from other included studies. The three RCTs included 230 children seen at primary PAUs in Australia, Canada, and the USA. One RCT compared a single intramuscular dose of 0.6 mg/kg dexamethasone, given shortly after arrival in the assessment unit, versus placebo.[8] The other RCTs compared 0.15 mg/kg oral dexamethasone[9] and 0.6 mg/kg intramuscular dexamethasone[10] versus placebo in children ready for discharge from the assessment unit. **Symptom improvement:** One RCT (96 children) found that intramuscular dexamethasone (0.6 mg/kg) versus placebo significantly improved the croup score within 5 hours (change in croup score: –2.9 dexamethasone *v* –1.3 placebo).[8] **Admission to hospital:** One RCT (96 children) found that intramuscular dexamethasone (0.6 mg/kg) versus placebo given shortly after arrival in the assessment unit significantly reduced admissions to hospital (RR of admission compared with placebo 0.25, 95% CI 0.13 to 0.49; NNT to prevent 1 additional admission 2, 95% CI 1 to 3).[8] **Reattendance:** For the week after discharge, all three RCTs (total 230 children) found that dexamethasone versus placebo significantly reduced rates of reattendance to any medical practitioner or institution during the week following treatment (RR for reattendance compared with placebo 0.33, 95% CI 0.19 to 0.56; NNT to prevent 1 additional child reattending 12, 95% CI 6 to 60).[8–10]

Harms: None reported.

Comment: The children were observed for up to 5 hours in a PAU before discharge was decided. Some children were treated with nebulised adrenaline (epinephrine).[10]

OPTION NEBULISED STEROIDS VERSUS PLACEBO IN PAEDIATRIC ASSESSMENT UNITS

RCTs have found that nebulised steroids versus placebo reduce the likelihood of a poor response within 2–5 hours by more than 50%, and reduce the risk of hospital admission. They found no significant difference in reattendance to any medical practitioner or institution after 1 week.

Benefits: We found three systematic reviews (search dates 1997,[6] 1997,[7] and not stated[11]), which included four RCTs comparing nebulised steroids versus placebo for children with croup in paediatric assessment units (PAUs — see glossary, p 328).[8,12–14] However, the reviews combined the results with RCTs of hospital based treatment. **Symptom improvement:** The four relevant RCTs (250 children) evaluated treatment in assessment units.[8,12–14] They compared a single dose of inhaled steroids versus placebo, given after humidified oxygen. Combined data from the three RCTs which dichotomised outcomes into either good (improvement in croup score of 2 or more) or poor response, showed a significantly reduced likelihood of a poor response within 2–5 hours after treatment (RR 0.44, 95% CI 0.29 to 0.67).[12–14] **Admission to hospital:** The four RCTs found that nebulised steroids halved the rate of admission (RR 0.55, 95% CI 0.38 to 0.81; NNT to prevent 1 additional admission 4, 95% CI 3 to 8).[8,12–14] **Reattendance:** The four RCTs found no evidence of a significant difference in rates of further admission (RR 0.74, 95% CI 0.26 to 2.08) or consultations with other health practitioners (RR 0.86, 95% CI 0.34 to 2.19) during the week after discharge from the assessment unit.[8,12–14]

Harms: Nebulised steroids appear to be well tolerated. In one of these four RCTs, two neutropenic children suffered bacterial tracheitis after treatment with nebulised dexamethasone.[14]

Comment: We found insufficient evidence to compare regimens of nebulised steroids. In the RCTs, children were observed for up to 5 hours in the assessment unit and all received humidified air or oxygen; in one RCT, both groups also received oral dexamethasone (0.6 mg/kg).[13] One pilot RCT (17 children in hospital) compared inhaled steroid (fluticasone propionate 1000 μg, 2 doses) versus placebo delivered by a metered dose inhaler and spacing device, as a potential treatment that could be given at home.[15] It found no evidence of benefit, but was too small to rule out a clinically significant effect. We found another systematic review (search date 1997) that did not analyse separately data from trials of nebulised steroids versus placebo.[6]

OPTION SYSTEMIC VERSUS NEBULISED STEROIDS IN PAEDIATRIC ASSESSMENT UNITS

RCTs have found that systemic dexamethasone and nebulised budesonide are equally effective in reducing symptoms. One RCT has found that oral dexamethasone versus nebulised budesonide reduces the rate of admission.

Benefits: We found one systematic review (search date 1997[7], 1 RCT[16]) and two additional RCTs.[8,17] The RCTs (280 children with acute croup attending an assessment unit) compared oral dexamethasone (0.6 mg/kg) versus nebulised budesonide (2 mg),[16,17] and intramuscular dexamethasone (0.6 mg/kg) versus nebulised budesonide (4 mg).[8] The RCTs found no significant difference between nebulised budesonide and systemic dexamethasone in rates of symptom resolution or reattendance after discharge, although fewer children on oral dexamethasone were admitted (RR oral *v* nebulised steroids 0.53, 95% CI 0.34 to 0.81).[8]

Harms: None reported.

Comment: None.

OPTION **NEBULISED ADRENALINE (EPINEPHRINE) IN PAEDIATRIC ASSESSMENT UNITS**

One small RCT has found that nebulised adrenaline versus placebo, given in the assessment unit to children suffering from croup, significantly improves symptoms within 30 minutes. Symptoms returned to pre-intervention severity in a third of children within 2 hours. One small RCT found no difference between nebulised adrenaline and inhaled helium–oxygen mixture in symptoms, although may have lacked power to detect a clinically important difference.

Benefits: We found no systematic review. **Versus placebo:** We found one RCT (54 children with stridor at rest seen in an assessment unit) comparing nebulised racemic adrenaline (0.5 mg/kg diluted to 2 mL with 0.9% sodium chloride) versus saline placebo.[18] It found a significant improvement in croup scores 30 minutes after treatment with adrenaline (mean scores 2.0 *v* 3.6 on placebo; CI not reported; $P < 0.01$). The trial found no significant reduction in duration of stay in the assessment unit (mean stay [range]: 11.5 h [5–21 h] *v* 13.3 h [6–24 h]). **Versus helium–oxygen mixture:** We found one RCT (29 children with mild to moderate croup) comparing 100% oxygen driven nebulised adrenaline (in 2.5 mL normal saline) versus a mixture of 70% helium and 30% oxygen alone.[19] Both treatments were given continuously for 3 hours and preceded by cool humidified oxygen and intramuscular dexamethasone (0.6 mg/kg). The RCT found no significant difference with nebulised racemic adrenaline versus helium–oxygen mixture in symptom improvement (measured as croup score; $P = 0.29$, mean changes and CI not reported). The RCT might have lacked power to detect clinically important differences.

Harms: We found no evidence of a significant difference in adverse effects after treatment with adrenaline or placebo. Of the children who had improved by 30 minutes, a considerable proportion relapsed, although there was no significant difference in the rate of relapse (return of croup scores to the pretreatment value) between the two groups (35% with adrenaline v 25% with placebo; RR adrenaline v placebo 1.41, 95% CI 0.36 to 5.51). This raises the question of whether children given nebulised adrenaline and then discharged may come to harm when symptoms recur. No children discharged in the RCT reattended for further treatment.[18] Children were observed for a minimum of 5 hours (up to 24 h). During this time, 40% of treated children and 48% of controls were given a further dose of adrenaline, whereas 52% of treated children and 58% of controls received oral betamethasone (6 mg) before final discharge. These differences were not significant. The RCT comparing nebulised racemic adrenaline versus the helium oxygen mixture did not report on harms.[19] However, one participant from each treatment group was excluded because they needed rescue doses of racemic adrenaline.

Comment: **Adrenaline combined with steroids:** We found no RCTs. Two prospective cohort studies assessed 115 children treated with nebulised adrenaline and dexamethasone (0.6 mg/kg) in an assessment unit. Of the 55–66% who responded satisfactorily, all were discharged after 3–4 hours of observation, and none reattended for further medical care within 24–48 hours.[20,21]

QUESTION What are the effects of treatment in hospital?

OPTION INHALATION OF HUMIDIFIED AIR/OXYGEN IN HOSPITAL

The effectiveness of inhaling humidified air/oxygen has not been evaluated adequately.

Benefits: We found no systematic review. We found one RCT (16 children) comparing up to 12 hours of care in a humidified atmosphere (air with relative humidity 87–95%) versus normal care.[22] It found no significant difference in recovery rates (mean croup scores at 6 h were 3.1 *v* 3.8).

Harms: None reported.

Comment: The study was not blinded, and selection, performance, and detection biases remain possible.

OPTION SYSTEMIC STEROIDS IN HOSPITAL

RCTs have found that giving systemic corticosteroids to children admitted with croup significantly improves symptoms by 12 hours and reduces hospital stay. Limited evidence suggests that a single dose of oral dexamethasone 0.3 mg/kg is as effective as 0.6 mg/kg in children admitted with croup.

Benefits: We found two systematic reviews (search dates 1999[23] and not stated[11]), which combined data from 11 relevant RCTs (904 children), and we found one additional RCT not included in either review (41 children).[24] The most common regimen was intramuscular or oral dexamethasone (0.3–0.6 mg/kg) as a single dose on admission or repeated over 24–48 hours. **Symptom improvement:** RCTs that evaluated symptomatic improvement at 12–24 hours found that significantly more children responded to steroids than to placebo (response defined as ≥ 2 points improvement of croup score; RR of response 1.23, 95% CI 1.13 to 1.33; NNT to achieve response in 1 additional child 7, 95% CI 5 to 10). **Hospital stay:** Four RCTs evaluated duration of hospital stay. Three found a significant reduction in hospital stay on dexamethasone compared with placebo (median stay 20 *v* 13 h,[17] mean stay 91 *v* 49 h[25] and 9 *v* 3 days[24]). The fourth RCT found no significant difference.[26] **Intubation rates:** Seven RCTs in the systematic review and two subsequent RCTs gave data on intubation rates.[17,23,24] Children given systemic steroids were less at risk of intubation than children taking placebo (RR 0.21, 95% CI 0.06 to 0.69). This combined estimate is dominated by one small study with a much higher than average rate of intubation (5/32 children).[24]

Harms: Systemic steroids seem to be well tolerated. We found three RCTs (130 children) reporting rates of secondary bacterial infection.[24,26,27] These reported nine cases of pneumonia, one of septicaemia, one of bacterial tracheitis, one of otitis media, and one of sinusitis. Six cases were in treated children and seven were in controls (RR for infection compared with placebo 0.94, 95% CI 0.33 to 2.69).

Comment: A significant reduction in time to symptom resolution may not reduce hospital stay, which is influenced by hospital policies and referral patterns, availability of treatment in the community, parental access to transportation and communications, and the tendency to discharge children at a certain time each day.[28]

OPTION HIGH VERSUS LOW DOSE SYSTEMIC STEROID REGIMENS IN HOSPITAL

Limited evidence suggests that a single dose of oral dexamethasone 0.3 mg/kg is as effective as 0.6 mg/kg in children admitted with croup.

Benefits: We found one systematic review (search date 1997),[7] which included one RCT (120 children admitted with croup) comparing different single doses of oral dexamethasone (0.6 *v* 0.3 mg/kg and 0.3 *v* 0.15 mg/kg).[25] It found no significant differences in rate of improvement in croup score, duration of hospital stay, or intubation rates. However, children given the lower dose of dexamethasone were more likely to be given nebulised adrenaline (epinephrine) than were those given the higher dose (RR 2.32, 95% CI 1.02 to 5.28). We found no studies comparing other systemic regimens.

Harms: None reported.

Comment: None.

OPTION NEBULISED STEROIDS IN HOSPITAL

RCTs have found that children admitted with croup given corticosteroids versus placebo improve more rapidly, leave hospital sooner, and are less likely to reattend. We found insufficient evidence on the effect of nebulised steroids on intubation rates.

Benefits: We found one systematic review (search date not stated,[11] 4 RCTs,[17,29–31] 252 children admitted to hospital with croup) comparing nebulised steroids with placebo. However, that review combined the results with RCTs conducted in paediatric assessment units (see glossary, p 328). **Symptom improvement:** One RCT evaluated budesonide 1 mg, two doses, 30 minutes apart.[29] The risk of an inadequate response by 2 hours was significantly reduced (RR 0.40, 95% CI 0.19 to 0.83; NNT to prevent 1 additional inadequate response 2, 95% CI 1 to 8). **Hospital stay:** Another RCT compared nebulised budesonide 2 mg initially, followed by 1 mg every 12 hours, versus placebo, and found a significant reduction in hospital stay (mean stay 36 *v* 55 h).[30] The third RCT compared budesonide 2 mg single dose versus placebo and reported a significant reduction in the number of children staying in hospital for more than 24 hours (RR 0.37, 95% CI 0.16 to 0.88; NNT 3, 95% CI 2 to 14).[17] **Intubation rates:** Three RCTs found that there was no significant effect on intubation rates (RR of intubation 0.18, 95% CI 0.01 to 3.67).[17,29,30] **Relapse rate:** The fourth RCT compared nebulised budesonide 2 mg versus placebo given every 12 hours while in hospital.[31] It found that budesonide accelerated clinical improvement (decrease in croup score by ≥ 2 points) compared with placebo ($P = 0.013$), and reduced the rate of further medical attendance during the 3 days after discharge (reattendance rate 1/34 with budesonide *v* 7/32 with placebo; CI not reported; $P = 0.02$).

Harms: Nebulised steroids seem to be well tolerated. Two RCTs reported adverse effects. One RCT reported one episode of nausea and one episode of distress caused by firm application of the face mask for 10 minutes.[30] The other RCT reported emotional distress in 6 of 42 children treated with budesonide nebulisers and 9 of 40 children treated with placebo.[31] In four children with severe croup (1 treated with budesonide and 3 with placebo), this led to interventional treatment outside of the protocol (nebulised adrenaline [epinephrine]).

Comment: The optimal regimen of nebulised steroids has not yet been established.

OPTION SYSTEMIC VERSUS NEBULISED STEROIDS IN HOSPITAL

We found no RCTs undertaken outside of paediatric assessment units of oral versus nebulised steroids for croup.

Benefits: We found no systematic review and no RCTs investigating the effects of oral versus nebulised steroids in hospital. We found limited evidence that systemic steroids may reduce admission rates if given in the paediatric assessment units (see glossary, p 328) (see benefits of systemic versus nebulised steroids in paediatric assessment units, p 323).

Harms: We found no evidence.

Comment: None.

OPTION NEBULISED ADRENALINE (EPINEPHRINE) IN HOSPITAL

One small RCT found that nebulised adrenaline versus placebo given by intermittent positive pressure ventilation to children suffering from croup significantly improved symptoms within 30 minutes. Symptoms returned to pre-intervention severity in a third of children within 2 hours. Two further RCTs found no significant difference between nebulised adrenaline and placebo, but may have lacked power to detect clinically important differences.

Benefits: We found no systematic review. **Versus placebo:** We found three RCTs (53 children admitted to hospital with croup) comparing nebulised adrenaline versus placebo. Two RCTs did not show improvement with adrenaline, but were too small to exclude a clinically important difference.[32,33] The other small RCT compared aerosolised racemic adrenaline versus 0.9% saline, both delivered by intermittent positive pressure breathing.[5] Children given adrenaline experienced greater reductions in croup score. The reduction was greatest within 30 minutes of treatment and was not apparent at 2 hours (mean croup scores at 30 min 1.7 *v* 3.1). **Nebuliser versus intermittent positive pressure breathing:** We found one RCT (14 children) comparing nebulised adrenaline delivered by intermittent positive pressure breathing versus nebulised adrenaline alone.[34] It found no significant difference in resolution of symptoms (mean croup scores at 30 min 3.1 *v* 2.4). **L-adrenaline versus racemic adrenaline:** We found one RCT (31 children) comparing racemic adrenaline versus L-adrenaline.[35] It found no significant difference in croup scores (mean scores at 30 min 3.8 *v* 4.8).

Harms: There was no significant difference in the risk of cardiovascular adverse effects with L-adrenaline or racemic adrenaline. Three children receiving racemic adrenaline were intubated (RR of intubation with racemic *v* L-adrenaline 6.59, 95% CI 0.37 to 118).[35] Children given nebulised adrenaline need medical observation because symptoms may return to pretreatment severity (see harms of nebulised adrenaline in paediatric assessment units, p 324).

Comment: Racemic adrenaline comprises equal amounts of D- and L-isomers and was historically chosen in favour of the more readily available L-form in the belief that it caused fewer adverse cardiovascular effects.

OPTION NEBULISED ADRENALINE (EPINEPHRINE) VERSUS STEROIDS IN HOSPITAL

We found no good evidence to compare the effectiveness of nebulised adrenaline and steroids.

Benefits: We found one systematic review (search date 1997),[7] which identified one RCT (66 children admitted to hospital with croup) comparing nebulised adrenaline (4 mg) versus nebulised budesonide (2 mg).[36] It found no significant difference in duration of hospital stay (mean difference in hospital stay, adrenaline *v* budesonide, –5.8 h, 95% CI –22.8 h to +11.2 h) or in croup scores (mean change –2.9 *v* –1.7; CI not reported; P = 0.08). We found no RCTs comparing nebulised adrenaline versus oral steroids.

Harms: None reported.

Comment: Nebulised adrenaline and steroids may have an additive effect through different modes of action, although whether this leads to improved outcomes is unknown.

GLOSSARY

Primary paediatric assessment unit (PAU) An emergency room or accident and emergency department with the facilities to monitor closely the clinical condition of a child with acute onset of inspiratory stridor.

Substantive changes

Nebulised adrenaline (epinephrine) in paediatric assessment units One new RCT;[19] conclusions unchanged.

REFERENCES

1. Denny FW, Murphy TF, Clyde WA Jr, et al. Croup: an 11-year study in a pediatric practice. *Pediatrics* 1983;71:871–876.
2. Phelan PD, Landau LI, Olinsily A. *Respiratory illness in children*. 2nd ed. Oxford: Blackwell Science, 1982:32–33.
3. Van Bever HP, Wieringa MH, Weyler JJ, et al. Croup and recurrent croup: their association with asthma and allergy. *Eur J Pediatr* 1999;158:253–257.
4. McEniery J, Gillis J, Kilham H, et al. Review of intubation in severe laryngotracheobronchitis. *Pediatrics* 1991;87:847–853.
5. Westley CR, Cotton EK, Brooks JG. Nebulized racemic epinephrine by IPPB for the treatment of croup: a double-blind study. *Am J Dis Child* 1978;132:484–487.
6. Ausejo M, Saenz A, Pham B, et al. The effectiveness of glucocorticoids in treating croup: meta-analysis. *BMJ* 1999;319:595–600. Search

date 1997; primary sources Cochrane Controlled Trials Register, Embase, Medline, and letters to authors.

7. Ausejo M, Saenz A, Pham B, et al. Glucocorticoids for Croup. In: The Cochrane Library, Issue 1, 2001. Oxford: Update Software. Search date 1997; primary sources Cochrane Controlled Trials Register, Embase, Medline, and letters to authors. Substantially amended June 1999.
8. Johnson DW, Jacobson S, Edney PC, et al. A comparison of nebulised budesonide, intramuscular dexamethasone, and placebo for moderately severe croup. *N Engl J Med* 1998;339:498–503.
9. Geelhoed GC, Turner J, Macdonald WBG. Efficacy of a small single dose of oral dexamethasone for outpatient croup: a double blind placebo controlled clinical trial. *BMJ* 1996;313:140–142.
10. Cruz MN, Stewart G, Rosenberg N. Use of dexamethasone in the outpatient management of acute laryngotracheitis. *Pediatrics* 1995;96:220–223.
11. Griffin S, Ellis S, Fitzgerald-Barron A, et al. Nebulised steroid in the treatment of croup: a systematic review of randomised controlled trials. *Br J Gen Pract* 2000;50:135–141. Search date not stated; primary sources Cinahl, Cochrane Controlled Trials Register, Embase, Medline, hand searching of article bibliographies and pharmaceutical industry database.
12. Klassen TP, Feldman ME, Watters LK, et al. Nebulized budesonide for children with mild-to-moderate croup. *N Engl J Med* 1994;331:285–289.
13. Klassen TP, Watters LK, Feldman ME, et al. The efficacy of nebulized budesonide in dexamethasone-treated outpatients with croup. *Pediatrics* 1996;97:463–466.
14. Johnson DW, Schuh S, Koren G, et al. Outpatient treatment of croup with nebulized dexamethasone. *Arch Pediatr Adolesc Med* 1996;150:349–355.
15. Jan Roorda R, Walhof CM. Effects of inhaled fluticasone propionate administered with metered dose inhaler and spacer in mild to moderate croup: a negative preliminary report. *Pediatr Pulmonol* 1998;25:114–117.
16. Klassen TP, Craig WR, Moher D, et al. Nebulized budesonide and oral dexamethasone for the treatment of croup: a randomized controlled trial. *JAMA* 1998;279:1629–1632.
17. Geelhoed GC, Macdonald WB. Oral and inhaled steroids in croup: a randomized, placebo-controlled trial. *Pediatr Pulmonol* 1995;20:355–361.
18. Kristjansson S, Berg-Kelly K, Winso E. Inhalation of racemic adrenaline in the treatment of mild and moderately severe croup. Clinical symptom score and oxygen saturation measurements for evaluation of treatment effects. *Acta Paediatr* 1994;83:1156–1160.
19. Weber JE, Chudnofsky CR, Younger JG, et al. A randomised comparison of helium-oxygen mixture (Heliox) and racemic epinephrine for the treatment of moderate to severe croup. *Pediatrics* 2001;107:E96.
20. Ledwith CA, Shea LM, Mauro RD. Safety and efficacy of nebulized racemic epinephrine in conjunction with oral dexamethasone and mist in the outpatient treatment of croup. *Ann Emerg Med* 1995;25:331–337.
21. Kunkel NC, Baker MD. Use of racemic epinephrine, dexamethasone, and mist in the outpatient management of croup. *Pediatr Emerg Care* 1996;12:156–159.
22. Bourchier D, Dawson KP, Fergusson DM. Humidification in viral croup: a controlled trial. *Aust Paediatr J* 1984;20:289–291.
23. Kairys SW, Olmstead EM, O'Connor GT. Steroid treatment of laryngotracheitis: a meta-analysis of the evidence from randomized trials. *Pediatrics* 1989;83:683–693. Search date June 1999; primary sources Medline, Embase, and Cochrane Library.
24. Sumboonnanonda A, Suwanjutha S, Sirinavin S. Randomized controlled trial of dexamethasone in infectious croup. *J Med Assoc Thai* 1997;80:262–265.
25. Geelhoed GC, Macdonald WBG. Oral dexamethasone in the treatment of croup: 0.15 mg/kg versus 0.3 mg/kg versus 0.6 mg/kg. *Pediatr Pulmonol* 1995;20:362–368.
26. Super DM, Cartelli NA, Brooks LJ, et al. A prospective randomized double-blind study to evaluate the effect of dexamethasone in acute laryngotracheitis. *J Pediatr* 1989;115:323–329.
27. Kuusela AL, Vesikari T. A randomized double-blind, placebo-controlled trial of dexamethasone and racemic epinephrine in the treatment of croup. *Acta Paediatr Scand* 1988;77:99–104.
28. Kemper KJ. Medically inappropriate hospital use in a pediatric population. *N Engl J Med* 1988;318:1033–1037.
29. Husby S, Agertoft L, Mortensen S, et al. Treatment of croup with nebulised steroid (budesonide): a double blind, placebo controlled study. *Arch Dis Child* 1993;68:352–355.
30. Godden CW, Campbell MJ, Hussey M, et al. Double blind placebo controlled trial of nebulised budesonide for croup. *Arch Dis Child* 1997;76:155–158.
31. Roberts GW, Master VV, Staugas RE, et al. Repeated dose inhaled budesonide versus placebo in the treatment of croup. *J Paediatr Child Health* 1999;35:170–174.
32. Gardner HG, Powell KR, Roden VJ, et al. The evaluation of racemic epinephrine in the treatment of infectious croup. *Pediatrics* 1973;52:52–55.
33. Taussig LM, Castro O, Beaudry PH, et al. Treatment of laryngotracheobronchitis (croup). *Am J Dis Child* 1975;129:790–793.
34. Fogel JM, Berg IJ, Gerber MA, et al. Racemic epinephrine in the treatment of croup: nebulization alone versus nebulization with intermittent positive pressure breathing. *J Pediatr* 1982;101:1028–1031.
35. Waisman Y, Klein BL, Boenning DA, et al. Prospective randomized double-blind study comparing L-epinephrine and racemic epinephrine aerosols in the treatment of laryngotracheitis (croup). *Pediatrics* 1992;89:302–306.
36. Fitzgerald D, Mellis C, Johnson M, et al. Nebulized budesonide is as effective as nebulized adrenaline in moderately severe croup. *Pediatrics* 1996;97:722–725.

Martin Osmond
Associate Professor of Pediatrics
University of Ottawa, Ottawa, Canada

Competing interests: None declared.

Depression in children and adolescents

Search date January 2002

Philip Hazell

QUESTIONS

INTERVENTIONS

See glossary, p 338

Key Messages

- **Cognitive therapy** One systematic review in children and adolescents with mild to moderate depression has found that cognitive behavioural therapy versus non-specific supportive therapies significantly improves symptoms (NNT 4 95% CI 3 to 5).
- **Electroconvulsive therapy** We found no RCTs on electroconvulsive therapy in children and adolescents with depression.
- **Interpersonal therapy (adolescents)** Two RCTs found that interpersonal therapy versus clinical monitoring or waiting list control significantly increased the number of adolescents with mild to moderate depression who recovered over 12 weeks.
- **Intravenous clomipramine** One small RCT found that in non-suicidal adolescents, intravenous clomipramine versus placebo significantly reduced depression scores at 6 days.
- **Lithium** One RCT found no significant difference with lithium versus placebo in global assessment or depression scores after 6 weeks in children with depression and family history of bipolar affective disorder. Lithium was associated with adverse effects.

Clin Evid 2002;8:330–339.

- **Long term effects of different treatments** We found no systematic review or RCTs looking at long term outcomes of interventions for depression in children and adolescents.
- **Monoamine oxidase inhibitors** One RCT found insufficient evidence on moclobemide versus placebo in children aged 9–15 years with major depression and some with a comorbid disorder. We found no RCTs of non-reversible monoamine oxidase inhibitors in children or adolescents.
- **Oral tricyclic antidepressants (adolescents)** One systematic review found no significant difference with oral tricyclic antidepressants (amitriptyline, desipramine, imipramine, nortriptyline) versus placebo in depression scores in adolescents and children with depression. Subgroup analyses found that oral tricyclic antidepressants versus placebo significantly reduced symptoms in adolescents but not in children. The review also found that oral tricyclic antidepressants were associated with adverse effects.
- **Oral tricyclic antidepressants (children)** Subgroup analyses in one systematic review found no significant difference with oral tricyclic antidepressants (amitriptyline, desipramine, imipramine, nortriptyline) versus placebo in children with depression. The review also found that oral tricyclic antidepressants were associated with adverse effects.
- **Selective serotonin reuptake inhibitors** One RCT found no significant difference with fluoxetine versus placebo in depression symptoms or psychological functioning in adolescents with depression after 8 weeks. Another RCT found that in children and adolescents with major depression fluoxetine versus placebo significantly improved depressive symptoms after 8 weeks. One RCT found that in adolescents with major depression, paroxetine versus placebo significantly improved remission after 8 weeks. Fluoxetine and paroxetine were associated with adverse effects. We found no RCTs on other selective serotonin reuptake inhibitors.
- **St John's Wort** We found no RCTs on St John's Wort (*Hypericum perforatum*) in children or adolescents with depression.
- **Venlafaxine** One RCT found no significant difference with venlafaxine versus placebo in improvement of depressive symptoms in children and adolescents with major depression after 6 weeks.
- **Family therapy; group treatments other than cognitive behavioural therapy** We found insufficient evidence in children and adolescents about the effects of these interventions.

DEFINITION Compared with adult depression, depression in children (6–12 years) and adolescents (13–18 years) may have a more insidious onset, may be characterised more by irritability than sadness, and occurs more often in association with other conditions such as anxiety, conduct disorder, hyperkinesis, and learning problems.[1]

INCIDENCE/ PREVALENCE Estimates of prevalence of depression among children and adolescents in the community range from 2–6%.[2,3] Prevalence tends to increase with age, with a sharp rise around onset of puberty. Pre-adolescent boys and girls are affected equally by the condition, but depression is seen more frequently among adolescent girls than boys.[4]

AETIOLOGY/ RISK FACTORS The aetiology is uncertain, but may include childhood events and current psychosocial adversity.

PROGNOSIS In children and adolescents, the recurrence rate of depressive episodes first occurring in childhood or adolescence is 70% by 5 years, which is similar to the recurrence rate in adults, but it is not clear if this is related to severity of depression.[4] Young people experiencing a moderate to severe depressive episode may be more likely than adults to have a manic episode within the next few years.[4,5] Trials of treatment for child and adolescent depression have found high rates of spontaneous remission (as much as two thirds of people in some inpatient studies).

AIMS To improve mood, social and occupational functioning, and quality of life; to reduce morbidity and mortality; to prevent recurrence of depressive disorder; and to minimise adverse effects of treatment.

OUTCOMES In children and adolescents there are developmentally specific pseudo-continuous self report measures such as the Children's Depression Rating Scale and the Children's Depression Inventory, although some studies of adolescents use scales developed for use in adults such as the Hamilton Rating Scale for Depression. Parent report pseudo-continuous measures such as the Children's Depression Inventory for Parents are also used. Categorical outcomes are sometimes expressed as people no longer meeting specified criteria for depression on a structured psychiatric interview such as the Kiddie-SADS, which combines data from children and their parents. Global improvement in symptoms as judged by an investigator is sometimes reported using the Clinical Global Impressions scale or the Clinical Global Assessment scale. Severity of depression is defined in some studies using cut-off scores on pseudo-continuous measures, such as the Children's Depression Rating scale and the Children's Depression Inventory, but is often not stated.

METHODS *Clinical Evidence* update search and appraisal January 2002, plus additional references identified by contributor.

QUESTION What are the effects of treatments?

OPTION TRICYCLIC ANTIDEPRESSANTS

One systematic review found no significant difference with oral tricyclic antidepressants (amitriptyline, desipramine, imipramine, nortriptyline) versus placebo in depression scores in children and adolescents with depression. Subgroup analyses found that oral tricyclic antidepressants versus placebo significantly reduced symptoms in adolescents but not in children. The review also found that oral tricyclic antidepressants were associated with adverse effects. One small RCT found that in non-suicidal adolescents, intravenous clomipramine versus placebo significantly reduced depression scores at 6 days.

Benefits: **Oral tricyclic antidepressants:** We found one systematic review (search date 2000, 13 RCTs, 506 children and adolescents aged 6–18 years, severity of depression not stated) comparing oral tricyclic antidepressants (amitriptyline, desipramine, imipramine, and nortriptyline) versus placebo.[6] The systematic review found no significant difference in overall improvement (depression checklist scores) with tricyclic antidepressants versus placebo (OR 0.84, 95% CI 0.56 to 1.25). Subgroup analyses found a significant reduction in symptoms with tricyclic antidepressants versus placebo in adolescents (7 RCTs: effect size SMD –0.47, 95% CI –0.92 to –0.02) but no significant difference in children (3 RCTs: effect size SMD –0.15, 95% CI –0.64 to +0.34). **Pulsed intravenous clomipramine:** See glossary, p 338. We found one RCT (16 non-suicidal adolescent outpatients, aged 14–18 years, with major depression [21-item Hamilton Rating Scale for Depression score ≥ 18]) comparing intravenous clomipramine (200 mg) versus placebo.[7] The RCT found that intravenous clomipramine versus placebo significantly decreased depression scores at 6 days (decrease in Hamilton Rating Scale for Depression score from baseline of ≥ 50%: 7/8 people with iv clomipramine *v* 3/8 with placebo).[7]

Harms: **Oral tricyclic antidepressants:** The systematic review found that tricyclic antidepressants were more commonly associated with vertigo (OR 8.47, 95% CI 1.40 to 51.0), orthostatic hypotension (OR 4.77, 95% CI 1.11 to 20.5), tremor (OR 6.29, 95% CI 1.78 to 22.17), and dry mouth (OR 5.19, 95% CI 1.15 to 23.5) than placebo.[6] The review found no significant differences for other adverse effects (tiredness [OR 1.52, 95% CI 0.63 to 3.67], sleep problems [OR 1.87, 95% CI 0.84 to 4.14], headache [OR 1.15, 95% CI 0.68 to 1.95], palpitations [OR 1.20, 95% CI 0.17 to 8.68], perspiration [OR 2.01, 95% CI 0.39 to 10.44], constipation [OR 1.94, 95% CI 0.72 to 5.24], or problems with micturition [OR 0.30, 95% CI 0.01 to 7.89]. **Pulsed intravenous clomipramine:** The RCT did not report any adverse effects.[7]

Comment: We found single case reports and case series of toxicity and mortality from tricyclic antidepressants in overdose and therapeutic doses. Further research is needed to determine long term effects of intravenous clomipramine.

OPTION MONOAMINE OXIDASE INHIBITORS

One RCT found insufficient evidence on moclobemide versus placebo in children aged 9–15 years with major depression and some with a comorbid disorder. We found no RCTs on non-reversible monoamine oxidase inhibitors in children or adolescents.

Benefits: We found no systematic review. **Reversible monoamine oxidase inhibitors:** We found one RCT (20 Turkish children aged 9–15 years with major depression, including 13 children with a comorbid disorder) comparing moclobemide versus placebo for 5 weeks.[8] The RCT found significant improvement with moclobemide versus placebo in one clinician rated scale (Clinical Global Impressions-investigator assessment of severity of depression, adverse effects, and global recovery) after 5 weeks but not on parent rated (Children's Depression Inventory for Parents) and self reported measures (Children's Depression Inventory).[8] **Non-reversible monoamine oxidase inhibitors:** We found no RCTs.

Harms: The RCT found no significant difference with moclobemide versus placebo in adverse effects assessed using Clinical Global Impression of adverse effects scale and self assessed adverse effects forms.[8] We found no information on the safety of moclobemide usage in children younger than 9 years.

Comment: The small sample size limits the conclusions that may be drawn from the one RCT.

OPTION SELECTIVE SEROTONIN REUPTAKE INHIBITORS

One RCT found no significant difference with fluoxetine versus placebo in depression symptoms or psychological functioning in adolescents with depression after 8 weeks. Another RCT found that in children and adolescents with major depression, fluoxetine versus placebo significantly improved depressive symptoms after 8 weeks. One RCT found that in adolescents with major depression, paroxetine versus placebo significantly improved remission after 8 weeks. Fluoxetine and paroxetine were associated with adverse effects. We found no RCTs on other selective serotonin reuptake inhibitors.

Benefits: **Fluoxetine:** We found one systematic review (search date 1998,[9] 2 RCTs[10,11]), which did not pool results. The first RCT (40 adolescents, aged 13–18 years, of whom 30 completed the trial, severity of depression not stated) found no significant difference after 8 weeks with fluoxetine (20–60 mg) versus placebo in mean number of depression symptoms or psychosocial functioning (Clinical Global Impressions scale).[11] The second RCT (96 children and adolescents aged 7–17 years with major depression) found fluoxetine (20 mg) versus placebo significantly improved depressive symptoms after 8 weeks in terms of Clinical Global Impressions scale (27/48 [56%] improved with fluoxetine *v* 16/48 [33%] with placebo; RR of failure to recover 0.66, 95% CI 0.45 to 0.96) and self reported Children's Depression Rating Scale (34% improved *v* 18%; P < 0.01), but did not improve other measures.[11] **Paroxetine:** We found one RCT (180 adolescents, aged 12–18 years, of whom 133 completed the trial, severity of depression score of at least 12 on the Hamilton Rating Scale for Depression and < 60 on the Children's Global Assessment scale) comparing paroxetine (20–40 mg) versus placebo versus imipramine for 8 weeks on end point response (Hamilton Rating Scale for Depression score ≤ 8 or a 50% reduction from baseline score) and change from baseline score (Hamilton Rating Scale for Depression). The RCT did not include a direct statistical comparison of paroxetine versus imipramine.[12] The RCT found that paroxetine versus placebo significantly improved remission (Hamilton Rating Scale for Depression: AR for failure to recover 37% with paroxetine *v* 54% with placebo; ARI 17%; no CI available; RR 0.68, 95% CI 0.49 to 0.95; P = 0.02). Among adolescents who completed treatment, paroxetine versus placebo significantly improved remission (Clinical Global Impressions scale of 133 people completing the study: AR for remission 66% with paroxetine *v* 48% with placebo; ARR 18%; P = 0.02). **Other selective serotonin reuptake inhibitors:** We found no RCTs.

Harms: **Fluoxetine:** One RCT found significantly more weight loss with fluoxetine versus placebo (data not provided).[10] The other RCT did not report on adverse effects.[11] **Paroxetine:** The RCT reported more serious adverse events with paroxetine (12%) versus placebo (2%).[12] The most frequent adverse effects were somnolence (17% with paroxetine *v* 3% with placebo) and tremor (11% with paroxetine *v* 2% with placebo) but no statistical analyses were reported.

Comment: There is insufficient information provided in one of the RCTs[10] to make an informed comparison with the other RCT.[11]

OPTION VENLAFAXINE

One RCT found no significant difference with venlafaxine versus placebo in improvement of depressive symptoms in children and adolescents with major depression after 6 weeks.

Benefits: We found one systematic review (search date 1998,[9] 1 RCT[13]). The RCT (33 children and adolescents aged 8–17 years with major depression and on psychotherapy) compared venlafaxine (37.5–75.0 mg/day in divided doses) versus placebo for 6 weeks.[13] It found no significant difference with venlafaxine versus placebo in improvement of depressive symptoms (Children's Depression Inventory, Hamilton Rating Scale for Depression, Children's Depression Rating Scale).

Harms: The RCT reported nausea in a subgroup of participants aged ≥ 13 years.[13]

Comment: The RCT lacked power to rule out a clinically important difference.

OPTION LITHIUM

One RCT found no significant difference with lithium versus placebo in global assessment or depression scores after 6 weeks in children with depression and family history of bipolar affective disorder. Lithium was associated with adverse effects.

Benefits: We found no systematic review. We found one RCT (30 children, aged 6–12 years, with depression and family history of bipolar affective disorder) comparing lithium versus placebo for 6 weeks.[14] The RCT found no significant difference with lithium versus placebo in global assessment (0 is worst, 100 is best) or depression scores (9 depression items of the Kiddie-SADS interview).

Harms: Of the 17 children randomised to lithium treatment, four were withdrawn because of adverse effects (3 had confusion, 1 had nausea and vomiting).[14]

Comment: The RCT lacked power to rule out a clinically important difference.

OPTION ST JOHN'S WORT (*HYPERICUM PERFORATUM*)

We found no RCTs on St John's Wort (*H perforatum*) in children or adolescents with depression.

Benefits: We found no RCTs on St John's Wort (*H perforatum*) in children or adolescents with depression.

Harms: We found no RCTs.

Comment: None.

OPTION ELECTROCONVULSIVE THERAPY

We found no RCTs on electroconvulsive therapy in children and adolescents with depression.

Benefits: We found no RCTs on electroconvulsive therapy in children and adolescents with depression.

Harms: We found no specific evidence on harms in children or adolescents. Known adverse effects in adults include memory impairment.

Comment: None.

OPTION SPECIFIC PSYCHOLOGICAL TREATMENTS

One systematic review has found that cognitive behavioural therapy increases the rate of resolution of the symptoms of depression compared with non-specific supportive therapies for children and adolescents with mild to moderate depression. We found limited evidence from two small RCTs about interpersonal therapy versus clinical monitoring alone or placement on a waiting list. We found insufficient evidence that family therapy or group treatments other than cognitive behavioural therapy are effective treatments for depression in children and adolescents.

Benefits: **Cognitive behavioural therapy:** See glossary, p 338. We found one systematic review (search date 1997, 6 RCTs, 376 people) of cognitive behavioural therapy versus other treatments ranging from waiting list control to supportive psychotherapy.[15] Cognitive behavioural therapy increased the rate of resolution of symptoms of depression (OR 3.2, 95% CI 1.9 to 5.2; NNT 4, 95% CI 3 to 5): a finding consistent with three non-systematic meta-analytic studies.[16–18] **Interpersonal therapy:** See glossary, p 338. We found two RCTs comparing 12 weekly sessions of interpersonal therapy versus clinical monitoring or waiting list control in adolescents with depression. The first RCT (48 adolescents aged 12–18 years with major depressive disorder) found that interpersonal therapy versus clinical monitoring significantly increased the number of adolescents who recovered (Hamilton Rating Scale for Depression < 6 or Beck Depressive Inventory < 9) (18/24 [75%] with interpersonal therapy *v* 11/24 [46%] with clinical monitoring alone; RR 1.64, 95% CI 1.00 to 2.68; ARR 0.29, 95% CI 0.03 to 0.56).[19] The second RCT (46 adolescents with major depression) comparing interpersonal therapy versus being on a waiting list found no significant difference in proportion of adolescents not manifesting severe depression (defined by a cut-off score on the Children's Depression Inventory) (17/19 [89%] with interpersonal therapy *v* 12/18 [67%] with waiting list; RR 1.33, 95% CI 0.94 to 1.93; ARR 0.22, 95% CI –0.03 to +0.49). However, if the Children's Depression Inventory score was considered as a continuous measure, the mean Children's Depression Inventory score was significantly lower after interpersonal therapy versus waiting list (P < 0.01).[20] **Systemic behavioural family therapy:** See glossary, p 338. We found one RCT (78 adolescents with major depressive disorder) comparing family therapy versus non-specific supportive therapy. The RCT found no significant difference in remission rates (combination of no longer meeting DSM-III-R criteria for major depression as determined by the Kiddie-SADS interview and Beck Depression Inventory score < 9: 29% with family therapy *v* 34% with non-specific supportive therapy).[21] **Group administered cognitive behavioural therapy:** We found one RCT (123 adolescents aged 14–18 years with major depression or dysthymia) comparing group administered cognitive behavioural therapy versus waiting list. It found that cognitive behavioural therapy significantly increased the remission rate (Longitudinal Interval Follow-up Evaluation interview for DSM-III-R diagnoses: 46/69 [67%] with group cognitive behavioural therapy *v* 13/27 [48%] on a waiting list; $P < 0.05$).[22] **Group therapeutic support versus group social skills training:** We found one RCT (66 adolescents aged 13–17 years, of whom 47 completed the protocol; 58 with major depression, 8 with dysthymia) comparing group therapeutic support versus group social skills training. In 26 adolescents (pretreatment scores in the clinical range for the Kiddie-SADS, Child Depression Inventory, and a self esteem instrument), the RCT found no significant difference in remission rates (score of < 4 on Kiddie-SADS dysphoria and anhedonia symptoms: 8/16 [50%] with group therapeutic support *v* 4/10 [40%] with group social skills training).[23]

Harms: The RCTs did not report any adverse effects.[16–23] We found no report of harms specifically for children and adolescents. In adults, there have been case reports suggesting that "imaginal flooding" (a form of cognitive behavioural therapy) worsens symptoms, leading for calls for caution in the use of this treatment.

Comment: Large RCTs are needed in more representative groups of people in a range of clinical settings including primary care. In the first RCT of interpersonal therapy, sessions were augmented by telephone contact.

QUESTION Which treatments are most effective at improving long term outcome?

We found no systematic review or RCTs looking at long term outcomes of interventions for depression in children and adolescents.

Benefits: We found no systematic review and no RCTs. We found no RCTs comparing structured psychotherapy with pharmacotherapy in children and adolescents. We found no RCTs comparing combined pharmacotherapy and psychotherapy with either treatment alone. We found no RCTs comparing different psychotherapies.

Harms: We found no RCTs.

Comment: We found one prospective cohort study, in which adolescents with depression had been randomised to cognitive behavioural therapy (see glossary, p 338), systemic behavioural family therapy, or non-directive supportive therapy. After the initial trial phase of 16 weeks, they were allowed booster treatments and also had access to open treatment in any modality for the 2 years of follow up. They were assessed at 3 monthly intervals for the first 12 months and then again at 24 months. The study found no significant difference between the groups. Of 106 adolescents, 38% experienced sustained recovery, 21% experienced persistent depression, and 41% had a relapsing course.[24]

GLOSSARY

Cognitive behavioural therapy A brief (20 sessions over 12–16 wks) structured treatment aimed at changing the dysfunctional beliefs and negative automatic thoughts that characterise depressive disorders.[25] Cognitive behavioural therapy requires a high level of training in the therapist, and has been adapted for children and adolescents suffering depression. A course of treatment is characterised by 8–12 weekly sessions, in which the therapist and the child collaborate to solve current difficulties. The treatment is structured and often directed by a manual. Treatment generally includes cognitive elements, such as the challenging of negativistic thoughts, and behavioural elements, such as structuring time to engage in pleasurable activity.

Interpersonal therapy A standardised form of brief psychotherapy (usually 12–16 weekly sessions) intended primarily for outpatients with unipolar non-psychotic depressive disorders. It focuses on improving the individual's interpersonal functioning and identifying the problems associated with the onset of the depressive episode.[26] In children and adolescents, interpersonal therapy has been adapted for adolescents to address common adolescent developmental issues, for example separation from parents, exploration of authority in relationship to parents, development of dyadic interpersonal relationships, initial experience with the death of a relative or friend, and peer pressure.

Non-directive supportive therapy Helping people to express feelings and clarify thoughts and difficulties; therapists suggest alternative understandings and do not give direct advice but try to encourage people to solve their own problems.

Pulsed intravenous clomipramine An intravenous loading procedure for clomipramine.

Systemic behavioural family therapy A combination of two treatment approaches that have been used effectively for dysfunctional families. In the first phase of treatment, the therapist clarifies the concerns that brought the family into treatment, and provides a series of reframing statements designed to optimise engagement in therapy and identification of dysfunctional behaviour patterns (systemic therapy). In the second phase, the family members focus on communication and problem solving skills and the alteration of family interactional patterns (family behaviour therapy).

Substantive changes

Tricyclic antidepressants Updated systematic review;[6] conclusions unchanged.
Selective serotonin reuptake inhibitors One new RCT on paroxetine;[12] additional information.

REFERENCES

1. Costello EJ, Angold A, Burns BJ, et al. The Great Smoky Mountains Study of Youth. Goals, design, methods, and the prevalence of DSM-III-R disorders. *Arch Gen Psychiatry* 1996;53:1129–1136.
2. Costello EJ. Developments in child psychiatric epidemiology. *J Am Acad Child Adolesc Psychiatry* 1989;28:836–841.
3. Lewinsohn PM, Rohde P, Seely JR. Major depressive disorder in older adolescents: prevalence, risk factors, and clinical implications. *Clin Psychol Rev* 1998;18:765–794.
4. Birmaher B, Ryan ND, Williamson DE, et al. Childhood and adolescent depression: a review of the past 10 years, Part I. *J Am Acad Child Adolesc Psychiatry* 1996;35:1427–1439.
5. Geller B, Fox LW, Fletcher M. Effect of tricyclic antidepressants on switching to mania and on the onset of bipolarity in depressed 6- to 12-year-olds. *J Am Acad Child Adolesc Psychiatry* 1993;32:43–50.
6. Hazell P, O'Connell D, Heathcote D, et al. Tricyclic drugs for depression in children and adolescents. In: The Cochrane Library, Issue 2, 2002. Oxford:

Update Software. Search date 2000; primary sources Medline, Excerpta Medica, and Cochrane trials database.

7. Sallee FR, Vrindavanam NS, Deas-Nesmith D, et al. Pulse intravenous clomipramine for depressed adolescents: double-blind, controlled trial. *Am J Psychiatry* 1997;154:668–673.
8. Avci A, Diler RS, Kibar M, et al. Comparison of moclobemide and placebo in young adolescents with major depressive disorder. *Ann Med Sci* 1999;8:31–40.
9. Williams JW, Mulrow CD, Chiquette E, et al. A systematic review of newer pharmacotherapies for depression in adults: evidence report summary. *Ann Intern Med* 2000;132:743–756. Search date 1998; primary sources Medline, Embase, Psychlit, Lilacs, Psyindex, Sigle, Cinahl, Biological Abstracts, Cochrane Controlled Trials, hand searches, and personal contacts.
10. Simeon JG, Dinicola VF, Ferguson HB, et al. Adolescent depression: a placebo-controlled fluoxetine treatment study and follow-up. *Prog Neuropsychopharmacol Biol Psychiatry* 1990;14:791–795.
11. Emslie GJ, Rush AJ, Weinberg WA, et al. A double-blind, randomized, placebo-controlled trial of fluoxetine in children and adolescents with depression. *Arch Gen Psychiatry* 1997;54:1031–1037.
12. Keller MB, Ryan ND, Strober M, et al. Efficacy of paroxetine in the treatment of adolescent major depression: a randomized, controlled trial. *J Am Acad Child Adolesc Psychiatry* 2001;40:762 772.
13. Mandoki MW, Tapia MR, Tapia MA, et al. Venlafaxine in the treatment of children and adolescents with major depression. *Psychopharmacol Bull* 1997;33:149–154.
14. Geller B, Cooper TB, Zimerman B, et al. Lithium for prepubertal depressed children with family history predictors of future bipolarity: a double-blind, placebo-controlled study. *J Affect Disord* 1998;51:165–175.
15. Harrington R, Whittaker J, Shoebridge P, et al. Systematic review of efficacy of cognitive behavioural therapies in childhood and adolescent depressive disorder. *BMJ* 1998;316:1559–1563. Search date 1997; primary sources Medline, Psychlit, Cochrane, and hand searches of reference lists, book chapters, conference proceedings, and relevant journals in the field.
16. Lewinsohn PM, Clarke GN. Psychosocial treatments for adolescent depression. *Clin Psychol Rev* 1999;19:329–342.
17. Reinecke MA, Ryan NE, DuBois DL. Cognitive-behavioral therapy of depression and depressive symptoms during adolescence: a review and meta-analysis. *J Am Acad Child Adolesc Psychiatry* 1998;37:26–34.
18. Mendez Carrillo FX, Moreno PJ, Sanchez-Meca J, et al. Effectiveness of psychological treatment for child and adolescent depression: a qualitative review of two decades of research. *Psicol Conductual* 2000;8:487–510.
19. Mufson L, Weissman MM, Moreau D, et al. Efficacy of interpersonal psychotherapy for depressed adolescents. *Arch Gen Psychiatry* 1999;56:573–579.
20. Rossello J, Bernal G. The efficacy of cognitive-behavioral and interpersonal treatments for depression in Puerto Rican adolescents. *J Consult Clin Psychol* 1999;67:734–745.
21. Brent DA, Holder D, Kolko D, et al. A clinical psychotherapy trial for adolescent depression comparing cognitive, family, and supportive therapy. *Arch Gen Psychiatry* 1997;54:877–885.
22. Clarke GN, Rohde P, Lewinsohn PM, et al. Cognitive-behavioral treatment of adolescent depression: efficacy of acute group treatment and booster sessions. *J Am Acad Child Adolesc Psychiatry* 1999;38:272–279.
23. Fine S, Forth A, Gilbert M, et al. Group therapy for adolescent depressive disorder: a comparison of social skills and therapeutic support. *J Am Acad Child Adolesc Psychiatry* 1991;30:79–85.
24. Birmaher B, Brent DA, Kolko D, et al. Clinical outcome after short-term psychotherapy for adolescents with major depressive disorder. *Arch Gen Psychiatry* 2000;57:29–36.
25. Haaga DAF, Beck AT. Cognitive therapy. In: Paykel ES, ed. *Handbook of affective disorders.* Edinburgh: Churchill Livingstone, 1992;511–523.
26. Klerman GL, Weissman H. Interpersonal psychotherapy. In: Paykel ES, ed. *Handbook of affective disorders.* Edinburgh: Churchill Livingstone, 1992;501–510.

Philip Hazell
Conjoint Professor of Child and Adolescent Psychiatry/Director Child and Youth Mental Health Service
University of Newcastle
New South Wales
Australia

Competing interests: The author has been paid a fee by Pfizer, the manufacturer of sertraline, for speaking to general practitioners about the evidence for the treatment of depression in young people. The author's service has been in receipt of funding from Eli Lilly to participate in a relapse prevention trial of tomoxetine for attention deficit hyperactivity disorder.

Gastro-oesophageal reflux in children

Search date May 2002

Yadlapalli Kumar and Rajini Sarvananthan

QUESTIONS

INTERVENTIONS

*Not widely licensed for use in children. Clinical use in adults has been restricted because of heart rhythm abnormalities.

Key Messages

- **Cisapride** One systematic review found no significant difference with cisapride versus placebo in clinical symptoms. Cisapride is not widely licensed for use in children and has been withdrawn or its use restricted in several countries because of an association with heart rhythm abnormalities.
- **Domeperidone** One small RCT in children aged 5 months to 11 years found insufficient evidence about the effects of domperidone versus placebo.
- **Feed thickeners** We found no clear evidence about the effects of feed thickeners. One small RCT in infants aged 1–16 weeks found no significant difference in regurgitation reported by parents with carob flour thickened feeds versus placebo thickened feeds. Another small RCT in infants aged 5–11 months found that carob flour versus traditional formula thickened with rice flour significantly reduced gastro-oesophageal reflux symptoms and episodes of vomiting.
- **H_2 antagonists** One small RCT in children aged 1 month to 14 years found that cimetidine (an H_2 antagonist) versus placebo significantly improved clinical or endoscopic features of gastro-oesophageal reflux complicated by oesophagitis over 12 weeks (NNT 2, 95% CI 2 to 5).
- **Metoclopramide** Three small RCTs found insufficient evidence about the effects of metoclopramide versus placebo. One small RCT found insufficient evidence about the effects of metoclopramide versus sodium alginate or versus placebo.
- **Positioning (left lateral or prone)** Small crossover RCTs in children aged under 6 months found limited evidence that prone or left lateral positioning versus supine positioning improved oesophageal pH variables. Both positions may be associated with sudden infant death syndrome.
- **Sodium alginate** One small RCT in children aged under 2 years found that sodium alginate versus placebo for 8 days significantly reduced episodes of regurgitation reported by parents. One small RCT in children aged 4 months to 17 years found insufficient evidence about the effects of sodium alginate versus metoclopramide or versus placebo.
- **Proton pump inhibitors; surgery (fundoplication)** We found no RCTs on the effects of these interventions.

Clin Evid 2002;8:340–347.

DEFINITION Gastro-oesophageal reflux disease is the passive transfer of gastric contents into the oesophagus due to transient or chronic relaxation of the lower oesophageal sphincter.[1] A survey of 69 children (median age 16 months) with gastro-oesophageal reflux disease attending a tertiary referral centre found that presenting symptoms were recurrent vomiting (72%), epigastric and abdominal pain (36%), feeding difficulties (29%), failure to thrive (28%), and irritability (19%).[2] Over 90% of children with gastro-oesophageal reflux disease have vomiting before 6 weeks of age.[1]

INCIDENCE/ PREVALENCE Gastro-oesophageal regurgitation is considered a problem if it is frequent, persistent, and is associated with other symptoms such as increased crying, discomfort with regurgitation, and frequent back arching.[1,3] A cross-sectional survey of parents of 948 infants attending 19 primary care paediatric practices found that regurgitation of at least one episode a day was reported in 51% of infants aged 0–3 months. "Problematic" regurgitation occurred in significantly fewer infants (14% *v* 51 %; $P < 0.001$).[3] Peak regurgitation reported as "problematic" was reported in 23% of infants aged 6 months.[3]

AETIOLOGY/ RISK FACTORS Risk factors for gastro-oesophageal reflux disease include immaturity of the lower oesophageal sphincter, chronic relaxation of the sphincter, increased abdominal pressure, gastric distension, hiatus hernia, and oesophageal dysmotility.[1] Premature infants and children with severe neurodevelopmental problems or congenital oesophageal anomalies are particularly at risk.[1]

PROGNOSIS Regurgitation is considered benign, and most cases resolve spontaneously by 12–18 months of age.[4] In a cross-sectional survey of 948 parents, the peak age for reporting four or more episodes of regurgitation was at 5 months of age (23%), which decreased to 7% at 7 months ($P < 0.001$). The prevalence of "problematic" regurgitation also reduced from 23% in infants aged 6 months to 3.25% in infants aged 10–12 months.[3] Rare complications of gastro-oesophageal reflux disease include oesophagitis with haematemesis and anaemia, respiratory problems (such as cough, apnoea, and recurrent wheeze), and failure to thrive.[1] A small comparative study (40 children) suggested that, when compared with healthy children, infants with gastro-oesophageal reflux disease had slower development of feeding skills and had problems affecting behaviour, swallowing, food intake, and mother–child interaction.[5]

AIMS To relieve symptoms, maintain normal growth, prevent complications such as oesophagitis, and minimise adverse effects of treatment.

OUTCOMES Clinical condition (in terms of improvement in symptoms of vomiting and regurgiation); growth; parental distress; incidence of complications (e.g. oesophagitis). Reflux Index, a measure of the percentage of time with a low oesophageal pH (frequently < pH 4), is a surrogate outcome often used in RCTs. Clinical interpretation of the resulting data is problematic.

METHODS *Clinical Evidence* update search and appraisal May 2002. The authors also searched Cinahl for studies on incidence and prevalence.

Gastro-oesophageal reflux in children

QUESTION What are the effects of treatment for symptomatic gastro-oesophageal reflux?

OPTION DIFFERENT SLEEP POSITIONS

Three crossover RCTs in children aged under 6 months found limited evidence that prone or left lateral positioning versus supine positioning improved oesophageal pH variables. Both positions may be associated with sudden infant death syndrome.

Benefits: We found no systematic review or RCTs on the effect of posture on clinical symptoms, but found three small crossover RCTs on effect of posture on oesophageal pH variables such as the reflux index.[6–8] The first RCT (crossover, 24 infants, age < 5 months) assessed four sleep positions (supine, prone, left lateral, right lateral) over 48 hours; for the first 24 hours the infant was held horizontally, for the remaining 24 hours the infant's head was elevated.[6] It found that the prone and left lateral positions versus the supine and right lateral positions significantly reduced the reflux index over 48 hours ($P < 0.001$); it found no significant difference in the reflux index with horizontal positioning versus head elevation.[6] The second RCT (crossover, 15 infants, age < 6 months) alternated placing infants for 2 hours in a prone position (head elevated in a harness) and placing infants for 2 hours in a supine position (in an infant seat where the head and trunk were elevated to 60°) after a feed of apple juice.[7] It found that prone positioning versus supine positioning significantly reduced the reflux index over 72 normal hours ($P < 0.001$).[7] The third RCT (crossover, 18 infants, < 37 wks gestation but > 7 days old) compared prone versus left lateral versus right lateral positions over 24 hours. It found that prone and left lateral positions versus right lateral position significantly reduced reflux index ($P < 0.001$), the number of reflux episodes ($P < 0.001$), and duration of longest reflux episode ($P < 0.001$).[8]

Harms: The RCTs gave no information on adverse effects (see comment below).[6–8]

Comment: All three RCTs measured the surrogate outcome of reflux index, and it is difficult to interpret the clinical importance of the observed changes.[6–8] The results of these RCTs should be interpreted with caution as oesophageal pH variable may change over time, and the results were not assessed prior to crossover. Both prone and left lateral positioning have been associated with an increased risk of sudden infant death syndrome (see sudden infant death syndrome for prone positioning, p 396). One large, prospective cohort study found that the left lateral sleeping position compared with the supine position increased the risk of sudden infant death syndrome (at 2 months, adjusted OR 6.6, 95% CI 1.7 to 25.2).[9]

OPTION FEED THICKENERS

We found no clear evidence. One small RCT in infants aged 1–16 weeks found no significant difference between carob flour thickened feeds and placebo thickened feeds in regurgitation reported by parents. One small

RCT in infants aged 5–11 months found that carob flour versus traditional formula thickened with rice flour significantly reduced gastro-oesophageal reflux symptoms and episodes of vomiting.

Benefits: We found no systematic review. **Versus placebo:** We found one RCT (20 infants aged 1–16 wks with regurgitation > 5 times daily, receiving formula feeds, parental reassurance and prone positioning) comparing caraob flour thickened feeds versus placebo.[10] It found that when feeds were thickened with carob flour versus placebo thickener (Saint John's bread, which is free of fibre and polysaccharides) fewer children had regurgitation (as documented by parental diary) after 1 week of treatment, but the difference was not significant (mean regurgitation score 2.2 with carob flour *v* 3.3 with placebo; $P = 0.14$).[10] **Versus each other:** We found one RCT (24 infants, age 5–11 months, crossover), which found that, after 2 weeks, carob flour versus traditional formula thickened with rice significantly reduced a symptom score (mean relative reduction 70% with carob flour *v* 49% with traditional formula plus rice; $P < 0.01$) and the frequency of vomiting recorded by parents ($P < 0.05$).[11]

Harms: One RCT (24 children, age 0–6 months with gastro-oesophageal reflux disease) assessing the effects of feed thickeners on cough found that feeds thickened with dry rice cereal versus isocaloric unthickened feeds significantly increased coughing after feeding (mean cough salvos/h 3.1 with thickened feeds *v* 2.0 with unthickened feeds; $P = 0.034$).[12]

Comment: The clinical significance of changes in regurgitation scores in the first RCT is unclear.[10] The results of the crossover RCT comparing carob flour versus traditional formula should be treated with caution as symptoms may change over time and the results were not assessed prior to crossover.[11]

OPTION SODIUM ALGINATE

One small RCT in children aged under 2 years found that sodium alginate versus placebo significantly reduced the frequency of episodes of regurgitation reported by parents. Another small RCT in childrean aged 4 months to 17 years found no significant difference in oseophageal pH variables with sodium alginate, metoclopramide or placebo, but may have been too small to exclude a clinically important difference.

Benefits: We found no systematic review, but found two RCTs.[13,14] The first RCT (20 children, mean age 28 months) found that sodium alginate versus lactose powder placebo for 8 days significantly reduced the frequency from of regurgitation episodes reported by parents (frequency relative to untreated level 25–33% with sodium alginate *v* 0% with placebo). Sodium alginate versus placebo also significantly improved oesophageal pH variables (Euler-Byrne index and reflux time, $P < 0.05$). The second RCT (30 children aged 4 months to 17 years) found no significant difference in the frequency of regurgitation episodes over 24 hours with sodium alginate; metoclopramide; or placebo given before a meal (episode defined as pH < 4) or in the reflux index over 24 hours (reported as non-significant; no further data provided). The RCT may have been too small to exclude a clinically important difference.[14]

Harms: The RCTs found no adverse effects.[13,14]

Comment: The high sodium content of sodium alginate may be inappropriate in preterm babies.[15]

OPTION CISAPRIDE

One systematic review found no significant difference with cisapride versus placebo in the proportion of children with improved symptoms at the end of treatment. Cisapride has been withdrawn or its use restricted in several countries because of an association with heart rhythm abnormalities.

Benefits: We found one systematic review (search date 2000, 8 RCTs).[16] It found no significant difference between cisapride versus placebo in the proportion of children whose symptoms had improved at the end of treatment (7 RCTs, 236 children; 51/123 [41%] with cisapride *v* 64/113 [57%] with placebo; RR 0.72, 95% CI 0.54 to 0.96), but found that cisapride significantly reduced the reflux index (5 RCTs, 176 children; WMD –6.49, 95% CI –10.13 to –2.85). Confidence in these results is reduced by several potential sources of bias: improvement was assessed by a variety of scales; in some RCTs the "same or worse" category included the subcategory of "slight improvement" and significant heterogeneity was found between studies on pooling results for symptom improvement; the review found evidence suggesting publication bias favouring RCTs with positive outcomes; and the reflux index is poorly correlated with clinical symptoms and the clinical importance of changes in reflux index are unclear.

Harms: The review found a non-significant increase in adverse effects with cisapride versus placebo (4 RCTs, 190 children; 56/95 [59%] with cisapride *v* 45/95 [47%] with placebo; RR 1.19, 95% CI 0.96 to 1.47), but did not describe specific adverse effects.[16] See comment below.

Comment: Cisapride has been withdrawn or its use restricted in several countries because of an increased frequency of heart rhythm abnormalities that are associated with sudden death.[17] One case control study (201 children, age 1–12 months) found that cisapride significantly prolonged the QTc interval on electrocardiogram in a subgroup of infants younger than 3 months, but in older infants the difference was not significant.[18] A second case control study (252 infants) found similar results.[19] A third case control study (120 children) found prolonged QT interval in some normal children with or without cisapride.[20] Gastrointestinal adverse effects (borborygmi, cramps, and diarrhoea) occured in 2% of infants.[18] Rash, pruritus, urticaria, bronchospasm, extrapyramidal effects, headache, dose-related increases in urinary frequency, hyperprolactinaemia, and reversible liver function abnormalities were extremely rare.[18] Most macrolide antibiotics and cimetidine elevate plasma cisapride levels and may increase the clinical risk.[18]

OPTION DOMPERIDONE New

One small RCT in children aged 5 months to 11 years found no significant difference in symptoms or reflux index with domperidone versus placebo, but may have been too small to exclude a clinically important difference.

Benefits: We found no systematic review. One small RCT (17 children, age 5 months to 11 years) found no significant difference in symptoms (vomiting, spitting, irritability, heartburn, coughing, choking) assessed by daily parent record or reflux index after 4 weeks treatment with domperidone versus placebo.[21] The RCT may have been too small to exclude a clinically important difference.

Harms: The RCT found that four children taking domperidone had mild self limiting diarrhoea compared with two children taking placebo.[21]

Comment: None.

OPTION H_2 ANTAGONISTS

One small RCT in children aged 1 month to 14 years found that cimetidine versus placebo significantly improved gastro-oesophageal reflux complicated by oesophagitis in children. We found no RCTs of ranitidine in children.

Benefits: We found no systematic review but found two small RCTs.[22,23] The first RCT (double blind, 37 children aged 1 month to 14 years with gastro-oesophageal reflux disease complicated by oesophagitis) found that cimetidine (30–40 mg/kg daily) versus placebo significantly reduced the proportion of children with gastro-oesophageal reflux over 12 weeks (ARR 51%, 95% CI 21% to 81%; NNT 2, 95% CI 2 to 5). Improvement was defined in terms of either clinical or endoscopic findings.[22] A second RCT (27 children, aged 3–14 years with gastro-oesophageal reflux disease) compared different doses of cimetidine but reported only physiological outcomes (gastric pH, gastric acid suppression).[23] We found no RCTs of ranitidine in children.

Harms: The RCTs found no adverse effects.[22,23]

Comment: Cimetidine has been reported to cause bradycardia in a small subgroup of people and may increase cisapride plasma levels.[18] Uncontrolled studies of ranitidine have reported bronchospasm, acute dystonic reactions, sinus node dysfunction, bradycardia, and vasovagal reactions.[18]

OPTION METOCLOPRAMIDE New

One small crossover RCT in infants aged 1–9 months found that metoclopramide versus placebo significantly reduced the reflux index over 2 weeks, but found no significant difference in average daily symptoms. Another small RCT in infants aged under 1 year found no significant difference in the reflux index at 14 days with metoclopramide versus placebo. A third RCT in children aged 4 months to 17 years found no significant difference in oseophageal pH variables with sodium alginate, metoclopramide or placebo, but may have been too small to exclude a clinically important difference.

Benefits: We found no systematic review but found three RCTs.[14,24,25] The first RCT (crossover; 30 infants aged 1–9 months receiving formula feed) found that metoclopramide (1 mg/kg four times daily) versus placebo significantly reduced the reflux index over 2 weeks ($P < 0.001$), but found no significant difference in average daily symptoms (see comment below).[24] A second RCT (44 infants aged under 1 year) found no significant difference in the reflux index at 14 days with metoclopramide (0.2 mg three times daily) versus placebo before a meal.[25] A third RCT (30 infants aged 4 months to 17 years) compared three treatments: metoclopramide; sodium alginate; and placebo (see sodium alginate, p 343)[14]

Harms: The RCTs gave no information on adverse effects.[14,24,25]

Comment: The results of the crossover RCT should be treated with caution as it did not assess the effects of metoclopramide versus placebo before crossover.[24] In the second RCT 5/44 (11%) of infants withdrew from the study, three because of lack of efficacy and two for unknown reasons; the results given are not intention to treat.[25] One observational study (42 infants), which assessed the effect of metoclopramide (0.2 mg or 0.3 mg) on pH parameters, found that metoclopramide was associated with dystonia in one infant and increased irritability in three infants.[26]

OPTION PROTON PUMP INHIBITORS

We found no RCTs about proton pump inhibitors for gastro-oesophageal reflux in children.

Benefits: We found no systematic review or RCTs on proton pump inhibitors for gastro-oesophageal reflux in children. One small case series did not report clinical outcomes.[27]

Harms: We found no systematic review or RCTs.

Comment: Proton pump inhibitors have been reported to cause hepatitis, and omeprazole chronically elevates serum gastrin.[27]

OPTION SURGERY

We found no RCTs about surgery for gastro-oesophageal reflux in children.

Benefits: We found no systematic review or RCT comparing surgery versus medical interventions, or one surgical procedure versus another.

Harms: A retrospective review (106 children) of modified Nissen's fundoplication found a failure rate of 8% and, when neurologically impaired children were included, a long term mortality of 8%.[28] If only neurologically normal children were considered, the mortality was 2% in the immediate postoperative period and 3% on long term follow up (3 deaths in 62 children; all deaths were in children with congenital abnormalities).

Comment: We found a cohort study of 22 children who had undergone anterior gastric fundoplication.[29] Twenty children (91%) remained asymptomatic at 2 years. Complications of surgical treatment include dumping, retching, intestinal obstruction, "gas bloat", and recurrence of gastro-oesophageal reflux disease.[15]

Substantive changes

Sodium alginate One new RCT[14]; conclusions unchanged.

REFERENCES

1. Herbst JJ. *Textbook of Gastroenterology and Nutrition in Infancy*. 2nd ed. New York: Raven Press, 1989:803–813.
2. Lee WS, Beattie RM, Meadows N, et al. Gastro-oesophageal reflux: Clinical profiles and outcome. *J Paediatr Child Health* 1999;35:568–571.
3. Nelson SP , Chen EH, Syniar GM, et al. Prevalence of symptoms of gastroesophageal reflux during infancy. *Arch Pediatr Adolesc Med* 1997;151:569–572.
4. Vandenplas Y, Belli D, Benhamou P, et al. A critical appraisal of current management practices for infant regurgitation — recommendations of a working party. *Eur J Pediatr* 1997;156:343–357.
5. Mathisen B, Worrall L, Masel J, et al. Feeding problems in infants with gastro-oesophageal reflux disease: a controlled study. *J Paediatr Child Health* 1999;35:163–169.
6. Tobin JM, McCloud P, Cameron DJS. Posture and gastro-oesophageal reflux: a case for left lateral positioning. *Arch Dis Child* 1997;76:254–258.
7. Orenstein SR, Whitington PF. Positioning for prevention of infant gastroesophageal reflux. *J Pediatr* 1983;103:534–537.
8. Ewer AK, James ME, Tobin JM. Prone and left lateral positioning reduce gastro-oesophageal reflux in preterm infants. *Arch Dis Child Fetal Neonatal Ed* 1999;81:F201–205.
9. Dwyer T, Ponsonby AB, Newman NM, et al. Prospective cohort study of prone sleeping position and sudden infant death syndrome. *Lancet* 1991;337:1244–1247.
10. Vandenplas Y, Hachimi-Idrissi S, Casteels A, et al. A clinical trial with an "anti-regurgitation" formula. *Eur J Pediatr* 1994;153:419–423.
11. Borrelli O, Salvia G, Campanozzi A, et al. Use of a new thickened formula for treatment of symptomatic gastroesophageal reflux in infants. *Ital J Gastroenterol Hepatol* 1997;29:237–242.
12. Orenstein SR, Shalaby TM, Putnam PE. Thickening feedings as a cause of increased coughing when used as therapy for gastroesophageal reflux in infants. *J Pediatr* 1992;121:913–915.
13. Buts JP, Barudi C, Otte JB. Double-blind controlled study on the efficacy of sodium alginate (Gaviscon) in reducing gastroesophageal reflux assessed by 24 hour continuous pH monitoring in infants and children. *Eur J Pediatr* 1987;146:156–158.
14. Forbes D, Hodgson M, Hill, R. The effects of gaviscon and metoclopramide in gastroesophageal reflux in children. *J Pediatr Gastroenterol Nutr* 1986;5:556–559.
15. Davies AEM, Sandhu BK. Diagnosis and treatment of gastro-oesophageal reflux. *Arch Dis Child* 1995;73:82–86.
16. Augood C, MacLennan S, Gilbert R, et al. Cisapride treatment for gastro oesophageal reflux. In: The Cochrane Library, Issue 2, 2002. Oxford: Update Software. Search date 2000; primary sources Cochrane Central Trials Register, Cochrane Specialised Trials register of the Cochrane Upper Gastrointestinal and Pancreatic Diseases Group, Medline, Embase, Science Citation Index, and hand searched reference lists.
17. WHO Pharmaceuticals Newsletter, No.3, 2000. http://www.who.int/medicines/library/pnewslet/pn32000.html (last accessed 12/09/2002).
18. Vandenplas Y, Belli DC, Benatar A, et al. The role of cisapride in the treatment of pediatric gastroesophageal reflux. *J Pediatr Gastroenterol Nutr* 1999;28:518–528.
19. Benatar A, Feenstra A, Decraene T, et al. Effects of cisapride on corrected QT interval, heart rate, and rhythm in infants undergoing polysomnography. *Pediatrics* 2000;106(6):E85.
20. Ramirez-Mayans J, Garrido-Garcia LM, Huerta-Tecanhuey A, et al. Cisapride and QTc interval in children. *Pediatrics* 2000;106:1028–1030.
21. Bines JE, Quinlan JE, Treves S, et al. Efficacy of domperidone in infants and children with gastroesophageal reflux. *J Pediatr Gastroenterol Nutr* 1992;14:400–405.
22. Cucchiara S, Gobio-Casali L, Balli F, et al. Cimetidine treatment of reflux esophagitis in children: An Italian multicentre study. *J Pediatr Gastroenterol Nutr* 1989;8:150–156
23. Lambert J, Mobassaleh M, Grand RJ. Efficacy of cimetidine for gastric acid suppression in pediatric patients. *J Pediatr* 1992;120:474–478.
24. Tolia V, Calhoun J, Kuhns L, et al. Randomized, double-blind trial of metoclopramide and placebo for gastroesophageal reflux. *J Pediatr* 1989;115:141–145.
25. Bellisant E, Duhamel JF, Guillot M, et al. The triangular test to assess the efficacy of metoclopramide in gastroesophageal reflux. *Clin Pharm Ther* 1997;61:377–384.
26. Hyams JS, Leichtner AM, Zamett LO, et al. Effect of metoclopramide on prolonged intraoesophageal pH testing in infants with gastroesophageal reflux. *J Pediatr Gastroenterol Nutr* 1986;5 :716–720.
27. Gunasekaran TS, Hassall EG. Efficacy and safety of omeprazole for severe gastroesophageal reflux in children. *J Pediatr* 1993;123:148–154.
28. Spillane AJ, Currie B, Shi E. Fundoplication in children: Experience with 106 cases. *Aust NZ J Surg* 1996;66:753–756.
29. Bliss D, Hirschl R, Oldham K, et al. Efficacy of anterior gastric fundoplication in the treatment of gastroesophageal reflux in infants and children. *J Paediatr Surg* 1994;29:1071–1075.

Yadlapalli Kumar
Consultant Paediatrician
Royal Cornwall Hospital, Treliske Truro Cornwall, UK

Rajini Sarvananthan
Lecturer in Paediatrics
Universiti Kebangsaan Malaysia, Malaysia

Competing interests: None declared.

Infantile colic

Search date May 2002

Teresa Kilgour and Sally Wade

QUESTIONS

INTERVENTIONS

See glossary, p 357

Key Messages

- **Car ride stimulation** One RCT found no evidence that car ride stimulation reduced maternal anxiety and hours of infant crying over 2 weeks more than reassurance and support alone.
- **Casein hydrolysate milk** RCTs found insufficient evidence about the effects of replacing cows' milk formula with casein hydrolysate hypoallergenic formula.
- **Cranial osteopathy** We found no RCTs about the effects of cranial osteopathy in infants with colic.
- **Dicycloverine** One systematic review found limited evidence that dicycloverine (dicyclomine) versus placebo reduced crying in infants with colic. RCTs found that dicycloverine versus placebo increased drowsiness, constipation, and loose stools, but the difference did not reach significance. Case reports of harms in infants have included breathing difficulties, seizures, syncope, asphyxia, muscular hypotonia, and coma.
- **Focused counselling** One RCT found no evidence that counselling mothers about specific management techniques (responding to crying with gentle soothing motion, avoiding over stimulation, using a pacifier, and prophylactic carrying) reduced maternal anxiety and hours of infant crying over 2 weeks more than reassurance and support alone. Another small RCT found that focused counselling versus substitution of soya or cows' milk with casein hydrolysate formula significantly decreased duration and extent of crying.
- **Herbal tea** One small RCT found that herbal tea (containing extracts of camomile, vervain, liquorice, fennel, and balm mint in a sucrose solution) versus sucrose solution significantly improved symptoms of colic rated by parents at 7 days.

- **Increased carrying** One RCT found no significant difference in daily crying time with carrying the infant, even when not crying, for at least an additional 3 hours a day versus a general advice group (to carry, check baby's nappy, feed, offer pacifier, place baby near mother, or use background stimulation such as music). The "advice to carry" group carried their babies for 4.5 hours daily compared with 2.6 hours daily in the general advice group.
- **Infant massage** One RCT found no significant difference with massage versus a crib vibrator in colic related crying or parental rating of symptoms of infantile colic, but it may have lacked power to detect a clinically important difference.
- **Low lactose (lactase treated) milk** RCTs found no significant difference in duration of crying with low lactose treated milk versus untreated milk.
- **Reduction of stimulation of the infant** One RCT found limited evidence that advice to reduce stimulation (by not patting, lifting, or jiggling the baby, or by reducing auditory stimulation) versus an empathetic interview significantly reduced crying after 7 days in infants under 12 weeks.
- **Simethicone (activated dimeticone)** One RCT found no significant difference with simethicone (activated dimeticone) versus placebo in the presence of colic when rated by carers. A second RCT found no significant difference with simethicone versus placebo in improvement as rated by parental interview, 24 hour diary, or behavioural observation. A third, poor quality RCT found that simethicone versus placebo significantly reduced the number of crying attacks on days 4–7 of treatment.
- **Soya based infant feeds** One small RCT found that soya based infant feeds versus standard cows' milk formula significantly reduced the duration of crying.
- **Spinal manipulation** Two RCTs found inconclusive results about the effects of spinal manipulation.
- **Sucrose solution** One small crossover RCT found limited evidence that sucrose solution versus placebo significantly improved symptoms of colic as rated by parents after 12 days.
- **Whey hydrolysate milk** One RCT found limited evidence that replacing cows' milk formula with whey hydrolysate formula significantly reduced crying recorded in a parental diary.

DEFINITION Infantile colic is defined as excessive crying in an otherwise healthy baby. The crying typically starts in the first few weeks of life and ends by 4–5 months. Excessive crying is defined as crying that lasts at least 3 hours a day, for 3 days a week, for at least 3 weeks.[1]

INCIDENCE/ PREVALENCE Infantile colic causes 1/6 (17%) families to consult a health professional. One systematic review of 15 community based studies found a wide variation in prevalence, which depended on study design and method of recording.[2] The two best prospective studies identified by the review yielded prevalence rates of 5% and 19%.[2] One RCT (89 breast and formula fed infants) found that, at 2 weeks of age, the prevalence of crying more than 3 hours a day was 43% among formula fed infants and 16% among breastfed infants. The prevalence at 6 weeks was 12% (formula fed) and 31% (breast fed).[3]

AETIOLOGY/ RISK FACTORS The cause of infantile colic is unclear and, despite its name, might not have an abdominal cause. It may reflect part of the normal distribution of infantile crying. Other possible explanations are painful intestinal contractions, lactose intolerance, gas, or parental misinterpretation of normal crying.[1]

PROGNOSIS Infantile colic improves with time. One study found that 29% of infants aged 1–3 months cried for more than 3 hours a day, but by 4–6 months of age the prevalence had fallen to 7–11%.[4]

AIMS To reduce infant crying and distress, and the anxiety of the family, with minimal adverse effects of treatment.

OUTCOMES Duration of crying or colic, as measured on dichotomous, ordinal, or continuous scales; parents' perceptions of severity (recorded in a diary).

METHODS *Clinical Evidence* update search and appraisal May 2002. The contributors also searched Cinahl for publications using reduction in crying or colic as the main outcome. Trials were excluded for the following reasons: infants studied had normal crying patterns, infants were older than 6 months, interventions lasted less than 3 days, trials had no control groups or had low scores on the Jadad Scale (see glossary, p 357).[5]

QUESTION **What are the effects of treatments for infantile colic?**

OPTION **DICYCLOVERINE**

One systematic review found limited evidence that dicycloverine (dicyclomine) versus placebo reduces crying in infants with colic. RCTs found that dicycloverine versus placebo increased drowsiness, constipation, and loose stools, but the difference did not reach significance. Case reports of harms in infants have included breathing difficulties, seizures, syncope, asphyxia, muscular hypotonia, and coma.

Benefits: We found two systematic reviews.[1,6] The first systematic review (search date 1996)[1] identified five RCTs (134 infants) comparing the effect of dicycloverine (see glossary, p 357) versus placebo on crying or the presence of colic. It found that dicycloverine (most frequently 5 mg 4 times daily) versus placebo significantly reduced crying (SMD 0.46, 95% CI 0.33 to 0.60). The clinical importance of this result is unclear (see comment below).[6] The second systematic review (search date 1999)[6] identified three RCTs included in the first systematic review,[1] but did not pool the results because the RCTs used different outcome measures. One RCT identified by the reviews found that dicycloverine versus placebo (cherry syrup) significantly reduced colic (elimination of colic: 63% with dicycloverine *v* 25% with placebo; RR 0.50, 95% CI 0.28 to 0.88; NNT 3, CI not provided).[7] The other two RCTs identified by the reviews used definitions of colic that included symptoms but not duration and frequency, and reported results in terms of clinical scores. Both RCTs found significantly better mean clinical scores with dicycloverine versus placebo.[6]

Harms: Two of five RCTs[8,9] in the systematic reviews[1,6] compared harms of dicycloverine versus placebo. The first RCT (crossover design, 30 infants) found more drowsiness with dicycloverine versus placebo (4/30 [13%] *v* 1/30 [3%]; ARI +10%, 95% CI –4% to +24%).[8] The second RCT (crossover design, 25 infants) found more loose stools or constipation in infants on dicycloverine versus placebo (3/25 [12%] *v* 1/25 [4%]; ARI +8%, 95% CI −7% to +23%).[9] Case reports of harms in infants have included breathing difficulties, seizures, syncope, asphyxia, muscular hypotonia, and coma.[10]

Comment: The review is limited because it pooled different outcome measures from RCTs and included crossover studies.[1] The crossover design is unlikely to provide valid evidence because infantile colic has a naturally variable course, and the effects of dicycloverine may continue even after a washout period.[11] Only one RCT identified by the reviews stated measures to make the control syrup taste the same as the drug syrup.[8]

OPTION SIMETHICONE (ACTIVATED DIMETICONE)

One RCT found no significant difference with simethicone (activated dimeticone) versus placebo in the presence of colic when rated by carers. A second RCT found no significant difference with simethicone versus placebo in improvement as rated by parental interview, 24 hour diary, or behavioural observation. A third, poor quality RCT found that simethicone versus placebo significantly reduced the number of crying attacks on days 4–7 of treatment.

Benefits: We found two systematic reviews (search dates 1996[1], 1999[6], same 3 RCTs in each review, 136 infants) comparing the effect of simethicone (see glossary, p 357) versus placebo on the duration of crying or the presence of colic.[6] The first RCT (double blind, crossover, 83 infants aged 2–8 wks) compared 0.3 mL of simethicone versus placebo before feeds.[12] It found no significant difference in colic when rated by carers (28% improved with simethicone *v* 37% with placebo *v* 20% with both; effect size for simethicone versus placebo: −0.10, 95% CI −0.27 to +0.08). The second RCT (double blind, crossover trial, 27 infants aged 2–8 wks) found no difference with simethicone versus placebo in improvement as rated by parental interview, 24 hour diary, or behavioural observation (effect size +0.06, 95% CI −0.17 to +0.28).[13] The third RCT (26 infants aged 1–12 wks) was of unsatisfactory quality; it reported no details on how cases of colic were defined.[14] It found that simethicone versus placebo significantly reduced the number of crying attacks on days 4–7 of treatment (effect size 0.54, 95% CI 0.21 to 0.87).[14]

Harms: None of the RCTs reported adverse effects with either simethicone or placebo.[12–14]

Comment: The crossover design of two of the RCTs limits their validity and clinical utility because infantile colic has a naturally variable course, and the effects of simethicone may continue even after a washout period.[12,13]

OPTION REPLACEMENT OF COWS' MILK WITH SOYA BASED INFANT FEEDS

One small RCT found that soya based infant feeds versus cows' milk reduced the duration of crying in infants with colic.

Benefits: We found two systematic reviews (search dates 1996[1] and 1999,[6] 2 RCTs). One RCT (19 infants) found that soya based infant feeds (see glossary, p 357) versus standard cows' milk formula reduced the duration of crying (4.3–12.7 h with soya based infant feeds *v* 17.3–20.1 h with cows' milk; mean difference –10.3 h, 95% CI –16.0 to –4.0 h).[15] The other RCT only considered infants admitted to hospital for colic and used weak methods (Jadad [see glossary, p 357] score 1).[16]

Harms: None reported in the RCTs.[15,16]

Comment: In the first RCT, mothers were not told which milk the babies received, but differences between the milks may have been detected from smell and texture.[15]

OPTION REPLACEMENT OF COWS' MILK WITH CASEIN HYDROLYSATE MILK

Two RCTs found insufficient evidence of the effects of casein hydrolysate milk versus cows' milk formula in infants with colic.

Benefits: We found two systematic reviews (search dates 1996[1] and 1999[6]), which identified the same two RCTs. The first RCT (double blind, crossover, 17 infants) studied the effect of each of three changes of infant diet over 4 days.[17] Bottle fed infants received casein hydrolysate milk (see glossary, p 357) and cows' milk alternately. By the third change, there was no notable difference in the incidence of colic between groups. A total of 8/17 (47%) infants left the study before completion. The second RCT (122 infants) compared bottle fed infants (38 infants) given casein hydrolysate milk (active diet) versus cows' milk formula, and breast fed infants (77 infants) with mothers on a hypoallergenic diet (see glossary, p 357) (active diet) versus controls on an unmodified diet.[18] Fifty four infants received the active diet, but the RCT did not specify which of these were bottle fed and which were breast fed. The RCT pooled the results of breast and bottle fed babies and found that the active diet versus control diet reduced infant distress as measured by parents on a validated chart. The number of bottle fed infants was too small to establish or exclude important effects in infants bottle fed casein hydrolysate milk versus cows' milk.

Harms: None reported in the RCTs.[17,18]

Comment: None.

OPTION — REPLACEMENT OF COWS' MILK FORMULA BY WHEY HYDROLYSATE FORMULA

One RCT found limited evidence that replacing cows' milk formula with whey hydrolysate formula reduced infant colic.

Benefits: We found two systematic reviews (search dates 1996[1] and 1999[6]) and one subsequent RCT.[19] The systematic reviews found no RCTs of adequate quality. The subsequent, double blind RCT (43 infants) found that whey hydrolysate formula (see glossary, p 357) (23 infants) versus standard cows' milk formula reduced the time that babies cried each day, measured by a validated parental diary (crying reduced by 63 min/day, 95% CI 1 to 127 min/day).[19]

Harms: None identified in the subsequent RCT.[19]

Comment: In the subsequent RCT, parents may not have been blind to the intervention. When asked, six indicated that they were aware of allocation, but two of these falsely identified the formula. When these infants' results were removed from the analysis, the crying time with whey hydrolysate formula versus standard cows' milk formula was significantly reduced by 58 minutes daily ($P = 0.03$).[19]

OPTION — LOW LACTOSE (LACTASE TREATED) MILK

Four RCTs found no significant difference in duration of crying with low lactose (lactase treated) milk versus untreated milk in infants with colic.

Benefits: We found two systematic reviews (search dates 1996[1] and 1999,[6] 2 RCTs) and two additional RCTs.[20,21] The first RCT in the systematic reviews (double blind, crossover, 10 weaned infants) compared four interventions: bottle feeding using pooled breast milk; low lactose (lactase treated) breast milk; cows' milk, and low lactose (lactase treated) cows' milk.[22] It found no evidence that low lactose milk reduced the timing, severity, or duration of colic recorded by parents. The second RCT (12 breast fed infants) in the reviews compared low lactose versus placebo drops given within 5 minutes of feeding and found no significant differences for time spent feeding, sleeping, or crying.[1,6] The first additional RCT (crossover, 13 infants) compared low lactose milk versus placebo treated milk.[20] It found no significant difference in crying time with low lactose milk versus placebo milk (1.1 h/day, 95% CI 0.2 to 2.1 h/day). The second additional RCT (crossover, 53 infants) found that low lactose formula/breast milk versus untreated formula/breast milk reduced cry time after crossover at 25 days, but the difference was not significant (median 11.0 h with lactase *v* 14.1 h with no lactase; median difference in crying time 23%; $P = 0.09$).[21]

Harms: None reported in the RCTs.[1,6,20,21]

Comment: It is difficult to make firm conclusions from these RCTs.[1,6,20–22] The babies were not selected on the basis of confirmed lactose intolerance. The crossover design of three of the RCTs limits their validity and clinical utility because infantile colic has a naturally variable course.[20–22]

OPTION SUCROSE SOLUTION

One small crossover RCT found that sucrose solution versus placebo significantly increased parent rated improvement in symptoms of infantile colic after 12 days.

Benefits: We found one systematic review (search date 1999, 1 small crossover RCT).[6] The RCT (19 infants) compared 2 mL of 12% sucrose solution versus placebo given to babies when they continued to cry despite comforting.[23] Parents, blind to the intervention, scored the effect of the treatment on a scale of 1–5. Treatments were crossed over after 3–4 days and again after 6–8 days. The RCT found that sucrose versus placebo significantly increased parent rated improvement after 12 days (12/19 [63%] with sucrose *v* 1/19 [5%] with placebo; ARI 58%, 95% CI 10% to 89%; NNT 2, 95% CI 1 to 10; RR 12, 95% CI 3 to 19).

Harms: None reported in the RCT.[23]

Comment: None.

OPTION HERBAL TEA

One small RCT found that herbal tea (containing extracts of chamomile, vervain, licorice, fennel, and balm mint in a sucrose solution) versus sucrose solution alone reduced parent rated symptoms of infantile colic.

Benefits: We found two systematic reviews (search dates 1996[1] and 1999,[6] 1 RCT[24]). The RCT compared herbal tea (containing extracts of chamomile, vervain, licorice, fennel, and balm mint in a sucrose solution) (33 infants) versus sucrose solution alone (35 infants) given by parents up to three times daily in response to episodes of colic.[24] Coding was only known to the pharmacist and the taste and smell of the tea and placebo were similar. Parents rated the response using a symptom diary. The RCT found that, at 7 days, herbal tea eliminated colic more frequently than sucrose solution (number of infants colic free: 19/33 [58%] with herbal tea *v* 9/35 [26%] with sucrose; ARI 32%, 95% CI 7% to 53%; RR 2.2, 95% CI 1.3 to 3.1; NNT 3, 95% CI 2 to 14).

Harms: None reported in the RCT.[24]

Comment: The RCT did not state the exact proportion of the herbs used in the preparation.[24]

OPTION BEHAVIOURAL MODIFICATION

One RCT found no significant difference in maternal anxiety or hours of infant crying over 2 weeks with focused counselling or car ride stimulation plus non-specific reassurance versus non-specific reassurance alone. Another small RCT found that focused counselling versus substitution of soya or cows' milk with casein hydrolysate formula significantly decreased duration and extent of crying. One RCT found limited evidence that advice to reduce stimulation (by not patting, lifting, or jiggling the baby, or by reducing auditory stimulation) versus an empathetic interview significantly reduced crying after 7 days in infants

under 12 weeks. One RCT found no significant difference in daily crying time with carrying the infant, even when not crying, for at least an additional 3 hours a day versus a general advice group (to carry, check baby's nappy, feed, offer pacifier, place baby near mother, or use background stimulation such as music).

Benefits: We found two systematic reviews (search dates 1996[1] and 1999,[6] 4 RCTs). **Focused counselling or car ride stimulation plus non-specific reassurance versus non-specific reassurance alone:** See glossary, p 357. One RCT (38 infants) identified by the reviews assessed maternal anxiety and the hours of crying each day by questionnaire. It found no evidence that counselling mothers about specific management techniques (responding to crying with gentle soothing motion, avoiding over stimulation, using a pacifier, and prophylactic carrying) or car ride stimulation reduced maternal anxiety and hours of infant crying over 2 weeks more than reassurance and support alone.[25] **Focused counselling versus elimination of cows' milk protein:** One RCT (20 infants) found that counselling parents to respond to their baby's cries by feeding, holding, offering a pacifier, stimulating, or putting the baby down to sleep, decreased duration and extent of crying significantly more than substitution of soya or cows' milk with casein hydrolysate formula (mean decrease in crying, recorded by parent diary, 2.1 h/day with counselling *v* 1.2 h/day with dietary change; P = 0.05).[26] **Increased carrying versus general advice:** The third RCT (66 infants) randomised mothers of babies with colic to carry their infant, even when not crying, for at least an additional 3 hours a day or to a general advice group (to carry, check baby's nappy, feed, offer pacifier, place baby near mother, or use background stimulation such as music). The "advice to carry" group carried their babies for 4.5 hours daily compared with 2.6 hours daily in the general advice group. There was no effect on daily crying time (mean difference 3 min less, 95% CI 37 min less to 32 min more).[27] **Reducing stimulation versus non-specific interview:** The fourth RCT (42 infants, median age 10 wks) allocated mothers of infants to advice to reduce stimulation (mothers were advised to reduce stimulation by not patting, lifting, or jiggling the baby, or reducing auditory stimulation) versus an empathetic interview. For infants under 12 weeks, advice to reduce stimulation versus no advice improved a change rating scale for more infants (after 7 days: 14/15 [93%] improved with advice *v* 6/12 [50%] with control; ARI 43%, 95% CI 8% to 49%; RR 1.9, 95% CI 1.2 to 2.0; NNT 2, 95% CI 2 to 13).[28] Improvement in the change rating scale was defined as a score of +2 or better on a scale from –5 to +5 that was meant to indicate perceived change in crying since the start of the trial. It is unclear whether this scale has been validated (see comment below).

Harms: None reported in the RCTs identified by the reviews.[1,6]

Comment: Behavioural modification involves interventions to change the way in which parents respond to their babies crying from colic. Mothers given advice to reduce stimulation were also given permission to leave their infants if they felt they could no longer tolerate the crying. It is unclear whether the improved change score represents a true change in the hours that the baby cried, or altered maternal perception.

OPTION CRANIAL OSTEOPATHY

We found no RCTs on the effects of cranial osteopathy in infants with colic.

Benefits: We found no systematic review and no RCTs on the effects of cranial osteopathy (see glossary, p 357) in infants with colic.

Harms: We found no RCTs.

Comment: None.

OPTION INFANT MASSAGE

One RCT found no significant difference with massage versus a crib vibrator for colic related crying or parental rating of symptoms of infantile colic, but it may have lacked power to detect a clinically important difference.

Benefits: We found no systematic review. **Versus usual care:** We found no RCTs. **Versus other care:** We found one RCT (58 infants, 47% with colic; see comment below comparing massage versus a crib vibrator over a 4 week period).[29] Infant massage (performed 3 times daily) included gentle stroking of the skin over different parts of the head, body, and limbs, using olive oil and while maintaining eye contact. The crib vibrator was used for 25 minute periods at least three times daily (see comment below). Colic symptom ratings were obtained from parental diaries of crying. The RCT found no significant difference with massage versus a crib vibrator for colic related crying or parental rating of symptoms (AR for less crying: 64% *v* 52%; P = 0.24, CI not provided).[29]

Harms: None reported in the RCT.[29]

Comment: Only 47% of infants in the RCT had colic, so the results may not apply to infants with colic.[29] The use of a crib vibrator as a control intervention is based on an earlier study in which a similar device was as effective as parental reassurance (see glossary, p 357) and support. It is unclear whether reduced crying in this RCT reflects the natural course of infantile colic or the specific effect of interventions. The RCT may have lacked power to detect clinically important effects.

OPTION SPINAL MANIPULATION

Two RCTs found insufficient evidence about the effects of spinal manipulation.

Benefits: We found no systematic review. We found two RCTs that assessed spinal manipulation (see glossary, p 357).[30,31] **Versus simethicone (activated dimeticone):** One RCT (41 infants) compared 2 weeks of spinal manipulation versus 2 weeks of daily treatment with simethicone (see glossary, p 357); parents recorded length of crying in a colic diary.[30] It found that spinal manipulation versus simethicone significantly reduced crying (mean reduction in crying for days 4–7: 2.4 h with spinal manipulation *v* 1.0 h with simethicone; P = 0.04; CI not provided).[30] Parents were not blinded to treatment. **Versus holding:** One RCT (86 infants) compared spinal palpation by a chiropractor versus holding of the infant by a nurse (3 times over 8 days).[31] The parents, who were blind to the intervention, rated symptom severity on a five point scale and recorded crying in a diary. The RCT found no difference with spinal palpation versus holding for crying reduction (by day 8, mean reduction 3.1 h for both groups; P = 0.98, CI not provided).

Harms: None were reported in the RCTs.[30,31]

Comment: It is unclear whether reduced crying reflected effects of interventions or spontaneous improvement.

GLOSSARY

Casein hydrolysate milk Contains casein protein; it is used in the same way as soya based infant feeds.

Cranial osteopathy Involves gentle manipulation of the tissues of the head by an osteopath.

Dicycloverine (dicyclomine) This has direct antispasmodic action on the gastrointestinal tract and anticholinergic effects, which are similar to atropine.

Hypoallergenic diet In bottle fed infants, a hypoallergenic diet uses a casein hydrolysate formula. In breast fed infants, a hypoallergenic diet involves a maternal diet, free of artificial colourings, preservatives, and additives, and low in common allergens (e.g. milk, egg, wheat, and nuts).

Jadad Scale This measures factors that impact on trial quality. Poor description of the factors, rated by low figures, are associated with greater estimates of effect. The scale includes three items: was the study described as randomised? (0–2); was the study described as double blind? (0–2); was there a description of withdrawals and drop outs? (0–1).[5]

Reassurance Informing the parent that infantile colic is a self limiting condition resolving by 3–4 months of age, and is not caused by disease or any fault in parental care.

Simethicone (activated dimeticone) It has defoaming properties, which can aid dispersion of gas in the gastrointestinal tract.

Soya based infant feeds Contain proteins from soya beans; the feeds are used as lactose free vegetable milks for those with lactose or cow's milk protein intolerance.

Spinal manipulation Chiropractic manual treatment of the infant's vertebral column.

Whey hydrolysate milk Contains whey protein; it is used in the same way as soya based infant feeds.

Substantive changes

Low lactose (lactase treated) milk One new RCT;[22] conclusions unchanged.

REFERENCES

1. Lucassen, PLB, Assendelf, WJJ, Gubbels JW, et al. Effectiveness of treatments for infantile colic: a systematic review. *BMJ* 1998;316:1563–1569. Search date 1996: primary sources Cochrane Controlled Trials Register, Embase, Medline, and hand searches of reference lists.
2. Lucassen PLBJ, Assendelft WJJ, Van Eijk JTHM, et al. Systematic review of the occurrence of infantile colic in the community. *Arch Dis Child* 2001; 84:398–403. Search date 1998; primary sources Embase and Medline.
3. Lucas A, St James-Roberts I. Crying, fussing and colic behaviour in breast and bottle-fed infants. *Early Hum Dev* 1998;53:9–19.
4. St James-Roberts I, Halil A. Infant crying patterns in the first year: normal community and clinical findings. *J Child Psychol Psychiatry* 1991;32:951–968.
5. Jadad AR, Moore RA, Carroll D, et al. Assessing the quality of reports of randomized clinical trials: is blinding necessary? *Control Clin Trials* 1996;17:1–12.
6. Garrison MM, Christakis DA. A systematic review of treatments for infant colic. *Pediatrics* 2000;106:184–190. Search date 1999; primary sources Medline, Cochrane Clinical Trials Registry, hand searches of reference lists, and authors.

7. Weissbluth M, Christoffel KK, Davis AT. Treatment of infantile colic with dicyclomine hydrochloride. *J Pediatr* 1984:104:951–955.
8. Hwang CP, Danielsson B. Dicyclomine hydrochloride in infantile colic. *BMJ* 1985;291:1014.
9. Gruinseit F. Evaluation of the efficacy of dicyclomine hydrochloride ("Merbentyl") syrup in the treatment of infantile colic. *Curr Med Res Opin* 1977;5:258–261.
10. Williams J, Watkin Jones R. Dicyclomine: worrying symptoms associated with its use in some small babies. *BMJ* 1984;288:901.
11. Fleiss JL. The crossover study. In: Fleiss JL, ed. *The design and analysis of clinical experiments*. New York: Wiley and Sons, 1986.
12. Metcalf TJ, Irons TG, Sher LD, et al. Simethicone in the treatment of infantile colic: a randomized, placebo-controlled, multicenter trial. *Pediatrics* 1994;94:29–34.
13. Danielsson B, Hwang CP. Treatment of infantile colic with surface active substance (simethicone). *Acta Paediatr Scand* 1985;74:446–450.
14. Sethi KS, Sethi JK. Simethicone in the management of infant colic. *Practitioner* 1988;232:508.
15. Campbell JPM. Dietary treatment of infantile colic: a double-blind study. *J R Coll Gen Pract* 1989;39:11–14.
16. Lothe L, Lindbert T, Jakobsson I. Cow's milk formula as a cause of infantile colic: a double-blind study. *Pediatrics* 1982;70:7–10.
17. Forsythe BWC. Colic and the effect of changing formulas: a double blind, multiple-crossover study. *J Pediatr* 1989;115:521–526.
18. Hill DJ, Hudson IL, Sheffield LJ, et al. A low allergen diet is a significant intervention in infantile colic: results of a community based study. *J Allergy Clin Immunol* 1995;96:886–892.
19. Lucassen LB, Assendelft WJ, Gubbels LW, et al. Infantile colic: crying time reduction with a whey hydrolysate; a double blind, randomized placebo-controlled trial. *Pediatrics* 2000;106:1349–1354.
20. Kearney PJ, Malone AJ, Hayes T, et al. A trial of lactase in the management of infant colic. *J Hum Nutr Diet* 1998;11:281–285.
21. Kanabar D, Randhawa M, Clayton P. Improvement of symptoms of infant colic following reduction of lactose load with lactase. *J Hum Nutr Diet* 2001,14;359–363.
22. Stahlberg MR, Savilahti E. Infantile colic and feeding. *Arch Dis Child* 1986;61:1232–1233.
23. Markestad T. Use of sucrose as a treatment for infant colic. *Arch Dis Child* 1997;77:356–357.
24. Weizman Z, Alkrinawi S, Goldfarb D, et al. Herbal teas for infantile colic. *J Pediatr* 1993;123:670–671.
25. Parkin PC, Schwartz CJ, Manuel BA. Randomised controlled trial of three interventions in the management of persistent crying of infancy. *Pediatrics* 1993;92;197–201.
26. Taubman B. Parental counselling compared with elimination of cow's milk or soy milk protein for the treatment of infant colic syndrome: a randomized trial. *Pediatrics* 1988;81:756–761.
27. Barr RG, McMullen SJ, Spiess H, et al. Carrying as a colic "therapy": a randomized controlled trial. *Pediatrics* 1991;87:623–630.
28. McKenzie S. Troublesome crying in infants: effect of advice to reduce stimulation. *Arch Dis Child* 1991;66:1461–1420.
29. Huhtala V, Lehtonen L, Heinonen R, et al. Infant massage compared with crib vibrator in the treatment of colicky infants. *Pediatrics* 2000;105:e84.
30. Wiberg JMM, Nordsteen J, Nilsson N. The short term effect of spinal manipulation in the treatment of infant colic: a randomized controlled clinical trial with a blinded observer. *J Manip Physiol Therap* 1999;22:517–522.
31. Olafsdottir E, Forshei S, Fluge G, et al. Randomised controlled trial of infant colic treated with chiropractic spinal manipulation. *Arch Dis Child* 2001;84:138–141.

Teresa Kilgour
Staff Grade Community Paediatrician
City Hospitals Sunderland
Sunderland
UK

Sally Wade
Staff Grade Community Paediatrician
Archer Street Clinic
Darlington
UK

Competing interests: None declared.

Measles

Search date November 2001

Anna Donald and Vivek Muthu

QUESTIONS

INTERVENTIONS

See glossary, p 367

Key Messages

Live combined measles, mumps, and rubella (MMR) vaccine; live monovalent measles vaccine

- Large cohort studies, large cross-sectional time series, and population surveillance data from different countries have all found that combined measles, mumps, and rubella (MMR) and live monovalent measles vaccination programmes reduce the risk of measles infection to near zero, especially in populations in which vaccine coverage is high.
- We found no RCTs comparing the effects of MMR versus no vaccination or placebo on measles infection rates. Such trials are likely to be considered unethical because of the large body of whole-population evidence finding benefit from vaccination.
- Unlike live monovalent measles vaccine, MMR additionally vaccinates against mumps and rubella, which themselves cause serious complications (mumps causes orchitis, pancreatitis, infertility, meningoencephalitis, deafness, and congenital fetal abnormalities; rubella causes deafness, blindness, heart defects, liver, spleen and brain damage, and stillbirth).
- One systematic review, one RCT, one large population based survey and one population based study found no evidence of MMR being associated with acute developmental regression compared with placebo or no vaccine. Large cross-sectional time series have consistently found no evidence of MMR or live monovalent measles vaccine being associated with autism.
- One large, long term population surveillance study and one population based case control study found no evidence that either the monovalent measles vaccine or MMR was associated with inflammatory bowel disease. One large cohort study and two population based case control studies found no association of inflammatory bowel disease with the monovalent vaccine.
- One systematic review and one additional RCT have found that MMR and monovalent measles vaccine are associated with a small and similar risk of self limiting fever within 3 weeks of vaccination compared with 100% risk of acute fever in people with measles.

Measles

DEFINITION Measles is an infectious disease caused by a ribonucleic acid (RNA) paramyxomavirus. The illness is characterised by an incubation period of 10–12 days; a prodromal period of 2–4 days with upper respiratory tract symptoms; Koplik's spots on mucosal membranes and high fever; followed by further fever; and a widespread maculopapular rash that persists for 5–6 days.[1]

INCIDENCE/ PREVALENCE Measles incidence varies widely according to vaccination coverage. Worldwide, there are an estimated 30 million cases of measles each year,[2] but an incidence of only 0–10/100 000 people in countries with widespread vaccination programmes such as the USA, UK, Mexico, India, China, Brazil, and Australia.[3] In the USA, before licensure of effective vaccines, greater than 90% of people were infected by the age of 15 years, whereas after licensure in 1963, incidence fell by about 98%.[1] Mean annual incidence in Finland was 366/100 000 in 1970,[4] but declined to about zero by the late 1990s.[5] Similarly, annual incidence declined to about zero in Chile, the English speaking Caribbean, and Cuba during the 1990s with introduction of vaccination programmes.[6,7]

AETIOLOGY/ RISK FACTORS Measles is spread through airborne droplets that persist for up to 2 hours in closed areas following the presence of an infected person. Measles is highly contagious. As with other infectious diseases, other risk factors include overcrowding, low herd immunity, and immunosuppression. People with immunosuppression, children of less than 5 years of age, and adults of more than 20 years of age have a higher risk of severe complications and death, although these also occur in healthy people (see prognosis below).[1] Newborn babies have a lower risk of measles than older infants because of the presence of protective maternal antibodies, although in recent US outbreaks, maternal antibody protection was lower than expected.[1]

PROGNOSIS The World Health Organization estimated that in the year 2000, measles caused 777 000 deaths and a burden of disease of 27.5 million disability adjusted life years.[8] **Disease in healthy people:** In developed countries, most prognostic data come from the pre-vaccination era and from subsequent outbreaks in non-vaccinated populations. In the USA, measles is complicated in about 30% of reported cases. From 1989–1991 in the USA, measles resurgence among young children (< 5 years) who had not been immunised led to 55 622 cases with more than 11 000 hospital admissions and 125 deaths.[1] Measles complications include diarrhoea (8%), otitis media (7%), pneumonia (6%), death (0.1–0.2%), acute encephalitis (about 0.1% followed by death in 15% and permanent neurological damage in about 25%), seizures (with or without fever in 0.6–0.7%), idiopathic thrombocytopenia (1/6000 reported cases), and subacute sclerosing panencephalitis causing degeneration of the central nervous system and death 7 years after measles infection (range 1 month to 27 years; 0.5–1.0/ 100 000 reported cases).[1,9] Measles during pregnancy results in higher risk of premature labour, spontaneous abortion, and low birth weight infants. An association with birth defects remains uncertain.[1]

Disease in malnourished or immunocompromised people: In malnourished or immunocompromised people, particularly those with vitamin A deficiency, measles case fatality can be as high as 25%. Worldwide, measles is a major cause of blindness and causes 5% of deaths in young children (< 5 years).[1,10]

AIMS Preventing measles with minimum adverse effects.

OUTCOMES **Prevention, benefits:** Clinically apparent measles and measles related complications, including death. We have included a proxy outcome (seroconversion — see glossary, p 367) because it is so highly correlated with vaccine efficacy.[11] **Prevention, harms:** Acute fever, febrile seizures, inflammatory bowel disease, developmental regression, autism and clinical measles after seroconversion.

METHODS *Clinical Evidence* search and appraisal November 2001. The authors also searched World Health Organization, US Communicable Disease Control, and UK Public Health Laboratory Service websites and hand searched national and international policy documents. In the benefits section, we have included RCTs and stronger observational studies, given that RCTs have long been considered unethical for assessing the clinical efficacy of measles vaccines (see benefits, p 361). In the harms section, we have included RCTs and robust observational studies (see harms, p 363). In the comment section, we have included weaker studies (see comment, p 366). We have included only those studies of the combined measles, mumps, and rubella vaccine (see glossary, p 367) that used the Schwarz strain of the measles virus and only those studies of the monovalent measles vaccine (see glossary, p 367) that considered live attenuated strains of the virus, because of the relative inefficacy of measles vaccines using killed strains.

QUESTION **What are the effects of interventions to prevent measles infection?**

OPTION **MEASLES VACCINATION**

We found no RCTs comparing measles infection rates following the combined measles, mumps, and rubella (MMR) vaccine versus placebo or versus monovalent vaccine alone. We found strong evidence from national population surveillance that both MMR and monovalent measles vaccination virtually eliminate risk of measles and measles complications. We found no evidence that MMR or live monovalent measles vaccines are associated with autism or inflammatory bowel disease. We found consistent evidence from RCTs and cohort studies that MMR and live monovalent measles vaccines are associated with small, similar risks of self limiting fever within 3 weeks of vaccination. Measles causes acute fever in 100% of infected children.

Benefits: **Monovalent measles vaccine or combined MMR vaccine versus placebo or no vaccine:** See glossary, p 367. We found two early RCTs of monovalent measles vaccine versus placebo or no vaccine in the UK[12] and USA.[13] Both found efficacy rates of 95% or greater for vaccines using live attenuated Schwarz[12] and Edmonston[13] strains of the measles virus (Schwarz RCT: 9538 children received live vaccine, 16 239 unvaccinated; Edmonston RCT: 1308 live vaccine, 1271 placebo). We found no RCTs comparing the clinical effects of MMR versus no vaccine or placebo. Such studies have been considered unethical because of previous evidence of the efficacy of measles vaccine and harms of measles infection. We found two RCTs that compared seroconversion (see glossary, p 367) rates of MMR versus placebo.[14,15] The first compared MMR versus placebo in 282 previously non-immune children (92% of whom were ≤1 year old). At 8 weeks, almost all children receiving MMR seroconverted for measles, whereas none of the children receiving placebo seroconverted (measles seroconversion rate 99%–100% with MMR, depending on vaccine batch used).[14] The second trial examined seroconversion with MMR vaccine in 1481 children (1232 MMR, 249 placebo), of whom 446 in the vaccine group were naïve to measles, mumps, and rubella.[15] In this subgroup, seroconversion rates at 8 weeks approached 100%, whereas none of the previously non-immune placebo group seroconverted for measles. One large, retrospective cohort study of the entire US population from 1985–1992 compared measles infection rates in children who were vaccinated versus children whose parents had declined vaccination (17 390 cases from a vaccinated population of 51 264 140 to 52 377 192 from 1985–1992; 2827 cases from an unvaccinated population of 234 040 to 245 887 from 1985–1992).[16] The study did not state what proportion of vaccinated children received monovalent versus MMR vaccine, although MMR was already widely used in the USA by 1985. The study found that although overall measles incidence was low because of herd immunity (see glossary, p 367), vaccination reduced measles infection compared with no vaccination (RR unvaccinated *v* vaccinated 4–170, depending on age group and year of survey). One large, prospective cohort study followed up 9274 children who had been enrolled in a placebo controlled trial of live monovalent measles vaccine in 1964 (36 530 children aged 10 months to 2 years; Schwarz strain vaccine).[17] The cohort study found that by 1990, over a period of 15 years (12–27 years after the trial) and after controlling for subsequent vaccination in initial placebo groups, but not controlling for growing herd immunity following mass vaccination, measles incidence was higher in the unvaccinated group (AR 0.3/1000 person years with vaccine *v* 1/1000 person years with no vaccine; $P < 0.001$). One systematic review (search date not stated, 10 cohort studies, 2 case control) and one subsequent cohort study examined effects of live monovalent measles vaccination on mortality. The review found that live, standard titre monovalent measles vaccination in seven developing countries reduced all-cause mortality by 30–80%, depending on follow up period and country.[18] The more recent study compared a group of children in Bangladesh vaccinated with live, Schwarz strain monovalent measles vaccine versus age matched, unvaccinated children (8135 matched pairs).[19] It found similar results (16 270 children aged 9–60 months; RR for death at 3 years' follow up vaccinated *v* unvaccinated 0.54, 95% CI 0.45 to 0.65). We found many population based studies from different countries with different healthcare systems and different socioeconomic and demographic distributions. These studies have consistently found measles vaccination coverage to be associated with a steep decline in measles. One cross-sectional time series from the World Health Organization found a global decline in reported measles incidence (which underestimates true incidence) from about 4 500 000 a year in 1980 to about 1 000 000 a year in 2000.[20] The decline was associated with the rise in reported measles vaccination coverage from about 10% in 1980 to about 80% in 2000. One population-based time series of measles incidence from Finland found that in a population of about 5 million people following the introduction of a live monovalent vaccination programme (1975–1981), the number of new measles cases each year fell from an average of 2074 cases in 1977–1981 to 44 cases in 1985. New cases declined to about zero by the mid 1990s. Shortly after introducing the MMR programme in Finland in 1982, rubella and mumps incidence also fell to about zero.[4] One cross-sectional study in a Brazilian city, which was repeated before and after a measles vaccination campaign in 1987 (8163 people, strain not stated) found that reported measles incidence fell from 222/100 000 in 1987 to 2.7/100 000 in 1988.[21] **MMR versus monovalent measles vaccine:** We found no RCTs comparing clinical effects of MMR versus monovalent vaccine in children of the same age. We found one RCT that compared live Schwarz strain monovalent measles vaccine given at 9 months of age followed by MMR at 15 months (442 children) versus MMR only (no prior vaccination) at 12 months (495 children).[22] Pre-vaccination measles seropositivity was higher in the younger, monovalent vaccine group, perhaps because of maternal antibody persistence (pre-vaccine, 8.1% sero-positive in monovalent group *v* 1.4% in MMR group; $P < 0.0001$). After 60 months' follow up, measles infection rates were higher with monovalent vaccination followed by MMR compared with MMR alone (AR for infection 2.7% with monovalent plus MMR *v* 0% with MMR; ARR 2.7%; CI not stated; $P < 0.0001$); however, effects may be confounded by the different timing of the vaccinations. We found two RCTs that compared seroconversion rates following live MMR versus Schwarz strain monovalent measles vaccine. The first trial (420 children with no clinical history of measles or mumps, mean age about 15 months) found similar seroconversion rates in both groups after 6 weeks (96.8% with monovalent measles *v* 92.6% with MMR).[23] The second RCT (319 children, mean age 13 months) also found similar seroconversion rates in both groups at 6 weeks (92% with Schwarz strain monovalent measles vaccine *v* 93% with MMR).[24]

Harms:

Acute fever and febrile convulsions: We found one systematic review and four RCTs examining fever as an outcome of vaccination in otherwise healthy children. Results should be interpreted in light of the 100% prevalence of acute fever in children with measles infection. The systematic review (search date 1998) reported that up to 5% of non-immune people develop moderate to high fever (≥38.6°C) within 7–21 days of vaccination.[25] The first RCT (cross-over design) compared the acute harms of MMR versus placebo in 1162 homozygous and heterozygous twins (460 children aged 1 year, of whom 1.3% had been previously vaccinated; 702 aged ≥ 2 years, 95% of whom had been previously vaccinated or experienced measles).[26] One member of each twin pair was randomly selected and allocated to MMR vaccination followed 3 weeks later by placebo, or vice versa. The other twin was allocated to the opposite combination. The trial found that among children aged 14–18 months, MMR was more likely to cause fever than placebo within 21 days (AR fever, 12% in MMR group *v* 4% in placebo group; OR for fever ≥39.5°C 2.83, 95% CI 1.47 to 5.45; OR for fever ≥38.5°C 3.28, 95% CI 2.23 to 4.82; OR for fever ≥37.5°C 2.66, 95% CI 1.66 to 3.08). The second and third RCTs, which compared MMR versus Schwarz strain monovalent measles vaccine in infants with no history of measles, found no difference in fever rates between the two groups.[23,24] The fourth RCT compared Schwarz strain monovalent measles vaccine given at 9 months followed by MMR at 15 months versus MMR alone at 12 months.[22] It found similar rates of fever for monovalent measles vaccine and initial MMR, although results may be confounded by the age difference between the two groups (AR for fever 8.7% with monovalent vaccine *v* 11.2% with MMR; P value not provided). One retrospective cohort study in 679 942 children from four US health maintenance organisations found that children who had received MMR were more likely to experience febrile convulsions at 1–2 weeks after MMR than children of the same age who had not been vaccinated, although the estimated increase in absolute risk was small (RR for febrile seizure 8–14 days after vaccination 2.83, 95% CI 1.44 to 5.55; ARI of febrile seizure, estimated by comparison with background seizure risk in all children aged 12–24 months, 0.025%; NNH 4000; CI not provided).[27] However, the study found no increase in risk within the first week or from 2–4 weeks following vaccination (RR for first wk 1.73, 95% CI 0.72 to 4.15; RR for 15–30 days 0.97, 95% CI 0.49 to 1.95). Seven years' follow up of 543 children with febrile convulsions in the initial month of follow up (22 following MMR, 521 who had not been vaccinated) found no difference between MMR versus no vaccination for subsequent seizure (RR 0.56, 95% CI 0.07 to 4.20). Similarly, among 271 children with febrile convulsion in one of the four participating health maintenance organisations, the study found no evidence that MMR vaccination prior to seizure increased risk of learning disability or developmental delay compared with no vaccination prior to seizure (RR after adjusting for age at first febrile seizure 0.56, 95% CI 0.07 to 4.20). We found one study that reported results of population based surveillance of harms of MMR in all 1.8 million people vaccinated over a 14 year period in Finland.[28] Surveillance was passive, relying on healthcare personnel to be aware of the surveillance programme and to report adverse events that they felt might be associated with MMR. Throughout the surveillance period, the programme was advertised in seminars, the media, and medical press. Acute reactions were more likely to have been reported than long term effects. The study found that fever was associated with MMR in 277 children (AR 0.02%). Children with fever not brought to the attention of health professionals would have escaped detection. Febrile seizure was reported in 52 cases (AR 0.003%), of which 28 cases could have been caused by MMR according to predefined clinical and serological criteria (AR 0.002%). **Developmental regression or autism:** The RCT comparing harms of MMR versus placebo found no evidence that MMR was associated with acute developmental regression (see glossary, p 367).[26] We found one systematic review of observational studies of different kinds that found no association between MMR and autism.[29] The review included two large cross-sectional time series. Neither found evidence that MMR is associated with autism, but that incidence of autism has been increasing independently of MMR coverage. The first study examined MMR vaccine coverage (see glossary, p 367) among children aged 14–17 months enrolled in Californian kindergartens and born between 1980 and 1994, and autism caseloads referred to the state developmental services department over the same period.[30] The study found that MMR coverage at 24 months rose slightly (from 72% in 1980 to 82% in 1994; 14% proportional rise); however, referral rates for new autism cases increased disproportionately in the same period (from 44/100 000 births in 1980 to 208/100 000 live births in 1994; 373% proportional rise). Referral rates to the department may not accurately reflect incidence of autistic syndromes. The second study, which took its data from a national UK general practice registry, found that the risk of autism among boys increased in the period from 1988–1993, whereas MMR coverage remained almost constant at about 97% over the same period (AR of first diagnosis of autism aged 2–5 years 0.008%, 95% CI 0.004% to 0.014% for cohort born in 1988 *v* 0.029%, 95% CI 0.020% to 0.043% for cohort born in 1993).[31] A third population based study identified 498 children diagnosed with autism born in eight health districts in the UK between 1979 and 1998.[32] The study found that incidence of autism increased over this period. However, there was no step increase or change in the rate of increase of incidence following the start of the MMR vaccination programme or after MMR coverage levelled off at almost 100%. The long term population based passive surveillance study from Finland similarly reported no cases of developmental regression in 1.8 million people vaccinated with MMR.[28] It also reported no cases of autism in the long term, although the study may have limited reliability for detecting long term adverse effects. **Inflammatory bowel disease:** We found one systematic review (search date 1998) of six large observational studies from different developed countries.[25] The review found no evidence of an association between inflammatory bowel disease and MMR and measles vaccines. We found three additional studies. The first was a retrospective cohort study comparing rates of ulcerative colitis, Crohn's disease, and inflammatory bowel disease (assessed by postal questionnaire) in 7616 people who had received live monovalent measles vaccination versus those who had not received measles vaccination by the age of 5 years (mean age at vaccination 17.6 months, standard deviation 7.4 months). People were those available from an original population based cohort of 16 000 children born in the first week of 1970 in the UK.[33] The study found no difference for risk of ulcerative colitis, Crohn's disease, or inflammatory bowel disease between people (aged 26 years at the time of the study) who had received monovalent measles vaccine and those who had not, whether or not the result was adjusted for sex, socioeconomic status, and crowding (AR for Crohn's disease 0.25% with vaccine *v* 0.31% without, adjusted OR 0.7, 95% CI 0.3 to 1.6; AR for ulcerative colitis 0.16% with vaccine *v* 0.27% without, adjusted OR 0.6, 95% CI 0.2 to 1.6; AR for inflammatory bowel disease 0.41% with vaccine *v* 0.58% without, adjusted OR 0.6, 95% CI 0.3 to 1.2). The second (the long term, prospective population based passive surveillance study from Finland) reported no cases of inflammatory bowel disease associated with vaccination in 1.8 million people vaccinated with MMR followed up for 14 years.[28] The third was a case control study of 142 people with definite or probable inflammatory bowel disease from members of four US health maintenance organisations (67 people with ulcerative colitis and 75 with Crohn's disease).[34] Cases were identified by computerised search of electronic records and manual abstraction of medical records (from 1958–1989 for 3 organisations and from 1979–1989 for 1; people who were not organisation members between 6 months of age and disease onset were excluded). The study found that people with inflammatory bowel disease were not more likely to have received MMR than people without inflammatory bowel disease taken from the same health maintenance organisation and matched for sex and year of birth (OR for Crohn's disease 0.40, 95% CI 0.08 to 2.00; OR for ulcerative colitis 0.80, 95% CI 0.18 to 3.56; OR for all inflammatory bowel disease 0.59, 95% CI 0.21 to 1.69). The study similarly found no evidence of an association between all measles containing vaccines, Crohn's disease, ulcerative colitis, or all inflammatory bowel disease. **Measles risk after seroconversion:** One systematic review of cohort studies (search date 1995) examined risk of measles infection at least 21 days after vaccine induced seroconversion (monovalent or polyvalent vaccine).[11] It identified 10 studies that met inclusion criteria. In the subset of six cohort studies examining live vaccine, where vaccination status was cross checked against medical records, risk of clinical measles infection in children who had seroconverted after vaccination was about zero (0 infections out of 2061 people exposed; 95% CI not provided).

Comment: **Benefits:** Many case control studies conducted during measles outbreaks have found that live measles vaccination (monovalent or MMR) protects against infection, with protective efficacy of about 95% or higher. Given the evidence for benefit already described, we have not included further details of these studies. In addition, and although not the focus of this topic, it should be noted that the MMR vaccine also protects people from mumps and rubella, which cause serious complications in non-immune people (mumps causes orchitis, pancreatitis, meningoencephalitis, deafness, and congential fetal abnormalities; congenital rubella infection causes deafness, blindness, heart defects, liver, spleen and brain damage, and stillbirth). **Harms:** In addition to the more reliable evidence described above, we found two case series. The first was a time sensitive, population based series of 473 children with childhood autism (see glossary, p 367) or atypical autism (see glossary, p 367) born between 1979 and 1998 and registered in five health districts in London, UK.[35] Of these children, 118 had documented evidence of developmental regression. The study found no trends for risk of developmental regression with respect to year of birth from 1979–1998, although MMR vaccination was introduced in 1988. The study found that MMR vaccination was just as likely to precede or follow documented parental concerns about development, suggesting that the temporal relation of vaccination and onset of developmental problems was not compatible with a causal association (443 children with autism in whom timing of first parental concerns recorded; 26% vaccinated prior to parental concern about development *v* 26% vaccinated after parental concerns expressed; P = 0.83). The second series raised the question of a possible relation between MMR and developmental disorder in 12 children with bowel symptoms.[36] The series was retrospective (parents surveyed up to 8 years after vaccination); small; lacked a control group, and was selective in its sample. For these reasons, we found that the study does not establish MMR as a cause of inflammatory bowel disease, autism or developmental regression and that its hypothesis has been satisfactorily tested by scientifically reliable studies (see harm section above).

GLOSSARY

Acute developmental regression Rapid loss of acquired developmental skills.
Atypical autism shares clinical features with autism but does not meet ICD-10 or DSM-IV diagnostic criteria.
Childhood autism ICD-10 or DSM-IV autism (comprising communication difficulties, problems with social interaction, and behavioural problems) in children aged under 3 years.
Combined measles, mumps, and rubella (MMR) vaccine Vaccine with components that aim to raise immunity to measles, mumps, and rubella infections. Contains live attenuated measles virus (Schwarz strain).
Herd immunity Background level of immunity in the community. A high level of herd immunity reduces risk of infection even in non-immune individuals, because there is no pool of at risk individuals who may transmit the infectious agent.
Live monovalent vaccine Commonly known as the single measles vaccine. Uses live, attenuated virus (most commonly Schwarz strain), and only to bring about measles immunity.
Seroconversion Development in the blood of specific antimeasles antibody. Seroconversion is a proxy for clinical efficacy.
Vaccine coverage Prevalence of vaccination in the community.

REFERENCES

1. Center for Disease Control. Epidemiology and Prevention of Vaccine-preventable Diseases. Atlanta: CDC, 2000.
2. http://www.unicef.org/programme/health/document/meastrat.pdf
3. http://www.who.int/vaccines-surveillance/graphics/htmls/meainc.htm
4. Peltola H, Heinonen P, Valle M, et al. The elimination of indigenous measles, mumps and rubella from Finland by a 12-year, two-dose vaccination program. *N Eng J Med* 1994;331:1397–1402.
5. Peltola H, Davidkin I, Valle M, et al. No measles in Finland. *Lancet* 1997;350:1364–1365.
6. de Quadros CA, Olive J, Hersh BS, et al. Measles elimination in the Americas: evolving strategies. *JAMA* 1996;275:224–229.
7. Pan American Health Organization. Surveillance in the Americas. *Weekly Bulletin* 1995;1.
8. World Health Report, 2001: Statistical annex. Geneva: WHO, 2001.
9. Miller E, Waight P, Farrington CP, Andrews N, Stowe J, Taylor B. Idiopathic thrombocytopenic purpura and MMR vaccine. *Arch Dis Child* 2001;84:227–229.
10. http://www.who.int/child-adolescent-health/OVERVIEW/Child_Health/child_epidemiology.htm
11. Anders J, Jacobson R, Poland G, Jacobson RSJ, Wollan PC. Secondary failure rates of measles vaccines: a metaanalysis of published studies. *Pediatr Infect Dis J* 1996;15:62–66. Search date 1995; primary sources Medline (English language only) and hand searching of references cited in initial search and references cited within first generation references.
12. Measles Vaccination subcommittee of the Committee on Development of Vaccines and Immunisation Procedures. Clinical trial of live measles vaccine given alone and live vaccine preceded by killed vaccine. Fourth report to the Medical Research Council. *Lancet* 1977;2:571–575.

13. Guinee VF, Henderson DA, Casey HL, et al. Cooperative measles vaccine field trial. I. Clinical efficacy. *Pediatrics* 1966;37:649–665.
14. Bloom JL, Schiff GM, Graubarth H, et al. Evaluation of a trivalent measles, mumps, rubella vaccine in children. *J Pediatr* 1975;87:85–87.
15. Schwarz AJ, Jackson JE, Ehrenkranz J, Ventura A, Schiff GM, Walters VW. Clinical evaluation of a new measles–mumps–rubella trivalent vaccine. *Am J Dis Child* 1975;129:1408–1412.
16. Salmon DA Haber M, Gangarosa E, Phillips L, Smith NJ, Chen RT. Health consequences of religious and philosophical exemptions from immunization laws: individual and societal risk of measles. *JAMA* 1999;282:47–53.
17. Ramsay ME, Moffatt D, O'Connor M. Measles vaccine: a 27-year follow up. *Epidemiol Infect* 1994;112:409–412.
18. Aaby P, Samb B, Simondon F, Seck AM, Knudsen K, Whittle H. Non-specific beneficial effect of measles immunisation: analysis of mortality studies from developing countries. *BMJ* 1995;311:481–485. Search date not stated; primary source Medline.
19. Koenig MA, Khan B, Wojtynak B. Impact of measles vaccination on childhood mortality in rural Bangladesh. *Bull World Health Organization* 1990;68:441–447.
20. http://www.who.int/vaccines-surveillance/graphics/htmls/IncMeas.htm
21. Pannuti CS, Moraes JC, Souza VA, Camargo MC, Hidalgo NT. Measles antibody prevalence after mass immunization in Sao Paulo, Brazil. *Bull World Health Organization* 1991;69:557–560.
22. Ceyhan M, Kanra G, Erdem G, Kanra B. Immunogenicity and efficacy of one dose measles–mumps–rubella (MMR) vaccine at twelve months of age as compared to monovalent measles vaccination at nine months followed by MMR revaccination at fifteen months of age. *Vaccine* 2001;19:4473–4478.
23. Edees S, Pullan CR, Hull D. A randomised single blind trial of a combined mumps measles rubella vaccine to evaluate serological response and reactions in the UK population. *Public Health* 1991;105:91–97.
24. Robertson CM, Bennet VJ, Jefferson N, Mayon-White RT. Serological evaluation of a measles, mumps, and rubella vaccine. *Arch Dis Child* 1988;63:612–616.
25. Duclos P, Ward BJ. Measles vaccines: a review of adverse events. Drug Safety 1998;6:435–454. Search date 1998; primary sources Stratton RS, Howe CJ, Johnston Jr RB. Adverse events associated with childhood vaccines: evidence bearing on causality. Washington DC: National Academy Press 1994 for papers published before 1994; for articles published after 1994 primary sources WHO Collaborating Centre for International Drug Monitoring Database; discussion groups; advisory committee documents and other unspecified databases.
26. Virtanen M, Peltola H, Paunio M, Heinonen OP. Day-to-day reactogenicity and the healthy vaccinee effect of measles–mumps–rubella vaccination. *Pediatrics* 2000;106:e62.
27. Barlow WE, Davis RL, Glasser JW. The risk of seizures after receipt of whole cell pertussins or measles mumps and rubella vaccine. *N Eng J Med* 2001;345:656–661.
28. Patja A, Davidkin I, Kurki T, Kallio MJ, Valle M, Peltola H. Serious adverse events after measles–mumps–rubella vaccination during a fourteen year prospective follow up. *Pediatr Infect Dis J* 2000;19:1127–1134.
29. Institute of Medicine. Immunization safety review: measles–mumps–rubella vaccine and austism. Washington DC: National Academy Press, 2001.
30. Dales L, Hammer SJ, Smith N. Time trends in autism and in MMR immunization coverage in California. *JAMA* 2001;285:1183–1185.
31. Kaye JA, del Mar Melero-Montes M, Jick H. Mumps, measles, and rubella vaccine and the incidence of autism recorded by general practitioners: a time trend analysis. *BMJ* 2001;322:460–463.
32. Taylor B, Miller E, Farrington CP, et al. Autism and measles, mumps, and rubella vaccine: no epidemiological evidence for a causal association. *Lancet* 1999;353:2026–
33. Morris DL, Montgomery SM, Thompson NP. Measles vaccination and inflammatory bowel disease: A National British Cohort study. *Am J Gastroenterol* 2000;95:3507–3512.
34. Davis RL, Kramarz P, Bohlke K, et al. Measles–mumps–rubella and other measles containing vaccines do not increase risk for inflammatory bowel disease: A case control study from the Vaccine Safety Datalink project. *Arch Pediatr Adolesc Med* 2001;155:354–359.
35. Taylor B, Miller E, Lingam R, Andrews N, Simmons A, Stowe J. Measles, mumps, and rubella vaccination and bowel problems or developmental regression in children with autism: a population study. *BMJ* 2002;324:393–396.
36. Wakefield AJ, Murch SH, Anthony A, et al. Ileal–lymphoid–nodular hyperplasia, non-specific colitis, and pervasive developmental disorder in children. *Lancet* 1998; 351:637–641.

Anna Donald

Vivek Muthu

Bazian Ltd
London
UK

Competing interests: None declared.

Nocturnal enuresis

Search date October 2001

Sara Bosson and Natalie Lyth

QUESTIONS

INTERVENTIONS

Key Messages

- **Age to start treatment** We found no RCTs on the best age to start treatment in children with nocturnal enuresis. Anecdotal experience suggests that reassurance is sufficient below the age of 7 years.
- **Carbamazepine** One small RCT found that carbamazepine versus placebo significantly increased the number of dry nights over 30 days in children aged over 7 years with nocturnal enuresis caused by detrusor instability.
- **Desmopressin (intranasal)** One systematic review has found that intranasal desmopressin versus placebo significantly reduces bedwetting by at least one night/week, and increases the chance of attaining 14 consecutive dry nights.
- **Dry bed training (in the long term)** One systematic review has found that significantly more children achieved 14 consecutive dry nights with dry bed training versus no treatment, but found no significant difference in the proportion of dry nights in the long term.
- **Enuresis alarm (in the long term)** One systematic review has found that significantly more children achieve 14 consecutive dry nights with enuresis alarms versus no treatment, and that 31–61% of children were still dry at 3 months. The review found that children using an alarm were 9 times less likely to relapse than children taking desmopressin. One RCT found that significantly more children achieved 4 weeks of dryness with alarm plus intranasal desmopressin (40 μg) versus alarm alone.
- **Indometacin** One small RCT found that indometacin (indomethacin) versus placebo significantly increased the number of dry nights in children aged over 6 years with primary nocturnal enuresis.

Nocturnal enuresis

- **Laser acupuncture** One RCT found no significant difference in the number of wet nights in children aged over 5 years with laser acupuncture versus intranasal desmopressin.
- **Standard home alarm clock (in the long term)** One RCT found that significantly more children achieved 14 consecutive dry nights with standard home alarm clock versus waking after 3 hours' sleep, but found no significant difference in the proportion of dry nights at 3 months.
- **Tricyclic drugs** One systematic review has found that tricyclic drugs (imipramine, desipramine) versus placebo significantly increase the chance of attaining 14 consecutive dry nights. It found no significant difference with imipramine versus an alarm during the treatment period but found that children using an enuresis alarm had fewer wet nights per week after the treatment had stopped. The review found that tricyclic drugs versus placebo increased adverse effects such as anorexia, anxiety reaction, constipation, depression, diarrhoea, dizziness, drowsiness, dry mouth, headache, irritability, lethargy, sleep disturbance, upset stomach, and vomiting.
- **Ultrasound** We found no RCTs on use of ultrasound. One small controlled trial in children aged 6–14 years found that ultrasound versus control significantly increased the proportion of dry nights for up to 12 months.

DEFINITION Nocturnal enuresis is the involuntary discharge of urine at night in the absence of congenital or acquired defects of the central nervous system or urinary tract in a child aged 5 years or older.[1] Disorders that have bedwetting as a symptom (termed "nocturnal incontinence") can be excluded by a thorough history, examination, and urinalysis. "Monosymptomatic" nocturnal enuresis is characterised by night time symptoms only and accounts for 85% of cases. Nocturnal enuresis is defined as primary if the child has never been dry for a period of more than 6 months, and secondary if such a period of dryness preceded the onset of wetting.

INCIDENCE/ PREVALENCE Between 15% and 20% of 5 year olds, 7% of 7 year olds, 5% of 10 year olds, 2–3% of 12–14 year olds, and 1–2% of people aged 15 years and over wet the bed twice a week on average.[2]

AETIOLOGY/ RISK FACTORS Nocturnal enuresis is associated with several factors, including small functional bladder capacity, nocturnal polyuria, and arousal dysfunction. Linkage studies have identified associated genetic loci on chromosomes 8q, 12q, 13q, and 22q11.[3–6]

PROGNOSIS Nocturnal enuresis has widely differing outcomes, from spontaneous resolution to complete resistance to all current treatments. About 1% of adults remain enuretic. Without treatment, about 15% of children with enuresis become dry each year.[7]

AIMS To stay dry on particular occasions (e.g. when visiting friends); to reduce the number of wet nights; to reduce the impact of the enuresis on the child's lifestyle; to initiate successful continence; to avoid relapse, with minimal adverse effects.

OUTCOMES Rate of initial success (defined as 14 consecutive dry nights); average number of wet nights per week; number of relapses after initial success; average number of wet nights after treatment has ceased.

METHODS *Clinical Evidence* search and appraisal October 2001.

QUESTION **What are the effects of treatments for short term relief of symptoms?**

OPTION **DESMOPRESSIN**

One systematic review has found that intranasal desmopressin versus placebo significantly reduces bedwetting by at least one night per week and increases the chance of attaining 14 consecutive dry nights. The review found insufficient evidence on lower versus higher doses of desmopressin and oral versus nasal administration of desmopressin.

Benefits: We found one systematic review (search date 1997).[8] **Versus placebo:** The review identified 16 RCTs comparing the effect of intranasal desmopressin (10–40 μg) versus placebo on mean number of wet nights per week. It found that each dose of desmopressin versus placebo significantly reduced bedwetting by at least one night per week (desmopressin 20 μg; RR –1.56, 95% CI –1.94 to –1.19). Three RCTs found that desmopressin versus placebo significantly increased the chance of attaining 14 consecutive dry nights (overall RR with desmopressin *v* placebo 4.6, 95% CI 1.4 to 15.0) (see table 1, p 376). **Other comparisons:** The review found insufficient evidence on lower versus higher doses of desmopressin and oral versus nasal administration of desmopressin.[8]

Harms: The systematic review reported nasal discomfort, headache, nosebleeds, bad taste, rash, sight disturbance, and anorexia.[8] Rarely, water intoxication has been reported.

Comment: The systematic review included only studies of interventions used to remedy either primary or secondary nocturnal enuresis (incontinence was excluded by medical examination or explicitly mentioned in the inclusion/exclusion criteria of included RCTs), and included a systematic measurement of baseline wetting and outcomes. Many of the included RCTs were of poor quality.

OPTION **TRICYCLIC DRUGS**

One systematic review has found that tricyclic drugs (imipramine, desipramine) versus placebo significantly increase the chance of attaining 14 consecutive dry nights. It found no significant difference with imipramine versus an alarm during the treatment period, but found that children using an enuresis alarm have one fewer wet night per week after the treatment had stopped. The review found that tricyclic drugs versus placebo increased adverse effects such as anorexia, anxiety reaction, constipation, depression, diarrhoea, dizziness, drowsiness, dry mouth, headache, irritability, lethargy, sleep disturbance, upset stomach, and vomiting.

Benefits: We found one systematic review (search date 1997, 22 RCTs, 1100 children).[9] Many of the trials were of poor quality. **Versus placebo:** The review identified 10 RCTs comparing effect of imipramine versus placebo on mean number of wet nights per week. It found that imipramine versus placebo reduced bedwetting by one night per week (WMD –0.84 nights, 95% CI –1.21 to –0.47 nights). It also found that tricyclic drugs (imipramine, desipramine) versus placebo significantly increased the chance of attaining 14 consecutive dry nights (imipramine, 4 RCTs: RR 5.0, 95% CI 2.4 to 10.4; desipramine, 1 RCT: RR 3.6, 95% CI 1.07 to 11.81) (see table 1, p 376). **Versus alarms:** The review (3 small RCTs, 103 children) found no significant difference in mean number of wet nights per week with imipramine versus an alarm during the treatment period.[9] However, two of the three RCTs found that when the treatment had stopped, children using an enuresis alarm had one fewer wet night per week (WMD 1.03 nights, 95% CI 0.19 to 1.87 nights).[9]

Harms: The systematic review reported more adverse effects with tricyclic drugs versus placebo. These included anorexia, anxiety reaction, burning sensation, constipation, depression, diarrhoea, dizziness, drowsiness, dry mouth, headache, irritability, lethargy, sleep disturbance, upset stomach, and vomiting.[9] The review also found that, when reported, tricyclic drugs were associated with more adverse effects than desmopressin (tricyclic drugs 83/480 [17.3%] *v* desmopressin 41/579 [7.1%]). Tricyclic drugs have been reported as fatal in overdose.

Comment: We found no good studies directly comparing tricyclic drugs versus desmopressin.

OPTION INDOMETACIN

One small RCT found that indometacin versus placebo significantly increased the number of dry nights in children aged over 6 years with primary nocturnal enuresis.

Benefits: We found no systematic review but found one RCT.[13] The RCT (85 children aged over 6 years with primary nocturnal enuresis) compared desmopressin versus indometacin (indomethacin) versus placebo. It found that indometacin suppository versus placebo significantly increased the number of dry nights over 3 weeks (mean number of dry nights 8.9 with indometacin *v* 3.8 with placebo; $P < 0.005$).[13]

Harms: The RCT did not report any adverse effects.

Comment: None.

OPTION CARBAMAZEPINE

One small RCT found that carbamazepine versus placebo significantly increased the number of dry nights over 30 days in in children aged over 7 years with nocturnal enuresis caused by detrusor instability.

Benefits: We found no systematic review but found one RCT.[14] The RCT (double blind crossover study, 26 children aged 7–15 years with detrusor instability on videocystourethrography) found that carbamazepine versus placebo significantly increased the number of dry nights over 30 days (mean number of dry nights 18.8 with carbamazepine *v* 3.9 with placebo; $P < 0.001$).

Harms: The RCT did not report any adverse effects.[14]

Comment: The study population had proven detrusor instability. It may not be possible to generalise these results to all children with nocturnal enuresis.

QUESTION What are the effects of long term treatments?

OPTION ALARMS AND DRY BED TRAINING

One systematic review has found that significantly more children achieve 14 consecutive dry nights with enuresis alarms versus no treatment, and that 31–61% were still dry at 3 months. The review found that children using an alarm were 9 times less likely to relapse than children taking desmopressin. One RCT found that significantly more children achieved 14 consecutive dry nights with a standard home alarm clock to wake the child immediately before their usual time of enuresis versus waking after 3 hours' sleep, but found no significant difference in the proportion of dry nights at 3 months. One RCT found that significantly more children achieved 4 weeks of dryness with an alarm plus intranasal desmopressin (40 μg) versus an alarm alone. Another systematic review has found that significantly more children achieve 14 consecutive dry nights with dry bed training plus an alarm versus no treatment. It found insufficient evidence on the effect of dry bed training plus alarm versus alarm alone.

Benefits: **Alarm versus no treatment:** We found one systematic review (search date 1997).[10] It found that significantly more children achieved 14 consecutive dry nights with alarm versus no treatment (4 RCTs; RR 3.7, 95% CI 2.6 to 5.3), and that 31–61% were still dry at 3 months (see table 1, p 376). **Standard home alarm clock versus waking:** We found one RCT.[11] It found that significantly more children achieved 14 consecutive dry nights with a standard home alarm clock to wake the child immediately before their usual time of enuresis versus waking after 3 hours' sleep (RR 1.3, 95% CI not stated; $P = 0.03$), but found no significant difference in the proportion of dry nights at 3 months (see table 1, p 376). **Alarm plus desmopressin versus alarm alone:** We found one RCT.[15] It found that significantly more children achieved 4 weeks of dryness with alarm plus intranasal desmopressin (40 μg) versus alarm alone (27/36 [75%] with an alarm plus desmopressin *v* 16/35 [46%] with an alarm alone; $P < 0.005$). **Dry bed training versus no treatment:** We found one systematic review (search date 1996).[12] It found that significantly more children achieved 14 consecutive dry nights with dry bed training versus no treatment (1 RCT; RR 2.5, 95% CI 0.55 to 11.4) (see table 1, p 376). **Dry bed training plus alarm versus no treatment:** We found one systematic review (search date 1996).[12] It found that significantly more children achieved 14 consecutive dry nights with dry bed training plus an alarm versus no treatment (1 RCT; RR 10, 95% CI 2.69 to 37.24) (see table 1, p 376). **Dry bed training plus alarm versus alarm alone:** We found one systematic review (search date 1997).[10] It found that children using an alarm alone were as likely as those using an alarm plus dry bed training to achieve 14 consecutive dry nights, but the confidence intervals were wide.

Harms: One systematic review found that adverse effects of alarms were limited to minor inconvenience because of malfunction or disturbance.[12] No adverse effects were reported in the two RCTs.[11,15]

Comment: None.

OPTION ULTRASOUND

We found no RCTs of ultrasound in children with primary nocturnal enuresis. We found one small controlled trial in children aged 6–14 years which found that ultrasound versus control significantly reduced the number of wet nights.

Benefits: We found no RCTs of ultrasound in children with primary nocturnal enuresis.

Harms: We found no RCTs.

Comment: We found one controlled trial (35 children with primary nocturnal enuresis, aged 6–14 years) comparing ultrasound (27 children) versus control (8 children treated without the apparatus being switched on).[16] Ultrasound treatment was applied daily to lumbosacral skin for 10 sessions. The controlled trial found that ultrasound versus control significantly reduced the number of wet nights per week at 1 week, 3 months, 6 months, and 12 months after treatment ($P < 0.05$ at all times). The study did not find any adverse effects. It is not clear why this prospective study has such a difference in population size between ultrasound and control groups.[16]

OPTION LASER ACUPUNCTURE

One RCT found no significant difference with laser acupuncture versus intranasal desmopressin in reduction of wet nights in children aged over 5 years with primary nocturnal enuresis.

Benefits: We found no systematic review. **Versus no treatment:** We found no RCTs. **Versus intranasal desmopressin:** We found one RCT (40 children aged > 5 years with primary nocturnal enuresis) comparing laser acupuncture versus intranasal desmopressin (20–40 μg for 3 months).[17] Laser acupuncture was applied to seven pre-defined acupuncture areas for 30 seconds per session for 10–15 sessions. Complete response was defined as a reduction in the number of wet nights of at least 90%. At 6 months, the RCT found no significant difference with laser acupuncture versus intranasal desmopressin in the reduction of wet nights (complete responders: 65% with laser acupuncture *v* 75% with desmopressin).

Harms: The RCT did not find any adverse effects with either laser acupuncture or intranasal desmopressin.[17]

Comment: Laser acupuncture treatment may not be widely available.

QUESTION What is the best age to start treatment?

We found no RCTs on the best age to start treatment in children with nocturnal enuresis. Anecdotal experience suggests that reassurance is sufficient below the age of 7 years.

Benefits: We found no RCTs on the best age to start treatment in children with nocturnal enuresis (see comment below).

Harms: We found no RCTs.

Comment: Anecdotal experience suggests that reassurance is sufficient below the age of 7 years. Behavioural treatments, such as alarms, require motivation and commitment from the child and a parent. Anecdotal experience suggests that children under the age of 7 years may not exhibit the commitment needed. Minimum ages for which drugs are licensed vary among countries.

REFERENCES

1. Forsythe WI, Butler R. 50 years of enuretic alarms; a review of the literature. *Arch Dis Child* 1991;64:879–885.
2. Blackwell C. *A guide to enuresis: a guide to treatment of enuresis for professionals*. Bristol: Eric, 1989.
3. Eiberg H. Total genome scan analysis in a single extended family for primary nocturnal enuresis: evidence for a new locus (ENUR 3) for primary nocturnal enuresis on chromosome 22q11. *Eur Urol* 1998;33:34–36.
4. Eiberg H. Nocturnal enuresis is linked to a specific gene. *Scand J Urol Nephrol* 1995;173(suppl):15–17.
5. Arnell H, Hjalmas M, Jagervall G, et al. The genetics of primary nocturnal enuresis: inheritance and suggestion of a second major gene on chromosome 12q. *J Med Genet* 1997;34:360–365.
6. Eiberg H, Berendt I, Mohr J. Assignment of dominant inherited nocturnal enuresis (ENUR 1) to chromosome 13q. *Nat Genet* 1995;10:354–356.
7. Forsythe WI, Redmond A. Enuresis and spontaneous cure rate of 1129 enuretics. *Arch Dis Child* 1974;49:259–263.
8. Glazener CMA, Evans JHC. Desmopressin for nocturnal enuresis in children. In: The Cochrane Library, Issue 3, 2001. Oxford: Update Software. Search date 1997; primary sources Medline, Embase, Amed, Assia, Bids, Cinahl, Psychlit, Sigle, and DHSS data.
9. Glazener CMA, Evans JHC. Tricyclic and related drugs for nocturnal enuresis in children. In: The Cochrane Library, Issue 3, 2001. Oxford: Update Software. Search date 1997; primary sources Medline, Embase, Amed, Assia, Bids, Cinahl, Psychlit, Sigle, and DHSS data.
10. Glazener CMA, Evans JHC. Alarm interventions for nocturnal enuresis in children (Cochrane Review). In: The Cochrane Library, Issue 3, 2001. Oxford: Update Software. Search date 1997; primary sources Medline, Embase, Amed, Assia, Bids, Cinahl, Psychlit, Sigle, and DHSS data.
11. El-Anany FG, Maghraby HA, Shaker SED, Abdel-Moneim AM. Primary nocturnal enuresis: a new approach to conditioning treatment. *Urology* 1999;53:405–409.
12. Lister-Sharp D, O'Meara S, Bradley M, Sheldon TA. University of York. NHS Centre for Reviews and Dissemination. August 1997. *A systematic review of the effectiveness of interventions for managing childhood nocturnal enuresis*. CRD Report 11. Search date 1996; primary sources Cochrane Library, Medline, Embase, and Psychlit.
13. Sener F, Hasanoglu E, Soylemezoglu O. Desmopressin versus indomethacin treatment in primary nocturnal enuresis and the role of prostaglandins. *Urology* 1998:52:878–881.
14. Al Waili NS. Carbamazepine to treat primary nocturnal enuresis: double-blind study. *Eur J Med Res* 2000;5:40–44.
15. Bradbury M. Combination therapy for nocturnal enuresis with desmopressin and an alarm device. *Scand J Urol Nephrol Suppl* 1997;183:61–63.
16. Kosar A, Akkus S, Savas S, *et al*. Effect of ultrasound in the treatment of primary nocturnal enuresis. *Scand J Urol Nephrol* 2000;34:361–365.
17. Radmayr C, Schlager A, Studen M, Bartsch G. Prospective Randomised trial using laser acupuncture versus desmopressin in the treatment of nocturnal enuresis. *Eur Urol* 2001;40:201–205.

Sara Bosson
Staff Grade Community Paediatrician
Weston Area Health Trust
Weston-Super-Mare
UK

Natalie Lyth
Associate Specialist Child Health
Northallerton Health Service Trust
Northallerton
UK

Competing interests: SB, none declared. NL has been reimbursed for attending a symposium by Ferring Pharmaceuticals, the manufacturer of desmotabs.

TABLE 1 **Treatments for enuresis: advantages and disadvantages (see text, p 371–373).**

	Initial success (14 consecutive dry nights)	Long term success	Evidence	Advantages	Disadvantages
Desmopressin[8]	RR *v* placebo 4.6, 95% CI 1.4 to 15.0	No better than placebo	Meta-analysis of 3 RCTs	Effective within days, few adverse effects with appropriate pretreatment advice	Case reports of water intoxication
Tricyclic drugs[9]	RR *v* placebo 5.0, 95% CI 2.4 to 10.4	No better than placebo (RR 1.1)	Meta-analysis of 4 RCTs	Effective within days	Risk of lethal overdose, frequent significant adverse effects
Alarm[10]	RR *v* no treatment 3.7, 95% CI 2.6 to 5.3	31–61% still dry at 3 months. Nine times less likely relapse than with desmopressin	Meta-analysis of 4 RCTs	Safe	Takes longer to become dry, needs good cooperation from child and family
Standard home alarm clock[11]	77.1% *v* 61.8% with waking after 3 hours' sleep (RR 1.3; $P = 0.03$)	No better at 3 months than waking after 3 hours' sleep (66% dry *v* 56%; $P = 0.19$)	1 RCT, 125 people	Safe, does not require bed wetting to initiate alarm	None reported
Dry bed training[12]	RR *v* no treatment 2.5, 95% CI 0.55 to 11.4	No better than no treatment (RR 0.4, 95% CI 0.14 to 1.13)	1 good quality RCT, 45 people	Safe	Requires high degree of motivation
Dry bed training plus alarm[12]	RR *v* no treatment 10, 95% CI 2.69 to 37.24	No better than alarm alone (RR 1.0, 95% CI 0.7 to 1.5)	1 RCT, 45 people	Safe	Requires an even greater input from the family than either treatment alone

Recurrent idiopathic epistaxis (nosebleeds)

Search date February 2002

Gerald McGarry

QUESTIONS

INTERVENTIONS

Key Messages

Treatments

- **Antiseptic cream versus cautery** We found no placebo controlled trials. One small RCT found no significant difference with chlorhexidine/neomycin cream versus silver nitrate cautery in reduction of nosebleeds after 8 weeks. Some children found the smell and taste of the antiseptic cream unpleasant. All children found cautery painful despite the use of local anaesthesia.
- **Cautery plus antiseptic cream versus antiseptic cream alone** We found no placebo controlled trials. One small RCT found insufficient evidence about the effects of silver nitrate cautery plus chlorhexidine/neomycin cream versus antiseptic cream alone.
- **Antiseptic cream versus other creams/ointments; cautery versus no treatment** We found no RCTs about the effects of these interventions.

Clin Evid 2002;8:377–379.

Recurrent idiopathic epistaxis (nosebleeds)

DEFINITION Recurrent idiopathic epistaxis is recurrent, self limiting, nasal bleeding in children for which no specific cause has been identified. There is no consensus on how frequent or severe recurrences need to be.

INCIDENCE/ PREVALENCE A cross sectional study of 1218 children (aged 11–14 years) found that 9% had frequent episodes of epistaxis.[1] It is likely that most epistaxis in children is not brought to the attention of health professionals, and that only the most severe episodes are considered for treatment.

AETIOLOGY/ RISK FACTORS In children, most epistaxis occurs from the anterior part of the septum in the region of Little's area.[2] Initiating factors include local inflammation, mucosal drying, and local trauma (including nose picking).[2] Epistaxis caused by other specific local (e.g. tumours) or systemic factors (e.g. clotting disorders) is not considered here.

PROGNOSIS Recurrent epistaxis is less common in adolescents over 14 years and many children "grow out" of this problem.

AIMS To reduce the number and severity of epistaxis episodes.

OUTCOMES Number and severity of epistaxis episodes.

METHODS *Clinical Evidence* search and appraisal February 2002.

QUESTION **What are the effects of treatments in children with recurrent idiopathic epistaxis?**

OPTION **ANTISEPTIC CREAMS**

We found no placebo controlled trials. One small RCT comparing chlorhexidine/neomycin cream versus silver nitrate cautery found no significant difference in reduction of nosebleeds. Some children found the smell and taste of antiseptic cream unpleasant. All children found cautery painful despite the use of local anaesthesia.

Benefits: We found no systematic review. **Versus other creams/ointments:** We found no RCTs. **Versus cautery:** We found one small RCT (48 children), which compared antiseptic cream (chlorhexidine hydrochloride 0.1%, neomycin sulphate 3250 U/g) applied to both nostrils twice daily for 4 weeks versus silver nitrate cautery.[3] Cautery was undertaken in secondary care using silver nitrate applied on a stick to prominent vessels or bleeding points. The children were aged 3–14 years, and had at least one episode of epistaxis in the previous 4 weeks and a "history of repeated epistaxis". After 8 weeks, the RCT found no significant difference between treatments. About half of the children in both groups had complete resolution (no bleeding in past 4 wks: 12/24 with antiseptic cream *v* 13/24 with cautery; RR 0.92, 95% CI 0.54 to 1.59). Rates of other outcomes were also similar between groups at 8 weeks: partial success (50% reduction in number of bleeds in past 4 wks: 4/24 with antiseptic cream *v* 3/24 with cautery), failure (less than 50% reduction in number of bleeds in past 4 wks: 7/24 with antiseptic cream *v* 6/24 with cautery), and lost to follow up at 8 weeks (1/24 with antiseptic cream *v* 2/24 with cautery). **Plus cautery:** See silver nitrate cautery, p 379.

Harms: No adverse reactions were observed with antiseptic cream, but some children found the smell and taste unpleasant (data not provided). Chlorhexidine/neomycin cream may cause occasional skin reactions. Some commercial antiseptic creams contain arachis (peanut) oil. All children undergoing cautery experienced pain even with the use of 5% cocaine as a local anaesthetic.[3]

Comment: See comment under silver nitrate cautery, p 379.

OPTION SILVER NITRATE CAUTERY

We found no placebo controlled trials. One small RCT comparing cautery versus antiseptic cream found no significant difference in reduction of nosebleeds (see antiseptic creams, p 378). One small RCT compared silver nitrate cautery plus a cream containing chlorhexidine/neomycin versus antiseptic cream alone. The RCT included too few children to allow conclusions to be drawn.

Benefits: We found no systematic review. **Versus no treatment:** We found no RCTs. **Versus antiseptic cream:** See antiseptic creams, p 378. **Plus antiseptic cream:** One RCT (40 adults, 24 children) compared once only silver nitrate cautery plus chlorhexidine hydrochloride 0.1%/neomycin sulphate 3250 U/g cream twice daily for 2 weeks with antiseptic cream alone. The study included too few children to allow conclusions to be drawn.[4]

Harms: The RCT did not report harms.[4] Recognised complications of cautery include pain and septal perforation, although the incidence of septal perforation following unilateral cautery in children is not known (see harms of antiseptic creams, p 379).

Comment: Both trials involving silver nitrate cautery were undertaken in the context of secondary care.[3,4] Silver nitrate cautery is also used in primary care. It is unknown if complication rates differ. Simultaneous bilateral cautery in children is not recommended because of an expected increased risk of perforation.

REFERENCES

1. Rodeghiero F, Castaman G, Dini E. Epidemiological investigation of the prevalence of von Willebrand's disease. *Blood* 1987;69:454–459.
2. Watkinson JC. Epistaxis. In: Kerr AG, Mackay IS, Bull TR, eds. *Scott-Brown's Otolaryngology, Volume 4 Rhinology*. Oxford: Butterworth-Heinemann, 1997;18:1–19.
3. Ruddy J, Proops DW, Pearman K, Ruddy H. Management of epistaxis in children. *Int J Paediatr Otorhinolaryngol* 1991;21:139–142.
4. Murthy P, Nilssen ELK, Rao S, McClymont LG. A randomised clinical trial of antiseptic nasal carrier cream and silver nitrate cautery in the treatment of recurrent anterior epistaxis. *Clin Otolaryngol* 1999;228–231.

Gerald McGarry
Consultant Otorhinolaryngologist
Honorary Clinical Senior Lecturer
Glasgow Royal Infirmary
Glasgow
UK

Competing interests: None declared.

Reducing pain during blood sampling in infants

Search date January 2002

Linda Franck and Ruth Gilbert

QUESTIONS

INTERVENTIONS

To be covered in future updates

Interventions in children over 1 year old

See glossary, p 393

Key Messages

Interventions to reduce pain during blood sampling in infants

- **Automated devices versus manual lancets** RCTs in preterm and term infants have found that automated devices versus manual lancets for heel puncture are less painful, cause less bruising, and reduce the time needed to obtain a sample.
- **Breast milk** RCTs found no evidence that breast milk or breastfeeding versus water reduced pain responses or crying in neonates undergoing heel puncture.

Clin Evid 2002;8:380–395.

- **Holding in term infants** One RCT found that holding the baby with skin to skin contact versus being swaddled in a crib significantly reduced crying and grimacing during heel puncture (NNT 3, 95% CI 2 to 13).
- **Holding plus sucrose versus holding alone for heel puncture** One RCT in term infants having heel puncture found that sucrose did not appear to increase the benefit of holding.
- **Manual lancets versus automated lancets** RCTs in preterm and term infants have found that manual lancets versus automated devices for heel puncture are more painful, cause more bruising, and increase the time taken to obtain a sample.
- **Multiple doses of sweet solution** One small RCT in preterm infants having heel puncture found no significant difference with multiple versus single doses of sucrose in pain scores.
- **Oral glucose for heel puncture and venepuncture** RCTs have found that oral glucose 30% versus water or versus no treatment significantly reduces pain responses and the duration of crying in preterm and term infants having heel puncture, and significantly reduces pain responses in term infants having venepuncture.
- **Oral glucose or sucrose versus any topical anaesthesia** We found no RCTs comparing oral glucose versus topical anaesthesia. One RCT found insufficient evidence about the effects of oral sucrose versus EMLA in children having venepuncture.
- **Oral sucrose for heel puncture** Systematic reviews and additional RCTs in preterm and term infants have found that oral sucrose 12–70% versus water or no treatment significantly reduces pain responses (particularly the duration of crying) during heel puncture.
- **Oral sucrose for venepuncture** RCTs have found that oral sucrose 24–30% versus water or no treatment significantly reduces pain responses (particularly the duration of crying) during venepuncture.
- **Oral sucrose plus pacifier versus pacifier or sucrose alone** One RCT in preterm infants found no significant difference in pain score during heel puncture between a pacifier dipped in sucrose versus a pacifier alone.
- **Oral sucrose versus oral glucose for venepuncture** One RCT found no significant difference in pain scores during venepuncture with sucrose 30% versus glucose 30%.
- **Other sweeteners for heel puncture** RCTs have found that other sweeteners (hydrogenated glucose; or an artificial sweetener, 10 parts cyclamate and 1 part saccharin) versus water significantly reduce pain scores and the percentage of time spent crying during heel puncture.
- **Other sweeteners for venepuncture** We found no RCTs of other sweeteners for venepuncture.
- **Pacifiers for heel puncture and venepuncture** RCTs in term and preterm infants have found that pacifiers given prior to heel puncture versus no treatment reduce pain responses. One RCT in term infants having venepuncture found that pacifiers versus water or versus no treatment significantly reduced pain responses.
- **Pacifier plus music versus pacifier alone for heel puncture** One RCT in preterm infants found no significant difference in pain score with pacifiers plus music versus pacifiers alone during heel puncture.

Reducing pain during blood sampling in infants

- **Prior stressful handling** One RCT found that handling (as if being prepared for a lumbar puncture) versus no handling significantly increased pain and crying for up to 2 minutes after heel puncture (NNH 5, 95% CI 3 to 17).
- **Prone position** One RCT found no significant difference in pain score with prone position versus side or supine position during heel puncture.
- **Rocking** One RCT found limited evidence that rocking by the examiner versus no intervention reduced pain in neonates undergoing heel puncture. Another RCT found no significant difference in pain response with simulated rocking by a mechanical device versus water given before heel puncture.
- **Swaddling** RCTs found no significant difference in pain responses from swaddling or positioning during heel puncture.
- **Topical anaesthetics for heel puncture** Systematic reviews and additional RCTs have found no evidence of reduced pain responses, particularly crying, in infants who received either lidocaine or lidocaine plus prilocaine cream (EMLA®) versus placebo prior to heel puncture.
- **Topical lidocaine–prilocaine emulsion for venepuncture** RCTs found limited evidence that lidocaine–prilocaine emulsion (EMLA®) versus placebo reduced pain responses to venepuncture.
- **Topical tetracaine (amethocaine) for venepuncture** RCTs found that tetracaine (amethocaine) versus placebo reduced pain scores and the number of infants who cried during venepuncture.
- **Tucking arms and legs in preterm infants** RCTs found limited evidence that pain responses were reduced by tucking the arms and legs into a mid-line flexed position during heel puncture.
- **Venepuncture versus heel puncture** RCTs have found that venepuncture versus heel puncture significantly reduces pain responses (particularly crying) during blood sampling, and also reduces the need for repeat punctures.
- **Warming prior to heel puncture** One RCT in term infants found no benefit of warming prior to heel puncture.

DEFINITION Methods of sampling blood in infants include heel puncture, venepuncture, and arterial puncture. Heel puncture involves lancing of the lateral aspect of the infant's heel, squeezing the heel, and collecting the pooled capillary blood. Venepuncture involves aspirating blood through a needle in a peripheral vein. Arterial blood sampling is not discussed in this review.

INCIDENCE/ PREVALENCE Almost every infant in the developed world undergoes heel puncture to screen for metabolic disorders (e.g. phenylketonuria). Many infants have repeated heel punctures or venepunctures to monitor blood glucose or haemoglobin. Preterm or ill neonates receiving intensive care may have 1–21 painful procedures a day.[1–3] Heel punctures comprise 61–87% and venepuncture comprise 8–13% of the invasive procedures performed on ill infants. Analgesics are rarely given specifically for blood sampling procedures, but 5–19% of infants receive analgesia for other indications.[2,3] In one study, comfort measures were provided during 63% of venepunctures and 75% of heel punctures.[3]

AETIOLOGY/ RISK FACTORS Blood sampling in infants can be difficult to perform, particularly in preterm or ill infants. Young infants may have increased sensitivity and more prolonged responses to pain than older age groups.[4] Factors that may affect the infant's pain responses include post-conceptional age, previous pain experience, and procedural technique.

PROGNOSIS Pain caused by blood sampling is associated with acute behavioural and physiological deterioration.[4] Other adverse effects of blood sampling include bleeding, bruising, haematoma, and infection. Extremely rarely, heel puncture can result in cellulitis, osteomyelitis, calcaneal spurs, and necrotising chondritis.[5–7]

AIMS To obtain an adequate blood sample with minimal pain for the infant and minimal adverse effects of treatments.

OUTCOMES We found no easily administered, widely accepted assessment of pain in infants. Where available, we have analysed the proportion of infants crying at all, or the duration of crying. Other pain related responses measured in the studies included facial expressions (the number of specific expressions, or the duration of those expressions), heart rate, and transcutaneous oxygen saturation levels. Studies used composite scales composed of behavioural and cardiorespiratory, or both, signs of pain related distress, only some of which have been validated. We have not pooled differences in pain related responses or for different pain scales.

METHODS *Clinical Evidence* search and appraisal January 2002, and additional hand searches to January 2002.

QUESTION What are the effects of interventions to reduce pain related distress during blood sampling in infants?

OPTION VENEPUNCTURE VERSUS HEEL PUNCTURE

Three RCTs have found that venepuncture versus heel puncture significantly reduces pain responses (particularly crying) during blood sampling, and also reduces the need for repeat punctures.

Benefits: We found one systematic review (search date 2001,[8] 3 RCTs;[9–11] 264 full term healthy neonates). All three RCTs found that venepuncture versus heel puncture significantly reduced pain responses, but each study used different measures of pain responses. Two of the RCTs found that fewer infants either cried after the procedure or had not stopped crying by 60 seconds with venepuncture compared with heel puncture (36/110 [33%] with venepuncture *v* 28/127 [22%] with heel puncture; RR 0.61, 95% CI 0.50 to 0.76; NNT 4, 95% CI 3 to 7).[9,11] All three RCTs found that venepuncture versus heel puncture significantly reduced the number of repeat punctures required to obtain an adequate sample (16/93 [17%] with venepuncture *v* 64/111 [58%] with heel puncture; RR 0.30, 95% CI 0.18 to 0.49).[8]

Harms: One of the RCTs reported bruising in a single infant following heel puncture and higher maternal anxiety during venepuncture than during heel puncture.[10] Too few infants were studied to detect infection or rare complications.

Comment: Of the three RCTs, only one reported adequate concealment of randomisation and blinded assessment of pain responses.[9] All three RCTs compared blood sampling procedures performed by a single individual in each study. We also found one clinical controlled trial (66 children) comparing venepuncture versus heel puncture (with spring loaded lancet using blinded assessment of pain responses).[12] The study found that infants cried less after venepuncture than after heel puncture (mean difference 66 s, 95% CI 26 s to 107 s). Failure to obtain a sample was more frequent with venepuncture than with heel puncture (6/36 [17%] with venepuncture *v* 0/30 [0%] with heel puncture; ARR 17%, 95% CI 3% to 30%).[12] There was significant heterogeneity between studies for repeat punctures.

OPTION ORAL SWEET SOLUTIONS

In term and preterm infants undergoing heel puncture or venepuncture, RCTs have found that oral sucrose or glucose versus water or no treatment significantly reduce pain responses (particularly the duration of crying). RCTs have found that other sweeteners (hydrogenated glucose; or an artificial sweetener, 10 parts cyclamate and 1 part saccharin) versus water significantly reduce pain scores and the percentage of time spent crying. We found no RCTs of other sweeteners for venepuncture. One small RCT found no significant difference between multiple and single doses of sucrose in pain scores in preterm infants having heel puncture. We found no clear evidence that any one sugar is superior to the others, or evidence about the optimum concentration for pain relief. One RCT in children having venepuncture found limited evidence that crying was significantly reduced in babies given sucrose alone or sucrose plus EMLA versus EMLA alone. We found no RCTs comparing oral glucose versus topical anaesthesia.

Benefits: **Sucrose for heel puncture:** We found four systematic reviews (search dates 1995,[13] 2001,[14] 1998,[15] 2000;[16] 10 RCTs[17–26]) and 9 additional RCTs[27–35] of oral sucrose (0.05–2.00 mL of 7.5–70%) versus water or no treatment in newborns undergoing heel puncture. The 19 RCTs included 1209 term and preterm neonates.[17–35] All six RCTs in preterm neonates found that sucrose (24–70%) versus water significantly reduced pain responses and pain scores.[18,21,22,26,33,34] The time spent crying during the procedure was significantly reduced (by 30 s), and the total duration of crying was significantly reduced (by 39 s).[18,22] Of the 16 trials in term neonates, seven RCTs found that sucrose (12–70%) versus water significantly reduced pain scores.[19,23,26,31,32,34,35] Seven RCTs found that sucrose versus water decreased the percentage of time spent crying.[17,19,23,27–29,32] Seven RCTs found significantly reduced crying time (mean or median differences 16–90 s).[20,22,25,30–32,35] In one RCT, a significant difference was found only for neonates given 50% sucrose and not for those given lower concentrations.[20] One RCT used a low concentration of sucrose (2 mL of 7.5%) and found no significant difference in duration of crying.[24] **Glucose for heel puncture:** We found four systematic reviews (search dates 1995,[13] 2001,[14] 1998,[15] 2000;[16] 2 RCTs[17,36]) and two additional RCTs.[11,37] Three RCTs included 412 term infants given 1–2 mL of 10–30% glucose versus water or no treatment prior to heel puncture.[11,17,36] Two RCTs found fewer infants cried at all with 30% glucose versus water,[11] no treatment,[36] or 10% glucose.[36] One RCT comparing glucose versus no treatment found that 30% glucose significantly reduced crying time (75% decrease) but 10% glucose did not significantly reduce crying time (50% decrease) compared with no treatment.[36] One RCT comparing 12% glucose versus water found no significant difference (mean crying time 56 s with glucose *v* 60 s with water).[17] One crossover trial of 17 preterm infants compared 10% glucose with no treatment. Mean pain scores were significantly reduced [Premature Infant Pain Profile (see glossary, p 393)] reduced by 2.5; $P < 0.001$).[37] **Other sweeteners for heel puncture:** We found three systematic reviews (search dates 1995,[13] 2001,[14] 1998;[15] 1 RCT[23]) and one additional RCT.[38] The RCT in the reviews comparing hydrogenated glucose versus water found significant decreases in pain score, duration of first cry and percentage of time spent crying, but no significant difference versus sucrose (25% or 50%).[23] The additional RCT (120 term infants) comparing an artificial sweetener (10 parts cyclamate and 1 part saccharin) versus water found small but significant differences in percentage of time crying and pain scores.[38] **Sucrose for venepuncture:** We found two systematic reviews (search dates 1995,[13] 2001;[14] 1 RCT[39]) and two additional RCTs[40,41] comparing sucrose versus water in 201 term neonates having venepuncture. The RCT from the reviews (28 preterm neonates) found that 24% sucrose versus water reduced mean crying time (mean duration of crying, 19 s in 8 preterm neonates given 24% sucrose *v* 73 s in 12 neonates given water). The RCT found that mean crying time was not significantly reduced with 12% sucrose versus water (8 neonates, 63 s).[39] The additonal RCTs found significantly reduced duration of crying and pain scores with 24–30% sucrose versus water or no treatment.[40,41] **Glucose for venepuncture:** We found two RCTs that compared 2 mL of 30% glucose versus water in term infants undergoing venepuncture.[11,40] One RCT (60 infants) found significantly reduced pain scores but no difference in the proportion of infants crying (46% with glucose *v* 39% with water).[11] The other RCT (75 infants) found significantly reduced median pain scores with glucose versus water or no treatment (median pain score difference 2, glucose 5, water 7, 95% CI 1 to 4; $P = 0.005$).[40] **Other sweeteners for venepuncture:** We found no RCTs of other sweeteners for venepuncture. **Concentration of glucose or sucrose for heel puncture and venepuncture:** We found two systematic reviews (search dates 2001[14] and 1998;[15] 1 RCT[36]) and six additional RCTs of the effects of glucose or sucrose concentration in heel puncture.[17,20,23,30,36,40] We found no studies of the effects of glucose or sucrose concentration in venepuncture. Three RCTs in term neonates compared different concentrations of sucrose during heel puncture.[17,20,23] One RCT (75 neonates) found that increasing concentrations of sucrose (2 mL of 12.5%, 25%, and 50%) produced significantly greater reductions in the duration of crying.[20] The other two trials found no difference in crying duration with different sucrose concentrations (56 infants in total, given 2 mL of 25–50% or 12–25% sucrose).[17,23] Three RCTs compared different concentrations of glucose during heel puncture.[30,36,40] One RCT (60 term and preterm infants) compared 1 mL of 10% versus 1 mL of 30% glucose; the study found no significant difference in the duration of crying or the proportion of babies who cried at all (no crying in 40% with 10% glucose *v* 53% with 30% glucose; $P > 0.05$).[36] **Multiple doses of sweeteners:** We found one RCT (32 preterm neonates, mean gestation 31 wks) that compared a single dose (0.5 mL) of 24% sucrose 2 minutes before heel puncture versus three doses given 2 minutes prior, immediately before the procedure, and during the procedure.[33] Pain scores measured at five points during the procedure were significantly different only at the latest time. **Sucrose versus glucose for heel puncture or venepuncture** We found one RCT (113 term infants undergoing heel puncture) comparing glucose versus sucrose. The study found that 30% sucrose versus 30% glucose reduced crying time by a mean of 30 seconds ($P = 0.006$).[30] Another RCT (150 term infants undergoing venepuncture) found no significant difference with 30% sucrose versus 30% glucose on pain scores.[40] **Repeated doses for repeated blood sampling:** We found no RCTs. **Sucrose versus topical anaesthesia:** See topical anathesia, p 387. **Glucose versus topical anaesthesia:** We found no RCTs. **Sucrose plus pacifier versus pacifier or sucrose alone:** See pacifiers, p 389.

Harms: No adverse effects from oral sucrose or glucose administered to full term or preterm infants were reported in any of the RCTs. The safety of repeated oral administration of sucrose or glucose has not been adequately investigated. Theoretical adverse effects include hyperglycaemia and necrotising enterocolitis.

Comment: Some studies were crossover RCTs, which might produce biased estimates of the effect of sucrose if neonates become habituated to pain or if the washout period between interventions is too short.[18,22,34] Only some RCTs reported adequate allocation concealment.[11,18,19,21,31,33,40] In one study it was uncertain whether infants were randomly allocated.[28] Most had blinded measurement of at least some of the pain responses, particularly crying, on the basis of independent audio or video tape recordings. One RCT had no blinded outcome assessment.[22] We found inadequate evidence about the benefits or harms of repeated administration of sucrose or glucose for repeated blood sampling.

OPTION BREAST MILK

Four RCTs found no evidence that breast milk or breast feeding (1 RCT) versus water reduced pain responses or crying in neonates undergoing heel puncture.

Benefits: We found one systematic review (search date 1998,[15] 2 RCTs,[25,36] 126 preterm and term neonates undergoing heel puncture) and two subsequent RCTs (147 term infants)[38,35] comparing breast milk

(1–2 mL) versus water. None found a significant effect of breast milk on duration of crying[25,35,36,38] or proportion of infants not crying.[36] One RCT (62 term infants) found no significant effect of breastfeeding versus water on duration of crying.[35] We found no RCTs on the effects of breast milk during venepuncture.

Harms: None reported.

Comment: Concealment of allocation was not clearly stated in any RCT. Assessment of pain responses was blind in two RCTs[35,38] and not clearly stated in the other two.[25,36]

OPTION TOPICAL ANAESTHETICS

Systematic reviews and additional RCTs found no evidence of reduced pain responses, particularly crying, in infants who received either lidocaine or lidocaine plus prilocaine cream (EMLA) versus placebo prior to heel puncture. Four RCTs found limited evidence that EMLA versus placebo reduced pain responses to venepuncture. Two RCTs found that tetracaine (amethocaine) gel versus placebo reduced pain scores and the number of infants who cried during venepuncture; one RCT found no evidence of reduced crying for heel puncture. One RCT in children having venepuncture found that crying time was significantly reduced in babies given EMLA versus water and found limited evidence that EMLA alone reduced crying less than sucrose or EMLA plus sucrose. We found no RCT comparing topical anaesthesia versus oral glucose or versus pacifiers.

Benefits: **Lidocaine (lignocaine) or EMLA for heel puncture:** We found three systematic reviews (search dates 1996[42] and 1998,[15] 1998;[43] 5 RCTs[44–48]) and one additional RCT,[1] comparing lidocaine or EMLA versus placebo in neonates undergoing heel puncture. Treatments were usually given 30–60 minutes before heel puncture, with the exception of one RCT that randomised infants to eight application times (10–120 min before heel puncture).[47] The five studies used different assessments of pain responses. Three RCTs included 186 preterm neonates[1,44,45] and three RCTs included 192 infants who were mainly term neonates.[46–48] None of the RCTs found a significant difference with lidocaine or EMLA versus placebo on pain scores. One RCT found no significant difference with EMLA versus placebo in the proportion of infants who cried during the procedure (54/56 [96%] *v* 52/54 [96%]).[47] **EMLA for venepuncture:** We found two systematic reviews (search dates 1996[42] and 1998;[15] 2 RCTs[49,50]) and two additional RCTs[51,52] that compared EMLA versus placebo in infants having venepuncture. One RCT (120 term infants) found that EMLA versus placebo significantly reduced the duration of crying (median 12 s *v* 31 s; $P < 0.05$) and pain score at 15 seconds after venepuncture (NFCS score (see glossary, p 393) 287 *v* 374; $P = 0.02$), but found no significant difference in pain score 60 seconds after venepuncture.[49] The second RCT (60 children) found that 19/28 in the EMLA group and 14/28 in the placebo group did not cry at all during the procedure. The study did not measure duration of cry or pain score.[50] The third RCT (41 infants and toddlers) found a significant difference in mean behavioural pain score with EMLA versus placebo ($P < 0.01$).[51] The fourth RCT (19 preterm infants) found that

EMLA versus placebo did not significantly reduce pain scores (NFCS score, mean difference 0, 95% CI −2.00 to +1.75) or the total duration of crying (median difference between EMLA and placebo −22 s, 95% CI −96 s to +24 s).[52] **Tetracaine (amethocaine) versus placebo:** We found three RCTs (in term and preterm infants reporting blinded assessments of pain scores and crying) comparing tetracaine (amethocaine) versus placebo.[53–55] Two RCTs involved 80 preterm and term neonates undergoing venepuncture.[53,54] Tetracaine significantly reduced the pain scores in infants having venepuncture and reduced the proportion who cried (4/19 [21%] with tetracaine *v* 15/20 [75%] with placebo; ARR 54% 95% CI 2% to 80%; NNT 2, 95% CI 1 to 4).[53,54] One RCT (60 neonates, median gestation 36 wks, undergoing heel puncture using an automated device) found that the tetracaine group had a lower pain score, and fewer infants cried with tetracaine than with placebo, but neither difference was significant (20/30 [67%] with tetracaine *v* 13/29 [45%]; ARI 22%, 95% CI −4% to +47%).[55] **Topical anaesthetic versus sucrose:** We found one RCT (55 venepunctures in 51 term neonates) that compared four treatments: EMLA alone; 24% sucrose alone; EMLA plus sucrose ; and water.[41] Crying was taped and assessed blind to treatment. Crying time was significantly higher in babies given water versus EMLA alone (P = 0.008) or versus sucrose with or without EMLA (P = 0.001). EMLA alone was reported to be less effective than sucrose alone or EMLA plus sucrose, but analyses were not presented. We found no studies of topical anaesthetic versus sweet solutions for heel puncture. **Topical anaesthetic versus glucose:** We found no RCTs. **Topical anaesthetic versus pacifiers:** We found no RCTs.

Harms: We found six RCTs (250 infants) that reported the absence of adverse reactions to EMLA, or to placebo, or no difference in minor, transient local reactions.[1,46–48,51,52] One cohort study (500 neonates) found unusual cutaneous effects associated with EMLA in four neonates under 32 weeks' gestation.[56] Methaemoglobinaemia can occur with the prilocaine constituent of EMLA. Levels of methaemoglobin over 25–30% can cause clinical symptoms of hypoxia.[57] We found one systematic review (search date 1996, 12 RCTs or cohort studies, > 355 neonates)[42] and two subsequent RCTs (167 neonates)[1,57] of EMLA for heel puncture, venepuncture, circumcision, or lumbar puncture. All but one of these studies found mean methaemoglobin levels less than 1.5% in neonates given EMLA. The other RCT (47 preterm and term infants given EMLA) found that the highest mean methaemoglobin levels (2.3%, range 0.6–6.2%) occurred after 15 days of repeated doses of EMLA.[56] A systematic review found two case reports of neonates who were treated with oxygen at methaemoglobin levels of 12% and 16%.[42] No local skin reactions were seen after application of tetracaine or placebo in the 140 neonates studied.

Comment: Some of the studies reported adequate concealment of allocation.[46,47,49,52–55] Three RCTs used video taped recordings of pain responses to blind assessors to the intervention.[49,51–53,55] In the other RCTs, although placebo ointment was used, pain responses were assessed by observers at the time of the procedure, rather than by scoring of video film. Deduction of treatment allocation may have been possible in the EMLA studies because of the smell and skin blanching caused by EMLA. One study excluded 25% of children who had high behaviour scores before puncture, and presented results only for selected subgroups.[51] The findings of this study may be difficult to generalise.

OPTION PACIFIERS

Eight RCTs found reduced pain responses in term and preterm infants given pacifiers compared with no treatment prior to heel puncture. Two RCTs in preterm neonates having heel puncture found that pacifiers plus sucrose or glucose versus pacifiers alone similarly reduced pain responses. One RCT found significant reduction in pain responses in term infants given a pacifier compared with water or no treatment during venepuncture. We found no RCTs comparing pacifiers versus topical anaesthesia.

Benefits: **Pacifier alone for heel puncture:** We found two systematic reviews (search dates 2001[14] and 1998;[15] 1 RCT[58]) and seven additional RCTs comparing pacifiers (see glossary, p 393) versus no treatment (445 infants of which 271 were preterm).[32,37,58–62] Pacifiers were given 2–5 minutes before heel puncture. Four RCTs were crossover trials.[37,58–60] All Four RCTs found that pacifiers versus no pacifiers significantly reduced pain responses[37,58,61] or the percentage of time spent in a distressed, fussy, or awake state.[60,61] In the three RCTs in term infants, those given a pacifier cried for significantly less time,[32,59,62] spent less time in fussy or awake states,[62] or had reduced pain score.[59] However, reductions were not significant for all measures of pain: in one study, grimacing was not significantly reduced by the pacifier[32] and in another, the pain score was similar during the procedure but fell more quickly in babies given pacifiers.[59] **Pacifier plus sucrose for heel puncture:** We found one RCT (crossover, 122 preterm neonates having heel puncture) that compared a pacifier dipped in 24% sucrose versus dipped in water.[58] The study found no significant difference in pain responses (mean Premature Infant Pain Profile score [see glossary, p 393]) between the interventions. **Pacifier plus glucose for heel puncture:** We found one RCT (crossover, 17 preterm infants) that compared a pacifier dipped in 10% glucose versus no treatment, 10% glucose alone, or pacifier alone.[37] Mean pain score was reduced (reduction in mean PIPP score: 3.6; $P = 0.001$) compared to no treatment, but was similar to glucose alone or pacifier alone. **Pacifier plus music for heel puncture:** One RCT (28 term and preterm infants) found no significant difference between pacifiers plus music versus pacifiers alone for pain score assessed at all time points except 4 minutes after heel puncture ($P < 0.001$).[59] **Pacifier plus multimodal sensory stimulation:** We found one RCT (crossover, 17 preterm infants) that found a pacifier plus multimodal sensory stimulation (pacifer plus glucose, massage, visual, and auditory stimulation) during heel puncture significantly reduced the pain score when compared with no treatment (mean PIPP score reduction: 7.15; $P < 0.001$) and when compared with glucose plus pacifer, pacifier alone, or glucose alone (mean PIPP score reduction: 2.6–4.55; P < 0.01 for each of the 3 comparisons).[37] **Pacifier for venepuncture:** We found one RCT (100 term infants undergoing venepuncture) comparing pacifiers in infants given pacifier or pacifier plus sucrose versus no treatment or 2 mL water orally.[39] The study found a significant reduction in the pain score during the procedure (median difference in 10 point pain score was 5 for pacifiers alone *v* water and 6 for pacifiers plus sucrose *v* water; P < 0.0001). **Pacifier versus topical anaesthestic:** We found no RCTs.

Harms: No adverse effects were reported in any of these studies.

Comment: None of the studies explicitly defined the method of allocation to pacifier or no treatment. Three RCTs blinded assessors to the intervention by analysing audio tapes of crying during the procedure.[37,60,62] Measurement of pain responses on the basis of facial expressions were not blinded to the pacifiers or music intervention.

OPTION HOLDING

One RCT in term infants found that holding the baby with skin to skin contact versus being swaddled in a crib significantly reduced crying and grimacing during heel puncture. One RCT in term infants having heel punture found that sucrose did not appear to modify the effect of holding.

Benefits: We found no systematic review but found two RCTs (124 term infants undergoing heel puncture).[19,63] The first RCT (30 infants) compared holding the baby with skin to skin contact versus being swaddled in a crib.[63] Crying and grimacing were significantly reduced in the babies held skin to skin (proportion crying during procedure 8% *v* 45%; ARR 37%; CI not provided; NNT 3, 95% CI 2 to 13). The second RCT (94 term newborns) compared sucrose, sucrose plus holding, holding with water, and water alone for heel puncture.[19] Pain scores and duration of crying decreased in the holding group compared with no holding and in the sucrose groups compared with no sucrose, but the differences were of borderline significance. There was no evidence of an interaction between sucrose and holding (P = 0.37).

Harms: None reported.

Comment: Assessment of crying was based on analysis of audio or video tape recordings and was blind to the sucrose intervention but not to holding.[19,63] Assessments based on facial expressions were not blind to the intervention.

OPTION ROCKING

One RCT of rocking versus no intervention in neonates undergoing heel puncture found limited evidence that rocking reduced pain. Another RCT found no significant difference in pain response.

Benefits: We found no systematic review but found two RCTs, comparing rocking versus no intervention.[21,62] One RCT (44 preterm infants, 25–34 wks gestation) compared 0.05 mL water given before heel puncture versus simulated rocking using a respirator attached to an air mattress.[21] The study found no significant differences for facial expressions of pain. The other RCT (40 term neonates) compared no intervention with being held vertically and rocked by the examiner.[62] The study found that rocking reduced the duration of crying (P = 0.05) during the procedure and the risk of persistent crying (2/20 [10%] with rocking *v* 9/20 [45%] with no intervention; ARR 35%; CI not provided; NNT 3, 95% CI 2 to 10).

Harms: None reported.

Comment: The method of allocation to rocking or standard care was adequate in one study[21] and unclear in the other.[61] Both studies used blinded assessment of pain responses based on video[21] and audio tape[62] recordings.

OPTION POSITION, SWADDLING, AND PRIOR HANDLING

Two RCTs found limited evidence that pain responses were reduced by tucking the arms and legs into a mid-line flexed position during heel puncture, or by avoiding stressful handling before heel puncture. Two RCTs found no difference in pain responses from positioning or swaddling during heel puncture.

Benefits: We found no systematic review but found four RCTs comparing positioning, swaddling, or stressful handling versus no intervention.[58,64–66] One crossover RCT (122 preterm infants, 25–34 wks gestation, undergoing heel puncture) compared prone position versus side or supine position. The study found no significant difference in the mean pain score.[58] One RCT (crossover, 15 preterm neonates) compared swaddling immediately after heel puncture versus standard care (no swaddling).[64] No significant difference in facial expressions of pain or arousal state were detected. Another RCT (crossover, 30 preterm neonates, 25–35 wks gestation) compared facilitative tucking during and after heel puncture (defined as the gentle containment of arms and legs in a flexed, mid-line position) with no intervention.[65] The study found a significant reduction in the total crying time and time to quietening (mean cry duration 2.2 *v* 0.3 min; P < 0.001). The fourth RCT (48 mainly preterm infants, mean gestation 35 wks) compared stressful handling (as if being prepared for a lumbar puncture) with avoidance of handling for 10 minutes prior to heel puncture.[66] The study found that prior handling increased facial expressions of pain, the proportion of time crying, and crying at all during the 2 minutes after heel puncture (21/21 [100%] handled babies cried *v* 21/27 [78%] non-handled babies; ARR 22%; CI not provided; NNT 5, 95% CI 3 to 17).

Harms: No adverse events were reported for any of these interventions.

Comment: None of the studies explicitly reported the method of allocation to the interventions and only the study comparing handling versus no handling assessed pain responses blind to the intervention.[66]

OPTION WARMING

One RCT found no effect of warming prior to heel puncture

Benefits: We found one systematic review (search date 1998,[15] 1 RCT[67]) that compared 57 term infants undergoing heel puncture on 80 occasions with an automated lancet with (41 infants) or without (40 infants) prior warming of the heel. The heel was warmed for 10 minutes with a gel pack at 40°C. A slightly higher proportion of infants grimaced and cried with warming versus not warming (14/41 [34%] *v* 10/40 [25%]; RR 1.4, 95% CI 0.7 to 2.7). Sampling time was slightly longer in the warmed heels (median time 44 s, interquartile range 25–62 s *v* 40 s, interquartile range 28–72 s), but the number of repeat punctures was slightly lower (5/41 [12%] *v* 8/40 [20%]; RR 0.6, 0.2 to 1.7).

Harms: We found no evidence about harms.

Comment: Method of allocation was not reported and assessment of outcomes was not blind to the intervention.

OPTION DEVICES FOR HEEL PUNCTURE

Four RCTs in preterm and term infants found that automated devices for heel puncture are less painful and cause less bruising than manual lancets and that samples are obtained more quickly. Two RCTs in preterm infants compared automated devices. One found no differences and the other found one device reduced sampling time and the need for repeat punctures.

Benefits: We found no systematic review but found four RCTs (70 preterm infants and 76 term infants) that compared spring loaded, automated devices with manual lancets.[68–71] One RCT (70 infants) found that fewer punctures occurred over 2–21 days in preterm infants randomised to repeated sampling using an automated device versus a manual lancet (mean difference in total number of punctures: 37, 95% CI 24 to 50).[68] The automated group had less bruising of the heel (27/32 [84%] with automated *v* 38/38 [100%] with manual; ARR 16%, 95% CI 4% to 28%; NNT 7), and inflammation of the heel (17/32 [53%] with automated *v* 30/38 [79%] with manual; ARR 26%, 95% CI 4% to 48%; NNT 4). One RCT (36 term infants) found a non-significant reduction in the risk of repeated puncture for a single sample (2/18 [11%] with automated *v* 3/18 [17%] with manual; ARR 6%, 95% CI –17% to +28%) and a significant increase in the proportion of infants who did not cry (5/18 [28%] with automated *v* 0/18 [0%] with manual; ARI 28%, 95% CI 5% to 50%; NNT 4).[69] One RCT found no difference in the time spent crying during a single procedure, but sampling was quicker with the automated device (mean difference 92 s, 95% CI 29 s to 154 s).[70] One RCT found a decreased duration of crying and sampling with the automated device than manual lancet (the results are being translated and will be presented in future *Clinical Evidence* updates).[71] Two further RCTs in preterm infants compared two types of automated devices used on 344 occasions in 108 infants.[72,73] In one RCT (187 samplings), lack of pain assessed by facial expression was similar in both groups (32/87 [37%] with the

Tenderfoot Preemie® v 33/83 [40%] with the Autolet®; ARR 3%, 95% CI –12% to +18%).[72] The sampling time was similar (57 infants: median time 5.0 s with Tenderfoot Preemie® v 6.43 s with Autolet®; $P < 0.05$). The risk of haemolysis was similar (12/60 [20%] with the Tenderfoot Preemie® v 17/61 [28%] with the Autolet®; ARR 8%, 95% CI –7% to +23%). Fewer repeat samples were needed with the Tenderfoot Preemie® (17/90 [19%] v 40/97 [41%]; ARR 22%, 95% CI 10% to 35%). The other RCT found a shorter collection time with the Tenderfoot Preemie® versus the Monolet® (mean 3.9 s v 5.4 s), fewer punctures to obtain a sample (mean 1 v 2.1), and fewer repeat samples (0/49 [0%] v 6/40 [15%]; ARR 15%, 95% CI 5% to 25%).[73]

Harms: Manual lancets carry a risk of accidental injury to patients and staff.

Comment: Two RCTs allocated babies sealed envelopes with the device allocation.[71,73] Allocation method was not clearly reported in any of the other studies. Three RCTs attempted to blind some of the outcome measures to the procedure.[68,69,71]

GLOSSARY

Hydrogenated glucose syrup An aqueous solution of hydrogenated part hydrolysed starch composed of a mixture of mainly maltitol with sorbitol and hydrogenated oligosaccharides and polysaccharides. Preparations containing a minimum 98% maltitol are known as maltitol syrup.

NFCS score Facial Coding System used to evaluate pain responses in full term and preterm infants. Presence or absence is recorded of six facial actions (e.g. eyes squeezed shut, deepening of the naso-labial furrow).

Pacifier A device with a teat that a baby sucks on for comfort. Some pacifiers can deliver a liquid to the baby. Also known as a "dummy", "soother", or "plug" in some countries.

Premature Infant Pain Profile score A seven item composite scale that scores behavioural and cardiorespiratory pain responses coded 0 to 3 (maximum score 21).

Stressful handling A term used to describe the undressing of an infant and holding in a fixed position, as if being prepared for a lumbar puncture.

REFERENCES

1. Stevens B, Johnston C, Taddio A, et al. Management of pain from heel lance with lidocaine–prilocaine (EMLA) cream: is it safe and efficacious in preterm infants? *J Dev Behav Pediatr* 1999;20:216–221.
2. Johnston CC, Collinge JM, Henderson SJ, Anand KJ. A cross-sectional survey of pain and pharmacological analgesia in Canadian neonatal intensive care units. *Clin J Pain* 1997;13:308–312.
3. Porter FL, Anand KJS. Epidemiology of pain in neonates. *Res Clin Forum* 1998;20:9–18.
4. Anand K, Stevens BJ, McGrath PJ. *Pain in neonates*. Amsterdam: Elsevier Science BV, 2000.
5. Meehan RM. Heel sticks in neonates for capillary blood sampling. *Neonatal Network* 1998;17:17–24.
6. Lilien LD, Harris VJ, Ramamurthy RS, Pildes RS. Neonatal osteomyelitis of the calcaneus: complications of heel puncture. *J Pediatr* 1976;88:478–480.
7. Blumenfeld TA, Turi GK, Blanc WA. Recommended site and depth of newborn heel skin punctures based on anatomical measurements and histopathology. *Lancet* 1979;1:230–233.
8. Shah V, Ohlsson A. Venepuncture versus heel lance for blood sampling in term neonates. In: The Cochrane Library, Issue 1, 2002. Oxford: Update Software 2001. Search date 2001; primary sources Cochrane Library, Medline, Embase, and Cinahl.
9. Larsson BA, Tannfeldt G, Lagercrantz H, Olsson GL. Venepuncture is more effective and less painful than heel lancing for blood tests in neonates. *Pediatrics* 1998;101:882–886.
10. Shah VS, Taddio A, Bennett S, Speidel BD. Neonatal pain response to heel stick vs venepuncture for routine blood sampling. *Arch Dis Child Fetal Neonatal Ed* 1997;77:F143–F144.
11. Eriksson M, Gradin M, Schollin J. Oral glucose and venepuncture reduce blood sampling pain in newborns. *Early Hum Dev* 1999;55:211–218.
12. Logan PW. Venepuncture versus heel prick for the collection of the Newborn Screening Test. Australian. *Aust J Adv Nurs* 1999;17:30–36.
13. Stevens B, Taddio A, Ohlsson A, Einarson T. The efficacy of sucrose for relieving procedural pain in neonates: a systematic review and meta-analysis. *Acta Paediatr* 1997;86:837–842. Search date 1995; primary sources Medline, Embase,

Reference Update, and hand searches of personal files, bibliographies, most recent neonatal and pain journals, and conference proceedings.

14. Stevens B, Yamada J, Ohlsson A. Sucrose for analgesia in newborn infants undergoing painful procedures. In: The Cochrane Library, Issue 1, 2002. Oxford: Update Software. Search date 2001; primary sources Medline, Embase, Reference Update, Cochrane Library, and hand searches of personal files, bibliographies, recent neonatal and pain journals, and conference proceedings.
15. Ohlsson A, Taddio A, Jadad AR, Stevens B. Evidence-based decision making, systematic reviews and the Cochrane collaboration: implications for neonatal analgesia. In: Anand K, Stevens B, McGrath PJ, eds. *Pain in Neonates*. Amsterdam: Elsevier Science BV, 2000:251–268. Search date 1998; primary sources Medline, Cochrane Library, hand searches of personal files, and reference lists.
16. Bauer K, Versmold H. Oral sugar solutions in pain therapy of neonates and premature infants. *Z Geburtshilfe Neonatol* 2001;205:80–85 Search date 2000; primary source PubMed.
17. Abad Massanet F, Diaz Gomez NM, Domenech Martinez E, Robayna Curbelo M, Rico Sevillano J. Analgesic effect of oral sweet solution in newborns. *An Esp Pediatr* 1995;43:351–354.
18. Bucher HU, Moser T, von Siebenthal K, Keel M, Wolf M, Duc G. Sucrose reduces pain reaction to heel lancing in preterm infants: a placebo-controlled, randomized and masked study. *Pediatr Res* 1995;38:332–335.
19. Gormally S, Barr RG, Wertheim L, et al. Contact and nutrient caregiving effects on newborn infant pain responses. *Dev Med Child Neurol* 2001;43:28–38.
20. Haouari N, Wood C, Griffiths G, Levene M. The analgesic effect of sucrose in full term infants: a randomised controlled trial. *BMJ* 1995;310:1498–1500.
21. Johnston CC, Stremler RL, Stevens BJ, Horton LJ. Effectiveness of oral sucrose and simulated rocking on pain response in preterm neonates. *Pain* 1997;72:193–199.
22. Ramenghi LA, Wood CM, Griffith GC, Levene MI. Reduction of pain response in premature infants using intraoral sucrose. *Arch Dis Child Fetal Neonatal Ed* 1996;74:F126–F128.
23. Ramenghi LA, Griffith GC, Wood CM, Levene MI. Effect of non-sucrose sweet tasting solution on neonatal heel prick responses. *Arch Dis Child Fetal Neonatal Ed* 1996;74:F129–F131.
24. Rushforth JA, Levene MI. Effect of sucrose on crying in response to heel stab. *Arch Dis Child* 1993;69:388–389.
25. Ors R, Ozek E, Baysoy G, et al. Comparison of sucrose and human milk on pain response in newborns. *Eur J Pediatr* 1999;158:63–66.
26. Gibbins SA. Efficacy and safety of sucrose for procedural pain relief in preterm and term neonates. *Dissert Abstract Int* 2001;62–04B:1804.
27. Blass EM, Hoffmeyer LB. Sucrose as an analgesic for newborn infants. *Pediatrics* 1991;87:215–218.
28. Blass EM. Pain-reducing properties of sucrose in human newborns. *Chem Senses* 1995;20:29–35.
29. Blass EM. Milk-induced hypoalgesia in human newborns. *Pediatrics* 1997:99:825–829.
30. Isik U, Ozek E, Bilgen H, Cebeci, D. Comparison of oral glucose and sucrose solutions on pain response in neonates. *J Pain* 2000;1:275–278.
31. Overgaard C, Knudsen A. Pain-relieving effect of sucrose in newborns during heel prick. *Biol Neonate* 1999;75:279–284.
32. Blass EM, Watt LB. Suckling- and sucrose-induced analgesia in human newborns. *Pain* 1999;83:611–623.
33. Johnston CC, Stremler R, Horton L, Friedman A. Effect of repeated doses of sucrose during heel stick procedure in preterm neonates. *Biol Neonate* 1999;75:160–166.
34. Mellah D, Gourrier E, Merbouche S, et al. Analgesia with saccharose during heel capillary prick. A randomized study in 37 newborns of over 33 weeks of amenorrhea. *Arch Pediatr* 1999;6:610–616 [in French].
35. Bilgen H, Ozek E, Cebeci D, Ors R. Comparison of sucrose, expressed breast milk, and breast-feeding on the neonatal response to heel prick. *J Pain* 2001;2:301–305.
36. Skogsdal Y, Eriksson M, Schollin J. Analgesia in newborns given oral glucose. *Acta Paediatr* 1997;86:217–220.
37. Bellieni CV, Buonocore G, Nenci A, et al. Sensorial saturation: an effective analgesic tool for heel-prick in preterm infants: a prospective randomized trial. *Biol Neonate* 2001;80:15–18.
38. Bucher HU, Baumgartner R, Bucher N, Seiler M, Fauchere JC. Artificial sweetener reduces nociceptive reaction in term newborn infants. *Early Hum Dev* 2000:59:51–60.
39. Abad F, Diaz NM, Domenech E, Robayna M, Rico J. Oral sweet solution reduces pain-related behaviour in preterm infants. *Acta Paediatr* 1996;85:854–858.
40. Carbajal R, Chauvet X, Couderc S, Olivier-Martin M. Randomised trial of analgesic effects of sucrose, glucose, and pacifiers in term neonates. *BMJ* 1999;319:1393–1397.
41. Abad F, Diaz-Gomez NM, Domenech E, et al. Oral sucrose compares favourably with lidocaine–prilocaine cream for pain relief during venepuncture in neonates. *Acta Paediatr* 2001;90:160–165.
42. Taddio A, Ohlsson A, Einarson TR, Stevens B, Koren G. A systematic review of lidocaine–prilocaine cream (EMLA) in the treatment of acute pain in neonates. *Pediatrics* 1998;101:E1. Search date 1996; primary sources Medline, Embase, Reference Update, and hand searches of personal files and meeting proceedings.
43. Essink-Tjebbes CM, Hekster YA, Liem KD, Van Dongen RTM. Topical use of local anesthetics in neonates. *Pharm World Sci* 1999;21:173–176. Search date 1998; primary source Medline.
44. Ramaioli F, Amice De D, Guzinska K, Ceriana P, Gasparoni A. EMLA cream and the premature infant. *Int Monitor Reg Anaesthesia* 1993;59. [Abstract]
45. Stevens B, Johnston C, Taddio A, Koren G, Aranda J. *The safety and efficacy of EMLA for heel lance in premature neonates*. International Association for the Study of Pain, 8th World Congress on Pain, Vancouver, Canada 1996;239:181–182.
46. Rushforth JA, Griffiths G, Thorpe H, Levene MI. Can topical lignocaine reduce behavioural response to heel prick? *Arch Dis Child Fetal Neonatal Ed* 1995;72:F49–F51.
47. Larsson BA, Jylli L, Lagercrantz H, Olsson GL. Does a local anaesthetic cream (EMLA) alleviate pain from heel-lancing in neonates? *Acta Anaesthesiol Scand* 1995;39:1028–1031.
48. Wester U. Analgesic effect of lidocaine ointment on intact skin in neonates. *Acta Paediatr* 1993;82:791.
49. Larsson BA, Tannfeldt G, Lagercrantz H, Olsson GL. Alleviation of the pain of venepuncture in neonates. *Acta Paediatr* 1998;87:774–779.

50. Lindh V, Wiklund U, Hakansson S. Assessment of the effect of EMLA during venipuncture in the newborn by analysis of heart rate variability. *Pain* 2000;86:247–254.
51. Robieux I, Kumar R, Radhakrishnan S, Koren G. Assessing pain and analgesia with a lidocaine–prilocaine emulsion in infants and toddlers during venipuncture. *J Pediatr* 1991;118:971–973.
52. Acharya AB, Bustani PC, Phillips JD, Taub NA, Beattie RM. Randomised controlled trial of eutectic mixture of local anaesthetics cream for venepuncture in healthy preterm infants. *Arch Dis Child Fetal Neonatal Ed* 1998;78:F138–F142.
53. Jain A, Rutter N. Does topical amethocaine gel reduce the pain of venepuncture in newborn infants? A randomised double blind controlled trial. *Arch Dis Child Fetal Neonatal Ed* 2000;83:F207–F210.
54. Moore J. No more tears: a randomized controlled double-blind trial of Amethocaine gel vs. placebo in the management of procedural pain in neonates. *J Adv Nurs* 2001;34:475–482.
55. Jain A, Rutter N, Ratnayaka M. Topical amethocaine gel for pain relief of heel prick blood sampling: a randomised double blind controlled trial. *Arch Dis Child Fetal Neonatal Ed* 2001;84:F56–F59.
56. Gourrier E, Karoubi P, el Hanache A, et al. Use of EMLA cream in a department of neonatology. *Pain* 1996;68:431–434.
57. Brisman M, Ljung BM, Otterbom I, Larsson LE, Andreasson SE. Methaemoglobin formation after the use of EMLA cream in term neonates. *Acta Paediatr* 1998;87:1191–1194.
58. Stevens B, Johnston C, Franck L, et al. The efficacy of developmentally sensitive interventions and sucrose for relieving procedural pain in very low birth weight neonates. *Nurs Res* 1999;48:35–43.
59. Bo LK, Callaghan P. Soothing pain-elicited distress in Chinese neonates. *Pediatrics* 2000:105:E49.
60. Corbo MG, Mansi G, Stagni A, et al. Nonnutritive sucking during heelstick procedures decreases behavioral distress in the newborn infant. *Biol Neonate* 2000;77:162–167.
61. Field T, Goldson E. Pacifying effects of nonnutritive sucking on term and preterm neonates during heelstick procedures. *Pediatrics* 1984;74:1012–1015.
62. Campos RG. Rocking and pacifiers: two comforting interventions for heelstick pain. *Res Nurs Health* 1994;17:321–331.
63. Gray L, Watt L, Blass EM. Skin-to-skin contact is analgesic in healthy newborns. *Pediatrics* 2000;105(1):e14.
64. Fearon I, Kisilevsky BS, Hains SMJ, Muir DW, Tranmer J. Swaddling after heel lance: age-specific effects on behavioural recovery in preterm infants. *J Dev Behav Pediatr* 1997;18:222–232.
65. Corff KE, Seideman R, Venkataraman PS, Lutes L, Yates B. Facilitated tucking: a nonpharmacologic comfort measure for pain in preterm neonates. *J Obstet Gynecol Neonatal Nurs* 1995;24:143–147.
66. Porter FL, Wolf CM, Miller JP. The effect of handling and immobilization on the response to acute pain in newborn infants. *Pediatrics* 1998;102:1383–1389.
67. Barker DP, Willetts B, Cappendijk VC, Rutter N. Capillary blood sampling: should the heel be warmed? *Arch Dis Child Fetal Neonatal Ed* 1996;74:F139–F140.
68. Vertanen H, Fellman V, Brommels M, Viinikka L. An automatic incision device for obtaining blood samples from the heels of preterm infants causes less damage than a conventional manual lancet. *Arch Dis Child Fetal Neonatal Ed* 2001;84:F53–F55.
69. Harpin VA, Rutter N. Making heel pricks less painful. *Arch Dis Child* 1983:226–228
70. Paes B, Janes M, Vegh P, LaDuca F, Andrew MA. Comparative study of heel-stick devices for infant blood collection. *Am J Dis Child* 1993;147:346–348.
71. Cologna M, Sperandio L. The effect of two different methods of heel lancing on pain reaction in preterm neonates. *Assistenza Infermieristica e Ricerca:AIR* 1999;18:185–192.
72. Barker DP, Latty BW, Rutter N. Heel blood sampling in preterm infants: which technique? *Arch Dis Child Fetal Neonatal Ed* 1994;71:F206–F208.
73. Kellam B, Sacks LM, Waller et al. Tenderfoot Preemie vs. a manual lancet: a clinical evaluation. *Neonatal Network* 2001;20:31–36.

Linda Franck
Professor of Children's Nursing Research
King's College School of Nursing and Midwifery
and Great Ormond Street Hospital for Children NHS Trust
London
UK

Ruth Gilbert
Senior Lecturer in Clinical Epidemiology/Honorary Consultant Paediatrician
Centre for Evidence-Based Child Health
Institute of Child Health
London
UK

Competing interests: None declared.

Sudden infant death syndrome

Search date November 2001

David Creery and Angelo Mikrogianakis

QUESTIONS

INTERVENTIONS

*Observational evidence only, RCTs unlikely to be conducted.

See glossary, p 401.

Key Messages

- **Advice to avoid bed sharing** One observational study found that a campaign to reduce a number of sudden infant death syndrome (SIDS) risk factors, which included advice to avoid bed sharing, was followed by a reduced incidence of SIDS. RCTs are unlikely to be conducted.
- **Advice to avoid over heating or over wrapping** One non-systematic review of observational studies and one additional observational study found that campaigns to reduce a number of SIDS risk factors, which included over wrapping, were followed by a reduced incidence of SIDS. RCTs are unlikely to be conducted.
- **Advice to avoid prone sleeping** One non-systematic review of observational studies and 11 additional observational studies found that campaigns involving advice to encourage non-prone sleeping positions were followed by a reduced incidence of SIDS. RCTs are unlikely to be conducted.
- **Advice to avoid tobacco smoke exposure** One non-systematic review of observational studies and three additional observational studies found that campaigns to reduce a number of SIDS risk factors, which included tobacco smoke exposure, were followed by a reduced incidence of SIDS. RCTs are unlikely to be conducted.
- **Advice to breast feed** One non-systematic review of observational studies and and two additional observational studies found that campaigns to reduce a number of SIDS risk factors, which included advice to breast feed, were followed by a reduced incidence of SIDS. RCTs are unlikely to be conducted.
- **Advice to avoid soft sleeping surfaces; advice to promote soother use** We found no evidence on the effects of these interventions in the prevention of SIDS.

DEFINITION Sudden infant death syndrome (SIDS) is the sudden death of an infant aged under 1 year that remains unexplained after review of the clinical history, examination of the scene of death, and postmortem.

INCIDENCE/ PREVALENCE The incidence of SIDS has varied over time and among nations (incidence per 1000 live births of SIDS in 1996: Netherlands 0.3; Japan 0.4; Canada 0.5; England and Wales 0.7; USA 0.8; and Australia 0.9).[1]

AETIOLOGY/ RISK FACTORS By definition, the cause of SIDS is not known. Observational studies have found an association between SIDS and a number of risk factors including prone sleeping position,[2,3] prenatal or postnatal exposure to tobacco smoke,[4] soft sleeping surfaces,[5,6] hyperthermia/overwrapping (see web extra tables A, B, and C at www.clinicalevidence.com),[7,8] bed sharing (particularly with mothers who smoke),[9,10] lack of breastfeeding,[11,12] and soother use (see glossary, p 401).[7,13]

PROGNOSIS Although by definition prognosis is not applicable for an affected infant, the incidence of SIDS is increased in the siblings of that infant.[14,15]

AIMS To reduce the incidence of SIDS, with minimal adverse effects from interventions.

OUTCOMES The incidence of SIDS; the adverse effects of interventions, measured directly or by quality of life questionnaires.

METHODS *Clinical Evidence* search and appraisal November 2001.

QUESTION **What are the effects of interventions to reduce the risk of sudden infant death syndrome?**

OPTION **ADVICE TO AVOID PRONE SLEEPING**

One non-systematic review and 11 observational studies found that campaigns involving advice to encourage non-prone sleeping positions were followed by a reduced incidence of sudden infant death syndrome.

Benefits: **Randomised studies:** We found no systematic review and no RCTs comparing advice to avoid prone sleeping positions (see glossary, p 401) versus no such advice (see comment below). **Observational studies following national advice campaigns:** We found one non-systematic review (3 observational studies, one of which has also been reported separately[16]),[12] and 11 additional observational studies following national advice campaigns (see comment below).[9,17–27] The review and additional observational studies describe eight campaigns that delivered advice to avoid prone positioning alone (see table 1, p 403),[17–19,21,22,24-26] and six campaigns that provided advice to avoid a combination of different risk factors including prone positioning (see table 2, p 404).[9,12,16,20,23,27] The review and additional observational studies all found that the incidence of sudden infant death syndrome

(SIDS) was reduced following the campaigns (see table 1, p 403 and table 2, p 404). One of the additional observational studies found that the incidence of prone positioning decreased significantly following the campaign (from 54% before campaign to 5% after campaign; $P < 0.001$).[27]

Harms: No frequencies of adverse effects of non-prone positioning were reported in 12 observational studies of advice to avoid prone sleeping.[9,12,16–27] One study found no increase in the risk of inhaling vomitus associated with non-prone positioning.[26] Two observational studies have documented a temporal relationship between advice to avoid prone sleeping and an increase in the incidence of occipital plagiocephaly without synostosis (see glossary, p 401), whereas the incidence of other forms of plagiocephaly with synostosis remained constant.[28,29]

Comment: The review of SIDS risk factor reduction campaigns in Norway, Denmark, and Sweden reported that the campaign in Norway provided advice to avoid prone sleeping plus advice to avoid tobacco smoke exposure.[12] However, the original paper describing the Norwegian campaign reported that this campaign only provided advice to avoid prone sleeping.[16] One of the additional observational studies reported that the incidence of SIDS was declining before the campaign started and, hence, the reduction attributable to advice provided by the campaign is not clear.[9,20] A second additional observational study did not report how advice was provided, exactly which SIDS risk factors were targeted, and did not describe details of the advice given to avoid exposure to cigarette smoke (i.e. prenatally, postnatally or both; maternal smoking alone or smoking by other household members as well).[23] A third additional observational study did not specify whether the advice to stop smoking was given to mothers or other family members and what advice was given regarding the avoidance of over heating.[27] Systematic reviews of observational studies have found an association between prone sleeping position and an increased risk of SIDS, leading to the initiation of non-prone sleep campaigns in several countries.[2,3] RCTs investigating the effects of advice to avoid prone positioning may be considered unethical given the existing observational evidence; they would also be difficult to conduct given the extremely large units of randomisation required and the high level of public awareness regarding the risks of prone positioning for sleep.

OPTION ADVICE TO AVOID TOBACCO SMOKE EXPOSURE

One non-systematic review and three observational studies found that campaigns to reduce a number of sudden infant death syndrome risk factors, which included tobacco smoke exposure, were followed by a reduced incidence of sudden infant death syndrome.

Benefits: **Randomised studies:** We found no systematic review and no RCTs comparing advice to avoid tobacco smoke exposure versus no such advice (see comment below). **Observational studies following national advice campaigns:** We found one non-systematic review (3 observational studies, one of which has also been reported separately[16]),[12] and three additional observational studies following national advice campaigns (see table 2, p 404).[9,20,23,27] The review and additional observational studies found that the campaigns were all followed by a reduced incidence of sudden infant death syndrome during the data collection periods (see table 2, p 404). However, the campaigns included advice in addition to the avoidance of tobacco smoke exposure, and in some countries the incidence of sudden infant death syndrome had started to fall before the campaign started (see comment under advice to avoid prone sleeping, p 398). The first additional observational study found that the population attributable risk (see glossary, p 401) for sudden infant death syndrome associated with maternal smoking alone was 44% (prevalence 19%; OR 5.17), and for maternal smoking plus bed sharing was 33% (prevalence 5%; OR 11.1). The third additional observational study found that the percentage of mothers not smoking during pregnancy increased significantly following the campaign (from 77% before campaign to 82% after campaign; $P < 0.01$).[27]

Harms: We found no evidence on harms associated with a reduction in infant tobacco smoke exposure.

Comment: The sudden infant death syndrome reduction attributable to a reduction in maternal smoking is unclear. RCTs investigating the effects of advice to reduce infant tobacco smoke exposure would be difficult to conduct given the extremely large units of randomisation required and the high level of public awareness regarding the risks of tobacco smoke exposure.

OPTION ADVICE TO AVOID SOFT SLEEPING SURFACES

We found no evidence on advice to avoid soft sleeping surfaces in the prevention of sudden infant death syndrome.

Benefits: We found no systematic review, RCTs, or observational studies (see comment below).

Harms: We found no evidence on harms associated with advice to avoid soft sleeping surfaces.

Comment: RCTs investigating the effects of advice to avoid soft sleeping surfaces would be difficult to conduct given the extremely large units of randomisation required.

OPTION ADVICE TO AVOID OVER HEATING OR OVER WRAPPING

One non-systematic review and one observational study found that campaigns to reduce a number of sudden infant death syndrome risk factors, which included over wrapping, were followed by a reduced incidence of sudden infant death syndrome.

Benefits: **Randomised studies:** We found no systematic review and no RCTs comparing advice to avoid over heating or over wrapping (see glossary, p 401) versus no such advice (see comment below). **Observational studies following national advice campaigns:** We found one non-systematic review (3 observational studies, one of which has also been reported separately[16]),[12] and one additional observational study following national advice campaigns (see table 2, p 404).[27] Two of the national advice campaigns reported in the review and the additional observational study provided advice to avoid over heating or over wrapping plus advice to avoid other sudden infant death syndrome risk factors (see comment under advice to avoid prone sleeping, p 398).[12,27] The third campaign reported by the review did not provide advice on over heating or over wrapping.[12,16] The review and additional observational study found that the campaigns were all followed by a reduction in the incidence of sudden infant death syndrome during the data collection periods (see table 2, p 404).

Harms: We found no evidence on harms associated with advice to avoid over heating or over wrapping.

Comment: RCTs investigating the effects of advice to avoid over heating or over wrapping would be difficult to conduct given the extremely large units of randomisation required.

OPTION ADVICE TO AVOID BED SHARING

One observational study found that a campaign to reduce a number of sudden infant death syndrome risk factors, which included advice to avoid bed sharing, was followed by a reduced incidence of sudden infant death syndrome.

Benefits: **Randomised studies:** We found no systematic review and no RCTs comparing advice to avoid bed sharing versus no such advice (see comment below). **Observational studies following national advice campaigns:** We found one observational study, which reported the results of a national campaign that provided advice to avoid bed sharing, to avoid prone sleeping (see glossary, p 401), to avoid exposing infants to tobacco smoke from any source either during pregnancy or for the first year of life, and to breast feed if possible (see comment below) (see table 2, p 404).[9,20] The observational study found that the incidence of sudden infant death syndrome reduced following the campaign, (see table 2, p 404) and that the population attributable risk (see glossary, p 401) for sudden infant death syndrome associated with maternal smoking plus bed sharing was 33% (prevalence 4.8%; OR 11.1).

Harms: We found no evidence on harms associated with advice to avoid bed sharing.

Comment: The observational study reported that advice to avoid bed sharing was introduced after the main campaign had started.[9,20] The study also reported that the incidence of sudden infant death syndrome was declining before the campaign started and, hence, the reduction attributable to advice provided by the campaign is not clear. RCTs investigating the effects of advice to avoid bed sharing would be difficult to conduct given the extremely large units of randomisation required.

OPTION ADVICE TO BREAST FEED

One non-systematic review and two observational studies found that campaigns to reduce a number of sudden infant death syndrome risk factors, which included advice to breast feed, were followed by a reduced incidence of sudden infant death syndrome.

Benefits: **Randomised evidence:** We found no systematic review and no RCTs comparing advice to encourage breast feeding versus no such advice in order to reduce the incidence of sudden infant death syndrome (see comment below). **Observational studies following national advice campaigns:** We found one non-systematic review (3 observational studies, one of which has also been reported separately[16]),[12] and two additional observational studies following national advice campaigns (see table 2, p 404).[9,20,27] The review and additional observational studies found that the campaigns were all followed by a reduced incidence of sudden infant death syndrome during the data collection periods (see table 2, p 404). However, the campaigns included advice other than advice to encourage breast feeding, and in some countries the incidence of sudden infant death syndrome had started to fall before the campaign started (see comment under advice to avoid tobacco smoke exposure, p 399). The second additional observational study found that the incidence of no breastfeeding decreased significantly following the campaign (from 21% before campaign to 7% after campaign; $P < 0.001$).[27]

Harms: We found no evidence on harms associated with advice to encourage breast feeding.

Comment: RCTs investigating the effects of promotion of breast feeding would be unethical given the evidence of benefits associated with breast feeding.

OPTION ADVICE TO PROMOTE SOOTHER USE

We found no evidence on advice to promote soother use in the prevention of sudden infant death syndrome.

Benefits: We found no systematic review, RCT, or observational studies (see comment below).

Harms: We found no evidence on harms associated with advice to promote soother use (see glossary, p 401).

Comment: RCTs investigating the effects of advice to promote soother use would be difficult to conduct given the extremely large units of randomisation required.

GLOSSARY

Occipital plagiocephaly with/without synostosis Flattening of the occipital bone with/without a malformation of the corresponding cranial suture line.

Over wrapping Wrapping/bundling of infants in excessive amounts of clothing or bedding as to result in sweating and/or significantly raised core temperatures.

Population attributable risk A measure of the disease rate in exposed people compared with that in unexposed people, multiplied by the prevalence of exposure to the risk factor in the population.

Prone sleeping Sleeping on one's front.

Soother (dummy, pacifier) An object placed in the infant's mouth for the sole purpose of providing comfort.

Sudden infant death syndrome

REFERENCES

1. Canadian Bureau of Reproductive and Child Health / Laboratory Centre for Disease Control / Canadian Perinatal Surveillance System (CPSS); Fact sheet: http://www.hc-sc.gc.ca/hpb/lcdc/brch/factshts/sids_e.html
2. Beal SM, Finch CF. An overview of retrospective case-control studies investigating the relationship between prone sleeping position and SIDS. *J Paediatr Child Health* 1991;27:334–339.
3. American Academy of Pediatrics AAP Task Force on Infant Positioning and SIDS. Positioning and SIDS. *Pediatrics* 1992;89(6 pt 1):1120–1126.
4. Anderson HR, Cook DG. Passive smoking and sudden infant death syndrome: review of the epidemiological evidence. *Thorax* 1997;52:1003–1009.
5. Mitchell EA, Thompson JM, Ford RP, Taylor BJ. Sheepskin bedding and the sudden infant death syndrome. New Z Cot Death Study Group. *J Pediatr* 1998;133:701–704.
6. Ponsonby AL, Dwyer T, Gibbons LE, Cochrane JA, Wang YG. Factors potentiating the risk of sudden infant death syndrome associated with the prone position. *N Engl J Med* 1993;329:377–382.
7. Fleming PJ, Blair PS, Bacon C, et al. Environment of infants during sleep and risk of the sudden infant death syndrome: results of the 1993–5 case-control study for confidential enquiry into stillbirths and deaths on infancy. Confidential Enquiry into Stillbirths and Deaths Regional Coordinators and Researchers. *BMJ* 1997;313:85–89.
8. Ponsonby AL, Dwyer T, Gibbons LE, Cochrane JA, Jones ME, McCall MJ. Thermal environment and sudden infant death syndrome: case-control study. *BMJ* 1992;304:277–282.
9. Mitchell EA, Tuohy PG, Brunt JM, et al. Risk factors for sudden infant death syndrome following the prevention campaign in New Zealand: a prospective study. *Pediatrics* 1997;100:835–840.
10. Scragg R, Mitchell EA, Taylor BJ, et al. Bed sharing, smoking, and alcohol in the sudden infant death syndrome. New Zealand Cot Death Study Group. *BMJ* 1993;307:1312–1318.
11. Mitchell EA, Taylor BJ, Ford RP, Stewart AW, Becroft DM, Thompson JM, et al. Four modifiable and other major risk factors for cot death: the New Zealand study. *J Paediatr Child Health* 1992;28(suppl 1):S3–S8.
12. Wennergren G, Alm B, Oyen N, et al. The decline in the incidence of SIDS in Scandinavia and its relation to risk-intervention campaigns. Nordic Epidemiological SIDS Study. *Acta Paediatrica* 1997;86:963–968.
13. L'Hoir MP, Engelberts AC, van Well GT, et al. Risk and preventive factors for cot death in The Netherlands, a low-incidence country. *Eur J Pediatr* 1998;157:681–688.
14. Oyen N, Skjaerven R, Irgens LM. Population-based recurrence risk of sudden infant death syndrome compared with other infant and fetal deaths. *Am J Epidemiol* 1996;144:300–305.
15. Guntheroth WG, Lohmann R, Spiers PS. Risk of sudden infant death syndrome in subsequent siblings. *J Pediatr* 1990;116:520–524.
16. Haaland K, Thoresen M. Crib death, sleeping position and temperature. *Tidsskr Nor Laegeforen* 1992;112:1466–1470. [Norwegian].
17. Schellscheidt J, Ott A, Jorch G. Epidemiological features of sudden infant death after a German intervention campaign in 1992. *Eur J Pediatr* 1997;156:655–660.
18. Skadberg BT, Morild I, Markestad T. Abandoning prone sleeping: Effect on the risk of sudden infant death syndrome. *J Pediatr* 1998;132:340–343.
19. Wigfield RE, Fleming PJ, Berry PJ, Rudd PT, Golding J. Can the fall in Avon's sudden infant death rate be explained by changes in sleeping position? *BMJ* 1992;304:282–283.
20. Mitchell EA, Aley P, Eastwood J. The national cot death prevention program in New Zealand. *Aust J Public Health* 16:158–161.
21. Markestad T, Skadberg B, Hordvik E, Morild I, Irgens LM. Sleeping position and sudden infant death syndrome (SIDS): effect of an intervention programme to avoid prone sleeping. *Acta Paediatr* 1995;84:375–378.
22. Vege A, Rognum TO, Opdal SH. SIDS – Changes in the epidemiological pattern in Eastern Norway 1984–1996. *Forensic Sci Int* 1998;93:155–166.
23. Adams EJ, Chavez GF, Steen D, Shah R, Iyasu S, Krous HF. Changes in the epidemiologic profile of sudden infant death syndrome as rates decline among California infants: 1990–1995. *Pediatrics* 1998;102:1445–1451.
24. Mitchell EA, Ford RP, Taylor BJ, et al. Further evidence supporting a causal relationship between prone sleeping position and SIDS. *J Paediatr Child Health* 1992;28(suppl 1):S9–12.
25. Dwyer T, Ponsonby AL, Blizzard L, Newman NM, Cochrane JA. The contribution of changes in the prevalence of prone sleeping position to the decline in sudden infant death syndrome in Tasmania. *JAMA* 1995;273:783–789.
26. Spiers PS, Guntheroth WG. Recommendations to avoid the prone sleeping position and recent statistics for sudden infant death syndrome in the United States. *Arch Pediatr Adolesc Med* 1994;148:141–146.
27. Kiechl-Kohlendorfer U, Peglow UP, Kiechl S, Oberaigner W, Sperl W. Epidemiology of sudden infant death syndrome (SIDS) in the Tyrol before and after an intervention campaign. *Wien Klin Wochenschr* 2001;113:27–32.
28. Kane AA, Mitchell LE, Craven KP, et al. Observations on a recent increase in plagiocephaly without synostosis. *Pediatrics* 1996; 97:877–885.
29. Gonzalez de Dios J, Moya M, Jimenez L, et al. Increase in the incidence of occipital plagiocephaly. *Rev Neurol* 1998;27:782–784.

David Creery

Angelo Mikrogianakis

Children's Hospital of Eastern Ontario
Ottawa
Canada

Competing interests: None declared.

TABLE 1 **Observational studies following national campaigns providing advice to avoid prone sleeping positions (see text, p 397).**

Country/reference	Dissemination	SIDS incidence/1000 live births (95% CI)		Number of infants	Risk of prone sleeping after campaign (95% CI)
		From	To		
Germany (West)	Not specified	1.56	0.92	59 cases, 156 controls	OR 11.7 (5.3 to 26.2)
North Rhine Westphalia[17]		2.17	1.33		
Norway[18]	Health professional education Media campaign	3.5 (2.64 to 4.36)	0.3 (0.05 to 0.54)	6 cases, 493 controls	OR 42.0 (5 to 390)
UK, Avon[19]	Maternal education Health professional education	3.5	1.7	32 cases, 70 controls 152 population based controls	NA
Norway/Hordaland[21]	Health professional education Media campaign	3.5	1.6	30 cases, 123 controls	OR 11.3 (3.6 to 36.5)
Norway[22]	Health professional education Media campaign	2	0.6	200 cases	NA
New Zealand[24]	Maternal education Health professional education Media campaign	4	3.1	485 cases, 1800 controls	NA
Australia[25]	Maternal education Health professional education	3.8 (3.5 to 4.2)	1.5 (0.9 to 2.2)	449 cases	NA
USA[26]	Media campaign	2.36	2.02	233 cases	NA

SIDS, sudden infant death syndrome; NA, not available.

TABLE 2 **Observational studies following national campaigns providing advice to avoid a number of sudden infant death syndrome risk factors including prone sleeping positions (see text, p 397–401).**

Country/year of start	Data collection	Advice to: *avoid* or [encourage]	Dissemination	SIDS incidence/1000 live births (95% CI)		Number of infants	Risk (95% CI)
				From	To		
Norway 1989[12,16]	1992–1995	*prone sleeping*	Newspapers National media broadcasts Midwives Other healthcare professionals Presentation at a SIDS prevention conference	2.3	0.6	244 cases 869 controls	Adjusted OR prone sleeping 5.4 (2.8 to 10.5)
Denmark 1991[12]	1992–1995	*prone sleeping* *tobacco smoke* *over wrapping*	Not described	1.6	0.2	244 cases 869 controls	Adjusted OR prone sleeping 5.4 (2.8 to 10.5)
Sweden 1992[12]	1992–1995	*prone sleeping* *tobacco smoke* *over wrapping* [breastfeeding]	Not described	1.0	0.4		

TABLE 2 continued

Country/year of start	Data collection	Advice to: *avoid* or [encourage]	Dissemination	SIDS incidence/1000 live births (95% CI) From	To	Number of infants	Risk (95% CI)
New Zealand 1990[9,20]	1991–1993	*prone sleeping* *tobacco smoke*(any source; during pregnancy/first year of life) *bed sharing* [breastfeeding]	Parents antenatal classes Postnatal wards Healthcare professionals Conferences Journals Public newspapers TV programmes	4.1	2.1	127 cases 922 controls	Not reported
California, 1990–1995[23]		*prone sleeping* *cigarette smoking*	Public	2.69 (black infants) 1.04 (other infants)	2.15 (black infants) 0.61 (other infants)	3508 cases	Not reported
Austria 1994–1995[27]		*prone sleeping* *smoking* *over heating* [breastfeeding]	Parents antenatal classes, maternity wards, routine health checks Public newspapers Radio/TV	1984–1994: 1.83	1995: 0.4 1996–1998 unchanged	160 cases	Not reported

SIDS, sudden infant death syndrome.

Urinary tract infection

Search date January 2002

James Larcombe

QUESTIONS

INTERVENTIONS

See glossary, p 418

Key Messages

Treatment of acute infection

- **Antibiotics versus placebo** Placebo controlled trials of antibiotics for symptomatic acute urinary tract infection in children are considered unethical.
- **Co-trimoxazole (3 day course)** One systematic review found no significant difference in cure rate between a 3 day and a conventional (7–10 day) course of co-trimoxazole.

- **Immediate empirical versus delayed antibiotic treatment** We found no RCTs on the effects of giving early empirical treatment versus awaiting the results of microscopy or culture in acute urinary tract infection in children. One RCT found no significant difference in risk of renal scarring with antibiotic (cephalosporins) treatment within 24 hours versus 24 hours after the onset of fever in children under 2 years with urinary tract infections.
- **Longer versus short courses of initial intravenous antibiotics** Two RCTs found no significant difference with long (7–10 days) versus short (3 days) course of initial intravenous antibiotic (ceftriaxone) treatment on development of renal scarring in children with acute pyelonephritis.
- **Longer versus short courses of oral antibiotics** One systematic review identified two RCTs that found significantly higher cure rate (eradication of causative organism on follow up culture) with longer (10 days) versus shorter (single dose/1 day) courses of oral antibiotics (amoxicillin, cefadroxil) in children with urinary tract infections. Another systematic review in children and adolescents aged < 18 years with uncomplicated cystitis found that conventional (≥ 5 days) versus short courses (≤ 4 days) significantly increased cure rate, but the difference disappeared when single dose studies were excluded. The difference in cure rate between short and conventional courses remained significant for amoxicillin (NNT 8, 95% CI 5 to 25) but not co-trimoxazole.
- **Oral versus initial intravenous antibiotics** One RCT found no significant difference with oral versus initial intravenous antibiotics (cephalosporins) in duration of fever, reinfection, renal scarring, or extent of scarring in children aged 2 years or younger with first confirmed urinary tract infection. The RCT found weak evidence from a post hoc subgroup analysis in children with grades III–IV reflux that renal scarring at 6 months may be more common with oral versus initial intravenous treatment.
- **Prolonged delay in treatment (> 7 days)** One systematic review found a significant difference in cure rate between a single dose and a conventional (10 day) course of amoxicillin. Five retrospective studies found that medium to long term delays (4 days to 7 years) in treatment may be associated with an increased risk of renal scarring.
- **Single dose amoxicillin** One systematic review found a significant difference in cure rate between a conventional (10 day) course versus a single dose of amoxicillin.

Diagnostic imaging in children with first urinary tract infection

- **Routine diagnostic imaging in all children with first urinary tract infection** We found no RCTs. One systematic review of descriptive studies found no evidence of benefit from routine diagnostic imaging of all children with a first urinary tract infection. We found indirect evidence suggesting that children at increased risk of morbidity may benefit from investigation.

Prevention of recurrence

- **Immunotherapy** One systematic review in premature and in low birth weight neonates has found that intravenous immunoglobulins versus placebo significantly reduce the occurrence of serious infections, including urinary tract infections, (NNT 24, 95% CI 15 to 83). One RCT found that pidotimod (an immunotherapeutic agent) versus placebo significantly reduced urinary tract infection recurrence in children.

- **Prophylactic antibiotics** One systematic review and an additional RCT found limited evidence that prophylactic antibiotics (co-trimoxazole, nitrofurantoin) versus placebo or no treatment reduced urinary tract infection recurrence in children. One RCT found that nitrofurantoin versus trimethoprim significantly reduced recurrence of urinary tract infection over 6 months (NNT 5, 95% CI 3 to 33) but also found that significantly more children discontinued treatment with nitrofurantoin versus trimethoprim because of adverse effects (NNH 5, 95% CI 3 to 13). We found no RCTs evaluating the optimum duration of prophylactic antibiotics.
- **Surgical correction of minor functional anomalies** We found no RCTs. One observational study suggested that children with minor anomalies do not develop renal scarring and therefore may not benefit from surgery.
- **Surgical correction of moderate to severe bilateral vesicoureteric reflux (grades III–IV) with bilateral nephropathy** One small RCT found a steady, but not significant, decline in glomerular filtration rate over 10 years with medical treatment versus surgery in children with moderate to severe bilateral vesicoureteric reflux.
- **Surgical correction of moderate to severe vesicoureteric reflux with adequate glomerular filtration rate (similar benefits to medical management)** One systematic review and one subsequent RCT found that, although surgery abolished reflux, there was no significant difference between surgical versus medical management (prophylactic antibiotic treatment) in preventing recurrence or complications from urinary tract infection after 6 months to 5 years in children with moderate to severe vesicoureteric reflux.

DEFINITION Urinary tract infection (UTI) is defined by the presence of a pure growth of more than 10^5 colony forming units of bacteria per mL. Lower counts of bacteria may be clinically important, especially in boys and in specimens obtained by urinary catheter. Any growth of typical urinary pathogens is considered clinically important if obtained by suprapubic aspiration. In practice, three age ranges are usually considered on the basis of differential risk and different approaches to management: children under 1 year; young children (1–4, 5, or 7 years, depending on the information source); and older children (up to 12–16 years). Recurrent UTI is defined as a further infection by a new organism. Relapsing UTI is defined as a further infection with the same organism.

INCIDENCE/ PREVALENCE Boys are more susceptible before the age of 3 months; thereafter the incidence is substantially higher in girls. Estimates of the true incidence of UTI depend on rates of diagnosis and investigation. At least 8% of girls and 2% of boys will have a UTI in childhood.[1]

AETIOLOGY/ RISK FACTORS The normal urinary tract is sterile. Contamination by bowel flora may result in urinary infection if a virulent organism is involved or if the child is immunosuppressed. In neonates, infection may originate from other sources. *Escherichia coli* accounts for about three quarters of all pathogens. *Proteus* is more common in boys (about 30% of infections). Obstructive anomalies are found in 0–4% and vesicoureteric reflux in 8–40% of children being investigated for their first UTI.[2] Although vesicoureteric reflux is a major risk factor for adverse outcome, other as yet unidentified triggers may also need to be present.

PROGNOSIS After first infection, about half of girls have a further infection in the first year and three quarters within 2 years.[3] We found no figures for boys, but a review suggests that recurrences are common under 1 year of age but rare subsequently.[4] Renal scarring occurs in 5–15% of children within 1–2 years of their first UTI, although 32–70% of these scars are noted at the time of initial assessment.[2] The incidence of renal scarring rises with each episode of infection in childhood.[5] An RCT comparing oral versus intravenous antibiotics found retrospectively that new renal scarring after a first UTI was more common in children with vesicoureteric reflux than in children without reflux (logistic regression model: AR of scarring 16/107 [15%] with reflux *v* 10/165 [6%] without reflux; RR 2.47, 95% CI 1.17 to 5.24).[6] A study (287 children with severe vesicoureteric reflux treated either medically or surgically for any UTI) evaluated the risk of renal scarring with serial DMSA (see glossary, p 418) scintigraphy over 5 years. It found that younger children (< 2 years) were at greater risk of renal scarring than older children regardless of treatment allocation for the infection (AR for deterioration in DMSA scan over 5 years 21/86 [24%] for younger children *v* 27/201 [13%] for older children; RR 1.82, 95% CI 1.09 to 3.03).[7] Renal scarring is associated with future complications: poor renal growth; recurrent adult pyelonephritis (see glossary, p 418); impaired glomerular function; early hypertension; and end stage renal failure.[8–11] A combination of recurrent urinary infection, severe vesicoureteric reflux, and the presence of renal scarring at first presentation is associated with the worst prognosis.

AIMS To relieve acute symptoms; to eliminate infection; and to prevent recurrence, renal damage, and long term complications.

OUTCOMES **Short term:** clinical symptoms and signs (dysuria, frequency, and fever); urine culture; incidence of new renal scars. **Long term:** incidence of recurrent infection; prevalence of renal scarring; renal size and growth; renal function; prevalence of hypertension and renal failure.

METHODS *Clinical Evidence* search and appraisal January 2002.

QUESTION What are the effects of treatment of acute urinary tract infection in children?

OPTION ANTIBIOTICS VERSUS PLACEBO

Placebo controlled trials of antibiotics for symptomatic acute urinary tract infections in children are considered unethical.

Benefits: We found no RCTs. Placebo controlled trials of antibiotics for symptomatic acute urinary tract infection in children are considered unethical.

Harms: We found no RCTs.

Comment: Placebo controlled trials would be considered unethical because there is a strong consensus that antibiotics are likely to be beneficial. The improved response seen with longer versus shorter courses of antibiotics is indirect evidence that antibiotics are likely to be more effective than no treatment.

OPTION IMMEDIATE EMPIRICAL VERSUS DELAYED ANTIBIOTIC TREATMENT

We found no RCTs on the effects of giving early empirical treatment versus awaiting the results of microscopy or culture in acute urinary tract infection in children. One RCT found no significant difference in risk of renal scarring with antibiotic (cephalosporins) treatment within 24 hours versus 24 hours after the onset of fever in children under 2 years with urinary tract infections. Five retrospective studies found that medium to long term delays (4 days in acute infection, 7 years in chronic infection) in treatment may be associated with an increased risk of renal scarring.

Benefits: We found no RCTs comparing immediate empirical treatment versus treatment delayed while awaiting the results of microscopy or culture. We found one RCT that compared oral cefixime for 14 days (double dose on day 1) versus intravenous cefotaxime for 3 days plus oral cefixime for 11 days for urinary tract infection in children under 2 years. It found no evidence that children treated 24 hours after the onset of fever were at greater risk of renal scarring than children presenting within 24 hours (9/99 [9%] of children presenting before 24 h developed scarring *v* 19/159 [12%] of children presenting later; RR 1.3, 95% CI 0.6 to 2.7; $P = 0.29$). However, this incidental analysis was done retrospectively.[6]

Harms: The RCT did not report on any adverse effects.[6]

Comment: Five retrospective observational studies found increased rates of scarring in children in whom diagnosis was delayed between 4 days (in acute urinary tract infection) to 7 years (when a child presented with chronic non-specific symptoms).[2]

OPTION LONGER VERSUS SHORT COURSES OF ORAL ANTIBIOTICS

One systematic review identified two RCTs that found significantly higher cure rate (eradication of causative organism on follow up culture) with longer (10 days) versus shorter (single dose/1 day) courses of oral antibiotics (amoxicillin, cefadroxil) in children with urinary tract infections. Another systematic review in children and adolescents aged < 18 years with uncomplicated cystitis found that conventional (≥ 5 days) versus short courses (≤ 4 days) significantly increased cure rate, but the significant difference disappeared when single dose studies were excluded. The difference in cure rate between short and conventional courses remained significant for amoxicillin but not co-trimoxazole.

Benefits: We found two systematic reviews.[12,13] The first systematic review (search date not stated, 14 RCTs) compared short course (single dose to 4 days) versus longer courses (7–10 days) of a range of antibiotics.[12] It found two RCTs that were adequately powered to find an effect. One RCT (49 children) compared amoxicillin (amoxycillin) single dose versus 10 day regimen, and the other RCT compared cefadroxil 1 day versus 10 day regimen.[14,15] Both RCTs found that longer courses cured (eradication of causative organism on 4 days' follow up culture) significantly more children (results from the higher quality RCT:[14] AR of failure to cure 14/38 [37%] with short course *v* 2/27 [7%] with long course; ARI short *v* long course 29%; RR 4.6; 95% CI not provided; $P < 0.01$). The remaining 12 RCTs found no significant difference between long versus short courses but were too small to rule out a clinically important difference (see comment below). The second systematic review (search date 1999, 22 RCTs, 1279 children and adolescents aged < 18 years with uncomplicated cystitis) compared the effects of short courses (≤ 4 days) versus conventional courses (≥ 5 days) of antibiotics on cure rates. Treatment failure was defined as positive at culture > 3 days but < 30 days after enrolment.[13] There was significant heterogeneity between studies (see comment below). The meta-analysis included the two RCTs[14,15] identified by the first systematic review.[12] Overall, the review found that conventional course versus shorter course of antibiotics significantly increased cure rate but the test for heterogeneity was significant (22 RCTs: difference in cure rate, 6.4%, 95% CI 1.9% to 10.9%; NNT with conventional course to prevent treatment failure 16, 95% CI 9 to 53). However, when single dose studies were excluded, there was no significant difference (13 RCTs; difference in cure rate +4.3%, 95% CI −0.95% to +9.48%).[13] The difference in cure rate remained significant when only the RCTs comparing the same antibiotic in the short and conventional courses were included (17 RCTs: 7.9%, 95% CI 2.1% to 13.8%; NNT with conventional course to prevent treatment failure 13, 95% CI 6 to 35). The difference in cure rate between a single dose and a 10 day course of amoxicillin remained significant (4 RCTs: 13%, 95% CI 4% to 24%; NNT with conventional course to prevent treatment failure 8, 95% CI 5 to 25) but not between a 3 day and a conventional (7–10 day) course of co-trimoxazole (+6.2%, 95% CI −3.7% to +16.2%).

Harms: The two RCTs identified by the first systematic review[12] did not report comparative harms for long versus short courses of antibiotics nor for immediate versus delayed treatment.[14,15] The second systematic review reported that dose related adverse effects, such as neutropenia with β-lactam antibiotics, seemed to increase in frequency with the length of administration.[13]

Comment: The first systematic review[12] rigorously evaluated the methods of the included studies. It found that few studies accounted for confounding factors such as age, sex, and previous urinary tract infections. Those that considered these did so by selecting one subgroup only and not by stratifying children according to these factors. This limits the generalisability of the results. The 12 trials that found no evidence of a difference between long and short courses were too small to exclude a clinically important effect. The second systematic review[13] based its findings on a meta-analysis of 22 studies conforming to its entry criteria. The studies differed in the lengths of treatment and antibiotics used, the definitions of cure, relapse, reinfection, and the diagnostic criteria for pyelonephritis (see glossary, p 418) or complicated urinary tract infection.

Some studies also compared dissimilar or variable antibiotics in the control (standard treatment length) group, though excluding these did not seem to affect the overall results. Comparisons were made both for the whole group and for subgroups. To reduce the problem of differences in study design biasing the results of the meta-analysis, treatment groups were compared with fixed or random effects models (a decision based on statistical analysis of the heterogeneity of the groups).

OPTION ORAL VERSUS INITIAL INTRAVENOUS ANTIBIOTICS

One RCT found no significant difference with oral versus initial intravenous antibiotics (cephalosporins) in duration of fever, reinfection rate, renal scarring, or extent of scarring in children aged 2 years or younger with first confirmed urinary tract infection. The RCT found weak evidence from a post hoc subgroup analysis in children with grades III-IV reflux that renal scarring at 6 months may be more common with oral versus initial intravenous treatment.

Benefits: We found one RCT (309 children, aged ≤ 2 years, fever > 38.2 °C, with a first urinary tract infection confirmed from catheter specimen) sufficiently powered to produce meaningful results. The RCT compared oral cefixime for 14 days (double dose on day 1) versus initial intravenous cefotaxime for 3 days plus 11 days of oral cefixime.[6] It found no significant difference between treatments in mean duration of fever (24.7 h with oral treatment *v* 23.9 h with initial iv; P = 0.76), reinfection rate (132/153 [86%] with oral treatment *v* 134/153 [88%] with initial iv treatment; P = 0.28), incidence of renal scarring (intention to treat analysis: 15/153 [10%] with oral treatment [21 children not scanned and counted as having no scarring] *v* 11/153 [7%] with initial iv treatment [13 children not scanned]; P = 0.21), and mean extent of scarring (8% of renal parenchyma with oral treatment *v* 9% with initial iv treatment). The RCT found weak evidence from a post hoc subgroup analysis in children with grades III-IV reflux (see glossary, p 418) that renal scarring at 6 months may be more common with oral versus initial intravenous treatment (new renal scarring within 6 months: 8/24 [33%] after oral antibiotics *v* 1/22 [5%] after iv antibiotics; ARI 29%, 95% CI 8% to 49%; NNH 3, 95% CI 2 to 13).[6]

Harms: The RCT did not report on adverse effects.[6]

Comment: The trial excluded 3/309 children because investigators considered that the severity of symptoms in these children warranted intravenous treatment.[6]

OPTION LONGER VERSUS SHORT COURSES OF INITIAL INTRAVENOUS ANTIBIOTICS

Two RCTs found no significant difference with longer (7–10 days) versus short (3 days) course of initial intravenous antibiotics (ceftriaxone) in the development of renal scarring in children with acute pyelonephritis.

Benefits: We found two RCTs comparing the effect of a long versus short course of initial intravenous antibiotics (ceftriaxone) on development of renal scarring in children with acute pyelonephritis (see glossary, p 418). One RCT (220 children aged 3 months to 16 years with positive urine culture and acute renal lesions on initial DMSA scintigraphy) compared a 10 day versus a 3 day course of initial intravenous ceftriaxone (50 mg/kg/day) followed by oral cefixime (4 mg/kg twice daily) to complete a 15 day course.[16] Scintigraphy was repeated after 3 months. Renal scars were defined as persistent or partially resolved changes in the same location as the lesions on the original DMSA. The RCT found no significant difference with a 10 day versus a 3 day course of initial antibiotic treatment in development of renal scarring at 3 months (AR 36/110 [33%] children with 10 day course *v* 40/110 [36%] children with 3 day course; RR 1.10; 95% CI 0.77 to 1.60). The development of renal scarring was unaffected by age, sex, duration of fever before treatment, degree of inflammation, presence of vesicoureteric reflux, or recruitment centre. The second RCT (92 children aged 6 weeks to 13 years, with a clinical diagnosis of acute pyelonephritis, positive urine culture, and abnormal DMSA scan) compared a 7 day versus a 3 day course of initial intravenous ceftizoxime followed by oral cefixime.[17] The DMSA scan was repeated after 6 months for detection of total or partial persistence of renal abnormalities. The RCT found no significant difference with a 3 day versus a 7 day course of initial intravenous antibiotic treatment on renal abnormalities at 6 months (11/44 [25%] children with 3 day course *v* 8/43 [19%] children with 7 day course; RR 1.34, 95% CI 0.60 to 3.01).

Harms: The two RCTs did not assess harms.[16,17]

Comment: Unlike the studies of long versus short courses of oral treatment and the study of oral versus intravenous antibiotics, there were few exclusions for severe presentation. In the larger study, 206 children failed to meet the strict entry criteria,[16] but there were then no further exclusions. Eleven of 103 children were excluded in the smaller study.[17]

QUESTION Which children with a first urinary tract infection benefit from diagnostic imaging?

We found no RCTs. One systematic review of descriptive studies found no evidence of benefit from routine diagnostic imaging of all children with a first urinary tract infection. We found indirect evidence suggesting that children at increased risk of morbidity may benefit from investigation.

Benefits: We found no RCTs on diagnostic imaging of children with a first urinary tract infection.

Harms: We found no RCTs. Potential harms include those relating to radiation, invasive procedures, and allergic reactions to contrast media.

Comment: We found one systematic review (search date 1994, 63 descriptive studies) that found no direct evidence that routine diagnostic imaging in children with urinary tract infection was effective.[2] The quality of studies was generally poor, and none included clinically important long term outcome measures. The studies reported no evidence of harms. Subgroups of children at high risk of morbidity, including those with vesicoureteric reflux, may benefit from early investigation.[2] However, it may be difficult to identify such children clinically.[18] One prospective study found that presentation with pyelonephritic symptoms in children of all ages is associated with high rates of renal abnormalities (abnormal initial scans in 34/65 [52%] children).[19] Another prospective study found that the highest rates of renal scarring after pyelonephritis occurred between 1 and 5 years of age.[20] A further prospective study by the same team found that children aged over 1 year had more abnormalities on DMSA scans at 3 months after an episode of pyelonephritis (54/129 [42%] of older children *v* 22/91 [24%] younger children; RR 1.73; 95% CI: 1.14 to 2.63).[16] They noted conflicting results in previous literature on this subject.[16] The study also found that girls were more likely than boys to develop scarring on DMSA scan at 3 months after an episode of pyelonephritis (67/171 [39%] girls *v* 9/49 [18%] boys; RR 2.13; 95% CI 1.15 to 3.96).[20]

QUESTION **What are the effects of interventions to prevent recurrence?**

OPTION **PROPHYLACTIC ANTIBIOTICS**

One systematic review and an additional RCT found limited evidence that prophylactic antibiotics (co-trimoxazole, nitrofurantoin) versus placebo or no treatment reduced urinary tract infection recurrence in children. One RCT found that nitrofurantoin versus trimethoprim significantly reduced recurrence of urinary tract infection over 6 months but also found that significantly more children discontinued treatment with nitrofurantoin versus trimethoprim because of adverse effects. We found no RCTs evaluating the optimum duration of prophylactic antibiotics.

Benefits: **Versus no prophylaxis:** We found one systematic review (search date 2001)[21] and one additional RCT.[22] The systematic review (3 RCTs, 151 children aged < 18 years at risk of recurrent urinary tract infection [UTI] but without a renal tract abnormality or major neurological, urological, or muscular disease) compared the effects of antibiotics (nitrofurantoin, co-trimoxazole) versus placebo or no treatment on risk of recurrent UTI.[21] There was variation between the RCTs in the duration of antibiotic prophylaxis (10 wk to 12 months) and method of concealment (see comment below). The review found that antibiotics versus placebo or no treatment significantly reduced the risk of recurrent UTI (RR 0.36, 95% CI 0.16 to 0.77).[21] The additional RCT (double blind, crossover trial, 18 girls [1 with vesicoureteric reflux], aged 3–13 years) found that antibiotics (nitrofurantoin) versus no antibiotics significantly reduced recurrent UTI (2 episodes in 1 year with antibiotics *v* 35 episodes without antibiotics; $P < 0.01$); see comment below.[19] **Comparison of antibiotics:** We found one systematic review (search date 2001, 1 RCT) comparing nitrofurantoin versus trimethoprim.[21] It found that nitrofurantoin versus trimethoprim significantly reduced recurrence of UTI over 6 months (RR 0.48, 95% CI 0.25 to 0.92; NNT 5, 95% CI 3 to 33). **Duration of prophylaxis:** We found no RCTs evaluating the optimum length of prophylaxis even in children with vesicoureteric reflux (although 2 studies of prolonged acute treatment were identified).[23]

Harms: **Versus no prophylaxis:** No adverse effects were reported in the RCTs included in the systematic review.[21] The additional RCT found no adverse effects with nitrofurantoin.[22] **Comparison of antibiotics:** One RCT found that significantly more children discontinued treatment with nitrofurantoin versus trimethoprim because of adverse effects including nausea, vomiting, or stomach ache (RR 3.17, 95% CI 1.36 to 7.37; NNH 5, 95% CI 3 to 13).[21] Potential harms include those of using long term antibiotics. One study found that although gastrointestinal flora were affected by treatment, *E coli* (cultured from rectal swabs from 70% of children) remained sensitive to the prophylactic antibiotic co-trimoxazole).[24] However, another study found that children who had recently received co-trimoxazole for 4 or more weeks were more likely to have resistant *E coli* isolates than those who had received no antibiotics (OR 23.4, 95% CI 12.0 to 47.6).[25]

Comment: The systematic review was thorough but the RCTs it identified had weak methods.[21] None of the RCTs included in the systematic review used intention to treat analyses. Only one had adequate concealment and one specified the outcome measures. The additional RCT was a crossover study that did not include a washout period and had a withdrawal rate of 20%. It did not report the results for the period before the crossover separately.[22] It may not be possible clinically to identify children who are at high risk of recurrent UTIs and long term damage.[26] Routine prophylaxis until the results of investigations are known may, therefore, be warranted, but we found no good evidence about the benefits or harms of antibiotic prophylaxis.

OPTION IMMUNOTHERAPY

One systematic review in premature and in low birth weight neonates has found that intravenous immunoglobulins versus placebo significantly reduce the occurrence of serious infections, including urinary tract infections. One RCT found that pidotimod (an immunotherapeutic agent) versus placebo significantly reduces urinary tract infection recurrence in children.

Benefits: **Intravenous immunoglobulin:** We found one systematic review (search date 1997, 15 RCTs), which compared intravenous immunoglobulin (see glossary, p 418) prophylaxis with placebo or no treatment.[27] It found that intravenous immunoglobulin prophylaxis significantly reduced serious infections, including urinary tract infections (UTIs), in preterm and in low birth weight neonates (RR 0.80, 95% CI 0.68 to 0.94; NNT 24, 95% CI 15 to 83).[27] The dose varied from 120 mg/kg to 1 g/kg. The number of treatments varied from one to seven. The specific effect on UTIs was not reported. **Other immunotherapeutic agents:** We found one RCT (double blind, 60 children aged 2–8 years with recurrent UTI) comparing pidotimod versus placebo added to standard antibiotic treatment.[28] The study included a further 60 day phase, using half dose pidotimod versus half dose placebo. The RCT found that pidotimod significantly reduced clinical recovery time in the acute situation (5 episodes of relapsing infection in 4/30 children with pidotimod *v* 19 episodes in

13/30 children with placebo; OR 0.17, 95% CI 0.04 to 0.61).[28] An open pilot study (40 children) compared nitrofurantoin with an antigenic extract of *E coli*.[29] No significant difference was found between the two treatments during active treatment or during the subsequent 6 months.

Harms: Parenteral treatment can cause pain, and there is an unmeasured risk from the administration of blood products.[27] **Intravenous immunoglobulin:** The systematic review found that prophylactic use of intravenous immunoglobulin was not associated with any short term serious adverse effects.[27] **Other immunotherapeutic agents:** In the RCT of pidotimod, the only adverse effects recorded were thought to be attributable to concomitant antibiotic treatment.[28] The open pilot study found no significant difference in withdrawal rates between the antigenic extract of *E coli* (1/22 [5%]) and nitrofurantoin (1/18 [6%]).[29]

Comment: **Intravenous immunoglobulin:** We found no evidence for or against the suggestion that preparations with specific antibodies against common pathogens are more beneficial.[30] The greatest benefits were noted in units with higher nosocomial infection rates (see glossary, p 418). It remains unclear whether intravenous immunoglobulin is only justified where infection control policies have failed to reduce the infection rate.[27] Preterm and low birth weight neonates might have greater immune deficiency than other neonates and might be expected to gain more from treatment with immunoglobulin. **Other immunotherapeutic agents:** We found one non-randomised age matched study in 10 otherwise healthy girls (aged 5–11 years) with recurrent UTI who were given intramuscular injections of inactivated uropathogenic bacteria (Solco-Urovac preparation). It found that the girls who had received the inactivated uropathogenic bacteria had significantly reduced frequency of subsequent UTI compared with 10 other age matched girls with UTI who had not received the inactivated bacteria preparation.[31] This study is limited by its non-randomised design and small sample size. We found another study (40 children aged 3–12 years with recurrent UTI caused by *E coli* and no anatomical or functional impairments of the urinary tract) comparing prophylactic antibiotics (amoxicillin with clavulanic acid or cephalosporins) versus prophylactic antibiotics plus an immunomodulator with *E coli* antigens (Uro-Vaxom) for 3 months followed up for 3 months after the end of treatment.[32] The method of randomisation was not stated. The study found that urinary sIgA levels, initially low in both groups were significantly raised 3 months after the end of treatment in the active treatment group but not in the control group. It also found that antibiotics plus immunomodulator versus antibiotics alone reduced recurrences over 6 months (recurrences, 2/25 [8%] with antibiotics plus immunomodulator *v* 8/13 [61%] with antibiotics alone).[32]

OPTION SURGICAL CORRECTION FOR ANOMALIES OBSTRUCTING MICTURITION

We found no RCTs. One observational study suggested that children with minor anomalies do not develop renal scarring and therefore may not benefit from surgery.

Benefits: We found no systematic review or RCTs.

Harms: Potential harms include the usual risks of surgery.

Comment: One small prospective study (271 children) suggested that children with minor anomalies do not develop renal scarring and therefore may not benefit from surgery.[33] Renal scars were present in more children with moderate degrees of vesicoureteric reflux than in children with minor anomalies (8/20 [40%] *v* 0/6 [0%]). In the presence of major anomalies, the prevention of UTIs is not the prime motive of surgical intervention.

OPTION SURGICAL CORRECTION FOR VESICOURETERIC REFLUX

One systematic review and one subsequent RCT found that, although surgery abolished reflux, there was no significant difference between surgical versus medical management (prophylactic antibiotic treatment) in preventing recurrence or complications from urinary tract infections after 6 months to 5 years in children with moderate to severe vesicoureteric reflux. One small RCT found a steady but not statistically significant decline in glomerular filtration rate over 10 years with medical treatment versus surgery in children with moderate to severe bilateral vesicoureteric reflux.

Benefits: **Versus medical management:** We found one systematic review[34] and two subsequent RCTs.[35,36] The systematic review (search date 1988, 4 RCTs, 830 children with moderate to severe [grades III-V —see glossary, p 418] vesicoureteric reflux) compared surgical correction versus medical management (continuous prophylactic antibiotics).[34] It found that surgery abolished reflux, but found no significant differences in rates of subsequent urinary tract infection, renal function, incidence of new renal scars, hypertension, or end stage renal failure among groups over a period of 6 months to 5 years. The first subsequent RCT (132 children aged ≤ 10 years with grades III-V vesicoureteric reflux, glomerular filtration rate ≥ 70 mL/min per $1.73m^2$) compared surgery versus medical management (prophylactic antibiotics) over 5 years. The RCT found no significant difference in development of new renal scarring with surgery versus medical management but found that surgery versus medical management reduced the incidence of pyelonephritis (see glossary, p 418) (pyelonephritis in 5/64 [8%] with surgery *v* 15/68 [22%] treated medically; ARR 14%, 95% CI 2% to 19%; RRR 65%, 95% CI 10% to 87%).[36] The second subsequent RCT (25 boys and 27 girls aged 1–12 years with bilateral vesicoureteric reflux [grades III-V] and bilateral nephropathy, glomerular filtration rate ≥ 20 mL/min per $1.73\ m^2$) compared corrective surgery versus medical management (prophylactic antibiotics: co-trimoxazole, trimethoprim, or nitrofurantoin) over 4 years.[35] It found no significant difference in development of new scars between medical treatment versus corrective surgery after 4 years (AR 7/54 [13%] kidneys with medical treatment *v* 8/50 [16%] kidneys with corrective surgery; RR 0.81, 95% CI 0.32 to 2.07).[35] **Longer term outcome:** We found one RCT (25 boys and 27 girls aged 1–12 years with bilateral vesicoureteric reflux [grades III-V] and bilateral nephropathy) with

10 year' follow up.[35] It found a steady decline in glomerular filtration rate over 10 years in children on medical treatment versus surgery (see table 1, p 420). There was no statistically significant difference between medical treatment versus surgery, but the study was underpowered to show an effect.

Harms: **Versus medical management:** The review gave no information on surgical complications, and none of the individual studies were designed to compare rates of adverse effects.[34] In one arm of the subsequent RCT, 7/9 children who had postoperative obstruction developed evidence of renal scarring on DMSA scintigraphy. This may have negated an otherwise beneficial effect of surgery over medical management.[36]

Comment: **Versus medical management:** The best results were obtained by centres handling the greatest number of children.[37] Surgery is usually considered only in children with more severe vesicoureteric reflux (grades III-V), who are less likely to experience spontaneous resolution.[4,38] **Longer term outcome:** The RCT involving children with bilateral moderate to severe vesicoureteric reflux and nephropathy found that, over a period of 4 years, 20/54 (37%) kidneys of children in the medical group had spontaneous resolution to no, or minimal, vesicoureteric reflux (grades 0 or I) and 47/50 (94%) kidneys had uncomplicated corrections in the surgical group (ARI 57%, 95% CI 47% to 69%).[35] We found one prospective cohort study (226 children aged 5 days to 12 years who presented with urinary tract infection and were found to have grades III–IV vesicoureteric reflux) with follow up of 10–41 years.[8] It found that surgery was associated with a higher rate of resolution of reflux compared with medical treatment (AR of resolution from age 8–14 years on micturating cystourethrography: 29/33 [88%] with surgery *v* 134/193 [69%] treated medically; ARI 19%, 95% CI 6% to 31%). The study did not compare clinical outcomes.[8]

GLOSSARY

Intravenous immunoglobulins (normal immunoglobulins for intravenous use) Immunoglobulin preparations derived from donated human plasma containing antibodies prevalent in the general population.

Nosocomial infection Definitions vary but typically an infection arising at least 48–72 hours after admission to hospital. The infection may have been acquired from other people, hospital staff, the hospital environment, or from within people themselves.

Pyelonephritis Inflammation of the kidney and its pelvis because of bacterial infection.

Severity of vesicoureteric reflux:

Grade I Reflux into ureters only.

Grade II Reflux into ureters, pelvis, and calyces.

Grade III Mild to moderate dilatation or tortuosity of ureters and mild to moderate dilatation of pelvis, but little or no forniceal blunting.

Grade IV As grade III, but with complete obliteration of forniceal angles, yet maintenance of papillary impressions in calyces.

Grade V Gross dilatation of ureters, pelvis, and calyces, and papillary impressions in calyces obliterated.

Substantive changes

Long versus short courses of oral antibiotics One new systematic review;[13] conclusions unchanged.

Long versus short courses of initial intravenous treatment New comparison.[16,17]

Prophylactic antibiotics, versus no prophylaxis One new systematic review;[21] conclusions unchanged.

Surgical correction for vesicoureteric reflux One new RCT;[35] conclusions unchanged.

REFERENCES

1. Stark H. Urinary tract infections in girls: the cost-effectiveness of currently recommended investigative routines. *Pediatr Nephrol* 1997;11:174–177.
2. Dick PT, Feldman W. Routine diagnostic imaging for childhood urinary tract infections: a systematic overview. *J Pediatr* 1996;128:15–22. Search date 1994; primary sources Medline, Current Contents, and hand searches of article bibliographies.
3. Smellie JM, Katz G, Gruneberg RN. Controlled trial of prophylactic treatment in childhood urinary tract infection. *Lancet* 1978;ii:175–178.
4. Jodal U, Hansson S, Hjalmas K. Medical or surgical management for children with vesico-ureteric reflux? *Acta Paediatr Suppl* 1999;431:53–61.
5. Jodal U. The natural history of bacteriuria in childhood. *Infect Dis Clin North Am* 1987;1:713–729.
6. Hoberman A, Wald ER, Hickey RW, et al. Oral versus initial intravenous therapy for urinary tract infections in young febrile children. *Pediatrics* 1999;104:79–86.
7. Piepsz A, Tamminen-Mobius T, Reiners C, et al. Five-year study of medical and surgical treatment in children with severe vesico-ureteric reflux dimercaptosuccinic acid findings. International Reflux Study Group in Europe. *Eur J Pediatr* 1998;157:753–758.
8. Smellie JM, Prescod NP, Shaw PJ, et al. Childhood reflux and urinary infection: a follow-up of 10–41 years in 226 adults. *Pediatr Nephrol* 1998;12:727–736.
9. Berg UB. Long-term follow-up of renal morphology and function in children with recurrent pyelonephritis. *J Urol* 1992;148:1715–1720.
10. Martinell J, Claeson I, Lidin-Janson G, et al. Urinary infection, reflux and renal scarring in females continuously followed for 13–38 years. *Pediatr Nephrol* 1995;9:131–136.
11. Jacobson S, Eklof O, Erikkson CG, et al. Development of hypertension and uraemia after pyelonephritis in childhood: 27 year follow up. *BMJ* 1989;299:703–706.
12. Moffatt M, Embree J, Grimm P, et al. Short course antibiotic therapy for urinary tract infections in children: a methodological review of the literature. *Am J Dis Child* 1988;142:57–61. Search date and primary sources not stated.
13. Tran D, Muchant DG, Aronoff SC. Short-course versus conventional length antimicrobial therapy for uncomplicated lower urinary tract infections in children: a meta-analysis of 1279 patients. *J Pediatr* 2001;139;93–99.
14. Avner ED, Ingelfinger JR, Herrin JT, et al. Single-dose amoxicillin therapy of uncomplicated pediatric urinary tract infections. *J Pediatr* 1983;102:623–627.
15. McCracken GH, Ginsburg CM, Namasonthi V, et al. Evaluation of short-term antibiotic therapy in children with uncomplicated urinary tract infection. *Pediatrics* 1981;67:796–801.
16. Benador D, Neuhaus TJ, Papazyan J-P, et al. Randomised controlled trial of three day versus 10 day intravenous antibiotics in acute pyelonephritis: effect on renal scarring. *Arch Dis Child* 2001;84;241–246.
17. Levtchenko E, Lahy C, Levy J, et al. Treatment of children with acute pyelonephritis: a prospective randomized study. *Paediatric Nephrology* 2001;16;878–884.
18. Smellie JM, Normand ICS, Katz G. Children with urinary infection: a comparison of those with and those without vesicoureteric reflux. *Kidney Int* 1981;20:717–722.
19. Benador D, Benador N, Slozman D, et al. Are younger patients at higher risk of renal sequelae after pyelonephritis? *Lancet* 1997;349:17–19.
20. Rosenberg AR, Rossleigh MA, Brydon MP, et al. Evaluation of acute urinary tract infection in children by dimercaptosuccinic acid scintography: a prospective study. *J Urol* 1992;148:1746–1749.
21. Williams GJ, Lee A, Craig JC. Long-term antibiotics for preventing recurrent urinary tract infection in children. In: The Cochrane Library, Issue 4, 2001. Oxford: Update Software.
22. Lohr JA, Nunley DH, Howards SS, et al. Prevention of recurrent urinary tract infections in girls. *Pediatrics* 1977;59:562–565.
23. Garin EH, Campos A, Homsy Y. Primary vesico-ureteral reflux: a review of current concepts. *Pediatr Nephrol* 1998;12:249–256.
24. Smellie JM, Gruneberg RN, Leakey A, et al. Long term low dose co-trimoxazole in prophylaxis of childhood urinary tract infection: clinical aspects/bacteriological aspects. *BMJ* 1976;2:203–208.
25. Allen UD, MacDonald N, Fuite L, et al. Risk factors for resistance to "first-line" antimicrobials among urinary tract isolates of *Escherichia coli* in children. *CMAJ* 1999;160:1436–1440.
26. Greenfield SP, Ng M, Gran J. Experience with vesicoureteric reflux in children: clinical characteristics. *J Urol* 1997;158:574–577.
27. Ohlsson A, Lacy JB. Intravenous immunoglobulin for preventing infection in pre-term and/or low-birth-weight infants. In: The Cochrane Library, Issue 4, 2001. Oxford: Update Software. Search date 1997; primary sources Medline, Embase, Cochrane Library, Reference Update, Science Citation Index, and hand searches of reference lists of identified RCTs and personal files.
28. Clemente E, Solli R, Mei V, et al. Therapeutic efficacy and safety of pidotimod in the treatment of urinary tract infections in children. *Arzneim Forsh* 1994;44:1490–1494.

29. Lettgen B. Prevention of urinary tract infections in female children. *Curr Ther Rcs* 1996;57:464–475.
30. Weisman LE, Cruess DF, Fischer GW. Opsonic activity of commercially available standard intravenous immunoglobulin preparations. *Paediatr Inf Dis J* 1994;13:1122–1125.
31. Nayir A, Emre S, Sirin A, et al. The effects of vaccination with inactivated uropathogenic bacteria in recurrent urinary tract infections of children. *Vaccine* 1995;13:987–990.
32. Czerwionka-Szarflarska M, Pawlowska M. Uro-vaxom in the treatment of recurrent urinary tract infections in children. *Pediatria Polska* 1996;71:599–604.
33. Pylkannen J, Vilska J, Koskimies O. The value of childhood urinary tract infection in predicting renal injury. *Acta Paediatr Scand* 1981;70:879–883.
34. Shanon A, Feldman W. Methodological limitations in the literature on vesicoureteric reflux: a critical review. *J Pediatr* 1990;117:171–178. Search date 1988; primary source Medline.
35. Smellie JM, Barratt TM, Chantler C, et al. Medical versus surgical treatment in children with severe bilateral vesicoureteric reflux and bilateral nephropathy: a randomized controlled trial. *Lancet* 2001;357:1329–1333.
36. Weiss R, Duckett J, Spitzer A. Results of a randomized clinical trial of medical versus surgical management of infants and children with grades III and IV primary vesico-ureteral reflux (United States): the international reflux study in children. *J Urol* 1992;148:1667–1673.
37. Smellie JM. Commentary: management of children with severe vesicoureteral reflux. *J Urol* 1992;148:1676–1678.
38. Sciagra R, Materassi M, Rossi V, et al. Alternative approaches to the prognostic stratification of mild to moderate primary vesicoureteral reflux in children. *J Urol* 1996;155:2052–2056.

James Larcombe
General Practitioner and Regional Research Fellow
NHSE Northern and Yorkshire
Sedgefield
UK

Competing interests: None declared.

TABLE 1 **Average glomerular filtration rates in children with bilateral vesicoureteric reflux and bilateral nephropathy at the commencement of the study, at 4 years and at 10 years after randomisation to medical or surgical management (see text, p 418).[35]**

Mean GFR (mL/min)	At entry	At 4 years	At 10 years
Medical management	72.4	70.2	68.3
Surgical management	71.7	73.7	74.1
Difference in change in GFR from entry (95% CI)	–	+7.1% (–6.4% to +20.6%)	+8.9% (–10.3% to +28.2%)

GFR, glomerular filtration rate.

Acute appendicitis

Search date November 2001

John Simpson and William Speake

QUESTIONS

INTERVENTIONS

To be covered in future updates
Antibiotic regimens and dosages for appendicectomy
Stump inversion at time of appendicectomy
Diagnosis of appendicitis

See glossary, p 426.

Key Messages

Treatments

- **Adjuvant antibiotics** One systematic review and one subsequent RCT in children and adults with simple or complicated appendicitis undergoing appendicectomy have found that prophylactic antibiotics versus no antibiotics significantly reduce wound infections and intra-abdominal abscesses.
- **Adjuvant antibiotics (in children with complicated appendicitis)** Subgroup analysis from one systematic review has found that antibiotics versus no antibiotics significantly reduce the number of wound infections in children with complicated appendicitis.
- **Adjuvant antibiotics (in children with simple appendicitis)** Subgroup analysis from one systematic review has found no significant difference in the number of wound infections with antibiotics versus no antibiotics in children with simple appendicitis. One subsequent RCT in children with simple appendicitis found no significant difference with antibiotic prophylaxis versus no antibiotic prophylaxis in wound infections, but the RCT may have been too small to exclude a clinically important difference.
- **Antibiotics versus surgery** One RCT in adults with suspected appendicitis found that conservative treatment with antibiotics versus appendicectomy significantly reduced both postoperative pain and postoperative morphine consumption. However, it found that 35% of people following conservative management were readmitted within 1 year with acute appendicitis and subsequently had an appendicectomy.

- **Laparoscopic surgery versus open surgery (in children)** One systematic review has found that laparoscopic surgery versus open surgery significantly reduces the number of wound infections and the length of hospital stay, but found no significant difference in postoperative pain, time to mobilisation, or numbers of intra-abdominal abscesses. One subsequent RCT in children aged 7–15 found no significant difference with laparoscopic surgery versus open surgery in length of hospital stay, time to return to normal activity, or numbers of wound infections.
- **Laparoscopic surgery versus open surgery (in adults)** One systematic review has found that laparoscopic surgery versus open surgery significantly reduces the number of wound infections, pain on the first postoperative day, the duration of hospital stay, and the time taken to return to work, but significantly increases the number of postoperative intra-abdominal abscesses.
- **Surgery versus no treatment** We found no RCTs of surgery versus no surgery.

DEFINITION Acute appendicitis is acute inflammation of the vermiform appendix.

INCIDENCE/ PREVALENCE The incidence of acute appendicitis is falling, although the reason for this is unclear. The reported lifetime risk of appendicitis in the USA is 8.7% in males and 6.7% in females,[1] and there are about 60 000 cases reported annually in England and Wales. Appendicitis is the commonest surgical emergency requiring operation.

AETIOLOGY/ RISK FACTORS The aetiology of appendicitis is uncertain although various theories exist. Most relate to luminal obstruction, which prevents escape of secretions and inevitably leads to a rise in intraluminal pressure within the appendix. This can lead to subsequent mucosal ischaemia, and the stasis provides an ideal environment for bacterial overgrowth. Potential causes of the obstruction are faecoliths, often due to constipation, lymphoid hyperplasia, or caecal carcinoma.[2]

PROGNOSIS The prognosis of untreated appendicitis is unknown, although spontaneous resolution has been reported in at least 1/13 (8%) episodes.[3] The recurrence of appendicitis following conservative management,[3,4] and recurrent abdominal symptoms in certain patients,[5] suggests that chronic appendicitis and recurrent acute or subacute appendicitis may also exist.[6] The standard treatment for acute appendicitis is appendicectomy. The mortality from acute appendicitis is less than 0.3%, rising to 1.7% following perforation.[7] The most common complication of appendicectomy is wound infection occurring in between 5 and 33% of cases.[8] Intra-abdominal abscess formation occurs less frequently in 2% of appendicectomies.[9] A perforated appendix in childhood does not appear to have subsequent negative consequences on female fertility.[10]

AIMS To reduce pain; prevent postoperative infection; shorten hospital stay; and hasten return to normal activity.

OUTCOMES Wound infection rates; intra-abdominal infection rates; postoperative pain; return of bowel function; return to normal activity; mortality.

METHODS *Clinical Evidence* search and appraisal November 2001. In addition the authors searched the Cochrane Library, Issue 1, 2002.

QUESTION What are the effects of treatment for acute appendicitis?

OPTION SURGERY VERSUS NO TREATMENT

We found no systematic review or RCTs of surgery versus no treatment.

Benefits: We found no systematic review or RCTs.

Harms: We found no good evidence.

Comment: An RCT in this area is unlikely to be conducted.

OPTION LAPAROSCOPIC SURGERY VERSUS OPEN SURGERY

One systematic review has found that in adults laparoscopic surgery versus open surgery significantly reduces the number of wound infections, pain on the first postoperative day, the duration of hospital stay, and the time taken to return to work, but significantly increases the number of postoperative intra-abdominal abscesses. The review has found that in children laparoscopic surgery versus open surgery significantly reduces the number of wound infections and the length of hospital stay, but found no significant difference in postoperative pain, time to mobilisation, or numbers of intra-abdominal abscesses. One subsequent RCT in children found no significant difference with laparoscopic surgery versus open surgery in length of hospital stay, time to return to normal activity, or numbers of wound infections.

Benefits: We found one systematic review[11] and one subsequent RCT.[12] The review (search date 2000, 45 RCTs, 4855 people) compared laparoscopic surgery versus open surgery. **In adults:** The systematic review (39 RCTs, 4550 people) found that laparoscopic surgery versus open surgery significantly reduced the number of wound infections (86/2213 [4%] with laparoscopic surgery *v* 161/2111 [8%] with open surgery; OR 0.47, 95% CI 0.36 to 0.62), but significantly increased the number of postoperative intra-abdominal abscesses (41/2239 [2%] with laparoscopic surgery *v* 13/2134 [< 1%] with open surgery; OR 2.77, 95% CI 1.61 to 4.77).[11] The review also found that laparoscopic surgery versus open surgery significantly reduced pain on the first postoperative day (measured using a 100 mm visual analogue scale, a reduction of 8 mm, 95% CI 3 to 13mm), significantly reduced the duration of hospital stay (difference of 0.7 days, 95% CI 0.4 to 1.0 days), and significantly reduced the time taken to return to work (difference of 3 days, 95% CI 1 to 5 days). **In children:** The systematic review (3 RCTs, 305 children aged 4–15 years) found that laparoscopic surgery versus open surgery significantly reduced the number of wound infections (0/153 [0%] with laparoscopic surgery *v* 12/152 [8%] with open surgery; OR.12, 95% CI 0.04 to 0.39), and significantly reduced the length of hospital stay (difference of –0.7 days, 95% CI –0.3 to –1.1 days).[11] The review reported that there were no intra-abdominal abscesses with either treatment. The review found no significant difference with laparoscopic surgery versus open surgery in postoperative pain (pain measured using a visual analogue scale; difference in visual analogue scale was –1 mm, 95% CI –8 to

+7 mm), and found no significant difference between treatments in the time to mobilisation (difference of –0.25 days, 95% CI –0.645 to +0.145 days). The subsequent RCT (43 children aged 7–15 years) compared laparoscopic surgery versus open surgery and found no significant difference in the length of hospital stay (3.1 days with laparoscopic surgery *v* 3.0 days with open surgery) or return to normal physical activity after 4 weeks.[12] The RCT found no wound infection occurred with either treatment.

Harms: A number of harms have been considered in the benefits section. The review and subsequent RCT did not report any further data on harms.[11,12]

Comment: The systematic review included people with a clinical diagnosis of acute appendicitis and provided no information on preoperative imaging or the use of perioperative antibiotics.[11] Analyses were performed on an intention to treat basis. Studies reporting a negative appendicectomy rate of more than 50% were excluded. The number of trials looking specifically at paediatric practice is small and, as in the adult studies, not all outcomes were assessed in all trials. The majority of the trials were unblinded and, in addition, strong heterogeneity was present for most of the analyses, although not for wound infections or intra-abdominal abscesses. The definition and reporting of additional operative or postoperative complications was inconsistent.

OPTION ANTIBIOTICS

One RCT found that conservative treatment with antibiotics versus appendicectomy significantly reduced both postoperative pain and postoperative morphine consumption. However, it found that 35% of people were readmitted within 1 year with acute appendicitis following conservative management and subsequently underwent appendicectomy.

Benefits: **Versus no treatment:** We found no systematic review and no RCTs. **Versus surgery:** We found one RCT (40 adults with suspected appendicitis), which compared antibiotic treatment (iv cefotaxime 2 g twice daily plus tinidazole 800 mg/day for 2 days followed by oral ofloxacin 200 mg twice daily plus tinidazole 500 mg twice daily for 8 days) versus open appendicectomy.[4] It found that people treated with antibiotics had significantly less pain in the period from 12 hours to 10 days following initiation of treatment compared with the operative group ($P < 0.01$; other data presented graphically) and significantly reduced morphine consumption ($P < 0.001$).

Harms: The RCT (40 adults) found that all people treated conservatively were discharged from hospital within 48 hours, except one who underwent surgery for generalised peritonitis following a perforation of the appendix 12 hours after randomisation to receive antibiotic treatment.[4] The RCT found that 7/20 (35%) people who received conservative management were readmitted with acute appendicitis and underwent appendicectomy within 1 year (mean 7 months, range 3–12 months). The RCT found that there was one wound infection in the surgically treated group, and that no deaths occurred with either treatment.

Comment: Inclusion criteria for the RCT included typical symptoms and signs of acute appendicitis, positive findings on ultrasound, and raised neutrophil/C-reactive protein levels on blood assays.

QUESTION What are the effects of adjuvant treatments for acute appendicitis?

OPTION ADJUVANT ANTIBIOTICS VERSUS PLACEBO/NO TREATMENT

One systematic review and one subsequent RCT in people with appendicitis have found that prophylactic antibiotics significantly reduce infections, although the situation in children is less clear. The review has found that in people with either simple or complicated appendicitis, perioperative systemic antibiotic prophylaxis versus no antibiotic prophylaxis significantly reduces numbers of wound infections and intra-abdominal abscesses, although subgroup analysis in people with complicated appendicitis found no significant difference in numbers of intra-abdominal abscesses. The review found limited evidence that in children with either simple or complicated appendicitis there was no significant difference in numbers of wound infections or intra-abdominal abscesses, although subgroup analysis found that in children with complicated appendicitis, antibiotic prophylaxis significantly reduced the number of wound infections. One subsequent RCT in children found no significant difference with antibiotic prophylaxis versus no antibiotic prophylaxis in wound infections.

Benefits: We found one systematic review (search date 2000, 44 RCTs or CCTs, 9298 adults and children undergoing appendicectomy with either simple appendicitis or complicated appendicitis [see glossary, p 426])[9] and one subsequent RCT, which compared antibiotic prophylaxis versus placebo or no prophylaxis.[13] The review found that perioperative systemic antibiotic prophylaxis versus no antibiotic prophylaxis significantly reduced the number of wound infections (20 RCTs/CCTs: 287/4326 [7%] with antibiotics *v* 632/4317 [15%] with no antibiotics; OR 0.32, 95% CI 0.24 to 0.42; see comment below), and significantly reduced the number of intra-abdominal abscesses (8 RCTs/CCTs: 16/2211 [< 1%] with antibiotics *v* 39/2257 [2%] with no antibiotics; OR 0.35, 95% CI 0.13 to 0.91).[9] Subgroup analysis found that in people with simple appendicitis antibiotic prophylaxis significantly reduced the number of wound infections (26 RCTs/CCTs: 113/2610 [4%] with antibiotics *v* 286/2707 [11%] with no antibiotics; OR 0.37, 95% CI 0.30 to 0.46); and significantly reduced the number of intra-abdominal abscesses (8 RCTs/CCTs: 9/1433 [< 1%] with antibiotics *v* 22/1535 [1%] with no antibiotics; OR 0.46, 95% CI 0.23 to 0.94), although subgroup analysis in people with complicated appendicitis found that antibiotic prophylaxis significantly reduced the number of wound infections (24 RCTs/CCTs: 121/645 [19%] with antibiotics *v* 175/507 [35%] with no antibiotics; OR 0.28, 95% CI 0.21 to 0.38), but found no significant difference in the number of intra-abdominal abcesses (3 RCTs/CCTs: 3/262 [1%] with antibiotics *v* 4/205 [2%] with no antibiotics; OR 0.54, 95% CI 0.12 to 2.43). The review also found no significant difference with topical antibiotics versus placebo in the number of wound infections (52/339 [15%] with topical antibiotics *v* 61/340 [18%] with placebo; OR 0.77, 95% CI 0.49 to 1.23). **In children:** The systematic review (7 RCTs, 987 children aged 0–15 years with either simple or complicated appendicitis) found no significant difference with perioperative systemic antibiotic prophylaxis versus no antibiotic prophylaxis in numbers of wound infections (23/548 [4%] with antibiotics *v* 34/542 [6%] with no antibiotics; OR 0.64, 95% CI 0.37 to 1.10), or in the number of intra-abdominal abcesses (1/142 [< 1%] with antibiotics *v* 5/141 [4%] with no antibiotics; OR 0.25, 95% CI 0.05 to 1.26; see comment below).[9] Subgroup analysis in children with simple appendicitis found no significant difference between treatments in numbers of wound infections (3 RCTs/CCTs: 7/347 [2%] with antibiotics *v* 8/357 [2%] with no antibiotics; OR 0.92, 95% CI 0.33 to 2.57), although in children with complicated appendicitis antibiotic prophylaxis significantly reduced the number of wound infections (3 RCTs/CCTs: 5/134 [4%] with antibiotics *v* 15/119 [13%] with no antibiotics; OR 0.31, 95% CI 0.12 to 0.77). The subsequent RCT (108 children with simple appendicitis) compared three treatments: no antibiotic; one antibiotic dose (1 g ceftriaxone); and 5 days of regular antibiotics (1 g ceftriaxone daily).[13] The RCT reported that only one wound infection occurred, and this was in a child who received no antibiotics (other numerical data not provided).

Harms: A number of harms have been considered in the benefits section. The review and RCT did not report any further data on harms.[9,13]

Comment: The systematic review did not distinguish between antibiotic regimens or between different antibiotic drugs.[9] These issues are being addressed in a systematic review to be published in the future. There were limited numbers of children in the systematic review and in the RCT; therefore, the results may lack statistical power.[9,13] The review found insufficient data to provide subgroup analysis for numbers of intra-abdominal abcesses in children with either simple or complicated appendicitis.[9] The benefit of antibiotics for simple appendicitis in children is unclear. The review did not report on preoperative imaging studies.[9]

GLOSSARY

Complicated appendicitis Perforated or gangrenous appendicitis.
Simple appendicitis Clinically normal or inflamed but not gangrenous or perforated appendix.

REFERENCES

1. Addiss DG, Shaffer N, Fowler BS, Tauxe RV. The epidemiology of appendicitis and appendectomy in the United States. *Am J Epidemiol* 1990;132:910–925.
2. Larner AJ. The aetiology of appendicitis. *Br J Hosp Med* 1988;39:540–542.
3. Cobben LP, de van Otterloo AM, Puylaert JB. Spontaneously resolving acute appendicitis: frequency and natural history in 60 patients. *Radiology* 2000;215:349–352.
4. Eriksson S, Granstrom L. Randomized controlled trial of appendicectomy versus antibiotic therapy for acute appendicitis. *Br J Surg* 1995;82:166–169.
5. Barber MD, McLaren J, Rainey JB. Recurrent appendicitis. *Br J Surg* 1997;84:110–112.
6. Mattei P, Sola JE, Yeo CJ. Chronic and recurrent appendicitis are uncommon entities often misdiagnosed. *J Am Coll Surg* 1994;178:385–389.
7. Velanovich V, Satava R. Balancing the normal appendectomy rate with the perforated appendicitis rate: implications for quality assurance. *Am Surg* 1992;58:264–269.
8. Krukowski ZH, Irwin ST, Denholm S, Matheson NA. Preventing wound infection after appendicectomy: a review. *Br J Surg* 1988;75:1023–1033.
9. Andersen BR, Kallehave FL, Andersen HK. Antibiotics versus placebo for prevention of

postoperative infection after appendectomy (Cochrane Review). In: The Cochrane Library, Issue 3, 2001. Oxford: Update Software. Search date 2000; primary sources Cochrane Controlled Trials Register, Medline, Embase, Cochrane Colorectal Cancer Group Specialised Register, and hand searches of reference lists of identified trials.
10. Andersson R, Lambe M, Bergstrom R. Fertility patterns after appendicectomy: historical cohort study. *BMJ* 1999;318:963–967.
11. Sauerland SR, Lefering, Neugebauer EAM. Laparoscopic versus open surgery for suspected appendicitis (Cochrane Review). In: The Cochrane Library, Issue 1, 2002. Oxford: Update Software. Search date 2000; primary sources The Cochrane Library, Medline, Embase, SciSearch, and Biosis.
12. Lavonius MI, Liesjarvi S, Ovaska J, Pajulo O, Ristkari S, Alanen M. Laparoscopic versus open appendectomy in children: a prospective randomised study. *Eur J Pediatr Surg* 2001;11:235–238.
13. Gorecki WJ, Grochowski JA. Are antibiotics necessary in nonperforated appendicitis in children? A double blind randomised controlled trial. *Med Sci Monit* 2001;7:289–292.

John Simpson
MRC Fellow

William Speake
Specialist Registrar
Division of Gastrointestinal Surgery
University Hospital Nottingham
UK

Competing interests: None declared.

Anal fissure

Search date January 2002

Marion Jonas and John Scholefield

QUESTIONS

INTERVENTIONS

See glossary, p 434

Key Messages

- **Anal advancement flap (as effective as internal anal sphincterotomy)** One RCT found no significant difference with lateral internal anal sphincterotomy versus anal advancement flap in patient satisfaction or fissure healing.
- **Anal stretch** One systematic review found no significant difference with internal anal sphincterotomy versus anal stretch in persistence of fissures, and that both procedures healed 70–95% of fissures. Anal stretch versus internal anal sphincterotomy significantly increased rates of flatus incontinence.
- **Botulinum A toxin-haemagglutinin complex (botulinum A toxin-hc)** RCTs have found that botulinum A toxin-hc versus placebo or topical glyceryl trinitrate (GTN) significantly increases fissure healing rates after 2 months, but found no significant difference with high dose versus low dose botulinum A toxin-hc in healing rates after 3 months.
- **Botulinum A toxin-hc plus topical isosorbide dinitrate** One RCT has found that botulinum A toxin-hc followed by three times daily application of topical isosorbide dinitrate versus botulinum A toxin-hc alone significantly increases fissure healing at 6 weeks.
- **Diltiazem** We found no placebo controlled RCTs. One small RCT found no significant difference with oral diltiazem versus topical diltiazem in fissure healing after 8 weeks.
- **Indoramin** One small RCT found no significant difference with oral indoramin versus placebo in fissure healing after 6 weeks.

Clin Evid 2002;8:428–435.

- **Internal anal sphincterotomy** One systematic review found no significant difference with internal anal sphincterotomy versus anal stretch in persistence of fissures, and that both procedures healed 70–95% of fissures. It found no significant difference with open versus closed internal sphincterotomy in persistence of fissures. One systematic review, one additional RCT, and one subsequent RCT found conflicting results for topical GTN versus internal sphincterotomy in fissure healing after 6–8 weeks.
- **Topical glyceral trinitrate (GTN)** One systematic review comparing topical GTN versus placebo identified two RCTs, which found that GTN significantly increased fissure healing after 8 weeks' treatment, and two RCTs, which found no significant difference in fissure healing after 4 weeks' treatment. One systematic review, one additional RCT, and one subsequent RCT found conflicting results for topical GTN versus internal sphincterotomy in fissure healing after 6–8 weeks. One systematic review found that botulinum A toxin-hc versus topical GTN significantly increased fissure healing rates after 2 months. One RCT found no significant difference with topical GTN versus a GTN patch in fissure healing after 8 weeks.

DEFINITION Anal fissure is a split or tear in the lining of the distal anal canal. It is a very painful condition often associated with fresh blood loss from the anus and perianal itching. **Acute anal fissures** have sharply demarcated, fresh mucosal edges, and often with granulation tissue at the base. **Chronic anal fissures** margins are indurated, there is less granulation tissue, and muscle fibres of the internal anal sphincter may be seen at the base. Fissures persisting for longer than 6 weeks are generally defined as chronic.

INCIDENCE/ PREVALENCE Anal fissures are common in all age groups, but we found no evidence to quantify the incidence.

AETIOLOGY/ RISK FACTORS Low intake of dietary fibre may be a risk factor for the development of acute anal fissures.[1] People with anal fissure often have raised resting anal canal pressures with anal spasm.[2,3] Men and women are equally affected by anal fissures, and up to 11% of women develop anal fissures after childbirth.[4]

PROGNOSIS Placebo controlled studies found that 70–90% of untreated "chronic" fissures did not heal during the study.[5,6]

AIMS To relieve symptoms (pain, bleeding, irritation); to heal the fissure; to minimise adverse effects of treatment.

OUTCOMES Number of people with fissure healing (intact anal mucosal lining); symptom score for intensity of symptoms of pain, bleeding, and irritation (typically a linear visual analogue scale that consists of an unmarked 100 mm horizontal line, the left end of which represents absence of symptoms and the right end represents the worst symptoms imaginable; a vertical mark is made across this line by the person with the fissure); number of people reporting adverse effects of treatment.

METHODS *Clinical Evidence* search and appraisal January 2002.

QUESTION What are the effects of treatments for chronic anal fissure?

OPTION TOPICAL GLYCERYL TRINITRATE

One systematic review comparing topical glyceryl trinitrate versus placebo identified two RCTs, which found that glyceryl trinitrate significantly increased fissure healing after 8 weeks' treatment, and two RCTs, which found no significant difference in fissure healing after 4 weeks' treatment. One systematic review, one additional RCT, and one subsequent RCT found conflicting results for topical glyceryl trinitrate versus internal anal sphincterotomy in fissure healing after 6–8 weeks. One systematic review found that botulinum A toxin-hc versus topical glyceryl trinitrate significantly increased fissure healing rates after 2 months. One RCT found no significant difference with topical glyceryl trinitrate versus a glyceryl trinitrate patch in fissure healing after 8 weeks.

Benefits: **Versus placebo:** We found one systematic review (search date not stated, 4 RCTs, 312 people; no statistical pooling of data provided).[7] The first RCT (80 people) identified by the review found that glyceryl trinitrate (GTN) (see glossary, p 434) versus placebo significantly increased the number of people with healed anal fissures (26/38 [68%] with GTN *v* 3/39 [8%] with placebo; RR 8.9, 95% CI 2.94 to 26.95), and significantly reduced median pain scores (pain scores measured using a linear analogue scale; median score 6.0, range 0–78 with GTN *v* median score 40.0, range 0–92 with placebo; $P < 0.05$) after 8 weeks' treatment.[5] The second RCT in the review compared three treatments: 0.2% GTN; escalating dose GTN (starting with 0.2% and increasing by 0.1% increments weekly to maximum 0.6%); and placebo.[6] It found that both GTN treatments combined versus placebo significantly increased anal fissure healing after 8 weeks' treatment and 2 weeks' follow up (31/46 [67%] with GTN *v* 7/22 [32%] with placebo; RR 2.1, 95% CI 1.11 to 4.03), but found no significant difference in pain scores (measured using a linear analogue scale; $P = 0.04$).[6] The third RCT (43 people) identified by the review found no significant difference with GTN versus placebo in the number of people with healed anal fissures after 4 weeks' treatment (11/24 [46%] with GTN *v* 3/19 [16%] with placebo; RR 2.0, 95% CI 0.65 to 6.45), and did not provide comparative data between treatments for pain scores.[8] The fourth RCT identified by the review found no significant difference with GTN versus placebo in the number of people with healed anal fissures after 4 weeks' treatment (29/59 [49%] with GTN *v* 31/60 [52%] with placebo; RR 0.95, 95% CI 0.67 to 1.36), and did not provide comparative data between treatments for pain scores.[9] **Versus internal sphincterotomy:** See glossary, p 434. We found one systematic review (search date not stated, 1 RCT, 82 people),[7] one additional RCT,[10] and one subsequent RCT.[11] The RCT (82 people with chronic anal fissures receiving stool softeners and fibre supplements) identified by the review found that internal sphincterotomy versus GTN ointment significantly improved fissure healing at 6 weeks (34/38 [89%] *v* 13/44 [30%]; ARI 60%, 95% CI 38% to 81%; RR 3.0, 95% CI 1.9 to 4.8).[12] The additional RCT (49 people with chronic anal fissure of duration 4 months receiving a high fibre diet and a laxative) found no significant difference with GTN ointment (0.2%) or GTN patch (10 mg) versus internal sphincterotomy in the number of people with healed fissures at 1 year (24/37 [65%] with GTN v 11/12 [92%] with internal sphincterotomy; RR 0.71, 95% CI 0.53 to 0.95).[10] The subsequent RCT (60 people) found that internal sphincterotomy versus GTN ointment significantly increased the number of people with healed anal fissures at 8 weeks (26/27 [96%] v 20/33 [61%]; RR 1.6, 95% CI 1.20 to 2.11).[11] (See benefits of surgical treatments), p 432. **Versus botulinum A toxin-hc:** See glossary, p 434. See benefits of botulinum A toxin-haemagglutinin complex, p 432. **Versus GTN patch:** We found one RCT (42 people), which found no significant difference with topical GTN (0.2% ointment applied twice daily) versus a GTN patch (10 mg/day) in fissure healing at 8 weeks (12/18 [67%] with topical GTN v 12/19 [60%] with a GTN patch; RR 1.1, 95% CI 0.66 to 1.70).[10]

Harms: Topical GTN caused headaches in 29–72% of people, compared to 21–27% with placebo.[5,6,8]

Comment: We found insufficient evidence about the optimal duration of topical GTN treatment. Recurrent fissures may occur after GTN treatment is discontinued.

OPTION DILTIAZEM *New*

One small RCT found no significant difference with oral diltiazem versus topical diltiazem in fissure healing after 8 weeks.

Benefits: We found no systematic review. **Versus placebo:** We found no RCTs. **Versus other treatments:** We found one RCT (50 people with chronic anal fissures), which found no significant difference with oral diltiazem (60 mg twice daily) versus 2% diltiazem gel topically (700 mg twice daily) in the number of people with healed fissures after 8 weeks' treatment (17/26 [65%] with oral diltiazem v 9/24 [38%] with diltiazem gel; RR 1.7, 95% CI 0.99 to 3.14).[13]

Harms: The RCT reported that oral diltiazem caused adverse effects in 8/24 (33%) people (nausea/vomiting in 3 people, headache in 2 people, rash in 2 people, altered sense of smell and taste in 1 person), and that topical diltiazem caused none of these adverse effects.[13]

Comment: We found insufficient evidence about the optimal duration of diltiazem treatment. The role of diltiazem in treating fissures previously failing to heal with glyceryl trinitrate is also unclear.

OPTION INDORAMIN *New*

One RCT found no significant difference with oral indoramin versus placebo in fissure healing after 6 weeks.

Benefits: We found no systematic review. **Versus placebo:** We found one RCT (23 people with chronic anal fissures), which found no significant difference with oral indoramin (20 mg twice daily) versus placebo in the number of people with healed fissures after 6 weeks (1/14 [7%] with indoramin *v* 2/9 [22%] with placebo; RR 0.3, 95% CI 0.03 to 3.05; see comment below).[14] The RCT did not provide comparative data between treatments for pain scores.

Harms: The RCT reported that indoramin caused adverse effects in 7/14 (50%) of people.[14]

Comment: The RCT reported that the single fissure that healed with indoramin recurred after 3 months.[14]

OPTION BOTULINUM A TOXIN-HAEMAGGLUTININ COMPLEX (BOTULINUM A TOXIN-HC)

RCTs have found that botulinum A toxin-hc versus placebo or topical glyceryl trinitrate significantly increases fissure healing rates after 2 months, and that botulinum A toxin-hc followed by three times daily application of topical isosorbide dinitrate versus botulinum A toxin-hc alone significantly increases fissure healing at 6 weeks. One RCT found no significant difference with high dose versus low dose botulinum A toxin-hc in healing rates after 3 months.

Benefits: **Versus placebo:** We found one systematic review (search date not stated, 1 RCT, 30 people with chronic idiopathic anal fissure).[7] The RCT identified by the review compared botulinum A toxin-hc (see glossary, p 434) (Botox preparation) versus placebo (saline) injection into the internal anal sphincter.[15] It found that botulinum A toxin-hc significantly increased healing rates (formation of a scar) after 2 months (11/15 [73%] with botulinum A toxin-hc *v* 2/15 [13%] with placebo; AR 60%, 95% CI 25% to 95%; RR 5.5, 95% CI 1.5 to 21). **Different doses:** We found no systemic review. We found one RCT (50 people with chronic anal fissure), which found no significant difference with higher dose (Dysport preparation, 40 units) versus lower dose (Dysport preparation, 20 units) botulinum A toxin-hc in healing rates after 3 months (20/25 [80%] *v* 19/25 [76%]; RR 1.1, 95% CI 0.78 to 1.41).[16] **Versus topical glyceryl trinitrate (GTN):** We found one systematic review (search date not stated, 1 RCT, 50 people with chronic anal fissure).[7] The RCT identified by the review found that botulinum A toxin-hc injection (20 units, Botox preparation) versus topical application of GTN 0.2% for 6 weeks significantly increased fissure healing rates at 2 months (96% with botulinum A toxin-hc *v* 60% with GTN; P = 0.005).[17] **Versus subsequent topical isosorbide dinitrate:** We found no systematic review. One RCT (30 people with anal fissures, which had failed to heal with topical isosorbide dinitrate alone) found that botulinum A toxin-hc injection (20 units) followed by three times daily application of topical isosorbide dinitrate (2.5 mg) versus botulinum A toxin-hc injection alone significantly increased the number of people with healed anal fissures at 6 weeks (10/15 [66%] with botulinum A toxin-hc plus isosorbide dinitrate *v* 3/15 [20%] with botulinum A toxin-hc alone; ARI 47%, 95% CI 11% to 82%; RR 3.3, 95% CI 1.14 to 9.75; NNT 3, 95% CI 2 to 5), but found no significant difference at 8 and 12 weeks after treatment.[18]

Harms: One RCT comparing different doses of botulinum A toxin-hc found flatus incontinence in 6% of people for less than 2 weeks, and faecal incontinence in 4% of people for 1 week.[16] Two RCTs reported no adverse effects associated with the use botulinum A toxin-hc.[15,17] Earlier pilot studies have also reported complications associated with the use of botulinum A toxin-hc, including pain, bleeding, sepsis associated with injection, and faecal incontinence, in up to 7% of people.[19,20]

Comment: Recurrent fissures may occur after treatment is discontinued. We found one cross sectional study (57 people with idiopathic anal fissure), which found that a higher dosage regimen (20 units Botox preparation) versus a lower dosage regimen (15 units Botox preparation) of botulinum A toxin-hc increased the number of people with healed fissures at 2 months (23/34 [68%] with high dose botulinum A toxin-hc *v* 10/23 [43%] with low dose botulinum A toxin-hc).[21]

OPTION SURGICAL TREATMENTS

One systematic review found no significant difference with internal anal sphincterotomy versus anal stretch in persistence of fissures, and that both procedures healed 70–95% of fissures. It found no significant difference with open versus closed internal sphincterotomy in persistence of fissures. The review found that anal stretch versus internal anal sphincterotomy significantly increased rates of flatus incontinence. One systematic review, one additional RCT, and one subsequent RCT found conflicting results for topical glyceryl trinitrate versus internal sphincterotomy in fissure healing after 6–8 weeks. One RCT found no significant difference with lateral internal sphincterotomy versus anal advancement flap in patient satisfaction or fissure healing.

Benefits: **Internal anal sphincterotomy:** We found one systematic review (search date not stated; data pooled for end points of persistence of fissure and postoperative incontinence of flatus, including 6 RCTs; 386 people), which compared internal anal sphincterotomy (see glossary, p 434) versus anal stretch (see glossary, p 434).[22] It found that both internal anal sphincterotomy and anal stretch healed 70–95% of fissures. The review found no significant difference with anal stretch versus internal anal sphincterotomy in persistence of fissure (6 RCTs; RR 1.16, 95% CI 0.65 to 2.08; see comment below), and no significant difference with open versus closed internal sphincterotomy in persistence of fissure (2 RCTs; RR 1.61, 95% CI 0.28 to 9.28; see comment below). See benefits of topical glyceryl trinitrate, p 430 **Anal advancement flap surgery:** We found no systematic review. We found one RCT (40 people), which found no significant difference with lateral internal sphincterotomy versus anal advancement flap (see glossary, p 434) in patient satisfaction or fissure healing (20/20 [100%] fissures healed after sphincterotomy *v* 17/20 [85%] following an advancement flap; P = 0.12).[23]

Harms: **Anal stretch versus sphincterotomy:** The systematic review found that anal stretch versus internal anal sphincterotomy significantly increased rates of flatus incontinence (4 RCTs; RR 6.63, 95% CI 2.06 to 21.3; see comment below), but found no significant difference with open versus closed lateral internal sphincterotomy in the risk of postoperative flatus incontinence (2 RCTs; RR 0.79, 95% CI 0.29 to 2.13; see comment below).[19] **Anal sphincterotomy versus anal advancement flap:** See harms of anal stretch for comparative harms, p 433. In a single RCT (40 people), no participant experienced incontinence after either anal sphincterotomy or after anal advancement flap.[23]

Comment: Only two outcomes were considered by the systematic review: persistence of the fissure and flatus incontinence.[22] Other outcomes (e.g. complications related to wound healing) may be relevant. The review reported that in contrast to the evidence from randomised studies, observational studies found that anal stretch (see glossary, p 434) versus internal anal sphincterotomy (see glossary, p 434) significantly increased rates of non-healing in four retrospective studies (RR 1.89, 95% CI 1.28 to 2.81).[22] The possibility of lower rates of fissure healing with anal advancement flap than with anal sphincterotomy requires further investigation.

GLOSSARY

Anal advancement flap Edges of the fissure are excised and healthy anal mucosa is mobilised to cover the defect.

Anal stretch Traditionally index and middle fingers of each hand inserted into the anal canal and pulled in opposite directions, the stretch held for 1 minute.

Botulinum A toxin-haemagglutinin complex (botulinum A toxin-hc) A formulation of botulinum A toxin and haemagglutinin for injection. Different preparations are used at different doses for the same indication and the strength (in units) of one preparation may not be equivalent to that of another preparation labelled as containing the same number of units.

Internal anal sphincterotomy Incision in the internal anal sphincter either posteriorly or laterally, but more commonly laterally, and usually "tailored" to the length of the fissure.

Topical glyceryl trinitrate (GTN) Usually applied as 0.2–0.3% ointment.

Substantive changes

Topical glyceryl trinitrate One new RCT[10] and one new systematic review;[7] conclusion unchanged.

REFERENCES

1. Jensen SL. Diet and other risk factors for fissure-in-ano. Prospective case control study. *Dis Colon Rectum* 1988;31:770–773.
2. Gibbons CP, Read NW. Anal hypertonia in fissures: cause or effect? *Br J Surgery* 1986;73:443–445.
3. Lund JN, Scholefield JH. Internal sphincter spasm in anal fissure. *Br J Surg* 1997;84:1723–1724.
4. Martin JD. Postpartum anal fissure. *Lancet* 1953;i:271–273.
5. Lund JN, Scholefield JH. A randomised, prospective, double-blind, placebo-controlled trial of glyceryl trinitrate ointment in the treatment of anal fissure. *Lancet* 1997;349:11–14.
6. Carapeti EA, Kamm MA, McDonald PJ, et al. Randomised controlled trial shows that glyceryl trinitrate heals anal fissures, higher doses are not more effective, and there is a high recurrence rate. *Gut* 1999;44:727–730.
7. Cook TA, Brading AF, Mortensen NJMcC. Review article: the pharmacology of the internal anal sphincter and new treatments of ano-rectal disorders. *Aliment Pharmacol Ther* 2001;15:887–898. Search date not stated; primary sources Medline and hand searches of reference lists from relevant papers.
8. Kennedy ML, Sowter S, Nguyen H, et al. Glyceryl trinitrate ointment for the treatment of chronic anal fissure: results of a placebo-controlled trial and long-term follow-up. *Dis Colon Rectum* 1999;42:1000–1006.
9. Altomare DF, Rinaldi M, Milito G, et al. Glyceryl trinitrate for chronic anal fissure: healing or headache? Results of a multicenter, randomized, placebo-controlled, double-blind trial. *Dis Colon Rectum* 2000;43:174–179; discussion 179–181.
10. Zuberi BF, Rajput MR, Abro H, et al. A randomized trial of glyceryl trinitrate ointment and nitroglycerin patch in healing of anal fissures. *Int J Colorectal Dis* 2000;15:243–245.
11. Evans J, Luck A, Hewett P. Glyceryl trinitrate vs. lateral sphincterotomy for chronic anal fissure: Prospective randomized trial. *Dis Colon Rectum* 2001;44:93–97.
12. Richard CS, Gregoire R, Plewes EA, et al. Internal sphincterotomy is superior to topical nitroglycerin

in the treatment of chronic anal fissure: results of a randomized, controlled trial by the Canadian Colorectal Surgical Trials Group. *Dis Colon Rectum* 2000;43:1048–1057; discussion 1057–1058.

13. Jonas M, Neal KR, Abercrombie JF, et al. A randomized trial of oral vs. topical diltiazem for chronic anal fissures. *Dis Colon Rectum* 2001;44:1074–1078.
14. Pitt J, Dawson PM, Hallan RI, et al. A double-blind randomized placebo-controlled trial of oral indoramin to treat chronic anal fissure. *Colorectal Dis* 2001;3:165–168.
15. Maria G, Cassetta E, Gui D, et al. A comparison of botulinum toxin and saline for the treatment of chronic anal fissure. *N Engl J Med* 1998;338:217–220.
16. Jost W, Schrank B. Chronic anal fissures treated wish botulinum toxin injections: a dose-finding study with Dysport. *Colorectal Dis* 1999;1:26–29.
17. Brisinda G, Maria G, Bentivoglio AR, et al. A comparison of injections of botulinum toxin and topical nitroglycerin ointment for the treatment of chronic anal fissure. *N Engl J Med* 1999;341:65–69.
18. Lysy J, Israelit-Yatzkan Y, Sestiery-Ittah M, et al. Topical nitrates potentiate the effect of botulinum toxin in the treatment of patients with refractory anal fissure. *Gut* 2001;48:221–224.
19. Jost WH, Schanne S, Mlitz H, et al. Perianal thrombosis following injection therapy into the external anal sphincter using botulinum toxin. *Dis Colon Rectum* 1995;38:781.
20. Jost WH. One hundred cases of anal fissure treated with botulin toxin: early and long-term results. *Dis Colon Rectum* 1997;40:1029–1032.
21. Maria G, Brisinda G, Bentivoglio AR, et al. Botulinum toxin injections in the internal anal sphincter for the treatment of chronic anal fissure: long-term results after two different dosage regimens. *Ann Surg* 1998;228:664–669.
22. Nelson R. Operative procedures for fissure in ano. In: The Cochrane Library, Issue 4, 2001. Oxford: Update Software. Search date not stated; primary sources Cochrane Library, Medline, the internet, and hand searches of cited reference lists from included reports.
23. Leong AF, Seow-Choen F. Lateral sphincterotomy compared with anal advancement flap for chronic anal fissure. *Dis Colon Rectum* 1995;38:69–71.

Marion Jonas
Specialist Registrar, General Surgery

John Scholefield
Professor of Surgery
University of Nottingham
Nottingham
UK

Competing interests: MJ none declared. JS Professor Scholefield have received commercial funding for research for attending symposium in this area.

Colonic diverticular disease

Search date January 2002

John Simpson and Robin Spiller

QUESTIONS

INTERVENTIONS

To be covered in future updates
Mesalazine in the treatment of diverticular disease

See glossary, p 443

Key Messages

Fibre to prevent complications of diverticular disease

- **Dietary fibre supplements** We found no RCTs of advice to consume a high fibre diet or of dietary fibre supplementation versus placebo.

Treatment of uncomplicated diverticular disease

- **Bran and ispaghula husk** Two small RCTs found no consistent effect of bran or ispaghula husk versus placebo on symptom relief after 12–16 weeks.
- **Elective surgery** We found no RCTs of elective colonic resection (open or laparoscopic).
- **Lactulose** One RCT found no significant difference with lactulose versus a high fibre diet in the number of people who considered themselves to be "much improved" (not defined) after 12 weeks.
- **Methylcellulose** One small RCT found no significant difference with methylcellulose versus placebo in mean symptom score after 3 months.
- **Rifaximin** One RCT found that oral rifaximin plus glucomannan versus glucomannan plus placebo significantly increases the number of people with uncomplicated diverticular disease who are symptom free after 12 months of treatment.

Clin Evid 2002;8:436–444.

Treatment of acute diverticulitis

- **Medical treatment** We found no RCTs of medical treatment versus placebo. One RCT comparing intravenous cefoxitin versus intravenous gentamicin plus intravenous clindamycin found no significant difference in rates of clinical cure. Observational studies in people with acute diverticulitis have found low mortality rates with medical treatment, but found that recurrence rates may be high.
- **Surgery** We found no RCTs of surgery versus no surgery or versus medical treatment. One RCT comparing acute resection versus no acute resection (involving a transverse colostomy) of the sigmoid colon found no significant difference in mortality rates. A second RCT comparing primary versus secondary sigmoid colonic resection found no significant difference in mortality rates, but found that primary resection significantly reduced rates of postoperative peritonitis (NNT 5, 95% CI 3 to 12) and emergency reoperation (NNT 7, 95% CI 4 to 35).

DEFINITION Colonic diverticula are mucosal out pouchings through the large bowel wall. They are often accompanied by structural changes (elastosis of the taenia coli, muscular thickening, and mucosal folding). They are usually multiple and occur most frequently in the sigmoid colon.

INCIDENCE/ PREVALENCE In the UK, the incidence of diverticulosis (see glossary, p 443) increases with age; about 5% of people are affected in their fifth decade of life and about 50% by their ninth decade.[1] Diverticulosis is common in developed countries, although there is a lower prevalence of diverticulosis in western vegetarians consuming a diet high in roughage.[2] Diverticulosis is almost unknown in rural Africa and Asia.[3]

AETIOLOGY/ RISK FACTORS There is an association between low fibre diets and diverticulosis of the colon.[3] Prospective observational studies have found that both physical activity and a high fibre diet are associated with a lower risk of developing diverticular disease (see glossary, p 443).[4,5] One case control study found an association between the ingestion of non-steroidal anti-inflammatory drugs and the development of severe diverticula complications including pericolic abscess, generalised peritonitis, bleeding, and fistula formation.[6] People in Japan, Singapore, and Thailand develop diverticula that affect predominantly the right side of the colon.[7]

PROGNOSIS Symptoms will develop in 10–25% of people with diverticula at some point in their lives.[1] It is unclear why some people develop symptoms and some do not. Even after successful medical treatment of acute diverticulitis (see glossary, p 443) almost two thirds of people suffer recurrent pain in the lower abdomen.[8] Recurrent diverticulitis is observed in 7–42% of people with diverticular disease, and once recovered from the initial attack the calculated yearly risk of suffering a further episode is 3%.[9] About half of recurrences occur within 1 year of the initial episode and 90% occur within 5 years.[10] Complications of diverticular disease (perforation, obstruction, haemorrhage, and fistula formation) are each seen in about 5% of people with colonic diverticula when followed up for between 10 and 30 years.[11] Intra-abdominal abscess formation may also occur.

AIMS	To reduce mortality, symptoms, and complications, with minimal adverse effects.
OUTCOMES	Subjective gastrointestinal symptoms assessed by the use of validated questionnaires. Admission and readmission rates as a result of diverticular disease and its complications. Incidence of diverticulitis, haemorrhage, perforation, abscess, fistula formation, and mortality. Stool weight and transit time are surrogate outcomes.
METHODS	*Clinical Evidence* update search and appraisal January 2002.

QUESTION What are the effects of a high fibre diet to prevent complications of diverticular disease?

We found no RCTs of advice to consume a high fibre diet or of dietary fibre supplementation versus placebo.

Benefits: We found no systematic review and no RCTs.

Harms: We found no evidence.

Comment: None.

QUESTION What are the effects of treatments for uncomplicated diverticular disease?

OPTION BRAN AND ISPAGHULA HUSK

Two RCTs found no consistent effect of bran or ispaghula husk versus placebo on symptom relief after 12–16 weeks.

Benefits: **Versus placebo:** We found no systematic review but found two RCTs of fibre supplements versus placebo.[12,13] The first RCT (76 people with uncomplicated diverticular disease (see glossary, p 443), no other gastrointestinal disorders, and no prior abdominal operations) compared three treatments: bran crispbread (6.99 g fibre daily); ispaghula husk drink (a bulk forming laxative; 9.04 g fibre daily); and placebo (2.34 g fibre daily).[12] It found no significant differences between the three treatments in pain score, lower bowel symptom score (combination of the pain score and sensation of incomplete emptying, straining, stool consistency, flatus, and aperients taken), or total symptom score (including nausea, vomiting, dyspepsia, belching, and abdominal distension; see comment below) after 16 weeks. The RCT also found that both active treatments versus placebo significantly improved straining at stool (bran *v* placebo, $P < 0.01$; ispaghula husk *v* placebo, $P < 0.001$; CI not provided), increased wet stool weight (both active treatments *v* placebo, $P < 0.001$; CI not provided) and stool frequency (both active treatments *v* placebo, $P < 0.001$; CI not provided), and significantly softened the stools (both active treatments *v* placebo, $P < 0.001$; CI not provided) after 16 weeks. The second RCT (18 people with radiologically confirmed diverticula and no other colonic disorder) compared bran crispbread (6.7 g fibre daily) versus placebo crispbread (0.6 g fibre daily).[13] It found that bran crispbread significantly improved total symptom score (RR and CI not provided; $P < 0.002$) and pain score (RR and CI not provided; $P < 0.02$), but found no significant difference in the scores for bowel dysfunction (passage of excessive wind per rectum, need to strain, frequency of evacuation, consistency of motion, presence of anal pain on defaecation, feeling of incomplete evacuation, presence of blood or mucus, use of laxatives) or dyspeptic symptoms (nausea, vomiting, heartburn, belching, and abdominal distension) after 3 months.

Harms: No significant adverse effects were reported in the RCTs.[12,13]

Comment: In the first RCT, 18/76 (24%) people withdrew from the trial and analysis of data was not by intention to treat.[12] The RCT did not specify the exact number of people receiving each treatment, thus precluding calculations of relative risk and confidence interval. People in both RCTs had been investigated to exclude coexisting abdominal pathology but the extent of the investigations was not stated.[12,13] Both studies were small in size, of short duration, and the difference in fibre content between control and treatment interventions was also small. Both treatment and control groups improved during the RCTs. One further RCT has been identified and is awaiting translation.[14]

OPTION METHYLCELLULOSE

One RCT found no significant difference with methylcellulose versus placebo on mean symptom score after 3 months.

Benefits: We found no systematic review but found one RCT (30 people with symptomatic diverticular disease [see glossary, p 443] and no other gastrointestinal disease) that compared methylcellulose (500 mg twice daily) versus placebo.[15] It found no significant difference between treatments on mean symptom score after 3 months (see comment below; mean symptom score 13.0 with methylcellulose *v* 16.7 with placebo; difference in means –3.7, 95% CI –8.9 to +1.5).

Harms: None reported.

Comment: The RCT used a categorical scale for a number of different symptoms where 1 = mild and 6 = severe.[15] The score used to assess symptoms and signs was not clearly described, but included barium enema results. The RCT was small, of short duration, and both the methylcellulose and placebo treatments were associated with an improvement in symptom scores. Diverticular disease was confirmed by barium enema but the extent of any other investigations to exclude comorbidity was not stated.

OPTION LACTULOSE

One RCT found no significant difference with lactulose versus a high fibre diet in the number of people who considered themselves to be "much improved" (not defined) after 12 weeks.

Benefits: We found no systematic review. **Versus placebo:** We found no RCTs. **Versus high fibre diet:** We found one RCT (43 people with diverticular disease (see glossary, p 443) and no other abdominal pathology) comparing lactulose (15 mL twice daily) versus a high fibre diet (30–40 g fibre daily).[16] It found no significant difference in the number of people who reported their symptoms to be much improved after 12 weeks (see comment below; 7/20 [35%] people with lactulose v 9/21 [43%] people with high fibre diet; RR 0.8, 95% CI 0.34 to 1.77).

Harms: The RCT found that a high fibre diet versus lactulose increased the number of people with new symptoms during the trial period, although the difference was not significant (12/21 [57%] people with high fibre diet v 9/20 [45%] people with lactulose; RR 1.3, 95% CI 0.70 to 2.34).[16] The symptoms were described as minor but no further details were provided. The RCT found that 2/20 (10%) people taking lactulose withdrew from the trial because of symptoms, one with abdominal pain and one with nausea.

Comment: Although "much improved" was used as an outcome by the RCT, this term was not clearly defined.[16] People were investigated to exclude coexisting abdominal pathology but the extent of the investigations was not stated.

OPTION ANTIBIOTICS (RIFAXIMIN)

One RCT has found that rifaximin plus glucomannan versus glucomannan plus placebo significantly increases the number of people who are symptom free after 12 months of treatment.

Benefits: We found no systematic review but found one RCT.[17] The RCT (168 people with uncomplicated diverticular disease [see glossary, p 443]) compared dietary fibre supplementation (glucomannan 2 g daily) plus oral rifaximin (400 mg twice daily) (see glossary, p 443) versus dietary fibre supplementation (glucomannan 2 g daily) plus placebo. Both treatments were given for 7 days each month for 1 year (see comment below). The RCT found that dietary fibre supplementation plus rifaximin significantly increased the number of people with no symptoms or only mild symptoms after 12 months of treatment (69% of people with rifaximin v 39% of people with placebo; $P = 0.001$; results presented graphically; absolute numbers not provided). The RCT found no significant difference between treatments in the severity of diarrhoea, tenesmus, or upper abdominal pain (absolute data and significance testing not provided).

Harms: The RCT did not report on harms.[17]

Comment: The RCT reported that 17/168 (10%) people did not complete the trial, although analysis was not by intention to treat.[17] For each treatment group, 2/84 (2%) people were withdrawn because of acute diverticulitis (see glossary, p 443).

OPTION ELECTIVE SURGERY

We found no RCTs of elective colonic resection (open or laparoscopic).

Benefits: We found no systematic review or RCTs.

Harms: We found no data on harms of elective surgery in people with diverticular disease (see glossary, p 443).

Comment: None.

QUESTION **What are the effects of treatments for acute diverticulitis?**

OPTION **MEDICAL TREATMENT**

We found no RCTs of medical treatment versus placebo. One RCT found no significant difference with intravenous cefoxitin versus intravenous gentamicin plus intravenous clindamycin in rates of clinical cure. Observational studies in people with acute diverticulitis have found low mortality rates with medical treatment but that recurrence rates may be high.

Benefits: We found no systematic review. **Versus placebo:** We found no RCTs. **Versus other medical treatments:** We found one RCT (51 people with a clinical diagnosis of acute diverticulitis (see glossary, p 443) who did not need immediate surgery) that compared intravenous cefoxitin (1–2 g every 6 h) versus intravenous gentamicin (1.7 mg/kg loading dose followed by 1–1.4 mg/kg every 8 h) plus intravenous clindamycin (total dose of 2400–2700 mg/day in 3 or 4 equal doses).[18] It found no significant difference in clinical cure rate (see comment below; 27/30 [90%] people with cefoxitin *v* 18/21 [86%] people with gentamicin plus clindamycin; RR 1.1, 95% CI 0.85 to 1.30).

Harms: In the RCT, toxicity (possibly antibiotic related) occurred with both treatments, although the numbers of people affected were not significantly different between treatments (2/30 [7%] people with cefoxitin *v* 3/21 [14%] people with gentamicin plus clindamycin; RR 0.47, 95% CI 0.09 to 2.56).[18]

Comment: Clinical cure was defined as complete resolution of symptoms and signs associated with diverticulitis plus discharge from hospital without recurrence for at least 6 weeks or plus having undergone an elective surgical procedure with primary anastomosis in the absence of colostomy without septic complications.[18] We found many observational studies of medical treatment for acute diverticulitis, with variable follow up periods (1–12 years), which consistently report low mortality rates (0–5%).[9,19–21] These observational trials also reported that 7–42% of people treated medically suffer recurrent episodes of acute diverticulitis.

OPTION **SURGERY**

One RCT found no significant difference with acute sigmoid colonic resection versus no acute resection (involving a transverse colostomy) in mortality rates. Subgroup analysis found that for people with purulent rather than faecal peritonitis, acute sigmoid colonic resection may increase mortality. A second RCT found no significant difference with primary versus secondary sigmoid colonic resection in mortality rates, but found that primary sigmoid colonic resection significantly reduced rates of postoperative peritonitis and emergency reoperation.

Benefits: We found no systematic review. **Surgery versus placebo or medical treatment:** We found no RCTs. **Open surgery versus other types of open surgery:** We found two RCTs.[22,23] The first

RCT (62 people with diffuse peritonitis complicating perforated acute diverticulitis (see glossary, p 443) of the left colon; median age 72 years) compared acute sigmoid colonic resection (with end colostomy of the proximal bowel and for the distal bowel formation of a mucus fistula or oversewing of the rectal stump) versus no acute resection (acute transverse colostomy, suture, and omental covering of a visible perforation).[22] The RCT found no significant difference with acute sigmoid colonic resection versus no acute resection in mortality within 30 days (8/31 [26%] people with acute resection *v* 6/31 [19%] people with no acute resection; RR 1.3, 95% CI 0.52 to 3.39). However, subgroup analysis of people with purulent peritonitis (46 people) found that acute sigmoid colonic resection versus no acute resection significantly increased post-operative mortality (6/25 [24%] people with acute resection *v* 0/21 [0%] people with no acute resection; ARI 24%, 95% CI 4.5% to 44%). Subgroup analysis of people with faecal peritonitis (16 people) found no significant difference with acute sigmoid colonic resection versus no acute resection in postoperative mortality (2/6 [33%] people with acute resection *v* 6/10 [60%] people with no acute resection; RR 0.6, 95% CI 0.16 to 1.92; see comment below). The second RCT (105 people with generalised peritonitis complicating sigmoid diverticulitis; mean age 66 years) compared primary versus secondary sigmoid colonic resection.[23] Primary resection involved surgical removal of the affected sigmoid colon plus either formation of an end colostomy or alternatively formation of a primary colorectal anastomosis with or without a proximal defunctioning colostomy. Secondary resection involved closing any visible bowel perforations initially plus the formation of a defunctioning colostomy. A second (definitive) procedure was then undertaken at a later date to perform a sigmoid colon resection plus a colorectal anastomosis with or without a defunctioning colostomy. The RCT found that primary versus secondary sigmoid colonic resection significantly reduced rates of postoperative peritonitis following the initial procedure (1/55 [2%] people with primary resection *v* 10/44 [23%] people with secondary resection; RR 0.09, 95% CI 0.01 to 0.70; NNT 5, 95% CI 3 to 12) and significantly reduced rates of emergency reoperation (2/55 [4%] people with primary resection *v* 9/48 [19%] people with secondary resection; RR 0.19, 95% CI 0.04 to 0.90; NNT 7, 95% CI 4 to 35). The RCT found no significant difference between treatments in mortality rate (13/55 [24%] people with primary resection *v* 9/48 [19%] people with secondary resection; RR 1.3, 95% CI 0.60 to 2.70; see comment below). **Open surgery versus laparoscopic surgery:** We found no RCTs.

Harms: The first RCT found no significant difference between treatments in rates of cardiopulmonary complications (13/31 [42%] with acute resection *v* 14/31 [45%] with no acute resection; RR 0.9, 95% CI 0.53 to 1.63), thromboembolism (3/31 [9.7%] with acute resection *v* 5/31 [16%] with no acute resection; RR 0.6, 95% CI 0.16 to 2.30), mental confusion (4/31 [13%] with acute resection *v* 4/31 [13%] with no acute resection; RR 1.0, 95% CI 0.27 to 3.65), or other complications (including wound dehiscence, wound infection but no dehiscence, intraperitoneal abscess formation, ileus, colocutaneous fistula, and revision of colostomy).[22] The second RCT found no significant difference between treatments in rates of wound complications (20/55 [36%] with primary resection *v* 23/48 [48%] with secondary resection; RR 0.8, 95% CI 0.48 to 1.20), rates of extra-abdominal septic complications (11/55 [20%] with primary resection *v* 12/48 [25%] with secondary resection; RR 0.8, 95% CI 0.39 to 1.65) or rates of extra-abdominal non-septic complications (26/55 [47%] with primary resection *v* 21/48 [44%] with secondary resection; RR 1.08, 95% CI 0.71 to 1.65).[23]

Comment: The first RCT was conducted in a single centre and took 14 years to recruit 62 people.[22] The second RCT was conducted in 17 centres and took 7 years to recruit 105 people.[23] Both studies were small and may have lacked the power to detect a significant difference between treatments. The high complication rates reported are not unexpected in predominantly elderly people following a perforation of the large bowel. The wide spectrum of presentation and operative treatment options for acute complicated diverticulitis makes RCTs difficult to perform.

GLOSSARY

Acute diverticulitis This condition occurs when a diverticulum becomes acutely inflamed. There may be general symptoms and signs of infection (including fever and rapid heart rate) with or without local symptoms and signs (pain and localised tenderness, usually in the lower left abdomen, sometimes with a mass that can be felt on abdominal or rectal examination).

Diverticular disease This term is used to describe diverticula associated with any symptoms.[24] Symptoms commonly include abdominal pain and alteration in bowel habit. Diverticular disease may be complicated by abscess formation, fistulae, perforation, obstruction, or haemorrhage.

Diverticulosis The presence of diverticula that are asymptomatic. Most people with sigmoid colonic diverticula have no symptoms.

Rifaximin A rifamycin antibacterial drug with antimicrobial actions similar to those of rifampicin. It is marketed predominantly in Italy.

REFERENCES

1. Parks TG. Natural history of diverticular disease of the colon. *Clin Gastroenterol* 1975;4:53–69.
2. Gear JS, Ware A, Fursdon P, et al. Symptomless diverticular disease and intake of dietary fibre. *Lancet* 1979;1:511–514.
3. Painter NS, Burkitt DP. Diverticular disease of the colon, a 20th century problem. *Clin Gastroenterol* 1975;4:3–21.
4. Aldoori WH, Giovannucci EL, Rimm EB, et al. Prospective study of physical activity and the risk of symptomatic diverticular disease in men. *Gut* 1995;36:276–282.
5. Aldoori WH, Giovannucci EL, Rimm EB, Wing AL, Trichopoulos DV, Willett WC. A prospective study of diet and the risk of symptomatic diverticular disease in men. *Am J Clin Nutr* 1994;60:757–764.
6. Campbell K, Steele RJ. Non-steroidal anti-inflammatory drugs and complicated diverticular disease: a case-control study. *Br J Surg* 1991;78:190–191.
7. Sugihara K, Muto T, Morioka Y, Asano A, Yamamoto T. Diverticular disease of the colon in Japan. A review of 615 cases. *Dis Colon Rectum* 1984;27:531–537.
8. Munson KD, Hensien MA, Jacob LN, Robinson AM, Liston WA. Diverticulitis. A comprehensive follow-up. *Dis Colon Rectum* 1996;39:318–322.
9. Haglund U, Hellberg R, Johnsen C, Hulten L. Complicated diverticular disease of the sigmoid colon. An analysis of short and long term outcome in 392 patients. *Ann Chir Gynaecol* 1979;68:41–46.
10. Parks TG, Connell AM. The outcome in 455 patients admitted for treatment of diverticular disease of the colon. *Br J Surg* 1970;57:775–778.
11. Boles RS, Jordon SM. The clinical significance of diverticulosis. *Gastroenterology* 1958;35:579–581.
12. Ornstein MH, Littlewood ER, Baird IM, Fowler J, North WR, Cox AG. Are fibre supplements really necessary in diverticular disease of the colon? A controlled clinical trial. *BMJ* 1981;282:1353–1356.
13. Brodribb AJ. Treatment of symptomatic diverticular disease with a high-fibre diet. *Lancet* 1977;1:664–666.
14. Darnis F, Souillac P. Treatment of functional colonic diseases and colonic diverticulosis. Comparative effects of bran and Kaologeais using a crossover method [in French]. *Med Chir Dig* 1980;9:435–437.
15. Hodgson WJ. The placebo effect. Is it important in diverticular disease? *Am J Gastroenterol* 1977;67:157–162.

16. Smits BJ, Whitehead AM, Prescott P. Lactulose in the treatment of symptomatic diverticular disease: a comparative study with high-fibre diet. *Br J Clin Pract* 1990;44:314–318.
17. Papi C, Ciaco A, Koch M, Capurso L. Efficacy of rifaximin in the treatment of symptomatic diverticular disease of the colon. A multicentre double-blind placebo-controlled trial. *Aliment Pharmacol Ther* 1995;9:33–39.
18. Kellum JM, Sugerman HJ, Coppa GF, et al. Randomized, prospective comparison of cefoxitin and gentamicin–clindamycin in the treatment of acute colonic diverticulitis. *Clin Ther* 1992;14:376–384.
19. Larson DM, Masters SS, Spiro HM. Medical and surgical therapy in diverticular disease: a comparative study. *Gastroenterology* 1976;71:734–737.
20. Sarin S, Boulos PB. Long-term outcome of patients presenting with acute complications of diverticular disease. *Ann R Coll Surg Engl* 1994;76:117–120.
21. Farthmann EH, Ruckauer KD, Haring RU. Evidence-based surgery: diverticulitis–a surgical disease? *Langenbecks Arch Surg* 2000;385:143–151.
22. Kronborg O. Treatment of perforated sigmoid diverticulitis: a prospective randomised trial. *Br J Surg* 1993;80:505–507.
23. Zeitoun G, Laurent A, Rouffet F, et al, and the French Association for Surgical Research. Multicentre, randomized clinical trial of primary versus secondary sigmoid resection in generalized peritonitis complicating sigmoid diverticulitis. *Br J Surg* 2000;87:1366–1374.
24. Kohler L, Sauerland S, Neugebauer E. Diagnosis and treatment of diverticular disease: results of a consensus development conference. The Scientific Committee of the European Association for Endoscopic Surgery. *Surg Endosc* 1999;13:430–436.

John Simpson

Robin Spiller
Division of Gastroenterology
University Hospital Nottingham
UK

Competing interests: None declared.

Colorectal cancer

Search date April 2002

Charles Maxwell-Armstrong and John Scholefield

QUESTIONS

INTERVENTIONS

To be covered in future updates
Surgery
Colonoscopic polypectomy
Immunotherapy
Specialist versus generalist surgical care
Liver resection for metastases

See glossary, p 450

Key Messages

- **Adjuvant chemotherapy** Three systematic reviews and one subsequent RCT have found that adjuvant chemotherapy significantly reduces mortality compared with surgery alone in people with Dukes' A, B, and C colorectal cancer. One RCT found that adding levamisole to adjuvant fluoruracil did not reduce mortality or recurrence rate compared with adjuvant fluorouracil alone in people with Dukes' A, B, and C colorectal cancer. One RCT found mortality or recurrence rates were similar with adjuvant fluorouracil plus high or low dose folinic acid in people with Dukes' A, B, and C colorectal cancer.
- **Preoperative radiotherapy** One systematic review found that preoperative radiotherapy reduced mortality and local recurrence compared with no radiotherapy, but a second systematic review and two subsequent RCTs found no significant difference with preoperative versus no radiotherapy. One RCT found that preoperative versus postoperative radiotherapy did not reduce mortality but preoperative radiotherapy significantly reduced local tumour recurrence. One systematic review has found that preoperative radiotherapy significantly increases postoperative morbidity.
- **Routine follow up** One systematic review and one additional RCT found conflicting evidence on the effects of routine follow up.
- **Total mesorectal excision** We found no RCTs of total mesorectal excision in people with rectal cancer. Observational studies suggest that total mesorectal excision may reduce the rate of local recurrence compared with conventional surgery.

Colorectal cancer

DEFINITION Colorectal cancer is a malignant neoplasm arising from the lining (mucosa) of the large intestine (colon and rectum). Nearly two thirds of colorectal cancers occur in the rectum or sigmoid colon. Colorectal cancer may be categorised as A, B, or C Dukes' (see glossary, p 450).

INCIDENCE/ PREVALENCE Colorectal cancer is the third most common malignancy in the developed world. It accounts for about 20 000 deaths each year in the UK and 60 000 deaths each year in the USA. Although the incidence of, and mortality from, colorectal cancer has changed little over the past 40 years, the incidence of the disease has fallen recently in both the UK and the USA.[1,2] In the UK, about a quarter of people with colorectal cancer present as emergencies with either intestinal obstruction or perforation.[3,4]

AETIOLOGY/ RISK FACTORS Colon cancer affects almost equal proportions of men and women, most commonly between the ages of 60 and 80 years. Rectal cancer is more common in men.[1] The pathogenesis of colorectal cancer involves genetic and environmental factors. The most important environmental factor is probably diet.[5]

PROGNOSIS Overall 5 year survival is about 50% and has not changed over the past 40 years. Disease specific mortality in both USA and UK cancer registries is decreasing but the reasons for this are unclear.[1,2] Surgery is undertaken with curative intent in over 80% of people, but about half suffer recurrence.

AIMS To reduce morbidity (e.g. bowel obstruction or perforation) and mortality associated with the tumour; to minimise adverse effects of treatment (e.g. avoiding permanent stoma by restoring intestinal continuity); to maximise quality of life.

OUTCOMES Survival; proportion of people with permanent stoma; incidence of local recurrence; rates of metastasis; adverse effects of treatment; quality of life.

METHODS *Clinical Evidence* update search and appraisal April 2002.

QUESTION What are the effects of adjuvant chemotherapy in people with colorectal cancer?

Three systematic reviews and one subsequent RCT have found that adjuvant chemotherapy significantly reduces mortality compared with surgery alone in people with Dukes' A, B, and C colorectal cancer. One RCT found that adding levamisole to adjuvant fluoruracil did not reduce mortality or recurrence rate compared with adjuvant fluorouracil alone in people with Dukes' A, B, and C colorectal cancer. One RCT found mortality or recurrence rates were similar with adjuvant fluorouracil plus high or low dose folinic acid in people with Dukes' A, B, and C colorectal cancer.

Benefits: **Versus placebo or no treatment:** We found three systematic reviews[6–8] and one subsequent RCT.[9] The first systematic review (search date 1993, 39 RCTs, 1673 people with Dukes' C colon cancer and 695 with Dukes' B or C rectal [see glossary, p 450]) found that adjuvant chemotherapy versus surgery alone significantly reduced mortality after 5 years (OR 0.91, 95% CI 0.83 to 0.99).[6] The second systematic review (search date not stated, 10 RCTs, 3088 people with Dukes' A, B, or C colorectal cancer) compared 1 week of portal vein infusion of fluorouracil within 5–7 days of surgery with no further treatment after surgery.[7] It found that portal vein infusion of fluorouracil significantly reduced mortality (6 year mortality 38% *v* 44%; RR 0.87, 95% CI 0.80 to 0.94; NNT 17, 95% CI 11 to 41). The third systematic review (search date not stated, 7 RCTs, 3437 people with Dukes' B or C colorectal cancer) compared adjuvant treatment with intravenous fluorouracil (plus leucovorin or levamisole) versus surgery alone.[8] It found that adjuvant fluorouracil based treatment significantly reduced mortality and significantly increased the number of people without recurrence at 5 years: 71% with fluorouracil based treatment *v* 64% with surgery alone; HR 0.76, 95% CI 0.68 to 0.85; recurrence free rate: 69% with fluorouracil based treatment *v* 58% with surgery alone; HR 0.68, 95% CI 0.60 to 0.76). The subsequent RCT (1029 people with Dukes' B or C colorectal cancer) compared adjuvant fluorouracil plus levamisole for 1 year versus surgery alone.[9] It found that adding fluorouracil and levamisole reduced mortality compared with surgery alone at 5 years (AR of survival 68% with fluorouracil based treatment *v* 58% with surgery alone; P = 0.007). **Fluorouracil plus levamisole versus fluorouracil alone:** We found one RCT (4927 people with Dukes' A, B, or C colorectal cancer and no residual disease following surgery) that compared chemotherapy with levamisole plus intravenous fluorouracil and folinic acid versus intravenous fluorouracil and folinic acid alone.[10] It found no significant difference in mortality or recurrence rate after 3 years (mortality: OR 1.10, 95% CI 1.00 to 1.22; recurrence: OR 1.00, 95% CI 0.97 to 1.13). **Low versus high dose folinic acid:** We found one RCT (4927 people with Dukes' A, B, or C colorectal cancer and no residual disease following surgery) that compared high dose folinic acid with low dose folinic acid in people given intravenous fluoruracil.[10] It found no significant difference in mortality or recurrence rate after 3 years (mortality: OR 1.04, 95% CI 0.94 to 1.15; recurrence: OR 1.00, 95% CI 0.91 to 1.09).

Harms: We found little good evidence on the harms of adjuvant chemotherapy in the treatment of colorectal cancer. In the first systematic review, the incidence of severe adverse effects (stomatitis, diarrhoea, nausea, and leukopenia) with fluorouracil and levamisole ranged from 10–30%, with life threatening toxicity occurring in about 5% of people.[6] For every 10 people treated, about three will experience an additional, severe adverse effect.[10,11]

Comment: In the UK, people aged over 75 years are not routinely considered for chemotherapy because of its potential toxicity, although we found no evidence to support or refute this policy.

QUESTION **What are the effects of preoperative radiotherapy in people with rectal cancer?**

Two systematic reviews and two subsequent RCTs found conflicting results about the effects of preoperative radiotherapy on mortality and recurrence compared with surgery alone. One RCT found that preoperative versus postoperative radiotherapy did not reduce mortality but preoperative radiotherapy significantly reduced local tumour recurrence. One systematic review has found that preoperative radiotherapy significantly increases postoperative morbidity.

Benefits: **Versus surgery alone:** We found two systematic reviews[12,13] and two subsequent RCTs.[14,15] The first systematic review (search date 1999, 14 RCTs, 5974 people) found that preoperative radiotherapy versus no preoperative radiotherapy significantly reduced mortality and local recurrence at 5 years (mortality: OR 0.84, 95% CI 0.72 to 0.98, NNT 25; local recurrence: 11 RCTs, 4494 people, OR 0.49, 95% CI 0.38 to 0.62, NNT 10).[12] It found no significant difference in risk of distant metastases at 5 years (OR 0.93, 95% CI 0.73 to 1.18). The second systematic review (search date not stated, 19 RCTs, 6623 people) found no significant difference with preoperative radiotherapy versus no preoperative radiotherapy in yearly death rates (RR 0.94; P = 0.09; CI not stated).[13] The first subsequent RCT (1861 people) compared preoperative radiotherapy plus total mesorectal excision versus total mesorectal excision alone.[14] It found that radiotherapy did not reduce mortality or overall recurrence rate at 2 years (mortality: HR 1.02, 95% CI 0.83 to 1.25; recurrence: 16% with radiotherapy *v* 21% with surgery alone; HR 1.21, 95% CI 0.97 to 1.52). The second subsequent RCT (557 people) found that radiotherapy versus surgery did not significantly reduce mortality or distant metastasis, but significantly reduced local recurrence after 10 years (mortality: HR 0.87, 95% CI 0.71 to 1.08; distant metastasis: HR 0.97, 95% CI 0.73 to 1.28; local recurrence: 0.46, 95% CI 0.31 to 0.69).[15] **Versus postoperative radiotherapy:** We found one RCT (415 people with Dukes' [see glossary, p 450] B or C rectal carcinoma) that compared preoperative radiotherapy (25.5 Gy in 1 wk) with postoperative radiotherapy (60.0 Gy over 7–8 wks).[16] It found no significant difference in 5 year survival, but preoperative radiotherapy significantly reduced local tumour recurrence after 5 years (survival: P = 0.5; results presented graphically; absolute numbers not provided; local recurrence: 13% with preoperative *v* 22% with postoperative radiotherapy; RR 0.59, 95% CI 0.37 to 0.91; NNT 11, 95% CI 7 to 49).

Harms: **Versus surgery alone:** We found one systematic review (search date 1998, 19 RCTs, 5110 people) of harms associated with preoperative adjuvant radiotherapy.[17] It found that preoperative radiotherapy increased early postoperative morbidity and mortality. Early harms included diarrhoea, wound infections (20% with preoperative radiotherapy *v* 10% with surgery alone), bowel obstruction, cardiovascular problems, and pain. In people with low rectal tumours who underwent abdominoperineal excision, preoperative radiotherapy versus surgery alone increased the rate of perineal wound breakdown (20% *v* 10%). Two RCTs (1027 people) identified by the review found that preoperative radiotherapy versus surgery alone significantly increased the risk of venous thromboembolism, fracture of the hip, intestinal obstruction, postoperative fistulae, cardiovascular events, and thrombotic events.[18] One observational study (171 people) found that preoperative radiotherapy versus surgery increased bowel frequency and urgency, impairing social life in about 30% of people.[19] One RCT (1531 people) found that preoperative radiotherapy versus surgery alone increased perioperative blood loss and perineal complications, but found no significant difference in perioperative mortality (mean perioperative blood loss 100 mL greater with radiotherapy; perineal complication rate 29% *v* 18%; P = 0.008).[20] **Versus postoperative**

radiotherapy: We found one systematic review (search date 1998, 9 RCTs) of harms associated with preoperative versus postoperative radiotherapy.[17] It found that postoperative versus preoperative radiotherapy increased anastomotic complications (breakdown and stricture formation).

Comment: There is limited evidence of modest improvement in survival following preoperative radiotherapy compared with surgery alone for rectal cancer. There is some evidence of an improvement in local recurrence but the risk of local recurrence for Dukes' A tumours is so low that preoperative radiotherapy is unlikely to provide much absolute benefit. There are unresolved issues about preoperative staging of rectal cancers and case selection for preoperative radiotherapy.

QUESTION What are the effects of routine follow up in people with colorectal cancer?

One systematic review and one additional RCT found conflicting evidence on the effects of routine follow up.

Benefits: We found one systematic review[21] and one additional RCT.[22] The systematic review (search date not stated, 5 RCTs, 1055 people; see comment below) compared intensive follow up versus less intensive or no follow up.[21] Four of the RCTs identified by the review found no significant difference in mortality, and one RCT found that intensive follow up significantly reduced mortality (absolute numbers not provided). The additional RCT (1418 people who had undergone removal of adenomatous polyps) compared follow up colonoscopy at 1 and 3 years versus 3 years only.[22] Follow up at 1 and 3 years significantly increased the number of people found to have new polyps (42% *v* 32%; RR of detection 1.3, 95% CI 1.1 to 1.6), but found no significant difference in the proportion of detected polyps with advanced pathology (about 3% in both groups; RR 1.0, 95% CI 0.5 to 2.2).

Harms: We found no evidence about harms.

Comment: In the systematic review, intensive follow up and less intensive follow up were not clearly defined.[21] One included RCT (212 people being followed up after treatment for colorectal cancer) found that follow up increased feelings of reassurance but not quality of life.[23] Most people in the trial said that they would still prefer follow up even if it did not lead to earlier detection of recurrence. Current follow up regimens are variable in frequency and intensity. We found no evidence on whether follow up should be stopped in elderly people (aged > 75 years), although many people with colorectal cancer are in this age group. The role of carcino-embryonic antigen monitoring is also uncertain.

QUESTION What are the effects of total mesorectal excision in people with rectal cancer?

We found no RCTs of total mesorectal excision in people with rectal cancer. Observational studies suggest that total mesorectal excision may reduce the rate of local recurrence compared with conventional surgery.

Colorectal cancer

Benefits: We found no systematic review or RCTs.

Harms: Following total mesorectal excision (see glossary, p 450) more people experienced increased stool frequency compared with techniques leaving a rectal stump (median 4–5 daily *v* 1–2 daily). Observational studies have found that there is a higher incidence of anastomotic leakage with total mesorectal excision (11–15% *v* 8–10%).[24]

Comment: One observational study (441 people) compared local recurrence rates before and after the introduction of total mesorectal excision (see table 1, p 452).[25] It found that local recurrence rates 1 year after surgery fell after the introduction of total mesorectal excision (4% before total mesorectal excision *v* 9% after). Several other observational studies have found similar results (see table 1, p 452).[24,26,27] Total mesorectal excision requires coloanal anastomosis, which may be important in the surgical treatment of rectal cancer.[25,26,28] Many surgeons routinely use a temporary defunctioning stoma after total mesorectal excision in an attempt to reduce the clinical consequences of anastomotic leakage.[25]

GLOSSARY

Dukes' classification Dukes' original classification of the pathological stages of carcinoma of the colon and rectum includes three stages: A, limited to mucosa and submucosa; B, penetration of the entire bowel wall and serosa or pericolic fat; C, stages A and B, and invasion into the regional draining lymph node system.[29] More recently, stage D has been proposed to classify patients with advanced and widespread regional involvement (metastasis).

Total mesorectal excision Removal of the entire rectal mesentery along with the rectum by sharp dissection.

Substantive changes

Adjuvant chemotherapy One new systematic review;[8] conclusions unchanged.
Adjuvant chemotherapy One new RCT;[9] conclusions unchanged.
Preoperative radiotherapy for rectal cancer One new systematic review and two new subsequent RCTs;[13–15] conclusions unchanged.

REFERENCES

1. Office of Population Censuses and Surveys. *Mortality statistics, cause, England and Wales 1993*. dh22. London: HMSO, 1995.
2. Miller BA, Ries LA, Hankey BF, et al. *Cancer statistics review 1973–1989*. Rockville, MD: National Institutes of Health, National Cancer Institute. Report No: NIH-NCI 92–2789.
3. Mella J, Biffen A, Radcliffe AG, et al. A population based on audit of colorectal cancer management in two United Kingdom health districts. *Br J Surg* 1997;84:1731–1736.
4. Scholefield JH, Robinson MHE, Mangham C, et al. Screening for colorectal cancer reduces emergency admissions. *Eur J Surg Oncol* 1998;24:47–50.
5. Kune G, ed. *Causes and control of colorectal cancer: a model for cancer prevention*. Boston: Kluwer Academic Publishers, 1996.
6. Dube S, Heyen F, Jenicek M. Adjuvant chemotherapy in colorectal carcinoma. Results of a meta analysis. *Dis Colon Rectum* 1997;40:35–41. Search date 1993; primary source Medline.
7. Liver Infusion Meta-analysis Group. Portal vein chemotherapy for colorectal cancer: a meta-analysis of 4000 patients in 10 studies. *J Natl Cancer Inst* 1997;89:497–505. Search date not stated; primary sources Medline, Cancerlit, Excerpta Medica, and hand searched books, journals, and registers of trials.
8. Sargent DJ, Goldberg RM, Jacobson SD, et al. A pooled analysis of adjuvant chemotherapy for resected colon cancer in elderly patients. *N Eng J Med* 2001;345:1091–1097. Search date not stated; primary sources Medline, bibliographies, and early trials leaders.
9. Taal BG, Van Tinteren H, Zoetmulder FA, et al. Adjuvant 5FU plus levamisole in colonic or rectal cancer: improved survival in stage II and III. *B J Cancer* 2001;85:1437–1443.
10. QUASAR Collaborative Group. Comparison of fluorouracil with additional levamisole, higher dose folinic acid or both as adjuvant chemotherapy for colorectal cancer: a randomised trial. *Lancet* 2000;355:1588–1596.
11. International Multicenter Pooled Analysis of Colon Cancer Trials (IMPACT) Investigators. Efficacy of adjuvant fluorouracil and folinic acid in colon cancer. *Lancet* 1995;345:939–944.

12. Camma C, Giunta M, Pagliaro L. Preoperative radiotherapy for resectable rectal cancer. A meta analysis. *JAMA* 2000:284:1008–1015. Search date 1999; primary sources Medline, Cancerlit, and hand searched reference lists. No company sponsorship stated.
13. Colorectal Cancer Collaborative Group. Adjuvant radiotherapy for rectal cancer: a systematic overview of 8507 patients from 22 randomised trials. *Lancet* 2001;358:1291–1304. Search date not stated; primary sources details not stated, based on the Early Breast Cancer Trialists' Collaborative Groups' methods who identified studies from: lists prepared by three international cancer research groups, hand searching meeting abstracts, consulting experts, and a computer aided literature search.
14. Kapiteijn E, Marijnen CA, Nagtegaal ID, et al. Preoperative radiotherapy combined with total mesorectal excision for resectable rectal cancer. *N Eng J Med* 2001;345:638–646.
15. Martling A, Holm T, Johansson H, et al. The Stockholm II trial on preoperative radiotherapy in rectal carcinoma: long-term follow-up of a population-based study. *Cancer* 2001;92:896–902.
16. Jansson-Frykholm G, Glimelius B, Pahlman L. Preoperative or postoperative irradiation in adenocarcinoma of the rectum. Final treatment results of a randomised trial and an evaluation of late secondary effects. *Dis Colon Rectum* 1993;36:564–572.
17. Ooi B, Tjandra J, Green M. Morbidities of adjuvant chemotherapy and radiotherapy for resectable rectal cancer: an overview. *Dis Colon Rectum* 1999;42:403–418. Search date 1998; primary source Medline.
18. Holm T, Singnomklao T, Rutqvist LE, et al. Adjuvant preoperative radiotherapy in patients with rectal carcinoma. Adverse effects during long term follow-up of two trials. *Cancer* 1996;78:968–976.
19. Dahlberg M, Glimelius B, Graf W, et al Preoperative irradiation affects functional results after surgery for rectal cancer: results from a randomised study. *Dis Colon Rectum* 1998;41:543–549.
20. Marijnen CAM, Kapiteijn E, Van de Velde CJH, et al. Acute side effects and complications after short-term preoperative radiotherapy combined with total mesorectal excision in primary rectal cancer: Report of a multicenter randomised trial. *J Clin Onc* 2002;20:817–825.
21. Kievit J. Colorectal cancer follow up: a reassessment of empirical evidence on effectiveness. *Eur J Surg Oncol* 2000;26:322–328. Search date not stated; primary source Medline. No company sponsorship stated.
22. Winawer SJ, Zauber AG, O'Brien MJ, et al. Randomised comparison of surveillance intervals after colonoscopic removal of newly diagnosed adenomatous polyps: the national polyp study workgroup. *N Engl J Med* 1993;328:901–906.
23. Stiggelbout AM, de Haes JCJM, Vree R, et al. Follow up of colorectal cancer patients: quality of life and attitudes towards follow up. *Br J Cancer* 1997;75:914–920.
24. Karanja ND, Corder AP, Bearn P, et al. Leakage from stapled low anastomosis after total mesorectal excision for carcinoma of the rectum. *Br J Surg* 1994;81:1224–1226.
25. McFarlane JK, Ryall RDH, Heald RJ. Mesorectal excision for rectal cancer. *Lancet* 1993;341:457–460.
26. Enker WE, Thaler HT, Cranor ML, et al. Total mesorectal excision in the operative treatment of carcinoma of the rectum. *J Am Coll Surg* 1995;181:335–346.
27. Singh S, Morgan MBF, Broughton M, et al. A ten-year prospective audit of outcome of surgical treatment for colorectal carcinoma. *Br J Surg* 1995;82:1486–1490.
28. Arbman G, Nilsson E, Hallbook O, et al. Local recurrence following total mesorectal excision for rectal cancer. *Br J Surg* 1996;83:375–379.
29. Dukes CE. The classification of cancer of the rectum. *J Pathol Bacteriol* 1932;35:323–332.

Charles Maxwell-Armstrong
Resident Surgical Officer
St Mark's Hospital
London
UK

John Scholefield
Professor of Surgery
University Hospital
Nottingham
UK

Competing interests: None declared.

TABLE 1 Effects of total mesorectal excision: results of non-randomised studies (see text, p 450).

Ref	Dukes' stage (number of people)	Intervention	Recurrence at 5 years (95% CI): Local	Recurrence at 5 years (95% CI): Overall	RRR of death by 5 years (95% CI)	Incidence of anastomic leak (95% CI)
24	B (88) C (73)	TME	5% (0% to 7.5%)	18% (10% to 25%)	78% (68% to 88%)	11% clinical 6.4% radiological
25	B (99) C (147)	TME	7.3%	23%	74%	NA
26	A, B, and C (158 in total)	TME	8%	24%	60%	10%
27	A (67) B (89) C (100)	TME Non-TME	6% at 1 year 14% at 1 year	NA	NA	8% (57% stoma rate) 9% (15% stoma rate)

NA, not applicable; TME, total mesorectal excision.

Helicobacter pylori infection

Search date April 2002

Brendan Delaney, Paul Moayyedi, and David Forman

QUESTIONS

INTERVENTIONS

See glossary, p 464

Key Messages

- **H pylori eradication for gastric B cell lymphoma** We found no RCTs of *H pylori* eradication treatment in people with B cell gastric lymphoma. Observational studies found limited evidence that 60–93% of people with localised, low grade B cell lymphoma respond to *H pylori* eradication treatment, avoiding the need for radical surgery, radiotherapy, or chemotherapy.

Helicobacter pylori infection

- ***H pylori* eradication for healing and preventing recurrence of duodenal ulcer** Systematic reviews and one subsequent RCT have found that *H pylori* eradication versus acid suppression or antisecretory treatment increases the proportion of ulcers healed at 6 weeks and reduces 1 year recurrence. One systematic review found that *H pylori* eradication versus ulcer healing alone or versus ulcer treatment plus subsequent acid suppression maintenance treatment significantly reduced the risk of rebleeding (*v* ulcer treatment alone, NNT 6, 95% CI 4 to 11; *v* ulcer treatment plus acid suppression, NNT 25, 95% CI 13 to 167).
- ***H* pylori eradication for healing and preventing recurrence of gastric ulcer** One systematic review has found that *H pylori* eradication treatment versus antisecretory treatment significantly reduces recurrent ulcers at 1 year (NNT 3, 95% CI 2 to 4). Observational evidence identified by the review found that eradication treatment heals 83% of gastric ulcers within 6 weeks of starting treatment. We found no RCTs of *H pylori* eradication treatment on preventing complications of gastric ulcers.
- ***H pylori* eradication for non-ulcer dyspepsia** One systematic review in people with non-ulcer dyspepsia has found that *H pylori* eradication versus placebo significantly reduces dyspeptic symptoms at 3–12 months (NNT 15, 95% CI 10 to 31).
- ***H pylori* eradication for prevention of gastric cancer (adenocarcinoma)** We found no RCTs of *H pylori* eradication in people at risk of gastric cancer. One RCT in people with gastric atrophy or intestinal metaplasia found that *H pylori* eradication versus no eradication increased the regression of high risk lesions. We found consistent evidence from observational studies of an association between *H pylori* infection and increased risk of distal gastric adenocarcinoma of the stomach.
- ***H pylori* eradication in people with gastro-oesophageal reflux disease** One RCT in people with gastro-oesophageal reflux disease found no significant difference with *H pylori* eradication treatment versus placebo in symptomatic relapse.
- ***H pylori* eradication rather than empirical acid suppression for uninvestigated dyspepsia** One RCT found that *H pylori* eradication versus placebo significantly increased relief from dyspeptic symptoms after 1 year (NNT 9, 95% CI 5 to 554).
- ***H pylori* eradication rather than endoscopy in people with uninvestigated dyspepsia not at risk of malignancy** One systematic review and one subsequent RCT have found no significant difference between *H pylori* testing plus eradication versus management based on initial endoscopy in dyspepsia after 1 year.
- **One triple regimen versus another** We found no systematic review or RCTs of the effects of different triple regimens on dyspeptic symptom scores, proportion of subjects with symptoms, quality of life, or mortality. One systematic review has found that clarithromycin 500 mg twice daily versus clarithromycin 250 mg twice daily plus a proton pump inhibitor plus amoxicillin significantly increases *H pylori* eradication (NNT 11, 95% CI 6 to 38), but found no significant difference between clarithromycin 500 mg twice daily versus clarithromycin 250 mg twice daily plus a proton pump inhibitor plus metronidazole in *H pylori* eradication rates. Another systematic review has found that a triple regimen containing ranitidine bismuth plus clarithromycin plus metronidazole versus a triple regimen containing ranitidine bismuth plus clarithromycin plus amoxicillin significantly increases eradication at 5–7 days.

- **Three day quadruple regimen (*v* 1 wk triple regimen)** One RCT comparing a 3 day quadruple regimen versus a 1 week triple regimen found no significant difference in *H pylori* eradication at 6 weeks, but found that people taking the 3 day quadruple regimen experienced significantly fewer days of adverse effects.
- **Triple regimen (*v* dual regimen)** We found no systematic review or RCTs of the effects of dual regimen versus triple regimens on dyspeptic symptom scores, proportion of subjects with symptoms, quality of life, or mortality. One systematic review has found that dual versus triple regimens eradicate *H pylori* from fewer people.
- **Two week triple regimen (*v* 1 wk triple regimen)** One systematic review found that 14 days versus 7 days treatment with proton pump inhibitor based triple regimens significantly increased *H pylori* cure rates (NNT 11, 95% CI 7 to 33).

DEFINITION *H pylori* is a Gram negative flagellated spiral bacterium found in the stomach. Infection with *H pylori* is predominantly acquired in childhood. The organism is associated with lifelong chronic gastritis and may cause other gastroduodenal disorders.

INCIDENCE/ PREVALENCE *H pylori* prevalence rates vary with birth cohort and social class in the developed world. Prevalence rates in many developed countries tend to be much higher (50–80%) in those born prior to 1950 in comparison to rates (< 20%) in those born more recently. In many developing countries the infection has a high prevalence (80–95%) irrespective of the period of birth.[1] Adult prevalence is believed to represent the persistence of a historically higher rate of infection acquired in childhood, rather than increasing acquisition of infection during life.

AETIOLOGY/ RISK FACTORS Overcrowded conditions associated with childhood poverty lead to increased transmission and higher prevalence rates. Adult reinfection rates are low — less than 1% a year.[1]

PROGNOSIS *H pylori* infection is believed to be causally related to the development of duodenal and gastric ulceration, gastric B cell lymphoma, and distal gastric cancer. About 15% of people infected with *H pylori* will develop a peptic ulcer, and 1% of people will develop gastric cancer during their lifetime.[2] *H pylori* infection is not associated with a specific type of dyspeptic symptom.

AIMS Improvement in dyspeptic symptoms; reduction in peptic ulcer complications; reduced mortality from peptic ulcer complications of gastric cancer; improved quality of life.

OUTCOMES Dyspeptic symptom scores and proportion of subjects with symptoms; quality of life; mortality.

METHODS *Clinical Evidence* update search and appraisal April 2002.

QUESTION **What are the effects of *H pylori* eradication treatment in people with a proven duodenal ulcer?**

Systematic reviews and one subsequent RCT have found that *H pylori* eradication versus acid suppression or antisecretory treatment increases the proportion of ulcers healed at 6 weeks and reduces 1 year

recurrence. One systematic review found that *H pylori* eradication versus ulcer healing alone or versus ulcer treatment plus subsequent acid suppression maintenance treatment significantly reduced the risk of rebleeding.

Benefits: **Endoscopic healing:** We found three systematic reviews,[3–5] and one subsequent RCT,[6] of *H pylori* eradication treatment in people with proven duodenal ulcers. The first systematic review (search date 1994, 7 RCTs) found in indirect comparisons that triple regimens (see glossary, p 465) versus acid suppressing drugs alone healed more duodenal ulcers at 6 weeks (299/310 [96%] with triple regimens *v* 191/251 [76%] with omeprazole alone).[3] The review analysed single arms from different RCTs, and as a result the comparison loses some of the benefits of randomisation. The second systematic review (search date 1995, 15 RCTs that directly compared treatments) found that triple regimens versus antisecretory treatment increased healing rates (91–97% with triple regimens *v* 20–90% with antisecretory drugs; no statistical comparison performed).[4] The third systematic review (search date 1996, 7 RCTs conducted in the USA, 989 *H pylori* positive people with duodenal ulcer given dual regimen) assessed ulcer healing in people receiving *H pylori* eradication treatment.[5] It found that most duodenal ulcers were endoscopically healed 6 weeks after the start of eradication treatment (68%, 95% CI 65% to 71% with eradication treatment). The review provided no comparative information on the ulcer healing rate in people given control treatment. The subsequent RCT (277 people with active duodenal ulcer) compared eradication treatment (metronidazole plus amoxicillin [amoxycillin] plus omeprazole) for 2 weeks followed by omaprazole 20 mg until the ulcer had healed versus omeprazole 20 mg twice daily until the ulcer had healed.[6] It found no significant difference between eradication treatment versus omeprazole alone in healing of duodenal ulcer at 4 weeks (84% *v* 92%; P = 0.07). The RCT assessed the two groups for a further 2 years (see prevention of recurrence below).[6] **Prevention of recurrence:** We found two systematic reviews,[3,4] and one subsequent RCT,[6] that compared the effects of eradication treatment versus antisecretory drugs alone on ulcer recurrence 1 year after treatment. The first systematic review (search date 1994) made indirect comparisons by analysing single arms from different RCTs, and as a result the comparison loses some of the benefits of randomisation.[3] The second systematic review (search date 1995, 20 RCTs) directly compared any type of eradication treatment versus antisecretory treatment.[4] Both systematic reviews found that eradication treatment versus antisecretory treatment reduced ulcer recurrence at 1 year (see table 1, p 467). In the subsequent RCT above, the 250 people whose ulcers had healed by 16 weeks entered the next phase of the study, which lasted 2 years.[6] In the first year, people in the omeprazole alone group were given omeprazole 20 mg and people receiving eradication treatment were given placebo. In the second year, both groups received no treatment and were observed. The RCT found no significant difference on intention to treat analysis (see glossary, p 465) in ulcer recurrence between eradication versus omeprazole after 1 year (10/139 [7%] with eradication *v* 15/137 [11%] with omeprazole; RR 0.66, 95% CI 0.30 to 1.38). A completer analysis

(173 people) found that eradication treatment versus omeprazole alone significantly reduced ulcer recurrence (5/86 [6%] with eradication *v* 39/87 [45%] with omeprazole; RR 0.87, 95% CI 0.70 to 0.96; NNT 3, 95% CI 2 to 4) but found no significant difference in dyspeptic symptoms requiring further treatment (0/86 [0%] with eradication *v* 12/87 [14%] with omeprazole; RR 1.0, 95% CI 0.7 to 1.0; NNT 8, 95% CI 5 to 13) after 2 years. **Prevention of bleeding:** We found one systematic review (search date 2000, 4 RCTs, 262 people)[7] that compared *H pylori* eradication versus ulcer treatment alone or versus ulcer treatment plus subsequent acid suppression maintenance treatment. The review found that *H pylori* eradication versus ulcer treatment alone significantly reduced the risk of rebleeding (6/133 [4.5%] with eradication *v* 28/129 [22%] with ulcer treatment alone; RR 0.24, 95% CI 0.11 to 0.53; NNT 6, 95% CI 4 to 11), and *H pylori* eradication versus ulcer treatment plus acid suppression also significantly reduced the risk of rebleeding (4/257 [1.6%] with eradication *v* 12/213 [5.6%] with ulcer treatment plus acid suppression; RR 0.3, 95% CI 0.09 to 0.77; NNT 25, 95% CI 13 to 167). **Prevention of perforation or obstruction:** We found no systematic review and no RCTs.

Harms: One systematic review (search date 1995) found that minor adverse effects are common with bismuth (see glossary, p 464) (40% of people), metronidazole (39%), clarithromycin (22%), and tinidazole (7%).[8] Discontinuation of treatment because of severe adverse effects is rare (bismuth 4%, metronidazole 2%, clarithromycin 1%, and tinidazole < 1%).

Comment: Indirect comparison is a weak form of evidence.[3] The characteristics of the people, settings, and procedures in the different RCTs may not be comparable. We excluded analyses that grouped people by *H pylori* status at the end of the trial. Observational evidence from RCTs suggests that duodenal ulcer recurrence rates 1 year after treatment are lower in people with successful *H pylori* eradication treatment (in the review of US RCTs: 20%, 95% CI 14% to 26%, in people cured of *H pylori v* 56%, 95% CI 50% to 61%, for people remaining infected).[5] The recurrence rate in non-US trials was lower than the recurrence rate found in the US trials (6% for people cured of *H pylori*). The difference in recurrence rates between US and non-US studies may be explained partially by the marked loss to follow up in the US trials (9–41%). However, countries with low prevalence of *H pylori* infection also have a low prevalence of duodenal ulcers, but a greater proportion of those ulcers arise from causes other than *H pylori*; therefore, eradication may be less effective where *H pylori* prevalence is low. Poor adherence to *H pylori* eradication treatment and the use of less effective regimens may lead to increased antibiotic resistance in *H pylori*, but we found no direct evidence to support this. The harms of *H pylori* eradication treatment are mainly the minor short term effects of the antibiotics, particularly nausea from metronidazole or clarithromycin, and diarrhoea. Bismuth may turn the stools black.

QUESTION **What are the effects of *H pylori* eradication treatment for people with a proven gastric ulcer?**

One systematic review has found that *H pylori* eradication treatment versus antisecretory treatment significantly reduces recurrent ulcers at 1 year. Observational evidence identified by the review found that eradication treatment heals 83% of gastric ulcers within 6 weeks of starting treatment. We found no RCTs of *H pylori* eradication treatment on preventing complications of gastric ulcers.

Benefits: **Endoscopic healing:** We found one systematic review (search date 1995, 6 RCTs) that compared eradication treatment versus no eradication treatment but did not analyse endoscopic healing of gastric ulcers.[4] **Prevention of recurrence:** The systematic review found that *H pylori* eradication treatment versus 4–6 weeks antisecretory treatment significantly reduced recurrent ulcers at 1 year (6 RCTs; RR 0.18, 95% CI 0.1 to 0.3; NNT 3, 95% CI 2 to 4).[4] **Prevention of complications:** We found no systematic review or RCTs.

Harms: See harms under effects of eradication treatment, p 457 for *H pylori* in people with a proven duodenal ulcer.

Comment: We found one systematic review (search date 1995, 14 cohort studies of people with uncomplicated gastric ulcer) that analysed the *H pylori* eradication arm.[4] It found that 6 weeks after the start of *H pylori* eradication treatment, 83% (95% CI 78% to 88%) of gastric ulcers were healed. Indirect comparison is a weak form of evidence. The characteristics of the people, settings, and procedures in the different RCTs may not be comparable.

QUESTION **What are the effects of *H pylori* eradication treatment in people with proven gastro-oesophageal reflux disease?**

One RCT in people with gastro-oesophageal reflux disease found no significant difference with *H pylori* eradication treatment versus placebo in symptomatic relapse.

Benefits: We found no systematic review but found one RCT (190 *H pylori* positive people with gastro-oesophageal reflux disease but no duodenal ulcer) comparing *H pylori* eradication treatment versus placebo, which found no significant difference in symptomatic relapse (83% in both groups; difference 0%, 95% CI −11% to +11%).[9]

Harms: We found insufficient evidence about the harms of *H pylori* eradication treatment in people with gastro-oesophageal reflux disease. Case control studies have found an increased risk of reflux symptoms after *H pylori* eradication.[10] However, discontinuation of acid suppression treatment after *H pylori* eradication might have unmasked symptoms of co-existing gastro-oesophageal reflux disease. Two RCTs in people with duodenal ulcer compared the effects of *H pylori* eradication treatment versus placebo on heartburn symptoms, but no analysis by intention to treat was reported.[11,12] One RCT (2324 people from the general population who tested positive for *H pylori*) found no significant difference *between H pylori* eradication versus placebo in reflux symptoms at 2 years.[13]

Comment: None.

QUESTION **What are the effects of *H pylori* eradication treatment in people with B cell lymphoma of the stomach?**

We found no RCTs of *H pylori* eradication treatment in people with B cell gastric lymphoma. Observational studies found limited evidence that 60–93% of people with localised, low grade B cell lymphoma respond to *H pylori* eradication treatment, avoiding the need for radical surgery, radiotherapy, or chemotherapy.

Benefits: We found no systematic review and no RCTs.

Harms: We found no RCTs.

Comment: Treatment options for primary gastric lymphoma include surgery, radiotherapy, chemotherapy, and *H pylori* eradication. We found no direct comparative studies. We found six prospective cohort studies of *H pylori* eradication in people with localised, low grade lymphomas.[14] Tumour regression occurred in 60–93% of people, but responses were sometimes delayed and some people relapsed within 1 year of treatment. A further large, but still uncontrolled study (28/34 patients with gastric B cell lymphoma were found to be *H pylori* positive and were given eradication treatment) found that 14/28 people (50%, 95% CI 31 to 69%) achieved complete remission at 18 months' follow up.[15]

QUESTION **What are the effects of *H pylori* eradication treatment in people at risk of gastric cancer?**

We found no RCTs of *H pylori* eradication in people at risk of gastric cancer. One RCT in people with gastric atrophy or intestinal metaplasia found that *H pylori* eradication versus no eradication increased the regression of high risk lesions. We found consistent evidence from observational studies of an association between *H pylori* infection and increased risk of distal gastric adenocarcinoma.

Benefits: **General population:** We found no systematic review and no RCTs of *H pylori* eradication treatment to prevent gastric cancer (adenocarcinoma). **In people at high risk of gastric cancer:** We found no systematic review and no RCTs of the effects of *H pylori* eradication on the development of gastric cancer in people at high risk. One RCT (852 people with gastric atrophy or intestinal metaplasia found at screening endoscopy) compared four treatments: *H pylori* eradication treatment; β carotene; ascorbic acid; and placebo.[16] It found that *H pylori* eradication treatment versus no eradication treatment increased lesion regression (calculated by multivariate modelling) for both atrophy (RR 4.8, 95% CI 1.6 to 14.2) and intestinal metaplasia (RR 3.1, 95% CI 1.0 to 9.3; no absolute numbers provided).

Harms: We found no RCTs in people at risk of gastric cancer.

Comment: We found one systematic review of nested case control studies (search date 1999, 12 studies, 1228 cases, 3406 controls).[17] In the absence of trial data, this is the best evidence of an association between *H pylori* infection and gastric cancer. The review found that overall there was a significant association between *H pylori* infection and the subsequent development of gastric cancer (OR 2.36, 95% CI 1.98 to 2.81). However, the review was able to use the individual study data to address two important sub-analyses. First, the review found no significant association between *H pylori* and cardia cancer (OR 0.99, 95% CI 0.72 to 1.35), but did find a significant association for non-cardia cancer (OR 2.97, 95% CI 2.34 to 3.77). Second, the review found a strong interaction with age and time from sample collection. *H pylori* does not colonise areas of cancer, intestinal metaplasia, or atrophy, and antibodies may be lost with increasing age. Prospective studies with a short time period between the collection of the serum sample and the development of the cancer, or retrospective studies, may underestimate the association. The review found a significant association between *H pylori* and non-cardia (distal) cancer where the time from sampling to cancer was more than 10 years (OR 5.93, 95% CI 3.41 to 10.3).

QUESTION **What are the effects of *H pylori* eradication treatment in people with proven non-ulcer dyspepsia?**

One systematic review in people with non-ulcer dyspepsia has found that *H pylori* eradication versus placebo significantly reduces dyspeptic symptoms at 3–12 months.

Benefits: We found one systematic review (search date 2000, 9 RCTs, 2541 people), which found that *H pylori* eradication versus placebo significantly improved recurrent dyspeptic symptoms at 3–12 months (AR of recurrent symptoms 896/1401 [64%] with eradication treatment *v* 820/1140 [72%] with placebo; RR 0.91, 95% CI 0.86 to 0.96; NNT 15, 95% CI 10 to 31).[18] Three RCTs (839 people) in the systematic review found no significant difference between *H pylori* eradication treatment versus placebo on quality of life at 12 months (WMD –0.25, 95% CI –3.49 to +2.99).[18]

Harms: See harms under effects of eradication treatment, p 457 for *H pylori* in people with a proven duodenal ulcer. We found two RCTs that assessed whether *H pylori* eradication treatment increases the prevalence of oesophagitis in people with non-ulcer dyspepsia.[19,20] They found no significant difference with *H pylori* eradication treatment versus placebo in endoscopically assessed oesophagitis (5.7% with eradication treatment *v* 2.9% with placebo; ARI +2.8%, 95% CI –0.5% to +6.0%; RR 2.1, 95% CI 0.9 to 4.6). No trial evaluated individual dyspeptic symptoms, so the effect on reflux symptoms cannot be estimated separately from epigastric pain.

Comment: None.

QUESTION What are the effects of *H pylori* eradication treatment in people with uninvestigated dyspepsia?

One RCT has found that *H pylori* eradication versus placebo significantly increased relief from dyspeptic symptoms after 1 year. One systematic review and one subsequent RCT in people with uninvestigated dyspepsia have found no significant difference between *H pylori* testing plus eradication versus management based on initial endoscopy in dyspepsia after 1 year.

Benefits: **H pylori eradication versus placebo:** We found one RCT (294 people with dyspeptic symptoms and confirmed *H pylori* infection) that found *H pylori* eradication versus placebo significantly increased relief from dyspeptic symptoms at 1 year (61/145 [42%] *v* 80/149 [54%]; RR 0.78, 95% CI 0.61 to 0.99; NNT 9, 95% CI 5 to 554).[21] **Initial *H pylori* testing plus eradication versus management based on initial endoscopy:** We found one systematic review (search date 1999, 3 RCTs, 1366 people; see comment below) comparing *H pylori* testing plus eradication versus management based on initial endoscopy.[22] It found no significant difference between *H pylori* testing plus eradication versus endoscopy based management in dyspepsia at 1 year (140/414 [34%] *v* 137/414 [33%]; RR 1.02, 95% CI 0.85 to 1.23). It found that *H pylori* testing plus eradication versus endoscopy based management significantly reduced the proportion of people requiring endoscopy (169/500 [34%] at 2–6 wks after eradication treatment *v* 486/489 [99%] with prompt endoscopy; RR 0.34, 95% CI 0.30 to 0.39). One subsequent RCT (708 people aged < 55 years referred for endoscopic investigation of dyspepsia by their primary care physician) found no significant difference with *H pylori* eradication versus endoscopy in dyspeptic symptoms at 1 year (260/293 [89%] with *H pylori* eradication *v* 249/291 [86%] with endoscopy; RR 1.03, 95% CI 0.97 to 1.1).[23] Only 8.2% of people initially randomised to *H pylori* eradication had an endoscopy in the following year.

Harms: The systematic review gave no information on adverse effects.[22] Two of the RCTs in the review found that a small number of people given *H pylori* eradication treatment discontinued treatment because of short term adverse effects, that were not specified (14/104 [13%] people in the first RCT in the review[24] and 4/80 [5%] in the second RCT[25]).

Comment: The results of the systematic review may not be applicable to all people with dyspepsia. People with "alarm" symptoms (dysphagia, weight loss, jaundice, epigastric mass, or anaemia), or over the age of 55 years, with either continuous epigastric pain or first onset of symptoms in the previous year, may have a significant risk of upper gastro-intestinal malignancy and may benefit from prompt endoscopy. Two of the RCTs in the review were conducted in a hospital setting and the third, conducted in primary care, is not yet published in full.[26] One of the RCTs in the review, conducted in a hospital setting, stipulated that all eligible people with dyspepsia who were consulting with a general medical practitioner should be included, but the other entered only routine referrals. The results of the review might not apply directly to primary care, where people with less severe dyspepsia might be treated and *H pylori* eradication rates might be lower, and the reassuring or anxiety provoking effect of specialist consultation might not be replicated.[22]

QUESTION Do eradication treatments differ in their effects?

OPTION DUAL VERSUS TRIPLE REGIMENS

We found no systematic review or RCTs of the effects of dual versus triple regimens on dyspeptic symptom scores, proportion of subjects with symptoms, quality of life, or mortality. One systematic review has found that dual versus triple regimens eradicate *H pylori* from fewer people.

Benefits: **Duodenal ulcer complication rates:** We found no systematic review and no RCTs. **Eradication rates:** We found one systematic review (search date 1995; 19 RCTs of omeprazole plus amoxicillin [amoxycillin] versus containing bismuth; 17 RCTs of dual regimens containing a proton pump inhibitor versus triple regimens [see glossary, p 465]).[8] No formal meta-analysis was performed, but dual regimens versus triple regimens (two antibiotics plus either a proton pump inhibitor or bismuth) eradicated *H pylori* from fewer people (results presented graphically).

Harms: See harms under effects of eradication treatment, p 457 for *H pylori* in people with a proven duodenal ulcer.

Comment: Systematic reviews of *H pylori* eradication treatment are difficult to interpret because they rarely pool RCTs in an analysis that maintains the randomised comparison. Instead, all treatment arms for one combination from any trial are pooled together, which greatly weakens the evidence. Many RCTs have additional methodological problems, such as lack of a gold standard for defining cure, and many are published only as an abstract. A systematic review comparing eradication treatments for *H pylori* eradication is in progress.[26] Factors that might influence the choice of eradication treatment for an individual also include ease of adherence, potential harms, allergy or sensitivity, drug resistance, and cost.

OPTION WHAT ARE THE EFFECTS OF DIFFERENT TRIPLE REGIMENS?

We found no systematic review or RCTs of the effects of different triple regimens on dyspeptic symptom scores, proportion of subjects with symptoms, quality of life, or mortality. One systematic review has found that clarithromycin 500 mg twice daily versus clarithromycin 250 mg twice daily plus a proton pump inhibitor plus amoxicillin significantly increases *H pylori* eradication, but found no significant difference between clarithromycin 500 mg twice daily versus clarithromycin 250 mg twice daily plus a proton pump inhibitor plus metronidazole in *H pylori* eradication rates. Another systematic review has found that a triple regimen containing ranitidine bismuth plus clarithromycin plus metronidazole versus a triple regimen containing ranitidine bismuth plus clarithromycin plus amoxicillin significantly increases eradication at 5–7 days.

Benefits: **Duodenal ulcer complication rates:** We found no systematic review and no direct comparison of the effect of different triple regimens (see glossary, p 465) on complication rates. **Eradication rates:** We found four systematic reviews comparing different triple regimens, two of which included indirect comparisons between RCTs (see table 2, p 468).[8,27–29] The first systematic review (search date 1998, 4 RCTs with direct, head-to-head comparisons of eradication regimens) found that clarithromycin 500 mg twice daily versus clarithromycin 250 mg twice daily in combination with a proton pump inhibitor (see glossary, p 464) and amoxicillin (amoxycillin) significantly increased *H pylori* eradication (90% with clarithromycin 500 mg *v* 80% with 250 mg; RR 0.89, 95% CI 0.81 to 0.97; NNT 11, 95% CI 6 to 38).[27] The review found no significant difference between clarithromycin 500 mg twice daily and clarithromycin 250 mg twice daily in combination with a proton pump inhibitor and metronidazole in eradication rates (89% with clarithromycin 500 mg twice daily *v* 87% with 250 mg twice daily; RR 0.98, 95% CI 0.93 to 1.04). The second systematic review (search date 2000, 8 RCTs, 1139 people with direct comparisons of eradication regimens) found that ranitidine bismuth (see glossary, p 464) 400 mg daily plus clarithromycin 250 mg plus metronidazole 400 mg twice daily versus ranitidine 400 mg daily plus clarithromycin 500 mg twice daily plus amoxicillin 1000 mg twice daily significantly increased eradication at 5–7 days (499/565 [88%] *v* 467/574 [81%]; RR 1.09, 95% CI 1.03 to 1.14).[28] The limited evidence from two systematic reviews with indirect comparisons found the highest eradication rates (85–90%) with omeprazole (20 mg daily, or equivalent) plus a combination of two of the following: amoxicillin (1–1.5 g daily), metronidazole (1.2 g daily), or clarithromycin (500 mg daily) with metronidazole or 1 g daily with amoxicillin (see comment below).[8,27] **Antibiotic resistance:** We found one systematic review (search date 1995, 19 RCTs, 1006 people with metronidazole sensitive *H pylori*, 452 with metronidazole resistant *H pylori*)[8] and one subsequent RCT[30] that assessed the efficacy of metronidazole (or other nitroimidazole) based triple and quadruple regimens with strains of *H pylori* that were resistant in the laboratory. The review found that nitroimidazole based regimens achieved *H pylori* eradication in significantly fewer people with strains showing nitroimidazole resistance in the laboratory than in people with sensitive strains (99%, 95% CI 97% to 100% eradication in people with sensitive strains *v* 69%, 95% CI 60% to 77% in people with resistant strains).[8]

Harms: See harms under effects of eradication treatment, p 457 for *H pylori* in people with a proven duodenal ulcer.

Comment: Indirect comparison is a weak form of evidence.[8,27] The characteristics of the people, settings, and procedures in the different RCTs may not be comparable. The systematic review assessing nitroimidazole resistance concluded that clinically important reduction of eradication rates is unlikely with a proportion of resistant strains below 15–25%.[8] Systematic reviews of *H pylori* eradication treatments are difficult to interpret (see dual versus triple regimens, p 462).

OPTION DURATION OF *H PYLORI* ERADICATION TREATMENT

One systematic review found that 14 days versus 7 days treatment with proton pump inhibitor based triple regimens treatment significantly increased *H pylori* cure rates (NNT 11, 95% CI 7 to 33). One subsequent RCT comparing a 3 day quadruple regimen versus a 1 week triple regimen found no significant difference in *H pylori* eradication at 6 weeks, but found that people taking the 3 day quadruple regimen experienced significantly fewer days of adverse effects.

Benefits: **Duodenal ulcer complication rates:** We found no systematic review and no RCTs. **Eradication rates:** We found one systematic review[31] and one subsequent RCT.[32] The review (search date 1999, 7 RCTs, 906 people) compared 14 days treatment with proton pump inhibitor based triple regimens (see glossary, p 465) versus 7 days treatment with proton pump inhibitor based triple regimens.[31] It found that 14 day treatment versus 7 day treatment significantly increased *H pylori* cure rates (339/470 [72.1%] *v* 353/436 [81.0%]; RR 0.89, 95% CI 0.83 to 0.96; NNT 11 95% CI 7 to 33). One subsequent RCT (118 people with active duodenal ulcer at endoscopy) compared a 3 day quadruple regimen (lansoprazole plus clarithromycin plus metronidazole plus bismuth subcitrate) versus a 7 day triple regimen (lansoprazole plus clarithromycin plus metronidazole).[32] It found no significant difference in *H pylori* eradication at 6 weeks (50/58 [86.2%] with 3 day quadruple regimen *v* 52/60 [86.7%] with 7 day triple regimen; RR 0.99, 95% CI 0.79 to 1.09).

Harms: See harms under effects of eradication treatment, p 457 for *H pylori* in people with a proven duodenal ulcer. The RCT, comparing a 3 day quadruple regimen versus a 1 week triple regimen, found that people taking the 3 day regimen experienced significantly fewer days of bitter taste, bowel disturbance, malaise, and dark stools (mean 2.54 days with 3 day quadruple regimen *v* mean 4.58 days with 7 day triple regimen; $P < 0.001$).[32] The systematic review found insufficient data to report harms.[31]

Comment: The systematic review only considered regimens containing clarithromycin plus either metronidazole or amoxycillin.[31] The risk of failure of a 7 day regimen as opposed to a 14 day regimen in any particular individual will relate to the local prevalence of antibiotic resistance, as 14 day regimens may overcome resistance to one of the antibiotics used. As longer regimens cost more and have a longer duration of minor side effects, the balance between local failure rate and cost must be decided on the basis of locally validated data.

GLOSSARY

Bismuth A compound containing bismuth, such as bismuth subsalicilate or ranitidine bismuth citrate.

Dual regimen *H pylori* eradication regimen consisting of two components.

Intention to treat analysis All subjects analysed according to the group to which they were randomised rather than some other grouping, such as post-treatment *H pylori* status, or an analysis based merely on those who completed the study.

MALT "Mucosa-associated lymphoid tissue" is constitutionally found in the intestine but not in the stomach. MALT lymphoma is also known as B cell gastric lymphoma.
Proton pump inhibitor A drug that directly inhibits the mechanism within the stomach that secretes acid, such as esomeprazole, lansoprazole, omeprazole, or rabeprazole.
Triple regimen *H pylori* eradication regimen consisting of three components. The original "triple regimen" was bismuth subsalicilate, metronidazole, and either amoxicillin (amoxycillin) or tetracycline. Now the term usually applies to a proton pump inhibitor plus two antibiotics.

Substantive changes

***H pylori* eradication in people with proven duodenal ulcer: prevention of bleeding** One new systematic review;[7] conclusions unchanged.
***H pylori* eradication in people with uninvestigated dyspepsia** Two new RCTs;[21,23] conclusions unchanged.
Duration of treatment One new systematic review;[31] found that 14 days treatment with triple regimen versus 7 days treatment significantly increases *H pylori* cure rates.

REFERENCES

1. Axon AT. *Helicobacter pylori* infection. *J Antimicrob Chemother* 1993;32(suppl A):61–68.
2. Graham DY. Can therapy ever be denied for *Helicobacter pylori* infection? *Gastroenterology* 1997;113:S113 S117.
3. Moore RA. *Helicobacter pylori* and peptic ulcer. Cortecs Diagnostics and the Health Technology Association. Oxford, 1995. Search date 1994; primary sources Medline and survey of pharmaceutical companies. http://www.jr2.ox.ac.uk/bandolier/bandopubs/hpyl/hpall.html (last accessed 27 March 2001).
4. Penston JG. Review article: Clinical aspects of *Helicobacter pylori* eradication therapy in peptic ulcer disease. *Aliment Pharmacol Ther* 1996;10:469–486. Search date 1995; primary sources Medline and conference abstracts.
5. Laine L, Hopkins RJ, Girardi LS. Has the impact of *Helicobacter pylori* therapy on ulcer recurrence in the United States been overstated? A meta-analysis of rigorously designed trials. *Am J Gastroenterol* 1998;93:1409–1415. Search date 1996; primary sources Medline, conference abstracts, and pharmaceutical companies (US trials only).
6. Bytzer P, Aalykke C, Rune S, et al. Eradication of *Helicobacter pylori* compared with long-term acid suppression in duodenal ulcer disease. A randomised trial with 2-year follow up. *Scand J Gastroenterol* 2000;10:1023–1032.
7. Sharma VK, Sahai AV, Corder FA, et al. *Helicobacter pylori* eradication is superior to ulcer healing with or without maintenance therapy to prevent further ulcer haemorrhage. *Aliment Pharm Ther* 2001;15:1939–1947. Search date 2000; primary sources Medline and conference abstracts.
8. Penston JG, McColl KEL. Eradication of *Helicobacter pylori*: an objective assessment of current therapies. *Br J Clin Pharmacol* 1997;43:223–243. Search date 1995; primary sources Medline and conference abstracts.
9. Moayyedi P, Bardhan C, Young L, et al. *Helicobacter pylori* eradication does not exacerbate reflux symptoms in gastroesophageal reflux disease. *Gastroenterology* 2001;121:1120–1126.
10. Labenz J, Blum AL, Bayerdorffer E, et al. Curing *Helicobacter pylori* infection in patients with duodenal ulcer may provoke reflux esophagitis. *Gastroenterology* 1997;112:1442–1447.
11. Vakil N, Hahn B, McSorley D. Recurrent symptoms and gastro-oesophageal reflux disease in patients with duodenal ulcer treated for *Helicobacter pylori* infection. *Aliment Pharmacol Ther* 2000;14:45–51.
12. Fallone CA, Barkun AN, Friedman G, et al. Is *Helicobacter pylori* eradication associated with gastroesophageal reflux disease? *Am J Gastroenterol* 2000;95:914–920.
13. Moayyedi P, Feltbower R, Brown J, et al. Effect of population screening and treatment for *Helicobacter pylori* on dyspepsia and quality of life in the community: a randomised controlled trial. *Lancet* 2000;355:1665–1669.
14. Roher HD, Vereet PR, Wormer O, et al. *Helicobacter pylori* in the upper gastrointestinal tract: medical or surgical treatment of gastric lymphoma? *Langenbeck's Arch Surg* 2000;385:97–105. Search date not stated; primary sources Medline and hand searches.
15. Steinbach G, Ford R, Glober G, et al. Antibiotic treatment of gastric lymphoma of mucosa-associated lymphoid tissue. An uncontrolled trial. *Ann Intern Med* 1999;131:88–95.
16. Correa P, Fontham ETH, Bravo JC, et al. Chemoprevention of gastric dysplasia: Randomized trial of antioxidant supplements and anti-*Helicobacter pylori* therapy. *J Natl Cancer Inst* 2000;92:1881–1888.
17. *Helicobacter* and Cancer Collaborative Group. Gastric cancer and *Helicobacter pylori*: a combined analysis of 12 case control studies nested within prospective cohorts. *Gut* 2001;49:347–353. Search date 1999; primary sources Medline and contact with investigators.
18. Soo S, Moayyedi P, Deeks J, et al. Eradication *Helicobacter pylori* for non-ulcer dyspepsia. In: The Cochrane Library, Issue 3, 2001. Oxford: Update Software. Search date 2000; primary sources Medline, Embase, Science Citation Index, conference abstracts, and survey of experts.

19. Blum AL, Talley NJ, O'Morain C, et al. Lack of effect of treating *Helicobacter pylori* infection in patients with nonulcer dyspepsia. *N Engl J Med* 1998;339:1875–1881.
20. Koelz HR, Arnold R, Stolte M, et al. Treatment of *Helicobacter pylori* (HP) does not improve symptoms of functional dyspepsia. *Gastroenterology* 1998;114:A182.
21. Chiba N, Veldhuyzen van Zanten SJO, Paul Sinclair, et al. Treating *Helicobacter pylori* infection in primary care patients with uninvestigated dyspepsia: the Canadian adult dyspepsia empiric treatment *Helicobacter pylori* positive (CADET-Hp) randomised controlled trial. *BMJ* 2002;324:1012.
22. Delaney BC, Innes MA, Deeks J, et al. Initial management strategies for dyspepsia. In: The Cochrane Library, Issue 3, 2001. Oxford: Update Software. Search date 1999; primary sources Medline, Embase, Science Citation Index, conference abstracts, and survey of experts.
23. McColl KEL, Murray LS, Gillen D, et al. Randomised trial of endoscopy with testing for *Helicobacter pylori* compared with non-invasive *H pylori* testing alone in the management of dyspepsia. *BMJ* 2002;324:999.
24. Lassen AT, Pedersen FM, Bytzer P, et al. *Helicobacter pylori* "test and eradicate" or prompt endoscopy for management of dyspeptic patients. A randomised controlled trial with one year follow-up. *Lancet* 2000;356:455–460.
25. Heaney A, Collins JSA, Watson RGP, et al. A prospective randomised trial of a "test and treat" policy versus endoscopy based management in young *Helicobacter pylori* positive patients with ulcer-like dyspepsia, referred to a hospital clinic. *Gut* 1999;45:186–190.
26. Forman D, Bazzoli F, Bennett C, et al. Therapies for the eradication of *Helicobater pylori*. Protocol for a Cochrane Review. In: The Cochrane Library, Issue 4, 2001. Oxford: Update Software.
27. Pipkin GA, Dixon JS, Williamson R, et al. Clarithromycin dual therapy regimens for eradication of *Helicobacter pylori*: a review. *Helicobacter* 1997;2:159–171. Search date 1997; primary sources Medline and conference abstracts.
28. Huang JQ, Hunt RH. The importance of clarithromycin dose in the management of *Helicobacter pylori* infection: a meta-analysis of triple therapies with a proton pump inhibitor, clarithromycin and amoxycillin or metronidazole. *Aliment Pharmacol Ther* 1999;13:719–729. Search date 1998; primary sources Medline and conference abstracts.
29. Janssen M, Van Oijen A, Verbeek A, et al. A systematic comparison of triple therapies for treatment of *Helicobacter pylori* infection with proton pump inhibitor/ranitidine bismuth citrate plus clarithromycin and either amoxicillin or a nitroimidazole. *Aliment Pharmacol Ther* 2001;15:613–624. Search date 2000; primary sources Medline and hand searches of reference lists and meetings abstracts.
30. Lind T, Peal MFU. The Mach 2 study: role of omeprazole in eradication of *Helicobacter pylori* with 1-week triple therapies. *Gastroenterology* 1999;116:248–253.
31. Calvet X, Garcia N, Lopez T, et al. A meta-analysis of short versus long therapy with a proton pump inhibitor, Clarithromycin and either Metronidazole or amoxycillin for treating *Helicobacter pylori* infection. *Aliment Pharm Ther* 200;14:603–609. Search date 1999; primary sources Medline and conference proceedings.
32. Wong B, Wang W, Wong W, et al. Three-day iansoprazole quadruple therapy for *Helicobacter pylori*-positive duodenal ulcers: a randomised controlled study. *Aliment Pharmacol Ther* 2001;15:843–849.

Brendan Delaney
Department of Primary Care and General Practice
University of Birmingham
Birmingham
UK

Paul Moayyedi
City Hospital NHS Trust
Birmingham
UK

David Forman
Cochrane Upper Gastrointestinal and Pancreatic Disease Collaborative Review Group
University of Leeds
Leeds
UK

Competing interests: PM has acted as an independent medical advisor for AstraZeneca and has received lecture fees from AstraZeneca, Wyeth, Byk Gulden, Abbott, and Eisai. DF has received lecture fees from AstraZeneca. BD has received lecture fees from AstraZeneca and Axcan Pharma.

TABLE 1 **Results of systematic reviews that compared the effects of eradication treatment versus non-eradication treatment on the rate of ulcer recurrence 1 year after treatment (see text, p 456).[3,4]**

Reference	Treatment		Ulcer recurrence by 1 year	
	Eradication	Control	Eradication	Control
3	Bismuth, tetracycline, metronidazole, and ranitidine or omeprazole	Histamine receptor antagonist alone 4–6 weeks	13/148 (8.8%) 7 RCTs	100/121 (83%) 5 RCTs
4 (20 RCTs)	Any type of eradication treatment	Antisecretory treatment	128/1059 (12%)	575/988 (58%)

TABLE 2 ***H pylori* eradication rates for triple regimens containing bismuth versus triple regimens containing proton pump inhibitors (see text, p 463).[8,27–29]**

Regimen	Source	Eradication rate (95% CI)
Bismuth triple regimens		
Bismuth, metronidazole, amoxicillin/tetracycline	1 SR (7979 people)[10]	78%* (77% to 79%)
Ranitidine, bismuth citrate, clarithromycin	1 SR (1475 people)[29]	85%* (83% to 87%)
Ranitidine bismuth citrate triple regimens		
RBC, clarithromycin 500 mg bd, amoxicillin 1000 mg bd	1 SR (1139 people)[31]	81%† (77% to 84%)
RBC, clarithromycin 250 mg bd, metronidazole 400 mg bd		88%† (85% to 91%)
PPI triple regimens		
Triple therapy (PPI, 2 antibiotics)	1 SR (3389 people)[10]	86%* (85% to 87%)
Clarithromycin 250 mg bd, PPI, amoxicillin	1 SR (385 people)[30]	80%†
Clarithromycin 500 mg bd, PPI, amoxicillin		89%†
Clarithromycin 250 mg bd, PPI, metronidazole		90%†
Clarithromycin 500 mg bd, PPI, metronidazole		87%†

*Rates are indirect comparisons based on pooled results from many different RCTs; †Rates represent direct comparisons. bd, twice daily; PPI, proton pump inhibitor; RBC, ranitidine bismuth citrate; SR, systematic review.

Stomach cancer

Search date May 2002

Peter McCulloch

QUESTIONS

INTERVENTIONS

Likely to be beneficial
Complete surgical resection* . .471
Subtotal gastrectomy (as effective as total gastrectomy) for resectable distal tumours . . .471

Unknown effectiveness
Conservative (as effective as radical) lymphadenectomy . .473
Adjuvant chemotherapy 474

Likely to be ineffective or harmful
Removal of adjacent organs. . .472

To be covered in future updates
Adjuvant radiotherapy
Endoscopic mucosal resection for early gastric cancer
Addition of bacterial and fungal extracts to adjuvant chemotherapy
Regional chemotherapy

* Observational evidence only; RCTs unlikely to be conducted.

See glossary, p 477

Key Messages

- **Adjuvant chemotherapy** Systematic reviews and subsequent RCTs have found limited evidence that adjuvant chemotherapy versus surgery alone significantly increases survival. RCTs in people from Japan have found conflicting results on the effects of adjuvant chemotherapy versus surgery alone on survival. Two RCTs found that adjuvant chemotherapy versus surgery alone significantly increased postoperative complications. The size of any benefit remains uncertain, and many recent adjuvant chemotherapy regimens have not been evaluated fully in RCTs.
- **Complete surgical resection** RCTs of complete surgical excision are unlikely to be conducted. Observational studies and multivariate analysis of RCTs have found a strong association between survival and complete excision of the primary tumour.
- **Conservative (as effective as radical) lymphadenectomy** Two RCTs comparing conservative versus radical lymphadenectomy found no significant difference in 5 year survival rates. One RCT found that radical versus conservative lymphadenectomy significantly increased perioperative mortality.
- **Removal of adjacent organs** One RCT found no significant difference with radical gastrectomy plus splenectomy versus radical gastrectomy alone in 5 year survival rates or postoperative mortality. The RCT found that radical gastrectomy plus splenectomy versus radical gastrectomy alone significantly increased the number of postoperative infections. Retrospective analyses of observational studies and RCTs in people with stomach cancer found that removal of additional organs (spleen and distal pancreas) versus no organ removal increased morbidity and mortality.

■ **Subtotal gastrectomy (as effective as total gastrectomy) for resectable distal tumours** RCTs in people with primary tumours in the distal stomach have found no significant difference with total versus subtotal gastrectomy in 5 year survival or postoperative mortality.

DEFINITION Stomach cancer is usually an adenocarcinoma arising in the stomach and includes tumours arising at or just below the gastro-oesophageal junction (type II and III junctional tumours). Tumours are staged according to degree of invasion and spread (see table 1, p 480).

INCIDENCE/ PREVALENCE The incidence of stomach cancer varies among countries and by sex (incidence per 100 000 population a year in Japanese men is about 80, Japanese women 30, British men 18, British women 10, white American men 11, white American women 7).[1] Incidence has declined dramatically in North America, Australia, and New Zealand since 1930, but the decline in Europe has been slower.[2] In the USA, stomach cancer remains relatively common among particular ethnic groups, especially Japanese–Americans and some Hispanic groups. The incidence of cancer of the proximal stomach and gastro-oesophageal junction is rising rapidly in most Western countries; the reasons for this are poorly understood.[3,4]

AETIOLOGY/ RISK FACTORS Distal stomach cancer is strongly associated with lifelong infection with *Helicobacter pylori* and poor dietary intake of antioxidant vitamins (A, C, and E).[5,6] In Western Europe and North America, distal stomach cancer is associated with relative socioeconomic deprivation. Proximal stomach cancer is strongly associated with smoking (OR about 4),[7] and is probably associated with gastro-oesophageal reflux, obesity, high fat intake, and medium to high socioeconomic status.

PROGNOSIS Invasive stomach cancer (stages T2–T4) is fatal without surgery. Mean survival without treatment is less than 6 months from diagnosis.[8,9] Intramucosal or submucosal cancer (stage T1) may progress slowly to invasive cancer over several years.[10] In the USA, over 50% of people recently diagnosed with stomach cancer have regional lymph node metastasis or involvement of adjacent organs. The prognosis after macroscopically and microscopically complete resection (R0) is related strongly to disease stage (see glossary, p 477), particularly penetration of the serosa (stage T3) and lymph node involvement. Five year survival rates range from over 90% in intramucosal cancer to about 20% in people with stage T3N2 disease (see table 1, p 480). In Japan, the 5 year survival rate for people with advanced disease is reported to be about 50%, but the explanation for the difference remains unclear. Comparisons between Japanese and Western practice are confounded by factors such as age, fitness, and disease stage, as well as by tumour location, because many Western series include gastro-oesophageal junction adenocarcinoma with a much lower survival after surgery.

AIMS To prevent progression; extend survival; and relieve symptoms, with minimal adverse effects.

OUTCOMES Survival; quality of life; adverse effects of treatment.

METHODS *Clinical Evidence* update search and appraisal May 2002. Hand searches of conference proceedings and consultations with experts were used to identify relevant studies.

QUESTION What are the effects of radical versus conservative surgical resection?

OPTION COMPLETE VERSUS INCOMPLETE TUMOUR RESECTION

Observational studies and multivariate analysis of RCTs have found a strong association between survival and complete excision of the primary tumour.

Benefits: We found no systematic review or RCTs directly comparing complete versus incomplete tumour resection or positive versus clear microscopic resection margins (see comment below). Multivariate risk factor analysis of RCTs and retrospective cohort studies found that failure to achieve microscopically clear resection margins was associated with a poor outcome independently of other indicators of tumour spread and behaviour.[11–13]

Harms: We found no systematic review or RCTs.

Comment: Current consensus is that improving long term survival is best achieved by complete resection of the primary tumour with microscopic confirmation of clear resection margins ("curative" gastrectomy). We found two observational studies of surgery versus no surgery.[8,9] They found that people who did not undergo resection (generally those with the most advanced disease and highest comorbidity) had a near zero 5 year survival in all case series, and mean survival without treatment from time of diagnosis was found to be less than 6 months. In view of this evidence it is unlikely that an RCT of surgery versus no surgery or complete versus incomplete tumour removal would be carried out. In people with similar stage weight loss and performance status, macroscopically incomplete tumour resection (palliative gastrectomy) was associated with twice the survival time of non-resection and with better quality of life owing to relief of tumour symptoms.[14]

OPTION TOTAL VERSUS SUBTOTAL GASTRECTOMY FOR RESECTABLE DISTAL TUMOURS

Two RCTs in people with primary tumours in the distal stomach found no significant difference with total versus subtotal gastrectomy in 5 year survival or postoperative mortality.

Benefits: We found no systematic review, but found two RCTs (787 people) comparing total versus subtotal (see glossary, p 477) gastrectomy.[15–18] Neither RCT used blinded allocation. **Five year survival:** The first RCT (648 people aged < 76 years with a resectable tumour and a macroscopic proximal margin of more than 6 cm) compared total versus subtotal gastrectomy.[17,18] All people involved in the RCT had a regional lymphadenectomy (D2). The RCT found no significant difference in the incidence of microscopic resection margin involvement (15/315 [4.8%] with subtotal gastrectomy *v* 6/303 [2.0%] with total gastrectomy; ARI +2.8%, 95% CI –0.1% to +9.6%) or in 5 year survival (Kaplan–Meier 5 year survival estimates 65% for subtotal *v* 62% for total gastrectomy; HR 0.89, 95% CI 0.68 to 1.17). Multivariate analysis found that after adjustment for covariates, the type of stomach surgery had no significant effect on 5 year survival (HR 1.01, 95% CI 0.76 to 1.33). The second RCT (169 people with potentially curable distal stomach cancer) compared total versus subtotal gastrectomy and found no significant difference in 5 year survival (48% in each group; CI not provided).[15,16] **Nutritional function and quality of life:** These outcomes were better with distal subtotal gastrectomy versus total gastrectomy.[19–22]

Harms: **Postoperative morbidity:** Morbidity included intra-abdominal sepsis, chest infections, wound sepsis, and fistulae. The first RCT found that subtotal versus total gastrectomy reduced postoperative morbidity, although the difference was not significant (29/320 [9%] with subtotal gastrectomy *v* 40/304 [13%] with total gastrectomy; RR 0.67, 95% CI 0.44 to 1.08), and mean duration of hospital stay (13.8 days for subtotal *v* 15.4 days for total gastrectomy).[17,18] The second RCT also found no significant difference in postoperative morbidity (32/93 [34%] for subtotal gastrectomy *v* 25/76 [32%] for total gastrectomy; RR 1.05, 95% CI 0.68 to 1.60).[15,16] **Postoperative mortality:** The first RCT found no significant difference in postoperative mortality (4/320 [1%] with subtotal gastrectomy *v* 7/304 [2%] with total gastrectomy; RR 0.54, 95% CI 0.16 to 1.84). The second RCT also found no significant difference in postoperative mortality (3/93 [3.2%] with subtotal gastrectomy *v* 1/76 [1.3%] with total gastrectomy; RR 2.45, 95% CI 0.26 to 23.01). Nearly all non-randomised studies that we identified reported higher mortality with total gastrectomy versus subtotal gastrectomy, but total gastrectomy tended to be performed in people with more extensive disease.

Comment: Infiltration of the proximal resection margin by microscopic tumour deposits is perceived as a problem in people with poorly differentiated "diffuse" cancer of the distal stomach undergoing distal subtotal gastrectomy. Some surgeons have therefore recommended total gastrectomy "de principe" (see glossary, p 477) for these tumours. The two RCTs have found similar survival after total and subtotal gastrectomy in people with primary tumours in the distal stomach.[15–18] Both RCTs recruited otherwise fit people, which may explain the low postoperative mortality. The lack of any evidence of survival benefit, and the poorer nutritional and quality of life outcomes, argue against total gastrectomy where subtotal distal gastrectomy is technically possible with an adequate margin.

OPTION REMOVAL OF ADJACENT ORGANS

One RCT found no significant difference with radical gastrectomy plus splenectomy versus radical gastrectomy alone in 5 year survival rates or postoperative mortality. The RCT found that radical gastrectomy plus splenectomy versus radical gastrectomy alone significantly increased the

number of postoperative infections. Retrospective analyses of observational studies and RCTs in people with stomach cancer found that removal of additional organs (spleen and distal pancreas) versus no organ removal increased morbidity and mortality.

Benefits: We found no systematic review. We found one RCT (187 people, aged 25–80 years), which compared radical (D2) gastrectomy plus splenectomy versus radical gastrectomy alone.[23] It found no significant difference in 5 year survival rates (42% with gastrectomy plus splenectomy *v* 36% with gastrectomy alone; $P > 0.5$; absolute numbers not provided).

Harms: The RCT (187 people) found that gastrectomy plus splenectomy versus radical gastrectomy alone significantly increased the number of postoperative infections (including fever > 38 °C, $P < 0.04$; pulmonary infections, $P < 0.008$; subphrenic abscesses, $P < 0.05$), but found no significant difference in postoperative mortality (4/90 [4%] with gastrectomy plus splenectomy *v* 3/97 [3%] with gastrectomy alone; RR 1.40, 95% CI 0.33 to 6.24).[23] Retrospective analyses of RCTs and cohort studies in which removal of the spleen and distal pancreas had been performed routinely during radical total (see glossary, p 477) gastrectomy (D2) (see table 2, p 480), and at the surgeon's discretion during non-radical total gastrectomy (D1), found that removal of the spleen or distal pancreas was associated with increased perioperative mortality (OR about 2) and no evidence of improved long term survival.[24,25]

Comment: Some advocates of radical surgery have suggested routine removal of the spleen and distal pancreas to ensure complete regional lymph node dissection during total gastrectomy. Current consensus is that removal of adjacent organs is justified only when necessary to ensure complete tumour removal, or when required because of trauma during surgery.

OPTION RADICAL VERSUS CONSERVATIVE LYMPHADENECTOMY

Two RCTs comparing radical versus conservative lymphadenectomy found no significant difference in 5 year survival rates. One RCT found that radical versus conservative lymphadenectomy significantly increased mortality.

Benefits: **Radical (D2, D3) versus conservative lymphadenectomy (D1):** We found no systematic review but found four RCTs comparing radical (regional and local) removal of perigastric lymph nodes (see glossary, p 477) versus conservative (local) removal of lymph nodes.[26–29] The first RCT (711 people) found no significant difference in 5 year survival rates (45% with conservative lymphadenectomy *v* 47% with radical lymphadenectomy; ARR +2%, 95% CI –5.6% to +9.6%).[26] The second RCT (400 people) also found no significant difference in 5 year survival rates (35% with conservative lymphadenectomy *v* 33% with radical lymphadenectomy; HR 1.1, 95% CI 0.87 to 1.39).[27] The other two smaller RCTs (55 people[28] and 43 people[29]) did not report evaluable 5 year survival rates. Subgroup analysis from the second RCT found a possible advantage for D2 resection in people with stage II and IIIA disease (corresponding to T1N2M0, T2N1M0, T3N0M0, T2N2M0, T3N1M0, and

T4N0M0), particularly in those people who did not have additional organ removal.[27] **Para-aortic (D4) versus regional and local (D3, D2) lymphadenectomy:** We found one small pilot study for an RCT (70 people with stomach cancer that had spread to the serosa or adjacent organs, T3 or T4) performed in Japan that compared removal of local, regional, and para-aortic lymph nodes versus removal of only local and regional lymph nodes (see glossary, p 477).[30] This pilot study was too small to detect clinically important differences in survival.

Harms: The four RCTs comparing radical versus conservative lymphadenectomy found increased perioperative mortality with the more extensive operation.[26–29] The second RCT (400 people) found significantly higher mortality with D2 versus D1 resection (13% with D2 resection *v* 6% with D1 resection; $P < 0.04$).[27] In the first RCT (711 people) the difference in mortality nearly achieved significance (10% with D2 *v* 6% with D1; $P = 0.06$).[26] In both of these large RCTs the excess mortality was associated closely with greater frequency of pancreatic and splenic removal with D2 resection.[26,27]

Comment: The RCTs were conducted by surgeons with limited prior experience and training in D2 resection, and results may have been affected by both learning curve effects[31] and failure to apply the assigned treatment (contamination and non-compliance).[32] One large prospective cohort study (1654 people with gastric cancer) found no benefit from D2 resection (defined within this study as > 25 lymph nodes removed; 300 people) versus D1 resection (≤ 25 nodes removed; 1096 people) in the entire cohort of people with gastric cancer after 10 years' follow up. Subgroup analysis found that there may be a beneficial effect of D2 versus D1 resection in the subgroup of people with stage II tumours (230 people; RR of long term survival 1.8, 95% CI 1.3 to 2.7).[33] Cohort studies comparing radical versus conservative lymphadenectomy are affected by numerous biases, particularly selection bias, where surgeons reserve D2 surgery for younger or fitter people, or where recent D2 operations are compared with historical D1 controls; definition differences (in the meaning of "limited" and "extended"); and stage migration bias (see glossary, p 477). These biases make the interpretation of observational data difficult.

QUESTION What are the effects of adjuvant chemotherapy?

Four systematic reviews and two subsequent RCTs have found limited evidence that adjuvant chemotherapy versus surgery alone significantly increases survival. RCTs in people from Japan have found conflicting results on the effects of adjuvant chemotherapy versus surgery alone on survival. Two RCTs found that adjuvant chemotherapy versus surgery alone significantly increased postoperative complications. The size of any benefit remains uncertain, and many more recent adjuvant chemotherapy regimens have not been evaluated fully in RCTs.

Benefits: **Adjuvant chemotherapy versus surgery alone:** We found four systematic reviews[34–37] and two subsequent RCTs[38,39] that compared adjuvant chemotherapy (see glossary, p 477) versus surgery alone. The first review (search date 1991, 11 RCTs, 2096 people) found that adjuvant chemotherapy versus surgery alone reduced the risk of death by the end of follow up, but the result was not significant (OR 0.88, 95% CI 0.78 to 1.08).[34] This review was criticised for involving trials that included people with known residual tumour after surgery and trials that also included immunotherapy and intraperitoneal delivery of the adjuvant treatment. A subsequent update of the review found that adjuvant chemotherapy versus surgery alone significantly reduced the risk of death by the end of follow up (OR 0.82, 95% CI 0.68 to 0.97).[40] The second review (search date 1999, 13 RCTs, 1990 people in non-Asian countries) excluded trials of people with known residual tumour after surgery or that also included immunotherapy and intraperitoneal treatment.[35] The review found that adjuvant chemotherapy versus surgery alone significantly reduced the risk of death (595/979 [61%] with adjuvant chemotherapy *v* 660/1011 [65%] with surgery alone; RR 0.93, 95% CI 0.87 to 0.99; NNT 22, 95% CI 12 to 353). The third review (search date 2000, 20 RCTs, 3658 people; see comment below) included most of the RCTs from the first two reviews, but also included two subsequent RCTs.[36] It found that adjuvant chemotherapy versus surgery alone significantly reduced the risk of death (HR 0.82, 95% CI 0.75 to 0.89). The fourth systematic review (search date 1998, 60 RCTs plus 92 non-randomised studies; 12 367 people) found that adjuvant chemotherapy versus surgery alone significantly improved survival (21 RCTs, 3692 people; OR 0.84, 95% CI 0.74 to 0.96).[37] Subgroup analysis found that adjuvant chemotherapy versus surgery alone significantly improved survival in people from Asian countries (OR 0.58, 95% CI 0.44 to 0.76), but found no significant difference in people from Western countries (OR 0.96, 95% CI 0.83 to 1.12). The first subsequent RCT (137 people with gastric adenocarcinoma and positive lymph nodes) compared adjuvant chemotherapy versus surgery alone and found that adjuvant chemotherapy significantly increased median survival time (31 months, range 7–60 months with adjuvant chemotherapy *v* 18 months, range 2–60 months with surgery alone; $P < 0.01$; HR for death 1.96, 95% CI 1.32 to 2.92).[38] The second subsequent RCT (556 people) compared adjuvant chemotherapy plus radiotherapy (4500 cGy in 25 fractions) versus surgery alone.[39] It found that adjuvant chemotherapy plus radiotherapy significantly increased median survival time (36 months with adjuvant chemotherapy plus radiotherapy *v* 27 months with surgery alone; HR for death 1.35, 95% CI 1.09 to 1.66; $P = 0.005$; see comment below). **Japanese RCTs:** We found 10 Japanese RCTs comparing adjuvant chemotherapy versus surgery alone.[41–44] One recent RCT (579 people after curative gastrectomy for early cancer, stage T1 or T2) compared adjuvant chemotherapy (mitomycin, fluorouracil, uracil, tegafur) versus surgery alone.[41] It found no significant difference in cancer related mortality after a median follow up of 72 months (47/288 [16%] with adjuvant chemotherapy *v* 59/291 [20%] with surgery alone; OR 0.77, 95% CI 0.50 to 1.17). A second recent RCT (435 people with stage II or III cancer) compared surgery plus intraperitoneal chemotherapy (using cisplatin alone) versus surgery plus intraperitoneal chemotherapy (using cisplatin plus tegafur-uracil, an orally administered derivative of 5-fluorouracil, and found no significant difference in 3 year survival rates or disease free survival rates.[43] A third recent RCT (139 people) compared three groups: surgery plus hyperthermic intraperitoneal chemotherapy; surgery plus normothermic intraperitoneal chemotherapy; and surgery alone.[44] It found that surgery plus hyperthermic chemotherapy (mitomycin C plus cisplatin at 42 °C) versus surgery alone significantly increased overall 5 year survival rates (P = 0.01; result presented graphically), and that surgery plus hyperthermic chemotherapy versus surgery plus normothermic chemotherapy (mitomycin C plus cisplatin at 37 °C) also significantly increased overall 5 year survival rates (P = 0.05; result presented graphically). Subgroup analysis found that these results were consistent for people with advanced disease (T3 or node positive), but in people with less advanced disease (T2 or node negative) found no significant difference in overall 5 year survival rates. Of the seven older RCTs published before 1985, only one found a significant benefit for chemotherapy.[42] This RCT (120 people) compared three groups: adjuvant chemotherapy with mitomycin alone versus adjuvant chemotherapy with mitomycin plus cytarabine plus fluorouracil versus surgery alone. It found that adjuvant chemotherapy with mitomycin plus cytarabine plus fluorouracil versus both other treatments significantly improved survival. The other six RCTs found no significant difference between adjuvant chemotherapy versus surgery alone in survival. **Adjuvant chemotherapy in palliative care:** We found no systematic review, but found one RCT.[45] The RCT (386 people including 74 people found to have inoperable gastric cancer at time of operation) compared three groups: no preoperative adjuvant chemotherapy; preoperative intravenous chemotherapy; and preoperative superselective intra-arterial chemotherapy.[45] Subgroup analysis of the 74 people with inoperable gastric cancer found that selective intra-arterial chemotherapy versus both other treatments significantly increased the number of people surviving up to 1 year (11/20 [55%] with intra-arterial chemotherapy *v* 0/43 [0%] with both other treatments; NNT 2, 95% CI 1 to 3). The median survival was 91 days with no adjuvant treatment, 96 days with intravenous treatment, and 401 days with intra-arterial treatment.[45]

Harms: Two RCTs reported toxicity (mainly nausea and vomiting) in 53% of people.[46,47] Serious toxicity was usually because of cardiac or cumulative haematological problems; treatment related mortality was 1–2%. We found no definitive evidence from completed studies to justify the concern that preoperative chemotherapy increases postoperative morbidity or mortality. Two RCTs found significant increases in some types of postoperative complications after intraperitoneal chemotherapy (pain, intra-abdominal sepsis without anastamotic leak, bleeding, and fistula formation),[48,49] but a more recent RCT in people from Japan found no such increase.[44] Adjuvant chemotherapy plus radiotherapy produced a treatment related mortality of only 1%, but 41% of people had grade III or IV toxicity.

Comment: The four systematic reviews included several trials in common.[34–37] Only published trials were included. All included trials were reported in English. There was no evidence of publication bias. No statistical heterogeneity of effects was found by the first two systematic reviews, but random effects meta-analysis was used, which may give a conservative estimate of the treatment effect.[34,35] The third systematic review is difficult to interpret.[36] Some of the results, included in the meta-analysis as if they were independent trials, seem to be duplicate versions of the same RCT.[50,51] This systematic review found significant heterogeneity between results of RCTs ($P = 0.028$), but a fixed effects model was used. These factors reduce confidence in the published estimate of effect. The significant effect observed by all four systematic reviews might indicate a small but real effect or alternatively the impact of undetected biases. It is also possible that certain subgroups of people may respond differently to other subgroups. Subgroup analysis in the second systematic review[35] suggested an effect only in RCTs in which at least two thirds of people had node positive disease, but the power was insufficient to draw definite conclusions and the result was not confirmed in the third systematic review.[36] In the second subsequent RCT, 54% of people received surgery less radical than a D1 resection.[39] Many more recent adjuvant chemotherapy regimens have not been evaluated fully in RCTs. Japanese adjuvant chemotherapy regimens often contain bacterial or fungal extracts. We found some evidence from one well designed RCT that addition of these substances to combined surgery and chemotherapy was associated with improved 5 year survival;[52] this will be reviewed in a future update. The quality of surgery in the RCT comparing adjuvant chemotherapy plus radiotherapy versus surgery alone was deficient by all current standards, and further studies are needed to determine whether the benefits found would be reproduced following more adequate resection.[39] The RCT of adjuvant chemotherapy in palliative care identified people before surgery who seemed to have no tumour spread, but who during surgery were found to have tumour spread.[45] The analysis applied to only 19% of those randomised and may not be generalised to all people with inoperable gastric cancer. One further meta-analysis has been identified, which will be incorporated in this review at a subsequent update.[53]

GLOSSARY

Adjuvant chemotherapy Treatment with cytotoxic drugs given in addition to surgery in an attempt to achieve cure.

Disease stage Surgical and microscopic assessment of the primary tumour. Microscopic spread to distant sites can be detected only by radical surgery, creating a potential bias.

Perigastric lymph nodes Lymph nodes that lie adjacent to the stomach.

Regional lymph nodes Lymph nodes that lie along the blood vessels that supply the stomach.

Stage migration bias Apparent increase in stage specific survival without influencing overall survival caused by recategorisation of the stage after removal of diseased lymph nodes.

Subtotal distal gastrectomy Removal of lower part (usually two thirds or four fifths) of the stomach.

Total gastrectomy Removal of the whole stomach.

Total gastrectomy "de principe" Total gastrectomy where it is not technically necessary to remove a distal tumour; this technique is used to minimise the risk of resection line involvement or later second cancer of the gastric stump.

Substantive changes

Adjuvant chemotherapy One new RCT;[44] conclusions unchanged.

Removal of adjacent organs One new RCT;[23] conclusions unchanged.

REFERENCES

1. Whelan SL, Parkin DM, Masuyer E, eds. *Trends in cancer incidence and mortality* (IARC scientific publication no. 102). Lyon: IARC Scientific Publications, 1993.
2. Cancer Research Campaign. *Factsheet 18*. London: Cancer Research Campaign, 1993.
3. Powell J, McConkey CC. Increasing incidence of adenocarcinoma of the gastric cardia and adjacent sites. *Br J Cancer* 1990;62:440–443.
4. Devesa SS, Blot WJ, Fraumeni JF Jr. Changing patterns in the incidence of esophageal and gastric carcinoma in the United States. *Cancer* 1998;83:2049–2053.
5. EUROGAST study group. An international association between *Helicobacter pylori* infection and gastric cancer. *Lancet* 1993;341:1359–1362.
6. Buiatti E, Palli D, Decarli A, et al. A case-control study of gastric cancer and diet in Italy. II Association with nutrients. *Int J Cancer* 1990;45:896–901.
7. Rios-Castellanos E, Sitas F, Shepherd NA, et al. Changing pattern of gastric cancer in Oxfordshire. *Gut* 1992;33:1312–1317.
8. Boddie AW Jr, McMurtrey MJ, Giacco GG, et al. Palliative total gastrectomy and esophagogastrectomy: an evaluation. *Cancer* 1983;51:1195–2000.
9. McCulloch P. Should general surgeons treat gastric carcinoma? An audit of practice and results. *Br J Surg* 1994;81:417–420.
10. Kohli Y, Kawai K, Fujita S. Analytical studies of the growth of human gastric cancer. *J Clin Gastroenterol* 1981;3:129–133.
11. Maruyama K, Okabayashi K, Kinoshita T. Progress in gastric cancer surgery in Japan and its limits of radicality. *World J Surg* 1987;11:418–425.
12. Jakl RJ, Miholic J, Koller R, et al. Prognostic factors in adenocarcinoma of the cardia. *Am J Surg* 1995;169:316–319.
13. Allum WH, Hallissey MT, Kelly KA. Adjuvant chemotherapy in operable gastric cancer: 5 year follow-up of the first British Stomach Cancer Group trial. *Lancet* 1989;1:571–574.
14. Haugstvedt T. Benefits of resection in palliative surgery. *Dig Surgery* 1994;11:121–125.
15. Gouzi JL, Huguier M, Fagniez PL, et al. Gastrectomie totale contre gastrectomie partielle pour adeno-cancer de l'antre. Une etude francaise prospective controlee. *Ann Chir* 1989;43:356–360.
16. Gouzi JL, Huguier M, Fagniez PL, et al. Total versus subtotal gastrectomy for adenocarcinoma of the gastric antrum. A French prospective controlled study. *Ann Surg* 1989;209:162–166.
17. Bozzetti F, Marubini E, Bonfanti G, et al. Total versus subtotal gastrectomy: surgical morbidity and mortality rates in a multicenter Italian randomized trial. *Ann Surg* 1997;226:613–620.
18. Bozzetti F, Marubini E, Bonfanti G, et al. Subtotal versus total gastrectomy for gastric cancer: five-year survival rates in a multicenter randomized Italian trial. *Ann Surg* 1999;230:170–178.
19. Davies J, Johnston D, Sue-Ling H, et al. Total or subtotal gastrectomy for gastric carcinoma? A study of quality of life. *World J Surg* 1998;22:1048–1055.
20. Wu CW, Hsieh MC, Lo SS, et al. Quality of life of patients with gastric adenocarcinoma after curative gastrectomy. *World J Surg* 1997;21:777–782.
21. Svedlund J, Sullivan M, Liedman B, et al. Quality of life after gastrectomy for gastric carcinoma: controlled study of reconstructive procedures. *World J Surg* 1997;21:422–433.
22. Roder JD, Stein HJ, Eckel F, et al. Quality of life after total and subtotal gastrectomy for gastric carcinoma. *Dtsch Med Wochenschr* 1996;121:543–549.
23. Csendes A, Burdiles P, Rojas J, et al. A prospective randomised study comparing D2 total gastrectomy versus D2 total gastrectomy plus splenectomy in 187 patients with gastric carcinoma. *Surgery* 2002;131:401–407.
24. Bonenkamp JJ, Songun I, Hermans J, et al. Randomised comparison of morbidity after D1 and D2 dissection for gastric cancer in 996 Dutch patients. *Lancet* 1995;345:745–748.
25. Cuschieri A, Fayers P, Fielding J, et al. Postoperative morbidity and mortality after D1 and D2 resections for gastric cancer: preliminary results of the MRC randomised controlled surgical trial. *Lancet* 1996;347:995–999.
26. Bonenkamp JJ, Hermans J, Sasako M, et al. Extended lymph-node dissection for gastric cancer. Dutch Gastric Cancer Group. *N Engl J Med* 1999;340:908–914.
27. Cuschieri A, Weedon S, Fielding J, et al. Patient survival after D1 and D2 resections for gastric cancer: long-term results of the MRC randomised surgical trial. *Br J Cancer* 1999;79:1522–1530.
28. Robertson CS, Chung SC, Woods SD, et al. A prospective randomised trial comparing R1 subtotal gastrectomy with R3 total gastrectomy for antral cancer. *Ann Surg* 1994;220:176–182.
29. Dent DM, Madden MV, Price SK. Randomised comparison of R1 and R2 gastrectomy for gastric carcinoma. *Br J Surg* 1988;75:110–112.
30. Maeta M, Yamashiro H, Saito H, et al. A prospective pilot study of extended (D3) and superextended para-aortic lymphadenectomy (D4) in patients with T3 or T4 gastric cancer managed by total gastrectomy. *Surgery* 1999;125:325–331.
31. Parikh D, Chagla L, Johnson M, et al. D2 gastrectomy: lessons from a prospective audit of the learning curve. *Br J Surg* 1996;83:1595–1599.
32. Bunt AMG, Hermans J, Boon MC, et al. Evaluation of the extent of lymphadenectomy in a randomised trial of Western versus Japanese style surgery in gastric cancer. *J Clin Oncol* 1994;12:417–422.
33. Siewert JR, Bottcher K, Stein HJ, et al. Relevant prognostic factors in gastric cancer: ten-year results of the German Gastric Cancer Study. *Ann Surg* 1998;228:449–461.
34. Hermans J, Bonenkamp JJ, Ban MC, et al. Adjuvant therapy after curative resection for gastric cancer: a meta-analysis of randomised trials. *J Clin Oncol* 1993;11:1441–1447. Search date 1991; primary sources Medline and hand searched references.
35. Earle CC, Maroun JA. Adjuvant chemotherapy after curative resection for gastric cancer in non-Asian patients: revisiting a meta-analysis of randomised

trials. *Eur J Cancer* 1999;35:1059–1064. Search date 1999; primary sources Medline and Cancerlit.

36. Mari E, Floriani I, Tinazzi A, et al. Efficacy of adjuvant chemotherapy after curative resection for gastric cancer: a meta-analysis of published randomised trials. A study of the GISCAD (Gruppo Italiano per lo Studio dei Carcinomi dell'Apparato Digerente). *Ann Oncol* 2000;11:837–843. Search date 2000; primary sources Medline, Embase, Cancerlit, and hand searched references.
37. Janunger KG, Hafstrom L, Nygren P, et al. A systematic overview of chemotherapy effects in gastric cancer. *Acta Oncol* 2001;40:309–326. Search date 1998; primary sources Medline, Cancerlit, and the Cochrane Library.
38. Neri B, Cini G, Andreoli F, et al. Randomized trial of adjuvant chemotherapy versus control after curative resection for gastric cancer: 5-year follow-up. *Br J Cancer* 2001;84:878–880.
39. MacDonald JS, Smalley SR, Benedetti J, et al. Chemoradiotherapy after surgery compared with surgery alone for adenocarcinoma of the stomach or gastro-oesophageal junction. *N Engl J Med* 2001;345:725–730.
40. Hermans J, Bonenkamp H. In reply [letter]. *J Clin Oncol* 1994;12:879–880.
41. Nakajima T, Nashimoto A, Kitamura M, et al. Adjuvant mitomycin and fluorouracil followed by oral uracil plus tegafur in serosa-negative gastric cancer: a randomised trial. Gastric Cancer Surgical Study Group. *Lancet* 1999;354:273–277.
42. Nakajima T, Fukami A, Takagi K, et al. Adjuvant chemotherapy with mitomycin C and with a multi drug combination of mitomycin, fluoro-uracil and cytosine arabinoside, after curative resection of gastric cancer. *Jpn J Clin Oncol* 1990;10:187–194.
43. Yoshino K, Fujita M, Hirata K, et al. Interim report on JFMTC Study no. 21 on the effectiveness of UFT as an adjuvant therapy for semi-advanced cancer of the stomach. *Gan To Kagaku Ryoho* 2000;27:263 270.
44. Yonemura Y, De Aretxabala X, Fujimura T, et al. Intraoperative chemohyperthermic peritoneal perfusion as an adjuvant to gastric cancer: final results of a randomized controlled study. *Hepato-gastroenterology* 2001;48:1776–1782.
45. Shchepotin IB, Chorny V, Hanfelt J, et al. Palliative superselective intra-arterial chemotherapy for advanced nonresectable gastric cancer. *J Gastrointest Surg* 1999;3:426–431.
46. Coombes RC, Schein PS, Chilvers CE, et al. A randomised trial comparing adjuvant 5-fluoro-uracil, doxorubicin and mitomycin C with no treatment in operable gastric cancer. International Collaborative Cancer Group. *J Clin Oncol* 1990;8:1362–1369.
47. Hallissey MT, Dunn JA, Ward LC, et al. The second British Stomach Cancer Group trial of adjuvant radiotherapy or chemotherapy in advanced gastric cancer: 5 year follow-up. *Lancet* 1994;343:1309–1312.
48. Rosen HR, Jatzko G, Repse S, et al. Adjuvant intraperitoneal chemotherapy with carbon-adsorbed mitomycin in patients with gastric cancer: results of a randomized multicenter trial of the Austrian Working Group for Surgical Oncology. *J Clin Oncol* 1998;16:2733–2738.
49. Yu W, Whang I, Averbach A, et al. Morbidity and mortality of early postoperative intraperitoneal chemotherapy as adjuvant therapy for gastric cancer. *Am Surg* 1998;64:1104–1108.
50. Alcobendas F, Milla A, Estape J, et al. Mitomycin C as an adjuvant in resected gastric cancer. *Ann Surg* 1983;198:13–17.
51. Grau JJ, Estape J, Alcobendas F. Positive results of adjuvant mitomycin C in resected gastric cancer: a randomised trial on 134 patients. *Eur J Cancer* 1993;29A:340–342.
52. Nakazato H, Koike A, Saji S, et al. Efficacy of immunochemotherapy as adjuvant treatment after curative resection of gastric cancer. Study Group of Immunochemotherapy with PSK for Gastric Cancer. *Lancet* 1994;343:1122–1126.
53. Panzini I, Gianni L, Fattori P, et al. Adjuvant chemotherapy in gastric cancer: a meta-analysis of randomized trials and a comparison with previous meta-analyses. *Tumori* 2002;88:21–27.

Peter McCulloch
Senior Lecturer in Surgery
University Hospital Aintree and University of Liverpool
Liverpool
UK

Competing interests: None declared.

TABLE 1 **Staging of stomach cancer (see text, p 470).**

Stage	Description
T1	Involvement of mucosa +/– submucosa
T2	Involvement of muscularis propria
T3	Involvement of serosa but no spread to adjacent organs
T4	Involvement of adjacent organs
N0	No lymph node involvement
N1	Local (perigastric) nodes involved
N2	Regional nodes involved
N3	More distant intra-abdominal nodes involved
M0	No metastases
M1	Metastases

TABLE 2 **Different types of surgical resection for stomach cancer (see text, p 473).**

Resection	Description
R0	Removal of all detectable tumour, with a margin of healthy tissue confirmed microscopically: synonymous with "curative" resection.
R1	Incomplete removal, with histological evidence of cancer at the resection margin.
R2	Incomplete removal, with macroscopically obvious remnants of the main tumour: synonymous with "palliative" resection.
D1	Removal of all or part of the stomach, together with local (perigastric) nodes.
D2	Removal of all or part of the stomach, together with local and regional nodes, which lie along the branches of the coeliac axis.
D3/D4	More radical lymph node resection, including removal of para-aortic nodes and nodes within the small bowel mesentery.

Chronic suppurative otitis media

Search date November 2001

Jose Acuin

QUESTIONS

INTERVENTIONS

Key Messages

- We found no RCTs with long term follow up.

Adults

- **Ear cleansing** We found no RCTs of ear cleansing (aural toilet) versus no treatment.
- **Oral and intravenous antibiotics** RCTs found insufficient evidence about the effects of oral and intravenous antibiotics versus placebo or no treatment. One systematic review found that systemic antibiotics were significantly less effective than topical antibiotics in reducing otoscopic features of chronic suppurative otitis media. We found no evidence about long term treatment.
- **Topical antibiotics** RCTs found limited evidence that topical quinolone antibiotics versus placebo improved otoscopic appearances. RCTs found no clear evidence of significant differences between topical antibiotics. Case studies have associated topical non-quinolone antibiotics with ototoxicity, affecting mainly vestibular function, although RCTs have found few adverse events associated with short term use. One systematic review found that topical antibiotics were significantly more effective than systemic antibiotics at reducing otoscopic features of chronic suppurative otitis media.

- **Topical antiseptics** We found no RCTs comparing topical antiseptics versus placebo or no treatment. One RCT compared topical antiseptics plus ear cleansing under microscopic control versus topical antibiotics alone versus oral antibiotics. It found no significant difference in the rate of persistent activity on otoscopy. However, the RCT was too small to exclude a clinically important difference.
- **Topical steroids** We found no RCTs comparing topical steroids versus placebo or no treatment.
- **Tympanoplasty with or without mastoidectomy** We found no RCTs comparing tympanoplasty with or without mastoidectomy versus no surgery for chronic suppurative otitis media without cholesteatoma.

Children

- **Ear cleansing** One systematic review found no significant difference in persistent otorrhoea or tympanic perforations with a simple form of ear cleansing versus no ear cleansing.
- **Oral and intravenous antibiotics** RCTs found insufficient evidence about the effects of systemic antibiotics in children with chronic suppurative otitis media.
- **Topical antibiotics** We found no RCTs comparing topical antibiotics versus placebo. One small and brief RCT found no significant difference in the proportion of ears with unchanged otorrohoea on otoscopy with a topical antibiotic plus steroid mixture plus ear cleansing versus ear cleansing alone. However, the confidence interval was wide and a clinically important difference cannot be excluded.
- **Topical antiseptics** RCTs found no significant reduction in otorrhoea with topical antiseptics versus placebo after 2 weeks. One RCT found no significant difference in otorrhoea with topical antiseptics versus topical antibiotic plus steroid. However, the RCTs were too small to exclude a clinically important effect.
- **Topical steroids** We found no RCTs comparing topical steroids versus placebo.
- **Tympanoplasty with or without mastoidectomy** We found no RCTs comparing tympanoplasty with or without mastoidectomy versus no surgery for chronic suppurative otitis media without cholesteatoma.

DEFINITION Chronic suppurative otitis media is a persistent inflammation of the middle ear or mastoid cavity. Synonyms include "chronic otitis media (without effusion)", chronic mastoiditis, and chronic tympanomastoiditis. Chronic suppurative otitis media is characterised by recurrent or persistent ear discharge (otorrhoea) over 2–6 weeks through a perforation of the tympanic membrane. Typical findings also include thickened granular middle ear mucosa, mucosal polyps, and cholesteatoma (see glossary, p 493) within the middle ear. Chronic suppurative otitis media is differentiated from chronic otitis media with effusion, in which there is an intact tympanic membrane with fluid in the middle ear but no active infection. Chronic suppurative otitis media does not include chronic perforations of the eardrum, that are dry, or only occasionally discharge, and have no signs of active infection.

INCIDENCE/ PREVALENCE The worldwide prevalence of chronic suppurative otitis media is 65–330 million people. Between 39–200 million (60%) suffer from significant hearing impairment. Otitis media has been estimated to cause 28 000 deaths and loss of over 2 million Disability Adjusted

Life Years (see glossary, p 493) in 2000,[1] 94% of which are in developing countries. Most of these deaths are presumably due to chronic suppurative otitis media because acute otitis media is a self limiting infection. Estimates of prevalence are shown in web extra table A at www.clinicalevidence.com.[2–33]

AETIOLOGY/ RISK FACTORS Chronic suppurative otitis media is assumed to be a complication after an initial episode of acute otitis media, but the risk factors for development of chronic suppurative otitis media are not clear. Frequent upper respiratory tract infections and poor socioeconomic conditions (overcrowded housing,[34] hygiene, and nutrition) may be related to the development of chronic suppurative otitis media.[35,36] Improvement of housing, hygiene and nutrition in Maori children was associated with a halving of the prevalence of chronic suppurative otitis media between 1978 and 1987.[37] For risk factors see acute otitis media, p 251.

PROGNOSIS Most children with chronic suppurative otitis media have mild to moderate hearing impairment (about 26–60 dB increase in hearing thresholds) based on surveys among children in Africa, Brazil,[38] India,[39] and Sierra Leone,[40] and among the general population in Thailand.[41] In many developing countries, chronic suppurative otitis media represents the most frequent cause of moderate hearing losses (40–60 dB).[42] Persistent hearing loss during the first 2 years of life may increase learning disabilities and poor scholastic performance.[43] Spread of infection may lead to life threatening complications such as intracranial infections and acute mastoiditis.[44] The frequency of serious complications has fallen 10-fold to about 0.24% in Thailand and 1.8% in Africa. This is believed to be associated with increased use of antibiotic treatment, tympanoplasty, and mastoidectomy (see glossary, p 494).[45–47] Cholesteatoma is another serious complication that has been found in a variable proportion of people with chronic suppurative otitis media (range 0–60%).[48–51] In the West, the incidence of cholesteatoma is low (in 1993 in Finland the age standardised incidence of cholesteatoma was 8 new cases per 100 000 population/year).[52]

AIMS To improve symptoms of otorrhoea; heal perforations; improve hearing; and reduce complications, with minimum adverse effects of treatment.

OUTCOMES **Dichotomous variables:** Proportion of people with otorrhoea measured subjectively or by otoscopy; with tympanic perforation; hearing loss; intra- and extracranial complications; death; or adverse effects. The correlation between subjective cessation of otorrhoea and otoscopic findings was poor in one RCT.[53] Many RCTs used compound outcomes (e.g. otoscopic finding of otorrhoea or otoscopic finding of inflammation in the middle ear). **Continuous variables:** Duration of otorrhoea free periods; severity of hearing loss.

METHODS *Clinical Evidence* search and appraisal November 2001. We found one systematic review (search date 1996, 24 RCTs, 1660 people) of treatments for chronic suppurative otitis media.[54] It did not analyse results for children and adults separately. We have excluded all studies that included both adults (aged ≥ 16) and children (aged ≤ 10),[55–58] or which failed to specify the age of participants.[59,60]

The RCTs varied in their definitions of chronic suppurative otitis media and measurements of severity. All RCTs were brief (7 days to 3 wks). Most had inadequate methods (see main text for descriptions). Participants with cholesteatoma were excluded from most, but not all, trials.

QUESTION **What are the effects of treatments for chronic suppurative otitis media in adults?**

OPTION **EAR CLEANSING (AURAL TOILET)**

We found no RCTs of ear cleansing versus no treatment in adults.

Benefits: We found one systematic review (search date 1996), which found no RCTs in adults of ear cleansing versus no treatment.[54]

Harms: We found no RCTs.

Comment: Techniques of ear cleansing vary considerably. In western countries, microsuction of the external and middle ear under microscopic control by a trained operator is the standard method of ear cleansing. Microscopic examination of the ear with ear cleansing is an important aspect of diagnosis of persistent otorrhoea; RCTs against no treatment would probably be considered unethical.

OPTION **TOPICAL ANTIBIOTICS**

We found no RCTs with long term follow up. Two RCTs found limited direct evidence that topical quinolone antibiotics versus placebo improved otoscopic appearances in adults with chronic suppurative otitis media. Six RCTs found no clear evidence of significant differences between topical antibiotics in adults. We found limited and indirect evidence that topical non-quinolone antibiotics plus topical steroid improved otoscopic appearances. One RCT found that topical non-quinolone antibiotic plus steroid versus topical steroid alone significantly improved otoscopic assessment of otorrhoea and inflammation in the middle ear. Short term topical antibiotics have been associated with few adverse events in RCTs; uncontrolled case studies have associated topical non-quinolone antibiotics with ototoxicity affecting mainly vestibular function. Topical antibiotics appear more effective than systematic antibiotics.

Benefits: **Topical antibiotics versus placebo:** We found no systematic review but found two small RCTs in adults.[61,62] Both RCTs found that quinolone topical antibiotics versus placebo improve otorrhoea, but both RCTs had weak methods. The first RCT (50 adults with chronic suppurative otitis media but no cholesteatoma [see glossary, p 493] in a hospital clinic in Thailand) found that, after 7 days, topical ciprofloxacin in saline (5 drops 0.25g/L 3 times daily for 7 days) versus topical saline significantly reduced the proportion of people with persistent signs on otoscopic examination (3/19 [16%] *v* 14/16 [88%]; OR 0.06, 95% CI 0.02 to 0.23).[60] The RCT lasted only 7 days, had 30% drop outs (15/50), and did not clearly describe the methods of randomisation and allocation concealment. The second RCT (51 adults with chronic suppurative otitis media without cholesteatoma in a hospital clinic in Israel, 60 ears) compared 3 weeks' treatment with topical ciprofloxacin versus topical tobramycin versus a dilute antiseptic solution (1% aluminium acetate), which functioned as a placebo. The RCT found that ciprofloxacin versus control significantly reduced the proportion of people with unimproved otorrhoea (4/19 [21%] with ciprofloxacin *v* 10/17 [59%] with the control; OR 0.21, 95% CI 0.06 to 0.80; NNT 3, 95% CI 2 to 18), but tobramycin versus control did not significantly reduce otorrhoea (5/18 [28%] with tobramycin *v* 10/17 [59%] with the control; OR 0.29, 95% CI 0.08 to 1.09). This RCT randomised people to treatments, but presented results for ears. The 1% aluminium acetate used as a control may not have been an inert control (see topical antiseptics, p 491). **Topical antibiotic versus other topical antibiotic:** We found one systematic review (search date 1996,[54] 4 RCTs, 406 adults) and two subsequent RCTs (see table 1, p 497).[62,67] Three RCTs found no clear difference in the otoscopic response with a topical quinolone (ciprofloxacin) versus a topical non-quinolones (gentamicin, tobramycin and polymyxin–neomycin–hydrocortisone). The three RCTs comparing different topical non-quinolone antibiotics found no significant difference in the proportion of people who still had a wet ear on otoscopy at the end of treatment (see table 1, p 497).[69–71] **Topical antibiotics plus topical steroids versus placebo:** We found one systematic review (search date 1996,[54] 2 RCTs,[53,68] 196 people) of combined topical antibiotics plus steroid for 4–6 weeks versus various control treatments. Both RCTs found that topical antibiotics plus steroid versus control treatment significantly reduced persistent otorrhoea. The first RCT (123 adults with chronic suppurative otitis media, no cholesteatoma, and no open mastoid cavity) found significantly fewer people had active otoscopic appearances after treatment with gentamicin plus hydrocortisone than with placebo (active appearance: 33/64 [52%] people with treatment *v* 44/59 [75%] with placebo; OR 0.38, 95% CI 0.18 to 0.78; NNT 5).[20] Similar results were found in 42 other people who had an open mastoid cavity. The second RCT (31 adults) also compared gentamicin plus hydrocortisone for 4 weeks versus placebo and found a significant reduction in the proportion of people with active ears on otoscopy at the end of treatment (6/17 [35%] with treatment *v* 11/14 [79%] with placebo; OR 0.18, 95% CI 0.05 to 0.75; NNT 3).[68] **Topical antibiotic plus steroid versus topical steroid:** The systematic review[54] found one RCT (64 adults),[69] which compared topical gentamicin plus hydrocortisone versus topical betamethasone for 3 weeks. It found significantly fewer people with persistent activity on otoscopy at the end of treatment (6/30 [20%] with gentamicin–hydrocortisone *v* 17/24 [71%] with betamethasone; ARR 51%, 95% CI 24% to 77%; OR 0.13, 95% CI 0.04 to 0.38; NNT 2). **Topical antibiotics versus systemic antibiotics:** see topical antiseptics). Topical antibiotic versus other topical antibiotic: We found one systematic review (search date 1996, 4 RCTs, 406 adults) and two subsequent RCTs (see table 1, p 497).[62,67] Three RCTs found no clear difference in the otoscopic response with a topical quinolone (ciprofloxacin) versus a topical non-quinolones (gentamicin, tobramycin and polymyxin–neomycin–hydrocortisone). The three RCTs comparing different topical non-quinolone antibiotics found nc significant difference in the proportion of people who still had a wet ear on otoscopy at the end of treatment (see table 1, p 497).[69–71] **Topical antibiotics plus topical steroids versus placebo:** We found one systematic review (search date 1996,[54] 2 RCTs,[53,68] 196 people) of combined topical antibiotics plus steroid for 4–6 weeks versus various control treatments. Both RCTs found that topical antibiotics plus steroid versus control treatment significantly reduced persistent otorrhoea. The first RCT (123 adults with chronic suppurative otitis media, no cholesteatoma, and no open mastoid cavity) found significantly fewer people had active otoscopic appearances after treatment with gentamicin plus hydrocortisone than with placebo (active appearance: 33/64 [52%] people with treatment *v* 44/59 [75%] with placebo; OR 0.38, 95% CI 0.18 to 0.78; NNT 5).[20] Similar results were found in 42 other people who had an open mastoid cavity. The second RCT (31 adults) also compared gentamicin plus hydrocortisone for 4 weeks versus placebo and found a significant reduction in the proportion of people with active ears on otoscopy at the end of treatment (6/17 [35%] with treatment *v* 11/14 [79%] with placebo; OR 0.18, 95% CI 0.05 to 0.75; NNT 3).[68] **Topical antibiotic plus steroid versus topical steroid:** The systematic review[54] found one RCT (64 adults),[69] which compared topical gentamicin plus hydrocortisone versus topical betamethasone for 3 weeks. It found significantly fewer people with persistent activity on otoscopy at the end of treatment (6/30 [20%] with gentamicin–hydrocortisone *v* 17/24 [71%] with betamethasone; ARR 51%, 95% CI 24% to 77%; OR 0.13, 95% CI 0.04 to 0.38; NNT 2). **Topical antibiotics versus systemic antibiotics:**[54] The adverse events included Candida infections, dizziness, itching, stinging, and ear ache. One subsequent small RCT found no reported adverse events with topical ciprofloxacin used for 7 days in 19 ears.[61] Another subsequent RCT (322 people) found no significant difference in the number of adverse events with topical ciprofloxacin versus topical polymyxin-B plus neomycin plus hydrocortisone (24/165 [15%] with ciprofloxacin *v* 12/153 [8%]; OR 1.95, 95% CI 0.97 to 3.89).[67] Vertigo was reported by two people with topical ciprofloxacin and by none using topical polymyxin-B plus neomycin plus hydrocortisone. **Ototoxic effects of topical antibiotics:** We found one systematic review[54] and two subsequent RCTs[61,56] in adults and childrenthat examined hearing before and after topical antibiotics. The systematic review (search date 1996, 11 RCTs)[54] found negligible or no changes in hearing levels after topical antibiotics. Three RCTs in adults and children[61,55,56] found no case of worsened hearing in those who were given topical ciprofloxacin or topical aminoglycoside. One RCT[67] found deterioration of the audiogram in only one person with topical polymyxin-B plus neomycin plus hydrocortisone after 6–12 days (0/157 with topical ciprofloxacin *v* 1/138 with topical polymyxin-B plus neomycin plus hydrocortisone; OR 0.12, 95% CI 0.002 to 5.99).

Comment: There is consensus that topical antibiotics must be combined with thorough ear cleansing to be effective. We found no evidence about long term effects on reducing complications. The comparative RCTs were small and their quality variable. We found no clear evidence from RCTs of ototoxicity from any topical antibiotic. However, this evidence is based only on the assessment of audiograms after short term exposure to the antibiotics, and uncontrolled case studies have reported ototoxicity associated with use of some topical non-quinolone antibiotics for 7–120 days.[70–72] Most of the people in the observational studies had vestibular rather than cochlear symptoms, suggesting that the evidence from audiograms and hearing tests may not exclude ototoxicity. Most topical non-quinolone antibiotics have license restrictions against prolonged use, or use in people with perforation of the ear drum.

OPTION TOPICAL ANTISEPTICS (ALUMINIUM ACETATE, BORAX, BORIC ACID, HYDROGEN PEROXIDE, IODINE POWDER)

We found no systematic review and no RCTs comparing topical antiseptics versus placebo or no treatment. One RCT in adults found no significant difference with topical antiseptics plus ear cleansing under microscopic control versus topical antibiotics versus oral antibiotics. The RCT was too small to establish or exclude a clinically important effect from topical antiseptics in adults.

Benefits: **Topical antiseptics versus placebo:** We found no systematic review and no RCT. **Topical antiseptics versus antibiotics:** We found one systematic review (search date 1996,[54] 1 RCT,[73] 51 people). The RCT (51 adults) found no significant difference with topical antiseptics (boric acid and iodine powder plus ear cleansing under microscopic vision) versus topical antibiotics (gentamicin or chloramphenicol) versus oral antibiotics (cefalexin [cephalexin], flucloxacillin, cloxacillin, or amoxycillin [amoxycillin] according to bacterial sensitivity) in the rate of persistent activity on otoscopy (13/20 [65%] with topical antiseptics *v* 15/18 [83%] with topical antibiotics *v* 8/13 [62%] with oral antibiotics; for topical antiseptic versus topical antibiotic, OR 0.40, 95% CI 0.10 to 1.66).[73]

Harms: Adverse effects included dizziness and local pain. The systematic review found negligible or no changes in hearing acuity after topical treatment.[54]

Comment: The available evidence from RCTs in adults is insufficient to establish or exclude a clinically important effect from topical antiseptics.

OPTION TOPICAL STEROIDS

We found no RCTs in adults comparing topical steroids versus placebo or versus no treatment.

Benefits: We found no systematic review or RCTs.

Harms: We found no systematic review or RCT.

Comment: Topical steroids have been used in combination with topical antibiotics (see topical antibiotics, p 484).

OPTION ORAL AND INTRAVENOUS ANTIBIOTICS

We found limited evidence about the effects of oral and intravenous antibiotics in adults with chronic suppurative otitis media. Oral antibiotics appear less effective than topical antibiotics. We found no clear evidence from RCTs that different systemic antibiotics differ in their effectiveness. We found no evidence about long term outcomes.

Chronic suppurative otitis media

Benefits: **Systemic antibiotics versus placebo in people receiving no other treatment:** We found one systematic review (search date 1996), which found no RCTs investigating the effects of systemic antibiotics in adults receiving no other treatment.[54] **Additional systemic antibiotics versus placebo in people receiving other non-antibiotic treatments:** We found one systematic review (search date 1996,[54] 1 RCT,[74] 26 adults) of systemic antibiotics versus placebo in people receiving other forms of treatment. The RCT[74] (26 adults having mastoidectomy/tympanoplasty [see glossary, p 494]) found a significant difference with intravenous ceftazidime versus no antibiotic in the proportion of people with otorrhoea on otoscopy or with positive *Pseudomonas aeruginosa* cultures (1/14 [7%] *v* 7/12 [58%]; OR 0.10, 95% CI 0.02 to 0.51). The RCT used computer generated random numbers but ended up with unbalanced groups with more people in the antibiotic arm having only tympanoplasty. **Additional systemic antibiotics versus placebo/no treatment in people receiving topical antibiotics:** We found one systematic review (search date 1996,[54] 2 RCTs,[75,76] 100 adults) of systemic antibiotic versus no systemic antibiotic in people treated with topical antibiotics. The first RCT found no significant difference with topical ciprofloxacin with and without oral ciprofloxacin (5/20 [25%] with oral ciprofloxacin *v* 3/20 [15%] with no oral ciprofloxacin; OR 1.84, 95% CI 0.40 to 8.49).[76] The second RCT found no significant difference with topical gentamicin–hydrocortisone with and without oral metronidazole (6/14 [43%] with metronidazole v 6/16 [38%] without metronidazole; OR 1.24, 95% CI 0.29 to 5.23).[75] **Oral plus topical non-quinolone antibiotics versus topical quinolone antibiotics:** We found one RCT (80 adults, 89 ears),[78] which found that topical ofloxacin (0.3%) versus oral amoxicillin (amoxycillin) plus topical chloramphenicol reduced the proportion of people with persistent symptoms or signs (ear pain, discharge or inflammation on otoscopic examination) after 2 weeks (33% of ears with ofloxacin v 63% of ears with oral amoxicillin plus topical chloramphenicol; absolute number of ears examined not stated; $P < 0.001$). The RCT randomised people, but analysed the number of ears with persistent otorrhoea. **Systemic antibiotics versus topical antibiotics:** We found one systematic review[54] (search date 1996, 5 RCTs, 271 adults) (see table 2, p 498).[73–83] All RCTs found a better response with topical than with systemic antibiotics. The topical antibiotics used were ofloxacin, ciprofloxacin, gentamicin, and chloramphenicol; the systemic antibiotics were oral cefalexin, cloxacillin, amoxicillin, ofloxacin, ciprofloxacin, co-amoxiclav, and intramuscular gentamicin. The systematic review found that, overall, topical antibiotics were more effective than systemic antibiotics at reducing otoscopic features of chronic suppurative otitis media by the end of the trials (34/153 [22%] with topical antibiotics *v* 77/138 [56%] with systemic antibiotics; OR 0.23, 95% CI 0.14 to 0.37; NNT 3 people). **Systemic antibiotics versus topical antiseptics:** We found one systematic review (search date 1996, 2 RCTs, 152 people).[54] The first RCT (51 adults) found no significant difference with oral antibiotics (cefalexin, flucloxacillin, cloxacillin, or amoxicillin according to bacterial sensitivity) versus topical antiseptics (boric acid and iodine powder plus ear cleansing under microscopic vision) versus topical antibiotics (gentamicin or chloramphenicol) in the rate of persistent activity on otoscopy (8/13 [62%] with oral antibiotics *v* 13/20 [65%] with topical antiseptics *v* 15/18 [83%] with topical antibiotics; for oral antibiotic *v* topical antiseptic, OR 0.87, 95% CI 0.21 to 3.61).[73] The second RCT (119 people with an age range from 11–79 years) found no significant difference with topical hydrogen peroxide or boric acid for 10–20 days versus various systemic antibiotics (choice based on sensitivity results, administered orally or iv) in the proportion with otoscopically persistent discharge or inflamed mucosa at the end of treatment (33/71 [46%] with systemic antibiotic *v* 29/48 [60%] with topical antiseptic; OR 0.58, 95% CI 0.28 to 1.19). The confidence interval is too large to exclude a clinically important difference. **Systemic antibiotics versus other systemic antibiotics:** We found one systematic review (search date 1996,[54] 1 RCT, 75 adults) and one subsequent RCTs (see comment below).[77] The RCT in the systematic review found no clear evidence of differences in effectiveness between oral ciprofloxacin (500 mg twice daily) and amoxicillin-clavulanate (500 mg 3 times daily) in persistent otoscopic activity (16/40 [40%] with ciprofloxacin *v* 22/35 [63%] with amoxicillin–clavulanate; OR 0.41, 0.16 to 1.00). One subsequent RCT (190 adults) found no significant difference with oral cefotiam hexetil versus amoxicillin–clavulanate in persistent otoscopic abnormality at the end of treatment (37/94 [39%] with cefotiam *v* 33/94 [35%] with amoxicillin–clavulanate; OR 1.20, 95% CI 0.67 to 2.16).[77]

Harms: The systematic review found that adverse effects of systemic antibiotics include Candida infections, headache, nausea, and allergic reactions.[54] One RCT found ototoxicity (defined as an elevation in bone conduction thresholds and/or speech reception thresholds of ≥ 5 dB) with amoxicillin–chloramphenicol but not with ciprofloxacin (absolute numbers not stated).[78]

Comment: We found two further, recent RCTs comparing quinolone versus non-quinolone antibiotics; they are being translated and their results may be included in future *Clinical Evidence* updates.[79,80]

OPTION MASTOIDECTOMY AND/OR TYMPANOPLASTY

We found no RCTs comparing tympanoplasty with or without mastoidectomy versus no surgery for chronic suppurative otitis media without cholesteatoma.

Benefits: We found no systematic review and no RCTs.

Harms: We found no RCTs.

Comment: We found no evidence from RCTs in adults, but found numerous retrospective studies. One retrospective study (41 people with bilateral chronic suppurative otitis media operated at one unit in Italy) compared hearing in ears that had previous tympanoplasty versus hearing in contralateral ears treated without surgery.[84] The hearing in both operated and non-operated ears progressively deteriorated, but the rate of decline was significantly lower in operated ears. Tympanoplasty can be combined with mastoidectomy when the possibility of restoring some functional hearing without jeopardising surgical clearance of the disease exists. Observational studies have found that the success of surgery depends on several factors (age, technical skill of the surgeon,[85] availability of remnant eardrum and ossicles,[86] type of mastoidectomy performed). Success in sealing a tympanic perforation with a graft can be 90–95%. Correction of hearing deficit can occur in about 50–70% of operated ears.[87–89]

QUESTION **What are the effects of treatments for chronic suppurative otitis media in children?**

OPTION **EAR CLEANSING**

One systematic review has found no evidence from two RCTs that a simple form of ear cleansing is better than no ear cleansing at improving the symptoms of chronic suppurative otitis media in children.

Benefits: **Versus no treatment:** We found one systematic review (search 1996,[54] 2 RCTs,[90,91] 658 children), which found that a simple form of ear cleansing versus no ear cleansing had no significant effect over 3–16 weeks on either the proportion of children with persistent otorrhoea (2 RCTs; 125/170 [74%] with ear cleansing *v* 91/114 [80%] with no treatment; OR 0.63, 95% CI 0.36 to 1.12) or the proportion with persistent tympanic perforations (1 RCT;[91] 125/144 [87%] *v* 63/73 [87%]; OR 1.04, 95% CI 0.46 to 2.38).

Harms: The review did not provide any evidence about the adverse effects of ear cleansing.

Comment: A synonym for ear cleansing is "aural toilet". Techniques of ear cleansing vary considerably. In western countries, microsuction of the external and middle ear under microscopic control by a trained operator is a standard method of ear cleansing. In developing countries (and in the 2 RCTs[90,91]) cleansing of the external auditory canal may be performed by parents, carers, or unaffected schoolchildren by dry mopping with cotton wool on orange sticks around four times daily. Both RCTs were performed in areas with a high prevalence of chronic suppurative otitis media (Solomon Islands[90] and Kenya[91]). The first RCT randomised 134 children but analysed ears. It followed all the randomised children for 6 weeks and presented results as number of ears with persistent otorrhoea.[90] The second RCT randomised 145 schools but analysed the numbers of children with persistent otorrhoea.[91] It followed children for 16 weeks, but analysed results only for the 72% of the children who completed the RCT. Neither study described allocation concealment methods. In one RCT,[23] the randomisation process was described but outcome assessors were not blinded to treatment allocation. The meta-analysis in the systematic review[54] combined results from the first RCT for the numbers of ears with persistent signs at 6 weeks with results from the second RCT for the number of children with persistent signs after 16 weeks; there was significant heterogeneity between the two RCTs in the effect of ear cleansing on otorrhoea ($P = 0.02$). Overall, we found no good evidence of benefit from simple ear cleansing, but the evidence is not strong enough to exclude a clinically important benefit.

OPTION TOPICAL ANTIBIOTICS

We found no RCTs about the effects of topical antibiotics in children with chronic suppurative otitis media. One small and brief RCT found no significant difference with a topical antibiotic plus steroid mixture plus ear cleansing versus ear cleansing alone, but the confidence interval was wide and a clinical important effect cannot be excluded.

Benefits: **Topical antibiotics alone:** We found one systematic review (search date 1996, no RCTs exclusively in children) and no subsequent RCTs.[54] **Topical antibiotics plus topical steroids versus placebo:** We found one systematic review (search date 1996,[54] 1 RCT,[90] 50 children, 67 ears) of combined topical antibiotics plus steroid (topical framycetin, gramicidin, and dexamethasone: Sofradex®) versus ear cleansing only. The RCT found no significant difference with topical antibiotics plus steroid versus ear cleansing only in the proportion of ears with unchanged otorrhoea on otoscopy after 6 weeks (17/41 [42%] with Sofradex plus ear cleansing v 13/26 [50%] with ear cleansing alone; OR 0.71, 95% CI 0.27 to 1.90). **Combined topical antibiotic plus steroid versus either component alone:** The systematic review found no RCTs.[54]

Harms: The RCT did not provide any evidence about harms.[54]

Comment: The RCT[23] found no difference in effectiveness between topical antibiotics with steroids and ear cleansing alone, but this study was small, did not report methods for allocation concealment and blinding, and randomised children but analysed ears. We found no evidence about long term effects on reducing complications. We found no clear evidence from RCTs of ototoxicity from any topical antibiotic. However, this evidence is based only on the assessment of audiograms after short term exposure to the antibiotics, and uncontrolled case studies have reported ototoxicity associated with use of some topical non-quinolone antibiotics for 7–120 days.[92–94] Most of the people in the observational studies had vestibular rather than cochlear symptoms, suggesting that the evidence from audiograms and hearing tests may not exclude ototoxicity. Most topical non-quinolone antibiotics have license restrictions against prolonged use, or use in people with perforation of the eardrum.

OPTION TOPICAL ANTISEPTICS (ALUMINIUM ACETATE, BORAX, BORIC ACID, HYDROGEN PEROXIDE, IODINE POWDER)

Two RCTs in children found no significant reduction of otorrhoea with topical antiseptics versus placebo. One RCT in children found no significant difference between topical antiseptics and topical antibiotic plus steroid. The RCTs were too small to exclude a clinically important effect.

Benefits: **Topical antiseptics versus placebo:** We found no systematic review but found two RCTs.[90,95] The first RCT (60 children with otorrhoea in a hospital clinic in South Africa, 67 ears) compared aluminium acetate solutions of varying concentrations (full strength [13%] *v* a quarter strength [3.25%] *v* a tenth strength [1.3%]).[95] The dilute solution was thought to be inactive. Results were obtained for 56 (84%) ears. The RCT found larger proportions of dry ears after 2 weeks with the two stronger solutions but the overall differences between the groups could have occurred by chance (21/26 [81% of ears] responded with full strength *v* 15/20 [75%] with a quarter strength *v* 5/10 [50%] with a tenth strength; Fisher exact P = 0.18). The second RCT (43 children, 58 ears) found no significant difference with topical antiseptic (boric acid 2% in 20% alcohol, 3 drops to each ear, 4/day after ear cleansing) versus ear cleansing alone in the proportion of children with unchanged otoscopic appearance after 6 weeks (12/32 [38%] with topical antiseptic *v* 13/26 [50%] with ear cleansing alone; OR 0.61, 95% CI 0.22 to 1.71).[90] **Topical antiseptics versus topical antibiotic plus steroid:** We found one systematic review (search date 1996,[54] 1 RCT,[90] 55 children, 73 ears), which found no significant difference with topical antiseptic (boric acid 2% in 20% alcohol, 3 drops to each ear, four times daily after ear cleansing) versus topical antibiotic plus steroid (framycetin, gramicidin, dexamethasone: Sofradex®) in the rate of persistent otorrhoea (12/32 [38%] with topical antiseptic *v* 17/41 [41%] with topical antibiotic plus steroid; OR 0.85, 95% CI 0.33 to 2.17).

Harms: Adverse effects included dizziness and local pain. The systematic review found negligible or no changes in hearing acuity after topical treatment.[54]

Comment: We found small studies that found no difference in the short term effects of topical antiseptics versus systemic antibiotics (see systemic antibiotics, p 492). The available evidence is insufficient to establish or exclude a clinically important effect from topical antiseptics.

OPTION TOPICAL STEROIDS

We found no RCTs comparing topical steroids versus placebo or no treatment in children.

Benefits: We found no systematic review or RCT.

Harms: We found no RCTs.

Comment: None.

OPTION ORAL AND INTRAVENOUS ANTIBIOTICS

RCTs found insufficient evidence of the effects of systemic antibiotics in children with otitis media.

Benefits: **Systemic antibiotics versus placebo in children receiving no other treatment:** We found one systematic review (search date 1996),[54] which found no RCTs investigating the effects of systemic antibiotics in children receiving no other treatment. **Additional systemic antibiotics versus placebo in children receiving other non-antibiotic treatments:** We found one systematic review (search date 1996,[54] 1 RCT,[96] 33 children). The RCT (33 children having ear cleansing by suctioning and debridement for 1–2 wks) found a significant reduction with intravenous antibiotic (mezlocillin or ceftazidime for 3–21 days) versus no antibiotic in otoscopic persistent otorrhoea detected at otoscopy after 6 months (0/21 [0%] with iv antibiotic *v* 11/12 [92%]; OR 0.02, 95% CI 0.004 to 0.08). **Additional systemic antibiotics versus placebo/no treatment in children receiving topical antibiotics:** We found one systematic review (search date

1996,[54] 1 RCT[90]). The RCT (62 children, 81 ears, all treated with ear cleansing plus Sofradex® drops) found no significant difference with oral clindamycin versus no clindamycin (15 mg/kg/day) on the proportion of ears with unchanged otoscopic otorrhoea after 6 weeks (23/40 [58%] with clindamycin *v* 17/41 [41%] without clindamycin; OR 1.88, 95% CI 0.79 to 4.48).[90] **Systemic antibiotics versus topical antibiotics:** We found one systematic review (search date 1996, no RCTs) and no subsequent RCT.[54] **Systemic antibiotics versus topical antiseptics:** We found one systematic review (search date 1996, no RCT).[54] **Systemic antibiotics versus other systemic antibiotics:** We found one systematic review (search date 1996,[54] 1 RCT, 36 children) and one subsequent RCT.[97] The systematic review found no evidence of differences in effectiveness between intravenous mezlocillin versus intravenous ceftazidime (otoscopic evidence of otorrhoea at the end of treatment: 0/17 [0%] with mezlocillin *v* 0/19 [0%] with ceftazidime).

Harms: The systematic review found that (in all age groups) adverse effects of systemic antibiotics include Candida infections, headache, nausea, and allergic reactions.[54]

Comment: We found no clear evidence from RCTs that systemic antibiotics differ in their effectiveness. The studies in children found similar results to those in adults.

OPTION MASTOIDECTOMY AND/OR TYMPANOPLASTY

We found no RCTs in children comparing tympanoplasty with or without mastoidectomy versus no surgery for chronic suppurative otitis media without cholesteatoma (see glossary, p 493).

Benefits: We found no systematic review and no RCT.

Harms: We found no RCTs.

Comment: We found no evidence from RCTs, but found numerous retrospective studies. Tympanoplasty is often combined with mastoidectomy whenever the possibility of restoring some functional hearing without jeopardising surgical clearance of the disease exists. Observational studies have found that the success of surgery depends on several factors (age, technical skill of the surgeon,[98] presence of middle ear discharge,[99] type of mastoidectomy performed, and technique of middle ear construction[100]). Success in sealing a tympanic perforation with a graft can be 90–95%. Correction of hearing deficit can occur in about 50–70% of operated ears.[101–103]

GLOSSARY

Cholesteatoma An accumulation of epithelial debris in the middle ear cavity that can arise congenitally or can be acquired. The tissue is probably derived from skin. It grows slowly but can erode and destroy adjacent structures (ossicles, the mastoid, the inner ear, or the bone leading to the intracranial cavity) potentially leading to persistent pain and otorrhoea, hearing loss, dizziness, facial nerve paralysis, and intracranial infection.

Disability Adjusted Life Year (DALY) A measure of the impact of a condition, designed to include the loss attributable to premature death and the loss caused by a disability of known duration and severity. One DALY is equivalent to the loss of 1 year of healthy life.

Chronic suppurative otitis media

Ear cleansing Also known as aural toilet.

Mastoidectomy A general term used to describe various surgical procedures that are usually used to remove abnormal parts of the mastoid bone and surrounding structures, or to allow access to the middle ear.

Tympanoplasty A general term used to describe various surgical repairs of the eardrum or ossicles of the middle ear to improve hearing in people with conductive deafness.

REFERENCES

1. World Health Report, 2000. http://www.who.int/whr/2001/archives/2000/en/pdf/Annex4-en.pdf. (last accessed 20/2/2002)
2. Bastos I, Reimer A, Ingvarsson L, Andreasson L. Chronic otitis media and hearing loss among school children in a refugee camp in Angola. *J Audiol Med* 1995;4:1–11.
3. Bastos I, Reimer A, Lundgren K. Chronic otitis media and hearing loss in otitis in urban schoolchildren in Angola – a prevalence study. *J Audiol Med* 1993;2:129–140.
4. Manni JJ. Lema PN. Otitis media in Dar es Salaam, Tanzania. *J Laryngol Otol* 1987;101:222–228.
5. Bastos I, Mallya J, Ingvarsson L, Reimer A, Andreasson L. Middle ear disease and hearing impairment in northern Tanzania. A prevalence study of schoolchildren in the Moshi and Monduli districts. *Int J Pediatr Otorhinolaryngol* 1995;32:1–12.
6. McPherson B, Holborow CA. A study of deafness in West Africa: the Gambian Hearing Health Project. *Int J Pediatr Otorhinolaryngol* 1985;10:115–135.
7. Pisacane A, Ruas I. Bacteriology of otitis media in Mozambique. *Lancet* 1982;1:1305.
8. Halama AR, Voogt GR, Musgrave GM. Prevalence of otitis media in children in a black rural community in Venda (South Africa). *Int J Pediatr Otorhinolaryngol* 1986;11:73–77.
9. Hatcher J, Smith A, Mackenzie I, et al. A prevalence study of ear problems in school children in Kiambu district, Kenya, May 1992. *Int J Pediatr Otorhinolaryngol* 1995;33:197–205.
10. Okeowo PA. Observations on the incidence of secretory otitis media in children. *J Trop Pediatr* 1985;31:295–298.
11. Bal I, Hatcher J. Results of Kenyan Prevalence Survey. *Her Net News* 1992;4:1–2. In Berman S. Otitis media in developing countries. *Pediatrics* 1996;1:126–130.
12. Cohen D, Tamir D. The prevalence of middle ear pathologies in Jerusalem school children. *Am J Otol* 1989;19:456–459.
13. Podoshin L, Fradis M, Ben-David Y, Margalit A, Tamir A, Epstein L. Cholesteatoma: an epidemiologic study among members of kibbutzim in northern Israel. *Ann Otol Rhinol Laryngol* 1986;95:365–368.
14. Bafaqeeh SA, Zakzouk S, Muhaimed HA, Essa A. Relevant demographic factors and hearing impairment in Saudi children: epidemiological study. *J Laryngol Otol* 1994;108:294–298.
15. Noh KT, Kim CS. The changing pattern of otitis media in Korea. *Int J Pediatr Otorhinolaryngol* 1985;9:77–87.
16. Kim CS, Jung HW, Yoo KY. Prevalence and risk factors of chronic otitis media in Korea: results of a nation-wide survey. *Acta Otolaryngol* 1993;113:369–375.
17. Jacob A, Rupa V, Job A, Joseph A. *Hearing impairment and otitis media in a rural primary school in South India. Int* J Pediatr Otorhinolaryngol 1997;39:133–138.
18. Elango S, Purohit GN, Hashim M, Hilmi R. Hearing loss and ear disorders in Malaysian school children. *Int J Pediatr Otorhinolaryngol* 1991;22:75–80.
19. Liming L, Weihua C, Fujie X. Disability among the elderly in China: analysis of the national sampling survey of disability in 1987. *Chin Med J* 1997;110:236–237.
20. Dang Hoang S, Nhan Trung S, Le T, et al. Prevalence of chronic otitis media in a randomly selected population sampled in two communities in Southern Vietnam. Proceedings of Copenhagen Otitis Media Conference, June 1–5, 1997;Abstr 13.
21. Garrett J, Stewart J. Hearing loss and otitis media in Guam: impact of professional services. *Asia Pac J Public Health* 1989;3:213–218.
22. Dever G, Stool S, Manning S, Stewart J. Otitis oceania: middle ear disease in the Pacific basin. *Ann Otol Rhinol Laryngol* 1990;99(suppl 149):25–27.
23. Elango S, Purohit GN, Hashim M, Hilmi R. Hearing loss and ear disorders in Malaysian school children. *Int J Pediatr Otorhinolaryngol* 1991;22:75–80.
24. Eason R, Harding F, Nicholson R, Nicholson D, Pada J, Gathercole J. Chronic suppurative otitis media in the Solomon Islands: a prospective microbiological, audiometric and therapeutic survey. *N Z Med J* 1986;99:812–815.
25. Dever G, Stool S, Manning S, Stewart J. Otitis oceania: middle ear disease in the Pacific basin. *Ann Otol Rhinol Laryngol* 1990;99(suppl 149):25–27.
26. Bastos I Reimer A, Andreasson L. Middle ear disease and hearing loss among urban children and orphans in Bauru, Brazil. A prevalence study. *J Audiol Med* 1994.
27. Browning GG, Gatehouse S. *The prevalence of middle ear disease in the adult British population. Clin* Otolaryngol 1992;17:317–321.
28. Alho OP, Jokinen K, Laitakari K, Palokangas J. Chronic suppurative otitis media and cholesteatoma. Vanishing diseases among Western populations? *Clin Otolaryngol* 1997;22:358–361.
29. Pedersen CB, Zachau-Christiansen B. Chronic otitis media and sequelae in the population of Greenland. *Scand J Soc Med* 1988;16:15–19.
30. Nelson SM, Berry RI. Ear disease and hearing loss among Navajo children – a mass survey. *Laryngoscope* 1994;94:316–323.
31. Canterbury D. Changes in hearing status of Alaskan natives. *Ann Otol Rhinol Laryngol* 1990;99(suppl):22–23.
32. Sunderman J, Dyer H. Chronic ear disease in Australian aborigines. *Med J Aust* 1984;140:708–711.
33. Nelson SM, Berry RI. Ear disease and hearing loss among Navajo children – a mass survey. *Laryngoscope* 1994;94:316–323.
34. Homoe P. Otitis media in Greenland. Studies on historical, epidemiological, microbiological, and immunological aspects. *Int J Circumpolar Health* 2001;60(suppl 2):1–54.
35. Tos M. Sequelae of secretory otitis media and the relationship to chronic suppurative otitis media. *Ann Otol Rhino Laryngol* 1990;99:18–19.
36. Daly KA, Hunter LL, Levine SC, Lindgren BR, Giebink GS. Relationships between otitis media sequelae and age. *Laryngoscope* 1998;108:1306–1310.

37. New Zealand Health Technology Assessment Clearing House. Screening programmes for the detection of otitis media with effusion and conductive hearing loss in pre–school and new entrant school children: A critical appraisal of the literature (NZHTA REPORT 3). Christchurch, New Zealand, June 1998. http://nzhta.chmeds.ac.nz/screen.htm (last accessed February 2002). Search date 1998; primary sources English language articles in Medline, Cinahl, HealthSTAR, Current Contents (combined files), Cochrane Library Database of Abstracts of Reviews of Effectiveness, NHS Economic Evaluation Database, New Zealand Bibliographic Network, New Zealand Ministry of Health publications, United States National Institute of Health publications, Catalogues of New Zealand medical libraries, and publications and current projects by the International Network of Agencies for Health Technology Assessment (INAHTA).
38. Bastos I. Otitis media and hearing loss among children in developing countries. Malmo, Sweden: University of Malmo, 1994.
39. Jacob A, Rupa V, Job A, Joseph A. Hearing impairment and otitis media in a rural primary school in south India. *Int J Pediatr Otorhinolaryngol* 1997;39:133–138.
40. Seely DR, Gloyd SS, Wright AD, Norton SJ. Hearing loss prevalence and risk factors among Sierra Leonean Children. *Arch Otolaryngol Head Neck Surg* 1995;121:853–858.
41. Antarasena S, Antarasena N, Lekagul S, Lutadul D. The epidemiology of deafness in Thailand. *Otolaryngol Head Neck Surg* 1988;3:9–13.
42. Muya EW, Owino O. *Special Education in Africa: Research Abstracts*. Nairobi:UNESCO;1986.
43. Teele DW, Klein JO, Chase C, Menyuk P, Rosner BA. Otitis media in infancy and intellectual ability, school achievement, speech, and language at age 7 years. Greater Boston Otitis Media Study Group. *J Infect Dis* 1990;162:685–694.
44. Osma U, Cureoglu S, Hosoglu S. The complications of chronic otitis media: report of 93 cases. *J Laryngol Otol* 2000;114:97–100.
45. Kenna M. Incidence and prevalence of complications of otitis media. *Ann Otol Rhinol Laryngol* 1990;99(suppl 149):38–39.
46. Berman S. Otitis media in developing countries. *Pediatrics* 1995;96:126–131.
47. Sorensen H. Antibiotics in suppurative otitis media. *Otolaryngol Clin North Am* 1977;10:45–50.
48. Mahoney JL. Mass management of otitis media in Zaire. *Laryngoscope* 1980;90:1200–1208.
49. Noh KT, Kim CS. The changing pattern of otitis media in Korea. *Int J Pediatr Otorhinolaryngol* 1985;9:77–87.
50. Nelson SM, Berry RI. Ear disease and hearing loss among Navajo children – a mass survey. *Laryngoscope* 1994;94:316–323.
51. Muhaimeid H, Zakzouk S, Bafaqeeh SA. Epidemiology of chronic suppurative otitis media in Saudi children. *Int J Pediatr Otorhinolaryngol* 1993;26:101–108.
52. Alho OP, Jokinen K, Laitakari K, Palokangas J. Chronic suppurative otitis media and cholesteatoma. Vanishing diseases among Western populations? *Clin Otolaryngol Allied Sci* 1997;22:358–361.
53. Browning GG, Gatehouse S, Calder IT. Medical management of active chronic otitis media: a controlled study. *J Laryngol Otol* 1988;102:491–495.
54. Acuin J, Smith A, Mackenzie I. Interventions for chronic suppurative otitis media. In: The Cochrane Library. Issue 4, 2001. Oxford: Update Software. Search date 1996; primary sources Medline, Hearing network database, handsearches, and experts.
55. Ozagar A, Koc A, Ciprut A, Tutkun A, Akdas F, Sehitoglu MA. Effects of topical otic preparations on hearing in chronic otitis media. *Otolaryngol Head Neck Surg* 1997;117:405–408.
56. De Miguel Martinez I, Vasallo M Jr, Ramos MA. Antimicrobial therapy in chronic suppurative otitis media. *Acta Otorrinolaringol Esp* 1999;50:15–19.
57. Rotimi V, Olabiyi D, Banjo T, Okeowo P. Randomised comparative efficacy of clindamycin, metronidazole, and lincomycin, plus gentamicin in chronic suppurative otitis media. *West Afr J Med* 1990;9:89–97.
58. Tutkun A, Ozagar A, Koc A, Batman C, Uneri C, Sehitoglu MA. Treatment of chronic ear disease – Topical ciprofloxacin vs topical gentamicin. *Arch Otolaryngol Head Neck Surg* 1995;121:1414–1416.
59. Tong MC, Woo JK, van Hasselt CA. A double-blind comparative study of ofloxacin otic drops versus neomycin-polymyxin B-hydrocortisone otic drops in the medical treatment of chronic suppurative otitis media. *J Laryngol Otol* 1996;110:309–314.
60. Clayton M, Osborne J, Rutherford D, Rivron R. A double-blind, randomized, prospective trial of a topical antiseptic versus a topical antibiotic in the treatment of otorrhea. *Clin Otolaryngol* 1990;15:7–10.
61. Kasemsuwan L, Clongsuesuek P. A double blind, prospective trial of topical ciprofloxacin versus normal saline solution in the treatment of otorrhoea. *Clin Otolaryngol* 1997;22:44–46.
62. Fradis M, Brodsky A, Ben David J, Srugo I, Larboni J, Podoshin L. Chronic otitis media treated topically with ciprofloxacin or tobramycin. *Arch Otolaryngol Head Neck Surg* 1997;123:1057–1060.
63. Gyde MC, Randall RF. Comparative double-blind study of trimethoprim-sulfacetamide-polymyxin B and of gentamicine in the treatment of otorrhoea. *Ann Otolaryngol Chir Cervicofac* 1978;95:43–55.
64. Gyde M. A double-blind comparative study of trimethoprim-polymyxin B versus trimethoprim-sulfacetamide-polymyxin B otic solutions in the treatment of otorrhea. *J Laryngol Otol* 1981;95:251–259.
65. Gyde MC, Norris D, Kavalec EC. The weeping ear: clinical re-evaluation of treatment. *J Int Med Res* 1982;10:333–340.
66. Llorente J, Sabater F, Maristany M, et al. Multicenter comparative study of the effectiveness and tolerance of topical ciprofloxacine (0.3%) versus topical gentamicine (0.3%) in the treatment of chronic suppurative otitis media without cholesteatoma. *An Otorrinolaringol Ibero Am* 1995;5:521–533.
67. Miro N, Perello E, Casamitjana F, Maiz J, et al. Controlled multicenter study on chronic suppurative otitis media treated with topical applications of ciprofloxacin 0.2% solution in single-dose containers or combination of polymyxin B, neomycin, and hydrocortisone suspension. *Otolaryngol Head Neck Surg* 2000; 23:617–623.
68. Picozzi G, Browning G, Calder I. Controlled trial of gentamicin and hydrocortisone ear drops in the treatment of active chronic otitis media. *Clin Otolaryngol* 1983;8:367–368.
69. Crowther JA, Simpson D. Medical treatment of chronic otitis media: steroid or antibiotic with steroid ear-drops? *Clin Otolaryngol* 1991;6:142–144.
70. Marias J, Rutka JA. Ototoxicity and topical eardrops. *Clin Otolaryngol* 1998;23:360–367.
71. Leliever WC. Topical gentamicin-induced positional vertigo. *Otolaryngol Head Neck Surg* 1985;93:553–555.
72. Longridge NS. Topical gentamicin vestibular toxicity. *J Otolaryngol* 1994;23:444–446.
73. Browning G. Picozzi G, Calder I, Sweeney G. Controlled trial of medical treatment of active chronic otitis media. *BMJ* 1983;287:1024.

74. Lildholdt T, Felding J, Juul A, Kristensen S, Schouenborg P. Efficacy of perioperative ceftazidime in the surgical treatment of chronic otitis media due to *Pseudomonas aeruginosa*. *Arch Otorhinolaryngol* 1986;243:167–169.
75. Picozzi G, Browning G, Calder I. Controlled trial of gentamicin and hydrocortisone ear drops with and without systemic metronidazole in the treatment of active chronic otitis media. *Clin Otolaryngol* 1984;9:305.
76. Esposito S, D'Errico G, Montanaro C. Topical and oral treatment of chronic otitis media with ciprofloxacin. *Arch Otolaryngol Head Neck Surg* 1990;116:557–559.
77. Cannoni M, Bonfils P, Sednaoui P, Sevenier F, Joubert-Collin M, Nisse-Durgeat S. Cefotiam hexetil versus amoxicillin/clavulanic acid for the treatment of chronic otitis media in adults. *Medecine et Maladies Infectieuses* 1997;27:915–921.
78. Supiyaphun P, Kerekhanjanarong V, Koranasophonepun J, Sastarasadhit V. Comparison of ofloxacin otic solution with oral amoxycillin plus chloramphenicol ear drop in treatment of chronic suppurative otitis media with acute exacerbation. *J Med Assoc Thai* 2000;83:61–68.
79. Sanchez Gonzalez, Galindo T. An open, comparative study of treatment of chronic middle ear otitis with levofloxacine vs amoxycillin/clavulanate. *Invest Med Int* 2001;28:33–36.
80. Baba S, Ito H, Kinoshita H, et al. Comparative study of cefmetazole and cefazolin in the treatment of suppurative otitis media. *Jpn J Antibiot* 1982;35:1523–1552.
81. Esposito S, D'Errico G, Montanaro C. Topical and oral treatment of chronic otitis media with ciprofloxacin. *Arch Otolaryngol Head Neck Surg* 1990;116:557–559.
82. Povedano Rodriguez V, Seco Pinero M, Jurado Ramos A, Lopez Villarejo P. Eficacia del ciprofloxacino topico en el tratamiento de la otorrea cronica. *Acta Otorrinolaryngologica Espa ola* 1995;46:15–18.
83. Yuen P, Lau S, Chau P, Hui Y, et al. Ofloxacin eardrop treatment for active chronic suppurative otitis media: prospective randomized study. *Am J Otol* 1994;15:670–673.
84. Colletti V, Fiorino FG, Indelicato T. Surgery vs natural course of chronic otitis media. Long term hearing evaluation. *Acta Otolaryngol* 1991;111:762–768.
85. Soldati D, Mudry A. Cholesteatoma in children: techniques and results. *Int J Pediatr Otorhinolaryngol* 2000;52:269–276.
86. Chang CC, Chen MK. Canal-wall-down tympanoplasty with mastoidectomy for advanced cholesteatoma. *J Otolaryngol* 2000;29:270–273.
87. Vartiainen E, Kansanen M. Tympanomastoidectomy for chronic otitis media without choleasteatoma. *Otolaryngol Head Neck Surg* 1992;106:230–234.
88. Mishiro Y, Sakagami M, Takahashi Y, Kitahara T, Kajikawa H, Kubo T. Tympanoplasty with and without mastoidectomy for non-cholesteatomatous chronic otitis media. *Eur Arch Otorhinolaryngol* 2001;258:13–15.
89. Berenholz LP, Rizer FM, Burkey JM, Schuring AG, Lippy WH. Ossiculoplasty in canal wall down mastoidectomy. *Otolaryngol Head Neck Surg* 2000;123:30–33.
90. Eason R, Harding E, Nicholson R, Nicholson D, Pada J, Gathercole J. Chronic suppurative otitis media in the Solomon Islands: a prospective, microbiological, audiometric and therapeutic survey. *N Z Med J* 1986;99:812–815.
91. Smith A, Hatcher J, Mackenzie I, et al. Randomised controlled trial of treatment of chronic suppurative otitis media in Kenyan schoolchildren. *Lancet* 1996;348:1128–1133.
92. Marias J, Rutka JA. Ototoxicity and topical eardrops. *Clin Otolaryngol* 1998;23:360–367.
93. Leliever WC. Topical gentamicin-induced positional vertigo. *Otolaryngol Head Neck Surg* 1985;93:553–555.
94. Longridge NS. Topical gentamicin vestibular toxicity. *J Otolaryngol* 1994;23:444–446.
95. Thorp MA, Gardiner IB, Prescott CA. Burow's solution in the treatment of active mucosal chronic suppurative otitis media: determining an effective dilution. *J Laryngol Otol* 2000;114:432–436.
96. Fliss D, Dagan R, Houri Z, Leiberman A. Medical management of chronic suppurative otitis media without cholesteatoma in children. *J Pediatr* 1990;116:991–996.
97. Somekh E, Cordova Z. Ceftazidime versus aztreonam in the treatment of pseudomonal chronic suppurative otitis media in children. *Scand J Infect Dis* 2000;32:197–199.
98. Soldati D, Mudry A. Cholesteatoma in children: techniques and results. *Int J Pediatr Otorhinolaryngol* 2000;52:269–276.
99. Tos M, Stangerup SE, Orntoft S. Reasons for reperforation after tympanoplasty in children. *Acta Otolaryngol Suppl* 2000;543:143–146.
100. Darrouzet V, Duclos JY, Portmann D, Bebear JP. Preference for the closed technique in the management of cholesteatoma of the middle ear in children: a retrospective study of 215 consecutive patients treated over 10 years. *Am J Otol* 2000;21:474–481.
101. Vartiainen E., Kansanen M. Tympanomastoidectomy for chronic otitis media without choleasteatoma. *Otolaryngol Head Neck Surg* 1992;106:230–234.
102. Mishiro Y, Sakagami M, Takahashi Y, Kitahara T, Kajikawa H, Kubo T. Tympanoplasty with and without mastoidectomy for non-cholesteatomatous chronic otitis media. *Eur Arch Otorhinolaryngol* 2001;258:13–15.
103. Berenholz LP, Rizer FM, Burkey JM, Schuring AG, Lippy WH. Ossiculoplasty in canal wall down mastoidectomy. *Otolaryngol Head Neck Surg* 2000;123:30–33.

Jose Acuin
Associate Professor
De La Salle University Health Sciences Campus
Dasmarinas Cavite
Philippines

Competing interests: None declared

TABLE 1 RCTs of topical antibitoics versus each other (see text, p 484).

Reference	Population with CSOM People/ears Age Setting	Comparison	Absolute results*	OR
Different topical non-quinolone antibiotics versus each other				
Gyde 1978[63]	Adults, 57 ears France Variable duration	Topical 0.3% gentamicin *v* topical trimethoprim-sulfacetamide-polymyxin B	4/30 (13%) 5/27(19%)	1.47 (0.36 to 6.03)
Gyde 1981[64]	27 ears France 7–14 days	Topical trimethoprim-sulfacetamide-polymyxin B *v* topical trimethoprim-polymyxin B	4/13 (31%) 8/14 (57%)	0.36 (0.08 to 1.59)
Gyde 1982[65]	14 adults France 30–40 years 2 weeks	Topical 0.3% gentamicin *v* topical colistin-neomycin-hydrocortisone	1/8 (13%) 1/6 (17%)	0.73 (0.04 to 13.45)
Topical quinolone versus topical non-quinolone antibiotics				
Llorente 1995[66]	308 adults Spain 30 days	Topical 0.3% ciprofloxacin *v* topical 0.3% gentamicin	8/159 (5%) 9/149 (6%)	0.82 (0.31 to 2.19)
Miro 2000[67]	322 adults 14–71 years Spain 6–12 days	Topical ciprofloxacin *v* topical polymyxin B-neomycin-hydrocortisone	22/168 (13%) 37/154 (24%)	0.48 (0.28 to 0.85) ITT 0.67 (0.30 to 1.51) on protocol
Fradis[62]	40 adults Clinics in Israel 3 weeks	Topical ciprofloxacin *v* topical tobramycin	10/19 (53%) *v* 8/18 (44%)	1.38 (0.39 to 4.91)

*Outcomes for all RCTs are the proportion of people with wet ear on otoscopic examination and with negative culture, usually measured at the end of treatment.

COSM, chronic suppurtive otitis media; ITT; intention to treat analysis; OR odds ration.

TABLE 2 RCTs of topical antibiotics versus systemic antibiotics (see text, p 488).

References	Population with chronic suppurative otitis media	Comparison	Persistent otorrhoea	
			Absolute results	OR
Browning 1983[73]	Adults Scottish hospital clinic	Topical gentamicin or chloramphenicol *v* various systemic antibiotics	11/18 (61%) *v* 8/13 (62%)	0.98 (0.23 to 4.15)
Esposito 1990[76]	60 adults 5–10 days	Topical cipofloxacin *v* oral ciprofloxacin	3/20 (15%) *v* 12/20 (60%)	0.15 (0.04 to 0.54)
Esposito 1992[81]	60 adults 5–10 days	Topical ciprofloxacin *v* im gentamicin	5/30 (17%) *v* 17/30 (57%)	0.15 (0.05 to 0.49)
Povedano 1995[82]	60 adults 10 days	Topical ciprofloxacin *v* oral ciprofloxacin	5/30 (17%) *v* 15/30 50%)	0.23 (0.08 to 0.56)
Yuen 1994[83]	60 adults 7 days	Topical ciprofloxacin *v* oral amoxicillin/clavulanate	7/30 (57%) *v* 20/30 (67%)	0.18 (0.07 to 0.49)

im, intramuscular.

Menière's disease

Search date February 2002

Adrian James and Marc Thorp

QUESTIONS

INTERVENTIONS

TREATMENT OF ACUTE ATTACKS
Unknown effectiveness
Anticholinergics. 501
Benzodiazepines 501
Betahistine. 501

PROPHYLACTIC TREATMENT
Unknown effectiveness
Diuretics. 502
Trimetazidine 502
Betahistine (for vertigo or tinnitus) 503
Dietary modification 504
Systemic aminoglycosides 504
Psychological support 504
Vestibular rehabilitation 505

Unlikely to be beneficial
Betahistine (for hearing loss) . .503

Likely to be ineffective or harmful
Lithium. 503

To be covered in future updates
Vasodilators (isoxsuprine)
Antipsychotics (prochlorperazine, sulpiride)
Phosphodiesterase inhibitors (ibudilast)
Surgical management

See glossary, p 505

Key Messages

Treatments for acute attacks

- **Anticholinergics; benzodiazepines; betahistine** We found no RCTs on the effects of these interventions.

Prophylactic interventions

- **Betahistine (for hearing loss)** RCTs found no significant difference with betahistine versus placebo in hearing as assessed by changes in pure tone audiograms.
- **Betahistine (for vertigo or tinnitus)** RCTs found insufficient evidence about the effects of betahistine versus placebo on the frequency and severity of attacks of vertigo, tinnitus, and on aural fullness.
- **Diuretics** One RCT found insufficient evidence on the effects of diuretics versus placebo.
- **Lithium** Small crossover RCTs in people with possible Menière's disease found no difference with lithium versus placebo in vertigo, tinnitus, aural fullness, or hearing, and found that lithium was associated with tremor, thirst, and polyuria in some people.
- **Trimetazidine** We found no RCTs comparing trimetazidine versus placebo. RCTs in people with definite or possible Menière's disease found no significant difference with trimetazidine versus betahistine in hearing or tinnitus, and found conflicting evidence on the effects of trimetazidine versus betahistine on vertigo.

Menière's disease

- **Dietary modification; psychological support; systemic aminoglycosides; vestibular rehabilitation** We found no RCTs on the effects of these interventions in preventing attacks of vertigo or tinnitus.

DEFINITION Menière's disease is characterised by recurrent episodes of spontaneous rotational vertigo and sensorineural hearing loss with tinnitus, and a feeling of fullness or pressure in the ear. It may be unilateral or bilateral. Acute episodes can occur in clusters of about 6–11 a year, although remission may last several months.[1] The diagnosis is made clinically.[2] It is important to distinguish Menière's disease from other types of vertigo that might occur independently with hearing loss and tinnitus, and respond differently to treatment (e.g. benign positional vertigo, acute labyrinthitis). Strict diagnostic criteria help. In this review we applied the classification of the American Academy of Otolaryngology–Head and Neck Surgery to RCTs to indicate the diagnostic rigour used in RCTs (see table 1, p 507).

INCIDENCE/ PREVALENCE Menière's disease is most common between 40–60 years of age, although younger people can be affected.[6,7] In Europe, the incidence is about 50–200/100 000 a year. A survey of general practitioner records of 27 365 people in the UK found an incidence of 43 affected people in a 1 year period (157/100 000).[8] Diagnostic criteria were not defined in this survey. A survey of over 8 million people in Sweden found an incidence of 46/100 000 a year with diagnosis strictly based on the triad of vertigo, hearing loss, and tinnitus.[9] From smaller studies, the incidence appears lower in Uganda[10] and higher in Japan (350/100 000 based on a national survey of hospital attendances during a single week).[7]

AETIOLOGY/ RISK FACTORS Menière's disease is associated with endolymphatic hydrops (raised endolymph pressure in the membranous labyrinth of the inner ear),[11] but a causal relationship between Menière's disease and endolymphatic hydrops remains unproven.[12] Specific disorders associated with hydrops (such as temporal bone fracture, syphilis, hypothyroidism, Cogan's syndrome, and Mondini dysplasia [see glossary, p 505]) can produce similar symptoms to Menière's disease.

PROGNOSIS Menière's disease is progressive, but fluctuates unpredictably. It is difficult to distinguish natural resolution from the effects of treatment. Significant improvement of vertigo is usually seen in the placebo arm of RCTs.[13,14] Acute attacks of vertigo often increase in frequency during the first few years after presentation then decrease in frequency in association with sustained deterioration in hearing.[6] In most people, vertiginous episodes eventually cease completely.[15] In one 20 year cohort study in 34 people, 28 (82%) people had at least moderate hearing loss (mean pure tone hearing loss > 50 dB)[1] and 16 (47%) developed bilateral disease. Symptoms other than hearing loss improve in 60–80% of people irrespective of treatment.[16]

AIMS To prevent attacks of Menière's disease; to reduce the severity of vertigo in acute attacks; to relieve chronic symptoms of hearing loss and tinnitus; to improve quality of life, with minimum adverse effects of treatment.

OUTCOMES Frequency and severity of acute attacks of vertigo; hearing acuity; severity of tinnitus; sensation of aural fullness; functional impairment and quality of life; adverse effects of treatment.

METHODS *Clinical Evidence* update search and appraisal February 2002. We excluded studies with loss to follow up over 20%. We excluded RCTs that did not use American Academy of otolaryngology–Head and Neck Surgery diagnostic criteria.[3–5]

QUESTION What are the effects of treatments for acute attacks?

OPTION ANTICHOLINERGIC DRUGS

We found no RCTs of anticholinergics for acute attacks of Menière's disease.

Benefits: We found no systematic review and no RCTs.

Harms: We found one non-randomised trial that gave no information on adverse effects (see comment below).[17]

Comment: The non-randomised trial (37 people with definite Menière's disease) compared an anticholinergic (glycopyrrolate 2 mg twice daily as required) versus placebo for 4 weeks.[17] It found that glycopyrrolate versus placebo significantly reduced a symptom score based on a validated scale,[18] including questions about the severity of vertigo and its impact on quality of life (Dizziness Handicap Inventory change from baseline to end of trial: 76 to 37 with glycopyrrolate *v* 73 to 75 with placebo; $P < 0.001$). The lack of randomisation means that this result should be interpreted with caution.

OPTION BENZODIAZEPINES

We found no RCTs of benzodiazepines for acute attacks of Menière's disease.

Benefits: We found no systematic review or RCTs.

Harms: We found no evidence.

Comment: None.

OPTION BETAHISTINE

We found no RCTs about the effects of betahistine for acute attacks of Menière's disease.

Benefits: We found no systematic review or RCTs.

Harms: We found no evidence.

Comment: One observational study held in 1940 found that intravenous histamine was associated with a reduced severity of acute attacks of Menière's disease.[19]

QUESTION **What are the effects of prophylactic interventions for Menière's disease?**

OPTION **DIURETICS**

One RCT found insufficient evidence on the effect of diuretics versus placebo to reduce vertigo and tinnitus in Menière's disease. It found no significant difference between diurectic versus placebo in hearing over 17 weeks.

Benefits: We found no systematic review but found one RCT (33 people with possible Menière's disease) of a diuretic (triamterene 50 mg plus hydrochlorothiazide 25 mg) versus placebo.[20] It found no significant audiological change in hearing over 17 weeks ($P > 0.2$).

Harms: The RCT gave no information on adverse effects.[20]

Comment: In the RCT, frequency of vertigo attacks was reduced and tinnitus was unchanged, but valid statistical analyses cannot be performed because only the mean of categorical data was presented.[20] An RCT of hydrochlorothiazide plus betahistine is being translated.[21]

OPTION **TRIMETAZIDINE**

We found no RCTs comparing trimetazidine versus placebo to prevent attacks of Menière's disease. Two RCTs found conflicting evidence about the effects of trimetazidine versus betahistine on vertigo in Menière's disease. The RCTs found no significant difference in hearing or tinnitus with trimetazidine versus betahistine.

Benefits: We found no systematic review. **Versus placebo:** We found no RCTs. **Versus betahistine:** We found two RCTs.[22,23] The first RCT (20 people with definite or probable Menière's disease) compared trimetazidine (20 mg three times daily) versus betahistine (8 mg three times daily) over 3 months.[22] It found no significant difference in hearing, tinnitus, aural fullness, or quality of life (RR improved quality of life 1.0, 95% CI 0.34 to 2.93). Trimetazidine versus betahistine significantly increased the number of people reporting that the duration of vertigo was "substantially better or cured" (RR 1.8, 95% CI 1.0 to 3.2) or reporting that the intensity of vertigo was "substantially better or cured" (RR 1.7, 95% CI 1.0 to 2.8). Trimetazidine versus betahistine also improved the global impression of vertigo scale significantly more than betahistine, but it is not clear if this scale has been validated (RR 2.5, 95% CI 1.17 to 5.3).[22] The second RCT (45 people with possible Menière's disease) of trimetazidine (20 mg three times daily) versus betahistine (12 mg three times daily) over 2 months found no significant difference in hearing or tinnitus.[23] A beneficial effect of trimetazidine on vertigo intensity was reported but is not confirmed by analysis of the available data ($P = 0.23$; 2-sided Fisher's exact test).

Harms: No significant adverse effects were reported in the RCTs.[22,23]

Comment: None.

OPTION BETAHISTINE

One systematic review found insufficient evidence about the effects of betahistine versus placebo in preventing attacks in Menière's disease. Two RCTs found conflicting evidence about the effects of betahistine versus trimetazidine on vertigo in Menière's disease. The RCTs found no difference in hearing or tinnitus with betahistine versus trimetazidine.

Benefits: **Versus placebo:** We found one systematic review (search date 1999, 6 RCTs,[13,24–28] 162 people) of betahistine versus placebo in people with Menière's disease.[29] The review did not perform a meta-analysis because of trial heterogeneity.[29] The first RCT identified by the review (30 people with possible Menière's disease) found that, after 6 weeks, betahistine (8 mg three times daily) versus placebo significantly reduced the severity of vertigo ($P = 0.0001$), tinnitus ($P = 0.001$), and aural fullness ($P = 0.02$); it did not report the number of people with each outcome.[24] The second RCT identified by the review (35 people with possible Menière's disease, crossover design) found that betahistine (24 mg three times daily in a slow release formulation) versus placebo for 16 weeks had no significant effect on tinnitus ($P = 0.68$) or aural fullness ($P = 0.63$).[13] Vertigo was not adequately assessed. The third small RCT identified by the review (16/36 people had a possible diagnosis of Menière's disease) found that betahistine (18 mg twice daily) versus placebo for 2 weeks had no significant effect on the number of people reporting improved vertigo (RR 1.17, 95% CI 0.86 to 1.58) or tinnitus (RR 2.4, 95% CI 0.11 to 51.32).[25] The fourth RCT identified by the review (10 people with possible Menière's disease) found that betahistine (8 mg three times daily) versus placebo had no significant effect over 6–12 months on the number of people with improved vertigo (RR 5.0, 95% CI 0.3 to 84), tinnitus, or aural fullness.[26] None of the RCTs found any change in pure tone audiograms.[13,24–26] The remaining two RCTs identified by the review reported insufficient detail to confirm reliably that the participants had Menière's disease.[27,28] **Versus trimetazidine:** See benefits of trimetazidine, p 502.

Harms: None of the RCTs identified by the review reported any significant adverse effects.[24–28] Because of its histaminergic action, betahistine is usually avoided in asthma and peptic ulcer disease.

Comment: Crossover studies are difficult to interpret if used to evaluate the effects of treatments on conditions that fluctuate in intensity or if interventions have prolonged effects.[30] Menière's disease is not a stable condition and it is unknown if any effects of betahistine are prolonged. An RCT of hydrochlorothiazide plus betahistine is being translated.[21]

OPTION LITHIUM

Two crossover RCTs found no difference in vertigo, tinnitus, aural fullness, or hearing with lithium versus placebo and found that lithium was associated with tremor, thirst, and polyuria in some people.

Benefits: We found no systematic review but found two crossover RCTs (50 people with possible Menière's disease) of lithium versus placebo.[31,32] They found no difference in vertigo, tinnitus, aural fullness, or hearing, but no analysable results were presented.

Harms: In the RCTs, serum lithium concentration was checked every 2 weeks to reduce the risk of adverse effects.[31,32] Two people withdrew from one RCT because of adverse effects from lithium (tremor, thirst, polyuria).[31]

Comment: The crossover RCT design may be inappropriate because Menière's disease is not stable and it is not clear that the lithium is free of any other effects.[31,32] Dosage was adjusted to maintain serum lithium concentration between 0.7–1.1 mmol/L.

OPTION DIETARY MODIFICATION

We found no RCTs about the effects of dietary modification in preventing attacks of Menière's disease.

Benefits: We found no systematic review or RCTs.

Harms: We found no good evidence.

Comment: It has been suggested that a low salt diet reduces endolymphatic pressure in endolymphatic hydrops,[33] but we found no RCTs of dietary modification.

OPTION SYSTEMIC AMINOGLYCOSIDES

We found no RCTs about the effects of systemic aminoglycosides in preventing attacks of Menière's disease.

Benefits: We found no systematic review or RCTs.

Harms: Systemic aminoglycosides are associated with a risk of severe disruption of balance (including oscillopsia) and sensorineural hearing loss.[34]

Comment: Aminoglycosides have been used in severe bilateral Menière's disease,[35–37] but we found no evidence from RCTs to support or to refute this.

OPTION PSYCHOLOGICAL SUPPORT

We found no RCTs about psychological support, such as reassurance, to prevent attacks of Menière's disease.

Benefits: We found no systematic review or RCTs.

Harms: We found no good evidence.

Comment: We found no good evidence about the effect of psychological support on Menière's disease. However, symptomatic improvement is seen with all treatments, including placebo[16,31] or being put on a waiting list for surgery.[38] Improvements noted after these types of psychological support have not been distinguished from improvements attributable to the natural history of Menière's disease.

OPTION VESTIBULAR REHABILITATION

We found no RCTs about the effects of vestibular rehabilitation exercises on Menière's disease.

Benefits: We found no systematic review or RCTs.

Harms: We found no good evidence.

Comment: Improvements noted after vestibular rehabilitation (see glossary, p 505) have not been distinguished from spontaneous improvement of Menière's disease.

GLOSSARY

Cogan's syndrome Episodic vertigo of the Menière's type, hearing loss, and interstitial keratitis, without syphilis.[5]
Mondini dysplasia A congenital deformity of the cochlea in which only the basal turns are present.
Vestibular rehabilitation Involves a series of exercises intended to improve the sense of balance through controlled movements of the head and body.[39] They are usually recommended for stable vestibular disorders.[40]

REFERENCES

1. Friberg U, Stahle J, Svedberg A. The natural course of Menière's disease. *Acta Otolaryngol Suppl* 1984;406:72–77.
2. Kitahara M. Concepts and diagnostic criteria of Menière's disease. In: Kitahara M, ed. *Menière's disease.* Tokyo: Springer–Verlag, 1990:3–12.
3. Alford BR. Menière's disease: criteria for diagnosis and evaluation of therapy for reporting. Report of subcommittee on equilibrium and its measurement. *Trans Am Acad Ophthalmol Otolaryngol* 1972;76:1462–1464.
4. Pearson BW, Brackmann DE. Committee on hearing and equilibrium guidelines for reporting treatment results in Menière's disease. *Otolaryngol Head Neck Surg* 1985;93:578–581.
5. Committee on hearing and equilibrium. Guidelines for the diagnosis and evaluation of therapy in Menière's disease. *Otolaryngol Head Neck Surg* 1995;113:181–185.
6. Moffat DA, Ballagh RH. Menière's Disease. In: Kerr AG, Booth JB, eds. *Scott-Brown's Otolaryngology.* 6th ed. Oxford, Butterworth-Heinemann, 1997:3/19/1–50.
7. Watanabe I. Incidence of Menière's disease, including some other epidemiological data. In: Oosterveld WJ, ed. *Menière's disease: A comprehensive appraisal.* Chichester: John Wiley & Sons Ltd, 1983:9–23.
8. Cawthorne T, Hewlett AB. Menière's disease. *Proc Royal Soc Med* 1954;47:663–670.
9. Stahle J, Stahle C, Arenberg IK. Incidence of Menière's disease. *Arch Otolaryngol* 1978;104:99–102.
10. Nsamba C. A comparative study of the aetiology of vertigo in the African. *J Laryngol Otol* 1972;86:917–925.
11. Hallpike C, Cairns H. Observations on the pathology of Menière's syndrome. *J Laryngol Otol* 1938;53:625–655.
12. Ruckenstein MJ, Harrison RV. Cochlear pathology in Menière's disease. In: Harris JP, ed. *Menière's disease.* The Hague: Kugler Publications, 1999:195–202.
13. Schmidt JT, Huizing EH. The clinical drug trial in Menière's disease with emphasis on the effect of betahistine SR. *Acta Otolaryngol* 1992;497(suppl):1–189.
14. Moser M, Ranacher G, Wilmot TJ, et al. A double-blind clinical trial of hydroxyethylrutosides in Menière's disease. *J Laryngol Otol* 1984;98:265–272.
15. Silverstein H, Smouha E, Jones R. Natural history versus surgery for Menière's disease. *Otolaryngol Head Neck Surg* 1989;100:6–16.
16. Torok N. Old and new in Menière's disease. *Laryngoscope* 1977;87:1870–1877.
17. Storper IS, Spitzer JB, Scanlan M. Use of glycopyrolate in the treatment of Menière's disease. *Laryngoscope* 1998;108:1442–1445.
18. Jacobson GP, Newman CW. The development of the Dizziness Handicap Inventory. *Arch Otolaryngol Head Neck Surg* 1990;116:424–427.
19. Sheldon CH, Horton BT. Treatment of Menière's disease with histamine administered intravenously. *Proceedings of the Staff Meetings of the Mayo Clinic* 1940;15:17–21.
20. van Deelen GW, Huizing EH. Use of a diuretic (Dyazide) in the treatment of Menière's disease. A double-blind cross-over placebo-controlled study. *ORL J Otorhinolaryngol Relat Spec* 1986;48:287–292.
21. Petermann W, Mulch G. Long-term therapy of Menière's disease. Comparison of the effects of betahistine dihydrochloride and hydrochlorothiazide [in German]. *Fortschr Medizin* 1982;100:431–435.
22. Kluyskens P, Lambert P, D'Hooge D. Trimetazidine contre betahistine dans le vertiges vestibulaires. *Ann Otolaryngol Chir Cervicofac* 1990;107(suppl 1):11–19.
23. Martini A, De Domenico F. Trimetazidine versus betahistine in Menière's disease. A double blind method [in French]. *Ann Otolaryngol Chir Cervicofac* 1990;107(suppl 1):20–27.
24. Salami A, Dellepiane M, Tinelle E, et al. Studio a doppia cecita' tra cloridrato di betaistina e placebo nel trattamento delle sindromi Menieriformi. *Valsalva* 1984;60:302–312.

25. Okamato K, Hazeyama F, Taira T, et al. Therapeutic results of betahistine in Menière's disease with statistical analysis. *Iryo* 1968;22:650–666.
26. Ricci V, Sittoni V, Nicora M. Valutazione terapeutica e tollerabilita del chloridrato di betaistina (Microser) in confronto a placebo nella malattia di Meniere. *Riv Ital Ornitolog Audiolog Foniat* 1987;7:347–350.
27. Burkin A. Betahistine treatment of Menière's syndrome. *Clin Med* 1967;74:41–48.
28. Elia JC. Double-blind evaluation of a new treatment for Menière's syndrome. *JAMA* 1966;196:187–189.
29. James AL, Burton MJ. Betahistine for Menière's disease or syndrome. In: The Cochrane Library, Issue 2, 2001. Oxford: Update Software. Search date 1999; primary sources Cochrane Controlled Trials Register, Medline, Embase, Index Medicus, and hand searching of reference lists.
30. Fleiss JL. The crossover study. In: *The design and analysis of clinical experiments*. Chichester: John Wiley & Sons, 1984.
31. Thomsen J, Bech P, Prytz S, et al. Menière's disease: lithium treatment (demonstration of placebo effect in a double blind cross-over trial). *Clin Otolaryngol* 1979;4:119–123.
32. Thomsen J, Bech P, Geisler A, et al. Lithium treatment of Menière's disease: results of a double-blind cross-over trial. *Acta Otolaryngol* 1976;82:294–296.
33. Furstenburg AC, Richardson G, Lathrop FD. Menière's disease. Addenda to medical therapy. *Arch Otolaryngol* 1941;34:1083–1092.
34. Balyan FR, Taibah A, De Donato G, et al. Titration streptomycin therapy in Meniere's disease: long-term results. *Otolaryngol Head Neck Surg* 1998;118:261–266.
35. Wilson WR, Schuknecht HF. Update on the use of streptomycin therapy for Menière's disease. *Am J Otol* 1980;2:108–111.
36. Graham MD. Bilateral Menière's disease. Treatment with intramuscular titration streptomycin sulfate. *Otolaryngol Clin North Am* 1997;30:1097–1100.
37. Shea JJ, Ge X, Orchik DJ. Long-term results of low dose intramuscular streptomycin for Menière's disease. *Am J Otol* 1994;15:540–544.
38. Kerr AG, Toner JG. A new approach to surgery for Menière's disease: talking about surgery. *Clin Otolaryngol* 1998;23:263–264.
39. Dix MR. The rationale and technique of head exercises in the treatment of vertigo. *Acta Otorhinolaryngol Belg* 1979;33:370–384.
40. Clendaniel RA, Tucci DL. Vestibular rehabilitation strategies in Menière's disease. *Otolaryngol Clin North Am* 1997;30:1145–1158.

Adrian James
Department of Otolaryngology
Radcliffe Infirmary
Oxford
UK

Marc Thorp
Department of Otolaryngology
University of Toronto
Toronto
Canada

Competing interests: None declared.

TABLE 1 American Academy of Otolaryngology–Head and Neck Surgery definition of the certainty of diagnosis of Menière's disease (see text, p 500).[3–5]

Certain	Definite Menière's plus postmortem confirmation
Definite	Two or more episodes of vertigo* plus audiometrically confirmed sensorineural hearing loss plus tinnitus or aural fullness plus other causes excluded
Probable	One episode of vertigo* plus audiometrically confirmed sensorineural hearing loss plus tinnitus or aural fullness plus other causes excluded
Possible	Episodes of vertigo* with no hearing loss, or sensorineural hearing loss with dysequilibrium; other causes excluded

*Defined as spontaneous, rotational vertigo lasting more than 20 minutes.

Middle ear pain and trauma during air travel

Search date March 2002

Simon Janvrin

QUESTIONS

INTERVENTIONS

Key Messages

- **Oral decongestants in adults** Two RCTs found limited evidence that oral pseudoephedrine versus placebo significantly reduced ear pain and hearing loss during air travel in adult passengers with a history of ear pain during air travel.
- **Oral decongestants in children** One small RCT found no significant difference with oral pseudoephedrine versus placebo in ear pain at take off or landing in children up to the age of 6 years.
- **Topical nasal decongestants in adults** One small RCT found insufficient evidence about the effects of topical nasal decongestants versus placebo during air travel.

Clin Evid 2002;8:508–510.

Middle ear pain and trauma during air travel

DEFINITION The effects of air travel on the middle ear can include tympanic membrane pain, vertigo, hearing loss, and perforation.

INCIDENCE/ PREVALENCE The prevalence of symptoms depends on the altitude, type of aircraft, and characteristics of the passengers. One point prevalence study found that 20% of adult and 40% of child passengers had negative pressure in the middle ear after flight, and that 10% of adults and 22% of children had auroscopic evidence of damage to the tympanic membrane.[1] We found no data on the incidence of perforation, which seems to be extremely rare in commercial passengers.

AETIOLOGY/ RISK FACTORS During aircraft descent, the pressure in the middle ear drops relative to that in the ear canal. A narrow, inflamed, or poorly functioning Eustachian tube impedes the necessary influx of air. As the pressure difference between the middle and outer ear increases, the tympanic membrane is pulled inward.

PROGNOSIS In most people symptoms resolve spontaneously. Experience in military aviation shows that most ear drum perforations will heal spontaneously.[2]

AIMS To prevent ear pain and trauma during air travel.

OUTCOMES Incidence and severity of pain and hearing loss; incidence of perforation of tympanic membrane.

METHODS *Clinical Evidence* search and appraisal March 2002.

QUESTION What are the effects of preventive interventions?

OPTION ORAL DECONGESTANTS

We found limited evidence from two RCTs suggesting that oral pseudoephedrine versus placebo may reduce the incidence of pain and hearing loss during flight in adult passengers with a history of ear pain during. One small RCT found no evidence of benefit in children up to the age of 6 years.

Benefits: We found no systematic review. We found three RCTs. Two RCTs (350 adult passengers) compared oral pseudoephedrine (120 mg given 30 mins before flight) versus placebo.[3,4] All people had a history of ear pain during air travel. Those with acute or chronic ear problems were excluded. A total of 272 passengers completed the post flight questionnaires. The RCTs found that pseudoephedrine versus placebo significantly reduced pain and hearing loss (incidence of symptoms in combined treatment groups: 33% *v* 64%; RR 0.51, 95% CI 0.31 to 0.84). The third RCT (50 children up to the age of 6 years) compared oral pseudoephedrine versus placebo.[5] It found no significant difference in ear pain between children taking treatment versus placebo at either take off or landing.

Harms: "Dry mouth or drowsiness" was reported by 7–15% of adult participants taking pseudoephedrine versus 2% on placebo.[3,4] More children taking pseudoephedrine were drowsy on take off compared with placebo (60% *v* 13%).[5]

Comment: None.

OPTION TOPICAL NASAL DECONGESTANTS

We found insufficient evidence on the effects of topical decongestants in this setting.

Benefits: We found no systematic review. We found one RCT comparing oxymetazoline nasal spray versus placebo nasal spray in 83 people during air travel.[3] It found no significant difference in reported ear pain between the two groups.

Harms: Nasal irritation was reported by 14% of people taking oxymetazoline. The rate in people taking placebo was not reported.

Comment: The RCT was too small to rule out an effect of topical decongestants.

REFERENCES

1. Stangerup S-E, Tjernstrom O, Klokke M, Harcourt J, Stokholm J. Point prevalence of barotitis in children and adults after flight, and the effect of autoinflation. *Aviat Space Environ Med* 1998;69:45–49.
2. O'Reilly BJ. Otorhinolaryngology. In: Ernsting J, Nicholson AN, Rainford DJ, eds. *Aviation Medicine*. 3rd edition. Oxford: Butterworth-Heinemann, 1999:319–336.
3. Jones JS, Sheffield W, White LJ, Bloom MA. A double-blind comparison between oral pseudoephedrine and topical oxymetazoline in the prevention of barotrauma during air travel. *Am J Emerg Med* 1998;16:262–264.
4. Csortan E, Jones J, Haan M, Brown M. Efficacy of pseudoephedrine for the prevention of barotrauma during air travel. *Ann Emerg Med* 1994;23:1324–1327.
5. Buchanan BJ, Hoagland J, Fischer PR. Pseudoephedrine and air travel-associated ear pain in children. *Arch Pediatr Adolesc Med* 1999;153:466–468.

Simon Janvrin
Civil Aviation Authority
West Sussex
UK

Competing interests: None declared.

Otitis media with effusion

Search date March 2002

Ian Williamson

QUESTIONS

INTERVENTIONS

Covered elsewhere in *Clinical Evidence*

See acute otitis media, p 251

Key Messages

- **Antihistamines plus oral decongestants** One systematic review found no significant difference between antihistamines plus oral decongestants versus placebo in clearance of effusion after 4 weeks.
- **Antimicrobial drugs (possible short term benefit)** One systematic review found limited evidence that antimicrobial drugs versus placebo or no treatment significantly increased resolution of effusion at up to 1 month. However, a subsequent systematic review found no significant difference with antimicrobial drugs versus placebo. Timing to outcome of included RCTs was unclear. Adverse effects of antibiotics (mainly nausea, vomiting, and diarrhoea) have been reported in 2–32% of children.
- **Autoinflation with nasal balloon (short term benefit)** One systematic review has found that autoinflation with a nasal balloon versus no treatment significantly improves effusion. Some children may find autoinflation difficult.
- **Change in modifiable risk factors** We found no RCTs on the effects of avoiding risk factors such as passive smoking and bottle feeding in preventing otitis media with effusion.
- **Mucolytics** One systematic review found no significant difference between 1–3 month courses of carbocisteine versus placebo or no treatment in resolution of effusion. Three small RCTs of bromhexine versus placebo found conflicting results.

Otitis media with effusion

- **Oral steroids** One systematic review found no significant difference between oral steroids versus placebo in clearance of effusion after 2 weeks. Oral steroids may cause behavioural changes, increased appetite, and weight gain.
- **Topical steroids** One small RCT found limited evidence that topical steroids plus antibiotics improved short term symptoms as compared with antibiotics alone. It did not report on adverse events.
- **Grommets with or without adenoidectomy; other autoinflation devices; tonsillectomy** We found insufficient evidence on the effects of these interventions.

DEFINITION Otitis media with effusion (OME), or "glue ear", is serous or mucoid but not mucopurulent fluid in the middle ear. Children usually present with hearing loss and speech problems. In contrast to those with acute otitis media (see topic, p 251), children with OME do not suffer from acute ear pain, fever, or malaise. Hearing loss is usually mild and often identified when parents express concern regarding their child's behaviour, school performance, or language development.

INCIDENCE/ PREVALENCE One study in the UK found that, at any time, 5% of children aged 2–4 years have persistent (at least 3 months) bilateral hearing loss associated with OME. The prevalence declines considerably beyond age 6 years.[1] About 80% of children aged 10 years have been affected by OME at some time in the past. OME is the most common reason for referral for surgery in children in the UK. Middle ear effusions also occur infrequently in adults after upper respiratory tract infection or after air travel.

AETIOLOGY/ RISK FACTORS Contributory factors include upper respiratory tract infection and narrow upper respiratory airways. Prospective case control studies have identified risk factors, including age 6 years or younger at first onset, daycare centre attendance, high number of siblings, low socioeconomic group, frequent upper respiratory tract infection, bottle feeding, and household smoking.[2,3] Most factors are associated with about twice the risk of developing OME.[4]

PROGNOSIS In 5% of preschool children, OME (identified by tympanometric screening) persists for at least 1 year.[5,6] One large cohort study (534 children) found that middle ear disease increased reported hearing difficulty at age 5 years (OR 1.44, 95% CI 1.18 to 1.76) and was associated with delayed language development in children up to age 10 years.[7]

AIMS To improve hearing and wellbeing; to avoid poor behavioural, speech, and educational development; to prevent recurrent earache and otitis media.

OUTCOMES Resolution of effusion (both speed and completeness) assessed by otoscopy, tympanometry, or global clinical assessment; hearing impairment, assessed by audiometry or tympanometry (although the positive predictive value of these tests has been reported as low as 49%);[8] developmental and behavioural tests; language and speech development; adverse effects of treatment. Patient centred outcomes in children with OME (e.g. disability or quality of life) need further development and evaluation.

METHODS *Clinical Evidence* update search and appraisal March 2002.

QUESTION What are the effects of preventive interventions?

OPTION MODIFYING RISK FACTORS

We found no RCTs that evaluated interventions to modify risk factors for otitis media with effusion, such as passive smoking and bottle feeding.

Benefits: We found no systematic review or RCTs of interventions aimed at modifying risk factors for otitis media with effusion.

Harms: We found insufficient data.

Comment: There is good epidemiological evidence that the risk of otitis media with effusion is increased by passive smoking,[2] bottle feeding,[3] low socioeconomic group, and exposure to a large number of other children.[8] Feasible preventive interventions may include strategies to reduce household smoking and encourage breast feeding.

QUESTION What are the effects of treatments?

OPTION ANTIMICROBIAL DRUGS

One systematic review found limited evidence that antibiotics improved short term outcomes. A second subsequent systematic review found no significant difference between antibiotics and placebo, but timing of outcome was unclear. Adverse effects with antibiotics (mainly nausea, vomiting, and diarrhoea) were reported in 2–32% of children.

Benefits: We found two systematic reviews.[8,9] The first systematic review (search date 1992, 10 blinded RCTs, 1041 children with otitis media with effusion, age range not stated) compared antimicrobial drugs (amoxicillin [amoxycillin] with or without clavulanic acid, cefaclor, erythromycin, sulphisoxazole, sulfamethoxazole [suphamethoxazole], or trimethoprim) versus placebo or versus no treatment.[8] Treatment duration varied from 2–5 weeks. Follow up was from 10–60 days. At up to 1 month, resolution of effusion (assessed by pneumatic otoscopy, tympanometry, and audiometry) was significantly more likely with antimicrobial treatment (pooled ARR for non-resolution versus placebo or no treatment 14%, 95% CI 4% to 24%; NNT 7). The second subsequent systematic review (search date 1997, 8 placebo controlled RCTs, 1292 children with otitis media with effusion, age range not stated) compared antibiotics versus placebo and found no significant effect on cure rate (cure rate 179/813 [22%] for antibiotics *v* 85/479 [18%] for placebo; ARI of cure +4.3%, 95% CI –0.1% to +8.6%).[9] The timing to outcomes of included RCTs was unclear.

Harms: The systematic reviews did not report rates of adverse events in children on placebo or no treatment. Adverse events on antibiotics were frequent. For amoxicillin, diarrhoea was reported in 20–30% and rashes in 3–5% of children. For co-amoxiclav, diarrhoea was reported in 9%, nausea and vomiting in 4%, and skin rashes and urticaria in 3% of children.[8,10] For antibiotics overall, nausea and vomiting, diarrhoea, or both were reported in 2–32% of children, and cutaneous reactions in less than 5%.[10] Adherence to lengthy courses of antibiotics was poor. Prescribing antibiotics for minor illness encouraged further consultations[11] and antibiotic resistance.[12]

Comment: In the second systematic review the timing to outcomes was not clear and has some studies in common with the first review.[9] The systematic review included in previous *Clinical Evidence* updates has been excluded because we decided that the subsequent review had eclipsed it,[9] and we had concerns about the inclusion of non-placebo controlled studies in the review.[13] The first systematic review included non-placebo controlled studies, and concerns have been raised about the studies included and methods used.[8]

OPTION CORTICOSTEROIDS

One systematic review found no evidence on the long term effects of oral steroids in children with otitis media with effusion. One small RCT found limited evidence that topical steroids plus antibiotics improved symptoms compared with antibiotics alone. Short courses of oral steroids can cause behavioural changes such as increased appetite and weight gain.

Benefits: We found one systematic review (search date 2000).[14] **Oral steroids versus placebo:** The systematic review identified three placebo controlled RCTs of oral steroids (either prednisone or dexamethasone) versus placebo (108 children with otitis media with effusion). Presence of effusion was assessed clinically by pneumatic otoscopy, tympanometry, and audiometry after 7–14 days of treatment. There was no significant difference in mean improvement at 2 weeks after treatment (AR of clearance compared with placebo 21%, 95% CI –3% to +44%). There were no available summary data beyond 6 weeks. **Corticosteroid plus antibiotic versus antibiotic alone:** The systematic review identified four RCTs (292 children) comparing antibiotic (cefixime, amoxycillin [amoxycillin], or sulfisoxazole) plus oral steroids (bethamethasone or prednisone) versus antibiotic alone. Time to measurement of results varied from 1 week to 2 months. There was a significant difference in clearance rates with combined treatment versus antibiotic alone (ARR for non-clearance *v* antibiotic alone at 2 wks 32%, 95% CI 20% to 50%), but there was significant heterogeneity between studies ($P < 0.01$). **Topical steroids:** The systematic review identified one RCT (61 children with chronic middle ear infection, ages 3–11 years), which found that intranasal steroids plus antibiotics versus either antibiotics alone or placebo spray significantly reduced effusions at 4 and 8 weeks (CI not provided; $P < 0.05$). It found that at 12 weeks intranasal steroids plus antibiotics significantly improved symptoms compared with antibiotics alone but not compared with antibiotics plus placebo.[15]

Harms: Short courses of oral steroids can cause behavioural changes, increased appetite, and weight gain. Idiosyncratic reactions have been reported, such as avascular necrosis of the femoral head and fatal varicella infections.

Comment: The trials were small. Use of secondary care populations weakens the applicability of results to primary care.

OPTION ANTIHISTAMINES AND DECONGESTANTS

One systematic review found no benefit from antihistamines and decongestants versus placebo in clearance of effusion in children with otitis media with effusion after 4 weeks.

Benefits: We found one systematic review (search date 1992, 4 placebo controlled RCTs, 1202 infants and older children, age range not stated).[8] Treatment lasted for 4 weeks. Meta-analysis found that combined antihistamine–decongestants versus placebo had no significant effect on effusion clearance rate, as assessed by history, otoscopy, and tympanometry (hierarchical Bayes meta-analysis: change in probability –0.009, 95% CI –0.036 to +0.054).

Harms: Adverse effects of antihistamines include hyperactivity, insomnia, drowsiness, behavioural change, blood pressure variability, and seizures. One RCT in healthy volunteers found that decongestant nose drops given for 3 weeks or more led to iatrogenic rhinitis.[16]

Comment: The RCTs included clinically heterogeneous groups (e.g. infants and older children) and selected individuals from ambulatory care or waiting lists. There were too few children with allergies for subgroup analysis.

OPTION MUCOLYTICS

One systematic review found that 1–3 month courses of carbocisteine or carbocisteine lysine compared with placebo or no treatment had no significant effect on resolution of effusion. Three small RCTs found conflicting results on the effects of bromhexine.

Benefits: We found one systematic review (search date 1993, 6 RCTs, 428 children ages 3–11 years and 2 adults) comparing carbocisteine, carbocisteine lysine, or both, versus placebo or no treatment.[17] Treatment lasted for 15–90 days. Meta-analysis found a greater frequency of complete resolution with mucolytics, but this did not quite reach significance (178 children; 80/81 [99%] with treatment v 54/98 [55%] with placebo; OR 2.25, 95% CI 0.97 to 5.22). Three small RCTs (155 children and 195 ears) comparing another mucolytic, bromhexine, versus placebo found conflicting results.[18–20]

Harms: The review gave no information on adverse effects.[17] Reported adverse effects of carbocisteine include gastric irritation, nausea, and rashes.

Comment: The RCTs were heterogeneous in their clinical outcomes and treatment duration.

OPTION AUTOINFLATION

One systematic review has found benefit from autoinflation using a nasal balloon, although some children may find autoinflation difficult. The value of all methods of autoinflation has not yet been adequately evaluated.

Benefits: We found one systematic review (search date not stated, 6 RCTs, age range not stated) comparing autoinflation versus no treatment.[21] Improvement was variously defined as being effusion free, improved tympanogram, or improvement in hearing. The RCTs assessing different treatment effects yielded different results. However, trials evaluating nasal balloons in children found a homogeneous effect size (3 RCTs, 386 children). Children treated with a purpose manufactured nasal balloon were more likely than control children to improve within 1 week to 3 months using tympanometric and audiometric criteria (OR 3.53, 95% CI 2.03 to 6.14).[21]

Harms: We found no reports of serious adverse effects.

Comment: The Eustachian tubes can be inflated by several methods, including blowing up a balloon through a plastic tube inserted into the nostril. In one RCT, 12% of children aged 3–10 years were unable to use the balloon.[22] Most trials appeared not to use intention to treat analysis, and beneficial effects were noted only when adherence was 70% or greater. The evidence is suboptimal because different methods were used, outcome assessments were not blinded, and follow up was short. Other methods of autoinflation (such as inflating a carnival blower through the nostril or forcible exhalation through the nostrils, with closed mouth, into an anaesthetic mask with a flowmeter attachment) have not been adequately evaluated.

OPTION SURGERY

One systematic review found limited evidence that surgery (insertion of grommets, adenoidectomy, or both) resulted in short term hearing gain. Grommets and adenoidectomy alone were of similar effectiveness. A subsequent RCT found that grommets and adenoidectomy combined was more effective than adenotonsillectomy or grommets either alone or combined. Three subsequent RCTs found no benefit in language development with grommets. We found no good evidence on the effects of tonsillectomy.

Benefits: We found one systematic review (search date 1992, 19 RCTs) of surgery in children with otitis media with effusion.[23] Nine RCTs reported the data per child (1508 children) and 10 reported data per ear (1452 children). None were placebo controlled, although some used children as their own controls. Outcomes were mean change in audiometry, tympanometry, and clinical and otoscopic evidence of otitis media with effusion. The review concluded that evidence for the effectiveness of surgical interventions was still confused. **Grommets:** The review reported a mean 12 dB improvement in hearing after insertion of grommets (CI not provided).[23] However, the authors concluded that this was difficult to interpret clinically. We found three subsequent RCTs.[24–26] The first RCT (187 children aged 16–24 months) compared treatment with ventilation tubes versus watchful waiting.[24] It found that verbal comprehension improved more in the children treated with ventilation tubes (significance not reported) and that expressive language improved, by 1 month, more in the children treated with ventilation tubes (significance not reported). However, the trial reported that the groups were not equivalent at baseline, with an initially higher level of educational development in children in the watchful waiting group. The second RCT (429 children aged ≤3 years) compared early versus delayed insertion of tympanostomy tubes.[25] It found no significant effect on language development measured on a range of scales. The third RCT (182 children, mean age 2.9 years) found that early insertion of bilateral grommets significantly reduced behavioural problems at 9 months compared with watchful waiting (24 withdrawals from watchful waiting, 8 from early surgery, no intention to treat analysis: Richman behaviour check list 25/84 [30%] *v* 31/66 [47%]; RR 0.63, 95% CI 0.30 to 0.96).[26] **Grommets plus adenoidectomy:** The review found that adenoidectomy gave little additional benefit over grommets alone in terms of mean hearing gain, which varied from 1.1–2.6 dB.[23] A subsequent RCT (228 children, ages 2–9 years) compared adenotonsillectomy or adenoidectomy (analysed together) versus neither procedure.[27] All children had a grommet inserted into one ear. Outcomes were mean audiometric change, and tympanometric and otoscopic clearance assessed over 6 months to 10 years after treatment. The trial found improved tympanometric and otoscopic clearance when combining adenoidectomy with grommets versus grommets alone or no surgery. Median duration of glue ear assessed tympanometrically was reduced from 7.8 years without treatment to 4.9 years with grommets, 4 years with adenoidectomy, and 2.8 years with adenoidectomy and grommets combined. The difference between duration for adenoidectomy alone and grommets alone was not significant (CI not provided; P = 0.2), but all other comparisons were significant. **Tonsillectomy:** The review found no good RCTs of tonsillectomy alone in otitis media with effusion.[23]

Harms: We found one systematic review (search date 1999), which found that transient otorrhoea was common postoperatively (7 studies, 1522 children: incidence 16%, 95% CI 14% to 18%) and later (23 studies, 5491 people: incidence 26%, 95% CI 25% to 27%).[28] Recurrent ear discharge was also common (7 studies, 1144 children: incidence 7.4%, 95% CI 6% to 9%) and often became chronic (3 studies, 451 children: incidence 3.8%, 95% CI 2% to 6%). A systematic review of observational and experimental studies (search date 1998) of the complications following grommet insertion found a reported prevalence of tympanosclerosis in 39–65% of ventilated ears as opposed to 0–10% of untreated ears.[29] Partial atrophy was noted in 16–73% of ears treated and in 5–31% of those untreated. Atelectasis ranged from 10–37% of ears treated as opposed to 1–20% of those untreated, and attic retraction between 10–52% and 29–40%, respectively. The average hearing loss associated with these abnormalities was less than 5 dB. **Adenoidectomy:** Deaths have been reported in 1/16 700–25 000 children when combined with tonsillectomy (no figures provided for adenoidectomy alone) and postoperative haemorrhage occurred in 0.5%.[30]

Comment: About half of children who have grommets inserted will undergo reinsertion within 5 years.[31] Resolution after surgery takes longer in younger children and in those whose parents smoke, irrespective of treatment.[26]

REFERENCES

1. Williamson IG, Dunleavey J, Bain J, Robinson D. The natural history of otitis media with effusion: a three year study of the incidence and prevalence of abnormal tympanograms in four SW Hampshire infant and first schools. *J Laryngol Otol* 1994;108:930–934.
2. Strachan DP, Cook DG. Health effects of passive smoking. 4. Passive smoking, middle ear disease and adenotonsillectomy in children. *Thorax* 1998;53:50–56. Search date 1997; primary sources Medline and Embase.

3. Paradise JL, Rockette HE, Colborn DK, et al. Otitis media in 2253 Pittsburgh area infants: prevalence and risk factors during the first two years of life. *Pediatrics* 1997;99:318–333.
4. Haggard M, Hughes E. *Objectives, values and methods of screening children's hearing – a review of the literature*. London: HMSO, 1991.
5. Zeilhuis GA, Rach GH, Broek PV. Screening for otitis media with effusion in pre-school children. *Lancet* 1989;1:311–314.
6. Fiellau-Nikolajsen M. Tympanometry in three year old children: prevalence and spontaneous course of MEE. *Ann Otol Rhinol Laryngol* 1980;89(suppl 68):233–237.
7. Bennett KE, Haggard MP. Behaviour and cognitive outcomes in middle ear disease. *Arch Dis Child* 1999;80:28–35.
8. Stool SE, Berg SO, Berman S, et al. *Otitis media with effusion in young children: clinical practice guideline number 12.* AHCPR Publication 94–0622. Rockville, Maryland: Agency for Health Care Policy and Research, Public Health Service, United States Department of Health and Human Services, July, 1994. Search date 1992; primary sources online database of National Library of Medicine and 10 specialised bibliographic databases.
9. Cantekin EI, McGuire TW. Antibiotics are not effective for otitis media with effusion: reanalysis of meta-analysis. *Otorhinolaryngol Nova* 1998;8:214–222. Search date 1997; primary sources RCTs in refereed journals and proceedings published between 1980 and 1997 in English language publications.
10. Computerised clinical information system. Denver, Colorado: Micromedex Inc, June 1993.
11. Little P, Gould C, Williamson I, Warner G, Gantley M, Kinmonth AL. Reattendance and complications in a randomised trial of prescribing strategies for sore throat: the medicalising effect of prescribing antibiotics. *BMJ* 1997;315:350–352.
12. Wise R, Hart T, Cars O, et al. Antimicrobial resistance is a major threat to public health [Editorial]. *BMJ* 1998;317:609–610.
13. Williams RL, Chalmers TC, Strange KC, Chalmers FT, Bowlin SJ. Use of antibiotics in preventing recurrent acute otitis media and in treating otitis media with effusion: a meta-analytic attempt to resolve the brouhaha. *JAMA* 1993;270:1344–1351. Search date 1993; primary sources Medline and Current Contents.
14. Butler CC, van der Voort JH. Oral or nasal steroids for hearing loss associated with otitis media with effusion in children. In: The Cochrane Library, Issue 1, 2002. Oxford: Update Software. Search date 2000; primary sources Cochrane Controlled Trials Register, Embase, and Medline.
15. Tracy TM, Demain JG, Hoffman KM, Goetz DW. Intranasal beclomethasone as an adjunct to treatment of chronic middle ear effusion. *Ann Allergy Asthma Immunol* 1998;80:198–206.
16. Graf P. Rhinitis medicamentosa: aspects of pathophysiology and treatment. *Eur J Allergy Clin Immunol* 1997;52(Suppl 40):28–34.
17. Pignataro O, Pignataro LD, Gallus G, Calori G, Cordaro CI. Otitis media with effusion and S-carboxymethylcysteine and/or its lysine salt: a critical overview. *Int J Pediatr Otorhinolaryngol* 1996;35:231–241. Search date 1993; primary sources Medline, Embase, and Biosis.
18. Van der Merwe J, Wagenfeld DJ. The negative effects of mucolytics in otitis media with effusion. *S Afr Med J* 1987;72:625–626.
19. Stewart IA, Guy AM, Allison RS, Thomson NJ. Bromhexine in the treatment of otitis media with effusion. *Clin Otolaryngol* 1985;10:145–149.
20. Roydhouse N. Bromhexine for otitis media with effusion. *N Z Med J* 1981;94:373–375.
21. Reidpath DD, Glasziou PP, Del Mar C. Systematic review of autoinflation for treatment of glue ear in children. *BMJ* 1999;318:1177–1178. Search date not stated; primary sources Medline, Cochrane Library, and pharmaceutical company database.
22. Blanshard JD, Maw AR, Bawden R. Conservative treatment of otitis media with effusion by autoinflation of the middle ear. *Clin Otolaryngol* 1993;18:188–192.
23. University of York. Centre for Reviews and Dissemination. 1992. The treatment of persistent glue ear in children. Effective Health Care 1(4). Search date 1992; primary sources BIDS, Medline, and Embase.
24. Rovers MM, Stratman H, Ingels K, van der Wilt GJ, van den Broek P, Zielhuis GA. The effect of ventilation tubes on language development in infants with otitis media with effusion: a randomised trial. *Pediatrics* 2000;106:3–42.
25. Paradise J, Feldman HM, Campbell TF, et al. Effect of early or delayed insertion of tympanostomy tubes for persistent otitis media on developmental outcomes at the age of three years. *N Engl J Med* 2001;344:1179–1187.
26. Wilks J, Maw R, Peters TJ, Harvey I, Golding J. Randomised controlled trial of early surgery versus watchful waiting for glue ear: The effect on behavioural problems in pre-school children. *Clin Otol Allied Sci* 2000;25:209–214.
27. Maw R, Bawden R. Spontaneous resolution of severe chronic glue ear in children and the effect of adenoidectomy, tonsillectomy, and insertion of ventilation tubes. *BMJ* 1993;306:756–760.
28. Kay DJ, Nelson M, Rosenfeld RM. Meta-analysis of tympanostomy tube sequelae. *Otolaryngol Head Neck Surg* 2001;124:374–380. Search date 1999; primary sources Medline and hand searches.
29. Schilder AG. Assessment of complications of the conditions and of the treatment of otitis media with effusion. *Int J Pediatr Otolaryngol* 1999;49(Suppl 1):S247–S251. Search date 1998; primary sources not stated.
30. Yardley MP. Tonsillectomy, adenoidectomy and adenotonsillectomy; are they safe day case procedures. *J Laryngol Otol* 1992;106:299–300.
31. Maw AR. Development of tympanosclerosis in children with otitis media with effusion and ventilation tubes. *J Laryngol Otol* 1991;105:614–617.

Ian Williamson
Senior Lecturer in Primary Medical Care
The University of Southampton
Southampton
UK

Competing interests: None declared.

Recurrent tonsillitis

Search date December 2001

William McKerrow

QUESTIONS

INTERVENTIONS

Unknown effectiveness

To be covered in future updates

Intermittent antibiotics

Long term antibiotics

Key Messages

- **Tonsillectomy versus antibiotics** We found no RCTs evaluating tonsillectomy in adults. One RCT in children with severe tonsillitis found limited evidence that tonsillectomy versus antibiotics may reduce throat infections in the first 2 years after treatment, but found no significant difference at 3 years.

DEFINITION Tonsillitis is infection of the parenchyma of the palatine tonsils. Recurrent severe tonsillitis results in significant morbidity, including time lost from school or work. The definition of severe recurrent tonsillitis is arbitrary, but criteria used recently as a measure of severity were five or more episodes of true tonsillitis a year, symptoms for at least a year, and episodes that are disabling and prevent normal functioning.[1]

INCIDENCE/PREVALENCE Recurrent sore throat has an incidence in general practice in the UK of 100/1000 population a year.[2] Acute tonsillitis is more common in childhood.

AETIOLOGY/RISK FACTORS Common bacterial pathogens include β haemolytic and other streptococci. Bacteria are cultured successfully only from a minority of people with tonsillitis. The role of viruses is uncertain.

PROGNOSIS We found no good data on the natural history of tonsillitis or recurrent sore throat in children or adults. Participants in RCTs who were randomised to medical treatment (courses of antibiotics as required) have shown a tendency towards improvement over time.[3,4]

AIMS To abolish tonsillitis; to reduce the frequency and severity of recurrent throat infections; to improve general wellbeing, behaviour, and educational achievement, with minimal adverse effects.

OUTCOMES Number and severity of episodes of tonsillitis or sore throat; requirement for antibiotics and analgesics; time off work or school; behaviour, school performance, general wellbeing; morbidity and mortality of surgery; and adverse effects of drugs.

METHODS *Clinical Evidence* search and appraisal December 2001.

QUESTION **Is tonsillectomy effective in severe tonsillitis in children and adults?**

OPTION **TONSILLECTOMY VERSUS ANTIBIOTICS**

Limited evidence from one RCT suggests that tonsillectomy may benefit some children with severe tonsillitis. We found no good evidence on tonsillectomy in adults. We found that many important outcome measures have not been considered.

Benefits: We found two systematic reviews (search dates 1997[5] and 1998[6]). **Children:** Both reviews identified the same two RCTs as being the only ones that met quality inclusion criteria.[3,4] The smaller RCT involved 91 children who fulfilled criteria for "severe tonsillitis" (7 episodes in the preceding year, or 5 episodes/year in the preceding 2 years, or 3 episodes/year in the preceding 3 years).[3] The children were randomised to tonsillectomy alone (27 children), adenotonsillectomy (16 children), or intermittent courses of antibiotics as needed (48 children). Sixteen children were withdrawn from the non-surgical group by their parents and had surgery, and children who developed infections after surgery received antibiotics as necessary for each episode of infection. Secondary outcome measures such as time off school were also considered. The authors concluded that children undergoing tonsillectomy experienced significantly fewer throat infections than those on antibiotics, amounting to an average of three fewer throat infections in the first 2 years, but by the third year the difference was no longer significant. The larger RCT (246 "less severely affected children") is published only in abstract form.[4] Some children in this study also underwent adenoidectomy. The limited data available provide no evidence of a difference between surgical and medical treatment. The second review concluded that it was not possible to determine the effectiveness of tonsillectomy from these RCTs.[6] **Adults:** The reviews found no RCTs that evaluated tonsillectomy in adults with recurrent tonsillitis or sore throats.

Harms: **Tonsillectomy:** The risks of tonsillectomy include those associated with general anaesthesia and those specific to the procedure. The overall complication rate in the smaller RCT[3] was 14% (all were "readily managed or self limiting") compared with 2–8% in one Scottish tonsillectomy audit.[7] Haemorrhage, either primary (in the immediate postoperative period) or secondary, occurred in 4% of children studied in the larger RCT[4] and fewer than 1% of children in the Scottish tonsillectomy audit.[7] **Antibiotics:** In the smaller RCT, erythematous rashes occurred in 4% of children in the non-surgical group while taking penicillin.[3] Other adverse effects of antibiotics include allergic reactions and the promotion of resistant bacteria. One RCT found that, for people with milder episodes of sore throat, the prescribing of antibiotics compared with no initial prescription increased the proportion of people who returned to see their physician in the short term because of sore throat (716 people with sore throat and an abnormal physical sign; return rate 38% with initial antibiotics *v* 27% without; adjusted HR for return 1.39, 95% CI 1.03 to 1.89).[8]

Comment: **Background:** Tonsillectomy is one of the most frequently performed surgical procedures in the UK, particularly in children, and accounts for about 20% of all operations performed by otolaryngologists.[7] Adenoidectomy is now performed with tonsillectomy only when there is a specific indication to remove the adenoids as well as the tonsils. **Quality of the evidence:** In the smaller RCT,[3] there were significant baseline differences between groups before treatment, and the authors pooled the results of tonsillectomy and adenotonsillectomy, making it impossible to assess the effectiveness of tonsillectomy alone. **Gaps in the evidence:** We found no RCT that found improved general wellbeing, development, or behaviour despite suggestions that these are influenced by tonsillectomy.[7] **New techniques:** Diathermy tonsillectomy and adjuvant treatment[9] may reduce adverse effects and are currently being studied.

REFERENCES

1. Management of Sore Throat and Indications for Tonsillectomy. National Clinical Guideline No 34. Scottish Intercollegiate Guidelines Network, Royal College of Physicians, 9 Queen Street, Edinburgh EH2 1JQ.
2. Shvartzman P. Careful prescribing is beneficial. *BMJ* 1994;309:1101–1102.
3. Paradise JL, Bluestone CD, Bachman RZ, et al. Efficacy of tonsillectomy for recurrent throat infection in severely affected children. *N Engl J Med* 1984;310:674–683.
4. Paradise JL, Bluestone CD, Rogers KD, et al. Comparative efficacy of tonsillectomy for recurrent throat infection in more versus less severely affected children [abstract]. *Pediatric Res* 1992;31:126A.
5. Marshall T. A review of tonsillectomy for recurrent throat infection. *Br J Gen Pract* 1998;48:1331–1335. Search date 1997; primary sources Cochrane Library and Medline.
6. Burton MJ, Towler B, Glasziou P. Tonsillectomy versus non-surgical treatment for chronic/recurrent

acute tonsillitis. In: The Cochrane Library, Issue 2, 2001. Oxford: Update Software. Search date 1998; primary sources Medline, Embase, Cochrane Controlled Trials Register, and hand searched references.

7. Blair RL, McKerrow WS, Carter NW, Fenton A. The Scottish tonsillectomy audit. *J Laryngol Otol* 1996;110(suppl 20):1–25.
8. Little P, Gould C, Williamson I, Warner G, Gantley M, Kinmouth, AL. Reattendance and complications in a randomised trial of prescribing strategies for sore throat: the medicalising effect of prescribing antibiotics. *BMJ* 1997;315:350–352.
9. Steward DL, Chung SJ. The role of adjuvant therapies and techniques in tonsillectomy. *Curr Opin Otolaryngol Head Neck Surg* 2000;8:186–192.

William McKerrow
Raigmore Hospital
Inverness
UK

Competing interests: None declared.

Tinnitus

Search date February 2002

Angus Waddell and Richard Canter

QUESTIONS

INTERVENTIONS

See glossary, p 531

Key Messages

- **Ginkgo biloba** One systematic review and one subsequent RCT found no significant difference with ginkgo biloba versus placebo in tinnitus symptoms.
- **Psychotherapy** We found limited evidence from two systematic reviews that psychotherapy may improve symptom scores of people with chronic tinnitus, but weakness of methods used in the reviews, and in the studies they included, means that the effects of psychotherapy remain unclear.
- **Tocainide** One RCT found no significant difference with tocainide versus placebo in improving symptoms, but found evidence that tocainide caused significantly more adverse effects after 30 days treatment (NNH 2, 95% CI 1 to 8).
- **Tricyclic antidepressants** One RCT in people with depression and chronic tinnitus found limited evidence that tricyclic antidepressants (nortriptyline) versus placebo improved tinnitus related disability, audiometric tinnitus loudness matching, and symptoms of depression, but found no significant difference in tinnitus severity. We found no evidence about the effects of tricyclic antidepressants in people with chronic tinnitus without depressive symptoms.
- **Acupuncture; antiepileptics; baclofen; benzodiazepines; cinnarizine; electromagnetic stimulation; hyperbaric oxygen; hypnosis; low power laser; nicotinamide; tinnitus masking devices; zinc** We found insufficient evidence about the effects of these interventions.

Tinnitus

DEFINITION Tinnitus is defined as the perception of sound, which does not arise from the external environment, from within the body (e.g. vascular sounds) or from auditory hallucinations related to mental illness. This review concerns the management of chronic tinnitus, where tinnitus is the only, or the predominant symptom, in an affected person.

INCIDENCE/ PREVALENCE Up to 18% of the general population in industrialised countries are mildly affected by chronic tinnitus, and 0.5% report tinnitus having a severe effect on their ability to lead a normal life.[1]

AETIOLOGY/ RISK FACTORS Tinnitus may occur as an isolated idiopathic symptom or in association with any type of hearing loss. Tinnitus may be a particular feature of presbyacusis, noise induced hearing loss, Menière's disease (see glossary, p 531) (see benefits under Menière's disease, p 499), or the presence of an acoustic neuroma. In people with toxicity from aspirin or quinine, tinnitus can occur while hearing thresholds remain normal. Tinnitus is also associated with depression, although it may be unclear whether the tinnitus is a manifestation of the depressive illness or a factor contributing to its development.[2]

PROGNOSIS Tinnitus may have an insidious onset, with a long delay before clinical presentation. It may persist for many years or decades, particularly when associated with a sensorineural hearing loss. In Menière's disease both the presence and intensity of tinnitus can fluctuate. Tinnitus may cause disruption of sleep patterns, an inability to concentrate, and depression.[3]

AIMS To reduce the loudness and intrusiveness of the tinnitus and to reduce its impact on daily life, with minimum adverse effects from treatment.

OUTCOMES The number of people with resolution of tinnitus; tinnitus loudness (assessed by visual analogue scale, symptom scores, or by audiometric matching); impact of tinnitus measured by estimates of interference with activities of daily life or with emotional state.

METHODS *Clinical Evidence* search and appraisal February 2002. We identified a few non-English language articles that require translation and, where appropriate, their results will be included in future *Clinical Evidence* updates.

QUESTION What are the effects of treatments for chronic tinnitus?

OPTION TRICYCLIC ANTIDEPRESSANTS

One RCT in people with depression and chronic tinnitus found limited evidence that tricyclic antidepressants (nortriptyline) versus placebo improved tinnitus related disability, audiometric tinnitus loudness matching, and symptoms of depression, but found no significant difference in tinnitus severity. We found no evidence about the effects of tricyclic antidepressants in people with chronic tinnitus without depressive symptoms.

Benefits: We found two systematic reviews (search dates 1998[4] and 1995[5]; 1 RCT). The RCT (92 people with tinnitus and depression or depressive symptoms but no bipolar disorder or other mental health diagnosis) identified by the reviews found that nortriptyline (titrated to maintain therapeutic blood levels) versus placebo significantly improved measures of depression, a tinnitus related disability score and audiometric tinnitus loudness matching (16–11 dB with nortriptyline *v* 19–18 dB with placebo; P = 0.006), but found no significant difference on the reporting of tinnitus severity after 6 weeks (43% of people improved with nortriptyline *v* 30% with placebo; P = 0.2; raw data not provided).[6]

Harms: Harms were not reported by the RCT.[6] Other studies have established that adverse effects of nortriptyline include dry mouth, blurred vision, and constipation (see harms of tricyclic antidepressants under depression, p 951).

Comment: We found no evidence about the effect of tricyclic antidepressants in people with chronic tinnitus who do not have depression or depressive symptoms.

OPTION BENZODIAZEPINES

We found insufficient evidence about the effects of benzodiazepines.

Benefits: We found one systematic review (search date 1995)[5] and one RCT. The RCT (40 people) identified by the review found that alprazolam (initially 0.5 mg/night) versus placebo significantly improved reported tinnitus severity after 12 weeks (13/17 [76%] improved with alprazolam *v* 1/19 [5%] with placebo; ARR 71%; RR 14.5, 95% CI 2.1 to 53), but interpretation of these results is difficult (see comment below).[7]

Harms: The RCT reported that two (10%) people receiving alprazolam withdrew from the trial because of excessive tiredness.[7] Long term use of benzodiazepines can lead to dependence (see harms of benzodiazepines under generalised anxiety disorder, p 974).

Comment: The RCT used dose adjustment of alprazolam but no dose adjustment of placebo, potentially biasing the results because of a difference in the attention given to people in the two groups.[7] Another systematic review (search date 1998) found three other studies that used weaker methods; none of the studies provided evidence that benzodiazepines versus placebo improved the impact of tinnitus.[4]

OPTION ANTIEPILEPTICS

We found insufficient evidence about the effects of antiepileptics.

Benefits: We found one systematic review (search date 1995, 1 RCT)[5] and one subsequent RCT.[8] The RCT (48 people) identified by the review found no significant difference with carbamazepine (150 mg three times daily for 30 days) versus placebo on reported tinnitus severity after 30 days treatment (2/24 [8%] improved with carbamazepine *v* 3/24 [13%] with placebo; ARR 4.2%; RR 0.67, 95% CI 0.12 to 3.6).[9] The subsequent RCT (31 people) used a crossover design and did not report results before the crossover (see comment below).[8]

Harms: The RCT identified by the review found that carbamazipine versus placebo significantly increased the number of people reporting adverse effects (including dizziness, nausea, and headaches; 25/34 [63%] with carbamazepine *v* 1/24 [4%] with placebo; RR 17.6, 95% CI 2.6 to 121; NNH 1, 95% CI 1 to 2). The subsequent RCT did not report harms (see harms of lamotrigine under epilepsy, p 1313).

Comment: A second systematic review found five RCTs comparing antiepileptic treatment versus placebo; all the RCTs included were small and brief.[4] The subsequent RCT found no significant difference with lamotrigine (25 mg/day for 2 wks, 50 mg/day for 2 wks, and then 100 mg/day for 4 wks) versus placebo in tinnitus loudness or annoyance measured on a visual analogue scale (11/31 [35%] people improved with lamotrigine *v* 6/31 [19%] people with placebo; ARI 16%; RR 1.8, 95% CI 0.78 to 4.34).[8]

OPTION NICOTINAMIDE

We found insufficient evidence about the effects of nicotinamide.

Benefits: We found one systematic review (search date 1998; 1 RCT)[4]. The RCT (48 people) identified by the review found no significant difference with nicotinamide (70 mg three times daily for 30 days) versus placebo on reported subjective improvement after 30 days treatment (2/24 [8%] people improved with nicotinamide *v* 3/24 [13%] with placebo; ARR 4%; RR 0.7, 95% CI 0.1 to 3.6).[10]

Harms: The RCT found no significant difference with nicotinamide versus placebo in the number of people reporting headache (4/24 [16%] with nicotinamide *v* 1/24 [4%] with placebo; RR 4.0, 95% CI 0.5 to 33.2) or the number of people reporting dizziness (2/24 [8%] *v* 0/24 [0%]).[10]

Comment: None.

OPTION CINNARIZINE

We found insufficient evidence about the effects of cinnarizine.

Benefits: We found one systematic review (search date 1998; 1 RCT)[4]. The RCT (30 people) identified by the review found no significant difference with cinnarizine (25 mg three times daily for 10 wks) versus placebo on reported subjective improvement (1/10 [10%] people improved with cinnarizine *v* 1/20 [5%] people with placebo; ARR 5%; RR 2.0, 95% CI 0.14 to 29; see comment below).[11]

Harms: The RCT did not report harms.[11]

Comment: The RCT did not specify the follow up period.[11]

OPTION ZINC

We found insufficient evidence about the effects of zinc.

Benefits: We found one systematic review (search date 1998; 1 RCT)[4]. The RCT (50 people) identified by the review found no significant difference with zinc (100 mg three times daily for 8 wks) versus placebo on reported tinnitus severity after 8 weeks treatment (2/23 [9%] people improved with zinc v 2/25 [8%] people with placebo; ARR 1%; RR 1.1, 95% CI 0.16 to 7).[12]

Harms: The RCT did not report harms.[12]

Comment: None.

OPTION BACLOFEN

We found insufficient evidence about the effects of baclofen.

Benefits: We found one systematic review (search date 1998; 1 RCT)[4]. The RCT (63 people) identified by the review found no significant difference with baclofen (10 mg twice daily increasing to 30 mg twice daily for 3 wks) versus placebo on reported subjective improvement (3/31 [10%] improved with baclofen v 1/32 [3%] with placebo; ARR 7%; RR 3.1, 95% CI 0.34 to 28; see comment below).[13]

Harms: The RCT did not report harms.[13]

Comment: The RCT did not specify the follow up period.[13]

OPTION TOCAINIDE

One RCT found no significant difference with tocainide versus placebo in improving symptoms, but found evidence that tocainide caused significantly more adverse effects after 30 days' treatment.

Benefits: We found one systematic review (search date 1995; 2 RCTs)[5]. The first RCT (40 people) identified by the review used a crossover design and did not give details of the washout period or the results before the crossover (see comment below).[14] The second RCT (48 people) identified by the review found no significant difference with tocainide (300 mg three times daily for 30 days) versus placebo on the number of people with improved symptoms after 30 days' treatment (1/24 [4%] with tocainide v 3/24 [13%] with control; ARR 8%; RR 0.33, 95% CI 0.04 to 3.0).[15]

Harms: The second RCT identified by the review found that tocainide versus placebo significantly increased the number adverse effects (11/24 [45.8%] v 2/24 [8.3%]; ARI 37%; RR 5.5, 95% CI 1.4 to 22.2; NNH 2, 95% CI 1 to 8).[15] The main adverse effects reported were rash (6/24 [25%] with tocainide v 1/24 [4%] with placebo), dizziness (3/24 [12%] with tocainide v 0/24 [0%] with placebo), and tremor (2/24 [8%] with tocainide v 0/24 [0%] with placebo).

Comment: The first RCT found no significant difference with oral tocainide (400 mg/day rising to 2.4 g/day for 4 wks) versus placebo in symptom scores (10/40 [25%] improved with tocainide *v* 4/40 [10%] with placebo; ARR 15%; RR 2.5, 95% CI 0.85 to 7.3).

OPTION ACUPUNCTURE

We found insufficient evidence about the effects of acupuncture.

Benefits: We found one systematic review (search date 1998, 6 studies, 185 people).[16] The review included one pseudo-randomised RCT,[17] two non-blinded RCTs,[11,18] two crossover RCTs,[19,20] and one blinded parallel group RCT.[21] All studies were small and brief. The blinded parallel group RCT (54 people) found no significant difference with acupuncture (25 sessions over 2 months) versus sham acupuncture (superficial penetration at random non-acupuncture points) in tinnitus loudness on a pooled visual analogue score (4% improvement with acupuncture *v* 1% deterioration with placebo).[21] The crossover RCTs did not report results before the crossover (see comment below).

Harms: The review did not report on adverse effects.[16]

Comment: The first crossover RCT (14 people) found that acupuncture versus sham acupuncture significantly increased the number of who people reported a reduction in tinnitus loudness after one session of treatment (5/14 [36%] with acupuncture *v* 0/14 [0%] with sham acupuncture; P = 0.05).[19] The second crossover RCT (20 people) found no significant difference with acupuncture versus placebo on a pooled visual analogue score of subjective tinnitus severity after 3 weeks (P = 0.22).[20]

OPTION PSYCHOTHERAPY

We found limited evidence from two systematic reviews that psychotherapy may improve symptom scores of people with chronic tinnitus, but weak methods used in the reviews and in the studies they included, means that the effects of psychotherapy remain unclear.

Benefits: We found two systematic reviews (search date 1995, 13 studies including non-randomised studies;[5] search date 1998, 8 RCTs, 269 people;[22] see comment below) of psychological treatments for tinnitus.[5,22] Both reviews used weak methods to calculate effect sizes. The first review pooled results from studies of widely differing designs and made comparisons between treated groups from different studies.[5] The second systematic review searched only Medline and Psychological Abstracts and excluded all non-English language papers.[22] The analysis pooled results from cognitive behavioural treatment, relaxation therapy, counselling, and stress management. It also compared treated groups from different studies. It calculated significant effect sizes for reduction of subjective loudness (SMD 0.68, 95% CI 0.62 to 0.74) and tinnitus annoyance (SMD 0.83, 95% CI 0.82 to 0.84).

Harms: Neither review reported on harms.[5,22]

Comment: Despite many studies on psychotherapeutic measures to treat tinnitus, the evidence for benefit remains limited. Many of the RCTs suffer from weak methods, high withdrawal rates, and pooled or surrogate outcome measures. The systematic reviews used weak methods;[5,22] pooling study results across arms of trials loses the benefits of randomisation and increases the risk of bias.

OPTION ELECTROMAGNETIC STIMULATION/EAR CANAL MAGNETS

We found insufficient evidence about the effects of magnets and electromagnetic stimulation.

Benefits: **Electromagnetic stimulation:** We found no systematic review, but found three small RCTs (136 people) comparing electromagnetic stimulation versus placebo.[23–25] The first RCT (58 people) found that electromagnetic stimulation versus placebo significantly increased the number of people who had improved tinnitus (14/31 [45%] *v* 2/23 [9%]; RR 5.2, 95% CI 1.3 to 20.6; see comment below).[24] The second RCT (48 people) found no significant difference with electromagnetic stimulation versus placebo in tinnitus sensation levels after 1 week (6/24 [25%] *v* 6/24 [25%]; RR 0.4, 95% CI 0.38 to 2.66).[23] The third RCT (20 people; see comment below) used a crossover design and did not report results before the crossover.[25] **Magnets:** We found no systematic review but found one RCT (49 people).[26] The RCT found no significant difference with a simple ear canal magnet versus placebo on tinnitus symptoms after 4 weeks treatment (7/26 [27%] with magnet *v* 4/23 [17%] with placebo; RR 1.5, 95% CI 0.53 to 4.5).

Harms: The RCTs reported no adverse effects associated with electromagnetic stimulation.[23–25]

Comment: The first RCT, which did not specify the length of follow up, reported that 4/58 (7%) people withdrew from the trial and that the analysis was not by intention to treat.[24] The crossover RCT found no significant difference with electrical suppression versus a placebo device in reduction in tinnitus severity (2/20 [10%] active device *v* 4/20 [20%] with placebo device; P = NS).[25]

OPTION HYPNOSIS

We found insufficient evidence about the effects of hypnosis.

Benefits: We found one systematic review (search date 1995)[5] and one additional RCT.[27] The review identified two studies, which were of insufficient quality for inclusion.[28,29] The additional RCT (92 people who were preselected to be suggestible to hypnosis) found no significant difference with three sessions teaching self hypnosis versus control (a single counselling session) on symptom severity scores after 3 months (24/44 [55%] improved with hypnosis *v* 23/42 [55%] with counselling; RR 1.0, 95% CI 0.68 to 1.46). The RCT also found no significant difference in the number of people reporting worsened tinnitus (11/44 [25%] with hypnosis *v* 14/42 [32%] with counselling; RR 0.8, 95% CI 0.4 to 1.5).

Harms: No adverse effects were reported.[5,27]

Comment: None.

OPTION **LOW POWER LASER**

We found insufficient evidence about the effects of low power laser.

Benefits: We found no systematic review but found one RCT.[30] The RCT (49 people) found no significant difference with laser (50 mW directed towards the mastoid bone) versus placebo in the number of people with improved tinnitus symptoms after 1 month (2/25 [8%] with laser *v* 7/24 [29%] with placebo; RR 0.27, 95% CI 0.06 to 1.2).[30]

Harms: No adverse effects were reported.[30]

Comment: None.

OPTION **TINNITUS MASKING DEVICES**

We found insufficient evidence about the effects of tinnitus masking devices.

Benefits: **Masking devices versus no treatment:** We found one systematic review (search date 1998, 1 RCT).[4] The RCT (75 people with tinnitus but no hearing difficulties) compared two types of tinnitus masking device versus a non-blinded control group. It found that either type of masking device versus control significantly improved symptoms (chi squared analysis $P < 0.01$; no supporting data given).[31]

Harms: The systematic review and RCT did not report on harms.[4,31]

Comment: Masking devices have been widely prescribed but we could find no evidence to support their use.

OPTION **GINKGO BILOBA** New

One systematic review and one subsequent RCT found no significant difference with ginkgo biloba versus placebo in tinnitus symptoms.

Benefits: We found one systematic review[32] and one subsequent RCT.[33] The systematic review (search date 1998, 5 RCTs)[32] contained three RCTs of insufficient quality for inclusion in this review. Of the remaining two trials identified by the review, the first (crossover RCT, 20 people) found no significant difference with ginkgo biloba extract (29.2 mg/day for 2 wks) versus placebo in tinnitus symptoms (see comment below).[34] The second RCT (99 people) compared ginkgo biloba extract (120 mg/day for 12 wks) versus placebo.[35] The RCT found an improvement in measured tinnitus loudness from 42 dB to 39 dB with ginkgo biloba extract versus no improvement in the control group (significance not stated; additional numerical data not provided). The subsequent RCT (1121 people) compared ginkgo biloba (50 mg three times daily for 12 wks) versus placebo.[33] It found no significant difference in the number of people reporting subjective improvement after 12 weeks treatment (34/360 [9.4%] with ginkgo biloba *v* 35/360 [9.7%] with placebo; ARI 0.3%, 95% CI –4.7 to 4.2).

Harms: The subsequent RCT reported gastrointestinal upset (3%), dizziness (1%), and mouth dryness (1%) in both treatment and control groups.[33]

Comment: The crossover RCT identified by the review did not specify the length of follow up.[34]

OPTION HYPERBARIC OXYGEN New

We found no evidence about the effects of hyperbaric oxygen.

Benefits: We found no systematic review or RCTs.

Harms: We found no evidence.

Comment: None.

GLOSSARY

Menière's disease A condition characterised by episodic vertigo, tinnitus, and sensorineural hearing loss.

REFERENCES

1. Coles RR. Epidemiology of tinnitus (1). *J Laryngol Otol* 1984;9(suppl):7–15.
2. Sullivan MD, Katon W, Dobie R, et al. Disabling tinnitus: association with affective disorder. *Gen Hosp Psychiatry* 1988;10:285–291.
3. Zoger S, Svedlund J, Holgers KM. Psychiatric disorders in tinnitus patients without severe hearing impairment: 24 month follow-up of patients at an audiological clinic. *Audiology* 2001;40:133–140.
4. Dobie RA. A review of randomized clinical trials in tinnitus. *Laryngoscope* 1999;109:1202–1211. Search date 1998; primary sources Medline and handsearches.
5. Schilter B, Jäger B, Heerman R, et al. Pharmacological and psychological treatment options in chronic subjective tinnitus: a meta-analysis of effective treatments. *HNO* 2000;48:589–597. Search date 1995; primary sources Medline, Psyindex, Psychlit, and handsearches including German, English, and French language papers.
6. Dobie RA, Sakai CS, Sullivan MD, et al. Antidepressant treatment of tinnitus patients: report of a randomized clinical trial and clinical prediction of benefit. *Am J Otol* 1993;14:18–23.
7. Johnson RM, Brummett R, Schleuning A. Use of alprazolam for relief of tinnitus. A double-blind study. *Arch Otolaryngol Head Neck Surg* 1993;119:842–845.
8. Simpson JJ, Gilbert AM, Weiner GM, et al. The assessment of lamotrigine, an antiepileptic drug, in the treatment of tinnitus. *Am J Otol* 1999;20:627–631.
9. Hulshof JH, Vermeij P. The value of carbamazepine in the treatment of tinnitus. *ORL J Otorhinolaryngol Relat Spec* 1985;47:262–266.
10. Hulshof JH, Vermeij P. The effect of nicotinamide on tinnitus: a double-blind controlled study. *Clin Otolaryngol* 1987;12:211–214.
11. Podoshin L, Ben-David Y, Fradis M, et al. Idiopathic subjective tinnitus treated by biofeedback, acupuncture and drug therapy. *Ear Nose Throat J* 1991;70:284–289.
12. Paaske PB, Pedersen CB, Kjems G, et al. Zinc in the management of tinnitus. Placebo-controlled trial. *Ann Otol Rhinol Laryngol* 1991;100:647–649.
13. Westerberg BD, Roberson JB Jr, Stach BA. A double-blind placebo-controlled trial of baclofen in the treatment of tinnitus [see comments]. *Am J Otol* 1996;17:896–903.
14. Lenarz T. Treatment of tinnitus with lidocaine and tocainide. *Scand Audiol Suppl* 1986;26:49–51.
15. Hulshof JH, Vermeij P. The value of tocainide in the treatment of tinnitus. *Arch Otolaryngol* 1985;241:279–283.
16. Park J, White AR, Ernst E. Efficacy of acupuncture as a treatment for tinnitus: a systematic review. *Arch Otolaryngol Head Neck Surg* 2000;126:489–492. Search date 1998; primary sources Medline, Cochrane Controlled Trials Register, Embase, and Ciscom.
17. Axelsson A, Andersson S, Gu LD. Acupuncture in the management of tinnitus: a placebo-controlled study. *Audiology* 1994;33:351–360.
18. Furugard S, Hedin PJ, Eggertz A, et al. Acupuncture worth trying in severe tinnitus. *Lakartidningen* 1998;95:1922–1928.
19. Marks NJ, Emery P, Onisiphorou C. A controlled trial of acupuncture in tinnitus. *J Laryngol Otol* 1984;98:1103–1109.
20. Hansen PE, Hansen JH, Bentzen O. Acupuncture therapy of chronic unilateral tinnitus. A double-blind cross-over study. *Ugeskr Laeger* 1981;143:2888–2890.
21. Vilholm OJ, Moller K, Jorgensen K. Effect of traditional Chinese acupuncture on severe tinnitus: a double-blind, placebo-controlled, clinical investigation with open therapeutic control. *Br J Audiol* 1998;32:197–204.
22. Andersson G, Lyttkens L. A meta-analytic review of psychological treatments for tinnitus. *Br J Audiol* 1999;33:201–210. Search date August 1998; primary sources Medline and psychological abstracts.
23. Fiedler SC, Pilkington H, Willatt DJ. Electromagnetic stimulation as a treatment of tinnitus: a further study. *Clin Otolaryngol* 1998;23:270.
24. Roland NJ, Hughes JB, Daley MB, et al. Electromagnetic stimulation as a treatment of tinnitus: a pilot study. *Clin Otolaryngol* 1993;18:278–281.
25. Dobie RA, Hoberg KE, Rees TS. Electrical tinnitus suppression: a double-blind crossover study. *Otolaryngol Head Neck Surg* 1986;95:319–333.

26. Coles R, Bradley P, Donaldson I, et al. A trial of tinnitus therapy with ear-canal magnets. *Clin Otolaryngol* 1991;16:371–372.
27. Mason JD, Rogerson DR, Butler JD. Client centred hypnotherapy in the management of tinnitus - is it better than counselling? *J Laryngol Otol* 1996;110:117–120.
28. Attias J, Shemesh Z, Sohmer H, et al. Comparison between self-hypnosis, masking and attentiveness for alleviation of chronic tinnitus. *Audiology* 1993;32:205–212.
29. Halama P. Erfahrungen mit der Hypnose-Therapie bei ambulaten Patienten, die unter Tinnitus leiden. Vergleichende Pilotstudie. *Experimental Klin Hypnose* 1992;8:49–69.
30. Mirz F, Zachariae R, Andersen SE, et al. The low-power laser in the treatment of tinnitus. *Clin Otolaryngol* 1999;24:346–354.
31. Stephens SDG, Corcoran AL. A controlled study of tinnitus masking. *Br J Audiol* 1985;19:159–167.
32. Ernst E, Stevinson C. Ginkgo biloba for tinnitus: a review. *Clin Otolaryngol* 1999;24:164–167. Search date 1998; primary sources Medline, Embase, The Cochrane Library, contact with manufacturers, and hand search of reference lists.
33. Drew S, Davies E. Effectiveness of ginkgo biloba in treating tinnitus: double blind, placebo controlled trial. *BMJ* 2001;322:73–75.
34. Holger K-M, Axelsson A, Pringle I. Ginkgo Biloba extract for the treatment of tinnitus. *Audiology* 1994;33:85–92.
35. Morgenstern C, Biermann E. Ginkgo-Spezialextrakt Egb 761 in der Behandlung des Tinnitus aurium. *Fortschr Med* 1997;115:7–11.

Angus Waddell
Southwest Training Scheme in Otolaryngology
University of Bristol
Bristol
UK

Richard Canter
Royal United Hospital NHS Trust and University of Bath
Bath
UK

Competing interests: None declared.

Wax in ear

Search date December 2001

George Browning

QUESTIONS

INTERVENTIONS

*Although many practitioners consider these to be standard treatments, we found no RCTs of these

See glossary, p 536

Key Messages

- **Ear syringing** There is consensus that ear syringing is effective but we found no RCTs comparing ear syringing versus no treatment or versus alternative treatment. A survey found that 38% of 274 general practitioners performing ear syringing reported complications, including otitis externa, perforation of the tympanic membrane, damage to the skin of the external canal, tinnitus, pain, and vertigo.
- **Manual removal (other than ear syringing)** We found no RCTs about mechanical methods of removing ear wax.
- **Wax softeners** One small RCT, in people with impacted wax, found that wax softeners versus no treatment reduced the risk of persisting impaction after 5 days treatment (NNT 5 ears, 95% CI 3 to 34). Five RCTs trials found no consistent evidence that any one type of wax softener was superior to the others. RCTs found insufficient evidence to assess the effects of wax softeners prior to syringing.

Wax in ear

DEFINITION	Ear wax is normal and becomes a problem only if it produces deafness, pain, or other aural symptoms. Ear wax may also need to be removed if it prevents inspection of the ear drum. The term "impacted" is used in different ways, and can merely imply the co-existence of wax obscuring the ear drum with symptoms in that ear.[1,2]
INCIDENCE/ PREVALENCE	We found four surveys of the prevalence of impacted wax (see glossary, p 536) (see table 1, p 537).[3–6] The prevalence was higher in men than in women, in the elderly than in the young, and in people with intellectual impairment.[7] One survey found that 289 Scottish general practitioners each saw an average of nine people a month requesting removal of ear wax.[1]
AETIOLOGY/ RISK FACTORS	Factors that prevent the normal extrusion of wax from the ear canal (e.g. wearing a hearing aid, using cotton buds) increase the chance of ear wax accumulating.
PROGNOSIS	Most ear wax emerges from the external canal spontaneously. Without impaction or adherence to the drum, there is likely to be minimal, if any, hearing loss. One survey of 21 unselected outpatients with completely obstructing wax (see glossary, p 536) found that the average improvement in hearing following syringing was 5.5 dB (95% CI 0.6 to 10.5 dB).[1]
AIMS	To relieve symptoms or to allow examination by completely removing impacted wax or obstructing wax; and to soften impacted wax to ease mechanical removal.
OUTCOMES	Proportion of people (or ears) with relief of hearing loss or discomfort; total removal of wax; proportion of people requiring further intervention to improve symptoms; ease of mechanical removal measured, for example, by the volume of water used to accomplish successful syringing.
METHODS	*Clinical Evidence* search and appraisal December 2001. A search for surveys of the prevalence of ear wax was performed in Medline and Embase in July 2001.

QUESTION What are the effects of methods to remove ear wax?

OPTION WAX SOFTENERS

One small RCT found limited evidence that using a wax softener versus no treatment significantly increased the proportion of ears that were completely cleared of wax after 5 days treatment. Five RCTs found no consistent evidence that any one type of wax softener was superior to the others. There is insufficient evidence to address the effects of wax softeners prior to syringing.

Benefits: We found no systematic review. **Versus placebo:** We found one RCT (113 people with impacted wax (see glossary, p 536) in one or both ears) (see table 2, p 538).[2] The ears were randomly allocated to treatment by the nursing staff with sterile water, sodium bicarbonate, a proprietary softening agent (arachis oil/chlorobutanol [chlorbutanol]/*p*-dichlorobenzene), or no treatment. Participants and nurses were blinded to the active treatment allocation. The people were recruited from a hospital for the elderly. People already using ear drops and people with known pathology of the ear canal or ear drum were excluded. Of those recruited, 13 left hospital and three died before completing the trial. Analysis of the remaining 97 people (155 ears) found that the risk of persisting impaction at the end of the trial was reduced by any active form of treatment compared with no treatment (AR of persistent impaction: 26/38 [68%] ears with no treatment *v* 55/117 [47%] ears with any active treatment; ARR 21%, 95% CI 3% to 35%; RR 1.31, 95% CI 1.06 to 1.75; NNT 5, 95% CI 3 to 34). **Versus other wax softeners:** We found five trials comparing wax softeners (see table 2, p 538).[2,8–11] Only two were RCTs[2,11] and the other ones did not state allocation stereotypes or were quasi-randomised trials. The trials were conducted in a variety of settings. They varied in size from 35 people to 286 ears. The most common outcomes were a subjective assessment of the amount of wax remaining, the need for syringing, the perceived ease of syringing, or the result of syringing. The trials found no consistent evidence that any one type of wax softener was clinically superior to any other. **Prior to syringing:** We found four RCTs comparing wax softeners given prior to ear syringing[12–15] and one quasi-randomised trial.[16] All had design deficiencies that could lead to bias. Two of the RCTs found differences in effectiveness between wax softeners, and the other RCTs two found no overall difference (see table 3, p 540). One quasi-randomised trial found no difference between water instilled for 15 minutes and oil instilled nightly for 3 days.[16]

Harms: Seven RCTs did not report complications or adverse effects. Two found single cases of irritation, itch, or buzzing.[8,9] One RCT found that the frequency of adverse effects was similar in people using arachis oil/chlorobutanol/*p*-dichlorobenzene versus a proprietary agent (Otocerol® — the composition of which was not stated — [see table 3, p 540]).[11]

Comment: We found no good evidence about the optimal duration of treatment. Most trials did not use rigorous methods of randomisation, and did not include control for degree of occlusion at randomisation. Many trials were sponsored by companies that manufactured only one of the products being tested, but the possibility of publication bias has not been assessed. The inclusion criteria for the RCTs were not always clear: many stated that the participants had impacted wax without defining how this was assessed. The RCT that included a no treatment group found that 32% of ears with impacted wax showed spontaneous resolution after 5 days.[2]

OPTION MECHANICAL METHODS

We found no good evidence about the benefits or harms of mechanical removal of wax. There is a consensus that ear syringing is effective but we found no RCTs comparing ear syringing versus no treatment or versus alternative treatment.

Benefits: We found no systematic review and no RCTs comparing mechanical methods intended to remove ear wax with no treatment or alternative treatment.

Wax in ear

Harms: A survey found that 38% of 274 general practitioners performing ear syringing reported complications, including otitis externa, perforation of the tympanic membrane, damage to the skin of the external canal, tinnitus, pain, and vertigo.[1] We found no study of the incidence of these complications, or the effect of training and experience. People may experience dizziness during syringing or when wax is removed by suction.

Comment: There is consensus that syringing is effective and that training can reduce complications, but we found no evidence. Other mechanical techniques include manual removal under direct vision, with or without a microscope, using suction, probes, or forceps. These methods require specific training and access to appropriate equipment.

GLOSSARY

Impacted wax Wax that has been compressed in the ear canal, completely obstructing the lumen. In practice, many RCTs define impaction as the presence of symptoms associated with obstructing wax.

Obstructing wax Wax that obscures direct vision of the ear drum.

REFERENCES

1. Sharp JF, Wilson JA, Ross L, Barr-Hamilton RM. Ear wax removal: a survey of current practice. *BMJ* 1990;301:1251–1252.
2. Keane EM, Wilson H, McGrane D, Coakley D, Walsh JB. Use of solvents to disperse ear wax. *Br J Clin Pract* 1995;49:7–12.
3. Kalantan KA, Abdulghani H, Al-Taweel AA, Al-Serhani AM. Use of cotton tipped swab and cerumen impaction. *Ind J Otol* 1999;5:27–31.
4. Minja BM, Machemba A. Prevalence of otitis media, hearing impairment and cerumen impaction among school children in rural and urban Dar es Salaam, Tanzania. *Int J Pediatr Otorhinolaryngol* 1996;37:29–34.
5. Swart SM, Lemmer R, Parbhoo JN, Prescolt CAJ. A survey of ear and hearing disorders amongst a representative sample of Grade 1 school children in Swaziland. *Int J Pediatr Otorhinolaryngol* 1995;32:23–34.
6. Lewis-Cullinan C, Janken JK. Effect of cerumen removal on the hearing ability of geriatric patients. *J Adv Nurs* 1990;15:594–600.
7. Brister F, Fullwood HL, Ripp T, Blodgett C. Incidence of occlusion due to impacted cerumen among mentally retarded adolescents. *Am J Ment Defic* 1990;15:594–600.
8. Dummer DS, Sutherland IA, Murray JA. A single-blind, randomized study to compare the efficacy of two ear drop preparations ("Andax" and "Cerumol") in the softening of ear wax. *Curr Med Res Opin* 1992;13:26–30.
9. Lyndon S, Roy P, Grillage MG, Miller AJ. A comparison of the efficacy of two ear drop preparations ("Aurax" and "Earex") in the softening and removal of impacted ear wax. *Curr Med Res Opin* 1992;13:21–25.
10. Fahmy S, Whitefield M. Multicentre clinical trial of Exterol as a cerumenolytic. *Br J Clin Pract* 1982;36:197–204.
11. Jaffe G, Grimshaw J. A multicentric clinical trial comparing Otocerol with Cerumol as cerumenolytics. *J Int Med Res* 1978;6:241–244.
12. Singer AJ, Sauris E, Viccellio AW. Ceruminolytic effects of docusate sodium: A randomized controlled trial. *Ann Emerg Med* 2000;36:228–232.
13. Amjad AH, Scheer AA. Clinical evaluation of cerumenolytic agents. *Eye Ear Nose Throat Mon* 1975;54:76–77.
14. Chaput de Saintonge DM, Johnstone CI. A clinical comparison of triethanolamine polypeptide oleate-condensate ear drops with olive oil for the removal of impacted wax. *Br J Clin Pract* 1973;27:454–455.
15. Fraser JG. The efficacy of wax solvents: in vitro studies and a clinical trial. *J Laryngol Otol* 1970;84:1055–1064.
16. Eekhof JA, de Bock GH, Le Cessie S, Springer MP. A quasi-randomised controlled trial of water as a quick softening agent of persistent earwax in general practice. *Br J Gen Pract.* 2001;51:635–637.

George Browning
Professor of Otorhinolaryngology
MRC Institute of Hearing Research
Glasgow
UK

Competing interests: None declared.

TABLE 1 Surveys of the prevalence of impacted wax in specified populations (see text, p 534).[3–6]

Reference	Where	Who	% with impacted wax
Kalantan et al[3]	Saudi Arabia	1278 people attending primary care centre (any reason)	25%
Minja et al[4]	Tanzania	802 primary school children	16%
Swart et al[5]	Swaziland	Infant school children	7%
Lewis-Cullinan et al[6]	USA	Hospitalised elderly people (all causes except intensive care)	35%

TABLE 2 **Effects of wax softeners: results of comparative RCTs** **(see text, p 534).**

Ref	Wax softener	Administration	Selection characteristic; setting	Number of people (ears)	Randomisation; blinding	Outcome	Results	Adverse effects
2	(a) Arachis oil Chlorobutanol *p*-dichlorobenzene (Cerumol®) (b) Sodium bicarbonate (in glycerol) (c) Sterile water (d) Nothing	4 drops twice a day for 5 days	Impacted ear(s); hospital	113 recruited; 97 completed (155)	Randomisation (technique not described) Double blind (active treatments)	Residual wax; 3 tiered clinical rating scale	Treatment better than no treatment; no difference between agents	None
8	(a) Ethyleneoxide-polyoxypropylene glycol Choline salicylate (b) Arachis oil Chlorobutanol *p*-dichlorobenzene (Cerumol®)		Impacted or hardened wax; general practice	50 (100)	Not stated; single blind	Wax amount, colour,and consistency; objective hearing; global impression of efficiency	No difference	Two irritation with (a); one itch, one buzzing with (b)
9	(a) Ethyleneoxide-polyoxypropylene glycol, Choline salicylate (b) Arachis oil Almond oil Rectified camphor oil	Drops to fill ear twice a day for 4 days	Symptoms requiring wax softener; general practice	36 (72)	Not stated; not blind	Need for syringing; ease of syringing; global impression of efficiency	(a) better than (b); easy removal: 37/38 *v* 19/30	One irritation with (b); one disliked smell
10	(a) 5% urea hydrogen peroxide in glycerol (b) Glycerol	5–10 drops twice a day for a week	Ear wax problems; ENT dept	40 (80)	Alternation; double blind	Need for syringing; ease of syringing	(a) better than glycerol; success: 35/40 *v* 20/40	None

TABLE 2 continued

Ref	Wax softener	Administration	Selection characteristic; setting	Number of people (ears)	Randomisation; blinding	Outcome	Results	Adverse effects
10	(a) 5% urea hydrogen peroxide in glycerol (b) Arachis oil, Chlorobutanol, *p*-dichlorobenzene (Cerumol®)	5–10 drops twice a day for a week	Ear wax problems; ENT department	50 (100)	Alternation; double blind	Need for syringing; ease of syringing	(a) better than (b); success: 47/50 *v* 24/50	None
11	(a) 5% urea hydrogen peroxide in glycerol (b) Arachis oil, Chlorobutanol, *p*-dichlorobenzene	5–10 drops twice a day for a week	Ear wax problems; general practice	160 (286)	Alternation; double blind	Need for syringing; ease of syringing	(a) better than (b); success: 146/157 *v* 93/129	None
11	(a) Otocerol® (b) Arachis oil, Chlorobutanol, *p*-dichlorobenzene (Cerumol®)	Three consecutive nights	For whom a wax softener would normally be prescribed; general practice	106 (not stated)	Random allocation; double blind	3 tiered clinical rating scale	No difference overall; 38/53 *v* 33/53	Pain; irritation; giddiness; smell (Otocerol® 7/53 Cerumol® 10/53)
12	(a) Triethalonamine polypeptide (b) Docusate sodium (Waxol®)							

ENT, ear, nose and throat.

TABLE 3 **Effects of wax softeners prior to syringing: results of comparative RCTs (see text, p 534).**

Ref	Wax softener	Administration	Selection characteristic; setting	Number of people (ears)	Randomisation; blind	Outcome	Results	Adverse effects
13	(a) Triethanolamine polypeptide oleate condensate (b) Carbamide peroxide	One dose 30 minutes before syringing	Hard or impacted wax; setting unclear	80 (not stated)	Random allocation; double blind	Result of syringing; 4 tiered clincal rating scale	(a) better than (b); success: 33/40 *v* 7/40 but (b) normally used as multiple installations	Not reported
14	(a) Triethanolamine polypeptide oleate condensate (b) Olive oil	One dose 20 minutes before syringing	Impacted wax suitable for syringing; hospital outpatient dept	67 (not stated)	Random order; double blind	3 tiered clinical rating scale	No difference overall (20/32 *v* 21/35); (a) needed less water	None
12	(a) Triethylamine polypeptide (b) Docusate sodium (Waxol®)	One dose 15 minutes before syringing	Partial or totally accluding wax	50 (50)	Random order; non-blinded	Visualisation of tympanic membrane	(b) better than (a) (22/27 *v* 8/23)	None
16	(a) Water, cotton ear plug® (b) Oil, cotton ear plug	(a) 15 minutes® (b) nightly for 3 days	Persistent wax after five syringing attemps; general practice	130 (224)	Quasi-randomised (year of birth); not blind	Number of attemps needed to clear	No difference; however, statistical tests performed may have been inadequate	Not addressed
15	(a) Arachis oil Chlorobutanol p-dichlorobenzene (Cerumol®) (b) Docusate sodium (Waxsol®) (c) Olive oil *v* (d) Sodium bicarbonate (in glycerol)	Ear canal filled for 15 minutes, once daily every 3 days	Bilateral hard and occluding wax; geriatric hospital	124 (248)	Each participant was allocated (d) in one randomly chosen ear and treatment in the other ear. Double blind.	Failed forceful syringing	(a) better than (d), 1/24 *v* 5/24	Red canals

Cardiovascular disease in diabetes

Search date April 2002

Janine Malcolm, Hilary Meggison, and Ronald Sigal

QUESTIONS

In people with diabetes mellitus what are the effects of:

INTERVENTIONS

See glossary, p 561

Key Messages

- **Angiotensin converting enzyme (ACE) inhibitor versus β blockers (as initial treatment in hypertension)** One RCT found that an ACE inhibitor captopril versus β blockers or diuretic significantly reduced myocardial infarction, stroke, or death (NNT 15, 95% CI 8 to 105). One large RCT found no significant difference with the ACE inhibitor captopril versus the β blocker atenolol in the number of cardiovascular events over about 8 years.

Cardiovascular disease in diabetes

- **ACE inhibitor versus calcium channel blocker (as initial treatment in hypertension)** One systematic review in people with type 2 diabetes has found that ACE inhibitors versus calcium channel blockers as initial treatment for hypertension significantly reduce cardiovascular events (NNT 13, 95% CI 7 to 25).
- **Angiotensin II receptor antagonist versus β blocker** Subgroup analysis of one RCT in people with diabetes and left ventricular hypertrophy found that after 4 years, losartan versus atenolol significantly reduced primary cardiovascular composite outcomes (cardiovascular mortality, stroke, myocardial infarction) (NNT 19, 95% CI 11 to 142)
- **Antihypertensive treatment** One RCT in people with diabetes and high blood pressure (BP 165–220/ < 95 mm Hg) found that hypertensive treatment (nitrendipine or enalapril with or without hydrochlorothiazide) versus placebo significantly reduced all cardiovascular events over a median of 2 years (NNT 13, 95% CI 10 to 31) but found no significant reduction in overall mortality. One RCT in people aged 55–80 years with diabetic nephropathy and hypertension found no significant difference with amlodipine versus placebo and with irbesartan versus placebo or amlodipine in cardiovascular composite end points (non-fatal myocardial infarction, heart failure). One RCT in people with diabetes, hypertension, and microalbuminuria found no significant reduction in non-fatal cardiovascular events with irbesartan versus placebo. One systematic review in people aged over 50 years has found that blood pressure lowering in people with diabetes significantly reduces mortality and stroke but had no significant effect on myocardial infarction. One RCT in people with diabetes aged over 55 years with additional cardiac risk factors, previously diagnosed coronary vascular disease, or both, has found that the ACE inhibitor ramipril versus placebo significantly reduces major cardiovascular events (NNT 22, 95% CI 14 to 43) and overall mortality (NNT 32, 95% CI 19 to 98) within 4.5 years. One RCT in people with diabetes and baseline blood pressure less than 140/90 mm Hg found that intensive (target diastolic BP 10 mm Hg below baseline) versus moderate (diastolic BP 80–89 mm Hg) blood pressure lowering significantly reduces cerebral vascular accidents (NNT 27, 95% CI 14 to 255) but found no significant difference for cardiovascular death, myocardial infarction, congestive heart failure, or all cause mortality.
- **Antiplatelet treatment** One RCT in men aged 40–80 years with diabetes has found that aspirin versus placebo significantly reduces the risk of first acute myocardial infarction within 5 years (NNT 16, 95% CI 12 to 47). Another RCT in people with diabetes and prior cardiovascular disease found no significant difference with aspirin versus placebo in the risk of acute myocardial infarction or overall mortality within 5 years. Subgroup analysis in one RCT of people presenting with unstable angina or acute myocardial infarction without ST elevation found that the addition of a glycoprotein IIb/IIIa inhibitor (tirofiban) to heparin significantly reduced the risk of death or myocardial infarction at 180 days (NNT 13, 95% CI 7 to 146). One systematic review has found that aspirin versus placebo significantly reduces the risk of morbidity and death from cardiovascular disease within 2 years (NNT 26, 95% CI 17 to 66) in people with diabetes and other risk factors for a cardiovascular event.
- **Blood glucose control** RCTs found that glucose lowering with insulin, sulphonylureas, or metformin may reduce the risk of first acute myocardial infarction. One large RCT in people with acute myocardial infarction found that intensive insulin treatment versus standard treatment significantly reduced mortality at 3.4 years.

- **Coronary artery bypass graft (CABG) versus percutaneous transluminal coronary angioplasty (PTCA)** One large RCT in people with diabetes and multivessel coronary artery disease has found that CABG versus PTCA significantly reduces mortality or myocardial infarction within 8 years (NNT 7, 95% CI 4 to 20). Another RCT found a non-significant reduction in mortality with CABG versus PTCA at 4 years. A third RCT in people with diabetes and multivessel coronary artery disease found no significant difference between CABG and PTCA with stent in short term outcome (to time of discharge) but at 1 year after the procedure there was significantly greater cumulative incidence of combined death, myocardial infarction, or repeat CABG or PTCA.
- **Lipid regulating agents (statins and fibrates)** One systematic review found that in people with diabetes, lovastatin or gemfibrozil versus placebo did not significantly reduce non-fatal myocardial infarction and death from coronary artery disease. One RCT in people aged 35–65 years with type 2 diabetes and hyperlipidaemia found that bezafibrate versus placebo significantly reduced myocardial infarction or new ischaemic changes on electrocardiogram within 3 years (NNT 6, 95% CI 5 to 20). Another RCT in people with diabetes aged 40–80 years found a significant decrease in all cause mortalilty, non-fatal myocardial infarction, coronary heart disease death, total stroke, or any revascularisation with simvastatin versus placebo. It found significant risk reduction in people with diabetes and previous coronary heart disease (NNT 23, 95% CI 12 to 897) and in people with diabetes and no prior coronary heart disease (NNT 21, 95% CI 14 to 40). Three RCTs identified by a systematic review found that statins versus placebo significantly decreased cardiovascular event rates (person years needed to treat 120, 95% CI 61 to 4856). One RCT including people with diabetes found a borderline significant difference in relative risk of coronary heart disease death or non-fatal acute myocardial infarction with gemfibrozil versus placebo. One RCT found that in people with type 2 diabetes, dyslipidaemia and at least one coronary lesion, fenofibrate versus placebo did not significantly reduce myocardial infarction or death. One RCT found that in people aged 21–74 years with diabetes who had previously undergone coronary artery bypass grafting, aggressive versus moderate lipid lowering did not significantly reduce the four year life event rate relative risk for myocardial infarction or death.
- **Lower target blood pressures** Large RCTs including people with diabetes and hypertension have found that tighter control of blood pressure with target diastolic blood pressures of less than or equal to 80 mm Hg reduces the risk of major cardiovascular events.
- **PTCA versus thrombolysis** One RCT in people with diabetes and prior acute myocardial infarction found that at 30 days there was a lower rate of composite endpoint (death, reinfarction or disabling stroke) but the difference was not significant.
- **Screening for high cardiovascular risk** We found no RCTs on screening people with diabetes for cardiovascular risk.
- **Smoking cessation** We found no RCTs on promotion of smoking cessation. Observational evidence and extrapolation from people without diabetes suggest that promotion of smoking cessation is likely to reduce cardiovascular events.
- **Stent plus glycoprotein IIb/IIIa inhibitors in people undergoing PTCA** RCTs in people with diabetes undergoing PTCA have found that the combination of stent and a glycoprotein IIb/IIIa inhibitor (abciximab) significantly reduces restenosis rates and serious morbidity.

Cardiovascular disease in diabetes

DEFINITION **Diabetes mellitus:** See definition under glycaemic control in diabetes, p 578. **Cardiovascular disease:** Atherosclerotic disease of the heart and/or the coronary, cerebral, or peripheral vessels leading to clinical events such as acute myocardial infarction (see glossary, p 561), congestive heart failure, sudden cardiac death, stroke, gangrene, and/or need for revascularisation procedures.

INCIDENCE/ PREVALENCE Diabetes mellitus is a major risk factor for cardiovascular disease. In the USA, 60–75% of people with diabetes die from cardiovascular causes.[1] The annual incidence of cardiovascular disease is increased in people with diabetes (men: RR 2–3; women: RR 3–4, adjusted for age and other cardiovascular risk factors).[2] About 45% of middle aged and older white people with diabetes have evidence of coronary artery disease compared with about 25% of people without diabetes in the same populations.[2] In a Finnish population based cohort study (1059 people with diabetes and 1373 people without diabetes, aged 45–64 years), the 7 year risk of acute myocardial infarction was as high in adults with diabetes without previous cardiac disease (20.2/100 person years) as it was in people without diabetes with previous cardiac disease (18.8/100 person years).[3]

AETIOLOGY/ RISK FACTORS Diabetes mellitus increases the risk of cardiovascular disease. Cardiovascular risk factors in people with diabetes include conventional risk factors (age, prior cardiovascular disease, cigarette smoking, hypertension, dyslipidaemia, sedentary lifestyle, family history of premature cardiovascular disease) and more diabetes specific risk factors (elevated urinary protein excretion, poor glycaemic control). Conventional risk factors for cardiovascular disease contribute to increasing the relative risk of cardiovascular disease in people with diabetes to about the same extent as in those without diabetes (see aetiology under primary prevention, p 95). One prospective cohort study (164 women and 235 men with diabetes, mean age 65 years; 437 women and 1099 men without diabetes, mean age 61 years followed for mortality for a mean 3.7 years following acute myocardial infarction) found that more people with diabetes died compared with people without diabetes (116/399 [29%] *v* 204/1536 [13%]; RR 2.2, 95% CI 1.8 to 2.7).[4] It also found that the mortality risk after myocardial infarction associated with diabetes was higher for women than for men (adjusted HR 2.7, 95% CI 1.8 to 4.2 for women *v* 1.3, 95% CI 1 to 1.8 for men). Physical inactivity is a significant risk factor for cardiovascular events in both men and women. One cohort study of women with diabetes found that participation in little (< 1 h/wk) or no physical activity compared with physical activity for at least 7 hours a week was associated with doubling of the risk of a cardiovascular event.[5] Another cohort study (1263 men with diabetes, mean follow up 12 years) found that low baseline cardiorespiratory fitness compared with moderate or high fitness increased overall mortality (RR 2.9, 95% CI 2.1 to 3.6); and overall mortality was higher in those reporting no recreational exercise in the previous 3 months compared with those reporting any recreational physical activity in the same period (RR 1.8, 95% CI 1.3 to 2.5).[6] The absolute risk of cardiovascular disease is almost the same in women as in men with diabetes. Diabetes specific cardiovascular risk factors include the duration of diabetes during adulthood (the years of exposure to diabetes before age 20 years add little to the risk of cardiovascular disease); raised blood glucose concentrations (reflected in fasting blood glucose or HbA1c [see glossary, p 561]); and any degree of microalbuminuria (albuminuria 30–299 mg/24 h).[7] People with diabetes and microalbuminuria have a higher risk of coronary morbidity and mortality than people with normal levels of urinary albumin and a similar duration of diabetes (RR 2–3).[8,9] Clinical proteinuria increases the risk of major cardiac events in type 2 diabetes (RR 3)[10] and in type 1 diabetes (RR 9)[7,11,12] compared with individuals with the same type of diabetes having normal albumin excretion. An epidemiological analysis of people with diabetes enrolled in the Heart Outcomes Prevention Evaluation (HOPE) clinical trial (3498 people with diabetes and at least 1 other cardiovascular risk factor; age > 55 years, of whom 1140 [32%] had microalbuminuria at baseline; 5 years' follow up) found higher risk for major cardiovascular events in those with microalbuminuria (albumin : creatinine ratio [ACR] ≥ 2.0 mg/mmol) compared with those without microalbuminuria (adjusted RR 1.97, 95% CI 1.68 to 2.31); and for all cause mortality (RR 2.15, 95% CI 1.78 to 2.60). It also found an association between ACR and the risk of major cardiovascular events (ACR 0.22 to 0.57 mg/mmol: RR 0.85, 95% CI 0.63 to 1.14; ACR 0.58 to 1.62 mg/mmol: RR 1.11, 95% CI 0.86 to 1.43; ACR 1.62 to 1.99 mg/mmol: RR 1.89, 95% CI 1.52 to 2.36).[13]

PROGNOSIS Diabetes mellitus increases the risk of mortality or serious morbidity after a coronary event (RR 1.5–3).[2,3,14,15] This excess risk is partly accounted for by increased prevalence of other cardiovascular risk factors in people with diabetes. A systematic review (search date 1998) found that, in people with diabetes admitted to hospital for acute myocardial infarction, "stress hyperglycaemia" versus lower blood glucose levels was associated with increased mortality in hospital (RR 1.7, 95% CI 1.2 to 2.4).[16] One large prospective cohort study (91 285 men aged 40–84 years, 5 years' follow up) found higher all cause and coronary heart disease mortality in men with diabetes versus men without coronary artery disease or diabetes (age adjusted RR 3.3, 95% CI 2.6 to 4.1 in men with diabetes and without coronary artery disease *v* RR 2.3, 95% CI 2.0 to 2.6 in healthy people; RR 5.6, 95% CI 4.9 to 6.3 in men with coronary artery disease but without diabetes *v* RR 2.2, 95% CI 2.0 to 2.4 in healthy people; RR 12.0, 95% CI 9.9 to14.6 in men with both risk factors *v* RR 4.7, 95% CI 4.0 to 5.4 in healthy people). Multivariate analysis did not materially alter these associations.[17] These findings support previous studies. Diabetes mellitus alone is associated with a twofold increase in risk for all cause death, a threefold increase in risk of death from coronary heart disease and, in people with pre-existing coronary heart disease, a 12-fold increase in risk of death from coronary heart disease compared with people with neither risk factor.[17]

AIMS To reduce mortality and morbidity from cardiovascular disease, with minimum adverse effects.

OUTCOMES Incidence of fatal or non-fatal acute myocardial infarction; congestive heart failure; sudden cardiac death; coronary revascularisation; stroke; gangrene; angiographic evidence of coronary, cerebral, vascular, or peripheral arterial stenosis.

METHODS *Clinical Evidence* update search and appraisal April 2002. We searched for systematic reviews and RCTs with at least 10 confirmed clinical cardiovascular events among people with diabetes. Studies reporting only intermediate end points (e.g. regression of plaque on angiography, lipid changes) were not included. Most of the evidence comes from subgroup analyses of large RCTs that included people with diabetes. As with all subgroup analyses, and studies with small numbers, these results must be interpreted as suggestive rather than definitive.

QUESTION **What are the effects of screening for high cardiovascular risk in people with diabetes?**

We found no large RCTs on screening people with diabetes for cardiovascular risk.

Benefits: We found no systematic review and no large RCTs.

Harms: We found no RCTs.

Comment: Screening for conventional risk factors as well as regular determination of HbA1c (see glossary, p 561), lipid profile, and urinary albumin excretion will identify people at high risk.[18,19] Consensus opinion in the USA recommends screening for cardiovascular disease with exercise stress testing in previously sedentary adults with diabetes who are planning to undertake vigorous exercise programmes.[18,20] We found no evidence that such testing prevents cardiac events.

QUESTION **What are the effects of promoting smoking cessation in people with diabetes?**

We found no RCTs on promotion of smoking cessation specifically in people with diabetes. Observational evidence and extrapolation from people without diabetes suggest that promotion of smoking cessation is likely to reduce cardiovascular events.

Benefits: We found no systematic review or RCTs on promotion of smoking cessation specifically in people with diabetes.

Harms: We found no RCTs.

Comment: Observational studies have found that cigarette smoking is associated with increased cardiovascular death in people with diabetes. In people without diabetes, smoking cessation has been found to be associated with reduced risk. People with diabetes are likely to benefit from smoking cessation at least as much as people who do not have diabetes but have other risk factors for cardiovascular events (see smoking cessation under secondary prevention of ischaemic cardiac events, p 129).

QUESTION What are the effects of controlling blood pressure in people with diabetes?

OPTION ANTIHYPERTENSIVE TREATMENT VERSUS NO ANTIHYPERTENSIVE TREATMENT

One RCT in people with diabetes and high blood pressure (BP 165–220/< 95 mm Hg) found that hypertensive treatment (nitrendipine or enalapril with or without hydrochlorothiazide) versus placebo significantly reduced all cardiovascular events over a median of 2 years but found no significant reduction in overall mortality. One RCT in people aged 30–70 years with diabetic nephropathy and hypertension found no significant difference in cardiovascular composite end points (non-fatal myocardial infarction, heart failure) with amlodipine versus placebo and with irbesartan versus placebo or amlodipine. The RCT found a higher incidence of hyperkalemia resulting in discontinuation of treatment with irbesartan versus placebo, or amlodipine. One RCT in people with diabetes, hypertension, and microalbuminuria found no significant reduction in non-fatal cardiovascular events with irbesartan versus placebo. One systematic review found that lowering blood pressure significantly reduced mortality and stroke but found no significant effect of blood pressure lowering on myocardial infarction. One RCT in people with diabetes aged over 55 years with additional cardiac risk factors, previously diagnosed coronary vascular disease, or both, has found that the angiotensin converting enzyme inhibitor ramipril versus placebo significantly reduces major cardiovascular events and overall mortality within 4.5 years. One RCT in people with diabetes and baseline blood pressure less than 140/90 mm Hg found that intensive (target diastolic BP 10 mm Hg below baseline) versus moderate (diastolic BP 80–89 mm Hg) blood pressure lowering significantly reduces cerebral vascular accidents but found no significant difference for cardiovascular death, myocardial infarction, congestive heart failure, or all cause mortality.

Benefits: **Primary prevention:** See table 1, p 565. We found one systematic review (published 1997, but withdrawn from the Cochrane Library and currently being updated)[21] and three subsequent RCTs.[22–24] The first subsequent RCT (4695 people, 495 with diabetes, aged ≥ 60 years with blood pressure 165–220/< 95 mm Hg) found that antihypertensive treatment (nitrendipine or enalapril with or without hydrochlorothiazide) versus placebo reduced all cardiovascular events over a median of 2 years (13/252 [5.2%] with antihypertensive treatment *v* 31/240 [12.9%] with placebo; ARR 8%, 95% CI 3% to 10%; RR 0.4, 95% CI 0.21 to 0.75; NNT 13, 95% CI 10 to 31), but had no significant effect on overall mortality (16/252 [6.3%] for antihypertensive treatment *v* 26/240 [10.8%] for controls; ARR +4.5%, 95% CI –0.7% to +7.4%; RR 0.59, 95% CI 0.32 to 1.06).[22] The second subsequent RCT (1715 people with nephropathy due to type 2 diabetes and hypertension, aged 30–70 years) found no significant difference in cardiovascular composite end points (non-fatal myocardial infarction, heart failure) with irbesartan versus placebo (NNT 68, 95% CI –29 to +16; NS), amlodipine versus placebo (NNT 37, 95% CI –45 to +13; NS), or irbesartan versus amlodipine (NNT 79, 95% CI –28 to +17; NS).[23]

The third subsequent RCT (590 people with type 2 diabetes, microalbuminuria, and hypertension, mean age 58 years) found a non-significant reduction in non-fatal cardiovascular events with irbesartan (300 mg) versus placebo (8/194 [4.1%] v 17/201 [8.5%]; NNT 23, 95% CI –236 to +11).[24] **Primary and secondary prevention:** See table 3, p 568. We found one systematic review (search date not stated, 6 RCTs, 7572 people with diabetes out of 15 367 people aged > 50 years)[25] and two subsequent RCTs.[26,27] The systematic review found that lowering blood pressure significantly reduced mortality (10 deaths/1000 person-years in treatment arms v 19 deaths/1000 person years in control arms; RR 0.51 95% CI 0.38 to 0.69) and stroke (8/1000 person years in treatment arms *v* 14/1000 person years in control arms; RR 0.61, 95% CI 0.46 to 0.83), but found no significant effect of blood pressure lowering on myocardial infarction (14/1000 person years in treatment arms *v* 16/1000 person years in control arms; rate ratio 0.76, 96% CI 0.51 to 1.01).[25] The first subsequent RCT (3577 people with diabetes out of 9541 people aged ≥ 55 years with at least 1 of the following risk factors: diagnosed coronary vascular disease, current smoker, hypercholesterolaemia, hypertension, or microalbuminuria) compared ramipril (10 mg) versus placebo and vitamin E versus placebo over 4.5 years in a 2 x 2 factorial design (see table 3, p 568).[26] It found that ramipril versus placebo significantly reduced major cardiovascular events (coronary vascular disease death, acute myocardial infarction, or stroke 277/1808 [15.3%] with ramipril *v* 351/1769 [19.8%] with placebo; RR 0.75, 95% CI 0.64 to 0.88; ARR 4.5%; NNT 22 meaning that 22 older people with diabetes and additional risk factors need to be treated for 4.5 years to prevent 1 major cardiovascular event, 95% CI 14 to 43), and death from any cause (196/1808 *v* 248/1769; RR 0.76, 95% CI 0.67 to 0.92; ARR 3.2%; NNT 32, 95% CI 19 to 98). The relative effect of ramipril was present in all subgroups regardless of hypertensive status, microalbuminuria, type of diabetes, and nature of diabetes treatment (diet, oral agents, or insulin). Vitamin E versus placebo had no significant effect on morbidity or mortality.[26] The second subsequent RCT compared intensive (target diastolic BP 10 mm Hg below baseline) versus moderate diastolic blood pressure control (diastolic BP 80–89 mm Hg) in normotensive (BP < 140/90) people with diabetes (480 people, 243 randomised to placebo, mean age 58.5 years; 118 to nisoldipine, mean age 59.1 years; and 119 to enalapril, mean age 59.4 years) over 5.3 years.[27] It found that people randomised to intensive treatment had a significantly lower incidence of cerebral vascular accidents compared to people receiving moderate treatment (4/237 [1.7%] *v* 13/243 [5.4%]; OR 3.29, CI 1.06 to 10.25; NNT 27, 95% CI 14 to 255). It found no significant differences in cardiovascular death, myocardial infarction, congestive heart failure, or all cause mortality.[27] **Secondary prevention:** We found one systematic review (search date 1997, but withdrawn from the Cochrane Library and currently being updated).[21]

Harms: **Primary prevention:** One RCT did not report any adverse effect.[22] The second RCT reported that participants (15.4 % with treatment v 22.8% with placebo) had serious adverse effects but did not state what they were.[24] The third RCT reported a higher incidence of hyperkalemia resulting in discontinuation of treatment with irbesartan versus amlodipine or placebo (11/579 [1.9%] with irbesartan v 3/567 [0.5%] with amlodipine v 2/569 [0.4%] with placebo; P = 0.01 for both comparisons).[23] **Primary and secondary prevention:** One RCT found that cough was 5% more frequent with angiotensin converting enzyme inhibitor (ramipril) versus placebo.[26] One systematic review and one RCT did not report on adverse effects.[25,27]

Comment: None.

OPTION DIFFERENT ANTIHYPERTENSIVE DRUGS

One systematic review in people with type 2 diabetes has found that angiotensin converting enzyme inhibitors versus calcium channel blockers as initial treatment for hypertension significantly reduces cardiovascular events. Subgroup analysis of one RCT in people with a mean age of 76 years with diabetes and hypertension found no significant difference in major cardiovascular events over 4 years with angiotensin converting enzyme inhibitors versus calcium channel blockers versus β blockers or diuretics. One RCT found that an angiotensin converting enzyme inhibitor captopril versus diuretics or β blockers significantly reduced myocardial infarction, stroke, or death (NNT 15, 95% CI 8 to 105). One large RCT found no significant difference with the angiotensin converting enzyme inhibitor captopril versus the β blocker atenolol in the number of cardiovascular events over about 8 years. Subgroup analysis of one RCT in people aged 55–80 years with diabetes and left ventricular hypertrophy found that after 4 years, losartan versus atenolol significantly reduced primary cardiovascular composite outcomes (cardiovascular mortality, stroke, myocardial infarction).

Benefits: We found one systematic review (search date 2000, 4 RCTs, 2180 people with diabetes aged 51–68 years)[28] and two subsequent RCTs.[29,30] The systematic review compared angiotensin converting enzyme (ACE) inhibitors (captopril, enalapril, fosinopril) versus other antihypertensive drugs (diuretics, β blockers, or calcium channel blockers; 1047 people).[28] **ACE inhibitors versus calcium channel blockers:** We found one systematic review,[28] which found two RCTs[31,32] comparing ACE inhibitors (enalapril, fosinopril) versus calcium channel blockers (amlodipine, nisoldipine) in people with diabetes, and one subsequent RCT[29] comparing ACE inhibitors (enalapril, lisinopril) versus calcium channel blockers (felodipine, isradipine) versus conventional treatment (β blockers [atenolol, metoprolol, pindolol] or hydrochlorothiazide plus amiloride). The two RCTs in the systematic review found that ACE inhibitors versus calcium channel blockers significantly reduced combined cardiovascular events (cardiovascular death, acute myocardial infarction, congestive heart failure, stroke, pulmonary infarction, angina) (34/424 [8%] with ACE inhibitors *v* 70/426 [16%] with calcium channel blockers; ARR 8%, 95% CI 4% to 13%; RR 0.49, 95% CI 0.33 to 0.72; NNT 13, 95% CI 7 to 25). ACE inhibitors versus calcium channel blockers also reduced the three outcomes of death, acute myocardial infarction, and stroke, but the reductions were not significant. The subsequent RCT (6614 people, 719 with diabetes, mean age 76 years, mean blood pressure 190/ 99 mm Hg) found (among the subgroup of people with diabetes) no significant difference in the incidence of major cardiovascular events over 4 years (64.2 events/1000 person years with ACE inhibitors *v* 67.7 with calcium channel blockers *v* 75.0 with the conventional agents — β blockers or diuretics).[29] **ACE inhibitors versus diuretics:** We found one systematic review,[28] which found no RCTs specifically comparing ACE inhibitors versus diuretics in people with diabetes, but found one RCT (572 people, 6.1 years) comparing ACE inhibitors versus alternative treatment that included β blockers, combination β blockers and diuretics, and diuretics in people with and without diabetes.[33] It found that captopril versus diuretics or β blockers reduced the number of people who experienced acute myocardial infarction, stroke, or death (43/263 [18%] with diuretics/β blockers *v* 30/309 [10%] with captopril; ARR 6.6%, 95% CI 1.1% to 12.2%; NNT 15, 95% CI 8 to 105).[28] **ACE inhibitors versus β blockers:** We found one systematic review,[28] which included one RCT (758 people, 456 cardiovascular events) comparing an ACE inhibitor (captopril) versus a β blocker (atenolol) over 8.4 years.[34] The RCT found no significant difference between captopril versus atenolol in the number of cardiovascular events (102/400 [25.5%] with captopril v 75/358 [20.9%] with atenolol; ARI +5%, 95% CI –1% to +11%; RR 1.22, 95% CI 0.94 to 1.58). **Angiotensin II receptor antagonists versus β blockers:** Subgroup analysis of the results of the third RCT (1195 people with diabetes out of 9193 people, aged 55–80 years)[35] comparing losartan (586 people) versus atenolol (609 people) in people with left ventricular hypertrophy showed that after a 4 year follow up, losartan versus atenolol significantly reduced the primary cardiovascular composite end points (cardiovascular mortality, stroke, and myocardial infarction occurred in 103/586 [17.6%] with losartan group v 139/609 [22.8%] with atenolol; NNT19, 95% CI 11 to 142).[35] **Other comparisons:** We found no systematic review but found one RCT.[30] The RCT (people aged ≥ 55 years, with hypertension and either previous coronary vascular disease or at least 1 additional coronary vascular disease risk factor) compared chlortalidone (chlorthalidone), doxazosin, amlodipine, and lisinopril.[30] After 3.3 years' follow up, the RCT found no significant difference between doxazosin (3183 people with diabetes) and chlortalidone (5481 people) in the primary outcome (fatal coronary heart disease or non-fatal acute myocardial infarction), but the doxazosin arm was terminated because of an excess risk of combined coronary vascular disease events (coronary heart disease death, non-fatal acute myocardial infarction, stroke, revascularisation procedures, angina, congestive heart failure, and peripheral vascular disease) compared with chlortalidone (OR 1.24, 95% CI 1.12 to 1.38). The RCT is still in progress.[30]

Harms: **ACE inhibitors versus calcium channel blockers:** The systematic review gave no information on adverse effects.[28] In one RCT, people taking atenolol gained more weight than those taking captopril (3.4 kg with atenolol *v* 1.6 kg with captopril; P = 0.02).[34] Over the first 4 years of the trial, people allocated to atenolol had higher mean HbA1c (see glossary, p 561) (7.5% *v* 7.0%; P = 0.004), but no significant difference was found between groups over the subsequent 4 years. There was no difference between atenolol and captopril in rates of hypoglycaemia, lipid concentrations, tolerability, blood pressure lowering, or prevention of disease events. **Angiotensin II receptor antagonists versus β blockers:** The RCT found that discontinuation of treatment because of adverse effects was less common with losartan versus atenolol (2/586 *v* 9/609). Adverse events occurring with significantly different frequency in losartan versus atenolol were bradycardia (1% v 9%; $P < 0.0001$), cold extremities (4% v 6%; $P < 0.0001$), albuminuria (5% v 6%; $P = 0.0002$), hyperglycaemia (5% v 7%; $P = 0.007$), asthenia/fatigue (15% v 17%; $P = 0.001$), back pain (12% v 10%; $P = 0.004$), dyspnoea (10% v 14%; $P = 0.002$).[35]

Comment: We found evidence that ACE inhibitors are superior to calcium channel blockers as initial treatment. We found no clear evidence directly comparing ACE inhibitors and diuretics. It is unclear whether ACE inhibitors and β blockers are equivalent. In most RCTs, combination treatment with more than one agent was required to achieve target blood pressures. One large RCT found that the ACE inhibitor ramipril, which reduces urinary protein excretion, also reduced cardiovascular morbidity and mortality in older diabetic people with other cardiac risk factors.[26] However, the relative cardioprotective effect was present to the same extent in people with or without microalbuminuria. The evidence suggests that thiazide diuretics, β blockers, and ACE inhibitors significantly reduce cardiovascular events in people with diabetes and are probably superior to calcium channel blockers as initial treatment for hypertension.

OPTION TARGET BLOOD PRESSURE

Large RCTs including people with diabetes and hypertension have found that tighter control of blood pressure with target diastolic blood pressures of less than or equal to 80 mm Hg reduces the risk of major cardiovascular events.

Benefits: We found no systematic review but found several RCTs with large numbers of participants with diabetes (see table 1, p 565 and table 2, p 567).[34,36,37] One large RCT (1148 people with type 2 diabetes and with hypertension managed with atenolol or captopril) found that tight blood pressure control (≤ 150/≤ 85 mm Hg) versus less tight control (≤ 180/≤105 mm Hg) reduced incidence of any diabetes related end points and diabetes related deaths (see glossary, p 561) (primarily cardiovascular deaths, stroke, and microvascular disease).[34,37] See UKPDS hypertension study in table 1, p 565. Another RCT found half the risk of major cardiovascular events with a target diastolic blood pressure of 80 mm Hg or less versus 90 mm Hg or less.[36] See HOT study in table 1, p 565.

Harms: We found no good evidence of a threshold below which it is harmful to lower blood pressure.

Comment: Aggressive lowering of blood pressure in people with diabetes and hypertension reduces cardiovascular morbidity and mortality. In most trials, combination treatment with more than one agent was required to achieve target blood pressures.

Cardiovascular disease in diabetes

QUESTION What are the effects of treating hyperlipidaemias in people with diabetes?

OPTION LIPID REGULATING AGENTS

A systematic review found that in people with diabetes, lovastatin or gemfibrozil versus placebo did not significantly reduce non-fatal myocardial infarction and death from coronary artery disease. One RCT in people aged 35–65 years with type 2 diabetes and hyperlipidaemia found that bezafibrate versus placebo significantly reduced myocardial infarction or new ischaemic changes on electrocardiogram within 3 years. Another RCT in people with diabetes aged 40–80 years found a significant decrease in all cause mortalilty, non-fatal myocardial infarction, coronary heart disease death, total stroke, or any revascularisation with simvastatin versus placebo. It found significant risk reduction in people with diabetes and previous coronary heart disease and in people with diabetes and no prior coronary heart disease. Three RCTs identified by a systematic review found that statins versus placebo significantly decreased cardiovascular event rates. One RCT including people with diabetes found a borderline significant difference in relative risk of coronary heart disease death or non-fatal acute myocardial infarction with gemfibrozil versus placebo. One RCT found that in people with type 2 diabetes, dyslipidaemia and at least one coronary lesion, fenofibrate versus placebo did not significantly reduce myocardial infarction or death. One RCT found that in people aged 21–74 years with diabetes who had previously undergone coronary artery bypass grafting, aggressive versus moderate lipid lowering did not significantly reduce the 4 year life event rate relative risk for myocardial infarction or death.

Benefits: **Primary prevention**: We found one systematic review (search date 2000,[25] 2 RCTs[38,39]), one additional RCT,[40] and one subsequent RCT[41] comparing lipid lowering agents versus placebo (see table 1, p 565). The systematic review pooled the results from two RCTs (290 people with diabetes, mean age 49 and 58 years) comparing lovastatin or gemfibrozil versus placebo for 5 years.[41] The review found that lovastatin or gemfibrozil versus placebo decreased non-fatal myocardial infarction and death from coronary artery disease by 11 events per 1000 person years, but this decrease was not statistically significant (8 *v* 19 events/1000 person years; summary rate ratio 0.44, 95% CI 0.17 to 1.20, person years needed to treat 97, 95% CI 45 to not meaningful).[25] The additional RCT (164 men and women with type 2 diabetes, aged 35–65 years; baseline lipids included one or more of the following: total cholesterol 5.2–8.0 mmol/L, serum triglyceride 1.8–8.0 mmol/L, high density lipoprotein cholesterol ≤ 1.1 mmol/L, or total to high density lipoprotein cholesterol ratio ≥ 4.7mmol/L) compared bezafibrate versus placebo for 3 years.[40] The RCT found that bezafibrate versus placebo significantly reduced myocardial infarction or new ischaemic changes on electocardiogram (5/64 [7.8%] *v* 16/64 [25%]; NNT 6, 95% CI 5 to 20). The subsequent RCT (5963 men and women with diabetes, aged 40–80 years, among whom 3982 had no previous coronary heart disease) compared simvastatin versus placebo for the primary prevention of coronary heart disease, stroke, and revascularisation over 5 years.[41] The RCT found a significant decrease in outcomes (all cause mortalilty, non-fatal myocardial infarction, coronary heart disease death, total stroke, or any revascularisation) with simvastatin versus placebo, even though by the end of the study 38% of those allocated placebo were taking a non-study statin. The risk reduction was similar for people with diabetes and previous coronary heart disease (325/972 [33.4%] with simvastatin *v* 381/1009 [37.8%] with placebo; ARR 4.3%, NNT 23, 95% CI 12 to 897) and people with diabetes and no prior coronary heart disease (276/2006 [13.8%] with simvastatin *v* 367/1976 [18.6%] with placebo; ARR 4.8%, NNT 21, 95% CI 14 to 40; see comment below).[41] **Secondary prevention:** See table 2, p 567. We found one systematic review (search date 2000, 2313 people with diabetes, mean age 58 years, 5 RCTs[42–46]).[25] Three RCTs[42,43,45] included in the review found that statins (pravastatin, simvastatin) versus placebo significantly decreased cardiovascular event rates (34 events with statins *v* 44 events with placebo per 1000 person years; RR 0.77 95% CI 0.62 to 0.96; person years needed to treat 120, 95% CI 61 to 4856).[25] One RCT included in the systematic review (4444 men and women aged 35–70 years with previous acute myocardial infarction [see glossary, p 561] or angina pectoris, total cholesterol concentrations of 5.5–8.0 mmol/L, and triglycerides ≤ 2.5 mmol/L) compared simvastatin versus placebo over a median of 5.4 years.[42] Simvastatin dosage was initially 20 mg daily, with blinded dosage titration up to 40 mg daily, according to cholesterol response during the first 6–18 weeks. The relative risk of main end points in people with diabetes treated with simvastatin were as follows: total mortality 0.57 (95% CI 0.30 to 1.08); major cardiovascular events 0.45 (95% CI 0.27 to 0.74); and any atherosclerotic event 0.63 (95% CI 0.43 to 0.92).[26] The second RCT included in the review (4159 men and women aged 21–75 years, 3–20 months after acute myocardial infarction and with total cholesterol < 6.2 mmol/L, triglycerides < 3.92 mmol/L, and low density lipoprotein cholesterol 3.0–4.5 mmol/L) compared pravastatin 40 mg daily versus placebo over a median of 5 years.[45] Among the people with diabetes, the relative risk of major coronary events (death from coronary disease, non-fatal acute myocardial infarction, coronary artery bypass graft, or percutaneous transluminal coronary angioplasty) was 0.75 (95% CI 0.57 to 1.0). The third RCT included in the review (9014 men and women aged 31–75 years with acute myocardial infarction or unstable angina, plasma total cholesterol 4.0–7.0 mmol/L, and plasma triglycerides < 5.0 mmol/L) compared pravastatin 40 mg daily versus placebo for a mean of 6.1 years.[43] Among the 782 participants with diabetes, the relative risk of coronary heart disease death or non-fatal acute myocardial infarction was 0.84 (95% CI 0.59 to 1.10). The fourth RCT included in the review (2531 men aged < 74 years with previous coronary vascular disease, acute myocardial infarction, angina, revascularisation, or angiographically documented coronary stenosis; high density lipoprotein cholesterol ≤ 1.0 mmol/L, low density lipoprotein cholesterol ≤ 3.6 mmol/L, and triglycerides ≤ 3.4 mmol/L) compared gemfibrozil 1200 mg daily with placebo for a median of 5.1 years (treatment was intended to raise high density lipoprotein cholesterol levels rather than reduce low density lipoprotein cholesterol).[44] Among the 627 participants with diabetes, the relative risk of coronary heart disease death or non-fatal acute myocardial infarction was 0.76 (95% CI 0.57 to 1.0). **Mixed primary and secondary prevention:** See table 3, p 568. We found three RCTs.[41,46,47] The first RCT (305 men and 113 women; mean age 57 years; with type 2 diabetes; HbA1c [see glossary, p 561] ≤170% of the upper limit of normal; at least 1 visible coronary lesion on angiogram; high density lipoprotein cholesterol/cholesterol ratio ≥4 plus either an low density lipoprotein cholesterol of 3.5–4.5 mmol/L and triglycerides ≤5.2 mmol/L, or triglycerides 1.7–5.2 mmol/L and low density lipoprotein cholesterol of 4.5 mmol/L; 50% had no previous clinical history of coronary artery disease) that compared the effect of fenofibrate 200 mg daily versus placebo on progression of coronary artery disease in type 2 diabetes for a minimum of 3 years.[47] The RCT found that, after 39 months on treatment and 6 additional months' follow up, fenofibrate versus placebo did not significantly reduce the number of people who either had myocardial infarction or died (15/207 [7.2%] with fenofibrate *v* 21/211 [9.9%] with placebo; ARR 2.7%, 95% CI −2.8% to +8.3%; RR 0.73, 95% CI 0.39 to 1.37).[47] The second RCT (1351 people, 116 with type 2 diabetes, aged 21–74 years, mean age 63.1 years) compared the effects of aggressive lipid lowering (lovastatin and cholestyramine as necessary to achieve and low density lipoprotein cholesterol of 1.55–2.20 mmol, 60–85 mg/dL) versus moderate lipid lowering (the same medication to achieve and low density lipoprotein cholesterol of 3.36–3.62 mmol/L, 130–140 mg/dL), in people who had undergone coronary artery bypass grafting 1–11 years previously (mean 4.3 years post coronary artery bypass grafting).[46] The RCT found a reduction in the 4 year event rate for death in those randomised to aggressive cholesterol lowering treatment versus moderate treatment (6.5 *v* 9.6; RR 0.67, 99% CI 0.12 to 3.75) and a reduction in the 4 year event rate for myocardial infarction in those allocated to aggressive versus moderate treatment groups (4.8 *v* 11.6; RR 0.40, 99% CI 0.07 to 2.47). None of these findings were statistically significant.[46]

Harms: The RCTs found no significant differences in adverse outcomes between placebo and treatment groups.

Comment: We found one RCT that is of major importance.[41] This study is interesting as it was not necessary to have an abnormal lipid profile or prior vascular disease to be enrolled in the study and provides the first clear evidence that statin treatment is effective for primary prevention of cardiovascular disease.[41] The RCT comparing aggressive versus moderate lipid lowering had limited power because of the small number of patients enrolled with diabetes.[46] Most published clinical trials with sufficient power to detect effects on cardiovascular events have enrolled comparatively few people with diabetes or have excluded them altogether. The available evidence is therefore based almost entirely on subgroup analyses of larger trials. Several large ongoing trials are evaluating the effects of fibrates in people with diabetes.

QUESTION **What are the effects of antiplatelet drugs in people with diabetes?**

OPTION **PROPHYLACTIC ASPIRIN**

One RCT in men aged 40 to 80 years with diabetes has found that aspirin versus placebo significantly reduces the risk of first acute myocardial infarction within 5 years. Another RCT in people with diabetes and prior cardiovascular disease found no significant difference with aspirin versus placebo in the risk of acute myocardial infarction or overall mortality within 5 years. One systematic review has found that aspirin versus placebo significantly reduces the risk of morbidity and death from cardiovascular disease within 2 years in people with diabetes and other risk factors for a cardiovascular event.

Benefits: **Primary prevention:** We found no systematic review but found two RCTs. In the only large primary prevention RCT, comparing aspirin versus placebo and reporting results for people with diabetes, 22 701 US male physicians aged 40–80 years were assigned to aspirin 325 mg every other day or to placebo, and followed for an average of 5 years.[48] The trial found that, after 5 years, among the 533 physicians with diabetes, aspirin versus placebo reduced the risk of acute myocardial infarction (see glossary, p 561) (11/275 [4%] with aspirin *v* 26/258 [10.1%] with placebo; RR 0.39, 95% CI 0.20 to 0.79; NNT 16, 95% CI 12 to 47). A second RCT comparing aspirin with placebo did not specify the number of people with diabetes, but it did report that aspirin reduced acute myocardial infarction to a similar degree in the subgroup of people with diabetes and in the overall trial population (RR 0.85).[36] **Primary and early secondary prevention:** We found one RCT (3711 people with diabetes, 30% with type 1 diabetes, 48% with prior cardiovascular disease).[49] It compared aspirin (650 mg daily) versus placebo and followed the participants for a mean of 5 years. It found a non-significant reduction in overall mortality in those treated with aspirin (RR 0.91, 95% CI 0.75 to 1.11). Acute myocardial infarction occurred in 289 people (16%) in the aspirin group and 336 (18%) in the placebo group (ARR 2%, 95% CI 0.1% to 4.9%). Fifty people would need to be treated for 5 years with aspirin 650 mg daily to prevent one additional acute myocardial infarction. **Secondary prevention:** We found one systematic review (search date 1990, 145 RCTs of antiplatelet treatment, primarily aspirin).[50] Results for people with diabetes are tabulated (see table 2, p 567).

Harms: In the large trial comparing aspirin versus placebo for primary and secondary prevention, fatal or non-fatal stroke occurred in 5% on aspirin and 4.2% on placebo (P = NS).[35] There was no significant increase with aspirin in the risks of vitreous, retinal, gastrointestinal, or cerebral haemorrhage. In the systematic review, doses of aspirin ranged from 75–1500 mg daily. Most trials used aspirin 75–325 mg daily. Doses higher than 325 mg daily increased the risk of haemorrhagic adverse effects without improving preventive efficacy. No difference in efficacy or adverse effects was found in the dose range 75–325 mg.[50]

Comment: We found insufficient evidence to define precisely which people with diabetes should be treated with aspirin. The risk of cardiovascular disease is very low before age 30 years; most white adults with diabetes aged over 30 years are at increased risk of cardiovascular disease. Widely accepted contraindications to aspirin treatment include aspirin allergy, bleeding tendency, anticoagulant treatment, recent gastrointestinal bleeding, and clinically active liver disease.[18,51]

OPTION GLYCOPROTEIN IIB/IIIA INHIBITORS

Subgroup analysis in one RCT of people presenting with unstable angina or acute myocardial infarction without ST elevation found that the addition of a glycoprotein IIb/IIIa inhibitor (tirofiban) to heparin significantly reduced the risk of death or myocardial infarction at 180 days.

Benefits: We found one RCT (1570 people, including 228 men and 134 women with diabetes, mean age 65 years, presenting with unstable angina or acute myocardial infarction [see glossary, p 561] without ST elevation, all started on aspirin at time of randomisation) comparing addition of a glycoprotein IIb/IIIa inhibitor (tirofiban) to heparin versus heparin alone.[68] Subgroup analysis at 180 days in people with diabetes found that addition of tirofiban to heparin versus heparin alone reduced the number of deaths or myocardial infarctions (19/169 [11.2%] with tirofiban plus heparin *v* 37/193 [19.2%] with heparin alone; ARR 8.0%, 95% CI 0.7% to 15.3%; NNT 13, 95% CI 7 to 146). **Adjunct to percutaneous coronary revascularisation**: See benefits of intracoronary stenting plus glycoprotein IIb/IIIa inhibitors, p 560.

Harms: The RCT found no significant difference between tirofiban plus heparin and aspirin versus heparin and aspirin alone in risk of bleeding (9.5% with tirofiban plus heparin and aspirin *v* 8.3% with heparin and aspirin alone).[68]

Comment: None.

QUESTION What are the effects of blood glucose control in prevention of cardiovascular disease in people with diabetes?

RCTs found that glucose lowering with insulin, sulphonylureas, or metformin may reduce the risk of first acute myocardial infaction. One large RCT in people with acute myocardial infarction found that intensive insulin treatment versus standard insulin treatment significantly reduced mortality at 3.4 years

Benefits: **Primary prevention:** See table 1, p 565. We found no systematic review but found three RCTs of intensive versus conventional treatment of hyperglycaemia and the microvascular and macrovascular complications of diabetes.[53,54,66,67] One RCT (3867 people, newly diagnosed with type 2 diabetes, median age 54 years, fasting blood glucose 6.1 to 15 mmol/L after 3 months dietary treatment) compared conventional treatment (1138 people treated with diet only, drugs added if fasting blood glucose > 15.0 mmol/L or hyperglycaemic symptoms occurred) versus intensive treatment (1573 people treated with sulphonylureas, 1156 people treated with insulin).[66] It found that intensive treatment reduced the risk of acute myocardial infarction (14.7/1000 person years for intensive *v* 17.4/1000 person years for conventional; RR 0.84, 95% CI 0.71 to 1.0), diabetes related outcomes (see glossary, p 561) (RR 0.88, 95% CI 0.80 to 0.99; NNT 39 for 5 years to prevent 1 additional diabetes related outcome), and improved glycaemic control (HbA1c [see glossary, p 561] 7% with intensive treatment *v* 7.9% with conventional treatment), but found no significant difference for risks of stroke and amputation.[66] The second RCT (753 people with newly diagnosed type 2 diabetes, > 120% of ideal body weight) compared intensive treatment with metformin (aiming for fasting blood glucose < 6 mmol/L) versus conventional treatment (mainly diet alone).[67] It found that metformin versus conventional treatment significantly reduced the risk of a diabetes related outcome (32%, 95% CI 13 to 47; P =0.002) and diabetes related death (see glossary, p 561) (42%, 95% CI 0 to 63; P = 0.017).[67] The third RCT (1441 people with type 1 diabetes aged 13–39 years and free of cardiovascular disease, hypertension, hypercholesterolaemia, and obesity at baseline) compared conventional versus intensive treatment, followed for a mean of 6.5 years (3.5–9 years) for atherosclerosis related events.[53] It found that major macrovascular events were almost twice as frequent in the conventionally treated group (40 events) as in the intensive treatment group (23 events), although the differences were not significant (ARR 2.2%; RR 0.59, 95% CI 0.32 to 1.1). **Secondary prevention:** See table 2, p 567. We found no systematic review but found two RCTs.[55–57] One small RCT (153 men with type 2 diabetes, mean age 60 years, many of whom had previous cardiovascular events) compared standard insulin (once daily) with intensive treatment with a stepped plan designed to achieve near normal blood sugar levels.[55] After 27 months, the rate of new cardiovascular events was not significantly different between the groups (24/75 [32%] with intensive treatment *v* 16/80 [20%] with standard insulin; RR 1.6, 95% CI 0.92 to 2.5). In the second RCT (620 people, mean age 68 years, 63% men, 84% with type 2 diabetes) with random blood glucose greater than or equal to 11 mmol/L were randomised within 24 hours of an acute myocardial infarction to either standard treatment or intensive insulin treatment.[56,57] The intensive insulin group received an insulin-glucose infusion for 24 hours followed by subcutaneous insulin four times daily for at least 3 months. The standard treatment group received insulin only when it was clinically indicated. HbA1c fell significantly with intensive insulin treatment (absolute fall of 1.1% with intensive treatment *v* 0.4% with standard treatment at 3 months and 0.9% *v* 0.4% at 12 months). Intensive treatment lowered mortality (ARs 19% *v* 26% at 1 year and 33% *v* 44% at a mean of 3.4 years; RR 0.72, 95% CI 0.55 to 0.92; NNT 9 treated for 3.4 years to prevent 1 additional premature death). The absolute reduction in the risk of mortality was particularly striking in people who were not previously using insulin and had no more than one of the following risk factors before the acute myocardial infarction that preceded randomisation: age 70 years or over, history of previous acute myocardial infarction, history of congestive heart failure, current treatment with digitalis. In this low risk subgroup, the ARR was 15% (NNT 7 for 3.4 years).

Harms: Sulphonylureas and insulin, but not metformin, increased the risks of weight gain and hypoglycaemia. On an intention to treat basis, the proportions of people per year with severe hypoglycaemic episodes were 0.7%, 1.2%, 1%, 2%, and 0.6% for the conventional chlorpropamide, glibenclamide, insulin, and metformin groups, respectively. These frequencies of hypoglycaemia were much lower than those observed with intensive treatment in people with type 1 diabetes.[53,54] One RCT found no evidence that any specific treatment (insulin, sulphonylurea, or metformin) increased overall risk of cardiovascular disease.[66,67]

Comment: The role of intensive glucose lowering in primary prevention of cardiovascular events remains unclear. However, such treatment clearly reduces the risk of microvascular disease and does not increase the risk of cardiovascular disease. The potential of the larger primary prevention RCT to demonstrate an effect of tighter glycaemic control was limited by the small difference achieved in median HbA1c between intensive and conventional treatment.[53,54] In contrast, in another primary prevention trial, a larger 1.9% difference in median HbA1c was achieved between groups, but the young age of the participants and consequent low incidence of cardiovascular events limited the power of the study to detect an effect of treatment on incidence of cardiovascular disease.[53,54] The study of insulin in type 2 diabetes[55] included men with a high baseline risk of cardiovascular events and achieved a 2.1% absolute difference in HbA1c. The RCT was small and the observed difference between groups could have arisen by chance. The design of the trial of intensive versus standard glycaemic control following acute myocardial infarction does not distinguish whether the early insulin infusion or the later intensive subcutaneous insulin treatment was the more important determinant of improved survival in the intensively treated group.[57] The possibility that oral hypoglycaemics may be harmful after acute myocardial infarction cannot be ruled out. The larger primary prevention trial found no evidence that oral hypoglycaemics increase cardiovascular mortality.[66,67]

QUESTION **What are the effects of revascularisation procedures in people with diabetes**

OPTION CORONARY ARTERY BYPASS VERSUS PERCUTANEOUS TRANSLUMINAL ANGIOPLASTY

One large RCT in people with diabetes and multivessel coronary artery disease has found that coronary artery bypass graft (CABG) versus percutaneous transluminal coronary angioplasty (PTCA) significantly reduces mortality or myocardial infarction within 8 years. Another RCT found a non-significant reduction in mortality with CABG versus PTCA at 4 years. A third RCT in people with diabetes and multivessel coronary artery disease found no significant difference between CABG and PTCA with

stent in short term outcome (to time of discharge), but at 1 year after the procedure there was significantly greater cumulative incidence of combined death, myocardial infarction, or repeat CABG or PTCA.

Benefits: We found no systematic review but found three RCTs (see table 2, p 567).[52,58,59] Two RCTs compared CABG versus PTCA, without stenting or a glycoprotein IIb/IIIa inhibitor,[52,58] and one RCT compared CABG versus PTCA with stenting.[59] The first RCT (1829 people with 2 or 3 vessel coronary disease, 353 with diabetes, mean age 62 years) found that, after a mean of 7.7 years, CABG versus PTCA significantly reduced the number of people who died or suffered Q-wave myocardial infarction (60/173 [34.7%] with CABG *v* 85/170 [50%] with PTCA; ARR 15%, 95% CI 5% to 26%; RR 0.69, 95% CI 0.54 to 0.89; NNT 7, 95% CI 4 to 20). This survival benefit was confined to those receiving at least one internal mammary graft. The second RCT (1054 people, 125 with diabetes, 94 men and 31 women, mean age 61 years) found a non-significant reduction in number of people who had died at 4 years' follow up with CABG versus PTCA (8/63 [12.5%] *v* 14/62 [22.6%]; ARR 9.9%, 95% CI –3.4% to +23.1%; NNT 10; NS).[58] The third RCT (1205 people with 2 or 3 vessel coronary disease, 208 with diabetes 112 randomised to PTCA with stent, 96 to CABG, mean age 62 years) found no significant difference in people with diabetes treated with CABG or PTCA in short term risks (up to discharge) of composite end point of death, myocardial infarction, repeat CABG, and repeat PTCA (11/112 [9.8%] with PTCA *v* 9/96 [9.4%] with CABG; NNT 224; NS). However at 1 year, the RCT found significantly higher incidence of the composite end point with PTCA/stent versus CABG (41/112 [36%] with PTCA/stent *v* 15 /96 [15.6%] with CABG, NNT 5, 95% CI 4 to 11).[59]

Harms: In the first RCT, in-hospital mortality among people with diabetes was 1.2% after CABG versus 0.6% after PTCA. Myocardial infarction during the initial hospitalisation was three times more common after CABG than after PTCA (5.8% *v* 1.8%). None of these differences were found to be significant.[52] The third RCT found a significant increase in risk of stroke with CABG versus PTCA with stent in people with diabetes (4 *v* 0; P = 0.04).[59]

Comment: None.

OPTION PERCUTANEOUS TRANSLUMINAL CORONARY ANGIOPLASTY VERSUS THROMBOLYSIS

One RCT in people with diabetes and prior acute myocardial infarction found that at 30 days there was a lower rate of composite end point (death, reinfarction, or disabling stroke) but the difference was not significant.

Benefits: We found no systematic review but found one RCT.[69] The RCT (1138 people with acute myocardial infarction presenting within 12 h of chest pain onset, 177 with diabetes mean age of 65 years) compared percutaneous transluminal coronary angioplasty (PTCA) versus thrombolysis (alteplase).[69] At 30 days, fewer people with diabetes assigned to PTCA experienced the composite end point of death, reinfarction, or disabling stroke, but the difference was not significant (11/99 [11%] with PTCA *v* 13/78 [17%] with alteplase; ARR +5.6%, 95% CI –4.8 to +15.9%). The RCT found no significant difference in 30 day mortality among people with diabetes (8/99 [8.1%] after PTCA *v* 5/78 [6.4%] after alteplase) (see table 2, p 567).[69]

Harms: See harms of coronary artery bypass versus PTCA, p 559.

Comment: None.

OPTION INTRACORONARY STENTING PLUS GLYCOPROTEIN IIB/IIIA INHIBITORS

RCTs in people with diabetes undergoing percutaneous transluminal coronary angioplasty have found that the combination of stent and a glycoprotein IIb/IIIa inhibitor (abciximab) significantly reduces restenosis rates and serious morbidity.

Benefits: We found no systematic review but found two RCTs (see table 2, p 567).[60–63] The first RCT (2792 people, 638 with diabetes, mean age 61 years, 38% female, all undergoing percutaneous transluminal coronary angioplasty or directional atherectomy without stenting) compared placebo plus standard dose heparin versus abciximab plus standard dose heparin versus abciximab plus low dose heparin. Abciximab was given as a bolus with 12 hour infusion. The primary indications for intervention were unstable angina (51%), stable ischaemia (33%), and recent acute myocardial infarction (16%). A total of 44% had a prior coronary intervention, 56% had multivessel disease, and 74% a history of hypertension. Abciximab versus placebo reduced the combined end point of death or acute myocardial infarction (see glossary, p 561) in both standard dose and low dose heparin arms (at 30 days by > 60% and at 6 months by > 50%). Abciximab reduced the rate of restenosis in people without diabetes (HR 0.78), but not in people with diabetes. The second RCT (2401 people; 491 with diabetes; mean age 60 years; 29% female, 69% hypertensive, 30% recent smokers, 48% prior acute myocardial infarction, 10% prior coronary artery bypass) compared stent plus placebo (173 people) versus stent plus abciximab (162 people) versus balloon angioplasty plus abciximab (156 people). The RCT found significant differences between stent plus abciximab versus the other two groups for death or large acute myocardial infarction at 12 months (4.9% with stent plus abciximab *v* 8.3% with percutaneous transluminal coronary agnioplasty plus abciximab *v* 13.9% with stent plus placebo), and for subsequent revascularisation rates (13.7% with stent and abciximab *v* 25.3% with percutaneous transluminal coronary agnioplasty plus abciximab *v* 22.4% with stent plus placebo).[61–63] We found an analysis of individual people results (1462 people with diabetes) of these two trials and a third, earlier trial.[64] It found that abciximab reduced overall mortality (26/540 [4.8%] *v* 21/844 [2.5%]; ARR 2.3%; NNT 43, 95% CI 23 to 421).

Harms: There was slightly greater bleeding in people given abciximab than in those given placebo (4.3% *v* 3.0% for major bleeding; 6.9% *v* 6.3% for minor bleeding; 0% *v* 0.17% for intracranial haemorrhage). None of these differences were significant.[65]

Comment: For people with diabetes undergoing percutaneous procedures, the combination of stent and glycoprotein IIb/IIIa inhibitor reduces restenosis rates and serious morbidity. It is unclear whether these adjunctive treatments would reduce morbidity, mortality, and restenosis associated with percutaneous revascularisation procedures to the levels seen with coronary artery bypass. There was imbalance of the baseline characteristics among the study groups of the second RCT.[61] However, in a multivariate analysis, the treatment effects remained after adjusting for baseline differences.

GLOSSARY

Acute myocardial infarction is infarction that occurs when circulation to a region of the heart is obstructed and necrosis is occurring; clinical symptoms include severe pain, pallor, perspiration, nausea, dyspnoea, and dizziness. Myocardial infarction is gross necrosis of the myocardium as a result of interruption of blood supply usually caused by atherosclerosis of the coronary arteries; myocardial infarction without pain or other symptoms (silent infarction) is common in people with diabetes

Diabetes related death includes fatal acute myocardial infarction or sudden death; fatal stroke; death from peripheral vascular disease; death from renal disease; death from hypoglycaemia or hyperglycaemia.

Diabetes related outcomes include the first occurrence of non-fatal acute myocardial infarction, heart failure, or angina; non-fatal stroke, amputation, renal failure, retinal photocoagulation or vitreous haemorrhage; cataract extraction or blindness in one eye.

HbA1c The haemoglobin A1c test is the most common laboratory test of glycated haemoglobin (haemoglobin that has glucose irreversibly bound to it). HbA1c provides an indication of the "average" blood glucose over the last 3 months. The HbA1c is a weighted average over time of the blood glucose level; many different glucose profiles can produce the same level of HbA1c.

Substantive changes

Antihypertensives versus no treatment: primary prevention Two new RCTs;[23,24] conclusions unchanged.

Antihypertensives versus no treatment: primary and secondary prevention One new systematic review[25] and one new RCT;[27] conclusions unchanged.

Different antihypertensive drugs: angiotensin II receptor antagonists versus β blockers One new RCT;[35] new comparison.

Lipid regulating agents: primary prevention One new systematic review[25] and one new RCT[41]. The RCT provided new evidence for the value of lipid lowering treatment for primary prevention in a wider range of people than previous research would have justified.

Lipid regulating agents: secondary prevention One new systematic review[25] and one new RCT;[41] the RCT included prespecified subgroup analyses looking separately at those with and without previous heart disease.

Lipid regulating agents: mixed primary and secondary prevention One new RCT;[46] conclusions unchanged.

Coronary artery bypass versus percutaneous transluminal angioplasty One new RCT;[59] conclusions unchanged.

REFERENCES

1. Geiss LS, Herman WH, Smith PJ. Mortality in non-insulin-dependent diabetes. In: Harris MI, ed. *Diabetes in America*. 2nd ed. Bethesda, MD: National Institutes of Health, 1995:233–255.
2. Wingard DL, Barrett-Connor E. Heart disease and diabetes. In: Harris MI, ed. *Diabetes in America*. 2nd ed. Bethesda, MD: National Institutes of Health, 1995:429–448.

3. Haffner SM, Lehto S, Ronnemaa T, et al. Mortality from coronary heart disease in subjects with type 2 diabetes and in nondiabetic subjects with and without prior myocardial infarction. *N Engl J Med* 1998;339:229–234.
4. Mukamai KJ, Nesto RW, Cohen MC, et al. Impact of diabetes on long-term survival after acute myocardial infarction. *Diabetes Care* 2001;24:1422–1427.
5. Hu FB, Stampfer MJ, Solomon C, et al. Physical activity and risk for cardiovascular events in diabetic women. *Ann Intern Med* 2001;134:96–105.
6. Wei M, Gibbons LW, Kampert JB, Nichaman MZ, Blair SN. Low cardiorespiratory fitness and physical inactivity as predictors of mortality in men with type 2 diabetes. *Ann Intern Med* 2000;132:605–611.
7. Krolewski AS, Warram JH, Freire MB. Epidemiology of late diabetic complications. A basis for the development and evaluation of preventive programs. *Endocrinol Metab Clin North Am* 1996;25:217–242.
8. Messent JW, Elliott TG, Hill RD, et al. Prognostic significance of microalbuminuria in insulin-dependent diabetes mellitus: a twenty-three year follow-up study. *Kidney Int* 1992;41:836–839.
9. Dinneen SF, Gerstein HC. The association of microalbuminuria and mortality in non-insulin-dependent diabetes mellitus: a systematic overview of the literature. *Arch Intern Med* 1997;157:1413–1418. Search date 1995; primary sources Medline, SciSearch, and hand searching of bibliographies.
10. Valmadrid CT, Klein R, Moss SE, Klein BE. The risk of cardiovascular disease mortality associated with microalbuminuria and gross proteinuria in persons with older-onset diabetes mellitus. *Arch Intern Med* 2000;160:1093–1100.
11. Borch Johnsen K, Andersen PK, Deckert T. The effect of proteinuria on relative mortality in type 1 (insulin-dependent) diabetes mellitus. *Diabetologia* 1985;28:590–596.
12. Warram JH, Laffel LM, Ganda OP, et al. Coronary artery disease is the major determinant of excess mortality in patients with insulin-dependent diabetes mellitus and persistent proteinuria. *J Am Soc Nephrol* 1992;3(suppl 4):104–110.
13. Gerstein Hertzel C, Johannes FE, Qilong Yi, et al. Albuminuria and risk of cardiovascular events, death and heart failure in diabetic and nondiabetic individuals. *JAMA* 2001;286:421–426.
14. Behar S, Boyko V, Reicher-Reiss H, et al. Ten-year survival after acute myocardial infarction: comparison of patients with and without diabetes. SPRINT Study Group. Secondary Prevention Reinfarction Israeli Nifedipine Trial. *Am Heart J* 1997;133:290–296.
15. Mak KH, Moliterno DJ, Granger CB, et al. Influence of diabetes mellitus on clinical outcome in the thrombolytic era of acute myocardial infarction: GUSTO-I Investigators: global utilization of streptokinase and tissue plasminogen activator for occluded coronary arteries. *J Am Coll Cardiol* 1997;30:171–179.
16. Capes SE, Hunt D, Malmberg K, et al. Stress hyperglycaemia and increased risk of death after myocardial infarction in patients with and without diabetes: a systematic overview. *Lancet* 2000;355:773–778. Search date 1998; primary sources Medline, Science Citation Index, hand searches of bibliographies of relevant articles, and contact with experts in the field.
17. Lotufo PA, Gazziano M, Chae CU, et al. Diabetes and all-cause coronary heart disease mortality among US male physicians. *Arch Intern Med* 2001;161:242–247.
18. Meltzer S, Leiter L, Daneman D, et al. Clinical practice guidelines for the management of diabetes in Canada. *Can Med Assoc J* 1998;159(suppl 8):1–29.
19. American Diabetes Association. Clinical practice recommendations 2000. *Diabetes Care* 2000;23(suppl 1):1–116.
20. American Diabetes Association. Diabetes mellitus and exercise. *Diabetes Care* 2000;23(suppl 1):50–54.
21. Fuller J, Stevens LK, Chaturvedi N, et al. Antihypertensive therapy in preventing cardiovascular complications in people with diabetes mellitus. In: The Cochrane Library, Issue 3, 2001. Oxford, Update Software. Search date not stated; primary sources Medline, Embase, and hand searches of specialist journals in cardiovascular disease, stroke, renal disease, and hypertension. Review subsequently withdrawn by The Cochrane Library and is currently being updated.
22. Tuomilehto J, Rastenyte D, Birkenhäger WH, et al. Effects of calcium-channel blockade in older patients with diabetes and systolic hypertension. *N Engl J Med* 1999;340:677–684.
23. Lewis EJ, Hunsicker LG, et al. Renoprotective effect of the angiotensin receptor antagonist irbesartan in patients wit nephropathy due to type 2 diabetes. *NEJM* 2001:345:851–860.
24. Parving HH, Lehnert H, et al. The effect of irbesartan on the development of diabetic nephropathy in patients with type 2 diabetes. *NEJM* 2001;345:870–878.
25. Huang ES, Meigs JB, Singer DE. The effect of interventions to prevent cardiovascular disease in patients with type 2 diabetes mellitus. *American J Med* 2001;111:633–642.
26. Heart Outcomes Prevention Evaluation (HOPE) Study Investigators. Effects of ramipril on cardiovascular and microvascular outcomes in people with diabetes mellitus: results of the HOPE study and the MICRO-HOPE substudy. *Lancet* 2000;355:253–259.
27. Schrier RW, Estacio RO, et al. Effects of aggressive blood pressure control in normotensive type 2 diabetic patients on albuminuria, retinopathy and strokes. *Kidney International* 2002;6:1086–1097.
28. Pahor M, Psaty BM, Alderman MH, et al. Therapeutic benefits of ACE inhibitors and other antihypertensive drugs in patients with type 2 diabetes. *Diabetes Care* 2000;23:888–892. Search date 2000; primary source Medline.
29. Lindholm LH, Hansson L, Ekbom T, et al. Comparison of antihypertensive treatment in preventing cardiovascular events in elderly diabetic patients: results from the Swedish trial in old patients with hypertension–2. *J Hypertens* 2000;18:1671–1675.
30. ALLHAT Collaborative Research Group. Major cardiovascular events in hypertensive patients randomised to doxazosin vs chlorthalidone: the antihypertensive and lipid-lowering treatment to prevent heart attack trial (ALLHAT). *JAMA* 2000;283:1967–1975.
31. Tatti P, Pahor M, Byington RP, et al. Outcome results of the Fosfinopril versus Amlodipine Cardiovascular Events randomised Trial (FACET) in patients with hypertension and NIDDM. *Diabetes Care* 1998;21:597–603.
32. Estacio RO, Jeffers BW, Hiatt WR, et al. The effect of nisoldipine as compared with enalapril on

cardiovascular events in patients with non-insulin-dependent diabetes and hypertension. *N Engl J Med* 1998;338:645–652.
33. Niskanen L, Hedner T, et al. Reduced cardiovascular morbidity and mortality in hypertensive diabetic patients on first line therapy with an ACE inhibitor compared with diuretic beta blocker based treatment regiment, a sub analysis of the captopril prevention project. *Diabetes Care* 2001;24:2091–2096.
34. UK Prospective Diabetes Study Group. Efficacy of atenolol and captopril in reducing risk of macrovascular and microvascular complications in type 2 diabetes: UKPDS 39. *BMJ* 1998;317:713–720.
35. Dahlof B, Devereux RB, et al. Cardiovascular morbidity and mortality in the losartan intervention for endpoint reduction in hypertension study (LIFE): a randomized trial against atenolol. *Lancet* 2002;359:995–1003.
36. Hansson L, Zanchetti A, Carruthers SG, et al. Effects of intensive blood-pressure lowering and low-dose aspirin in patients with hypertension: principal results of the Hypertension Optimal Treatment (HOT) randomised trial. *Lancet* 1998;351:1755–1762.
37. UK Prospective Diabetes Study Group. Tight blood pressure control and risk of macrovascular and microvascular complications in type 2 diabetes: UKPDS 38. *BMJ* 1998;317:703–713.
38. Downs JR, Clearfield M, Weis S, et al. Primary prevention of acute coronary events with lovastatin in men and women with average cholesterol levels: results of AFCAPS/TexCAPS. Air Force/Texas Coronary Atherosclerosis Prevention Study. *JAMA* 1998;279:1615–1622.
39. Koskinen P, Manttari M, Manninen V, et al. Coronary heart disease incidence in NIDDM patients in the Helsinki Heart Study. *Diabetes Care* 1992;15:820–825.
40. Elkeles RS, Diamond JR, Poulter C, et al. Cardiovascular outcomes in type 2 diabetes. A double-blind placebo-controlled study of bezafibrate: the St Mary's, Ealing, Northwick Park Diabetes Cardiovascular Disease Prevention (SENDCAP) Study. *Diabetes Care* 1998;21:641–648.
41. Heart Protection Study Collaborative Group. MRC/BHF Heart Protection Study of cholesterol lowering with simvastatin in 20 536 high-risk individuals: a randomised placebo-controlled trial. *Lancet* 2002;360:7–22.
42. Pyorala K, Pedersen TR, Kjekshus J, et al. Cholesterol lowering with simvastatin improves prognosis of diabetic patients with coronary heart disease. A subgroup analysis of the Scandinavian Simvastatin Survival Study (4S). *Diabetes Care* 1997;20:614–620.
43. The Long-term Intervention with Pravastatin in Ischemic Disease (LIPID) Study Program. Prevention of cardiovascular events and death with pravastatin in patients with coronary heart disease and a broad range of initial cholesterol levels. *N Engl J Med* 1998;339:1349–1357.
44. Rubins HB, Robins SJ, Collins D, et al. Gemfibrozil for the secondary prevention of coronary heart disease in men with low levels of high-density lipoprotein cholesterol. Veterans Affairs High-Density Lipoprotein Cholesterol Intervention Trial Study Group. *N Engl J Med* 1999;341:410–418.
45. Sacks FM, Pfeffer MA, Moye LA, et al. The effect of pravastatin on coronary events after myocardial infarction in patients with average cholesterol levels. Cholesterol and Recurrent Events Trial investigators. *N Engl J Med* 1996;335:1001–1009.
46. Hoogwerf BJ, Waness A, et al. Effects of aggressive cholesterol lowering and low dose anticoagulation on clinical and angiographic outcomes in patients with diabetes. *Diabetes*1999;48:1289–1294.
47. Anonymous. Effect of fenofibrate on progression of coronary-artery disease in type 2 diabetes: The Diabetes Atherosclerosis Interventions Study, a Randomized Study. *Lancet* 2001;357:905–910.
48. Steering Committee of the Physicians' Health Study Research Group. Final report on the aspirin component of the ongoing Physicians' Health Study. *N Engl J Med* 1989;321:129–135.
49. ETDRS Investigators. Aspirin effects on mortality and morbidity in patients with diabetes mellitus. *JAMA* 1992;268:1292–1300.
50. Collaborative overview of randomised trials of antiplatelet therapy–I: Prevention of death, myocardial infarction, and stroke by prolonged antiplatelet therapy in various categories of patients. Antiplatelet Trialists' Collaboration. *BMJ* 1994;308:81–106. Search date 1990; primary sources Medline, Current Contents, manual searches of journals, reference lists from clinical trials and review articles, and enquiry among colleagues and manufacturers of antiplatelet agents for unpublished studies.
51. American Diabetes Association. Aspirin therapy in diabetes. *Diabetes Care* 1997;20:1772–1773.
52. The BARI Investigators. Seven-year outcome in the Bypass Angioplasty Revascularization Investigation (BARI) by treatment and diabetic status. *J Am Coll Cardiol* 2000;35:1122–1129.
53. DCCT Research Group. Effect of intensive diabetes management on macrovascular events andrisk factors in the Diabetes Control and Complications Trial. *Am J Cardiol* 1995;75:894–903.
54. DCCT Research Group. The effect of intensive treatment of diabetes on the development and progression of long-term complications in insulin-dependent diabetes mellitus. *N Engl J Med* 1993;329:977–986.
55. Abraira C, Colwell J, Nuttall F, et al. Cardiovascular events and correlates in the Veterans Affairs Diabetes Feasibility Trial: Veterans Affairs Cooperative Study on glycemic control and complications in type II diabetes. *Arch Intern Med* 1997;157:181–188.
56. Malmberg K, Ryden L, Efendic S, et al. Randomised trial of insulin-glucose infusion followed by subcutaneous insulin treatment in diabetic patients with acute myocardial infarction (DIGAMI study): effects on mortality at 1 year. *J Am Coll Cardiol* 1995;26:57–65.
57. Malmberg K. Prospective randomised study of intensive insulin treatment on long term survival after acute myocardial infarction in patients with diabetes mellitus. DIGAMI (Diabetes Mellitus, Insulin Glucose Infusion in Acute Myocardial Infarction) Study Group. *BMJ* 1997;314:1512–1515.
58. Kurbaan AS, Bowker TJ, Ilsley CD, et al. Difference in the mortality of the CABRI diabetic and nondiabetic populations and its relation to coronary artery disease and the revascularization mode. *Am J Cardiol* 2001;87:947–950.
59. Abizaid A, Costa MA, et al. Clinical and economic impact of diabetes mellitus on percutaneous and surgical treatment of multivessel coronary disease patients indights form the arterial revascularization therapy study (ARTS) trial. Circulation 2001;104:533–538.
60. Kleiman NS, Lincoff AM, Kereiakes DJ, et al. Diabetes mellitus, glycoprotein IIb/IIIa blockade, and heparin: evidence for a complex interaction in a multicenter trial. EPILOG Investigators. *Circulation* 1998;97:1912–1920.

61. Marso SP, Lincoff AM, Ellis SG, et al. Optimizing the percutaneous interventional outcomes for patients with diabetes mellitus: results of the EPISTENT (Evaluation of platelet IIb/IIIa inhibitor for stenting trial) diabetic substudy. *Circulation* 1999;100:2477–2484.
62. The EPISTENT Investigators. Randomised placebo-controlled and balloon-angioplasty-controlled trial to assess safety of coronary stenting with use of platelet glycoprotein-IIb/IIIa blockade. The EPISTENT Investigators. Evaluation of platelet IIb/IIIa inhibitor for stenting. *Lancet* 1998;352:87–92.
63. Topol EJ, Mark DB, Lincoff AM, et al. Outcomes at 1 year and economic implications of platelet glycoprotein IIb/IIIa blockade in patients undergoing coronary stenting: results from a multicentre randomised trial. EPISTENT Investigators. Evaluation of Platelet IIb/IIIa Inhibitor for Stenting. *Lancet* 1999;354:2019–2024. [Published erratum appears in *Lancet* 2000;355:1104].
64. The EPIC Investigation. Use of a monoclonal antibody directed against the platelet glycoprotein IIb/IIIa receptor in high-risk coronary angioplasty. *N Engl J Med* 1994;330:956–961.
65. Bhatt DL, Marso SP, Lincoff AM, et al. Abciximab reduces mortality in diabetics following percutaneous coronary intervention. *J Am Coll Cardiol* 2000;35:922–928.
66. UK Prospective Diabetes Study Group. Intensive blood-glucose control with sulphonylureas or insulin compared with conventional treatment and risk of complications in patients with type 2 diabetes (UKPDS 33). *Lancet* 1998;352:837–853.
67. UK Prospective Diabetes Study Group. Effect of intensive blood-glucose control with metformin on complications in overweight patients with type 2 diabetes (UKPDS 34). *Lancet* 1998;352:854–865.
68. Theroux P, Alexander J, Pharand C, et al. Glycoprotein IIb/IIIa receptor blockade improves outcomes in diabetic patients presenting with unstable angina/Non-ST-elevation myocardial infarction results from the platelet receptor inhibitor in ischemic syndrome management in patients limited by unstable signs and symptoms. *Circulation* 2000;102:2466–2472.
69. Hasdai D, Granger CB, Srivatsa S, et al. Diabetes mellitus and outcome after primary coronary angioplasty for acute myocardial infarction: lessons from the GUSTO-IIb angioplasty study. *J Am Coll Cardiol* 2000;35:1502–1512.

Janine Malcolm
Fellow, Endocrinology and Metabolism

Hilary Meggison
Fellow, Endocrinology and Metabolism

Ottawa Hospital
Ottawa
Canada

Ronald Sigal
Assistant Professor of Medicine and Human Kinetics
University of Ottawa
Ottawa
Canada

Competing interests: RS has received speaker's fees from Aventis (manufacturer of glyburide, metformin, glimepiride, ramipril, and insulin glargine), Novo Nordisk (manufacturer of insulin and repaglinide), and Pfizer (manufacturer of atorvastatin). He has received reimbursement for travel expenses from Bristol-Myers Squibb (manufacturer of pravastatin), Aventis, and Pfizer, and has received consulting fees from Pfizer. HM and JM none declared.

TABLE 1 **Primary prevention of cardiovascular events in people with diabetes: evidence from systematic reviews and randomised trials (see text, p 547).**

Study	Interventions	Study type	Duration (years)	Outcome	Events / Sample size (%)*		NNT	95% CI for NNT
					Intervention	Control		
Antihypertensive medication								
UKPDS Hypertension Study[34,37]	"Tight" target BP (≤ 150/≤ 85) with captopril or atenolol *v* "less tight" target (≤ 180/ ≤ 105)	RCT	8.4	AMI (fatal or non-fatal) Stroke Peripheral vascular events	107/758 (14%) 38/758 (5.0%) 8/758 (1.1%)	83/390 (21%) 34/390 (8.7%) 8/390 (2.1%)	14 27 ND	9 to 35 18 to 116 ND
HOT[36]	Felodipine and ACE inhibitor, or β blocker, with 3 distinct target BPs	RCT	3.8	AMI (fatal or non-fatal), stroke (fatal or non-fatal), or other cardiovascular death	22/499 (4.4%) Target diastolic BP 80 mmHg	45/501 (9.0%) Target diastolic BP 90 mmHg	22	16 to 57
FACET[31]	Fosinopril *v* amlodipine	RCT	2.9	AMI, stroke, or admission to hospital for angina	14/189 (7.4%) Fosinopril	27/191 (14%) Amlodipine	15	10 to 199
ABCD[32]	Enalapril *v* nisoldipine	RCT	5	AMI (fatal or non-fatal)	5/235 (2.1%) Enalapril	25/235 (11%) Nisoldipine	12	10 to 19
Syst-Eur[22]	Nitrendipine; enalapril ± hydrochlorothiazide (20 mm Hg BP lowering) *v* placebo	RCT	2	MI, CHF, or sudden cardiac death	13/252 (5%)	31/240 (13%)	13	10 to 31

TABLE 1 continued

Lipid-regulating agents								
AFCAPS/TexCAPS[38]	Lovastatin	RCT	5	MI, unstable angina, or sudden cardiac death	4/84 (4.8%)	6/71 (8.5%)	27	NS
SENDCAP[40]	Bezafibrate	RCT	3	MI or new ischaemic changes on ECG	5/64 (7.8%)	16/64 (25%)	6	5 to 20
Helsinki[39]	Gemfibrozil	RCT	5	MI or cardiac death	2/59 (3.4%)	8/76 (10.5%)	14	NS
HPS[41]	Simvastatin *v* placebo	RCT	5	CHD, stroke, revascularisation	133/1455 (9.1%)	197/1457 (13.5%)	23	15 to 48
Blood glucose control								
UKPDS[66]	Intensive treatment with insulin and/or sulphonylurea *v* conventional treatment	RCT	5	MI (fatal or non-fatal)	387/2729 (14.2%)	186/1138 (16.3%)	46	NS
UKPDS[67]	Intensive treatment with metformin *v* conventional treatment	RCT	5	MI (fatal or non-fatal)	39/342 (11%)	73/411 (18%)	16	10 to 71
DCCT[53,54]	Intensive insulin treatment in type 1 diabetes	RCT	6.5	Major macrovascular events‡	23/711 (3.2%)	40/730 (5.5%)	45	28 to 728
Aspirin								
Physicians' Health Study[48]	Aspirin	RCT	5	MI (fatal or non-fatal)	11/275 (4.0%)	26/258 (10%)	16	12 to 47
ETDRS (mixed primary and secondary prevention)[49]	Aspirin	RCT	5	MI (fatal or non-fatal)	289/1856 (15.6%)	336/1855 (18.1%)	39	21 to 716

*People with diabetes only. ‡Combined MI (fatal or non-fatal), sudden cardiac death, revascularisation procedure, angina with coronary artery disease confirmed by angiography or by non-invasive testing, stroke, lower limb amputation, peripheral arterial events requiring revascularisation, claudication with angiographic evidence of peripheral vascular disease. ACE, angiotensin converting enzyme; AMI, acute myocardial infarction; BP, blood pressure; CHD, coronary heart disease; CHF, chronic heart failure; CVD, cardiovascular disease; ECG, electrocardiogram; MI, myocardial infarction; ND, no data; NNT, number needed to treat; NS, not significant; RCT, randomised

TABLE 2 Secondary prevention of cardiovascular events in people with diabetes (see text, p 552).

Study	Interventions	Study Type	Duration (years)	Outcome	Events / sample size (%)*		NNT	95% CI for NNT
					Intervention	Control		
Lipid-regulating agents								
4S[42]	Simvastatin	RCT	5.4	CHD death or non-fatal MI	24/105 (23%)	44/97 (45%)	5	3 to 10
CARE[45]	Pravastatin	RCT	5	Coronary disease death, non-fatal MI, or revascularisation	81/282 (29%)	112/304 (37%)	12	7 to 194
LIPID[43]	Pravastatin	RCT	6.1	CHD death or non-fatal MI	76/396 (19%)	88/386 (23%)	28	NS
Veterans[44]	Gemfibrozil	RCT	5.1	CHD death or non-fatal MI	88/309 (29%)	116/318 (37%)	13	7 to 144
Blood glucose control								
DIGAMI[56,57]	Insulin infusion followed by intensive insulin treatment *v* usual care	RCT	3.4	Overall mortality	102/306 (33%)	138/314 (44%)	9	6 to 33
Antiplatelet treatments								
Antiplatelet trialists[50]	Aspirin *v* placebo	SR	Median 2 years	CVD mortality and morbidity	415/2248 (19%)	502/2254 (22%)	26	17 to 66
PRISM-PLUS[68]	Tirofiban plus heparin *v* heparin alone	RCT	180 days	Death or MI	Tirofiban plus heparin 16/169 (11.2%)	Heparin alone 37/193 (19.2%)	13	7 to 146
Revascularisation								
ARTS[59]	CABG *v* PTCA and stent	RCT	1	Death, MI, revascularisation	CABG 15/96 (15.6%)	PTCA and stent 41/112 (36.6%)	5	3 to 11
GUSTO IIb[69]	PTCA *v* alteplase	RCT	2	Death, non-fatal reinfarction, or disabling stroke	PTCA 11/99 (11%)	Alteplase 13/78 (16%)	18	NS
BARI[52]	CABG *v* PTCA	RCT	7.7	Death or non-fatal Q wave MI	CABG 60/173 (35%)	PTCA 85/170 (50%)	7	4 to 21
CABRI[58]	CABG *v* PTCA	RCT	4	Death	CABG 8/63 (12.7%)	PTCA 14/62 (22.6%)	10	NS
EPIC[64]/EPILOG[60]/ EPISTENT[61–63]	Abciximab *v* control	Pooled	1	Overall death rate	26/540 (4.8%)	21/844 (2.5%)	43	23 to 422
EPIC[64]/EPILOG[60]/ EPISTENT[61–63]	Abciximab *v* control	Pooled	1	Death or non-fatal MI	185/540 (34%)	246/844 (29%)	20	9 to 1423

*People with diabetes only. CABG, coronary artery bypass grafting; CHD, coronary heart disease; CVD, cardiovascular disease; MI, myocardial infarction;

TABLE 3 Mixed primary and secondary prevention of cardiovascular events in people with diabetes (see text, p 547).

Interventions	Study type	Duration (years)	Outcome	Events / sample size (%) (people with diabetes only) Intervention	Control	NNT	95% CI for NNT
Antihypertensive medication							
ACE inhibitors *v* diuretics or calcium channel blockers[28]	Meta-analysis	2.8 to 6.2	CVD death, MI, CHF, angina, or stroke.	ACE inhibitor 158/733	Diuretics or calcium channel blockers 266/789	6	4 to 8
Captopril *v* diuretics and/or β blockers[33]	RCT	6	Fatal and non-fatal MI, stroke, CV deaths	39/309 (13%)	67/263 (26%)	15	9 to 93
Enalapril or nisoldipine *v* placebo[27]	RCT	5	AMI (fatal or non-fatal)	68/237 (29%)	66/243 (27%)	65	11 to 16
Enalapril *v* placebo[27]	RCT	5	AMI (fatal or non-fatal)	67/237 (28%)	67/234 (29%)	72	11 to 15
Losarten v atenolol[35]	RCT	4	CV death, stroke, MI	39/586 (7%)	53/609 (9%)	47	20 to 109
Ramipril 10 mg daily versus placebo[26]	RCT	4.5	MI, stroke, or CVD. Overall mortality	277/1808 (15%) 196/1808 (11%)	351/1769 (20%) 240/1769 (14%)	22 32	14 to 43 19 to 98
Lipid-regulating agents							
Micronised fenobibrate *v* placebo[47]	RCT	3.8 (including 6 months' follow up)	Death or MI	15/207 (7.2%)	21/111(10%)	37	NS

*People with diabetes only. ACE, angiotensin-converting enzyme; CHF, congestive heart failure; CVD, cardiovascular disease; MI, myocardial infarction; NS, not significant.

Foot ulcers and amputations in diabetes

Search date May 2002

Dereck Hunt and Hertzel Gerstein

QUESTIONS

INTERVENTIONS

See glossary, p 576

Key Messages

Preventive interventions

- **Education (ulcer recurrence and major amputation)** We found no RCTs on the effects of education on prevention of diabetic foot complications. One non-randomised trial found that specific foot care education versus routine diabetes care education significantly decreased ulcer recurrences (NNT 10, 95% CI 6 to 26) and major amputations (NNT 14, 95% CI 8 to 50) after 2 years.
- **Screening and referral to foot care clinics (major amputations in those at high risk)** One RCT identified by a systemic review has found that a diabetes screening and protection programme (involving referral to a foot clinic) versus usual care significantly reduces the risk of major amputation after 2 years (NNT 91, 95% CI 53 to 250).
- **Therapeutic footwear (ulcer recurrence)** One RCT found no significant difference in foot ulceration rates between therapeutic footwear (fitted with cork or polyurethane inserts) versus usual footwear in people with diabetes and previous foot ulcer but without severe deformity. One non-randomised controlled trial identified by a systematic review found that therapeutic footwear (made according to the Towey guidelines) versus ordinary shoes significantly reduced the recurrence of ulceration after 1 year (NNT 4, 95% CI 2 to 14).

Clin Evid 2002;8:569–577.

Therapeutic interventions

- **Cultured human dermis (non-infected foot ulcer healing)** One systematic review found that cultured human dermis (Dermagraft, weekly for 8 wks) versus control increased ulcer healing by 21% at 12 weeks in people with non-infected diabetic foot ulcer, but the result did not reach significance.
- **Human skin equivalent (chronic neuropathic non-infected foot ulcer healing)** One RCT found that human skin equivalent (Graftskin applied weekly for maximum of 5 wks) versus saline moistened gauze significantly increased ulcer healing rates in people with chronic neuropathic non-infected foot ulcers (NNT 6, 95% CI 3 to 20).
- **Pressure off-loading with non-removable cast (non-infected foot ulcer healing)** One RCT identified by a systematic review has found that pressure off-loading with total contact casting versus traditional dressing changes significantly improves non-infected diabetic foot ulcer healing (NNT 2, 95% CI 1 to 3). RCTs have found that pressure off-loading with either total contact casting or non-removable fibreglass casts versus removable casts or shoes significantly improves non-infected diabetic foot ulcer healing at 12 weeks.
- **Systemic hyperbaric oxygen (infected ulcers)** One RCT in people with severely infected foot ulcers found that systemic hyperbaric oxygen plus usual care versus usual care alone significantly reduced the risk of foot amputation after 10 weeks (NNT 5, 95% CI 2 to 23). Another small, short term RCT found no significant difference in the risk of major amputation after 2 weeks.
- **Topical growth factors (non-infected foot ulcer healing)** One systematic review found inconsistent evidence about the effects of four different topical growth factors versus placebo on ulcer healing rates in people with non-infected diabetic foot ulcers.

DEFINITION Diabetic foot ulceration is full thickness penetration of the dermis of the foot in a person with diabetes. Ulcer severity is often classified using the Wagner system. Grade 1 ulceration refers to superficial ulcers that involve the full skin thickness but not any underlying tissues. Grade 2 ulceration refers to deeper ulcers that penetrate down to ligaments and muscle, but do not involve bone or have any abscess formation. Grade 3 ulceration refers to deep ulcers that have evidence of cellulitis or abscess formation, and are often complicated with osteomyelitis. Ulcers with evidence of localised gangrene are classified as Grade 4 and Grade 5 ulcers have extensive gangrene involving the entire foot.

INCIDENCE/ PREVALENCE Studies conducted in Australia, Finland, the UK, and the USA have reported the annual incidence of foot ulcers among people with diabetes as 2.5–10.7%, and the annual incidence of amputation as 0.25–1.8%.[1–10]

AETIOLOGY/ RISK FACTORS Long term risk factors for foot complications, including foot ulcers and amputation, include duration of diabetes, poor glycaemic control, and the presence of microvascular complications (retinopathy, nephropathy, and neuropathy). However, the strongest predictors for development of foot complications are altered foot sensation and previous foot ulcer.[1–8]

PROGNOSIS People with diabetes are at risk of developing complications in the lower extremities. These include foot ulcers, infections, and vascular insufficiency. Amputation of a lower extremity is indicated if complications are severe or do not improve with appropriate treatment. As well as affecting quality of life, these complications form a large proportion of the healthcare costs of diabetes. For people with healed diabetic foot ulcers, the 5 year cumulative rate of ulcer recurrence is 66% and of amputation is 12%.[11]

AIMS To prevent diabetic foot complications, including ulcers and amputations; and to improve ulcer healing and prevent amputations where ulcers already exist, with minimum adverse effects.

OUTCOMES Rates of development or recurrence of foot ulcers or major foot lesions; rate of amputation (surgical removal of all or part of the lower extremity: minor amputations involve partial removal of a foot, including toe or forefoot resections; and major amputations are above or below knee amputations); time ulcers take to heal, or the proportion healed in a given period; rates of hospital admission; rates of foot infection; adverse effects of treatment.

METHODS *Clinical Evidence* update search and appraisal May 2002.

QUESTION What are the effects of preventive interventions?

OPTION SCREENING AND REFERRAL TO FOOT CARE CLINIC

One RCT identified by a systemic review has found that a diabetes screening and protection programme (involving referral to a foot clinic) versus usual care significantly reduces the risk of major amputation after 2 years.

Benefits: We found one systematic review (search date 1998, 1 RCT, 2002 people attending a general diabetes clinic).[12] The RCT compared a diabetes screening and protection programme versus usual care over 2 years.[13] People in the diabetes screening and protection programme were screened for deficits in pedal pulses, light touch, and vibration sensation. People with persistent abnormal findings were referred to the diabetic foot clinic if they had a history of foot ulcer, were found to have a low ankle-brachial index (< 0.75), or were noted to have foot deformities. The clinic provided podiatry and protective shoes as well as education regarding foot care. Usual care consisted of the normal follow up for people in the clinic who could be referred to the foot care clinic if a healthcare professional requested this. The RCT found that significantly more people receiving usual care versus diabetes screening and protection programme needed major amputation (12/1000 [1.2%] *v* 1/1000 [0.1%]; ARI 1.1%, 95% CI 0.4% to 1.9%; NNT 91, 95% CI 53 to 250).

Harms: The RCT gave no information on harms.[13]

Comment: None.

OPTION THERAPEUTIC FOOTWEAR

One RCT found no significant difference in foot ulceration rates between therapeutic footwear (fitted with cork or polyurethane inserts) versus usual footwear in people with diabetes and previous foot ulcer but

without severe deformity. One non-randomised controlled trial identified by a systematic review found that therapeutic footwear (made according to the Towey guidelines) versus ordinary shoes significantly reduced the recurrence of ulceration after 1 year.

Benefits: We found one RCT (400 people with diabetes mellitus and previous foot ulcer but without severe deformity, mean age 62 years) comparing extra-depth and extra-width therapeutic shoes fitted with customised cork inserts versus therapeutic shoes fitted with polyurethane inserts versus usual footwear for 2 years.[14] The RCT found no significant difference in foot ulceration rates between therapeutic footwear and usual footwear (foot ulceration rates 15% with cork insert *v* 14% with polyurethane insert *v* 17% with usual footwear; RR cork insert *v* usual footwear 0.88, 95% CI 0.51 to 1.52; RR polyurethane insert *v* usual footwear 0.85, 95% CI 0.48 to 1.48).

Harms: The RCT did not report any adverse effects.[14]

Comment: We found one systematic review (search date 1998),[12] which identified one non-randomised controlled trial.[15] The trial alternately allocated 69 people with a previous diabetic foot ulcer to either an intervention group (in which people received therapeutic shoes) or to a control group (in which people continued to wear their ordinary shoes).[15] Therapeutic shoes were manufactured according to the Towey guidelines (super depth to fit customised insoles and toe deformities, and made with soft thermoformable leather along with semirocker soles). All participants received information on foot care and footwear. After 1 year, the study found that wearing therapeutic shoes versus ordinary shoes significantly reduced ulcer recurrence (27% with intervention *v* 58% with control; RR 0.47; ARR 31%, 95% CI 7% to 55%; NNT 4, 95% CI 2 to 14). The controlled trial did not report any adverse effects associated with therapeutic shoes. Alternate allocation increases the possibility of bias from confounding factors for the two treatment groups.

OPTION EDUCATION

We found no RCTs on the effects of education on prevention of diabetic foot complications. One non-randomised trial found that specific foot care education versus routine diabetes care education significantly reduced ulcer recurrences and major amputations after 2 years.

Benefits: We found no RCTs on effects of education on prevention of diabetic foot complications.

Harms: We found no RCTs.

Comment: We found one systematic review (search date 1998)[16] and one non-randomised controlled trial.[17] The trial (227 people who presented with foot infection, ulcer, or for assistance after a previous amputation, allocated according to their social security number) evaluated the effect of providing a single, 1 hour educational class on diabetic foot complications and important components of foot care versus routine diabetes education with respect to diet, weight, exercise, and medication.[17] Surgical treatment was provided for all people when necessary. Follow up at 2 years found that allocation to the specific educational session significantly reduced ulcer recurrences (4.5% for education *v* 14.7% for control group; RR 0.31; ARR 10%, 95% CI 4% to 16%; NNT 10, 95% CI 6 to 26) and major amputation (2.8% for education *v* 10.2% for control group; RR 0.28; ARR 7%, 95% CI 2% to 13%; NNT 14, 95% CI 8 to 50). Allocation by social security number may introduce systematic biases and could create confounding factors between the two groups.

QUESTION What are the effects of therapeutic interventions?

OPTION PRESSURE OFF-LOADING

One RCT identified by a systematic review has found that pressure off-loading with total contact casting versus traditional dressing changes significantly improves non-infected diabetic foot ulcer healing. RCTs have found that pressure off-loading with either total contact casting or non-removable fibreglass casts versus removable casts or shoes significantly improves non-infected diabetic foot ulcer healing at 12 weeks.

Benefits: We found one systematic review (search date 1998,[16] 1 RCT,[18] 40 people with diabetes and plantar foot ulcers but free of signs of infection or gangrene, told to minimise weight bearing), and two subsequent RCTs evaluating pressure off-loading (see glossary, p 576) versus controls.[19,20] **Versus traditional dressing changes:** The RCT identified in the systematic review compared total contact casting versus traditional dressing changes.[18] Casts were applied by an experienced physiotherapist, changed after 5–7 days, and then every 2–3 weeks until healing occurred. Control participants were provided with accommodative footwear and crutches or a walker, and were instructed to complete wet to dry dressing changes 2–3 times daily. The RCT found that total contact casting versus traditional dressing changes significantly increased ulcer healing (91% for total contact casting *v* 32% for traditional dressing; ARR 59%, 95% CI 31% to 87%; NNT 2, 95% CI 1 to 3) and reduced infection ($P < 0.05$).[18] **Versus removable casts/shoes:** One RCT (63 people with diabetes mellitus and non-infected neuropathic plantar foot ulcers) compared total contact casting versus using a removable cast walker versus using a half-shoe.[19] All participants had weekly visits for wound care and debridement and were followed up for 12 weeks. It found that total contact casting versus removable cast walkers or half-shoes significantly increased ulcer healing at 12 weeks (89% with contact casting *v* 61% with removable cast walker or half-shoe; ARR 28%, 95% CI 5% to 51%; NNT 4, 95% CI 2 to 19).[19] Another RCT (50 people with diabetes mellitus and non-infected neuropathic plantar foot ulcers) compared non-removable fibreglass casts versus specialised cloth shoes with rigid soles and off-loading insoles over 30 days. All participants had dressing changes every 2 days. It found that non-removable fibreglass casts versus specialised cloth shoes significantly improved ulcer healing (50% of ulcers healed with fibreglass casts *v* 21% with specialised cloth shoes; ARR 29%, 95% CI 1.4% to 57%; NNT 4, 95% CI 2 to 72).[20] **Versus topical growth factors:** See glossary, p 576. We found no RCTs.

Harms: The RCT identified in the systematic review found that 3/21 (14%) people treated with total contact casting developed fungal infections that required topical treatment. These events did not prevent continued casting.[18] No adverse effects were observed in the two subsequent RCTs.[19,20]

Comment: Total contact casting is the application of a layer of plaster over the foot and lower leg designed to distribute pressure evenly over the entire plantar aspect of the foot to reduce exposure of plantar ulcers to pressure, even when the person is walking. Soft tissue infections and osteomyelitis are contraindications to total contact casting.

OPTION CULTURED HUMAN DERMIS

One systematic review found a non-significant increase in ulcer healing at 12 weeks with cultured human dermis (Dermagraft, weekly for 8 wks) versus control in people with non-infected diabetic foot ulcer.

Benefits: We found one systematic review (search date 1998, 2 unblinded RCTs) comparing topical application of cultured human dermis (see glossary, p 576) versus controls in people attending hospital outpatient clinics with diabetic foot ulcers who were free of signs of infection or severe vascular compromise.[16] All participants received wound debridement and were encouraged to avoid weight bearing on the affected limb. The systematic review found a non-significant increase in ulcer healing at 12 weeks with cultured human dermis (Dermagraft, weekly for 8 wks) versus control (+21% increase in ulcer healing at 12 wks, 95% CI −13% to +36%).

Harms: One RCT identified by the systematic review found no significant difference between cultured human dermis and controls in rates of ulcer infections, and no effect on haematology or serum chemistry values or glycaemic control. The other RCT found no significant differences in wound infection rates.[16]

Comment: Cultured human dermis (Dermagraft) may not be widely available.

OPTION HUMAN SKIN EQUIVALENT — New

One RCT found that human skin equivalent (Graftskin applied weekly for a maximum of 5 wks) versus saline moistened gauze significantly increased ulcer healing rates in people with chronic neuropathic non-infected foot ulceration.

Benefits: We found one RCT (208 people aged 18–80 years with diabetes mellitus and chronic neuropathic non-infected foot ulceration) comparing human skin equivalent (see glossary, p 576) (Graftskin applied weekly for a maximum of 5 wks) versus saline moistened gauze (applied weekly). It found that ulcer healing was significantly higher with human skin equivalent versus saline moistened gauze after 12 weeks (56% with human skin equivalent *v* 38% with saline moistened gauze; ARI 18%, 95% CI 5% to 33%; RR 1.5, 95% CI 1.1 to 2.0; NNT 6, 95% CI 3 to 20).[21]

Harms: The RCT found no significant adverse effects. Wound infections and cellulitis were equally frequent. Osteomyelitis and amputations were less frequent in people receiving human skin equivalent (osteomyelitis: 2.7% with human skin equivalent *v* 10.4% with saline moistened gauze; amputations: 6.3% with human skin equivalent *v* 15.6% with saline moistened gauze).

Comment: Human skin equivalent may not be widely available.

OPTION TOPICAL GROWTH FACTORS

One systematic review found inconsistent evidence about the effects of four different topical growth factors versus placebo on ulcer healing rates in people with non-infected diabetic foot ulcers.

Benefits: We found one systematic review (search date 1998, 6 double blind RCTs) comparing four different topical growth factors (see glossary, p 576) versus placebo in people attending hospital outpatient clinics with diabetic foot ulcers who were free of signs of infection or severe vascular compromise.[16] All participants received wound debridement and were encouraged to avoid weight bearing on the affected limb. The systematic review did not pool the results from the six RCTs.[16] One RCT (65 people) found that treatment with an arginine-glycine aspartic (RGD) acid matrix twice weekly for up to 10 weeks versus placebo significantly increased healing rates (non-healing: 65% with matrix *v* 92% with placebo; RR 0.71; ARR 27%, 95% CI 6% to 48%; NNT 4, 95% CI 2 to 15).[22] The second RCT (118 people) found that treatment with platelet derived growth factors (30 µg/g once daily for up to 20 wks) increased healing rates (non-healing: 52% with platelet derived growth factors *v* 75% with placebo; RR 0.69; ARR 23%, 95% CI 5% to 41%; NNT 5, 95% CI 3 to 14).[23] A third RCT (382 people) found that treatment with platelet derived growth factors (100 µg/g once daily for up to 20 wks) significantly increased healing rates (non-healing: 50% *v* 65% with placebo; RR 0.77; ARR 15%, 95% CI 2% to 28%; NNT 7, 95% CI 4 to 42).[24] This RCT found no benefit with lower doses (30 µg/g once daily for up to 20 wks) of platelet derived growth factors versus placebo (non-healing: 64% with platelet derived growth factors *v* 65% with placebo). Two RCTs evaluated a growth factor derived from thrombin induced human platelets (CT-102) applied twice weekly. One small RCT (13 people) found no significant effect on healing rates (non-healing: 29% with thrombin induced human platelets growth factor *v* 83% with placebo; RR 0.34; ARR +55%, 95% CI −2% to +81%).[25] The second, larger RCT (81 people) found a significant increase in healing rates (non-healing: 20% with thrombin induced human platelets growth factor *v* 71% with placebo; RR 0.28; ARR 51%, 95% CI 19% to 84%; NNT 2, 95% CI 1 to 5).[26] The sixth RCT (17 people) found no significant difference with recombinant basic fibroblast growth factor versus control treatment.[27] The systematic review reported less frequent ulcer site infections with topical growth factors versus placebo.

Harms: The systematic review reported no growth factor related adverse effects.[16]

Comment: These therapeutic agents are not widely available and may be expensive. There has been little long term follow up of people treated with these growth factors.

OPTION SYSTEMIC HYPERBARIC OXYGEN

One RCT in people with severely infected foot ulcers found that systemic hyperbaric oxygen plus usual care versus usual care alone significantly reduced the risk of foot amputation after 10 weeks. Another small, short term RCT found no significant difference in the risk of major amputation after 2 weeks.

Benefits: We found one systematic review (search date 1998, 1 RCT)[16] and one additional RCT.[28] The RCT in the systematic review (70 people with severe infected diabetic foot ulcers with full thickness gangrene or abscess, or a large infected ulcer that had not healed after 30 days) compared systemic hyperbaric oxygen (see glossary, p 576) (daily 90 min sessions at 2.2–2.5 atmospheres) plus usual care (aggressive debridement, broad spectrum iv antibiotics, revascularisation if indicated, and optimised glycaemic control) versus usual care alone.[29] After 10 weeks, rates of major amputation were significantly lower in the intervention group (8.6% with intervention *v* 33% with control; RR 0.26, 95% CI 16 to 92; ARR 24%, 95% CI 4% to 45%; NNT 5, 95% CI 2 to 23). The additional RCT (30 people with chronic infected foot ulcers) compared usual treatment (including debridement, iv antibiotics, and optimised glycaemic control) versus usual treatment plus four treatments with hyperbaric oxygen over 2 weeks. It found no significant reduction of the risk of major amputation in the intervention group (ARR +33%, 95% CI –1.6% to +68%).[28]

Harms: In the larger RCT, two people developed symptoms of barotraumatic otitis, but this did not interrupt treatment.[29]

Comment: The additional RCT may have been too small to rule out a clinically important effect.

GLOSSARY

Cultured human dermis consists of neonatal fibroblasts cultured *in vitro* onto a bioabsorbable mesh to produce a living, metabolically active tissue containing normal dermal matrix proteins and cytokines.

Human skin equivalent consists of two allogenic layers containing human skin cells. One layer is formed by dermal cells (human fibroblasts) and the second layer is formed by epidermal cells. Human skin equivalent produces cytokines and growth factors involved in the skin healing process.

Pressure off-loading refers to the use of different techniques designed to minimise the amount of force applied to the ulcer site.

Systemic hyperbaric oxygen refers to exposing a patient to a high oxygen, high pressure environment designed to improve oxygen delivery to the ulcer site.

Topical growth factors are synthetically produced factors specifically designed to promote cellular proliferation or matrix production at an ulcer site.

Substantive changes

Therapeutic footwear One new RCT;[14] conclusions unchanged.

REFERENCES

1. Rith-Najarian SJ, Stolusky T, Gohdes DM. Identifying diabetic patients at high risk for lower-extremity amputation in a primary health care setting. *Diabetes Care* 1992;15:1386–1389.
2. Veves A, Murray HJ, Young MJ, et al. The risk of foot ulceration in diabetic patients with high foot pressure: a prospective study. *Diabetologia* 1992;35:660–663.
3. Young MJ, Breddy JL, Veves, et al. The prediction of diabetic neuropathic foot ulceration using vibration perception thresholds: a prospective study. *Diabetes Care* 1994;17:557–560.
4. Humphrey ARG, Dowse GK, Thoma K, et al. Diabetes and nontraumatic lower extremity amputations. Incidence, risk factors, and prevention: a 12 year follow-up study in Nauru. *Diabetes Care* 1996;19:710–714.
5. Lee JS, Lu M, Lee VS, et al. Lower-extremity amputation: incidence, risk factors, and mortality in the Oklahoma Indian diabetes study. *Diabetes* 1993;42:876–882.
6. Lehto S, Ronnemaa T, Pyorala K, et al. Risk factors predicting lower extremity amputations in patients with NIDDM. *Diabetes Care* 1996;19:607–612.
7. Moss SE, Klein R, Klein B. Long-term incidence of lower-extremity amputations in a diabetic population. *Arch Fam Med* 1996;5:391–398.
8. Nelson RG, Gohdes DM, Everhart JE, et al. Lower-extremity amputations in NIDDM: 12 year follow-up study in Pima Indians. *Diabetes Care* 1988;11:8–16.
9. Boyko ED, Ahroni JH, Stensel V, et al. A prospective study of risk factors for diabetic foot ulcer. The Seattle diabetic foot study. *Diabetes Care* 1999;22:1036–1042.
10. Abbott CA, Carrington AL, Ashe H, et al. The North-West Diabetes Foot Care Study: incidence of, and risk factors for, new diabetic foot ulceration in a community-based patient cohort. *Diabet Med* 2002;19:377–384.
11. Apelqvist J, Larsson J, Agardh CD. Long-term prognosis for diabetic patients with foot ulcers. *J Intern Med* 1993;233:485–491.
12. Mason J, O'Keeffe C, McIntosh A, et al. A systematic review of foot ulcer in patients with type 2 diabetes mellitus. I: prevention. *Diabet Med* 1999;16:801–812. Search date 1998; primary sources Cochrane Controlled Trials Register, Medline, Embase, Cinahl, Healthstar, Psychlit, Science Citation, Social Science Citation, Index to Scientific and Technical Conference Proceedings (ISI), HMIC database, and Sigle.
13. McCabe CJ, Stevenson RC, Dolan AM. Evaluation of a diabetic foot screening and protection programme. *Diabet Med* 1998;15:80–84.
14. Reiber GE, Smith DG, Wallace C, et al. Effect of therapeutic footwear on foot reulceration in patients with diabetes: a randomized controlled trial. *JAMA* 2002;287:2552–2558.
15. Uccioli L, Faglia E, Monticone G, et al. Manufactured shoes in the prevention of diabetic foot ulcers. *Diabetes Care* 1995;18:1376–1378.
16. Mason J, O'Keeffe C, Hutchinson A, et al. A systematic review of foot ulcer in patients with type 2 diabetes mellitus. II: treatment. *Diabet Med* 1999;16:889–909. Search date 1998; primary sources Cochrane Controlled Trials Register, Medline, Embase, Cinahl, Healthstar, Psychlit, Science Citation, Social Science Citation, Index to Scientific and Technical Conference Proceedings (ISI), HMIC database, and Sigle.
17. Malone JM, Snyder M, Anderson G, et al. Prevention of amputation by diabetic education. *Am J Surg* 1989;158:520–524.
18. Mueller MJ, Diamond JE, Sinacore DR, et al. Total contact casting in treatment of diabetic planter ulcers. *Diabetes Care* 1989;12:384–388.
19. Armstrong DG, Nguyen HC, Lavery LA, et al. Off-loading the diabetic foot wound: a randomized clinical trial. *Diabetes Care* 2001;24:1019–1022.
20. Caravaggi C, Faglia E, De Giglio R, et al. Effectiveness and safety of a nonremovable fiberglass off-bearing cast versus a therapeutic shoe in the treatment of neuropathic foot ulcers: a randomized study. *Diabetes Care* 2000;23:1746–1751.
21. Veves A, Falanga V, Armstrong DG, et al. Graftskin, a human skin equivalent, is effective in the management of noninfected neuropathic diabetic foot ulcers: a prospective randomized multicenter clinical trial. *Diabetes Care* 2001;24:290–295.
22. Steed DL, Ricotta JJ, Prendergast JJ, et al. Promotion and acceleration of diabetic ulcer healing by arginine-glycine-aspartic acid (RGD) peptide matrix. *Diabetes Care* 1995;18:39–46.
23. Steed DL, and the Diabetic Ulcer Study Group. Clinical evaluation of recombinant human platelet-derived growth factor for the treatment of lower extremity diabetic ulcers. *J Vasc Surg* 1995;21:71–81.
24. Wieman TJ, Smiell JM, Su Y. Efficacy and safety of a topical gel formulation of recombinant human platelet-derived growth factor-BB (Becaplermin) in patients with chronic neuropathic diabetic ulcers. *Diabetes Care* 1998;21:822–827.
25. Steed D, Goslen J, Holloway G, et al. Randomized prospective double-blind trial in healing chronic diabetic foot ulcers. *Diabetes Care* 1992;15:1598–1604.
26. Holloway G, Steed D, DeMarco M, et al. A randomized controlled dose response trial of activated platelet supernatant, topical CT-102 in chronic, non-healing diabetic wounds. *Wounds* 1993;5:198–206.
27. Richard J, Richard C, Daures J, et al. Effect of topical basic fibroblast growth factor on the healing of chronic diabetic neuropathic ulcer of the foot. *Diabetes Care* 1995;18:64–69.
28. Doctor N, Pandya S, Supe A. Hyperbaric oxygen therapy in diabetic foot. *J Postgrad Med* 1992;38:112–114.
29. Faglia E, Favales F, Aldeghi A, et al. Adjunctive systemic hyperbaric oxygen therapy in treatment of severe prevalently ischemic diabetic foot ulcer. *Diabetes Care* 1996;19:1338–1343.

Dereck Hunt
Assistant Professor of Medicine

Hertzel Gerstein
Professor of Medicine
McMaster University
Hamitlon, Ontario, Canada

Competing interests: None declared.

Glycaemic control in diabetes

Search date September 2001

William Herman

QUESTIONS

INTERVENTIONS

Key Messages

Intensive control of hyperglycaemia in people aged 13–75 years

- One systematic review and large subsequent RCTs in people with type 1 or type 2 diabetes have found strong evidence that intensive versus conventional glycaemic control significantly reduces the development and progression of microvascular and neuropathic complications. A second systematic review has found that intensive versus conventional treatment is associated with a small reduction in cardiovascular risk.
- RCTs have found that intensive treatment increases the incidence of hypoglycaemia and weight gain, without adverse impact on neuropsychological function or quality of life.
- The benefit of intensive treatment is limited by the complications of advanced diabetes (such as blindness, end stage renal disease, or cardiovascular disease), major comorbidity, and reduced life expectancy.
- Large RCTs have found that diabetic complications increase with HbA1c concentrations above the non-diabetic range.

Intensive control of hyperglycaemia in people with frequent severe hypoglycaemia

- The benefits of intensive treatment of hyperglycaemia are described above.
- It is difficult to weigh the benefit of reduced complications against the harm of increased hypoglycaemia. The risk of intensive treatment is increased by a history of severe hypoglycaemia or unawareness of hypoglycaemia, advanced autonomic neuropathy or cardiovascular disease, and impaired ability to detect or treat hypoglycaemia (such as altered mental state, immobility, or lack of social support). For people likely to have limited benefit or increased risk with intensive treatment, it may be more appropriate to negotiate less intensive goals for glycaemic management that reflect the person's self determined goals of care and willingness to make lifestyle modifications.

DEFINITION Diabetes mellitus is a group of disorders characterised by hyperglycaemia (definitions vary slightly, one current US definition is fasting plasma glucose ≥ 7.0 mmol/L or ≥ 11.1 mmol/L 2 h after a 75 g oral glucose load, on 2 or more occasions). Intensive treatment is designed to achieve blood glucose values as close to the non-diabetic range as possible. The components of such treatment are education, counselling, monitoring, self management, and pharmacological treatment with insulin or oral antidiabetic agents to achieve specific glycaemic goals.

INCIDENCE/ PREVALENCE Diabetes is diagnosed in around 5% of adults aged 20 years or older in the USA.[1] A further 2.7% have undiagnosed diabetes on the basis of fasting glucose. The prevalence is similar in men and women, but diabetes is more common in some ethnic groups. The prevalence in people aged 40–74 years has increased over the past decade.

AETIOLOGY/ RISK FACTORS Diabetes results from deficient insulin secretion, decreased insulin action, or both. Many processes can be involved, from autoimmune destruction of the β cells of the pancreas to incompletely understood abnormalities that result in resistance to insulin action. Genetic factors are involved in both mechanisms. In type 1 diabetes there is an absolute deficiency of insulin. In type 2 diabetes, insulin resistance and an inability of the pancreas to compensate are involved. Hyperglycaemia without clinical symptoms but sufficient to cause tissue damage can be present for many years before diagnosis.

PROGNOSIS Severe hyperglycaemia causes numerous symptoms, including polyuria, polydipsia, weight loss, and blurred vision. Acute, life threatening consequences of diabetes are hyperglycaemia with ketoacidosis or the non-ketotic hyperosmolar syndrome. There is increased susceptibility to certain infections. Long term complications of diabetes include retinopathy (with potential loss of vision), nephropathy (leading to renal failure), peripheral neuropathy (increased risk of foot ulcers, amputation, and Charcot joints), autonomic neuropathy (cardiovascular, gastrointestinal, and genitourinary dysfunction), and greatly increased risk of atheroma affecting large vessels (macrovascular complications of stroke, myocardial infarction, or peripheral vascular disease). The physical, emotional, and social impact of diabetes and demands of intensive treatment can also create problems for people with diabetes and their families. One systematic review (search date 1998) of observational studies in people with type 2 diabetes found a positive association between increased blood glucose concentration and mortality.[2] It found no minimum threshold level.

AIMS To slow development and progression of the microvascular, neuropathic, and cardiovascular complications of diabetes, while minimising adverse effects of treatment (hypoglycaemia and weight gain) and maximising quality of life.

OUTCOMES Quality of life; short term burden of treatment; long term clinical complications; risks and benefits of treatment. Both the development of complications in people who have previously been free of them, and the progression of complications, are used as outcomes.

Scales of severity are used to detect disease progression (e.g. 19 step scales of diabetic retinopathy; normoalbuminuria, microalbuminuria, and albuminuria for nephropathy; absence or presence of clinical neuropathy).

METHODS *Clinical Evidence* search and appraisal September 2001.

QUESTION What are the effects of intensive versus conventional glycaemic control?

One systematic review and three subsequent RCTs in people with type 1 and type 2 diabetes have found that intensive treatment compared with conventional treatment reduces development and progression of microvascular and neuropathic complications. A second systematic review in people with type 1 diabetes, and two additional RCTs in people with type 2 diabetes, found no evidence that intensive treatment increased adverse cardiovascular outcomes. Intensive treatment reduces the number of macrovascular events but has no significant effect on the number of people who develop macrovascular disease. Intensive treatment is associated with hypoglycaemia and weight gain, but does not seem to affect neuropsychological function or quality of life adversely.

Benefits: **Microvascular and neuropathic complications:** We found one systematic review (search date 1991, 16 small RCTs of type 1 diabetes)[3] and three subsequent long term RCTs [4–6] that found the relative risks of retinopathy, nephropathy, and neuropathy were all significantly reduced by intensive treatment versus conventional treatment (see table 1, p 586). In one subsequent RCT (1441 people with type 1 diabetes) about half had no retinopathy and half had mild retinopathy at baseline.[4] At 6.5 years, intensive treatment significantly reduced the progression of retinopathy and neuropathy. After a further 4 years the benefit was maintained, regardless of whether people stayed in the groups to which they were initially randomised.[7] The difference in the median HbA1c concentration for people initially randomised to intensive or conventional care narrowed. The proportion of people with worsening retinopathy and nephropathy was also significantly lower for those who had received intensive treatment. However, another subsequent RCT compared a conventional dietary treatment policy with two different intensive treatment policies based on sulphonylurea and insulin (3867 people with newly diagnosed type 2 diabetes, age 25–65 years, fasting plasma glucose 6.1–15.0 mmol/L after 3 months' dietary treatment, no symptoms of hyperglycaemia, follow up 10 years).[6] HbA1c rose steadily in both groups. Intensive treatment was associated with a significant reduction in any diabetes related end point (40.9 *v* 46.0 events/1000 person years; RRR 12%, 95% CI 1% to 21%), but no significant effect on diabetes related deaths (10.4 *v* 11.5 deaths/1000 person years; RRR +10%, 95% CI −11% to +27%) or all cause mortality (17.9 *v* 18.9 deaths/1000 person years; RRR +6%, 95% CI −10% to +20%). Secondary analysis found that intensive treatment was associated with a significant reduction in microvascular end points (8.6 *v* 11.4/1000 person years; RRR 25%, 95% CI 7% to 40%) compared with conventional treatment (see table 1, p 586).[6] **Cardiovascular outcomes:**

We found one systematic review[8] and two additional RCTs.[5,6] The systematic review (search date 1996, 6 RCTs, 1731 people with type 1 diabetes followed for 2–8 years) found that intensive insulin treatment versus conventional treatment decreased the number of macrovascular events (OR 0.55, 95% CI 0.35 to 0.88), but had no significant effect on the number of people developing macrovascular disease (OR 0.72, 95% CI 0.44 to 1.17) or on macrovascular mortality (OR 0.91, 95% CI 0.31 to 2.65).[8] The additional RCTs included people with type 2 diabetes.[5,6] In the first RCT the number of major cerebrovascular, cardiovascular, and peripheral vascular events in the intensive treatment group was half that of the conventional treatment group (0.6 *v* 1.3 events/100 person years), but the event rate in this small trial was low and the results were not significant.[5] In the second RCT, intensive treatment versus conventional treatment was associated with a non-significant reduction in the risk of myocardial infarction (AR 387/2729 [14%] with intensive treatment *v* 186/1138 [16%] with conventional treatment; RRR +13%, 95% CI –2% to +27%), a non-significant increase in the risk of stroke (AR 148/2729 [5.4%] *v* 55/1138 [4.8%]; RRI +12%, 95% CI –17% to +51%), and a non-significant reduction in the risk of amputation or death from peripheral vascular disease (AR 29/2729 [1.1%] *v* 18/1138 [1.6%]; RRR +33%, 95% CI –20% to +63%).[6]

Harms: **Hypoglycaemia:** We found one systematic review[9] and three additional RCTs.[5,6,10] The systematic review (search date not stated, 14 RCTs with at least 6 months' follow up and monitoring of HbA1c, 2067 people with type 1 diabetes followed for 0.5–7.5 years) found that the median incidence of severe hypoglycaemia was 7.9 episodes/100 person years among intensively treated people and 4.6 episodes/100 person years among conventionally treated people (OR 3.0, 95% CI 2.5 to 3.6). The risk of severe hypoglycaemia was associated with the degree of HbA1c lowering in the intensive treatment groups ($P = 0.005$). The three additional RCTs included people with type 2 diabetes with lower baseline rates of hypoglycaemia. In the first RCT (110 people), there was no significant difference in rates of hypoglycaemia between groups.[5] In the second RCT (3867 people), the rates of major hypoglycaemic episodes per year were 0.7% with conventional treatment, 1.0% with chlorpropamide, 1.4% with glibenclamide, and 1.8% with insulin. People in the intensive treatment group had significantly more hypoglycaemic episodes than those in the conventional group ($P < 0.0001$).[6] In the third RCT (1704 overweight people) major hypoglycaemic episodes occurred in 0.6% of overweight people in the metformin treated group.[10] **Weight gain:** Four RCTs found more weight increase with intensive treatment than with standard treatment.[4–6,11] One RCT found weight remained stable in people with type 1 diabetes in the conventional treatment group, but body mass index increased by 5.8% in the intensive treatment group (95% CI not presented; $P < 0.01$).[11] In the second RCT (1441 people with type 1 diabetes) intensive treatment was associated with increased risk of developing a body weight more than 120% above the ideal (12.7 cases/100 person years with intensive treatment *v* 9.3 cases/100 person years with conventional treatment; RR 1.33). At 5 years, people treated intensively gained

4.6 kg more than people treated conventionally (CI not provided for weight data).[4] In the third RCT, the increase in body mass index from baseline to 6 years was not significant in either group (intensive treatment group 20.5 to 21.2 kg/m^2, conventional treatment group 20.3–21.9 kg/m^2).[5] In the fourth RCT, weight gain at 10 years was significantly higher in people with type 2 diabetes in the intensive treatment group compared with people in the conventional treatment group (mean 2.9 kg; $P < 0.001$), and people assigned insulin had a greater gain in weight (4.0 kg) than those assigned chlorpropamide (2.6 kg) or glibenclamide (1.7 kg).[6] We found one systematic review (search date 1996, 10 RCTs)[12] and one subsequent RCT[10] comparing metformin and sulphonylurea. Meta-analysis in the review found that sulphonylurea was associated with an increase in weight from baseline and metformin with a decrease (difference 2.9 kg, 95% CI 1.1 kg to 4.4 kg). In the subsequent RCT, overweight participants randomly assigned to intensive blood glucose control with metformin had a similar change in body weight to the conventional treatment group, and less increase in mean body weight than people receiving intensive treatment with sulphonylureas or insulin.[10] **Neuropsychological impairment:** We found no systematic review on neuropsychological impairment, but found two RCTs.[13–16] One RCT (102 people) compared intensified with standard treatment in people with type 1 diabetes. It found no cognitive impairment associated with hypoglycaemia after 3 years.[13,14] The second RCT found that intensive treatment did not affect neuropsychological performance.[15] People who had repeated episodes of hypoglycaemia did not perform differently from people who did not have repeated episodes.[16] **Quality of life:** We found three RCTs that reported quality of life in people undergoing intensive versus conventional treatment.[17–19] Together, they suggested that quality of life is lowered by complications, but is not lowered directly by intensive versus conventional treatment. The first RCT (1441 people) found that intensive treatment did not reduce quality of life in people with type 1 diabetes.[17] Severe hypoglycaemia was not consistently associated with a subsequent increase in distress caused by symptoms or decline in the quality of life. However, in the primary prevention intensive treatment group, repeated severe hypoglycaemia (3 or more events resulting in coma or seizure) tended to increase the risk of distress caused by symptoms. The second RCT (77 adolescents with type 1 diabetes) found after 1 year that behavioural intervention plus intensive diabetes management versus intensive diabetes management alone significantly improved quality of life, diabetes and medical self efficacy, and HbA1c (7.5% *v* 8.5%; $P = 0.001$).[18] The behavioural intervention included six small group sessions and monthly follow up aimed at social problem solving, cognitive behaviour modification, and conflict resolution. The third RCT of intensive versus conventional treatment of type 2 diabetes assessed quality of life in two large cross sectional samples at 8 and 11 years after randomisation (disease specific measures in 2431 people and generic measures in 3104 people), and also in a small cohort (diabetes specific quality of life measures in 374 people 6 months after randomisation and annually thereafter for 6 years).[19] The cross-sectional studies found no significant effect of intensive versus conventional treatment on scores for mood, cognitive mistakes, symptoms, work satisfaction, or general health. The longitudinal study also found no significant difference in quality of life scores other than a small increase in the number of symptoms in people allocated to conventional than to intensive treatment. In the cross sectional studies, people who had macrovascular or microvascular complications in the past year had lower quality of life than people without complications. People treated with insulin who had two or more hypoglycaemic episodes during the previous year reported more tension, more overall mood disturbance, and less work satisfaction than those with no hypoglycaemic attacks (after adjusting for age, time from randomisation, systolic blood pressure, HbA1c, and sex). It was unclear whether frequent hypoglycaemic episodes affected quality of life, or whether people with certain personality traits or symptoms simply reported increased numbers of hypoglycaemic attacks.

Comment: We found one follow up study in people with type 1 diabetes 11.4 years after randomisation.[20] In people originally randomised to intensive treatment, it found that the fall in systolic blood pressure with upright posture (one measure of cardiovascular sympathetic dysfunction) and cardiovascular parasympathetic autonomic dysfunction (regardless of how it was measured) developed at a significantly slower pace.[20]

QUESTION What is the optimum target blood glucose?

Large RCTs in people with type 1 and type 2 diabetes have found that risk of development or progression of complications increases progressively as HbA1c increases above the non-diabetic range.

Benefits: We found no systematic review but found two large RCTs.[4,6] The first RCT (1441 people with type 1 diabetes) found that lower HbA1c was associated with a lower risk of complications.[4,21] The second RCT (3867 people with type 2 diabetes) found that, as concentrations of HbA1c were reduced, the risk of complications fell but the risk of hypoglycaemia increased.[6,19] A further analysis of the second RCT (3642 people who had HbA1c measured 3 months after the diagnosis of diabetes and who had complete data whether or not they were randomised in the trial) found that each 1% reduction in mean HbA1c was associated with reduced risk of any diabetes related microvascular or macrovascular event (RR 0.79, 95% CI 0.76 to 0.83), diabetes related death (RR 0.79, 95% CI 0.73 to 0.85), all cause mortality (RR 0.86, 95% CI 0.81 to 0.91), microvascular complications (RR 0.63, 95% CI 0.59 to 0.67), and myocardial infarction (RR 0.86, 95% CI 0.79 to 0.92).[22] These prospective observational data suggested that there is no lower glycaemic threshold for the risk of complications; the better the glycaemic control, the lower the risk of complications. They also suggested that the rate of increase of risk for microvascular disease with hyperglycaemia is greater than that for macrovascular disease.

Harms: Both RCTs found that hypoglycaemia was increased by intensive treatment.[19,21]

Comment: It is difficult to weigh the benefit of reduced complications against the harm of increased hypoglycaemia. The balance between benefits and harms of intensive treatment in type 1 diabetes may be less favourable in children under 13 years or in older adults, and in people with repeated severe hypoglycaemia or unawareness of hypoglycaemia. Similarly, the balance between benefits and harms of intensive treatment in type 2 diabetes may be less favourable in people over 65 years or in those with longstanding diabetes. The benefit of intensive treatment is limited by the complications of advanced diabetes (such as blindness, end stage renal disease, or cardiovascular disease), major comorbidity, and reduced life expectancy. The risk of intensive treatment is increased by a history of severe hypoglycaemia or unawareness of hypoglycaemia, advanced autonomic neuropathy or cardiovascular disease, and impaired ability to detect or treat hypoglycaemia (such as altered mental state, immobility, or lack of social support). For people likely to have limited benefit or increased risk with intensive treatment, it may be more appropriate to negotiate less intensive goals for glycaemic management that reflect the person's self determined goals of care and willingness to make lifestyle modifications.

REFERENCES

1. Harris MI, Flegal KM, Cowie CC, et al. Prevalence of diabetes, impaired fasting glucose, and impaired glucose tolerance in US adults: the third national health and nutrition examination survey, 1988–1994. *Diabetes Care* 1998;2:518–524.
2. Groeneveld Y, Petri H, Hermans J, et al. Relationship between blood glucose level and mortality in type 2 diabetes mellitus: a systematic review. *Diabet Med* 1999;16:2–13. Search date 1998; primary source Medline.
3. Wang PH, Lau J, Chalmers TC. Meta-analysis of effects of intensive blood glucose control on late complications of type I diabetes. *Lancet* 1993;341:1306–1309. Search date 1991; primary source Medline.
4. The Diabetes Control and Complications Trial Research Group. The effect of intensive treatment of diabetes on the development and progression of long-term complications in insulin-dependent diabetes mellitus. *N Engl J Med* 1993;329:977–986.
5. Ohkubo Y, Kishikawa H, Arake E, et al. Intensive insulin therapy prevents the progression of diabetic microvascular complications in Japanese patients with non-insulin-dependent diabetes mellitus: a randomized prospective 6-year study. *Diabetes Res Clin Pract* 1995;28:103–117.
6. UK Prospective Diabetes Study Group. Intensive blood-glucose control with sulphonylureas or insulin compared with conventional treatment and risk of complications in patients with type 2 diabetes. *Lancet* 1998;352:837–853.
7. The DCCT/Epidemiology of Diabetes Interventions and Complications Research Group. Retinopathy and nephropathy in patients with type 1 diabetes four years after a trial of intensive therapy. *N Engl J Med* 2000;342:381–389.
8. Lawson ML, Gerstein HC, Tsui E, et al. Effect of intensive therapy on early macrovascular disease in young individuals with type 1 diabetes. *Diabetes Care* 1999;22:B35–B39. Search date 1996; primary sources Medline, Citation Index, reference lists, and personal files.
9. Egger M, Smith GD, Stettler C, et al. Risk of adverse effects of intensified treatment in insulin-dependent diabetes mellitus: a meta-analysis. *Diabet Med* 1997;14:919–928. Search date not stated; primary sources Medline, reference lists, and specialist journals.
10. UK Prospective Diabetes Study Group. Effect of intensive blood-glucose control with metformin on complications in overweight patients with type 2 diabetes. *Lancet* 1998;352:854–865.
11. Reichard P, Berglund B, Britz A, et al. Intensified conventional insulin treatment retards the microvascular complications of insulin-dependent diabetes mellitus (IDDM): the Stockholm diabetes intervention study (SDIS) after 5 years. *J Intern Med* 1991;30:101–108.
12. Johansen K. Efficacy of metformin in the treatment of NIDDM. *Diabetes Care* 1999;22:33–37. Search date 1996; primary sources current list of medical literature, Index Medicus, Medline, Embase, and hand searched references.
13. Reichard P, Nilsson BY, Rosenqvist U. The effect of long-term intensified insulin treatment on the development of microvascular complications of diabetes mellitus. *N Engl J Med* 1993;29:304–309.
14. Reichard P, Berglund A, Britz A, et al. Hypoglycaemic episodes during intensified insulin treatment: increased frequency but no effect on cognitive function. *J Intern Med* 1991;229:9–16.
15. The Diabetes Control and Complications Trial Research Group. Effects of intensive diabetes therapy on neuropsychological function in adults in the diabetes control and complications trial. *Ann Intern Med* 1996;124:379–388.
16. Austin EJ, Deary IJ. Effects of repeated hypoglycaemia on cognitive function. A psychometrically validated reanalysis of the diabetes control and complications trial data. *Diabetes Care* 1999;22:1273–1277.
17. The Diabetes Control and Complications Trial Research Group. Influence of intensive diabetes treatment on quality-of-life outcomes in the diabetes control and complications trial. *Diabetes Care* 1996;19:195–203.
18. Grey M, Boland EA, Davidson M, Li J, Tamborlane W. Coping skills training for youth with diabetes

mellitus has long-lasting effects on metabolic control and quality of life. *J Pediatr* 2000;137:107–113.

19. UK Prospective Diabetes Study Group. Quality of life in type 2 diabetic patients is affected by complications but not by intensive policies to improve blood glucose or blood pressure control (UKPDS 37). *Diabetes Care* 1999;22:1125–1136.
20. Reichard P, Jensen-Urstad K, Ericsson M, Jensen-Urstad M, Lindblad LE. Automonic neuropathy – a complication less pronounced in patients with type 1 diabetes mellitus who have lower blood glucose levels. *Diabet Med* 2000;17:860–866.
21. The Diabetes Control and Complications Trial Research Group. The absence of a glycaemic threshold for the development of long-term complications: the perspective of the diabetes control and complications trial. *Diabetes* 1996;45:1289–1298.
22. Stratton IM, Adler AI, Neil HAW, et al, on behalf of the UK Prospective Diabetes Study Group. Association of glycaemia with macrovascular and microvascular complications of type 2 diabetes (UKPDS 35): prospective observational study. *BMJ* 2000;321:405–412

William Herman
Professor of Internal Medicine and Epidemiology
University of Michigan Medical Center
Ann Arbor Michigan
USA

Competing interests: None declared.

TABLE 1 **Risk (odds ratio) for development or progression of microvascular, nephropathic, and neuropathic complications with intensive versus conventional treatment. Odds ratio, number needed to treat, and confidence intervals were all calculated from data in papers (see text, p 580).**

	Systematic Review[3]	DCCT[4]	Kumamoto[5]	UKPDS[6]
Studies	16 RCTs	RCT	RCT	RCT
Number of participants	ND	1441	110	3867
Type of diabetes	Type 1	Type 1	Type 2	Type 2*
Follow up	8–60 months	6.5 years	6 years	10 years
Change in HbA1c	1.4%	2.0%	2.0%	0.9%
Progression of retinopathy				
OR (95% CI)	0.49 (0.28 to 0.85)	0.39 (0.28 to 0.55)	0.25 (0.09 to 0.65)	0.66 (0.48 to 0.92)
NNT (95% CI) over duration of study	ND	5 (4 to 7)	4 (3 to 11)	10 (6 to 50)
Development of retinopathy				
OR (95% CI)	ND	0.22 (0.14 to 0.36)	ND	ND
NNT (95% CI) over duration of study	ND	6 (5 to 7)	ND	ND
Development or progression of nephropathy				
OR (95% CI)	0.34 (0.20 to 0.58)	0.50 (0.39 to 0.63)	0.26 (0.09 to 0.76)	0.54 (0.25 to 1.18)
NNT (95% CI) over duration of study	ND	7 (6 to 11)	5 (4 to 19)	ND
Development or progression of neuropathy				
OR (95% CI)	ND	0.36 (0.24 to 0.54)	ND	0.42 (0.23 to 0.78)
NNT (95% CI) over duration of study	ND	13 (11 to 18)	ND	5 (3 to 16)

*All participants had fasting plasma glucose > 6.0 mmol/L on two occasions: 93% had fasting plasma glucose ≥ 7.0 mmol/L (American Diabetes Association criterion) and 86% had fasting plasma glucose ≥ 7.8 mmol/L (World Health Organization criterion). CI, confidence interval; ND, no data.

Search date May 2002

David Arterburn

QUESTIONS

INTERVENTIONS

To be covered in future updates
Ephedrine-caffeine; olestra; acarbose; cholecystokinin agonists; neuropeptide Y antagonists; β3 adrenergic agonists; leptin; growth hormone; surgery.

Covered elsewhere in *Clinical Evidence*
Non-drug therapy: see changing behaviour, p 37
Weight loss: see primary prevention, p 95

See glossary, p 597

Key Messages

- **Dexfenfluramine** One systematic review found that dexfenfluramine versus placebo promotes weight loss in healthy obese adults. Dexfenfluramine has been associated with valvular heart disease and pulmonary hypertension and is no longer marketed for use in obesity.
- **Diethylpropion** One systematic review found that diethylpropion versus placebo promotes modest weight loss in healthy obese adults. We found two case reports describing pulmonary hypertension and psychosis with diethylpropion. We found insufficient evidence on weight regain and long term safety. Diethylpropion is no longer marketed in Europe for use in obesity because of a possible link between diethylpropion and heart and lung problems that could not be totally excluded.
- **Fenfluramine** One systematic review found that fenfluramine versus placebo promotes modest weight loss in healthy obese adults. Fenfluramine has been associated with valvular heart disease and pulmonary hypertension and is no longer marketed for use in obesity.
- **Fenfluramine plus phentermine** One RCT found that fenfluramine plus phentermine versus placebo promoted weight loss. The combination of fenfluramine plus phentermine has been associated with valvular heart disease and pulmonary hypertension and is no longer marketed for use in obesity.

- **Fluoxetine** One systematic review found that fluoxetine versus placebo promotes modest weight loss in healthy obese adults. We found insufficient evidence on weight regain and long term safety of fluoxetine in obesity. One systematic review of antidepressant treatment has found an association between selective serotonin reuptake inhibitors and uncommon but serious adverse events including bradycardia, bleeding, granulocytopenia, seizures, hyponatraemia, hepatotoxicity, serotonin syndrome and extrapyramidal effects.
- **Mazindol** One systematic review found that mazindol versus placebo promotes modest weight loss in healthy obese adults. We found one case report of pulmonary hypertension diagnosed 1 year after stopping treatment with mazindol. We found one clinical evaluation of mazindol in people with stable cardiac disease that found an association between mazindol and cardiac events such as atrial fibrillation. We found insufficient evidence on weight regain and long term safety.
- **Orlistat** Systematic reviews and subsequent RCTs have found that in addition to a low calorie diet, orlistat versus placebo modestly increases weight loss in adults with obesity. Adverse effects such as oily spotting from the rectum, flatulence, and faecal urgency occurred in up to 27% of people taking orlistat. We found insufficient evidence on weight regain and long term safety.
- **Phentermine** One systematic review found that phentermine versus placebo promotes modest weight loss in healthy obese adults. We found insufficient evidence on weight regain and long term safety. Phentermine is no longer marketed in Europe for use in obesity because a link between phentermine and heart and lung problems could not be totally excluded.
- **Phenylpropanolamine** One systematic review found that phenylpropanolamine versus placebo promotes modest weight loss in healthy obese adults. One case control study found that phenylpropanolamine significantly increased risk of haemorrhagic stroke in the first 3 days of use. Phenylpropanolamine is no longer marketed for use in obesity.
- **Sibutramine** A systematic review and RCTs have found that sibutramine versus placebo promotes modest weight loss in healthy, obese adults (body mass index 25–40 kg/m^2) with diabetes, hyperlipidaemia and hypertension. One RCT has found that sibutramine is more effective than placebo for weight maintenance after weight loss in healthy, obese adults but weight regain occurs when sibutramine is discontinued. Sibutramine is no longer marketed in Italy for use in obesity because of concerns about severe adverse reactions including tachycardia, hypertension, arrhythmia, and two deaths due to cardiac arrests. One RCT found that sibutramine achieved greater weight loss than either orlistat or metformin.
- **Sibutramine plus orlistat** One RCT found no significant change in mean body weight over a 16 week period with sibutramine plus orlistat versus sibutramine alone.

DEFINITION Obesity is a chronic condition characterised by an excess of body fat. It is most often defined by the body mass index (BMI) (see glossary, p 597), a mathematical formula that is highly correlated with body fat. BMI is weight in kilograms divided by height in metres squared (kg/m^2). In the USA and UK, people with BMIs between 25–30 kg/m^2 are categorised as overweight, and those with BMIs above 30 kg/m^2 are categorised as obese.[1] Nearly 5 million US adults used prescription weight loss medication in 1996–1998. A quarter of users were not overweight, suggesting that weight loss medication may be inappropriately used. This is thought to be especially the case among women, white people, and Hispanic people.[2]

INCIDENCE/ PREVALENCE Obesity has increased steadily in many countries since 1900. In the UK in 1994, it was estimated that 13% of men and 16% of women were obese.[1,3] In the past decade alone, the prevalence of obesity in the USA has increased from 12% in 1991 to 27% in 1999.[4]

AETIOLOGY/ RISK FACTORS The cause of obesity includes both genetic and environmental factors. Obesity may also be induced by drugs (e.g. high dose glucocorticoids), or be secondary to a variety of neuroendocrine disorders such as Cushing's syndrome and polycystic ovary syndrome.[5]

PROGNOSIS Obesity is a risk factor for several chronic diseases, including hypertension, dyslipidaemia, diabetes, cardiovascular disease, sleep apnoea, osteoarthritis, and some cancers.[1] The relation between increasing body weight and mortality is curvilinear, with mortality rate increasing in people with low body weight. Whether this is caused by increased mortality risk at low body weights or by unintentional weight loss is not clear.[6] Results from five prospective cohort studies and 1991 national statistics suggest that the number of annual deaths attributable to obesity among US adults is about 280 000.[7]

AIMS To achieve realistic gradual weight loss and prevent the morbidity and mortality associated with obesity, without undue adverse effects.

OUTCOMES We found no studies that used the primary outcomes of functional morbidity or mortality. Proxy measures include mean weight loss (kg), number of people losing 5% or more of baseline body weight, and number of people maintaining weight loss.

METHODS *Clinical Evidence* update search and appraisal May 2002.

QUESTION What are the effects of drug treatments in adults?

OPTION SIBUTRAMINE

A systematic review and RCTs have found that that sibutramine versus placebo promotes modest weight loss in healthy obese adults (body mass index 25–40 kg/m^2) with diabetes, hyperlipidaemia, and hypertension. One RCT has found that sibutramine is also more effective than placebo for weight maintenance after weight loss in healthy obese adults but weight regain occurs when sibutramine is discontinued. Sibutramine is no longer marketed in Italy for use in obesity because of concerns about severe adverse reactions including tachycardia, hypertension, arrhythmia, and two deaths due to cardiac arrests. One RCT found that sibutramine achieved greater weight loss than either orlistat or metformin. Another RCT found no significant change in mean body weight over a 16 week period with sibutramine plus orlistat versus sibutramine alone.

Benefits: **Sibutramine:** We found one systematic review (search date 2000, 11 RCTs),[8] six additional RCTs,[9–14] and five subsequent RCTs[15–19] comparing sibutramine versus placebo (see table 1, p 601). The systematic review pooled data for groups of RCTs with similar follow up.[8] The review found that sibutramine (10–20 mg daily) reduced weight more than placebo after 8 weeks (3 RCTs, 106 people, WMD sibutramine v placebo –3.4 kg, 95% CI –4.22 kg to –2.58 kg).[8] The review also pooled analyses of two 6 month trials (207 people) and found that sibutramine (10–20 mg daily) achieved weight loss of 5% or greater more frequently than placebo (RR for > 5% weight loss: sibutramine v placebo 2.1, 95% CI 1.7 to 2.6).[8] One RCT (485 healthy, obese adults) comparing sibutramine (10 or 15 mg daily) versus placebo for 52 weeks found that sibutramine reduced weight more than placebo (–4.4 kg v –6.4 kg v –1.6 kg; $P < 0.01$ sibutramine 10 mg or 15 mg v placebo).[11] A second RCT compared intermittent sibutramine (15 mg daily for wks 1–12, 19–30, and 37–48) versus continuous sibutramine (15 mg daily) versus placebo for 48 weeks. The RCT found no significant difference between intermittent and continuous sibutramine: both regimens reduced weight more than placebo (1001 healthy obese adults, –3.3 kg v –3.8 kg v +0.2 kg; $P < 0.001$ intermittent or continuous sibutramine v placebo).[10] Five RCTs found that maximal weight loss with sibutramine may be achieved as early as 12 weeks and longer duration trials suggest that weight loss continues until 24 weeks.[9–11,14,17] One RCT (605 healthy, obese adults) evaluated sibutramine for weight maintenance for 2 years.[12] People received sibutramine (10 mg daily) plus diet for 6 months; 467 people with more than 5% weight loss were then randomly assigned to sibutramine (10 mg daily) or placebo for an additional 18 months. The RCT found that a greater proportion of people maintained 80% or more of their original weight loss at 24 months with sibutramine versus placebo (43% with sibutramine v 16% with placebo; $P < 0.001$). Weight regain occurred when sibutramine was discontinued (73% of initial weight loss regained over 18 months).[12] Another RCT followed people for 6 months after discontinuation of sibutramine and reported 43% weight regain.[19] Three RCTs in obese adults with type 2 diabetes[13,16,18] and one RCT in obese adults with hyperlipidaemia[15] have found a significant decrease in weight with sibutramine versus placebo when used in addition to dietary modification. Two other RCTs in obese adults with hypertension have found a significant decrease in weight with sibutramine versus placebo.[9,17] **Versus orlistat or metformin**: We found one RCT (150 obese women) comparing sibutramine (20 mg daily) versus orlistat (120 mg 3 times daily) versus metformin (850 mg twice daily) for 6 months.[20] All people were also instructed to follow a reduced calorie diet. The RCT found that sibutramine achieved greater weight loss than either orlistat or metformin (–13.0 kg with sibutramine v –8.0 kg with orlistat v –9.0 kg with metformin; $P < 0.0001$). **Sibutramine plus orlistat**: We found one RCT (42 women who had completed 1 year of sibutramine plus lifestyle modification), which compared sibutramine (10–15 mg daily) plus orlistat (120 mg 3 times daily) versus sibutramine plus placebo.[21] Mean body weight did not change significantly in either group over a 16 week period (+0.1 kg with combined treatment v +0.5 kg with sibutramine plus placebo).

Harms: **Sibutramine:** We found no evidence about safety beyond 2 years of treatment. Sibutramine was withdrawn from the market in Italy in 2002 in response to 50 reported adverse reactions, including seven severe adverse reactions (tachycardia, hypertension, and arrhythmia) and two deaths due to cardiac arrests. To date, none of the other regulatory agencies including the Medicines Control Agency, UK; the Food & Drug Administration, USA; Health, Canada; and the Therapeutics Goods Administration, Australia have taken any regulatory actions against the drug.[22] **Versus orlistat or metformin**: One RCT reported dry mouth, insomnia, constipation, and hypertension with sibutramine and abdominal discomfort with orlistat and metformin.[20] **Sibutramine plus orlistat**: One RCT reported that people who received sibutramine plus orlistat experienced more soft stools (50%), bowel movements (50%), and oily evacuation (42.9%) than those who received sibutramine alone (9.1% with sibutramine plus orlistat, 9.1% with sibutramine alone, and 0% with placebo; $P < 0.05$).[21]

Comment: None.

OPTION PHENTERMINE

One systematic review found that phentermine versus placebo promotes modest weight loss in healthy obese adults. We found insufficient evidence on weight regain and long term safety. Phentermine is no longer marketed in Europe for use in obesity because a link between phentermine and heart and lung problems could not be totally excluded.

Benefits: We found one systematic review (search date 1999, 6 RCTs) comparing phentermine (15–30 mg daily) versus placebo in healthy, obese adults with mean follow up of 13.2 weeks (range 2–24 wks).[23] The mean numbers of people in each arm were 32 (range 15–76) for phentermine and 29.4 (range 12–74) for placebo. The review found that phentermine produced significant weight loss (effect size < 0.8 [information presented graphically]; difference in weight loss between phentermine and placebo in the 6 RCTs ranged from 0.6–6.0 kg). The review also compared phentermine versus other agents (diethylpropion, dexfenfluramine, fenfluramine, fluoxetine, mazindol, orlistat, phenylpropanolamine, and sibutramine) and found no significant difference in effect size between phentermine and the other agents (based on 95% CIs).[23]

Harms: The systematic review did not make any comment on adverse effects.[23] We found no evidence of serious adverse reactions. Phentermine given alone has not been associated with valvular heart disease.[24] A European Commission review of the risks and benefits of phentermine concluded that randomised trials do not adequately show efficacy for weight loss. Although no new safety problems were identified with phentermine, the Commission commented that a link between phentermine and "heart and lung problems could not be totally excluded". As a result of this report and subsequent regulatory actions, phentermine has been withdrawn from the market in Europe.[25]

Comment: Most of the people treated with phentermine received additional lifestyle treatment.[23] High withdrawal rates have been reported for phentermine.

OPTION MAZINDOL

One systematic review found that mazindol versus placebo promotes modest weight loss in healthy obese adults. We found one case report of pulmonary hypertension diagnosed 1 year after stopping treatment with mazindol. We found one clinical evaluation of mazindol in people with stable cardiac disease that found an association between mazindol and cardiac events such as atrial fibrillation. We found insufficient evidence on weight regain and long term safety.

Benefits: We found one systematic review (search date 1999, 22 RCTs) comparing mazindol (1–3 mg daily) versus placebo in healthy obese adults with mean follow up of 11.0 weeks (range 2–20 wks).[23] The mean number of people in each arm was 24 (range 8–50) for mazindol and 18 (range 8–30) for placebo. The review found that mazindol produced weight loss that was significantly different from placebo (effect size < 0.8 [information presented graphically]; difference in weight loss between mazindol and placebo in the 22 RCTs ranged from 0.1–7.3 kg). The review also compared mazindol versus other agents (diethylpropion, dexfenfluramine, fenfluramine, fluoxetine, orlistat, phenylpropanolamine, phentermine, and sibutramine) and found no significant difference in effect size between mazindol and the other agents except sibutramine and fenfluramine (based on 95% CIs).[23]

Harms: The systematic review did not comment on adverse effects.[23] We found a single case report of pulmonary hypertension diagnosed 12 months after stopping mazindol that had been taken for 10 weeks.[26] One clinical evaluation in people with stable cardiac disease found an association between mazindol and cardiac events (3 episodes of atrial fibrillation and 2 of syncope in 15 people receiving mazindol for 12 wks).[27] The frequency of serious adverse events with this agent remains unclear.

Comment: None.

OPTION DIETHYLPROPION

One systematic review found that diethylpropion versus placebo promotes modest weight loss in healthy obese adults. We found two case reports describing pulmonary hypertension and psychosis with diethylpropion. We found insufficient evidence on weight regain and long term safety. Diethylpropion is no longer marketed in Europe for use in obesity because a link between diethylpropion and heart and lung problems could not be totally excluded.

Benefits: We found one systematic review (search date 1999, 9 RCTs) comparing diethylpropion (75 mg daily) versus placebo in healthy, obese adults with mean follow up of 17.6 weeks (range 6–52 wks).[23] The mean number of people in each arm was 22 (range 5–32) for diethylpropion and 18 (range 4–29) for placebo. The review found that diethylpropion produced weight loss that was significantly different from placebo (effect size < 0.8 [information presented graphically]; difference in weight loss between diethylpropion and placebo in the 9 RCTs ranged from 1.6–11.5 kg). The review also compared diethylpropion versus other agents (dexfenfluramine, fenfluramine, fluoxetine, mazindol, orlistat, phenylpropanolamine, phentermine, and sibutramine) and found no significant difference in effect size between diethylpropion and the other agents (based on 95% CIs).[23]

Harms: The systematic review did not comment on adverse effects.[23] Case reports have described pulmonary hypertension and psychosis in users of diethylpropion.[28,29] The frequency of serious adverse events with this agent remains unclear. A European Commission review of the risks and benefits of diethylpropion concluded that randomised trials do not adequately show efficacy for weight loss. Although no new safety problems were identified with diethylpropion, the Commission commented that a link between diethylpropion and "heart and lung problems could not be totally excluded". As a result of this report and subsequent legal actions, diethylpropion has been withdrawn from the market in Europe.[25]

Comment: None.

OPTION FLUOXETINE

One systematic review found that fluoxetine versus placebo promotes modest weight loss in healthy obese adults. We found insufficient evidence on weight regain and long term safety of fluoxetine in obesity. One systematic review of antidepressant treatment has found an association between selective serotonin reuptake inhibitors and uncommon but serious adverse events including bradycardia, bleeding, granulocytopenia, seizures, hyponatraemia, hepatotoxicity, serotonin syndrome, and extrapyramidal effects.

Benefits: We found one systematic review (search date 1999) comparing fluoxetine (32.5–60.0 mg daily) versus placebo.[23] This review included 11 RCTs in healthy, obese adults with mean follow up of 27.5 weeks (range 6–60 wks). The mean number of people in each arm was 55.2 (range 9–136) for fluoxetine and 55.7 (range 9–136) for placebo. The review found that fluoxetine produced significant weight loss (effect size < 0.8 [information presented graphically]; difference in weight loss between fluoxetine and placebo in the 11 RCTs ranged from 0.2–7.4 kg). The review also compared fluoxetine versus other agents (diethylpropion, dexfenfluramine, fenfluramine, mazindol, orlistat, phenylpropanolamine, phentermine, and sibutramine) and found no significant difference in effect size between fluoxetine and the other agents except sibutramine and fenfluramine (based on 95% CIs).[23]

Harms: One systematic review did not comment on adverse effects.[23] One RCT (not included in the systematic review[23]) comparing fluoxetine versus placebo for obesity reported more frequent gastrointestinal symptoms, sleep disturbance, sweating, tremor, amnesia, and thirst in the active treatment groups (frequency of events not provided).[30] One systematic review (search date 1998) of antidepressant treatment found that selective serotonin reuptake inhibitors were associated with a 10–15% incidence of anxiety, diarrhoea, dry mouth, headache, and nausea. The review also found an association between selective serotonin reuptake inhibitors and uncommon but serious adverse events including bradycardia, bleeding, granulocytopenia, seizures, hyponatraemia, hepatotoxicity, serotonin syndrome, and extrapyramidal effects (see glossary, p 598).[31]

Comment: None.

OPTION FENFLURAMINE OR DEXFENFLURAMINE

One systematic review found that fenfluramine, dexfenfluramine, or fenfluramine plus phentermine versus placebo promotes modest weight loss in healthy obese adults. Dexfenfluramine, fenfluramine, and fenfluramine plus phentermine have been associated with valvular heart disease and pulmonary hypertension and are no longer marketed for use in obesity.

Benefits: **Fenfluramine:** We found one systematic review (search date 1999) comparing fenfluramine (39–120 mg daily) versus placebo.[23] This review included 14 RCTs in healthy obese adults with mean follow up of 9.7 weeks (range 4–18 wks). The mean number of people in each arm was 20 (range 5–58) for fenfluramine and 21.2 (range 6–68) for placebo. The review found that fenfluramine produced significant weight loss (effect size > 0.8 [information presented graphically]; difference in weight loss between fenfluramine and placebo in the 14 RCTs ranged from 0.1–5.0 kg). The review found no significant difference in effect size between fenfluramine and the other agents but fenfluramine produced significantly better weight loss compared with other agents except sibutramine (based on 95% CIs). **Dexfenfluramine:** We found one systematic review (search date 1999) comparing dexfenfluramine (30–130 mg daily) versus placebo.[23] This review included 14 RCTs in healthy, obese adults with mean follow up of 30 weeks (range 4–56 wks). The mean number of people in each arm was 46.6 (range 5–295) for dexfenfluramine and 44.1 (range 5–268) for placebo. The review found that dexfenfluramine produced weight loss that was significantly different from placebo (effect size < 0.8 [information presented graphically]; difference in weight loss between dexfenfluramine and placebo in the 14 RCTs ranged from 0.2–10.0 kg). The review found no significant difference in effect size between dexfenfluramine and the other agents except sibutramine and fenfluramine (based on 95% CIs). **Fenfluramine plus phentermine:** We found one RCT (121 people, 30–80% overweight), which found that a combination of phentermine (15 mg daily) plus fenfluramine (60 mg daily) reduced weight more than placebo after treatment for 6 months (–14.3 kg with phentermine plus fenfluramine *v* –4.6 kg with placebo; mean difference –9.7 kg, 95% CI –12.0 to –7.4 kg). The trial found that weight loss ceased at 18 weeks of treatment; weight regain was noted after 60 weeks of treatment.[32]

Harms: **Dexfenfluramine, fenfluramine, fenfluramine plus phentermine:** These agents have been associated with valvular heart disease and primary pulmonary hypertension,[33,34] and are no longer marketed.[35] One 25 centre retrospective cohort study in 1473 people found prevalence rates and relative risk of aortic regurgitation of 8.9% with dexfenfluramine (RR 2.18, 95% CI 1.32 to 3.59; NNH 20) and 13.7% with phentermine plus fenfluramine (RR 3.34, 95% CI 2.09 to 5.35; NNH 10) compared with 4.1% with no treatment.[36] At 1 year follow up using repeat echocardiography of 1114 people (75.6% of people recruited), more of the dexfenfluramine and fenfluramine plus phentermine group had decreased aortic regurgitation versus controls (6.4% with dexfenfluramine *v* 1.7% controls; P < 0.001; 4.5% with fenfluramine plus phentermine; P = 0.03).[37] One prospective study (1072 people) found no significant increase in the risk of valvular heart disease in people taking dexfenfluramine for less than 3 months compared with those taking placebo (sustained release dexfenfluramine RR 1.6, 95% CI 0.8 to 3.4; regular dexfenfluramine RR 1.4, 95% CI 0.7 to 3.0, when compared with placebo).[38] At 1 year follow up, repeat echocardiography of 914 people (83.5% of people recruited) revealed more people had a reduction in aortic regurgitation in both dexfenfluramine groups versus placebo (5.1% sustained release dexfenfluramine; P = 0.002 and 6.4% regular dexfenfluramine; P < 0.001).[39] One case control study (95 people with primary pulmonary hypertension and 355 matched controls) found a history of fenfluramine use was associated with increased risk of primary pulmonary hypertension (OR 6.3, 95% CI 3.0 to 13.2). The odds ratio was higher among people who had taken fenfluramine in the past year (OR 10.1, 95% CI 3.4 to 29.9), and among people treated for more than 3 months (OR 23.1, 95% CI 6.9 to 77.7).[40]

Comment: None.

OPTION PHENYLPROPANOLAMINE

One systematic review found that phenylpropanolamine versus placebo promotes modest weight loss in healthy obese adults. One case control study found that phenylpropanolamine significantly increased risk of haemorrhagic stroke in the first 3 days of use. Phenylpropanolamine is no longer marketed for use in obesity.

Benefits: We found one systematic review (search date 1999) comparing phenylpropanolamine (57–75 mg daily) versus placebo.[23] This review included 7 RCTs in healthy obese adults with mean follow up of 7.4 weeks (range 2–14 wks). The mean number of people in each arm was 23.5 (range 8–36) for phenylpropanolamine and 22.4 (range 10–36) for placebo. The review found that phenylpropanolamine produced significant weight loss (effect size < 0.8 [information presented graphically]; difference in weight loss between phenylpropanolamine and placebo in the 7 RCTs ranged from 0.3–2.0 kg). The review also compared phenylpropanolamine versus other agents (diethylpropion, dexfenfluramine, fenfluramine, fluoxetine, mazindol, orlistat, phentermine, and sibutramine) and found no significant difference in effect size between phenylpropanolamine and the other agents except sibutramine and fenfluramine (based on 95% CIs).[23]

Harms: A case control study (men and women aged 18–49 years) found that phenylpropanolamine used as an appetite suppressant increased the risk of haemorrhagic stroke within the first 3 days of use (adjusted OR 15.9, lower confidence limit 2.04; $P = 0.013$). For the association between phenylpropanolamine in appetite suppressants and risk for haemorrhagic stroke among women, the adjusted odds ratio was 16.6 (lower confidence limit 2.2; $P = 0.011$).[41] Phenylpropanolamine is no longer marketed for use in obesity.[42]

Comment: None.

OPTION ORLISTAT

Systematic reviews and subsequent RCTs have found that in addition to a low calorie diet, orlistat versus placebo modestly increases weight loss in adults with obesity. Adverse effects such as oily spotting from the rectum, flatulence, and faecal urgency occurred in up to 27% of people taking orlistat. We found insufficient evidence on weight regain and long term safety.

Benefits: We found two systematic reviews (search dates 2000),[43,44] one licensing review[45] and three additional RCTs.[46–48] The most comprehensive of the three reviews included 14 RCTs and pooled data for groups of RCTs with similar study designs.[44] Studies were excluded if they did not analyse separately people who were not overweight or obese. The 11 published RCTs in the systematic review (5124 adults with mean body mass index [see glossary, p 597] > 30 kg/m^2) found no significant difference in weight after 12 weeks between orlistat (50–60 mg 3 times daily) plus reduced calorie diet versus placebo plus diet (2 RCTs: WMD −1.24 kg, 95% CI −2.65 kg to +0.16 kg).[44] However, higher dose orlistat (120 mg 3 times daily) was associated with greater weight loss than placebo at 12 weeks (1 RCT: mean weight loss 4.74 kg with orlistat *v* 2.98 kg with placebo; CI not provided; $P = 0.001$).[44] The two included 6 month trials were not pooled. In the first, 119 people received orlistat (120 mg 3 times daily) or placebo. All people received a calorie restricted diet. At 6 months, orlistat reduced weight more than placebo (mean weight loss: 10.75 kg with orlistat *v* 7.34 kg with placebo; $P < 0.05$).[49] The second RCT with 6 months' follow up compared orlistat (30, 60, 120, or 240 mg 3 times daily) versus placebo among 605 people on a reduced calorie diet. All doses of orlistat significantly increased weight loss at 6 months compared with placebo (weight loss from baseline: 6.5% with placebo *v* 8.5% with orlistat 30 mg; P value not provided; *v* 8.8% with orlistat 60 mg; $P \leq 0.002$; *v* 9.8% with orlistat 120 mg; $P \leq 0.001$; *v* 9.3% with orlistat 240 mg; $P \leq 0.001$).[50] Pooled analysis of four trials with 1 year follow up (2111 people) found that orlistat

(120 mg 3 times daily) reduced weight more than placebo (WMD for weight change with orlistat *v* placebo −2.90 kg, 95% CI −3.61 kg to −2.19 kg).[44] Two RCTs were not included in the 1 year pooled analysis. In these trials, 901 people were placed on a reduced calorie diet and were also randomised to orlistat (120 mg 3 times daily) versus placebo. Both found that orlistat increased weight loss compared with placebo (AR for > 10% weight loss from baseline at 1 year: 35% with orlistat *v* 21% with placebo; P = 0.02;[51] 30% with orlistat *v* 16% with placebo; P < 0.001[52]). The review found similar results at 2 years. Two trials were pooled examining change in body weight at 2 years using orlistat (120 mg 3 times daily) versus placebo. People taking orlistat had significantly greater weight loss (WMD −3.19 kg, 95% CI −4.25 kg to −2.12 kg).[44] We found one RCT that compared effects of orlistat (30, 60, and 120 mg 3 times daily) versus placebo on weight regain after 6 months of diet plus exercise counselling.[44] It found that orlistat reduced weight regain compared with placebo (P < 0.001 for orlistat 120 mg *v* placebo). We identified three additional RCTs.[46 48] The first (46 people) compared orlistat (120 mg 3 times daily) versus placebo for 52 weeks. Orlistat reduced weight more than placebo (mean weight reduction at 6 months 8.6 kg with orlistat *v* 5.5 kg with placebo; P value and CI not provided). The second additional RCT (376 adults with type 2 diabetes, hypercholesterolaemia, or hypertension) found that dietary counselling plus orlistat (120 mg 3 times daily) versus placebo significantly increased the proportion of people who lost 5% or more of their initial body weight (54% with orlistat *v* 41% with placebo; P < 0.001), but did not significantly increase weight reduction of 10% or more (AR 19% *v* 14.6%).[47] The third additional RCT (294 people with hypercholesterolaemia) compared orlistat (120 mg 3 times daily) versus placebo for 24 weeks. Mean weight loss for the orlistat group was 4.66 kg versus 1.88 kg for the placebo group (P < 0.001).[48]

Harms: Common adverse events such as oily spotting from the rectum, flatulence, and faecal urgency were more common with orlistat than placebo (22–27% with orlistat *v* 1–7% with placebo).[53] Subsequent RCTs have identified similar rates of gastrointestinal adverse events. The review found that gastrointestinal adverse events were more common with orlistat than placebo and that orlistat was also associated with lower serum levels of fat soluble vitamins, such that vitamin supplements were sometimes deemed necessary.[44]

Comment: People in six of the seven trials in one systematic review were selected for participation after losing weight on a preliminary low calorie diet with placebo for 4–5 weeks before randomisation.[53] Because of the high rates of gastrointestinal adverse effects associated with orlistat, authors have queried whether blinded evaluation is possible. At the end of a "double blinded" 16 week trial, 22/26 people correctly identified their treatment group.[21]

GLOSSARY

Body mass index Expressed as weight in kilograms divided by height in metres squared (kg/m^2). In the USA and UK, individuals with body mass indexes of 25–30 kg/m^2 are considered overweight; those with body mass indexes above 30 kg/m^2 are considered obese.

Extrapyramidal effects Include acute dystonia, a Parkinsonism-like syndrome, and akathisia.

Serotonin syndrome Clinical features include agitation, ataxia, diaphoresis, diarrhoea, fever, hyper-reflexia, myoclonus, shivering, and changes in mental status. The occurrence and severity of syndrome does not seem to be dose related.

Substantive changes

Sibutramine Five new RCTs;[15–19] conclusions unchanged.
Phentermine One new systematic review;[23] conclusions unchanged.
Mazindol One new systematic review;[23] conclusions unchanged.
Diethylpropion One new systematic review;[23] now categorised as Trade off between benefits and harms.
Fluoxetine One new systematic review;[23] now categorised as Trade off between benefits and harms.
Fenfluramine One new systematic review;[23] conclusions unchanged.
Phenylpropanolamine One new systematic review;[23] conclusions unchanged.
Orlistat One new RCT;[48] conclusions unchanged.

REFERENCES

1. National Institutes of Health. Clinical guidelines on the identification, evaluation, and treatment of overweight and obesity in adults: the Evidence Report. Bethesda, Maryland: US Department of Health and Human Services, 1998.
2. Khan LK, Serdula MK, Bowman BA, et al. Use of prescription weight loss pills among U.S. adults in 1996–1998. *Ann Int Med* 2001;134:282–286.
3. University of York, NHS Centre for Reviews and Dissemination. A systematic review of the interventions for the prevention and treatment of obesity, and the maintenance of weight loss. York, England: NHS Centre for Reviews and Dissemination, 1997. Search date 1995; primary sources Medline, Embase, Bids, Dare, Psychlit, bibliographies of review articles, and contributions from peer reviewers.
4. Prevalence of overweight and obesity among adults: United States, 1999. US Department of Health and Human Services, Centers for Disease Control and Prevention. Hyattsville, MD: National Center for Health Statistics; 2000.
5. Bray GA. Obesity: etiology. UpToDate [serial on CD-ROM] 2000;8(1). UpToDate Inc, Wellesley, Massachusetts, USA.
6. Bray GA. Obesity: overview of therapy for obesity. UpToDate [serial on CD-ROM] 2000;8(1). UpToDate Inc, Wellesley, Massachusetts, USA.
7. Allison DB, Fontaine KR, Manson JE, et al. Annual deaths attributable to obesity in the United States. *JAMA* 1999;282:1530–1538.
8. University of York, NHS Centre for Reviews and Dissemination. A systematic review of the clinical effectiveness of sibutramine and orlistat in the management of obesity. York, UK: NHS Centre for Reviews and Dissemination, 2000. Search date 2000.
9. McMahon FG, Fujioka K, Singh BN, et al. Efficacy and safety of sibutramine in obese white and African American patients with hypertension: a 1-year, double-blind, placebo-controlled multicenter trial. *Arch Int Med* 2000;160:2185–2191.
10. Wirth A, Krause J. Long-term weight loss with sibutramine: a randomized controlled trial. *JAMA* 2001;286:1331–1339.
11. Smith IG, Goudler MA. Randomized placebo-controlled trial of long-term treatment with sibutramine in mild to moderate obesity. *J Fam Pract* 2001;50:505–512.
12. James WP, Astrup A, Finer N, et al. Effect of sibutramine on weight maintenance after weight loss: a randomized trial. STORM Study Group. Sibutramine Trial of Obesity Reduction and Maintenance. *Lancet* 2000;356:2119–2125.
13. Fujioka K, Seaton TB, Rowe E, et al. Weight loss with sibutramine improves glycaemic control and other metabolic parameters in obese patients with type 2 diabetes. *Diabetes Obes Metab* 2000;2:175–187.
14. Apfelbaum M, Vague P, Ziegler O, et al. Long-term maintenance of weight loss after a very-low calorie diet: a randomized blinded trial of the efficacy and tolerability of sibutramine. *Am J Med* 1999;106:179–184.
15. Dujovne CA, Zavoral JH, Rowe E, et al. Effects of sibutramine on body weight and serum lipids: a double-blind, randomized, placebo-controlled study in 322 overweight and obese patients with dyslipidemia. *Am Heart J* 2001;142:489–497.
16. Gokcel A, Karakose H, Ertorer EM, et al. Effects of sibutramine in obese female subjects with type 2 diabetes and poor blood glucose control. *Diabetes Care* 2001;24:1957–1960.
17. McMahon FG, Weinstein SP, Rowe E, et al. Sibutramine is safe and effective for weight loss in obese patients whose hypertension is well controlled with angiotensin-converting enzyme inhibitors. *J Hum Hypertens* 2002;16:5–11.
18. Serrano-Rios M, Melchionda N, Moreno-Carretero E. Role of sibutramine in the treatment of obese type 2 diabetic patients receiving sulphonylurea therapy. *Diabet Med* 2002;19:119–124.
19. Fanghanel G, Cortinas L, Sanchez-Reyes L, et al. Second phase of a double-blind study clinical trial on sibutramine for the treatment of patients suffering from essential obesity: 6 months after treatment cross-over. *Int J Obesity* 2001;25:741–747.
20. Gokcel A, Gumurdulu Y, Karakose H, et al. Evaluation of the safety and efficacy of sibutramine, orlistat, and metformin in the treatment of obesity. *Diabetes Obes Metab* 2002;4:49–55.
21. Wadden TA, Berkowitz RI, Womble LG, et al. Effects of sibutramine plus orlistat in obese women following 1 year of treatment by sibutramine alone: a placebo-controlled trial. *Obes Res* 2000;8:431–437.
22. Health Sciences Authority. Centre for Pharmaceutical Administration. Drug Alerts.

Updates Report on Sibutramine. Information page. http://www.hsa.gov.sg/hsa/CPA/CPA_pharma_drugalerts.htm#12 (last accessed 3 Sept 2002).
23. Haddock CK, Poston WSC, Dill PL, et al. Pharmacotherapy for obesity: a quantitative analysis of four decades of published randomized clinical trials. *Int J Obes* 2002;26:262–273. Search date 1999; primary sources Medline, PsychInfo, handsearching, and personal contact with individual authors.
24. Gaasch WH, Aurigemma GP. Valvular heart disease induced by anorectic drugs. UpToDate [serial on CD-ROM] 2000;8(3). UpToDate Inc, Wellesley, Massachusetts, USA.
25. Medicines Control Agency. Committee on Safety in Medicines. Important safety message: European withdrawal of anorectic agents/appetite suppressants: new legal developments, no new safety issues: licences for phentermine and amfepramone being withdrawn May 2001. Information page. http://www.mca.gov.uk/ourwork/monitorsafequalmed/safetymessages/anorectic.htm (last accessed 3 Sept 2002).
26. Hagiwara M, Tsuchida A, Hyakkoku M, et al. Delayed onset of pulmonary hypertension associated with an appetite suppressant, mazindol: a case report. *Jpn Circ* 2000;64:218–221.
27. Bradley MH, Blum NJ, Scheib RJ. Mazindol in obesity with known cardiac disease: a clinical evaluation. *J Int Med Res* 1974;2:347–349.
28. Thomas SH, Butt AY, Corris PA, et al. Appetite suppressants and primary pulmonary hypertension in the United Kingdom. *Br Heart J* 1995;74:660–663.
29. Little JD, Romans SE. Psychosis following readministration of diethylpropion: a possible role for kindling? *Int Clin Psychopharmacol* 1993;8:67–70.
30. Goldstein DJ, Rampey AH Jr, Enas GG, et al. Fluoxetine: a randomized clinical trial in the treatment of obesity. *Int J Obes* 1994;18:129–135.
31. Mulrow CD, Williams JW Jr, Trivedi M, et al. Treatment of depression – newer pharmacotherapies. *Psychopharmacol Bull* 1998;34:409–795. Search date 1998; primary sources the Cochrane Collaboration Depression, Anxiety and Neurosis (CCDAN) Review Group register of trials, and bibliographies of trial and review articles.
32. Weintraub M. Long term weight control study: the National Heart, Lung, and Blood Institute funded multimodal intervention study. *Clin Pharmacol Ther* 1992;51:581–646.
33. Poston WS, Foreyt JP. Scientific and legal issues in fenfluramine/dexfenfluramine litigation. *J Texas Med* 2000;96:48–56.
34. Connolly HM, Crary JL, McGoon MD, et al. Valvular heart disease associated with fenfluramine-phentermine. *N Engl J Med* 1997;337:581–588.
35. Scheen AJ, Lefebvre PJ. Pharmacological treatment of obesity: present status. *Int J Obes Relat Metab Disord* 1999;23(suppl 1):47–53.
36. Gardin JM, Schumacher D, Constantine G, et al. Valvular abnormalities and cardiovascular status following exposure to dexfenfluramine and phentermine/fenfluramine. *JAMA* 2000;283:1703–1709.
37. Gardin JM, Weissman NJ, Leung C, et al. Clinical and echocardiographic follow-up of patients previously treated with dexfenfluramine or phentermine/fenfluramine. *JAMA* 2001;286:2011–2014.
38. Weissman NJ, Tighe JF, Gottdiener JS, et al. An assessment of heart-valve abnormalities in obese patients taking dexfenfluramine, sustained-release dexfenfluramine, or placebo. Sustained release dexfenfluramine study group. *N Engl J Med* 1998;339:725–732.
39. Weissman NJ, Panza JA, Tighe JF, et al. Natural history of valvular regurgitation 1 year after discontinuation of dexfenfluramine therapy. *Ann Intern Med* 2001;134:267–273.
40. Abenhaim L, Moride Y, Brenot F, et al. Appetite-suppressant drugs and the risk of primary pulmonary hypertension. International primary pulmonary hypertension study group. *N Engl J Med* 1996;335:609–616.
41. Horwitz RI, Brass LM, Kernan WN, et al. Phenylpropanolamine and risk of hemorrhagic stroke: final report of the hemorrhagic stroke project. http://www.fda.gov/ohrms/dockets/ac/00/backgrd/3647b1_tab19.doc (last accessed 3 Sept 2002).
42. Food and Drug Administration. Center for Drug Evaluation and Research. Phenylpropanolamine (PPA) information page. http://www.fda.gov/cder/drug/infopage/ppa/ (last accessed 3 September 2002).
43. Lucas KH, Kaplan-Machlis B. Orlistat: a novel weight loss therapy. *Ann Pharmacother* 2001;35:314–328. Search date 2000; primary sources Medline, Roche Laboratories, organisational guidelines, National Institutes of Health and Food and Drug Administration web sites, Doctor's Guide online, and reference sections of published articles.
44. O'Meara S, Riemsma R, Shirran L, et al. A rapid and systematic review of the clinical effectiveness and cost-effectiveness of orlistat in the management of obesity. *Health Technol Assess* 2001;5:1–81. Search date 2000; primary sources Amed, Biosis, British Nursing Index, the Cochrane Library, Cinahl, Dare, DH-Data, EconLit, Embase, Health Management Information Service, HTA database, Index to Scientific and Technical Proceedings, King's Fund database, Medline, National Research Register, NEED, Health Economic Evaluations Database, Science Citation Index, Social Science Citation Index, Internet searches, reference lists of relevant reviews, and contact with the authors of conference abstracts.
45. European Agency for the Evaluation of Medicinal Products. Committee for proprietary medicinal products. European public assessment report (EPAR) – Xenical. London: European Agency for the Evaluation of Medicinal Products, 1998.
46. James WPT, Avenell A, Broom J, et al. A one-year trial to assess the value of orlistat in the management of obesity. *Int J Obes Relat Metab Disord* 1997;21(suppl 3):S24–S30.
47. Lindgarde F. The effect of orlistat on body weight and coronary heart disease risk profile in obese patients: the Swedish Multimorbidity Study. *J Int Med* 2000;248:245–254.
48. Muls E, Kolanowski J, Scheen A, et al. The effects of orlistat on weight and on serum lipids in obese patients with hypercholesterolemia: a randomized, double-blind, placebo-controlled, multicentre study. *Int J Obes* 2001;25:1713–1721.
49. Micic D, Ivkovic-Lazar T, Dragojevic R, et al. Orlistat, a gastrointestinal lipase inhibitor, in therapy of obesity with concomitant hyperlipidemia. *Med Pregl* 1999;52:323–333.
50. Van Gaul LF, Broom JI, Enzi G, et al. Efficacy and tolerability of orlistat in the treatment of obesity: a 6-month dose-ranging study. *Eur J Clin Pharmacol* 1998;54:125–132.
51. Finer N, James WPT, Kopelman PG, et al. One-year treatment of obesity: a randomized,

double-blind, placebo-controlled, multicentre study of orlistat, a gastrointestinal lipase inhibitor. *Int J Obes* 2000;24:306–313.
52. Sjostrom L, Rissanen A, Anderson T, et al. Randomised placebo-controlled trial of orlistat for weight loss and prevention of weight regain in obese patients. *Lancet* 1998;352:167–173.
53. Anonymous. Orlistat: no hurry. *Can Fam Physician* 1999;45:2331–2351. Search date 1999; primary sources Medline, Embase, Reactions, the Cochrane Library, hand searches of international journals, the Prescribe Library, and clinical pharmacology reference texts, and personal contact with Produits Roche, the European Medicines Evaluation Agency, and Food and Drug Administration committees.

David Arterburn
Health Services Research Fellow
Health Services Research and Development
VA Puget Sound Health Care System
Department of Veterans Affairs
Seattle
USA

Competing interests: None declared. The views expressed in this article are those of the authors and do not necessarily represent the views of the US Department of Veterans Affairs.

TABLE 1 Unpooled RCTs comparing sibutramine versus placebo for weight loss (see text, p 589).

Trial duration	Study	Number of people	Special population	Lifestyle modification	Intervention	Mean weight change (kg)	P value
24 weeks	15	322	Obese with hyperlipidaemia	Diet	Placebo	–0.6	
					Sibutramine 20 mg daily	–4.9	$P < 0.05$
	13	175	Obese with type 2 diabetes	Diet	Placebo	–0.4	
					Sibutramine 20 mg daily	–3.7	$P < 0.05$
	16	60	Obese with type 2 diabetes	Diet	Placebo	0.91	
					Sibutramine 10 mg daily	–9.61	$P < 0.0001$
	18	134	Obese with type 2 diabetes	Diet	Placebo	–1.7	
					Sibutramine 15 mg daily	–4.5	$P < 0.001$
48 weeks	10	1001	Healthy, obese	None	Placebo	0.2	
					Continuous sibutramine 15 mg daily	–3.8	$P < 0.001$
					Intermittent sibutramine 15 mg daily	–3.3	$P < 0.001$
52 weeks	11	485	Healthy, obese	Diet	Placebo	–1.6	
					Sibutramine 10 mg daily	–4.4	$P < 0.01$
					Sibutramine 15 mg daily	–6.4	$P < 0.001$
	17	220	Obese with hypertension	Diet	Placebo	–0.4	
					Sibutramine 20 mg daily	–4.5	$P < 0.05$
	9	224	Obese with hypertension	Diet	Placebo	–0.5	
					Sibutramine 20 mg daily	–4.4	$P < 0.05$

Primary hypothyroidism

Search date December 2001

Lars Kristensen and Birte Nygaard

QUESTIONS

INTERVENTIONS

CLINICAL (OVERT) HYPOTHYROIDISM

Beneficial

Unknown effectiveness

SUBCLINICAL HYPOTHYROIDISM

Unknown effectiveness

*No RCT evidence, but there is clinical consensus that levothyroxine is beneficial in clinical (overt) hypothyroidism.

See glossary, p 607

Key Messages

- Treating clinical (overt) or subclinical hypothyroidism with thyroid hormone (levothyroxine; L-thyroxine) can induce hyperthyroidism (reduced thyroid stimulating hormone).

Clinical (overt) hypothyroidism

- **Levothyroxine (L-thyroxine)** We found no RCTs on the effects of levothyroxine (L-thyroxine) versus placebo, but there is consensus that treatment is beneficial. Treating clinical (overt) hypothyroidism with thyroid hormone (levothyroxine; L-thyroxine) can induce hyperthyroidism (reduced thyroid stimulating hormone).
- **Levothyroxine (L-thyroxine) plus liothyronine** One small RCT found that levothyroxine plus liothyronine versus levothyroxine alone improved some participant measures of mood and physical symptoms. Another RCT found insufficient evidence about the effects of combination treatment with levothyroxine plus liothyronine.

Subclinical hypothyroidism

- **Levothyroxine (L-thyroxine)** One RCT in women with biochemically defined subclinical hypothyroidism found that levothyroxine (L-thyroxine) versus placebo improved dry skin, cold intolerance, or constipation at 1 year, but the RCT was small and the difference was not significant. Two RCTs found inconclusive results about the effect of levothyroxine versus placebo on cognitive function. Treating subclinical hypothyroidism with thyroid hormone (levothyroxine; L-thyroxine) can induce hyperthyroidism (reduced thyroid stimulating hormone).

DEFINITION Hypothyroidism is characterised by low levels of blood thyroid hormone. **Clinical (overt) hypothyroidism** is diagnosed on the basis of characteristic clinical features consisting of mental slowing, depression, dementia, weight gain, constipation, dry skin, hair loss, cold intolerance, hoarse voice, irregular menstruation, infertility, muscle stiffness and pain, bradycardia, hypercholesterolaemia, combined with a raised blood level of thyroid stimulating hormone (TSH) (serum TSH levels > 12 mU/L), and a low serum thyroxine (T4) level (serum T_4 < 60 nmol/L). **Subclinical hypothyroidism** is diagnosed when serum TSH is raised (serum TSH > 4 mU/L) but serum thyroxine (T4—see glossary, p 607) is normal and there are no symptoms or signs, or only minor symptoms or signs, of thyroid dysfunction. **Primary hypothyroidism** is seen after destruction of the thyroid gland because of autoimmune causes (the majority), or iatrogenic causes such as surgery, radioiodine, and radiation (the minority). **Secondary hypothyroidism** is seen after damage of the pituitary gland or hypothalamic function resulting in insufficient production of TSH. Secondary hypothyroidism is not covered in this review.

INCIDENCE/ PREVALENCE Hypothyroidism is more common in women than in men (in the UK female : male ratio of 6 : 1). A study (2779 people in UK with a median age of 58 years) found the incidence of clinical (overt) hypothyroidism was 40/10 000 women a year and 6/10 000 men a year. The prevalence was 9.3% in women and 1.3% in men.[1] In areas with high iodine intake the incidence of hypothyroidism can be higher than in areas with normal to subnormal iodine intake. In Denmark, where there is moderate iodine insufficiency, the overall incidence of hypothyroidism is 1.4/10 000 a year increasing to 8/10 000 a year in people older than 70 years of age.[2] The incidence of subclinical hypothyroidism increases with age; up to 10% of women over the age of 60 years have subclinical hypothyroidism (evaluated from data from the Netherlands and USA).[3,4]

AETIOLOGY/ RISK FACTORS Primary thyroid gland failure can occur as a result of chronic autoimmune thyroiditis, postradioactive iodine treatment, or thyroidectomy. Other causes include drug adverse effects (e.g. amiodarone and lithium), transient hypothyroidism due to silent thyroiditis, subacute thyroiditis, or postpartum thyroiditis.

PROGNOSIS Hypothyroidism results in mental slowing, depression, dementia, weight gain, constipation, dry skin, hair loss, cold intolerance, hoarse voice, irregular menstruation, infertility, muscle stiffness and pain, bradycardia, and hypercholesterolaemia. In people with subclinical hypothyroidism, the risk of developing overt hypothyroidism is described in the UK Whickham Survey (25 years' follow up; for women: OR 8, 95% CI 3 to 20; for men: OR 44, 95% CI 19 to 104; if both a raised TSH and positive antithyroid antibodies were present; for women: OR 38, 95% CI 22 to 65; for men: OR 173, 95% CI 81 to 370). For women, it found an annual risk of 4.3% a year (if both raised serum TSH and antithyroid antibodies were present), 2.6% a year (if raised serum TSH was present alone); the minimum number of people with raised TSH and antithyroid antibodies who would need treating to prevent this progression to clinical (overt) hypothyroidism in one person over 5 years is 5 to 8.[1]

Cardiovascular disease: A large cross-sectional study (25 862 participants with serum TSH between 5.1–10 mU/L) found significantly higher mean total cholesterol concentrations in hypothyroid people compared with euthyroid people (5.8 *v* 5.6 mmol/L).[3] Another study (124 elderly women with subclinical hypothyroidism, 931 euthyroid women) found a significantly increased risk of myocardial infarction in women with subclinical hypothyroidism (OR 2.3, 95% CI 1.3 to 4.0) and for aortic atherosclerosis (OR 1.7, 95% CI 1.1 to 2.6).[4] **Mental health:** Subclinical hypothyroidism is associated with depression.[5] People with subclinical hypothyroidism may have depression that is refractory to both antidepressant drugs and thyroid hormone alone. Memory impairment, hysteria, anxiety, somatic complaint, and depressive features without depression have been described in people with subclinical hypothyroidism.[6]

AIMS To eliminate the symptoms of hypothyroidism and maximise quality of life.

OUTCOMES Quality of life and neuropsychological impairments (evaluated by congestive functions tests, memory tests, reaction time, self rating mood scales, and depression scores); cardiovascular disease (episodes of atrial fibrillation and ischaemic events); changes in body composition (measured by osteodensitometry or bioimpedance measurements); prevention of progression from subclinical to overt hypothyroidism; adverse effects of treatments (bone mass, fracture rate, development of hyperthyroidism).

METHODS *Clinical Evidence* search and appraisal December 2001, with an additional manual search of reference lists.

QUESTION **What are the effects of treatments for clinical (overt) hypothyroidism?**

OPTION **LEVOTHYROXINE (L-THYROXINE) FOR CLINICAL (OVERT) HYPOTHYROIDISM**

We found no RCTs on levothyroxine (L-thyroxine) versus placebo in people with clinical (overt) hypothyroidism, but clinical consensus suggests that treatment is beneficial.

Benefits: We found no RCTs comparing levothyroxine versus placebo in people with clinical hypothyroidism.

Harms: We found no RCTs comparing levothyroxine versus placebo in people with clinical hypothyroidism. A risk of levothyroxine treatment is over treatment (leading to subclinical hyperthyroidism [decreased serum thyroid stimulating hormone but no symptoms] or to clinical hyperthyroidism). **Fracture rate:** One longitudinal observational study (1180 people on levothyroxine followed for an average of 8.6 years) found no significant increase in fracture rate with levothyroxine versus control.[7] **Bone mass:** One systematic review of cross-sectional RCTs on changes in bone mass (search date not stated, 13 RCTs, total of 441 premenopausal women and 317 postmenopausal women on prolonged levothyroxine treatment with reduced serum TSH concentration but normal T4 and T3 [see glossary, p 607] values).[8] In premenopausal women (average age 40 years, treated with levothyroxine 164 µg daily for 8.5 years leading to suppressed serum TSH) the review found a non-significant reduction in bone mass with levothyroxine versus control after 8.5 years (2.7% less bone mass with levothyroxine versus control; NS). In postmenopausal women (average age 61.2 years, treated with levothyroxine 171 µg daily for 9.9 years leading to suppressed serum TSH), it found that levothyroxine versus control significantly increased bone loss after 9.9 years (9.0% less bone mass with levothyroxine *v* control, 95% CI 2.4% to 15.7%). **Atrial fibrillation:** One observational study found that in people aged over 60 years taking levothyroxine, a low serum TSH concentration (≤0.1 mU/L) was associated with an increased risk of atrial fibrillation (diagnosed by electrocardiogram) at 10 years (incidence of atrial fibrillation, 28% in people with low TSH *v* 11% in people with normal TSH values; RR 3.1, 95% CI 1.7 to 5.5).[9]

Comment: None.

OPTION **LEVOTHYROXINE (L-THYROXINE) PLUS LIOTHYRONINE FOR CLINICAL (OVERT) HYPOTHYROIDISM**

One small RCT in people with clinical (overt) hypothyroidism found that levothyroxine (L-thyroxine) plus liothyronine versus levothyroxine alone improved some measures of mood and physical symptoms. Another RCT found insufficient evidence about the effects of levothyroxine plus liothyronine.

Benefits: We found no systematic review but found two small RCTs evaluating the effect of levothyroxine plus liothyronine in people with clinical (overt) hypothyroidism. **Quality of life:** The first RCT (crossover design, 33 people with clinical hypothyroidism, mean dose of levothyroxine at baseline 175 µg [range 100–300 µg]) compared effects of levothyroxine versus levothyroxine plus liothyronine for two 5 week periods (during one period the people received the usual dose of levothyroxine and in the other period 50 µg of levothyroxine was replaced with 12.5 µg of liothyronine in randomised order).[10] The RCT found that levothyroxine plus liothyronine versus levothyroxine alone significantly improved some measures of mood and physical symptoms on a participant rated 100 mm visual analogue scale (10/15 [67%] measures significantly improved *v* 5/15 [33%]; NS), but found no consistent effect on investigator assessment of cognitive performance or mood scores. At the end of the study, participants were asked which treatment they preferred: 20 people preferred combination treatment with levothyroxine plus liothyronine, 11 had no preference, and two preferred levothyroxine alone.[10] The second RCT (double blind, crossover design, 87 people aged 29–76 years) compared levothyroxine (200–300 µg) versus combination of levothyroxine (150–200 µg) plus liothyronine (50–100 µg).[11] Each participant received 2 months' treatment with each regime. The RCT found that 48% of participants had no preference between treatments, 33%

preferred levothyroxine alone, and 18% preferred the combination (measured using a participant completed questionnaire; statistical significance not stated). The RCT did not conduct any evaluations of cognitive function, mood, or physical symptoms.[11] No conclusions can be drawn from these findings.

Harms: The first RCT did not report adverse effects apart from 2/33 (6%) people feeling slightly nervous with the combination of levothyroxine plus liothyronine, and one person withdrawing from the study after becoming anxious during levothyroxine plus liothyronine treatment.[10] The second RCT found a higher incidence of adverse effects (including palpitations, irritability and nervousness, tremor, perspiration, and loss of appetite) with levothyroxine plus liothyronine treatment versus levothyroxine alone (40/87 [46%] *v* 9/87 [10%] ARI 36%, 95% CI 22% to 49%; NNH 3).[11] In the second RCT, the total dose of thyroid hormone (levothyroxine and liothyronine) was higher than the dose used in the first RCT.

Comment: None.

QUESTION What are the effects of treatments for subclinical hypothyroidism?

OPTION LEVOTHYROXINE (L-THYROXINE) FOR SUBCLINICAL HYPOTHYROIDISM

One RCT in women with biochemically defined subclinical hypothyroidism found that levothyroxine (L-thyroxine) versus placebo improved dry skin, cold intolerance, or constipation at 1 year, but the RCT was small and the improvement was not significant. Two RCTs found inconclusive results about the effect of levothyroxine versus placebo on cognitive function in people with subclinical hypothyroidism.

Benefits: We found no systematic review, but found three RCTs evaluating the effect of levothyroxine in people with subclinical hypothyroidism.[12–14] **General symptoms:** We found one RCT (33 women with increased thyroid stimulating hormone [TSH], normal serum thyroxine and normal free T4 and [T3—see glossary, p 607]). Women also had an average of two of the following symptoms: muscle cramps, dry skin, cold intolerance, fatigue, or constipation. Physical examination revealed no signs of hypothyroidism, apart from dry or coarse skin, which was present in about 50% of women in each group. The RCT compared effects of levothyroxine (0.05 mg daily) versus placebo on general symptoms (evaluated by a questionnaire in participants stating if they were feeling better, unchanged, or worse) for 1 year. It found that levothyroxine versus placebo improved overall symptoms but the difference was not significant (8/17 [47%] people with levothyroxine *v* 3/16 [19%] people with placebo; $P = 0.14$, recalculated by *Clinical Evidence*).[12] **Cognitive function:** We found two RCTs. The first RCT (double blind crossover design, 17 women, aged 51–73 years, with increased TSH, normal T4 and T3, and without clinical evidence of thyroid disease) compared the effect of levothyroxine (0.1 mg daily) versus placebo on cognitive function and subjective rating after 6 months.[13] A beneficial effect was defined as a significantly better score with treatment versus pretreatment score in two or more psychometric tests. It found that 4/17 (24%) tests were significantly better after levothyroxine treatment versus pretreatment scores. No firm conclusions could be drawn from these findings. The second RCT (37 people, aged > 55 years, TSH >6.0 mU/L, normal T4 and T3, and thyroxine binding globulin) compared levothyroxine (0.025 μg daily for 4 wks then 0.05 μg daily) versus placebo for 10 months. It found no significant difference with levothyroxine versus placebo on any outcome except in one psychometric memory score, based on a battery of cognitive function tests evaluating memory.[14] No firm conclusions could be drawn from these findings.

Harms: One RCT did not report on adverse effects.[12] In the second RCT, 2/20 (10%) people receiving levothyroxine withdrew from the trial because of nervousness and palpitations.[13] In the third RCT, 2/18 (11%) people taking levothyroxine withdrew because of complications (1 had increased angina and 1 had new onset of atrial fibrillation).[14]

Comment: **Muscular function:** We found one observational study (33 people with increased TSH; normal levels of free T_4; and neuromuscular symptoms including fatigue, muscle cramps, muscle weakness, and abnormal sensation of burning or tingling significantly more frequent than control). It found a significant improvement in symptoms after levothyroxine treatment versus pretreatment ($P = 0.0001$).[15] We found no studies evaluating the muscular strength in people with subclinical hypothyroidism.

GLOSSARY

T3 is used as an abbreviation for endogenous tri-iodothyronine in medical and biochemical reports.

T4 is used as an abbreviation for endogenous thyroxine in medical and biochemical reports.

REFERENCES

1. Vanderpump MP, Tunbridge WM, French JM, et al. The incidence of thyroid disorder in the community: A twenty-year follow-up of the Whickham survey. *Clin Endocriniol (Oxf)* 1995;43:55–68.
2. Laurberg P, Bülow Pedersen I, Pedersen KM, Vestergaard H. Low incidence rate of overt hypothyroidism compared with hyperthyroidism in an area with moderately low iodine intake. *Thyroid* 1999;9:33–38.
3. Canaris GJ, Manowitz NR, Mayor G, Ridgway C. The Colorado thyroid disease prevalence study. *Arch Intern Med* 2000;160:526–533.
4. Hak AE, Pols HA, Visser TJ, Drexhage HA, Hofman A, Witteman JC. Subclinical hypothyroidism is an independent risk factor for atherosclerosis and myocardial infarction in elderly women: the Rotterdam Study. *Ann Intern Med* 2000;132:270–278.
5. Haggerty JJ, Stern RA, Mason GA, Beckwith J, Morey CE, Prange AJ. Subclinical hypothyroidism: a modifiable risk factor for depression? *Am J Psychiatry* 1993;150:508–510.
6. Monzani F, Del Guerra P, Caraccio N, et al. Subclinical hypothyroidism: neurobehavioral features and beneficial effect of L-thyroxine treatment. *Clin Investig* 1993;71:367–371.
7. Leese GP, Jung RT, Guthrie C, Waugh N, Browning MCK. Morbidity in patients on L-thyroxine: a comparison of those with a normal TSH to those with a suppressed TSH. *Clin Endocrinol* 1992;37:500 503.
8. Faber J, Galløe AM. Changes in bone mass during prolonged subclinical hyperthyroidism due to L-thyroxine treatment: a meta analysis. *Eur J Endocrinol* 1994;130:350–356. Search date not stated; primary sources Medline and handsearching of references from literature and abstracts published at international endocrinological meetings 1985–1992.
9. Sawin CT, Geller A, Wolf PA, et al. Low serum thyrotropin concentrations as a risk factor for atrial fibrillation in older persons. *N Engl J Med* 1994;331:1249–1252.
10. Bunevicius R, Kazanavicius G, Zalinkevicius R, Prange AJ. Effects of thyroxine as compared with thyroxine plus triiodothyronine in patients with hypothyroidism. *N Engl J Med* 1999;340:424–470.
11. Smith RN, Taylor SA, Massey JC. Controlled clinical trial of combined triiodothyronine and thyroxine in the treatment of hypothyroidism. *BMJ* 1970;4:145–148.
12. Cooper DS, Halpern R, Wood LC, Levin AA, Ridgway EC. L-thyroxine therapy in subclinical hypothyroidism. *Ann Intern Med* 1984;101:18–24.

13. Nyström E, Caidahl K, Fager C, Wikkelsö C Lundberg PA, Lindstedt G. A double-blind cross-over 12 months study of L-thyroxine treatment of women with subclinical hypothyroidism. *Clin Endocrinol* 1988;29:63–76.
14. Jaeschke R, Guyatt G, Gerstein H, et al. Does treatment with L-thyroxine influence health status in middle-aged and older adults with subclinical hypothyroidism? *J Gen Intern Med* 1996;11:771–773.
15. Monza ni F, Caraccio N, Del Guerra P, Casolaro A, Ferrannini E. Neuromuscular symptoms and dysfunction in subclinical hypothyroid patients: beneficial effect of L-T4 replacement therapy. *Clin Endocrinol* 1999;51:237–242.

Lars Kristensen
Associate Professor, MD, Dr Med Sci

Birte Nygaard
MD, PhD

University of Copenhagen
Herlev Copenhagen
Denmark

Competing interests: None declared

Acute anterior uveitis

Search date February 2002

André Curi, Kimble Matos, and Carlos Pavesio

QUESTIONS

INTERVENTIONS

Unknown effectiveness

To be covered in future updates

Mydriatics
Oral steroids
Slow taper of drug treatment
Subconjunctival steroid injection
Treatment of chronic iridocyclitis

See glossary, p 613

Key Messages

- **Non-steroidal eye drops** RCTs found no significant difference in the proportion of people judged to be clinically cured with non-steroidal versus placebo eye drops and with non steroidal versus steroid eye drops.
- **Steroid eye drops** One small RCT found no significant difference in symptom severity after 14 or 21 days with steroid eye drops (betamethasone phosphate/clobetasone butyrate) versus placebo. Two RCTs found no significant difference with prednisolone versus rimexolone in the number of anterior chamber cells per examination field (a marker of disease severity in acute anterior uveitis). Two other RCTs found that prednisolone versus loteprednol significantly increased the proportion of people with less than five anterior chamber cells per examination field after 28 days. RCTs found that rimexolone and loteprednol were less likely than prednisolone to increase intraocular pressures, although differences were not significant.

Acute anterior uveitis

DEFINITION Anterior uveitis is inflammation of the uveal tract, and includes iritis and iridocyclitis. It can be classified according to its clinical course into acute or chronic anterior uveitis, or according to its clinical appearance into granulomatous or non-granulomatous anterior uveitis. Acute anterior uveitis is characterised by an extremely painful red eye, often associated with photophobia and occasionally with decreased visual acuity. Chronic anterior uveitis is defined as inflammation lasting over 6 weeks. It is usually asymptomatic, but many people have mild symptoms during exacerbations.

INCIDENCE/ PREVALENCE Acute anterior uveitis is rare, with an annual incidence of 12/100 000 population.[1] It is more common in Finland (annual incidence 22.6/100 000, prevalence 68.7/100 000), probably owing to genetic factors such as the high frequency of HLA-B27 in the Finish population.[2] It has equal sex incidence, and less than 10% of cases occur before the age of 20 years.[2,3]

AETIOLOGY/ RISK FACTORS No cause is identified in 60–80% of people with acute anterior uveitis. Systemic disorders that may be associated with acute anterior uveitis include ankylosing spondylitis; Reiter's syndrome; juvenile chronic arthritis; Kawasaki syndrome; infectious uveitis; Behçet's syndrome; inflammatory bowel disease; interstitial nephritis; sarcoidosis; multiple sclerosis; Wegener's granulomatosis; Vogt-Koyanagi-Harada syndrome; and masquerade syndromes (see glossary, p 613). Acute anterior uveitis also occurs in association with HLA-B27 expression not linked to any systemic disease, and may also be the manifestation of an isolated eye disorder such as Fuchs' iridocyclitis, Posner-Schlossman syndrome, or Schwartz syndrome. Acute anterior uveitis may also occur following surgery or as an adverse drug or hypersensitivity reaction.[2,3]

PROGNOSIS Acute anterior uveitis is often self limiting, but we found no evidence about how often it resolves spontaneously, in which people, or over what length of time. Complications include posterior synechiae (see glossary, p 613), cataract, glaucoma, and chronic uveitis. In a study of 154 people (232 eyes) with acute anterior uveitis (119 people HLA-B27 positive), visual acuity was better than 20/60 in 209/232 (90%) eyes, 20/60 or worse in 23/232 (10%) eyes, and worse than 20/200 (classified as legally blind) in 11/232 (5%) eyes.[4]

AIMS To reduce inflammation; to relieve pain; and to prevent complications and loss of visual acuity, with minimal adverse effects.

OUTCOMES Degree of inflammation using scores that register cell counts and flare in the anterior chamber; keratic precipitates; ciliary flush; and severity of symptoms (photophobia and pain).

METHODS *Clinical Evidence* search and appraisal February 2002.

QUESTION What are the effects of topical anti-inflammatory eye drops?

OPTION TOPICAL STEROID TREATMENTS

One small RCT found no significant difference with steroid (betamethasone phosphate/clobetasone butyrate) versus placebo eye drops in symptom severity after 14 or 21 days. Two RCTs found no significant difference with prednisolone versus rimexolone in the number of anterior chamber cells per examination field. Two other RCTs found that prednisolone versus loteprednol significantly increased the number of people with fewer than five anterior chamber cells per examination field after 28 days. RCTs found that rimexolone and loteprednol were less likely than prednisolone to be associated with increased intraocular pressure, although differences were not statistically significant.

Benefits: We found no systematic review. **Versus placebo:** We found one RCT (60 people) that compared three treatments: betamethasone phosphate 1% (2 drops every 2 h); clobetasone butyrate 0.1% (2 drops every 2 h); and placebo.[5] The RCT found no significant difference with steroid (betamethasone phosphate/clobetasone butyrate) versus placebo eye drops in symptom severity after 14 or 21 days (results presented graphically; see comment below). **Versus each other:** We found four RCTs.[6,7] Two RCTs (183 people and 93 people) compared prednisolone 1% versus rimexolone 1% eye drops.[6] The larger RCT found no significant difference in the number of anterior chamber cells per examination field (a marker of disease severity in acute anterior uveitis) after 28 days (see comment below; difference in mean number of anterior chamber cells 0.2, 95% CI not provided; P = 0.16). The smaller RCT found similar results.[6] Two RCTs (170 people and 70 people) compared prednisolone 1% versus loteprednol 0.5% eye drops.[7] The larger RCT found that prednisolone significantly increased the number of people with fewer than five anterior chamber cells per examination field after 28 days (77/89 [87%] with prednisolone *v* 58/81 [72%] with loteprednol; RR 1.20, 95% CI 1.03 to 1.42; NNT 7, 95% CI 4 to 35). The smaller RCT found similar results.[7] **Versus topical non-steroidal treatments:** See topical non-steroidal treatments, p 612.

Harms: Adverse effects of topical steroid eye drops include local irritation, hyperaemia, oedema, and blurred vision. Rarely, topical eye drops have been associated with glaucoma, cataract, and herpes simplex keratitis. In the RCTs, adverse events were generally mild, resolved without treatment, and did not result in permanent damage.[5–7] In the smaller RCT comparing loteprednol versus prednisolone eye drops, 4/70 (6%) people were withdrawn because of adverse effects: cystoid macular oedema and ocular symptoms in the loteprednol group, and interstitial keratitis and increase in age-related macular degeneration in the prednisolone group.[7] **Raised intraocular pressure:** Clinically significant increases in intraocular pressure (defined as > 10 mmHg from baseline) were found more frequently with prednisolone versus rimexolone and with prednisolone versus loteprednol, although the differences were not found to be statistically significant (11/94 [12%] people with prednisolone v 6/89 [7%] people with rimexolone; RR 1.73, 95% CI 0.70 to 4.50;[6] 6/91 [7%] people with prednisolone v 1/84 [1%] people with loteprednol; RR 5.5, 95% CI 0.7 to 45.0[7]).

Comment: In the RCT comparing steroid eye drops versus placebo, 12/60 (20%) people did not complete the trial and analysis of data was not by intention to treat.[5] Of these, 4/12 people were withdrawn from the placebo group because of the severity of their anterior uveitis. The trial was too small to rule out any clinically important effect of topical steroids. In the larger of the two RCTs comparing prednisolone versus rimexolone eye drops, 23/183 (13%) people did not complete the trial and analysis of data was not by intention to treat.[6] Topical steroids have been standard treatment for anterior uveitis since the early 1950s, especially for people with acute or severe uveitis.

OPTION TOPICAL NON-STEROIDAL TREATMENTS

RCTs have found no significant difference between non-steroidal versus placebo eye drops and between non-steroidal versus steroid eye drops in the number of people judged as being clinically cured.

Benefits: We found no systematic review. **Versus placebo:** We found one RCT (100 people) that compared three treatments: non-steroidal (tolmetin 5%), steroid (prednisolone 0.5%), and placebo (sterile saline 0.9%) eye drops (see versus topical steroids below).[8] Participants were asked to instil two drops every 2 hours during the waking period plus atropine 1% eye drops daily. The RCT found no significant difference with non-steroidal versus placebo eye drops in the number of people judged as clinically cured after 21 days (15/32 [47%] people with tolmetin v 16/32 [50%] people with placebo; RR 0.9, 95% CI 0.6 to 1.6). **Versus topical steroids:** We found three RCTs.[8–10] The first RCT (71 people) compared three treatments: prednisolone disodium phosphate 0.5%; betamethasone disodium phosphate 0.1%; and tolmetin sodium dihydrate 5%.[9] Participants were asked to instil one drop every 2 hours during the waking period, and all received atropine 1% eye drops once daily. The RCT found no significant difference with non-steroidal (tolmetin sodium dihydrate) versus steroid (prednisolone disodium phosphate/betamethasone disodium phosphate) eye drops in the number of people judged as clinically cured after 21 days (see comment below; 12/21 [57%] people with tolmetin sodium dihydrate v 31/39 [79%] with prednisolone disodium phosphate/betamethasone disodium phosphate; RR 1.4, 95% CI 0.9 to 2.1). The second RCT (49 people) compared non-steroidal (indometacin [indomethacin] 0.1%) versus steroid (dexamethasone 1%) eye drops administered six times daily.[10] Most participants (equal numbers in each group) also received atropine eye drops three times daily. The RCT found no significant difference in the number of people judged to be clinically cured after 14 days (see comment below; 12/25 [48%] people with indometacin v 18/24 [75%] people with dexamethasone; RR 0.6, 95% CI 0.4 to 1.0). The third RCT (100 people) compared three treatments: steroid (prednisolone 0.5%), non-steroidal (tolmetin 5%), and placebo eye drops (sterile saline 0.9%) (see versus placebo above).[8] It found no significant difference with non-steroidal versus steroid eye drops in the number of people judged as clinically cured after 21 days (see comment below; 15/32 [47%] people with tolmetin *v* 22/32 [69%] people with prednisolone; RR 0.7, 95% CI 0.4 to 1.1).

Harms: See topical steroid treatments, p 611. In the RCT comparing non-steroidal versus steroidal eye drops, 6/20 (30%) people receiving non-steroidal eye drops reported a transient stinging sensation in their eyes.[9] In the RCT comparing indometacin 0.1% versus dexamethasone 1% eye drops, more people receiving indometacin reported eye irritation, although the difference was not significant (7/25 [28%] people with indometacin *v* 3/24 [13%] people with dexamethasone; RR 2.2, 95% CI 0.7 to 7.8).[10]

Comment: Two RCTs used "clinical cure" as an outcome measure, although neither defined this term.[8,9] The RCT comparing non-steroidal versus placebo eye drops reported that 6/71 (8%) people did not complete the trial,[8] and the first RCT comparing non-steroidal versus steroid eye drops reported that 11/71 (15%) people did not complete the trial.[9] Neither of these RCTs analysed data by intention to treat. The second RCT comparing non-steroidal versus steroid eye drops defined "clinical cure" as absence of clinical signs or symptoms suggestive of inflammation.[10]

GLOSSARY

Masquerade syndromes Comprise a group of disorders that occur with intraocular inflammation and are often misdiagnosed as a chronic idiopathic uveitis.

Posterior synechiae Adhesions between the iris and the lens capsule.

REFERENCES

1. Darrel RW, Wagner HP, Kurland CT. Epidemiology of uveitis: incidence and prevalence in a small urban community. *Arch Ophthalmol* 1962;68:501–514.
2. Paivonsalo-Hietanen T, Tuominen J, Vaahtoranta-Lehtonen H, Saari KM. Incidence and prevalence of different uveitis entities in Finland. *Acta Ophthalmol Scand* 1997;75:76–81.
3. Rosenbaum JT. Uveitis. An internist's view. *Arch Intern Med* 1989;149:1173–1176.
4. Linssen A, Meenken C. Outcomes of HLA-B27-positive and HLA-B27-negative acute anterior uveitis. *Am J Ophthalmol* 1995;120:351–361.
5. Dunne JA, Travers JP. Topical steroids in anterior uveitis. *Trans Ophthalmol Soc UK* 1979;99:481–484.
6. Foster CS, Alter G, DeBarge RL, et al. Efficacy and safety of rimexolone 1% ophthalmic suspension vs prednisolone acetate in the treatment of uveitis. *Am J Ophthalmol* 1996;122:171–182.
7. The Loteprednol Etabonate US Uveitis Study Group. Controlled evaluation of loteprednol etabonate and prednisolone acetate in the treatment of acute anterior uveitis. *Am J Ophthalmol* 1999;127:537–544.
8. Young BJ, Cunninghan WF, Akingbehin T. Double-masked controlled clinical trial of 5% tolmetin versus 0.5% prednisolone versus 0.9% saline in acute endogenous nongranulomatous anterior uveitis. *Br J Ophthalmol* 1982;66:389–391.
9. Dunne JA, Jacobs N, Morrison A, Gilbert DJ. Efficacy in anterior uveitis of two known steroids and topical tolmetin. *Br J Ophthalmol* 1985;69:120–125.
10. Sand BB, Krogh E. Topical indometacin, a prostaglandin inhibitor, in acute anterior uveitis. A controlled clinical trial of non-steroid versus steroid anti-inflammatory treatment. *Acta Ophthalmol* 1991;69:145–148.

André Curi
Clinical Research Fellow

Kimble Matos
Research Fellow

Carlos Pavesio
Consultant Ophthalmic Surgeon
Moorfields Eye Hospital
London, UK

Competing interests: None declared.

Age related macular degeneration

Search date March 2002

Jennifer Arnold and Shirley Sarks

QUESTIONS

INTERVENTIONS

See glossary, p 625

Key Messages

Prevention

- **Laser to drusen** We found insufficient evidence that drusen reduction by laser prevents late age related macular degeneration (AMD) — choroidal neovascularisation or geographic atrophy. One RCT and three pilot studies for RCTs found that laser treatment versus no laser treatment to eyes with high risk drusen significantly improved visual acuity after 2 years (NNT 9, 95% CI 6 to 25). A second RCT found that visual acuity with laser treatment versus no laser treatment only improved in a subgroup of eyes with a reduction in the number of drusen of greater than 50%. It also found that, in eyes with unilateral (but not bilateral) drusen, laser versus no treatment significantly increased the short term incidence of choroidal neovascularisation.

Treatment

- **External beam radiation** One large RCT in people with exudative AMD comparing low dose external beam radiation versus placebo has found no significant difference in the number of people with moderate visual loss after 1 year. Smaller RCTs comparing both low and high dose external beam radiation versus placebo or no treatment found conflicting evidence. We found insufficient evidence on long term safety, although RCTs found no evidence of toxicity to the optic nerve or retina after 12–24 months.
- **Photodynamic treatment with verteporfin** Two RCTs in selected people with exudative AMD found that photodynamic treatment with verteporfin versus placebo significantly reduced the risk of moderate and severe visual loss after 1–2 years. In the first RCT, subgroup analysis suggests the benefit is greatest in people with predominantly classic lesions on fluorescein angiography. In the second RCT, a more modest benefit was seen in the second year of treatment in people with only occult (no classic) lesions on fluorescein angiography. Both RCTs found that photodynamic treatment with verteporfin was associated with an initial loss of vision and photosensitive reactions in a small number of people.
- **Proton beam and scleral plaque radiotherapy** Non-randomised pilot studies found inconclusive evidence about proton beam and scleral plaque (local) radiotherapy used in a variety of dosing and timing schedules.
- **Subcutaneous interferon alfa-2a** One large RCT found that subcutaneous interferon alfa-2a versus placebo increased visual loss after 1 year, although the difference was not significant, and found evidence of serious ocular and systemic adverse effects.
- **Submacular surgery** We found insufficient evidence on the effects of submacular surgery. Case series have found that rates of recurrent choroidal neovascularisation are high, and there is a clinically important risk of ocular complications resulting in visual loss and a need for further surgical intervention.
- **Thermal laser photocoagulation** Four large RCTs in people with exudative AMD and well demarcated lesions have found that thermal laser photocoagulation versus no treatment significantly decreases the rate of severe visual loss after 2–3 years and preserves contrast sensitivity. Choroidal neovascularisation recurs within 2 years in about half of those treated. Photocoagulation may reduce visual acuity initially.

DEFINITION Age related macular degeneration (AMD) is the late stage of age related maculopathy (see glossary, p 625). AMD has two forms: atrophic (or dry) AMD, characterised by geographic atrophy (see glossary, p 625); and exudative (or wet) AMD, characterised by choroidal neovascularisation (see glossary, p 625), which eventually causes a disciform scar.

INCIDENCE/ PREVALENCE AMD is a common cause of blindness registration in industrialised countries. Atrophic AMD is more common than the more sight threatening exudative AMD, affecting about 85% of people with AMD.[1] End stage (blinding) AMD is found in about 2% of all people aged over 50 years, and incidence rises with age (0.7–1.4% of people aged 65–75 years; 11–19% of people aged > 85 years).[2–4]

AETIOLOGY/ RISK FACTORS Age is the strongest risk factor. Ocular risk factors for the development of exudative AMD include the presence of soft drusen (see glossary, p 625), macular pigmentary change, and choroidalneovascularisation in the other eye. Systemic risk factors include hypertension, smoking, and a family history of AMD.[5–8] Diet and exposure to ultraviolet light are suspected as aetiological agents, but this remains unproved.

PROGNOSIS AMD impairs central vision, which is required for reading, driving, face recognition, and all fine visual tasks. **Atrophic AMD** progresses slowly over many years, and time to legal blindness (see glossary, p 625) is highly variable (usually about 5–10 years).[9,10] **Exudative AMD** is more often threatening to vision; 90% of people with severe visual loss owing to AMD have the exudative type. This condition usually manifests with a sudden worsening and distortion of central vision. A modelling exercise (derived primarily from cohort studies) found the risk of developing exudative AMD in people with bilateral soft drusen was 1–5% at 1 year and 13–18% at 3 years.[11] The observed 5 year rate in a population survey was 7%.[12] Most eyes (estimates vary from 60–90%) with exudative AMD progress to legal blindness and develop a central defect (scotoma) in the visual field.[13–16] Peripheral vision is preserved, allowing the person to be mobile and independent. The ability to read with visual aids depends on the size and density of the central scotoma and the degree to which the person retains sensitivity to contrast. Once exudative AMD has developed in one eye, the other eye is at high risk (cumulative estimated incidence: 10% at 1 year, 28% at 3 years, and 42% at 5 years).[5]

AIMS To minimise loss of visual acuity and central vision; to preserve the ability to read with or without visual aids; to optimise quality of life; to minimise adverse effects of treatment.

OUTCOMES Visual acuity; rates of legal blindness; contrast sensitivity; quality of life; visual fields; rate of adverse effects of treatment. Visual acuity is measured using special eye charts, usually the Early Treatment of Diabetic Retinopathy Study chart, although many studies do not specify which chart was used. Stable vision is usually defined as loss of two lines or less on the Early Treatment of Diabetic Retinopathy Study chart. Moderate and severe visual loss is defined as a loss of greater than three and six lines, respectively. Loss of vision to legal blindness (< 20/200) is also used as an outcome. A reading of 20/200 (or 6/60 in metric) on the Snellen chart means that a person can see at 20 feet (or 6 m) what a normally sighted person can see at 200 feet (or 60 m).

METHODS *Clinical Evidence* update search and appraisal March 2002.

QUESTION What are the effects of interventions to prevent age related macular degeneration?

OPTION LASER TO DRUSEN

One RCT and three pilot studies for RCTs found that laser versus no treatment improved visual acuity. A second RCT found no significant difference with laser versus no treatment in the number of eyes with an increased visual acuity of one line or more on the Early Treatment of Diabetic Retinopathy Study chart after 1 year; however, subgroup analysis

found that, in eyes with a reduction of 50% or more in the number of drusen after laser treatment, visual acuity improved significantly. It also found that, in eyes with unilateral (but not bilateral) drusen, laser versus no treatment significantly increased the short term incidence of choroidal neovascularisation. We found insufficient evidence that laser induced drusen reduction results in a decreased incidence of late age related macular degeneration — choroidal neovascularisation or geographic atrophy.

Benefits: We found no systematic review. **Versus no treatment:** We found two RCTs and three pilot studies for RCTs.[17–22] The first RCT (229 eyes, 75 people with unilateral drusen (see glossary, p 625) and 77 people with bilateral drusen; see comment below) compared three treatments: diode laser (see glossary, p 625) treatment at a threshold level (visible burns; 56 eyes); diode laser treatment at a subthreshold level (invisible burns; 49 eyes); and no laser treatment (91 eyes).[17] It found that laser treatment at either level (threshold or subthreshold) versus no laser treatment significantly increased the number of eyes with improved visual acuity (defined as an improvement of ≥ 2 lines on the Early Treatment of Diabetic Retinopathy Study [ETDRS] chart) after 2 years (12/105 [11%] with laser treatment *v* 0/91 [0%] with no treatment; NNT 9, 95% CI 6 to 25). The RCT found no significant difference with threshold versus subthreshold treatment in the number of eyes with improved visual acuity after 2 years (8/56 [14%] with threshold laser treatment *v* 4/49 [8%] with subthreshold treatment; RR 1.8, 95% CI 0.56 to 5.50). The second RCT (120 eyes with unilateral drusen, 312 eyes with bilateral drusen, 276 people; see comment below) compared argon-green laser versus no laser treatment.[18,19] It found no significant difference with laser treatment versus no treatment in the number of eyes with an increased visual acuity of one line or more on the ETDRS chart after 1 year (60/167 [36%] with laser treatment *v* 48/183 [26%] with no laser treatment; RR 1.4, 95% CI 1.0 to 1.88), and no significant difference in the number of eyes with decreased visual acuity of one line or more on the ETDRS chart after 1 year (44/167 [26%] with laser treatment *v* 65/183 [36%] with no laser treatment; RR 0.7, 95% CI 0.54 to 1.02). Subgroup analysis found that significantly more eyes with a reduction of 50% or more in the number of drusen versus eyes with less than 50% reduction in the number of drusen after laser treatment had an increase in visual acuity of one line or more on the ETDRS chart after 1 year (36/77 [48%] with 50% or more reduction *v* 24/90 [27%] with less than 50% reduction; RR 1.8, 95% CI 1.16 to 2.66). The first pilot study for an RCT (27 people aged 46–81 years with age related macular degeneration and symmetrical drusen in both eyes) compared laser treatment versus no treatment.[20] For each person, one eye was randomised to receive laser treatment and the other eye received no treatment. It found that visual acuity in the treated eye was better than the visual acuity in the control eye in 12 people, the same as the control eye in 13 people, and worse than the control eye in two people (P = 0.006; CI not provided; RR calculation not possible) after a mean of 3.2 years. Two other small pilot studies for RCTs found similar results.[21,22]

Harms: Macular laser treatment may induce choroidal neovascularisation (see glossary, p 625) and retinal atrophy. The first RCT found no significant difference with threshold versus non-threshold laser treatment in the number of eyes with choroidal neovascularisation after 24 months (7/59 [12%] with threshold laser treatment *v* 4/49 [8%] with subthreshold laser treatment; RR 1.5, 95% CI 0.45 to 4.68).[17] In the second RCT, early analysis found that in the subgroup of people with unilateral drusen, argon-green laser versus no laser treatment significantly increased the incidence of choroidal neovascularisation (estimated 12 month incidence 10/59 [17%] with laser treatment *v* 2/61 [3%] with no laser treatment; $P < 0.05$; CI not provided; see comment below).[19] In the subgroup of people with bilateral drusen, the second RCT found no significant difference with laser treatment versus no treatment in the estimated 12 month incidence of choroidal neovascularisation (5% with laser treatment *v* 2% with no laser treatment; RR 2.0, 95% CI 0.37 to 11.0). All RCTs sought to minimise choroidal neovascularisation by using low intensity and subthreshold lasers and by positioning laser burns at a distance (generally > 500 μm) from the fovea centre. Both RCTs found that laser induced retinal atrophy was uncommon, with 2/120 (2%) treated eyes affected in one study,[19] and 1/105 (1%) treated eyes affected in the other.[17]

Comment: The first RCT reported that 196/229 (86%) eyes completed 24 months' follow up, although it is not clear whether analysis of data was by intention to treat.[17] The second RCT ceased enrolment and treatment prematurely because of a higher incidence of choroidal neovascularisation within the first 12 months in people receiving laser treatment with unilateral (but not with bilateral) drusen.[18,19] The second RCT reported that 351/432 (81%) eyes completed 12 months' follow up, although analysis of data was not by intention to treat and people with choroidal neovascularisation were excluded.[18,19] We found no evidence of an effective treatment for the majority of people with exudative age related macular degeneration. There is now considerable interest in preventive strategies for people with high risk drusen. One model estimates that a preventive measure of 10% efficacy in people with bilateral drusen would more than double the prevention of legal blindness (see glossary, p 625) relative to current treatment.[23] Other RCTs of laser to drusen are either ongoing[24] or planned.[17,18]

QUESTION **What are the effects of treatments for exudative age related macular degeneration?**

OPTION **THERMAL LASER PHOTOCOAGULATION**

Four large RCTs in people with well demarcated exudative age related macular degeneration have found that thermal laser photocoagulation versus no treatment significantly decreases the rate of severe visual loss after 2–5 years, although two RCTs found an initial loss of visual acuity. The RCTs found that choroidal neovascularisation recurs in about half of those treated within 2 years. Of four smaller RCTs, one found that fovea sparing laser photocoagulation versus no treatment significantly increased the number of eyes with improved or maintained visual acuity

after 12 months, whereas the other three RCTs found no significant difference between scatter (non-confluent) laser versus no treatment in occult choroidal neovascularisation. Three RCTs found no significant difference with two different wavelengths of laser photocoagulation versus each other in visual acuity after a maximum of 5 years. One pilot study for an RCT in people with recurrent subfoveal choroidal neovascularisation following previous laser photocoagulation treatment found no significant difference with laser photocoagulation versus submacular surgery in the number of eyes with improved visual acuity after 2 years.

Benefits: We found no systematic review. **Versus no treatment:** We found four large unblinded multicentre RCTs in selected populations with exudative age related macular degeneration comparing laser photocoagulation versus no treatment (see table 1, p 628).[13–16,25-27] We also found four smaller RCTs that included a wider range of people.[28–31] All four large RCTs found that laser treatment versus no treatment clinically and statistically reduced the risk of severe visual loss (defined as loss of ≥ 6 lines on the special eye chart) after 3 years' follow up. Participants differed in terms of the position of the choroidal neovascularisation (see glossary, p 625) on the retina, whether far, near, or under the centre of fixation (extrafoveal,[13,15] juxtafoveal,[16,25] or subfoveal[14,26,27]). In the study of extrafoveal choroidal neovascularisation, a significant reduction in severe visual loss with laser photocoagulation treatment versus no treatment was found (either by intention to treat analysis or by treatment analysis), despite the fact that 22/117 (19%) eyes randomised to observation later received laser photocoagulation.[13,15] Re-analysis of data for people with juxtafoveal choroidal neovascularisation found that the significant reduction in severe visual loss with laser photocoagulation treatment versus no treatment after 3 years was limited to those people with pure classic choroidal neovascularisation (no occult element) on fluorescein angiography (237/496 [52%] of randomised eyes; OR 2.2, 95% CI 1.4 to 3.4). The two RCTs in people with subfoveal choroidal neovascularisation (new and recurrent disease) found a significant reduction in severe visual loss with laser photocoagulation treatment versus no treatment despite an immediate loss of vision in the treated groups (loss of an average of 3 lines on the special eye chart).[14] Of the four smaller RCTs, one RCT (127 eyes) found that fovea sparing laser photocoagulation versus no treatment significantly increased the number of eyes with improved or maintained visual acuity (defined as loss of < 3 lines on the Early Treatment of Diabetic Retinopathy Study chart) after 12 months (28/68 [41%] with laser treatment *v* 12/59 [20%] with no treatment; RR 2.0, 95% CI 1.13 to 3.61; NNT 5, 95% CI 3 to 16).[28] The other three RCTs found no significant difference between scatter (non-confluent) laser versus no treatment in occult choroidal neovascularisation (see comment below).[29–31] **Different wavelengths:** We found three RCTs that compared two wavelengths of laser photocoagulation (krypton-red or argon-green (see glossary, p 625)) versus each other for choroidal neovascularisation in age related macular degeneration.[32,33] All three RCTs found no significant difference between krypton-red versus argon-green laser photocoagulation in visual acuity after a maximum of 5 years.

Versus submacular surgery: See benefits of submacular surgery, p 622. **Effects in people with choroidal neovascularisation identified by indocyanine green angiography:** We found no RCTs. Uncontrolled case series in selected people have reported good outcomes.

Harms: Laser destroys new vessels and surrounding retina, and the resultant scar causes a corresponding defect in the central visual field. If the laser is applied to subfoveal lesions, or if the laser burn spreads to the fovea, visual acuity will be impaired; two of the RCTs described immediate loss of visual acuity with laser treatment (an average loss of 3 lines on the special eye chart).[14,27] We found no evidence of other adverse effects.

Comment: Three of the four small RCTs comparing scatter laser photocoagulation versus no treatment were too small to rule out any significant treatment effect.[29–31] The benefits of laser photocoagulation depend on accurate, complete treatment requiring high quality angiography and trained, experienced practitioners.[13–16,25–27] The risk of immediate loss of visual acuity with laser photocoagulation may limit its acceptability.

OPTION RADIOTHERAPY

One large RCT in people with exudative age related macular degeneration comparing low dose external beam radiation versus placebo found no significant difference in the number of people with moderate visual loss after 1 year. Smaller RCTs comparing both low and high dose external beam radiation versus placebo or no treatment found conflicting evidence. We found conflicting and inconclusive evidence from non-randomised pilot studies using proton beam and scleral plaque (local) radiotherapy in a variety of dosing and timing schedules. We found insufficient evidence on long term safety, although RCTs found no evidence of toxicity to the optic nerve or retina after 12–24 months.

Benefits: We found no systematic review. **Low dose external beam radiation:** We found three RCTs.[34–36] The first RCT (205 people with new subfoveal choroidal neovascularisation — see glossary, p 625) compared external beam radiation (8 fractions of 2 Gy/fraction) delivered to the macula versus placebo (8 fractions of 0 Gy/fraction).[34] It found no significant difference in the number of people with moderate visual loss (defined as loss of ≥ 3 lines on a special eye chart) after 1 year (51% with radiotherapy treatment *v* 53% with placebo; P = 0.88; CI not provided; absolute numbers not available; see comment below). No treatment benefit was detected for subgroups of people classified as having classic or occult lesions on the basis of fluorescein angiography (occult lesions: 47% with radiotherapy treatment *v* 49% with placebo; P = 0.80; classic/mixed lesions: 58% with radiotherapy treatment *v* 58% with placebo; P = 0.47; CI not provided; absolute numbers not available). The second RCT (83 people; see comment below) compared external beam radiation (7 fractions of 2 Gy/fraction) versus placebo (sham radiation).[35] It found no significant difference between treatments in visual acuity measured on an Early Treatment of Diabetic Retinopathy Study chart (mean number of lines lost: 4.14 with radiation treatment *v* 3.39 with placebo; P = 0.35; CI not provided) or in angiographic outcomes (lesion size/ progression of choroidal neovascularisation) after 12 months. The third RCT (101 people) compared external beam radiation (10 fractions of 2 Gy/fraction) versus observation and found that external beam radiation significantly reduced mean visual loss after 2 years (P < 0.0001; CI not provided; absolute numbers not available; visual acuity reported as logarithm of the minimum angle of resolution).[36] **High dose external beam radiation:** We found one RCT[37] and one pilot study for an RCT.[38] The RCT (74 people with new subfoveal choroidal neovascularisation) compared external beam radiation (4 fractions of 6 Gy/fraction) delivered to the macula versus observation.[37] It found no significant difference between treatments in the number of people with moderate or severe visual loss (defined as losses of 3 or 6 lines on a special eye chart) after 12 months (absolute numbers not available; 32.0% with radiotherapy *v* 52.2% observation; AR –20%, 95% CI –44% to +4%). The pilot study for an RCT (27 people) compared a single fraction external beam radiation (7.5 Gy) versus observation.[38] It found no significant difference between treatments in the number of people with stable vision (defined as a loss of < 3 lines on an Early Treatment of Diabetic Retinopathy Study chart) over a mean follow up of 17 months (range 7–32 months; 10/14 [71%] with radiotherapy *v* 5/13 [38%] with observation; RR 1.9, 95% CI 0.87 to 3.98). **Proton beam and scleral plaque radiotherapy:** We found conflicting and inconclusive evidence from non-randomised pilot studies using proton beam and scleral plaque (local) radiotherapy in a variety of dosing and timing schedules.

Harms: The first RCT comparing low dose external beam radiation versus placebo found no significant difference in cataract formation or dry eye symptoms after 12 months (see comment below).[34] Radiotherapy is potentially toxic to the retina, optic nerve, lens, and lacrimal system, with toxic effects sometimes manifesting up to 2 years after treatment.[39] The biological effects of external beam radiation, both benefit and harm, depend on the dose in each fraction, the number of fractions delivered, and the time between each fraction. Total doses of up to 25 Gy, delivered in daily fractions of 2 Gy or less, are generally claimed not to cause damage to the retina or optic nerve. Uncontrolled pilot studies suggest that the main risks using the present dosing and delivery techniques are cataract formation (2/41 [5] people in one series),[40] and transient dry eye symptoms (10/75 [13%] in a second case series).[41] One case series using total doses of 16–20 Gy in fraction sizes of 4–5 Gy found radiation toxicity of the optic nerve, retina, or choroid in 20/231 (9%) eyes after 12–24 months.[42] Another case series of proton beam radiation found radiation retinopathy in 11/27 (41%) eyes exposed to higher doses after 12 months.[43] A two centre case series of people treated with external beam radiation (5–10 fractions of 2 Gy/fraction) reported an abnormal choroidal vascular growth pattern associated with macular bleeding and exudation, and marked loss of visual acuity.[44] This change was detected in 12/95 (12%) people and 7/98 (7%) people after 3–12 months.

Comment: In the first RCT, we could not replicate the percentages presented in the paper from the raw data provided for cataract and dry eye symptom results.[34] In the second RCT, recruitment was ceased early (before estimated sample size of 100 people had been reached) because of small differences in outcomes between groups at 1 year.[35] Further RCTs are underway using both low and high dose external beam radiotherapy. Experience from pilot studies and case series suggests that, although higher radiation doses may be more effective in inducing regression of choroidal neovascularisation, they carry an increased risk of sight threatening toxicity. RCTs with less than 2 years' follow up may miss important adverse effects.

OPTION SUBMACULAR SURGERY

We found insufficient evidence on the effects of submacular surgery. Case series have found that rates of recurrent choroidal neovascularisation are high, and there is a clinically significant risk of ocular complications resulting in visual loss and the potential need for further surgical intervention.

Benefits: We found no systematic review. **Versus no treatment:** We found no RCTs. **Versus laser photocoagulation:** We found one pilot study for an RCT (70 people with recurrent subfoveal choroidal neovascularisation (see glossary, p 625) following previous laser photocoagulation treatment) that compared submacular surgery versus laser photocoagulation.[45] It found no significant difference between treatments in the number of eyes with improved visual acuity (defined as visual acuity better than or no more than one line worse than baseline as measured on a modified Bailey-Lovie chart) after 2 years (14/28 [50%] with surgery *v* 20/31 [65%] with laser treatment; RR 0.8, 95% CI 0.49 to 1.22). **Versus alternative surgical techniques:** We found one RCT (80 eyes with exudative age related macular degeneration) comparing submacular surgery (see glossary, p 626) plus subretinal injection of tissue plasminogen activator versus submacular surgery plus subretinal injection of a control solution (balanced salt solution).[46] It found no significant difference in the number of eyes with any visual improvement using an Early Treatment of Diabetic Retinopathy Study chart (5/40 [12%] with surgery plus tissue plasminogen activator *v* 6/40 [15%] with surgery plus control; RR 0.8, 95% CI 0.28 to 2.51) or with fluorescein angiographic evidence of active choroidal neovascularisation after 1 year (7/40 [18%] with surgery plus tissue plasminogen activator *v* 8/40 [20%] with surgery plus control; RR 0.9, 95% CI 0.35 to 2.18).

Harms: Submacular surgery may threaten vision itself or necessitate further surgical intervention. However, we found no information on the frequency of adverse events. The largest case series of people with age related and non-age related macular degeneration treated with submacular surgery reported cataract formation (in up to 40%), retinal detachment (5–8%), recurrent new vessel formation (18–35% within 12 months), and macular complications (haemorrhage and pucker; no rates provided).[47]

Comment: Most evidence for submacular surgery currently comes from small uncontrolled case series (< 50 people with age related macular degeneration) with short follow up times, often including people with other types of macular degeneration. These series found that few people with age related macular degeneration had improved vision with surgery.[39,47] Comparing results is difficult because of evolving surgical techniques, changes in outcome measures, and variations in follow up. Several large non-blinded RCTs are currently recruiting and will compare standardised surgical technique versus no treatment in new and haemorrhagic choroidal neovascularisation in people with age related macular degeneration (S Bressler, personal communication, 1999). Other surgical techniques are being developed in volunteers, including macular translocation and retinal pigment epithelial transplantation, but these have yet to be formally evaluated.

OPTION SUBCUTANEOUS INTERFERON ALFA-2A

One large RCT found that subcutaneous interferon alfa-2a (an antiangiogenesis drug) versus placebo increased visual loss, although the difference was not significant, and found evidence of serious ocular and systemic adverse effects.

Benefits: We found no systematic review. We found one RCT (481 people with subfoveal choroidal neovascularisation (see glossary, p 625) due to age related macular degeneration) comparing three doses of subcutaneous interferon alfa-2a (1.5, 3, and 6 million IU given 3 times weekly for 1 year) versus placebo.[47] It found that interferon alfa-2a at all doses versus placebo increased the number of people with a reduction in visual acuity of at least three lines on a Snellen chart after 52 weeks, although the difference was not significant (see comment below; 142/286 [50%] with interferon alfa-2a *v* 40/105 [38%] with placebo; RR 1.2, 95% CI 0.90 to 1.62).

Harms: Adverse effects of interferon alfa-2a were common and potentially severe in this RCT[47] and in other poorer quality RCTs. Effects included fatigue and influenza-like symptoms, gastrointestinal symptoms (including nausea, diarrhoea, and loss of appetite), and central and peripheral nervous system effects (including headaches and dizziness). Although at least one adverse event was reported in 90/105 (86%) people taking placebo, the proportion of people on active treatment who suffered adverse effects increased with dose, as did the severity of adverse effects. The RCT reported that 20/286 (7%) people receiving interferon alfa-2a developed interferon associated retinopathy (retinal haemorrhages or cotton wool spots).[48]

Comment: In the RCT, 90/481 (18%) of people did not complete the trial and analysis of data was not by intention to treat.[47] There is widespread interest in safe, effective antiangiogenesis drugs for prophylaxis in exudative age related macular degeneration. Several drugs are currently under preclinical and early phase clinical study. RCTs are currently investigating the use of intraocular or periocular steroids and antivascular endothelial growth factor.

OPTION PHOTODYNAMIC TREATMENT WITH VERTEPORFIN

Two RCTs in people with age related macular degeneration found that photodynamic treatment with verteporfin versus placebo significantly reduced the number of people with moderate or severe vision loss after 1–2 years. In the first RCT, subgroup analysis suggested the benefit is greatest in people with predominantly classic lesions on fluorescein angiography. Subgroup analysis in the second RCT suggested a more modest benefit in the second year of treatment in people with only occult (no classic) lesions on fluorescein angiography. Both RCTs found that photodynamic treatment with verteporfin was associated with an initial loss of vision and photosensitive reactions in a small number of people.

Benefits: We found one systematic review (search date 2000, 1 RCT, 609 people with new and recurrent subfoveal choroidal neovascularisation (see glossary, p 625) due to age related macular degeneration)[49] and one subsequent RCT.[50] The RCT included in the review compared photodynamic treatment (see glossary, p 625) with verteporfin (see glossary, p 626) (6 mg/m^2 body surface area) versus placebo (photodynamic treatment with 5% dextrose solution). Treatments were repeated as necessary every 3 months. Results were reported after 12 months[49] and, subsequently, after 24 months.[51] The RCT reported in the systematic review The RCT found that photodynamic treatment with verteporfin versus placebo significantly increased the number of people with stable vision after 12 months (defined as a loss of < 15 letters or 3 lines of vision on a special eye chart; 246/402 [61%] with photodynamic treatment with verteporfin *v* 96/207 [46%] with placebo; RR 1.3, 95% CI 1.12 to 1.56; NNT 7, 95% CI 5 to 15)[49] and after 24 months (213/402 [53%] with photodynamic treatment with verteporfin *v* 78/207 [38%] with placebo; RR 1.4, 95% CI 1.15 to 1.71; NNT 7, 95% CI 5 to 14).[51] Subgroup analysis found that benefit was greater in people with predominantly classic choroidal neovascularisation (see glossary, p 625) lesions (94/159 [59%] with photodynamic treatment with verteporfin *v* 26/83 [31%] with placebo; RR 1.9, 95% CI 1.34 to 2.66), and greatest in people with only classic lesions (65/93 [70%] photodynamic treatment with verteporfin *v* 14/49 [29%] with placebo; RR 2.5, 95% CI 1.54 to 3.88) after 24 months. The subsequent RCT (339 people with occult or classic choroidal neovascularisation due to age related macular degeneration; see comment below) found that photodynamic treatment with verteporfin (6 mg/m^2 body surface area) versus placebo (photodynamic treatment with 5% dextrose solution) significantly reduced the number of people with moderate vision loss (defined as a loss of ≥ 15 letters of vision or more on a special eye chart; 121/225 [54%] with photodynamic treatment with verteporfin *v* 76/114 [67%] with placebo; RR 0.8, 95% CI 0.68 to 0.96; NNT 8, 95% CI 5 to 39) and severe vision loss (defined as a loss of ≥ 30 letters of vision on a special eye chart; 67/225 [30%] with photodynamic treatment with verteporfin *v* 54/114 [47%] with placebo; RR 0.6, 95% CI 0.48 to 0.83; NNT 6, 95% CI 4 to 15) after 2 years.[50] Subgroup analysis of people with only occult choroidal neovascularisation (no classic lesions) on fluorescein angiography (166 [74%] people receiving photodynamic treatment with verteporfin and 92 [81%] people receiving placebo) found that photodynamic treatment with verteporfin versus placebo significantly reduced the number of people with moderate vision loss (91/166 [55%] with photodynamic treatment with verteporfin *v* 63/92 [68%] with placebo; RR 0.8, 95% CI 0.7 to 0.97) and with severe vision loss (48/166 [29%] with photodynamic treatment with verteporfin *v* 43/92 [47%] with placebo; RR 0.6, 95% CI 0.45 to 0.86; see comment below) after 2 years.

Harms: Verteporfin is a photosensitive dye and care must be taken to avoid leakage into surrounding tissues during infusion and exposure to bright light soon after treatment. Advice in the study was to avoid light for 48 hours but some photosensitive reactions were observed in treated people after 3–5 days.[49] The treatment was well tolerated but was more likely than the control intervention to cause a transient decrease in vision, injection site reactions, photosensitivity, and infusion related low back pain. Severe loss of vision (greater than 20 letters or 4 lines on a special eye chart) was recorded in 3/402 people (< 1%) in the first RCT[49,51] and 10/225 people (4%) in the subsequent RCT,[50] within 7 days of treatment, although some visual recovery occurred in most cases. The risk appears to be higher in people with occult and no classic choroidal neovascularisation. The possibility of rare but severe adverse events remains.

Comment: The subsequent RCT included a subset of people with only occult and no classic choroidal neovascularisation lesions.[50] Further analysis of this subgroup has suggested that the treatment effect recorded by the RCT may be influenced by baseline visual acuity and lesion size.[52]

GLOSSARY

Age related maculopathy Degenerative disease of the macula (centre of the retina): classified as early (marked by drusen and pigmentary change, and usually associated with normal vision) and late (when it is known as age related macular degeneration).

Choroidal neovascularisation New vessels in the choroid, classified by fluorescein angiography: in terms of its position in relation to the fovea — extrafoveal, juxtafoveal, or subfoveal; in terms of its appearance — classic (well defined) or occult (poorly defined); and in terms of its borders — well demarcated or poorly demarcated.

Drusen Small, yellow, bright objects, often near the macula, seen by ophthalmoscopy. They are located under the basement membrane of the retinal pigment epithelium. They are present in many older people with normal vision, but a greater number of large drusen indicate higher risk of subsequent loss of acuity from age related macular degeneration.

Geographic atrophy The end stage of atrophic age related macular degeneration with atrophy of the retina and inner choroidal layers at the macular leaving only the deep choroidal vessels visible.

Laser (diode, krypton, argon-green) Lasers used in ophthalmology that produce focused light of different specific wavelengths.

Legal blindness Visual acuity less than 20/200.

Photodynamic treatment A two step procedure of intravenous infusion of a photosensitive dye followed by application of a non-thermal laser that activates the dye. The treatment aims to cause selective closure of the choroidal new vessels.

Predominantly classic choroidal neovascularisation Choroidal neovascularisation in which more than 50% of lesion area consists of classic choroidal neovascularisation on fluorescein angiography.

Submacular surgery Removal of haemorrhage and/or choroidal neovascularisation after vitrectomy.
Verteporfin A photosensitive dye used in photodynamic treatment.

REFERENCES

1. Bressler SB, Bressler NM, Fine SL. Age-related macular degeneration. *Surv Ophthalmol* 1988;32:375–413.
2. Klein R, Klein BEK, Linton KLP. Prevalence of age-related maculopathy: the Beaver Dam Eye Study. *Ophthalmology* 1992;99:933–943.
3. Vingerling JR, Dielemans I, Hofman A, et al. The prevalence of age-related maculopathy in the Rotterdam study. *Ophthalmology* 1995;102:205–210.
4. Mitchell P, Smith W, Attebo K, et al. Prevalence of age-related maculopathy in Australia. The Blue Mountains Eye Study. *Ophthalmology* 1995;102:1450–1640.
5. Macular Photocoagulation Study Group. Risk factors for choroidal neovascularisation in the second eye of patients with juxtafoveal or subfoveal choroidal neovascularisation secondary to age-related macular degeneration. *Arch Ophthalmol* 1997;115:741–747.
6. Pieramici DJ, Bressler SB. Age-related macular degeneration and risk factors for the development of choroidal neovascularization in the fellow eye. *Curr Opin Ophthalmol* 1998;9:38–46.
7. Smith W, Assink J, Klein R, et al. Risk factors for age-related macular degeneration: pooled findings from three continents. *Ophthalmology* 2001;108:697–704.
8. Age-related Eye Disease Study Research Group. Risk factors associated with age-related macular degeneration. A case-control study in the age-related eye disease study: age-related eye disease study report number 3. *Ophthalmology* 2000;107:2224–2232.
9. Maguire P, Vine AK. Geographic atrophy of the retinal pigment epithelium. *Am J Ophthalmol* 1986;102:621–625.
10. Sarks JP, Sarks SH, Killingsworth M. Evolution of geographic atrophy of the retinal pigment epithelium. *Eye* 1988;2:552–577.
11. Holz FG, Wolfensberger TJ, Piguet B, et al. Bilateral macular drusen in age-related macular degeneration: prognosis and risk factors. *Ophthalmology* 1994;101:1522–1528.
12. Klein R, Klein BEK, Jensen SC, et al. The five-year incidence and progression of age-related maculopathy. The Beaver Dam Eye study. *Ophthalmology* 1997;104:7–21.
13. Macular Photocoagulation Study Group. Argon laser photocoagulation for neovascular maculopathy: Five-year results from randomized clinical trials. *Arch Ophthalmol* 1991;109:1109–1114.
14. Macular Photocoagulation Study Group. Laser photocoagulation of subfoveal neovascular lesions of age-related macular degeneration: updated findings from two clinical trials. *Arch Ophthalmol* 1993;111:1200–1209.
15. Macular Photocoagulation Study Group. Argon laser photocoagulation for neovascular maculopathy. Three-year results from randomized clinical trials. *Arch Ophthalmol* 1986;104:694–701.
16. Macular Photocoagulation Study Group. Laser photocoagulation for juxtafoveal choroidal neovascularisation. Five-year results from randomized clinical trials. *Arch Ophthalmol* 1994;112:500–509.
17. Olk, RJ, Friberg TR, Stickney KL, et al. Therapeutic benefits of infrared (810 nm) diode laser macular grid photocoagulation in prophylactic treatment of nonexudative age-related macular degeneration: two-year results of a randomized pilot study. *Ophthalmology* 1999;106:2082–2090.
18. Ho CA, Maguire MG, Yoken J, et al. The Choroidal Neovascularization Prevention Trial research group. Laser-induced drusen reduction improves visual function at 1 year. *Ophthalmology* 1999;106:1367–1373.
19. The Choroidal Neovascularization Prevention Trial research group. Laser treatment in eyes with large drusen. Short-term effects seen in a pilot randomized clinical trial. *Ophthalmology* 1998;105:11–23.
20. Little HL, Showman JM, Brown BW. A pilot randomized controlled study on the effect of laser photocoagulation of confluent soft macular drusen. *Ophthalmology* 1997;104:623–631.
21. Frennesson C, Nilsson SEG. Prophylactic laser treatment in early age-related maculopathy reduced the incidence of exudative complications. *Br J Ophthalmol* 1998;82:1169–1174.
22. Figueroa MS, Regueras A, Bertrand J, et al. Laser photocoagulation for macular soft drusen. Updated results. *Retina* 1997;17:378–384.
23. Lanchoney DM, Maguire MG, Fine SL. A model of the incidence and consequences of choroidal neovascularisation secondary to age-related macular degeneration. Comparative effects of current treatment and potential prophylaxis on visual outcomes in high-risk patients. *Arch Ophthalmol* 1998;116:1045–1052.
24. Owens SL, Guymer RH, Gross-Jendroska M, et al. Fluorescein angiographic abnormalities after prophylactic macular photocoagulation for high-risk age-related maculopathy. *Am J Ophthalmol* 1999;127:681–687.
25. Macular Photocoagulation Study Group. Occult choroidal neovascularization. Influence on visual outcome in patients with age-related macular degeneration. *Arch Ophthalmol* 1996;114:400–412.
26. Macular Photocoagulation Study Group. Persistent and recurrent neovascularization after laser photocoagulation for subfoveal choroidal neovascularization of age-related macular degeneration. *Arch Ophthalmol* 1994;112:489–499.
27. Macular Photocoagulation Study Group. Visual outcome after laser photocoagulation for subfoveal choroidal neovascularization secondary to age-related macular degeneration. The influence of initial lesion size and initial visual acuity. *Arch Ophthalmol* 1994;112:480–488.
28. Coscas G, Soubrane G, Ramahefasolo C, et al. Perifoveal laser treatment for subfoveal choroidal new vessels in age-related macular degeneration. Results of a randomized clinical trial. *Arch Ophthalmol* 1991;109:1258–1265.
29. Bressler NM, Maguire MG, Murphy PL, et al. Macular scatter ("grid") laser treatment of poorly demarcated subfoveal choroidal neovascularisation in age-related macular degeneration. Results of a randomised pilot trial. *Arch Ophthalmol* 1996;114:1456–1464.
30. Arnold J, Algan M, Soubrane G, et al. Indirect scatter laser photocoagulation to subfoveal choroidal neovascularization in age-related macular degeneration. *Graefes Arch Clin Exp Ophthalmol* 1997;235:208–216.

31. Barondes MJ, Pagliarini S, Chisholm IH, et al. Controlled trial of laser photocoagulation of pigment epithelial detachments in the elderly: 4 year review. *Br J Ophthalmol* 1992;76:5–7.
32. Macular Photocoagulation Study Group. Evaluation of argon green vs krypton red laser for photocoagulation of subfoveal choroidal neovascularisation in the Macular Photocoagulation Study. *Arch Ophthalmol* 1994;112:1176–1184.
33. Willan AR, Cruess AF, Ballantyne M. Argon green vs krypton red laser photocoagulation for extrafoveal choroidal neovascularization secondary to age-related macular degeneration: 3-year results of a multicentre randomized trial. *Can J Ophthalmol* 1996;31:11–17.
34. The Radiation Therapy for Age-related Macular Degeneration (RAD) study group. A prospective randomized double-masked trial on radiation therapy for neovascular age-related macular degeneration (RAD) study. *Ophthalmology* 1999;106:2239–2247.
35. Marcus DM, Sheils W, Johnson MH, et al. External beam irradiation of subfoveal choroidal neovascularization complicating age-related macular degeneration: one-year results of a prospective, double-masked, randomized clinical trial. *Arch Ophthalmol* 2001;119:171–180.
36. Kobayashi H, Kobayashi K. Age-related macular degeneration: long-term results of radiotherapy for subfoveal neovascular membranes. *Am J Ophthalmol* 2000;130:617–635.
37. Bergink GJ, Hoyng CB, Van der Maazen RW, et al. A randomized controlled clinical trial on the efficacy of radiation therapy in the control of subfoveal choroidal neovascularization in age-related macular degeneration: radiation versus observation. *Graefes Arch Clin Exp Ophthalmol* 1998;236:321–325.
38. Char DH, Irvine AI, Posner MD, et al. Randomized trial of radiation for age-related macular degeneration. *Am J Ophthalmol* 1999;127:574–578.
39. Ciulla TA, Danis RP, Harris A. Age-related macular degeneration: a review of experimental treatments. *Surv Ophthalmol* 1998;43:134–146.
40. Hart PM, Chakravarthy U, MacKenzie G, et al. Teletherapy for subfoveal choroidal neovascularisation of age-related macular degeneration: results of follow up in a non randomised study. *Br J Ophthalmol* 1996;80:1046–1050.
41. Finger PT, Berson A, Sherr D, et al. Radiation therapy for subretinal neovascularization. *Ophthalmology* 1996;103:878–889.
42. Mauget-Faysse M, Chiquet C, Milea D, et al. Long term results of radiotherapy for subfoveal choroidal neovascularisation in age-related macular degeneration. *Br J Ophthalmol* 1999;83:923–928.
43. Flaxel CJ, Fridrichsen EJ, Osborn Smith J, et al. Proton beam irradiation of subfoveal choroidal neovascularisation in age-related macular degeneration. *Eye* 2000;14:155–164.
44. Spaide RF, Leys A, Herrmann-Delemazure B, et al. Radiation-associated choroidal neovasculopathy. *Ophthalmology* 1999;106:2254–2260.
45. Submacular Surgery Trials Pilot Study Investigators. Submacular surgery trials randomized pilot trial of laser photocoagulation versus surgery for recurrent choroidal neovascularization secondary to age-related macular degeneration: I. Ophthalmic outcomes. Submacular surgery trials pilot study report number 1. *Am J Ophthalmol* 2000;130:387–407.
46. Lewis H, Van der Brug MS. Tissue plasminogen activator-assisted surgical excision of subfoveal choroidal neovascularization in age-related macular degeneration: a randomized, double-masked trial. *Ophthalmology* 1997;104:1847–1851.
47. Thomas MA, Dickinson JD, Melberg NS, et al. Visual results after surgical removal of subfoveal choroidal neovascular membranes. *Ophthalmology* 1994;101:1384–1396.
48. Pharmacological Therapy for Macular Degeneration study group. Interferon alfa-2a is ineffective for patients with choroidal neovascularization secondary to age-related macular degeneration: results of a prospective randomized placebo-controlled clinical trial. *Arch Ophthalmol* 1997;115:865–872.
49. Wormald R, Evans J, Smeeth L. Photodynamic therapy for neovascular age-related macular degeneration. In: The Cochrane Library, Issue 2, 2001. Oxford: Update Software. Search date 2000; primary sources Cochrane Controlled Trials Register, Cochrane Eyes and Vision Group Register, Medline, Embase, Science Citation Index, experts, and hand searched references.
50. Verteporfin In Photodynamic Therapy Study Group. Verteporfin therapy of subfoveal choroidal neovascularization in age-related macular degeneration: two-year results of a randomized clinical trial including lesions with occult with no classic choroidal neovascularization: verteporfin in photodynamic therapy report 2. *Am J Ophthalmol* 2001;131:541–560.
51. Treatment of age-related macular degeneration with photodynamic therapy (TAP) study group. Photodynamic therapy of subfoveal choroidal neovascularisation in age-related macular degeneration with verteporfin. Two-year results of 2 randomized clinical trials: TAP report 2. *Arch Ophthalmol* 2001;119:198–207.
52. Bressler NM. Verteporfin therapy of subfoveal choroidal neovascularization in age-related macular degeneration: two-year results of a randomized clinical trial including lesions with occult with no classic choroidal neovascularization-verteporfin in photodynamic therapy report 2. *Am J Ophthalmol* 2002;133:168–169.

Jennifer Arnold
Consultant Ophthalmologist
Marsden Eye Specialists
Parramatta New South Wales
Australia

Shirley Sarks
Honorary Senior Research Associate
Prince of Wales Medical Research Institute
Randwick New South Wales
Australia

Competing interests: JA was a clinical investigator in the study of photodynamic treatment using verteporfin, funded by Novartis/QLT, and has been supported by Novartis for attendance at conferences and symposia. SS none declared.

TABLE 1 Laser photocoagulation of choroidal neovascularisation versus observation in exudative age related macular degeneration: results of Macular Photocoagulation Study Group RCTs (see text, p 619).

Site of CNV (type of laser)	Number of eyes	Severe visual loss (6 or more lines)	Vision level treated *v* control	Rate of recurrence in treated eyes
Extrafoveal CNV (argon-blue-green)[13,15]	236	RR 1.5 at 6 months to 5 years; $P = 0.001$	≥20/40 at 3 years; 33% *v* 22%	54% at 5 years
Juxtafoveal CNV (krypton-red)[16,25]	496	RR 1.2 at 6 months to 5 years; $P = 0.04$	≥20/40 at 3 years; 13% *v* 7%	76% at 5 years (classic CNV only)
New subfoveal CNV (argon-green or krypton)[14,26,27]	373	20% treated *v* 37% control at 2 years; $P < 0.01$	> 20/200 at 4 years; 12% *v* 11%	44% at 3 years
Recurrent subfoveal CNV (argon-green or krypton)[14,26,27]	206	9% treated *v* 28% control at 2 years; $P = 0.03$	> 20/200 at 3 years; 25% *v* 12%	39% at 3 years

CNV, choroidal neovascularisation.

Bacterial conjunctivitis

Search date February 2002

Christine Chung, Elisabeth Cohen, and Justine Smith

QUESTIONS

INTERVENTIONS

Key Messages

- **Antibiotic treatment in culture positive bacterial conjunctivitis** One systematic review has found that antibiotics (polymyxin–bacitracin, ciprofloxacin, or ofloxacin) versus placebo significantly increase rates of both clinical and microbiological cure after 2–5 days. RCTs comparing different antibiotics versus each other found conflicting results for rates of clinical and microbiological cure.
- **Empirical antibiotic treatment of suspected bacterial conjunctivitis** One systematic review found limited evidence that topical norfloxacin versus placebo significantly increased rates of clinical and microbiological improvement or cure after 5 days. RCTs comparing different topical antibiotics versus each other found no significant difference in rates of clinical or microbiological cure. One RCT found no significant difference with topical polymyxin–bacitracin ointment versus oral cefixime in the number of people who improved clinically or microbiologically.

Bacterial conjunctivitis

DEFINITION Conjunctivitis is any inflammation of the conjunctiva, generally characterised by irritation, itching, foreign body sensation, and tearing or discharge. Bacterial conjunctivitis may usually be distinguished from other types of conjunctivitis by the presence of a yellow–white mucopurulent discharge. There is also usually a papillary reaction (small bumps with fibrovascular cores on the palpebral conjunctiva, appearing grossly as a fine velvety surface). Bacterial conjunctivitis is usually bilateral. This review covers only non-gonococcal bacterial conjunctivitis.

INCIDENCE/ PREVALENCE We found no good evidence on the incidence or prevalence of bacterial conjunctivitis.

AETIOLOGY/ RISK FACTORS Conjunctivitis may be infectious (caused by bacteria or viruses) or allergic. In adults, bacterial conjunctivitis is less common than viral conjunctivitis, although estimates vary widely (viral conjunctivitis has been reported to account for 8–75% of acute conjunctivitis).[1–3] *Staphylococcus* species are the most common pathogens for bacterial conjunctivitis in adults, followed by *Streptococcus pneumoniae* and *Haemophilus influenzae*.[4,5] In children, bacterial conjunctivitis is more common than viral, and is mainly caused by *H influenzae, S pneumoniae*, and *Moraxella catarrhalis*.[6,7]

PROGNOSIS Most bacterial conjunctivitis is self limiting. One systematic review (search date 2002) found clinical cure or significant improvement with placebo within 2–5 days in 64% of people (99% CI 54% to 73%).[8] Some organisms cause corneal or systemic complications, or both; otitis may develop in 25% of children with *H influenzae* conjunctivitis,[9] and systemic meningitis may complicate primary meningococcal conjunctivitis in 18% of people.[10]

AIMS To achieve rapid cure of inflammation, and to prevent complications, with minimum adverse effects of treatment.

OUTCOMES Time to cure or improvement. **Clinical signs/symptoms:** hyperaemia, discharge, papillae, follicles, chemosis, itching, pain, photophobia. Most studies used a numbered scale to grade signs and symptoms. Some studies also included evaluation by investigators and patients regarding success of treatment. **Culture results:** These are proxy outcomes usually expressed as the number of colonies, sometimes with reference to a threshold level. Results were often classified into categories such as eradication, reduction, persistence, and proliferation.

METHODS *Clinical Evidence* search and appraisal February 2002.

QUESTION **What are the effects of empirical treatment with antibiotics in adults and children with suspected bacterial conjunctivitis?**

One systematic review found limited evidence that topical norfloxacin versus placebo significantly increased rates of clinical and microbiological improvement or cure after 5 days. RCTs comparing different topical antibiotics versus each other found no significant

difference in rates of clinical or microbiological cure. One RCT found no significant difference with topical polymyxin–bacitracin ointment versus oral cefixime in the number of people who improved clinically or in bacteriological failure rates.

Benefits: **Versus placebo:** We found one systematic review (search date 2000, 1 RCT, 284 adults; 50% of participants were culture positive) comparing topical norfloxacin versus placebo.[8] It found that norfloxacin significantly increased rates of clinical and microbiological improvement or cure after 5 days (88%, 95% CI 81% to 93% with norfloxacin *v* 72%, 95% CI 63% to 79% with placebo; $P < 0.01$; see comment below). **Versus each other:** We found no systematic review but found 20 RCTs in adults and children (see web extra table A at www.clinicalevidence.com). These RCTs found no significant difference between different topical antibiotics versus each other in rates of clinical or microbiological cure. Six of the RCTs (evaluating lomefloxacin, fusidic acid, rifamycin, chloramphenicol, and tobramycin) found no significant difference between different antibiotics in effectiveness or tolerability (grading by patients).[11–16] One of the RCTs found no significant difference with polymyxin bacitracin ointment plus oral placebo versus topical placebo plus oral cefixime in the number of people who improved clinically or in bacteriological failure rates.[17]

Harms: The placebo controlled RCT identified by the review reported minor adverse events in 4.2% of people using norfloxacin and 7.1% using placebo (no statistical analysis available).[5] Placebo contained higher proportions of benzalkonium chloride (0.01% with placebo *v* 0.0025% with norfloxacin). One non-systematic review described complications of topical antibiotics.[18] These included four reported cases of idiosyncratic aplastic anaemia associated with topical chloramphenicol and three cases of Stevens–Johnson syndrome associated with topical sulphonamides. However, the review did not report the number of people using these drugs, making it difficult to exclude other possible causes of aplastic anaemia.

Comment: The placebo controlled RCT identified by the review did not address the effect of using topical antibiotics on antibiotic resistance, which would be of interest given the self limiting nature of the disease.[5] None of the trials specified their methods for selecting participants. The findings may not be generalisable to primary care populations. Most trials included children as well as adults, and the ratio of children to adults was usually not specified. The comparisons of lomefloxacin versus chloramphenicol and fusidic acid, and the comparison of norfloxacin versus fusidic acid, were single blind. Lomefloxacin and fusidic acid are not available in the USA, and chloramphenicol is rarely used in the USA because of reports of idiosyncratic aplastic anaemia.

QUESTION What are the effects of topical antibiotics in adults and children with culture positive bacterial conjunctivitis?

One systematic review has found that antibiotics (polymyxin–bacitracin, ciprofloxacin, or ofloxacin) versus placebo significantly increase rates of both clinical and microbiological cure. RCTs comparing different antibiotics versus each other found conflicting results for rates of clinical and microbiological cure.

Benefits: **Versus placebo:** Wc found one systematic review (search date 2000, 3 RCTs) in people with culture positive bacterial conjunctivitis, which compared antibiotics (polymyxin–bacitracin, ciprofloxacin, and ofloxacin) versus placebo.[8] The review identified no trials of gentamicin that included only culture proven conjunctivitis. The first RCT (84 children) identified by the review found that in children with culture proven *H influenzae* and *S pneumoniae* bacterial conjunctivitis topical polymyxin–bacitracin versus placebo significantly increased clinical cure after 3–5 days (62% with antibiotic *v* 28% with placebo; $P < 0.02$), but found no significant difference after 8–10 days (91% with antibiotic *v* 72% with placebo; $P > 0.05$).[19] The RCT found that topical polymyxin–bacitracin versus placebo significantly increased microbiological cure rates after both 3–5 days and 8–10 days. The RCT also found that when systemic antibiotics were given for concurrent problems, there was no significant difference in outcomes between treatments, although the numbers were too small to rule out a clinically important effect (see web extra table A at www.clinicalevidence.com). The second and third RCTs identified by the review did not specify the ages of participants. The second RCT (177 people) identified by the review found that ciprofloxacin versus placebo significantly improved microbiological cure rates after 3 days (132/140 [94%] with antibiotic *v* 22/37 [59%] with placebo; RR 1.59, 95% CI 1.21 to 2.08).[20] The third RCT (132 people) identified by the review found that ofloxacin versus placebo significantly increased clinical and microbiological improvement after 2 days (64% with ofloxacin *v* 22% with placebo; $P < 0.001$).[21] **Versus each other:** We found no systematic review but found six RCTs.[20,22–26] The first RCT (139 children) found that fusidic acid versus chloramphenicol significantly increased the number of children judged to have been clinically cured (85% with fusidic acid *v* 48% with chloramphenicol; $P < 0.0001$).[22] The second RCT (251 people) found no significant difference between ciprofloxacin versus tobramycin in reduction or eradication of bacteria after 7 days (94.5% with ciprofloxacin *v* 91.9% with tobramycin; $P > 0.5$).[20] The third RCT (141 children) found no significant difference between ciprofloxacin versus tobramycin in the number of children judged to have been clinically cured (87% with ciprofloxacin *v* 90% with tobramycin; $P > 0.05$) or in the number of children in whom microbiological eradication was achieved (90% with ciprofloxacin *v* 84% with tobramycin; $P = 0.29$) after 7 days.[23] The fourth RCT (156 children) compared three treatments: trimethoprim–polymyxin, gentamicin, and sulfacetamide (sulphacetamide).[24] It found no significant difference between any of the treatments in the number of children judged to have been clinically cured (84% with trimethoprim–polymyxin *v* 88% with gentamicin *v* 89% with sulfacetamide; $P > 0.1$), or in the number of children in whom microbiological eradication was achieved (83% with trimethoprim–polymyxin *v* 68% with gentamicin *v* 72% with sulfacetamide; $P > 0.1$) after 2–7 days. The fifth RCT (40 people) found no significant difference between lomefloxacin versus ofloxacin in the number of people whose symptoms and signs had resolved after 7 days (88% with lomefloxacin *v* 75% ofloxacin; $P < 0.08$).[25]The sixth RCT (121 people) found that topical netilmicin (0.3%) versus topical gentamicin (0.3%) administered as one or two drops to affected eyes four times daily significantly increased the number of people whose infections were judged to have resolved after both 5 and 10 days (P = 0.01 after 5 days; P = 0.001 after 10 days; other results presented graphically).[26]

Harms: Of the 116 children initially enrolled in the first placebo controlled RCT identified by the review, one was excluded because of possible allergic reaction to the ointment; the other exclusions were unrelated to adverse effects.[19] In RCTs that included people with both culture proved and suspected bacterial conjunctivitis, minor adverse events were reported with antibiotics: burning, bitter taste, pruritus, or punctate epithelial erosions (35% with tobramycin *v* 20% with ciprofloxacin; no statistical detail available),[27] bad taste (20% with norfloxacin *v* 6% with fusidic acid),[28] stinging (50% with norfloxacin *v* 37% with fusidic acid),[28] and burning (33% with gentamicin *v* 20% with lomefloxacin).[13] The RCT comparing topical netilmicin versus topical gentamicin found no significant difference in the number of people reporting adverse reactions to either drug (redness, itching, and burning).[26]

Comment: The third RCT identified by the review, which compared antibiotics versus placebo, is published only in abstract form.[21] A fourth RCT identified by the review is published in Japanese and is awaiting translation.[29] None of the RCTs addressed the effect on antibiotic resistance of using topical antibiotics in bacterial conjunctivitis, which would be of interest given the self limiting nature of the disease. Furthermore, they did not report on patient oriented outcomes or look at rates of reinfection.

REFERENCES

1. Wishart PK, James C, Wishart MS, Darougar S. Prevalence of acute conjunctivitis caused by chlamydia, adenovirus, and herpes simplex virus in an ophthalmic casualty department. *Br J Ophthalmol* 1984;68:653–655.
2. Fitch CP, Rapoza PA, Owens S, et al. Epidemiology and diagnosis of acute conjunctivitis at an inner-city hospital. *Ophthalmology* 1989;96:1215–1220.
3. Woodland RM, Darougar S, Thaker U, et al. Causes of conjunctivitis and keratoconjunctivitis in Karachi, Pakistan. *Trans R Soc Trop Med Hygiene* 1992;86:317–320.
4. Seal DV, Barrett SP, McGill JI. Aetiology and treatment of acute bacterial infection of the external eye. *Br J Ophthalmol* 1982;66:357–360.
5. Miller IM, Wittreich J, Vogel R, Cook TJ, for the Norfloxacin-Placebo Ocular Study Group. The safety and efficacy of topical norfloxacin compared with placebo in the treatment of acute bacterial conjunctivitis. *Eur J Ophthalmol* 1992;2:58–66.
6. Gigliotti F, Williams WT, Hayden FG, et al. Etiology of acute conjunctivitis in children. *J Pediatr* 1981;98:531–536.
7. Weiss A, Brinser JH, Nazar-Stewart V. Acute conjunctivitis in childhood. *J Pediatr* 1993;122:10–14.
8. Sheikh A, Hurwitz B, Cave J. Antibiotics versus placebo for acute bacterial conjunctivitis. In: The Cochrane Library, Issue 3, 2001. Oxford: Update Software. Search date 2000; primary sources Cochrane Controlled Trials Register, Medline, bibliographies of identified trials, Science Citation Index, and personal contacts with investigators and pharmaceutical companies.
9. Bodor FF. Conjunctivitis-otitis media syndrome: more than meets the eye. *Contemp Pediatr* 1989;6:55–60.
10. Barquet N, Gasser I, Domingo P, et al. Primary meningococcal conjunctivitis: report of 21 patients and review. *Rev Infect Dis* 1990;12:838–847.
11. Kettenmeyer A, Jauch A, Boscher M, et al. A double-blind double-dummy multicenter equivalence study comparing topical lomefloxacin 0.3% twice daily with norfloxacin 0.3% four times daily in the treatment of acute bacterial conjunctivitis. *J Clin Res* 1998;1:75–86.
12. Agius-Fernandez A, Patterson A, Fsadni M, et al. Topical lomefloxacin versus topical chloramphenicol in the treatment of acute bacterial conjunctivitis. *Clin Drug Invest* 1998;15:263–269.
13. Montero J, Casado A, Perea E, et al. A double-blind double-dummy comparison of topical lomefloxacin 0.3% twice daily with topical gentamicin 0.3% four times daily in the treatment of acute bacterial conjunctivitis. *J Clin Res* 1998;1:29–39.
14. Adenis JP, Arrata M, Gastaud P, et al. Etude randomisee multicentrique acide fusidique gel ophtalmique et rifamycine collyre dans les conjonctivites aigues. *J Fr Ophtalmol* 1989;12:317–322.
15. Huerva V, Ascaso FJ, Latre B, et al. Tolerancia y eficacia de la tobramicina topica vs cloranfenicol

en el tratamiento de las conjunctivitis bacterianas. *Ciencia Pharmaceutica* 1991;1:221–224.

16. Gallenga PE, Lobefalo L, Colangelo L, et al. Topical lomefloxacin 0.3% twice daily versus tobramycin 0.3% in acute bacterial conjunctivitis: a multicenter double-blind phase III study. *Ophthalmologica* 1999;213:250–257.
17. Wald ER, Greenberg D, Hoberman A.. Short term oral cefixime therapy for treatment of bacterial conjunctivitis. *Pediatr Infect Dis Jl* 2001;20:1039–1042.
18. Stern GA, Killingsworth DW. Complications of topical antimicrobial agents. *Int Ophthalmol Clin* 1989;29:137–142.
19. Gigliotti G, Hendley JO, Morgan J, et al. Efficacy of topical antibiotic therapy in acute conjunctivitis in children. *J Pediatr* 1984;104:623–626.
20. Leibowitz HM. Antibacterial effectiveness of ciprofloxacin 0.3% ophthalmic solution in the treatment of bacterial conjunctivitis. *Am J Ophthalmol* 1991;112:29S–33S.
21. Ofloxacin Study Group III. A placebo-controlled clinical study of the fluoroquinolone ofloxacin in patients with external infection. *Invest Ophthalmol Vis Sci* 1990;31:572.
22. Van Bijsterveld OP, El Batawi Y, Sobhi FS, et al. Fusidic acid in infections of the external eye. *Infection* 1987;15:16–19.
23. Gross RD, Hoffman RO, Lindsay RN. A comparison of ciprofloxacin and tobramycin in bacterial conjunctivitis is children. *Clin Pediatr* 1997;36:435–444.
24. Lohr JA, Austin RD, Grossman M, et al. Comparison of three topical antimicrobials for acute bacterial conjunctivitis. *Pediatr Infect Dis J* 1988;7:626–629.
25. Tabbara KF, El-Sheik HF, Monowarul Islam SM, Hammouda E. Treatment of acute bacterial conjunctivitis with topical lomefloxacin 0.3% compared to topical ofloxacin 0.3%. *Eur J Ophthalmol* 1999; 9:269–275.
26. Papa V, Aragona P, Scuderi AC, et al. Treatment of acute bacterial conjunctivitis with topical netilmicin. *Cornea* 2002;21:43–47.
27. Alves MR, Kara JN. Evaluation of the clinical and microbiological efficacy of 0.3% ciprofloxacin drops and 0.3% tobramycin drops in the treatment of acute bacterial conjunctivitis. *Revista Brasiliera de Oftalmol* 1993;52:371–377.
28. Wall AR, Sinclair N, Adenis JP. Comparison of Fucithalmic (fusidic acid viscous eye drops 1%) and Noroxin (norfloxacin ophthalmic solution 0.3%) in the treatment of acute bacterial conjunctivitis. *J Clin Res* 1998;1:316–325.
29. Mitsui Y, Matsuda H, Miyajima T, et al. Therapeutic effects of ofloxacin eye drops (DE-055) on external infection of the eye: multicentral double blind test. *J Rev Clin Ophthalmol* 1986;80:1813–1828.
30. The Trimethoprim-Polymyxin B Sulphate Ophthalmic Ointment Study Group. Trimethoprim-polymyxin B sulphate ophthalmic ointment versus chloramphenicol ophthalmic ointment in the treatment of bacterial conjunctivitis — a review of four clinical studies. *J Antimicrob Chemother* 1989;23:261–266.
31. Behrens-Baumann W, Quentin CD, Gibson JR, et al. Trimethoprim-polymyxin B sulphate ophthalmic ointment in the treatment of bacterial conjunctivitis: a double-blind study versus chloramphenicol ophthalmic ointment. *Curr Med Res Opin* 1988;11:227–231.
32. Van-Rensburg SF, Gibson JR, Harvey SG, Burke CA. Trimethoprim-polymyxin ophthalmic solution versus chloramphenicol ophthalmic solution in the treatment of bacterial conjunctivitis. *Pharmatherapeutica* 1982;3:274–277.
33. Gibson JR. Trimethoprim-polymyxin B ophthalmic solution in the treatment of presumptive bacterial conjunctivitis — a multicentre trial of its efficacy versus neomycin-polymyxin B-gramicidin and chloramphenicol ophthalmic solutions. *J Antimicrob Chemother* 1983;11:217–221.
34. Genee E, Schlechtweg C, Bauerreiss P, Gibson JR. Trimethoprim-polymyxin eye drops versus neomycin-polymyxin-gramicidin eye drops in the treatment of presumptive bacterial conjunctivitis — a double-blind study. *Ophthalmologica* 1982;184:92–96.
35. Malminiemi K, Kari O, Latvala M-L, et al. Topical lomefloxacin twice daily compared with fusidic acid in acute bacterial conjunctivitis. *Acta Ophthalmol Scand* 1996;74:280–284.
36. Carr WD. Comparison of Fucithalmic (fusidic acid viscous eye drops 1%) and Chloromycetin Redidrops (chloramphenicol eye drops 0.5%) in the treatment of acute bacterial conjunctivitis. *J Clin Res* 1998;1:403–411.
37. Horven I. Acute conjunctivitis. A comparison of fusidic acid viscous eye drops and chloramphenicol. *Acta Ophthalmol* 1993;71:165–168.
38. Hvidberg J. Fusidic acid in acute conjunctivitis. Single-blind, randomized comparison of fusidic acid and chloramphenicol viscous eye drops. *Acta Ophthalmol* 1987;65:43–47.
39. Uchida Y. Clinical efficacy of topical lomefloxacin (NY-198) in bacterial infections of the external eye. *Folia Ophthalmologica* 1991;42:59–70.

Christine Chung
Cornea Fellow

Elisabeth Cohen
Director
Cornea Service, Wills Eye Hospital
Jefferson Medical College
Philadelphia
USA

Justine Smith
Assistant Professor of Ophthalmology
Casey Eye Institute
Oregon Health & Science University
Portland
USA

Competing interests: None declared.

Diabetic retinopathy

Search date January 2002

Simon Harding

QUESTIONS

INTERVENTIONS

DIABETIC RETINOPATHY

Beneficial

Control of diabetes (see glycaemic control in diabetes, p 578)

Control of hypertension (see primary prevention, p 95)

Smoking cessation (see primary prevention, p 95)

Peripheral retinal laser photocoagulation in people with proliferative retinopathy . 637

Peripheral retinal laser photocoagulation in people with preproliferative *(moderate/severe non-proliferative)* retinopathy 637

Macular photocoagulation in people with clinically significant macular oedema 639

Likely to be beneficial

Grid photocoagulation to zones of retinal thickening in people with diabetic maculopathy 639

Unknown effectiveness

Macular photocoagulation in people with maculopathy but without clinically significant macular oedema 639

VITREOUS HAEMORRHAGE

Likely to be beneficial

Vitrectomy in people with severe vitreous haemorrhage and proliferative retinopathy (if performed early) 640

Unknown effectiveness

Vitrectomy in people with maculopathy 640

To be covered in future updates

Retinal detachment surgery in diabetic retinopathy

Cataract surgery in diabetic retinopathy

Octreotide

Aspirin

Covered elsewhere in *Clinical Evidence*

Prevention of diabetic retinopathy (see glycaemic control in diabetes, p 578)

In this topic terms used in the UK are written in normal text, and visual acuities are presented in units of metres; where terms used in the USA are different they are written in italics and visual acuities are presented in units of feet (see table 1, p 643).

See glossary, p 641

Key Messages

Diabetic retinopathy

- **Control of diabetes** (see glycaemic control in diabetes, p 578).
- **Control of hypertension** (see primary prevention, p 95).

- **Grid photocoagulation to zones of retinal thickening in people with diabetic maculopathy** One RCT found a significant improvement in visual acuity in eyes treated with grid photocoagulation versus untreated eyes at 12 months (NNT 4 eyes, 95% CI 3 to 8) and at 24 months (NNT 3 eyes, 95% CI 2 to 6). Photocoagulation versus no photocoagulation reduced the risk of moderate visual loss by 50–70%.
- **Macular photocoagulation in people with clinically significant macular oedema** One large RCT has found that laser photocoagulation to the macula versus no treatment reduces visual loss at 3 years in eyes with macular oedema and mild to moderate diabetic retinopathy (NNT 8, 95% CI 7 to 12), with some evidence of greater benefit in eyes with better vision. Subgroup analysis found that focal laser treatment was significantly more effective in reducing visual loss in eyes with clinically significant macular oedema, particularly in people in whom the centre of the macula was involved or imminently threatened.
- **Macular photocoagulation in people with maculopathy but without clinically significant macular oedema** The role of macular photocoagulation in this population remains unclear.
- **Peripheral retinal laser photocoagulation in people with preproliferative (moderate/severe non-proliferative) retinopathy** RCTs have found that peripheral retinal photocoagulation versus no treatment significantly reduces the risk of severe visual loss at 5 years. The people in these RCTs had maculopathy in addition to preproliferative retinopathy; the influence of this combination is unclear.
- **Peripheral retinal laser photocoagulation in people with proliferative retinopathy** RCTs have found that peripheral retinal photocoagulation versus no treatment significantly reduces the risk of severe visual loss at 2–3 years.
- **Smoking cessation** (see primary prevention, p 95).

Vitreous haemorrhage

- **Vitrectomy in people with maculopathy** The role of vitrectomy in this population remains unclear.
- **Vitrectomy in people with severe vitreous haemorrhage and proliferative retinopathy (if performed early)** One RCT found that early versus deferred (for 1 year) vitrectomy significantly reduced visual loss at 1, 2 and 3 years in eyes with severe vitreous haemorrhage and proliferative retinopathy (NNT 10 eyes, 95% CI 6 to 30). Subgroup analysis found significant benefit in people with type 1 diabetes but not those with type 2.

DEFINITION Diabetic retinopathy is characterised by varying degrees of microaneurysms, haemorrhages, exudates *(hard exudates)*, venous changes, new vessel formation, and retinal thickening. It can involve the peripheral retina or the macula, or both. The range of severity of retinopathy includes background *(mild non-proliferative)*, preproliferative *(moderate/severe non-proliferative)*, proliferative, and advanced retinopathy (see glossary, p 641). Involvement of the macula can be focal, diffuse, ischaemic (see glossary, p 641), or mixed.

INCIDENCE/ PREVALENCE Diabetic eye disease is the most common cause of blindness in the UK, responsible for 12% of registrable blindness in people aged 16–64 years.[1]

AETIOLOGY/ RISK FACTORS Risk factors include age, duration and control of diabetes, raised blood pressure, and raised serum lipids.[2]

PROGNOSIS Natural history studies from the 1960s found that at least half of people with proliferative diabetic retinopathy progressed to Snellen visual acuity (see glossary, p 641) of less than 6/60 (*20/200*) within 3–5 years.[3–5] After 4 years' follow up the rate of progression to less than 6/60 *(20/200)* visual acuity in the better eye was 1.5% in people with type 1 diabetes, 2.7% in people with non-insulin requiring type 2 diabetes, and 3.2% in people with insulin requiring type 2 diabetes.[6]

AIMS To prevent visual disability, partial sight, and blindness; to improve quality of life, with minimum adverse effects.

OUTCOMES Incidence of visual disability (visual acuity of 6/24 [*20/80*] or worse in the better eye), partial sight registration (visual acuity 6/60 [*20/200*] or worse in the better eye), and registrable blindness (visual acuity 3/60 [*10/200*] or worse in the better eye). Much of the published data used eyes as the unit of analysis rather than people. Significant loss of vision is often defined as loss of two or more Snellen lines of acuity (vision measured on standard Snellen chart) roughly equivalent to doubling of the visual angle (visual angle is the angle subtended at the eye of the smallest letter visible by that eye) — a measure used extensively in research.

METHODS *Clinical Evidence* search and appraisal January 2002. Additional papers were identified from manual searches. All trials with sufficient data to allow calculation of numbers needed to treat were included. Where no large trials were found, smaller, less detailed trials were included. Figures for numbers needed to treat and numbers needed to harm refer to the number of eyes rather than patients.

QUESTION What are the effects of treatment for diabetic retinopathy?

OPTION PERIPHERAL RETINAL LASER PHOTOCOAGULATION

RCTs have found that peripheral retinal photocoagulation versus no treatment reduces the risk of severe visual loss in eyes with various types of diabetic retinopathy (severe preproliferative [*severe non-proliferative*], proliferative, proliferative with high risk characteristics) and reduces the frequency of vitrectomy in people with severe preproliferative retinopathy (before new vessels have developed) or proliferative retinopathy without high risk characteristics. We found no evidence that one type of laser is better than another.

Benefits: **Peripheral photocoagulation versus no treatment:** We found no systematic review but found six RCTs[7–13] (see table 2, p 644) that recruited people with different grades of diabetic retinopathy, and compared different regimens of peripheral retinal photocoagulation versus no treatment or versus deferred treatment. Two RCTs recruited only people with proliferative diabetic retinopathy; both found that peripheral photocoagulation versus no treatment significantly reduced the risk of blindness after 2 or 3 years.[7,8] Two large RCTs recruited people with either preproliferative (*moderate/severe non-proliferative*) or proliferative retinopathy; both found that early photocoagulation versus no early photocoagulation decreased the risk of severe visual loss at 5 years, but in one of the RCTs the rate of severe visual loss was low and the effect was not significant.[9,10] A subgroup analysis[14] of one of these RCTs[10] found that the benefit was significant in people with type 2 diabetes and with severe preproliferative (*severe non-proliferative*) or early proliferative retinopathy without high risk characteristics (see glossary, p 641). The other two RCTs recruited only people with preproliferative (*non-proliferative*) diabetic retinopathy, but most of the people in these RCTs had diabetic maculopathy.[11,12] Both RCTs found that peripheral photocoagulation versus no treatment significantly reduced the risk of visual deterioration at 5 years. We found no RCTs of photocoagulation in people with severe preproliferative (*severe non-proliferative*) retinopathy, or in people with milder forms of background or preproliferative (*mild or moderate non-proliferative*) retinopathy who have not yet developed maculopathy. **Different types of laser:** We found no systematic review. A large multicentre RCT found no difference in effectiveness between krypton red and argon laser in the treatment of proliferative diabetic retinopathy with new vessels on the disc.[15] A smaller RCT compared argon versus double frequency lasers in 42 eyes with proliferative diabetic retinopathy and found no difference in rates of regression of new vessels after mean follow up of 29 months.[16]

Harms: Adverse effects include loss of visual field and visual acuity,[16–18] increased glare,[19] reduced contrast[19,20] and colour sensitivity,[21] temporary choroidal effusion, anterior uveitis, worsening macular oedema, and pain during treatment. Most studies were too small to provide accurate estimates of the frequency of these adverse effects, and they probably overestimate the risks because they used old treatment protocols. In one RCT, using an argon treatment protocol that has since been modified in current practice, constriction of visual field to within 45° of fixation occurred in 5% of eyes (NNH 20), constriction within 30° in 0%, and loss of vision by two or more Snellen lines in 3% (NNH 33).[9] **Fractionation:** One RCT found that adverse effects (including exudative retinal detachment, choroidal detachment, and angle closure) were reduced if photocoagulation was administered in multiple sessions spaced over time rather than in a single session.[22] **Different types of laser:** We found no clear evidence of different rates of complications with different lasers. Argon blue/green causes temporarily reduced colour sensation in treating surgeons. Dye laser[23] and orange laser (600 nm)[24] may be more painful than argon for peripheral retinal photocoagulation.[22] Several small studies found minimal or no difference in macular function after alternative lasers.

Comment: Limited prospective observational data suggest that peripheral retinal photocoagulation should be repeated until there is evidence of regression.[24] We found no evidence that theoretical advantages with certain lasers are reflected in significant improvements in clinical outcomes. Studies of visual field loss do not consider field loss before laser photocoagulation; one study found significant field loss in people with diabetes before laser compared with people without diabetes ($P < 0.01$).[25] We found one meta-analysis[26] of photocoagulation versus no treatment for diabetic retinopathy; its results are difficult to interpret because it was not based on a published systematic review, it did not include the largest RCT,[10] and it included one RCT of macular photocoagulation.[27]

OPTION MACULAR LASER PHOTOCOAGULATION FOR MACULOPATHY

RCTs have found that laser photocoagulation to the macula versus no treatment reduces visual loss at 2–3 years in eyes with macular oedema and mild to moderate or preproliferative *(moderate/severe non-proliferative)* diabetic retinopathy, with some evidence of greater benefit in eyes with better vision. Subgroup analysis in one large RCT found that focal laser treatment versus no treatment was significantly more effective in reducing visual loss in eyes with clinically significant macular oedema, particularly in people in whom the centre of the macula was involved or imminently threatened; the role of photocoagulation in other categories of maculopathy remains unclear. We found no evidence that one type of laser is better than another in diabetic maculopathy.

Benefits: **Macular photocoagulation versus no treatment:** We found no systematic review. We found three RCTs comparing macular argon laser photocoagulation versus no treatment in eyes with maculopathy, two using focal treatment to micoraneurysms,[27–29] and one using a grid to zones of thickened retina.[30] **Focal treatment to microaneurysms:** The first RCT (39 people with symmetrical macular oedema and preproliferative [*moderate/severe non-proliferative*] diabetic retinopathy) found that fewer people had visual deterioration after 2 years with photocoagulation versus no treatment, but the difference was not significant (visual deterioration of 30 completers: 7/30 [23%] eyes with laser *v* 13/30 [43%] eyes with no treatment; RR 0.54, 95% CI 0.25 to 1.16).[27] The second and much larger RCT (2244 people with macular oedema plus mild to moderate retinopathy) compared focal laser treatment (see glossary, p 641) using an argon laser versus observation.[29] At 3 years, treatment significantly reduced the risk of moderate visual loss (RR 0.50; NNT 8, 95% CI 7 to 12). Subgroup analysis found that focal laser treatment was significantly more effective in eyes with clinically significant macular oedema (see glossary, p 641), particularly in people in whom the centre of the macula was involved or imminently threatened.[13,31] The benefit was less in eyes with less extensive macular oedema; however, this may have been because both groups had low rates of visual loss from baseline. **Grid laser to zones of retinal thickening:** A single RCT (160 eyes with diffuse maculopathy with or without clinically significant macular oedema) found significant improvement in visual acuity in treated compared with untreated eyes at 12 months (RR 0.14; NNT 4, 95% CI 3 to 8) and at 24 months (RR 0.22; NNT 3, 95% CI 2 to 6).[30] Photocoagulation reduced the risk of moderate visual loss (defined as a doubling of the visual angle, equivalent to loss of about two Snellen lines) by 50–70%.[29,30] **Different types of laser:** We found no systematic review. Several small RCTs have found no difference between argon, diode, krypton red, and dye lasers in people with maculopathy.

Harms: Uncontrolled studies found loss of contrast sensitivity and visual acuity associated with direct application of the laser to the centre of the fovea. We found no accurate estimates of the frequency of adverse effects. **Focal treatment to microaneurysms:** The largest RCT found no significant difference in the frequency of immediate visual loss in treated compared with untreated participants.[29] One prospective observational study reported a 40% reduction in macular function in people undergoing focal argon paramacular treatment.[32] Other complications include laser damage to the centre of the fovea and induction of choroidal neovascularisation, but we found no good data on frequency. **Grid laser to zones of retinal thickening:** In the relevant RCT, paracentral grid like scotomas or haze were visible to most people treated with grid photocoagulation, but the data are insufficient to estimate the frequency of this effect.[30]

Comment: The benefits of laser photocoagulation are less notable in people with maculopathy than in those with proliferative retinopathy. RCTs are needed to compare efficacy and harm of focal and grid laser protocols. We found no evidence that theoretical advantages of certain types of laser result in significant improvements in clinical outcomes.

QUESTION **What are the effects of treatments for vitreous haemorrhage?**

OPTION **VITRECTOMY**

One RCT found that vitrectomy reduced visual loss if performed early in people with vitreous haemorrhage, especially in those with severe proliferative retinopathy. Its role in people with both vitreous haemorrhage and diabetic maculopathy remains unclear.

Benefits: We found no systematic review. **In retinopathy:** We found one RCT comparing early vitrectomy (see glossary, p 641) or deferral of vitrectomy for 1 year in 616 eyes with proliferative retinopathy and recent severe vitreous haemorrhage (see glossary, p 641) (reducing visual acuity to ≤2/60 [*5/200*]).[33] At 1, 2, and 3 years after treatment, eyes in the early treatment group were significantly more likely to have visual acuity of at least 6/12 (*20/40*) than those in the deferred treatment group (RRR for visual acuity of < 6/12 0.55; NNT 10, 95% CI 6 to 30). Subgroup analysis showed significant benefit in people with type 1 diabetes but not in those with type 2 diabetes. **In maculopathy:** We found no RCTs.

Harms: A retrospective study of 260 eyes treated with vitrectomy reported neovascular glaucoma in 6%, retinal detachment in 8%, and cataract in 27%.[34] Glaucoma was more likely in people with associated preoperative retinal detachment. In one RCT, the use of preoperative intravitreal tissue plasminogen activator failed to reduce the rate of complications in 56 patients undergoing vitrectomy for the complications of proliferative diabetic retinopathy.[35]

Comment: None.

GLOSSARY

Advanced retinopathy Retinopathy characterised by tractional retinal detachment (see below), vitreous haemorrhage obscuring fundus details, or both.

Background retinopathy *(mild non-proliferative)* Characterised by microaneurysms, small haemorrhages, and exudates *(hard exudates)*.

Clinically significant macular oedema Characterised by one or more of the following: retinal thickening at or within 500 μm of the centre of the fovea; exudates *(hard exudates)* at or within 500 μm of the centre of the fovea when accompanied by retinal thickening; one or more disc area(s) of thickening extending to within one disc diameter of the centre of the fovea. This is a clinical feature of maculopathy common to many eyes with maculopathy and indicates a significant threat to vision.

Diffuse exudative maculopathy Characterised by thickened oedematous retina at the fovea, often with cystic changes.

Focal exudative maculopathy Characterised by exudates *(hard exudates)* within one disc diameter of the centre of the fovea or circinate rings of exudates *(hard exudates)* within the macula.

Focal laser treatment Laser applied directly to microaneurysms.

Grid laser treatment Laser applied in a grid pattern to zones of retinal thickening and/or zones of capillary non-perfusion.

High risk characteristics (1) new vessels at the disc extending over at least a third of the disc area; and/or (2) new vessels at the disc extending over less than one third of the disc area or new vessels elsewhere extending over at least half of the disc area, both in the presence of vitreous or pre-retinal haemorrhage.

Ischaemic maculopathy Characterised by zones of capillary non-perfusion visible only on fluorescein angiography but often inferred from presence of deep blot haemorrhages within the fovea.

Preproliferative retinopathy Mild, moderate, or severe *(moderate or severe non-proliferative)* depending on number/location of lesions; characterised by cotton wool spots, deep round haemorrhages, venous beading, loops and reduplication, and intraretinal microvascular anomalies.

Proliferative retinopathy Characterised by new vessels at the disc or elsewhere.

Snellen visual acuity The Snellen chart usually includes letters, numbers, or pictures printed in lines of decreasing size, which are read or identified from a fixed distance; distance visual acuity is usually measured from a distance of 6 metres *(20 feet)*. The Snellen visual acuity is written as a fraction: 6/18 means that from 6 metres away the best line that can be read is a line that could normally be read from a distance of 18 metres away.

Tractional retinal detachment Fibrous scar tissue between the vitreous humour and retina pulls the retina away from the underlying retinal pigment epithelium. This type of retinal detachment is most common in the proliferative diabetic retinopathy.

Vitrectomy The vitreous is the normally clear gelatinous material that fills most of the inside of the eye. The vitreous can be affected by bleeding, inflammatory cells, debris, or scar tissue. Vitrectomy involves removal of the abnormal vitreous material.

Vitreous haemorrhage Bleeding into the vitreous of the eye from blood vessels arising from the retina.

REFERENCES

1. Evans J, Rooney C, Ashwood F, Dattani N, Wormald R. Blindness and partial sight in England and Wales: April 1990–March 1991. *Health Trends* 1996;28:5–12.
2. Ebeling P, Koivisto VA. Occurrence and interrelationships of complications in insulin-dependent diabetes in Finland. *Acta Diabetol* 1997;34:33–38.
3. Beetham WP. Visual prognosis of proliferating diabetic retinopathy. *Br J Ophthalmol* 1963;47:611–619.
4. Caird FI, Burditt AF, Draper GJ. Diabetic retinopathy: a further study of prognosis for vision. *Diabetes* 1968;17:121–123.
5. Deckert T, Simonsen SE, Poulsen JE. Prognosis of proliferative retinopathy in juvenile diabetes. *Diabetes* 1967;10:728–733.

6. Klein R, Klein BEK, Moss SE. The Wisconsin epidemiologic study of diabetic retinopathy: an update. *Aust NZ J Ophthalmol* 1990;18:19–22.
7. British Multicentre Study Group. Proliferative diabetic retinopathy: treatment with xenon arc photocoagulation. *BMJ* 1977;i:739–741.
8. Hercules BL, Gayed II, Lucas SB, Jeacock J. Peripheral retinal ablation in the treatment of proliferative diabetic retinopathy: a three-year interim report of a randomised, controlled study using the argon laser. *Br J Ophthalmol* 1977;61:555–563.
9. Diabetic Retinopathy Study Research Group. DRS group 8: photocoagulation treatment of proliferative diabetic retinopathy. *Ophthalmology* 1981;88:583–600.
10. Flynn HW Jr, Chew EY, Simons BD, Barton FB, Remaley NA, Ferris FL III, and The Early Treatment Diabetic Retinopathy Study Research Group. Pars plana vitrectomy in the Early Treatment Diabetic Retinopathy Study. ETDRS report number 17. *Ophthalmology* 1992;99:1351–1357.
11. British Multicentre Study Group. Photocoagulation for diabetic maculopathy: a randomized controlled clinical trial using the xenon arc. *Diabetes 1983*;32:1010–1016.
12. Patz A, Schatz H, Berkow JW, Gittelsohn AM, Ticho U. Macular edema — an overlooked complication of diabetic retinopathy. *Trans Am Acad Ophthalmol Otol* 1973;77:34–42.
13. Early Treatment Diabetic Retinopathy Study Research Group. Early photocoagulation for diabetic retinopathy: ETDRS report 9. *Ophthalmology* 1991;98:766–785.
14. Ferris F. Early photocoagulation in patients with either type I or type II diabetes. *Trans Am Ophthalmol Soc* 1996;94:505–537.
15. Bandello F, Brancato R, Lattanzio R, Trabucchi G, Azzolini C, Malegori A. Double-frequency Nd:YAG laser vs argon-green laser in the treatment of proliferative diabetic retinopathy: randomized study with long-term follow-up. *Lasers Surg Med* 1996;19:173–176.
16. Blankenship GW. A clinical comparison of central and peripheral argon laser panretinal photocoagulation for proliferative diabetic retinopathy. *Ophthalmology* 1988;95:170–177.
17. Pearson AR, Tanner V, Keightey SJ, Casswell AG. What effect does laser photocoagulation have on driving visual fields in diabetics? *Eye* 1998;12:64–68.
18. Theodossiadis GP. Central visual field changes after panretinal photocoagulation in proliferative diabetic retinopathy. *Ophthalmologica* 1990;201:71–78.
19. Mackie SW, Walsh G. Contrast and glare sensitivity in diabetic patients with and without pan-retinal photocoagulation. *Ophthalmic Physiol Opt* 1998;18:173–181.
20. Khosla PK, Rao V, Tewari HK, Kumar A. Contrast sensitivity in diabetic retinopathy after panretinal photocoagulation. *Ophthalmic Surg* 1994;25:516–520.
21. Birch J, Hamilton AM. Xenon arc and argon laser photocoagulation in the treatment of diabetic disc neovascularization. Part 2: effect on colour vision. *Trans Ophthalmol Soc UK* 1981;101:93–99.
22. Doft BH. Single versus multiple treatment sessions of argon laser panretinal photocoagulation for proliferative diabetic retinopathy. *Ophthalmology* 1982;89:772–779.
23. Seiberth V, Schatanek S, Alexandridis E. Panretinal photocoagulation in diabetic retinopathy: argon versus dye laser coagulation. *Graefes Arch Clin Exp Ophthalmol* 1993;231:318–322.
24. Cordeiro MF, Stanford MR, Phillips PM, Shilling JS. Relationship of diabetic microvascular complications to outcome in panretinal photocoagulation treatment of proliferative diabetic retinopathy. *Eye* 1997;11:531–536.
25. Buckley S. Field loss after pan retinal photocoagulation with diode and argon lasers. *Doc Ophthalmol* 1992;82:317–322.
26. Duffy SW, Rohan TE, Altman DG. A method for combining matched and unmatched binary data: application to randomized, controlled trials of photocoagulation in the treatment of diabetic retinopathy. *Am J Epidemiol* 1989;130:371–378.
27. Blankenship GW. Diabetic macular edema and argon laser photocoagulation: a prospective randomized study. *Ophthalmology* 1979;86:69–75.
28. The krypton argon regression neovascularization study research group. Randomized comparison of krypton versus argon scatter photocoagulation for diabetic disc neovascularization: the krypton argon regression neovascularization study report number 1. *Ophthalmology* 1993;100:1655–1664.
29. Early Treatment Diabetic Retinopathy Study Research Group. Photocoagulation for diabetic macular edema. *Arch Ophthalmol* 1985;103:1796–1806.
30. Olk RJ. Modified grid argon (blue-green) laser photocoagulation for diffuse diabetic macular edema. *Ophthalmology* 1986;93:938–950.
31. Anonymous. Focal photocoagulation treatment of diabetic macular edema: relationship of treatment effect to fluorescein angiographic and other retinal characteristics at baseline: ETDRS report 19. *Arch Ophthalmol* 1995;113:1144–1155.
32. Ciavarella P, Moretti G, Falsini B, Porciatti V. The pattern electroretinogram (PERG) after laser treatment of the peripheral or central retina. *Curr Eye Res* 1997;16:111–115.
33. Diabetic Retinopathy Vitrectomy Study Group. Early vitrectomy for severe vitreous hemorrhage in diabetic retinopathy. Four-year results of a randomized trial: diabetic retinopathy vitrectomy study report 5. *Arch Ophthalmol* 1990;108:958–964.
34. Sima P, Zoran T. Long-term results of vitreous surgery for proliferative diabetic retinopathy. *Doc Ophthalmol* 1994;87:223–232.
35. Le Mer Y, Korobelnik, JF, Morel C, Ullern M, Berrod JP. TPA-assisted vitrectomy for proliferative diabetic retinopathy: results of a double-masked, multicenter trial. *Retina* 1999;19:378–382.

Simon Harding
Consultant Ophthalmologist
St Paul's Eye Unit Royal Liverpool
University Hospital
Liverpool
UK

Competing interests: None declared.

TABLE 1 Equivalent UK and US terminology where different (see text, p 635).

UK terminology	US terminology
Background retinopathy	*Mild non-proliferative retinopathy*
Preproliferative retinopathy	*Moderate non-proliferative retinopathy*
Severe preproliferative retinopathy	*Severe non-proliferative retinopathy*
Exudate	*Hard exudate*
Snellen visual acuity measured in metres (e.g. 6/24)	*Snellen visual acuity measured in feet (e.g. 20/80)*

TABLE 2 RCTs of peripheral photocoagulation versus no treatment in people with diabetic retinopathy (see text, p 637).

Ref	Number of people (eyes)	Degree of retinopathy*			Comparison	Outcome (at time)	Result* (analyses by number of eyes) (95% CI in parentheses)
		Preproliferative (Non-proliferative)	Proliferative	Diabetic maculopathy			
7	100 (200)	No	All (bilateral)		Peripheral xenon arc *v* no treatment	Blindness by last assessment (mean around 2 years)	5/100 *v* 17/100 RR 0.29 (0.11 to 0.77) NNT 9 (5 to 31)
8	94 (188)	No	All (bilateral)		Peripheral argon laser *v* no treatment	Blindness (3 years)	7/94 (7%) *v* 36/94 (38%) RR 0.19 (0.09 to 0.41) NNT 3 (3 to 6)
9	1742 (3484)	Yes if bilateral	Yes	Yes	Peripheral + focal photocoagulation *v* no treatment	Severe visual loss (5 years)	90/650 (14%) *v* 171/519 (33%) RR 0.42 (0.34 to 0.53) NNT 6 (5 to 7)
13	3711 (7422)	Yes	Yes	Yes	Various early photocoagulation regimens *v* deferred photocoagulation	Severe visual loss (5 years)	2.6% *v* 3.7%† HR 0.77 (0.56 to 1.06)
10	As above	As above	As above	As above	As above	Vitrectomy rate‡ (5 years)	2.3% *v* 4.0%†
11	99 (198)	Yes	No	All	Peripheral xenon arc *v* no treatment	Visual deterioration (5 years)	19/60 (32%) *v* 39/60 (55%) RR 0.49 (0.32 to 0.74) NNT 3 (2 to 7)
12	63 (126)	Yes if bilateral	No	Yes	Peripheral laser *v* no treatment	Visual deterioration (26 months)	4/63 (6%) *v* 40/63 (63%) RR 0.10 (0.04 to 0.26) NNT 2 (2 to 3)

In these columns, a blank means that the RCT did not explicitly state if included people had that characteristic. "All": only people with that characteristic were included; "Yes": some people with that characteristic were included; "No": all people with that characteristic were explicitly excluded.
*Where necessary, relative risks were calculated by *Clinical Evidence* using absolute risks stated in each RCT.
†The RCT reported percentages and did not provide absolute numbers. Hazard ratio taken from the published report is based on Cox proportional hazards model.
‡The indication for vitrectomy changed halfway through the RCT. Initially vitrectomy was performed only after onset of severe visual loss. Later, it was performed 1–6 months after severe vitreous haemorrhage.

Glaucoma

Search date December 2001

Rajiv Shah and Richard Wormald

QUESTIONS

INTERVENTIONS

To be covered in future updates

Treating ocular hypertension in people without established glaucoma
Early detection of glaucoma (opportunistic case finding, population screening)

* No placebo controlled RCTs but strong consensus that treatments are effective

See glossary, p 651

Key Messages

Primary open angle glaucoma

- **Laser trabeculoplasty (versus medical treatment)** One RCT found that combined treatment with initial laser trabeculoplasty followed by medical treatment versus medical treatment alone significantly reduced intraocular pressure and deterioration in optic disc appearance, and significantly improved visual fields after a mean of 7 years.
- **Laser trabeculoplasty (versus surgical treatment)** RCTs found that laser trabeculoplasty reduced intraocular pressures significantly less than surgical trabeculectomy, and found conflicting results for changes in visual acuity after 5–7 years.
- **Surgical trabeculectomy** RCTs found that surgical trabeculectomy versus medical treatment significantly reduced both visual field loss and intraocular pressures, but found no significant difference between treatments in visual acuity after about 5 years. RCTs found that surgical trabeculectomy versus laser trabeculoplasty significantly reduced intraocular pressure, but found conflicting results for changes in visual acuity after 5–7 years.

Clin Evid 2002;8:645–652.

- **Topical medical treatment** One systematic review found limited evidence that topical medical treatments versus placebo significantly reduced intraocular pressure after a minimum of 3 months, but found no significant difference between treatments in visual field loss on long term follow up. The systematic review did not clearly define the medical treatments involved.

Normal tension glaucoma

- **Lowering intraocular pressure** One RCT found that surgical and/or medical treatment significantly reduced progression of visual field loss after 8 years (NNT 5, 95% CI 3 to 9), but found that surgery significantly increased cataract formation.

Acute angle closure glaucoma

- **Medical treatments of acute angle closure glaucoma** We found no placebo controlled RCTs, but strong consensus suggests that medical treatments are effective. One RCT found no significant difference in intraocular pressure after 2 hours with low dose pilocarpine versus an intensive pilocarpine regimen versus pilocarpine ocular inserts. We found no RCTs of other medical treatments.
- **Surgical treatments of acute angle closure glaucoma** We found no placebo controlled RCTs, but strong consensus suggests that surgical treatments are effective. One RCT found no significant difference with surgical iridectomy versus laser iridotomy in visual acuity or intraocular pressure after 3 years.

DEFINITION Glaucoma is a group of diseases characterised by progressive optic neuropathy. It is usually bilateral but asymmetric and may occur at any point within a wide range of intraocular pressures. All forms of glaucoma show optic nerve cupping with pallor, associated with peripheral visual field loss. **Primary open angle glaucoma** occurs in people with an open drainage angle and no secondary identifiable cause. **Normal tension glaucoma** occurs in people with intraocular pressures that are consistently below 21 mmHg (a point two standard deviations above the population mean). **Acute angle closure glaucoma** is a rapid and severe rise in intraocular pressure caused by physical obstruction of the anterior chamber drainage angle.

INCIDENCE/ PREVALENCE Glaucoma occurs in 1–2% of white people aged over 40 years, rising to 5% at 70 years. Primary open angle glaucoma accounts for two thirds of those affected, and normal tension glaucoma for about a quarter.[1,2] In black people glaucoma is more prevalent, presents at a younger age with higher intraocular pressures, is more difficult to control, and is the main irreversible cause of blindness.[1,3] Glaucoma related blindness is responsible for 8% of new blind registrations in the UK.[4]

AETIOLOGY/ RISK FACTORS The major risk factor for developing primary open angle glaucoma is raised intraocular pressure. Lesser risk factors include family history and ethnic origin. The relationship between systemic blood pressure and intraocular pressure may be an important determinant of blood flow to the optic nerve head and, as a consequence, may represent a risk factor for glaucoma.[5] Systemic hypotension, vasospasm (including Raynaud's disease and migraine), and a history of major blood loss have been reported as risk factors for normal tension glaucoma in hospital based studies. Risk factors for acute angle closure glaucoma include family history, female sex, being long sighted, and cataract. A recent systematic review failed to find any evidence supporting the theory that routine pupillary dilatation with short acting mydriatics was a risk factor for acute angle closure glaucoma.[6]

PROGNOSIS Advanced visual field loss is found in about 20% of people with primary open angle glaucoma at diagnosis,[7] and is an important risk factor for glaucoma related blindness.[8] Blindness results from gross loss of visual field or loss of central vision. Once early field defects have appeared, and where the intraocular pressure is greater than 30 mmHg, untreated people may lose the remainder of the visual field in 3 years or less.[9] As the disease progresses, people with glaucoma have difficulty moving from a bright room to a darker room, and judging steps and kerbs. Progression of visual field loss is often slower in normal tension glaucoma. Acute angle glaucoma leads to rapid loss of vision, initially from corneal oedema and subsequently from ischaemic optic neuropathy.

AIMS To prevent progression of visual field loss and to minimise adverse effects of treatment.

OUTCOMES Visual acuity; visual fields. Optic disc cupping and intraocular pressure are surrogate outcomes.

METHODS *Clinical Evidence* search and appraisal December 2001.

QUESTION **What are the effects of treatments for established primary open angle glaucoma?**

OPTION **TOPICAL MEDICAL TREATMENT**

One systematic review found limited evidence that topical medical treatments versus placebo significantly reduce intraocular pressure after a minimum of 3 months, but found no significant difference between treatments in visual field loss on long term follow up. The systematic review did not clearly define the medical treatments involved.

Benefits: We found one systematic review (search date 1991, 16 placebo controlled RCTs, 86 comparative RCTs, 5000 people).[10] **Intraocular pressure:** The review found that medical treatment versus placebo significantly reduced mean intraocular pressure after a minimum of 3 months (see comment below; 16 placebo controlled RCTs; mean reduction in intraocular pressure 4.9 mmHg, 95% CI 2.5 mmHg to 7.3 mmHg). **Visual field loss:** The review found no significant difference with medical treatment versus placebo in visual field loss after long term follow up (see comment below; 3 RCTs, 302 people; pooled OR for any worsening of visual field loss 0.75, 95% CI 0.42 to 1.35).

Harms: Systemic adverse effects of topical treatments are uncommon but may be serious, including exacerbation of chronic obstructive airways disease after use of non-selective topical β blockers. Non-selective topical β blockers can also cause systemic hypotension and reduction in resting heart rate, and are contraindicated in people with cardiac failure.[11]

Comment: We could not identify the types of participants, types of topical medical treatments, or the definition of long term follow up from the systematic review.[10] Two RCTs sponsored by the US National Institutes of Health are underway and have not yet reported any results: The Early Manifest Glaucoma Study and the Ocular Hypertension Treatment Study. The European Glaucoma Prevention Study is also due to present its findings soon.

OPTION LASER TRABECULOPLASTY

One RCT found that combined treatment with initial laser trabeculoplasty followed by medical treatment versus medical treatment alone significantly reduced intraocular pressure and deterioration in optic disc appearance, and significantly improved visual fields after a mean of 7 years. Two RCTs found that surgical trabeculectomy versus laser trabeculoplasty reduced intraocular pressures, but found conflicting results for changes in visual acuity.

Benefits: We found no systematic review, but found three RCTs.[12–14] **Versus medical treatment:** The first RCT (203 people) found that combined treatment (initial laser trabeculoplasty followed by medical treatment) versus medical treatment alone significantly reduced intraocular pressure (1.2 mmHg greater reduction in intraocular pressure with combined treatment; $P = 0.001$; CI not provided), significantly (statistically, not clinically) improved visual fields (0.6 dB greater improvement with combined treatment; $P < 0.001$; CI not provided), and significantly reduced deterioration in optic disc appearance ($P = 0.005$; CI not provided) after a mean of 7 years.[12] **Versus surgical treatment:** See benefits of surgical trabeculectomy, p 648.

Harms: Adverse effects of laser trabeculoplasty are mild and include a transient rise in intraocular pressure (>5 mmHg in 91/271 participants) and formation of peripheral anterior synechiae (in 93/271 participants).[12]

Comment: The first RCT was a multicentre trial with multiple observers, although it is not clear whether these observers were masked to the intervention.[12]

OPTION SURGICAL TRABECULECTOMY

Two RCTs found that surgical trabeculectomy versus medical treatment significantly reduced both visual field loss and intraocular pressures, but found no significant difference between treatments in visual acuity. Two RCTs found that surgical trabeculectomy versus laser trabeculoplasty reduced intraocular pressure, but found conflicting results for changes in visual acuity. One RCT in people with normal tension glaucoma found that treatment including trabeculectomy versus no treatment significantly increased cataract formation after 8 years, and observational studies have found a reduction in central vision with surgical trabeculectomy.

Benefits: We found no systematic review. **Versus medical treatment:** We found two RCTs.[13,15] One RCT (116 people) compared trabeculectomy (followed by medical treatment when indicated) versus medical treatment (followed by trabeculectomy when medical treatment failed).[15] It found no significant difference between treatments in visual acuity (P = 0.44; other results presented graphically; CI not provided), but found that trabeculectomy versus medical treatment significantly reduced visual field loss (P = 0.03; other results presented graphically; CI not provided) after a mean of 4.6 years. The second RCT (186 people) compared three treatments: medical treatment (pilocarpine ± timolol ± a sympathomimetic), laser trabeculoplasty, and surgical trabeculectomy.[13] It found that surgical trabeculectomy versus both other treatments significantly reduced intraocular pressures (P = 0.0001; other results presented graphically; CI not provided), but found no significant difference between any of the treatments in visual acuity (results presented graphically) after 5 years. **Versus initial laser trabeculoplasty:** We found two RCTs.[13,14] One RCT (776 eyes with advanced glaucoma; 451 black people, 325 white people) compared surgical trabeculectomy versus laser trabeculoplasty as initial treatments.[14] Initial surgical trabeculectomy was followed by laser trabeculoplasty and repeat surgical trabeculectomy as required; initial laser trabeculoplasty was followed by surgical trabeculectomy as required. The RCT found that in black people initial laser trabeculoplasty versus surgical trabeculectomy significantly improved vision (both visual acuity and visual field; P < 0.01; other results presented graphically; CI not provided), although in white people the RCT found no significant difference between treatments in vision (results presented graphically) after 7 years. The RCT also found that in both black people and white people surgical trabeculectomy versus laser trabeculoplasty reduced intraocular pressure (significance not reported and results presented graphically). The second RCT is described above.[13]

Harms: Surgical trabeculectomy is associated with a reduction in central vision. In one study, 83% of participants lost two lines of Snellen visual acuity.[16] One RCT in people with normal tension glaucoma has found that treatment including trabeculectomy versus no treatment significantly increased cataract formation after 8 years, (see harms of lowering intraocular pressure in normal tension glaucoma, p 650).[17,18]

Comment: None.

QUESTION What are the effects of lowering intraocular pressure in people with normal tension glaucoma?

One RCT found that surgical and/or medical treatment significantly reduced progression of visual field loss after 8 years, but surgery significantly increased cataract formation.

Benefits: We found no systematic review. We found one RCT (140 eyes in 140 people), which compared treatment to reduce intraocular pressure by 30% (with drugs or trabeculectomy, or both; 61 eyes) versus no treatment (79 eyes).[17] Progression of visual field loss was defined in terms of deepening of an existing scotoma, a new or expanded field defect coming close to central vision, or a fresh scotoma in a previously normal part of the visual field. Optic disc changes were photographed and independently assessed by two ophthalmologists. The RCT found that treatment significantly reduced progression of visual field loss after 8 years (7/61 [12%] eyes with treatment *v* 28/79 [35%] eyes with no treatment; RR 0.32, 95% CI 0.15 to 0.70; NNT 5, 95% CI 3 to 9).

Harms: The RCT found that treatment (drugs ± trabeculectomy) versus no treatment significantly increased cataract formation after 8 years (23/61 [38%] with treatment *v* 11/79 [14%] with no treatment; RR 2.71, 95% CI 1.4 to 5.1; NNH 4, 95% CI 2 to 10).[17] Subgroup analysis found that the excess risk of cataract formation was confined to those people treated surgically (P = 0.0001; CI not provided). See harms of surgical trabeculectomy, p 650.

Comment: A companion paper[18] to the RCT[17] suggests that the favourable effect of intraocular pressure lowering treatment versus no treatment is evident only when the cataract inducing effect of trabeculectomy is removed. Not all cases of normal pressure glaucoma progress when untreated (40% at 5 years).[18]

QUESTION What are the effects of treatment for acute angle closure glaucoma?

OPTION MEDICAL TREATMENTS

We found no RCTs of pilocarpine versus placebo in acute angle closure glaucoma. One RCT found no significant difference between low dose pilocarpine versus an intensive pilocarpine regimen versus pilocarpine ocular inserts in intraocular pressure after 2 hours. We found no RCTs of other medical treatments for acute angle closure glaucoma.

Benefits: **Pilocarpine versus placebo:** We found no RCTs (see comment below). **Low dose pilocarpine versus intensive pilocarpine:** We found no systematic review, but found one RCT (77 eyes) that compared three groups: initial treatment with low dose pilocarpine (2% pilocarpine drops applied to the eye twice in 1 h), intensive pilocarpine (4% pilocarpine drops applied to the eye every 5 min for 1 h or longer), and pilocarpine ocular inserts (releasing 40 μg pilocarpine/h).[19] All of the people in the RCT also received treatment with intravenous acetazolamide (500 mg iv). The RCT found no significant difference in intraocular pressures after 2 hours (statistical data not provided).

Harms: The RCT reported that ocular inserts were associated with local discomfort (statistical data not provided).[19]

Comment: RCTs of pilocarpine versus placebo would be considered unethical. There is a strong consensus that medical treatments that involve pressure lowering drugs (especially those that can be given parenterally, such as iv acetazolamide) are effective in acute angle closure glaucoma. We found no evidence from RCTs to support this view.

OPTION SURGICAL IRIDECTOMY AND LASER IRIDOTOMY

One RCT found no significant difference with surgical iridectomy versus laser iridotomy in visual acuity or intraocular pressure after 3 years.

Benefits: **Surgical or laser procedure versus placebo:** We found no RCTs. **Surgical peripheral iridectomy versus Nd:YAG laser iridotomy:** We found no systematic review, but found one RCT (48 people with uniocular acute angle closure glaucoma) that compared peripheral iridectomy versus Nd:YAG laser iridotomy (see glossary, p 651).[20] It found no significant difference in visual acuity (0.30 logMAR units with peripheral iridectomy *v* 0.57 logMAR units with laser iridotomy; statistical data not provided) and no significant difference in intraocular pressure (intraocular pressure < 21 mmHg: 15/21 [70%] with peripheral iridectomy *v* 19/27 [72%] with laser iridotomy; RR 1.02, 95% CI 0.71 to 1.46) after 3 years.

Harms: Surgical iridectomy (see glossary, p 651) involves opening the eye with risk of serious complications, including intraocular infection or haemorrhage. We found no published evidence quantifying these risks. Nd:YAG laser iridotomy is associated with haemorrhage from the iris, pressure spikes, and corneal oedema.[21] Nd:YAG and argon laser iridotomy can produce focal, non-progressive lens opacity.[22] In one RCT, iris haemorrhage was more common with the Nd:YAG laser but pupil distortion, iritis, and late blockage were more common with the argon laser.[23]

Comment: Management of acute angle closure glaucoma is aimed at restoring flow of aqueous humour to the anterior chamber angle and adjacent trabecular meshwork. One RCT found that the mean number of laser burns required to penetrate the iris was six with the Nd:YAG laser and 73 with the argon laser.[23]

GLOSSARY

Laser iridotomy Involves making a hole in the base of the iris (without opening the eye) using either an argon or Nd:YAG laser.

Surgical iridectomy Opening the eye at the corneal limbus and removing a triangle of tissue from the base of the iris.

REFERENCES

1. Sommer A, Tielsch JM, Katz J, et al. Relationship between intraocular pressure and primary open angle glaucoma among white and black Americans. *Arch Ophthalmol* 1991;109:1090–1095.
2. Coffey M, Reidy A, Wormald R, Xian WX, Wright L, Courtney P. The prevalence of glaucoma in the west of Ireland. *Br J Ophthalmol* 1993;77:17–21.
3. Leske MC, Connell AM, Wu SY, et al. Incidence of open-angle glaucoma: the Barbados Eye Studies. The Barbados Eye Studies Group. *Arch Ophthalmol* 2001;119:89–95.
4. Government Statistical Service. *Causes of blindness and partial sight amongst adults.* London: HMSO, 1988.
5. Tielsch JM, Katz J, Quigley HA, et al. Diabetes, intraocular pressure, and primary open-angle glaucoma in the Baltimore Eye Survey. *Ophthalmology* 1995;102:48–53.
6. Pandit RJ, Taylor R. Mydriasis and glaucoma: exploding the myth. A systematic review. *Diabet Med* 2000;17:693–699.
7. Sheldrick JH, Ng C, Austin DJ, Rosenthal AR. An analysis of referral routes and diagnostic accuracy in cases of suspected glaucoma. *Ophthalmic Epidemiol* 1994;1:31–38.
8. Fraser S, Bunce C, Wormald R, Brunner E. Deprivation and late presentation of glaucoma: case-control study. *BMJ* 2001;322:639–643.
9. Jay JL, Murdoch JR. The rates of visual field loss in untreated primary open angle glaucoma. *Br J Ophthalmol* 1993;77:176–178.
10. Rossetti L, Marchetti I, Orzalesi N, Scorpiglione N, Torri V, Liberati A. Randomised clinical trials on medical treatment of glaucoma: are they appropriate to guide clinical practice? *Arch Ophthalmol* 1993;111:96–103. Search date 1991; primary source Medline.
11. Diamond JP. Systemic adverse effects of topical ophthalmic agents: implications for older patients. *Drugs Aging* 1997;11:352–360.
12. Glaucoma Laser Trial Group. The glaucoma laser trial (GLT) and glaucoma laser trial follow-up study: results. *Am J Ophthalmol* 1995;120:718–731.
13. Migdal C, Gregory W, Hitchins R, Kolker AE. Long-term functional outcome after early surgery compared with laser and medicine in open angle glaucoma. *Ophthalmology* 1994;101:1651–1657.
14. The Advanced Glaucoma Intervention Study (AGIS): 4. Comparison of treatment outcomes within race. Seven year results. *Ophthalmology* 1998;105:1146–1164.
15. Jay JL, Allan D. The benefit of early trabeculectomy versus conventional management in primary open angle glaucoma relative to severity of disease. *Eye* 1989;3:528–535.

16. Costas UP, Smith M, Spaeth GL, Gondham S, Markovitz B. Loss of vision after trabeculectomy. *Ophthalmology* 1993;100:599–612.
17. Collaborative normal-tension glaucoma study group. Comparison of glaucomatous progression between untreated patients with normal-tension glaucoma and patients with therapeutically reduced intraocular pressure. *Am J Ophthalmol* 1998;126:487–497.
18. Collaborative normal-tension glaucoma study group. The effectiveness of intraocular pressure reduction in the treatment of normal-tension glaucoma. *Am J Ophthalmol* 1998;126:498–505.
19. Edwards RS. A comparative study of Ocusert Pilo 40, intensive pilocarpine and low-dose pilocarpine in the initial treatment of primary acute angle-closure glaucoma. *Curr Med Res Opin* 1997;13:501–509.
20. Fleck BW, Wright E, Fairley EA. A randomised prospective comparison of operative peripheral iridectomy and Nd:YAG laser iridotomy treatment of acute angle closure glaucoma: 3 year visual acuity and intraocular pressure control outcome. *Br J Ophthalmol* 1997;81:884–888.
21. Fleck BW, Dhillon B, Khanna V, Fairley E, McGlynn C. A randomised, prospective comparison of Nd:YAG laser iridotomy and operative peripheral iridectomy in fellow eyes. *Eye* 1991;5:315–321.
22. Pollack IP, Robin AL, Dragon DM, et al. Use of neodymium:YAG laser to create iridotomies in monkeys and humans. *Trans Am Ophthalmol Soc* 1984;82:307–328.
23. Moster MR, Schwartz LW, Spaeeth GL, Wilson RP, McAllister JA, Poryzees EM. Laser iridectomy. A controlled study comparing argon and neodymium:YAG. *Ophthalmology* 1986;93:20–24.

Rajiv Shah
Glaucoma Fellow

Richard Wormald
Consultant Ophthalmic Surgeon
Moorfields Eye Hospital
London
UK

Competing interests: None declared.

Ocular herpes simplex

Search date April 2002

Nigel Barker

QUESTIONS

INTERVENTIONS

See glossary, p 660

Key Messages

Treating epithelial disease

- **Debridement** One systematic review has found no significant difference between debridement versus placebo in the proportion of people healed, but has found that debridement plus antiviral treatment versus debridement alone significantly increases the number of people healed after 7 and 14 days. The outcome measure "healed" was not clearly defined.
- **Interferons** One systematic review has found that topical interferon versus placebo significantly increases the number of people healed after 7 and 14 days. The review found no significant difference between topical interferon versus a topical antiviral agent in the number of people healed after 7 days, but found that topical interferon significantly increased the number of people healed after 14 days.
- **Topical antiviral agents** One systematic review has found that idoxuridine or vidarabine versus placebo significantly increases the number of people healed after 14 days, and that trifluridine or aciclovir (acyclovir) versus idoxuridine significantly increases the number of people healed after 7 and 14 days.

Treating stromal keratitis

- **Oral aciclovir** One RCT in people receiving topical corticosteroids plus antiviral treatment found no significant difference between oral aciclovir versus placebo in rates of treatment failure at 16 weeks.
- **Topical corticosteroids** One RCT in people receiving topical antiviral treatment found that topical corticosteroids versus placebo significantly reduced the progression and shortened the duration of stromal keratitis.

Preventing ocular herpes simplex

- **Long term (1 year) oral aciclovir** One large RCT in people with at least one previous episode of epithelial or stromal keratitis found that long term oral aciclovir versus placebo significantly reduced the risk of recurrences after 1 year.
- **Short term (3 wks) oral aciclovir** One RCT in people with epithelial keratitis receiving topical trifluridine found no significant difference between short term prophylaxis with oral aciclovir versus placebo in the rate of stromal keratitis or iritis at 1 year.

Preventing ocular herpes simplex in people with corneal grafts

- **Oral aciclovir** One small RCT found limited evidence that prophylactic use of oral aciclovir significantly reduced recurrences and improved graft survival.

DEFINITION Ocular herpes simplex is usually caused by herpes simplex virus type 1 (HSV-1) but also occasionally by the type 2 virus (HSV-2). Ocular manifestations of HSV are varied and include blepharitis (inflammation of the eyelids), canalicular obstruction, conjunctivitis, epithelial keratitis (see glossary, p 660), stromal keratitis (see glossary, p 660), iritis, and retinitis. HSV infections are classified as neonatal, primary (HSV in a person with no previous viral exposure), and recurrent (previous viral exposure with humoral and cellular immunity present).

INCIDENCE/PREVALENCE Infections with HSV are usually acquired in early life. A US study found antibodies against HSV-1 in about 50% of people with high socioeconomic status and 80% of people with low socioeconomic status by age 30 years.[1] However, only about 20–25% of people with HSV antibodies had any history of clinical manifestations of ocular or cutaneous herpetic disease.[2] Ocular HSV is the most common cause of corneal blindness in high income countries and is the most common cause of unilateral corneal blindness in the world.[3] A 33 year study of the population of Rochester, Minnesota, found the annual incidence of new cases of ocular herpes simplex was 8.4/100 000 (95% CI 6.9 to 9.9) and the annual incidence of all episodes (new and recurrent) was 20.7/100 000 (95% CI 18.3 to 23.1).[4] The prevalence of ocular herpes was 149 cases/100 000 population (95% CI 115 to 183). Twelve per cent of people had bilateral disease.

AETIOLOGY/RISK FACTORS Epithelial keratitis results from productive, lytic viral infection of the corneal epithelial cells. Stromal keratitis and iritis are thought to result from a combination of viral infection and compromised immune mechanisms. Observational evidence (346 people with ocular HSV in the placebo arm of an RCT) has found that the risk of developing stromal keratitis was 4% in people with no previous history of stromal keratitis (RR 1.0) as compared with 32% (RR 10, 95% CI 4.32 to 23.38; $P < 0.001$) with previous stromal keratitis, but that a history of epithelial keratitis was not a risk factor for recurrent epithelial keratitis.[5] Age, sex, ethnicity, and previous experience of non-ocular HSV disease were not associated with an increased risk of recurrence.[5]

PROGNOSIS HSV epithelial keratitis tends to resolve within 1–2 weeks. In a trial of 271 people treated with topical trifluorothymidine and randomly assigned to receive either oral aciclovir or placebo, the epithelial lesion had resolved completely or was at least less than 1 mm after 1 week of treatment with placebo in 89% of people and after 2 weeks in 99% of people.[6] Stromal keratitis or iritis occurs in about 25% of people following epithelial keratitis.[7] The effects of HSV stromal keratitis include scarring, tissue destruction, neovascularisation, glaucoma, and persistent epithelial defects. Rate of recurrence of ocular herpes for people with one episode is 10% at 1 year, 23% at 2 years, and 50% at 10 years.[8] The risk of recurrent ocular HSV infection (epithelial or stromal) has also been found to increase with the number of previous episodes reported (2 or 3 previous episodes: RR 1.41, 95% CI 0.82 to 2.42; 4 or more previous episodes: RR 2.09, 95% CI 1.24 to 3.50).[5] Of corneal grafts performed in Australia over a 10 year period, 5% were in people with visual disability or with actual or impending corneal perforation following stromal ocular herpes simplex. The recurrence of HSV in a corneal graft has a major effect on graft survival. The Australian Corneal Graft Registry has found that, in corneal grafts performed for HSV keratitis, there was at least one HSV recurrence in 58% of corneal grafts that failed over a follow up period of 9 years.[9]

AIMS To reduce the morbidity of HSV keratitis and iritis; to reduce the risk of recurrent disease after a first episode; to reduce the risk of recurrent disease; and to improve corneal graft survival after penetrating keratoplasty (see glossary, p 660).

OUTCOMES Healing time; severity and duration of symptoms; severity of complications; rates of recurrence; corneal graft survival.

METHODS *Clinical Evidence* update search and appraisal April 2002.

QUESTION What are the effects of treatments for epithelial ocular herpes simplex?

OPTION TOPICAL ANTIVIRAL AGENTS

One systematic review has found that antiviral treatment (idoxuridine or vidarabine) versus placebo significantly increases the number of people healed after 14 days. The review also found that either trifluridine or aciclovir (acyclovir) versus idoxuridine significantly increases the number of people healed after 7 and 14 days, but found no significant difference with vidarabine versus idoxuridine in the number of people healed after 7 or 14 days. The review included "healed" as an outcome measure without clearly defining this term.

Benefits: We found one systematic review (search date 2000, 96 RCTs, 4991 people; see comment below).[10] **Versus placebo:** The review found that idoxuridine versus placebo significantly increased the number of people healed after 7 days (10 RCTs; OR 4.05, 95% CI 2.60 to 6.30; see comment below) and after 14 days (2 RCTs; OR 4.17, 95% CI 1.33 to 13.00).[10] The review also compared vidarabine versus placebo and found no significant difference in the number of people healed after 7 days (numerical data not provided), but found that vidarabine significantly increased the number of people healed after 14 days (1 RCT; OR 5.40, 95% CI 1.42 to 20.5). **Versus each other:** The review found that trifluridine versus idoxuridine significantly increased the number of people healed after 7 days (3 RCTs; OR 4.74, 95% CI 2.52 to 8.91) and after 14 days (4 RCTs; OR 6.83, 95% CI 3.02 to 15.5).[10] The review also found that aciclovir versus idoxuridine significantly increased the number of people healed after 7 days (8 RCTs; OR 5.33, 95% CI 3.33 to 8.53) and after 14 days (11 RCTs; OR 3.71, 95% CI 2.27 to 6.08), but that there was no significant difference with vidarabine versus idoxuridine in the number of people healed after 7 days (3 RCTs; OR 1.24, 95% CI 0.72 to 2.00) or after 14 days (3 RCTs; OR 1.24, 95% CI 0.65 to 2.37). **Antiviral treatment plus physical debridement:** See benefits of debridement, p 656.

Harms: The review did not report harms.[10]

Comment: The review included "healed" as an outcome measure without clearly defining this term.[10] It reported that the number of people involved in the comparison of vidarabine versus placebo was small, although it did not provide any absolute numbers.

OPTION DEBRIDEMENT

One systematic review has found no significant difference between debridement versus placebo in the number of people healed after 7 or 14 days. The review found that debridement plus antiviral treatment versus debridement alone significantly increased the number of people healed after both 7 and 14 days, and that debridement plus antiviral treatment versus antiviral treatment alone significantly increased the number of people healed after 7 days but not after 14 days. The review included "healed" as an outcome measure without clearly defining this term.

Benefits: We found one systematic review (search date 2000, 96 RCTs, 4991 people).[10] **Debridement alone:** The review compared different types of physicochemical debridement versus placebo and found no significant difference in the number of people healed after 7 days (2 RCTs; OR 1.62, 95% CI 0.72 to 3.61; see comment below) or after 14 days (1 RCT; OR 2.12, 95% CI 0.38 to 12.0).[10] **Debridement plus antiviral treatment:** The review found that physicochemical debridement plus an antiviral agent versus physicochemical debridement alone significantly increased the number of people healed after 7 days (7 RCTs; OR 2.08, 95% CI 1.17 to 3.71) and after 14 days (2 RCTs; OR 10.81, 95% CI 1.81 to 64.5).[10] The review also found that physicochemical debridement plus an antiviral agent versus antiviral treatment alone significantly increased the number of people healed after 7 days (7 RCTs;

OR 2.01, 95% CI 1.21 to 3.34), but found no significant difference in the number of people healed after 14 days (significance testing not provided). One RCT identified by the review compared debridement plus aciclovir versus debridement plus idoxuridine and found no significant difference in the number of people healed after 7 or 14 days (significance testing not provided).

Harms: The review reported that epithelial keratitis (see glossary, p 660) occurred in some people after physicochemical debridement alone (absolute numbers not provided), and limited the use of this treatment.[10]

Comment: The review found that all methods of debriding the corneal epithelium produced similar rates of re-epithelialisation.[10] The variety of treatments used in the review limits the applicability of the summary results. The review included "healed" as an outcome measure without clearly defining this term.

OPTION INTERFERONS

One systematic review has found that topical interferon versus placebo significantly increases the number of people healed after both 7 and 14 days. The review found no significant difference between topical interferon versus a topical antiviral agent in the number of people healed after 7 days, but found that topical interferon significantly increased the number of people healed after 14 days. The review also found that topical interferon plus a topical antiviral agent versus a topical antiviral agent alone significantly increased the number of people healed after 14 days. The review included "healed" as an outcome without clearly defining this term.

Benefits: We found one systematic review (search date 2000, 96 RCTs, 4991 people).[10] **Versus placebo:** The review found that topical interferon versus placebo significantly increased the number of people healed after 7 days (3 RCTs; OR 2.09, 95% CI 1.15 to 3.81; see comment below) and after 14 days (2 RCTs; OR 3.43, 95% CI 1.30 to 9.02).[10] **Different concentrations:** The review found no significant difference with low concentration interferon (< 1 MU/mL) versus higher concentrations of interferon in the number of people healed after 7 days (1 RCT; OR 0.21, 95% CI 0.02 to 2.42).[10] **Versus topical antivirals:** The review found no significant difference with topical interferon versus topical antiviral agents in the number of people healed after 7 days (2 RCTs; OR 1.18, 95% CI 0.29 to 4.75), but found that topical interferon versus a topical antiviral agent significantly increased the number of people healed after 14 days (3 RCTs; OR 3.48, 95% CI 1.06 to 11.4).[10] **Topical interferons plus antiviral agents:** The review found that topical interferon plus a topical antiviral agent versus a topical antiviral agent alone (usually trifluridine) significantly increased the number of people healed after 7 days (8 RCTs; OR 13.3, 95% CI 7.41 to 23.9) but found no significant difference in the number of people healed after 14 days (5 RCTs; OR 2.62, 95% CI 0.91 to 7.57).[10]

Harms: The review did not report on harms.[10]

Comment: The review included "healed" as an outcome measure without clearly defining this term.[10]

QUESTION **What are the effects of treatments for stromal ocular herpes simplex?**

OPTION **TOPICAL CORTICOSTEROIDS**

One RCT in people receiving topical antiviral treatment found that topical corticosteroids versus placebo significantly reduced the progression and shortened the duration of stromal keratitis.

Benefits: We found one RCT (106 people; see comment below) comparing topical prednisolone sodium phosphate (in decreasing concentrations over 10 wks) versus placebo.[11] All participants received topical trifluridine. It found that prednisolone versus placebo significantly reduced the persistence or progression of stromal inflammation and shortened the duration of stromal keratitis (see glossary, p 660) (median 26 days with corticosteroid *v* median 72 days with placebo; difference in medians 46 days, 95% CI 14 to 58 days).

Harms: The RCT found that adverse events were recorded in nine people given steroids.[11] Four people developed dendritic epithelial keratitis (see glossary, p 660) and were removed from the trial. Four people developed toxic responses to trifluridine after week 5. These people were not withdrawn but the trifluridine was stopped. One person developed an epithelial defect and was withdrawn. Adverse events were reported in six people receiving placebo. All six were withdrawn from the study (1 person developed dendritic keratitis, 3 people developed an epithelial defect, and 2 people developed allergic conjunctivitis attributed to trifluorothymidine within the first 9 days of the trial).

Comment: The trial did not specify whether or not intention to treat analysis was performed.[11]

OPTION **ORAL ACICLOVIR**

One RCT in people receiving topical corticosteroids plus antiviral treatment found no significant difference between oral aciclovir versus placebo in rates of treatment failure at 16 weeks.

Benefits: We found one RCT (104 people with herpes simplex virus stromal keratitis [see glossary, p 660] receiving concomitant topical corticosteroids and trifluridine) of oral aciclovir versus placebo.[12] The primary outcome was time to treatment failure (assessed using 8 criteria). The RCT found no significant difference between aciclovir versus placebo in median time to treatment failure (84 days with aciclovir *v* 62 days with placebo; P = 0.46; CI not reported), and no significant difference in reported rates of treatment failure by week 16 (38/51 [75%] with aciclovir *v* 39/53 [74%] with placebo; RR 1.01, 95% CI 0.78 to 1.24).

Harms: The RCT found that two people in the placebo group developed adverse effects attributed to trifluridine (epithelial keratopathy in 1 person and an allergic reaction in the other).[12] Other adverse effects reported included pneumonia with possible pulmonary embolus (1 person), congestive heart failure (1 person), diarrhoea (1 person), oedema of the lower extremities (1 person), and anaemia (1 person). Adverse reactions reported in the aciclovir group included toxicity to trifluorothymidine (1 person) and headache (1 person).

Comment: None.

QUESTION What are the effects of interventions used as prophylaxis for people with ocular herpes simplex?

OPTION ORAL ACICLOVIR

One large RCT in people with at least onc previous episode of epithelial or stromal keratitis found that long term (1 year) oral aciclovir versus placebo significantly reduced the risk of recurrences after 1 year. One RCT in people with epithelial keratitis receiving topical trifluridine found no significant difference between short term prophylaxis (3 wks) with oral aciclovir versus placebo in the rate of stromal keratitis or iritis at 1 year.

Benefits: We found no systematic review. We found two RCTs.[6,13] The first RCT (703 immunocompetent people aged ≥12 years who had epithelial or stromal ocular herpes simplex virus in one or both eyes within the preceding 12 months) compared oral aciclovir (400 mg twice daily for 1 year) versus placebo.[13] It found that aciclovir treatment significantly reduced the risk of any type of recurrence after 1 year (19% with aciclovir *v* 32% with placebo; RR 0.55, 95% CI 0.41 to 0.75). Prespecified subgroup analysis (337 people with at least 1 previous episode of stromal keratitis) found that aciclovir versus placebo significantly reduced the risk of stromal keratitis (see glossary, p 660), but only in people who had at least one prior episode (14% with aciclovir *v* 28% with placebo; RR 0.48, 95% CI 0.29 to 0.80). The RCT found no rebound in the rate of ocular herpes simplex virus in thc 6 months after stopping treatment with aciclovir. The second RCT (287 people with epithelial keratitis (see glossary, p 660) all treated with topical trifluridine) compared a 3 week course of oral aciclovir versus placebo.[6] It found no significant difference in the rate of stromal keratitis or iritis (11% with aciclovir *v* 10% with placebo; RR 1.04, 95% CI 0.52 to 2.10), and no significant difference in the cumulative probability of developing stromal keratitis or iritis at 1 year of follow up (12% with aciclovir *v* 11% with placebo; P = 0.92; CI not reported).

Harms: One RCT found that adverse effects (mostly gastrointestinal problems) were uncommon and occurred with similar frequency in both groups.[13] Thirty two people (15 aciclovir *v* 17 placebo) discontinued treatment because of adverse effects. The most common adverse effect reported was gastrointestinal upset (7 aciclovir *v* 9 placebo).

Comment: None.

QUESTION What are the effects of antiviral prophylaxis on corneal graft survival?

OPTION ORAL ACICLOVIR

One small RCT found limited evidence that prophylactic use of oral aciclovir significantly reduced recurrences and improved graft survival.

Benefits: We found no systematic review. We found one small non-blinded RCT (22 people, 23 eyes, who had received keratoplasty [see glossary, p 660]), which compared oral aciclovir (800 or 1000 mg, 4 or 5 times orally daily, tapered during the first 12 months, for a maximum of 15 months) versus usual care.[14] Oral aciclovir was started before surgery or on the first day after surgery. The RCT found that oral aciclovir versus usual care significantly reduced the number of recurrences of ocular herpes simplex after a mean follow up of 17 months in people receiving aciclovir and 21 months in those receiving placebo (0% with aciclovir *v* 44% with placebo; $P < 0.01$), and also that aciclovir versus usual care significantly reduced the number of eyes with graft failure (14% with aciclovir treated eyes *v* 56% with placebo; $P < 0.05$; CI not provided).

Harms: None reported.

Comment: None.

GLOSSARY

Epithelial keratitis Inflammation of the cells that form the surface layer of the cornea.

Keratoplasty A procedure in which diseased corneal tissue is removed and replaced by donor corneal material.

Stromal keratitis Inflammation of the middle layer of the cornea. The stroma forms 90% of the corneal substance. It lies between the epithelium and Bowman's membrane anteriorly and Desçemet's membrane and the endothelium posteriorly.

REFERENCES

1. Nahmias AJ, Lee FK, Beckman-Nahmias S. Sero-epidemiological and sociological patterns of herpes simplex virus infection in the world. *Scand J Infect Dis Suppl* 1990;69:19–36.
2. Kaufman HE, Rayfield MA, Gebhardt BM. Herpes simplex viral infections. In: Kaufman HE, Baron BA, McDonald MB, eds. *The Cornea*. 2nd ed. Woburn, MA: Butterworth-Heinemann, 1997.
3. Dawson CR, Togni B. Herpes simplex eye infections: clinical manifestations, pathogenesis, and management. *Surv Ophthalmol* 1976;21:121–135.
4. Liesegang TJ, Melton LJ III, Daly PJ, et al. Epidemiology of ocular herpes simplex. Incidence in Rochester, Minnesota, 1950 through 1982. *Arch Ophthalmol* 1989;107:1155–1159.
5. Herpetic Eye Disease Study Group. Predictors of recurrent herpes simplex virus keratitis. *Cornea* 2001;20:123–128.
6. The Herpetic Eye Disease Study Group. A controlled trial of oral acyclovir for the prevention of stromal keratitis or iritis in patients with herpes simplex virus epithelial keratitis. The Epithelial Keratitis Trial. *Arch Ophthalmol* 1997;115:703–712.
7. Wilhelmus KR, Coster DJ, Donovan HC, et al. Prognosis indicators of herpetic keratitis. Analysis of a five-year observation period after corneal ulceration. *Arch Ophthalmol* 1981;99:1578–1582.
8. Liesegang TJ. Epidemiology of ocular herpes simplex. Natural history in Rochester, Minnesota, 1950 through 1982. *Arch Ophthalmol* 1989;107:1160–1165.
9. Williams KA, Muehlberg SM, Lewis RF, et al. *The Australian Corneal Graft Registry:1996 Report*. Adelaide: Mercury Press, 1997.
10. Wilhelmus KR. Interventions for herpes simplex virus epithelial keratitis (Cochrane Review). In: The Cochrane Library, Issue 3, 2001. Oxford: Update Software. Search date 2000; primary sources Medline, Central, Embase, Index medicus, Excerpta Medica Ophthalmology, Cochrane Eyes and Vision Group specialised register, The Cochrane Controlled Trials Register, hand searching of reference lists of primary reports, review articles, and corneal textbooks, and conference proceedings pertaining to ocular virology.
11. Wilhelmus KR, Gee L, Hauck WW, et al. Herpetic Eye Disease Study. A controlled trial of topical corticosteroids for herpes simplex stromal keratitis. *Ophthalmology* 1994;101:1883–1895.

12. Barron BA, Gee L, Hauck WW, et al. Herpetic Eye Disease Study. A controlled trial of oral acyclovir for herpes simplex stromal keratitis. *Ophthalmology* 1994;101:1871–1882.
13. Herpetic Eye Disease Study Group. Acyclovir for the prevention of recurrent herpes simplex virus eye disease. *N Engl J Med* 1998;339: 300–306.
14. Barney NP, Foster CS. A prospective randomized trial of oral acyclovir after penetrating keratoplasty for herpes simplex keratitis. *Cornea* 1994;13:232–236.

Nigel Barker
Consultant Ophthalmologist
Specialist Eye Centre
Christ Church
Barbados

Competing interests: None declared.

Trachoma

Search date October 2001

Denise Mabey and Nicole Fraser-Hurt

QUESTIONS

INTERVENTIONS

INTERVENTIONS TO PREVENT SCARRING TRACHOMA BY REDUCING ACTIVE TRACHOMA

Likely to be beneficial

TREATMENT OF SCARRING TRACHOMA

Likely to be beneficial

See glossary, p 668

Key Messages

Interventions to prevent scarring trachoma by reducing active trachoma

- **Antibiotics (versus placebo or no treatment)** One unpublished systematic review found limited evidence from low powered RCTs that antibiotics versus control significantly reduced active trachoma after 3 and 12 months. One additional RCT has found that topical tetracycline plus face washing versus no intervention significantly reduced the proportion of children with trachoma after 3 months.
- **Oral azithromycin (versus topical tetracycline)** One unpublished systematic review found limited evidence from three RCTs that oral azithromycin versus topical tetracycline significantly reduced active trachoma after 3 months. These RCTs were low powered or of unusual design, and at 12 months the difference between treatments disappeared. One subsequent RCT found that oral azithromycin versus topical tetracycline significantly increased clinical resolution of trachoma at 10 weeks and 6 months.
- **Promotion of face washing plus topical tetracycline** One RCT identified by two systematic reviews found that promotion of face washing plus topical tetracycline versus topical tetracycline alone significantly reduced the rate of severe trachoma after 1 year, but found no significant difference in the overall rate of trachoma. However, the RCT was too small to rule out a clinically important effect. One additional large RCT has found that face washing alone versus no intervention did not significantly reduce the proportion of children with trachoma after 3 months, although face washing plus topical tetracycline versus no intervention significantly reduced the proportion of children with trachoma after 3 months.

Clin Evid 2002;8:662–672.

Treatment of scarring trachoma

- **Bilamellar tarsal rotation (versus other eyelid surgery), when performed by an experienced operator** We found no RCTs on the effects of surgery to improve visual acuity in people with scarring trachoma. In people with major trichiasis, one RCT found limited evidence that tarsal rotation versus eversion splinting, tarsal advance or tarsal grooving significantly increased operative success after 2 weeks, but found no significant difference between tarsal rotation versus tarsal advance and rotation in operative success after 2 weeks. A second RCT found that tarsal rotation versus tarsal advance and rotation significantly increased operative success after 25 months. In people with minor trichiasis, one RCT found that tarsal rotation versus cryoablation or electrolysis significantly increased operative success after 25 months.

DEFINITION **Active trachoma** is chronic inflammation of the conjunctiva caused by infection with *Chlamydia trachomatis*. The World Health Organization classification for active trachoma defines mild trachoma (grade TF) as the presence of five or more follicles in the upper tarsal conjunctiva of at least 0.5 mm diameter. Severe trachoma (grade TI) is defined as pronounced inflammatory thickening of the upper tarsal conjunctiva that obscures more than half of the normal deep vessels. **Scarring trachoma** is caused by repeated active infection by *C trachomatis* in which the upper eyelid is shortened and distorted (entropion) and the lashes abrade the eye (trichiasis). Blindness results from corneal opacification, which is related to the degree of entropion/trichiasis.

INCIDENCE/ PREVALENCE Trachoma is the world's leading cause of preventable blindness and is second only to cataract as an overall cause of blindness.[1] Globally, active trachoma affects an estimated 150 million people, most of them children. About 5.5 million people are blind or at risk of blindness as a consequence of trachoma. Trachoma is a disease of poverty regardless of geographical region. Scarring trachoma is prevalent in large regions of Africa, the Middle East, south-west Asia, the Indian subcontinent, and Aboriginal communities in Australia, and there are also small foci in Central and South America.[1] In areas where trachoma is constantly present at high prevalence, active disease is found in more than 50% of preschool children and may have a prevalence of 60–90%.[2] The prevalence of active trachoma decreases with increasing age, with less than 5% of adults showing signs of active disease.[2] Although similar rates of active disease are observed in male and female children, the later sequelae of trichiasis, entropion, and corneal opacification are more common in women than men.[2] As many as 75% of women and 50% of men over the age of 45 years may show signs of scarring disease.[3]

AETIOLOGY/ RISK FACTORS Active trachoma is associated with young age and with situations in which there is close contact between people. Discharge from the eyes and nose may be a source of further reinfection.[4] Sharing a bedroom with someone who has active trachoma is a risk factor for infection.[5] Facial contact with flies is held to be associated with active trachoma, but studies reporting this relationship employed weak methods.[6]

PROGNOSIS Corneal damage from trachoma is caused by multiple processes. Scarring may cause an inadequate tear film and a dry eye may be more susceptible to damage from inturned lashes, leading to corneal opacification. The prevalence of scarring and consequent blindness increases with age and, therefore, is most commonly seen in older adults.[7]

AIMS To prevent active trachoma; to reduce the rate of progression to scarring; to relieve entropion and trichiasis in people with scarring trachoma; to minimise side effects of treatment.

OUTCOMES Rates of active trachoma; clinical signs of active trachoma using the World Health Organization grading scale; laboratory evidence of *C trachomatis* infection; eyelid position; degree of entropion/trichiasis.

METHODS *Clinical Evidence* search and appraisal October 2001.

QUESTION **What are the effects of interventions to prevent scarring trachoma by reducing active trachoma?**

OPTION **PUBLIC HEALTH**

One RCT identified by two systematic reviews found that promotion of face washing plus topical tetracycline versus topical tetracycline alone significantly reduced the rate of severe trachoma after 1 year, but found no significant difference in the overall rate of trachoma. However, the RCT was too small to rule out a clinically important effect. One additional RCT found that face washing alone versus no intervention did not significantly reduce the proportion of children with trachoma, although face washing plus topical tetracycline versus no intervention significantly reduced the proportion of children with trachoma. A pilot study for an RCT included in the systematic reviews found that fly control using insecticide versus no intervention significantly reduced the incidence of trachoma.

Benefits: We found two systematic reviews[8,9] and one additional RCT.[10] The first systematic review (search date 1999) identified one RCT and one pilot study for an RCT.[8] The second systematic review (search date 1999) identified the same RCT and pilot study as the first review plus two subsequent RCTs (see comment below).[9] **Promotion of face washing:** Both reviews identified one RCT (1417 children aged 1–7 years in 6 villages) that compared promotion of face washing plus 30 days of daily topical tetracycline (ointment) versus 30 days of daily topical tetracycline alone.[11] It found that promotion of face washing plus topical tetracycline increased the likelihood of children having a clean face on at least two of three follow up visits, although the result was not significant (OR for having a clean face with face washing plus topical tetracycline *v* topical tetracycline alone 1.6, 95% CI 0.94 to 2.74). The RCT also found that promotion of face washing plus topical tetracycline versus topical tetracycline alone significantly reduced the risk of severe trachoma after 1 year (OR for severe trachoma 0.62, 95% CI 0.40 to 0.97), but found that this reduction was not significant for all grades of trachoma combined (OR for mild and severe trachoma 0.81, 95% CI 0.42 to 1.59). The RCT found that when all participants from intervention and control villages were pooled, children who had a sustained clean face were significantly less likely to have active trachoma than those who had ever had a dirty face (OR 0.58, 95% CI 0.47 to 0.72). The additional RCT (1143 children in 36 communities) compared three groups: daily face washing (performed by a teacher); daily face washing (performed by a teacher) plus daily topical tetracycline (as drops for 1 wk each month); and no intervention.[10] Trachoma was defined as the presence of at least one follicle or some papillae on the upper tarsal plate (this study predated the present World Health Organization definition of trachoma). Losses to follow up were treated as being trachoma positive. The RCT found no significant difference between face washing alone versus no intervention in the number of children with trachoma after 3 months (191/246 [78%] with face washing alone *v* 160/211 [76%] with no intervention; RR 1.0; CI not provided). It also found that face washing plus tetracycline drops versus no intervention significantly reduced the number of children with trachoma after 3 months (215/312 [69%] with face washing plus topical tetracycline *v* 160/211 [78%] with no intervention; RR 0.9; CI not provided).[10] **Fly control using insecticide:** The reviews identified one pilot study for an RCT (414 children < 10 years) that compared spraying of deltamethrin for 3 months versus no intervention in two pairs of villages.[6] One pair received the intervention or none in the wet season and one pair received the intervention or none in the dry season. There were a total of 191 children under 10 years of age in the control villages and 223 children in the intervention villages. The pilot study found that spraying of deltamethrin significantly reduced the number of new cases of trachoma (World Health Organization classification) after 3 months (RR 0.25, 95% CI 0.09 to 0.64).

Harms: The reviews and additional RCT did not report adverse effects.[8–10]

Comment: Cluster randomisation used in the RCTs and the pilot study limits the power to detect differences between groups, and makes interpretation of the results for individual children difficult.[6,10,11] The RCT comparing promotion of face washing plus topical tetracycline versus topical tetracycline alone was too small to rule out a clinically important effect.[11] The two subsequent RCTs identified by the second systematic review compared antibiotics versus health education plus face washing, and it was not possible to extract data relating to the health education and face washing interventions separately.[9] The additional RCT predates the simplified World Health Organization classification of trachoma, limiting the applicability of the results.[10]

OPTION ANTIBIOTICS

One unpublished systematic review found limited evidence from low powered RCTs that antibiotics versus control significantly reduced active trachoma after 3 and 12 months. One additional RCT found that topical tetracycline plus face washing versus no intervention significantly reduced the proportion of children with trachoma after 3 months. The same review found limited evidence from three RCTs that oral azithromycin versus topical tetracycline significantly reduced active trachoma after 3 months. Those RCTs were low powered or of unusual

design, and at 12 months the difference between treatments disappeared. One subsequent RCT found that oral azithromycin versus topical tetracycline significantly increased clinical resolution of trachoma at 10 weeks and 6 months.

Benefits: **Versus placebo or no treatment:** We found one unpublished systematic review (search date 1999, 11 RCTs)[12] and one additional RCT.[10] The review identified eight RCTs that compared antibiotics (topical or oral) versus control (no treatment, placebo, or a monthly vitamin tablet)(see table 1, p 670).[13–20] The review found that antibiotics versus control significantly reduced active trachoma (assessed clinically) after 3 months (8 RCTs; OR 0.43, 95% CI 0.35 to 0.52) and after 12 months (5 RCTs; OR 0.47, 95% CI 0.38 to 0.60; see comment below). The review found no significant difference between treatments in *C trachomatis* infection rates based on bacteriological testing after 3 months (3 RCTs; OR 0.63, 95% CI 0.38 to 1.05), but found that antibiotics significantly reduced infection rates after 12 months (1 RCT; OR 0.27, 95% CI 0.11 to 0.67). For the additional RCT see benefits of public health interventions, p 664. **Oral versus topical antibiotics:** We found one unpublished systematic review (search date 1999, 3 RCTs, 6226 people; see comment below)[12] and one subsequent RCT.[21] The review found that oral azithromycin versus topical tetracycline significantly reduced active trachoma after 3 months (3 RCTs, 6226 people; OR 0.82, 95% CI 0.71 to 0.94), but found no significant difference between treatments in rates of active trachoma after 12 months (1 RCT; 5573 people; OR 0.88, 95% CI 0.77 to 1.01) (see table 2, p 671).[12] The review also found that oral azithromycin versus topical tetracycline significantly reduced bacteriologically defined infection after both 3 months (OR 0.49, 95% CI 0.39 to 0.62) and 12 months (OR 0.70, 95% CI 0.57 to 0.87) (see table 2, p 671). The subsequent RCT (314 children) compared a single dose of oral azithromycin versus topical tetracycline and found that oral azithromycin significantly increased the cure rate (defined as clinical resolution of trachoma) after 10 weeks (104/152 [68%] with azithromycin *v* 71/139 [51%] with tetracycline; RR 1.31, 95% CI 1.08 to 1.59) and after 6 months (135/154 [88%] *v* 103/141 [73%] with tetracycline; RR 1.19, 95% CI 1.06 to 1.34).[21]

Harms: None reported.

Comment: RCTs conducted prior to 1987 may use definitions of trachoma that differ from the present World Health Organization definition.[10,13–19] **Versus placebo or no treatment:** The trials were undertaken in various settings, and most were in children attending boarding schools.[10,12] Several unusual study designs were used, for example family based treatment. The trials were all of moderate or poor quality and many had no intention to treat analysis. Antibiotic treatments included topical and oral doses. **Oral versus topical treatment:** Two of the RCTs were small (total 224 people) and low powered.[12] The third RCT compared mass treatment, in which people were treated irrespective of disease status and were randomly allocated by village (cluster randomisation).[12] Correlation analysis found some similarity between individuals within a cluster, limiting the validity of results. We found no evidence regarding the development of bacterial resistance.

QUESTION **What are the effects of surgical treatments for scarring trachoma (entropion and trichiasis)?**

We found no good evidence on the effects of surgery to improve visual acuity in people with scarring trachoma. In people with major trichiasis, one RCT found that tarsal rotation versus eversion splinting, tarsal advance, and tarsal grooving significantly increased operative success, but found no significant difference between tarsal rotation versus tarsal advance and rotation in operative success. A second RCT found that tarsal rotation versus tarsal advance and rotation significantly increased operative success. In people with minor trichiasis, one RCT found that tarsal rotation versus cryoablation or electrolysis significantly increased operative success. In people with major trichiasis, one RCT found no significant difference between village versus health centre based tarsal rotation surgery in operative success.

Benefits: We found no systematic review but found three RCTs.[25–27] In the two RCTs that compared surgical interventions versus each other, one experienced surgeon performed most of the operations.[25,26] Both of these RCTs defined operative success as no lashes in contact with the globe in primary position of gaze and complete lid closure with gentle voluntary effort. **Major trichiasis:** See glossary, p 668. The first RCT (165 Omani villagers, 165 eyelids) compared five surgical techniques: bilamellar tarsal rotation; eversion splinting; tarsal advance; tarsal grooving; and tarsal advance and rotation (see glossary, p 668).[25] It found that tarsal rotation versus eversion splinting, tarsal advance, and tarsal grooving significantly increased operative success after 2 weeks (30/44 [68%] with tarsal rotation *v* 8/25 [32%] with eversion splinting; RR 2.13, 95% CI 1.16 to 3.91; 30/44 [68%] with tarsal rotation *v* 11/41 [27%] with tarsal advance; RR 2.5, 95% CI 1.5 to 4.4; 30/44 [68%] with tarsal rotation *v* 3/32 [9%] with tarsal grooving; RR 7.3, 95% CI 2.4 to 21.8), but found no significant difference between tarsal rotation versus tarsal advance and rotation in operative success after 2 weeks (30/44 [68%] with tarsal rotation *v* 10/23 [43%] with tarsal advance and rotation; RR 1.57, 95% CI 0.94 to 2.6). However, analysis was not by intention to treat and the power of the trial was low. The second RCT (Omani villagers, 200 eyelids) compared bilamellar tarsal rotation versus tarsal advance and rotation.[26] It found that tarsal rotation significantly increased operative success after 25 months (HR for failure, tarsal advance and rotation *v* tarsal rotation 3.1, 95% CI 1.9 to 5.2). **Minor trichiasis:** See glossary, p 668. The second RCT (172 eyelids) compared three treatments: tarsal rotation; cryoablation; and electrolysis.[26] It found that tarsal rotation versus both other treatments significantly increased operative success after 25 months (HR of failure, electrolysis *v* tarsal rotation 6.1, 95% CI 2.9 to 12.8; HR of failure, cryoablation *v* tarsal rotation 7.5, 95% CI 3.6 to 15.4). **Location of surgery:** We found one RCT (158 people with major trichiasis), which compared village versus health centre based tarsal rotation surgery for major trichiasis.[27] It found that attendance rates were not significantly different between interventions (57/86 [66%] *v* 32/72 [44%]; RR 1.5, 95% CI not provided). The RCT also found that there was also no significant difference between interventions in operative success rate (defined as no evidence of trichiasis) after 3 months (intention to treat analysis by *Clinical Evidence*; 52/86 [60%] with village surgery *v* 30/72 [42%] with health centre surgery; RR 1.4, 95% CI not available).[27]

Harms: Adverse outcomes of interventions were corneal exposure, ulceration, phthisis bulbi (see glossary, p 668), and severe recurrent trichiasis.[25,28] In the two RCTs that compared different surgical techniques versus each other, major trichiasis and defective closure after surgical procedures for scarring trachoma were more common after eversion splinting, tarsal advance, and tarsal grooving than after bilamellar tarsal rotation and tarsal advance and rotation.[25,26] Cryoablation of the eyelashes can cause necrosis of the lid margin, corneal ulcers, and in the RCT in which cryoablation was used it was the only procedure associated with onset of phthisis bulbi (2 cases out of 57).[26] Further details of harms are summarised in table 3, p 672.

Comment: The pragmatic definitions of major trichiasis and minor trichiasis are limited to use in these trials.[25,26] In both RCTs comparing surgical interventions, one experienced operator performed most of the surgery. The evidence of both benefits and harms may not be applicable to different operators, or where the quality of surgical equipment does not match those in the trials. In the RCT comparing village based versus health centre based surgery, problems with the unit of randomisation prevented the calculation of confidence limits for the relative risks stated.

GLOSSARY

Bilamellar tarsal rotation The upper lid is cut full thickness horizontally in a line parallel and 3 mm from the eyelid margin and running from just lateral to the lacrimal punctum to the lateral canthus. Everting sutures are then placed through all layers of the lid to prevent the margin from turning inwards.

Eversion splinting The lid margin is split posterior to the lashes, the eversion of the anterior section is maintained by sutures tied over a roll of paraffin gauze.

Major trichiasis Lid closure complete; six or more lashes in contact with eyeball.

Minor trichiasis Lid closure complete; one to five lashes in contact with eyeball.

Phthisis bulbi A disorganised, shrunken eye that has no perception of light.

Tarsal advance The lid margin is split posterior to the lashes. The skin, lashes, and orbicularis are freed from the tarsal plate and retracted away from the cornea and are sutured back on to the tarsal plate, leaving a bare area of tarsus to act as the lid margin.

Tarsal advance and rotation The upper lid is everted over a speculum. The tarsal plate is fractured parallel to and 3 mm from the lid margin. In this operation the skin and orbicularis are not cut. The short portion of tarsal plate attached to the lid margin is then rotated through 180° and sutured into place to form the new lid margin.

Tarsal grooving A wedge of skin, orbicularis, and tarsus is removed parallel to the lid margin. Sutures through all layers act to evert the lid margin.

REFERENCES

1. Thylefors B, Negrel AD, Pararajasegaram R, et al. Global data on blindness. *Bull World Health Organ* 1995;73:115–121.
2. West SK, Munoz B, Turner VM, et al. The epidemiology of trachoma in central Tanzania. *Int J Epidemiol* 1991;20:1088–1092.
3. Courtright P, Sheppard J, Schachter J, et al. Trachoma and blindness in the Nile Delta: current patterns and projections for the future in the rural Egyptian population. *Br J Ophthalmol* 1989;73:536–540.
4. Bobo L, Munoz B, Viscidi R, et al. Diagnosis of *Chlamydia trachomatis* eye infection in Tanzania by polymerase chain reaction/enzyme immunoassay. *Lancet* 1991;338:847–850.
5. Bailey R, Osmond C, Mabey DCW, et al. Analysis of the household pattern of trachoma in a Gambian village using a Monte Carlo simulation procedure. *Int J Epidemiol* 1989;18:944–951.
6. Emerson PM, Lindsay SW, Walraven GE, et al. Effect of fly control on trachoma and diarrhoea. *Lancet* 1999;353:1401–1403.
7. Munoz B, West SK. The forgotten cause of blindness. *Epidemiol Rev* 1997;19:205–217.
8. Emerson PM, Cairncross S, Bailey RL, Mabey DC. Review of the evidence base for the "F" and "E" components of the SAFE strategy for trachoma control. *Trop Med Int Health* 2000;5:515–527. Search date 1999; primary sources Medline, BIDS, and hand searches of reference lists.
9. Pruss A, Mariotti SP. Preventing trachoma through environmental sanitation: a review of the evidence base. *Bull World Health Organ* 2000;78:258–266. Search date 1999; primary sources Medline, Healthstar, and hand searches of reference lists and selected conference proceedings.
10. Peach H, Piper S, Devanesen D, et al. Trial of antibiotic drops for the prevention of trachoma in school-age Aboriginal children. *Annual Report Menzies School for Health Research* 1986;74–76.
11. West S, Munoz B, Lynch M, et al. Impact of facewashing on trachoma in Kongwa, Tanzania. *Lancet* 1995;345:155–158.
12. Mabey D, Fraser-Hurt N. Antibiotics for trachoma (Protocol for a Cochrane Review). In: The Cochrane Library, Issue 4, 2000. Oxford: Update Software. Search date 1999; primary sources Medline, Embase, Cinalh, Science Citation Index, and personal contacts.
13. Attiah MA, el Kohly AM. Clinical assessment of the comparative effect of terramycin and GS 2989 in the mass treatment of trachoma. *Rev Int Trach Pathol Ocul Trop Subtrop Sante Publique* 1973;50:11–20.
14. Darougar S, Jones BR, Viswalingam N, et al. Family-based suppressive intermittent therapy of hyperendemic trachoma with topical oxytetracycline or oral doxycycline. *Br J Ophthalmol* 1980;64:291–295.
15. Dawson CR, Hanna L, Wood TR, et al. Controlled trials with trisulphapyrimidines in the treatment of chronic trachoma. *J Infect Dis* 1969;119:581–590.
16. Foster SO, Powers DK, Thygeson P. Trachoma therapy: a controlled study. *Am J Ophthalmol* 1966;61:451–455.
17. Hoshiwara I, Ostler HB, Hanna L, et al. Doxycycline treatment of chronic trachoma. *JAMA* 1973;224:220–223.
18. Shukla BR, Nema HV, Mathur JS, et al. Gantrisin and madribon in trachoma. *Br J Ophthalmol* 1966;50:218–221.
19. Woolridge RL, Cheng KH, Chang IH, et al. Failure of trachoma treatment with ophthalmic antibiotics and systemic sulphonamides used alone or in combination with trachoma vaccine. *Am J Ophthalmol* 1967;63(suppl):1577–1586.
20. Tabbara KF, Summanen P, Taylor PB, et al. Minocycline effects in patients with active trachoma. *Int Ophthalmol* 1988;12:59–63.
21. Bowman RJC, Sillah A, Van Dehn C, et al. Operational comparison of single-dose azithromycin and topical tetracycline for trachoma. *Investig Ophthalmol Visu Sci* 2000;41:4074–4079.
22. Dawson CR, Schachter J, Sallam S, et al. A comparison of oral azithromycin with topical oxytetracycline/polymyxin for the treatment of trachoma in children. *Clin Infect Dis* 1997;24:363–368.
23. Schachter J, West SK, Mabey D, et al. Azithromycin in control of trachoma. *Lancet* 1999;354:630–635.
24. Tabbara KF, Abu el Asrar A, al Omar O, et al. Single-dose azithromycin in the treatment of trachoma. A randomized, controlled study. *Ophthalmology* 1996;103:842–846.
25. Reacher MH, Huber MJE, Canagaratnam R, et al. A trial of surgery for trichiasis of the upper lid from trachoma. *Br J Ophthalmol* 1990;74:109–113.
26. Reacher MH, Munoz B, Alghassany A, et al. A controlled trial of surgery for trachomatous trichiasis of the upper lid. *Arch Ophthalmol* 1992;110:667–674.
27. Bowman RJ, Soma OS, Alexander N, et al. Should trichiasis surgery be offered in the village? A community randomised trial of village vs. health centre-based surgery. *Trop Med Internat Health* 2000;5:528–533.
28. Reacher MH, Taylor HR. The management of trachomatous trichiasis. *Rev Int Trach Pathol Ocul Trop Subtrop Sante Publique* 1990;67:233–262.

Nicole Fraser-Hurt
Epiconsult Ltd
Nhlangano
Swaziland

Denise Mabey
Guy's and St Thomas' Hospital Trust
London
UK

Competing interests: None declared.

TABLE 1 **Interventions to prevent scarring trachoma by reducing active trachoma: RCTs of antibiotics compared with no treatment, placebo, or a monthly vitamin tablet in people with active trachoma (see text, p 666).**

Study	Treatment	Route	Dose	Duration	Comparison
13	Tetracycline derivative GS2989	Topical	0.25%	Once every school day for 11 weeks	No treatment
13	Oxytetracycline	Topical	Not stated	Once every school day for 11 weeks	No treatment
14	Oxytetracycline	Topical	1%	Twice daily for 7 consecutive days every month for 12 months	Vitamin pills, orally, 1 dose every month for 12 months
14	Doxycycline	Oral	5 mg/kg	1 dose every month for 12 months	Vitamin pills, orally, 1 dose every month for 12 months
15	Trisulfapyrimidine	Oral	3.5 g/day	3 daily during 3 consecutive weeks	Lactose, orally, 3 daily for 3 weeks
15	Trisulfapyrimidine	Oral	3.5 g/day	3 daily during 3 consecutive weeks	Lactose, orally, 3 daily for 3 weeks
16	Sulfametopyridazine	Oral	0.5 g	Once daily for 5 consecutive days every week for 3 weeks	No treatment
16	Tetracycline	Topical	1%	3 times daily on 5 consecutive days every week for 6 weeks	No treatment
17	Doxycycline	Oral	2.5–4.0 mg/kg	Once daily for 5 consecutive days every week up to 28 doses in 40 days	Placebo once daily for 5 consecutive days every week up to 28 doses in 40 days
18	Sulfafurazole plus sulfadimethoxine	Topical plus oral	15%/100 mg/kg	Twice daily for 5 consecutive days every month for 5 months/biweekly for 5 months	No treatment
18	Sulfadimethoxine	Oral	100 mg/kg	Twice weekly or weekly dose for 5 months	No treatment
18	Sulfafurazole	Topical	15%	Twice daily for 5 consecutive days every month for 5 months	No treatment
19	Tetracycline	Topical	1%	Twice daily for 6 consecutive days every week for 6 weeks	No treatment
20	Minocycline	Oral	100 mg	Once daily on 5 consecutive days every week for 5 weeks	Placebo topically twice daily on 5 consecutive days every week for 5 weeks
20	Tetracycline	Topical	1%	Twice daily on 5 consecutive days every week for 5 weeks	Placebo topically twice daily on 5 consecutive days every week for 5 weeks

TABLE 2 **Interventions to prevent scarring trachoma by reducing active trachoma: RCTs comparing rates of active trachoma and bacteriological infection following oral azithromycin or topical tetracycline (see text, p 666).**

Study	Treatment	Dose	Duration	Comparison	Dose/duration
22	Azithromycin orally	20 mg/kg	1 dose, or 3 times 1 dose at weekly intervals, or 6 times 1 dose at 28 day intervals	1% topical oxytet/polymyxin plus oral placebo	Ointment once daily for 5 consecutive days monthly for 6 months
23	Azithromycin orally	20 mg/kg up to 1 g	Once a week for 3 weeks	1% topical oxytetracycline	Once daily for 6 weeks
	Women of childbearing age; erythromycin	500 mg twice daily or 250 mg four times daily	14 days	ND	ND
24	Azithromycin orally	20 mg/kg	1 dose	1% topical tetracycline	Twice daily for 5 consecutive days every week for 6 weeks

ND, no data.

TABLE 3 Summary of harms following surgery for scarring trachoma (see text, p 668).

	Bilamellar tarsal rotation	Tarsal advance and rotation	Eversion splinting	Tarsal advance	Tarsal grooving
Reference[26]					
Major trichiasis	4/150	4/101	ND	ND	ND
Defective closure	2/150	1/101	ND	ND	ND
Reference[28]					
Major trichiasis	1/44	1/23	7/25	10/41	11/32
Defective closure	2/44	0/23	0/25	0/41	5/32

ND, no data.

Chickenpox

Search date March 2002

George Swingler and Jimmy Volmink

QUESTIONS

INTERVENTIONS

See glossary, p 678

Key Messages

Prevention

- **Aciclovir in people with immunocompromise other than HIV** We found no RCTs.
- **High dose aciclovir (> 3200 mg/day) in people with HIV infection** One systematic review has found that high dose aciclovir (at least 3200 mg/day) versus placebo significantly reduces clinical chickenpox (NNT 23, 95% CI 17 to 39) and reduces all cause mortality over 22 months' treatment.
- **Live attenuated vaccine in healthy children** Two RCTs have found that live attenuated varicella vaccine versus placebo significantly reduces clinical chickenpox, with no significant increase in adverse effects.
- **Live attenuated vaccine in immunocompromised people** We found no RCTs in immunocompromised people on the effects of live attenuated varicella vaccine.
- **Varicella zoster immune globulin versus zoster immune globulin in immunocompromised children** One RCT in immunocompromised children exposed to a sibling with chickenpox found no significant difference with varicella zoster immune globulin versus zoster immune globulin in clinical chickenpox at 12 weeks.

Clin Evid 2002;8:673–679.

- **Zoster immune globulin versus human serum globulin in healthy children** One small RCT in children exposed to a sibling with chickenpox found that zoster immune globulin versus human immune serum globulin significantly reduced the number of exposed children with clinical chickenpox at 20 days.

Treatment

- **Intravenous aciclovir for treatment of chickenpox in children with malignancy** Two RCTs compared intravenous aciclovir versus placebo; one large RCT has found that aciclovir significantly reduces clinical deterioration (NNT 3, 95% CI 2 to 4), and the other small RCT found no significant difference in clinical deterioration.
- **Oral aciclovir in healthy people (given < 24 h of onset of the rash)** RCTs have found that oral aciclovir versus placebo given within 24 hours of onset of the rash significantly reduces the symptoms of chickenpox.
- **Oral aciclovir in healthy people (given > 24 h after the onset of the rash)** RCTs found that oral aciclovir versus placebo given beyond 24 hours after onset of rash did not significantly reduce the symptoms of chickenpox.

DEFINITION Chickenpox is due to primary infection with varicella zoster virus (VZV). In healthy people it is usually a mild self limiting illness, characterised by low grade fever, malaise, and a generalised, itchy vesicular rash.

INCIDENCE/ PREVALENCE Chickenpox is extremely contagious. Over 90% of unvaccinated people become infected, but at different ages in different parts of the world. Over 80% of people have been infected by the age of 10 years in the USA, UK, and Japan, but only by 30 years of age or older in India, Southeast Asia, and the West Indies.[1,2]

AETIOLOGY/ RISK FACTORS Chickenpox is caused by exposure to VZV.

PROGNOSIS **Infants and children:** In healthy children the illness is usually mild and self limited. In the USA, the death rates in children aged 1–14 years and infants with chickenpox are about 1.4/100 000 and 7/100 000, respectively.[3] In Australia, mortality in children aged between 1 and 11 years with chickenpox is about 0.5–0.6/100 000, and in infants with chickenpox it is about 1.2/100 000.[4] Bacterial skin sepsis is the most common complication in children under 5 years of age, and acute cerebellar ataxia is the most common complication in older children; both cause hospital admission in 2–3/10 000 children.[5] **Adults:** Mortality in adults is higher, at about 31/100 000.[3] Varicella pneumonia is the most common complication, causing 20–30 hospital admissions/10 000 adults.[5] Activation of latent VZV infection can cause acute infection, herpes zoster, which is also known as shingles (see postherpetic neuralgia, p 809). **Cancer chemotherapy:** One case series (77 children with cancer and chickenpox) found that more children receiving chemotherapy versus those in remission developed progressive chickenpox with multiple organ involvement (19/60 [32%] *v* 0/17 [0%]), and more children died (4/60 [7%] *v* 0/17 [0%]).[6] **HIV infection:** One retrospective case series found that one in four children with HIV who acquired chickenpox in hospital developed pneumonia and 5% died.[7] In a retrospective cohort study (73 children with HIV and chickenpox), infection beyond 2 months occurred in 10 children (14%) and recurrent VZV infections occurred in 38 children (55%).[8] Half of recurrent infections involved generalised rashes and the other half had zoster. **Newborns:** We found no cohort studies of untreated children with perinatal exposure to chickenpox. One cohort study (281 neonates receiving varicella zoster immune globulin [see glossary, p 678] because their mothers had developed a chickenpox rash during the month before or after delivery) found that 134 (48%) developed a chickenpox rash and 19 (14%) developed severe chickenpox.[9] Severe chickenpox occurred in neonates of mothers whose rash had started during the 7 days before delivery.

AIMS To prevent clinical chickenpox (characterised by a rash); to reduce the duration of illness and complications of chickenpox.

OUTCOMES Development of clinical chickenpox; duration of illness (onset of last new lesions, disappearance of fever); complications of chickenpox; mortality.

METHODS *Clinical Evidence* update search and appraisal March 2002. All identified RCTs with English abstracts were reviewed.

QUESTION What are the effects of treatments to prevent chickenpox?

OPTION LIVE ATTENUATED VARICELLA VACCINE

Two RCTs identified by a systematic review have found that live attenuated varicella vaccine versus placebo significantly reduces chickenpox in healthy children, with no significant increase in adverse effects. We found no RCTs in immunocompromised people.

Benefits: We found one systematic review (search date 2000, 10 RCTs, 14 non-randomised trials, 18 cohort studies), which did not perform meta-analysis.[10] **In healthy people:** Only two of the RCTs in the review reported clinical outcomes.[10] The first RCT (914 healthy children aged 1–14 years) found that live attenuated varicella vaccine versus placebo significantly reduced clinical chickenpox at 9 months (0/468 [0%] with vaccine *v* 38/446 [8.5%] with placebo; OR 0.0, 95% CI 0.0 to 0.09) and at 2 years (1/163 [1%] with vaccine *v* 21/161 [13%] with placebo; OR 0.05, 95% CI 0.01 to 0.35). The second RCT (327 healthy children aged 10–30 months) also found that live attenuated varicella vaccine versus placebo significantly reduced clinical chickenpox after a mean of 29 months (AR 5/166 [3.0%] *v* 41/161 [25%]; RR 0.12, 95% CI 0.05 to 0.29). **In immunocompromised people:** The review identified no RCTs assessing clinical outcomes in people receiving cancer chemotherapy, in people with HIV, or in those aged under 1 month or over 65 years.[10]

Harms: **In healthy people:** The second RCT in the review found that the only reported adverse effect with varicella vaccine was a non-significant increase in varicella-like papules or vesicles (AR 5.4% with vaccine *v* 3.7% with placebo; RR 1.45, 95% CI 0.53 to 4.0).[10] No children had fever or constitutional symptoms. One postmarketing analysis of a database of 89 753 vaccinated adults and children failed to find associations with any rare serious adverse events.[11] Another analysis found that the rate of serious adverse events was

2.9/100–000 doses.[12] **In immunocompromised people:** One RCT found that, of 22 children vaccinated at the start of cancer chemotherapy, three (14%) developed mild maculopapular rashes and fever 16, 24, and 40 days after vaccination, and one had an isolated fever 7 days after vaccination.[13]

Comment: A new systematic review of vaccines for preventing varicella in children and adults is under way.[14]

OPTION ACICLOVIR

One systematic review has found that high dose aciclovir (at least 3200 mg/day) versus placebo significantly reduces the risk of clinical chickenpox and reduces all cause mortality over 22 months' treatment in people with HIV infection. We found no RCTs in people with other forms of immunocompromise.

Benefits: **In people with HIV:** We found one systematic review (search date not stated, 8 RCTs, 1792 people with different stages of HIV, median CD4 count 34–607/mm^3) comparing high dose aciclovir versus placebo.[15] Three of the RCTs were unpublished, including two pharmaceutical company trials. It found that aciclovir (at least 3200 mg/day) versus placebo taken for up to 22 months significantly reduced clinical chickenpox (AR 14/895 [2%] with aciclovir *v* 54/897 [6%] with placebo; OR 0.29, 95% CI 0.13 to 0.63; NNT 23, 95% CI 17 to 39). All cause mortality was also reduced (HR 0.78, 95% CI 0.65 to 0.93; OR 0.75, 95% CI 0.57 to 1.00). We found no RCTs of lower doses of aciclovir in people with HIV. **In other immunocompromised people:** We found no RCTs of aciclovir in people with other forms of immunocompromise.

Harms: The systematic review did not assess adverse effects (see harms under aciclovir for treatment, p 678).

Comment: None.

OPTION ZOSTER IMMUNE GLOBULIN

One small RCT in healthy children found that zoster immune globulin versus immune serum globulin significantly reduced the number of children with clinical chickenpox. We found no RCTs of zoster immune globulin versus varicella zoster immune globulin in healthy children. In immunocompromised children, one RCT found no significant difference between zoster immune globulin and varicella zoster immune globulin in risk of clinical chickenpox.

Benefits: We found no systematic review. **Versus placebo:** We found no RCTs. **Versus immune serum globulin (ISG) in healthy children:** See glossary, p 678. We found one small RCT (12 healthy susceptible children exposed to a sibling with recent onset of chickenpox) comparing zoster immune globulin (ZIG) (see glossary, p 678) (2 mL/10 kg) versus ISG (2 mL/10 kg).[16] It found that ZIG significantly reduced the number of children with clinical chickenpox at 20 days (AR 0/6 [0%] *v* 6/6 [100%]; OR 0.0, 95% CI 0 to 0.28). **Versus ISG in immunocompromised children:** We found no RCTs. **Versus varicella zoster immune globulin (VZIG) in**

healthy children: We found no RCTs. **Versus VZIG in immunocompromised children:** See glossary, p 678. We found one RCT (164 immunocompromised children, mostly with leukaemia, exposed to a sibling with chickenpox) comparing ZIG (1.25 mL/10 kg) versus VZIG (1.25 mL/10 kg).[17] It found no significant difference in the number of children with clinical chickenpox at 12 weeks (AR 31/88 [37%] with ZIG *v* 36/81 [44%] with VZIG; RR 0.84, 95% CI 0.58 to 1.22). A second RCT compared high dose VZIG (2.5 mL/10 kg) versus low dose VZIG (1.25 mL/10 kg).[17] It found no significant difference in the number of children with clinical chickenpox at 12 weeks (AR 19/40 [47.5%] with low dose *v* 22/46 [48%] with high dose; RR 1.00, 95% CI 0.61 to 1.65).

Harms: None of the RCTs assessed adverse effects.

Comment: The imprecise estimates might not exclude clinically important differences, especially in the comparison of high dose versus low dose VZIG.[17]

QUESTION **What are the effects of treatments for chickenpox?**

OPTION **ACICLOVIR**

RCTs have found that oral aciclovir versus placebo significantly reduces the symptoms of chickenpox in healthy people when given within 24 hours of onset of the rash, but found no significant difference if started after 24 hours. Two RCTs compared intravenous aciclovir versus placebo in children with cancer; one large RCT has found that aciclovir significantly reduces clinical deterioration, whereas the other small RCT found no significant difference.

Benefits: **In healthy people:** We found one systematic review (search date 1997) in adults, which identified three RCTs and did not perform meta-analysis.[18] The first RCT (76 adults) compared aciclovir (800 mg five times daily) versus placebo given within 24 hours of the rash or 24 72 hours after the rash. It found that aciclovir given within 24 hours versus placebo significantly reduced the maximum number of lesions and the time to full crusting of lesions, but found no difference in time to full crusting of lesions if aciclovir was given after 24 hours. The two remaining RCTs (total of 168 healthy people) compared aciclovir versus placebo given to people more than 24 hours after the onset of the rash.[18] Neither found a significant difference in the time to last new lesions, and did not provide numerical information on the time to cessation of fever. We found three RCTs in children and adolescents (total of 888 healthy children and adolescents) comparing oral aciclovir versus placebo given within 24 hours of the onset of the rash.[19–21] The largest RCT (724 children) found that aciclovir (20 mg/kg four times daily) versus placebo significantly reduced the time to the last new lesions (median 1 day with aciclovir *v* 2 days with placebo; $P < 0.001$) and reduced the time to cessation of fever (median 1 day with aciclovir *v* 2 days with placebo; $P < 0.001$; CI not provided).[20] The second RCT (62 adolescents) found that aciclovir (800 mg four times daily) versus placebo significantly reduced the time to last new lesions (median 2.2

days with aciclovir *v* 3.2 days with placebo; $P < 0.001$; CI not provided).[19] The third RCT (102 children) found no significant difference between aciclovir (10–20 mg/kg four times daily) versus placebo in the time to last new lesions, but aciclovir significantly reduced the time to cessation of fever (median 1 day with aciclovir *v* 2 days with placebo; $P = 0.001$; CI not provided).[21] We found one RCT that included children, adolescents, and adults (77 people). It found that aciclovir started on the second versus the third day of the rash significantly reduced the time to the last new lesions in children (median 4 days *v* 5 days; $P < 0.04$; CI not provided) but found no significant difference in adolescents and adults.[22] Earlier treatment significantly reduced the time to cessation of fever in adolescents (median 2–3 days *v* 3–4 days; $P < 0.02$; CI not provided) but not in children and adults. **In immunocompromised people:** We found two placebo controlled RCTs of intravenous aciclovir in children with cancer receiving chemotherapy.[23,24] The largest RCT (50 children aged 1–14 years with chickenpox, 60% of whom had a rash for > 24 h) found that significantly less children receiving aciclovir versus placebo (500 mg/m^2) clinically deteriorated and had to be transferred to open aciclovir (1/25 [4%] with aciclovir *v* 12/25 [48%] with placebo; RR 0.08, 95% CI 0.01 to 0.59; NNT 3, 95% CI 2 to 4).[23] Analysis of the remaining children not moved to open aciclovir treatment found that aciclovir significantly reduced the time to full crusting of lesions (mean 5.7 *v* 7.1 days; $P < 0.013$; CI not provided), but found no significant difference in cessation of fever. The second RCT (20 children, mean age 6.4 years) comparing aciclovir (500 mg/m^2) versus placebo found no significant difference in the number of children who clinically deteriorated and who subsequently needed to receive open aciclovir (AR 1/8 [12.5%] with aciclovir *v* 5/12 [42%]; RR 0.30, 95% CI 0.04 to 2.1).[24] However, the RCT was too small to exclude a clinically important difference.

Harms: No serious harms were reported in any of the seven RCTs in healthy people, except for one child taking placebo who developed cerebellar ataxia. Of the three RCTs (total of 889 people) reporting possible adverse effects, none found significant differences between treatment and control groups, or unfavourable trends in children taking aciclovir.[19–21] Adverse effects assessed included gastrointestinal symptoms, leukopoenia, thrombocytopoenia, and abnormalities of liver enzymes.

Comment: The effect on the measured outcomes was small and of questionable clinical importance in healthy people who make an uneventful recovery without treatment. In the first RCT in immunocompromised children, the exclusion of the children taking placebo who clinically deteriorated from the subsequent analysis means that the effect of placebo may have been overestimated, diminishing the significance of differences between treatments.[23]

GLOSSARY

Immune serum globulin (ISG) Immunoglobulin prepared from pooled human plasma.

Varicella zoster immune globulin (VZIG) Prepared from units of donor plasma selected for high titres of antibodies to varicella zoster virus.

Zoster immune globulin (ZIG) Prepared from the plasma of donors convalescing from herpes zoster (sustainable supplies are difficult to obtain).

Substantive changes

Live attenuated varicella vaccine New systematic review;[10] conclusions unchanged.
Live attenuated varicella vaccine New analysis on harms;[12] conclusions unchanged.
Aciclovir, treatment New systematic review;[18] conclusions unchanged.
Aciclovir, treatment New RCT;[22] conclusions unchanged.

REFERENCES

1. Lee BW. Review of varicella zoster seroepidemiology in India and Southeast Asia. *Trop Med Int Health* 1998;3:886–890.
2. Garnett GP, Cox MJ, Bundy DA, et al. The age of infection with varicella-zoster virus in St Lucia, West Indies. *Epidemiol Infect* 1993;110:361–372.
3. Preblud SR. Varicella: complications and costs. *Pediatrics* 1986;78:728–735.
4. Scuffman PA, Lowin AV, Burgess MA. The cost effectiveness of varicella vaccine programs for Australia. *Vaccine* 1999;18:407–415.
5. Guess HA, Broughton DD, Melton LJ, et al. Population-based studies of varicella complications. *Pediatrics* 1986;78:723–727.
6. Feldman S, Hughes WT, Daniel CB. Varicella in children with cancer: seventy-seven cases. *Pediatrics* 1975;56:388–397.
7. Leibovitz E, Cooper D, Giurgiutiu D, et al. Varicella-zoster virus infection in Romanian children infected with the human immunodeficiency virus. *Pediatrics* 1993;92:838–842.
8. von Seidlein L, Gillette SG, Bryson Y, et al. Frequent recurrence and persistence of varicella-zoster virus infections in children infected with human immunodeficiency virus type 1. *J Pediatr* 1996;128:52–57.
9. Miller E, Cradock-Watson JE, Ridehalgh MK. Outcome in newborn babies given anti-varicella-zoster immunoglobulin after perinatal maternal infection with varicella-zoster virus. *Lancet* 1989;2:371–373.
10. Skull SA, Wang EE. Varicella vaccination: a critical review of the evidence. *Arch Dis Child* 2001;85:83–90. Search date 2000; primary sources Medline, Embase, The Cochrane Library, reference lists, the internet for position papers from health oganisations, and vaccine product information.
11. Black S, Shinefield H, Ray P, et al. Postmarketing evaluation of the safety and effectiveness of varicella vaccine. *Pediatr Infect Dis J* 1999;18:1041–1046.
12. Wise RP, Salive ME, Braun MM, et al. Postlicensure safety surveillance for varicella vaccine. *JAMA* 2000;284:1271–1279.
13. Cristofani LM, Weinberg A, Peixoto V, et al. Administration of live attenuated varicella vaccine to children with cancer before starting chemotherapy. *Vaccine* 1991;9:873–876.
14. Coole L, Law B, McIntyre P. Vaccines for preventing varicella in children and adults. (Protocol for a Cochrane Review). In: The Cochrane Library, Issue 1, 2002. Oxford: Update Software.
15. Ioannidis JP, Collier AC, Cooper DA, et al. Clinical efficacy of high-dose aciclovir in patients with human immunodeficiency virus infection: a meta-analysis of randomized individual patient data. *J Infect Dis* 1998;178:349–359. Search date not stated; primary sources Medline, handsearching of abstracts from meetings, trial directories, and communication with experts.
16. Brunell PA, Ross A, Miller LH, et al. Prevention of varicella by zoster immune globulin. *N Engl J Med* 1969;280:1191–1194.
17. Zaia JA, Levin MJ, Preblud SR, et al. Evaluation of varicella-zoster immune globulin: protection of immunosuppressed children after household exposure to varicella. *J Infect Dis* 1983;147:737–743.
18. Alfandari S. Second question: antiviral treatment of varicella in adult or immunocompromised patients. *Medecine et Maladies Infectieuses* 1998;28:722–729. Search date 1997; primary sources Medline, Embase, and handsearches of reference lists and selected journals.
19. Balfour HH Jr, Rotbart HA, Feldman S, et al. Aciclovir treatment of varicella in otherwise healthy adolescents. The Collaborative Aciclovir Varicella Study Group. *J Pediatr* 1992;120:627–633.
20. Dunkle LM, Arvin AM, Whitley RJ, et al. A controlled trial of aciclovir for chickenpox in normal children. *N Engl J Med* 1991;325:1539–1544.
21. Balfour HH Jr, Kelly JM, Suarez CS, et al. Aciclovir treatment of varicella in otherwise healthy children. *J Pediatr* 1990;116:633–639.
22. Balfour HH Jr, Edelman CK, Anderson RS, et al. Controlled trial of acyclovir for chickenpox evaluating time of initiation and duration of therapy and viral resistance. *Pediatr Infect Dis J* 2001;20:919–926.
23. Nyerges G, Meszner Z, Gyarmati E, et al. Aciclovir prevents dissemination of varicella in immunocompromised children. *J Infect Dis* 1988;157:309–313.
24. Prober CG, Kirk LE, Keeney RE. Aciclovir therapy of chickenpox in immunosuppressed children: a collaborative study. *J Pediatr* 1982;101:622–625.

George Swingler
School of Child
and Adolescent Health
Red Cross Children's Hospital
and the University of Cape Town;
and the South African Cochrane
Centre
Cape Town
South Africa

Jimmy Volmink
Director of Research and Analysis
Global Health Council
Washington DC
USA

Competing interests: None declared.

Congenital toxoplasmosis

Search date March 2002

Piero Olliaro

QUESTIONS

INTERVENTIONS

Unknown effectiveness

Key Messages

- **Spiramycin and other antiparasitic drugs** Two systematic reviews of cohort studies in women who seroconvert during pregnancy found insufficient evidence on the effects of current antiparasitic treatment versus no treatment on mother or baby. We found that the quality of evidence was poor (studies included in the systematic reviews were small; groups were not directly comparable; only two studies provided information about the control group; congenital infection was common in the treatment groups; and treatment was associated with reduced transmission in only five out of nine of the included studies); therefore, we are uncertain whether antiparasitic drugs are more beneficial than harmful.

Clin Evid 2002;8:680–683.

DEFINITION Toxoplasmosis is caused by the parasite *Toxoplasma gondii*. Infection is asymptomatic or unremarkable in immunocompetent individuals, but leads to a lifelong antibody response. During pregnancy, toxoplasmosis can be transmitted across the placenta and cause intrauterine death, neonatal growth retardation, mental retardation, ocular defects, and blindness in later life. Congenital toxoplasmosis (confirmed infection of the fetus or newborn) can present at birth, either as subclinical disease, which may evolve with neurological or ophthalmological disease later in life, or as a disease of varying severity, ranging from mild ocular damage to severe mental retardation.

INCIDENCE/ PREVALENCE We found few prospective population surveys of toxoplasma seroprevalence. Reported rates vary across and within countries, as well as over time. The risk of primary infection is highest in young people, including young women during pregnancy. We found no cohort studies describing annual seroconversion rates in women of childbearing age nor incidence of primary infection. One systematic review (search date 1996) identified 15 studies that reported rates of seroconversion ranging from 2.4–16/1000 in Europe and from 2–6/1000 in the USA.[1] France began screening for congenital toxoplasmosis in 1978, and during the period 1980–1995 the seroconversion rate during pregnancy was 4–5/1000.[2]

AETIOLOGY/ RISK FACTORS Toxoplasma infection is usually acquired by ingesting either sporocysts (from unwashed fruit or vegetables contaminated by cat faeces) or tissue cysts (from raw or undercooked meat). The risk of contracting toxoplasma infection varies with eating habits, contact with cats and other pets, and occupational exposure. Infection can also be acquired congenitally.

PROGNOSIS One systematic review of studies conducted from 1983–1996 found no population based prospective studies of the natural history of toxoplasma infection during pregnancy.[1] One systematic review (search date 1997) reported nine controlled, non-randomised studies, and found that untreated toxoplasmosis acquired during pregnancy was associated with infection rates in children of between 10–100%.[3] We found two European studies that correlated gestation at time of seroconversion with risk of transmission and severity of disease at birth.[4,5] Risk of transmission increased with gestational age at maternal seroconversion, reaching 70–90% for infections acquired after 30 weeks' gestation. In contrast, the risk of the infected infant developing clinical disease was highest when infection occurred early in pregnancy. The highest risk of early signs of disease (including chorioretinitis and hydrocephaly) was about 10%, and occurred with infection between 24 and 30 weeks' gestation.[5] Infants with untreated congenital toxoplasmosis and generalised neurological abnormalities at birth develop mental retardation, growth retardation, blindness or visual defects, seizures, and spasticity. Children with untreated subclinical infection at birth may develop cognitive and motor deficits and visual defects or blindness up to the age of 20 years. One case control study (845 school children in Brazil) found mental retardation and retinochoroiditis to be significantly associated with positive toxoplasma serology (population attributable risk 6–9%).[6]

Congenital toxoplasmosis

AIMS To prevent fetal transmission, congenital infection, ocular defects, and mental retardation in neonates and in later life, with minimum adverse effects.

OUTCOMES Incidence of spontaneous abortion, fetal infection, and overt neonatal disease (mental retardation and ocular defects); serological positivity in the newborn; adverse effects of treatment.

METHODS *Clinical Evidence* update search and appraisal March 2002.

QUESTION **What are the effects on mother and baby of antiparasitic treatment in women found to be seropositive for toxoplasma during pregnancy?**

We found no reliable evidence on the effects of treating women who seroconvert during pregnancy.

Benefits: We found two systematic reviews (search dates 1997).[3,7] The first identified no RCTs.[3] The second review identified nine small cohort studies comparing treatments (spiramycin alone, pyrimethamine-sulphonamides, or a combination of the two treatments) versus no treatment.[7] One study of case series of women treated with spiramycin or spiramycin plus pyrimethamine-sulphonamide found no evidence of difference in outcomes (fetal infection, overt neonatal disease) associated with treatment.[8] Comparing data from these studies was difficult because of different follow up periods.

Harms: Spiramycin and pyrimethamine-sulphonamides are reportedly well tolerated and non-teratogenic.[9] Sulpha drugs are known to carry a risk of kernicterus in the newborn and should be avoided if possible in the third trimester; there is also a risk of bone marrow suppression, which can be reduced through concomitant use of folic acid.[9]

Comment: We found that the quality of evidence was poor, so we are uncertain whether antiparasitic drugs are more beneficial than harmful. Studies included in the systematic review were small, groups were not directly comparable, only two studies provided information about the control group, congenital infection was common in the treatment groups, and treatment was associated with reduced transmission in only five out of nine of the included studies.[7] One decision analysis on screening for and treating intrauterine toxoplasma infection has suggested a theoretical risk that treatment may save the pregnancy without preventing infection in the neonate, leading to a net increase in congenital cases.[10] Drug regimens of co-trimoxazole (trimethoprim plus sulfamethoxazole [sulphamethoxazole]), atovaquone, or fluoroquinolones, which are either used or are being tested for secondary prophylaxis of toxoplasmosis in immunocompromised people (particularly those with HIV infection), have not been studied in pregnancy because their reproductive toxicity has not been properly documented. Finally, optimal duration of follow up is not established, although the longer the children are observed the higher the incidence of sequelae.

REFERENCES

1. Eskild A, Oxman A, Magnus P, et al. Screening for toxoplasmosis in pregnancy: what is the evidence of reducing a health problem? *J Med Screen* 1996;3:188–194. Search date February 1996; primary sources Medline, Cochrane Pregnancy and Childbirth Database, and hand searched references.
2. Carme B, Tirard-Fleury V. Toxoplasmosis among pregnant women in France: seroprevalence, seroconversion and knowledge levels: trends 1965–1995. *Med Malad Infect* 1996;26:431–436.
3. Wallon M, Liou C, Garner P, et al. Congenital toxoplasmosis: systematic review of evidence of efficacy of treatment in pregnancy. *BMJ* 1999;318:1511–1514. Search date 1997; primary sources Medline, Embase, Pascal, Biological Abstracts, and personal communications.
4. Foulon W, Villena I, Stray-Pedersen B, et al. Treatment of toxoplasmosis during pregnancy: a multicenter study of impact on fetal transmission and children's sequelae at age 1 year. *Am J Obstet Gynecol* 1999;180:410–415.
5. Dunn D, Wallon M, Peyron F, et al. Mother-to-child transmission of toxoplasmosis: risk estimates for clinical counselling. *Lancet* 1999;353:1829–1833.
6. Caiaffa WT, Chiari CA, Figueiredo AR, et al. Toxoplasmosis and mental retardation: report of a case-control study. *Mem Inst Oswaldo Cruz* 1993;88:253–261.
7. Peyron F, Wallon M, Liou C, et al. Treatments for toxoplasmosis in pregnancy. In: The Cochrane Library, Issue 2, 2000. Oxford: Update Software. Search date 1997; primary sources Medline, Embase, Pascal, Biological Abstracts, and the Cochrane Controlled Trials Register.
8. Vergani P, Ghidini A, Ceruti P, et al. Congenital toxoplasmosis: efficacy of maternal treatment with spiramycin alone. *Am J Reprod Immunol* 1998;39:335–340.
9. Garland SM, O'Reilly MA. The risks and benefits of antimicrobial therapy in pregnancy. *Drug Saf* 1995;13:188–205.
10. Bader TJ, Macones GA, Asch DA. Prenatal screening for toxoplasmosis. *Obstet Gynecol* 1997;90:457–464.

Piero Olliaro
Scientist/Manager
UNDP/World Bank/WHO Special Programme for Research and Training in Tropical Diseases CDS/TDR/World Health Organization
Geneva
Switzerland

Competing interests: None declared.

Diarrhoea

Search date January 2002
Guy de Bruyn

QUESTIONS

INTERVENTIONS

To be covered in future updates
Absorbent agents
Antisecretory agents
Bismuth subsalicylate

See glossary, p 690

Key Messages

- **Amino acid oral rehydration solution (ORS) (*v* standard ORS)** Small RCTs have found that amino acid ORS versus standard ORS reduces the total volume and duration of diarrhoea.
- **Antimotility agents** RCTs have found that loperamide hydrochloride and loperamide oxide versus placebo significantly reduce the time to relief of symptoms, but frequently cause constipation. We found insufficient evidence about the effects of other antimotility agents.
- **Bicarbonate free ORS (*v* standard ORS)** One RCT found no significant difference in total stool output or duration of diarrhoea with standard ORS plus bicarbonate versus an otherwise identical ORS in which the bicarbonate was replaced with chloride. Three RCTs found no significant difference in the duration or volume of diarrhoea with standard ORS plus bicarbonate versus an otherwise identical ORS in which the bicarbonate was replaced with citrate.
- **Empirical antibiotic treatment in community acquired diarrhoea** RCTs have found that ciprofloxacin versus placebo reduces the duration of community acquired diarrhoea by 1 to 2 days. RCTs comparing empirical treatment with other antibiotics versus placebo found conflicting results. In one RCT, significantly more people taking lomefloxacin versus placebo had adverse effects (33% with lomefloxacin *v* 3% with placebo), and 2/44 (5%) of people taking lomefloxacin had anaphylaxis.

Clin Evid 2002;8:684–692.

- **Empirical antibiotic treatment in travellers' diarrhoea** One systematic review and one additional RCT have found that empirical use of antibiotics versus placebo significantly increases cure rate at 3–6 days. Adverse effects varied with each antibiotic and occurred in 2–18% of people.
- **Reduced osmolarity ORS (*v* standard ORS)** Three RCTs comparing reduced osmolarity ORS versus standard ORS found a small and inconsistent effect on total volume of stool and duration of diarrhoea.
- **Rice based ORS (*v* standard ORS)** One systematic review has found that rice based ORS versus standard ORS significantly reduces the 24 hour stool volume.

DEFINITION Diarrhoea is watery or liquid stools, usually with an increase in stool weight above 200 g daily and an increase in daily stool frequency.

INCIDENCE/ PREVALENCE An estimated 4000 million cases of diarrhoea occurred worldwide in 1996, resulting in 2.5 million deaths.[1] In the USA, the estimated incidence for infectious intestinal disease is 0.44 episodes per person a year, or one episode per person every 2.3 years, resulting in about one consultation with a doctor per person every 28 years.[2] A recent community study in the UK reported an incidence of 19 cases per 100 person years, of which 3.3 cases per 100 person years resulted in consultation with a general practitioner.[3] The epidemiology of travellers' diarrhoea (in people who have crossed a national boundary) is not well understood. Incidence is higher in travellers visiting developing countries, but it varies widely by location and season of travel.[4]

AETIOLOGY/ RISK FACTORS The cause of diarrhoea depends on geographic location, standards of food hygiene, sanitation, water supply, and season. Commonly identified causes of sporadic diarrhoea in adults in developed countries include *Campylobacter*, *Salmonella*, *Shigella*, *Escherichia coli*, *Yersinia*, protozoa, and viruses. No pathogens are identified in more than half of people with diarrhoea. In returning travellers, about 80% of episodes are caused by bacteria such as enterotoxigenic *E coli*, *Salmonella*, *Shigella*, *Campylobacter*, *Vibrio*, enteroadherent *E coli*, *Yersinia*, and *Aeromonas*.[5]

PROGNOSIS In developing countries, diarrhoea is reported to cause more deaths in children under 5 years of age than any other condition.[1] Few studies have examined which factors predict poor outcome in adults. In developed countries, death from infectious diarrhoea is rare, although serious complications, including severe dehydration and renal failure, can occur and may necessitate admission to hospital. Elderly people and those in long term care have an increased risk of death.[6]

AIMS To reduce the infectious period, length of illness, risk of dehydration, risk of transmission to others, and rates of severe illness; and to prevent complications and death.

OUTCOMES Time from start of treatment to last loose stool; number of loose stools a day; stool volume; time to first formed stool; duration of diarrhoea; duration of excretion of organisms; presence of bacterial resistance; relief of cramps, nausea and vomiting; incidence of vomiting; incidence of severe illness; and rate of hospital admission.

METHODS *Clinical Evidence* update search and appraisal January 2002.

QUESTION What are the effects of empirical antibiotic treatment in travellers' diarrhoea?

One systematic review and one additional RCT have found that empirical use of antibiotics versus placebo significantly increases the cure rate of travellers' diarrhoea. Antibiotic treatment is associated in some people with prolonged presence of bacterial pathogens in the stool and development of resistant strains.

Benefits: We found one systematic review[7] and one additional RCT.[8] The systematic review (search date 1999, 12 RCTs, 1474 people with travellers' diarrhoea, including students, package tourists, military personnel, and volunteers) compared empirical use of antibiotics versus placebo.[7] Antibiotics evaluated included aztreonam, bicozamycin, ciprofloxacin, co-trimoxazole (trimethoprim–sulfamethoxazole [sulphamethoxazole]; TMP–SMX), fleroxacin, norfloxacin, ofloxacin, and trimethoprim, which were given for durations varying from a single dose to 5 days. The review found that antibiotics significantly increased the cure rate at 72 hours (defined as cessation of unformed stools or > 1 unformed stool/24 h without additional symptoms; OR 5.9, 95% CI 4.1 to 8.6). The additional RCT (598 people, 70% of whom had travelled recently) compared norfloxacin versus placebo. It found that norfloxacin significantly increased the number of people cured after 6 days (34/46 [74%] with norfloxacin *v* 18/48 [38%] with placebo; RR 1.97, 95% CI 1.32 to 2.95).[8]

Harms: The systematic review found that adverse effects varied with each antibiotic, and ranged in frequency from 2–18%.[7] Gastrointestinal symptoms (cramps, nausea, and anorexia), dermatological symptoms (rash), and respiratory symptoms (cough and sore throat) were most frequently reported. One small RCT included in the review found that significantly more people taking ciprofloxacin developed resistant isolates at 48 hours (ciprofloxacin *v* placebo; ARI 50%, 95% CI 15% to 85%).[7] Another RCT (181 adults with acute diarrhoea) reported three cases of continued excretion of *Shigella* in people taking co-trimoxazole versus one person taking placebo.[9] Two of these isolates became resistant to the drug, although the participants were clinically well.[7] Other RCTs found no post-treatment resistance, or did not report it.[7] The additional RCT found that people with salmonella infection treated with norfloxacin versus placebo had significantly prolonged excretion of *Salmonella* species (median time to clearance of *Salmonella* species from stools: 50 days with norfloxacin *v* 23 days with placebo; CI not provided).[8] In addition, 6/9 *Campylobacter* isolates obtained after treatment had developed resistance to norfloxacin.

Comment: Only 3/10 trials using the duration of diarrhoea as an outcome reported adequate statistical data for the duration of diarrhoea after initiation of treatment.[8] This limits the applicability of the results.

QUESTION What are the effects of empirical antibiotic treatment in community acquired diarrhoea?

RCTs have found that ciprofloxacin reduces the duration of community acquired diarrhoea by 1 to 2 days. RCTs comparing empirical treatment with other antibiotics versus placebo either found no effect or did not report time to cure.

Benefits: We found no systematic review. We found 10 RCTs in nine reports (1848 people)[10–18] comparing one or more antibiotics with placebo (see table 1, p 692). RCTs were conducted in 13 sites in 12 countries. Five RCTs were conducted in developed countries, and the remainder in developing countries. The largest study included 332 adults (in hospital for the treatment of their diarrhoeal illness) in a multicentre trial of fleroxacin.[10] Eight RCTs evaluated quinolones, four evaluated co-trimoxazole, one evaluated clioquinol, and one evaluated nifuroxazide.[10–18] Entry criteria varied among RCTs, and treatment duration ranged from a single dose to 5 days. Six RCTs found that antibiotics reduced illness duration or decreased number of liquid stools at 48 hours,[12,13,15–18] whereas three RCTs found no reduction in illness duration.[10,11,14] One RCT found reduced duration of diarrhoea for ciprofloxacin but not for co-trimoxazole.[13]

Harms: Adverse effects varied by agent. In one RCT (88 people) comparing lomefloxacin versus placebo, 33% of lomefloxacin treated people reported adverse effects compared with 3% taking placebo (ARI 31%, 95% CI 17% to 46%).[11] Two people taking lomefloxacin were withdrawn from the trial after developing anaphylactic reactions. In the same RCT, 18% of treated people developed isolates resistant to lomefloxacin. In the multicentre RCT (173 people with acute diarrhoea) of ciprofloxacin and co-trimoxazole, five people with *Campylobacter* isolated from stools (2 treated with ciprofloxacin, 3 treated with co-trimoxazole) developed isolates resistant to the treatment antibiotic.[15] In the largest RCT (508 adults), three deaths occurred (2 with fleroxacin *v* 1 with placebo).[16] Two of the deaths occurred from hypovolaemic shock (1 with fleroxacin *v* 1 with placebo).

Comment: The main pathogenic organisms found in each study varied and may partly explain variations in effect. Reported outcomes varied between trials, which precludes direct comparisons or summaries of treatment effect.

QUESTION What are the effects of oral rehydration for severe diarrhoea?

We found no direct studies of oral rehydration compared with placebo or no treatment. Numerous RCTs compared one type of rehydration with another. One small RCT comparing intravenous rehydration versus rehydration through a nasogastric tube found no difference in duration or volume of diarrhoea. Two RCTs comparing amino acid oral rehydration solution (ORS) versus standard ORS have found that amino acid ORS reduces the total volume and duration of diarrhoea. One small RCT found no significant effect of replacing ORS bicarbonate with chloride, and

three RCTs found no effect of replacing ORS bicarbonate with citrate. Three RCTs found a small and inconsistent effect on total volume of stool and duration of diarrhoea with reduced osmolarity ORS versus standard ORS. One systematic review has found that rice based ORS compared with standard ORS reduces the 24 hour stool volume.

Benefits: Effects of oral rehydration solutions in severe diarrhoea (see web extra table A at www.clinicalevidence.com).[19–29] **Versus no rehydration:** We found no systematic review or RCTs. **Versus intravenous rehydration:** We found no systematic review. We found one small RCT (20 adults with cholera and severe dehydration) comparing enteral rehydration through a nasogastric tube versus intravenous rehydration.[19] Both groups received initial intravenous fluids for up to 90 minutes. The RCT found no significant difference in the total duration of diarrhoea (44 h with iv fluids *v* 37 h with nasogastric fluids; difference +7 h, 95% CI –6 to +20 h), total volume of stool passed (8.2 L *v* 11 L; difference –2.8 L, 95% CI –8 L to +3 L), or duration of *Vibrio* excretion (1.1 days *v* 1.4 days; difference 0.3 days, 95% CI 0 days to 1 day). **Amino acid ORS:** We found no systematic review. We found three RCTs (48 adults,[20] 97 men,[21] 108 men[22]) comparing amino acid ORS versus the standard ORS (see glossary, p 690). In the two RCTs where intravenous rehydration was given, amino acid ORS versus standard ORS reduced the total duration of diarrhoea and the total volume of stool.[20,21] **Bicarbonate free ORS:** We found no systematic review. We found one small RCT (60 people with cholera and severe dehydration) comparing standard ORS plus bicarbonate versus an otherwise identical ORS in which the bicarbonate was replaced with chloride.[23] The RCT found no significant difference in total stool output or duration of diarrhoea. **Citrate ORS:** We found no systematic review. We found three RCTs (367 people) comparing citrate versus standard/bicarbonate ORS.[24–26] None of the RCTs found a significant difference between treatments in the duration or volume of diarrhoea. **Reduced osmolarity ORS:** We found no systematic review. We found three RCTs, which found a small and inconsistent effect on total volume of stool and duration of diarrhoea.[27–29] **Rice based ORS:** We found one systematic review (search date 1998, 22 RCTs) in people with cholera and non-cholera diarrhoea.[30] The review found that in adults and children with cholera, rice based ORS versus standard ORS significantly reduced the 24 hour stool volume (adults: 4 RCTs, WMD –51 mL/kg, 95% CI –66 mL/kg to –35 mL/kg; children: 5 RCTs, WMD –67 mL/kg, 95% CI –94 mL/kg to –41 mL/kg). One RCT found that both rice based ORS and low sodium rice based ORS reduced stool output compared with standard ORS (4 L for rice based ORS *v* 5 L for standard ORS, $P < 0.02$; 3 L for low sodium rice based ORS *v* 5 L for standard ORS, $P < 0.05$).[29]

Harms: **Versus amino acid ORS:** One RCT (108 men) reported no episodes of hypernatraemia or hyponatraemia in people taking a modified ORS or standard ORS.[22] **Citrate versus bicarbonate ORS:** One RCT (130 people with cholera) reported that more people taking citrate ORS had an unpleasant taste than those taking bicarbonate ORS (29% of people *v* 13% of people).[25] In another RCT, 2/115 people taking an effervescent citrate ORS had an unpleasant taste (results not reported for bicarbonate ORS).[26] **Versus reduced osmolarity ORS:** Reduced osmolarity ORS significantly increased the risk of non-symptomatic hyponatraemia (OR 2.1, 95% CI 1.1 to 4.1).[27] In RCTs evaluating symptomatic hyponatraemia, no cases were reported.[27,28]

Comment: All people with cholera received antibiotic treatment in addition to fluid treatment. Oral tetracycline or doxycycline were widely used, and were initiated at varying intervals after the start of oral fluid treatment. Response to ORS in people with cholera may not be comparable to those with less severe forms of diarrhoea. No studies were found comparing oral rehydration with no rehydration, as these would be unethical.

QUESTION What are the effects of antimotility agents for acute diarrhoea in adults?

RCTs have found that, in people with acute diarrhoea, loperamide hyrochloride, and loperamide oxide significantly reduce the time to relief of symptoms, but may cause constipation. We found insufficient evidence about the effects of other antimotility agents.

Benefits: We found no systematic review. **Difenoxin:** We found no RCTs of sufficient quality. **Diphenoxylate:** One RCT (152 adults with acute diarrhoea for < 24 h) comparing diphenoxylate–atropine versus placebo found that diphenoxylate significantly reduced the number of bowel actions in the 24 hours after treatment ($P = 0.05$).[31] The RCT found no significant difference in median time to last loose stool (25 h *v* 30 h; $P = 0.29$). **Lidamidine:** We found two RCTs comparing lidamidine (loading dose of 2–4 mg, then subsequent doses 6/h or as required) versus placebo. The first RCT (30 adults with acute diarrhoea) found that lidamidine reduced the stool weight after 29 hours (435 g with lidamidine 4 mg *v* 364 g with lidamidine 2 mg *v* 576 g with placebo).[32] The second RCT (105 adults with acute diarrhoea) found that lidamidine reduced the number of loose stools after 72 hours (8.5 stools *v* 3.9 stools; P values not provided).[33] **Loperamide hydrochloride:** We found four RCTs comparing loperamide hydrochloride (loading dose of 4 mg, then 2 mg with each loose stool) versus placebo.[33–36] Two of the RCTs (409 people[34] and 261 people[35] with acute diarrhoea) found that loperamide significantly reduced the median time to complete relief of symptoms, which was defined as the time between taking the loading dose of loperamide and the time after which one pasty, watery, or loose stool was passed (189 people: 27 h with loperamide *v* 45 h with placebo, $P = 0.006$;[34] 123 people: 18 h with loperamide *v* 37 h with placebo, $P = 0.007$).[35] The third RCT (50 people) found that loperamide versus placebo significantly reduced the number of stools for the first 2 days, but subsequently the difference was not significant.[36] The fourth RCT (105 adults with acute diarrhoea) found no significant difference in the number of stools passed within 72 hours.[33] **Loperamide oxide:** We found five RCTs (409 people,[34] 261 people,[35] 230 people,[37] 242 people,[38] 258 people[39] with acute diarrhoea) comparing loperamide oxide (loading dose 1–8 mg, followed by 0.5–4 mg with each loose stool) versus placebo. All RCTs found that loperamide oxide significantly reduced the time to complete relief of symptoms.

Harms: **Lidamidine:** Constipation occurred in more people taking lidamidine versus placebo (1/35 [3%] *v* 0/35 [0%]).[33]. **Loperamide hydrochloride:** Two RCTs (409 people[34] and 261 people[35]) found that constipation was significantly more frequent in people taking loperamide versus placebo (25% *v* 7%; ARI 18%, 95% CI 8% to 28%; NNH 5, 95% CI 3 to 12;[34] 22% *v* 10%; ARI 12%, 95% CI 5% to 29%; NNH 5, 95% CI 3 to 18[35]). **Loperamide oxide:** One RCT (409 people) found that significantly more people taking loperamide oxide had constipation (24% with loperamide oxide *v* 7% with placebo; ARI 17%, 95% CI 7% to 27%; NNH 5, 95% CI 3 to 14).[34] Another RCT (230 people) found that symptom scores for tiredness and sleepiness were significantly higher in people taking loperamide oxide 1 mg versus placebo (P = 0.01).[37]

Comment: The RCTs used different outcome measures, making it difficult to summarise and compare results.

GLOSSARY

Standard ORS An oral rehydration solution that includes citrate 10 mmol/L and glucose 111 mmol/L, and has an osmolarity of 311 mmol/L.

Substantive changes

Antibiotics for community acquired diarrhoea New RCT;[18] conclusion unchanged.
Antimotility agents for acute diarrhoea New RCT;[39] conclusion unchanged.

REFERENCES

1. *The World Health Report 1997*. Geneva: World Health Organization, 1997:14–22.
2. Garthwright WE, Archer DL, Kvenberg JE. Estimates of incidence and costs of intestinal infectious diseases in the United States. *Public Health Rep* 1988;103:107–115.
3. Wheeler JG, Sethi D, Cowden JM, et al. Study of infectious intestinal disease in England: rates in the community, presenting to general practice, and reported to national surveillance. *BMJ* 1999;318:1046–1050.
4. Cartwright RY, Chahed M. Foodborne diseases in travellers. *World Health Stat Q* 1997;50:102–110.
5. DuPont HL, Ericsson C. Prevention and treatment of traveller's diarrhoea. *N Engl J Med* 1993;328:1821–1927.
6. Lew JF, Glass RI, Gangarosa RE, et al. Diarrheal deaths in the United States 1979 through 1987. *JAMA* 1991;265:3280–3284.
7. De Bruyn G, Hahn S, Borwick A. Antibiotic treatment for travellers' diarrhoea (Cochrane Review). In: The Cochrane Library, Issue 4, 2001. Oxford: Update Software. Search date 1999; primary sources The Cochrane Collaboration Trials Register (Issue 3, 1998), Medline, Embase, and hand searching and contact with experts.
8. Wistrom J, Jertborn M, Ekwall E, et al. Empiric treatment of acute diarrheal disease with norfloxacin: a randomized, placebo-controlled study. Swedish Study Group. *Ann Intern Med* 1992;117:202–208.
9. Ericsson CD, Johnson PC, DuPont HL, et al. Ciprofloxacin or trimethoprim–sulfamethoxazole as initial therapy for travelers' diarrhea. *Ann Intern Med* 1987;106:216–220.
10. De la Cabada FJ, DuPont HL, Gyr K, et al. Antimicrobial therapy of bacterial diarrhea in adult residents of Mexico – lack of an effect. *Digestion* 1992;53:134–141.
11. Ellis-Pegler RB, Hyman LK, Ingram RJ, et al. A placebo controlled evaluation of lomefloxacin in the treatment of bacterial diarrhoea in the community. *J Antimicrob Chemother* 1995;36:259–263.
12. Pichler HE, Diridl G, Stickler K, et al. Clinical efficacy of ciprofloxacin compared with placebo in bacterial diarrhea. *Am J Med* 1987;82(suppl 4A):329–332.
13. Goodman LJ, Trenholme GM, Kaplan RL, et al. Empiric antimicrobial therapy of domestically acquired acute diarrhea in urban adults. *Arch Intern Med* 1990;150:541–546.
14. Noguerado A, Garcia-Polo I, Isasia T, et al. Early single dose therapy with ofloxacin for empirical treatment of acute gastroenteritis: a randomised, placebo-controlled double-blind clinical trial. *J Antimicrob Chemother* 1995;36:665–672.
15. Dryden MS, Gabb RJ, Wright SK. Empirical treatment of severe acute community-acquired gastroenteritis with ciprofloxacin. *Clin Infect Dis* 1996;22:1019–1025.
16. Butler T, Lolekha S, Rasidi C, et al. Treatment of acute bacterial diarrhea: a multicenter

international trial comparing placebo with fleroxacin given as a single dose or once daily for 3 days. *Am J Med* 1993;94(3A):187S–194S.
17. Lolekha S, Patanachareon S, Thanangkul B, et al. Norfloxacin versus co-trimoxazole in the treatment of acute bacterial diarrhoea: a placebo controlled study. *Scand J Infect Dis* 1988;56(suppl):35–45.
18. Bouree P, Chaput JC, Krainik F, et al. Double-blind controlled study of the efficacy of nifuroxazide versus placebo in the treatment of acute diarrhea in adults. *Gastroenterol Clin Biol* 1989;13:469–472.
19. Pierce NF, Sack RB, Mitra RC, et al. Replacement of water and electrolyte losses in cholera by an oral glucose-electrolyte solution. *Ann Intern Med* 1969;70:1173–1181.
20. Nalin DR, Cash RA, Rahman M, et al. Effect of glycine and glucose on sodium and water absorption in patients with cholera. *Gut* 1970;11:768–772.
21. Patra FC, Sack DA, Islam A, et al. Oral rehydration formula containing alanine and glucose for treatment of diarrhoea: a controlled trial. *BMJ* 1989;298:1353–1356.
22. Khin-Maung-U, Myo-Khin, Nyunt-Nyunt-Wai, et al. Comparison of glucose/electrolyte and maltodextrin/glycine/glycyl-glycine/electrolyte oral rehydration solutions in cholera and watery diarrhoea in adults. *Ann Trop Med Parasitol* 1991;85:645–650.
23. Sarker SA, Mahalanabis D. The presence of bicarbonate in oral rehydration solution does not influence fluid absorption in cholera. *Scand J Gastroenterol* 1995;30:242–245.
24. Mazumder RN, Nath SK, Ashraf H, et al. Oral rehydration solution containing trisodium citrate for treating severe diarrhoea: controlled clinical trial. *BMJ* 1991;302:88–89.
25. Hoffman SL, Moechtar MA, Simanjuntak CH, et al. Rehydration and maintenance therapy of cholera patients in Jakarta: citrate-based versus bicarbonate-based oral rehydration salt solution. *J Infect Dis* 1985;152:1159–1165.
26. Ahmed SM, Islam MR, Butler T. Effective treatment of diarrhoeal dehydration with an oral rehydration solution containing citrate. *Scand J Infect Dis* 1986;18:65–70.
27. Alam NH, Majumder RN, Fuchs GJ. Efficacy and safety of oral rehydration solution with reduced osmolarity in adults with cholera: a randomised double-blind clinical trial. *Lancet* 1999;354:296–299.
28. Faruque ASG, Mahalanabis D, Hamadani JD, et al. Reduced osmolarity oral rehydration salt in cholera. *Scand J Infect Dis* 1996;28:87–90.
29. Bhattacharya MK, Bhattacharya SK, Dutta D, et al. Efficacy of oral hyposmolar glucose-based and rice-based oral rehydration salt solutions in the treatment of cholera in adults. *Scand J Gastroenterol* 1998;33:159–163.
30. Fontaine O, Gore SM, Pierce NF. Rice-based oral rehydration solution for treating diarrhoea. In: The Cochrane Library, Issue 3, 2000. Oxford: Update Software. Search date 1998; primary sources Medline, Embase, Lilacs, Cochrane Controlled Trials Register, and Cochrane Infectious Diseases Group.
31. Lustman F, Walters EG, Shroff NE, et al. Diphenoxylate hydrochloride (Lomotil®) in the treatment of acute diarrhoea. *Br J Clin Pract* 1987;41:648–651.
32. Heredia Diaz JG, Alcantara I, Solis A. Evaluation of the safety and effectiveness of WHR-1142A in the treatment of non-specific acute diarrhea. *Rev Gastroenterol Mex* 1979;44:167–73 [in Spanish].
33. Heredia Diaz JG, Kajeyama Escobar ML. Double-blind evaluation of the effectiveness of lidamidine hydrochloride (WHR-1142A) vs. loperamide vs. placebo in the treatment of acute diarrhea. *Salud Publica Mex* 1981;23:483–491 [in Spanish].
34. Hughes IW. First line treatment in acute non-dysenteric diarrhoea: clinical comparison of loperamide oxide, loperamide and placebo. *Br J Clin Pract* 1995;49:181–185.
35. Van den Eynden B, Spaepen W. New approaches to the treatment of patients with acute, nonspecific diarrhea: a comparison of the effects of loperamide and loperamide oxide. *Curr Ther Res* 1995;56:1132–1141.
36. Van Loon FPL, Bennish ML, Speelman P, et al Double blind trial of loperamide for treating acute watery diarrhoea in expatriates in Bangladesh. *Gut* 1989;30:492–495.
37. Dettmer A. Loperamide oxide in the treatment of acute diarrhea in adults. *Clin Ther* 1994;16:972–980.
38. Dreverman JWM, Van der Poel AJM. Loperamide oxide in acute diarrhoea: a double-blind, placebo-controlled trial. *Aliment Pharmacol Ther* 1995;9:441–446.
39. Cardon E, Van Elsen J, Frascio M, et al. Gut-selective opiates: the effect of loperamide oxide in acute diarrhoea in adults. The Diarrhoea Trialists Group. *Eur J Clin Res* 1995;7:135–144.

Guy de Bruyn
Fellow in Program in Infectious Diseases
University of Washington and Fred
Hutchinson Cancer Research Centre
Seattle, Washington
USA

Competing interests: None declared.

TABLE 1 **Effects of empirical antibiotic treatment of community acquired diarrhoea: results of placebo controlled RCTs** **(see text, p 687).**

Intervention	Total number of participants	Mean duration of diarrhoea from start of treatment*		Difference between means (95% CI)†
		Placebo group	Intervention group	
Lomefloxacin 400 mg daily for 5 days[11]	84	3.2 days	4.4 days	+1.2 days (0.1 day to 2.5 days)
Ofloxacin 400 mg single dose[14]	117	3.4 days	2.5 days	–0.9 days (–1.8 days to 0.0 days)
Co-trimoxazole 800/160 mg bd for 3 days[10]	287	30.2 h	24.4 h	–5.8 h
Cloquinol 250 mg tds for 3 days[10]	287	30.2 h	25.5 h	–4.7 h
Enoxacin 400 mg bd for 5 days[10]	137	44.9 h	38.9 h	–6.0 h
Co-trimoxazole 160/800 mg bd for 5 days[10]	137	44.9 h	42.3 h	–2.6 h
Ciprofloxacin 500 mg bd for 5 days[12]	162	2.9 days	1.5 days	–1.4 days
Ciprofloxacin 500 mg bd for 5 days[13]	173	3.4 days	2.4 days	–1.0 day
Co-trimoxazole 160/800 mg bd for 5 days[13]	173	3.4 days	NA	NA
Ciprofloxacin 500 mg bd for 5 days[15]	85	4.6 days	2.2 days	–2.4 days
Nifuroxazide 400 mg bd for 5 days[18]	88	3.3 days	2.1 days	–1.2 days

†If available from published data. *Two other RCTs[16,17] did not report mean duration of diarrhoea.
bd, twice daily; h, hours; NA, not available from published data; tds, three times daily.

HIV infection

Search date March 2002

Margaret Johnson, Andrew Phillips, David Wilkinson, and Bazian Ltd (temporary contributors)

QUESTIONS

INTERVENTIONS

Key Messages

Prevention

- **Early diagnosis and treatment of sexually transmitted diseases (STDs)** One RCT has found that early diagnosis and treatment of STDs significantly reduces the risk of acquiring HIV infection over 2 years.
- **Postexposure prophylaxis in healthcare workers** One case control study found limited evidence suggesting that postexposure prophylaxis with zidovudine may reduce the risk of HIV infection over 6 months. Evidence from other settings suggests that combining several antiretroviral drugs is likely to be more effective than zidovudine alone.
- **Presumptive mass treatment of STDs** One RCT found no significant difference with presumptive, mass treatment for STDs versus no treatment in the incidence of HIV over 20 months.

Clin Evid 2002;8:693–701.

HIV infection

Treatment

- **Early versus delayed antiretroviral treatment** We found no RCTs evaluating delayed versus early treatment with two or three drug regimens. RCTs conducted when zidovudine was the only drug available found no significant difference between immediate versus delayed treatment in survival at 1 year.
- **Three drug antiretroviral regimens** Two RCTs have found that using a protease inhibitor plus two nucleoside analogue drugs versus two nucleoside analogue drugs alone halves the risk of new AIDS diseases or death over about 1 year. Both RCTs found that the risk of serious adverse effects was similar with three versus two drug regimens. Triple therapy is likely to reduce the risk of drug resistance compared with double therapy.
- **Two drug antiretroviral regimens/single drug antiretroviral regimens** Large RCTs, with follow up of 1–3 years, have found that two drug regimens (zidovudine plus another nucleoside analogue or protease inhibitor drug) versus zidovudine alone significantly reduce the risk of new AIDS defining illnesses and death. Adverse events were common in all treatment groups.

DEFINITION HIV infection refers to infection with the human immunodeficiency virus type 1 or type 2. Clinically, this is characterised by a variable period (average around 8–10 years) of asymptomatic infection, followed by repeated episodes of illness of varying and increasing severity as immune function deteriorates. The type of illness varies greatly by country, availability of specific treatments for HIV, and prophylaxis for opportunistic infections.

INCIDENCE/ PREVALENCE Worldwide estimates suggest that, by December 1999, about 50 million people had been infected with HIV, about 16 million people had died as a result, and about 16 000 new HIV infections were occurring each day.[1] About 90% of HIV infections occur in the developing world.[1] Occupationally acquired HIV infection in healthcare workers has been documented in 95 definite and 191 possible cases, although this is likely to be an underestimate.[2]

AETIOLOGY/ RISK FACTORS The major risk factor for transmission of HIV is unprotected heterosexual or homosexual intercourse. Other risk factors include needlestick injury, sharing drug injecting equipment, and blood transfusion. An HIV infected woman may also transmit the virus to her baby. This has been reported in 15–30% of pregnant women with HIV infection. Not everyone who is exposed to HIV will become infected, although risk increases if exposure is repeated, at high dose, or through blood. There is at least a 2–5 times greater risk of HIV infection among people with sexually transmitted diseases.[3]

PROGNOSIS Without treatment, about half of people infected with HIV will become ill and die from AIDS over about 10 years.

AIMS To reduce transmission of HIV; to prevent or delay the onset of AIDS, as manifested by opportunistic infections and cancers; to increase survival; to minimise loss of quality of life caused by inconvenience and adverse effects of current regimens.

OUTCOMES Incidence of HIV infection, new AIDS diseases, and adverse events; mortality; quality of life.

METHODS *Clinical Evidence* update search and appraisal March 2002. In addition, we contacted experts in the field, and reviewed abstract books and CDs for conferences held since 1995. Trials were included if they were designed to detect differences in clinical end points. We have included evidence on single and two drug antiretroviral regimens, because it may be useful in countries where three drug treatment is not currently widely available.

QUESTION **What are the effects of preventive interventions?**

OPTION **EARLY DETECTION AND TREATMENT OF SEXUALLY TRANSMITTED DISEASES**

One RCT has found that early diagnosis and treatment of sexually transmitted diseases significantly reduces the incidence of HIV infection.

Benefits: We found no systematic review. One RCT randomised 12 communities in Tanzania (about 12 000 people) to intervention or no intervention.[4] Intervention consisted of diagnosis and treatment of sexually transmitted diseases (STDs) at a local health centre (within 90 min walking distance), provision of free condoms during the current STD episode, and health education by healthcare workers trained in STD case management. The RCT found that intervention reduced the risk of acquiring HIV over 2 years (RR 0.58, 95% CI 0.42 to 0.79).

Harms: Syndromic case management (treating people for the most likely causes of their symptoms and signs) may result in wrong or unnecessary treatment. The RCT gave no information on this.[4]

Comment: There is a clear biological mechanism for the synergistic effect of STDs on HIV transmission, and for STD control as an HIV control strategy. The inflammation associated with STDs increases HIV shedding in genital secretions, and treating STDs reduces this inflammation.[5] Syndromic management of STDs is more commonly used in developing countries. In developed countries a microbiological diagnosis is usually made, allowing specific treatment. The trial, randomised by the community and analysed by the individual, uses regression analysis in an attempt to overcome the associated cluster bias, but it is unclear whether this is successful.

OPTION **PRESUMPTIVE SEXUALLY TRANSMITTED DISEASE TREATMENT**

One RCT found no evidence of benefit from presumptive, mass treatment for sexually transmitted diseases.

Benefits: We found no systematic review. One RCT randomised 10 communities in Uganda (about 12 000 people) to intervention or no intervention.[6] Intervention consisted of treating all adults with several drugs for sexually transmitted diseases (STDs) every 10 months. Although prevalence of some STDs fell in intervention communities, there was no significant difference in the incidence of HIV between intervention and control communities over 20 months of follow up (incidence of HIV in both groups about 1.5/100 person years; RR intervention *v* control 0.97, 95% CI 0.81 to 1.16).

Harms: Mass treatment means that many uninfected people will be unnecessarily treated for STDs, exposing them to risks of adverse drug reactions and drug resistance. The RCT gave no information on this.[6]

Comment: The trial's negative finding has several possible explanations other than ineffectiveness of the intervention: a high incidence of symptomatic STDs between rounds of mass treatment; a low population attributable risk for treatable STDs; and intense exposure to HIV. The trial, randomised by the community and analysed by the individual, uses regression analysis in an attempt to overcome the associated cluster bias, but it is unclear whether this is successful. As many as 80% of STDs are unrecognised or asymptomatic.[7]

QUESTION What are the effects of postexposure prophylaxis in healthcare workers?

One case control study found that, in people exposed to HIV, those who became infected were less likely to have received postexposure prophylaxis with zidovudine. Evidence from other settings suggests that combined treatment with several antiretroviral drugs is likely to be more effective than treatment with zidovudine alone.

Benefits: We found no systematic review or RCTs. **Zidovudine alone:** One case control study from the USA and France evaluated outcomes in 31 health workers who acquired HIV infection after occupational exposure, and outcomes in 679 controls who did not acquire HIV infection despite occupational exposure.[8] This study included people followed up for at least 6 months after exposure. HIV infection was less likely in people who received postexposure prophylaxis compared with those who did not (reduction in OR by 81%, 95% CI 43% to 94%). It found that the risk of seroconversion increased with severity of exposure; for example, a penetrating injury with a hollow, bloody needle carried the greatest risk. **Zidovudine plus other antiretroviral drugs:** We found no studies of postexposure prophylaxis using combinations of antiretroviral drugs.

Harms: Short term toxicity (including fatigue, nausea, and vomiting) and gastrointestinal discomfort have been reported by 50–75% of people taking zidovudine and caused 30% to discontinue postexposure prophylaxis.[9] Treatment studies suggest that the frequency of adverse effects is higher in people taking a combination of antiretroviral drugs (reported in 50–90%), which may reduce adherence to postexposure prophylaxis (24–36% discontinued). The risk of drug interactions is also increased. Severe adverse effects, including hepatitis and pancytopenia, have been reported in people taking combination postexposure prophylaxis, but the incidence is not known.

Comment: Case control studies are considered sufficient because experimental studies are hard to justify ethically, and are logistically difficult because of the low rate of seroconversion in those exposed. A summary of 25 studies (22 seroconversions in 6955 exposed people) found that the risk of HIV transmission after percutaneous exposure was 0.32% (95% CI 0.18% to 0.45%) and that the risk after mucocutaneous exposure was 0.03% (95% CI 0.006% to 0.19%).[2] Indirect evidence for postexposure prophylaxis comes from animal studies[8] and from a placebo controlled RCT of zidovudine in pregnant women,[10] which found reduced frequency of mother to child HIV transmission, presumed to be caused in part by postexposure prophylaxis. RCTs have found that combinations of two, three, or more antiretroviral drugs are more effective than single drug regimens in suppressing viral replication. There is also an unquantified risk that zidovudine alone may not prevent transmission of zidovudine resistant strains of HIV. This constitutes the rationale for combining antiretroviral drugs for postexposure prophylaxis.

QUESTION **What are the effects of different antiretroviral treatment regimens?**

OPTION **TWO DRUG VERSUS ONE DRUG ANTIRETROVIRAL REGIMENS**

Large RCTs, with follow up of 1–3 years, have found that two drug regimens (zidovudine plus another nucleoside analogue or protease inhibitor drug) versus zidovudine alone reduce the risk of new AIDS defining illnesses and death. Adverse events were common in all treatment groups.

Benefits: We found one systematic review (search date not stated, 6 RCTs, 7700 people),[11] two additional RCTs,[12,13] and one subsequent RCT[14] comparing two drug versus one drug regimens. The review compared zidovudine/didanosine or zidovudine/zalcitabine versus zidovudine alone.[11] Participants entered the trials with various stages of infection and were followed for an average of 29 months, during which time 2904 people developed progressive disease and 1850 died. The combined versus single drug regimens significantly delayed disease progression (RR with addition of didanosine 0.74, 95% CI 0.67 to 0.82; RR with addition of zalcitabine 0.86, 95% CI 0.78 to 0.94) and death (RR with addition of didanosine 0.72, 95% CI 0.64 to 0.82; RR with addition of zalcitabine 0.87, 95% CI 0.77 to 0.98). After 3 years, the estimated percentages of people who were alive and without a new AIDS event were 53% for zidovudine plus didanosine versus 49% for zidovudine plus zalcitabine versus 44% for zidovudine alone; the percentages alive were 68% versus 63% versus 59%. The first additional RCT (940 people) comparing zalcitabine plus saquinavir (a protease inhibitor) versus either drug as monotherapy found that combination treatment significantly reduced clinical disease (RR 0.51, 95% CI 0.36 to 0.72) or death (RR 0.32, 95% CI 0.16 to 0.64) at 1 year.[12] The second additional RCT (1895 people with CD4 positive T cell counts 25–250/mm^3) found that adding lamivudine (a nucleoside analogue) to regimens containing zidovudine (zidovudine alone in 62%, zidovudine plus didanosine or zalcitabine in the rest) significantly reduced the risk of AIDS or death over about 1 year (HR 0.42, 95% CI 0.32 to 0.57).[13] The subsequent RCT (996 people who had never received antiretroviral treatment) compared zidovudine plus indinavir (a protease inhibitor) versus either zidovudine or indinavir alone.[14] It found that combination treatment versus zidovudine alone significantly reduced the rate of progression to AIDS after a median follow up of 1 year (combination *v* zidovudine; RR 0.30, 95% CI 0.18 to 0.50). It found no significant difference between combination treatment versus indinavir alone (RR 0.77, 95% CI 0.72 to 2.32). We found one additional RCT, which was stopped prematurely because of low study size and power (see comment below).[15]

Harms: Adverse effects such as anaemia and neutropenia were common in all groups in all of the RCTs cited above. Up to a third of participants experienced a serious adverse event, with the highest rates in those with lower CD4 counts. Adverse events led to cessation of blind treatment in about a third of participants. The addition of didanosine to zidovudine versus zidovudine alone increased the risks of nausea (RR 1.8, 95% CI 1.1 to 2.9), abdominal pain (RR 1.6, 95% CI 1.0 to 2.7), and pancreatitis (RR 4.6, 95% CI 1.0 to 22.0). Addition of zalcitabine increased the risk of neuropathy (RR 2.2, 95% CI 1.4 to 3.6).[11] Addition of lamivudine did not significantly increase the rate of adverse events.[13] The subsequent RCT found that frequent adverse effects in all three treatment groups were abdominal pain, fever, asthenia/fatigue, and malaise.[14] Both indinavir alone and indinavir plus zidovudine versus zidovudine significantly increased the risk of kidney stone formation (40/332 [12%] with indinavir or indinavir plus zidovudine *v* 13/332 [4%] with zidovudine; RR 3.08, 95% CI 1.72 to 5.29; NNH 12, 95% CI 6 to 36). Overall, 2.9% of people permanently discontinued some or all of their study treatment because of adverse effects, prior to an AIDS related clinical event.[16]

Comment: We found one RCT (256 people with HIV but not AIDS and with CD4 count 300–500/mm^3) comparing zidovudine plus zalcitabine versus zidovudine alone.[15] It found no significant difference between treatments for AIDS defining events after a median 634 days' follow up (10 AIDS events in total). However, clinically important differences could not be excluded because recruitment and follow up were terminated prematurely and the study size did not meet planned power requirements. Two drug regimens often allow substantial residual viral replication in an environment where drug resistant variants have selective advantage. Resistance to these drugs tends to develop over several months to years.[16] The relevance of this is not fully understood but prior use of, and measurable resistance to, nucleoside analogue reverse transcriptase inhibitors tends to be associated with poorer virological response to new regimens that include drugs of this class.[17–19]

OPTION THREE DRUG REGIMENS CONTAINING A PROTEASE INHIBITOR VERSUS TWO DRUG REGIMENS

Two RCTs have found that using a protease inhibitor with two nucleoside analogue drugs versus two nucleoside analogue drugs alone halves the risk of new AIDS diseases or death over about 1 year. Both RCTs found that the risk of serious adverse effects was similar with three versus two drug regimens.

Benefits: We found no systematic review but found two RCTs, both with less than 2 years of follow up. The first RCT (1156 people previously treated with zidovudine; CD4 counts < 200/mm^3) compared zidovudine/lamivudine/indinavir versus zidovudine/lamivudine.[20] It found that triple therapy significantly reduced the rates of AIDS or death (ARR 5%; RR 0.50, 95% CI 0.33 to 0.76). The second RCT (3485 people with CD4 counts of 50–350/mm^3 who had never received zidovudine) compared zidovudine/zalcitabine/saquinavir versus zidovudine/zalcitabine or zidovudine/saquinavir.[21] It also found that triple therapy significantly reduced the risk of AIDS or death (RR of AIDS or death 0.50; CI not reported; P = 0.0001). Health related quality of life did not change significantly over 48 weeks for those in the triple therapy group (change from baseline –0.4 points for physical health summary and +1.4 for mental health summary); a deterioration occurred in both dual therapy groups (–2.5 and +0.1, respectively, for zalcitabine/saquinavir and –2.2 and +0.3, respectively, for zidovudine/saquinavir).[22]

Harms: In the first RCT, about a fifth of participants in both groups experienced serious adverse events.[20] The most common were non-specific discomfort, malaise, fever, headache, nausea, and vomiting. The addition of indinavir to zidovudine/lamivudine reduced the risk of neutropenia (5% *v* 15%; P < 0.001), but increased the risk of hyperbilirubinaemia (6% *v* 1%; P < 0.001) and renal colic/renal stone formation (4% *v* 1%; CI not reported; P = 0.001). In the second RCT, about 25% of people in each group had nausea, 10% diarrhoea, 10% vomiting, 10% headache, 4% abdominal pain, and 3% peripheral neuropathy.[21] There was no significant difference between people taking three versus two drugs in other adverse effects (fever, asthenia, anorexia, rash, pruritus, myalgia, insomnia, anaemia, buccal mucosa ulceration, and dyspepsia).

Comment: Longer term follow up of people taking protease inhibitors has found abnormal fat distribution, hyperglycaemia, and raised triglyceride and cholesterol concentrations. The clinical significance of these changes is uncertain. Many drugs interact with protease inhibitors because of inhibition of cytochrome P450.

OPTION EARLY VERSUS DEFERRED ANTIRETROVIRAL TREATMENT

One systematic review compared early versus deferred antiretroviral treatment, but the RCTs were all started when zidovudine was the only drug available. Overall, they found no significant difference in the risk of AIDS free survival or overall survival with extended follow up. We found no RCTs exploring this question with two or three drug regimens.

Benefits: We found one systematic review (search date not stated, 5 RCTs, 7722 people with asymptomatic HIV mainly with CD4 counts > 200/mm^3) comparing zidovudine given immediately versus zidovudine deferred until the early signs of AIDS.[23] It found that immediate versus deferred treatment significantly increased AIDS free survival at 1 year (78/4431 [1.76%] with immediate zidovudine *v* 131/3291 [3.98%] with deferred zidovudine; OR 0.52, 95% CI 0.39 to 0.68), but the difference was not significant at the end of the RCTs (median follow up of 50 months; 1026/4431 [23.2%] with immediate zidovudine *v* 882/3291 [26.8%] with deferred zidovudine; OR 0.96, 95% CI 0.87 to 1.05). Overall survival was similar in the two groups at 1 year (24/4431 [5.4%] with immediate zidovudine *v* 18/3291 [5.5%] with deferred zidovudine; OR 1.22, 95% CI 0.67 to 2.25) and at the end of the RCTs (734/4431 [16.6%] with immediate zidovudine *v* 617/3291 [18.7%] with deferred zidovudine; OR 1.04, 95% CI 0.93 to 1.16).

Harms: A meta-analysis presented pooled toxicity data in terms of events per 100 patient years.[24] In asymptomatic people, early treatment conferred a small but significant increase in the risk of anaemia (RR of haemoglobin < 8.0 g/dL; early *v* deferred treatment 2.1, 95% CI 1.1 to 4.1; AR 0.4 events per 100 person years). There was also a small increase in risk of neutropenia with early treatment (AR 1.1 events per 100 person years; CI not reported; P = 0.07). In symptomatic people, the excess incidence of severe anaemia probably reflected the high doses of zidovudine (1200–1500 mg/day; RR of severe anaemia, high *v* low dose 3.6, 95% CI 1.3 to 10). The authors advised that the toxicity results should be interpreted cautiously, because the results varied considerably.

Comment: No new trials on this question are ongoing. With three drug regimens, rates of AIDS and death are currently low and treatment is known to be beneficial up to and over a 2 year period (see three drug regimens, p 698). Many people feel sufficiently certain about when to start treatment — based on evidence about HIV pathogenesis, resistance, immune regeneration with treatment, and long term adverse effects — and so would not consider randomisation to immediate versus deferred treatment. Decisions on when to initiate multidrug treatment are currently based on our understanding of how HIV induces immune damage, the capacity for immune regeneration while on treatment, the toxicity and inconvenience of treatment, and the risk of resistance, rather than on results of RCTs.

REFERENCES

1. United Nations AIDS website: http://www.unaids.org.
2. Public Health Laboratory Services. *Occupational transmission of HIV. Summary of published reports.* London: PHLS, December 1997.
3. Centres for Disease Control and Prevention. HIV prevention through early detection and treatment of other sexually transmitted diseases – United States. *MMWR Morb Mortal Wkly Rep* 1998;47:RR12.
4. Grosskurth H, Mosha F, Todd J, et al. Impact of improved treatment of sexually transmitted diseases on HIV infection in rural Tanzania: randomised controlled trial. *Lancet* 1995;346:530–536.
5. Cohen MS, Hoffman IF, Royce RA, et al. Reduction of concentration of HIV-1 in semen after treatment of urethritis: implications for prevention of sexual transmission of HIV-1. *Lancet* 1997;349:1868–1873.
6. Wawer MJ, Sewankambo NK, Serwadda D, et al. Control of sexually transmitted diseases for AIDS prevention in Uganda: a randomised community trial. *Lancet* 1999;353:525–535.
7. Wilkinson D, Abdool Karim SS, Harrison A, et al. Unrecognised sexually transmitted infections in rural South African women: a hidden epidemic. *Bull World Health Organ* 1999;77:22–28.
8. Centers for Disease Control and Prevention. Public health service guidelines for the management of health-care worker exposures to HIV and recommendations for post exposure prophylaxis. *MMWR Morb Mortal Wkly Rep* 1998;47:RR7.
9. Cardo DM, Culver DH, Ciesielski CA, et al. Case-control study of HIV seroconversion in health care workers after percutaneous exposure. *N Engl J Med* 1997;337:1485–1490.
10. Connor EM, Sperling RS, Gelber R, et al. Reduction of maternal–infant transmission of human immunodeficiency virus type 1 with zidovudine treatment: paediatric AIDS clinical trials group protocol 076 study group. *N Engl J Med* 1994;331:1173–1180.
11. HIV Trialists' Collaborative Group. Zidovudine, didanosine, and zalcitabine in the treatment of HIV infection: meta-analyses of the randomised evidence. *Lancet* 1999;353:2014–2015. Search date not stated; primary sources Medline, hand searches of conference proceedings, and personal contact with investigators and pharmaceutical companies.
12. Haubrich R, Lalezari J, Follansbee SE, et al. Improved survival and reduced clinical progression in HIV-infected patients with advanced disease treated with saquinavir plus zalcitabine. *Antivir Ther* 1998;3:33–42.
13. CAESAR Co-ordinating Committee. Randomized trial of addition of lamivudine or lamivudine plus loviride to zidovudine-containing regimens for patients with HIV-1 infection: the CAESAR trial. *Lancet* 1997;349:1413–1421.
14. Lewi DS, Suleiman JM, Uip DE, et al. Randomized, double-blind trial comparing indinavir alone, zidovudine alone and indinavir plus zidovudine in antiretroviral therapy-naïve HIV-infected individuals

with CD4 cells counts between 50 and 250/mm³. *Rev Inst Med Trop Sao Paulo* 2000;42:27–36.
15. Moyle GJ, Bouza E, Antunes F, et al. Zidovudine monotherapy versus zidovudine plus zalcitabine combination therapy in HIV-positive persons with CD4 cell counts 300–500 cells/mm³: a double-blind controlled trial. The M50003 Study Group Coordinating and Writing Committee. *Antivir Ther* 1997;2:229–236.
16. Brun-Vezinet F, Boucher C, Loveday C, et al. HIV-1 viral load, phenotype, and resistance in a subset of drug-naïve participants from the Delta trial. *Lancet* 1997;350:983–990.
17. D'Aquila RT, Johnson VA, Welles SL, et al. Zidovudine resistance and HIV-1 disease progression during antiretroviral therapy. *Ann Intern Med* 1995;122:401–408.
18. Ledergerber B, Egger M, Opravil M, et al. Clinical progression and virological failure on highly active antiretroviral therapy in HIV-1 patients: a prospective cohort study. *Lancet* 1999;353:863–868.
19. Staszewski S, Miller V, Sabin CA, et al. Virological response to protease inhibitor therapy in an HIV clinic cohort. *AIDS* 1999;13:367–373.
20. Hammer SM, Squires KE, Hughes MD, et al. A controlled trial of two nucleoside analogues plus indinavir in persons with HIV infection and CD4 cell counts of 200/mm³ or less. *N Engl J Med* 1997;337:725–733.
21. Stellbrink H-J, Hawkins D, Clumeck N, et al. Randomized, multicentre phase III study of saquinavir plus zidovudine plus zalcitabine in previously untreated or minimally pretreated HIV-infected patients. *Clin Drug Invest* 2000;20:295–307.
22. Revicki DA, Moyle G, Stellbrink HJ, et al. Quality of life outcomes of combination zalcitabine–zidovudine, saquinavir–zidovudine, and saquinavir–zalcitabine–zidovudine therapy for HIV-infected adults with CD4 cell counts between 50 and 350/mm³. *AIDS* 1999;13:851–858.
23. Darbyshire J, Foulkes M, Peto R, et al. Immediate versus deferred zidovudine (AZT) in asymptomatic or mildly symptomatic HIV infected adults. In: The Cochrane Library, Issue 4, 2000. Oxford: Update Software. Search date not stated; primary sources Medline, hand searches of conference abstracts, and contact with investigators and pharmaceutical companies.
24. Ioannidis JP, Cappelleri JC, Lau J, et al. Early or deferred zidovudine therapy in HIV-infected patients without an AIDS-defining illness: a meta-analysis. *Ann Intern Med* 1995;122:856–866. Search date 1994; primary sources Medline, AIDSLine, AIDSTrials, AIDSDrugs, CHEMID, hand searches of current contents, and international conferences on AIDS.

Margaret Johnson
Consultant in HIV Medicine
Royal Free Hospital
London
UK

Andrew, Phillips
Professor
Royal Free Centre for
HIV Medicine and
Department of Primary Care and
Population Sciences
Royal Free and
University College Medical School
London
UK

David Wilkinson
Professor
Pro Vice Chancellor and Vice President
Division of Health Sciences
University of South Australia
Adelaide
Australia

Bazian Ltd (temporary contributors)
London
UK

Competing interests: DW, none declared. MJ and AP have received reimbursement for attending and speaking at symposia, funds for research and members of staff, and fees for consulting from various pharmaceutical companies producing antiretroviral drugs, including Abbott, Boehringer Ingleheim, Agouron, GlaxoSmithKline, Bristol-Myers Squibb, Roche, and DuPont.

Influenza

Search date March 2002

Timothy Uyeki, Andrea Winquist, and Bazian Ltd (temporary contributors)

QUESTIONS

INTERVENTIONS

Key Messages

- **All antivirals (reduction of serious influenza complications)** We found insufficient evidence about the effects of antiviral agents on reducing serious complications of influenza, but we found strong evidence that influenza immunisation reduces the risk of complications and death in people at high risk for complications from influenza, including elderly people (see influenza vaccine under community acquired pneumonia, p 1546).
- **Oral amantadine for early treatment of influenza A in adults (duration of symptoms reduced)** One systematic review and three additional RCTs have found that oral amantadine versus placebo reduces the duration of influenza A symptoms by about 1 day. We found insufficient evidence about adverse effects in this setting. We found no good evidence of benefit if amantadine is started more than 2 days after symptom onset.
- **Orally inhaled zanamivir for early treatment of influenza A and B in adults (duration of symptoms reduced)** One systematic review has found that orally inhaled zanamivir versus placebo reduces the duration of influenza symptoms by about 1 day. Adverse effects were similar in people taking zanamivir and in people taking placebo. We found no good evidence of benefit if zanamivir is started more than 2 days after symptom onset.

Clin Evid 2002;8:702–708.

- **Oral oseltamivir for early treatment of influenza A and B in adults (duration of symptoms reduced)** Two RCTs have found that oral oseltamivir versus placebo reduces the duration of influenza symptoms by about 1 day. Oral oseltamivir versus placebo increases the incidence of nausea and vomiting. We found no good evidence of benefit if oseltamivir is started more than 1.5 days after symptom onset.
- **Oral rimantadine for early treatment of influenza A in adults (duration of symptoms reduced)** One systematic review has found that oral rimantadine versus placebo reduces the duration of influenza A symptoms by about 1 day. We found insufficient evidence about adverse effects in this setting. We found no good evidence of benefit if rimantadine is started more than 2 days after symptom onset.

DEFINITION Influenza is caused by infection with influenza viruses. Uncomplicated influenza is characterised by the abrupt onset of fever, chills, non-productive cough, myalgias, headache, nasal congestion, sore throat, and fatigue.[1] Influenza is usually diagnosed clinically. Not all people infected with influenza viruses become symptomatic. People infected with other pathogens may have symptoms identical to those of influenza.[2] The percentage of infections resulting in clinical illness can vary from about 40–85%, depending on age and pre-existing immunity to the virus.[3] Influenza can be confirmed by viral culture, immunofluorescence staining, enzyme immunoassay, or rapid diagnostic testing of nasopharyngeal, nasal or throat swab specimens, or by serologic testing of paired sera. Some rapid tests detect influenza A only, some detect and distinguish between influenza A and B, whereas others detect but do not distinguish between influenza A and B.

INCIDENCE/ PREVALENCE In temperate areas of the Northern Hemisphere, influenza activity typically peaks between late December and early March, whereas in temperate areas of the Southern Hemisphere influenza activity typically peaks between May and September. In tropical areas, influenza can occur throughout the year.[2] The annual incidence of influenza varies yearly, and depends partly on the underlying level of population immunity to circulating influenza viruses.[1] One localised study in the USA found that serological conversion with or without symptoms occurred in 10–20% a year, with the highest infection rates in people aged under 20 years.[4] Attack rates are higher in institutions and in areas of overcrowding.[5]

AETIOLOGY/ RISK FACTORS Influenza viruses are transmitted primarily from person to person through respiratory droplets disseminated during sneezing, coughing, and talking.[1,6]

PROGNOSIS The incubation period of influenza is 1–4 days and infected adults are usually contagious from the day before symptom onset until 5 days after symptom onset. The signs and symptoms of uncomplicated influenza usually resolve within a week, although cough and fatigue may persist.[1] Complications include otitis media, bacterial sinusitis, secondary bacterial pneumonia, and, less commonly, viral pneumonia and respiratory failure. Complications are also caused by exacerbation of underlying disease.[1,2] In the USA each year, over 110 000 admissions to hospital and about 20 000 deaths are related to influenza.[2] The risk of hospitalisation is highest in people 65 years or older, in very young children, and in those with chronic medical conditions.[1,7,8] Over 90% of influenza related deaths during recent seasonal epidemics in the USA have been in people 65 years or older.[1] During influenza pandemics, morbidity and mortality may be high in younger age groups.[1] Severe illness is more common with influenza A infections than influenza B infections.[1]

AIMS To reduce the duration and severity of influenza signs and symptoms, the risk of complications, and to minimise adverse effects of treatment.

OUTCOMES Severity and duration of symptoms; frequency and severity of complications of influenza; adverse effects of treatment.

METHODS *Clinical Evidence* update search and appraisal March 2002. The authors searched Medline (1966–2001; major MeSH topics: amantadine and influenza, rimantadine and influenza; keywords: zanamivir, 4-guanidino-Neu5Ac2en, GG167, oseltamivir, GS4104, and Ro64-0796). Meeting abstracts were used to identify unpublished studies of zanamivir and oseltamivir. We included only systematic reviews and double blind RCTs of treatment versus placebo for naturally occurring influenza. We excluded RCTs and reviews of chemoprophylaxis of influenza, experimentally induced influenza, and reviews that combined RCTs of more than one agent. We only assessed people with laboratory confirmed influenza. For amantadine and rimantadine, we included only RCTs of influenza A. For zanamivir and oseltamivir, we included studies of influenza A or B. For zanamivir, we included only RCTs of orally inhaled drug and excluded intranasal drops plus oral inhalation unless oral inhalation results were reported separately. For amantadine, rimantadine, and oseltamivir we included only RCTs of oral administration. We excluded RCTs primarily on children younger than 18 years, those that used an antipyretic rather than a placebo as control, RCTs in which the delay from symptom onset to starting treatment was unclear, and RCTs without quantitative measures of clinical effectiveness.

QUESTION What are the effects of antiviral treatment of influenza in adults?

OPTION ORAL AMANTADINE

One systematic review and additional RCTs have found that oral amantadine versus placebo reduces the duration of influenza A symptoms by about 1 day. We found insufficient evidence to assess adverse effects in this setting.

Benefits: We found one systematic review (search date 1997, 7 RCTs, 531 otherwise healthy people)[9] and three additional RCTs[10–12] of oral amantadine (usually started within 48 h of symptom onset) versus placebo for the treatment of influenza A (see web extra table A at www.clinicalevidence.com). The review found that amantadine significantly reduced the duration of fever (temperature > 37.0°C reduced by 1 day, 95% CI 0.7 to 1.3). We found no RCTs of the effect of amantadine in preventing serious complications of influenza, such as pneumonia or exacerbation of chronic diseases. We found no RCTs of amantadine for treatment of influenza A in pregnant women, those with chronic disease, or in immunised people.

Harms: The review found no significant difference in the frequency of adverse effects between amantadine and placebo groups. However, the included RCTs contained little information about the relative adverse effects of amantadine compared with placebo when used for treatment of influenza A (see web extra table A at www.clinicalevidence.com).[13–15] More evidence is available about the harms of amantadine when used for prophylaxis of influenza A (see comment below).

Comment: *In vitro* studies have found that amantadine has specific antiviral activity against influenza A, but not influenza B viruses.[16] The RCTs used different outcome measures, so summarising results is difficult. Only one RCT examined amantadine in elderly people.[12] All RCTs considered only people with laboratory confirmed influenza A, so the analyses were not by intention to treat. The proportion of influenza A isolates from the general population exhibiting resistance to amantadine has remained low.[17,18] Amantadine resistant influenza A viruses have not been found to be more virulent than non-resistant viruses.[2] The limited evidence from elderly and high risk groups makes it difficult to generalise results to these populations. A systematic review found that use of amantadine versus placebo for prophylaxis of influenza A is associated with an increased incidence of gastrointestinal and central nervous system adverse effects.[9]

OPTION ORAL RIMANTADINE

One systematic review has found that oral rimantadine versus placebo reduces the duration of influenza A symptoms by about 1 day. We found insufficient evidence about adverse effects in this setting.

Benefits: We found one systematic review (search date 1997, 3 RCTs, 104 otherwise healthy adults)[9] and one small additional RCT[19] of rimantadine (usually started within 48 h of symptom onset) versus placebo for the treatment of influenza A (see web extra table A at www.clinicalevidence.com). The review found that rimantadine versus placebo significantly reduced the duration of fever (temperature > 37.0°C reduced by 1.3 days, 95% CI 0.8 to 1.8). We found no RCTs of rimantadine for treatment of influenza A in people over 65 years of age, in pregnant women, in those with chronic disease, or in immunised people. We found no RCTs of the effect of rimantadine in preventing serious complications of influenza, such as pneumonia or exacerbation of chronic diseases.

Harms: The review found insufficient evidence about the adverse effects of rimantadine versus placebo in people with influenza A.[9] One non-systematic review (340 adults) of rimantadine treatment versus placebo found that more people taking rimantadine had central nervous system symptoms, most commonly insomnia (10.8% *v* 8.6%; P value not provided); and gastrointestinal symptoms, most commonly abdominal pain and nausea (6.0% *v* 2.3%; P value not provided).[20] Additional evidence is available about adverse effects of rimantadine when used for prophylaxis of influenza A (see comment below).

Comment: *In vitro* studies have found that rimantadine has specific antiviral activity against influenza A, but not influenza B viruses.[16] The RCTs used different outcome measures so summarising results is difficult. Additional studies of rimantadine have been performed in

Russia, but information in English is limited.[21] Viruses that are resistant to rimantadine show cross-resistance to amantadine, and *vice versa*.[17] Influenza A viruses resistant to rimantadine have not been found to be more virulent than non-resistant viruses.[2] The proportion of influenza A isolates from the general population exhibiting resistance to rimantadine (or amantadine) has remained low.[17,18] The limited evidence from elderly and high risk groups makes it difficult to generalise results to these populations. A systematic review found that use of rimantadine versus placebo for prophylaxis of influenza A is associated with an increased incidence of gastrointestinal adverse effects.[9]

OPTION ORALLY INHALED ZANAMIVIR

One systematic review has found that orally inhaled zanamivir versus placebo reduces the duration of influenza symptoms by about 1 day. Adverse effects were similar in people taking zanamivir versus placebo.

Benefits: We found one systematic review (search date 2000, 5 RCTs, 1498 people with influenza)[22] and two additional RCTs (78 people with influenza)[23,24] that compared inhaled zanamivir (usually started within 48 h of symptom onset) versus placebo (see web extra table B at www.clinicalevidence.com). Some of the RCTs included small numbers of people 65 years or older, and people with chronic cardiac or respiratory illness.[24–27] The review found that zanamivir versus placebo significantly reduced the time to alleviation of symptoms (median time reduced by 1.4 days, 95% CI 0.8 to 1.9 days). The first additional RCT (27 people with influenza) found no significant difference between zanamivir versus placebo in the time to alleviation of symptoms (median time reduced by 4.5 days, $P = 0.3$).[24] The second additional RCT (51 people with influenza) found that zanamivir versus placebo reduced the time to alleviation of symptoms by 0.5 days (P value not provided).[23] The review performed a meta-analysis including one RCT (313 people with influenza) and subgroups of people at high risk from four of the original RCTs (171 people).[28] It found no significant difference between zanamivir versus placebo in the time to alleviation of symptoms (484 people; median time reduced by 1.67 days, 95% CI −0.02 to +3.37 days).[28] We found no RCTs of the effect of zanamivir in preventing serious complications of influenza, such as pneumonia or exacerbation of chronic diseases.

Harms: Adverse effects were similar in people taking zanamivir compared with placebo (the inhaled lactose vehicle alone) (see web extra table B at www.clinicalevidence.com).[22] Use of zanamivir has been associated with bronchospasm and worsening of underlying respiratory disease (see comment below).[29]

Comment: Zanamivir is administered as an orally inhaled powder. *In vitro* studies have found that zanamivir has antiviral activity against both influenza A and B viruses.[30] RCTs have predominantly included people with influenza A (≥ 85%). Because of the short period that zanamivir has been available, and the lack of optimal assays to detect resistant strains, we found insufficient evidence to comment on the development of viral resistance to zanamivir.[2,31–36] The observational evidence that zanamivir is associated with bronchospasm and worsening of underlying respiratory disease suggests that zanamivir should not usually be recommended for people with underlying airways disease because of the risk of serious events.[29]

OPTION ORAL OSELTAMIVIR

Two RCTs have found that oral oseltamivir versus placebo reduces the duration of influenza symptoms by about 1 day, but increases the incidence of nausea and vomiting.

Benefits: We found no systematic review of oseltamivir used to treat influenza. We found two RCTs of oseltamivir versus placebo.[37,38] People in both RCTs were selected with a temperature of 38.0°C or greater. Both RCTs found that oseltamivir (started within 36 h of symptom onset) versus placebo significantly reduced the duration of influenza symptoms by about 1 day (see web extra table B at www.clinicalevidence.com). We found no RCTs of oseltamivir for influenza in people 65 years or older, in pregnant women, in people with chronic disease, or in vaccinated people. We found no RCTs of the effect of oseltamivir in preventing serious complications of influenza, such as pneumonia, or exacerbation of chronic diseases.

Harms: Nausea and vomiting were significantly more common in people receiving oseltamivir versus placebo.[37,38]

Comment: Studies in mice and ferrets have found that oseltamivir has *in vitro* activity against both influenza A and B viruses.[39] The RCTs predominantly included people with influenza A (97%).[37,38] Because of the short period that oseltamivir has been available, and the lack of optimal assays to detect resistant strains, we found insufficient evidence to comment on the development of viral resistance to oseltamivir.[2,32,36,40]

REFERENCES

1. Cox NJ, Fukuda K. Influenza. *Infect Dis Clin North Am* 1998;12:27–38.
2. Bridges CB, Fukuda K, Uyeki TM, et al. Prevention and control of influenza: recommendations of the Advisory Committee on Immunization Practices (ACIP). *MMWR* 2002;51(No. RR-3).
3. Fox JP, Cooney MK, Hall CE, et al. Influenza virus infections in Seattle families, 1975–1979. II. Pattern of infection in invaded households and relation of age and prior antibody to occurrence of infection and related illness. *Am J Epidemiol* 1982;116:228–242.
4. Sullivan KM, Monto AS, Longini IM. Estimates of the US health impact of influenza. *Am J Public Health* 1993;83:1712–1716.
5. Kilbourne ED. *Influenza*. New York: Plenum Medical Book Co, 1987:269–270.
6. Tablan OC, Anderson LJ, Arden NH, et al. Hospital Infection Control Practices Advisory Committee. Guideline for prevention of nosocomial pneumonia. *Infect Control Hosp Epidemiol* 1994;15:587–604.
7. Neuzil KM, Mellen BG, Wright PF, et al. The effect of influenza on hospitalizations, outpatient visits, and courses of antibiotics in children. *N Engl J Med* 2000;342:225–231.
8. Izurieta HS, Thompson WW, Kramarz P, et al. Influenza and the rates of hospitalization for respiratory disease among infants and young children. *N Engl J Med* 2000;342:232–239.
9. Jefferson TO, Demicheli V, Deeks JJ, et al. Amantadine and rimantadine for preventing and treating influenza A in adults. In: The Cochrane Library, Issue 1, 2002. Oxford: Update Software. Search date 1997; primary sources Medline, Cochrane Controlled Trials Register, Embase, reviews of references of identified trials, and letters to manufacturers and authors.
10. Baker LM, Shock MP, Iezzoni DG. The therapeutic efficacy of Symmetrel (amantadine hydrochloride) in naturally occurring influenza A2 respiratory illness. *J Am Osteopath Assoc* 1969;68:1244–1250.
11. Galbraith AW, Schild AW, Schild GC, et al. The therapeutic effect of amantadine in influenza occurring during the winter of 1971–1972 assessed by double-blind study. *J R Coll Gen Pract* 1973;23:34–37.
12. Walters HE, Paulshock M. Therapeutic efficacy of amantadine HCl. *Mo Med* 1970;67:176–179.
13. Kitamoto O. Therapeutic effectiveness of amantadine hydrochloride in influenza A2: double-blind studies. *Jpn J Tuberc Chest Dis* 1968;15:17–26.
14. Kitamoto O. Therapeutic effectiveness of amantadine hydrochloride in naturally occurring Hong Kong influenza: double-blinded studies. *Jpn J Tuberc Chest Dis* 1971;17:1–7.

15. Van Voris LP, Betts RF, Hayden FG, et al. Successful treatment of naturally occurring influenza A/USSR/77 H1N1. *JAMA* 1981;245:1128–1131.
16. Tominack RL, Hayden FG. Rimantadine hydrochloride and amantadine hydrochloride use in influenza A virus infections. *Infect Dis Clin North Am* 1987;1:459–478.
17. Belshe RB, Burk B, Newman F, et al. Resistance of influenza A viruses to amantadine and rimantadine: results of one decade of surveillance. *J Infect Dis* 1989;159:430–435.
18. Ziegler T, Hemphill ML, Ziegler M-L, et al. Low incidence of rimantadine resistance in field isolates of influenza A viruses. *J Infect Dis* 1999;180:935–939.
19. Rabinovich S, Baldini JT, Bannister R. Treatment of influenza: the therapeutic efficacy of rimantadine HCl in a naturally occurring influenza A2 outbreak. *Am J Med Sci* 1969;257:328–335.
20. Soo W. Adverse effects of rimantadine: summary from clinical trials. *J Respir Dis* 1989;10(suppl.):S26–S31.
21. Zlydnikov DM, Kubar OI, Kovaleva TP, et al. Study of rimantadine in the USSR: a review of the literature. *Rev Infect Dis* 1981;3:408–421.
22. Burls A, Clark W, Stewart A, et al. *Zanamivir for the treatment of influenza in adults, West Midlands Development and Evaluation Service*. Birmingham, 2000. Report for the National Institute for Clinical Excellence (NICE). Available at http://www.nice.org.uk (last accessed 03/09/2002). Search date 2000; primary sources Cochrane Library, Medline, Embase, Science Citation Index, GlaxoSmithKline, Clinical Trials Register, hand searching of Scrip, FDA submissions and conference abstracts, and information submitted by GlaxoSmithKline to NICE.
23. Matsumoto K, Ogawa N, Nerome K, et al. Safety and efficacy of the neuraminidase inhibitor zanamivir in treating influenza virus infection in adults: results from Japan. *Antiviral Ther* 1999;4:61–68.
24. Boivin G, Goyette N, Hardy I, et al. Rapid antiviral effect of inhaled zanamivir in the treatment of naturally occurring influenza in otherwise healthy adults. *J Infect Dis* 2000;181:1471–1474.
25. The MIST (Management of Influenza in the Southern Hemisphere Trialists) Study Group. Randomized trial of efficacy and safety of inhaled zanamivir in treatment of influenza A and B infections. *Lancet* 1998;352:1877–1881.
26. Lalezari J, Klein T, Stapleton J, et al. The efficacy and safety of inhaled zanamivir in the treatment of influenza in otherwise healthy and "high risk" individuals in North America [abstract]. *J Antimicrob Chemother* 1999;44(suppl. A):42.
27. Makela MJ, Pauksens K, Rostila T, et al. Clinical efficacy and safety of the orally inhaled neuraminidase inhibitor zanamivir in the treatment of influenza: a randomized, double-blind, placebo-controlled European study. *J Infect* 2000;40:42–48.
28. National Institute for Clinical Excellence. *Zanamivir for the treatment of influenza in adults*. Supplement to the assessment report: 2000. Available at http://www.nice.org.uk (last accessed 3 Sept 2002).
29. Henney JE. Revised labeling for zanamivir. *JAMA* 2000;284:1234.
30. Woods JM, Bethell RC, Coates JAV, et al. 4-guanidino-2,4-dideoxy-2,3-dehydro-N-acetylneuraminic acid is a highly effective inhibitor of both the sialidase (neuraminidase) and growth of a wide range of influenza A and B viruses *in vitro*. *Antimicrob Agents Chemother* 1993;37:1473–1479.
31. Read RC. Letter to the Editor. *Lancet* 1999;353:668–669.
32. Tisdale M. Monitoring of viral susceptibility: new challenges with the development of influenza NA inhibitors. *Rev Med Virol* 2000;10:45–55.
33. Barnett JM, Cadman A, Gor D. Zanamivir susceptibility monitoring and characterization of influenza virus clinical isolates obtained during phase II clinical efficacy studies. *Antimicrob Agents Chemother* 2000;44:78–87.
34. Gubareva LV, Kaiser L, Brenner MK, et al. Evidence for zanamivir resistance in an immunocompromised child infected with influenza B virus. *J Infect Dis* 1998;178:1257–1262.
35. Gubareva LV, Webster RG, Hayden FG. Detection of influenza virus resistance to neuraminidase inhibitors by an enzyme inhibition assay. *Antiviral Res* 2002;53:47–61.
36. Zambon M, Hayden FG. Position statement: global neuraminidase inhibitor susceptibility network. *Antiviral Res* 2001;49:147–156.
37. Treanor JJ, Hayden FG, Vrooman PS, et al. Efficacy and safety of the oral neuraminidase inhibitor oseltamivir in treating acute influenza: a randomized controlled trial. *JAMA* 2000;283:1016–1024.
38. Nicholson KG, Aoki FY, Osterhaus ADME, et al. Efficacy and safety of oseltamivir in treatment of acute influenza: a randomized controlled trial. *Lancet* 2000;355:1845–1850.
39. Mendel DB, Tai CY, Escarpe PA, et al. Oral administration of a prodrug of the influenza virus neuraminidase inhibitor GS4071 protects mice and ferrets against influenza infection. *Antimicrob Agents Chemother* 1998;42:640–646.
40. Gubareva LV, Webster RG, Hayden FG. Detection of influenza virus resistance to neuraminidase inhibitors by an enzyme inhibition assay. *Antiviral Res* 2002;53:47–61.

Timothy Uyeki
Medical Epidemiologist
Centers for Disease Control and Prevention
National Center for Infectious Diseases
Division of Viral and Rickettsial Diseases
Influenza Branch
Atlanta, Georgia
USA

Andrea Winquist
Medical Epidemiologist
Centers for Disease Control and Prevention
Epidemiology Program Office
Division of Applied Public Health Training
State Branch
Atlanta, Georgia
USA

Competing interests: None declared.

Search date November 2001

Diana Lockwood

QUESTIONS

INTERVENTIONS

PREVENTION

Beneficial

Bacillus Calmette Guerin (BCG) vaccine 711

BCG plus killed *Mycobacterium leprae* 711

Likely to be beneficial

ICRC vaccine 711

Unknown effectiveness

Mycobacterium w vaccine 711

TREATMENT

Beneficial

Dapsone plus rifampicin for paucibacillary leprosy* 713

Rifampicin plus dapsone plus clofazimine for multibacillary leprosy* 714

Unlikely to be beneficial

Single dose versus multiple dose treatment for single skin lesion leprosy (both increase cure rates but multiple more than single dose) 715

To be covered in future updates

Treatment of reactions

*Observational evidence only, RCTs unlikely to be conducted.

See glossary, p 716

Key Messages

Prevention

- **Bacillus Calmette-Guerin (BCG) vaccine** One RCT and three population based controlled clinical trials found that BCG vaccination versus no intervention or placebo significantly reduced the incidence of leprosy for up to 16 years. The degree of protection varied between countries, with higher protection in Uganda than Burma (now Myanmar).
- **BCG plus killed Mycobacterium leprae** One RCT found that in people with a BCG scar, BCG plus killed *M leprae* versus placebo significantly reduced the incidence of leprosy over 5–9 years. In people without a BCG scar, the RCT found that the addition of *M leprae* to BCG did not significantly reduce the incidence of leprosy. Another RCT found that BCG plus killed *M leprae* versus saline significantly reduced the incidence of leprosy over about 7 years.
- **ICRC vaccine** One RCT found that ICRC vaccine versus placebo significantly reduced the incidence of leprosy over about 7 years. The effect was higher than that observed with BCG alone, and similar to that observed with BCG plus killed *M leprae*.
- **Mycobacterium w vaccine** One RCT found that *Mycobacterium w* vaccine versus placebo marginally reduced the incidence of leprosy over about 7 years.

Treatment

- **Dapsone plus rifampicin for paucibacillary leprosy** We found no systematic review or RCT on multidrug treatment for paucibacillary leprosy. We found no RCT comparing dapsone plus rifampicin versus dapsone alone. Observational studies found that in people taking dapsone plus rifampicin for 6 months, up to 38% of lesions had resolved at 1 year and relapse rates were low for up to 8 years.
- **Rifampicin plus dapsone plus clofazimine for multibacillary leprosy** We found no systematic review or RCT. We found no RCT comparing rifampicin plus clofazimine plus dapsone versus dapsone alone, or versus dapsone plus rifampicin. Observational studies found that multidrug treatment for 24 months improved skin lesions and was associated with a low relapse rate.
- **Single dose versus multiple dose treatment for single skin lesion leprosy** One RCT found that 6 months treatment with rifampicin monthly plus dapsone daily significantly increased the cure rate at 18 months compared with a single dose of rifampicin plus minocycline plus ofloxacin (NNT 13, 95% CI 8 to 40). Some improvement occurred in 99% of people in both groups. Adverse effects were similar with both regimens.

DEFINITION Leprosy is a chronic granulomatous disease caused by *Mycobacterium leprae*, and primarily affects the peripheral nerves and skin. The clinical outcome of infection is determined by the individual's immune response to *M leprae*. A spectrum of disease types are seen. At the tuberculoid end of the Ridley–Jopling scale, cell mediated immunity is good and there are few skin lesions. At the lepromatous end of the scale there is diminished reactivity for *M leprae* resulting in uncontrolled bacterial multiplication, and skin and mucosal infiltration. Peripheral nerve damage occurs across the spectrum. Between the poles are the unstable borderline tuberculoid and borderline lepromatous forms. Classification is based on the clinical appearance and bacterial index of lesions (see glossary, p 716). The World Health Organization field classification (see glossary, p 716) is based on the number of skin lesions: single lesion leprosy (1 lesion), paucibacillary leprosy (2–5 skin lesions), and multibacillary leprosy (> 5 skin lesions).[1]

INCIDENCE/ PREVALENCE Worldwide, about 720 000 new cases of leprosy are reported each year,[2] and about 2 million people have leprosy related disabilities. Six major endemic countries (India, Brazil, Myanmar, Madagascar, Nepal, and Mozambique) account for 88% of all new cases. Cohort studies show a peak of disease presentation between 10–20 years of age.[3] After puberty there are twice as many male as female cases.

AETIOLOGY/ RISK FACTORS *M leprae* is discharged from the nasal mucosa of people with untreated lepromatous leprosy, and transmitted through the nasal mucosa of recipients with subsequent spread of mycobacteria to skin and nerves. It is a hardy organism and has been shown to survive in the Indian environment for many months.[4] Risk factors include household contact with a person with leprosy. We found no good evidence of a relationship between HIV infection, nutrition, and socio-economic status.[5]

PROGNOSIS Complications of leprosy include nerve damage, immunological reactions, and bacillary infiltration. In the absence of treatment, tuberculoid and some borderline tuberculoid infections will eventually resolve spontaneously. Other people with borderline tuberculoid and borderline lepromatous leprosy slowly develop lepromatous infection. Many people have peripheral nerve damage at the time of diagnosis, ranging from 15% in Bangladesh[6] to 55% in Ethiopia.[7] Immunological reactions can occur with or without antibiotic treatment. Further nerve damage occurs through immune mediated reactions (Type 1) and neuritis (see glossary, p 716). Erythema nodosum leprosum (see glossary, p 716) (Type 2 reaction) is an immune complex mediated reaction causing fever, malaise, and neuritis, which is reported to occur in 20% of people with lepromatous leprosy and 5% with borderline lepromatous leprosy.[8] Secondary impairments (wounds, contractures, and digit resorption) occur in 33–56% of people with established nerve damage.[9] We found no recent information on mortality.

AIMS **Vaccines:** To prevent leprosy. **Treatment:** To treat infection and improve skin lesions; to prevent relapse and complications (nerve damage and erythema nodosum leprosum).

OUTCOMES **Prevention:** Incidence of leprosy (RCTs should have a long follow up period as the incubation period can be 2–15 years, depending on disease type). **Treatment:** Clinical improvement, relapse rate, quality of life, adverse effects of treatment, and mortality.

METHODS *Clinical Evidence* search and appraisal November 2001. A search was performed for cohort studies of dapsone plus rifampicin. Additional references were identified from reference lists.

QUESTION What are the effects of measures to prevent leprosy? New

OPTION BACILLUS CALMETTE-GUERIN (BCG)

We found no systematic review but found three large controlled clinical trials and two RCTs. One RCT and three controlled clinical trials found that BCG vaccination versus no intervention or placebo significantly reduced the incidence of leprosy. The degree of protection varied between countries, with higher protection in Uganda than Burma (now Myanmar). Two RCTs found BCG plus killed *M leprae* versus placebo reduced the incidence of leprosy. However, in one of these RCTs that stratified people according to the presence of a BCG scar, leprosy was only reduced in people with a scar. One RCT found that both the *Mycobacterium w* and ICRC vaccine versus placebo reduced the incidence of leprosy, although the reduction with *Mycobacterium w* was only marginal.

Benefits: We found no systematic review. We found three large controlled clinical trials and two RCTs carried out in leprosy endemic areas with clinical leprosy as the outcome measure and follow up for 5–16 years (see web extra table A at www.clinicalevidence.com).[10–14] **BCG alone versus no treatment:** We found two controlled clinical trials.[10,12] The first controlled trial conducted in Uganda (quasi-randomised; 19 323 children with Heaf grade (see glossary, p 716) 0, 1, or 2; most of them < 10 years of age; range 0–16 years; follow up 14 years) found that BCG significantly reduced the incidence of leprosy (143/9036 [1.6%] with BCG *v* 19/9052 [0.2%] with no treatment; RR 0.13, 95% CI 0.08 to 0.21; NNT 73, 95% CI 62 to 93).[10] The second trial conducted in Burma, now Myanmar (14 435 children aged 0–14 years, follow up 13–16 years) compared two different BCG vaccines, each containing different concentrations of bacilli versus no treatment.[12] The BCG with the highest concentration of bacilli significantly reduced the incidence of leprosy over 14 years (3.8/1000 person years (see glossary, p 716) with BCG *v* 5.4/1000 person years for controls; RRR 30%, 95% CI 19% to 40%). It also found that protection was higher in boys than girls (35% with boys *v* 23% with girls). However, the BCG containing a lower concentration of bacilli had no significant protective effect (5.0/1000 person years with BCG *v* 5.6/1000 person years; RRR 11%, 95% CI –3% to 23%). **BCG alone versus placebo:** We found one controlled clinical trial[11] and one RCT.[13] The controlled clinical trial conducted in Papua New Guinea (stratified, quasi-randomised; 5356 children aged < 14 years, follow up for 13–16 years) compared BCG versus saline. It found that BCG reduced the incidence of leprosy (2.8/1000 person years with BCG *v* 5.4/1000 person years with saline; RRR 48%, 95% CI 34% to 59%), and significantly reduced mortality (cause of mortality not known; 442/2707 [16.3%] with BCG *v* 489/2649 [18.5%] with saline; RR 0.89, 95% CI 0.79 to 0.99; NNT 47, 95% CI 24 to 997). No significant differences in protective effect were found between females (RRR 50%, 95% CI 29% to 65%) and males (RRR 46%, 95% CI 25% to 61%). Protection was greater for those under 15 years of age at vaccination compared with those more than 15 years (54% for < 15 years *v* 34% for > 15 years).[11] The RCT, conducted in India (randomised, double blind, 171 400 healthy people aged 1–65 years, follow up for 6–7 years), compared five treatments: ICRC vaccine (see glossary, p 716) (22 541 people); *Mycobacterium w* vaccine (33 720 people); BCG (38 213 people); BCG plus killed *M leprae* (38 229 people); and normal saline (38 697 people). It found that BCG versus saline significantly reduced the incidence of leprosy (RRR 34.1%, 95% CI 13.5% to 49.8%).[13] **BCG plus killed *M leprae* versus placebo:** We found two RCTs.[13,14] The first RCT conducted in Malawi (double blind, 121 020 healthy people without history of previous leprosy or tuberculosis, severe malnutrition, or other severe illness, aged ≥ 3 months, follow up for 5–9 years) stratified people according to the presence of previous BCG vaccination scar. Those without a BCG scar (66 155 people) received BCG or BCG plus killed *M leprae*.[14] Those with a scar or a doubtful scar (54 865 people) received either BCG, BCG plus killed *M leprae*, or placebo. In people with a BCG scar, the RCT found that BCG or BCG plus killed *M leprae* versus placebo significantly reduced the incidence of leprosy (combined analysis for BCG or BCG plus killed *M leprae* versus placebo; RR 0.51, 95% CI 0.26 to 0.99; P = 0.04). However, in people without a scar, it found no significant difference in the incidence of leprosy with the addition of killed *M leprae* to BCG (RR 1.06, 95% CI 0.62 to 1.82; P = 0.82). No significant differences were found between a higher versus standard dose of *M leprae*. The second RCT conducted in India found that BCG plus killed *M leprae* versus placebo significantly reduced the incidence of leprosy (RRR 64.0%,

95% CI 50.4% to 73.9%).[13] **ICRC vaccine versus placebo:** One RCT conducted in India (see BCG alone *v* placebo above) found that ICRC vaccine versus normal saline significantly reduced the incidence of leprosy (RRR 65.5%, 95% CI 48.0% to 77.0%).[13] ***Mycobacterium w* versus placebo:** One RCT conducted in India (see BCG alone *v* placebo above) found that *Mycobacterium w* vaccine versus normal saline reduced the incidence of leprosy (RRR 25.7%, 95% CI 1.9% to 43.8%).[13]

Harms: The RCT conducted in India found that "fluctuant lymphadenitis" was minimal with all four vaccines used, and no other adverse effects were observed (numbers not provided).[13] The remaining trials did not report on harms.[10–12,14]

Comment: **BCG plus killed *M leprae* versus placebo:** The RCT conducted in India found that both BCG plus killed *M leprae* and ICRC vaccines had the highest efficacy. The RCT included a statistical adjustment for the multiple comparisons against placebo.[13] Follow up times varied between studies; therefore incidence rates were used to present results.[13,14] In the trial in Malawi, 7/82 people (9%) tested positive for the HIV.[14] Eleven different batches of BCG were used. The number of people lost to follow up was high (26%), and the sample size may have been insufficient to rule out clinically important effects, given that there were multiple comparisons against placebo.[14]

QUESTION What are the effects of treatments for paucibacillary leprosy? New

OPTION DAPSONE PLUS RIFAMPICIN

We found no systematic review or RCT on multidrug treatment for paucibacillary leprosy. We found no RCT comparing dapsone plus rifampicin versus dapsone alone. Observational studies found that in people taking dapsone plus rifampicin, up to 38% of lesions had resolved at 1 year and relapse rates were low.

Benefits: We found no systematic review or RCT. We found seven observational studies assessing the affects of multidrug treatment (dapsone 100 mg/day plus rifampicin 600 mg monthly for 6 months) with follow up from 6 months to 10 years (see table 1, p 718 and table 2, p 719).[15–22] **Skin lesions:** Three observational studies reported resolution of lesions (see comment below) (see table 1, p 718).[15–19] One study (499 people) found that resolution of lesions occurred in 38% of people after 1 year;[16] another (50 people) found that resolution occurred in 8% of people after 6 months.[15] The number of people with lesions that were clinically active after treatment ranged from 2–44%.[15–17] **Nerve impairment:** Two studies reported the outcome of nerve impairment (see table 1, p 718).[17,19] One (499 people) found that new disabilities occurred in 2.5% of people, and worsening of existing disabilities occurred in 3.3% after 4 years.[19] The other study (130 people) found that the visible disabilities (World Health Organization grade II (see glossary, p 716)) increased from 4% at enrolment to 7% after 8–10 years' follow up.[17] **Relapse rates:** Six observational studies reported relapse rates over a 3–8 year follow up period (see table 2, p 719).[17–22] They reported relapse rates ranging from 0 in Ethiopia[18] to 2.5% over 4 years in Malawi (see table 2, p 719).[19] The risk of relapse ranged from 0.66/1000 person years in China[22] to 6.5/1000 person years in Malawi.[19]

Harms: None of the studies formally monitored adverse effects. In one study, hepatitis due to rifampicin developed in 1/130 (0.8%) people (the method of diagnosis was not stated).[17] In another study 1/503 (0.2%) people suffered an "allergic reaction" to rifampicin and dapsone (details not provided).[16]

Comment: The studies used different methods of assessment making it difficult to compare results. The combination of dapsone plus rifampicin for paucibacillary leprosy was introduced by the World Health Organization in 1982 without formal trials comparing it against dapsone. Studies had shown that 30% of *M leprae* isolates were resistant to dapsone;[23] therefore, a multidrug regime was introduced urgently. It is clinically difficult to differentiate relapse from reaction in paucibacillary leprosy.

QUESTION What are the effects of treatments for multibacillary leprosy? New

OPTION RIFAMPICIN PLUS DAPSONE PLUS CLOFAZIMINE

We found no systematic review or RCTs. We found no RCTs comparing rifampicin plus clofazimine plus dapsone versus dapsone alone, or versus dapsone plus rifampicin. Observational studies found that multidrug treatment improved skin lesions and was associated with a low relapse rate.

Benefits: We found no systematic review or RCTs. We found six observational studies assessing the effects of multidrug treatment (monthly supervised rifampicin 600 mg and clofazimine 300 mg, plus daily unsupervised dapsone 100 mg and clofazimine 500 mg) for 24 months.[17,18,20,22,24,25] **Skin lesions:** One study in Thailand (53 people) found that 29% lesions were still active at 3 years (see table 3, p 720).[17] **Nerve impairment:** The study in Thailand found that the proportion of people with visible deformity (World Health Organization grade II (see glossary, p 716)) increased from 8% at enrolment to 13% at 8–10 years' follow up.[17] **Relapse:** Six observational studies reported relapse rates (see table 4, p 720),[17,18,20,22,24,25] which varied from 0 in Ethiopia to 20.4 per 100 person years (see glossary, p 716) in India. In the study conducted in India, the overall relapse rate was 20/260 (7.7%) over about 8 years (2.04/1000 person years), and 18/20 (90%) relapses were in people with a bacterial index (see glossary, p 716) greater than 4 at the start of treatment.[24]

Harms: Most studies did not report on adverse effects. Skin pigmentation may occur with clofazimine, which may be especially problematic in people with fair skin.

Comment: Only one study[24] stratified its results according to bacterial index. The World Health Organization study group on chemotherapy recommended that treatment be given for 24 months.[26] In 1998, the 7th Expert committee gave the option of reducing the length of treatment from 24 months to 12 months.[1] We found no controlled trial to support this recommendation. We found one RCT (93 people with untreated lepromatous leprosy), which compared dapsone (50 mg/day) plus daily rifampicin (450 mg) versus dapsone (50 mg/day) plus monthly rifampicin (1200 mg) for the first 6 months of treatment.[27] It found no significant difference in clinical improvement between daily versus monthly rifampicin (40/47 [85%] with daily rifampicin *v* 43/46 [91%]; RR 0.91, 95% CI 0.62 to 1.03). Adverse effects were more common with daily versus monthly rifampicin, causing discontinuation in 8.5% of people with daily rifampicin versus 0% with monthly rifampicin.[27]

QUESTION What are the effects of treatments for single skin lesion leprosy? New

OPTION SINGLE DOSE TREATMENTS

One RCT found that 6 months treatment with rifampicin monthly plus dapsone daily significantly increased the cure rate compared with a single dose of rifampicin plus minocycline plus ofloxacin at 18 months. Adverse effects were similar with both regimens.

Benefits: We found no systematic review. We found one RCT (1483 people with single skin lesions typical of paucibacillary leprosy; see comment below) comparing a single administration of rifampicin (600 mg) plus ofloxacin (400 mg) plus minocycline (100 mg) versus multidrug treatment dapsone (100 mg/day) plus rifampicin monthly (600 mg) for 6 months.[28] Outcomes measured at 18 months were based on a scoring system involving five measurements: disappearance of the lesion, reduction in hypopigmentation, reduction in the degree of infiltration, reduction in the size of the lesion, and improvement in sensation in the lesion. Treatment failure was defined as no change or increase of the clinical score, and marked improvement was defined as a difference of 13 between the baseline and 18 month scores. The RCT found that multidrug versus single dose treatment significantly increased the proportion of people with marked improvement (392/684 [57.3%] with multidrug *v* 361/697 [51.8%] with single dose; P = 0.04), and with complete cure (374/684 [54.7%] *v* 327/697 [46.9%]; RR 1.17, 95% CI 1.05 to 1.28; NNT 13, 95% CI 8 to 40). There were 12 treatment failures (6 in each group) and 99.1% of people in both groups had some improvement by the end of the study.[28]

Harms: Allergic reactions (which were not specified) occurred in seven people (6 taking multidose *v* 1 taking single dose treatment), and gastrointestinal effects occurred in five people (2 taking multidose *v* 3 taking single dose treatment). There was no significant difference in the number of type 1 reactions (see glossary, p 716) (7/697 [1.0%] with single dose treatment *v* 3/684 [0.4%] with multidose; ARI +0.6%, 95% CI –0.2% to +3.4%).

Comment: The RCT did not specify its diagnostic criteria and did not confirm the clinical diagnosis. The follow up of only 18 months for people in the single dose treated group is short for detection of relapses. Some infections in this group would have resolved spontaneously, and the absence of a control group means that the treatment effect cannot be estimated.[28] Single dose treatments have previously been assessed in people with paucibacillary leprosy. One RCT (622 people in Zaïre) compared two single dose regimens: rifampicin (40 mg/kg) plus clofazimine (1200 mg) versus rifampicin (40 mg/kg) plus clofazimine (100 mg) plus dapsone (100 mg) plus ethionamide (500 mg). It found that the overall relapse rate was 20.4/1000 person years (see glossary, p 716), which was substantially higher than the relapse rate found for 6 months' treatment with dapsone plus rifampicin (see dapsone plus rifampicin, p 713), or rifampicin plus dapsone plus clofazimine (see rifampicin plus dapsone plus clofazimine, p 714). However, single dose treatment has operational advantages in the field, particularly when people live in remote areas and are unable to attend a clinic for several months.[29]

GLOSSARY

Bacteriological index A measure of the density of *M leprae* in the skin. Slit skin smears are made at several sites, the smears are stained and examined microscopically. The number of bacteria per high power field is scored on a logarithmic scale (0–6) and the index calculated by dividing the total score by the numbers of sites sampled.

Heaf grade 0 = 0–4 mm in duration; 1 = 5–9; 2 = 10–14; 3 = 15–19; 4 = ≥20. A grade 3 or 4 test generally indicates infection with *M tuberculosis*, although the cut off point varies between countries.

ICRC vaccine A vaccine developed at the Indian Cancer Research Centre.

Neuritis Inflammation of a nerve presenting with any of the following: spontaneous nerve pain, paraesthesia, tenderness, sensory, motor, or autonomic impairment.

Person years at risk The number of new cases of disease in a specified time period divided by the number of person years at risk during that period (average number at risk of relapse multiplied by the length of observation)

Type 1 (reversal) reaction A delayed type hypersensitivity reaction occurring at sites of *M leprae* antigen. It presents with acutely inflamed skin lesions and acute neuritis (nerve tenderness with loss of function)

Type 2 reaction or Erythema Nodosum Leprosum (ENL) An immunological complication of multibacillary leprosy presenting with short lived and recurrent crops of tender erythematous subcutaneous nodules which may ulcerate. There may be signs of systemic involvement with fever, inflammation in lymph nodes, nerves, eyes, joints, testes, fingers, toes, or other organs.

World Health Organization disability grading These are simple gradings for use in the field, mainly for collection of general data regarding disabilities.[1] Grade 0 = no anaesthesia, no visible deformity or damage; Grade 1 = anaesthesia present, but no visible deformity or damage; Grade 2 = visible deformity or damage present.

REFERENCES

1. WHO Expert Committee on Leprosy. *World Health Organ Tech Rep Ser* 1988;768:1–51.
2. World Health Organization. Leprosy global situation. *Wkly Epidemiol Rec* 2002;77:1–8.
3. Fine PE. Leprosy: the epidemiology of a slow bacterium. *Epidemiol Rev* 1982;4:161–188.
4. Desikan KV, Sreevatsa. Extended studies on the viability of *Mycobacterium leprae* outside the human body. *Lepr Rev* 1995;66:287–295.
5. Lienhardt C, Kamate B, Jamet P, et al. Effect of HIV infection on leprosy: a three-year survey in Bamako, Mali. *Int J Lepr Other Mycobact Dis* 1996;64:383–391.
6. Croft RP, Richardus JH, Nicholls PG, et al. Nerve function impairment in leprosy: design, methodology, and intake status of a prospective cohort study of 2664 new leprosy cases in Bangladesh (The Bangladesh Acute Nerve Damage Study). *Lepr Rev* 1999;70:140–159.

7. Saunderson P, Gelore S, Desta K, et al. The pattern of leprosy-related neuropathy in the AMFES patients in Ethiopia: definitions, incidence, risk factors and outcome. *Lepr Rev* 2000;71:285–308.
8. Pfaltzgraff R, Ramu G. Clinical leprosy. In: Hastings R ed. *Leprosy*. Edinburgh, Churchill Livingstone, 1994:237–287.
9. van Brakel WH. Peripheral neuropathy in leprosy and its consequences. *Lepr Rev* 2000;71:S146–S153.
10. Brown JA, Stone MM, Sutherland I. BCG vaccination of children against leprosy in Uganda: results at end of second follow-up. *Br Med J* 1968;1:24–27.
11. Bagshawe A, Scott GC, Russell DA, et al. BCG vaccination in leprosy: final results of the trial in Karimui, Papua New Guinea, 1963–79. *Bull World Health Organ* 1989;67:389–399.
12. Lwin K, Sundaresan T, Gyi MM, et al. BCG vaccination of children against leprosy: fourteen-year findings of the trial in Burma. *Bull World Health Organ* 1985;63:1069–1078.
13. Gupte MD, Vallishayee RS, Anantharaman DS, et al. Comparative leprosy vaccine trial in south India. *Indian J Lepr* 1998;70:369–388.
14. Karonga Prevention Trial Group. Randomised controlled trial of single BCG, repeated BCG, or combined BCG and killed *Mycobacterium leprae* vaccine for prevention of leprosy and tuberculosis in Malawi. *Lancet* 1996;348:17–24.
15. Kar PK, Arora PN, Ramasastry CV, et al. A clinicopathological study of multidrug therapy in borderline tuberculoid leprosy. *J Indian Med Assoc* 1994;92:336–337.
16. Boerrigter G, Ponnighaus JM, Fine PE. Preliminary appraisal of a WHO-recommended multiple drug regimen in paucibacillary leprosy patients in Malawi. *Int J Lepr Other Mycobact Dis* 1988;56:408–417.
17. Dasananjali K, Schreuder PA, Pirayavaraporn C. A study on the effectiveness and safety of the WHO/MDT regimen in the northeast of Thailand; a prospective study, 1984–1996. *Int J Lepr Other Mycobact Dis* 1997;65:28–36.
18. Gebre S, Saunderson P, Byass P. Relapses after fixed duration multiple drug therapy: the AMFES cohort. *Lepr Rev* 2000;71:325–331.
19. Boerrigter G, Ponnighaus JM, Fine PE, et al. Four-year follow-up results of a WHO-recommended multiple drug regimen in paucibacillary leprosy patients in Malawi. *Int J Lepr Other Mycobact Dis* 1991;59:255–261.
20. Schreuder PA. The occurrence of reactions and impairments in leprosy: experience in the leprosy control program of three provinces in northeastern Thailand, 1987–1995 [correction of 1978–1995]. I. Overview of the study. *Int J Lepr Other Mycobact Dis* 1998;66:149–158.
21. Chopra NK, Agarawal JS, Pandya PG. A study of relapse in paucibacillary leprosy in a multidrug therapy project, Baroda District, India. *Lepr Rev* 1990;61:157–162.
22. Li HY, Hu LF, Hauang WB, et al. Risk of relapse in leprosy after fixed duration multi-drug therapy. *Int J Lepr Other Mycobact Dis* 1997;65:238–245.
23. Ji B. Drug resistance in leprosy – a review. *Lepr Rev* 1985;56:265–278.
24. Girdhar BK, Girdhar A, Kumar A. Relapses in multibacillary leprosy patients: effect of length of therapy. *Lepr Rev* 2000;71:144–153.
25. Shaw IN, Natrajan MM, Rao GS, et al. Long-term follow up of multibacillary leprosy patients with high BI treated with WHO/MDT regimen for a fixed duration of two years. *Int J Lepr Other Mycobact Dis* 2000;68:405–409.
26. Chemotherapy of leprosy. Report of a WHO study group. WHO Technical Report Series, No 847, 1994
27. Yawalkar SJ, McDougall AC, Languillon J, et al. Once-monthly rifampicin plus daily dapsone in initial treatment of lepromatous leprosy. *Lancet* 1982;1:1199–1202.
28. Single-lesion Multicentre Trial Group. Efficacy of single-dose multidrug therapy for the treatment of single-lesion paucibacillary leprosy. *Ind J Leprosy* 1997.
29. Pattyn SR. A randomized clinical trial of two single-dose treatments for paucibacillary leprosy. *Lepr Rev* 1994;65(1):45–57.

Diana Lockwood
Consultant Leprologist
London School of Hygiene & Topical Medicine and The Hospital for Tropical Diseases
London
UK

Competing interests: None declared.

TABLE 1 **Dapsone plus rifampicin in paucibacillary leprosy — clinical outcomes (see text, p 711).**

Ref	Location	Cohort size	Follow up (years)	Skin lesions	Nerve impairment
16, 19	Malawi	499	1[16] 4[19]	**At 1 year[16]** *Not evident:* 180/473 (38.0%)[16] *Visible but not active:* 282/473 (59.6%)[16] *Visible and active:* 11/473 (2.3%)[16]	**At 4 years[19]** *New disabilities:* 12/484 (2.5%)[16] *Worsening of existing disabilities:* 16/484 (3.3%)[16]
15	India	50	0.5	*Inactive:* 4/50 (8%) *Marked improvement:* 16/50 (32%) *Regression (active):* 22/50 (44%) *Increased activity:* 8/50 (16%)	No data
17	Thailand	130	8–10	*Clinically active after treatment:* 27/123 (22%)	*Grade 2 disability:* At enrolment, 4% At follow up, 7% (absolute numbers not provided)

TABLE 2 Dapsone plus rifampicin in paucibacillary leprosy — relapse rates (see text, p 711).

Ref	Location	Cohort size	Treatment	Follow up (years)	Relapse rate
20	Thailand	420	MDT	About 5	8/393 (2.0%) 4.1/1000 PYAR (estimated as timescale not definite)
19	Malawi	499	MDT	4	12/484 (2.5%) 6.5/1000 PYAR
21	India	11 095	MDT (723 people received a second course)	3	21/10 995 (0.19%) PYAR not calculable as relapse rate for people receiving two courses was not presented separately
22	China	878 (who had not previously received chemotherapy)	MDT	5	0.66/1000 PYAR
17	Thailand	124	MDT	Mean 8.2	2/112 [1.8%] 2.0/1000 PYAR
18	Ethiopia	246	MDT	Mean 4.1	0

MDT, multidrug treatment; PYAR, person-years at risk.

TABLE 3 Dapsone/rifampicin in multibacillary leprosy — clinical outcomes (see text, p 714).

Ref	Location	Cohort size	Skin lesions	Nerve impairment
17	Thailand	53	Clinically active at about 3 years: 14/49 (29%)	Grade 2 disability: Start of treatment: 8% End of treatment: 13%

TABLE 4 Dapsone plus rifampicin in multibacillary leprosy — relapse rates (see text, p 714).

Ref	Location	Cohort size	Follow up (years)	Relapse rate
20	Thailand	220	3	2/198 (1.0%) 3.3/1000 PYAR
22	China	2318	10	0/1000 PYAR
17	Thailand	53 (12 with BI ≥ 5 at enrolment	8 (range 2–10)	0/1000 PYAR
18	Ethiopia	256 (57 people with BI > 4 at enrolment)	4.3 (range 0–8.6) 38% followed up for ≥ 5 years	0/1000 PYAR
24	India	260	Range 1–8	20/260 (7.6%) 20.4/1000 PYAR 18/20 (90%) with BI > 4 at enrolment
25	India	65	Range 1–8	1/46 (2.1%) 0.023/1000 PYAR

BI, bacterial index; PYAR, person years at risk.

Lyme disease

Search date May 2002

Edward Hayes

QUESTIONS

INTERVENTIONS

Beneficial

Three doses of recombinant Osp–A Lyme disease vaccine with adjuvant in immunocompetent people aged 15–70 years exposed to North American strains of *Borrelia burgdorferi* 724

Prophylactic treatment of tick bite....725

Likely to be beneficial

Penicillin (better than placebo for Lyme arthritis)....726

Doxycycline (as effective as amoxicillin and probenecid for Lyme arthritis)....726

*Ceftriaxone (more effective than penicillin for Lyme arthritis)..726

*Cefotaxime (more effective than penicillin for Lyme arthritis)..726

*Cefotaxime (more effective than penicillin for late neurological Lyme disease)....728

Unknown effectiveness

Lyme disease vaccine in Europe or Asia....725

Ceftriaxone (in late neurological Lyme disease)....728

Likely to be ineffective or harmful

Oral antibiotic treatment of people with Lyme arthritis plus neuroborreliosis....726

Ceftriaxone plus doxycycline (in people with late neurological Lyme disease who had been previously treated)....728

*Based on subgroup analysis of RCTs

See glossary, p 729

Key Messages

Administration of Lyme disease vaccine

- **Lyme disease vaccine in Europe or Asia** We found no evidence about the effectiveness of recombinant outer surface protein A (Osp–A) vaccine in European or Asian populations. There is heterogeneity of the species that cause Lyme disease in Europe and Asia. The vaccine may not be as effective in European or Asian populations as it is in North American.
- **Three doses of recombinant Osp–A Lyme disease vaccine with adjuvant in immunocompetent people aged 15–70 years exposed to North American strains of Borrelia burgdorferi** One RCT has found that a vaccine (consisting of recombinant outer surface protein A [Osp–A] of *Borrelia burgdorferi* combined with adjuvant) versus placebo significantly reduces the incidence of Lyme disease in people at high risk of developing Lyme disease within North America (NNT 110, 95% CI 80 to 167 after 3 doses).

Clin Evid 2002;8:721–733.

Prophylactic treatment of tick bite

- **Prophylactic treatment of tick bite** Combined results from RCTs have found that prophylactic antibiotics versus placebo for the treatment of tick bite reduce the incidence of Lyme disease.

Treatment of Lyme arthritis

- **Cefotaxime (more effective than penicillin for Lyme arthritis)** One RCT found weak evidence from subgroup analysis of people with Lyme arthritis that cefotaxime versus penicillin significantly increased the number of people with full recovery at 2 years (NNT 4, 95% CI 2 to 10).
- **Ceftriaxone (more effective than penicillin for Lyme arthritis)** One RCT found weak evidence from subgroup analysis of people with Lyme arthritis that ceftriaxone versus penicillin significantly improved symptoms at 3 months (NNT 2, 95% CI 1 to 4).
- **Doxycycline (as effective as amoxicillin and probenecid for Lyme arthritis)** One RCT in people with Lyme arthritis has found no significant difference between doxycycline versus amoxicillin plus probenicid in resolution of Lyme arthritis.
- **Oral antibiotic treatment of people with Lyme arthritis plus neuroborreliosis** Some people have developed symptoms of neuroborreliosis after oral antibiotic treatment of Lyme arthritis.
- **Penicillin (better than placebo for Lyme arthritis)** One RCT in people with Lyme arthritis has found that penicillin versus placebo significantly increases resolution of Lyme arthritis at 3 weeks (NNT 2, 95% CI 1 to 8).

Treatment of late neurological Lyme disease

- **Cefotaxime (more effective than penicillin for late neurological Lyme disease)** One RCT found weak evidence from subgroup analysis of people with late Lyme disease that cefotaxime versus penicillin significantly increased the number of people with full recovery at 2 years (NNT 4, 95% CI 3 to 12).
- **Ceftriaxone (in late neurological Lyme disease)** One RCT found weak evidence from subgroup analysis in people with late neurological Lyme disease and found that there was no significant difference between ceftriaxone versus cefotaxime in the proportion of people who were asymptomatic at 8 months after treatment.
- **Ceftriaxone plus doxycycline (in people with late neurological Lyme disease who had been previously treated)** One RCT comparing ceftriaxone plus doxycycline versus placebo in people with previously treated Lyme disease and persistent neurological symptoms found no significant difference in health related quality of life at interim analysis at 180 days; therefore the RCT was terminated.

DEFINITION Lyme disease is an inflammatory illness resulting from infection with spirochetes of the *Borrelia burgdorferi* genospecies transmitted to humans by ticks. Some infected people have no symptoms. The characteristic manifestation of early Lyme disease is erythema migrans: a circular rash at the site of the infectious tick attachment that expands over a period of days to weeks in 80–90% of people with Lyme disease. Early disseminated infection may cause secondary erythema migrans, disease of the nervous system (facial palsy or other cranial neuropathies, meningitis, and radiculoneuritis), musculoskeletal disease (arthralgia) and, rarely, cardiac disease (myocarditis or transient atrioventricular block). Untreated or inadequately treated Lyme disease can cause late disseminated manifestations weeks to months after infection. These late manifestations include arthritis, polyneuropathy, and encephalopathy. Diagnosis of Lyme disease is based primarily on clinical findings and a high likelihood of exposure to infected ticks. Serological testing may be helpful in people with endemic exposure who have clinical findings consistent with later stage disseminated Lyme disease.

INCIDENCE/ PREVALENCE Lyme disease occurs in temperate regions of North America, Europe, and Asia. It is the most commonly reported vector borne disease in the USA, with over 16 000 cases reported a year.[1] Most cases occur in the northeastern and northcentral states, with a reported annual incidence in endemic states as high as 67.9/100 000 people.[1] In highly endemic communities, the incidence of Lyme disease may exceed 1000/100 000 people a year.[2] In some countries of Europe, the incidence of Lyme disease has been estimated to be over 100/100 000 people a year.[3] Foci of Lyme disease have been described in northern forested regions of Russia, in China, and in Japan.[4] Transmission cycles of *B burgdorferi* have not been described in tropical areas or in the Southern hemisphere.[4]

AETIOLOGY/ RISK FACTORS Lyme disease is caused by infection with any of the *B burgdorferi* sensu lato genospecies. Virtually all cases of Lyme disease in North America are the result of infection with *B burgdorferi*. In Europe, Lyme disease may be caused by *B burgdorferi*, *B garinii,* and *B afzelii*. The infectious spirochetes are transmitted to humans through the bite of certain *Ixodes* ticks.[4] Humans who have frequent or prolonged exposure to the habitats of infected *Ixodes* ticks are at highest risk of acquiring Lyme disease. Individual risk depends on the likelihood of being bitten by infected tick vectors, which varies with the density of vector ticks in the environment, the prevalence of infection in ticks, and the extent of a person's contact with infected ticks. The risk of Lyme disease is often concentrated in focal areas. In the USA, risk is highest in certain counties within northeastern and northcentral states during the months of April to July.[2] People become infected when they engage in activities in wooded or bushy areas that are favourable habitats for ticks, and deer and rodent hosts.

PROGNOSIS Lyme disease is rarely fatal. Untreated Lyme arthritis resolves at a rate of 10–20% a year; over 90% of facial palsies due to Lyme disease resolve spontaneously, and most cases of Lyme carditis resolve without sequelae.[5] However, untreated Lyme disease can result in arthritis (50% of untreated people), meningitis or neuropathies (15% of untreated people), carditis (5–10% of untreated people with erythema migrans) and, rarely, encephalopathy.

AIMS To prevent Lyme disease; to ameliorate or eliminate the symptoms of established Lyme disease; to reduce sequelae, with minimal adverse effects.

OUTCOMES **For prophylaxis:** incidence of Lyme disease, adverse events. **For treatment:** incidence, prevalence, or severity of symptoms and signs of short term manifestations; long term sequelae of infection; quality of life.

METHODS *Clinical Evidence* update search and appraisal May 2002. Additional searches of author's files.

QUESTION What are the effects of measures to prevent Lyme disease?

OPTION LYME DISEASE VACCINE

One RCT has found that recombinant outer surface lipoprotein A (Osp–A) vaccine versus placebo significantly reduces the incidence of Lyme disease in immunocompetent adults 15 years or older in North America who are at high risk of Lyme disease. We found no evidence about the effectiveness of this vaccine in Europe or Asia, where a greater variety of *B burgdorferi* genospecies cause Lyme disease.

Benefits: We found no systematic review but found one RCT (10 936 people, aged 15–70 years, living in endemic areas in the USA) that compared a vaccine made of recombinant outer surface lipoprotein A (Osp–A) plus adjuvant (see glossary, p 729) versus placebo.[6] People in the RCT were self selected and were at high risk of Lyme disease. The RCT found that, compared with placebo, the vaccine significantly reduced laboratory confirmed Lyme disease after two doses in the first year (AR of developing Lyme disease 22/5469 [0.4%] with vaccine *v* 43/5467 [0.8%] with placebo; RR 0.51, 95% CI 0.31 to 0.85; NNT 260, 95% CI 146 to 1046). After a third dose 1 year later, there was a greater reduction of the incidence of laboratory confirmed Lyme disease (16/5469 [0.3%] with vaccine *v* 66/5467 [1.2%] with placebo; RR 0.24, 95% CI 0.14 to 0.42; NNT 110, 95% CI 80 to 167); asymptomatic infection was prevented completely (0/5469 [0%] with vaccine *v* 15/5467 [0.3%] with placebo; NNT 365, 95% CI 222 to 687).

Harms: We found nine RCTs evaluating adverse effects of Osp–A vaccines.[6–14] No serious adverse events were found to be causally related to the vaccine in any of these trials. The results are summarised in table 1 (see, p 731).

Comment: The rOsp–A vaccine is no longer commercially available. **Applicability of the evidence:** The absolute benefit of vaccination in the RCT was high (1 case of Lyme disease prevented for every 110 people vaccinated), which was partly because the people recruited into the RCT were self selected and had a very high incidence of Lyme disease in the untreated group.[6] If the risk of Lyme disease in the unvaccinated population was 100/100 000 people a year (comparable to the reported Lyme disease incidence in many endemic areas),[1,3] then about 1316 people would need to be vaccinated to prevent one case of Lyme disease. We found no evidence about the effectiveness of this vaccine in Europe or Asia, and no clinical evidence of efficacy in children. **Other RCTs:** One RCT evaluated the efficacy of recombinant Osp–A vaccine without adjuvant.[7] It found that the vaccine reduced the incidence of Lyme disease by 68% (95% CI 36% to 85%) after two doses in the first year. However, the criteria for confirming the diagnosis of Lyme disease were not clearly defined. Of 1734 suspected cases of Lyme disease in 2 years, only 499 were reviewed "in depth" by the Data and Safety Monitoring Board. The RCT reported an estimate of vaccine efficacy after a third dose of vaccine, but this dose was not part of the original RCT protocol, was given only to a subset of participants, and the criteria for selection of the subset who received the third dose were not specified. This RCT found that the efficacy of vaccine was highest in people aged less than 60 years, but results for this subgroup were not provided.[7]

QUESTION Prophylactic treatment of tick bite

One RCT and a meta-analysis by *Clinical Evidence* have found that prophylactic antibiotics versus placebo for the treatment of tick bite significantly reduce the incidence of Lyme disease.

Benefits: We found one systematic review[15] and one subsequent RCT[16] comparing prophylactic antibiotics versus placebo for the treatment of tick bite (see table 2, p 733). The review (search date 1995, 3 RCTs, 639 adults and children who recognised *Ixodes scapularis* tick bites in the preceding 72 h) found that prophylactic treatment with antibiotics (penicillin, amoxicillin [amoxycillin], and tetracycline were studied in the individual trials) versus placebo reduced the risk of developing clinical Lyme disease (erythema migrans), but the difference was not significant (0/308 [0%] with antibiotics *v* 4/292 [1.4%] with placebo; ARR 1.4%, 95% CI 0% to 3%; OR 0.0, 95% CI 0.0 to 1.5); P = 0.12).[15] The subsequent RCT (482 people ≥ 12 years old who had removed an attached *I scapularis* tick in the preceding 72 h) compared doxycycline (200 mg as a single dose) versus placebo.[16] It found that doxycycline versus placebo significantly reduced the number of people with erythema migrans at the site of the tick bite after 6 weeks (1/235 [0.4%] with doxycycline *v* 8/247 [3.2%] with placebo; ARR 2.8%, 95% CI 0.4% to 5.2%; NNT 36, 95% CI 20 to 250), and the number of people with any evidence of Lyme disease (erythema migrans at the site of the tick bite, or at other sites, or a viral-like illness with laboratory evidence of Lyme disease, 3/235 [1.3%] with doxycycline *v* 11/247 [4.5%] with placebo; ARR 3.2%, 95% CI 0.2% to 6.2%; NNT 31). Of 431 people who had serum samples tested at study entry and 3 and 6 weeks later, none had asymptomatic seroconversion for antibody to *B burgdorferi*. Erythema migrans at the site of the tick bite only occurred after the removed tick was in the nymph stage, was partially engorged, and was estimated to be attached for more than 72 hours. A subgroup analysis found that in people who removed partially engorged nymphal ticks, doxycycline versus placebo reduced erythema migrans at the site of the tick bite (AR 1/78 [1.3%] with doxycycline *v* 8/81 [9.9%] with placebo; ARR 8.6%, 95% CI 1.4% to 15.8%; NNT 12, 95% CI 7 to 71). Meta-analysis of the RCTs in the review and the subsequent RCT by *Clinical Evidence* found that antibiotics versus placebo significantly reduced the number of people with erythema migrans (1/543 [0.2%] *v* 12/539 [2.2%]; ARR 2%, 95% CI 0.7% to 3.3%; RR 0.19, 95% CI 0.05 to 0.72; NNT 49, 95% CI 30 to 135) and also reduced the number of people with any evidence of Lyme disease (3/543 [0.6%] *v* 18/539 [3.3%]; ARR 2%, 95% CI 1% to 4%; RR 0.25, 95% CI 0.09 to 0.69; see web extra figures A and B at www.clinicalevidence.com).

Harms: One RCT in the review reported a rash with penicillin (AR 1/27 [4%] with penicillin *v* 0/29 [0%] with placebo; NNH 27), and another RCT reported a rash with amoxicillin (AR 2/205 [1%] with amoxicillin *v* 0/182 [0%] with placebo; NNH 103).[16] The third RCT in the review reported no adverse effects among persons who had been treated with antibiotics. The RCT conducted after the review found that of the 309 people who recorded data on adverse events, significantly more people taking doxycycline versus placebo had nausea or vomiting (33/156 [21.0 %] with doxycycline *v* 6/153 [3.9%] with placebo; ARI 17.2%, 95% CI 9.8% to 24.6%; NNH 6).[16]

Comment: There is a possibility that people treated with antibiotics for tick bite may not develop erythema migrans but could progress to late stages of Lyme disease. However, none of the people who were treated with antibiotics in the RCTs had asymptomatic infection with *B burgdorferi*, or developed late manifestations of Lyme disease during follow up (ranging from 6 wks to up to 3 years). The most recent and largest RCT found that for a baseline risk of 1% for contracting Lyme disease in the control group, the number needed to treat for a single dose of doxycycline (200 mg) to prevent Lyme disease was 31 over a 6 week period. The same RCT found that the number needed to harm for nausea or vomiting from this treatment was six; therefore, about five people would develop nausea or vomiting for every person in whom Lyme disease was prevented. People in the RCT with adult and/or non-engorged ticks did not develop Lyme disease, although Lyme disease can occur following the bite of an engorged adult tick. If treatment was limited to people with engorged nymphal ticks (NNT 12), then two people would develop nausea and less than one person would develop vomiting for every person in whom Lyme disease was prevented.

QUESTION What are the effects of antibiotic treatment for Lyme disease arthritis?

One RCT has found that penicillin versus saline placebo significantly increases resolution of Lyme arthritis. Another RCT found no significant difference between doxycycline versus amoxicillin plus probenicid in resolving Lyme arthritis. Other RCTs have reported results for subgroups of people with Lyme arthritis and have found that ceftriaxone and cefotaxime may both be more effective than penicillin at improving Lyme arthritis. Some people have developed symptoms of neuroborreliosis after oral antibiotic treatment of arthritis.

Benefits: We found no systematic review. **People with Lyme arthritis:** We found two RCTs that selected people with Lyme disease arthritis and randomised them to different treatments.[20,21] The first RCT (40 people with Lyme disease arthritis) compared intramuscular benzathine penicillin (7.3 MU/wk for 3 wks) versus saline placebo.[20] It found that penicillin versus saline increased the number of people having complete resolution of the arthritis (AR 7/20 [35%] with penicillin *v* 0/20 [0%] with placebo; NNT 2, 95% CI 1 to 8). The second RCT (48 people with Lyme arthritis) compared oral doxycycline (100 mg twice daily for 30 days) versus oral amoxicillin (500 mg) plus probenicid (four times daily for 30 days).[22] After 3 months, an intention to treat analysis found similar rates of arthritis resolution in both groups (AR 18/25 [72%] with doxycyline v 16/23 [70%] with amoxicillin plus probenicid; RR 1.04, 95% CI 0.72 to 1.49). In the doxycycline group, one person had recurrence of arthritis and another developed polyneuropathy after treatment. In the amoxicillin plus probenicid group, one person had recurrent arthritis, two developed polyneuropathy, and two developed encephalopathy. **Subgroup analyses:** We found three other RCTs that recruited people with a variety of forms of late Lyme disease (including Lyme arthritis).[22–24] The first RCT (23 people with late Lyme disease, 70% with arthritis) compared ceftriaxone (2 g iv every 12 h for 14 days) versus penicillin (4 MU iv every 4 h for 10 days).[22] Ceftriaxone appeared to be more effective than penicillin, but the differences in rates of clinical improvement after 3 months were not significant (AR of improvement 12/13 [92%] with ceftriaxone v 5/10 [50%] with penicillin; RR 1.85, 95% CI 0.97 to 3.50). More of the subgroup of people with arthritis improved with ceftriaxone (AR 9/9 [100%] with ceftriaxone v 2/7 [29%] with penicillin; NNT 2, 95% CI 1 to 4). The second RCT (135 people with late Lyme disease, 73 with arthritis) compared cefotaxime (6 g/day for 8–10 days) versus penicillin G (20 MU/day for 8–19 days).[24] Two years after treatment, full recovery was more frequent with cefotaxime (AR 44/69 [64%] with cefotaxime v 25/66 [38%] with penicillin; RR 1.68, 95% CI 1.18 to 2.41; NNT 3, 95% CI 2 to 11). In the subgroup of people with arthritis, recovery was also increased by cefotaxime (17/39 [44%] with cefotaxime v 4/34 [12%] with penicillin; RR 3.7, 95% CI 1.4 to 9.9; NNT 4, 95% CI 2 to 10). The third RCT (62 people with disseminated Lyme disease, 13 people with Lyme arthritis) did not report separate results for the subgroup with arthritis. It compared intravenous ceftriaxone followed by oral amoxicillin plus probenicid versus oral cefixime plus probenicid.[25]

Harms: Some people have developed symptoms of neuroborreliosis (see glossary, p 729) after oral antibiotic treatment of arthritis. Jarisch-Herxheimer reactions (see glossary, p 729) have been described in people treated for late Lyme disease. This reaction was reported in 11/44 (25%) people treated with ceftriaxone,[22] in 10/66 (15%) treated with penicillin, and 19/69 (28%) treated with cefotaxime (RR with cefotaxime v with penicillin 1.8, 95% CI 0.9 to 3.6; NNH 8).[24] Possible "Herxheimer-like" reactions, including fever, transient rash, and worsening of symptoms or cardiac arrhythmia, were reported in an unspecified number of people treated with cefixime and probenicid, and with ceftriaxone followed by amoxicillin.[25] No significant differences were found in the risk of developing a prolonged form of such reactions for people receiving ceftriaxone plus amoxicillin versus cefixime plus probenecid (18/30 [60%] with ceftriaxone and amoxicillin treatment v 12/30 [40%] with cefixime and probenicid; RR 1.50, 95% CI 0.88 to 2.54). Other harms include those expected from the antibiotics. In RCTs including people with Lyme arthritis, the following adverse effects were reported: diarrhoea and skin rash with ceftriaxone;[22] shock and colitis with penicillin; anaphylaxis and colitis with cefotaxime;[22] rash and gastrointestinal effects with amoxicillin and probenicid;[21] diarrhoea and rash with cefixime; and nausea, diarrhoea, and rash with ceftriaxone followed by amoxicillin.[24]

Comment: Results of the RCTs that presented results for subgroups of people with Lyme arthritis should be interpreted with caution as people with arthritis were not randomly assigned to treatment groups. The RCTs were small, and the type, dose, and regimen of antibiotics used varied between trials. The enrolment criteria also varied between trials. Only one RCT had a placebo control.[21] The proportion of people who respond in comparative RCTs is difficult to interpret because, without a placebo comparison, it is unclear how many people would have responded without treatment.

QUESTION What are the effects of antibiotic treatments for late neurological Lyme disease?

One RCT comparing ceftriaxone plus doxycycline versus placebo in people with previously treated Lyme disease and persistent late neurological symptoms found no significant difference in health related quality of life at interim analysis at 180 days, and therefore was terminated. One small RCT that reported results for a subgroup of people with late neurological Lyme disease found weak evidence that cefotaxime may be more effective than penicillin in eliminating neurological symptoms. A small RCT of people with neuroborreliosis of varying durations found no significant difference between cefotaxime and ceftriaxone in the number of people asymptomatic after 8 months.

Benefits: We found no systematic review. **People with late neurological Lyme disease:** We found one RCT (129 people, 78 people seropositive for *B burgdorferi*, 51 people who were seronegative) comparing antibiotics (iv ceftriaxone 2 g/day for 30 days followed by oral doxycycline 100 mg twice daily for 60 days) versus placebo.[25] All participants had been previously treated for Lyme disease but had persistent symptoms including arthralgia, myalgia, neurocognitive changes, altered sensation, malaise, headache, and sleep disturbance. At 180 days, a planned interim analysis of 107 people found that the probability of finding a significant difference in health related quality of life (measured on the medical outcomes survey short form general health survey; SF-36) after full study enrolment was less than 5%, and the study was therefore terminated.[25] **Subgroup analyses:** We found two comparative RCTs that reported results for people with late neurological Lyme disease.[23,24,26] The first RCT (135 people with late Lyme disease, 93 with neuropathy) compared cefotaxime (6 g/day for 8–10 days) versus penicillin G (20 MU/day for 8–19 days).[23] Two years after treatment, cefotaxime versus penicillin significantly increased complete recovery (44/69 [64%] with cefotaxime *v* 25/66 [38%] with penicillin; RR 1.68, 95% CI 1.18 to 2.41; NNT 4, 95% CI 3 to 12). Similar results were reported for the subgroup with neuropathy (35/49 [71%] with cefotaxime *v* 20/44 [46%] with penicillin; RR 1.57, 95% CI 1.09 to 2.27; NNT 4). The second RCT (33 people with Lyme neuroborreliosis (see glossary, p 729) of varying duration) compared ceftriaxone (2 g iv/day for 10 days) versus cefotaxime (2 g iv every 8 h for 10 days).[26] Some of the people treated with ceftriaxone were asymptomatic prior to treatment, and so were excluded from analysis (3/17). Of the remaining people, most (17/30) had disease duration of over 30 days at study entry, and some (8/30) had a duration over 60 days. The RCT found no significant difference in the number of people who were asymptomatic after 8 months (8/14 [57%] with ceftriaxone *v* 9/16 [56%] with cefotaxime; RR 1.02, 95% CI 0.54 to 1.90).

Harms: See harms under treatments for Lyme disease arthritis, p 727. The RCT in people with previously treated Lyme disease found no significant difference in the overall rate of adverse events between the antibiotic and placebo groups. In the other clinical trials involving late neurological Lyme disease reported above, the following adverse effects were reported: shock and colitis with penicillin, and anaphylaxis and colitis with cefotaxime;[22] rash with cefotaxime, and fever, diarrhoea, and elevated liver enzymes with ceftriaxone.[26] One case control study found an association between biliary disease and ceftriaxone treatment of suspected late Lyme disease.[27]

Comment: The RCTs of untreated people either recruited people with late Lyme disease, some of whom had neurological manifestations, or people with Lyme neuroborreliosis, some of whom had late disease. Results presented for these subsets of study participants may be subject to undetected biases, because people with late neurological disease were not randomly assigned to treatment groups. None of these RCTs had a placebo treated control group. The antibiotics used in RCTs, as well as doses and schedules, varied between trials. The enrolment criteria also varied between trials.

GLOSSARY

Adjuvant A substance such as aluminium hydroxide included in a vaccine to enhance its effectiveness.

Jarisch-Herxheimer reaction An inflammatory reaction in tissues induced by antibiotic treatment of spirochetal diseases, and believed to be caused by an immunological reaction to the release of spirochetal antigens.

Neuroborreliosis Central or peripheral neuropathy resulting from infection with *Borrelia sp* spirochetes.

REFERENCES

1. Orloski KA, Hayes EB, Campbell GL, et al. Surveillance for Lyme disease – United States, 1992–1998. *Mor Mortal Wkly Rep* 2000;49(SS-3):1–11.
2. Centers for Disease Control. Recommendations for the use of Lyme disease vaccine: recommendations of the Advisory Committee on Immunization Practices (ACIP). *Mor Mortal Wkly Rep* 1999;48(RR-7):1–17, 21–25.
3. O'Connel S, Granstorm M, Gray JS, et al. Epidemiology of European Lyme borreliosis. *Zentralbl Bakteriol* 1998;287:229–240.
4. Dennis DT. Epidemiology, ecology, and prevention of Lyme disease. In: Rahn DW, Evans J, eds. *Lyme disease*. Philadelphia, PA, USA: American College of Physicians, 1998:7–34.
5. Rahn DW, Evans J, eds. *Lyme disease*. Philadelphia, PA, USA: American College of Physicians, 1998.
6. Steere AC, Sikand VJ, Meurice F, et al. Vaccination against Lyme disease with recombinant Borrelia burgdorferi outer-surface lipoprotein A with adjuvant. *N Engl J Med* 1998;339:209–215.
7. Sigal LH, Zahradnik JM, Lavin P, et al. A vaccine consisting of recombinant Borrelia burgorferi outer-surface protein A to prevent Lyme disease. *N Engl J Med* 1998;339:216–222.
8. Feder HM, Beran J, Van Hoecke C, et al. Immunogenicity of a recombinant Borrelia burgdorferi outer surface protein A vaccine against Lyme disease in children. *J Pediatr* 1999;135:575–579.
9. Keller D, Koster FT, Marks DH, et al. Safety and immunogenicity of a recombinant outer surface protein A Lyme vaccine. *JAMA* 1994;271:1764–1768.
10. Van Hoecke C, Comberbach M, De Grave D, et al. Evaluation of the saftey, reactogenicity and immonogenicity of three recombinant outer surface protein (OspA) Lyme vaccines in healthy adults. *Vaccine* 1996;14(17–18):1620–1626.
11. Beran J, De Clercq N, Dieussaert I, et al. Reactogenicity and immunogenicity of a Lyme disease vaccine in children 2–5 years old. *Clin Infec Dis* 2000;31:1504–1507.
12. Sikand VJ, Halsey N, Krause PJ, et al. Safety and immunogeniciy of a recombinant Borrelia burgdorferi outer surface protein A vaccine against

Lyme disease in health children and adolescents: a randomized controlled trial. *Pediatrics* 2001;108:123–128.
13. Van Hoecke C, Lebacq E, Beran J, et al. Alternative vaccination schedules (0, 1, and 6 months versus 0, 1, and 12 months) for a recombinant OspA Lyme disease vaccine. *Clin Infect Dis* 1999;28(6):1260–1264.
14. Schoen RT, Sikand VK, Caldwell MC, et al. Safety and immunogenicity profile of a recombinant outer-surface protein A Lyme disease vaccine: clinical trial of a 3-dose schedule at 0, 1, and 2 months. *Clin Ther* 22(3):315–325.
15. Warshafsky S, Nowakowski J, Nadelman RB, et al. Efficacy of antibiotic prophylaxis for prevention of Lyme disease. *J Gen Intern Med* 1996;11:329–333. Search date 1995; primary sources Medline and hand search of reference list for english language papers.
16. Nadelman RB, Nowakowski J, Fish D, et al, and Tick and Bite Study Group. Prophylaxis with single-dose doxycycline for the prevention of Lyme disease after an Ixodes scapularis tick bite. *New Engl J Med* 2001;345:79–84.
17. Costello CM, Steere AC, Pinkerton RE, et al. A prospective study of tick bites in an endemic area for Lyme disease. *J Infect Dis* 1989;159:136–139.
18. Shapiro ED, Gerber MA, Holabird NB, et al. A controlled trial of antimicrobial prophylaxis for Lyme disease after deer-tick bites. *New Engl J Med* 1992;327:1769–1773.
19. Agre F, Schwartz R. The value of early treatment of deer tick bites for the prevention of Lyme disease. *Am J Dis Children* 1993;147:945–947.
20. Steere AC, Green J, Schoen RT, et al. Succesful parenteral penicillin therapy of established Lyme arthritis. *N Engl J Med* 1985;312:869–874.
21. Steere AC, Levin RE, Molloy PJ, et al. Treatment of Lyme arthritis. *Arthr Rheum* 1994;37:878–888.
22. Dattwyler RJ, Halperin JJ, Volkman DJ, et al. Treatment of late Lyme borreliosis — randomized comparison of ceftriaxone and penicillin. *Lancet* 1998;1:1191–1194.
23. Hassler D, Zoller M, Haude H-D, et al. Cefotaxime versus penicillin in the late stage of Lyme disease — prospective, randomized therapeutic study. *Infection* 1990;18:16–20.
24. Oksi J, Nikoskelainen J, Vijanen MK. Comparison of oral cefixime and intravenous ceftriaxone followed by oral amoxicillin in disseminated Lyme borreliosis. *Eur J Clin Microbiol Infect Dis* 1998;17:715–719.
25. Klempner MS, Hu LT, Evans J, et al. Two controlled trials of antibiotic treatment in patients with persistent symptoms and a history of Lyme disease. *New Engl J Med* 2001;345(2):85–92.
26. Pfister H-W, Preac-Mursic V, Wilske B, et al. Randomized comparison of ceftriaxone and cefotaxime in Lyme neuroborreliosis. *J Infect Dis* 1991;163:311–318.
27. Ettestad PJ, Campbell GL, Welbel SF, et al. Biliary complications in the treatment of unsubstantiated Lyme disease. *J Infect Dis* 1995;171:356–361.

Edward Hayes
Chief, Epidemiology Section
US Centers for Disease Control and Prevention
Fort Collins Colorado
USA

Competing interests: None declared.

TABLE 1 **Adverse effects related to Lyme disease vaccine; results of RCTs (see text, p 724).[6–14]**

Ref	Study population	Regimen	Local effects	Systemic effects
Versus placebo comparisons				
6	10 936 people (15–70 years), 9998 evaluated for adverse effects	Osp–A 30 μg *v* placebo at 0, 1, and 12 months	Pain, redness, swelling: vaccine *v* placebo; all $P < 0.001$	**< 30 days** Myalgias, achiness, influenza-like illness, fever, chills (all $P < 0.001$) **> 30 days** Similar in both groups
12	4087 people (4–18 years)	Osp–A 30 μg *v* placebo at 0, 1, and 12 months	Pain, redness, swelling: vaccine *v* placebo; 78% *v* 55%; $P < 0.001$	Fever, fatigue, headache, rash, arthralgia: vaccine *v* placebo; 30% *v* 22%; $P < 0.001$
7	10 305 people (≥ 18 years)	Osp–A 30 μg *v* placebo at 0 and 1 month (7515 people had booster at 12 months)	Pain at injection site: vaccine *v* placebo *1st dose:* 0.3% *v* 0.04% *2nd dose:* 0.8% *v* 0.1% *3rd dose:* 1.5% *v* 0.2%	Musculoskeletal: vaccine *v* placebo *1st dose:* 6.4% *v* 1.3% *2nd dose:* 3.3% *v* 1.1% *3rd dose:* not stated
9	36 people (18–65 years)	Adjuvanted Osp–A 10 μg *v* unadjuvanted Osp–A 10 μg *v* placebo	Pain, tenderness, or both were more common with vaccine *v* placebo; small sample size	Small sample size

Ref	Population	Intervention	Local symptoms	Systemic symptoms
Dose versus dose comparisons				
11	91 children (2–5 years old)	Osp–A 15 μg *v* Osp–A 30 μg, both given at 0 and 1 month	Pain, redness, swelling: Osp–A 15 μg *v* Osp–A 30 μg; 77.2% *v* 77.8%; P > 0.05	Arthralgia, drowsiness, fever, irritability, rash: Osp–A 15 μg *v* Osp–A 30 μg; 47.8% *v* 38.9%; P > 0.05
8	250 children (5–15 years)	Osp–A 15 μg *v* Osp–A 30 μg, both with adjuvant and given at 0, 1, and 2 months	Redness, swelling, soreness: no significant difference between doses	Only significant difference was headache: Osp–A 15 μg *v* Osp–A 30 μg, 15% *v* 9%; P < 0.008
10	240 people (18–50 years)	Three formulations of the Osp–A vaccine	One or more of the symptoms of pain, redness, swelling, and induration occurred in up to 48.8% of people after any single dose	One or more of the symptoms of fever, headache, malaise, rash, arthralgia, were reported by ≤ 10.1% of people after any single dose
Different dosing schedules				
13	800 adults (15–50 years)	Osp–A vaccine given at 0, 1, and 6 months *v* at 0, 1, and 12 months	At least one local symptom occurred in 75% of people in each group	At least one systemic symptom occurred in 19% in both groups
14	956 adults (17–72 years)	Osp–A vaccine 30 μg given at 0, 1, and 12 months *v* at 0, 1, 2, and 12 months	Soreness was most common: in both groups 82.5% with 3 doses *v* 81.7% with 4 doses; NS	Fatigue was the most common symptom: 21.8% *v* 19.7%; NS. Arthralgia: 12.5% with 3 doses *v* 9.6% with 4 doses; P = 0.007

NS, not significant; ref, reference.

TABLE 2 **Prophylactic treatment of tick bite with antibiotics; results of placebo controlled RCTs (see text, p 725).[16,25–27]**

Ref	Population (all noticed tick bites < 72 h prior to study enrolment)	Intervention	Number of people with any evidence of Lyme disease (antibiotic *v* placebo)	Adverse effects (antibiotic *v* placebo)
16	482 people aged ≥ 12 years	Doxycycline (200 mg single dose) versus placebo	3/235 (1%) *v* 11/247 (4%); ARR 3.2%, 95% CI 0.2% to 6.2%	Nausea: 24/156 (15.4%) *v* 4/153 (2.6%); ARI 12.8%, 95% CI 6.4% to 19.2%; NNH 8, 95% CI 6 to 16 Vomiting: 9/156 (5.8%) *v* 2/153 (1.3%); ARI 4.5%, 95% CI 0.3% to 8.6%; NNH 23, 95% CI 12 to 303)
17	68 people aged ≥ 5 years	Penicillin (250 mg qds for 10 days) versus placebo	0/32 (0%) *v* 1/36 (3%); ARR 2.8%, 95% CI −3.0% to +8.5%	Rash: 1/27 (4%) *v* 0/29 (0%)
18	372 people of any age	Amoxicillin (250 mg tds for 10 days) versus placebo	0/205 (0%) *v* 2/182 (1%); ARR 1.1%, 95% CI −0.3% to +2.5%	Rash possibly due to amoxicillin: 2/205 (1%) *v* 0/182 (0%)
19	184 people aged 3–19 years	Penicillin (250 mg qds for 10 days in people < 9 years) or tetracycline (250 mg qds for 10 days in people > 9 years) versus placebo	0/89 (0%) *v* 4/90 (4%); ARR 4.4%, 95% CI 0.1% to 8.8%	Hives reported in one person who received placebo

qds, four times daily; ref, reference; tds, three times daily.

Malaria in endemic areas

Search date February 2002

Aika Omari and Paul Garner

QUESTIONS

INTERVENTIONS

To be covered in future updates
Artemotil
Anticonvulsants
Treatment in pregnancy

Covered elsewhere in *Clinical Evidence*
See Malaria: prevention in travellers, p 744.

See glossary, p 742

Key Messages

Medical treatments for falciparum malaria

- **Artemether versus quinine** Systematic reviews found no significant difference in mortality with artemether versus quinine.
- **Chloroquine versus quinine** Two RCTs in children found no significant difference in mortality with chloroquine versus quinine in The Gambia between 1988 and 1994 when chloroquine resistance was uncommon.
- **Desferrioxamine mesylate** One systematic review found limited evidence that desferrioxamine mesylate versus placebo reduced the risk of persistent seizures in children with cerebral malaria, but adverse effects were more common.
- **Dexamethasone** One systematic review has found no significant difference in mortality with dexamethasone versus placebo, but gastrointestinal bleeding and seizures were more common with dexamethasone.
- **Exchange blood transfusion** We found no RCTs on exchange blood transfusions.
- **High first dose quinine** Three RCTs found that an initial high dose of quinine versus the standard dose increased the speed of parasite clearance. The RCTs found no significant difference in mortality, but may have been underpowered to detect a clinically important difference. One RCT found that more participants experienced short term partial hearing loss with high versus standard dose quinine.

- **Initial blood transfusion** One systematic review found no significant difference in deaths in clinically stable children who received an initial blood transfusion for malaria anaemia, and found more adverse events.
- **Intramuscular versus intravenous quinine** One RCT in children found no significant difference with intramuscular versus intravenous quinine in recovery times or deaths in Kenya in 1990.
- **Quinine** We found no RCTs comparing quinine versus placebo or no treatment, but there is consensus that treatment is likely to be beneficial.
- **Rectal artemisinin versus quinine** One systematic review found no significant difference in mortality with rectal artemisinin versus quinine.
- **Sulfadoxine–pyrimethamine versus quinine** One RCT found that sulfadoxine–pyrimethamine versus quinine cleared parasites faster in children with complicated non-cerebral malaria in 1992–1994 in The Gambia, but found no significant difference in mortality.

DEFINITION Severe malaria is caused by the protozoan infection of red blood cells with *Plasmodium falciparum.* Clinically complicated malaria presents with life threatening conditions, which include coma, severe anaemia, renal failure, respiratory distress syndrome, hypoglycaemia, shock, spontaneous haemorrhage, and convulsions. The diagnosis of cerebral malaria should be considered where there is encephalopathy in the presence of malaria parasites. A strict definition of cerebral malaria requires the presence of unrousable coma, and no other cause of encephalopathy (eg. hypoglycaemia, sedative drugs) in the presence of *P falciparum* infection.[1] This review does not currently include the treatment of malaria in pregnancy.

INCIDENCE/ PREVALENCE Malaria is a major health problem in the tropics with 300–500 million clinical cases, and an estimated 1.1–2.7 million deaths each year as a result of severe malaria.[2] Over 90% of deaths occur in children below 5 years of age, mainly from cerebral malaria and anaemia.[2] In areas where malaria transmission is stable (endemic), those most at risk of acquiring severe malaria are children under 5 years old, because adults and older children have partial immunity that offers some protection. In areas where malaria transmission is unstable (non-endemic), severe malaria affects both adults and children. Non-immune travellers and migrants are also at risk from developing severe malaria.

AETIOLOGY/ RISK FACTORS Malaria is transmitted by the bite of infected female anopheline mosquitoes. Certain genes are associated with resistance to severe malaria. Human leukocyte antigens (HLA), namely HLA-Bw53 and HLA-DRB1*1302, protect against severe malaria. However, the associations of HLA antigens with severe malaria are limited to specific populations.[3,4] Haemoglobin S[3] and haemoglobin C[5] are also protective against severe malaria. Genes have also been associated with an increased susceptibility to severe malaria, such as the tumour necrosis factor gene (see aetiology under malaria: prevention in travellers, p 744).[6]

PROGNOSIS In children under 5 years of age with cerebral malaria, the estimated case fatality of treated malaria is 19%, although reported hospital case fatality may be as high as 10–40%.[1,7] Neurological sequelae persisting for more than 6 months occur in more than 2% of the survivors, and include ataxia, hemiplegia, speech disorders, behavioural disorders, epilepsy, and blindness. Severe malarial anaemia has a case fatality rate higher than 13%.[7] In adults, the mortality of cerebral malaria is 20%; this rises to 50% in pregnancy,[8] and neurological sequelae occur in about 3% of survivors.[8]

AIMS To prevent death and cure the infection; to prevent long term disability; to minimise neurological sequelae resulting from cerebral malaria, with minimal adverse effects of treatment.

OUTCOMES Death; parasite clearance at day 7 or 14; parasite clearance time (see glossary, p 742); fever clearance time (see glossary, p 742); time to walking and drinking; coma recovery time and neurological sequelae at follow up; adverse events.

METHODS *Clinical Evidence* search and appraisal February 2002. The World Health Organization criteria for severe malaria were applied to included RCTs.[1]

QUESTION What are the effects of medical treatments for complicated falciparum malaria in non-pregnant people?

OPTION QUININE VERSUS PLACEBO OR NO TREATMENT

Consensus statements recommend quinine for the treatment of severe falciparum malaria.

Benefits: We found no RCTs comparing quinine with placebo or no treatment.

Harms: We found two observational studies on hypoglycaemia secondary to quinine-induced hyperinsulinaemia. One study in people with severe malaria treated with quinine in Thailand found a correlation between plasma quinine and insulin levels during hypoglycaemic episodes ($P = 0.007$).[9] One prospective cohort study in Zaire (9 children and 19 adults) treated severe malaria with intravenous quinine (average dose 8.5 mg/kg base hourly). Nine people developed significant hypoglycaemia (glucose < 2.8 mmol/L), which was associated with inappropriately high plasma insulin levels.[10] It is not clear from these studies if hypoglycaemia was caused by malaria or by quinine administration.

Comment: RCTs of quinine versus placebo in severe malaria would be regarded as unethical. The use of quinine to treat severe malaria was established before modern trial methods were developed. In a case series in Singapore (1944–1945), 15 adults with acute severe malaria were treated with continuous intravenous quinine.[11] Thirteen recovered and two comatose people died. In a non-comparative study in Zaire (1987), intravenous quinine (10 mg/kg 8 hourly for 3 days) was administered to 34 children (7 months to 13 years) with severe or moderate falciparum malaria (see glossary, p 742).[12] One child who was comatose on admission died. The mean parasite clearance time (see glossary, p 742) was 59.6 hours. The mean fever clearance time (see glossary, p 742) was 44.1 hours. Thirty three children were clinically well and had negative blood slides on day 7. Reviews[13,14] and consensus statements[1,15,16] recommend quinine for treating severe falciparum malaria, particularly in chloroquine resistant areas.

OPTION CHLOROQUINE VERSUS QUININE

Two RCTs in children found no difference in mortality between chloroquine and quinine in the Gambia between 1988 and 1994 when chloroquine resistance was uncommon.

Benefits: We found no systematic review. We found two RCTs.[17,18] One RCT (50 Gambian children, age 1–10 years with severe malaria) compared intramuscular chloroquine (3.5 mg base/kg 6 hourly) versus intramuscular quinine (20 mg salt/kg immediately followed by 10 mg salt/kg 12 hourly) in 1988.[17] It found no significant difference in mortality (2/25 [8%] with chloroquine *v* 6/25 [24%] with quinine; RR 0.33, 95% CI 0.07 to 1.50) or fever resolution (37.7 h with chloroquine *v* 39.1 h with quinine; WMD −1.4 h, 95% CI −14.0 h to +11.2 h). Median time to full recovery from coma was 18 hours in both groups. Recovery time from prostration was similar in both groups (median time to standing: 42 h with chloroquine *v* 48 h with quinine). Recovery time to drinking was also similar in both groups (10 h with chloroquine *v* 11 h with quinine). The second RCT (92 Gambian children, aged 1–9 years) compared subcutaneous chloroquine (2.5 mg/kg 4 hourly) versus intramuscular quinine (10 mg/kg 8 hourly) in the treatment of complicated, non-cerebral malaria between 1992 and 1994.[18] One child in each group died. The fever clearance time (see glossary, p 742) was faster with chloroquine (median: 27 h [range 6–66 h] with chloroquine *v* 42 h [range 6–96 h] with quinine; $P = 0.02$).

Harms: In the first RCT, one child treated with chloroquine developed pruritus (chloroquine *v* quinine RR 3.0, 95% CI 0.13 to 70.3), whereas three children treated with quinine developed hypoglycaemia (chloroquine *v* quinine RR 0.14, 95% CI 0.01 to 2.63).[17]

Comment: The effects on mortality were inconclusive because of the small number of people in both trials. One RCT excluded participants with cerebral malaria who are an important group in children suffering from severe malaria.[18] Chloroquine resistance was documented in the second trial.[18] Chloroquine resistance has since become widespread in sub-Saharan Africa, resulting in more deaths and an increase in severe disease.[19]

OPTION SULFADOXINE–PYRIMETHAMINE VERSUS QUININE

One RCT found sulfadoxine–pyrimethamine cleared parasites faster than quinine in children with complicated non-cerebral malaria in 1992–1994 in The Gambia, but found no significant difference in mortality.

Benefits: We found no systematic review. We found one RCT (92 Gambian children aged 1–9 years with complicated, non-cerebral malaria, in 1992–1994) that compared intramuscular sulfadoxine–pyrimethamine (sulfadoxine 25 mg/kg plus pyrimethamine 1.25 mg/kg) versus intramuscular quinine (10 mg/kg 8 hourly) versus chloroquine.[18] It found no significant difference in mortality (2/36 [6%] with sulfadoxine–pyrimethamine *v* 1/28 [4%] with quinine; RR 1.56, 95% CI 0.15 to 16.3). Sulfadoxine–pyrimethamine cleared parasites faster than quinine (median [parasite clearance time—see glossary, p 742) 42 h [range 18–78h] *v* 66 h [range 30–90h]; $P < 0.001$).

Harms: One child treated with quinine developed an injection abscess (0/36 [0%] with sulfadoxine–pyrimethamine *v* 1/28 [3.6%] with quinine; RR 0.26, 95% CI 0.01 to 6.18).[18]

Comment: People with cerebral malaria, who form an important group in children suffering from severe malaria, were excluded from this RCT. Resistance to sulfadoxine–pyrimethamine was documented in the Gambia in 1991.[18]

OPTION INTRAMUSCULAR VERSUS INTRAVENOUS QUININE

One RCT in children found no difference between intramuscular and intravenous quinine in treating severe malaria in Kenya in 1990.

Benefits: We found no systematic review. We found one RCT (59 children < 12 years old), which compared high dose intramuscular versus high dose intravenous quinine (20 mg salt/kg loading immediately followed by 10 mg salt/kg 12 hourly) versus standard dose intravenous quinine in severe falciparum malaria (see glossary, p 742) in Kenya (1989–1990).[20] The RCT found no significant difference in mortality (3/20 [15%] deaths in the intramuscular quinine group *v* 1/18 [5.6%] in the intravenous quinine group; RR 2.7, 95% CI 0.3 to 23.7), in mean parasite clearance time (see glossary, p 742) (57 h with im quinine *v* 58 h with iv quinine; WMD –1.0 h, 95% CI –12.2 h to +10.2 h), in mean recovery times to drinking (47 h with im quinine *v* 32 h with iv quinine; WMD 15 h, 95% CI –5.6 h to 35.6 h), or in mean recovery times to walking (98 h with im *v* 96 h with iv quinine; WMD 2.0 h, 95% CI –24.5 h to +28.5 h).

Harms: Neurological sequelae were reported in two children in the im group, and one child in the iv group had transient neurological sequelae, which was not specified (2/20 [10%] with im quinine *v* 1/18 [5.6%] with iv quinine; RR 1.8, 95% CI 0.2 to 18.2).

Comment: Quinine concentration profiles were similar with both routes of administration, and peak concentrations were achieved soon after intramuscular injection. The sample size might have been insufficient to rule out important clinical differences.

OPTION HIGH FIRST DOSE OF QUININE VERSUS STANDARD DOSE QUININE

Three RCTs found that an initial high dose of quinine versus the standard dose increased the speed of parasite clearance. The RCTs found no significant difference in mortality, but may have been underpowered to detect a clinically important difference. One RCT found that more participants experienced short term partial hearing loss with high versus standard dose quinine.

Benefits: We found no systematic review. We found three RCTs comparing an initial high dose of quinine with other regimens.[20–22] The first RCT (59 Kenyan children with severe falciparum malaria (see glossary, p 742) aged ≤ 12 years) compared an initial high dose of intravenous quinine (20 mg salt/kg over 2 h, then 10 mg salt/kg 12 hourly) versus standard quinine dose (10 mg/kg salt over 2 h, then 5 mg/kg salt 12 hourly) versus intramuscular quinine between 1989 and 1990.[20] It found more children died with the standard dose, but the difference was not significant (1/18 [6%] with initial high dose of quinine v 4/21 [19%] with the standard dose; RR 0.29, 95% CI 0.04 to 2.38; see comment below). Mean parasite clearance was faster with the high dose (58 h with high dose v 77 h with standard dose, WMD –19 h, 95% CI –32.2 h to –5.8 h). The mean time taken to recover consciousness was similar in both groups (14 h with high dose v 13 h with standard dose; WMD 1 h, 95% CI –8.8 h to +10.8 h). It found no significant difference in the mean time taken to recover to drinking (32 h with high dose v 36 h with standard dose; WMD –4 h, 95% CI –16.6 h to +8.6 h). The second RCT (33 Kenyan people with severe malaria aged ≥ 14 years) compared initial high dose quinine (20 mg/kg over 4 h, 10 mg/kg every 8 h) versus the standard dose (10 mg/kg every 8 h) between 1989 and 1990.[21] It found no significant difference in mortality (1/17 [6%] with high dose v 1/16 [6%] with standard dose) or in mean fever clearance time (see glossary, p 742) (44.0 h with high dose v 51.4 h with standard dose; WMD –7.4 h, 95% CI –19.1 h to +4.3 h), but mean parasite clearance was slightly quicker with high dose quinine (42.2 h with high dose v 47.1 h with standard dose; WMD –4.9 h, 95% CI –10.8 h to +1.1 h). The third RCT (20 people from Cameroon with cerebral malaria; mean ages 24.3 years in high dose group and 22.8 in standard dose group) compared an initial high dose of quinine (16 mg/kg over 8 h, then 8 mg/kg 8 hourly) versus the standard dose (8 mg/kg 8 hourly) in 1991.[22] It found shorter coma duration (6.8 h with high dose v 13 h with standard dose; P = 0.003) and faster parasite clearance time (see glossary, p 742) (40.8 h with high dose v 52.2 h with standard dose; P = 0.05) with the initial high dose of quinine.

Harms: One RCT reported significantly more temporary (< 2 wk) partial hearing loss with the initial high dose of quinine (10/17 [59%] with high dose v 3/16 [19%] with standard dose; RR 3.14, 95% CI 1.05 to 9.38).[21]

Comment: The RCTs may have been too small to detect a clinically important difference.[20–22]

OPTION ARTEMETHER VERSUS QUININE

Systematic reviews have found no difference between artemether and quinine in preventing deaths in severe malaria.

Benefits: We found two systematic reviews.[23,24] The first review (search date not stated, 11 RCTs, 2264 people, including both children and adults) conducted a meta-analysis of individual patient data (7 RCTs, 1919 participants) comparing intramuscular artemether versus intravenous quinine (1 RCT used im quinine) in the treatment of severe falciparum malaria (see glossary, p 742).[23] Parasite clearance was faster with artemether (HR 0.62, 95% CI 0.56 to 0.69). It found that less people died with artemether but the difference was not significant (136/961 [14%] with artemether v 164/958 [17%] with quinine; OR 0.8, 95% CI 0.62 to 1.02). It found no significant difference in the speed of coma recovery (risk of quicker recovery with quinine, HR 1.09, 95% CI 0.97 to 1.22), fever clearance time (see glossary, p 742) (risk of quicker recovery with quinine, HR 1.01, 95% CI 0.90 to 1.15), or neurological sequelae (81/807 with artemether [10%] v 91/765 [12%] with quinine, OR 0.82, 95%

CI 0.59 to 1.15). The second review (search date 1999) compared intramuscular artemether versus intravenous quinine (11 RCTs, 2142 people).[24] It found a small but significant reduction in mortality with artemether (OR 0.72, 95% CI 0.57 to 0.91), but significance was sensitive to removing three RCTs with inadequate methods (OR 0.79, 95% CI 0.59 to 1.05). It found no difference in neurological sequelae at recovery (OR 0.80, 95% CI 0.52 to 1.25).

Harms: The review found no significant difference in neurological sequelae (see above).[23,24]

Comment: The combination of either death or neurological sequelae as an adverse outcome was lower in people treated with artemether (OR 0.77, 95% CI 0.62 to 0.96) in the individual patient data meta-analysis.[23]

OPTION RECTAL ARTEMISININ DERIVATIVES (ARTEMISININ OR ARTESUNATE) VERSUS QUININE

One systematic review has found no significant difference in mortality between rectal artemisinin and quinine.

Benefits: We found one systematic review (search date 1999, 3 RCTs, 2653 people), which compared rectal artemisinin versus quinine in severe malaria.[24] Two RCTs were conducted in Vietnam and one in Ethiopia (1996–1997). Meta-analysis found lower mortality with artemisinin (3 RCTs, 9/87 [10%] with artemisinin *v* 16/98 [16%] with quinine; RR 0.73, 95% CI 0.35 to 1.50) and quicker coma recovery time (2 RCTs, 59 people; WMD –9.0 h, 95% CI –19.7 h to 1.7 h), but the difference was not significant. Fever clearance time (see glossary, p 742) was not significantly different (no figures provided). We found no RCTs comparing rectal artesunate with quinine.

Harms: Artemisinin versus quinine significantly reduced the risk of hypoglycemia in one trial (3/30 [10%] with artemisinin *v* 19/30 [63.3%] with quinine; RR 0.16, 95% CI 0.05 to 0.48).[25]

Comment: The World Health Organization is currently conducting a trial of prompt administration rectal artesunate for severe malaria by paramedical staff before referral to hospital (P Olliaro, personal communication, 2002).

OPTION DESFERRIOXAMINE MESYLATE

One systematic review found limited evidence that the risk of persistent seizures was reduced with desferrioxamine mesylate, but adverse effects were more common.

Benefits: **Versus placebo:** We found one systematic review (search date 1998, 2 RCTs, 435 children > 6 years of age with cerebral malaria treated with quinine) of desferrioxamine mesylate (100 mg/kg/day iv for 72 h) versus placebo.[26] Both RCTs were conducted in Zambia (1990–1991). The review found no difference in overall mortality (39/217 [18%] with desferrioxamine *v* 28/218 [13%] with placebo;

RR 1.40, 95% CI 0.89 to 2.18) but results were heterogeneous. The review found that desferrioxamine mesylate significantly reduced the risk of persistent seizures (93/168 [55.4%] with desferrioxamine v 115/166 [69.3%] with placebo; RR 0.80, 95% CI 0.67 to 0.95).

Harms: In one RCT, desferrioxamine mesylate was associated with more episodes of phlebitis (26/172 [15%] with desferrioxamine v 20/172 [12%] with placebo; RR 1.30, 95% CI 0.76 to 2.24) and recurrent hypoglycaemia (43/172 [25%] with desferrioxamine v 29/172 [17%] with placebo; RR 1.48, 95% CI 0.97 to 2.26) than placebo.[27]

Comment: The trials were probably underpowered to detect a clinically significant difference in adverse events.

OPTION GLUCOCORTICOID DRUGS (DEXAMETHASONE)

One systematic review has found no significant difference in mortality between dexamethasone versus placebo, but gastrointestinal bleeding and seizures were more common with dexamethasone.

Benefits: **Versus placebo:** We found one systematic review (search date 1999, 2 RCTs, 143 people treated with quinine) of dexamethasone versus placebo over 48 hours.[28] One RCT was conducted in Indonesia and the other in Thailand. The review found no significant difference in mortality (14/71 [20%] with dexamethasone v 16/72 [25%] with placebo; RR 0.89, 95% CI 0.47 to 1.68). One RCT found a longer mean time between start of treatment and coma resolution with dexamethasone group (76 h with dexamethasone v 57 h with placebo; $P < 0.02$),[29] but the other RCT found no significant difference (83.4 h with dexamethasone v 80.0 h with placebo; WMD 3.4 h, 95% CI –31.3 h to +38.1 h).[30]

Harms: Gastrointestinal bleeding (7/71 [10%] with dexamethasone v 0/72 [0%] with placebo; RR 8.17, 95% CI 1.05 to 63.6) and seizures (11/71 [15.5%] with dexamethasone v 3/72 [4%] with placebo; RR 3.32, 95% CI 1.05 to 10.47) were more common with dexamethasone.[28]

Comment: No effect of steroids on mortality was demonstrated but the trial numbers are small. The effect of steroids on disability was not recorded as only short term outcomes were measured.

OPTION INITIAL BLOOD TRANSFUSION FOR TREATING MALARIAL ANAEMIA

One systematic review has found no significant difference in deaths, but more adverse events among clinically stable children who receive an initial blood transfusion for malaria anaemia.

Benefits: We found one systematic review (search date 1999, 2 RCTs, 230 children).[31] One RCT compared initial blood transfusion versus conservative treatment in Tanzanian children and the other RCT compared blood transfusion versus iron supplements in Gambian children. Both trials excluded children who were clinically unstable with respiratory distress or signs of cardiac failure. Meta-analysis found fewer deaths in the transfused children but the difference was not significant (1/118 [1%] with transfusion v 3/112 [3%] with control; RR 0.41, 95% CI 0.06 to 2.70).

Harms: Coma and convulsions occurred more often after transfusion (8/118 [6.8%] with transfusion *v* 0/112 [0%] without transfusion; RR 8.6, 95% CI 1.1 to 66).[31] Seven of the eight adverse events occurred in one RCT. Meta-analysis combining deaths and severe adverse events found no significant difference between transfused and non-transfused patients (8/118 [7%] with transfusion *v* 3/112 [3%] without transfusion; RR 2.5, 95% CI 0.7 to 9.3). Hepatitis B or HIV transmission were not reported.

Comment: Studies were small and loss to follow up was greater than 10%, both of which are both potential sources of bias. No results were available on adults. Significantly more children in the non-transfused group required transfusion in addition to the primary allocated intervention (1/118 [1%] with transfusion *v* 11/112 [10%] without transfusion; RR 0.12, 95% CI 0.02 to 0.68).

OPTION EXCHANGE BLOOD TRANSFUSION

We found no good evidence on exchange blood transfusions.

Benefits: We found no systematic review or RCTs on exchange blood transfusion in malaria.

Harms: We found no good evidence.

Comment: Two retrospective observational studies found no reduction of mortality in people with severe falciparum malaria (see glossary, p 742) treated with an exchange blood transfusion. One retrospective study (124 people) conducted in Europe (Germany, Austria, and Switzerland) of exchange transfusion found no difference in mortality (13/61 [21%] with exchange transfusion *v* 6/63 [9.5%] with usual care; OR 2.2, 95% CI 0.9 to 5.5).[32] However, the transfusion protocol was not standardised, the sample size was small, and observer bias was present. The second study (50 people with severe falciparum malaria) of exchange transfusion was conducted in Thailand. It found no significant effect on mortality (20/29 [69%] with exchange transfusion *v* 10/21 [48%] with no exchange; RR 1.4, 95% CI 0.9 to 2.4).[33] However, the mean admission parasitaemia and the proportion of people with greater than 10% parasitaemia was significantly higher in the exchange transfusion group.

GLOSSARY

Falciparum malaria Malaria resulting from an infection with *Plasmodium falciparum*, one of the four species of malaria parasites found in humans.

Fever clearance time The time between commencing treatment and the temperature returning back to normal.

Parasite clearance time (PCT) The time between commencing treatment and the first negative blood test. PCT 50 is the time taken for parasites to be reduced to 50% of first test value and PCT 90 is the time taken for parasites to be reduced to 10% of first test value.

REFERENCES

1. World Health Organization. Severe falciparum malaria. World Health Organization, Communicable Diseases Cluster. *Trans R Soc Trop Med Hyg* 2000;94 (suppl 1):S1–90.
2. World Health Organization. WHO Expert Committee on Malaria: Twentieth report. 1998 Geneva Switzerland. *World Health Organ Tech Rep Ser* 2000;892:i–v:1–74.

3. Hill AVS. Malaria resistance genes: a natural selection. *Trans R Soc Trop Med Hyg* 1992;86:225–226.
4. Hill AVS. Genetic susceptibility to malaria and other infectious diseases: from the MHC to the whole genome. *Parasitology* 1996;112:S75–84.
5. Modiano D, Luoni G, Sirima BS, et al. Haemoglobin C protects against clinical *Plasmodium falciparum* malaria. *Nature* 2001;414:305–308.
6. McGuire W, Hill AV, Allsopp CE, Greenwood BM, Kwiatkowski D. Variation in the TNF-alpha promoter region associated with susceptibility to cerebral malaria. *Nature* 1994;371:508–510.
7. Murphy SC, Breman JG. Gaps in the childhood malaria burden in Africa: Cerebral malaria, neurological sequelae, anemia, respiratory distress, hypoglycemia, and complications of pregnancy. *Am J Trop Med Hyg* 2001;64:S57–67.
8. White NJ. Malaria. In: Cook GC, ed. *Manson's tropical diseases*. 20th ed. London: WB Saunders 1996:1087–1164.
9. White N, Warrell D, Chanthavanich P, et al. Severe hypoglycemia and hyperinsulinemia in falciparum malaria. *N Engl J Med* 1983;309:61–66.
10. Okitolonda W, Delacollette C, Malengreau M, et al. High incidence of hypoglycaemia in African patients treated with intravenous quinine for severe malaria. *BMJ* 1987;295:716–718.
11. Strahan JH. Quinine by continuous intravenous drip in the treatment of acute falciparum malaria. *Trans R Soc Trop Med Hyg* 1948;41:669–76.
12. Greenberg AE, Nguyen-Dinh P, Davachi F, et al. Intravenous quinine therapy of hospitalized children with Plasmodium Falciparum malaria in Kinshasa, Zaire. *Am J Trop Med Hyg* 1988;40:360–364.
13. Hall AP. The treatment of severe falciparum malaria. *Trans R Soc Trop Med Hyg* 1977;71:367–378.
14. Warrell DA. Treatment of severe malaria. *J R Soc Med* 1989;82(suppl 17):44–50.
15. World Health Organization. The use of antimalarial drugs. Report of a WHO Informal consultation, 13–17 November 2000 (WHO/CDS/RBM/2001.33). Geneve: World Health Organization, 2001.
16. Looareesuwan S, Olliaro P, White NJ, Chongsuphajaisiddhi T, Sabcharoen A, Thimasarn K, et al. Consensus recommendation on the treatment of malaria in Southeast Asia. *Southeast Asian J Trop Med Public Health* 1998;29:355–360.
17. White NJ, Waller D, Kwiatkowski D, Krishna S, Craddock C, Brewster D. Open comparison of intramuscular chloroquine and quinine in children with severe chloroquine-sensitive falciparum malaria. *Lancet* 1989;2:1313–1316.
18. Giadom B, De Veer GE, van Hensbroek B, Corrah PT, Jaffar S, Greenwood BM. A comparative study of parenteral chloroquine, quinine and pyrimethamine-sulfadoxine in the treatment of Gambian children with complicated, non-cerebral malaria. *Ann Trop Paediatr* 1996:16;85–91.
19. Nuwaha F. The challenge of chloroquine-resistant malaria in sub-Saharan Africa. *Health Policy Plan* 2001;16:1–12.
20. Pasvol G, Newton CRJC, Winstanley PA, et al. Quinine treatment of severe falciparum malaria in African children: a randomized comparison of three regimens. *Am J Trop Med Hyg* 1991;45:702–713.
21. Tombe M, Bhatt KM, Obel AOK. Quinine loading dose in severe falciparum malaria at Kenyatta National Hospital, Kenya. *East Afr Med J* 1992;69:670–674.
22. Louis FJ, Fargier JJ, Maubort B, et al. Severe malaria attacks in adults in Cameroon: comparison of 2 therapeutic protocols using quinine via parenteral route. [French]. *Ann Soc Belg Med Trop* 1992;72:179–188.
23. Artemether Quinine Meta-analysis Study Group. A meta-analysis using individual patient data of trials comparing artemether with quinine in the treatment of severe falciparum malaria. *Trans R Soc Trop Med Hyg* 2001;95:637–50. Search date not stated; primary sources Medline, Cochrane, and discussions with an international panel of malaria clinical investigators.
24. McIntosh HM, Olliaro P. Artemisinin derivatives for treating severe malaria. In: The Cochrane Library, Issue 3, 2001. Oxford: Update Software. Search date 1999; primary sources Cochrane Infectious Diseases Group Trials Register, Medline, BIDS Science Citation Index, Embase, African Index Medicus, LILACS, handsearching of reference lists and conference abstracts, and contact with organisations and researchers in the field and pharmaceutical companies.
25. Birku Y, Makonnen F, Bjorkman A. Comparison of rectal artemisinin with intravenous quinine in the treatment of severe malaria in Ethiopia. *East Afr Med J* 1999;76:154–159.
26. Smith HJ, Meremikwu M. Iron chelating agents for treating malaria. In: The Cochrane Library, Issue 3, 2001. Oxford: Update Software. Search date 1998; primary sources Trials Register of the Cochrane Infectious Diseases Group, CCTR, Medline, Embase, and handsearching of reference lists.
27. Thuma PE, Mabeza GF, Biemba G, Bhat GJ, McLaren C, Moyo VM, et al. Effect of iron chelation therapy on mortality in children with cerebral malaria. *Trans R Soc Trop Med Hyg* 1998;92:214–218.
28. Prasad K, Garner P. Steroids for treating cerebral malaria (Cochrane Review). In: The Cochrane Library, Issue 3, 2001. Oxford: Update Software. Search date 1999; primary sources Trials Register of the Cochrane Infectious Diseases Group and the Cochrane Controlled Trials Register.
29. Warrell DA, Looareesuwan S, Warrell MJ, et al. Dexamethasone proves deleterious in cerebral malaria. A double-blind trial in 100 comatose patients. *N Engl J Med* 1982;306:313–319.
30. Hoffman SL, Rustama D, Punjabi NH, et al. High-dose dexamethasone in quinine-treated patients with cerebral malaria: a double blind, placebo-controlled trial. *J Infect Dis* 1988;158:325–331.
31. Meremikwu M, Smith HJ. Blood transfusion for treating malarial anaemia. In: The Cochrane Library, Issue 3, 2001. Oxford: Update Software. Search date 1999; primary sources the Trials Register of the Cochrane Infectious Diseases Group, Embase, African Index Medicus, LILACS, hand searching of reference lists, and contact with experts.
32. Burchard GD, Kroger J, Knobloch J, et al. Exchange blood transfusion in severe falciparum malaria: retrospective evaluation of 61 patients treated with, compared to 63 patients treated without exchange transfusion. *Trop Med Int Health* 1997;2:733–740.
33. Hoontrakoon S, Suputtamongkol Y. Exchange transfusion as an adjunct to the treatment of severe falciparum malaria. *Trop Med Int Health* 1998;3:156–161.

Aika Omari
Paul Garner
Professor of Medicine
Liverpool School of Tropical Medicine, Liverpool, UK

Competing interests: None declared.

Malaria: prevention in travellers

Search date March 2002

Ashley Croft

QUESTIONS

INTERVENTIONS

Key Messages

Non-drug preventive interventions

- **Aerosol insecticides** One large observational study in travellers found insufficient evidence on the effects of aerosol insecticides in preventing malaria. Two RCTs in malaria endemic areas found that indoor spraying of aerosol insecticides reduced clinical malaria.
- **Air conditioning and electric fans** One large observational study found that air conditioning significantly reduced the incidence of malaria. One small observational study found that electric fans reduced the number of culicine mosquitos in indoor spaces.
- **Full length clothing** One observational study found that wearing trousers and long sleeved shirts significantly reduced the incidence of malaria.

- **Insecticide treated clothing** Two RCTs in soldiers and refugee householders have found that permethrin treated fabric (clothing or sheets) significantly reduces the incidence of malaria.
- **Insecticide treated nets** We found no RCTs in travellers. One systematic review in residents of a malaria endemic area has found that nets treated with insecticide significantly reduce the number of mild episodes of malaria and reduced child mortality (NNT 180, CI not available).
- **Insecticide treated nets in pregnant travellers** We found no RCTs of the effects of insecticide treated nets on pregnant travellers. One RCT of pregnant residents found inconclusive evidence on the effects of permethrin treated nets in preventing malaria.
- **Insect repellents containing DEET in children** We found no RCTs on the effects of DEET in preventing malaria in child travellers. Case reports in young children found serious adverse effects with DEET.
- **Mosquito coils and vaporising mats** We found no systematic review and no RCTs of the effects of coils and vaporising mats in preventing malaria in travellers. One RCT of coils and one observational study of pyrethroid vaporising mats found that these devices reduced numbers of mosquitoes in indoor spaces.
- **Smoke** We found no RCTs of the effects of smoke in preventing malaria. One controlled clinical trial found that smoke repelled mosquitoes during the evening.
- **Topical insect repellents** We found no systematic review and no RCTs on the effects of topical insect repellents in preventing malaria. One very small crossover RCT found that DEET preparations protected against mosquito bites.
- **Biological control measures; insect buzzers and electrocuters; insecticides in airline pilots; insecticide treated clothing in pregnant travellers; topical insect repellents in pregnant travellers** We found no RCTs on the effects of these interventions.

Drug prophylaxis

- **Amodaquine** We found insufficient evidence on the effects of amodaquine on malaria in travellers. However, we found limited observational evidence that amodquine may cause liver damage and hepatitis.
- **Atovaquone plus proguanil** One RCT found no significant difference between atovaquone plus proguanil versus chloroquine plus proguanil in preventing malaria. One RCT found no difference between atovaquone plus proguanil versus mefloquine in preventing malaria.
- **Chloroquine** We found no RCTs about the effects of chloroquine in travellers. One RCT in Austrian workers residing in Nigeria found no significant difference between chloroquine versus sulfadoxine plus pyrimethamine in the incidence of malaria at 6–22 months.
- **Chloroquine plus proguanil** One RCT found no significant difference between chloroquine plus proguanil versus proguanil alone or versus chloroquine plus other antimalaria drugs in the incidence of *Plasmodium falciparum* malaria. One RCT found no significant difference between chloroquine plus proguanil versus atovaquone plus proguanil in preventing malaria.
- **Doxycycline in adults** Two RCTs in soldiers have found that doxycycline versus placebo significantly reduces the risk of malaria.

Malaria: prevention in travellers

- **Mefloquine in adults** One RCT in soldiers comparing mefloquine versus placebo found that mefloquine had a 100% protective efficacy. One RCT of mefloquine versus atovaquone plus proguanil found no cases of clinical malaria throughout the trial, but found a significantly higher rate of neuropsychiatric harm with mefloquine.
- **Pyrimethamine plus dapsone** We found no RCTs in travellers. One RCT in Thai soldiers comparing pyrimethamine plus dapsone versus proguanil plus dapsone found no significant difference in *P falciparum* infection rates over 40 days.
- **Sulfadoxine plus pyrimethamine** We found insufficient evidence on the effect of these drugs in travellers.
- **Antimalaria drugs in airline pilots or pregnant travellers; doxycycline in children; mefloquine in children** We found no RCTs on the effects of these interventions.

Vaccines

- We found no RCTs in travellers. One systematic review of antimalaria vaccines in residents of malaria endemic areas has found that the SPf66 vaccine versus placebo significantly reduces first attacks of malaria.

DEFINITION Malaria is caused by a protozoan infection of red blood cells with one of four species of the genus *Plasmodium*: *P falciparum*, *P vivax*, *P ovale,* and *P malariae*.[1] Clinically, malaria may present in different ways but is usually characterised by fever (which may be swinging), tachycardia, rigors, and sweating. Anaemia, hepatosplenomegaly, cerebral involvement, renal failure, and shock may occur.[2,3]

INCIDENCE/ PREVALENCE Each year there are 300–500 million clinical cases of malaria. About 40% of the world's population is at risk of acquiring the disease.[2,3] Each year 25–30 million people from non-tropical countries visit malaria endemic areas, of whom 10 000–30 000 contract malaria.[4,5] Most RCTs of malaria prevention have been carried out on soldiers and travellers. The results of these trials may not be applicable to people such as refugees and migrants, who are likely to differ in their health status and their susceptibility to disease and adverse drug effects.

AETIOLOGY/ RISK FACTORS Malaria is mainly a rural disease, requiring nearby standing water. It is transmitted by bites of infected female anopheline mosquitoes, mainly at dusk and during the night.[1,6–8] In cities, mosquito bites are usually from female culicine mosquitoes, which are not vectors of malaria.[9] Malaria is resurgent in most tropical countries and risk to travellers is increasing.[10] The sickle cell trait has been shown to convey some protection against malaria in non-immune carriers of that trait. Non-immune adults with the sickle cell trait who develop severe malaria have lower parasite densities, fewer complications (e.g. cerebral malaria), and a reduced mortality compared with adults without the trait.[11] There is little good evidence on the degree of protection afforded by the sickle cell trait.[12]

PROGNOSIS Ninety per cent of tourists and business travellers who contract malaria do not become ill until after they return home.[5] "Imported malaria" is easily treated if diagnosed promptly, and follows a serious course in only about 12% of people.[13,14] The most severe form is cerebral malaria, with a case fatality rate in adult travellers of 2–6% mainly because of delays in diagnosis.[3,15]

AIMS To reduce the risk of infection; to prevent illness and death, with minimal adverse effects of treatment.

OUTCOMES Rates of clinical malaria and death, and adverse effects of treatment. Proxy measures include numbers of mosquito bites and rates of mosquito catches in indoor areas. We found limited evidence linking numbers of mosquito bites and risk of malaria.[16]

METHODS *Clinical Evidence* update search and appraisal March 2002.

QUESTION **What are the effects of non-drug preventive interventions in adult travellers?**

OPTION **AEROSOL INSECTICIDES**

One large observational study in travellers found insufficient evidence on the effects of aerosol insecticides in preventing malaria. Two RCTs in malaria endemic areas found that indoor spraying of aerosol insecticides reduced clinical malaria.

Benefits: We found no systematic review or RCTs in travellers. We found one questionnaire survey (89 617 European tourists returning from East Africa), which found that commercially available personal aerosol insecticides did not significantly reduce the incidence of malaria ($P = 0.55$).[17] Two community RCTs found that indoor residual spraying of synthetic pyrethroids reduced clinical malaria in lifelong residents of malaria-endemic areas.[18,19]

Harms: We found no reports of adverse effects.

Comment: Historically, indoor residual spraying has not been recommended for short stay travellers, but we found no evidence to support this.

OPTION **BIOLOGICAL CONTROL MEASURES**

We found no evidence of the effects of biological control measures in preventing malaria.

Benefits: We found no systematic review or RCTs of biological control measures in preventing malaria. One systematic review (search date 1997) identified two cohort studies based on mosquito counts. It found no evidence that growing the citrosa plant and encouraging natural predation of insects by erecting bird or bat houses reduced bites to humans from infected anopheline mosquitoes.[20]

Harms: We found no evidence of harms.

Comment: The only known way to reduce mosquito populations naturally is to eliminate sources of standing water, such as blocked gutters, tree stump holes and discarded tyres, cans and bottles.[20]

OPTION AIR CONDITIONING AND ELECTRIC FANS

One large observational study in travellers found that air conditioning significantly reduced the incidence of malaria. One small observational study found that electric ceiling fans significantly reduced numbers of culicine but not anopheline mosquitoes in indoor spaces.

Benefits: We found no systematic review or RCTs. One questionnaire survey of 89 617 European tourists returning from East Africa found that sleeping in an air conditioned room significantly reduced the incidence of malaria ($P = 0.04$).[17] One cohort study (6 experimental huts in Pakistan villages) of various antimosquito interventions found that an electric ceiling fan run at high speed significantly reduced total catches of blood fed culicine mosquitoes ($P < 0.05$), but did not significantly reduce total catches of blood fed anopheline mosquitoes.[21]

Harms: We found no evidence of harms.

Comment: These studies support the finding that mosquitoes are reluctant to fly in windy conditions,[22] but suggest that anopheline mosquitoes are more tolerant of wind turbulence than are culicine mosquitoes.

OPTION INSECT BUZZERS AND ELECTROCUTERS

We found no evidence of the effects of insect electrocuters and ultrasonic buzzers in preventing malaria.

Benefits: We found no systematic review and no RCTs with clinical malaria as an outcome.

Harms: We found no evidence of harms.

Comment: We found one non-randomised controlled trial (18 houses in Gabon) of a commercially available ultrasound emitting device. The trial lasted 6 weeks and used total mosquito catches as an outcome.[23] Most mosquitoes were culicine. It found no significant difference between the ultrasound emitting device and a sham device in mosquito catches ($P = 0.48$).[23] See comment under biological control measures, p 747.

OPTION MOSQUITO COILS AND VAPORISING MATS

We found no systematic review and no RCTs of the effects of coils and vaporising mats in preventing malaria in travellers. One RCT of coils and one observational study of pyrethroid vaporising mats found that these devices reduced numbers of mosquitoes in indoor spaces.

Benefits: We found no systematic review and no RCTs that used clinical malaria as an outcome. We found one RCT (18 houses in Malaysia) of various mosquito coil formulations versus no treatment.[24] It found that treated coils reduced populations of culicine mosquitoes by 75%.[24] One systematic review (search date 1997) identified one observational study of pyrethroid vaporising mats in six experimental huts in a Pakistan village setting. It found that the mats reduced total catches of blood fed mosquitoes by 56%.[20]

Harms: We found no evidence of harms.

Comment: None.

OPTION SMOKE

We found no RCTs of the effects of smoke in preventing malaria in travellers. One controlled clinical trial found that smoke repelled mosquitoes during the evening.

Benefits: We found no systematic review and no RCTs of smoke in preventing malaria. One controlled clinical trial, in which five small fires were tended on five successive evenings in a village in Papua New Guinea, found a smoke specific and species specific effect from different types of smoke. Catches of one anopheline species were reduced by 84% by burning betelnut (95% CI 62% to 94%), 69% by burning ginger (95% CI 25% to 87%), and 66% by burning coconut husks (95% CI 17% to 86%).[25]

Harms: There may be an irritant and toxic effect of smoke on the eyes and respiratory system, but this effect was not quantified in the controlled clinical trial.[25]

Comment: None.

OPTION INSECTICIDE TREATED NETS

We found no systematic review and no RCTs in travellers. One systematic review in malaria endemic settings has found that insecticide treated nets prevent malaria and reduce child mortality.

Benefits: We found no systematic review and no RCTs in travellers. We found one systematic review (search date not stated) that identified 18 RCTs in malaria endemic settings (non-traveller children and adults).[26] It found that nets sprayed or impregnated with permethrin versus no nets or untreated nets reduced the number of mild episodes of malaria (ARR 39%, 95% CI 27% to 48%) and child mortality (RR 0.83, 95% CI 0.77 to 0.90 [CI calculated by *Clinical Evidence*] NNT 180; CI not available).

Harms: We found no evidence of harms.

Comment: Permethrin remains active for about 4 months.[6]

OPTION INSECTICIDE TREATED CLOTHING

Two RCTs have found that permethrin treated fabric (clothing or sheets) significantly reduces the risk of contracting malaria.

Benefits: We found no systematic review but found two RCTs. The first RCT (172 male Colombian soldiers patrolling a malaria endemic area for a mean of 4.2 wks) found that permethrin impregnated uniforms versus non-impregnated uniforms significantly reduced the incidence of malaria (3/86 [3%] *v* 12/86 [13%]; RR 0.25, 95% CI 0.07 to 0.85).[27] The second RCT (102 refugee households in north-western Pakistan) found that permethrin treated wraps and top sheets versus placebo significantly reduced the risk of falciparum malaria (RR 0.56, 95% CI 0.41 to 0.78).[28]

Harms: The first RCT also included an analysis of permethrin impregnated uniforms versus non-impregnated uniforms in 286 soldiers patrolling a leishmaniasis endemic area for a mean 6.6 weeks. It found that 2/229 (0.9%) participants wearing permethrin impregnated uniforms experienced irritation and itching. No comparative information was given for soldiers wearing non-impregnated uniforms.

Comment: In the first RCT, the entire uniform (hat, shirt, undershirt, trousers, socks) was treated with a single application of permethrin. All participants were instructed to wear uniform continuously, day and night, with the sleeves rolled down. Each participant washed his own uniform two to three times during the study, using soap and water, but uniforms were not reimpregnated with permethrin. Topical insect repellents were not used. Trials in soldiers may not be generalisable to other travellers.

OPTION FULL LENGTH CLOTHING

One observational study in travellers found that wearing trousers and long sleeved shirts significantly reduced the incidence of malaria.

Benefits: We found no systematic review or RCTs. We found one questionnaire survey (89 617 European tourists returning from East Africa), which found that wearing long sleeved shirts and trousers significantly reduced the incidence of malaria ($P = 0.02$).[17] **Other lifestyle changes:** We found no studies (see comment below).

Harms: None.

Comment: Lifestyle change implies not travelling to malaria endemic regions during the rainy season (when most malaria transmission occurs) and not going outdoors in the evening or at night. Travellers who take day trips from a malaria free city to a malaria endemic region may be at minimal risk if they return to the city before dusk.[29] Some authors suggest wearing long sleeved shirts and trousers at dusk and wearing light rather than dark colours, as insects prefer landing on dark surfaces.[9,29]

OPTION TOPICAL INSECT REPELLENTS

We found no systematic review and no RCTs on the effects of topical insect repellents in preventing malaria. One very small crossover RCT found that DEET preparations protected against mosquito bites.

Benefits: We found no systematic review and no RCTs of topical repellents in preventing malaria. One small crossover RCT (4 people), involving successive random exposure to *Aedes aegypti* mosquitoes, compared six different topical controlled release preparations of DEET. It found that all gave at least 95% protection against mosquito bites.[30] **Topical repellents plus insecticide treated clothing:** See insecticide treated clothing, p 749.

Harms: We found a case series of systemic toxic reactions (confusion, irritability, insomnia) in US national park employees after repeated and prolonged use of DEET.[31] We found 14 case reports of contact urticaria and irritant contact dermatitis (mostly in soldiers) as a result of DEET.[17] The risk of absorption is especially high if DEET is left in the antecubital fossa overnight.[32] It also degrades certain plastics, such as spectacle frames.[33]

Comment: DEET is a broad spectrum repellent effective against mosquitoes, biting flies, chiggers, fleas, and ticks, and has been used for 40 years.[20] Although most authorities would recommend the use of topical repellents in malaria endemic areas, the only evidence comes from small RCTs with non-clinical outcomes. Larger RCTs are needed to compare DEET with other topical repellents and placebo in preventing malaria.

QUESTION What are the effects of drug prophylaxis in adult travellers?

OPTION CHLOROQUINE

We found no RCTs in travellers of the effects of chloroquine. One RCT in Austrian workers residing in Nigeria found no significant difference between chloroquine versus sulfadoxine plus pyrimethamine in the incidence of malaria.

Benefits: We found no systematic review or RCTs in travellers. One RCT (173 Austrian industrial workers residing in Nigeria) found no significant difference between chloroquine versus sulfadoxine plus pyrimethamine in the incidence of malaria at 6–22 months.[34]

Harms: The RCT found that chloroquine was associated with insomnia in 3/87 (3%) people.[35] Two people withdrew from the study owing to adverse effects: one with skin rash and the other with visual disturbance. Retrospective questionnaire surveys suggested that severe adverse effects were rare at prophylactic dosages.[35]

Comment: Alcohol consumption, other medication, and comorbidities can modify the effects of antimalaria drugs.[36,37]

OPTION CHLOROQUINE PLUS PROGUANIL

RCTs found no evidence that chloroquine plus proguanil is more effective than proguanil alone or than chloroquine plus other antimalaria drugs.

Benefits: We found no systematic review but found two RCTs. **Versus chloroquine plus sulfadoxine plus pyrimethamine:** One open label RCT (767 Scandinavian travellers to East Africa) comparing chloroquine plus proguanil versus chloroquine plus sulfadoxine plus pyrimethamine found no significant difference in rates of *P falciparum* malaria (4/384 [1%] *v* 3/383 [0.7%] travellers; RR 1.3, 95% CI 0.3 to 5.9).[38] **Versus proguanil alone:** One RCT in Dutch travellers to Africa found no significant difference between chloroquine (300 mg) weekly plus proguanil (200 mg daily) versus proguanil alone in incidence of *P falciparum* malaria (risk per 100 person months: chloroquine plus proguanil 2.8, 95% CI 0.9 to 10.1 *v* proguanil 6.0, 95% CI 2.6 to 14.0).[39]

Harms: In the RCT in Scandinavian travellers, adverse effects associated with chloroquine plus proguanil were nausea (3%), diarrhoea (2%), and dizziness (1%).[38] One cohort study (470 British soldiers in Belize) found that the risk of mouth ulcers almost doubled with chloroquine plus proguanil compared with proguanil alone (P = 0.025).[40]

Comment: The rates of confirmed *P falciparum* malaria in both trials were so small that a clinically important effect cannot be excluded.

OPTION DOXYCYCLINE IN ADULTS

Two RCTs in soldiers have found that doxycycline versus placebo significantly reduces the risk of malaria. One RCT found that doxycycline was associated with nausea and vomiting, diarrhoea, cough, headache, and unspecified dermatological symptoms at 13 weeks. We found no evidence on long term safety.

Benefits: We found no systematic review but found two RCTs. The first RCT (136 Indonesian soldiers) compared doxycycline versus mefloquine versus placebo in a malaria endemic setting. It found that, in an area of drug resistance, doxycycline versus placebo significantly reduced the risk of malaria (AR 1/67 [2%] with doxycycline *v* 53/69 [77%] with placebo; RR 0.02, 95% CI 0.003 to 0.14; NNT 1, 95% CI 1 to 2).[41] The second RCT (300 Indonesian soldiers and immigrants with limited immunity) comparing azithromycin versus doxycycline versus placebo found that doxycycline versus placebo significantly reduced the incidence of malaria (2/75 [3%] cases of *P falciparum* malaria with doxycycline *v* 29/77 [38%] with placebo; RR 0.07, 95% CI 0.02 to 0.29 NNT 3, 95% CI 2 to 4; 1/75 [2%] cases of *P vivax* malaria with doxycycline *v* 27/77 [35%] with placebo; RR 0.04, 95% CI 0.01 to 0.28).[42]

Harms: The first RCT found that doxycycline was associated with gastrointestinal symptoms (including nausea and vomiting, abdominal pain, and diarrhoea) in 16/67 (24%) soldiers, unspecified dermatological problems in 22/67 (33%), cough in 21/67 (31%), and headache in 11/67 (16%) over 13 weeks.[41] One questionnaire survey (383 returned Australian travellers taking doxycycline) found that 40% reported nausea or vomiting, 12% reported diarrhoea, and 9% of female travellers reported vaginitis.[43] Evidence from case reports suggests that, in sunny conditions, up to 50% of travellers using doxycycline may experience photoallergic skin rash.[44]

Comment: Most drug trials in travellers have been in soldiers, and the results may not be generalisable to tourists or business travellers.[45,46] The first RCT was a three arm parallel RCT. It compared mefloquine (68 people) versus doxycycline (67 people) versus placebo (69 people). Only the comparison of doxycycline versus placebo is included here.[41]

OPTION MEFLOQUINE IN ADULTS

One systematic review of one RCT in soldiers has found that mefloquine versus placebo had a protective efficacy of 100%. One RCT of mefloquine versus atovaquone plus proguanil found no cases of clinical malaria throughout the trial, but found a significantly higher rate of neuropsychiatric harm with mefloquine.

Benefits: **Versus placebo:** We found one systematic review (search date 2000)[46] that identified one RCT (203 Indonesian soldiers) comparing mefloquine versus doxycycline versus placebo in a malaria endemic setting. It found that mefloquine versus placebo had a protective efficacy (100%, 95% CI 93% to 100%). **Versus atovaquone plus proguanil:** One RCT (976 people) comparing mefloquine versus atovaquone plus proguanil found no clinical cases of malaria among people in the trial.[47]

Harms: The systematic review found no significant difference between mefloquine versus alternative antimalaria prophylaxis (chloroquine or doxycycline) in withdrawal (29/863 [3%] with mefloquine *v* 20/798 [2%] with alternative prophylaxis; RR 1.32, 95% CI 0.75 to 2.31).[46] Commonly reported adverse effects associated with mefloquine were headache (16%), insomnia (15%), and fatigue (8%).[46] The review found over 500 case reports of mefloquine adverse events, including four reports of death. These reports suggest that mefloquine is a potentially harmful drug for tourists and business travellers and requires more careful evaluation through an RCT in these groups.[46] One subsequent RCT (1013 non-immune tourists and business travellers) compared mefloquine plus placebo versus atovaquone plus proguanil plus placebo.[47] It found no significant difference in the risk of adverse events (313/493 [63.5%] with atovaquone plus proguanil *v* 324/483 [67.1%] with mefloquine; ARR 2.6%, 95% CI –3.4% to +8.5%). However, when adverse effects specifically attributable to the study drug were analysed, there were significantly more adverse effects caused by mefloquine than atovaquone plus proguanil (204/483 [42%] with mefloquine *v* 149/493 [30%] with atovaquone plus proguanil; RR 1.40, 95% CI 1.18 to 1.66; NNH 9, 95% CI 6 to 17; see comment below). Specifically, mefloquine versus atovaquone plus proguanil increased the incidence of "strange or vivid dreams" (66/483 [14%] *v* 33/493 [7%]), insomnia (65/483 [13%] *v* 15/493 [3%]), dizziness or vertigo (43/483 [9%] *v* 11/493 [2%]), anxiety (18/483 [4%] *v* 3/493 [1%]), depression (17/483 [4%] *v* 3/493 [1%]), visual difficulties (16/483 [3%] *v* 8/493 [2%]), and headache (19/493 [4%] *v* 32/483 [7%]). Retrospective questionnaire surveys in tourists and business travellers found that sleep disturbance and psychosis were common.[47,48] One review of 74 dermatological case reports found that up to 30% of mefloquine users developed a maculopapular rash and 4–10% had pruritus.[49] Nine cohort studies in tourists found that more women than men experienced more adverse effects (including dizziness, sleep disturbance, headache, diarrhoea, and nausea) with mefloquine.[43,48,50–56] One retrospective questionnaire survey of 93 668 European travellers to East Africa found that elderly travellers experienced fewer adverse reactions (not specified) with mefloquine than younger travellers ($P < 0.05$).[57]

Comment: Trials in soldiers may not be generalisable to other travellers. The RCT in Indonesian soldiers was a three arm parallel RCT. It compared mefloquine (68 people) versus doxycycline (67 people) versus placebo (69 people). Only the comparison of mefloquine versus placebo is included here.[46] The subsequent RCT of mefloquine versus atovaquone plus proguanil suggested a higher rate of adverse effects with mefloquine than in previous studies, but this RCT only reported adverse events that occurred after starting active treatment, which was 3 weeks earlier in the mefloquine than in the atovaquone plus proguanil group.

Malaria: prevention in travellers

OPTION ATOVAQUONE PLUS PROGUANIL

One RCT found no significant difference between atovaquone plus proguanil versus chloroquine plus proguanil in preventing malaria in travellers.

Benefits: We found no systematic review and no placebo controlled RCTs, but found two RCTs against other prophylactic regimens. **Versus chloroquine plus proguanil:** One multicentre RCT (1083 travellers)[58] comparing atovaquone plus proguanil versus chloroquine plus proguanil found no significant difference in the incidence of malaria (1/511 [0.2%] cases of *P ovale* malaria with atovaquone plus proguanil *v* 3/511 [0.6%] cases of *P falciparum* malaria with chloroquine plus proguanil; ARR 0.4%; RR 0.33, 95% CI 0.03 to 3.16). **Versus mefloquine:** See benefits under mefloquine in adults, p 752.

Harms: The multicentre RCT found no significant difference between atovaquone plus proguanil versus chloroquine plus proguanil in one or more adverse events (311/351 [61%] with atovaquone plus proguanil *v* 329/511 [64%] with chloroquine plus proguanil; RR 0.95, 95% CI 0.85 to 1.04).[58] Common adverse effects were mainly gastrointestinal (atovaquone plus proguanil *v* chloroquine plus proguanil: diarrhoea 5% *v* 7%, mouth ulcers 4% *v* 5%, abdominal pain 3% *v* 6%, nausea 2% *v* 7%), neuropsychiatric (atovaquone plus proguanil *v* chloroquine plus proguanil: strange/vivid dreams 4% *v* 3%, dizziness 3% *v* 4%, insomnia 2% *v* 2%), and visual difficulties (2% *v* 2%).[58] See also harms under mefloquine in adults, p 753.

Comment: None.

OPTION AMODIAQUINE

We found insufficient evidence on the effects of amodiaquine on malaria in travellers. However, we found limited observationl evidence that amodiaquine may cause liver damage and hepatitis.

Benefits: We found no RCTs in travellers.

Harms: One retrospective cohort study in 10 000 British travellers taking prophylactic amodiaquine reported severe neutropenia in about 1/2000 users.[59] We found 28 case reports describing liver damage or hepatitis in travellers who had taken amodiaquine to treat or prevent malaria.[60–65]

Comment: None.

OPTION PYRIMETHAMINE PLUS DAPSONE

We found insufficient evidence on the effects of pryimethamine plus dapsone in travellers.

Benefits: We found no RCTs in travellers. One RCT in Thai soldiers comparing pyrimethamine plus dapsone versus proguanil/dapsone found no significant difference in *P falciparum* infection rates over 40 days.[66]

Harms: The RCT in Thai soldiers found that fewer than 2% reported any drug related symptoms from pyrimethamine plus dapsone.[66] One retrospective cohort study in 15 000 Swedish travellers taking pyrimethamine plus dapsone reported agranulocytosis in about 1/2000 users.[67]

Comment: None.

OPTION SULFADOXINE PLUS PYRIMETHAMINE

We found insufficient evidence on the effects of sulfadoxine plus pyrimethamine in travellers.

Benefits: We found no RCTs of sulfadoxine plus pyrimethamine alone. We found one RCT of sufladoxine plus pyrimethamine plus chloroquine versus chloroquine plus proguanil. See benefits of cholorquine plus proguanil, p 751.

Harms: One retrospective cohort study in 182 300 US travellers taking prophylactic sulfadoxine plus pyrimethamine reported severe cutaneous reactions (erythema multiforme, Stevens-Johnson syndrome, toxic epidermal necrolysis) in 1/5000–8000 users, with a mortality of about 1/11 000–25 000 users.[67]

Comment: None.

QUESTION What are the effects of antimalaria vaccines in travellers?

We found no RCTs in travellers of the effects of antimalaria vaccines. One systematic review of antimalaria vaccines in residents of malaria endemic areas has found that the SPf66 vaccine versus placebo significantly reduces first attacks of malaria.

Benefits: We found no systematic review or RCTs of antimalaria vaccines in travellers. One systematic review (search date 1999, 13 RCTs) of antimalaria vaccines in residents of malaria endemic areas found that the SPf66 vaccine versus placebo significantly reduced first attacks of *P falciparum* malaria (1039/3718 [28%] with SPf66 *v* 1108/3681 [30%] with placebo; RR 0.90, 95% CI 0.84 to 0.96).[68]

Harms: The systematic review found that, in all but one of the RCTs of the SPf66 vaccine, fewer than 10% of recipients reported a systemic reaction (fever, headache, gastric symptoms, muscle pain, dizziness), and fewer than 35% reported a local reaction (inflammation, nodules, pain, erythema, pruritus, induration, injection site warmth).[68] The remaining RCT found a larger proportion of local cutaneous reactions, although these resolved within 24 hours with symptomatic treatment. It also reported higher systemic reaction rates after vaccination (11–16%), although rates after placebo were also higher (10–13%). Surveillance was also more intense than in the other RCTs.

Comment: None.

QUESTION **What are the effects of antimalaria interventions in child travellers?**

OPTION **INSECT REPELLENTS CONTAINING DEET IN CHILDREN**

We found no RCTs on the effects of DEET in preventing malaria in child travellers. Case reports in young children found serious adverse effects with DEET.

Benefits: We found no systematic review or RCTs.

Harms: We found 13 case reports of encephalopathic toxicity in children aged under 8 years after excessive use (not clearly defined) of topical insect repellents containing DEET.[69,70]

Comment: Infants and young children have thinner skin and greater surface area to mass ratio.[71] Some authors advise that ethylhexanediol should be used as a topical insect repellent in preference to DEET in children aged 1–8 years, and that in infants only plant based topical repellents, such as citronella oil, are safe.[72] However, we found insufficient evidence about the effects of these alternative repellents.

OPTION **DOXYCYCLINE IN CHILDREN**

We found no RCTs in child travellers on the use of doxycycline. Case reports in young children found adverse effects with doxycycline.

Benefits: We found no systematic review or RCTs.

Harms: Case reports have found that doxycycline inhibits bone growth and discolours teeth in children aged under 12 years.[9,35]

Comment: None.

OPTION **MEFLOQUINE IN CHILDREN**

We found no systematic review and no RCTs of the effects of mefloquine in preventing malaria in child travellers.

Benefits: We found no systematic review or RCTs.

Harms: Three RCTs in children and adults with symptomatic *P falciparum* malaria found that mefloquine was associated with less vomiting, nausea, anorexia, diarrhoea, and dizziness in children than in adults.[73–75]

Comment: None.

QUESTION **What are the effects of antimalaria interventions in pregnant travellers?**

OPTION **INSECTICIDE TREATED NETS IN PREGNANT TRAVELLERS**

We found no RCTs of the effects of insecticide treated nets on pregnant travellers. One RCT of pregnant residents found conflicting evidence on the effects of permethrin treated nets in preventing malaria.

Benefits: We found no systematic review or RCTs in pregnant travellers. We found one RCT (341 pregnant women living in Thailand, 3 sites), which compared permethrin treated nets versus non-treated nets versus usual practice.[76] Two sites found no significant difference in the incidence of malaria with treated nets, whereas the third site found that treated nets significantly reduced the incidence of malaria.

Harms: We found no evidence relating to pregnant travellers. The RCT of permethrin treated nets in Thailand found no evidence of toxic effects to mother or fetus.[76]

Comment: Pregnant women are relatively immunosuppressed and are at greater risk of malaria than non-pregnant women.[77] Contracting malaria significantly increases the likelihood of losing the fetus.[78]

OPTION INSECTICIDE TREATED CLOTHING IN PREGNANT TRAVELLERS

We found no systematic review or RCTs in pregnant travellers of the effects of impregnated clothing.

Benefits: We found no systematic review or RCTs.

Harms: We found little evidence relating to pregnant travellers. **Permethrin:** One RCT (341 pregnant women living in Thailand) of permethrin treated nets found no evidence of toxic effects to mother or fetus.[76] **DEET:** See harms of topical insect repellents in pregnant travellers, p 757.

Comment: Pregnant women are relatively immunosuppressed and are at greater risk of malaria than non-pregnant women.[77] Contracting malaria significantly increases the likelihood of losing the fetus.[78]

OPTION TOPICAL INSECT REPELLENTS IN PREGNANT TRAVELLERS

We found no RCTs in pregnant travellers. It is unclear which topical insect repellents are safe in pregnancy.

Benefits: We found no systematic review or RCTs.

Harms: We found little evidence in pregnant travellers. **DEET:** We found one case report indicating an adverse fetal outcome (mental retardation, impaired sensorimotor coordination, craniofacial dysmorphology) in a child whose mother had applied DEET daily throughout her pregnancy.[79] One RCT in pregnant women (897 refugees in a Thai forest area of low malaria endemicity) comparing DEET (median dose 214.2 g per pregnancy) versus a cosmetic cream found no differences in weekly reporting of headache, dizziness, or nausea and vomiting. It also found no adverse effects on infant survival, growth, or development at either birth or 1 year (survival 95.2% with DEET v 94.0% without DEET, P = 0.57; mean weight at 1 year 7983 g with DEET v 7984 g without DEET).[80] Some animal studies have found that DEET crosses the placental barrier.[81] Animal studies of reproductive effects of DEET are inconclusive.[78,82]

Comment: The RCT in refugees reported that DEET significantly increased the number of women reporting skin warmth (359/449 [80%] with DEET *v* 258/448 [58%] with cosmetic cream; RR 1.39, 95%

CI 1.27 to 1.52.), although the clinical significance of this is unclear.[80] Pregnant women are relatively immunosuppressed and are at greater risk of malaria than non-pregnant women.[77] Contracting malaria significantly increases the likelihood of losing the fetus.[78] Some authors advise that only plant based topical insect repellents, such as citronella oil, are safe in pregnancy, because of a potential risk of mutagenicity from DEET.[72] However, we found no evidence on the effects of alternative repellents.

OPTION ANTIMALARIA DRUGS IN PREGNANT TRAVELLERS

We found no RCTs on the effects of antimalaria drugs in pregnant travellers. We found insufficient evidence on the safety of chloroquine, doxycycline, and mefloquine in pregnancy.

Benefits: We found one systematic review (search date 2000), which identified no RCTs in pregnant travellers. It identified 15 RCTs of antimalaria drugs in pregnancy: all in residents of malaria endemic settings.[83] It found that antimalaria prophylaxis versus no prophylaxis significantly reduced the number of women infected at least once (5/167 [3%] *v* 37/170 [22%]; RR 0.14, 95% CI 0.06 to 0.34) and significantly reduced the number of episodes of fever (22/119 [18%] with prophylaxis *v* 45/108 [42%] with no prophylaxis; RR 0.42, 95% CI 0.27 to 0.66). It found no significant difference between antimalaria prophylaxis versus no prophylaxis in the number of perinatal deaths (66/1494 [4%] *v* 64/1426 [4%]; RR 1.02, 95% CI 0.73 to 1.43) or preterm births (17/182 [9%] with prophylaxis *v* 22/175 [12%] with no prophylaxis; RR 0.75, 95% CI 0.42 to 1.35), but found that antimalaria prophylaxis versus no prophylaxis resulted in significantly higher birth weight in the infant (OR 0.53, 95% CI 0.32 to 0.81).[83]

Harms: **Chloroquine:** One RCT (1464 pregnant long term residents of Burkina Faso) gave no information on adverse effects.[84] **Doxycycline:** Case reports have found that doxycycline taken in pregnancy or while breast feeding may damage fetal or infant bones or teeth.[9,35] **Mefloquine:** One RCT (339 long term Thai residents) found that mefloquine versus placebo significantly increased the number of women reporting dizziness (28% with mefloquine *v* 14% with placebo; $P < 0.005$), but found no other significant adverse effects on the mother, the pregnancy, or on infant survival or development over 2 years' follow up.[85]

Comment: Pregnant women are relatively immunosuppressed and are at greater risk of malaria than non-pregnant women.[77] Contracting malaria significantly increases the likelihood of losing the fetus.[78] Mefloquine is secreted in small quantities in breast milk, but it is believed that levels are too low to harm infants.[35]

QUESTION What are the effects of antimalaria interventions in airline pilots?

OPTION INSECTICIDES IN AIRLINE PILOTS

We found no RCTs on the use of insecticides in airline pilots.

Benefits: We found no systematic review or RCTs.

Harms: We found no evidence of harms of insecticides in airline pilots.

Comment: None.

OPTION ANTIMALARIA DRUGS IN AIRLINE PILOTS

We found no RCTs of the effects of antimalaria drugs in airline pilots.

Benefits: We found no systematic review or RCTs. One retrospective questionnaire survey (28 Israeli pilots taking doxycycline and 15 non-aviator crew taking mefloquine) found no cases of malaria at 4 weeks.[86]

Harms: **Doxycycline:** One retrospective questionnaire survey (28 Israeli pilots) found that 39% experienced adverse effects from doxycycline (abdominal pain 7/28, fatigue 5/28).[86] **Mefloquine:** One placebo controlled RCT of adverse effects (23 trainee commercial pilots) found no evidence that mefloquine significantly affected flying performance (mean total number of errors recorded by the instrument coordination analyser 12.6 with mefloquine *v* 11.7 with placebo).[87] One retrospective questionnaire survey (15 Israeli non-aviator aircrew) found that 13% experienced adverse effects from mefloquine (dizziness, nausea, and abdominal pain in 2/15, abdominal discomfort in 1/15).[86]

Comment: None.

Substantive changes

Atovaquone plus proguanil New RCT;[47] conclusion unchanged but high rates of adverse events with mefloquine.

Topical insect repellents in pregnant travellers New RCT;[80] found no significant difference in adverse events with DEET versus cosmetic cream.

REFERENCES

1. White NJ. Malaria. In: Cook GC, ed. *Manson's tropical diseases*. 20th ed. London: WB Saunders, 1996:1087–1164.
2. World Health Organization. *The world health report 1997. Conquering suffering, enriching humanity*. Geneva: WHO Office of Information, 1997.
3. Murphy GS, Oldfield EC. Falciparum malaria. *Infect Dis Clin North Am* 1996;10:747–755.
4. Kain KC, Keystone JS. Malaria in travelers. Epidemiology, disease and prevention. *Infect Dis Clin North Am* 1998;12:267–284.
5. World Health Organization. *International Travel and Health*. Geneva: WHO, 1999.
6. Winstanley P. Malaria: treatment. *J R Coll Physicians Lond* 1998;32:203–207.
7. Baudon D, Martet G. Paludisme et voyageurs: protection et information [in French]. *Med Trop (Mars)* 1997;57:497–500.
8. *Health information for international travel, 1996–97*. Atlanta: US Department of Health and Human Services, Public Health Service, Centers for Disease Control and Prevention, National Center for Infectious Diseases, Division of Quarantine; 1997 HHS Publication No 95:8280.
9. Bradley DJ, Warhurst DC. Guidelines for the prevention of malaria in travellers from the United Kingdom. *Commun Dis Rep CDR Rev* 1997;7:R137–R152.
10. Krogstad DJ. Malaria as a reemerging disease. *Epidemiol Rev* 1996;18:77–89.
11. Hill AVS. Malaria resistance genes: a natural selection. *Trans R Soc Trop Med Hyg* 1992;86:225–232.
12. Fleming AF. Haematological diseases in the tropics. In: Cook GC, ed. *Manson's tropical diseases*. 20th ed. London: WB Saunders, 1996:101–173.
13. Olsen VV. Basic considerations in connection with malaria prophylaxis [in Danish]. *Ugeskr Læger* 1998;160:2410–2411.
14. Miller SA, Bergman BP, Croft AM. Epidemiology of malaria in the British Army from 1982–1986. *J R Army Med Corps* 1999;145:20–22.
15. Dolmans WMV, van der Kaay HJ, Leentvaar-Kuijpers A, et al. Malariaprofylaxe: adviezen wederom aangepast. *Ned Tijdschr Geneeskd* 1996;140:892–893.
16. Beier JC, Oster CN, Onyango FK, et al. *Plasmodium falciparum* incidence relative to entomological inoculation rates at a site proposed for testing malaria vaccines in western Kenya. *Am J Trop Med Hyg* 1994;50;529–536.
17. Schoepke A, Steffen R, Gratz N. Effectiveness of personal protection measures against mosquito bites for malaria prophylaxis in travelers. *J Travel Med* 1998;128:931–940.

18. Misra SP, Webber R, Lines J, et al. Spray versus treated nets using deltamethrin – a community randomized trial in India. *Trans R Soc Trop Med Hyg* 1999;93:456–457.
19. Rowland M, Mahmood P, Iqbal J, et al. Indoor residual spraying with alphacypermethrin controls malaria in Pakistan: a community-randomized trial. *Trop Med Int Health* 2000;5:472–481.
20. Fradin MS. Mosquitoes and mosquito repellents: a clinician's guide. *Ann Intern Med* 1998;128:931–940. Search date 1997; primary sources Medline, the Internet, the Extension Toxicology Network database, hand searches of reference lists, and contact with distributors of natural insect repellents.
21. Hewitt SE, Farhan M, Urhaman H, et al. Self-protection from malaria vectors in Pakistan: an evaluation of popular existing methods and appropriate new techniques in Afghan refugee communities. *Ann Trop Med Parasitol* 1996;90:337–344.
22. Service MW. *Mosquito ecology: field sampling methods*. 2nd ed. London: Chapman and Hall, 1993.
23. Sylla el-HK, Lell B, Krsmsner PG. A blinded, controlled trial of an ultrasound device as mosquito repellent. *Wein Klin Wochenschr* 2000;112:448–450.
24. Yap HH, Tan HT, Yahaya AM, et al. Field efficacy of mosquito coil formulations containing d-allethrin and d-transallethrin against indoor mosquitoes especially *Culex quinquefasciatus*. *Southeast Asian J Trop Med Public Health* 1990;21:558–563.
25. Vernède R, van Meer MMM, Aplers MP. Smoke as a form of personal protection against mosquitoes, a field study in Papua New Guinea. *Southeast Asian J Trop Med Public Health* 1994;25:771–775.
26. Lengeler C. Insecticide treated bednets and curtains for preventing malaria. In: The Cochrane Library, Issue 1, 2002. Oxford: Update Software. Search date not stated; primary sources Cochrane Infectious Diseases Group Trial Register, Medline, Embase, and hand searches of reference lists, relevant journals, and personal contact with funding agencies and manufacturers.
27. Soto J, Medina F, Dember N, Berman J. Efficacy of permethrin-impregnated uniforms in the prevention of malaria and leishmaniasis in Colombian soldiers. *Clin Infect Dis* 1995;21:599–602.
28. Rowland M, Durrani N, Hewitt S, et al. Permethrin-treated *chaddars* and top-sheets: appropriate technology for protection against malaria in Afghanistan and other complex emergencies. *Trans R Soc Trop Med Hyg* 1999;93:465–472.
29. Juckett G. Malaria prevention in travelers. *Am Fam Physician* 1999;59:2523–2530.
30. Gupta RK, Rutledge LC. Laboratory evaluation of controlled-release repellent formulations on human volunteers under three climatic regimens. *J Am Mosq Control Assoc* 1989;5:52–55.
31. McConnell R, Fidler AT, Chrislip D. Everglades National Park health hazard evaluation report. Cincinatti, Ohio: US Department of Health and Human Services, Public Health Service, 1986. NIOSH Health Hazard Evaluation Report No. HETA-83–085-1757.
32. Lamberg SI, Mulrennan JA. Bullous reaction to diethyl toluamide (DEET) resembling a blistering insect eruption. *Arch Dermatol* 1969;100:582–586.
33. Curtis CF, Townson H. Malaria: existing methods of vector control and molecular entomology. *Br Med Bull* 1998;54:311–325.
34. Stemberger H, Leimer R, Widermann G. Tolerability of long-term prophylaxis with Fansidar: a randomized double-blind study in Nigeria. *Acta Trop* 1984;41:391–399.
35. Petersen E. Malariaprofylakse. *Ugeskr Læger* 1997;159:2723–2730.
36. Gherardin T. Mefloquine as malaria prophylaxis. *Aust Fam Physician* 1999;28:310.
37. Schlagenhauf P. Mefloquine for malaria chemoprophylaxis 1992–1998: a review. *J Travel Med* 1999;6:122–133.
38. Fogh S, Schapira A, Bygbjerg IC, et al. Malaria chemoprophylaxis in travellers to east Africa: a comparative prospective study of chloroquine plus proguanil with chloroquine plus sulfadoxine-pyrimethamine. *BMJ* 1988;296:820–822.
39. Wetsteyn JCFM, de Geus A. Comparison of three regimens for malaria prophylaxis in travellers to east, central, and southern Africa. *BMJ* 1993;307:1041–1043.
40. Drysdale SF, Phillips-Howard PA, Behrens RH. Proguanil, chloroquine, and mouth ulcers. *Lancet* 1990;335:164.
41. Ohrt C, Richie TL, Widjaja H, et al. Mefloquine compared with doxycycline for the prophylaxis of malaria in Indonesian soldiers. A randomized, double-blind, placebo-controlled trial. *Ann Intern Med* 1997;126:963–972.
42. Taylor WR, Richie TL, Fryauff DJ, et al. Malaria prophylaxis using azithromycin: a double-blind, placebo-controlled trial in Irian Jaya, Indonesia. *Clin Infect Dis* 1999;28:74–81.
43. Phillips MA, Kass RB. User acceptability patterns for mefloquine and doxycycline malaria chemoprophylaxis. *J Travel Med* 1996;3:40–45.
44. Leutscher PDC. Malariaprofylakse. *Ugeskr Læger* 1997;159:4866–4867.
45. Anonymous. Mefloquine and malaria prophylaxis [letter]. *Drug Ther Bull* 1998;36:20–22.
46. Croft AMJ, Garner P. Mefloquine for preventing malaria in non-immune adult travellers. In: The Cochrane Library, Issue 1, 2001. Oxford: Update Software. Search date 2000; primary sources Cochrane Infectious Diseases Group Trial Register, Medline, Embase, Lilacs, Science Citation Index, hand searches of reference lists of articles, and personal contact with researchers in the subject of malaria chemoprophylaxis, and drug companies.
47. Overbosch D, Schilthuis H, Bienzle U, et al. Atovaquone-proguanil versus mefloquine for malaria prophylaxis in nonimmune travelers: results from a randomized double-blind study. *Clin Infect Dis* 2001;33:1015–1021.
48. Barrett PJ, Emmins PD, Clarke PD, Bradley DJ. Comparison of adverse events associated with use of mefloquine and combinations of chloroquine and proguanil as antimalarial prophylaxis: postal and telephone survey of travellers. *BMJ* 1996;313:525–528.
49. Smith HR, Croft AM, Black MM. Dermatological adverse effects with the antimalarial drug mefloquine: a review of 74 published case reports. *Clin Exp Dermatol* 1999;24:249–254.
50. Weinke T, Trautmann M, Held T, et al. Neuropsychiatric side effects after the use of mefloquine. *Am J Trop Med Hyg* 1991;45:86–91.
51. Bem L, Kerr L, Stuerchler D. Mefloquine prophylaxis: an overview of spontaneous reports of severe psychiatric reactions and convulsions. *J Trop Med Hyg* 1992;95:167–169.
52. Huzly D, Schönfeld C, Beurle W, et al. Malaria chemoprophylaxis in German tourists: a prospective study on compliance and adverse reactions. *J Travel Med* 1996;3:148–155.
53. Schlagenhauf P, Steffen R, Lobel H, et al. Mefloquine tolerability during chemoprophylaxis:

focus on adverse event assessments, stereochemistry and compliance. *Trop Med Int Health* 1996;1:485–494.
54. Handschin JC, Wall M, Steffen R, et al. Tolerability and effectiveness of malaria chemoprophylaxis with mefloquine or chloroquine with or without co-medication. *J Travel Med* 1997;4:121–127.
55. Van Riemsdijk MM, van der Klauw MM, van Heest JAC, et al. Neuro-psychiatric effects of antimalarials. *Eur J Clin Pharmacol* 1997;52:1–6.
56. Micheo C, Arias C, Rovira A. Adverse effects and compliance with mefloquine or chloroquine + proguanil malaria chemoprophylaxis. *Proceedings of the Second European Conference on Travel Medicine,* Venice, Italy, 2000:29–31.
57. Mittelholzer ML, Wall M, Steffen R, et al. Malaria prophylaxis in different age groups. *J Travel Med* 1996;4:219–223.
58. Hogh B, Clarke PD, Camus D, et al. Atovaquone-proguanil versus chloroquine-proguanil for malaria prophylaxis in non-immune travellers: a randomised, double-blind study. *Lancet* 2000;356:1888–1894.
59. Hatton CSR, Peto TEA, Bunch C, et al. Frequency of severe neutropenia associated with amodiaquine prophylaxis against malaria. *Lancet* 1986;1:411–414.
60. Neftel K, Woodtly W, Schmid M, et al. Amodiaquine induced agranulocytosis and liver damage. *BMJ* 1986;292:721–723.
61. Larrey D, Castot A, Pessayre D, et al. Amodiaquine-induced hepatitis. A report of seven cases. *Ann Intern Med* 1986;104:801–803.
62. Woodtli W, Vonmoos P, Siegrist P, et al. Amodiaquin-induzierte hepatitis mit leukopenie. *Schweiz Med Wochenschr* 1986;116:966–968.
63. Bernuau J, Larrey D, Campillo B, et al. Amodiaquine-induced fulminant hepatitis. *J Hepatol* 1988;6:109–112.
64. Charmot G, Goujon C. Hépatites mineures pouvant être duesà l'amodiaquine. *Bull Soc Pathol Exot* 1987;80:266–270.
65. Raymond JM, Dumas F, Baldit C, et al. Fatal acute hepatitis due to amodiaquine. *J Clin Gastroenterol* 1989;11:602–603.
66. Shanks GD, Edstein MD, Suriyamongkol V, et al. Malaria chemoprohylaxis using proguanil/dapsone combinations on the Thai-Cambodian border. *Am J Trop Med Hyg* 1992;46:6543–648.
67. Miller KD, Lobel HO, Satriale RF, et al. Severe cutaneous reactions among American travelers using pyrimethamine-sulfadoxine for malaria prophylaxis. *Am J Trop Med Hyg* 1986;35:451–458.
68. Graves P, Gelbland H. Vaccines for preventing malaria. In: The Cochrane Library, Issue 1, 2001. Oxford: Update Software. Search date 1999; primary sources Cochrane Infectious Diseases Group Trials Register, Cochrane Controlled Trial Register, Medline, Embase, hand searches of reference lists, and personal contact with organisations and researchers in the field.
69. Osimitz TG, Murphy JV. Neurological effects associated with use of the insect repellent *N,N*-diethyl-*m*-toluamide (DEET). *J Toxicol Clin Toxicol* 1997;35:435–441.
70. De Garbino JP, Laborde A. Toxicity of an insect repellent: *N,N*-diethyl-*m*-toluamide. *Vet Hum Toxicol* 1983;25:422–423.
71. Are insect repellents safe [editorial]? *Lancet* 1988;ii:610–611.
72. Bouchaud O, Longuet C, Coulaud JP. Prophylaxie du paludisme. *Rev Prat* 1998;48:279–286.
73. Smithuis FM, van Woensel JBM, Nordlander E, et al. Comparison of two mefloquine regimens for treatment of *Plasmodium falciparum* malaria on the northeastern Thai-Cambodian border. *Antimicrob Agents Chemother* 1993;37:1977–1981.
74. Ter Kuile FO, Dolan G, Nosten F, et al. Halofantrine versus mefloquine in treatment of multidrug-resistant falciparum malaria. *Lancet* 1993;341:1044–1049.
75. Luxemburger C, Price RN, Nosten F, et al. Mefloquine in infants and young children. *Ann Trop Paediatr* 1996;16:281–286.
76. Dolan G, ter Kuile FO, Jacoutot V, et al. Bed nets for the prevention of malaria and anaemia in pregnancy. *Trans R Soc Trop Med Hyg* 1993;87:620–626.
77. Suh KN, Keystone JS. Malaria prophylaxis in pregnancy and children. *Infect Dis Clin Pract* 1996;5:541–546.
78. Osimitz TG, Grothaus RH. The present safety assessment of DEET. *J Am Mosq Control Assoc* 1995;11:274–278.
79. Schaefer C, Peters PW. Intrauterine diethyltoluamide exposure and fetal outcome. *Reprod Toxicol* 1992;6:175–176.
80. McGready R, Hamilton KA, Simpson JA, et al. Safety of the insect repellent *N,N*-diethyl-*m*-toluamide (DEET) in pregnancy. *Am J Trop Med Hyg* 2001;65:285–289.
81. Blomquist L, Thorsell W. Distribution and fate of the insect repellent 14C-*N,N*-diethyl-*m*-toluamide in the animal body. II. Distribution and excretion after cutaneous application. *Acta Pharmacol Toxicol (Copenh)* 1977;41:235–243.
82. Samuel BU, Barry M. The pregnant traveler. *Infect Dis Clin North Am* 1998;12:325–354.
83. Garner PGü, Imezoglu AM. Prevention versus treatment for malaria in pregnant women. In: The Cochrane Library, Issue 2, 2001. Oxford: Update Software. Search date 2000; primary sources Cochrane Infectious Diseases Group Trial Register, Cochrane Controlled Trials Register, Medline, Embase, hand searches of reference lists, and personal contact with researchers.
84. Cot M, Roisin A, Barro D, et al. Effect of chloroquine chemoprophylaxis during pregnancy on birth weight: results of a randomized trial. *Am J Trop Med Hyg* 1992;46:21–27.
85. Nosten F, ter Kuile F, Maelankiri L, et al. Mefloquine prophylaxis prevents malaria during pregnancy: a double-blind, placebo-controlled study. *J Infect Dis* 1994;169:595–603.
86. Shamiss A, Atar E, Zohar L, Cain Y. Mefloquine versus doxycycline for malaria prophylaxis in intermittent exposure of Israeli Air Force aircrew in Rwanda. *Aviat Space Environ Med* 1996;67:872–873.
87. Schlagenhauf P, Lobel H, Steffen R, et al. Tolerance of mefloquine by Swissair trainee pilots. *Am J Trop Med Hyg* 1997;56:235–240.

Ashley Croft
Consultant in Public Health Medicine
Ministry of Defence, London, UK

Competing interests: None declared.

Mammalian bites

Search date November 2001

Iara Marques de Medeiros and Humberto Saconato

QUESTIONS

INTERVENTIONS

Likely to be beneficial
Education to prevent bites....764
Antibiotic prophylaxis........765
Debridement, irrigation, and decontamination* 766
Antibiotics for treatment of infectious complications of mammalian bites* 766

Unknown effectiveness
Education to prevent bites in specific occupational groups.764
Tetanus toxoid after mammalian bites.........764
Closure of cutaneous wounds .766
Antibiotics versus other antibiotics for treatment of infectious complications of mammalian bites..................766

To be covered in future updates
Prevention of human and animal rabies

*No RCT evidence but there is consensus that treatment is likely to be beneficial.

See glossary, p 767

Key Messages

- **Antibiotics for treatment of infectious complications of mammalian bites** We found no RCTs of antibiotics versus placebo for the treatment of infectious complications of mammalian bites. However, there is consensus that antibiotics are likely to be beneficial.
- **Antibiotic prophylaxis** Limited evidence from one systematic review found no significant difference with antibiotics versus control in the infection rate in people bitten by a dog, cat, or human in the preceding 24 hours. Meta-analysis according to the site of the wound found that antibiotics significantly reduced infections of the hand (NNT 4, 95% CI 2 to 50). One small RCT in the review found that in people with human bites, antibiotics versus control significantly reduced the rate of infection.
- **Antibiotics versus other antibiotics for treatment of infectious complications of mammalian bites** One RCT in people with infected and uninfected animal and human bites comparing penicillin with or without dicloxacillin versus amoxicillin/clavulanic acid found no significant difference in failure rate (which was undefined).
- **Closure of cutaneous wounds** One poor quality RCT comparing primary wound closure versus no closure in people with dog bites found no significant difference in the incidence of infection, but the RCT was too small to exclude clinically important effects.

Clin Evid 2002;8:762–768.

- **Debridement, irrigation, and decontamination** We found no systematic review, RCTs, or good cohort studies assessing debridement, irrigation, decontamination measures, and serum infiltration in the wound. However, there is consensus that such measures are likely to be beneficial.
- **Education to prevent bites** We found no RCTs of the effect of education programmes on the incidence of mammalian bites. One RCT found that an educational programme versus no education in school children significantly increased precautionary behaviour around dogs.
- **Education to prevent bites in specific occupational groups** We found no RCTs of education to prevent bites in specific occupational groups.
- **Tetanus toxoid after mammalian bites** We found no evidence on the effects of tetanus toxoid in preventing tetanus after human or animal bites.

DEFINITION Bite wounds are mainly caused by humans, dogs, or cats. They include superficial abrasions (30–43%), lacerations (31–45%), and puncture (see glossary, p 767) wounds (13–34%).[1]

INCIDENCE/ PREVALENCE In the USA, 17–18% of people with dog bites seek medical attention, and 1% require hospitalisation;[2,3] the incidence of dog bites is 3.5–4.7 million bites a year.[4] Children constitute 30–50% of all mammalian bite injuries.[5] In areas where domestic animal rabies has not been controlled, dogs account for 90% of the reported animal bites in humans. In contrast, in areas where domestic animal rabies is well controlled, dogs account for less than 5% of the reported animal bites.

AETIOLOGY/ RISK FACTORS Over 70% of cases, people are bitten by their own pets or by an animal known to them. Males are more likely to be bitten than females, and males are most likely to be bitten by dogs whereas females are more likely to be bitten by cats.[4] One study found that children under 5 years old were significantly more likely than older children to provoke animals prior to being bitten.[6] One study of infected dog and cat bites found that the most commonly isolated bacteria was *Pasteurella*, followed by *Streptococci*, *Staphylococci*, *Moraxella*, *Corynebacterium*, and *Neisseria*.[7] Mixed aerobic and anaerobic infection was more common than anaerobic infection alone.

PROGNOSIS In the USA, dog bites cause about 20 deaths a year.[8] In children, dog bites frequently involve the face, potentially resulting in severe lacerations, and scarring.[9] Rabies, a life threatening viral encephalitis, may be contracted as a consequence of being bitten or scratched by a rabid animal. More than 99% of human rabies is in developing countries where canine rabies is endemic.[10] In people bitten by a rabid animal and not treated, the risk of contracting rabies has been estimated to be 5–80%, depending on the animal species, severity of the bite, infectivity of the animal saliva, virus inoculum, host factors, and possibly the strain of rabies virus.[11,12] One study in the USA reported that the risk of rabies in 21 people with proven rabies exposure was between 5–15%.[13]

AIMS To reduce mammalian bites; to reduce complications after mammalian bites, with minimal adverse effects.

OUTCOMES Prevention of mammalian bites; prevention of infection after mammalian bites; cure rate of infection due to mammalian bites.

METHODS *Clinical Evidence* search and appraisal November 2001. In addition, we searched Web of Science (Science Citation Index to October 2001). Observational studies were used when systematic reviews or RCTs were not found.

QUESTION What are the effects of interventions to prevent mammalian bites?

OPTION EDUCATION

We found no RCTs of the effect of education programmes on the incidence of mammalian bites. One RCT found that an educational programme versus no education in school children significantly increased precautionary behaviour around dogs. We found no RCTs of education to prevent bites in specific occupational groups.

Benefits: We found no systematic review. **In the general population:** We found no RCTs on the effect of education programmes on the incidence of mammalian bites. One RCT (346 school children aged 7–8 years in 8 primary schools in Sydney, Australia) cluster randomised schools to either an educational programme or no education.[14] The educational programme consisted of one 30 minute lesson demonstrating behavioural techniques around dogs, such as how to recognise friendly, angry, or frightened dogs; how to approach dogs and owners when they wanted to pat a dog; and how to adopt a precautionary and protective body posture when approached or knocked over by a dog. After 10 days, children were videotaped for 10 minutes whilst playing in school grounds where a dog was leashed. The trial found that children in schools receiving education versus no education were significantly less likely to pat the dog without hesitation and try to excite it (118/149 [79%] *v* 18/197 [9%]; RR 0.16, 95% CI 0.064 to 0.20), and if they did it was only after considerable period of careful assessment. **In specific occupational groups:** We found no RCTs.

Harms: The RCT did not report on adverse effects.[14]

Comment: The trial was brief and reported only the proxy outcome of behaviour modification. The effect of such a programme on the incidence of dog bites in the long term is unclear.

QUESTION What are the effects of measures to prevent complications from mammalian bites?

OPTION TETANUS TOXOID

We found no evidence on the effects of tetanus toxoid in preventing tetanus after human or animal bites.

Benefits: We found no systematic review, RCTs, or cohort studies in human or animal bites.

Harms: We found no evidence.

Comment: General measures to prevent tetanus may be beneficial (cleaning the wound, removing debris, excision [except on the face], irrigation, and excision and removal of skin flaps around puncture wounds), but we found no RCTs to confirm or refute this view. We found no studies of the effects of passive immunisation using tetanus immunoglogulin.[15]

OPTION ANTIBIOTIC PROPHYLAXIS

Limited evidence from one systematic review found no significant difference between antibiotics versus control in the infection rate in people with dog, cat, or human bites. Meta-analysis according to the site of the wound found that antibiotics significantly reduced infections of the hand. One small RCT in the review found that in people with human bites, antibiotics versus control significantly reduced the rate of infection.

Benefits: We found one systematic review (search date 2000, 7 RCTs, 1 quasi-randomised controlled trial, 522 people bitten by dogs, cats, or humans in the preceding 24 h) comparing prophylactic antibiotics versus placebo or no treatment.[16] There was significant heterogeneity between trials. It found no significant difference between antibiotics versus placebo in the infection rate after dog, cat, and human bites (timescale not specified: OR 0.49, 95% CI 0.15 to 1.58). When the results were analysed for each wound site (hands, trunk, arms, or head/neck), antibiotics significantly reduced only infections of the hand (3 RCTs: 2% with antibiotics *v* 28% with control; OR 0.10, 95% CI 0.01 to 0.86; NNT 4, 95% CI 2 to 50). **Animal bites:** The review identified six RCTs (463 people) of dog bites, and found no significant difference between antibiotics versus control in the rate of infection (10/225 [4%] with antibiotics *v* 13/238 [5%] with control; OR 0.74, 95% CI 0.30 to 1.85). The review identified one small RCT of cat bites (12 people), which found no significant difference in the rate of infection between antibiotics versus control reduced (4/6 [67%] with antibiotics *v* 0/5 with control; $P < 0.06$).[16] **Human bites:** The review included one RCT of human bites (48 people with uncomplicated bites on the hand in the preceding 24 h) comparing oral cephalosporin versus intravenous cephalosporin plus penicillin versus placebo. All participants received debridement, irrigation, and sterile dressing and remained in hospital for 5 days. It found that antibiotics by either route versus placebo significantly reduced the number of people with wound infection (0/33 with oral or intravenous antibiotics *v* 7/15 [47%]; $P < 0.05$, timescale not stated).[16]

Harms: The review did not report on adverse effects.[16]

Comment: Most of the RCTs were small, and gave insufficient information about allocation concealment and randomisation. Some studies were not double blind, and four studies had withdrawal rates of greater than 10%.[16] The effects of antibiotic prophylaxis in preventing complications of mammalian bites remains unclear. Only a few studies analysed the effect of antibiotics on specific wound types (lacerations, [puncture—see glossary, p 767], or avulsions).[16]

OPTION **PRIMARY WOUND CLOSURE**

One poor quality RCT comparing primary wound closure versus no closure in people with dog bites found no significant difference in the incidence of infection, but the RCT was too small to exclude clinically important effects.

Benefits: We found no systematic review. We found one RCT (96 people bitten by dogs in the preceding 30 mins to 24 h) comparing primary wound closure versus no closure.[17] All wounds were debrided and irrigated, and tetanus immunisation was updated but no antibiotics were given. In uncomplicated lacerations, closure was performed by an experienced nurse; in complicated lacerations closure was performed by a specialist. The RCT found no difference between closed versus open wounds in the incidence of infection (timescale not stated: 7/92 [8%] with closed *v* 6/77 [8%] with open; RR 0.98, 95% CI 0.33 to 2.62). There were significantly more infections of the hand compared with the rest of the body (69% with hand *v* 31% with rest of body), but there was no difference between closure and non-closure groups in hand infections (5/9 [56%] with closure *v* 4/9 [44%] with non-closure). The rabies risk was not assessed.

Harms: The RCT did not report on adverse effects.[17]

Comment: Although the RCT found no increased risk of infection with primary wound closure, further RCTs are required to confirm this conclusion, and also to evaluate if wound closure may increase the risk of rabies.

OPTION **DEBRIDEMENT, IRRIGATION, AND DECONTAMINATION**

We found no systematic review, RCTs, or good cohort studies assessing debridement, irrigation, decontamination measures, and serum infiltration in the wound. However, there is consensus that such measures are likely to be beneficial.

Benefits: We found no systematic review, RCTs, or good cohort studies.

Harms: We found no evidence.

Comment: It would be regarded as unethical to conduct an RCT comparing debridement, irrigation, and decontamination versus no treatment.

QUESTION **What are the effects of treatments for the infectious complications of mammalian bites?**

OPTION **ANTIBIOTICS**

We found no RCTs of antibiotics versus placebo for the treatment of infectious complications of mammalian bites. One RCT in people with infected and uninfected animal and human bites comparing penicillin with or without dicloxacillin versus amoxicillin/clavulanic acid found no significant difference in failure rate (which was undefined).

Benefits: We found no systematic review. **Versus placebo:** We found no RCTs. **Versus other antibiotics:** We found one RCT (61 people bitten in the preceding 30 mins to 10 days; 48 by animals, 13 by humans) comparing penicillin with or without dicloxacillin versus amoxicillin (amoxycillin)/clavulanic acid.[10] Treatment was given for 5 days in people bitten less than 8 hours previously without clinical infection (34 people), and for 10 days in people bitten more than 8 hours previously or with clinical infection (27 people). All wounds received usual care, and were left closed or open at the discretion of the attending physician. Before inclusion, 27 people already had clinical signs of infection (see comment below). The RCT found no significant difference in failure rate (which was undefined) between penicillin/dicloxacillin versus amoxicillin/clavulanic acid (timescale not stated: 1/31 [3%] *v* 3/30 [10%]; RR 0.32, 95% CI 0.03 to 2.54).

Harms: Adverse effects were significantly more common in people using amoxicillin/clavulanic acid versus penicillin/dicloxacillin (13/31 [42%] *v* 3/30 [10%]; RR 4.2, 95% CI 1.5 to 7.4; NNH 3, 95% CI 2 to 19). Diarrhoea was the most common adverse event (9/31 [29%] with amoxicillin/clavulanic acid *v* 1/30 [3%] with penicillin/dicloxacillin; RR 8.71, 95% CI 1.34 to 23.3; NNH 4, 95% CI 1 to 79).[10]

Comment: Interpretation of the results is difficult as the main outcome measure of "failure rate" was not defined. Also, failure rates were not separated according to whether people had infected or uninfected wounds at inclusion.

GLOSSARY

Abrasion The scraping or rubbing away of a small area of skin or mucous membrane.

Laceration Occurs when the skin and/or soft tissues are torn by the crushing and shearing forces produced on impact; characterised by ragged, irregular margins, surrounding contusion, marginal abrasion, and tissue bridging in the wound depths.

Puncture A wound caused by perforation of the skin with a sharp point.

REFERENCES

1. Dire DJ. Emergency management of dog and cat bite wounds. *Emerg Med Clin North Am* 1992;10:719–736.
2. Sacks JJ, Kresnow M, Houston B. Dog bites: how big a problem? *Injury Prev* 1996;2:52–54.
3. Quinlan KP, Sacks JJ. Hospitalizations for dog bite injuries. *JAMA* 1999;281:232–233.
4. Overall KL, Love M. Dog bites to humans–demography, epidemiology, injury and risk. *JAMA* 2001;218:1923–1934.
5. Fishbein DB, Bernard KW. Rabies virus. In: *Mandell, Douglas and Bennett's Principles and practice of Infectious Diseases*. 4th ed. Vol 2:1527–1543.
6. Avner JR, Baker MD. Dog bites in urban children. *Pedriatrics* 1991;88:55–57.
7. Talan DA, Citron DM, Abrahamian FM, Moran GJ, Goldstein EJ. Bacteriologic analysis of infected dog and cat bites. Emergency Medicine Animal Bite Infection Study Group. *N Engl J Med* 1999;340:85–92.
8. Sacks JJ, Sattin RW, Bonzo SE. Dog bite-related fatalities from 1979 through 1988. *JAMA* 1989;262:1489–1492.
9. Karlson TA. The incidence of facial injuries from dog bites. *JAMA* 1984;251:3265–3267.
10. Goldstein EJC, Reinhardt JF, Murray PM, Finegold SM. Outpatient therapy of bite wounds. Demographic data, bacteriology, and prospective, randomized trial of amoxicillin/clavulanic acid versus penicillin +/- dicloxacillin. *Int J Dermatol* 1987;26:123–127.
11. Hattwick M, Gregg MB. The disease in man. In: Baer GM, ed. *The natural history of rabies*. New York: Academic Press, 1975:281–304.
12. Suntharasamai P, Warrell DA, Warrell MJ, et al. New purified Vero-cell vaccine prevents rabies in patients bitten by rabid animals. *Lancet* 1986;2:129–131.
13. Anderson LJ, Sikes RK, Langkop CW. Postexposure trial of a human diploid cell strain rabies vaccine. *J Infect Dis* 1980;142:133–138.

14. Chapman S, Cornwall J, Righetti J, Sung L. Preventing dog bites in children: randomised controlled trial of an educational intervention. *BMJ* 2000;320:1512–1513.
15. De Melker HE, De Melker RA. Dog bites: publications on risk factors, infections, antibiotics and primary wound closure. *Ned Tijdschr Geneesd* 1996;140:709–713.
16. Medeiros I, Saconato H. Antibiotic prophylaxis for mammalian bites (Cochrane Review). In: The Cochrane Library, Issue 2, 2001. Oxford: Update Software. Search date 2000; primary sources Medline, Embase, Lilacs, and the Cochrane Controlled Trials Register.
17. Maimaris C, Quinton DN. Dog-bite lacerations: a controlled trial of primary wound closure. *Arch Emerg Med* 1988;5:156–161.

Iara Marques de Medeiros

Humberto Saconato
Universidade Federal do Rio Grande do Norte
Natal
Brazil

Competing interests: None declared.

Meningococcal disease

Search date June 2002

J Correia and C A Hart

QUESTIONS

INTERVENTIONS

Likely to be beneficial
Prophylactic antibiotics in contacts* 771

Unknown effectiveness
Antibiotics for throat carriage (reduce carriage but unknown effect on risk of disease) . . .771
Pre-admission parenteral antibiotics in suspected cases* 772

To be covered in future updates
Vaccines (monovalent/multivalent, polysaccharide alone, or conjugate)
Treatment of meningococcal disease

*Based on observational evidence. RCTs unlikely to be conducted.

Key Messages

- **Antibiotics for throat carriage (reduce carriage but unknown effect on risk of disease)** RCTs have found that antibiotics versus placebo significantly increase the number of people with eradication of meningococcus in the throat. We found no evidence that eradicating throat carriage reduces the risk of meningococcal disease.
- **Pre-admission parenteral antibiotics in suspected cases** We found no RCTs on the effect of pre-admission antibiotics. It is unlikely that RCTs will be performed because of the unpredictably rapid course of meningococcal disease in some people, the intuitive risks involved in delaying treatment, and the relatively low risk of causing harm. Most of the observational studies we found show a trend toward benefit with antibiotics, but at least one found contradictory results.
- **Prophylactic antibiotics in contacts** We found no RCTs about the effects of prophylactic antibiotics on the incidence of meningococcal disease among contacts. RCTs are unlikely to be performed because the intervention has few associated risks whereas meningitis has high associated risks. Observational evidence suggests that antibiotics reduce the risk of meningococcal disease. We found no evidence to address the question of which contacts should be treated.

Meningococcal disease

DEFINITION Meningococcal disease is any clinical condition caused by *Neisseria meningitidis* (the meningococcus) groups A, B, C, or other serogroups. These conditions include purulent conjunctivitis, septic arthritis, meningitis, and septicaemia with or without meningitis.

INCIDENCE/ PREVALENCE Meningococcal disease is sporadic in temperate countries, and is most commonly caused by group B or C meningococci. The incidence in the UK varies from 2–8 cases/100 000 people a year,[1] and in the USA from 0.6–1.5/100 000 people.[2] Occasional outbreaks occur among close family contacts, secondary school pupils, and students living in halls of residence. Sub-Saharan Africa has regular epidemics due to serogroup A, particularly in countries lying between The Gambia in the west and Ethiopia in the east (the "meningitis belt"), where incidence during epidemics reaches 500/ 100 000 people.[3]

AETIOLOGY/ RISK FACTORS The meningococcus infects healthy people and is transmitted by close contact: probably by exchange of upper respiratory tract secretions (see table 1, p 776).[4–12] Risk of transmission is greatest during the first week of contact.[7] Risk factors include crowding and exposure to cigarette smoke.[13] Children younger than 2 years of age have the highest incidence, with a second peak between ages 15–24 years. There is currently an increased incidence of meningococcal disease among university students, especially among those in their first term and living in catered accommodation,[14] although we found no accurate numerical estimate of risk from close contact in, for example, halls of residence. Close contacts of an index case have a much higher risk of infection than do people in the general population.[7,10,11] The risk of epidemic spread is higher with groups A and C meningococci than with group B meningococci.[4–6,8] It is not known what makes a meningococcus virulent, but certain clones tend to predominate at different times and in different groups. Carriage of meningococcus in the throat has been reported in 10–15% of people; recent acquisition of a virulent meningococcus is more likely to be associated with invasive disease.

PROGNOSIS Mortality is highest in infants and adolescents, and is related to disease presentation: case fatality rates are 19–25% in septicaemia, 10–12% in meningitis plus septicaemia, and less than 1% in meningitis alone.[15–17]

AIMS To prevent disease in contacts.

OUTCOMES Rates of infection; rates of eradication of throat carriage; adverse effects of treatment.

METHODS *Clinical Evidence* update search and appraisal June 2002. In addition, the author drew from a collection of references from the pre-electronic data era.

QUESTION What are the effects of prophylactic antibiotics on risk of disease in people exposed to someone with meningococcal disease?

We found no RCTs on the effects of prophylactic antibiotics on the incidence of meningococcal disease among contacts. One observational study suggested that sulfaiazine reduced the risk of meningococcal disease over 8 weeks. We found no good evidence to address the question of which contacts should be treated.

Benefits: We found no systematic review and no RCTs examining the effect of prophylactic antibiotics in people who have been in contact with someone with meningococcal disease (see comment below). **Rifampicin:** We found only anecdotal data. **Phenoxymethylpenicillin:** We found one retrospective study, but the results of that study cannot be generalised beyond the sample tested.[18] **Sulfadiazine:** One observational cohort study of soldiers in temporary troop camps in the 1940s compared the incidence of meningococcal disease in camps where sulfadiazine (sulphadiazine) was given to everyone after a meningococcal outbreak versus incidence in camps where no prophylaxis was given. The study reported a higher incidence of meningococcal disease in soldiers not given prophylaxis (approximate figures 17/9500 [0.18%] *v* 2/7000 [0.03%] over 8 wks).[19]

Harms: **Rifampicin:** No excess adverse effects compared with placebo were found in RCTs on eradicating throat carriage of meningococcal disease.[20,21] However, rifampicin is known to cause various adverse effects, including turning urine and contact lenses orange, and inducing hepatic microsomal enzymes, potentially rendering oral contraception ineffective. Rifampicin prophylaxis may be associated with emergence of resistant strains.[22] **Sulfadiazine:** One in 10 soldiers experienced minor adverse events, including headache, dizziness, tinnitus, and nausea.[19]

Comment: RCTs addressing this question are unlikely to be performed because the intervention has few associated risks whereas meningococcal disease has high associated risks. RCTs would also need to be large to find a difference in incidence of meningococcal disease. In the sulfadiazine cohort study, the two infected people in the treatment group only became infected after leaving the camp.[19]

QUESTION What are the effects of antibiotics in people with throat carriage of meningococcal disease?

RCTs have found that antibiotics versus placebo significantly reduce throat carriage of meningococcus. We found no evidence that eradicating throat carriage reduces the risk of meningococcal disease.

Benefits: We found no systematic review. **Incidence of disease:** We found no RCTs or observational studies that examined whether eradicating throat carriage of meningococcus reduces the risk of meningococcal disease. **Throat carriage:** We found five placebo controlled RCTs that examined the effect of antibiotics on carriage of meningococcus in the throat (see table 2, p 777).[20,21,23–25] All trials reported that antibiotics (rifampicin, minocycline, or ciprofloxacin) achieved high rates of eradication (ranging from 90–97%), except one trial of rifampicin in students with heavy growth on culture, in which the rate of eradication was 73%.[20] Eradication rates on placebo ranged from 9–29%. We found seven RCTs that compared different antibiotic regimens (see table 3, p 778).[26–32] Three RCTs found no significant difference between rifampicin and minocycline, ciprofloxacin, or intramuscular ceftriaxone.[27,30,32] A fourth RCT randomised households to different treatments and found that intramuscular ceftriaxone versus rifampicin increased eradication rates.[29] However, that trial used cluster randomisation, and therefore the results should be interpreted with caution. Another trial found no significant difference between oral azithromycin versus rifampicin in eradicating meningococcal throat carriage.[31]

Harms: **Minocycline:** One RCT reported adverse effects (1 or more of nausea, anorexia, dizziness, and abdominal cramps) in 36% of participants.[23] **Rifampicin:** See harms of postexposure antibiotic prophylaxis, p 771. **Ciprofloxacin:** Trials of single dose prophylactic regimens reported no more adverse effects than comparators or placebo.[24,25,30] Ciprofloxacin is contraindicated in pregnancy and in children because animal studies have indicated a possibility of articular cartilage damage in developing joints.[33] **Ceftriaxone:** Two trials of ceftriaxone found no significant adverse effects.[29,30] In one trial, 12% of participants complained of headache.[31] Ceftriaxone is given as a single intramuscular injection. **Azithromycin:** No serious or moderate adverse effects were reported, but nausea, abdominal pain, and headache of short duration were reported equally in the azithromycin and rifampicin treated groups.[29]

Comment: Eradication of meningococcal throat carriage is a well accepted surrogate for prevention of meningococcal disease. It is unlikely that any RCT will be conducted on the efficacy of prophylactic antibiotics in preventing secondary community acquired meningococcal disease in household contacts, because the number of participants required would be large.

QUESTION What are the effects of pre-admission antibiotics in people with suspected meningococcal disease?

We found no RCTs on the effect of pre-admission antibiotics in meningococcal disease. Most observational studies we found suggest a trend toward benefit with antibiotics, but at least one found contradictory results.

Benefits: We found no systematic review and no RCTs on pre-admission antibiotics for suspected meningococcal disease. **Penicillin:** We found seven observational studies on the effect of pre-admission parenteral penicillin in people of all ages with confirmed, probable, or suspected meningococcal disease (see table 4, p 779).[34–40] We also found two reports of pooled data from six of the observational studies.[41,42] The first report (3 English observational studies,[34–36] 487 people) found that antibiotics significantly reduced mortality (OR 2.61, 95% CI 1.04 to 7.18).[41] However, the second report (664 people; the same people in the English studies[34–36] plus partial data from a Danish cohort[43]) found no significant benefit with antibiotics (outcomes not specified; OR 0.82, 95% CI 0.43 to

1.56).[42] We found one additional observational study that assessed the effect of antibiotics in people with suspected meningitis in an epidemic setting in sub-Saharan Africa.[44] The results were difficult to interpret and no conclusions can be drawn. **Other antibiotics:** We found six observational studies on the effect of giving pre-admission antibiotics other than penicillin to people with suspected meningococcal disease.[45–50] All described disease outcomes when a range of antibiotics (including both oral and parenteral drugs) were given to individuals (mainly children) from a few hours up to a week before being admitted to hospital to treat meningococcal disease. One large case series (667 people)[45] found no significant benefit with pre-admission antibiotics in terms of mortality or sequelae, but found that the duration of symptoms before admission was significantly longer in people receiving pre-admission antibiotics (CI not provided; $P < 0.001$). Other studies have found that prior antibiotics significantly reduced mortality ($P < 0.01$;[46] OR 0.06, 95% CI 0.01 to 0.024[47]), sequelae (OR 0.16, 95% CI 0.04 to 0.58),[47] and the risk of developing invasive disease in unsuspected cases (OR 0.26, 95% CI 0.08 to 0.81).[49] One study (288 children aged 3–36 months) found no significant benefit with antibiotics for meningitis caused by *N meningitidis*, but found significantly fewer complications (neurological or hearing problems, death) in children with pneumococcal meningitis (OR 0.14, 95% CI 0.02 to 0.79).[50] However, all of these results need careful interpretation (see comment below).

Harms: One study about the harms of penicillin found that anaphylaxis occurred in about 0.04% of cases, and fatal anaphylaxis occurred in about 0.002% of cases.[51] One of the studies reported a death from penicillin anaphylaxis.[47]

Comment: We found no studies about the relationship between early treatment with antibiotics and development of subsequent antibiotic resistance. Given the limitations of observational studies, the confounding effects of increased disease awareness (following media coverage or official recommendations) leading to early suspicion and diagnosis (by parents and doctors) and earlier referral, the evaluation of the effect of pre-admission penicillin on mortality is problematic. However, it is unlikely that RCTs on pre-admission antibiotics will be performed because of the unpredictably rapid course of disease in some people, the intuitive risks involved in delaying treatment, combined with a relatively low risk of causing harm. A systematic review of the effects of pre-admission antibiotics is under way.

REFERENCES

1. www.phls.co.uk/facts/meni.htm. Disease Facts: Meningococcal Disease.
2. Centers for Disease Control. Summary of notifiable diseases United States, 1997. *MMWR Morb Mortal Wkly Rep* 1998;46:1–87.
3. Hart CA, Cuevas LE. Meningococcal disease in Africa. *Ann Trop Med Parasitol* 1997;91:777–785.
4. French MR. Epidemiological study of 383 cases of meningococcus meningitis in the city of Milwaukee, 1927–1928 and 1929. *Am J Public Health* 1931;21:130–137.
5. Pizzi M. A severe epidemic of meningococcus meningitis in 1941–1942, Chile. *Am J Public Health* 1944;34:231–239.
6. Lee WW. Epidemic meningitis in Indianapolis 1929–1930. *J Prev Med* 1931;5:203–210.
7. De Wals P, Herthoge L, Borlée-Grimée I, et al. Meningococcal disease in Belgium. Secondary attack rate among household, day-care nursery and pre-elementary school contacts. *J Infect* 1981;3(suppl 1):53–61.
8. Kaiser AB, Hennekens CH, Saslaw MS, et al. Seroepidemiology and chemoprophylaxis of

disease due to sulphonamide resistant *Neisseria meningitidis* in a civilian population. *J Infect Dis* 1974;130:217–221.
9. Zangwill KM, Schuchat A, Riedo FX, et al. School-based clusters of meningococcal disease in the United States. *JAMA* 1997;277:389–395.
10. The Meningococcal Disease Surveillance Group. Meningococcal disease secondary attack rate and chemoprophylaxis in the United States. *JAMA* 1976;235:261–265.
11. Olcen P, Kjellander J, Danielson D, et al. Epidemiology of *Neisseria meningitidis*: prevalence and symptoms from the upper respiratory tract in family members to patients with meningococcal disease. *Scand J Infect Dis* 1981;13:105–109.
12. Hudson, PJ, Vogt PL, Heun EM, et al. Evidence for school transmission of *Neisseria meningitidis* during a Vermont outbreak. *Pediatr Infect Dis* 1986;5:213–217.
13. Stanwell-Smith RE, Stuart JM, Hughes AO, et al. Smoking, the environment and meningococcal disease: a case control study. *Epidemiol Infect* 1994;112:315–328.
14. Communicable Disease Surveillance Centre. Meningococcal disease in university students. *Commun Dis Rep CDR Wkly* 1998;8:49.
15. Andersen BM. Mortality in meningococcal infections. *Scand J Infect Dis* 1978;10:277–282.
16. Thomson APJ, Sills JA, Hart CA. Validation of the Glasgow meningococcal septicaemia prognostic score: a 10 year retrospective survey. *Crit Care Med* 1991;19:26–30.
17. Riordan FAI, Marzouk O, Thomson APJ, et al. The changing presentation of meningococcal disease. *Eur J Pediatr* 1995;154:472–474.
18. Hoiby EA, Moe PJ, Lystad A, et al. Phenoxymethyl-penicillin treatment of household contacts of meningococcal disease patients. *Antonie Van Leeuwenhoek* 1986;52:255–257.
19. Kuhns DW, Nelson CT, Feldman HA, et al. The prophylactic value of sulfadiazine in the control of meningococcic meningitis. *JAMA* 1943;123:335–339.
20. Deal WB, Sanders E. Efficacy of rifampicin in treatment of meningococcal carriers. *N Engl J Med* 1969;281:641–645.
21. Eickhoff TC. In vitro and in vivo studies of resistance to rifampicin in meningococci. *J Infect Dis* 1971;123:414–420.
22. Weidmer CE, Dunkel TB, Pettyjohn FS, et al. Effectiveness of rifampin in eradicating the meningococcal carrier state in a relatively closed population: emergence of resistant strains. *J Infect Dis* 1971;124:172–178.
23. Devine LF, Johnson DP, Hagerman CR, et al. The effect of minocycline on meningococcal nasopharyngeal carrier state in naval personnel. *Am J Epidemiol* 1971;93:337–345.
24. Renkonen OV, Sivonen A, Visakorpi R. Effect of ciproflaxacin on carrier rate of *Neisseria meningitidis* in army recruits in Finland. *Antimicrob Agents Chemother* 1987;31:962–963.
25. Dworzack DL, Sanders CC, Horowitz EA, et al. Evaluation of single dose ciprofloxacin in the eradication of *Neisseria meningitidis* from nasopharyngeal carriers. *Antimicrob Agents Chemother* 1988;32:1740–1741.
26. Artenstein MS, Lamson TH, Evans JR. Attempted prophylaxis against meningococcal infection using intramuscular penicillin. *Mil Med* 1967;132:1009–1011.
27. Guttler RB, Counts GW, Avent CK, et al. Effect of rifampicin and minocycline on meningococcal carrier rates. *J Infect Dis* 1971;124:199–205.
28. Blakebrough IS, Gilles HM. The effect of rifampicin on meningococcal carriage in family contacts in northern Nigeria. *J Infect* 1980;2:137–143.
29. Schwartz B, Al-Tobaiqi A, Al-Ruwais A, et al. Comparative efficacy of ceftriaxone and rifampicin in eradicating pharyngeal carriage of Group A *Neisseria meningitidis*. *Lancet* 1988;1:1239–1242.
30. Cuevas LE, Kazembe P, Mughogho GK, et al. Eradication of nasopharyngeal carriage of *Neisseria meningitidis* in children and adults in rural Africa: A comparison of ciprofloxacin and rifampicin. *J Infect Dis* 1995;171:728–731.
31. Girgis N, Sultan Y, Frenck RW Jr, et al. Azithromycin compared with rifampin for eradication of masopharyngeal colonization by *Neisseria meningitidis*. *Pediatr Infect Dis* J 1998;17:816–819.
32. Simmons G, Jones N, Calder L. Equivalence of ceftriaxone and rifampicin in eliminating nasopharyngeal carriage of serogroup B *Neisseria meningitidis*. *J Antimicrob Chemother* 2000;45:909–911.
33. Schulter G. Ciprofloxacin: a review of its potential toxicologic effects. *Am J Med* 1987(suppl 4A);82:91–93.
34. Strang JR, Pugh EJ. Meningococcal infections: reducing the case fatality rate by giving penicillin before admission to hospital. *BMJ* 1992;305:141–143.
35. Cartwright K, Reilly S, White D, et al. Early treatment with parenteral penicillin in meningococcal disease. *BMJ 1992*;305:143–147.
36. Gossain S, Constantine CE, Webberley JM. Early parenteral penicillin in meningococcal disease. *BMJ* 1992;305:523–524.
37. Woodward CM, Jessop EG, Wale MCJ. Early management of meningococcal disease. *Commun Dis Rep CDR Rev* 1995;5:R135–R137.
38. Sorensen HT, Nielsen GL, Schonheyder HC, et al. Outcome of pre-hospital antibiotic treatment of meningococcal disease. *J Clin Epidemiol* 1998;51:717–721.
39. Jolly K, Stewart G. Epidemiology and diagnosis of meningitis: results of a five-year prospective, population-based study. *Commun Dis Public Health* 2001;4:124–129.
40. Jefferies C, Lennon D, Stewart J, et al. Meningococcal disease in Auckland, July 1992 – June 1994. *N Z Med J* 1999;112:115–117.
41. Cartwright K, Strang J, Gossain S, et al. Early treatment of meningococcal disease [letter]. *BMJ* 1992;305:774.
42. Sorensen HT, Steffensen FH, Schonheyder HC, et al. Clinical management of meningococcal disease. Prospective international registration of patients may be needed. *BMJ* 1998;316:1016–1017.
43. Sorensen HT, Moller-Petersen J, Krarup HB, et al. Early treatment of meningococcal disease. *BMJ* 1992;305:774.
44. Wall RA, Hassan-King M, Thomas H, et al. Meningococcal bacteraemia in febrile contacts of patients with meningococcal disease. *Lancet* 1986;2:624.
45. Bohr V, Rasmussen N, Hansen B, et al. 875 cases of bacterial meningitis: diagnostic procedures and the impact of preadmission antibiotic therapy. Part III of a three-part series. *J Infect* 1983;7:193–202.
46. Goldacre MJ. Acute bacterial meningitis in childhood: aspects of pre-hospital care in 687 cases. *Arch Dis Child* 1977;52:501–503.
47. Barquet N, Domingo P, Cayla JA, et al. Meningococcal disease in a large urban population (Barcelona, 1987–1992): predictors of

dismal prognosis. Barcelona Meningococcal Disease Surveillance Group. *Arch Intern Med* 1999;159:2329–2340.
48. Morant GA, Diez DJ, Gimeno CC, et al. [An analysis of prior antibiotic treatment on the impact of meningococcal disease in children of the Valencian Community. The Study Group of Invasive Diseases]. *Anales Espanoles de Pediatria* 1999; 50;17–20.
49. Wang VJ, Malley R, Fleisher GR, et al. Antibiotic treatment of children with unsuspected meningococcal disease. *Arch Pediatr Adolesc Med* 2000;154:556–560.
50. Bonsu BK, Harper MB. Fever interval before diagnosis, prior antibiotic treatment, and clinical outcome for young children with bacterial meningitis. *Clin Infect Dis* 2001;32:566–572.
51. Idsoe O, Guthe T, Willcox RR, et al. Nature and extent of penicillin side-reactions, with particular reference to fatalities from anaphylactic shock. *Bull World Health Organ* 1968;38:159–188.

J Correia
Instituto Materno Infantil de Pernambuco
Recife
Brazil

C A Hart
Professor
Department of Medical Microbiology and Genitourinary Medicine
University of Liverpool
Liverpool
UK

Competing interests: None declared.

TABLE 1 Risk of infection among contacts (see text, p 770).

Group of meningococcus	Setting	Risk
A	Household contacts in Milwaukee, USA[4]	AR 1100/100 000; RR not possible to estimate
	General population in Santiago province, Chile	Attack rate in general population 23–262/100 000 (1941 and 1942)
	Household contacts in Chile[5]	Attack rate in household contacts 250/100 000 (2.5%) over both years
	General population in Indianapolis, USA[6]	AR 4500/100 000; RR not possible to estimate
B	Household contacts in Belgium[7]	RR 1245*
	Nursery schools[7]	RR 23*
	Day care centres[7]	RR 76*
C	Household contacts from two lower socioeconomic groups Dade County, Florida, USA[8]	Attack rate in two communities 13/100 000 population. Attack rate in household contacts 5/85 (582/100 000)
Unspecified	School based clusters in USA. Predominant meningococcal types: 13 clusters of Gp C, 7 Gp B, 1 Gp Y, 1 GpC/W135 (impossible to distinguish)[9]	RR 2.3*
	Household contacts from several states in USA, meningococcus types B and C predominantly[10]	RR 500–800*
	Household contact in Norway. Meningococcus types A, B, and C predominantly[11]	RR up to 4000*
	Schools in Vermont. Predominant meningococcus type C[12]	OR 14.1 (95% CI 1.6 to 127)

*Compared with the risk in the general population.

TABLE 2 **Effect of antibiotics on throat carriage: results of placebo controlled RCTs (see text, p 771).**

Antibiotic	Group of meningococcus	Participants	Eradication		RR (95% CI)
			Treatment (%)	Placebo (%)	
Rifampicin (oral)[20]	B, X, Z	30 students with heavy growth on culture	11/15 (73)	2/15 (13)	5.5 (1.5 to 21)
Rifampicin (oral)[21]	B, C, Y, Z29 E, W 135, NT	76 airforce recruits	36/38* (95)	3/22‡ (14)	7.0 (5.8 to 8.1)
Minocycline (oral)[23]	Predominantly Y (63%)	149 naval recruits	37/41 (90)†	14/48 (29)§	3.1 (2.6 to 3.6)
Ciprofloxacin (oral)[24]	Non-groupable (61%), B (17.5%)	120 army recruits in Finland	54/56 (97) 5 second samples missing	7/53 (13) 6 second samples missing or not a carrier	7.3 (6.5 to 8.1)
Ciprofloxacin (oral)[25]	B (41%), Z (33%)	46 healthy volunteers	22/23 (96) (1 did not adhere to treatment)	2/22 (9)	10.5 (8.9 to 12.1)

*9 lost to follow up. †37 either did not have meningococci prior to treatment or did not provide a full set of cultures. ‡7 lost to follow up. §23 either did not have meningococci prior to treatment or did not provide a full set of cultures.

TABLE 3 **Effects of antibiotics on throat carriage: results of comparative RCTs** **(see text, p 771).**

Antibiotic	Group of meningococcus	Participants	Rate of eradication (%)	RR (95% CI)
Phenoxymethylpenicillin (im)[26]	C (49%), B (33%), NG (17%)	Adults	41/118 (35)	No data
Erythromycin (oral)[26]	C	Adults	0/7 (0)	No data
Rifampicin (oral)[27]	B + C (31%), NG (69%)	Adults	43/51 (84)	0.89 (0.76 to 1.02)
Minocycline (oral)[27]	B + C (31%), NG (69%)	Adults	36/38 (95)	No data
Rifampicin (oral)[27]	A	Children	37/48 (77)	No data
Sulfadimidine (oral)[28]	A	Children	0/34 (0)	No data
Ceftriaxone (im)[29]	A	Adults and children	66/68 (97)	1.29 (1.10 to 1.49)
Rifampicin (oral)[29]	A	Adults and children	27/36 (75)	No data
Ceftriaxone (im)[30]	A	Adults and children	39/41 (95)	No data
Ciprofloxacin (oral)[30]	A	Adults and children	70/79 (89)	No data
Rifampicin (oral)[30]	A	Adults and children	85/88 (97)	No data
Azithromycin (oral)[31]	B (63%), A (37%)	Adults	56/60 (93)	No data
Rifampicin (oral)[31]	B (63%), A (37%)	Adults	56/59 (95)	No data
Ceftriaxone (im)[32]	B (54%), other serogroups (46%)	Adults and children	97/100 (97)	No data
Rifampicin (oral)[32]	B (51%), other serogroups (49%)	Adults and children	78/82 (95.1)	No data

im, intramuscular.

TABLE 4 Effects of early (pre-admission) parenteral penicillin: results of observational studies (see text, p 772).

Setting	Group of meningococcus	Participants	Parenteral penicillin (number of deaths/ number of people [%]) Given	Not given	RR (95% CI)
District general hospital in Darlington, UK (from 1986–1991)[34]	NR	46 people admitted to hospital with confirmed, probable, and possible MD, all age groups (52% < 5 years of age)	0/13 (0)	8/33 (24.3)	Incalculable
Three health districts in south-west England, UK (from 1982–1991)[35]	Mostly B and C	340* confirmed, probable, and possible cases of MD, all age groups (36% < 5 years of age)	5/93 (5.4)	22/246 (8.9)	RR 0.6 (0.23 to 1.54)
Worcester health district, England, UK (1986–1992)[36]	NR	102† confirmed, probable, and possible cases of MD; age distribution not reported	1/23 (4.4)	11/79 (13.9)	RR 0.31 (0.04 to 2.29)
District hospital in Wessex, England, UK (1990–1993)[37]	NR	68 cases of MD, all age groups (44% < 5 years of age)	0/13 (0)	3/55 (5.5)	Not calculated
County of North Jutland, Denmark‡[38]	NR	302 cases of MD seen by GPs before admission to hospital. All age groups.	9/44 (20.5)	16/258 (6.2)	Adjusted OR 3.2 (95% CI 0.9–10.6)§
Hospitals in Auckland, New Zealand (1992–1997)[40]	Predominantly B	106** confirmed or probable cases of MD, all age groups.	1/24 (4.2)	2/42 (4.9)	RR 0.85 (0.08 to 8.93)
Health district in England, UK (from 1994–1998)[39]‡‡	Mostly B (53%) and C (30%)	258†† confirmed, probable, and possible cases of MD; all age groups (49% < 5 years of age)	2/72 (2.8)	16/186 (8.6)	RR 0.32 (0.08 to 1.37)

*Number of individuals seen by their general practitioners (GPs) before admission; in one fatal case, there was no information on previous antibiotic use. †A total of 109 patients had their records reviewed, but seven were excluded from analysis because they had received oral penicillin. ‡A partial series of 177 cases from the Danish historical cohort was reported in 1992,[43] showing similar trends of excess mortality in the treated group OR 9.3 (95% CI 3.1 to 27.9). §Adjusted OR, multivariate analysis. **The only prospective study found; all others in the table are retrospective. ††The paper also reports meningitis of other aetiologies. Only those regarded as meningococcal disease are described here. ‡‡The only prospective study found. All others in the table are retrospective. CI, confidence interval; MD, meningococcal disease; NR, not reported.

Mother to child transmission of HIV

Search date January 2002

Jimmy Volmink

QUESTIONS

INTERVENTIONS

See glossary, p 785

Key Messages

- **Antiretroviral drugs** One systematic review has found that, in mothers with HIV, zidovudine versus placebo given to mothers significantly reduces the incidence of HIV in infants at follow up of about 3–18 months (NNT 9, 95% CI 7 to 14). One RCT has found that nevirapine versus zidovudine given to mothers with HIV and to their newborns significantly reduces the incidence of HIV in infants. One RCT has found that a longer versus a shorter course of zidovudine given to mother and infant significantly reduces the incidence of HIV in infants.
- **Avoiding breast feeding** One RCT in women with HIV who had access to clean water and health education has found that formula feeding versus breast feeding significantly reduces the incidence of HIV in infants after 24 months, without increasing infant mortality. However, in countries with high infant mortality, avoiding breast feeding may increase infant morbidity and mortality further.
- **Elective caesarean section** One RCT found limited evidence that elective caesarean section versus vaginal delivery in women with HIV reduced the incidence of HIV in infants at 18 months.
- **Immunotherapy** One RCT found no significant difference in the incidence of HIV in infants of mothers taking hyperimmune globulin (HIVIG) versus immunoglobulin without HIV antibody (IVIG), in addition to a standard zidovudine regimen, but may have been too small to exclude a clinically important difference.
- **Vaginal microbicides** We found insufficient evidence about the effects of vaginal microbicides on the transmission of HIV to infants.
- **Vitamin supplements** RCTs found no significant difference in the incidence of HIV at birth, 6 weeks or 3 months in the infants of pregnant women given vitamin A or multivitamins versus placebo.

Clin Evid 2002;8:780–787.

DEFINITION Mother to child transmission of HIV-1 (see glossary, p 785) infection can occur during pregnancy in the intrapartum period, or postnatally through breast feeding.[1] In contrast, HIV-2 (see glossary, p 785) is rarely transmitted from mother to child.[2] Infected children usually have no symptoms and signs of HIV at birth, but develop them over subsequent months or years.[3]

INCIDENCE/ PREVALENCE A review of 13 cohorts found that the risk of mother to child transmission of HIV is on average about 15–20% in Europe, 15–30% in the USA, and 25–35% in Africa.[4] One global report estimated that 620 000 children below the age of 15 years were infected with HIV during 1999, bringing the total number of children with HIV, acquired immune deficiency syndrome (AIDS), or both to 1.3 million worldwide.[5] Most of these children were infected from their mother and 90% live in sub-Saharan Africa.

AETIOLOGY/ RISK FACTORS Transmission of HIV to children is more likely if the mother has a high viral load.[1,6,7] Women with detectable viraemia (by p24 antigen or culture) have double the risk of transmitting HIV-1 to their infants than those who do not.[1] Breast feeding has also been shown in prospective studies to be a risk factor.[8,9] Other risk factors include sexually transmitted diseases, chorioamnionitis, prolonged rupture of membranes, and vaginal mode of delivery.[5,10–13]

PROGNOSIS About 25% of infants infected with HIV progress rapidly to AIDS or death in the first year. Some survive beyond 12 years of age.[3] One European study found a mortality of 15% in the first year of life and a mortality of 28% by the age of 5 years.[14]

AIMS To reduce mother to child transmission of HIV and improve infant survival, with minimal adverse effects.

OUTCOMES HIV infection status of the child; infant morbidity and mortality; maternal morbidity and mortality; adverse effects of treatment.

METHODS *Clinical Evidence* update search and appraisal January 2002.

QUESTION What are the effects of measures to reduce mother to child transmission of HIV?

OPTION ANTIRETROVIRAL DRUGS

One systematic review has found that zidovudine versus placebo significantly reduces the incidence of HIV in infants. One RCT has found that nevirapine versus zidovudine given to the mother and to her newborn significantly reduces the risk of HIV transmission. One RCT has found that longer versus shorter courses of zidovudine given to mother and infant significantly reduces the incidence of HIV in infants.

Benefits: **Zidovudine versus placebo:** We found one systematic review (search date not stated, 4 RCTs, 1585 women) that compared zidovudine versus placebo given to the mother before, during, or after labour (see table 1, p 787).[15] In one of the included RCTs, infants of mothers receiving zidovudine were also given zidovudine for 6 weeks after birth.[16] Meta-analysis found that zidovudine versus placebo significantly reduced the incidence of HIV in infants (AR 79/616 [13%] with zidovudine *v* 150/634 [24%]; RR 0.54,

95% CI 0.42 to 0.69; NNT 9, 95% CI 7 to 14). The results were still significant when the RCT of zidovudine that used the most intensive regimen[16] was excluded from the analysis (combined results for less intensive regimens versus placebo: AR 70/495 [14%] *v* 119/507 [23%]; RR 0.60, 95% CI 0.46 to 0.79; NNT 11, 95% CI 8 to 20).[17–19] The effect of zidovudine versus placebo was similar in reducing the incidence of HIV in infants from breast feeding and non-breast-feeding mothers (breast feeding RR 0.62, 95% CI 0.46 to 0.85; non-breast-feeding RR 0.50, 95% CI 0.30 to 0.85). **Zidovudine versus nevirapine:** The systematic review[15] identified one unblinded RCT (626 women from a predominantly breast feeding population in Uganda) that compared zidovudine versus nevirapine.[20] It found that nevirapine given to mothers as a single oral dose at the onset of labour, and to infants as a single dose within 72 hours of birth, versus zidovudine given orally to women during labour, and to their newborns for 7 days after birth, significantly reduced the number of infants with HIV at 14–16 weeks (AR 65/250 [26%] *v* 37/246 [15%]; RR 0.58, 95% CI 0.40 to 0.83). **Alternative zidovudine regimens:** One RCT (1437 women) compared four different zidovudine regimens; zidovudine was given to mothers from a specific time in gestation until delivery and to the infant until a specific age: "short–short" course (mother from 35 wks, infant for up to 3 days); "long–long" (mother from 28 wks, infant for up to 6 wks); "short–long" (mother from 35 wks, infant for up to 6 wks); and "long–short" (mother from 28 wks, infant for up to 3 days). The RCT found that a "long–long" course versus a "short–short" course significantly reduced the number of infants with HIV (AR 9/220 [4%] with long course *v* 24/229 [10%] with short course; RR 2.56, 95% CI 1.22 to 5.39). As the short–short regimen seemed not to reduce transmission of HIV, it was discontinued at the first interim analysis. The trial found no significant difference between a "long–long" versus "short–long" (26/401 [7%] with "long–long" *v* 29/338 [9%] with "short–long" course; RR 1.32, 95% CI 0.80 to 2.20) or versus a "long–short" (26/401 [7%] with "long–long" *v* 16/340 [5%] with "long–short" course; RR 0.73, 95% CI 0.40 to 1.33).[21]

Harms: **Zidovudine versus placebo:** The review found that intensive zidovudine versus placebo significantly increased the risk of neonatal haematological toxicity (RR 1.86, 95% CI 1.18 to 2.94; specific effects undefined), whereas no significant difference was found for less intensive regimens versus placebo (RR 0.77, 95% CI 0.44 to 1.35).[15] Infants who received the most intensive regimen, who were followed for 18 months, had mild reversible anaemia that resolved by 12 weeks of age.[22] The same trial in uninfected infants followed for a median of 4.2 years found no significant difference between zidovudine versus placebo in growth patterns, immunological parameters, or the occurrence of childhood cancers.[23] The RCT of combination antiretroviral treatment has reported no serious adverse drug reactions to date.[15] **Zidovudine versus nevirapine:** The RCT found no significant difference in serious adverse effects in mothers and infants (4.0% *v* 4.7% in mothers; 19.8% *v* 20.5% in infants up to 18 months of age).[23] **Alternative zidovudine regimens:** The RCT found that the rate of serious adverse events in mothers and infants was similar for all regimens. The rates of severe anaemia in infants were "long–long" (1%); "long–short" (0%); "short–long" (0.3%); and "short–short" (1.3%).[21]

Comment: The review[15] identified one RCT in progress in South Africa, Uganda, and Tanzania, comparing zidovudine plus lamivudine versus placebo. Preliminary results suggest that zidovudine plus lamivudine reduces the risk of HIV transmission at 6 weeks of age when given in the antenatal, intrapartum, and postpartum period (RR 0.52, 95% CI 0.35 to 0.76), and during the intrapartum and postpartum period (RR 0.66, 95% CI 0.46 to 0.94). The RCT found that zidovudine plus lamivudine given during the intrapartum period alone did not significantly affect the risk of transmission (RR 1.01, 95% CI 0.74 to 1.38).

OPTION ELECTIVE CAESAREAN SECTION

One RCT found limited evidence that elective caesarean section versus vaginal delivery significantly reduced the incidence of HIV in infants at 18 months.

Benefits: We found one systematic review (search date not stated, 1 RCT, 436 women) that compared elective caesarean section at 38 weeks versus vaginal delivery.[15] It found that caesarean section significantly reduced the number of infants with HIV at 18 months (AR 3/170 [3%] with caesarean section *v* 21/200 [11%] with vaginal delivery; RR 0.16, 95% CI 0.05 to 0.55; NNT 11, 95% CI 10 to 21).

Harms: No serious adverse effects were reported in either group. Postpartum fever was significantly more common in women having caesarean section versus vaginal delivery (15/225 [7%] with caesarean section *v* 2/183 [1%] with vaginal delivery; RR 6.1, 95% CI 1.5 to 22.0; NNH 18, 95% CI 16 to 50). Postpartum bleeding, intravascular coagulation, or severe anaemia occurred rarely in either group.

Comment: A total of 15% of the women withdrew from the trial or were lost to follow up. None of the women analysed breast fed, although this was not stated as specific exclusion criterion. More women who gave birth by caesarean section versus vaginal delivery had received zidovudine during pregnancy (70% with caesarean section *v* 58% with vaginal delivery); this means that the observed difference between groups may not have been exclusively due to the different delivery methods.

OPTION AVOIDING BREAST FEEDING

One RCT in women with HIV, who had access to clean water and health education, has found that formula feeding versus breast feeding significantly reduces the incidence of HIV in infants at 24 months without increasing mortality. However, in countries with high infant mortality, avoiding breast feeding may increase infant morbidity and mortality further.

Benefits: We found no systematic review. We found one RCT (425 HIV-1 [see glossary, p 785] seropositive women with access to clean water and health education in Kenya) that found that breast feeding versus formula feeding significantly increased the number of infants with HIV at 24 months (AR 61/197 [31%] with breast feeding *v* 31/205 [15%]; RR 2.0, 95% CI 1.4 to 3.0; NNT 6, 95% CI 4 to 13).[23] Although infants were breast fed throughout the trial duration, the greatest exposure to breast milk occurred during the first 6 months of life. The trial found no significant difference in mortality at 24 months with breast feeding versus formula feeding (AR 45/197 [23%] with breast feeding *v* 39/204 [19%] with formula feeding; RR 1.2, 95% CI 0.8 to 1.8).[24]

Harms: The RCT did not report on adverse effects (see comment below).

Comment: In countries with high infant mortality, avoiding breast feeding may further increase infant morbidity and mortality through its effect on nutrition, immunity, maternal fertility, and birth spacing. Access to clean water and education when using formula feeds may explain the similar mortality in breast fed and formula fed infants.

OPTION VAGINAL MICROBICIDES

We found insufficient evidence about the effects of vaginal microbicides on the incidence of HIV in infants.

Benefits: We found no systematic review or RCTs.

Harms: One non-randomised trial (see comment below) reported no adverse effects in mothers or in infants.

Comment: We found one non-randomised trial (2094 women) that compared vaginal cleansing (with 0.25% chlorhexidine) from admission in labour to delivery versus no vaginal cleansing.[25] Women were allocated to the treatment or control group on the basis of months of the year. The trial found no significant difference in the transmission of HIV after vaginal cleansing versus no cleansing (AR 136/505 [27%] with vaginal cleansing *v* 133/477 [28%] without vaginal cleansing; RR 0.1, 95% CI 0.8 to 1.2). The results should be interpreted with caution because HIV status was not determined in the 41% of infants who were lost to follow up, and the trial was not randomised and was, therefore, potentially biased.

OPTION IMMUNOTHERAPY

One RCT found no significant difference in the incidence of HIV in infants of mothers taking HIV hyperimmune globulin versus immunoglobulin without HIV antibody in addition to a standard zidovudine regimen, but may have been too small to exclude a clinically important difference.

Benefits: We found one systematic review (search date not stated, 1 RCT, 501 women)[15] that compared HIV hyperimmune globulin (HIVIG) versus immunoglobulin without HIV antibody (IVIG) given to women during pregnancy, the intrapartum period, and to their infants at birth. Women in both groups received a standard course of zidovudine and no infants were breast fed. The RCT found no significant difference in transmission of HIV between HIVIG versus IVIG regimens at 6 months of age (4.1% with HIVIG *v* 6.0% with IVIG; no CI available; P = 0.36).

Harms: The trial reported no significant adverse effects.[15]

Comment: The low overall transmission rate (5%) in this study was much lower than the anticipated rate of greater than 15% used to calculate the appropriate sample size. The trial is unable to exclude a clinically important effect of HIVIG on the number of children with HIV.[15]

OPTION VITAMIN SUPPLEMENTS

Two RCTs found that vitamin supplements versus placebo given to pregnant women had no significant effect on the incidence of HIV in their infants at birth, 6 weeks, or 3 months.

Benefits: We found no systematic review and two RCTs.[26,27] The first RCT (1083 women with HIV-1 [see glossary, p 785] between 12 and 27 weeks' gestation in Tanzania) compared vitamin A, multivitamin supplements (excluding vitamin A), or both versus placebo, using a factorial design.[26] It found no significant difference in the number of infants with HIV in women taking multivitamins or vitamin A versus placebo at birth (multivitamins *v* placebo: AR 38/376 [10%] *v* 24/363 [7%], RR 1.54, 95% CI 0.94 to 2.51; vitamin A *v* placebo: AR 38/380 [10%] *v* 24/358 [7%], RR 1.49, 95% CI 0.91 to 2.43) or at 6 weeks among infants free of infection at birth (multivitamins *v* placebo: 31/191 [16%] *v* 28/179 [16%], RR 1.04, 95% CI 0.65 to 1.66; vitamin A *v* placebo: 35/196 [18%] *v* 24/174 [14%], RR 1.30, 95% CI 0.80 to 2.09).[28] The second RCT (728 pregnant women with HIV in South Africa) compared vitamin A with placebo.[27] It found no significant difference in the number of children with HIV infection at 3 months (20% with vitamin A *v* 22% with placebo; no CI available). Mortality was similar in vitamin A and placebo groups at 1, 3, and 13 months of age.

Harms: Neither RCT reported adverse effects.[26,27] However, as vitamin A is potentially teratogenic, its use in pregnancy may lead to birth defects.[29,30]

Comment: The RCTs were performed because observational studies have found an association in pregnant women between transmission of HIV and low serum levels of vitamin A.[28]

GLOSSARY

Human immunodeficiency virus type 1 (HIV-1) is the most common cause of HIV disease throughout the world.

Human immunodeficiency virus type 2 (HIV-2) is predominantly found in West Africa and is more closely related to the simian immunodeficiency virus than to HIV-1.

Mother to child transmission of HIV

REFERENCES

1. John GC, Kreiss J. Mother-to-child transmission of human immunodeficiency virus type 1. *Epidemiol Rev* 1996;18:149–157.
2. Adjorlolo-Johnson G, De Cock KM, Ekpini E, et al. Prospective comparison of mother-to-child transmission of HIV-1 and HIV-2 in Abidjan, Ivory Coast. *JAMA* 1994;272:462–466.
3. Peckham C, Gibb D. Mother-to-child transmission of the human immunodeficiency virus. *N Engl J Med* 1995;333:298–302.
4. The Working Group on MTCT of HIV. Rates of mother-to-child transmission of HIV-1 in Africa, America and Europe: results of 13 perinatal studies. *J Acquir Immune Defic Syndr* 1995;8:506–510.
5. UNAIDS (Joint United Nations Programme on HIV/AIDS). *Report of the global HIV/AIDS epidemic*. June 2000. Geneva: UNAIDS; 2000. UNAIDS/00.13E.
6. Mofenson LM. Epidemiology and determinants of vertical HIV transmission. *Semin Pediatr Infect Dis* 1994;5:252–256.
7. Khouri YF, McIntosh K, Cavacini L, et al. Vertical transmission of HIV-1: correlation with maternal viral load and plasma levels of CD4 binding site anti-gp 120 antibodies. *J Clin Invest* 1995;95:732–737.
8. Dunn DT, Newell ML, Ades AE, et al. Risk of human immunodeficiency virus type-1 transmission through breastfeeding. *Lancet* 1992;240:585–588.
9. Miotti PG, Taha ET, Newton I, et al. HIV transmission through breastfeeding: a study in Malawi. *JAMA* 1999;282:744–749.
10. Nair P, Alger L, Hines S, et al. Maternal and neonatal characteristics associated with HIV infection in infants of seropositive women. *J Acquir Immune Defic Syndr* 1993;6:298–302.
11. Minkoff H, Burns DN, Landesman S, et al. The relationship of the duration of ruptured membranes to vertical transmission of human immunodeficiency virus. *Am J Obstet Gynecol* 1995;173:585–589.
12. European Collaborative Study. Risk factors for mother-to-child transmission of HIV-1. *Lancet* 1992;339:1007–1012.
13. Mofenson LM. A critical review of studies evaluating the relationship of mode of delivery to perinatal transmission of human immunodeficiency virus. *Pediatr Infect Dis J* 1995;14:169–176.
14. The European Collaborative Study. Natural history of vertically acquired human immunodeficiency virus-1 infection. *Pediatrics* 1994;94:815–819.
15. Brocklehurst P. Interventions aimed at decreasing the risk of mother-to-child transmission of HIV infection. In: The Cochrane Library, Issue 3, 2000. Oxford: Update Software. Search date not stated; primary sources Cochrane Pregnancy and Childbirth Group Trials Register and Cochrane Controlled Trials Register.
16. Connor EM, Sperling RS, Gelber RD, et al. Reduction of maternal-infant transmission of human immunodeficiency type 1 with zidovudine treatment. *N Engl J Med* 1994;311:1173–1180.
17. Shaffer N, Chuachoowong R, Mock PA, et al. Short-course zidovudine for perinatal HIV-1 transmission in Bangkok, Thailand: a randomised controlled trial. Bangkok Collaborative Perinatal HIV Transmission Study Group. *Lancet* 1999;353:773–780.
18. Wiktor SZ, Ekpini E, Karon JM, et al. Short-course oral zidovudine for prevention of mother-to-child transmission of HIV-1 in Abidjan, Cote d'Ivoire: a randomised trial. *Lancet* 1999;353:781–785.
19. Dabis F, Msellati P, Meda N, et al. Six-month efficacy, tolerance, and acceptability of a short regimen of oral zidovudine to reduce vertical transmission of HIV in breastfed children in Cote d'Ivoire and Burkina Faso: a double-blind placebo-controlled multicentre trial. DITRAME Study Group. Diminution de la Transmission Mere-Enfant. *Lancet* 1999;353:786–792.
20. Guay LA, Musoke P, Fleming T, et al. Intrapartum and neonatal single-dose nevirapine compared with zidovudine for prevention of mother-to-child transmission of HIV-1 in Kampala, Uganda: HIVNET 012 randomised trial. *Lancet* 1999;354:795–802.
21. Lallemant M, Jourdain G, Le Couer S, et al. A trial of shortened zidovudine regimens to prevent mother-to-child transmission of human immunodeficiency virus type 1. *N Engl J Med* 2000:343:982–991.
22. Sperling RS, Shapiro DE, McSherry GD, et al. Safety of the maternal-infant zidovudine regimen utilized in the Pediatric AIDS Clinical Trial Group 076 Study. *AIDS* 1998;12:1805–1813.
23. Culnane M, Fowler MG, Lee S, et al. Lack of long term effects of in utero exposure to zidovudine among uninfected children born to HIV-infected women. *JAMA* 1999;281:151–157.
24. Nduati R, John G, Mbori-Ngacha D, et al. Effect of breastfeeding and formula feeding on transmission of HIV-1: a randomized clinical trial. *JAMA* 2000;283:1167–1174.
25. Biggar RJ, Miotti PG, Taha TE, et al. Perinatal intervention trial in Africa: effect of a birth canal cleansing intervention to prevent HIV transmission. *Lancet* 1996;347:1647–1650.
26. Fawzi WW, Msamanga G, Hunter D, et al. Randomized trial of vitamin supplements in relation to vertical transmission of HIV-1 in Tanzania. *J Acquir Immune Defic Syndr* 2000;23:246–254.
27. Coutsoudis A, Pillay K, Spooner E, et al. Randomized trial testing the effect of vitamin A supplementation on pregnancy outcomes and early, mother-to-child HIV-1 transmission in Durban, South Africa. *AIDS* 1999;13:1517–1524.
28. Fawzi WW, Hunter DJ. Vitamins in HIV disease progression and vertical transmission. *Epidemiology* 1998;9:457–466.
29. Wiegand UW, Hartmann S, Hummler H. Safety of vitamin A: recent results. *Int J Vitam Nutr Res* 1998;68:411–416.
30. Bendich A, Langseth L. Safety of vitamin A. *Am J Clin Nutr* 1989;49:358–371.

Jimmy Volmink
Director of Research and Analysis
Global Health Council
Washington, DC
USA

Competing interests: None declared.

TABLE 1 **Placebo controlled trials of zidovudine to reduce mother to child transmission of HIV (see text, p 781).**

Ref	Participants	Maternal treatment	Infant treatment	Transmission rate	RR (95% CI)
Infants not breast fed					
16	477 women with confirmed HIV (60 centres in the USA and France)	*Antepartum* Orally 1 mg 5 times daily starting at 14–34 weeks' gestation *Intrapartum* 2 mg/kg iv over 1 hour then 1 mg/kg/hour until delivery	Orally 2 mg/kg every 6 hours for 6 weeks (given only to babies of mothers treated with ZDV)	At 18 months: placebo 26%, ZDV 8%	0.32 (0.18 to 0.59)
17	397 women with confirmed HIV-1 (2 centres in Bangkok and Thailand)	*Antepartum* Orally 300 mg twice daily from 36 weeks' gestation *Intrapartum* Orally 300 mg every 3 hours until delivery	Nil	At 6 months: placebo 19%, ZDV 9%	0.52 (0.30 to 0.85)
Infants breast fed					
18	280 women with confirmed HIV-1 (1 hospital in the Ivory Coast)	*Antepartum* Orally 300 mg twice daily from 36 weeks' gestation *Intrapartum* Orally 300 mg every 3 hours until delivery	Nil	At 3 months: placebo 25%, ZDV 16%	0.63 (0.38 to 1.05)
19	431 women with confirmed HIV-1 (Ivory Coast and Burkina Faso)	*Antepartum* Orally 250 or 300 mg twice daily from 36–38 weeks' gestation *Intrapartum* Orally single dose of 500 or 600 mg at onset of labour *Postpartum* Orally 250 or 300 mg twice daily for 7 days	Nil	At 6 months: placebo 28%, ZDV 18%	0.62 (0.40 to 0.95)

iv, intravenously; ref, reference; ZDV, zidovudine.

Opportunistic infections and HIV

Search date January 2002

John Ioannidis and David Wilkinson

QUESTIONS

INTERVENTIONS

To be covered in future updates

Opportunistic infections, treatment

Covered elsewhere in *Clinical Evidence*

Different antiretroviral regimens (see HIV infection, p 693)

See glossary, p 805

Key Messages

- **Aciclovir (for herpes simplex virus and varicella zoster virus)** One systematic review has found that aciclovir versus placebo significantly reduces herpes simplex virus and varicella zoster virus infection, and reduces overall mortality in people at different clinical stages of HIV infection. It found no reduction in cytomegalovirus.
- **Azithromycin (for *Mycobacterium avium* complex [MAC])** One RCT has found that azithromycin versus placebo significantly reduces the incidence of MAC.
- **Azithromycin (for PCP)** One RCT has found that azithromycin, either alone or in combination with rifabutin versus rifabutin alone, reduces the risk of PCP in people receiving standard PCP prophylaxis.
- **Clarithromycin (for MAC)** One RCT has found that clarithromycin versus placebo significantly reduces the incidence of MAC.
- **Clarithromycin plus ethambutol (for MAC in people with previous MAC)** RCTs have found that clarithromycin plus ethambutol, with or without rifabutin, significantly reduces the incidence of MAC.
- **Clofazimine or high dose clarithromycin (for MAC in people with previous MAC)** RCTs have found that clofazimine or high dose clarithromycin versus other combination treatment are associated with increased mortality.
- **Discontinuing prophylaxis for MAC in people with CD4 > 100/mm^3 on highly active antiretroviral treatment (HAART)** Two RCTs in people taking HAART found that discontinuation of prophylaxis for MAC disease did not increase the incidence of MAC disease.
- **Discontinuing prophylaxis for PCP and toxoplasmosis in people with CD4 > 200/mm^3 on HAART** One systematic review of two unblinded RCTs in people taking HAART found that discontinuation of prophylaxis did not increase the incidence of PCP. Two unblinded RCTs found that discontinuation of prophylaxis did not increase the incidence of toxoplasmosis.
- **Famciclovir (for recurrent herpes simplex virus)** One small RCT found that famciclovir versus placebo reduced the rate of viral shedding, but provided insufficient evidence on the effect of famciclovir on herpes simplex virus recurrence.
- **Fluconazole or itraconazole (invasive fungal disease)** RCTs in people with advanced HIV disease have found that both fluconazole and itraconazole versus placebo significantly reduce the incidence of invasive fungal infections. One RCT found that fluconazole versus clotrimazole reduced the incidence of invasive fungal disease and mucocutaneous candidiasis. One RCT found no difference between high and low dose fluconazole.
- **Isoniazid tuberculosis prophylaxis for 6–12 months (*v* combination treatment for 2 months — similar benefits, fewer harms)** RCTs found no evidence of a difference in effectiveness between regimens using combinations of tuberculosis drugs for 2–3 months and those using isoniazid alone for 6–12 months. One RCT found that multidrug regimens increased the number of people with adverse reactions resulting in cessation of treatment.
- **Itraconazole (for histoplasmosis)** We found no RCTs. One open label uncontrolled study found that itraconazole may be effective in preventing the relapse of histoplasmosis.
- **Itraconazole (for *Penicillium marneffei* and cryptococcal meningitis)** Two RCTs have found that itraconazole versus placebo significantly reduces the incidence of relapse of *P marneffei* infection and candidiasis. One RCT found that itraconazole versus fluconazole significantly reduced the relapse of cryptococcal meningitis.

- **Oral ganciclovir (in people with severe CD4 depletion)** One RCT has found that oral ganciclovir versus placebo significantly reduces the incidence of cytomegalovirus in people with severe CD4 depletion. It found that 25% of people who did not develop cytomegalovirus developed severe neutropenia. A second RCT found no significant differences.
- **Rifabutin plus either clarithromycin or azithromycin (for MAC)** One RCT has found that rifabutin plus clarithromycin versus rifabutin alone significantly reduces the incidence of MAC. Another RCT has found that rifabutin plus azithromycin versus azithromycin alone or rifabutin alone significantly reduces the incidence of MAC at 1 year.
- **Stopping prophylaxis for cytomegalovirus in people with CD4 > 100/mm³ on HAART** We found insufficient evidence on the effects of discontinuation of maintenance treatment for cytomegalovirus retinitis or other end organ disease in people taking HAART.
- **TMP/SMX (trimethoprim/sulfamethoxazole [sulphamethoxazole]—co-trimoxazole) (for PCP and toxoplasmosis)** Systematic reviews have found that TMP/SMX versus placebo or pentamidine significantly reduces the incidence of PCP or toxoplasmosis. Systematic reviews have found that TMP/SMX versus dapsone (with or without pyrimethamine) reduces the incidence of PCP, but found no difference in the incidence of toxoplasmosis. One systematic review and one subsequent RCT found no significant difference between high and low dose TMP/SMX for PCP prophylaxis, although adverse effects were more common with the higher dose.
- **Atovaquone (no difference from dapsone or aerosolised pentamidine for Pneumocystis carinii pneumonia [PCP] in people intolerant of TMP/SMX)** We found no RCTs of atovaquone versus placebo. RCTs found no significant difference in the incidence of PCP with atovaquone versus dapsone or versus aerosolised pentamidine.
- **Tuberculosis prophylaxis versus placebo** Systematic reviews have found that in people who are HIV and tuberculin skin test positive, antituberculosis prophylaxis versus placebo significantly reduces the frequency of tuberculosis over 2–3 years. The reviews have found no evidence of benefit in people who are HIV positive but tuberculin skin test negative. One RCT found that the benefit of prophylaxis diminished with time after treatment was stopped.
- **Valaciclovir (for cytomegalovirus)** One RCT has found that valaciclovir versus aciclovir reduces the incidence of cytomegalovirus, but is associated with increased mortality.

DEFINITION Opportunistic infections are intercurrent infections that occur in people infected with HIV. Prophylaxis aims to avoid either the first occurrence of these infections (primary prophylaxis) or their recurrence (secondary prophylaxis, maintenance treatment). This review includes *Pneumocystis carinii* pneumonia (PCP), *Toxoplasma gondii* encephalitis, *Mycobacterium tuberculosis*, *Mycobacterium avium* complex (MAC) disease, cytomegalovirus (CMV) disease (most often retinitis), infections from other herpes viruses (herpes simplex virus and varicella zoster virus), and invasive fungal disease (*Cryptococcus neoformans*, *Histoplasma capsulatum*, and *Penicillium marneffei* [see glossary, p 805]).

INCIDENCE/ PREVALENCE The incidence of opportunistic infections is high in people with immune impairment. Data available before the introduction of highly active antiretroviral treatment (HAART) suggest that, with a CD4 < 250/mm^3, the 2 year probability of developing an opportunistic infection is 40% for PCP, 22% for CMV, 18% for MAC, 6% for toxoplasmosis, and 5% for cryptococcal meningitis.[1] The introduction of HAART has reduced the rate of opportunistic infections. A recent cohort study found that the introduction of HAART decreased the incidence of PCP by 94%, CMV by 82%, and MAC by 64%, as presenting AIDS events. HAART decreased the incidence of events subsequent to the diagnosis of AIDS by 84% for PCP, 82% for CMV, and 97% for MAC.[2]

AETIOLOGY/ RISK FACTORS Opportunistic infections are caused by a wide array of pathogens and result from immune defects induced by HIV. The risk of developing opportunistic infections increases dramatically with progressive impairment of the immune system. Each opportunistic infection has a different threshold of immune impairment, beyond which the risk increases substantially.[1] Opportunistic pathogens may infect the immunocompromised host *de novo*, but usually they are simply reactivations of latent pathogens in such hosts.

PROGNOSIS Prognosis depends on the type of opportunistic infection. Even with treatment they may cause serious morbidity and mortality. Most deaths owing to HIV infection are caused by opportunistic infections.

AIMS To prevent the occurrence and relapse of opportunistic infections; to discontinue unnecessary prophylaxis; to minimise adverse effects of prophylaxis and loss of quality of life.

OUTCOMES First occurrence and relapse of opportunistic infections and adverse effects of treatments. We have not considered neoplastic diseases associated with specific opportunistic infections.

METHODS *Clinical Evidence* search and appraisal January 2002. We also reviewed abstract books/CDs for the following conferences held between 1995 and early 2001: European Clinical AIDS, HIV Drug Treatment, Interscience Conferences on Antimicrobial Agents and Chemotherapy, National Conferences on Human Retroviruses and Opportunistic Infections, and World AIDS Conference. We placed emphasis on systematic reviews and RCTs published after 1993. We considered observational evidence if no RCTs were available or if they covered a broader spectrum than randomised evidence.

QUESTION **What are the effects of prophylaxis for *Pneumocystis carinii* pneumonia and toxoplasmosis?**

John Ioannidis

OPTION **TMP/SMX**

Systematic reviews have found that TMP/SMX is more effective than pentamidine or placebo at reducing the incidence of *P carinii* pneumonia or toxoplasmosis. Two systematic reviews have found that TMP/SMX compared with dapsone (with or without pyrimethamine) reduces the incidence of *P carinii* pneumonia, but found no difference in the incidence

of toxoplasmosis. One systematic review and one subsequent RCT has found no significant difference between high and low dose TMP/SMX for *P carinii* pneumonia prophylaxis, although adverse effects are more common with the higher dose.

Benefits: We found two systematic reviews (search dates 1995[3] and not stated[4]). **TMP/SMX versus placebo:** The first systematic review (35 RCTs) found that prophylaxis with TMP/SMX (or aerosolised pentamidine) reduced the incidence of *P carinii* pneumonia (PCP) more than placebo (RR 0.32, 95% CI 0.23 to 0.46). There were no placebo controlled data on the incidence of toxoplasmosis. One subsequent RCT (545 people in sub-Saharan Africa with symptomatic disease, second or third clinical stage disease in the [WHO staging system (see glossary, p 805)] regardless of CD4 cell count) comparing TMP/SMX with placebo found no significant difference in incidence of PCP or toxoplasmosis.[5] **TMP/SMX versus pentamidine:** The first systematic review found that TMP/SMX versus aerosolised pentamidine significantly reduced the incidence of PCP (RR 0.58, 95% CI 0.45 to 0.75).[3] The second systematic review found that TMP/SMX was more effective at preventing toxoplasmosis than aerosolised pentamidine, but the result did not reach significance (RR 0.78, 95% CI 0.55 to 1.11).[4] **TMP/SMX versus dapsone (with or without pyrimethamine):** The first systematic review found that TMP/SMX compared with dapsone (with or without pyrimethamine) reduced the incidence of PCP, but the result did not reach significance (RR 0.61, 95% CI 0.34 to 1.10).[3] The second review found that TMP/SMX was significantly more effective in preventing PCP than dapsone/pyrimethamine (RR 0.49, 95% CI 0.26 to 0.92). It found no significant difference between TMP/SMX and dapsone/pyrimethamine in preventing toxoplasmosis (RR 1.17, 95% CI 0.68 to 2.04).[4] **High versus low dose TMP/SMX:** The first systematic review found no significant difference in the rate of PCP infection between lower dose (160/800 mg 3 times/wk or 80/400 mg daily) and higher dose (160/800 mg daily) of TMP/SMX (failure rate per 100 person years was 1.6, 95% CI 0.9 to 2.5 with lower dose *v* 0.5, 95% CI 0 to 2.9 with higher dose).[3] One subsequent RCT (2625 people) also found no significant difference in the rate of PCP infection in people receiving TMP/SMX 160/800 mg daily compared with three times weekly (3.5 *v* 4.1 per 100 person years; P = 0.16).[6]

Harms: **TMP/SMX:** The first systematic review found that severe adverse effects (predominantly rash, fever, and haematological effects leading to discontinuation within 1 year) occurred in more people taking higher doses of TMP/SMX than those taking lower doses (25% *v* 15%).[3] The RCT comparing high dose with low dose TMP/SMX found that discontinuation because of adverse effects was significantly more common in people taking high doses of TMP/SMX (RR 2.14; P < 0.001).[6] The RCT in sub-Saharan Africa found that people on TMP/SMX were less likely to suffer a serious event (death or hospital admission, irrespective of the cause) than those on placebo regardless of their initial CD4 cell count (84 *v* 124; HR 0.57, 95% CI 0.43 to 0.75; P < 0.001). Moderate neutropenia occurred more frequently with TMP/SMX (neutropenia AR 62/271 [23%] with TMP/SMX *v* 26/244 [10%] with placebo; RR 2.1, 95% 1.4 to 3.3;

NNH 8, 95% CI 5 to 14).[5] Two RCTs (largest 377 people) found that gradual initiation of TMP/SMX may improve tolerance of the regimen.[7,8] Two RCTs (238 people; 50 people) found no significant benefit from acetylcysteine in preventing TMP/SMX hypersensitivity reactions in HIV infected people.[9,10] **Dapsone:** The first systematic review found that adverse effects occurred in more people taking high doses than low doses of dapsone (29% *v* 12%).[2] A third systematic review (search date 1996, 16 trials, 4267 people) evaluating dapsone toxicity found no significant difference in mortality for dapsone (OR for mortality for dapsone *v* other prophylaxis 1.11, 95% CI 0.96 to 1.29).[11] **Pentamidine:** Bronchospasm occurred in 3% of people taking aerosolised pentamidine 300 mg monthly.[3]

Comment: **Concomitant coverage for toxoplasmosis:** Standard TMP/SMX prophylaxis or dapsone should offer adequate coverage for toxoplasmosis. Pentamidine has no intrinsic activity against *T gondii*. Toxoplasmosis risk is probably clinically meaningful only with CD4 < 100/mm^3 and positive toxoplasma serology.[1] **Role of highly active antiretroviral treatment (HAART):** We found more than 50 RCTs on the prophylaxis of PCP and/or toxoplasmosis, but their results should be interpreted with caution because they were conducted mostly before the advent and widespread use of HAART. Although this is unlikely to affect the comparative results, HAART has resulted in a large decrease in the rate of PCP, toxoplasmosis, and other opportunistic infections; therefore, the absolute benefits of these prophylactic regimens are probably smaller when used with HAART. **Prophylaxis in Africa:** Beneficial effects of TMP/SMX in Africa may be largely because of prophylaxis for bacterial infections rather than PCP. The largest trial conducted in Africa found that TMP/SMX significantly reduced mortality and hospital admissions.[5] However, a smaller trial (100 people) found no significant effect on mortality or hospital admission, although it may have lacked power to detect a significant difference (HR for death or hospital admission 1.10, 95% CI 0.57 to 2.13).[12]

OPTION ATOVAQUONE IN TMP/SMX INTOLERANT PEOPLE

RCTs found no significant difference between atovaquone, dapsone, or aerosolised pentamidine in preventing *Pneumocystis carinii* pneumonia. None of the interventions were compared to placebo.

Benefits: We found no systematic review. **Versus placebo:** We found no RCTs. **Versus dapsone:** One RCT (1057 people intolerant of TMP/SMX, of whom 298 had a history of *P carinii* pneumonia [PCP]) found no significant difference between atovaquone 1500 mg daily compared with dapsone 100 mg daily (15.7 *v* 18.4 cases of PCP per 100 person years; P = 0.20).[13] **Versus pentamidine:** One RCT (549 people intolerant of TMP/SMX) compared high dose with low dose atovaquone (1500 mg daily *v* 750 mg daily) with monthly aerosolised pentamidine (300 mg). It found no significant difference between the groups in the incidence of PCP (26% *v* 22% *v* 17%) or mortality (20% *v* 13% *v* 18%) after a median follow up of 11.3 months.[14]

Harms: The RCT comparing atovaquone with dapsone found that the overall risk of stopping treatment because of adverse effects was similar in the two arms (RR 0.94, 95% CI 0.74 to 1.19).[13] Atovaquone was stopped more frequently than dapsone in people who were receiving dapsone at baseline (RR 3.78, 95% CI 2.37 to 6.01; P < 0.001), and less frequently in people not receiving dapsone at baseline (RR 0.42, 95% CI 0.30 to 0.58; P < 0.001).

Comment: See role of highly active antiretroviral treatment in comment under TMP/SMX, p 793.

OPTION AZITHROMYCIN

One RCT found that azithromycin, either alone or in combination with rifabutin, reduces the risk of *Pneumocystis carinii* pneumonia compared with rifabutin alone in people receiving standard *Pneumocystis carinii* pneumonia prophylaxis.

Benefits: We found no systematic review. **Versus placebo:** We found no RCTs. **Versus other drugs:** We found one RCT (693 people) that compared azithromycin, rifabutin, and both drugs in combination in people who were already receiving standard *P carinii* pneumonia (PCP) prophylaxis. It found that azithromycin, either alone or in combination with rifabutin, reduced the risk of developing PCP by 45% when compared with rifabutin alone (P = 0.008).[15]

Harms: Gastrointestinal side effects are common with azithromycin, but they are usually mild and do not lead to stopping treatment. The addition of rifabutin significantly increased the risk of stopping treatment (RR 1.67; P = 0.03).[16]

Comment: See role of highly active antiretroviral treatment (HAART) in comment under TMP/SMX, p 793. The low incidence of PCP infection in people taking HAART means that the absolute benefit of prophylaxis is smaller.

QUESTION What are the effects of antituberculosis prophylaxis in people with HIV infection?

David Wilkinson

OPTION ANTITUBERCULOSIS PROPHYLACTIC REGIMENS VERSUS PLACEBO

Two systematic reviews have found that in people who are HIV and tuberculin skin test positive, antituberculosis prophylaxis reduces frequency of tuberculosis in the short term. The reviews found no evidence of benefit in people who are HIV positive but tuberculin skin test negative. One RCT found that the benefit of prophylaxis diminished with time after treatment was stopped.

Benefits: We found two systematic reviews. The first systematic review (search date 2000) identified seven RCTs in 4652 HIV positive adults from Haiti, Kenya, USA, Zambia, and Uganda.[17] All compared isoniazid (6–12 months) or combination treatment (3 months) with placebo. Mean follow up was 2–3 years, and the main outcomes, stratified by tuberculin skin test positivity, were tuberculosis (either microbiological or clinical) and death. Among tuberculin skin test positive adults, antituberculosis prophylaxis significantly reduced the incidence of tuberculosis (RR compared with placebo 0.24, 95% CI 0.14 to 0.40) and was associated with a non-significant reduction in the risk of death (RR compared with placebo 0.77, 95% CI 0.58 to 1.03). Among tuberculin skin test negative adults there was no significant difference in risk of tuberculosis (RR compared with placebo 0.87, 95% CI 0.56 to 1.36) or death (RR compared with placebo 1.07, 95% CI 0.88 to 1.30). The second review (search date not stated, 7 trials, 4529 people) compared isoniazid versus placebo only.[18] Among tuberculin skin test positive participants the incidence of tuberculosis was significantly reduced (RR compared with placebo 0.40, 95% CI 0.24 to 0.65), but again there was no significant difference among tuberculin skin test negative participants (RR compared with placebo 0.84, 95% CI 0.54 to 1.30). This review found no evidence of any impact on mortality.[18] One of the RCTs included in the systematic reviews (1053 Zambian adults; 161 tuberculin skin test positive, 517 negative, the rest unknown) comparing isoniazid versus rifampicin plus pyrazinamide versus placebo for up to 6 months recently published results at 3 years' follow up.[19] Many people taking placebo were offered isoniazid after randomisation. However, intention to treat analysis found that isoniazid or rifampicin plus pyrazinamide versus placebo significantly reduced the risk of tuberculosis at 2.5 years (cumulative AR not provided; RR 0.55, 95% CI 0.32 to 0.93), although the benefit diminished over this time (P = 0.01) We found one subsequent RCT published as a letter (see comment below).[20]

Harms: Data on adverse drug reactions were not always stratified by tuberculin skin test positivity. In the first review there was a significant increase in adverse drug reactions requiring cessation of treatment on isoniazid compared with placebo (RR 1.75, 95% CI 1.23 to 2.47).[17] In the second review, the estimated RR was 1.36 (95% CI 1.00 to 1.86).[18]

Comment: Without prophylaxis, people who are HIV and tuberculin skin test positive have a 50% or more lifetime risk of developing tuberculosis compared with a 10% lifetime risk in people who are HIV positive but tuberculin skin test negative.[21] Clinical features of tuberculosis may be atypical in people with HIV infection and diagnosis may be more difficult, disease progression more rapid, and outcome worse. The subsequent RCT published as a letter (237 HIV positive Haitian adults with negative tuberculin skin test) found no significant difference between isoniazid (300 mg) versus no treatment in mortality, or the incidence of AIDS or tuberculosis at 1 year.[20]

OPTION DIFFERENT ANTITUBERCULOSIS PROPHYLACTIC REGIMENS

RCTs found no evidence of a difference in effectiveness between regimens using combinations of tuberculosis drugs for 2–3 months and those using isoniazid alone for 6–12 months. One RCT found that multidrug regimens increased the number of people with adverse reactions resulting in cessation of treatment.

Benefits: We found no systematic review. We found six RCTs.[19,22–26] Three RCTs (750, 1583, and 393 people) compared isoniazid versus rifampicin/pyrazinamide in people who were HIV and tuberculin skin test positive.[22–24] All found no significant difference in rates of tuberculosis. The fourth RCT (1564 HIV and tuberculin skin test positive people from Uganda) compared three treatments (isoniazid alone, isoniazid plus rifampicin, and isoniazid, rifampicin, and pyrazinamide) versus placebo.[25] It found that the risk of tuberculosis was significantly reduced with isoniazid alone (RR compared with placebo 0.33, 95% CI 0.14 to 0.77), and with isoniazid and rifampicin combined (RR compared with placebo 0.40, 95% CI 0.18 to 0.86). However, it found only a non-significant trend towards reduction with isoniazid, rifampicin, and pyrazinamide combined (RR compared with placebo 0.51, 95% CI 0.24 to 1.08). The fifth RCT (133 adults, mixed tuberculin skin test positive and negative) comparing isoniazid for 12 months versus isoniazid plus rifampicin for 3 months found no significant difference in the incidence of tuberculosis (AR 4.2% with isoniazid *v* 2.1% with isoniazid plus rifampicin, RR 0.51, 95% CI 0.09 to 2.8).[26] The sixth RCT (1053 Zambian adults; 161 tuberculin skin test positive, 517 negative, the rest unknown) compared isoniazid for 6 months versus rifampicin plus pyrazinamide for 3 months versus placebo.[19] Many people in the placebo group were offered isoniazid after randomisation. However, intention to treat analysis found no significant difference between isoniazid versus rifampicin plus pyrazinamide in the rate of tuberculosis at any time during mean follow up of 3 years.

Harms: One RCT found that the proportion of people discontinuing treatment increased with the number of drugs given: isoniazid 1%, isoniazid plus rifampicin 2%, and all three drugs 6%.[23]

Comment: There is concern about emergence of rifampicin resistance if this drug is used in antituberculosis prophylaxis, although we found no reports of this. However, there is a theoretical risk that widespread, unsupervised use of isoniazid alone could promote resistance to this drug, although we found no evidence that this has happened.

QUESTION What are the effects of prophylaxis for disseminated *Mycobacterium avium* complex disease for people without previous *M avium* complex disease?

John Ioannidis

OPTION AZITHROMYCIN

One RCT has found that azithromycin significantly reduced the incidence of *M avium* complex more than placebo.

Benefits: We found no systematic review. One RCT (174 people with AIDS and CD4 < 100/mm^3) found that azithromycin reduced the incidence of *M avium* complex (MAC) more than placebo (11% *v* 25%; P = 0.004).[27]

Harms: Gastrointestinal side effects were more likely with azithromycin than with placebo (71/90 [79%] v 25/91 [28%]; NNH 2), but they were rarely severe enough to cause discontinuation of treatment (8% v 2% in the two arms; P = 0.14).[27]

Comment: Prospective cohort studies found that the risk of disseminated MAC disease increased substantially with a lower CD4 count and was clinically important only for CD4 < 50/mm^3.[1] **Role of highly active antiretroviral treatment (HAART):** Most of the RCTs of MAC prophylaxis were conducted before the widespread use of HAART. HAART reduces the absolute risk of MAC infection. The absolute risk reduction of prophylactic regimens may be smaller when used in people treated with HAART.

OPTION CLARITHROMYCIN

One RCT found that clarithromycin reduced the incidence of *Mycobacterium avium* complex compared with placebo.

Benefits: We found one systematic review (search date 1997) of prophylaxis and treatment of *M avium* complex (MAC).[28] It identified one RCT (682 people with advanced AIDS) that found that clarithromycin compared with placebo significantly reduced the incidence of MAC (6% v 16%; HR 0.31, 95% CI 0.18 to 0.53). It found no significant difference in the death rate (32% v 41%; HR 0.75; P = 0.026).[29]

Harms: Adverse effects led to discontinuation of treatment in slightly more people taking clarithromycin than placebo (8% v 6%; P = 0.45). More people taking clarithromycin suffered altered taste (11% v 2%) or rectal disorders (8% v 3%).[27]

Comment: Prospective cohort studies found that the risk of disseminated MAC disease increased substantially with a lower CD4 count and was clinically important only for CD4 < 50/mm^3.[1] See role of highly active antiretroviral treatment in comment under azithromycin, p 794.

OPTION COMBINATION TREATMENT

RCTs have found that clarithromycin alone and clarithromycin plus rifabutin both reduce the incidence of *Mycobacterium avium* complex compared with rifabutin alone. Azithromycin plus rifabutin reduce the incidence of *M avium* complex compared with azithromycin alone or rifabutin alone.

Benefits: **Clarithromycin plus rifabutin:** We found no systematic review. One RCT (1178 people with AIDS) compared rifabutin versus clarithromycin versus clarithromycin plus rifabutin.[30] It found that the risk of *M avium* complex (MAC) was significantly reduced in the clarithromycin alone group (RRR 44% for clarithromycin v rifabutin; P = 0.005) and the combination group when compared with rifabutin alone (RRR 57% for combination v rifabutin; P = 0.0003). There was no significant difference in the risk of MAC between the combination and clarithromycin arms (P = 0.36). **Azithromycin plus rifabutin:** One RCT (693 people) found that the combination of azithromycin plus rifabutin versus azithromycin alone significantly reduced the incidence of MAC at 1 year (15.3% with rifabutin *v* 7.6% for azithromycin *v* 2.8% with rifabutin plus azithromycin; $P = 0.008$ for rifabutin *v* azithromycin; $P = 0.03$ for combination *v* azithromycin).[16]

Harms: In one RCT, dose limiting toxicity was more likely with azithromycin plus rifabutin than with azithromycin alone (HR 1.67; $P = 0.03$).[16] In another RCT, adverse events occurred in 31% of people receiving the combination of clarithromycin and rifabutin compared with 16% on clarithromycin alone and 18% on rifabutin alone ($P < 0.001$).[28] Uveitis occurred in 42 people: 33 were on clarithromycin plus rifabutin, seven were on rifabutin alone, and two were on clarithromycin alone. **Uveitis:** We found one systematic review (search date 1994, 54 people with rifabutin associated uveitis).[31] It found that uveitis was dose dependent. It occurred from 2 weeks to more than 7 months after initiation of rifabutin treatment, and was more likely in people taking rifabutin and clarithromycin. In most people, uveitis resolved 1–2 months after discontinuation of rifabutin.

Comment: Prospective cohort studies found that the risk of disseminated MAC disease increased substantially with a lower CD4 count and was clinically important only for CD4 < 50/mm^3.[1] Clarithromycin may inhibit rifabutin metabolism; rifabutin may decrease levels of delavirdine and saquinavir. See role of highly active antiretroviral treatment in comment under azithromycin, p 794.

QUESTION **What are the effects of prophylaxis for disseminated *Mycobacterium avium* complex disease for people with previous *M avium* complex disease?**

John Ioannidis

OPTION **COMBINATION TREATMENT**

RCTs have found that clarithromycin and ethambutol, with or without rifabutin, reduce the incidence of *M avium* complex. Clofazimine and high dose clarithromycin are associated with increased mortality.

Benefits: We found no systematic review but found four RCTs. The first RCT (95 people) found that the combination of clarithromycin (1000 mg daily), clofazimine, and ethambutol was associated with significantly fewer relapses of *M avium* complex (MAC) than the combination of clarithromycin plus clofazimine without ethambutol (68% relapsed in 3 drug regimen *v* 12% in 2 drug regimen at 36 wks; $P = 0.004$).[32] The second RCT (106 people) found that the addition of clofazimine to clarithromycin and ethambutol did not improve clinical response and was associated with higher mortality.[33] The third RCT (144 people) found that the combination of clarithromycin, rifabutin, and ethambutol reduced the relapse rate of MAC compared with clarithromycin plus clofazimine.[34] The fourth RCT (198 people) found no significant difference in survival between people taking clarithromycin plus ethambutol and people taking clarithromycin plus ethambutol plus rifabutin.[35]

Harms: The second RCT, which added clofazimine to clarithromycin plus rifabutin, found a higher mortality in the clofazimine arm (62% with clofazimine *v* 38% without clofazimine; P = 0.012).[33] High doses of clarithromycin (1000 mg twice daily)[36,37] and clofazimine[33] were associated with increased mortality. One RCT (85 people) comparing clarithromycin 500 mg twice daily versus 1000 mg twice daily found that after a median follow up of 4.5 months, more people died with the higher dose (17/40 [43%] with 1000 mg twice daily *v* 10/45 [22%] with 500 mg twice daily; ARI 20%, 95% CI 0.2% to 33%; NNH 5, 95% CI 3 to 470).[36] A similar difference was seen in another RCT (154 people).[37] Combinations of drugs may lead to increased toxicity. Optic neuropathy may occur with ethambutol, but has not been reported in RCTs in people with HIV where the dose and symptoms were carefully monitored.[35,36]

Comment: The observed increased mortality associated with clofazimine and high doses of clarithromycin has led to avoidance of these drugs.

QUESTION What are the effects of prophylaxis for cytomegalovirus, herpes simplex virus, and varicella zoster virus?

John Ioannidis

OPTION GANCICLOVIR

One RCT has found that oral ganciclovir versus placebo significantly reduces the incidence of cytomegalovirus in people with severe CD4 depletion compared with placebo. It found that 25% of people who did not develop cytomegalovirus developed severe neutropenia. A second RCT found no significant differences.

Benefits: We found no systematic review. **Versus placebo:** We found two RCTs. The first RCT (725 people with a median CD4 count of $22/mm^3$) found that oral ganciclovir halved the incidence of cytomegalovirus (CMV) compared with placebo (event rate 16% *v* 30%; P = 0.001).[38] The second RCT (994 HIV-1 infected people with CD4 $< 100/mm^3$ and CMV seropositivity) found no difference in the rate of CMV in people taking oral ganciclovir compared with placebo (event rates 13.1 *v* 14.6 per 100 person years; HR 0.92, 95% CI 0.65 to 1.27).[39] Both RCTs found no significant difference in overall mortality.

Harms: In the first RCT, 25% of people who did not develop CMV developed severe neutropenia (and were then treated with granulocyte colony stimulating factor).[38]

Comment: Differences in the results of RCTs may have arisen by chance or owing to protocol variability; for example, no baseline ophthalmologic examinations were performed in the second trial.[39] The low incidence of CMV disease in people taking HAART, and the high rates of adverse events, means that the clinical value of oral ganciclovir in people who have not had active CMV disease is unclear.

OPTION ACICLOVIR AND VALACICLOVIR

One systematic review has found that aciclovir versus placebo does not reduce the incidence of cytomegalovirus disease, but significantly reduces herpes simplex virus and varicella zoster virus infection and overall mortality in people at different clinical stages of HIV infection. One RCT has found that valaciclovir reduces the incidence of cytomegalovirus disease more than aciclovir, but was associated with increased mortality.

Benefits: We found one systematic review of individual patient data (search date not stated, 8 RCTs) in people with asymptomatic HIV infection to full-blown AIDS.[40] It found no difference in protection against cytomegalovirus (CMV) disease between aciclovir compared with no treatment or placebo. However, aciclovir significantly reduced overall mortality (RR 0.81; $P = 0.04$) and herpes simplex virus (HSV) and varicella zoster virus (VZV) infections ($P < 0.001$ for both).[40] One RCT (1227 CMV seropositive people with CD4 < 100/mm^3) compared valaciclovir, high dose aciclovir, and low dose aciclovir. It found increased mortality in the valaciclovir group, which did not reach statistical significance ($P = 0.06$).[41] The CMV rate was lower in the valaciclovir group than the aciclovir groups (12% *v* 18%; $P = 0.03$).

Harms: One RCT found that toxicity and early medication discontinuations were significantly more frequent in the valaciclovir arm (1 year discontinuation rate: 51% for valaciclovir *v* 46% for high dose aciclovir *v* 41% for low dose aciclovir).[39]

Comment: The survival benefit with aciclovir is unclear. The absolute risk reduction may be higher in people who have frequent HSV or VZV infections.

OPTION FAMCICLOVIR

One small RCT found that famciclovir versus placebo reduced the rate of viral shedding, but provided insufficient evidence on the effect of famciclovir on herpes simplex virus recurrence.

Benefits: We found no systematic review. One small crossover placebo controlled RCT (48 people) found that famciclovir suppressed herpes simplex virus in people with frequent recurrences (herpes simplex virus was isolated in 9/1071 famciclovir days *v* 122/1114 placebo days; $P < 0.001$).[42] Breakthrough reactivations on famciclovir were short lived and often asymptomatic.

Harms: Famciclovir was well tolerated, and the incidence of adverse effects was similar in both groups.

Comment: The conclusions of this study are difficult to interpret. The randomisation process allocated participants to groups, but the intention to treat analysis involved the number of days with symptoms rather than the number of participants who improved. There was no assessment of statistical significance of clinical outcomes. The trial's analysis is impeded by a high withdrawl rate.

QUESTION **What are the effects of prophylaxis for invasive fungal disease in people without previous fungal disease?**

John Ioannidis

OPTION **AZOLES**

RCTs in people with advanced HIV disease have found that both fluconazole and itraconazole versus placebo significantly reduce the incidence of invasive fungal Infections. One RCT found that fluconazole reduced the incidence of invasive fungal disease and mucocutaneous candidiasis more than clotrimazole. One RCT found no difference between high and low dose fluconazole.

Benefits: We found no systematic review. **Fluconazole versus placebo:** One RCT (323 women with CD4 $\leq 300/mm^3$) found that fluconazole versus placebo significantly reduced the incidence of candidiasis (44% *v* 58% suffered at least one episode of candidiasis; RR 0.56, 95% CI 0.41 to 0.77).[43] **Itraconazole versus placebo:** One RCT (295 people with advanced HIV disease) found that itraconazole reduced the incidence of invasive fungal infections (6 *v* 19; P = 0.0007).[44] It found no significant effect on recurrent or refractory candidiasis. **High dose versus low dose fluconazole:** One RCT (636 people) compared fluconazole 200 mg daily with 400 mg once weekly and found no difference in the rate of invasive fungal infections over a follow up of 74 weeks (8% *v* 6%; ARR 2.2%, 95% CI –1.7% to +6.%). However, the incidence of candidiasis was twice as common in people taking the weekly dose.[45] **Fluconazole versus clotrimazole:** One RCT found that fluconazole reduced the incidence of invasive fungal disease and mucocutaneous candidal infections compared with clotrimazole (4% *v* 11%; relative hazard 3.3, 95% CI 1.5 to 7.6).[46] None of the above RCTs found any difference in mortality.

Harms: Congenital anomalies have occurred in a few children born to mothers receiving fluconazole. Itraconazole is embryotoxic and teratogenic in animals. Azoles may interact with antiretroviral regimens.[47] Azole drugs inhibit the metabolism of some drugs such as terfenadine. Theoretically they may increase the risk of sudden death because of ventricular tachycardia.

Comment: Azoles effectively reduce invasive fungal disease. Any absolute benefit is probably even lower in people treated with highly active antiretroviral treatment. Lack of evidence of any survival benefit, potential for complex drug interactions with current antiretroviral regimens, and potential for developing resistant fungal isolates, means that there is doubt about routine antifungal prophylaxis in HIV infected people without previous invasive fungal disease.

QUESTION What are the effects of prophylaxis for invasive fungal disease in people with previous fungal disease?

John Ioannidis

OPTION AZOLES

Two RCTs found that itraconazole versus placebo significantly reduced the incidence of relapse of *Penicillium marneffei* infection and candidiasis. One RCT found that itraconazole versus fluconazole significantly reduced the relapse of cryptococcal meningitis.

Benefits: We found no systematic review. **Itraconazole versus placebo:** One RCT (71 people with AIDS in Asia) found that itraconazole reduced the relapse of 805)*P marneffei* infection compared with placebo (0/36 [0%] *v* 20/35 [57%] relapsed within 1 year; $P < 0.001$).[48] A second RCT (44 people with HIV infection and candidiasis, treated with itraconazole 200 mg for 4 wks before randomisation) compared prophylaxis with itraconazole versus placebo for 24 weeks. It found that itraconazole reduced the number of people who relapsed (5/24 [21%] with itraconazole *v* 14/20 [70%] with placebo; ARR 49%, 95% CI 19% to 64%; NNT 2, 95% CI 2 to 5) and increased the time interval before relapse occurred (median time to relapse: itraconazole 8.0 wks *v* placebo 10.4 wks; $P = 0.001$).[49] **Itraconazole versus fluconazole:** One RCT (108 people with HIV infection) found that itraconazole reduced relapses of successfully treated cryptococcal meningitis more than fluconazole (13/57 [23%] *v* 2/51 [4%]; ARR 19%, 95% CI 6.2 to 31.7; RR 0.17, 95% CI 0.04 to 0.71; NNT 5, 95% CI 3 to 16).[50] The trial was stopped early because of the higher rate of relapse with fluconazole.

Harms: In one RCT, discontinuation of itraconazole occurred in two people because of skin rashes, one because of severe anaemia, and one because of gastrointestinal effects compared with none taking fluconazole.[50]

Comment: In addition to these studies, one open label uncontrolled study (44 people) found that itraconazole may be effective in preventing the relapse of histoplasmosis.[51] Recurrent infection is common in people with previous *C neoformans*, *H capsulatum,* and *P marneffei* infections. Maintenance for life may be needed in the presence of immune impairment.

QUESTION What are the effects of discontinuing prophylaxis against opportunistic pathogens in people on highly active antiretroviral treatment?

John Ioannìdis

OPTION DISCONTINUATION OF PROPHYLAXIS FOR *PNEUMOCYSTIS CARINII* PNEUMONIA AND TOXOPLASMOSIS IN PEOPLE WITH CD4 > 200/MM^3 ON HAART

One systematic review of two unblinded RCTs found that discontinuation of prophylaxis did not increase the incidence of *P carinii* pneumonia. Two unblinded RCTs found that discontinuation of prophylaxis did not increase the incidence of toxoplasmosis.

Benefits: ***P carinii*** **pneumonia (PCP):** We found onc systematic review (search date 2001, 2 RCTs, 3584 people, two non-randomised controlled trials, and 10 studies with other designs) about the cffccts of discontinuing prophylaxis.[52] The review found a low incidence of PCP in people discontinuing both primary and secondary prophylaxis after a mean of 1.5 years (7/3035 [0.23%] with discontinuing primary prophylaxis and 1/549 [0.18%] discontinuing secondary prophylaxis; mean annual incidence over 1.5 years 0.23%, 95% CI 0.10% to 0.46%; no statistical heterogeneity among studies). Neither of the two RCTs identified in the review found any cases of PCP after discontinuation (first RCT: 587 people with satisfactory response to highly active antiretroviral treatment [HAART], CD4 > 200/mm^3, and viral load < 5000 copies/mm^3 for > 3 months, AR for PCP or toxoplasma encephalitis at median 20 months = 0%, whether or not prophylaxis continued;[53] second RCT: 708 people taking HAART, CD4 > 200/mm^3 for 3 months, AR for PCP at 6 months = 0%).[54] **Toxoplasmosis:** We found two RCTs.[54,55] The first, which was included in the systematic review, found no cases of toxoplasma encephalitis at 6 months in people discontinuing prophylaxis (see PCP above).[54] The second RCT (302 people with a satisfactory response to HAART) compared discontinuation with continuation of toxoplasma prophylaxis.[55] After a median of 10 months it found no episodes of toxoplasma encephalitis in cither group.

Harms: The systematic review found no direct harms from discontinuing prophylaxis.[52]

Comment: The risk of PCP may increase again in people who do not respond to antiretroviral treatment. We found no direct evidence of the effects of different HAART regimens on the risk of PCP or toxoplasmosis. Antiretroviral regimens with different mechanisms of action may have different clinical effects on opportunistic infections and HIV disease progression, despite inducing satisfactory suppression of HIV-1 replication and adequate CD4 responses. Also, CD4 cell count is an incomplete marker of immune reconstitution. It is theoretically conceivable that people with the same CD4 count may have different immune deficits regarding control of PCP and other opportunistic pathogens. An extensive amount of research is being conducted on other parameters of immune reconstitution, but the clinical implications are uncertain at present. One decision analysis based on the systematic review suggested that in the long term, discontinuation of PCP prophylaxis in people who respond to HAART should result in fewer PCP episodes and fewer prophylaxis related adverse effects.[52]

OPTION DISCONTINUATION OF PROPHYLAXIS FOR *MYCOBACTERIUM AVIUM* COMPLEX DISEASE IN PEOPLE WITH CD4 > 100/MM³ ON HAART

Two RCTs found that discontinuation of prophylaxis for *M avium* complex disease did not increase the incidence of *M avium* complex disease.

Benefits: We found no systematic review. We found two RCTs. The first RCT (520 people without previous *M avium* complex [MAC] disease, with CD4 > 100/mm^3 in response to highly active antiretroviral treatment [HAART]) compared azithromycin with placebo.[56] There were no episodes of confirmed MAC disease in either group over a median follow up of 12 months. The second RCT (643 people with CD4 > 100/mm^3 in response to HAART) compared azithromycin 1200 mg once weekly versus placebo. Over a median follow up of 16 months there was no significant difference in the incidence of MAC between the groups (2/321 [0.62%] with placebo *v* 0/322 [0%] with azithromycin; difference 0.5 events per 100 person years, 95% CI –0.2 to +1.2 events per 100 person years).[57]

Harms: In both RCTs, adverse effects leading to discontinuation of treatment were more common with azithromycin than with placebo (7% *v* 1%; P = 0.002; 8% *v* 2%; P < 0.001).[56,57]

Comment: It is not clear whether different antiretroviral regimens have different clinical effects on opportunistic infections and on the need for specific prophylaxis.

OPTION DISCONTINUATION OF MAINTENANCE TREATMENT FOR CYTOMEGALOVIRUS IN PEOPLE WITH A CD4 > 100/MM³ ON HIGHLY ACTIVE ANTIRETROVIRAL TREATMENT

We found insufficient evidence on the effects of discontinuation of maintenance treatment for cytomegalovirus retinitis or other end organ disease.

Benefits: We found no systematic review or RCTs.

Harms: We found no evidence from systematic reviews or RCTs.

Comment: We found several small case series (see table 1, p 808).[58–66] The study with the longest follow up (mean 20.4 months) found no relapses in 41 people discontinuing maintenance treatment.[58] However, another study with mean follow up of 14.5 months found five (29%) relapses among 17 participants who withdrew from maintenance; all of them occurred after the CD4 cell count had dropped again to below 50/mm^3 (8 days/10 months after this event).[61] In one observational series, 12/14 participants (86%) had evidence of immune reconstitution retinitis even before starting withdrawal of prophylaxis.[60] Worsening uveitis was associated with a substantial vision loss (> 3 lines) in three participants. It is difficult to conduct a RCT of adequate sample size to exclude modest differences in relapse rates. The observational evidence suggests that withdrawal of cytomegalovirus (CMV) maintenance treatment may be considered in selected people in whom CMV disease is in remission, CD4 > 100mm^3, and HIV replication remains suppressed. We found no clear evidence on whether quantification of CMV viraemia should be considered in the decision to withdraw from maintenance. One small case series found that relapses were associated with a drop in the CD4 cell count.[61] However, we found no randomised or other reliable evidence of when CMV maintenance treatment should be reinstituted.

GLOSSARY

***Penicillium marneffei* infection** A common opportunistic infection in south-east Asia.

The WHO staging system for HIV infection and disease consists of a "clinical axis" that is represented by a sequential list of clinical conditions believed to have prognostic significance, which subdivides the course of HIV infection into four clinical stages; and a "laboratory axis" that subdivides each clinical stage into three strata according to CD4 cell count or total lymphocyte count.

REFERENCES

1. Gallant JE, Moore RD, Chaisson RE. Prophylaxis for opportunistic infections in patients with HIV infection. *Ann Intern Med* 1994;120:932–944.
2. Detels R, Tarwater P, Phair JP, et al. Effectiveness of potent antiretroviral therapies on the incidence of opportunistic infections before and after AIDS diagnosis. *AIDS* 2001;15:347–355.
3. Ioannidis JPA, Cappelleri JC, Skolnik PR, Lau J, Sacks HS. A meta-analysis of the relative efficacy and toxicity of *Pneumocystis carinii* prophylactic regimens. *Arch Intern Med* 1996;156:177–188. Search date 1995; primary sources Medline and conference abstracts.
4. Bucher HC, Griffith L, Guyatt GH, Opravil M. Meta-analysis of prophylactic treatments against *Pneumocystis carinii* pneumonia and toxoplasma encephalitis in HIV-infected patients. *J Acquir Immune Defic Syndr Hum Retrovirol* 1997;15:104–114. Search date not stated; primary sources Medline, Aidsline, Aidstrials, Aidsdrugs, screening the Proceedings of the International and European Conferences on AIDS, bibliographies of identified trials, and by contacting experts.
5. Anglaret X, Chene G, Attia A, et al. Early chemoprophylaxis with trimethroprim-sulphamethoxazole for HIV-1-infected adults in Abidjan, Cote d'Ivoire: a randomized trial. *Lancet* 1999;353:1463–1468.
6. El-Sadr W, Luskin-Hawk R, Yurik TM, et al. A randomized trial of daily and thrice weekly trimethoprim-sulfamethoxazole for the prevention of *Pneumocystis carinii* pneumonia in HIV-infected individuals. *Clin Infect Dis* 1999;29:775–783.
7. Leoung GS, Stanford JF, Giordano MF, et al. Trimethoprim-sulfamethoxazole (TMP-SMZ) dose escalation versus direct rechallenge for Pneumocystis carinii pneumonia prophylaxis in human immunodeficiency virus-infected patients with previous adverse reaction to TMP-SMZ. *J Infect Dis* 2001;184:992–997.
8. Para MF, Finkelstein D, Becker S, et al. Reduced toxicity with gradual initiation of trimethoprim-sulfamethoxazole for *Pneumocystis carinii* pneumonia. *J Acquir Immune Defic Syndr Hum Retrovirol* 2000;24:337–343.
9. Walmsley SL, Khorasheh S, Singer J, Djurdjev O. A randomized trial of N-acetylcysteine for prevention of trimethoprim-sulfamethoxazole hypersensitivity reactions in *Pneumocystis carinii* pneumonia prophylaxis (CTN057). Canadian HIV Trials Network 057 Study Group. *J Acquir Immune Defic Syndr Hum Retrovirol* 1998;19:498–505.
10. Akerlund B, Tynell E, Bratt G, Bielenstein M, Lidman C. N-acetylcysteine treatment and the risk of toxic reactions to trimethoprim-sulphamethoxazole in primary *Pneumocystis carinii* prophylaxis in HIV-infected patients. *J Infect* 1997;35:143–147.
11. Saillour-Glenisson F, Chene G, Salmi LR, et al. Effect of dapsone on survival in HIV-infected patients: a meta-analysis. *Rev Epidemiol Sante Publique* 2000;48:17–30. Search date 1996; primary sources Medline, Aidstrials, Aidsdrugs, registries of clinical trials, abstracts from international AIDS conferences and infectious diseases meetings, and consultation with active experts.
12. Maynart M, Lievre L, Sow PS, et al. Primary prevention with cotrimoxazole for HIV-1-infected adults: results of the pilot study in Dakar, Senegal. *J Acquir Immune Defic Syndr* 2001;26:130–136.

13. El Sadr WM, Murphy RL, Yurik TM, et al. Atovaquone compared with dapsone for the prevention of *Pneumocystis carinii* pneumonia in patients with HIV infection who cannot tolerate trimethoprim, sulfonamides, or both. Community Programs for Clinical Research on AIDS and the AIDS Clinical Trials Group. *N Engl J Med* 1998;339:1889–1895.
14. Chan C, Montaner J, Lefebre EA, et al. Atovaquone suspension compared with aerosolized pentamidine for prevention of *Pneumocystis carinii* in human immunodeficiency virus-infected subjects intolerant of trimethoprim or sulfonamides. *J Infect Dis* 1999;180:369–376.
15. Dunne MW, Bozzette S, McCutchan JA, et al. Efficacy of azithromycin in prevention of *Pneumocystis carinii* pneumonia: a randomized trial. California Collaborative Treatment Group. *Lancet* 1999;354:891–895.
16. Havlir DV, Dube MP, Sattler FR, et al. Prophylaxis against disseminated *Mycobacterium avium* complex with weekly azithromycin, daily rifabutin, or both. California Collaborative Treatment Group. *N Engl J Med* 1996;335:392–398.
17. Wilkinson D. Drugs for preventing tuberculosis in HIV infected persons. In: The Cochrane Library, Issue 4, 2001. Oxford: Update Software. Search date 2000; primary sources Cochrane Infectious Diseases Group Trials Register, Cochrane Controlled Trials Register Issue 3, Embase, and hand searched references.
18. Bucher HC, Griffith LE, Guyatt GH, et al. Isoniazid prophylaxis for tuberculosis in HIV infection: a meta-analysis of randomised controlled trials. *AIDS* 1999;13:501–507. Search date not stated; primary sources Medline, Embase, CAB Health, Biosis, Health Star, IDIS Drug File, DHSS-Data, Medical Toxicology and Health, Drug Information, Aidsline, Aidstrial, Aidsdrug, Cochrane Controlled Trials Register, hand searched references, and conference proceedings.
19. Quigley MA, Mwinga A, Hosp M, et al. Long-term effect of preventive therapy for tuberculosis in a cohort of HIV infected Zambian adults. *AIDS* 2001;15:215–222.
20. Fitzgerald DW, Severe P, Joseph P, et al. No effect of isoniazid prophylaxis for purified protein derivative negative HIV-infected adults living in a country with endemic tuberculosis: results of a randomised trial. *J AIDS* 2001;28:305–307.
21. Selwyn PA, Hartel D, Lewis VA, et al. A prospective study of the risk of tuberculosis among intravenous drug users with human immunodeficiency virus infection. *N Engl J Med* 1989;320:545–550.
22. Halsey NA, Coberly JS, Desmormeaux J, et al. Randomised trial of isoniazid versus rifampicin and pyrazinamide for prevention of tuberculosis in HIV-1 infection. *Lancet* 1998;351:786–792.
23. Mwinga A, Hosp M, Godfrey-Fausset P, et al. Twice weekly tuberculosis preventive therapy in HIV infection in Zambia. *AIDS* 1998;12:2447–2457.
24. Gordin F, Chaisson RE, Matts JP, et al. Rifampin and pyrazinamide vs isoniazid for prevention of tuberculosis in HIV-infected persons: an international randomized trial. *JAMA* 2000;283:1445–1450.
25. Whalen CC, Johson JL, Okwera A, et al. A trial of three regimens to prevent tuberculosis in Ugandan adults with the human immunodeficiency virus. *N Engl Med* 1997;337:801–808.
26. Alfaro EM, Cuadra F, Solera J, et al. Assessment of two chemoprophylaxis regimens for tuberculosis in HIV-infected patients. *Med Clin* 2000;115:161–165.
27. Oldfield EC, Fessel WJ, Dunne MW, et al. Once weekly azithromycin therapy for prevention of *Mycobacterium avium* complex infection in patients with AIDS: a randomized, double-blind, placebo-controlled multicenter trial. *Clin Infect Dis* 1998;26:611–619.
28. Faris MA, Raasch RH, Hopfer RL, Butts JD. Treatment and prophylaxis of disseminated *Mycobacterium avium* complex in HIV-infected individuals. *Ann Pharmacother* 1998;32:564–573. Search date 1997; primary sources Medline and Aidsline.
29. Pierce M, Crampton S, Henry D, et al. A randomized trial of clarithromycin as prophylaxis against disseminated *Mycobacterium avium* complex infection in patients with advanced immunodeficiency syndrome. *N Engl J Med* 1996;335:384–391.
30. Benson CA, Williams PL, Cohn DL, et al. Clarithromycin or rifabutin alone or in combination for primary prophylaxis of *Mycobacterium avium* complex disease in patients with AIDS: a randomized, double-blind, placebo-controlled trial. *J Infect Dis* 2000;181:1289–1297.
31. Tseng AL, Walmsley SL. Rifabutin-associated uveitis. *Ann Pharmacother* 1995;29:1149–1155. Search date 1994; primary sources Medline and hand searches of reference lists and conference abstracts.
32. Dube MP, Sattler FR, Torriani FJ, et al. A randomized evaluation of ethambutol for prevention of relapse and drug resistance during treatment of *Mycobacterium avium* complex bacteremia with clarithromycin-based combination therapy. *J Infect Dis* 1997;176:1225–1232.
33. Chaisson RE, Keiser P, Pierce M, et al. Clarithromycin and ethambutol with or without clofazimine for the treatment of bacteremic *Mycobacterium avium* complex disease in patients with HIV infection. *AIDS* 1997;11:311–317.
34. May T, Brel F, Beuscart C, et al. Comparison of combination therapy regimens for the treatment of human immunodeficiency virus-infected patients with disseminated bacteremia due to *Mycobacterium avium*. ANRS Trial 033 Curavium Group. Agence Nationale de Reserche sur le Sida. *Clin Infect Dis* 1997;25:621–629.
35. Gordin F, Sullam P, Shafran S, et al. A placebo-controlled trial of rifabutin added to a regimen of clarithromycin and ethambutol in the treatment of *M. avium* complex bacteremia. *Clin Infect Dis* 1999;28:1080–1085.
36. Cohn DL, Fisher EJ, Peng GT, et al. A prospective randomized trial of four three-drug regimens in the treatment of disseminated *Mycobacterium avium* complex disease in AIDS patients: excess mortality associated with high-dose clarithromycin. Terry Beirn Programs for Clinical Research on AIDS. *Clin Infect Dis* 1999;29:125–133.
37. Chaisson RE, Benson CA, Dube MP, et al. Clarithromycin therapy for bacteremic *Mycobacterium avium* complex disease: a randomized, double-blind, dose-ranging study in patients with AIDS. *Ann Intern Med* 1994;121:905–911.
38. Spector SA, McKinley GF, Lalezari JP, et al. Oral ganciclovir for the prevention of cytomegalovirus disease in persons with AIDS. Roche Cooperative Oral Ganciclovir Study Group. *N Engl J Med* 1996;334:1491–1497.
39. Brosgart CL, Louis TA, Hillman DW, et al. A randomized, placebo-controlled trial of the safety and efficacy of oral ganciclovir for prophylaxis of cytomegalovirus disease in HIV-infected individuals. Terry Beirn Community Programs for Clinical Research on AIDS. *AIDS* 1998;12:269–277.
40. Ioannidis JPA, Collier AC, Cooper DA, et al. Clinical efficacy of high-dose acyclovir in patients with

human immunodeficiency virus infection: a meta-analysis of randomized individual patient data. *J Infect Dis* 1998;178:349–359. Search date not stated; primary sources Medline, abstract searching from major meetings, trial directories, and communication with experts, investigators of the identified trials, and industry researchers.

41. Feinberg JE, Hurwitz S, Cooper D, et al. A randomized, double-blind trial of valaciclovir prophylaxis for cytomegalovirus disease in patients with advanced human immunodeficiency virus infection. AIDS Clinical Trials Group Protocol 204/Glaxo Wellcome 123–014 International CMV Prophylaxis Study Group. *J Infect Dis* 1998;177:48–56.
42. Schacker T, Hu HL, Koelle DM, et al. Famciclovir for the suppression of symptomatic and asymptomatic herpes simpiex virus reactivation in HIV-infected persons: a double-blind, placebo-controlled trial. *Ann Intern Med* 1998;128:21–28.
43. Schuman P, Capps L, Peng G, et al. Weekly fluconazole for the prevention of mucosal candidiasis in women with HIV infection: a randomized, double-blind, placebo-controlled trial. *Ann Intern Med* 1997;126:689–696.
44. McKinsey DS, Wheat LJ, Cloud GA, et al. Itraconazole prophylaxis for fungal infections in patients with advanced human immunodeficiency virus infection: randomized, placebo-controlled, double blind study. National Institute of Allergy and Infectious diseases Mycoses Study Group. *Clin Infect Dis* 1999;28:1049–1056.
45. Havlir DV, Dube MP, McCutchan JA, et al. Prophylaxis with weekly versus daily fluconazole for fungal infections in patients with AIDS. *Clin Infect Dis* 1998;27:253–256.
46. Powderly WG, Finkelstein DM, Feinberg J, et al. A randomized trial comparing fluconazole with clotrimazole troches for the prevention of fungal infections in patients with advanced human immunodeficiency virus infection. *N Engl J Med* 1995;332:700–705.
47. Tseng AL, Foisy MM. Management of drug interactions in patients with HIV. *Ann Pharmacother* 1997;31:1040–1058.
48. Supparatpinyo K, Perriens J, Nelson KE, Sirisanthana T. A controlled trial of itraconazole to prevent relapse of *Penicillium marneffei* infection in patients with the human immunodeficiency virus. *N Engl J Med* 1998;339:1739–1743.
49. Smith D, Midgley J, Gazzard B. A randomized, double blind study of itraconazole versus placebo in the treatment and prevention of oral or oesophageal candidosis in patients with HIV infection. *Int J Clin Pract* 1999;53:349–352.
50. Saag MS, Cloud GA, Graybill JR, et al. A comparison of itraconazole versus fluconazole as maintenance therapy for AIDS-associated cryptococcal meningitis. *Clin Infect Dis* 1999;28:291–296.
51. Wheat J, Hafner R, Wulfsohn M, et al. Prevention of relapse of histoplasmosis with itraconazole in patients with the acquired immunodeficiency syndrome. *Ann Intern Med* 1993;118:610–616.
52. Trikalinos TA, Ioannidis JPA. Discontinuation of *Pneumocystis carinii* prophylaxis in patients infected with human immunodeficiency virus: a meta-analysis and decision analysis. *Clin Infect dis* 2001;33:1901–1909. Search date 2001; Primary sources Medline, AIDSline, Embase, and abstracts from major meetings.
53. Lopez Bernaldo de Quiros JC, Miro JM, Pena JM, et al. A randomized trial of the discontinuation of primary and secondary prophylaxis against *Pneumocystis carinii* pneumonia after highly active antiretroviral therapy in patients with HIV infection. *N Engl J Med* 2001;344:159–167.
54. Mussini C, Pezzotti P, Govoni A, et al. Discontinuation of primary prophylaxis for *Pneumocystis carinii* pneumonia and toxoplasmic encephalitis in human immunodeficiency virus type I-infected patients: the changes in opportunistic prophylaxis study. *J Infect Dis* 2000;181:1635–1642.
55. Miro JM, Lopez JC, Podzamczer D, et al, and the GESIDA 04/98B study group. Discontinuation of toxoplasmic encephalitis prophylaxis is safe in HIV-1 and *T. gondii* co-infected patients after immunological recovery with HAART. Preliminary results of the GESIDA 04/98B study. In: Abstracts of the 7th Conference on Retroviruses and Opportunistic Infections, Alexandria, Virginia: Foundation for Retrovirology and Human Health. Abstract no. 230.
56. El-Sadr WM, Burman WJ, Grant LB, et al. Discontinuation of prophylaxis for *Mycobacterium avium* complex disease in HIV-infected patients who have a response to antiretroviral therapy. *N Engl J Med* 2000;342:1085–1092.
57. Currier JS, Williams PL, Koletar SL, et al. Discontinuation of Mycobacterium avium complex prophylaxis in patients with antiretroviral therapy-induced increases in CD4+ cell count. A randomized, double-blind, placebo-controlled trial. *Ann Intern Med* 2000;133:493–503.
58. Curi AL, Muralha A, Muralha L, Pavesio C. Suspension of anticytomegalovirus maintenance therapy following immune recovery due to highly active antiretroviral therapy. *Br J Ophthalmol* 2001;85:471–473.
59. Jouan M, Saves M, Tubiana R, et al. Discontinuation of maintenance therapy for cytomegalovirus in HIV-infected patients receiving highly active antiretroviral therapy. RESTIMOP study team. *AIDS* 2001;15:23–31.
60. Whitcup SM, Fortin E, Lindblad AS, et al. Discontinuation of anticytomegalovirus therapy in patients with HIV infection and cytomegalovirus retinitis. *JAMA* 1999;282:1633–1637.
61. Torriani FJ, Freeman WR, MacDonald JC, et al. CMV retinitis recurs after stopping treatment in virological and immunological failure of potent antiretroviral therapy. *AIDS* 2000;14:173–180.
62. Postelmans L, Gerald M, Sommereijns B, Caspers-Velu L. Discontinuation of maintenance therapy for CMV retinitis in AIDS patients on highly active antiretroviral therapy. *Ocul Immunol Inflamm* 1999;7:199–203.
63. Jabs DA, Bolton SG, Dunn JP, Palestine AG. Discontinuing anticytomegalovirus therapy in patients with immune reconstitution after combination therapy. *Am J Opthalmol* 1998;126:817–822.
64. Vrabec TR, Baldassano VF, Whitcup SM. Discontinuation of maintenance therapy in patients with quiescent cytomegalovirus retinitis and elevated CD4+ counts. *Ophthalmology* 1998;105:1259–1264.
65. McDonald JC, Torriani FJ, Morse LS, Karavellas MP, Reed JB, Freeman WR. Lack of reactivation of cytomegalovirus (CMV) retinitis after stopping CMV maintenance therapy in AIDS patients with sustained elevations in CD4 T cells in response to highly active antiretroviral therapy. *J Infect Dis* 1998;177:1182–1187.
66. Tural C, Romeu J, Sirera G, et al. Long-lasting remission of cytomegalovirus retinitis without maintenance therapy in human immunodeficiency virus-infected patients. *J Infect Dis* 1998;177:1080–1083.

John Ioannidis
Chairman
Department of Hygiene and Epidemiology
University of Ioannina School of Medicine
Ioannina
Greece

David Wilkinson
Professor
South Australian Centre for Rural and Remote
Health University of Adelaide and University of South Australia
Whyalla
Australia

Competing interests: None declared.

TABLE 1 Observational studies of discontinuation of cytomegalovirus maintenance treatment in people with previous cytomegalovirus disease (see text, p 804).

Reference	Criteria for discontinuation	Participants	Follow up (months)	Relapses
Torriani*[61]	CD4 >70	17	14.5 (mean)	5
Postelmans[62]	CD4 ≥ 75	8	8 (median)	0
Whitcup[60]	CD4 >150	14	16.4 (mean)	0
Jabs[63]	CD4 297 < (median)	15	8 (median)	0
Vrabec[64]	CD4 >100	8	11.4 (mean)	0
McDonald*[65]	183 (median)	11	5 (median)	0
Tural[66]	CD4 >150, VL < 200/mL –ve CMV by PCR	7	9 (median)	0
Curi[58]	CD4 > 143	41	20.4 (mean)	0
Jouan[59]	CD4 > 75 VL < 30 000/mL	48	11 (mean)	2

Studies with more than five people are included. CD4 count is measured in cells/mm^3. *McDonald et al is an early report of the same study followed by the Torriani et al report. All relapses in the latter report occurred in people who had already experienced a decrease of CD4 to < 50 cells/mm^3.
CMV, cytomegalovirus; PCR, polymerase chain reaction; VL, viral load (HIV-1 RNA in plasma).

Postherpetic neuralgia

Search date January 2002

Tim Lancaster, David Wareham, and John Yaphe

QUESTIONS

INTERVENTIONS

Key Messages

Preventing postherpetic neuralgia

- **Amitriptyline** One small RCT found that amitriptyline versus placebo started within 48 hours of rash onset and continued for 90 days reduced the prevalence of postherpetic neuralgia at 6 months, but the difference did not quite reach significance.
- **Corticosteroids** Systematic reviews have found conflicting evidence about the effects of corticosteroids alone on postherpetic neuralgia. One RCT found limited evidence that high dose steroids added to antiviral agents may be of short term benefit in acute herpes zoster, but found no significant effect on pain at 6 months. There is concern that corticosteroids may cause dissemination of herpes zoster.
- **Oral antiviral agents (aciclovir, famciclovir, valaciclovir, netivudine)** Systematic reviews have found that daily aciclovir versus placebo reduces the prevalence of postherpetic pain at 6 months by about 50%. One RCT found that famciclovir versus placebo significantly reduced mean pain duration after acute herpes zoster. One systematic review of one RCT found that valaciclovir versus aciclovir significantly reduced the prevalence of postherpetic neuralgia at 6 months (NNT 16, 95% CI 9 to 100). One RCT found no significant difference in outcomes between netivudine and aciclovir. One RCT found no significant difference in postherpetic neuralgia after 7 days with valaciclovir versus famciclovir.

Postherpetic neuralgia

- **Topical antiviral agents (idoxuridine)** One systematic review has found that idoxuridine versus placebo or versus oral aciclovir increases short term pain relief in acute herpes zoster, but has found no significant difference in pain at 6 months.
- **Adenosine monophosphate, amantadine; cimetidine; inosine pranobex; levodopa** RCTs found insufficient evidence on the effects of these interventions.

Treating established postherpetic neuralgia

- **Dextromethorphan** One RCT found no significant difference with dextromethorphan versus placebo in pain at 6 weeks.
- **Epidural morphine** One small RCT found that epidural morphine versus placebo reduced pain by more than 50% but the reduction was not maintained beyond 36 hours. Epidural morphine caused intolerable opioid effects in 75% of people.
- **Gabapentin** One systematic review has found that gabapentin versus placebo significantly relieves pain after 8 weeks treatment (NNT 5, 95% CI 3 to 13). One additional RCT found similar results.
- **Oxycodone (oral opioid)** One crossover RCT found that oral oxycodone versus placebo significantly reduced pain after 4–8 weeks, but was associated with more adverse effects.
- **Topical anaesthesia** One small RCT found that lidocaine patches versus placebo increased pain relief over 12 hours.
- **Topical counterirritants** One systematic found limited evidence that capsaicin versus placebo significantly improved pain relief, but also caused painful skin reactions.
- **Tricyclic antidepressants** One systematic review has found that tricyclic antidepressants (amitryptyline or desipramine) versus placebo significantly increase pain relief at 6 weeks.

DEFINITION Postherpetic neuralgia is pain that sometimes follows resolution of acute herpes zoster and healing of the zoster rash. It can be severe, accompanied by itching, and follows the distribution of the original infection. Herpes zoster is an acute infection caused by activation of latent varicella zoster virus (human herpes virus 3) in people who have been rendered partially immune by a previous attack of chickenpox. Herpes zoster infects the sensory ganglia and their areas of innervation. It is characterised by pain along the distribution of the affected nerve, and crops of clustered vesicles over the area.

INCIDENCE/ PREVALENCE In a UK general practice survey of 321 cases, the annual incidence of herpes zoster was 3.4/1000.[1] Incidence varied with age. Herpes zoster was relatively uncommon in people under the age of 50 years (< 2/1000 a year), but rose to 5–7/1000 a year in people aged 50–79 years, and 11/1000 in people aged 80 years or older. In a population based study of 590 cases in Rochester, Minnesota, USA, the overall incidence was lower (1.5/1000) but with similar increases in incidence with age.[2] Prevalence of postherpetic neuralgia depends on when it is measured after acute infection, and there is no agreed time point.

AETIOLOGY/ RISK FACTORS The main risk factor for postherpetic neuralgia is increasing age. In a UK general practice study (involving 3600–3800 people, 321 cases of acute herpes zoster) there was little risk in those under the age of 50 years, but postherpetic neuralgia developed in over 20% of people who had had acute herpes zoster aged 60–65 years and in 34% aged over 80 years.[1] No other risk factor has been found to predict consistently which people with herpes zoster will experience continued pain. In a general practice study in Iceland (421 people followed for up to 7 years after an initial episode of herpes zoster), the risk of postherpetic neuralgia was 1.8% (95% CI 0.6% to 4.2%) for people under 60 years of age and the pain was mild in all cases.[27] The risk of severe pain after 3 months in people aged over 60 years was 1.7% (95% CI 0% to 6.2%).

PROGNOSIS About 2% of people with acute herpes zoster in the UK general practice survey had pain for more than 5 years.[1] Prevalence of pain falls as time elapses after the initial episode. Among 183 people aged over 60 years in the placebo arm of a UK trial, the prevalence of pain was 61% at 1 month, 24% at 3 months, and 13% at 6 months after acute infection.[3] In a more recent RCT, the prevalence of postherpetic pain in the placebo arm at 6 months was 35% in 72 people over 60 years of age.[4]

AIMS To prevent or reduce postherpetic neuralgia by intervention during acute attack; to reduce the severity and duration of established postherpetic neuralgia, with minimal adverse effects of treatment.

OUTCOMES Prevalence of persistent pain 6 months after resolution of acute infection and healing of rash. We did not consider short term outcomes such as rash healing or pain reduction during the acute episode. It is difficult to assess the clinical significance of reported changes in "average pain"; therefore, we present data as dichotomous outcomes where possible (pain absent or greatly reduced, or pain persistent).

METHODS Our initial search was part of two systematic reviews of treatments for acute herpes zoster and postherpetic neuralgia on the basis of comprehensive searches of published and unpublished studies to 1993.[5,6] The details of the searches are described in the published reports. This search was updated by a *Clinical Evidence* search and appraisal in January 2002. Where meta-analyses from systematic reviews were available, they were taken to be the most reliable estimates of treatment effectiveness. In trials, the most common time point chosen for assessing the prevalence of persistent pain was 6 months, which we use in this review unless otherwise specified.

QUESTION **What are the effects of interventions during an acute attack of herpes zoster aimed at preventing postherpetic neuralgia?**

OPTION **ORAL ANTIVIRAL AGENTS (ACICLOVIR, FAMCICLOVIR, VALACICLOVIR, NETIVUDINE)**

Systematic reviews have found that daily aciclovir versus placebo reduces the prevalence of postherpetic pain at 6 months by about 50%. One systematic review has found that famciclovir versus placebo significantly reduces mean pain duration after acute herpes zoster. One

systematic review has found that valaciclovir versus aciclovir significantly reduces the prevalence of postherpetic neuralgia at 6 months. One RCT found no significant difference in effectiveness between netivudine and aciclovir. Another RCT found no significant difference between valaciclovir and famciclovir in the resolution of postherpetic neuralgia or in adverse effects over 7 days.

Benefits: **Aciclovir versus placebo:** We found three systematic reviews.[5,7,8] The most recent review (search date 1998) reported the results of older reviews.[7] The oldest review (search date 1993) pooled estimates from eight placebo controlled RCTs of aciclovir in both inpatient and general practice settings (932 people).[5] It found no significant pain reduction from aciclovir at 6 months (OR 0.70, 95% CI 0.47 to 1.06). The second systematic review (search date 1996) identified five placebo controlled RCTs (792 people) of oral aciclovir, including one not published at the time of the earlier systematic review.[8] It found that taking a minimum of 4 g aciclovir daily for at least 7 days significantly reduced the prevalence of postherpetic neuralgia at 6 months (OR for presence of pain 0.54, 95% CI 0.36 to 0.81; ARR 0.16; NNT 7; no CI available). **Famciclovir versus placebo:** We found one systematic review (search date 1998, 1 RCT, 419 people).[7] The multicentre RCT in the review compared two different doses of famciclovir in immunocompetent adults (age > 18 years) and defined duration of postherpetic neuralgia as time to pain resolution. It found that both doses of famciclovir versus placebo significantly reduced the duration of pain after acute herpes zoster (median duration of pain with 500 mg [138 people] 63 days, with 750 mg [135 people] 61 days, with placebo [146 people] 119 days; no CI available). **Aciclovir versus other antivirals:** We found one systematic review (search date 1998, 1 RCT, 1141 people).[7] The RCT in the review compared valaciclovir (a precursor of aciclovir) given three times daily for 7 or 14 days versus 7 days of aciclovir. When the results from the two valaciclovir regimens were combined, those treated with valaciclovir had a lower prevalence of pain at 6 months (AR 19.3% *v* 25.3%; RR 0.92; NNT 16, 95% CI 9 to 100). We found one double blind RCT of netivudine versus aciclovir (511 people), which found no significant difference in effectiveness between the two.[9] **Addition of amitriptyline:** We found no systematic review or RCTs. **Valaciclovir versus famciclovir:** We found no systematic review. One RCT (597 immunocompetent people aged ≥50 years) compared valaciclovir (1 g 3 times daily) versus famciclovir (500 mg 3 times daily) given within 72 hours of appearance of the rash for 7 days.[10] It found no significant difference in postherpetic neuralgia (HR 1.01, 95% CI 0.82 to 1.24).

Harms: The reviews found that the most common adverse events reported with aciclovir were headache and nausea. In placebo controlled trials, these effects occurred with similar frequency with treatment and placebo (headache 37% *v* 43%, nausea 13% *v* 14%). There were no major adverse events reported in the RCTs included in the systematic review.[5] In the RCTs, famciclovir, valaciclovir, and netivudine had similar safety profiles to aciclovir.[9,11,12] In the RCT comparing valaciclovir versus famciclovir the two drugs had similar safety profiles.[10]

Comment: We found no evidence on adherence, but it has been suggested that adherence to treatment may be better with the newer antiviral drugs because they are given one to three times daily compared with five times daily for aciclovir.

OPTION TOPICAL ANTIVIRAL AGENTS (IDOXURIDINE)

One systematic review has found that idoxuridine versus placebo or versus oral aciclovir increases short term pain relief in acute herpes zoster, but found no significant difference at 6 months.

Benefits: We found one systematic review (search date 1993, 4 RCTs, 431 people).[5] **Versus placebo:** Three RCTs (242 people) compared topical idoxuridine versus placebo. Pooled results were not reported because of heterogeneity and poor quality of the trials. Two of the RCTs found that treatment during an acute attack significantly increased pain relief at 1 month, but none of the three RCTs found any significant difference at 6 months. **Versus aciclovir:** One RCT found that topical idoxuridine versus oral aciclovir significantly increased pain relief at 1 month (OR 0.41, 95% CI 0.15 to 1.11), but found no significant difference in prevalence of pain at 6 months (RR 0.38, 95% CI 0.13 to 1.00).[13]

Harms: We found no reports of significant adverse effects from idoxuridine. Application beneath dressings may be cumbersome.

Comment: None.

OPTION CORTICOSTEROIDS

Systematic reviews have found conflicting evidence from RCTs about the effects of corticosteroids alone on postherpetic neuralgia. One RCT found limited evidence that high dose steroids added to antiviral agents may be of short term benefit in acute herpes zoster, but found no significant effect on pain at 6 months.

Benefits: **Corticosteroids alone:** We found two systematic reviews (search dates 1993 and 1998).[5,7] The earlier review (search date 1993) included RCTs of corticosteroids with conflicting results and concluded that it was not possible to assess the effect of corticosteroids.[5] The more recent review (search date 1998) identified one RCT (201 people) subsequent to the earlier review.[7] The RCT found no significant differences in pain at 3 or 6 months. **Corticosteroids plus aciclovir:** We found one systematic review (search date 1998, 2 RCTs, 608 people). The first RCT (400 people) randomised people into four active treatment groups: 7 days of aciclovir (101 people); 7 days of aciclovir plus 21 days of prednisolone (99 people); 21 days of aciclovir (101 people); or 21 days of aciclovir plus prednisolone (99 people).[14] It found no significant differences in relief of postherpetic neuralgia. The second RCT (208 people) had a factorial design, randomising people to 21 days of aciclovir plus prednisone (60 mg initially, tapered over 3 wks), prednisone plus placebo, aciclovir plus placebo, or two placebos. Although there was evidence of short term benefit from prednisone, there was no significant effect on pain prevalence at 6 months after disease onset.[15]

Harms: It is feared that corticosteroids might cause dissemination of herpes zoster. This effect was not reported in an RCT of prednisolone in the earlier systematic review.[5] In the RCT of aciclovir plus prednisone, two people receiving prednisone plus aciclovir placebo and one receiving aciclovir plus prednisone placebo developed cutaneous dissemination of lesions (see harms of corticosteroids under rheumatoid arthritis, p 1250).[15]

Comment: None.

OPTION TRICYCLIC ANTIDEPRESSANTS (AMITRIPTYLINE)

One small RCT found that amitriptyline versus placebo started within 48 hours of rash onset and continued for 90 days reduced the prevalence of postherpetic neuralgia at 6 months, but the difference did not quite reach significance.

Benefits: We found one systematic review (search date 1998, 1 RCT, 90 people).[7] The RCT in the review (72 people aged > 60 years)[4] found that amitriptyline 25 mg taken within 48 hours of rash onset and continued for 90 days versus placebo reduced the prevalence of postherpetic neuralgia at 6 months, but the result did not reach significance (AR 16% *v* AR 35%; RR 0.45; ARR +0.19, 95% CI –0.003 to +0.39).

Harms: The RCT did not report adverse effects.[4] In another RCT, amitriptyline was associated with adverse anticholinergic effects such as dry mouth, sedation, and urinary difficulties.[5]

Comment: Interpretation of the RCT is complicated because practitioners were allowed to decide whether an antiviral agent was prescribed as well as amitriptyline.[4] Blinding may also have been inadequate.

OPTION OTHER DRUG TREATMENTS

RCTs found insufficient evidence on the effects of other drug treatments in acute herpes zoster.

Benefits: We found one systematic review (search date 1993), which identified small, single RCTs of adenosine monophosphate, amantadine, and levodopa.[5] The RCTs found some short term benefit in treating herpes zoster. No benefit was found in small studies of cimetidine and inosine pranobex.[5]

Harms: We found no evidence.

Comment: None.

QUESTION What are the effects of interventions after the rash has healed to relieve established postherpetic neuralgia?

OPTION TRICYCLIC ANTIDEPRESSANTS

One systematic review has found that tricyclic antidepressants versus placebo significantly increase pain relief in postherpetic neuralgia. One additional RCT found no significant difference between fluphenazine plus amitriptyline versus amitriptyline alone in pain scores.

Benefits: We found one systematic review (search date 1993, 3 RCTs, 216 people)[6] and one additional RCT.[16] Two RCTs in the review compared amitriptyline versus placebo; the other RCT compared desipramine versus placebo. The review found that tricyclic antidepressants versus placebo taken for 3–6 weeks significantly improved pain relief from postherpetic neuralgia at the end of the treatment period (OR for complete or large reduction in pain at end of treatment period 0.15, 95% CI 0.08 to 0.27). The additional RCT (49 people) compared four groups: amitriptyline plus fluphenazine, amitriptyline alone, fluphenazine alone, and placebo.[16] It found that no significant difference between amitriptyline plus fluphenazine versus amitriptyline alone in pain scores. The trial may have lacked power to detect clinically important differences.

Harms: Tricyclic antidepressants are associated with anticholinergic adverse effects. In one RCT, amitriptyline versus placebo was associated with more adverse effects: dry mouth (AR 62% *v* 40%), sedation (AR 62% *v* 40%), and urinary difficulties (AR 12% *v* < 5%).[17] Syncope and heart block occurred in one person in a trial of desipramine in people with postherpetic neuralgia.[18] The additional RCT found that sleepiness was more common in people taking fluphenazine than those taking amitriptyline or placebo ($P < 0.05$).[16]

Comment: The adverse effects of tricyclic antidepressants are dose related; therefore, they may be less pronounced when used to treat postherpetic neuralgia, because lower doses are used compared with treating depression.

OPTION TOPICAL COUNTERIRRITANTS

One systematic review found limited evidence that the topical counterirritant, capsaicin, versus placebo significantly improved pain relief in postherpetic neuralgia, but also caused painful skin reactions.

Benefits: We found one systematic review (search date 1993, 2 placebo controlled RCTs, 205 people), which found that capsaicin versus placebo significantly improved pain relief (total 205 people; OR for complete or greatly reduced pain 0.29, 95% CI 0.16 to 0.54).[5]

Harms: Reported local skin reactions included burning, stinging, and erythema. These effects tended to subside with time and frequency of use.[19]

Comment: The difficulty in blinding studies with capsaicin because of skin burning may have caused over estimation of benefit.

OPTION TOPICAL ANAESTHESIA

One small RCT found that lidocaine patches versus placebo increased short term pain relief in postherpetic neuralgia.

Benefits: We found no systematic review. We found one small, placebo controlled RCT of lidocaine (lignocaine) patches (35 people).[20] Active patches reduced average pain scores on a visual analogue scale over 12 hours.

Harms: No systemic adverse effects were noted with lidocaine patches, and systemic absorption as determined by blood concentrations was minimal.[20]

Comment: None.

OPTION GABAPENTIN

One systematic review and one additional RCT have found that gabapentin versus placebo relieves pain in postherpetic neuralgia.

Benefits: We found one systematic review (search date 1999, 1 multicentre RCT, 229 people)[21] and one additional RCT.[22] The RCT in the review compared the anticonvulsant drug gabapentin versus placebo in people who remained on tricyclic antidepressants or opiates during the trial.[23] It found that gabapentin significantly reduced the number of people reporting pain after 8 weeks of treatment (for pain much or moderately reduced; RR 0.73; ARR 20%; NNT 5, 95% CI 3 to 13). The additional RCT (multicentre, 334 people) found that gabapentin (1800 mg or 2400 mg daily in 3 divided doses) versus placebo significantly reduced mean daily pain scores (pain reduction with gabapentin 1800 mg *v* placebo, 18.8%, 95% CI 10.9% to 26.8%; pain reduction with gabapentin 2400 mg *v* placebo, 18.7%, 95% CI 10.7% to 26.7%).[22]

Harms: The additional RCT found that gabapentin versus placebo increased somnolence, dizziness, ataxia, and peripheral oedema.[23] However, withdrawal rates were not significantly different.

Comment: None.

OPTION NARCOTIC ANALGESICS

One small crossover RCT found oral oxycodone versus placebo reduced pain from postherpetic neuralgia but was associated with more adverse effects. One small placebo controlled RCT found that epidural morphine was poorly tolerated and of little benefit. One RCT of the non-opioid dextromethorphan versus placebo found no evidence of benefit.

Benefits: We found no systematic review, but found three RCTs.[24–26] The first, a crossover RCT of oxycodone (50 people, 4 wks on each treatment) versus placebo found that oxycodone significantly improved pain on a visual analogue scale, but the data could not be converted into a dichotomous outcome. However, it found that 67% of people had a masked preference for oxycodone versus 11% for placebo.[24] The second, small, single blind, placebo controlled RCT found that epidural morphine versus placebo led to pain reduction of more than 50% in 2/11 (18%) people, but this could not be sustained beyond 36 hours.[25] A third, small, double blind, crossover RCT (18 people) found no evidence of pain relief from 6 weeks' treatment with dextromethorphan (a codeine analogue) versus placebo.[26]

Harms: The first RCT reported that oxycodone produced adverse effects such as constipation, nausea, and sedation with greater frequency than placebo (76% *v* 49%; RR 1.4, 95% CI 0.5 to 3.4).[24] Epidural morphine produced intolerable opioid effects in 6/8 (75%) people treated.[25] High dose dextromethorphan produced sedation and ataxia, causing 5/18 (28%) people to stop treatment.[26]

Comment: None.

REFERENCES

1. Hope-Simpson RE. Postherpetic neuralgia. *J R Coll Gen Pract* 1975;25:571–575.
2. Helgason S, Petursson G, Gudmundsson S, et al. Prevalence of postherpetic neuralgia after a first episode of herpes zoster prospective study with long term follow up. *BMJ* 2000;321:794–796.
3. Mckendrick MW, McGill JI, Wood MJ. Lack of effect of aciclovir on postherpetic neuralgia. *BMJ* 1989;298:431.
4. Bowsher D. The effects of pre-emptive treatment of postherpetic neuralgia with amitriptyline: a randomised, double-blind, placebo-controlled trial. *J Pain Symptom Manage* 1997;13:327–331.
5. Lancaster T, Silagy C, Gray S. Primary care management of acute herpes zoster: systematic review of evidence from randomised controlled trials. *Br J Gen Pract* 1995;45:39–45. Search date 1993; primary sources Medline, hand searched primary care journals, references from books, specialists, and makers of drugs in identified trials for published and unpublished data.
6. Volmink J, Lancaster T, Gray S, et al. Treatments for postherpetic neuralgia–a systematic review of randomised controlled trials. *Fam Pract* 1996;13:84–91. Search date 1993; primary sources Medline and Embase.
7. Alper BS, Lewis R. Does treatment of acute herpes zoster prevent or shorten postherpetic neuralgia? A systematic review of the literature. *J Fam Pract* 2000;49:255–264. Search date 1998; primary sources Medline, Cochrane Controlled Trials Register, hand searched reference lists, and web based searches.
8. Jackson JL, Gibbons R, Meyer G, et al. The effect of treating herpes zoster with oral aciclovir in preventing postherpetic neuralgia. A meta-analysis. *Arch Intern Med* 1997;157:909–912. Search date 1996; primary sources Medline, National Institute of Health database of funded studies, and Cochrane Controlled Trials Register.
9. Soltz-Szots J, Tyring S, Andersen PL, et al. A randomised controlled trial of aciclovir versus netivudine for treatment of herpes zoster. International zoster study group. *J Antimicrob Chemother* 1998;41:549–556.
10. Tyring SK, Beutner KR, Tucker BA, Anderson WC, Crooks RJ. Antiviral therapy for herpes zoster: Randomised, controlled clinical trial of valaciclovir and famciclovir therapy in immunocompetent patients aged 50 years and older. *Arch Fam Med* 2000;9:863–869.
11. Tyring S, Barbarash RA, Nahlik JE, et al. Famciclovir for the treatment of acute herpes zoster: effects on acute disease and postherpetic neuralgia. A randomised, double-blind, placebo-controlled trial. Collaborative famciclovir herpes zoster study group. *Ann Intern Med* 1995;123:89–96.
12. Beutner KR, Friedman DJ, Forszpaniak C, et al. Valaciclovir compared with aciclovir for improved therapy for herpes zoster in immunocompetent adults. *Antimicrob Agents Chemother* 1995;39:1546–1553.
13. Aliaga A, Armijo M, Camacho F, et al. A topical solution of 40% idoxuridine in dimethyl sulfoxide compared to oral aciclovir in the treatment of herpes zoster. A double-blind multicenter clinical trial [in Spanish]. *Med Clin (Barc)* 1992;98:245–249.
14. Wood MJ, Johnson RW, McKendrick MW, et al. A randomised trial of aciclovir for 7 days or 21 days with and without prednisolone for treatment of acute herpes zoster. *N Engl J Med* 1994;330:896–900.
15. Whitley RJ, Weiss H, Gnann JW Jr, et al. Aciclovir with and without prednisone for the treatment of herpes zoster. A randomized, placebo-controlled trial. The National Institute of Allergy and Infectious Diseases Collaborative Antiviral Study Group. *Ann Intern Med* 1996;125:376–383.
16. Graff-Radford S, Shaw LR, Naliboff BN. Amitriptyline and fluphenazine in the treatment of postherpetic neuralgia. *Clin J Pain* 2000;16:188–192.
17. Max MB, Schafer SC, Culnane M, et al. Amitriptyline, but not lorazepam, relieves postherpetic neuralgia. *Neurology* 1988;38:1427–1432.
18. Kishore-Kumar R, Max MB, Schafer SC, et al. Desipramine relieves postherpetic neuralgia. *Clin Pharmacol Ther* 1990;47:305–312.
19. Bernstein JE, Korman NJ, Bickers DR, et al. Topical capsaicin treatment of chronic postherpetic neuralgia. *J Am Acad Dermatol* 1989;21:265–270.

20. Rowbotham MC, Davies PS, Verkempinck C, et al. Lidocaine patch: double-blind controlled study of a new treatment method for postherpetic neuralgia. *Pain* 1996;65:39–44.
21. Collins SL, Moore RA, McQuay HJ, Wiffen P. Antidepressants and anticonvulsants for diabetic neuropathy and postherpetic neuralgia: a quantitative systematic review. *J Pain Symptom Manage* 2000;20:449–458. Search date 1999; primary sources Medline, Embase, the Cochrane Library, Oxford Pain Relief Database, and hand searches of reviews and reference lists.
22. Rice ASC, Maton S, Baronowski AP. Gabapentin in postherpetic neuralgia: A randomized, double blind, placebo controlled study. *Pain* 2001;94:215–224.
23. Rowbotham M, Harden N, Stacey B, et al. Gabapentin for the treatment of postherpetic neuralgia: a randomised controlled trial. *JAMA* 1998;280:1837–1842.
24. Watson CP, Babul N. Efficacy of oxycodone in neuropathic pain: a randomised trial in postherpetic neuralgia. *Neurology* 1998;50:1837–1841.
25. Watt JW, Wiles JR, Bowsher DR. Epidural morphine for postherpetic neuralgia. *Anaesthesia* 1996;51:647–651.
26. Nelson KA, Park KM, Robinovitz E, et al. High-dose oral dextromethorphan versus placebo in painful diabetic neuropathy and postherpetic neuralgia. *Neurology* 1997;48:1212–1218.
27. Helgason S, Petursson G, Gudmundsson S, et al. Prevalence of postherpetic neuralgia after a first episode of herpes zoster: prospective study with long term follow up. *BMJ* 2000;321:794.

Tim Lancaster
Reader in General Practice
Department of Primary Health Care
University of Oxford
Oxford
UK

David Wareham
Clinical Training Fellow & Honorary SpR in Medical Microbiology
Queen Mary University of London & Barts & The London NHS Trust
London
UK

John Yaphe
Department of Family Medicine
Rabin Medical Centre
Petach Tikvah
Israel

Competing interests: None declared.

Tuberculosis

Search date April 2002

Paul Garner and Alison Holmes

QUESTIONS

INTERVENTIONS

To be covered in future updates

Preventing tuberculosis in people without HIV infection

Covered elsewhere in *Clinical Evidence*

See preventing tuberculosis under HIV infection, p 693

See glossary, p 827

Key Messages

Treating newly diagnosed tuberculosis

- **Chemotherapy for less than 6 months** One systematic review in people with newly diagnosed tuberculosis found limited evidence that reducing the duration of chemotherapy to less than 6 months significantly increased relapse rates.
- **Comparative benefits of different regimens in multidrug resistant tuberculosis** We found no RCTs in people with newly diagnosed tuberculosis comparing different drug regimens for multidrug resistant tuberculosis.

- **Intermittent short course chemotherapy (as good as daily treatment)** Limited evidence from two RCTs in people with newly diagnosed tuberculosis found no significant difference in cure rates with daily versus twice or three times weekly short course chemotherapy regimens.
- **Pyrazinamide** RCTs found that, in people with newly diagnosed tuberculosis, regimens containing pyrazinamide versus other regimens speed up sputum clearance in the first 2 months, but have found conflicting evidence about effects on relapse rates.
- **Regimens containing quinolones** We found insufficient evidence in people with newly diagnosed tuberculosis comparing regimens containing quinolones versus existing regimens.
- **Short course chemotherapy (as good as longer courses)** RCTs in people with newly diagnosed tuberculosis found no evidence of a difference in relapse rates with standard short course (6 months) versus longer term (8–9 months) chemotherapy.

Treating multidrug resistant tuberculosis

- We found no good evidence comparing different drug regimens for multidrug resistant tuberculosis.

Improving adherence and reattendance

- **Cash incentives** One systematic review has found that cash incentives versus usual care significantly improve attendance among people living in deprived circumstances. Two subsequent RCTs found conflicting results on the effect of cash incentives on treatment completion.
- **Community health advisors** One RCT found that health advisors recruited from the community versus usual care significantly increased attendance for treatment.
- **Defaulter actions** RCTs have found that intensive action (repeated home visits and reminder letters) versus routine action (single reminder letter and home visit) for defaulters significantly improves completion of treatment.
- **Directly observed treatment** One systematic review and one additional RCT found no significant difference between directly observed treatment versus self treatment in cure or treatment completion; therefore, a policy of directly observed treatment for all people with tuberculosis is unlikely to be beneficial.
- **Health education by a nurse** One RCT found that health education by a nurse versus an educational leaflet significantly improved treatment completion.
- **Prompts and contracts to improve reattendance for Mantoux test reading** One RCT in healthy people found that telephone prompts to return for Mantoux test reading versus no prompts slightly increased the number of people who reattended, but the difference was not significant. Another RCT in healthy people found that a verbal commitment versus no commitment significantly increased reattendance for Mantoux reading.
- **Health education by a doctor; prompts to adhere to treatment; sanctions for non-adherence; staff training** We found insufficient evidence on the effects of these interventions.

DEFINITION Tuberculosis is caused by *Mycobacterium tuberculosis* and can affect many organs. Specific symptoms relate to site of infection and are generally accompanied by fever, sweats, and weight loss.

INCIDENCE/ PREVALENCE	About a third of the world's population is infected with *M tuberculosis*. The organism kills more people than any other infectious agent. The World Health Organization estimates that 95% of cases are in developing countries, and that 25% of avoidable deaths in developing countries are caused by tuberculosis.[1]
AETIOLOGY/ RISK FACTORS	Social factors include poverty, overcrowding, homelessness, and inadequate health services. Medical factors include HIV and immunosuppression.
PROGNOSIS	Prognosis varies widely and depends on treatment.[2]
AIMS	To cure tuberculosis; eliminate risk of relapse; reduce infectivity; avoid emergence of drug resistance; and prevent death.
OUTCOMES	*M tuberculosis* in sputum (smear examination and culture), symptoms, weight, cure, relapse rates, attendance, completion of treatment.
METHODS	*Clinical Evidence* update search and appraisal April 2002. Key words: tuberculosis, pulmonary, isoniazid, pyrazinamide, and rifampicin. We included all Cochrane systematic reviews and studies that were randomised or used alternate allocation, and had at least 1 year follow up after completion of treatment.

QUESTION **What are the effects of different drug regimens in people with newly diagnosed pulmonary tuberculosis?**

OPTION **SHORT COURSE CHEMOTHERAPY (6 MONTHS)**

RCTs found no evidence of a difference in relapse rates between standard short course (6 months) and longer term (8–9 months) chemotherapy in people with pulmonary tuberculosis. RCTs suggest that treatment with pyrazinamide in the first 2 months speeds up sputum clearance, but the evidence relating to its effect on relapse rates is conflicting.

Benefits: We found no systematic review, but found four RCTs.[3–6] **Versus longer courses:** We found two RCTs (1295 people with untreated, culture/smear positive pulmonary tuberculosis), which compared 6 versus 8–9 months of chemotherapy.[3,4] Participants were followed up for at least 1 year after treatment was completed. The trials were performed in the UK and in East and Central Africa, and used different combinations of isoniazid, rifampicin, ethambutol, streptomycin, and pyrazinamide for initial (first 2 months) and continuation treatment. The RCTs found no significant difference in relapse rates between short course and longer regimens. **Different short course regimens:** The second RCT found no significant difference between regimens using ethambutol or streptomycin as the fourth drug in the initial phase.[4] A 6 month regimen using rifampicin and isoniazid throughout was highly effective (relapse rate 2%) and significantly better than isoniazid alone in the 4 month continuation phase (relapse rate 9%). When treatment with isoniazid alone was prolonged in a 6 month continuation phase, the relapse rate was not significantly better than with 4 months' continuation.[3] **Pyrazinamide:** The second RCT found that sputum conversion was faster with regimens containing pyrazinamide for the first 2 months, but there was no significant difference in relapse rates at 3 years' follow up.[4] The third RCT (833 people) compared four different 6 month regimens and found that bacterial relapse was higher for those not receiving pyrazinamide in the 12 months after chemotherapy (12/160 [7.5%] v 8/625 [1.3%]).[5] The fourth RCT (497 people) of ongoing pyrazinamide found that relapse at 18 months was more likely in those not receiving pyrazinamide, but the difference was not significant (3.1% with pyrazinamide v 1.0% with no pyrazinamide).[6]

Harms: In the largest RCT, possible adverse reactions were reported in 24/851 people (3%), with six requiring modification of treatment.[3] Two people in the trial developed jaundice, one of whom died. **Pyrazinamide:** Adding pyrazinamide did not increase the incidence of hepatitis (4% with pyrazinamide and 4% with no pyrazinamide).[4] However, mild adverse effects were more common, including arthralgia, skin rashes, flu-like symptoms, mild gastrointestinal disturbance, vestibular disturbance, peripheral neuropathy, and confusion. Arthralgia was the most common adverse effect, reported in about 1% of people on pyrazinamide, but was mild and never required modification of treatment.[3,4]

Comment: In people treated previously, the organisms may have acquired drug resistance so short course chemotherapy may not be effective.

OPTION INTERMITTENT SHORT COURSE CHEMOTHERAPY

Two RCTs found no significant difference in cure rates between daily versus twice or three times weekly short course regimens, but the limited data available did not exclude a clinically important difference.

Benefits: We found one systematic review (search date 2001, 1 RCT, 399 people)[7] and one subsequent RCT (206 children).[8] The review compared three times weekly versus daily chemotherapy for 6 months in people with newly diagnosed pulmonary tuberculosis. One month after treatment was completed there was no significant difference in bacteriological cure rates (defined as negative sputum culture, 99.9% with three times weekly v with daily 100.0%) or relapse (5/186 [2.7%] people with three times weekly v 1/192 [0.5%] people with daily; RR 4.0, 95% CI 0.7 to 24.1).[7] The subsequent RCT comparing twice weekly versus daily chemotherapy found no significant difference in cure rates (85/89 [95%] people with twice weekly v 114/117 [97%] people with daily; RR 0.98, 95% CI 0.84 to 1.02).[8] At least 12 cohort studies have found cure rates of 80–100% with three times weekly regimens taken over 6–9 months.[7]

Harms: Intermittent treatment has the potential to contribute to drug resistance, but this was not shown in the studies.[7]

Comment: The RCTs had low event rates and were too small to exclude a clinically significant difference between the dosing regimens.

OPTION CHEMOTHERAPY FOR LESS THAN 6 MONTHS

One systematic review found limited evidence suggesting that reducing duration of treatment to less than 6 months significantly increased relapse rates.

Benefits: We found one systematic review (search date 1999, 7 RCTs, 2248 outpatients with newly diagnosed pulmonary tuberculosis), which compared a variety of shorter (minimum 2 months) and longer (maximum 12 months) drug regimens.[9] The trials included people in India, Hong Kong, Singapore, and Germany. The review found that a 3 month versus a 12 month regimen significantly increased relapse rates (5 RCTs: RR 3.03, 95% CI 2.08 to 4.40). One of the RCTs found that people given a 2 month regimen were significantly less likely to change or discontinue drugs than those given a 12 month regimen (6/299 [2.0%] *v* 17/299 [5.7%]; RR 0.35; 95% CI 0.14 to 0.88).[9]

Harms: The review found similar rates of adverse events or toxicity with both shorter and longer regimens.

Comment: The treatments were given under optimal conditions. In clinical practice adherence is likely to be lower, so relapse rates associated with the shorter regimens are likely to be higher than those in clinical trials.

OPTION REGIMENS CONTAINING QUINOLONES

We found insufficient evidence on regimens containing quinolones.

Benefits: We found no systematic review, but found two RCTs.[10,11] One RCT in Tanzania (200 people) comparing a regimen containing ciprofloxacin versus a regimen not containing a quinolone found that more people relapsed after the ciprofloxacin regimen, but the difference was not significant (RR of relapse at 6 months 16.0, 95% CI 0.9 to 278.0).[10] A relatively low dosage of ciprofloxacin was used (750 mg/day). The second RCT (160 people) compared a regimen containing ciprofloxacin versus a regimen without, and focused only on adverse effects (see harms below).[11]

Harms: Adverse effects, which were mild and responsive to symptomatic treatment, were similar in people taking quinolone regimens versus controls.[11]

Comment: Quinolones have good bactericidal activity *in vitro*. Some of the newer quinolones have enhanced antimycobacterial activity compared with ciprofloxacin.

QUESTION What are the effects of different drug regimens in people with multidrug resistant tuberculosis?

We found no RCTs comparing different drug regimens for multidrug resistant tuberculosis.

Benefits: We found no systematic review and no RCTs comparing different regimens in people with multidrug resistant tuberculosis.

Harms: We found no evidence.

Comment: Current clinical practice in multidrug resistant tuberculosis is to include at least three drugs to which the particular strain of tuberculosis is sensitive, using as many bactericidal agents as possible. People are observed directly and managed by a specialised clinician.

QUESTION **Which interventions improve adherence to treatment?**

OPTION **STAFF TRAINING**

We found insufficient evidence on the effects of staff training on adherence to treatment.

Benefits: We found one systematic review (search date 2000, 1 poorly randomised RCT; see comment below) comparing intensive staff supervision versus routine supervision at centres in Korea performing tuberculosis extension activities.[12] Centres were paired and randomised, and supervision was carried out by senior doctors. The review found that higher completion rates were achieved with intensive supervision (RR 1.2; CIs not estimated because of cluster design).

Harms: None reported.

Comment: The trial used cluster randomisation, but the unit of analysis was the individual.

OPTION **PROMPTS**

We found no RCTs about the effects of prompts on reattendance.

Benefits: We found one systematic review (search date 2000), which found no RCTs of prompts to return for treatment.[12]

Harms: None.

Comment: None.

OPTION **DEFAULTER ACTIONS**

One systematic review has found that intensive action for defaulter actions improves completion of treatment.

Benefits: We found one systematic review (search date 2000, 2 RCTs conducted in India).[12] The first RCT in the review found that up to four home visits to defaulters (see glossary, p 827) significantly improved completion of treatment compared with the routine policy of a reminder letter followed by one home visit (RR 1.32, 95% CI 1.02 to 1.71). The second RCT found that up to two reminder letters significantly improved completion of treatment (RR 1.21, 95% CI 1.05 to 1.39), even in people who were illiterate.

Harms: None reported.

Comment: None.

OPTION **CASH INCENTIVES**

One systematic review has found that cash incentives versus usual care improve attendance among people living in deprived circumstances. One subsequent RCT found that cash incentives improved treatment completion in intravenous drug users. Another subsequent RCT found no significant difference in treatment completion with immediate versus deferred cash incentives.

Benefits: **Versus no cash incentive:** We found one systematic review (search date 2000, 2 RCTs conducted in the USA)[12] and one subsequent RCT.[13] The first RCT in the review found that in homeless men, money ($5) versus usual care improved attendance at the first appointment (RR 1.6, 95% CI 1.3 to 2.0). The second RCT in the review (in migrants) found that combining cash ($10) with health education versus usual care improved attendance (RR 2.4, 95% CI 1.5 to 3.7).[12] The subsequent RCT (163 iv drug users) compared three groups: direct observation at a participant chosen site plus a $5 a visit incentive; direct observation at a designated site plus $5 a visit; and direct observation at a participant chosen site without a cash incentive. It found that both groups given cash incentives versus the group given no incentive were significantly more likely to complete treatment (28/53 [53%] with chosen site plus $5 *v* 2/55 [4%] with no cash incentive; OR 29.7, 95% CI 6.5 to 134.5; 33/55 [60%] with designated site plus $5 *v* 2/55 [4%] with no cash incentive; OR 39.7, 95% CI 8.7 to 134.5).[13] **Immediate versus deferred cash incentive:** We found one RCT (300 iv drug users), which compared three groups: treatment with direct observation by a nurse; treatment with self administration plus peer counselling and education; and routine care (see direct patient observation, p 826). Participants were further randomised to receive a $10 immediate versus deferred cash incentive.[14] The immediate payment was given at the end of each month when people completed a routine assessment for adherence and drug toxicity. The deferred payment was given either after the 6 months' treatment period or when the person withdrew from the study. The RCT found no difference between immediate versus deferred payments in treatment completion (125/150 [83%] *v* 112/150 [75%]; P = 0.09).[14]

Harms: The RCTs did not assess adverse effects.

Comment: None.

OPTION HEALTH EDUCATION

One RCT found that health education by a nurse improved treatment completion, with no evidence of benefit from health education by a doctor. One RCT in drug users found no significant effect of health education.

Benefits: We found one systematic review (search date 2000, 2 RCTs conducted in the USA).[12] The first RCT in the review compared three methods of health education versus an educational leaflet. Health education consisted of telephoning by a nurse, visiting by a nurse, or consultation by a clinic doctor. The trial found that treatment completion was significantly increased by the nurse telephone call versus the leaflet (75/80 [94%] *v* 55/77 [71%]; RR 1.30, 95% CI 1.18 to 1.37) and by the nurse visit versus the leaflet (75/79 [95%] *v* 55/77 [71%]; RR 1.33, 95% CI 1.20 to 1.38). However, consultation by the clinic doctor was not significantly better than the education leaflet (64/82 [78%] *v* 55/77 [71%]; RR 1.09, 95% CI 0.89 to 1.23). The second RCT in drug users found that 5–10 minutes of health education had no significant effect on whether people kept a scheduled appointment (RR 1.04, 95% CI 0.70 to 1.54).[12]

Harms: None measured.

Comment: Education is often part of a package of care that includes prompts and incentives, which makes it difficult to evaluate the independent effects of education.

OPTION SANCTIONS

We found no RCTs on the effect of sanctions.

Benefits: We found one systematic review (search date 2000), which identified no RCTs of sanctions.[12]

Harms: The use of sanctions may be ethically dubious.

Comment: In New York (USA), incarcerating people who did not comply with treatment was thought to increase compliance with the Department of Health's community tuberculosis treatment programme.[15]

OPTION COMMUNITY HEALTH ADVISORS

One RCT found that health advisors recruited from the community increased attendance for treatment.

Benefits: We found one systematic review (search date 2000, 1 RCT in homeless people).[12] It found that health advisors recruited from the community increased the number of people who kept their appointments (62/83 [75%] attended *v* 42/79 [53%]; RR 1.4, 95% CI 1.1 to 1.8).

Harms: None reported.

Comment: None.

OPTION DIRECT PATIENT OBSERVATION

One systematic review and one additional RCT found no significant difference between directly observed treatment versus self treatment in cure and completion rates.

Benefits: We found one systematic review (search date 2001, 4 RCTs, 1603 people)[16] and one additional RCT.[14] The review compared direct observation of people as they took their drugs (by a health professional, lay health worker, or family member) versus self administered treatment. Treatment for all studies was for 6 months, and cure was measured at the end of treatment (3 RCTs) or 1–2 months (1 RCT). The review found no significant difference between any directly observed treatment versus self treatment in cure (4 RCTs; RR 1.02, 95% CI 0.86 to 1.21) or cure plus treatment completion (4 RCTs; RR 1.06, 95% CI 1.00 to 1.13). When analysed by the person observing the treatment, there was no significant difference in cure and treatment completion between self treatment versus health professional, lay health worker, or family member. However, people given a choice of supervisor had significantly increased cure rates (1 RCT, 836 people; RR 1.13, 95% CI 1.04 to 1.24), and cure plus treatment completion (RR 1.11, 95% CI 1.03 to 1.18).[16] The additional RCT (300 iv drug users) compared three groups: treatment with direct observation by nurse, treatment with self administration plus peer counselling and education, and routine care. Participants were further randomised to receive a $10 immediate versus deferred cash incentive (see cash incentives, p 824).[14] It found no significant difference between observation or peer support versus self administration alone in treatment completion (observation *v* self administration alone, P = 0.86; peer support *v* self administration alone, P value not stated).[14]

Harms: Potential harms include reduced cooperation between patient and doctor, removal of individual responsibility, detriment to long term sustainability of antituberculosis programmes, and increased burden on health services to the detriment of care for other diseases. None of these has been adequately investigated.

Comment: Numerous observational studies have evaluated interventions described as directly observed treatment, but all were packages of interventions that included specific investment in antituberculosis programmes, such as strengthened drug supplies; improved microscopy services; and numerous incentives, sanctions, and other co-interventions that were likely to influence adherence.[17,18]

QUESTION Which interventions improve reattendance for Mantoux test reading?

OPTION PROMPTS AND CONTRACTS TO IMPROVE REATTENDANCE FOR MANTOUX TEST READING

Two RCTs found conflicting evidence on the effects of prompts and contracts on reattendance for Mantoux test reading.

Benefits: **Prompts:** We found one systematic review (search date 2000, 1 RCT, 701 healthy people).[12] The RCT compared an automatic telephone message prompt to return for Mantoux reading versus no prompt. It found that people were slightly more likely to return in the intervention group, but the difference was not significant (93% with intervention *v* 88% with no intervention; RR 1.05, 95% CI 1.00 to 1.10).[12] **Contracts:** We found no systematic review. One RCT in healthy students in the USA found that, compared with no commitment, reattendance for Mantoux reading was significantly improved by verbal commitments (RR 1.10, 95% CI 1.03 to 1.18) and by written commitments (RR 1.12, 95% CI 1.05 to 1.19).[19]

Harms: None reported.

Comment: None.

GLOSSARY

Defaulter actions Actions taken by health workers when people fail to attend for treatment of their tuberculosis.

Tuberculosis

Substantive changes

Directly observed treatment One new systematic review;[16] categorisation changed from "unknown effectiveness" to "unlikely to be beneficial".

REFERENCES

1. Global Tuberculosis Programme. *Treatment of tuberculosis*. Geneva: World Health Organization, 1997:WHO/TB/97.220.
2. Enarson D, Rouillon A. Epidemiological basis of tuberculosis control. In: Davis PD, ed. *Clinical tuberculosis*. 2nd ed. London: Chapman and Hall Medical, 1998.
3. East and Central African/British Medical Research Council Fifth Collaborative Study. Controlled clinical trial of 4 short-course regimens of chemotherapy (three 6-month and one 8-month) for pulmonary tuberculosis. *Tubercle* 1983;64:153–166.
4. British Thoracic Society. A controlled trial of 6 months chemotherapy in pulmonary tuberculosis, final report: results during the 36 months after the end of chemotherapy and beyond. *Br J Dis Chest* 1984;78:330–336.
5. Hong Kong Chest Service/British Medical Research Council. Controlled trial of four thrice weekly regimens and a daily regimen given for 6 months for pulmonary tuberculosis. *Lancet* 1981;1:171–174.
6. Farga V, Valenzuela P, Valenzuela MT, et al. Short-term chemotherapy of tuberculosis with 5-month regimens with and without pyrazinamide in the second phase (TA-82) [in Spanish]. *Rev Med Chil* 1986;114:701–705.
7. Mwandumba HC, Squire SB. Fully intermittent dosing with drugs for tuberculosis in adults. In: The Cochrane Library, Issue 1, 2002. Oxford: Update Software. Search date 2001; primary sources Cochrane Infectious Diseases Group Trials Register, Cochrane Controlled Trials Register, Medline, Embase, reference lists of article, and researchers contacted for unpublished trials.
8. Naude JMTW, Donald PR, Huseey GD, et al. Twice weekly vs. daily chemotherapy for childhood tuberculosis. *Pediatr Infect Dis* 2000;19:405–410.
9. Gelband H. Regimens of less than six months treatment for TB. In: The Cochrane Library, Issue 1, 2002. Oxford: Update Software. Search date 1999; primary sources Medline, Cochrane Parasitic Diseases Trials Register, contact with researchers, and hand searches of reference lists.
10. Kennedy N, Berger L, Curran J, et al. Randomized controlled trial of a drug regimen that includes ciprofloxacin for the treatment of pulmonary tuberculosis. *Clin Infect Dis* 1996;22:827–833.
11. Kennedy N, Fox R, Uiso L, et al. Safety profile of ciprofloxacin during long-term therapy for pulmonary tuberculosis. *J Antimicrob Chemother* 1993:32:897–902.
12. Volmink J, Garner P. Interventions for prompting adherence to tuberculosis treatment. In: The Cochrane Library, Issue 3, 2001. Oxford: Update Software. Search date 2000; primary sources Medline, Embase, Cochrane Controlled Trials Register 1998, Issue 3, Cochrane Collaboration Effective Professional Practice (CCEPP) Registry Trials, LILACS to 2000, hand searches of journals and reference lists, and contact with authors.
13. Malotte CK, Hollingshead JR, Larro M. Incentives vs. outreach workers for latent tuberculosis treatment in drug users. *Am J Prev Med* 2001;20:103–107.
14. Chaisson R, Barnes GL, Hackman JR, et al. A randomized, controlled trial of interventions to improve adherence to isoniazid therapy to prevent tuberculosis in injection drug users. *Am J Med* 2001;110:610–615.
15. Fujiwara PI, Larkin C, Frieden TR. Directly observed therapy in New York history, implementation, results and challenges. *Tuberculosis* 1997;18:135–148.
16. Volmink J, Garner P. Directly observed therapy for treating tuberculosis. In: The Cochrane Library, Issue 1, 2002. Oxford: Update Software. Search date 2001; primary sources, Cochrane Library, Medline, Embase, LILACS, hand searches of reference lists, and contact with experts in the field and relevant organisations.
17. Garner P. What makes DOT work? *Lancet* 1998;352:1326–1327.
18. Volmink J, Matchaba P, Garner P. Directly observed therapy and treatment adherence. *Lancet* 2000;355:1345–1350. Search date 1999; primary sources Medline, Embase, Cochrane Controlled Trials Register, and hand searches of reference lists.
19. Wurtele SK, Galanos AN, Roberts MC. Increasing return compliance in a tuberculosis detection drive. *J Behav Med* 1980;3:311–318.

Paul Garner
Professor
Liverpool School of Tropical Medicine
Liverpool
UK

Alison Holmes
Senior Lecturer
Hammersmith Hospital
Imperial College
London
UK

Competing interests: None declared.

Acute renal failure

Search date April 2002

John A Kellum, Martine Leblanc, and Ramesh Venkataraman

QUESTIONS

INTERVENTIONS

*We found insufficient evidence of effectiveness, but failure or delay in hydration results in harm.

See glossary, p 844

Key Messages

Acute renal failure prevention

- **Acetylcysteine** One small RCT found limited evidence that acetylcysteine versus placebo significantly reduced the incidence of acute renal failure induced by contrast media (NNT 6, 95% CI 3 to 21).
- **Calcium channel blockers for early allograft dysfunction** One large RCT found no significant difference with isradipine versus placebo in reducing graft dysfunction in renal transplantation. We found no RCTs of the effects of calcium channel blockers in other forms of acute renal failure.
- **Dopamine** One systematic review and one subsequent RCT have found that dopamine versus placebo does not prevent the onset of acute renal failure, the need for dialysis, or mortality.
- **Fluids** We found no RCTs of fluids versus no intervention to prevent acute renal failure. However, dehydration is an important risk factor for acute renal failure and recommended volumes of fluid have little potential for harm. One RCT found that hydration with 0.9% sodium chloride intravenous infusion versus 0.45% sodium chloride intravenous infusion significantly reduced the incidence of contrast media associated nephropathy.
- **Lipid formulations of amphotericin (better than standard formulations)** One RCT found limited evidence that lipid versus standard formulations of amphotericin may cause less nephrotoxicity. We found no evidence about the long term safety of lipid formulations of amphotericin.
- **Loop diuretics** One systematic review has found that loop diuretics versus fluids alone do not prevent acute renal failure. One RCT in people with acute tubular necrosis induced by contrast media found that diuretics versus 0.9% sodium chloride infusion significantly increased acute renal failure (NNH 4, 95% CI 2 to 17). Another RCT found that diuretics versus 0.9% sodium chloride infusion significantly increased acute renal failure after cardiac surgery (NNH 6, 95% CI 3 to 34).
- **Low osmolality contrast media (better than standard)** One systematic review comparing low osmolality contrast media versus standard contrast media has found that the development of acute renal failure or need for dialysis are rare events. However, nephrotoxicity (evaluated by serum creatinine) was less likely with low osmolality contrast media, especially in people with underlying renal impairments.
- **Mannitol** Small RCTs in people with traumatic rhabdomyolysis, or undergoing coronary artery bypass, vascular, or biliary tract surgery found that mannitol versus hydration alone did not reduce acute renal failure. One RCT found that mannitol versus 0.9% sodium chloride infusion increased the risk of acute renal failure, but the difference was not significant.
- **Natriuretic peptides** One large RCT found no significant difference with natriuretic peptides versus placebo in the prevention of acute renal failure induced by contrast media. Subgroup analysis in another RCT found that atrial natriuretic peptide versus placebo reduced dialysis free survival in non-oliguric people (NNH 8, 95% CI 4 to 36).
- **Single (better than multiple doses of aminoglycosides)** One RCT found that single daily dosing versus standard preparations and dosing of aminoglycosides significantly reduced nephrotoxicity (NNT 5, 95% CI 2 to 24).
- **Theophylline in acute renal failure induced by contrast media** RCTs found that theophylline versus placebo does not prevent acute renal failure induced by contrast media when people are adequately hydrated.

Acute renal failure in critically ill people

- **Biocompatible dialysis membranes (better than non-biocompatible membranes)** Limited evidence from RCTs suggests that biocompatible membranes versus non-biocompatible membranes reduce mortality.
- **Continuous versus intermittent renal replacement therapy** One systematic review of all prior randomised and observational studies comparing intermittent to continuous renal replacement therapies found no difference between therapies overall, but found a survival benefit with continuous renal replacement therapy when the analysis was restricted to the subgroup of studies that compared people with similar baseline severity of illness. Weaknesses in included studies preclude a definitive conclusion.
- **Dopamine** One systematic review found no significant difference in mortality, onset of acute renal failure or need for dialysis with dopamine versus control. One additional RCT found that low dose dopamine versus placebo did not reduce renal dysfunction. Dopamine has been associated with important adverse effects, including extravasation necrosis, gangrene, tachycardia, and conduction abnormalities.
- **Fenoldopam** We found no systematic review or RCTs about the effects of fenoldopam, but its use has been associated with hypotension.
- **High dose continuous replacement renal therapy (better than low dose)** One RCT found good evidence that high dose versus low dose continuous renal replacement therapy (haemofiltration) significantly reduces mortality (NNT 7, 95% CI 4 to 16). One RCT found evidence that high dose haemofiltration reduced mortality compared to low dose haemofiltration in continuous renal replacement therapy. A small prospective study found that intensive (daily) intermittent haemodialysis reduced mortality in people with acute renal failure when compared to conventional alternate-day haemodialysis.
- **Loop diurectics** RCTs in people with oliguric acute renal failure found no significant difference in renal recovery, number of days spent on dialysis, or mortality with loop diuretics versus placebo. Loop diuretics have been associated with toxicity and low renal perfusion.
- **Natriuretic peptides** RCTs have found no significant difference with atrial natriuretic peptide or ularitide (urodilantin) versus placebo in dialysis free survival in oliguric and non-oliguric people. One of the RCTs found that atrial natriuretic peptide may reduce survival in non-oliguric people.
- **Continuous versus bolus diuretics; combined diuretics and albumin** We found insufficient evidence on the effects of these interventions.

DEFINITION Acute renal failure (ARF) is characterised by abrupt and sustained decline in glomerular filtration rate (see glossary, p 845),[1] which leads to accumulation of urea and other chemicals in the blood. There is no clear consensus on a biochemical definition,[2] but most studies define it as a serum creatinine of 2–3 mg/dL (200–250 μmol/L), an elevation of more than 0.5 mg/dL (45 μmol/L) over a baseline creatinine below 2 mg/dL (170 μmol/L), or a twofold increase of baseline creatinine. "Severe" ARF has been defined as a serum concentration of creatinine above 5.5 mg/dL (500 μmol/L) or as requiring renal replacement therapy. ARF is usually classified according to the location of the predominant primary pathology (prerenal, intrarenal, and postrenal failure [see glossary, p 845]). People who are critically ill are those who are unstable and at imminent risk of death, which usually implies that they are people who need to be in, or have been admitted to, the intensive care unit (ICU).

INCIDENCE/ PREVALENCE Two prospective observational studies (2576 people) have found that established ARF affects nearly 5% of people in hospital and as many as 15% of critically ill people depending on the definitions used.[3,4]

AETIOLOGY/ RISK FACTORS **For acute renal failure prevention:** Risk factors for ARF that are consistent across multiple causes include hypovolaemia; hypotension; sepsis; pre-existing renal, hepatic, or cardiac dysfunction; diabetes mellitus; and exposure to nephrotoxins (e.g. aminoglycosides, amphotericin, immunosuppressive agents, non-steroidal anti-inflammatory drugs, angiotensin converting enzyme inhibitors, iv contrast media) (see table 1, p 848). Isolated episodes of ARF are rarely seen in critically ill people, but are usually part of multiple organ dysfunction syndromes (see glossary, p 845). ARF requiring dialysis is rarely seen in isolation (< 5% of people). The kidneys are often the first organs to fail.[10] In the perioperative setting, ARF risk factors include prolonged aortic clamping, emergency rather than elective surgery, and use of higher volumes (> 100 mL) of intravenous contrast media. One study (3695 people) using multiple logistic regression identified these independent risk factors: baseline creatinine clearance below 47 mL/minute (OR 1.20, 95% CI 1.12 to 1.30), diabetes (OR 5.5, 95% CI 1.4 to 21.0), and identified a marginal effect for doses of contrast media above 100 mL (OR 1.01, 95% CI 1.00 to 1.01). Mortality of people with ARF requiring dialysis was 36% during hospitalisation.[11] **For acute renal failure in critically ill people:** Prerenal ARF (see glossary, p 845) is caused by reduced blood flow to the kidney from renal artery disease, systematic hypotension, or maldistribution of blood flow. Intrarenal ARF (see glossary, p 845) is caused by parenchymal injury (acute tubular necrosis, interstitial nephritis, embolic disease, glomerulonephritis, vasculitis, or small vessel disease). Postrenal ARF is caused by urinary tract obstruction. Observational studies (in several hundred people from Europe, North America, and West Africa with ARF) found a prerenal cause in 40–80%, an intrarenal cause in 10–50%, and a postrenal cause in the remaining 10%.[12–17] Prerenal ARF is the commonest type of ARF in people who are critically ill,[12,18] but ARF in this context is usually part of multisystem failure, and most frequently because of acute tubular necrosis resulting from ischaemic or nephrotoxic injury, or both.[19,20]

PROGNOSIS One retrospective study (1347 people with ARF) found that mortality was less than 15% in people with isolated ARF.[21] One recent prospective study (> 700 people) found that in people with ARF, overall mortality and the need for dialysis was higher in an ICU than in a non-ICU setting, despite no significant difference between the groups in mean maximal serum creatinine (need for dialysis 71% in ICU *v* 18% in non-ICU; P < 0.001; mortality 72% in ICU *v* 32% in non-ICU; P = 0.001).[22]

AIMS **Prevention:** To preserve renal function. **Critically ill people:** To prevent death; to prevent complications of ARF (volume overload, acid–base disturbance, and electrolyte abnormalities); and to prevent the need for chronic dialysis, with minimum adverse effects.

OUTCOMES **Prevention:** Rates of ARF, nephrotoxicity (see glossary, p 845), or both. Surrogate outcomes were limited to measurements of biochemical evidence of organ function (serum creatinine or creatinine clearance) after the intervention. Surrogate markers such as urine output or renal blood flow were not considered as evidence of effectiveness. **Critically ill people:** Rate of death; rate of renal recovery; adverse effects of treatment. Extent of natriuresis is a proxy outcome.

METHODS *Clinical Evidence* update search and appraisal April 2002.

QUESTION What are the effects of interventions to prevent acute renal failure in people at high risk?

Ramesh Venkataraman, Martine Leblanc, and John A Kellum

OPTION FLUIDS

We found insufficient evidence on the effect of fluids in the prevention of acute renal failure compared to no intervention. However, dehydration is an important risk factor for acute renal failure and recommended volumes of fluid have little potential of harm. One RCT found that hydration with 0.9% sodium chloride infusion versus 0.45% sodium chloride infusion significantly reduced radiocontrast induced nephropathy. This effect was greater in women, people with diabetes, and those who received more than 250 mL of contrast.

Benefits: **Versus no treatment:** We found no RCTs comparing fluids with no intervention. RCTs have combined fluids (especially 0.45% sodium chloride infusion) with other active treatments. Comparisons between outcomes in these trials and historical untreated controls are difficult but suggest benefit from fluids.[23] In certain settings, such as traumatic rhabdomyolysis, early and aggressive fluid resuscitation has had dramatic benefits compared with historical controls.[24] **Versus other fluids:** We found one RCT (1620 people) comparing hydration using 0.9% sodium chloride infusion versus hydration with 0.45% sodium chloride infusion in radiocontrast induced nephropathy, in people who had a coronary angiography.[25] Radiocontrast induced nephropathy was defined as an increase in serum creatinine of more than 0.5 mg/dL (45 µmol/L) within 48 hours. The RCT found that hydration with 0.9% sodium chloride infusion versus 0.45% sodium chloride infusion, significantly reduced radiocontrast induced nephropathy (0.7% with physiologic saline [0.9% sodium chloride infusion] *v* 2% with 0.45% sodium chloride infusion; P = 0.04). Three predefined subsets of people (women, people with diabetes, and those who received > 250 mL of the contrast) benefited the most from 0.9% sodium chloride infusion hydration.

Harms: The volumes of fluids recommended, such as 1 L, and the rates of infusion (generally < 500 mL/h) have little potential for harm in most people. The RCT did not report data on harms.[25]

Comment: Hypovolaemia is a significant risk factor for acute renal failure. The provision of adequate maintenance fluids is considered important in preventing acute renal failure. Additional fluid loading may be useful because it assures adequate intravascular volume. It also stimulates urine output, theoretically limiting renal exposure time to higher concentrations of nephrotoxins.

OPTION LOOP DIURETICS

We found evidence from one systematic review that loop diuretics versus fluids alone are not effective and may be harmful in the prevention of acute renal failure. Two RCTs have found that diuretics versus 0.9% sodium chloride infusion seem to worsen outcome in acute tubular necrosis induced by contrast media and after cardiac surgery.

Benefits: We found one systematic review (search date 1997, 7 RCTs) comparing fluids alone versus diuretics in people at risk of acute renal failure from various causes.[26] It found no evidence of benefit associated with diuretics.

Harms: Diuretics seem to worsen outcomes in acute tubular necrosis induced by contrast media[23] and after cardiac surgery.[27] We found two RCTs addressing harms. The first RCT (78 people with chronic renal insufficiency who had a cardiac angiography, mean serum creatinine 2.1 ± 0.6 mg/dL or 186 ± 53 μmol/L) found that acute renal failure (defined as an increase in serum creatinine ≥ 0.5 mg/dL or 44 μmol/L at 48 h) was significantly more likely to occur when people were treated with furosemide (frusemide) (10/25 [40%] with furosemide *v* 3/28 [11%] with 0.9% sodium chloride infusion; RR 3.73, 95% CI 1.16 to 12.10; NNH 4, 95% CI 2 to 17).[19] The second RCT found that furosemide versus 0.9% sodium chloride was associated with the development of postcardiac surgery acute renal failure (6/41 [15%] with furosemide *v* 0/40 [0%] with sodium chloride; NNH 6, 95% CI 3 to 34).[27]

Comment: The trials addressing harms[23,27] provided a three-way comparison showing significant differences among the three groups ($P < 0.05$). Although they seem to have used the same control group for both comparisons, no adjustment was made or multiple comparisons.

OPTION MANNITOL

We found insufficient evidence provided by low powered RCTs addressing the effects of mannitol on the development of acute renal failure in people with traumatic rhabdomyolysis, or undergoing coronary artery bypass surgery, or vascular or biliary tract surgery. One RCT found that mannitol versus 0.9% sodium chloride increased the risk of acute renal failure, but the difference was not significant.

Benefits: We found no systematic review. Several small RCTs found no decrease in the incidence of acute renal failure (ARF) with mannitol over hydration alone in a variety of conditions, including coronary artery bypass surgery,[28] traumatic rhabdomyolysis,[29] vascular,[30] or biliary tract surgery.[31] One trial comparing 0.9% sodium chloride, furosemide, and mannitol (78 people with chronic renal insufficiency who had a cardiac angiography, mean serum creatinine 2.1 ± 0.6 mg/dL or 186 ± 53 µmol/L) found that ARF (defined as an increase in serum creatinine ≥ 0.5 mg/dL or 44 µmol/L at 48 h) was more likely to occur when people were treated with mannitol rather than with 0.9% sodium chloride (see harms below), although the difference was not significant.[24]

Harms: In ARF induced by contrast media, mannitol was not associated with a significantly increased risk of ARF compared with saline fluids (AR 7/25 [28%] with mannitol *v* 3/28 [11%] with physiologic saline; RR 2.61, 95% CI 0.76 to 9.03), but the sample size was small and it was not possible to exclude harms.[23]

Comment: Mannitol is an intravascular volume expander and may also function as a free radical scavenger, as well as an osmotic diuretic. A trial addressing the effect of mannitol on renal function[23] provided a three-way comparison showing significant differences among the three groups ($P < 0.05$). Although they seem to have used the same control group to compare both interventions, no adjustment was made for multiple comparisons.

OPTION DOPAMINE

We found good evidence that dopamine versus placebo is not effective in the prevention of acute renal failure.

Benefits: We found one systematic review (search date 1999, 17 RCTs, 854 people)[32] and one subsequent large RCT[33] using dopamine for the prevention of acute renal failure. The meta-analysis was adequately powered and suggested that dopamine versus placebo did not prevent mortality (4.7% with dopamine *v* 5.6% with placebo; RR 0.83, 95% CI 0.39 to 1.77), onset of acute renal failure (15.3% with dopamine *v* 19.5% with placebo; RR 0.79, 95% CI 0.54 to 1.13), or need for dialysis (13.9% with dopamine *v* 16.5% with placebo; RR 0.89, 95% CI 0.66 to 1.21).[32] The subsequent RCT, which is the largest to date (328 critically ill people with signs of sepsis), evaluated dopamine in early renal dysfunction (see glossary, p 845). It found that dopamine versus placebo had no significant effect on the development of acute renal failure (peak serum creatinine concentration during treatment was 2.7 ± 1.6 mg/dL [245 ± 144 µmol/L] in the dopamine group *v* 2.8 ± 1.6 mg/dL [249 ± 147 µmol/L] in the placebo group; $P = 0.93$), the requirement of dialysis (35/161 [22%] with dopamine *v* 40/163 [25%] with placebo; RR 0.89, 95% CI 0.58 to 1.30), intensive care unit length of stay (13 ± 14 days with dopamine *v* 14 ± 15 days with placebo; $P = 0.67$), hospital length of stay (29 ± 27 days with dopamine *v* 33 ± 39 days with placebo; $P = 0.29$), or mortality (69/161 [43%] with dopamine *v* 66/163 [40%] with placebo; RR 1.06, 95% CI 0.8 to 1.33).

Harms: One systematic review[26] and one large RCT in people with sepsis[33] found no evidence on harms. Dopamine has known adverse effects including extravasation necrosis, gangrene, tachycardia, headache, conduction abnormalities, and effects of prolactin.

Comment: The increase in urine output associated with dopamine is often thought to be caused exclusively by the increase in renal blood flow and, therefore, it may be confused with evidence of benefit. However, dopamine also has a significant diuretic effect.

OPTION DOPAMINE 1 RECEPTOR AGONISTS (FENOLDOPAM) New

We found no RCTs on the effects of fenoldopam in preventing acute renal failure from any cause.

Benefits: We found no systematic review or RCTs evaluating clinical outcomes.

Harms: Fenoldopam may cause hypotension and therefore can predispose to renal failure by reducing renal perfusion pressure.[34]

Comment: Although many small RCTs and one systematic review[35] have shown that fenoldopam increases renal blood flow,[36] renal plasma flow[37] and creatinine clearance,[38] we found no RCTs evaluating clinical outcomes.

OPTION NATRIURETIC PEPTIDES

One large RCT found that atrial natriuretic peptide versus placebo does not significantly reduce the incidence of acute renal failure induced by contrast media. We found insufficient evidence to evaluate the effect of natriuretic peptides for other forms of acute renal failure.

Benefits: We found no systematic review, but found one large RCT (247 people) evaluating three different doses of atrial natriuretic peptide (0.01, 0.05, and 0.1 μg/kg/min) versus placebo in the prevention of acute renal failure (ARF) induced by contrast media.[39] It found no difference in the incidence of ARF between groups (19% with placebo *v* 23 % with 0.01 μg/kg/min anaritide *v* 23% with 0.05 μg/kg/min anaritide *v* 25% with 0.10 μg/kg/min anaritide).

Harms: We found one RCT (504 people with early ARF). It found worse dialysis free survival in a subgroup of people (378 non-oliguric people) when treated with atrial natriuretic peptide versus placebo (survival rates 88/183 [48%] with atrial natriuretic peptide *v* 116/195 [59%] with placebo; RR 1.24, 95% CI 1.02 to 1.50; NNH 8, 95% CI 4 to 36).[40]

Comment: Natriuretic peptides (atrial natriuretic peptide and urodilantin) have also been evaluated in the treatment of ARF (see benefits of natriuretic peptides, p 844).

OPTION THEOPHYLLINE

RCTs found no evidence that theophylline versus placebo effective in preventing acute renal failure.

Benefits: We found no systematic review. We found one non-systematic review (3 RCTs, 177 people) of theophylline (a non-selective adenosine antagonist) for prevention of acute renal failure induced by contrast media.[41] It found that theophylline (810 mg/day) versus placebo provided no protection against acute renal failure (defined as increase in serum creatinine of > 0.5 mg/dL or > 44 μmol/L) when people are adequately hydrated (renal failure 5.7% with theophylline *v* 3.4% with placebo; no additional data available).

Harms: Theophylline has a narrow therapeutic index and known adverse effects (see harms of theophyllines under chronic obstructive pulmonary disease, p 1530).

Comment: We found no RCTs of selective adenosine antagonists or non-selective adenosine antagonists for other forms of acute renal failure.

OPTION CALCIUM CHANNEL BLOCKERS

One RCT found that isradipine versus placebo did not significantly reduce early allograft dysfunction in renal transplantation. We found no RCTs assessing the effects of calcium channel blockers in reducing other forms of acute renal failure.

Benefits: We found one RCT (210 people) of isradipine versus placebo on renal allograft function after transplantation.[42] Median serum creatinine levels at 3 months (185 μmol/L with isradipine *v* 220 μmol/L with placebo; P = 0.002) and 12 months (141 μmol/L with isradipine *v* 158 μmol/l with placebo; P = 0.021) were significantly better in the isradipine group. However, there was no significant difference in the incidence of graft dysfunction (34/98 [35%] with isradipine *v* 44/112 [39%] with placebo; RR 1.13, 95% CI 0.79 to 1.62) or in the severity or duration (isradipine 9.1, SD ± 8.7 days *v* placebo 9.3, SD ± 8.1 days) of graft dysfunction.

Harms: As a class, calcium channel blockers are associated with hypotension and bradycardia as well as numerous, less serious adverse effects. The incidence and nature of adverse effects varies between individual drugs (see harms of antihypertensive drug treatment, p 37).

Comment: None.

OPTION ACETYLCYSTEINE

One small RCT found that *N*-acetylcysteine versus placebo significantly reduced the risk of acute renal failure induced by contrast media.

Benefits: We found one RCT (83 people with chronic renal insufficiency) of acetylcysteine versus placebo to prevent of acute renal failure induced by contrast media.[43] It found that the incidence of acute renal failure (defined as an increase in serum creatinine ≥ 0.5 mg/dL or 44 μmol/L at 48 h) was significantly reduced (1/41 [2%] with acetylcysteine *v* 9/42 [21%] with placebo; RR 0.11, 95% CI 0.02 to 0.86; NNT 6, 95% CI 3 to 21).[43]

Harms: Acetylcysteine has been widely used to treat people with acetaminophen overdose, and has virtually no toxicity at therapeutic levels (see harms of paracetamol poisoning, p 1447).

Comment: The clinical relevance of a rise in serum creatinine of 0.5 mg/dL (44 μmol/L) at 48 hours, the study end point, is unclear. Long term follow up was not carried out and the study was too small to evaluate either dialysis or mortality as end points.

OPTION SINGLE VERSUS MULTIPLE DOSES OF AMINOGLYCOSIDES

One good quality RCT found that single versus multiple doses of aminoglycosides significantly reduced nephrotoxicity.

Benefits: We found one systematic review (search date 1995, 422 people, not limited to people in intensive care units).[44] It found equal antimicrobial efficacy (pooled risk ratio for bacteriological cure was 1.00, 95% CI 0.86 to 1.16 and pooled risk ratio for clinical cure was 0.97, 95% CI 0.91 to 1.05) and no difference in nephrotoxicity (see glossary, p 845) with single doses versus multiple doses of aminoglycosides (RR 0.78, 95% CI 0.31 to 1.94). One of the RCTs included in the review (85 people), which was highlighted for its scientific rigour, compared once daily versus three times daily dosing of gentamicin. It found equal efficacy but significantly less incidence of nephrotoxicity with single dosing (2/40 [5%] with single dosing *v* 11/45 [24%]; RR 0.21, 95% CI 0.05 to 0.87; NNT 5, 95% CI 2 to 24).[45] Nephrotoxicity was defined as an increase in serum creatinine of 0.5 mg/dL (45 μmol/L) or more.

Harms: The review found no evidence of greater harm from once daily aminoglycoside dosing (see RR of nephrotoxicity mentioned in benefits above).

Comment: The risk from aminoglycosides is highest in people with volume depletion, underlying renal, cardiac, or hepatic disease, or when combined with diuretics or other nephrotoxic agents (see glossary, p 845).

OPTION LIPID FORMULATIONS OF AMPHOTERICIN B VERSUS STANDARD FORMULATIONS

We found no RCTs. Lipid formulations of amphotericin B seem to cause less nephrotoxicity compared with standard formulations, but direct comparisons of long term safety are lacking.

Benefits: We found no systematic review and no RCTs.

Harms: We found no evidence of greater harms from lipid formulations of amphotericin B (see glossary, p 845). However, these formulations are still nephrotoxic and should be used with care.

Comment: A Phase II trial of a lipid formulation of amphotericin B (556 people) found an incidence of renal toxicity (defined by any increase in serum creatinine) of 24% (*v* 60–80% with standard formulation of amphotericin B). People with baseline serum creatinine in excess of 2.5 mg/dL (221 μmol/L) on standard amphotericin B showed a significant decrease in serum creatinine when transferred to the lipid formulation ($P < 0.001$).[46] One trial found that simply infusing amphotericin B in a lipid solution designed for parenteral nutrition did not result in any benefit and may be associated with pulmonary adverse effects.[47] Fluid loading can be useful in reducing the risk of acute renal failure from all nephrotoxins. Considerable variability may exist between individual lipid formulations of amphotericin B in terms of efficacy and safety.

OPTION **LOW OSMOLALITY VERSUS STANDARD CONTRAST MEDIA**

One systematic review has found that low versus standard osmolality contrast media are associated with less renal toxicity. The benefit was greatest in people with pre-existing renal impairment (especially those with diabetes mellitus).

Benefits: We found one systematic review (search date 1991, 31 RCTs, 5146 people) comparing low osmolality contrast media (see glossary, p 845) with standard contrast media.[48] Overall, low osmolality contrast media did not influence the development of acute renal failure or need for dialysis (these are rare events), but there was less nephrotoxicity (see glossary, p 845) with low osmolality contrast media, measured by serum creatinine. The overall benefit was small for people without prior renal failure (OR 0.75, 95% CI 0.52 to 1.10), and was greatest in people with underlying renal impairment (OR 0.50, 95% CI 0.36 to 0.68).

Harms: We found no evidence of increased harms with low osmolality contrast media.

Comment: Low osmolality contrast media are more expensive than standard contrast media. Acute renal failure induced by contrast media occurs most commonly in people with diabetic nephropathy (incidence nearly 50%, varies with the degree of baseline renal function).

QUESTION **What are effects of treatments for critically ill people with acute renal failure?**

Martine Leblanc, Ramesh Venkataraman, and John A Kellum

OPTION **CONTINUOUS VERSUS INTERMITTENT RENAL REPLACEMENT THERAPY**

Two systemic reviews found insufficient evidence to conclude whether continuous renal replacement therapy is associated with improved patient outcome compared to intermittent renal replacement therapy.

Benefits: We found two systematic reviews.[49,50] The more recent systematic review included all prior randomised and observational studies comparing intermittent to continuous renal replacement therapies (see glossary, p 845) (search date 1998, 13 studies, 3 RCTs, 1400 critically ill people with acute renal failure).[50] It found no significant difference in mortality (mortality with continuous *v* intermittent therapy: RR 0.93, 95% CI 0.79 to 1.09). Subgroup analysis adjusting by baseline severity of illness found a survival benefit with continuous renal replacement therapy (mortality: RR 0.48, 95% CI 0.34 to 0.69). A secondary analysis including all studies and adjusting for study quality found that continuous modalities significantly reduced mortality (RR 0.72, 95% CI 0.60 to 0.87).[50] The second systematic review (search date 1994, 15 observational studies, 1173 people)[49] has been eclipsed by the one described above.[50]

Harms: We found no good studies comparing the adverse effects of continuous renal replacement with intermittent renal replacement therapy (see glossary, p 845). The systematic reviews did not provide data on harms.[49,50] Heparin is often used with both intermittent and continuous renal replacement therapy, and may have adverse effects (see thromboembolism, p 209).[51] Hypotension is common with intermittent haemodialysis, whereas haemodynamic stability is better preserved with continuous renal replacement therapy.[52]

Comment: The evidence from the latest systematic review may be insufficient to draw conclusions regarding the preferred mode of renal replacement for critically ill people with acute renal failure. Only after adjusting for baseline severity, study quality, or both was the review able to show a benefit with continuous renal replacement therapies. The systematic review concluded that although there is a suggestion of benefit with continuous renal replacement therapy, there was insufficient data to draw reliable conclusions.[50]

OPTION HIGH DOSE VERSUS LOW DOSE CONTINUOUS RENAL REPLACEMENT THERAPY

One RCT has found that a higher versus a lower delivered dose of dialysis significantly improves survival in people with acute renal failure.

Benefits: We found no systematic review. We found a recent RCT (425 people)[53] comparing three doses of continuous replacement renal therapy (20, 35, and 45 mL/kg/h of haemofiltration in postdilution). Mortality was similar for the two high dose arms (60/139 [43%] with 35 mL/kg/h *v* 59/140 [42%] with 45 mL/kg/h), but was significantly higher in the low dose arm (86/146 [59%] with 20 mL/kg/h). Survival time analysis was adjusted for three way comparison (combined RR 1.38, 95% CI 1.14 to 1.67; NNT 7, 95% CI 4 to 16).

Harms: We found no evidence that the higher dialysis dose is associated with increased adverse effects (such as haemodynamic instability, intolerance, or bleeding). In a prospective study on daily intermittent haemodialysis,[54] there was no evidence of increased morbidity compared to alternate day dialysis. In particular, hypotension was less common with daily treatment.

Comment: There is no standard method to compare dialysis dosage between continuous and intermittent renal replacement therapies (see glossary, p 845), but urea kinetic modelling predicts that the doses used in this study would be impossible to achieve without continuous renal replacement therapy (see glossary, p 845).[55] In addition, the underlying mechanisms for solute removal are different based on the type of treatment applied (convection with haemofiltration versus diffusion with haemodialysis). This makes comparisons of elimination of diverse solutes difficult. However, a recent, small, prospective study (160 people) has found that a higher dose of dialysis delivered as daily intermittent haemodialysis versus alternate day haemodialysis sessions is associated with improved survival in people with acute renal failure (RR 0.59, 95% CI 0.39 to 91).[54] Although this study may have had low power to detect important differences and did not deliver the prescribed dialysis dose, it does support the concept that a dose–response relationship exists for dialysis in acute renal failure and suggests that the traditional, end stage renal disease based, dose recommendation may be too low.

OPTION BIOCOMPATIBLE VERSUS NON-BIOCOMPATIBLE DIALYSIS MEMBRANES

We found limited evidence from three out of four RCTs that biocompatible membranes versus non-biocompatible membranes may reduce mortality in critically ill people with acute renal failure.

Benefits: We found no systematic review, but found four RCTs (590 people)[56–59] comparing biocompatible (see glossary, p 844) (synthetic) versus non-biocompatible (cellulose based) dialysis membranes in critically ill people with all cause acute renal failure. Despite being described as randomised, two of the RCTs had important problems with their quality. The first RCT (52 people) found a better survival rate with biocompatible membranes (62% with biocompatible membranes *v* 35% with non-biocompatible membranes; P = 0.05) and a higher incidence of renal recovery at time of discharge with biocompatible membranes (AR for survival 23/37 [62%] with biocompatible membranes *v* 13/35 [37%] with non-biocompatible membranes; RR 1.67, 95% CI 1.02 to 2.76; NNT 4, 95% CI 3 to 51).[56] The second RCT (180 people) found 60% survival with biocompatible membranes versus 58% with bio-incompatible membranes (OR 1.07, 95% CI 0.54 to 2.11; P = 0.87), and identical rates of recovery of renal function between groups (57%).[57] However, the RCT was not analysed by intention to treat, and 12% of people were excluded after randomisation. Also, it was funded by makers of bio-incompatible membranes. The third RCT (106 people) compared two types of synthetic membranes to a semi-synthetic cellulose based membrane, and found no significant difference in survival at 80 days.[58] The fourth RCT (66 people)[59] did not find any difference in renal recovery or survival with biocompatible membranes versus non-biocompatible membranes (76% survival with cellulose acetate at 30 days *v* 73% with polysulfone; 58% renal recovery at 30 days with cellulose acetate *v* 39% with polysulfone). However, the RCT had insufficient power to detect clinically important differences in outcome.

Harms: Severe anaphylactoid reactions in people taking angiotensin converting enzyme inhibitors have been reported occasionally with certain synthetic biocompatible membranes (exact frequency unknown).[60]

Comment: One quasi randomised trial (alternate assignment)[61] extended recruitment from the original sample of 72 people with acute renal failure[62] to 153.[61] It found a significant difference in survival to discharge (57% with biocompatible membranes *v* 46% with non-biocompatible membranes; P = 0.03) and recovery of renal function (64% with biocompatible membranes *v* 43% with non-biocompatible membranes; P = 0.001).[57,58] This RCT found that mortality due to sepsis (by time of discharge) was lower with biocompatible membranes (12% with biocompatible membranes *v* 46% with non-biocompatible membranes; P = 0.016). One prospective observational cohort study (2410 people with chronic renal failure) found a 25% relative increase in mortality in people using non-biocompatible (cellulose based) versus biocompatible (synthetic) membranes (P < 0.001).[63] The ability of the membrane to cause immune activation depends on the structure of the material used.[64] We found no evidence that the results comparing synthetic and cellulose based materials can be extrapolated to highly substituted cellulose based ("semi-biocompatible") membranes. An RCT (43 people with end stage renal failure who were oliguric after undergoing cadaveric renal transplantation and were diagnosed as having delayed graft function) compared polysulfone biocompatible dialysis membrane versus cuprophane membrane as bioincompatible membrane. It found no significant differences in the mean time to graft recovery (14 days with polysulfone *v* 11 days with cuprophane; P = 0.18).[65] One quasi randomised clinical trial (using open randomisation list; 72 people with acute renal failure) found no significant difference on survival and renal recovery when treated either with a biocompatible low flux membrane or a biocompatible high flux membrane.[66] There were no significant differences in survival rates (7/38 [18.7%] with low flux *v* 7/34 [20.6%] with high flux; RR 0.90, 95% CI 0.35 to 2.3) or rates of recovery of renal function (10/38 [26.3%] with low flux *v* 8/34 [23.5%] with high flux; RR 1.1, 95% CI 0.5 to 2.5). No single study has been adequately powered to address this question.

OPTION DOPAMINE

One systematic review found no significant difference in mortality, onset of acute renal failure or need for dialysis with dopamine versus control. One additional RCT found that compared to placebo, low dose dopamine did not reduce renal dysfunction. Dopamine has been associated with important adverse effects, including extravasation necrosis, gangrene, tachycardia, and conduction abnormalities.

Benefits: We found one systematic review and one additional RCT.[32,33] The systematic review (search date 1999, 58 trials of which 17 were RCTs, 2149 people) found among the 24 studies reporting on clinical outcomes that dopamine produced no significant reduction of mortality (11 trials, 508 people; 4.7% with dopamine *v* 5.6% with control; RR 0.83, 95% CI 0.39 to 1.77), onset of acute renal failure (11 trials, 511 people; 15.3% with dopamine *v* 19.5% with control; RR 0.79, 95% CI 0.54 to 1.13), or need for dialysis with dopamine (10 trials, 618 people; 13.9% with dopamine *v* 16.5 with control; RR 0.89, 95% CI 0.66 to 1.21).[32] The additional RCT (multicentre, double blind, placebo controlled: 328 people with early renal dysfunction [see glossary, p 845] defined as oliguria [see glossary, p 845] or increase in serum creatinine) found that compared to placebo, low dose dopamine did not confer any protection from renal dysfunction (according to peak creatinine levels).[33]

Harms: Dopamine has recognised adverse effects, including extravasation necrosis, gangrene, tachycardia, headache, conduction abnormalities, and effects of prolactin. We found no good evidence about harms in this setting. The systematic review and the RCT did not provide data on harms.[32,33]

Comment: Studies using dopamine to prevent renal failure or to ameliorate the progression have not found any benefit (see prevention of acute renal failure, p 833).

OPTION LOOP DIURETICS

Two small RCTs found that loop diuretics versus placebo had no significant effect on renal recovery, the number of days spent on dialysis, or mortality. The RCTs lacked power to exclude a clinically important effect, and included people from a non-intensive care unit setting. Loop diuretics have been associated with toxicity and low renal perfusion.

Benefits: We found no systematic review. We found two RCTs (66 and 58 people; some in intensive care units, proportion unknown) comparing intravenous furosemide with placebo in people with oliguric acute renal failure of various causes.[67,68] In the second RCT, all people received one dose of furosemide 1 g and were then randomised to continued treatment or placebo. Neither RCT found significant differences in renal recovery (first RCT 19/33 [58%] with furosemide *v* 22/33 [67%] with placebo; RR 0.86, 95% CI 0.50 to 1.20;[67] second RCT 10/28 [36%] with furosemide *v* 12/28 [43%] with placebo; RR 0.83, 95% CI 0.37 to 1.45)[68] or mortality. The RCTs lacked power to exclude a clinically important effect of loop diuretics on these outcomes.

Harms: Ototoxicity can occur with high doses of loop diuretics. No adverse effects were reported in the first trial.[61] Deafness occurred in two people in the second trial; both were randomised to furosemide. Hearing loss was permanent in one of these people.[68] Diuretics may reduce renal perfusion and add a prerenal component to the renal failure, but the frequency of this event is uncertain.[69] See harms of loop diuretics, p 834.

Comment: None.

OPTION CONTINUOUS INFUSION VERSUS BOLUS INJECTION OF LOOP DIURETICS

We found no RCTs comparing continuous infusion versus bolus injection of loop diuretics.

Benefits: We found no systematic review and no RCTs in critically ill people with acute renal failure.

Harms: One small, crossover RCT (8 people with acute deterioration of chronic renal failure, mean creatinine clearance 0.28 mL/s) found that fewer people experienced myalgia when treated with continuous infusion than with bolus dosing of bumetanide (3/8 [38%] people with bolus dosing *v* 0/8 [0%] with continuous infusion).[70]

Comment: The small crossover trial found that continuous infusion resulted in a net increase in sodium excretion over 24 hours (mean increase in sodium excretion 48 mmol/day, 95% CI 16 mmol/day to 60 mmol/day; P = 0.01).

OPTION INTRAVENOUS ALBUMIN SUPPLEMENTATION PLUS LOOP DIURETICS

We found no RCTs on the effects of adding intravenous albumin to loop diuretic treatment in critically ill people with acute renal failure.

Benefits: We found no systematic review and no RCTs evaluating clinical outcomes in critically ill people with acute renal failure.

Harms: We found insufficient evidence in people with acute renal failure. One systematic review (30 RCTs, 1419 people, most without acute renal failure) found that albumin increased the risk of death in unselected critically ill people (mortality 98/704 [14%] with albumin *v* 58/715 [8%] with control; RR 1.68, CI 1.26 to 2.23). All of the included trials were small and combined highly heterogeneous populations.[71]

Comment: One crossover RCT (9 people with nephrotic syndrome) compared furosemide alone versus furosemide plus albumin versus albumin alone.[72] It found that furosemide was superior to albumin alone, and furosemide plus albumin resulted in the greatest urine and sodium excretion. The clinical significance of this finding is unclear.

OPTION NATRIURETIC PEPTIDES

RCTs have found that both atrial natriuretic peptide and ularitide (urodilantin) are ineffective in treating acute renal failure in oliguric and non-oliguric people. In addition, atrial natriuretic peptide is possibly harmful in non-oliguric people.

Benefits: We found no systematic review but found three RCTs.[40,73,74] One large RCT (504 people) found no overall difference in dialysis free survival with atrial natriuretic peptide versus placebo in people with acute renal failure.[40] Preplanned subgroup analysis suggested a possible benefit to people with oliguria (see glossary, p 845), and lower survival rates in non-oliguric people. However, a recent RCT (220 people)[73] in people with oliguric acute renal failure found no improvement in dialysis free survival with a 24 hour infusion of atrial natriuretic peptide compared to placebo. A third RCT compared ularitide ([orurodilantin] a natriuretic peptide with less system haemodynamic effects) in a dose finding (5, 20, 40, or 80 ng/kg/min ularitide), placebo controlled RCT (176 people). Ularitide did not reduce the requirement for dialysis (people who needed dialysis: 35% with 5 ng/kg/min ularitide *v* 36% with 20 ng/kg/min ularitide *v* 28% with 40 ng/kg/min ularitide *v* 41% with 80 ng/kg/min ularitide *v* 36% with placebo; P = non-significant).[74]

Harms: One RCT found that natriuretic peptide caused significant hypotension versus placebo (95% with natriuretic peptide *v* 55% with placebo; $P < 0.01$). Also, atrial natriuretic peptide may be associated with a worse outcome in people with non-oliguric renal failure (dialysis free survival in 378 non-oliguric people was 48% with anaritide *v* 59% with placebo; $P = 0.03$).[73] See harms of natriuretic peptides, p 836.

Comment: We found no evidence of any significant improvement of acute renal failure with atrial natriuretic peptide.

GLOSSARY

Biocompatible Artificial materials can induce an inflammatory response. This response can be humoral (including complement) or cellular. Materials are classified as biocompatible if they are less likely to induce an immune response or induce a less severe response compared with bio-incompatible materials. We found no standards by which this comparison can be made. Biocompatible dialysis membranes are made from synthetic materials, whereas bio-incompatible membranes are cellulose based.

Continuous renal replacement therapy Any extracorporeal blood purification treatment intended to substitute for impaired renal function over an extended period of time and applied for, or aimed at being applied for, 24 hours a day.

Early allograft dysfunction Renal dysfunction that occurs after renal transplantation, and which is usually secondary to ischaemic injury.

Early renal dysfunction An acute derangement in renal function that is still evolving.

Glomerular filtration rate The most basic aspect of renal function, glomerular filtration rate is the rate of elaboration of protein free plasma filtrate (ultrafiltration) across the walls of the glomerular capillaries.

Intermittent renal replacement therapy Renal support that is not, nor intended to be, continuous; usually prescribed for a period of 12 hours or less.

Intrarenal acute renal failure Caused by parenchymal injury, most commonly acute tubular necrosis, but also interstitial nephritis, embolic disease, glomerulonephritis, vasculitis, or small vessel disease.

Lipid formulations of amphotericin B Complexes of amphotericin B and phospholipids or sterols. This reduces the toxicity of amphotericin B while preserving its antifungal activity.

Low osmolality contrast media Contrast media with osmolality less than 300 mOsm/L.

Multiple organ dysfunction syndrome A syndrome of progressive organ failure, affecting one organ after another and believed to be the result of persistent or recurrent infection or inflammation.

Nephrotoxic agents Any agent that has the potential to produce nephrotoxicity.

Nephrotoxicity Renal parenchymal damage manifested by a decline in glomerular filtration rate, tubular dysfunction, or both.

Oliguria Urine output less than 5 mL/kg daily.

Postrenal (obstructive) acute renal failure Caused by urinary tract obstruction.

Prerenal (functional) acute renal failure Caused by renal hypoperfusion, secondary to renal artery disease, systemic hypotension, or maldistribution of blood flow.

REFERENCES

1. Nissenson AR. Acute renal failure: definition and pathogenesis. *Kidney Int Suppl* 1998;66:7–10.
2. Bellomo R, Ronco C. The changing pattern of severe acute renal failure. *Nephrology* 1991;2:602–610.
3. Hou SH, Bushinsky DA, Wish JB, et al. Hospital-acquired renal insufficiency: a prospective study. *Am J Med* 1983;74:243–248.
4. Brivet FG, Kleinknecht DJ, Loirat P, et al. Acute renal failure in intensive care units — causes, outcomes and prognostic factors of hospital mortality: a prospective multicenter study. *Crit Care Med* 1996;24:192–198.
5. Wiecek A, Zeier M, Ritz E. Role of infection in the genesis of acute renal failure. *Nephrol Dial Transplant* 1994;9(suppl 4):40–44.
6. Myers BD, Moran SM. Hemodynamically mediated acute renal failure. *N Engl J Med* 1986;314:97–100.
7. Ward MM. Factors predictive of acute renal failure in rhabdomyolysis. *Arch Intern Med* 1988;148:1553–1557.
8. Kahlmeter G, Dahlager JI. Aminoglycoside toxicity — a review of clinical studies published between 1975 and 1982. *J Antimicrob Chemother* 1984;13(suppl A):9–22. Search date 1982; primary sources Medline, Toxline, and personal contact with pharmaceutical companies.
9. Butler WT, Bennett JE, Alling DW, et al. Nephrotoxicity of amphotericin B, early and late events in 81 patients. *Ann Intern Med* 1964;61:175–187.
10. Tran DD, Oe PL, De Fijter CWH, et al. Acute renal failure in patients with acute pancreatitis: prevalence, risk factors, and outcome. *Nephrol Dial Transplant* 1993;8:1079–1084.
11. McCullough PA, Wolyn R, Rocher LL, et al. Acute renal failure after coronary intervention: incidence, risk factors, and relationship to mortality. *Am J Med* 1997;103:368–375.
12. Thadhani R, Pascual M, Bonventre JV. Acute renal failure. *N Engl J Med* 1996;334:1448–1460.
13. Kleinknecht D. Epidemiology in acute renal failure in France today. In: Biari D, Neild G, eds. *Acute renal failure in intensive therapy unit*. Berlin: Springer-Verlag, 1990:13–21.
14. Coar D. Obstructive nephropathy. *Del Med J* 1991;63:743–749.
15. Kaufman J, Dhakal M, Patel B, et al. Community acquired acute renal failure. *Am J Kidney Dis* 1991;17:191–198.

16. Bamgboye EL, Mabayoje MO, Odutala TA, et al. Acute renal failure at the Lagos University Teaching Hospital. *Ren Fail* 1993;15:77–80.
17. Nolan CR, Anderson RJ. Hospital-acquired acute renal failure. *J Am Soc Nephrol* 1998;9:710–718.
18. Cantarovich F, Bodin L. Functional acute renal failure. In: Cantarovich F, Rangoonwala B, Verho M, eds. *Progress in acute renal failure 1998*. Paris: Hoechst Marion Roussel, 1998:55–65.
19. Brezis M, Rosen S. Hypoxia of the renal medulla. Its implication for disease. *N Engl J Med* 1995;332:647–655.
20. Bonventre JV. Mechanisms of ischemic acute renal failure. *Kidney Int* 1993;43:1160–1178.
21. Turney JH, Marshall DH, Brownjohn AM, et al. The evolution of acute renal failure, 1956–1988. *QJM* 1990;74:83–104.
22. Liano F, Junco E, Pascual J, et al. The spectrum of acute renal failure in the intensive care unit compared to that seen in other settings. The Madrid Acute Renal Failure Study Group. *Kidney Int Suppl* 1998;53:16–24.
23. Solomon R, Werner C, Mann D, et al. Effects of saline, mannitol, and furosemide to prevent acute decreases in renal function induced by radiocontrast agents. *N Engl J Med* 1994;331:1416–1420.
24. Better OS, Stein JH. Early management of shock and prophylaxis of acute renal failure in traumatic rhabdomyolysis. *N Engl J Med* 1990;322:825–829.
25. Mueller C, Buerkle G, Buettner HJ, et al. Prevention of contrast media-associated nephropathy: randomized comparison of 2 hydration regimes in 1620 patients undergoing coronary angioplasty. *Arch Int Med* 2002;162:329–336.
26. Kellum JA. The use of diuretics and dopamine in acute renal failure: a systematic review of the evidence. *Crit Care* 1997;1:53–59. Search date 1997; primary sources Medline and hand searches of bibliographies of relevant articles.
27. Lassnigg A, Donner E, Grubhofer G, et al. Lack of renoprotective effects of dopamine and furosemide during cardiac surgery. *J Am Soc Nephrol* 2000;11:97–104.
28. Ip-Yam PC, Murphy S, Baines M, et al. Renal function and proteinuria after cardiopulmonary bypass: the effects of temperature and mannitol. *Anesth Analg* 1994;78:842–847.
29. Homsi E, Barreiro MF, Orlando JM, et al. Prophylaxis of acute renal failure in patients with rhabdomyolysis. *Ren Fail* 1997;19:283–288.
30. Beall AC, Holman MR, Morris GC, et al. Mannitol-induced osmotic diuresis during vascular surgery. *Arch Surg* 1963;86:34–42.
31. Gubern JM, Sancho JJ, Simo J, et al. A randomized trial on the effect of mannitol on postoperative renal function in patients with obstructive jaundice. *Surgery* 1988;103:39–44.
32. Kellum JA, Decker JM. The use of dopamine in acute renal failure: a meta-analysis. *Crit Care Med* 2001;29:1526–1531.
33. Bellomo R, Chapman M, Finfer S, et al. Low-dose dopamine in patients with early renal dysfunction: a placebo-controlled randomised trial. Australian and New Zealand Intensive Care Society (ANZICS) Clinical Trials Group. *Lancet* 2000;356:2139–2143.
34. Mathur VS, Swan SK, Lambrecht LJ, et al. The effects of fenoldopam, a selective dopamine receptor agonist, on systemic and renal hemodynamics in normotensive subjects. *Crit Care Med* 1999;27:1832–1837.
35. Chu VL, Cheng GW. Fenoldopam in the prevention of contrast media-induced acute renal failure. *Ann Pharmacother* 2001;35:1278–1282.
36. Mathur VS, Swan SK, Lambrecht LJ, et al. The effects of fenoldopam, a selective dopamine receptor agonist, on systemic and renal hemodynamics in normotensive subjects. *Crit Care Med* 1999;27:1832–1837.
37. Tumlin JA, Wang A, Murray PT, et al. Fenoldopam mesylate blocks reductions in renal plasma flow after radiocontrast dye infusion: a pilot trial in the prevention of contrast nephropathy. *Am Heart J* 2002;143:894–903.
38. Halpenny M, Lakshmi S, O' Donnell A, et al. Fenoldopam — renal and splanchnic effects in patients undergoing coronary bypass surgery. *Anesthesia* 2001;56:953–960.
39. Kurnik BR, Allgren RL, Genter FC, et al. Prospective study of atrial natriuretic peptide for the prevention of radiocontrast-induced nephropathy. *Am J Kidney Dis* 1998;31:674–680.
40. Allgren RL, Marbury TC, Rahman SN, et al. Anaritide in ATN. Auriculin anaritide ARF study group. *N Engl J Med* 1997;336:828–834.
41. Venkataraman R, Kellum JA. Novel approaches to the treatment of acute renal failure. *Expert Opin Invest Drugs* 2000;9:2579–2592.
42. Van Riemsdijk IC, Mulder PG, De Fijter JW, et al. Addition of Isradipine (lomir) results in a better renal function after kidney transplantation: a double-blind, randomized, placebo-controlled, multi-center study. *Transplantation* 2000;70:122–126.
43. Tepel M, Van der Giet M, Schwarzfeld C, et al. Prevention of radiographic-contrast-agent-induced reductions in renal function by acetylcysteine. *N Engl J Med* 2000;343:180–184.
44. Hatala R, Dinh TT, Cook DJ. Single daily dosing of aminoglycosides in immunocompromised adults: a systematic review. *Clin Infect Dis* 1997;24:810–815. Search date 1995; primary sources Medline, hand searches of selected infectious diseases journals and bibliographies of relevant articles, and personal contact with primary investigators of selected studies.
45. Prins JM, Buller HR, Kuijper EJ, et al. Once versus thrice daily gentamicin in patients with serious infections. *Lancet* 1993;341:335–339.
46. Walsh TJ, Hiemenz JW, Seibel NL, et al. Amphotericin B lipid complex for invasive fungal infections: analysis of safety and efficacy in 556 cases. *Clin Infect Dis* 1998;26:383–396.
47. Schoffski P, Freund M, Wunder R, et al. Safety and toxicity of amphotericin B in glucose 5% or intralipid 20% in neutropenic patients with pneumonia or fever of unknown origin: randomised study. *BMJ* 1998;317:379–384.
48. Barrett BJ, Carlisle EJ. Metaanalysis of the relative nephrotoxicity of high and low-osmolality iodinated contrast media. *Radiology* 1993;188:171–178. Search date 1991; primary sources Medline, Embase, hand searches of reference lists of selected articles, and personal contact with authors of selected primary studies and pharmaceutical companies manufacturing contrast media.
49. Jakob SM, Frey FJ, Uehlinger DE. Does continuous renal replacement therapy favourably influence the outcome of the patients? *Nephrol Dial Transplant* 1996;11:1250–1255. Search date 1994; primary sources not stated.
50. Kellum JA, Angus DC, Johnson JP, et al. Continuous versus intermittent renal replacement therapy: a meta-analysis. *Int Care Med* 2002;28:29–37.
51. Ronco C. Continuous renal replacement therapies for the treatment of acute renal failure in intensive care patients. *Clin Nephrol* 1993;40:187–198.
52. Heering P, Morgera S, Schmitz FJ, et al. Cytokine removal and cardiovascular hemodynamics in

septic patients with continuous venovenous hemofiltration. *Intensive Care Med* 1997;23:288–296.
53. Ronco C, Bellomo R, Homel P, et al. Effects of different doses in continuous veno-venous haemofiltration on outcomes of acute renal failure: a prospective randomised trial. *Lancet* 2000;356:26–30.
54. Schiffl H, Lang SM, Fischer R. Daily hemodialysis and the outcome of acute renal failure. *N Engl J Med* 2002;346:305–310.
55. Gotch FA, Sargent JA, Keen ML. Whither goest Kt/V? *Kidney Int* 2000;58(suppl 76):3–18.
56. Schiffl H, Lang SM, Konig A, et al. Biocompatible membranes in acute renal failure: prospective case-controlled study. *Lancet* 1994;344:570–572.
57. Jorres A, Gahl GM, Dobis C, et al. Haemodialysis-membrane biocompatibility and mortality of patients with dialysis-dependent acute renal failure: a prospective randomised multicentre trial. International Multicentre Study Group. *Lancet* 1999;354:1337–1341.
58. Gastaldello K, Melot C, Kahn RJ, et al. Comparison of cellulose diacetate and polysulfone membranes in the outcome of acute renal failure. A prospective randomized study. *Nephrol Dial Transplant* 2000;15:224–230.
59. Albright RC, Smelser JM, McCarthy JT, et al. Patient survival and renal recovery in acute renal failure: randomized comparison of cellulose acetate and polysulfone membrane dialyzers. *Mayo Clinic Proc* 2000;75:1141–1147.
60. Kammerl MC, Schaefer RM, Schweda F, et al. Extracorporal therapy with AN69 membranes in combination with ACE inhibition causing severe anaphylactoid reactions: still a current problem? *Clin Nephrol* 2000;53:486–488.
61. Himmelfarb J, Tolkoff RN, Chandran P, et al. A multicenter comparison of dialysis membranes in the treatment of acute renal failure requiring dialysis. *J Am Soc Nephrol* 1998;9:257–266.
62. Hakim RM, Wingard RL, Parker RA. Effect of the dialysis membrane in the treatment of patients with acute renal failure. *N Engl J Med* 1994;331:1338–1342.
63. Hakim RM, Held PJ, Stannard DC, et al. Effect of the dialysis membrane on mortality of chronic hemodialysis patients. *Kidney Int* 1996;50:566–570.
64. Kellum JA. Primum non nocere and the meaning of modern critical care. *Curr Opin Critical Care* 1998;4:400–405.
65. Woo YM, Craig AM, King BB, et al. Biocompatible membranes do not promote graft recovery following cadaveric renal transplantation. *Clin Nephrol* 2002;57:38–44.
66. Ponikvar JB, Rus RR, Kenda RB, et al. Low-flux versus high-flux synthetic dialysis membrane in acute renal failure: prospective randomized study. *Artif Organs* 2001;25:946–950.
67. Kleinknecht D, Ganeval D, Gonzales-Duque LA, et al. Furosemide in acute oliguric renal failure. A controlled trial. *Nephron* 1976;17:51–58.
68. Brown CB, Ogg CS, Cameron JS. High dose furosemide in acute renal failure: a controlled trial. *Clin Nephrol* 1981;15:90–96.
69. Kellum JA. Use of diuretics in the acute care setting. *Kidney Int* 1998;53(suppl 66):67–70.
70. Rudy DW, Voelker JR, Greene PK, et al. Loop diuretics for chronic renal insufficiency: a continuous infusion is more efficacious than bolus therapy. *Ann Intern Med* 1991;115:360–366.
71. The Albumin Reviewers. Human albumin solution for resuscitation and volume expansion in critically ill patients. In: The Cochrane Library, Issue 1, 2002. Oxford: Update Software. Search date 2001; primary sources The Cochrane Injuries Group Register, the Cochrane Library, Medline, Embase, Bids, Index to Scientific and Technical Proceedings, and hand searched references.
72. Fliser D, Zurbruggen I, Mutschler E, et al. Coadministration of albumin and furosemide in patients with the nephrotic syndrome. *Kidney Int* 1999;55:629–634.
73. Lewis J, Salem M, Chertow GM, et al. Atrial natriuretic factor in oliguric acute renal failure. Anaritide Acute Renal Failure study group. *Am J Kid Dis*. 2000;36:767–774.
74. Meyer M, Pfarr E, Schirmer G, et al. Therapeutic use of natriuretic peptide ularitide in acute renal failure. *Ren Fail* 1999;21:85–100.

John Kellum
Associate Professor
Department of Critical Care Medicine
University of Pittsburgh
Pittsburgh
USA

Martine Leblanc
Assistant Professor of Nephrology and Critical Care
Maisonneuve–Rosemont Hospital
University of Montreal
Montreal
Canada

Ramesh Venkataraman
Visiting Instructor
Department of Critical Care Medicine
University of Pittsburgh
Pittsburgh
USA

Competing interests: JK has been paid by Gambro Healthcare Inc for lecturing and running educational programmes on acute renal failure; ML and RV none declared.

TABLE 1 **Selected risk factors for acute renal failure (ARF) (see text, p 832).**

Risk factor	Incidence of ARF	Comments
Sepsis	Unknown	Sepsis seems to be a contributing factor in as many as 43% of ARF cases[5]
Aortic clamping	Approaches 100% when > 60 minutes[6]	Refers to cross-clamping (no flow) above the renal arteries
Rhabdomyolysis	16.5%[7]	None
Aminoglycosides	8–26%[8]	None
Amphotericin	88% with > 5 g total dose[9]	60% overall incidence of nephrotoxicity

Benign prostatic hyperplasia

Search date March 2002

Robyn Webber, Michael Barry, and Claus Roehrborn

QUESTIONS

INTERVENTIONS

Key Messages

- **α Blockers** Systematic reviews and two subsequent RCTs have found that α blockers are more effective than placebo for improving lower urinary tract symptoms. Systematic reviews and subsequent RCTs found no significant differences among different α blockers. Two RCTs found limited evidence that α blockers were more effective in improving symptoms than 5α reductase inhibitors. We found no direct comparison of α blockers with surgical treatment.
- **5α reductase inhibitors** One systematic review and one subsequent RCT have found that 5α reductase inhibitors are more effective than placebo for improving lower urinary tract symptoms and reducing complications in men with benign prostatic hyperplasia, especially in men with larger prostates. Two RCTs found limited evidence that 5α reductase inhibitors were less effective at improving symptoms than α blockers. We found no direct comparison of 5α reductase inhibitors with surgical treatment.
- **β–sitosterol plant extract** One systematic review found that β–sitosterol plant extract versus placebo significantly improved lower urinary tract symptoms in the short term.
- **Rye grass pollen extract** One systematic review found limited evidence that rye grass pollen extract versus placebo increased self rated improvement and reduced nocturia in the short term.
- **Saw palmetto plant extracts** One systematic review has found that self rated improvement is better in men taking saw palmetto compared with placebo. It found no significant difference in symptom scores between saw palmetto and finasteride.

Clin Evid 2002;8:849–863.

- **Transurethral microwave thermotherapy** RCTs have found that transurethral microwave thermotherapy versus sham treatment significantly reduces symptoms. One systematic review and one RCT found limited evidence that transurethral resection relieved short term symptoms more than transurethral microwave thermotherapy. One RCT found limited evidence that transurethral microwave thermotherapy improved symptoms more than α blockers over 18 months.
- **Transurethral resection** We found limited evidence from two RCTs that transurethral resection was more effective than watchful waiting for improving symptoms and reducing complications, and did not increase the risk of erectile dysfunction or incontinence. One systematic review found greater symptom improvement with transurethral resection versus visual laser ablation, but transurethral resection was associated with a higher risk of blood transfusion.
- **Transurethral resection versus less invasive surgical techniques** We found limited evidence from two RCTs that transurethral resection is more effective than watchful waiting for improving symptoms and reducing complications, and did not increase the risk of erectile dysfunction or incontinence. Two systematic reviews and subsequent RCTs found no significant differences between transurethral resection and transurethral incision or between transurethral resection and electrical vaporisation for symptoms. One systematic review found greater symptom improvement with transurethral resection versus visual laser ablation, but transurethral resection was associated with a higher risk of blood transfusion.
- **Transurethral resection versus transurethral needle ablation** We found limited evidence from one RCT that transurethral resection versus transurethral needle ablation reduced symptoms of benign prostatic hyperplasia, although transurethral needle ablation caused fewer adverse effects.

DEFINITION Benign prostatic hyperplasia is defined histologically. Clinically, it is characterised by lower urinary tract symptoms (urinary frequency, urgency, a weak and intermittent stream, needing to strain, a sense of incomplete emptying, and nocturia), and can lead to complications, including acute urinary retention.

INCIDENCE/ PREVALENCE Estimates of the prevalence of symptomatic benign prostatic hyperplasia range from 10–30% for men in their early 70s, depending on how benign prostatic hyperplasia is defined.[1]

AETIOLOGY/ RISK FACTORS The mechanisms by which benign prostatic hyperplasia causes symptoms and complications are unclear, although bladder outlet obstruction is an important factor.[2] The best documented risk factors are increasing age and functioning testes.[3]

PROGNOSIS Community and practice based studies suggest that men with lower urinary tract symptoms can expect slow progression of the symptoms.[4,5] However, symptoms can wax and wane without treatment. In men with symptoms of benign prostatic hyperplasia, rates of acute urinary retention range from 1–2% a year.[5–7]

AIMS To reduce or alleviate lower urinary tract symptoms; to prevent complications; and to minimise adverse effects of treatment.

OUTCOMES Burden of lower urinary tract symptoms; rates of acute urinary retention and prostatectomy; risks of adverse effects of treatment; and self rated improvement. Symptoms are measured using the validated International Prostate Symptom Score (IPSS), which includes seven questions measuring symptoms on an overall scale of 0–35, with higher scores representing more frequent symptoms.[8] Older studies used a variety of symptom assessment instruments, which makes comparisons difficult (the American Urological Association Symptom Index).

METHODS This review was originally based on ongoing Medline searches and prospective journal hand searches by the Patient Outcomes Research Team for Prostatic Diseases (Agency for Health Care Policy and Research grant number HS0839). *Clinical Evidence* update search and appraisal March 2002.

QUESTION What are the effects of medical treatments?

OPTION α BLOCKERS

Systematic reviews and two subsequent RCTs have found that α blockers are more effective than placebo for improving lower urinary tract symptoms in men with benign prostatic hyperplasia. Systematic reviews and subsequent RCTs found no significant differences among different α blockers. Two RCTs found limited evidence that α blockers were more effective in improving symptoms than 5α reductase inhibitors. We found no direct comparison of α blockers with surgical treatment.

Benefits: **Versus placebo:** We found two systematic reviews that examined effects of any α blocker (search dates 1998, 21 RCTs;[9] and 1999, 24 RCTs[10]), and one systematic review that examined effects of tamsulosin (search date 2000, 6 RCTs[11]). Most RCTs included in the first two reviews found a greater improvement in symptoms with α blockers than with placebo (results presented graphically or in tabular form; overall significance not stated). The largest RCT (2084 men with benign prostatic hyperplasia) compared terazosin at doses of up to 10 mg daily for 1 year versus placebo. Treatment achieved significantly greater mean improvement in International Prostate Symptom Score (IPSS) (–7.6 points from baseline with terazosin *v* –3.7 with placebo; mean change, terazosin *v* placebo –3.9 points, 95% CI –5.5 points to –3.3 points).[12] We found insufficient evidence on the effect of α blockers on complications of benign prostatic hyperplasia. One small RCT included in the reviews (81 men) found sustained release alfuzosin (5 mg twice daily) for 48 hours increased the ability to pass urine after catheter removal in men catheterised for acute retention from 5–29% (NNT 4).[13] The third review found that tamsulosin versus placebo (0.4 or 0.8 mg daily) improved symptoms and peak urine flow (WMD for mean change from baseline for Boyarsky symptom score for 0.4 mg tamsulosin *v* placebo was –1.1 points, 95% CI –1.49 to –0.72 points; for 0.8 mg tamsulosin *v* placebo was –1.6 points, 95% CI –2.3 to –1.0; WMD for change in peak urine flow from baseline for 0.4 mg tamsulosin 1.1 mL/s, 95% CI 0.59 mL/s to 1.51 mL/s; for 0.8 mg 1.1 mL/s, 95% CI 0.65 mL/s to 1.48 mL/s). The first subsequent RCT (795 men) compared controlled released versus standard doxazosin versus placebo.[14] It found that more men had a reduction from baseline in IPSS of at least 30% with either formulation of doxazosin compared with placebo (74.7% with doxazosin *v* 73.5% with doxazosin controlled release *v* 53.5% with placebo;

absolute figures not reported, significance not stated). The second subsequent RCT (536 men) compared prolonged release alfuzosin 10 mg versus placebo, and prolonged-release alfuzosin 15 mg versus placebo. It found that alfuzosin 10 and 15 mg significantly improved symptoms compared with placebo (mean change in IPSS from baseline at end point –3.6 points with alfuzosin 10 mg *v* –3.4 points with alfuzosin 15 mg *v* –1.6 points with placebo; alfuzosin 10 mg *v* placebo P = 0.001; alfuzosin 15 mg *v* placebo P = 0.004). There was no significant difference between 10 and 15 mg.[15] **Versus each other:** We found two systematic reviews (one comparing any α blockers, search date 1998, 3 RCTs;[9] one comparing tamsulosin versus other α blockers, search date 2000, 5 RCTs[11]). The most recent review did not pool results for comparisons between tamsulosin and all other α blockers.[11] It found no significant difference between tamsulosin (0.2 mg daily) and terazosin (2–5 mg daily) for improving IPSS and urine flow (4 RCTs; WMD for change in IPSS –0.72 points, 95% CI –2.54 points to +1.51 points; WMD for change in peak urine flow –0.26 mL/s, 95% CI –1.12 mL/s to +0.60 mL/s). It similarly found no significant differences between tamsulosin and alfuzosin or prazosin (tamsulosin *v* alfuzosin: 1 RCT; improvement in Boyarsky symptom score about 40% in each group; increase in peak urine flow about 16% in each group; tamsulosin *v* prazosin: 1 RCT; improvement in IPSS 26% with tamsulosin *v* 38% with prazosin; improvement in peak urine flow 15% with tamsulosin *v* 27% with prazosin, P reported as non-significant). We found three additional RCTs.[16,17] The first was of limited quality (see comment below) and compared terazosin versus alfuzosin.[16] It found no significant difference between treatments for change in IPSS score. The second and third RCTs (total of 1475 men) were combined in a meta-analysis, which found no significant difference between standard and controlled release doxazosin for IPSS improvement from baseline (–7.9 points with controlled release *v* –8.0 points with standard; adjusted mean difference –0.1 points, 95% CI –0.5 points to +0.3 points).[17] **Versus 5α reductase inhibitors:** We found no systematic review. We found two RCTs of limited quality (see comment below).[18,19] One RCT (1229 men with benign prostatic hyperplasia) compared finasteride versus an α blocker or versus both treatments combined.[18] It found that terazosin was associated with a greater reduction in symptoms than finasteride, regardless of prostate size (difference in mean IPSS scores at 1 year 2.9 points). There was no significant difference between treatment with both agents versus terazosin alone. The second RCT (1051 men) compared alfuzosin versus finasteride versus both drugs combined over 6 months.[19] It found that alfuzosin versus finasteride significantly decreased the mean IPSS score from baseline, and found no significant difference between alfuzosin alone versus combination treatment. **Versus transurethral microwave thermotherapy:** See transurethral microwave thermotherapy, p 858.

Harms: **Versus placebo:** The first systematic review found that withdrawals attributed to adverse events were similar for alfuzosin, tamsulosin (0.4 mg dose), and placebo (results were presented graphically; significance not stated).[9] There was little observable difference between the number of men experiencing dizziness with alfuzosin or tamsulosin compared with placebo (results presented graphically; significance not stated). However, more men experienced dizziness after terazosin and doxazosin than placebo (results presented graphically; significance not stated). Both selective and less selective α blockers may be associated with abnormal ejaculation: the risk of abnormal ejaculation was higher with tamsulosin than placebo (4.5% with tamsulosin *v* 1.0% with placebo).[20] A second systematic review (search date 2000; 6 RCTs) found no significant difference between tamsulosin and placebo for withdrawal due to adverse events (4 RCTs; RR 1.08, 95% CI 0.72 to 1.62).[11] However, it found that tamsulosin significantly increased abnormal ejaculation, rhinitis, and dizziness compared with placebo (abnormal ejaculation: 4 RCTs; AR 10.8% with tamsulosin *v* < 1% with placebo; RR 17.0, 95% CI 2.5 to 114.0; rhinitis: 4 RCTs; AR 11.2% with tamsulosin *v* 6% with placebo; RR 1.84, 95% CI 1.24 to 2.72; dizziness: 5 RCTs; AR 11.9% with tamsulosin *v* 7.8% with placebo; RR 1.50, 95% CI 1.13 to 1.98). **Versus each other:** The first systematic review found that risks of dizziness, asthenia, and postural hypotension were similar with tamsulosin versus a less selective α blocker, alfuzosin (1 RCT; dizziness 7%, asthenia 2%, and postural hypotension 2% of men in each group).[9] One systematic review (search date 2000, 5 RCTs) compared tamsulosin versus other α blockers.[11] It found that men taking tamsulosin (0.2 mg daily) were less likely to discontinue treatment due to adverse effects than men taking terazosin (4 RCTs; RR 0.15, 95% CI 0.04 to 0.57). Compared with alfuzosin or prazosin, tamsulosin (0.4 or 0.2 mg daily) was associated with greater all cause withdrawal from treatment, although the differences were not significant (tamsulosin *v* alfuzosin: 1 RCT; RR for withdrawal 1.46, 95% CI 0.66 to 3.25; tamsulosin *v* prazosin: 1 RCT; RR for withdrawal 2.87, 95% CI 0.65 to 12.65).[11] The review found no significant difference between tamsulosin and alfuzosin for dizziness (1 RCT: AR 6.8% with tamsulosin *v* 7.3% with alfuzosin, RR 0.94, 95% CI 0.39 to 2.29), asthenia (1 RCT: AR 3% with tamsulosin *v* 1.6% with alfuzosin; RR 1.88, 95% CI 0.35 to 10.08), but a lower incidence of headache with alfuzosin (1 RCT: AR 7.6% with tamsulosin *v* 3.2% with alfuzosin; RR 2.35, 95% CI 0.76 to 7.29).[11] The review found that risk of abnormal ejaculation increased with increasing dose of tamsulosin (0% with 0.2 mg daily; 18% with 0.8 mg daily; significance not stated).[11] **Versus 5α reductase inhibitors:** In the RCT comparing terazosin versus finasteride, dizziness was seen in 26% of men with terazosin (8% with finasteride), generalised weakness in 14% with terazosin (7% with finasteride), rhinitis in 7% with terazosin (3% with finasteride), and postural hypotension in 8% with terazosin (2% with finasteride), whereas sexual dysfunction was more common in men taking finasteride (impotence 9% with finasteride *v* 6% with terazosin).[18]

Comment: Men with severe symptoms can expect the largest absolute fall in their symptom scores with medical treatment.[12,21] Prazosin, terazosin, and doxazosin lower blood pressure and may be used to treat both hypertension and benign prostatic hyperplasia.[22] One RCT (not included in the reviews) comparing α blockers is limited by its small sample size, low drug doses, and unclear methods of randomisation and blinding.[16]

OPTION 5α REDUCTASE INHIBITORS

One systematic review and one subsequent RCT have found that 5α reductase inhibitors are more effective than placebo for improving lower urinary tract symptoms and reducing complications in men with benign prostatic hyperplasia, especially in men with larger prostates. Two RCTs found limited evidence that 5α reductase inhibitors were less effective at improving symptoms than α blockers. We found no direct comparison with surgical treatment.

Benefits: **Versus placebo:** We found one systematic review (search date 1999, 11 338 men, 12 RCTs),[10] two non-systematic reviews,[23,24] and one subsequent RCT (generating numerous publications).[7,25–28] The systematic review found that finasteride versus placebo significantly reduced symptom scores (10 RCTs, results presented in tabular form; 9/11 individual results significant, overall significance not stated).[10] The first non-systematic review (published in 1996) combined the results of six RCTs of finasteride.[23] Treatment versus placebo was associated with a significantly greater reduction in symptom scores (difference in symptom score –0.9 points, 95% CI –1.2 to –0.6 [range of score 0–30 points]). The benefit over placebo was greatest in men with larger prostates (≥ 40 g). The second non-systematic review (meta-analysis, published in 1997) combined the results of three placebo controlled RCTs of finasteride.[24] Finasteride reduced the 2 year risk of acute urinary retention requiring catheterisation from 2.7% to 1.1% (NNT 62), of progression to prostatectomy from 6.5% to 4.2% (NNT 44), and of either event from 7.5% to 4.9% (NNT 38). The subsequent RCT (3040 men with enlarged prostates and symptoms of benign prostatic hyperplasia) compared finasteride 5 mg daily versus placebo.[7] After 4 years of treatment, finasteride versus placebo significantly reduced symptoms (difference in symptom score –1.6 points, 95% CI –2.5 to –0.7 [range of score 0–34 points]). Finasteride versus placebo significantly reduced the risk of acute urinary retention (6.6% with finasteride v 2.8% with placebo; NNT 26, 95% CI 22 to 38), of prostatectomy (8.3% with finasteride v 4.2% with placebo; NNT 24, 95% CI 19 to 37), and of the risk of either event (13.2% with finasteride v 6.6% with placebo; NNT 15, 95% CI 12 to 20). There was a greater effect among men with higher concentrations of prostate specific antigen at baseline (3.3–12.0 ng/mL), reflecting larger prostates (risk of either acute urinary retention or of needing prostatectomy was 19.9% with placebo v 8.3% with finasteride; NNT 8, 95% CI 7 to 11).[24] This RCT also found that after 4 years, finasteride versus placebo produced a larger fall in International Prostate Symptom Score. The fall was greater for men with prostate specific antigen levels greater than 1.3 ng/mL than with men with prostate specific antigen levels equal to or lower than 1.3 ng/mL.[25] **Versus α blockers:** See α blockers, p 851. We found two RCTs. Neither RCT selected men on the basis of prostate size.[18,19] They found limited evidence that 5α reductase inhibitors were less effective at improving symptoms than α blockers.

Harms: The systematic review[10] reported that RCTs found increased rates of adverse effects with finasteride versus placebo in the first year. The most common adverse events associated with finasteride in the first year were decreased libido, impotence, and ejaculatory dysfunction. The largest RCT (3168 men) found decreased libido (4.0% *v* 2.8%; not significant; P value not stated), increased impotence (6.6% *v* 4.7%; significant; P value not stated), and ejaculatory dysfunction (2.1% *v* 0.6%; significant; P value not stated) versus placebo. Another large RCT (2342 men) found decreased libido (3.1% *v* 1.2%; significant; P value not stated), increased impotence (6.8% *v* 3.2%; significant; P value not stated), and increased ejaculatory dysfunction (2.3% *v* 0.5%; significant; P value not stated). The large subsequent 4 year RCT (3040 men) found that, after the first year of treatment, there was no significant difference in decreased libido (2.6% *v* 2.6%) or impotence (5.1% *v* 5.1%) between finasteride and placebo, but there was still a slightly greater rate of ejaculation disorder (0.2% *v* 0.1%, significance not tested).[7] Although finasteride reduced concentrations of prostate specific antigen by a mean of 50% (individual responses were highly variable), its use for up to 4 years did not change the rate of detection of prostate cancer compared with placebo.[7] **Versus α blockers:** See α blockers, p 851.

Comment: The meta-analysis of finasteride's impact on symptoms at 1–2 years found that finasteride was significantly more effective than placebo in men with larger prostates.[23] However, the absolute difference in mean decrease of symptom score from baseline between men with the smallest and largest prostates was only about one point. The relative effectiveness of finasteride versus placebo also seemed higher in men with slightly raised prostate specific antigen levels,[25] and it is assumed that the higher prostate specific antigen is a proxy for a larger prostate.

QUESTION What are the effects of surgical treatments?

OPTION TRANSURETHRAL RESECTION OF THE PROSTATE

We found limited evidence from two RCTs that transurethral resection was more effective than watchful waiting for improving symptoms and reducing complications, and did not increase the risk of erectile dysfunction or incontinence. Two systematic reviews and subsequent RCTs found no significant difference in symptoms between transurethral resection and transurethral incision or between transurethral resection and electrical vaporisation. One systematic review and subsequent RCTs found limited evidence that transurethral resection may improve symptoms more than visual laser ablation than but that transurethral resection may be associated with a higher risk of blood transfusion.

Benefits: **Versus watchful waiting:** We found no systematic review. We found two RCTs comparing transurethral resection (TURP) versus conservative treatment.[29,30] The first RCT (556 men with moderate symptoms of benign prostatic hyperplasia) compared TURP versus watchful waiting.[29] More men receiving TURP versus watchful waiting improved (90% with TURP *v* 39% with watchful waiting), and had reduced symptoms. After 5 years, the treatment failure rate was 10% with TURP versus 21% with watchful waiting (NNT 9, 95% CI 7 to 17), and 36% of men assigned to watchful waiting had crossed over to surgery.[31] Treatment failure was defined as death, acute urinary retention, high residual urine volume, renal azotaemia, bladder stones, persistent incontinence, or a high symptom score. The major categories of treatment failure reduced by TURP were acute urinary retention, development of a large bladder residual (> 350 mL), and deterioration to a severe symptom level. The second RCT (223 men) had a shorter duration of follow up (7.5 months).[30] It found that TURP versus monitoring significantly improved the International Prostate Symptom Score (IPSS) (difference in IPSS 10.4 points, 95% CI 8.5 points to 12.3 points). **Versus less invasive techniques:** We found three systematic reviews and four subsequent RCTs.[32–38] The first review (search date 1999, 9 RCTs) compared TURP versus transurethral incision.[32] Four RCTs (243 men) examined symptom scores at 12 months and found no significant difference (WMD +0.2 points, 95% CI –0.8 points to +1.1 points). The review found little good, long term evidence. The second review (search date 1999) compared TURP versus visual laser ablation (4 RCTs, 331 men) or laser contact vaporisation (1 RCT, 28 men).[33] The review did not perform a meta-analysis. The RCTs comparing TURP versus visual laser ablation found that TURP was more effective at reducing symptom score, but length of hospital stay was shorter with visual laser ablation. The largest RCT (151 men) found significantly better changes in symptom scores at 52 weeks' follow up with TURP (American Urological Association Index mean score reduced with TURP from 18.2 preoperatively to 5.1 *v* 18.1 to 7.7 with laser ablation). The RCT of TURP versus laser contact vaporisation (28 men, 3 treatment groups) found no significant difference in symptom scores or quality of life at 12 months' follow up.[33] Two subsequent RCTs found higher surgical re-treatment rates with laser ablation and with laser contact vaporisation (38% with visual laser ablation *v* 16% with TURP at 5 years[37] and 19% with laser contact vaporisation *v* 9% with TURP at 3 years[38]). One RCT (120 men) compared Holmium laser ablation versus TURP. It found no significant difference in symptom scores at 1 year (American Urological Association Index score Holmium 4.2 *v* TURP 4.8; P = 0.92).[36] The third systematic review (search date 1999, 5 RCTs, 454 men) compared TURP versus electrical vaporisation.[34] Meta-analysis of three RCTs found a greater improvement in symptom scores at 12–24 months with electrical vaporisation but the difference was not significant (figures reported as SMD +0.21, 95% CI –0.03 to +0.44). One of the RCTs reported a significant reduction in symptom score with electrical vaporisation and four found no significant difference. Two subsequent RCTs compared TURP and electrical vaporisation.[39,40] The first (100 men) found no significant difference between treatments in symptoms at 3 months after treatment (mean IPSS decreased from 21.6 points to 5.0 points with TURP *v* from 19.4 points to 4.0 points with vaporisation; CI and P value for direct comparison not stated).[39] The second RCT (185 men) also found no significant difference between treatments for symptoms at 12 months (mean decrease in IPSS from baseline 12.8 points for

TURP *v* 12.5 points for vaporisation; CI and P value not stated).[40] **Versus transurethral microwave thermotherapy and transurethral needle ablation:** See transurethral microwave thermotherapy, p 858, and transurethral needle ablation, p 859.

Harms: Analysis of administrative data found that mortality in the 30 days after TURP for benign prostatic hyperplasia ranged from 0.4% for men aged 65–69 years to 1.9% for men aged 80–84 years, and has fallen in recent years.[41] In one review of observational studies, TURP for benign prostatic hyperplasia was associated with immediate surgical complications in 12% of men, bleeding requiring intervention in 2%, erectile dysfunction in 14%, retrograde ejaculation in 74%, and incontinence in about 5%.[42–44] Analysis of claims data found a reoperation rate, implying need for retreatment, of about 1% a year.[41] However, in the only comparative trial, men randomised to prostatectomy did not seem to have a greater rate of erectile dysfunction or incontinence than men assigned to watchful waiting.[29,31] One systematic review found that visual laser ablation is associated with a lower risk of blood transfusion than TURP (RR 0.09, 95% CI 0.02 to 0.47; 0/145 [0%] with laser ablation *v* 15/146 [10%] with TURP), but a higher risk of urinary tract infection (RR 3.85, 95% CI 1.87 to 7.94; absolute figures not stated).[33] The largest RCT found fewer cases of blood transfusion with visual laser ablation versus TURP (0/76 [0%] with laser ablation *v* 12/75 [16%] with TURP). The third systematic review found that TURP and electrical vaporisation had similar risks of blood transfusion, irritative symptoms, and urinary tract infections although confidence intervals were large.[34] However, electrical vaporisation was associated with a significant increase in the risk of urinary retention (17.1% with electrical vaporisation *v* 3.8% with TURP; RR 3.64, 95% CI 1.68 to 7.92; absolute figures not stated) compared with TURP. One RCT (150 men) in the review reported more transient stress urinary incontinence with electrical vaporisation versus TURP (13/70 [19%] with electrical vaporisation *v* 0/80 [0%] with TURP). The first subsequent RCT (100 men) found that no-one having either TURP or electrical vaporisation required transfusion.[39] It also found no significant difference for rates of erectile dysfunction between the two groups (22% with TURP *v* 24% with vaporisation; P values and CI not stated).[40] However, the second subsequent RCT (185 men) found no significant difference between TURP and electrical vaporisation for rates of postoperative incontinence (6/92 [6.5%] with TURP *v* 5/93 [5.4%] with vaporisation; RR 1.2, 95% CI 0.4 to 3.8).[40] Rates of haemorrhage requiring blood transfusion and of urethral stricture were low in both groups and not significantly different (transfusion: 9/92 [9.8%] with TURP *v* 6/93 [6.5%] with vaporisation, RR 1.5, 95% CI 0.6 to 4.1; urethral stricture 7/92 [7.6%] with TURP *v* 5/93 [5.4%] with vaporisation, RR 1.4, 95% CI 0.5 to 4.3).[40]

Comment: Rapid changes in techniques and few controlled trials with adequate follow up make comparisons between TURP and newer surgical techniques difficult. In the first systematic review, RCTs were limited by sample size (total 350 men) and duration of follow up (maximum 24 months). The second review reported that RCTs of

TURP versus laser ablation were limited generally by small sample size, brief follow up, and lack of blinding.[33] The third review of TURP versus electrical vaporisation found that none of the RCTs were blinded or intention to treat, but four out of five RCTs had less than 10% loss to follow up.[34]

OPTION TRANSURETHRAL MICROWAVE THERMOTHERAPY

RCTs have found that transurethral microwave thermotherapy versus sham treatment significantly reduces symptoms of benign prostatic hyperplasia. One systematic review and one RCT found limited evidence that transurethral resection relieved short term symptoms better than thermotherapy. One RCT found limited evidence that thermotherapy improved symptoms more than α blockers over 18 months.

Benefits: **Versus sham treatment:** We found no systematic review. We found three small to medium sized RCTs comparing transurethral microwave thermotherapy (TUMT) versus sham treatment.[45–47] In the largest RCT (220 men), TUMT improved the International Prostate Symptom Score (IPSS) significantly more than sham treatment (5 points lower; $P < 0.05$).[45] In the second RCT (169 men), TUMT significantly improved IPSS more than sham treatment at 6 months ($P < 0.05$).[46] The third RCT (50 men) compared TUMT versus sham treatment. It found a greater reduction in symptom score with TUMT versus sham treatment (Masden symptom score reduction 7.3 with TUMT *v* 3.9 with sham treatment; significance was not tested). **Versus transurethral resection of the prostate:** We found one systematic review[34] (search date 1999, 3 RCTs, 200 men) comparing TUMT versus transurethral resection (TURP) and one additional RCT.[48] In the systematic review, symptom improvement was significantly better with TURP in one RCT ($P < 0.05$) but not significantly different in the other two.[34] The additional RCT (147 men) found better symptomatic outcomes with TURP (IPSS change *v* baseline at 1 year: 60% with TUMT *v* 85% with TURP; significance not stated).[48] **Versus α blockers:** One RCT (103 men) compared TUMT versus terazosin (up to 10 mg daily) and found significantly more improvement in symptoms after TUMT at 6 and 18 months (difference in IPSS at 18 months 35%; $P < 0.001$).[49,50]

Harms: Adverse events associated with TUMT varied among trials, but included the need for catheterisation for more than 1 week (8% with TUMT *v* 2% with sham treatment),[46] persistent irritative symptoms (22% with TUMT *v* 8% with sham treatment),[45] haematuria (14% with TUMT *v* 1% with sham treatment),[45] and sexual dysfunction (mostly haematospermia and other ejaculatory abnormalities, 29% with TUMT *v* 1% with sham treatment).[45] In one RCT, retrograde ejaculation was substantially less common after TUMT versus TURP (27% with TUMT *v* 74% with TURP).[51] The RCT (103 men) comparing TUMT versus α blockers found more adverse events in the α blocker group over the first 6 months (17 events between 52 men with α blockers *v* 7 events between 51 men with TUMT).[49,50] With α blockers the most common adverse events were dizziness (7 cases) and asthenia (4 cases); in the TUMT group they were urinary tract infection (3 cases).

Comment: TUMT can be performed in an outpatient setting, and uses heat generated by a microwave antennae in the urethra to coagulate prostate tissue. The long term effects of TUMT have not been adequately evaluated in controlled studies. The systematic review reported that trials were limited by small sample size, short duration of follow up (maximum 30 months), and large loss to follow up.

OPTION TRANSURETHRAL NEEDLE ABLATION

We found limited evidence from one RCT that transurethral resection versus transurethral needle ablation reduced symptoms of benign prostatic hyperplasia, although transurethral needle ablation caused fewer adverse effects.

Benefits: We found no systematic review. **Versus transurethral resection:** We found one RCT (121 men) comparing transurethral resection (TURP) versus transurethral needle ablation (TUNA).[52] The mean International Prostate Symptoms Score (IPSS) at 1 year was significantly lower with TURP than TUNA (IPSS 11.1 points with TUNA *v* 8.3 points with TURP; P = 0.04).

Harms: Compared with TURP, TUNA was associated with less retrograde ejaculation (38% with TURP *v* 0% with TUNA) and bleeding (100% with TURP *v* 32% with TUNA).[52]

Comment: TUNA can be performed in an outpatient setting, and uses radiofrequency energy through two intraprostatic electrodes to generate heat to coagulate prostate tissue. Anaesthesia requirements vary in reported studies. The long term effects of treatment have not been adequately evaluated.

QUESTION What are the effects of herbal treatments?

OPTION SAW PALMETTO PLANT EXTRACTS

One systematic review has found that self rated improvement is better in men taking saw palmetto compared with placebo. It found no significant difference in symptom scores between saw palmetto and finasteride.

Benefits: We found one systematic and one subsequent non-systematic review. The systematic review (search date 1997, 18 RCTs, 2939 men) included all saw palmetto preparations;[53] the non-systematic review (11 RCTs) included only one saw palmetto preparation.[54] **Versus placebo:** The systematic review found that more men reported self rated improvement with saw palmetto versus placebo (6 RCTs: RR 1.7, 95% CI 1.2 to 2.4). It found a significant difference in nocturia in men receiving saw palmetto compared with placebo (10 RCTs: WMD of 0.76 episodes/night, 95% CI 0.32 to 1.21).[53] The non-systematic review focused only on nocturia and found similar results.[54] **Versus 5α reductase inhibitors:** The systematic review (2 RCTs, 1440 men) found a greater improvement in symptom scores with finasteride versus saw palmetto but the difference was not significant (WMD +0.37, 95% CI –0.44 to +1.19).[53]

Harms: In the systematic review, withdrawal rates were significantly higher with saw palmetto versus placebo (9% with saw palmetto *v* 7% with placebo; P = 0.02), and not significantly different versus finasteride (9% with saw palmetto *v* 11% with finasteride; P = 0.87). The risk of erectile dysfunction was similar with saw palmetto versus placebo (1.1% with saw palmetto *v* 0.7% with placebo; P = 0.58), but was significantly lower versus finasteride (1.1% with saw palmetto *v* 4.9% with finasteride; P < 0.001).[53]

Comment: The RCTs were brief and few used a validated symptom score. Different preparations, which may not be equivalent, are available directly to consumers without prescription in many countries.

OPTION β–SITOSTEROL PLANT EXTRACT

One systematic review found that β–sitosterol plant extract versus placebo significantly improved lower urinary tract symptoms compared with placebo in the short term.

Benefits: **Versus placebo:** We found one systematic review (search date 1998, 4 RCTs, 519 men), which compared β–sitosterol versus placebo.[51] Trials lasted for 4–26 weeks. The review found that β–sitosterol significantly reduced the International Prostate Symptom Score (2 RCTs: WMD –4.9 points, 95% CI –6.3 to –3.5).

Harms: Gastrointestinal adverse effects occurred in more men taking β–sitosterol than placebo (1.6% with β–sitosterol *v* 0% with placebo; significance not stated). Impotence was also more common in men taking β–sitosterol (0.5% β–sitosterol *v* 0% with placebo; significance not stated). Withdrawal rates were similar in both groups (7.8% with β–sitosterol *v* 8.0% with placebo; significance not stated).[51]

Comment: The RCTs were limited by a short follow up period (maximum 26 wks). Different preparations are available, which may be of variable content, making it difficult to generalise results.

OPTION RYE GRASS POLLEN EXTRACT

One systematic review found limited evidence that rye grass pollen extract versus placebo increased self rated improvement and reduced nocturia compared with placebo in the short term.

Benefits: **Versus placebo:** We found one systematic review (search date 1997, 2 RCTs, 163 men), which compared rye grass pollen extract versus placebo.[55] It found that pollen extract versus placebo significantly increased self rated improvement (1 RCT, 60 men: 20/31 [65%] with pollen *v* 7/26 [27%] with placebo; RR 2.40, 95% CI 1.21 to 4.75; NNT 3, 95% CI 2 to 9), and significantly reduced nocturia (2 RCTs: 50/79 [63%] with pollen *v* 23/74 [31%] with placebo; RR 2.05, 95% CI 1.41 to 3.99). However, the results should be interpreted with caution (see comment below).[55]

Harms: The review found that nausea occurred in one man taking pollen extract (number in placebo group not stated). Withdrawal rates were not significantly different (4.8% with pollen *v* 2.7% with placebo; P = 0.26).[55]

Comment: Both RCTs were limited by small sample sizes and a short follow up period (12 and 24 wks). Concealment of treatment allocation was unclear. The composition of the preparations was unknown, making it difficult to generalise results.

Substantive changes

α Blockers One new systematic review and one new RCT;[11,15] conclusions unchanged.

TURP versus less invasive techniques Two new RCTs;[39,40] conclusions unchanged.

REFERENCES

1. Bosch JL, Hop WC, Kirkels WJ, et al. Natural history of benign prostatic hyperplasia: appropriate case definition and estimation of its prevalence in the community. *Urology* 1995;46(suppl A):34–40.
2. Barry MJ, Adolfsson J, Batista JE, et al. Committee 6: measuring the symptoms and health impact of benign prostatic hyperplasia and its treatments. In: Denis L, Griffiths K, Khoury S, et al, eds. *Fourth International Consultation on BPH, Proceedings*. Plymouth, UK: Health Publication Ltd, 1998:265–321.
3. Oishi K, Boyle P, Barry MJ, et al. Committee 1: Epidemiology and natural history of benign prostatic hyperplasia. In: Denis L, Griffiths K, Khoury S, et al, eds. *Fourth International Consultation on BPH, Proceedings*. Plymouth, UK: Health Publication Ltd, 1998:23–59.
4. Jacobsen SJ, Girman CJ, Guess HA, et al. Natural history of prostatism: longitudinal changes in voiding symptoms in community dwelling men. *J Urol* 1996;155:595–600.
5. Barry MJ, Fowler FJ, Bin L, et al. The natural history of patients with benign prostatic hyperplasia as diagnosed by North American urologists. *J Urol* 1997;157:10–15.
6. Jacobsen S, Jacobson D, Girman C, et al. Natural history of prostatism: risk factors for acute urinary retention. *J Urol* 1997;158:481–487.
7. McConnell J, Bruskewitz R, Walsh P, et al. The effect of finasteride on the risk of acute urinary retention and the need for surgical treatment among men with benign prostatic hyperplasia. *N Engl J Med* 1998;338:557–563.
8. Barry MJ, Fowler FJ Jr, O'Leary MP, et al. The American Urological Association symptom index for benign prostatic hyperplasia. *J Urol* 1992;148:1549–1557.
9. Djavan B, Marberger M. A meta-analysis on the efficacy and tolerability of α1-adrenoceptor antagonists in patients with lower urinary tract symptoms suggestive of benign prostatic obstruction. *Eur Urol* 1999;36:1–13. Search date 1998; primary source Medline.
10. Clifford GM, Farmer RDT. Medical therapy for benign prostatic hyperplasia: a review of the literature. *Eur Urol* 2000;38:2–19. Search date 1999; primary sources Medline, Embase, and the Cochrane Library.
11. Wilt TJ, MacDonald R, Nelson D. Tamsulosin for treating lower urinary tract symptoms compatible with benign prostatic obstruction: a systematic review of efficacy and adverse effects. *J Urol* 2002;167:177–183. Search date 2000; primary sources Medline, Embase, The Cochrane Library, Cochrane prostatic Disease and Urologic Malignancies Group Trial Register, and hand searched reference lists.
12. Roehrborn CG, Oesterling JE, Auerbach S, et al. The Hytrin community assessment trial study: a one–year study of terazosin versus placebo in the treatment of men with symptomatic benign prostatic hyperplasia. *Urology* 1996;47:159–168.
13. McNeil SA, Daruwala PD, Mitchell IDC, et al. Sustained-release alfuzosin and trial without catheter after acute urinary retention: a prospective placebo-controlled trial. *BJU Int* 1999;84:622–627.
14. Andersen M, Dahlstrand C, Hoye K. Double blind trial of the efficacy and tolerability of doxazosin in the gastrointestinal therapeutic system, doxazosin standard, and placebo in patients with benign prostatic hyperplasia. *Eur Urol* 2000;38:400–409.
15. Roehrborn CG. Efficacy and safety of once-daily alfuzosin in the treatment of lower urinary tract symptoms and clinical benign prostatic hyperplasia: a randomized, placebo-controlled trial. *Urology* 2001;58:953–959.
16. Fourcade RO. Efficiency and tolerance of terazosine in ambulatory patients with benign prostatic hypertrophy: comparative randomized and double-blind trial versus alfuzosin. *Prog Urol* 2000;10:246–253.
17. Kirby RS, Andersen M, Gratzke P, et al. A combined meta-analysis of double-blind trials of the efficacy and tolerability of doxazosin-gastrointestinal therapeutic system, doxazosin standard and placebo in patients with benign prostatic hyperplasia. *BJU Int* 2001;87:192–200.
18. Lepor H, Williford WO, Barry MJ, et al. The efficacy of terazosin, finasteride, or both in benign prostatic hyperplasia. Veterans' Affairs cooperative studies benign prostatic hyperplasia study group. *N Engl J Med* 1996;335:533–539.
19. Debruyne FMJ, Jardin A, Colloi D, et al. Sustained-release alfuzosin, finasteride and the combination of both in the treatment of benign prostatic hyperplasia. *Eur Urol* 1998;34:169–175.
20. Hofner K, Claes H, De Reijke TM, et al. Tamsulosin 0.4 mg once daily: effect on sexual function in patients with lower urinary tract symptoms suggestive of benign prostatic obstruction. *Eur Urol* 1999;36:335–341.
21. Mobley D, Dias N, Levenstein M. Effects of doxazosin in patients with mild, intermediate, and severe benign prostatic hyperplasia. *Clin Ther* 1998;20:101–109.
22. Kaplan S, Kaplan N. Alpha-blockade: monotherapy for hypertension and benign prostatic hyperplasia. *Urology* 1996;48:541–550.
23. Boyle P, Gould AL, Roehrborn CG. Prostate volume predicts outcome of treatment of benign prostatic hyperplasia with finasteride: meta-analysis of randomized clinical trials. *Urology* 1996;48:398–405.
24. Andersen J, Nickel J, Marshall V, et al. Finasteride significantly reduces acute urinary retention and

need for surgery in patients with symptomatic benign prostatic hyperplasia. *Urology* 1997;49:839–845.

25. Roehrborn CG, Boyle P, Bergner D, et al. Serum prostate specific antigen and prostate volume predict long-term changes in symptoms and flow rate: results of a four-year, randomised trial comparing finasteride and placebo. *Urology* 1999:54;663–669.
26. Roehrborn CG, McConnell JD, Lieber M, et al. Serum prostate-specific antigen concentration is a powerful predictor of acute urinary retention and the need for surgery in men with clinical benign prostatic hyperplasia. *Urology* 1999;53:473–480.
27. Roehrborn CG, Bruskewitz R, Nickel GC, et al. Urinary retention in patients with BPH treated with finasteride or placebo over 4 years. *Eur Urol* 2000;37:528–536.
28. Kaplan S, Garvin D, Gilhooly P, et al. Impact of baseline symptom severity on future risk of benign prostatic hyperplasia-related outcomes and long-term response to finasteride. *Urology* 2000;56:610–616.
29. Wasson J, Reda D, Bruskewitz R, et al. A comparison of transurethral surgery with watchful waiting for moderate symptoms of benign prostatic hyperplasia. *N Engl J Med* 1995;332:75–79.
30. Donovan JL, Peters T, Neal DE, et al. A randomized trial comparing transurethral resection of the prostate, laser therapy and conservative treatment of men with symptoms associated with benign prostatic enlargement: the ClasP study. *J Urol* 2000;164:65–70.
31. Flanigan RC, Reda DC, Wasson JH, et al. Five year outcome of surgical resection and watchful waiting for men with moderately symptomatic benign prostatic hyperplasia: a Department of Veterans' Affairs cooperative study. *J Urol* 1998;160:12–17.
32. Yang Q, Peters TJ, Donovan JL, et al. Transurethral incision compared with transurethral resection of the prostate for bladder outlet obstruction: a systematic review and meta-analysis of randomized controlled trials. *J Urol* 2001;165:1526–1532. Search date 1999; primary sources Medline, Embase, ISI, the Cochrane Library, and Cochrane Prostatic Diseases and Urologic Cancers Group Trial Register.
33. Wheelahan J, Scott NA, Cartmill R, et al. Minimally invasive laser techniques for prostatectomy: a systematic review. *BJU Int* 2000;86:805–815. Search date 1999; primary sources Medline, Embase, Current Contents, and the Cochrane Library.
34. Wheelahan J, Scott NA, Cartmill R, et al. Minimally invasive non-laser thermal techniques for prostatectomy: a systematic review. *BJU Int* 2000;86:977–988. Search date 1999; primary sources Medline, Embase, Current Contents, and the Cochrane Library.
35. Riehmann M, Knes JM, Heisey D, et al. Transurethral resection versus incision of the prostate: a randomized, prospective study. *Urology* 1995;45:768–775.
36. Gilling PJ, Mackey M, Cresswell M, et al. Holmium laser versus transurethral resection of the prostate: a randomized prospective trial with 1-year followup. *J Urol* 1999;162:1640–1644.
37. McAllister WJ, Absalom MJ, Mir K, et al. Does endoscopic laser ablation of the prostate stand the test of time? Five-year results test results from a multicentre randomised controlled trial of endoscopic laser ablation against transurethral resection of the prostate. *BJU Int* 2000;85:437–439.
38. Keoghane SR, Lawrence KC, Gray AM, et al. A double-blind randomized controlled trial and economic evaluation of transurethral resection vs contact laser vaporization for benign prostatic enlargement: a 3-year follow-up. *BJU Int* 2000;85:74–78.
39. Kupeli S, Yilmaz E, Soygur T, et al. Randomized study of transurethral resection of the prostate and combined transurethral resection and vaporization of the prostate as a therapeutic alternative in men with benign prostatic hyperplasia. *J Endourol* 2001;15:317–321.
40. Helke C, Manseck A, Hakenberg OW, et al. Is transurethral vaporesection of the prostate better than standard transurethral resection? *Eur Urol* 2001;39:551–557.
41. Lu-Yao GL, Barry MJ, Chang CH, et al. Transurethral resection of the prostate among Medicare beneficiaries in the United States: time trends and outcomes. *Urology* 1994;44:692–698.
42. McConnell JD, Barry MJ, Bruskewitz RC, et al. *Direct treatment outcomes–complications. Benign prostatic hyperplasia: diagnosis and treatment.* Clinical Practice Guideline, Number 8. Rockville, Maryland: Agency for Health Care Policy and Research, Public Health Service, US Department of Health and Human Services, 1994:91–98.
43. McConnell JD, Barry MJ, Bruskewitz RC, et al. *Direct treatment outcomes – sexual dysfunction. Benign prostatic hyperplasia: diagnosis and treatment.* Clinical Practice Guideline, Number 8. Rockville, Maryland: Agency for Health Care Policy and Research, Public Health Service, US Department of Health and Human Services, 1994:99–103.
44. McConnell JD, Barry MJ, Bruskewitz RC, et al. *Direct treatment outcomes – urinary incontinence. Benign prostatic hyperplasia: diagnosis and treatment.* Clinical Practice Guideline, Number 8. Rockville, Maryland: Agency for Health Care Policy and Research, Public Health Service, US Department of Health and Human Services, 1994:105–106.
45. Roehrborn C, Preminger G, Newhall P, et al. Microwave thermotherapy for benign prostatic hyperplasia with the Dornier Urowave: results of a randomized, double-blind, multicenter, sham-controlled trial. *Urology* 1998;51:19–28.
46. Larson T, Blute M, Bruskewitz R, et al. A high-efficiency microwave thermoablation system for the treatment of benign prostatic hyperplasia: results of a randomized, sham-controlled, prospective, double-blind, multicenter clinical trial. *Urology* 1998;51:731–742.
47. De la Rosette J, De Wildt M, Alivizatos G, et al. Transurethral microwave thermotherapy (TUMT) in benign prostatic hyperplasia: placebo versus TUMT. *Urology* 1994;44:58–63.
48. Francisca EA, D'Ancona FC, Meuleman EJ, et al. Sexual function following high energy microwave thermotherapy: results of a randomized controlled study comparing transurethral microwave thermotherapy to transurethral prostatic resection. *J Urol* 1999;161:486–490.
49. Djavan B, Roehrborn CG, Shariat S, et al. Prospective randomized comparison of high energy transurethral microwave thermotherapy versus alpha blocker treatment of patients with benign prostatic hyperplasia. *J Urol* 1999;161:139–143.
50. Djavan B, Seitz C, Roehrborn C, et al. Targeted transurethral microwave thermotherapy versus alpha-blockade in benign prostatic hyperplasia: outcomes at 18 months. *Urology* 2001;57:66–70.
51. Wilt TJ, Macdonald R, Ishani A. Beta-sitosterol for the treatment of benign prostatic hyperplasia: a systematic review. *BJU Int* 1999;83:976–983.

Search date 1998; primary sources Medline, Embase, Phytodok, and the Cochrane Library.

52. Bruskewitz R, Issa M, Roehrborn C, et al. A prospective, randomized 1-year clinical trial comparing transurethral needle ablation to transurethral resection of the prostate for the treatment of symptomatic benign prostatic hyperplasia. *J Urol* 1998;159:1588–1594.
53. Wilt T, Ishani A, Stark G, et al. Serenoa repens for benign prostatic hyperplasia. In: The Cochrane Library, Issue 2, 2002. Oxford: Update Software. Search date 1997; primary sources Medline, Embase, Phytodok, and the Cochrane Library.
54. Boyle P, Robertson C, Lowe F, et al. Meta-analysis of clinical trials of Permixon in the treatment of benign prostatic hyperplasia. *Urology* 2000;55:533–539.
55. Macdonald R, Ishani A, Rutks I, et al. A systematic review of Cernilton for the treatment of benign prostatic hyperplasia. *BJU Int* 2000;85:836–841. Search date 1997; primary sources Embase and the Cochrane Library. Additional Medline search 1998.

Robyn Webber
Consultant Urologist
Hairmyres Hospital
East Kilbride
Scotland

Michael Barry
General Medicine Unit
Massachusetts General Hospital
Boston
USA

Claus Rochrborn
Associate Professor
Department of Urology
The University of Texas Southwestern
Medical Center
Dallas
USA

Competing interests: MB, none declared. CR has received a fee for consulting, speaking, research, and running educational programmes for MSD, GlaxoSmithKline, Sanofi Synthélabo, and Urologix. RW has been reimbursed by MSD, the manufacturers of finostende, for attending several conferences.

Chronic prostatitis

Search date June 2002

Jeffrey Stern and Anthony Schaeffer

QUESTIONS

INTERVENTIONS

Key Messages

In men with chronic bacterial prostatitis

- **α Blockers (when added to antimicrobials)** We found limited evidence from one RCT suggesting that adding α blockers to antimicrobials versus antimicrobials alone may significantly improve symptoms and reduce recurrence.
- **Oral antimicrobial drugs** We found no RCTs of the effects of oral antimicrobial drugs. Retrospective cohort studies report cure rates of 0–88% depending on the drug used and the duration of treatment.
- **Local injection of antimicrobials; radical prostatectomy; transurethral resection** We found no RCTs on the effects of these interventions.

In men with chronic abacterial prostatitis

- **Allopurinol** One systematic review found limited evidence from one small RCT that allopurinol versus placebo significantly improved symptoms over about 8 months.
- **Anti-inflammatory medications (pentosan polysulfate sodium)** One RCT found no significant difference with pentosan polysulfate sodium versus placebo in symptoms, but the RCT may have been too small to rule out a clinically important difference.
- **α Blockers** One systematic review found limited evidence suggesting that α blockers versus placebo may significantly improve maximal flow time and pain.
- **5α-Reductase inhibitors** One systematic review of one small RCT found insufficient evidence on the effects of 5α reductase inhibitors.

- **Transurethral microwave thermotherapy** One systematic review found limited evidence from one RCT suggesting that transurethral microwave thermotherapy versus sham treatment may significantly improve quality of life at 3 months, and symptoms over 21 months.
- **Biofeedback; prostatic massage; Sitz bath** We found no good evidence on these interventions.

DEFINITION **Chronic bacterial prostatitis** is characterised by a positive culture of expressed prostatic secretions. It can be symptomatic (recurrent urinary tract infection, or suprapubic, lower back, or perineal pain), asymptomatic, or associated with minimal urgency, frequency, and dysuria. **Chronic abacterial prostatitis** is characterised by pelvic or perineal pain, often associated with urinary urgency, nocturia, weak urinary stream, frequency, dysuria, hesitancy, dribbling after micturition, interrupted flow, and inflammation (white cells) in prostatic secretions. Symptoms can also include suprapubic, scrotal, testicular, penile, or lower back pain or discomfort, known as prostodynia, in the absence of inflammation in prostatic secretions.

INCIDENCE/ PREVALENCE One US community based study (58 955 visits by men ≥ 18 years to office based physicians) estimated that 9% of men have a diagnosis of chronic prostatitis at any one time.[1] Another study found that, of men with genitourinary symptoms, 8% presenting to urologists and 1% presenting to primary care physicians are diagnosed with chronic prostatitis.[2] Most cases of chronic prostatitis are abacterial. Acute bacterial prostatitis, although easy to diagnose and treat, is rare.

AETIOLOGY/ RISK FACTORS Organisms commonly implicated in bacterial prostatitis include *Escherichia coli*, other Gram negative *Enterobacteriaceae*, occasionally *Pseudomonas* species, and rarely Gram positive enterococci. The cause of abacterial prostatitis is unclear, but autoimmunity could be involved.[3]

PROGNOSIS One recent study found that chronic abacterial prostatitis had an impact on quality of life similar to that from angina, Crohn's disease, or a previous myocardial infarction.[4]

AIMS To relieve symptoms and eliminate infection where present, with minimum adverse effects.

OUTCOMES Symptom improvement (symptom scores, bother scores); quality of life; urodynamics; rates of bacteriological cure (clearance of previously documented organisms from prostatic secretions).

METHODS *Clinical Evidence* search and appraisal June 2002. Additional author search of Medline up to July 1998.

QUESTION What are the effects of treatments for chronic bacterial prostatitis?

OPTION ORAL ANTIMICROBIAL DRUGS

We found no RCTs of the effects of oral antimicrobial drugs. Retrospective cohort studies report cure rates of 0–88% depending on the drug used and the duration of treatment.

Benefits: We found no systematic review and no RCTs. **Trimethoprim-sulfamethoxazole:** One non-systematic review identified 10 retrospective cohort studies in 135 men with bacteriologically confirmed prostatitis treated with trimethoprim-sulfamethoxazole (trimethoprim-sulphamethoxazole) (160 mg/800 mg twice daily for 10–140 days).[5] The studies reported cure rates of 0–71%. Over 30% of men were cured when treated for at least 90 days. **Quinolones:** One review summarised three retrospective cohort studies in 106 men treated with norfloxacin (400 mg twice daily for 10, 28, and 174 days).[6] The studies reported cure rates of 64–88%. We also found six retrospective cohort studies in 141 men treated with ciprofloxacin (250–500 mg twice daily for 14–259 days), with cure rates of 60–75%. **Amoxicillin/clavulanic acid and clindamycin:** One cohort study included 50 men who were resistant to empirical treatment with quinolone. The expressed prostatic secretions from 24 of these men exhibited high colony counts of Gram positive and Gram negative anaerobic bacteria, either alone (18 men) or in combination with aerobic bacteria (6 men). After treatment with either amoxicillin (amoxycillin)/clavulanic acid or clindamycin for 3–6 weeks, all men had a decrease or total elimination of symptoms and no anaerobic bacteria were detected in prostatic secretions.[7]

Harms: The studies of trimethoprim-sulfamethoxazole did not report adverse effects. In the other studies, toxicity from quinolones was rare. Late relapse (6–12 months after treatment) was common.

Comment: Higher cure rates with quinolones may be explained by greater penetration into the prostate.[8] We reviewed only studies that used standard methods to localise infection to the prostate.[9]

OPTION LOCAL INJECTION OF ANTIMICROBIALS

We found no RCTs on the local injection of antimicrobials.

Benefits: We found no systematic review and no RCTs.

Harms: Infection is a theoretical risk of this invasive procedure.

Comment: One small cohort study (24 men with refractory chronic bacterial prostatitis) found that eradication of infection was eventually achieved after an unstated period in 15 men with gentamicin (160 mg) plus cefazolin (cephazolin) (3 g) injected directly into the prostate through the perineum.[10]

OPTION α BLOCKERS

We found limited evidence from one RCT suggesting that adding α blockers to antimicrobials versus antimicrobials alone may significantly improve symptoms and reduce recurrence.

Benefits: We found no systematic review. We found no RCTs comparing α blockers versus placebo. We found one RCT (64 men with bacterial prostatitis; mean age 48 years) of α blockers (either 1–2 mg terazosin daily, 2.5 mg terazosin daily, or 2.5 mg alfuzosin once or twice daily) plus antimicrobials versus antimicrobials alone.[11] Men given α blockers plus antimicrobials versus antimicrobials alone had significantly higher rates of symptomatic improvement and significantly lower rates of recurrence (assessed by culture of expressed prostatic secretions; $P = 0.02$; no RR or CI provided; 5 people withdrew from treatment).

Harms: No adverse effects of α blockers were reported in this study.[11]

Comment: None.

OPTION **TRANSURETHRAL RESECTION**

We found no RCTs on the effects of transurethral resection.

Benefits: We found no systematic review, RCTs, or prospective cohort studies.

Harms: One RCT in men with benign prostatic hypertrophy found no difference in the incidence of impotence or urinary incontinence with transurethral resection or watchful waiting.[12]

Comment: One retrospective cohort study reported 40–50% cure rates in 50 men with chronic prostatitis treated with transurethral resection. However, proof of bacterial prostatitis was not obtained in many men.[13]

OPTION **RADICAL PROSTATECTOMY**

We found no RCTs on the effects of radical prostatectomy.

Benefits: We found no systematic review or RCTs.

Harms: Case series found that radical prostatectomy can cause impotence (9–75% depending upon age)[14] and varying degrees of urinary stress incontinence (8%).[15] Other potential harms include those associated with any open surgery.

Comment: We found one report of radical prostatectomy in two young men whose refractory bacterial prostatitis caused relapsing haemolytic crises.[16]

QUESTION **What are the effects of treatments for chronic abacterial prostatitis?**

OPTION **α BLOCKERS**

One systematic review found limited evidence suggesting that α blockers versus placebo may significantly improve maximal flow time and pain.

Benefits: We found one systematic review (search date 1999, 2 RCTs, 50 men).[17] The first RCT (20 people) identified by the review compared alfuzosin (2.5 mg three times daily) versus placebo. It found a significant improvement in maximal flow time with alfuzosin (with 15.4 mL/s to 20.3 mL/s alfuzosin *v* 13.9 mL/s to 15.6 mL/s with placebo; $P = 0.01$; RR not provided).[18] It found no significant difference in other outcomes (insufficient information was presented to assess comparative effects on symptom scores). The second RCT (30 people) identified by the review found that pain after prostatic massage significantly improved with α blockers (phenoxybenzaime 10 mg twice daily) versus placebo (at 6 wks; $P < 0.05$).

Harms: The first RCT reported a transient decrease in systolic blood pressure in four people and a slight decrease in libido in two people all treated with alfuzosin.[17]

Comment: None.

OPTION 5α REDUCTASE INHIBITORS

One systematic review of one small RCT found insufficient evidence on the effects of 5α reductase inhibitors.

Benefits: We found one systematic review (search date 1999, 1 RCT, 41 men) that compared finasteride versus placebo.[17] The RCT found that although symptom scores decreased significantly with finasteride after 1 year, there was no significant difference in pain with finasteride versus placebo.[19] The RCT was small and had low power (31/41 [75%] of men were allocated to finasteride *v* 10/41 [25%] of men to placebo).

Harms: Three people treated with finasteride reported partial impotence compared with none in the placebo group.[19]

Comment: Finasteride is known to decrease prostate volume (as it did in this study; $P < 0.03$), but it is unclear how this relates to symptoms of prostatitis.[19]

OPTION ANTI-INFLAMMATORY MEDICATIONS

One RCT found no significant difference with pentosan polysulfate sodium versus placebo in symptoms, but the RCT may have been too small to exclude a clinically important difference.

Benefits: We found one systematic review (search date 1999, 1 RCT, 30 men)[17] that compared pentosan polysulfate sodium (100 mg twice daily) versus placebo. Outcomes included symptom changes by physician rating, symptom score, and uroflowmetry. The RCT found no significant difference in either physician rated improvement (pentosan polysulfate sodium group 7/10 [70%] improved *v* placebo 5/14 [36%] improved; RR 2.0, 95% CI 0.87 to 4.4) or in local symptom scores (pentosan polysulfate sodium 5/10 [50%] improved *v* placebo 6/14 [43%] improved; RR 1.2, 95% CI 0.5 to 2.8).[20] Six people were excluded from the analysis for non-compliance or having bacterial prostatitis (analysis was not intention to treat). The RCT may have been to small to rule out important clinical differences.

Harms: Two people given pentosan polysulfate sodium reported diarrhoea. No people treated with placebo developed gastrointestinal adverse symptoms.

Comment: "Physician rated improvement" is not an objective measurement. There was no significant difference between experimental and control groups with other, more objective and standardised, outcomes.

OPTION TRANSURETHRAL MICROWAVE THERMOTHERAPY

One systematic review found limited evidence from one RCT suggesting that transurethral microwave thermotherapy versus sham treatment may significantly improve quality of life at 3 months and symptoms over 21 months.

Benefits: We found one systematic review (search date 1999,[17] 1 double blind RCT,[21] 20 men) that compared transurethral microwave thermotherapy versus sham treatment. It found a significant improvement in quality of life with thermotherapy versus sham treatment at 3 months (scale 0–10; quality of life improved from 4.4 to 3.0 with transurethral microwave thermotherapy *v* unchanged at 5.2 with sham treatment; $P < 0.05$). Significantly more men had improvement of a subjective global assessment by more than 50% over a mean of 21 months with thermotherapy versus sham treatment (7/10 [70%] *v* 1/10 [10%]; RR 7, 95% CI 1 to 47; NNT 2, 95% CI 2 to 6). The review found no good evidence on the effects of thermotherapy on cure or recurrence rate.

Harms: Four men complained of transient (resolved in 3 wks) adverse reactions, including haematuria (2 men), urinary tract infection, impotence, urinary retention, urinary incontinence, and premature ejaculation (each occurring in 1 man).[21] However, the RCT did not report if the men with adverse events were treated with active treatment or sham treatment.

Comment: Thermotherapy caused persistent elevation of leucocytes in the prostatic fluid, which could indicate tissue damage.

OPTION ALLOPURINOL

One systematic review found limited evidence from one small RCT that allopurinol versus placebo significantly improved symptoms over about 8 months.

Benefits: We found one systematic review (search date 2000,[22] 1 RCT,[23] 54 men). The RCT compared treatment with allopurinol (600 mg daily), allopurinol (300 mg daily), and placebo. Thirty four men (63%) completed the study, which lasted 240 days. All recorded data were used in the analysis. The RCT found allopurinol significantly reduced the "degree of discomfort" score (pretreatment score = 0; score –1.1 with allopurinol *v* placebo –0.2 with placebo; $P = 0.02$).[23]

Harms: None of the men receiving allopurinol reported any significant adverse events but the RCT did not explain what constitutes a significant adverse event; 55% of people on placebo and 68% of people on allopurinol completed the trial.[23]

Comment: The symptom score was not validated and the high withdrawal rate makes the results difficult to interpret.[23]

OPTION PROSTATIC MASSAGE

We found no RCTs on the effects of prostatic massage.

Benefits: We found no systematic review or RCTs.

Harms: We found no good evidence.

Comment: None.

OPTION SITZ BATHS

We found no RCTs on the effects of Sitz baths.

Benefits: We found no systematic review or RCTs.

Harms: We found no good evidence.

Comment: None.

OPTION BIOFEEDBACK

We found no RCTs on the effects of biofeedback.

Benefits: We found no systematic review or RCTs.

Harms: We found no good evidence.

Comment: None.

REFERENCES

1. Roberts RO, Lieber MM, Rhodes T, et al. Prevalence of a physician-assigned diagnosis of prostatitis: the Olmsted County study of urinary symptoms and health status among men. *Urology* 1998;51:578–584.
2. Collins MM, Stafford, RS, O'Leary MP, et al. How common is prostatitis? A national survey of physician visits. *J Urol* 1998;159:1224–1228.
3. Alexander RB, Brady F, Ponniah S. Autoimmune prostatitis: evidence of T cell reactivity with normal prostatic proteins. *Urology* 1997;50:893–899.
4. Wenninger K, Heiman JR, Rothman I, et al. Sickness impact of chronic nonbacterial prostatitis and its correlates. *J Urol* 1996;155:965–968.
5. Hanus PM, Danzinger LH. Treatment of chronic bacterial prostatitis. *Clin Pharm* 1984;3:49–55.
6. Naber KG, Sorgel F, Kees F, et al. Norfloxacin concentration in prostatic adenoma tissue (patients) and in prostatic fluid in patients and volunteers. 15th International Congress of Chemotherapy, Landsberg. In: Weidner N, Madsen PO, Schiefer HG, eds. *Prostatitis: etiopathology, diagnosis and therapy.* New York: Springer Verlag, 1987.
7. Szoke I, Torok L, Dosa E, et al. The possible role of anaerobic bacteria in chronic prostatitis. *Int J Androl* 1998;21:163–168.
8. Cox CE. Ofloxacin in the management of complicated urinary tract infections, including prostatitis. *Am J Med* 1980;87(suppl 6c):61–68.
9. Meares EM, Stamey TA. Bacteriologic localization patterns in bacterial prostatitis and urethritis. *Invest Urol* 1968;5:492–518.
10. Baret L, Leonare A. Chronic bacterial prostatitis: 10 years of experience with local antibiotics. *J Urol* 1998;140:755–757.
11. Barbalias GA, Nikiforidis G, Liatsikos EN. Alpha-blockers for the treatment of chronic prostatitis in combination with antibiotics. *J Urol* 1998;159:883–887.
12. Wasson JH, Reda DJ, Bruskewitz RC, et al. A comparison of transurethral surgery with watchful waiting for moderate symptoms of benign prostatic hyperplasia. *N Engl J Med* 1995;332:75–79.
13. Smart CJ, Jenkins JD, Lloyd RS. The painful prostate. *Br J Urol* 1975;47:861–869.
14. Quinlan DM, Epstein JI, Carter BS, et al. Sexual function following radical prostatectomy: influence of preservation of neurovascular bundles. *J Urol* 1991;145:998–1002.
15. Steiner MS, Morton RA, Walsh PC. Impact of radical prostatectomy on urinary continence. *J Urol* 1991;145:512–515.
16. Davis BE, Weigel JW. Adenocarcinoma of the prostate discovered in 2 young patients following total prostatovesiculectomy for refractory prostatitis. *J Urol* 1990;144:744–745.
17. Collins M, MacDonald R, Wilt T. Diagnosis and treatment of chronic abacterial prostatitis: a systematic review. *Ann Intern Med* 2000;133:367–368. Search date 1999; primary sources Medline, Cochrane Library, hand searches of bibliographies, and contact with an expert.
18. de la Rosette JJ, Karthaus HF, van Kerrebroeck PE, et al. Research in "prostatitis syndromes": the use of alfuzosin (a new alpha 1-receptor-blocking agent) in patients mainly presenting with micturition complaints of an irritative nature and confirmed urodynamic abnormalities. *Eur Urol* 1992;22:222–227.
19. Leskinen M, Lukkarinen O, Marttila T. Effects of finasteride in patients with inflammatory chronic

pelvic pain syndrome: a double-blind, placebo-controlled, pilot study. *Urology* 1999;53:502–505.
20. Wédren H. Effects of sodium pentosanpolysulphate on symptoms related to chronic non-bacterial prostatitis. *Scand J Urol Nephrol* 1987;21:81–88.
21. Nickel J, Sorensen R. Transurethral microwave thermotherapy for nonbacterial prostatitis: a randomized double-blind sham controlled study using new prostatitis specific assessment questionnaires. *J Urol* 1996;155:1950–1955.
22. McNaughton Collins M, MacDonald R, Wilt T. Interventions for chronic abacterial prostatitis. In: The Cochrane Library, Issue 2, 2002. Oxford: Update Software. Search date 2000; primary sources Medline, The Cochrane Library, hand searches of bibliographies of identified articles and reviews, and contact with an expert.
23. Persson B, Ronquist G, Ekblom M. Ameliorative effect of allopurinol on nonbacterial prostatitis: a parallel double-blind controlled study. *J Urol* 1996;155:961–964.

Anthony Schaeffer
Professor and Chair

Jeffrey Stern
Department of Urology
Northwestern University Medical School
Chicago
USA

Competing interests: AS has been reimbursed by Ortho McNeil for attending and speaking at several conferences. He has also received consulting fees from Bayer Corp and Johnson and Johnson. JS none declared.

Erectile dysfunction

Search date April 2002.

Michael O'Leary and Bazian Ltd (temporary contributors)

QUESTIONS

INTERVENTIONS

See glossary, p 879

Key Messages

- **Intracavernosal alprostadil** One large RCT found that intracavernosal alprostadil versus placebo significantly increased the chances of a satisfactory erection.
- **Intraurethral alprostadil** One large RCT (in men who had previously responded to alprostadil) found limited evidence that intraurethral alprostadil (prostaglandin E1) significantly increased the chances of successful sexual intercourse and at least one orgasm over 3 months. About a third of men suffered penile ache. We found no direct comparisons of intraurethral alprostadil with either intracavernosal alprostadil or oral drug treatments.
- **L-arginine** One small RCT found no significant difference in sexual function with L-arginine versus placebo, but it may have been too small to exclude a clinically important difference.
- **Penile prostheses, vacuum devices** We found insufficient evidence on the effects of penile prostheses and vacuum devices.
- **Sildenafil** One systematic review has found that sildenafil versus placebo significantly increases the number of men reporting improved erection (NNT 2, 95% CI 2 to 3) and successful intercourse. Additional RCTs have found similar results. We found no RCTs directly comparing sildenafil versus other treatments. Adverse effects, including headaches, flushing, and dyspepsia, are reported in up to a quarter of men. Deaths have been reported in men on concomitant treatment with oral nitrates.
- **Topical alprostadil** Two quasi randomised trials found limited evidence that topical alprostadil versus placebo increased the number of men with erections sufficient for intercourse.
- **Trazodone** One small RCT found no significant difference in erections or libido with trazodone versus placebo, but it may have been too small to exclude a clinically important difference.

Clin Evid 2002;8:872–880.

- **Yohimbine** One systematic review has found that yohimbine versus placebo significantly improves self reported sexual function and penile rigidity at 2–10 weeks. We found no RCTs directly comparing yohimbine versus other treatments. Transient adverse effects are reported in up to a third of men.

DEFINITION Erectile dysfunction has largely replaced the term "impotence". It is defined as the persistent inability to obtain or maintain sufficient rigidity of the penis to allow satisfactory sexual performance.

INCIDENCE/ PREVALENCE We found little good epidemiological information, but one cross sectional study found that age is the variable most strongly associated with erectile dysfunction, and that up to 30 million men in the USA may be affected.[1] Even among men in their 40s, nearly 40% report at least occasional difficulty obtaining or maintaining erection, whereas this approaches 70% in 70 year olds.

AETIOLOGY/ RISK FACTORS It is now believed that about 80% of cases of erectile dysfunction have an organic cause, the rest being psychogenic in origin. Risk factors include increasing age, smoking, and obesity. Erectile problems fall into three categories: failure to initiate; failure to fill, caused by insufficient arterial inflow into the penis to allow engorgement and tumescence because of vascular insufficiency; and failure to store because of veno-occlusive dysfunction.

PROGNOSIS We found no good evidence on prognosis in untreated organic erectile dysfunction.

AIMS To restore satisfactory erections, with minimal adverse effects.

OUTCOMES Patient and partner self reports of satisfaction and sexual function; objective tests of penile rigidity; adverse effects of treatment.

METHODS *Clinical Evidence* update search and appraisal April 2002.

QUESTION What are the effects of treatments?

OPTION YOHIMBINE

A systematic review has found that yohimbine is significantly more effective than placebo. We found no comparisons of yohimbine with other oral or local treatments. Transient adverse effects are reported in up to a third of men.

Benefits: We found one systematic review (search date 1997, 7 RCTs, 11–100 men with erectile dysfunction, defined variously as organic, psychogenic, and of unknown cause) comparing the α blocker, yohimbine, versus placebo.[2] Duration of treatment ranged from 2–10 weeks, and outcomes varied from self reported improvement in sexual function to objective tests of penile rigidity. The RCTs found positive responses in significantly more men taking yohimbine versus placebo (34–73% *v* 9–45%; OR 3.85, 95% CI 2.22 to 6.67; average absolute figures not provided). One subsequent placebo controlled, crossover trial (22 men, randomisation not mentioned) comparing yohimbine (single daily dose 100 mg for 30 days) versus placebo found no significant difference between treatments in erectile function.[3]

Harms: The review found that adverse events were reported in 10–30% of men receiving yohimbine versus 5–16% with placebo (significance not reported) and were generally mild, including agitation, anxiety, headache, mild increase in blood pressure, increased urinary output, and gastrointestinal upset.[2] In the small subsequent trial no men discontinued treatment.[3]

Comment: The end points in some of these trials were subjective and of questionable validity. The subsequent trial did not make clear if it was randomised or not.[3]

OPTION SILDENAFIL

One systematic review has found that sildenafil versus placebo significantly increases the number of men reporting improved erection and successful intercourse. Additional RCTs have found similar results. We found no RCTs directly comparing sildenafil versus other treatments. Adverse effects, including headaches, flushing, and dyspepsia, are reported in up to a quarter of men. Deaths have been reported in men on concomitant treatment with oral nitrates.

Benefits: We found one systematic review (search date 1999, 21 RCTs)[4] and four subsequent RCTs.[5–8] **In men with any cause of erectile dysfunction:** The systematic review (search date 1999, 16 RCTs, 3988 men) found that more men reported improvement of their erections with sildenafil than with placebo (ARI for improvement in erections, sildenafil *v* placebo 54%, 95% CI 48% to 59%; NNT for improved erections 2, 95% CI 2 to 3).[4] The review also examined the effects of sildenafil versus placebo on sexual function (using questions 3 and 4 of the international index of erectile dysfunction [see glossary, p 879]). All eight RCTs that reported this outcome found that sildenafil significantly improved sexual function compared with placebo. We found three subsequent RCTs. The first RCT (236 men) compared sildenafil (25–100 mg taken as needed before attempted intercourse) versus placebo.[5] After 12 weeks' treatment, sildenafil significantly improved sexual function (questions 3 and 4 of the international index of erectile dysfunction) and rate of successful intercourse attempts compared with placebo (mean improvement on question 3, 1.87 points with sildenafil *v* 0.68 points with placebo, $P < 0.0001$; mean improvement on question 4, 2.12 points with sildenafil *v* 0.86 points with placebo, $P < 0.0001$; rate of successful intercourse attempts 62% with sildenafil *v* 30% with placebo, $P < 0.0001$). The second RCT (152 men with erectile dysfunction and depressive symptoms) compared 12 weeks' treatment with sildenafil versus placebo.[6] It found that sildenafil significantly improved self reported improvement in erections, self reported improvement in ability to have intercourse, and improvement in sexual function (90% reported improvement in erections with sildenafil *v* 11% with placebo, P value not reported; 89% reported improvement in ability to have sexual intercourse with sildenafil *v* 13% with placebo, P value not reported; $P < 0.001$ in favour of sildenafil for difference in scores for questions 3 and 4 of the international index of erectile dysfunction). The third RCT (247 men) compared 12 weeks' treatment with sildenafil (25–100 mg) versus placebo. Compared with placebo, sildenafil significantly improved the primary outcomes of participant and partner rated ability to achieve and maintain erection and satisfaction with intercourse (questions 3, 4, and 7 of the international index of erectile dysfunction; P < 0.001 for all comparisons).[7] **In men with diabetes:** The systematic review (search date 1999, 2 RCTs)[4] found that sildenafil significantly improved erections compared with placebo (improved erections reported by 48–57% with sildenafil *v* 10% with placebo; P < 0.005).[4] We found one additional placebo controlled RCT (219 men).[8] It found that sildenafil (25–100 mg) improved participant rated improvement in erections and score on questions 3 and 4 of the international index of erectile dysfunction after 12 weeks (64.6% had improved erections with sildenafil *v* 10.5% with placebo, 95% CI presented graphically, P < 0.0001; mean improvement in question 3 score 3.42 with sildenafil *v* 1.86 with placebo; mean improvement in question 4 score 3.35 with sildenafil *v* 1.84 with placebo, P < 0.0001 for both comparisons). **In men with spinal cord injury:** The systematic review (search date 1999, 2 RCTs restricted to men with spinal cord injury) did not report trial results separately.[4] The first RCT (26 men with spinal cord injury between the sixth thoracic vertebra and the fifth lumbar vertebra)[9] compared sildenafil versus placebo. It found that sildenafil significantly improved erections (9/12 [75%] with sildenafil *v* 1/14 [7%] with placebo; RR 10.0, 95% CI 1.5 to 71). At 28 days, significantly more men in the treatment group reported improvements in quality of sex life (P = 0.001) and wished to continue treatment (P = 0.02).[9] The second RCT (178 men with erectile dysfunction secondary to spinal trauma) was a double blind crossover comparison of sildenafil versus placebo. It found that sildenafil improved sexual intercourse more than placebo (80% reported improved sexual intercourse with sildenafil *v* 10% with placebo).[4]

Harms: In one RCT included in the review, headache, flushing, and dyspepsia were reported in 6–18% of men taking sildenafil.[11] In a second included RCT in men with diabetes, cardiovascular event rates were similar in the two groups (4/136 [3%] sildenafil *v* 6/132 [5%] placebo; RR 0.6, 95% CI 0.2 to 2.2).[12] In an third included RCT in men with spinal cord injury, none discontinued treatment.[9] One subsequent RCT (236 men with any cause of erectile dysfunction) found that sildenafil was associated with facial flushing (25.2%), dizziness (6.7%), headache (5.9%), and palpitations (3.4%).[5] The second subsequent RCT found that headache, flushing, dyspepsia, and abnormal perception of colour or brightness were more common with sildenafil than placebo (20% *v* 6% for headache; 15% *v* 0% for dyspepsia; 15% *v* 1% for flushing; 8% *v* 1% for abnormal vision).[6] The third subsequent RCT found similar results.[7] Another study[13] reported specifically on adverse effects of sildenafil. It summarised results from a series of RCTs (4274 men aged 19–87 years with erectile dysfunction owing to a range of causes for > 6 months and a mean of 5 years). All men were treated for up to 6 months, and 2199 received further open label treatment for up to 1 year.[13] It found more adverse events with sildenafil versus placebo, including headache (16% *v* 4%; significance not reported), flushing (10% *v* 1%; significance not reported), and dyspepsia (7% *v* 2%; significance not reported). Similar proportions in both groups discontinued treatment (about 2.4%).[13] An important contraindication to prescribing sildenafil is concomitant use of oral nitrates. This combination results in precipitous hypotension. By 1999, about 60 deaths had been reported to the US Food and Drug Administration in men who had been given prescriptions for sildenafil, but it is not known whether any of the deaths were directly attributable to the drug. Long term (> 1 year) safety of sildenafil is unknown. One of the RCTs in men with psychogenic or mixed aetiology erectile found that adverse effect were mild and transient.[14]

Comment: None.

OPTION L-ARGININE

One small RCT found no evidence that L-arginine improved sexual function compared with placebo, although the trial was too small to rule out a clinically important difference.

Benefits: We found no systematic review. We found one small RCT (50 men with erectile dysfunction) comparing high dose L-arginine (5 g daily given orally) versus placebo.[15] It found no significant difference in sexual function between L-arginine and placebo, although the power of the study was not adequate to rule out a clinically important difference (sexual function improved in 9/29 [31%] men with L-arginine *v* 2/17 [12%] with placebo; RR 2.6, 95% CI 0.6 to 10.8).

Harms: The trial reported decreases in systolic or diastolic blood pressure, or both, although this caused no systemic effects and required no drug interruptions. The trial found some "fluctuation in heart rate", which was described as clinically insignificant. Nausea, vomiting, diarrhoea, headache, flushing, and numbness have been reported after the administration of L-arginine, although none of the men in this study reported any such complaints.

Comment: None.

OPTION TRAZODONE

One small RCT found no evidence that trazodone was more effective than placebo in men with erectile dysfunction, although the trial was too small to rule out a clinically important effect.

Benefits: We found no systematic review. One small crossover RCT (48 men with erectile dysfunction, washout period 3 wks) compared trazodone versus placebo.[16] Men were treated with either trazodone (50 mg) or placebo at bedtime for 3 months. It found no evidence that trazodone improved erections or libido (improved erections reported by 19% with trazodone *v* 24% with placebo, CI and P value not provided, described as NS; improved libido reported by 35% with trazodone *v* 20% with placebo; CI and P value not provided; described as NS).

Harms: The trial reported drowsiness (31% of men), dry mouth (1%), and fatigue (19%) with trazodone. Comparative rates for trazodone versus placebo were not available.

Comment: None.

OPTION INTRAURETHRAL ALPROSTADIL

One large RCT (in men who had previously responded to alprostadil) found limited evidence that intraurethral alprostadil (prostaglandin E1) significantly increased the chances of successful sexual intercourse and at least one orgasm over 3 months. About a third of men suffered penile ache. We found no direct comparisons of intraurethral alprostadil with either intracavernosal alprostadil or oral drug treatments.

Benefits: We found no systematic review. We found one RCT reported in full.[17] It began by testing the response to intraurethral alprostadil in 1511 men aged 27–88 years who had erectile dysfunction of organic cause for at least 3 months. In clinic testing, 66% had erections sufficient for intercourse. These 996 men were randomised to intraurethral alprostadil or placebo for use at home.[17] Over 3 months, those given alprostadil were more likely to report having successful sexual intercourse (65% with alprostadil *v* 19% with placebo; $P < 0.001$) and at least one orgasm (64% with alprostadil *v* 24% with placebo; $P < 0.001$). Subsequent RCTs, published only in abstract form, found slightly lower increased risks of achieving satisfactory erections of 30–48% with alprostadil.

Harms: The most common adverse effect was mild to moderate penile ache, occurring in about a third of men during clinic testing (36%) of whom only 36/1511 (2.4%) withdrew because of it.[17] We found no reports of priapism, penile fibrosis, or other serious adverse events.

Comment: The trial preselected men who had a good response to alprostadil before randomisation. This will tend to increase the size of the effect compared with placebo.

OPTION INTRACAVERNOSAL ALPROSTADIL

One large RCT found that intracavernosal injection of alprostadil (prostaglandin E1) significantly increased the chances of a satisfactory erection. We found no direct comparisons of intracavernosal alprostadil with either intraurethral or oral drug treatments. One small RCT found limited evidence that vacuum devices were as effective as intracavernosal alprostadil injections for rigidity but not for orgasm.

Benefits: We found no systematic review. We found one large multicentre trial (1128 men aged 20–79 years with all causes of erectile dysfunction, but excluding heavy smokers and men with uncontrolled hypertension or diabetes).[18] Of these, nearly 300 men were randomly assigned to double blind doses of placebo or 2.5, 5, 10, or 20 μg of alprostadil. Injections were given and outcome was assessed by an investigator or research nurse. None of the 59 men who received placebo had a response. There were significant differences in response between all doses versus placebo and a significant dose–response relationship. The remaining 884 men, including 52 who had taken part in the dose–response study, were enrolled in a single blind, dose escalation study (201 men) and an uncontrolled open label flexible dose study to assess efficacy, safety, and feasibility of self injection at home (683 men). Of the 13 762 injections for which men recorded their response, nearly 90% were followed by satisfactory sexual activity.[18] **Versus vacuum**

devices: One crossover RCT (50 men with erectile dysfunction, 44 of whom completed the study) compared intracavernosal self injections of alprostadil versus vacuum devices.[19] Outcome was assessed by a questionnaire given to men and their partners after 15 uses for each device, and couples were followed for 18–24 months. There was no significant difference in the ability to achieve an erection suitable for intercourse. However, the ability to attain orgasm was significantly better with alprostadil ($P < 0.05$). On a scale of 1 to 10, overall satisfaction was significantly better when using alprostadil, both for men (6.5 with alprostadil *v* 5.4 with vacuum device; $P < 0.05$) and partners (6.5 with alprostadil *v* 5.1 with vacuum device; $P < 0.05$). Younger men (< 60 years), and those with shorter duration of erectile dysfunction (< 12 months), favoured alprostadil ($P < 0.05$).

Harms: Penile pain was reported by a half of the men in the study of efficacy and safety of alprostadil injection, and priapism (prolonged erection for > 4 h) by 1%.[18] There was no significant difference in the frequency of adverse events between vacuum devices and alprostadil.[19]

Comment: Most men can be taught to inject themselves using small gauge needles. In the RCT comparing injections and vacuum devices, 80% of the 44 couples who completed the study were still using one or other treatment after 18–24 months.[19]

OPTION TOPICAL ALPROSTADIL

Two quasi randomised trials found limited evidence that topical alprostadil versus placebo increased the number of men with erections sufficient for intercourse.

Benefits: We found no systematic review. We found two quasi randomised trials (see comment below).[20,21] The first single blind trial (48 men with erectile dysfunction owing to organic, psychogenic, or mixed causes) compared topical alprostadil versus placebo.[20] Men were assigned in sequential order to either 0.5, 1, or 2.5 mg alprostadil gel (36 men) or placebo (12 men). One dose of alprostadil or placebo gel was applied to the glans and shaft of the penis and washed off after 3 hours. Significantly more men achieved an erection sufficient for intercourse with any dose of alprostadil versus placebo (25/36 [69%] with alprostadil *v* 2/12 [17%] with placebo; RR 4.2, 95% CI 1.8 to 5.5; NNT 2, 95% CI 1 to 8). The second RCT (62 men) compared alprostadil topically applied to the glans of the penis only versus placebo in a clinic setting. Significantly more men reported an erection deemed sufficient for vaginal penetration (12/31 [39%] *v* 2/29 [7%]; RR 5.6, 95% CI 1.4 to 23.0; NNT 3, 95% CI 2 to 9).[21]

Harms: Men receiving alprostadil to the glans and shaft of the penis were significantly more likely to have skin irritation than those on placebo (100% on 0.5 mg dose *v* 67% on placebo; no P value provided). Irritation was more severe with alprostadil than with placebo (measured by mean irritation score ranging from 0–2; 1.75 with

0.5 mg dose *v* 0.67 with placebo; $P < 0.0013$).[20] In the trial in which alprostadil was applied to the glans only, significantly greater erythema was reported with alprostadil versus placebo ($P < 0.001$; absolute figures not provided).[21] It reported that 3% of men had severe erythema.

Comment: Allocation of men in both trials was sequential and may mean that the groups were systematically different; the characteristics of each group were not reported.

OPTION VACUUM DEVICES

We found that vacuum devices have not been adequately assessed in RCTs. One small RCT found limited evidence that they were as effective as intracavernosal alprostadil (prostaglandin E1) injections for rigidity but not for orgasm.

Benefits: We found no systematic review. We found no RCTs versus placebo. **Versus intracavernosal injections:** See benefits of intracavernosal alprostadil, p 877.

Harms: We found insufficient evidence.

Comment: Vacuum devices may be less popular than injections because only the distal portion of the penis becomes firm, but they are presumed to be safe.[19]

OPTION PENILE PROSTHESES

We found no RCTs. Use of penile prostheses is usually considered only after less invasive treatments have failed.

Benefits: We found no RCTs. Anecdotal evidence suggests that patient satisfaction may be high, but we found no good studies.

Harms: One recent study found the morbidity of penile prostheses to be 9% (surgical revision 7%, mechanical failure 2.5%). Infection rates were between 2% and 7%.[22]

Comment: None.

GLOSSARY

Questions 3 and 4 of the international index of erectile dysfunction The questions have been validated for assessing the effects of sildenafil on sexual function. The questions ask "over the past 4 weeks, when you have attempted sexual intercourse, how often were you able to penetrate (enter) your partner?", and "over the past 4 weeks, during sexual intercourse, how often were you able to maintain your erection after you have penetrated (entered) your partner?" Questions are answered on a six point scale.

Substantive changes

Sildenafil New systematic review replaces existing RCTs.[4] Four additional RCTs identified;[5–8] conclusions unchanged.

REFERENCES

1. Feldman HA, Goldstein I, Dimitrios GH, et al. Impotence and its medical and psychosocial correlates: results of the Massachusetts male aging study. *J Urol* 1994;151:54–61.
2. Ernst E, Pittler MH. Yohimbine for erectile dysfunction: a systemic review and meta-analysis of randomized clinical trials. *J Urol*

1998;159:433–436. Search date 1997; primary sources Medline, Embase, The Cochrane Library, and hand searched references.
3. Teloken C, Rhoden EL, Sogari P, et al. Therapeutic effects of high dose yohimbine hydrochloride on organic erectile dysfunction. *J Urol* 1998;159:122–124.
4. Burls A., Gold L, Clark W. Systematic review of randomised controlled trials of sildenafil (Viagra) in the treatment of male erectile dysfunction. *Br J Gen Pract* 2001;51:1004–1012. Search date 1999; primary sources Medline, Embase, Psyclit, The Cochrane Library, National Research Register, Pharmline, PreMedline, Internet search engines, handsearch of general medical journals and reference lists, contact with the pharmaceutical company and experts in the field.
5. Chen KK, Hsieh JT, Huang ST, et al. ASSESS-3: a randomised, double-blind, flexible-dose clinical trial of the efficacy and safety of oral sildenafil in the treatment of men with erectile dysfunction in Taiwan. *Int J Impot Res* 2001;13:221–229.
6. Seidman SN, Roose SP, Menza MA, et al. Treatment of erectile dysfunction in men with depressive symptoms: results of a placebo-controlled trial with sildenafil citrate. *Am J Psychiatry* 2001;158:1623–1630.
7. Lewis R, Bennett CJ, Borkon WD, et al. Patient and partner satisfaction with Viagra (sildenafil citrate) treatment as determined by the Erectile Dysfunction Inventory of Treatment Satisfaction Questionnaire. *Urology* 2001;57:960–965.
8. Boulton AJ, Selam JL, Sweeney M, et al. Sildenafil citrate for the treatment of erectile dysfunction in men with Type II diabetes mellitus. *Diabetologia* 2001;44:1296–1301.
9. Derry FA, Dinsmore WW, Fraser M, et al. Efficacy and safety of oral sildenafil in men with erectile dysfunction caused by spinal cord injury. *Neurology* 1998;51:1629–1633.
10. Dinsmore WW, Hodges M, Hargreaves C, et al. Sildenafil citrate in erectile dysfunction: near normalization in men with broad spectrum erectile dysfunction compared with age-matched healthy control subjects. *Urology* 1999;53:800–805.
11. Goldstein I, Lue TF, Harin PN, et al, for the Sildenafil Study Group. Oral sildenafil in the treatment of erectile dysfunction. *N Engl J Med* 1998;338:1397–1404.
12. Rendell MS, Rajfer J, Wicker PA, et al. Sildenafil for treatment of erectile dysfunction in men with diabetes: a randomized controlled trial. *JAMA* 1999;281:421–426.
13. Morales A, Gingell C, Collins M, et al. Clinical safety of oral sildenafil citrate (Viagra) in the treatment of erectile dysfunction. *Int J Impot Res* 1998;10:69–74.
14. Olsson AM, Speakman MJ, Dinsmore WW, et al. Sildenafil citrate (Viagra) is effective and well tolerated for treating erectile dysfunction of psychogenic or mixed aetiology. *Int J Clin Pract* 2000;54:561–566.
15. Chen J, Wollman Y, Chernichovsky T, et al. Effect of oral administration of high-dose nitric oxide donor L-arginine in men with organic erectile dysfunction: results of a double-blind randomized placebo-controlled study. *BJU Int* 1999;83:269–273.
16. Costabile RA, Spevak M. Oral trazodone is not effective therapy for erectile dysfunction: a double blind placebo-controlled trial. *J Urol* 1999;161:1819–1822.
17. Padma-Nathan H, Hellstrom WJ, Kaiser FE, et al, for the Medicated Urethral System for Erection (MUSE) Study Group. Treatment of men with erectile dysfunction with transurethral alprostadil. *N Engl J Med* 1997;336:1–7.
18. PGE1 Study Group. Prospective, multicenter trials of efficacy and safety of intracavernosal alprostadil (prostaglandin E1) sterile powder in men with erectile dysfunction. *N Engl J Med* 1996;334:873–877.
19. Soderdahl DW, Thrasher JB, Hansberry KL, et al. Intracavernosal drug induced erection therapy vs external vacuum device in the treatment of erectile dysfunction. *Br J Urol* 1997;79:952–957.
20. McVary KT, Polepalle S, Riggi S, et al. Topical prostaglandin E1 SEPA gel for the treatment of erectile dysfunction. *J Urol* 1999;162:726–730.
21. Goldstein I, Payton TR, Schechter PJ. A double blind placebo controlled efficacy and safety study of topical gel formulation of 1% alprostadil (Topiglan) for the in office treatment of erectile dysfunction. *Urology* 2001;57:301–305.
22. Goldstein I, Newman L, Baum N, et al. Safety and efficacy outcome of Mentor α 1 inflatable penile prosthesis implantation for impotence treatment. *J Urol* 1997;157:833–839.

Michael O'Leary
Associate Professor
Department of Surgery
Harvard Medical School
Boston
USA

Bazian Ltd (temporary contributors)
London
UK

Competing interests: The author has received honoraria from Pfizer for educational programmes on sildenafil, and has received research support to study this agent.

Prostate cancer: metastatic

Search date January 2002

M Dror Michaelson, James A Talcott, and Matthew R Smith

QUESTIONS

INTERVENTIONS

* Categorisation based on observational evidence, RCTs unlikely to be conducted.

See glossary, p 889

Key Messages

In men with metastatic prostate cancer

- **Androgen deprivation** We found limited evidence from RCTs suggesting that androgen deprivation versus no initial treatment reduced mortality. One systematic review and one subsequent RCT found no evidence of a difference between different types of androgen deprivation (orchidectomy, diethylstillbestrol, and luteinsing hormone releasing hormone agonists).
- **Combined androgen blockade (androgen deprivation and non-steroidal antiandrogen) compared with androgen deprivation alone** Inconclusive evidence from four systematic reviews suggests that there could be a 2–5% improvement in 5 year survival associated with combined androgen blockade (androgen deprivation plus a non-steroidal antiandrogen) versus androgen deprivation alone.

Prostate cancer: metastatic

- **Deferred androgen deprivation** One small RCT without formal surveillance criteria, found that immediate androgen deprivation versus deferring androgen deprivation until disease progression becomes apparent in men with stage D1 prostate cancer after reduced prostatectomy significantly increased overall survival after a median of 7 years. Subgroup analysis from a large RCT found no significant difference in survivial after about 10 years. This RCT also found that deferred androgen deprivation resulted in higher rates of complications.
- **Intermittent androgen deprivation** We found no RCTs assessing the long term effects of intermittent versus continuous androgen deprivation on mortality, morbidity, or quality of life.

In men with symptomatic androgen independent metastatic prostate cancer

- **Bisphosphonates** One systematic review of two poor quality RCTs found insufficient evidence about the effects of bisphosphonates.
- **Chemotherapy (palliation but no evidence of an effect on survival)** RCTs have found that chemotherapy plus corticosteroids versus corticosteroids alone reduces pain, lengthens palliation, and improves quality of life, but found no improvement in overall survival.
- **External beam radiation (palliation but no evidence of an effect on survival)** We found no RCTs comparing external beam radiation versus palliative treatments other than radionuclides. Observational evidence suggests complete pain relief in about a quarter of people, and placebo controlled RCTs would probably be considered unethical. A systematic review of one RCT in men with symptomatic bone metastases found no difference in survival between external beam radiation versus strontium-89; however, strontium-89 was associated with significantly fewer new sites of pain, and reduced need for additional radiotherapy.
- **Radionuclides (palliation but no clear evidence of an effect on survival)** One systematic review found one small RCT in men with symptomatic bone metastases, which found no difference in survival between external beam radiation plus placebo versus external beam radiation plus strontium-89. However, strontium-89 significantly reduced the number of new sites of pain. A second RCT in men with symptomatic bone metastases found no difference in survival between external beam radiation versus strontium-89; however, strontium-89 was associated with significantly fewer new sites of pain, and reduced need for additional radiotherapy. One small subsequent RCT in men with painful bone metastases found that samarium-153 versus placebo significantly reduced pain scores. A second small subsequent RCT in a selected population found an improvement in survival with strontium-89 versus placebo, but the results are difficult to generalise.

DEFINITION See non-metastatic prostate cancer, p 891. Androgen independent metastatic disease is defined as disease that progresses despite androgen deprivation.

INCIDENCE/ PREVALENCE See non-metastatic prostate cancer, p 891.

AETIOLOGY/ RISK FACTORS See non-metastatic prostate cancer, p 891.

PROGNOSIS Prostate cancer metastasises predominantly to bone. Metastatic prostate cancer can result in pain, weakness, paralysis, and death.

AIMS	To reduce mortality and disability; to control symptoms and maximise quality of life; and to minimise adverse effects of treatment.
OUTCOMES	Survival; response in terms of symptoms and signs; quality of life; adverse effects of treatment.
METHODS	*Clinical Evidence* update search and appraisal January 2002.

QUESTION What are the effects of treatment for men with metastatic prostate cancer?

OPTION ANDROGEN DEPRIVATION

We found limited evidence from RCTs suggesting that androgen deprivation reduced mortality in men with metastatic prostate cancer. One systematic review and one subsequent RCT found no evidence of a difference in effectiveness between different methods of androgen deprivation (orchidectomy, diethylstilbestrol, and luteinising hormone releasing hormone agonists).

Benefits: **Versus no initial treatment:** We found no systematic review of androgen deprivation versus no initial treatment and no recent RCTs. Three RCTs (about 4000 men with all stages of prostate cancer) performed between 1959 and 1975 compared androgen deprivation (diethylstilbestrol [stilboestrol], orchidectomy [see glossary, p 889], or oestrogens) versus no initial treatment. They found no difference in overall survival. Re-analysis of updated data from these RCTs found a modest survival advantage with androgen deprivation.[1] The report did not provide statistical details. **Different types of androgen deprivation:** We found one systematic review (search date 1998, 24 RCTs, > 6600 men with metastatic prostate cancer).[2] It found no significant differences between treatment groups in overall progression free survival, time to progression, or overall survival in the most of the trials. It found no significant differences in 2 year survival between orchidectomy versus luteinising hormone releasing hormone agonists (HR 1.26, 95% CI 0.91 to 1.39), versus diethylstilbestrol (HR 0.98, 95% CI 0.76 to 1.27), or versus non-steroidal antiandrogen monotherapy (HR 1.22, 95% CI 0.99 to 1.50). One large subsequent RCT (915 men with advanced prostate cancer stage T0–4, M1 (see table 1 in non-metastatic prostate cancer, p 891) compared parenteral oestrogen versus total androgen ablation (orchidectomy or triptorelin). It found no significant difference in mortality at follow up (mortality at 18 months' median follow up 266/458 [58%] with oestrogen *v* 269/457 [59%] with total androgen ablation, RR 0.99, 95% 0.89 to 1.10).[3]

Harms: All forms of androgen deprivation are known to be associated with vasomotor flushing, loss of libido, gynaecomastia, weight gain, osteoporosis, and loss of muscle mass; we found insufficient prospective frequency data for these adverse effects. One RCT (915 men with metastatic prostate cancer) found that androgen deprivation by orchidectomy or by combination of gonadotrophin releasing hormone analogue with an antiandrogen induces significantly more hot flushes than polyestradiol phosphate (1 or more flushes,

336/452 [74.3%] *v* 135/449 [30.1%], RR 2.5, 95% CI 2.1 to 2.9, NNH 3, 95% CI 2 to 3).[4] Diethylstilbestrol is associated with an increased risk of cardiovascular events, gastric irritation, and allergic reactions, and for these reasons is not used routinely.[1] Orchidectomy has cosmetic and potential psychological consequences. Luteinising hormone releasing hormone agonists may cause an initial clinical flare owing to transient increases in androgen levels.

Comment: Androgen deprivation therapy has been used as the standard of care for men with metastatic disease because of the frequency and duration of effect; therefore, there are no contemporary randomised trials with a no treatment arm. The lack of apparent benefit in earlier trials[1] was probably because of the high cardiovascular event rate associated with high dose diethylstilbestrol.

OPTION IMMEDIATE VERSUS DEFERRED ANDROGEN DEPRIVATION

Subgroup analysis from one RCT found no evidence of improved survival from immediate treatment in men with asymptomatic bone metastases, although the risk of major complications increased with treatment deferred until disease progression. A small RCT in men with node positive disease after radical prostatectomy found significantly improved overall survival with immediate versus delayed treatment.

Benefits: We found no systematic review. We found two RCTs comparing immediate versus deferred deprivation (orchidectomy [see glossary, p 889] or luteinising hormone releasing hormone agonist).[5,6] Immediate androgen deprivation was initiated at diagnosis of prostate cancer; deferred androgen deprivation was initiated at the time of clinical disease progression. The first RCT (938 men with stage T2–4 disease, but no symptomatic metastases) did not have formal surveillance requirements or criteria for starting androgen deprivation in the deferred treatment group.[5] Subgroup analysis found no significant difference in mortality in people with confirmed metastatic prostate cancer (111/130 [85.4%] with immediate treatment *v* 113/131 [86.3%] with deferred treatment, RR 0.99, 95% CI 0.90 to 1.09). It found higher mortality in people with locally advanced disease with delayed versus immediate treatment, but the difference was not significant (150/256 [58.6%] with immediate treatment *v* 171/244 with deferred treatment [70.1%], RR 0.84, 95% CI 0.42 to 0.88). Overall results, including people with M0 or M1 cancer, found about a halving of the risk of major complications, including pathological fractures (11/469 [2.3%] with immediate treatment *v* 21/465 [4.5%] with deferred treatment; $P > 0.05$), spinal cord compression (9/469 [1.9%] with immediate treatment *v* 23/465 [4.9%] with deferred treatment; $P < 0.05$), ureteric obstruction (33/469 [7.0%] *v* 55/465 [11.8%]) and extraskeletal metastases (37/469 [7.9%] *v* 55/465 [11.8%]; $P < 0.05$). The trial did not make clear the time interval over which outcomes were recorded, although this seemed to be at least 10 years. A more recent, smaller RCT (98 men with node positive disease after radical prostatectomy) compared immediate androgen deprivation versus deferred therapy.[6] It found significant improvement in overall survival in the immediate treatment group after median follow up of 7.1 years (40/47 [85%] with immediate treatment *v* 33/51 [65%] with deferred treatment; ARR 20%, 95% CI 3% to 36%; RR 1.3, 95% CI 1.0 to 1.7).

Harms: We found no good prospective evidence on adverse effects of immediate compared to deferred androgen deprivation in men with metastatic prostate cancer.

Comment: A limitation of the first RCT was that about half the people who died in the deferred treatment arm did not receive androgen deprivation at all.[5] The high rate of complications in the deferred group suggests that men need careful surveillance for disease progression, with timely initiation of androgen deprivation before major complications. The smaller RCT had poorer survival in the deferred treatment arm compared with other contemporary series.[6]

OPTION COMBINED ANDROGEN BLOCKADE (ANDROGEN DEPRIVATION AND ANTIANDROGEN)

Inconclusive evidence from systematic reviews suggests that there could be a 2–5% improvement in 5 year survival associated with combined androgen blockade (androgen deprivation plus a non-steroidal antiandrogen) versus androgen deprivation alone.

Benefits: We found two systematic reviews.[7,8] The largest systematic review (search date not stated; identified 27 RCTs; 8275 people, most of whom had stage D2 disease [see table 1 in non-metastatic prostate cancer, p 891]) compared androgen deprivation (orchidectomy or luteinising hormone releasing hormone agonist) plus an antiandrogen versus androgen deprivation alone.[7] The review found no clearly significant difference in mortality (72.4% with androgen deprivation alone *v* 70.4% with combined blockage; RR 0.97, 95% CI 0.94 to 1.00). Exclusion of seven trials (1784 men) of cyproterone acetate (see comment below) found a small reduction in mortality from combined androgen blockade (75.3% with androgen deprivation alone *v* 72.4% combined with non-steroidal antiandrogens; ARR 2.9%; P = 0.005). The most recent review (search date not stated, 20 RCTs, 6320 men) compared androgen deprivation alone (orchidectomy or luteinising hormone releasing hormone agonist) versus androgen deprivation combined with non-steroidal antiandrogens (flutamide or nilutamide).[8] Overall, the review found a significant improvement in 5 year survival in men receiving combined androgen blockade (AR of death 69.9% *v* 75.1% with androgen deprivation alone; OR for survival at 5 years 1.29, 95% CI 1.11 to 1.50). No significant differences were seen at 1 or 2 years' follow up. Five years' follow up was only provided in 7/20 studies.

Harms: The most recent review found that combined androgen blockade using non-steroidal antiandrogens increases the risk of diarrhoea (10% *v* 2%), gastrointestinal pain (7% *v* 2%), and non-specific ophthalmologic events (29% *v* 5%).[8] Flutamide is also associated with a higher rate of anaemia (8% *v* 5%).[5]

Comment: Cyproterone acetate is a steroidal antiandrogen with intrinsic androgenic activity and lower antiandrogenic activity than non-steroidal antiandrogens.

OPTION **INTERMITTENT VERSUS CONTINUOUS ANDROGEN DEPRIVATION**

We found insufficient evidence on the effects of intermittent androgen deprivation in men with metastatic prostate cancer.

Benefits: We found no systematic review and no RCTs assessing the long term effects of intermittent androgen deprivation on mortality, morbidity, or quality of life.

Harms: We found insufficient evidence to assess harms.

Comment: None.

QUESTION **What are the effects of treatments for men with symptomatic androgen independent metastatic disease?**

OPTION **CHEMOTHERAPY**

RCTs have found that chemotherapy decreases pain and prolongs pain relief in some men with symptomatic androgen independent prostate cancer. We found no evidence that chemotherapy prolongs survival.

Benefits: We found no systematic review. We found three RCTs.[9–11] The first RCT (161 men with symptomatic androgen independent metastatic prostate cancer) compared mitoxantrone (mitozantrone) plus prednisone versus prednisone alone.[9] Men not on mitoxantrone were crossed over to mitoxantrone at disease progression or if non-responding at 6 weeks. It found that men receiving chemotherapy were significantly more likely to experience pain reduction (29% with chemotherapy plus prednisone *v* 12% with prednisone alone; P = 0.01), enjoy longer pain relief (43 *v* 18 wks; P < 0.0001), and show improvements in quality of life. There was no significant difference in overall survival. The second unblinded RCT (242 men) compared mitoxantrone plus hydrocortisone versus hydrocortisone alone. People were allowed alternative chemotherapy after disease progression.[10] It found no significant difference in survival (median duration 12.3 months with mitoxantrone plus hydrocortisone *v* 12.6 months with hydrocortisone; P = 0.77). However, pain and analgesic use were reduced after chemotherapy. The third RCT (458 men with prostate cancer and painful bone metastases) compared suramin plus hydrocortisone versus placebo plus hydrocortisone.[11] People on placebo were allowed to cross over to suramin at disease progression. It found that chemotherapy improved pain (pain response 43% with chemotherapy *v* 28% with placebo; P = 0.01). It found no significant effect on survival (median survival 286 days with suramin *v* 279 days with placebo; reported as non-significant but P value not provided).

Harms: The RCTs reported no treatment related deaths. There were nine episodes of febrile neutropenia (World Health Organization [WHO] grade 3 or 4) among 130 men treated with 796 courses of mitoxantrone.[9] Five men experienced cardiac arrhythmia or decreased left ventricular ejection fraction, including two who developed congestive heart failure.

Comment: A crossover design reduces the likelihood of reaching reliable conclusions about the effect of chemotherapy on survival, because most people allocated to placebo eventually received chemotherapy. Early, unpublished clinical trials suggested high response rates for taxane based chemotherapy and an intergroup RCT comparing it with established regimens is ongoing.

OPTION EXTERNAL BEAM RADIATION THERAPY

We found no RCTs comparing external beam radiation versus palliative treatments other than radionuclides. Observational evidence suggests complete pain relief in about a quarter of people, and placebo controlled RCTs would probably be considered unethical. A systematic review of one RCT in men with symptomatic bone metastases found no difference in survival between external beam radiation versus strontium-89; however, strontium-89 was associated with significantly fewer new sites of pain, and reduced need for additional radiotherapy.

Benefits: **Versus other no treatment or placebo:** We found one systematic review (search date 1996, 0 RCTs), which found no RCTs of external beam radiation versus no treatment or placebo.[12] We found no additional RCTs (see comment below). The systematic review reported changes from baseline in RCTs comparing external beam radiotherapy versus radionuclides and comparing different doses and schedules. The observational studies (11 studies, 1486 people) found complete pain relief in 27% (368/1373) of people and at least 50% pain relief in 42% (628/1486) of people treated with external beam radiotherapy (see comment below). **External beam versus radionuclides:** We found one systematic review (search date 1996, 1 RCT, 305 men).[12] The RCT (305 men) compared external beam radiation versus strontium-89.[13] It found that strontium-89 was associated with significantly fewer new sites of pain ($P < 0.05$) and significantly reduced need for additional radiotherapy ($P < 0.04$). However, it found no significant difference in survival (median survival 33 weeks with strontium-89 *v* 28 weeks with radiotherapy; $P = 0.10$).[12] **Different schedules and doses:** We found one systematic review (search date 1996, 9 RCTs, 1486 men with symptomatic bone metastases from a variety of malignancies).[12] The RCTs compared different radiation treatment fractionation schedules and doses of external beam radiation. It found minimal differences in pain relief between different fractionation schedules and doses.

Harms: The systematic review reported that adverse event reporting was poor.[12]

Comment: In men with painful bone metastases it would be considered unethical to compare external beam radiation with placebo or no treatment. It is reasonable to consider the effectiveness of no treatment to be zero as spontaneous remission has not been described in bone metastases from prostate cancer.

OPTION RADIONUCLIDE THERAPY

One systematic review found one small RCT in men with symptomatic bone metastases, which found no difference in survival between external beam radiation plus placebo versus external beam radiation plus

strontium-89. However, strontium-89 significantly reduced the number of new sites of pain. One small subsequent RCT in men with painful bone metastases found that samarium-153 versus placebo significantly reduced pain scores. A second small subsequent RCT in a selected population found an improvement in survival with strontium-89 versus placebo, but the results are difficult to generalise. One RCT in men with symptomatic bone metastases found no difference in survival between external beam radiation versus strontium-89; however, strontium-89 was associated with significantly fewer new sites of pain, and reduced need for additional radiotherapy.

Benefits: **Versus other palliative treatments:** We found one systematic review (search date 1996, 1 RCT, 126 men)[12] and two subsequent RCTs.[14,15] The RCT in the systematic review (126 men) compared external beam radiation plus strontium-89 versus external beam radiation plus placebo.[16] Although the RCT found no significant difference in overall survival or symptom relief, strontium-89 significantly reduced the number of new sites of pain ($P < 0.02$), and significantly reduced analgesic requirement (17% stopped taking analgesics with radionuclide *v* 2% on placebo; $P < 0.05$). The first subsequent RCT (118 people with painful bone metastases from multiple primaries) compared samarium-153 lexidronam 0.5 mCi/kg versus samarium-153 lexidronam 1 mCi/kg versus placebo over 4 weeks.[15] It found that samarium-153 1 mCi/kg significantly reduced pain scores versus placebo at weeks 1–4 ($P < 0.034$). Samarium-153 0.5 mCi/kg reduced pain scores significantly more than placebo at week 1 ($P = 0.044$) but not at other weeks ($P > 0.078$). The second subsequent RCT (72 men with androgen independent, metastatic prostate cancer who had initially responded to "induction" chemotherapy with ketoconazole and doxorubicin alternating with estramustine and vinblastine) compared maintenance chemotherapy (doxorubicin) with and without strontium-89.[14] From follow up of 67 people to death, it was estimated that strontium-89 significantly increased median overall survival (27.7 months with chemotherapy plus strontium-89 *v* 16.8 months with chemotherapy alone; $P < 0.002$) and significantly increased time to progression (13.9 months with chemotherapy plus strontium-89 *v* 7.0 months with chemotherapy alone; $P < 0.0001$) (see comment below). **Versus external beam radiation:** (See external beam versus radionuclides under benefits of external beam radiation therapy, p 887).

Harms: Strontium-89 was associated with thrombocytopenia (WHO grade 3 or 4) in 7–33% of men and leukopenia (WHO grade 3 or 4) in 3–12% of men.[12,17] Other radionuclides with selective bone localisation have similar rates of haematological toxicity. There was no significant difference between treatment schedules and doses of external beam radiation in rates of nausea, vomiting, or diarrhoea.[18]

Comment: The small RCT[17] included in previous versions of *Clinical Evidence* was removed because of its small size and weak methods. The results of the second subsequent RCT are difficult to generalise because they were in a selected population who had reacted favourably to an atypical chemotherapy regimen.[14]

OPTION BISPHOSPHONATES

We found insufficient evidence on the effects of bisphosphonates in men with prostate cancer.

Benefits: One systematic review (search date not stated, 2 RCTs, 156 men with prostate cancer and symptomatic bone metastases) found no reduction in bone pain with bisphosphonates.[19]

Harms: The systematic review identified 18 RCTs of bisphosphonates in men with bone metastases from a variety of cancers.[19] No RCT reported major toxicity. Treatment with pamidronate was associated with increased frequency of anterior uveitis and episcleritis.

Comment: Both RCTs in the systematic review[19] had weak methods; one did not use a pain scale, whereas the other assessed etidronate, a bisphosphonate that is pharmacologically unsuitable for treating bone metastases. One RCT found potential benefit of pamidronate in preventing bone loss in men receiving androgen deprivation therapy, but it was not designed to assess effect on disease progression.

GLOSSARY

Orchidectomy Also known as orchiectomy.

Substantive changes

Androgen deprivation: different types of androgen deprivation New systematic review.[2] It found no significant differences in 2 year survival between orchidectomy versus luteinising hormone releasing hormone agonists or versus non-steroidal antiandrogen monotherapy.

Androgen deprivation One RCT found that androgen deprivation by orchidectomy or by combination of gonadotrophin releasing hormone analogue with an antiandrogen induces significantly more hot flushes than polyestradiol phosphate.[4]

Radionuclide therapy versus other palliative treatments: One new RCT found that strontium-89 versus placebo reduced pain scores over 4 weeks.[15]

REFERENCES

1. Byar DP, Corle DK. Hormone therapy for prostate cancer: results of the Veterans Administration Cooperative Urologic Research Group studies. *NCI Monogr* 1988;7:165–170.
2. Seidenfeld J, Samson DJ, Hasselblad V, et al. Single-therapy androgen suppression in men with advanced prostate cancer: a systematic review and meta-analysis. *Ann Intern Med* 2000;132:566–577. Search date 1998; primary sources Medline, Cancerlit, Embase, The Cochrane Library, and Current Contents.
3. Hedlund PO, Henriksson P. Parenteral estrogen versus total androgen ablation in the treatment of advanced prostate carcinoma: effects on overall survival and cardiovascular mortality. *Urology* 2000;55:328–332.
4. Spetz A, Hammar M, Lindberg B, et al. Prospective evaluation of hot flashes during treatment with parenteral estrogen or complete androgen ablation for metastatic carcinoma of the prostate. *J Urol* 2001;166:517–520.
5. Medical Research Council Prostate Cancer Working Party Investigators Group. Immediate versus deferred treatment for advanced prostatic cancer: initial results of the Medical Research Council trial. *Br J Urol* 1997;79:235–246.
6. Messing EM, Manola J, Sarodsy M, et al. Immediate hormonal therapy compared with observation after radical prostatectomy and pelvic lymphadenectomy in men with node-positive prostate cancer. *N Engl J Med* 1999;341:1781–1789.
7. Prostate Cancer Clinical Trialists' Collaborative Group. Maximum androgen blockade in advanced prostate cancer: an overview of the randomized trials. *Lancet* 2000;355:1491–1498. Search date not stated; primary sources computerised literature search, proceedings of congresses, contacts with authors, trial groups, and pharmaceutical industry.
8. Schmitt B, Wilt TJ, Schellhammer PF, et al. Combined androgen blockade with non-steroidal antiandrogens for advanced prostate cancer: a systematic review. *Urology* 2001;57:727–732. Search date not stated; primary sources Blue Cross and Blue Shield Association's Technology Evaluation Center data set, Cochrane Controlled Trials Register, Cochrane Central Register, and the Veterans Administration Cochrane Prostate Disease and Urologic Malignancy Register.
9. Tannock IF, Osoba D, Stockler MR, et al. Chemotherapy with mitoxantrone plus prednisone

or prednisone alone for symptomatic hormone-resistant prostate cancer: a Canadian randomized trial with palliative end points. *J Clin Oncol* 1996;14:1756–1764.
10. Kantoff PW, Halabi S, Conaway M, et al. Hydrocortisone with or without mitoxantrone in men with hormone-refractory prostate cancer: results of the Cancer and Leukemia Group B 9182 Study. *J Clin Oncol* 1999;17:2506–2513.
11. Small EJ, Marshall E, Reyno L, et al. Suramin therapy for patients with symptomatic hormone-refractory prostate cancer: results of a randomised phase III trial comparing suramin plus hydrocortisone to placebo plus hydrocortisone. *J Clin Oncol* 2000;18:1440–1450.
12. McQuay HJ, Carroll D, Moore RA. Radiotherapy for painful bone metastases: a systematic review. *Clin Oncol (R Coll Radiol)* 1997;9:150–154. Search date 1996; primary sources Medline, the Oxford Pain Relief database, Embase, Cochrane Library, and reference lists.
13. Quilty PM, Kirk D, Bolger JJ, et al. A comparison of the palliative effects of strontium-89 and external beam radiotherapy in metastatic prostate cancer. *Radiother Oncol* 1994;31:33–40.
14. Tu S, Millikan RE, Mengistu B, et al. Bone-targeted therapy for advanced androgen-independent carcinoma of the prostate: a randomized Phase II trial. *Lancet* 2001;357:336–341.
15. Serafini AN, Houston SJ, Resche I, et al. Palliation of pain associated with metastatic bone cancer using samarium-153 lexidronam: a double-blind placebo-controlled clinical trial. *J Clin Oncol* 1998;16:1574–1581.
16. Porter AT, McEwan AJ, Powe JE, et al. Results of a randomized Phase-III trial to evaluate the efficacy of strontium-89 adjuvant to local field external beam irradiation in the management of endocrine resistant metastatic prostate cancer. *Int J Radiat Oncol Biol Phys* 1993;25:805–813.
17. Maxon HR, Schroder LE, Hertzberg VS, et al. Rhenium-186(Sn)HEDP for treatment of painful osseous metastases: results of a double-blind crossover comparison with placebo. *J Nucl Med* 1991;32:1877–1881.
18. Robinson RG, Preston DF, Schiefelbein M, et al. Strontium 89 therapy for the palliation of pain due to osseous metastases. *JAMA* 1995;274:420–424. Search date 1994; primary source Medline.
19. Bloomfield DJ. Should bisphosphonates be part of the standard therapy of patients with multiple myeloma or bone metastases from other cancers? An evidence-based review. *J Clin Oncol* 1998;16:1218–1225. Search date not stated; primary sources Medline, hand search of major cancer journals, reference lists, and contact with experts.

M Dror Michaelson
Instructor in Medicine
Massachusetts General Hospital
Boston
USA

James A Talcott
Assistant Professor of Medicine
Harvard Medical School
Boston
USA

Matthew R Smith
Assistant Professor
Massachusetts General Hospital
Boston
USA

Competing interests: None declared.

Prostate cancer: non-metastatic

Search date October 2001

Timothy Wilt

QUESTIONS

INTERVENTIONS

See glossary, p 900

Key Messages

Clinically localised prostate cancer

- **Androgen suppression** We found no RCTs assessing the effects of primary treatment with early androgen suppression in the absence of symptoms on length or quality of life in men with clinically localised prostate cancer. We found limited evidence from one RCT that androgen suppression with bicalutamide versus placebo reduced disease progression after a median of 2.6 years, but interpreting the results was difficult because men with prostate cancer of different stages were included in the trial.
- **External beam radiation** We found no RCTs comparing external beam radiation versus watchful waiting. Limited evidence from one small RCT suggests that external beam radiation versus radical prostatectomy may increase the risk of metastases.

- **Radical prostatectomy** One small RCT found no evidence that radical prostatectomy improved survival or reduced the risk of metastases compared with watchful waiting. Limited evidence from one RCT in men with clinically localised prostate cancer suggests that radical prostatectomy versus radiation treatment may reduce the risk of metastases (NNT 5, 95% CI 3 to 25). Radical prostatectomy carries the risks of major surgery and of sexual and urinary dysfunction.
- **Watchful waiting** One small RCT found no significant difference in survival between radical prostatectomy versus watchful waiting in men with clinically localised prostate cancer. We found no information from RCTs on quality of life.
- **Androgen suppression in asymptomatic men with raised prostate specific antigen concentrations after early treatment; brachytherapy; cryosurgery** We found no RCTs on the effects of these interventions.

Locally advanced prostate cancer

- **Androgen suppression in addition to early external beam radiation (improves survival compared with radiation and deferred androgen suppression)** One systematic review has found that immediate versus deferred androgen suppression in men with locally advanced disease treated with radiotherapy significantly increases survival at 5 years. One RCT found no difference in overall survival or local disease control after orchiectomy, whether or not it was combined with radiotherapy, but the results are difficult to interpret.
- **Androgen suppression initiated at diagnosis** RCTs found limited evidence that, in men with locally advanced disease, androgen suppression initiated at diagnosis versus deferred androgen suppression reduces complications and may improve survival.
- **Immediate androgen suppression after radical prostatectomy and pelvic lymphadenectomy in men with node-positive prostate cancer (compared with radical prostatectomy and deferred androgen suppression)** One RCT in men with node positive prostate cancer has found that immediate androgen suppression versus deferred androgen suppression after radical prostatectomy and pelvic lymphadenectomy significantly reduces mortality over a median of 7.1 years (NNT 4, 95% CI 3 to 33).

DEFINITION Prostatic cancer is staged according to two systems: the tumour, node, metastasis (TNM) classification system, and the American Urologic Staging system (see table 1, p 902). Non-metastatic prostate cancer can be divided into clinically localised disease and advanced disease. Clinically localised disease is prostate cancer thought to be confined to the prostate gland by clinical examination. Locally advanced disease is disease that has spread outside the capsule of the prostate gland but has not yet spread to other organs. Metastatic disease is prostate cancer that has spread outside the prostate gland to either local, regional, or systemic lymph nodes, seminal vesicles, or to other body organs (e.g. bone, liver, brain) and is not connected to the prostate gland. We consider clinically localised and locally advanced disease in a separate chapter from metastatic disease (see prostate cancer: metastatic, p 881).

INCIDENCE/ PREVALENCE Prostate cancer is the most common non-dermatological malignancy worldwide and is the second most common cause of cancer death in men in the USA.[1] There were an estimated 180 400 new cases and 31 900 deaths in the USA in 2000.[2] For a 50 year old man with a life expectancy of 25 years, the lifetime risk of microscopic prostate cancer is about 42%, the risk of clinically evident prostate cancer is 10%, and that of fatal prostate cancer is 3%.[3]

AETIOLOGY/ RISK FACTORS Risk factors include age, family history of prostate cancer, black race, and possibly higher dietary fat and calcium intake. In the USA, black men have about a 60% higher incidence rate than white men.[4] The prostate cancer incidence rate for black men living in the USA is about 90/100 000 (ages < 65 years) and about 1300/100 000 (ages 65–74 years). For white men, incidence rates are about 44/100 000 (ages < 65 years) and 900/100 000 (ages 65–74 years).

PROGNOSIS The chance that men with well to moderately differentiated, palpable, clinically localised prostate cancer will remain free of symptomatic progression is 70% at 5 years and 40% at 10 years.[5] The risk of symptomatic disease progression is higher in men with poorly differentiated prostate cancer.[6] One retrospective analysis of a large surgical series in men with clinically localised prostate cancer found that the median time from the increase in prostate specific antigen (PSA) concentration to the development of metastatic disease was 8 years. Time to PSA progression, PSA doubling time, and Gleason score (see glossary, p 900) were predictive of the probability and time to development of metastatic disease. Once men developed metastatic disease, the median actuarial time to death was less than 5 years.[7] Morbidity from local or regional disease progression includes haematuria, bladder obstruction, and lower extremity oedema. In the USA, population based studies found that death rates from prostate cancer have declined by only about 1/100 000 men since 1992, despite widespread testing for PSA and increased rates of radical prostatectomy (see glossary, p 900) and radiotherapy.[8,9] Regions of the USA with the greatest decreases in mortality are those with the lowest rates of testing for PSA and treatment with radical prostatectomy or radiation.[9] Countries with low rates of testing and treatment do not have consistently higher age adjusted rates of death from prostate cancer than countries with high rates of testing and treatment such as the USA.

AIMS To prevent premature death and disability, and to minimise adverse effects of treatment.

OUTCOMES Survival; time to progression; response in terms of symptoms and signs; quality of life; adverse effects of treatment. Where clinical outcomes are not available, surrogate outcomes have been used (PSA concentration; Gleason score for histological grade).

METHODS *Clinical Evidence* search and appraisal October 2001. Additional author search: Cochrane Library and Medline to 2001 for systematic reviews and RCTs, using the search strategy of the Department of Veterans' Affairs Coordinating Centre for the Cochrane Review Group on Prostatic Diseases.

QUESTION **What are the effects of treatments for clinically localised prostate cancer?**

OPTION **WATCHFUL WAITING**

One small RCT found no significant difference in survival with radical prostatectomy versus watchful waiting in men with clinically localised prostate cancer. We found no information from RCTs on quality of life.

Benefits: We found no recent systematic reviews, but found one overview that did not provide details of the studies included (search date 1993, 165 articles),[1] and one non-systematic decision analysis.[10] We found two more recent large cohort studies, which found that, in men managed with watchful waiting, 15 year disease specific survival was 80%: ranging from 95% for well differentiated to 30% for poorly differentiated cancers.[11,12] **Versus early androgen suppression:** We found no RCTs. **Versus radical prostatectomy:** See glossary, p 900. We found one RCT (see benefits of radical prostatectomy, p 894).[13]

Harms: Watchful waiting may avoid the risks of surgery but does not remove a cancer that is potentially curable and that may progress to cause death and disability. However, we found insufficient evidence to comment on whether early intervention reduces the risk of disease specific death and disability compared with watchful waiting.

Comment: There is about a 10 year lead time between the detection of cancers by raised prostate specific antigen concentrations and detection by digital rectal examination or the development of symptoms. This means that outcomes are likely to be similar in men with palpable tumours who are followed for 15 years and men whose tumours are detected because of raised prostate specific antigen concentrations who are followed for 25 years (lead time bias).

OPTION **RADICAL PROSTATECTOMY**

One small RCT found no evidence that radical prostatectomy improved survival compared with watchful waiting. Radical prostatectomy may reduce the risk of metastases compared with external beam radiation. Radical prostatectomy carries the risks of major surgery and of sexual and urinary dysfunction.

Benefits: We found no recent systematic reviews. **Versus watchful waiting:** One small RCT (142 men with clinically localised prostate cancer) compared radical prostatectomy (see glossary, p 900) versus watchful waiting. After a median follow up of 23 years (range 19–27 years), it found longer survival with prostatectomy but the difference was not significant (median survival 10.6 years with prostatectomy *v* 8 years with watchful waiting; no 95% CI provided).[13] Analysis was not by intention to treat. **Versus external beam radiation:** One RCT (97 men with clinically localised prostate cancer) compared radical prostatectomy versus external beam radiation. Men receiving prostatectomy had reduced risk of metastases (4/41 [9.8%] "treatment failures" with prostatectomy *v* 17/56 [30.4%] with radiation; RR 0.32, 95% CI 0.12 to 0.88; NNT 5, 95% CI 3 to 25).[14]

Harms: Fatal complications have been reported in 0.5–1% of men treated with radical prostatectomy and may exceed 2% in men aged 75 years and older.[15] Nearly 8% of men older than 65 years suffered major cardiopulmonary complications within 30 days of operation. The incidence of other adverse effects of surgery was over 80% for sexual dysfunction, 30% for urinary incontinence requiring pads or clamps to control wetness, 18% for urethral stricture, 3% for total urinary incontinence, 5% for faecal incontinence, and 1% for bowel injury requiring surgical repair.[1,16–18]

Comment: Both RCTs of radical prostatectomy took place before the advent of tests for prostate specific antigen and were too small to rule out a clinically important difference between groups. Radical prostatectomy may benefit selected groups of men with localised prostate cancer, particularly younger men with higher grade tumours, but the studies did not look for this effect. The available evidence suggests that in most men the benefits in quality adjusted life expectancy are at best small and sensitive to individual's preferences.[10] No differences have been found in the general health related quality of life among non-randomised groups treated with radical prostatectomy, radiation, or watchful waiting.[19] Two ongoing trials are comparing radical prostatectomy versus watchful waiting.[20,21]

OPTION EXTERNAL BEAM RADIATION

We found limited evidence from one small RCT that, compared with radical prostatectomy, external beam radiation increased the risk of metastases in men with clinically localised prostate cancer. We found no RCTs comparing external beam radiation versus watchful waiting. One RCT found that conformal radiotherapy reduced rates of radiation proctitis and rectal bleeding compared with conventional radiotherapy. We found no evidence of a difference in survival between conventional and conformal radiotherapy.

Benefits: **Versus watchful waiting:** We found no RCTs. **Versus radical prostatectomy:** See glossary, p 900. We found one RCT (see benefits of radical prostatectomy, p 894).[14] **Conformal versus conventional radiotherapy:** See glossary, p 900. One RCT (225 men with non-metastatic prostate cancer T1–T4, N0, or M0) compared conformal versus conventional radiotherapy.[22] Primary outcomes were adverse effects (see harms below). It did not report on survival, but found no significant difference in tumour control (by prostate specific antigen level) between treatments after a median follow up of 3.6 years.

Harms: The RCT of radiotherapy versus radical prostatectomy made no mention of adverse effects.[14] One survey of men treated with external beam radiation reported that 7% wore pads to control wetness, 23–32% were impotent, and 10% reported problems with bowel dysfunction.[23] Treatment related mortality was less than 0.5%.[1] External beam radiation requires that men return for daily outpatient treatment for up to 6 weeks. **Conventional versus conformal radiotherapy:** The RCT found that significantly fewer men treated with conformal radiation developed radiation induced proctitis and rectal bleeding. It found no differences between groups for adverse effects on the bladder.[22]

Comment: Up to 30% of men with clinically localised prostate cancer treated with radiotherapy still have positive biopsies 2–3 years after treatment.[24] One retrospective, non-randomised, multicentre pooled analysis found 5 year estimates of overall survival, disease specific survival, and freedom from biochemical failure (as defined by raised prostate specific antigen) to be 85%, 95%, and 66%, respectively. Estimated 5 year rates of no biochemical recurrence according to prostate specific antigen concentrations before treatment and Gleason scores (see glossary, p 900) ranged from 81% for pretreatment prostate specific antigen less than 10 ng/mL to 29% for prostate specific antigen of 20 ng/mL or more, and a Gleason score from 7–10.[25]

OPTION BRACHYTHERAPY

Systematic reviews found no RCTs on the effects of brachytherapy in men with clinically localised prostate cancer.

Benefits: We found three systematic reviews (search dates 1997,[26] 1999,[27] and 1999[28]), which identified no RCTs comparing brachytherapy (see glossary, p 900) alone or in combination with other treatments (androgen suppression (see glossary, p 900) or radiation).

Harms: In one review, complications reported from 13 case series and three cohort studies included acute urinary retention (1–14%), incontinence (5–6%), cystitis/urethritis (14%), urethral stricture (1%), proctitis (1–14%), and impotence (4–50%).[27]

Comment: One systematic review identified 13 case series and three cohort studies.[27] The studies used proxy outcomes (evidence of disease measure by prostate specific antigen [PSA] testing). Results varied considerably from one series to another and were highly dependent on tumour stage, grade, and pretreatment serum PSA levels. Results in men with T1 or T2 tumours, Gleason score (see glossary, p 900) of 6 or lower, and serum PSA level of 10 ng/mL or less were similar to those from case series of people undergoing radical prostatectomy (see glossary, p 900). One additional retrospective cohort study (1872 men) found that in low risk men (see table 1, p 902) (stage T1c, stage T2a, PSA concentration ≤ 10 ng/mL, and Gleason score ≤ 6) the chance of a high PSA concentration at 5 years was similar whether they were treated with radiation or brachytherapy implant (with or without preceding androgen suppression) or with radical prostatectomy. Men at intermediate or high risk (Gleason score > 6 or PSA > 10 ng/mL) were more likely to have high PSA concentration at 5 years with brachytherapy than with radical prostatectomy (RR of high PSA in men at intermediate risk 3.1, 95% CI 1.5 to 6.1; RR in men at high risk 3.0, 95% CI 1.8 to 5.0).[29] The study used proxy outcomes (PSA concentrations) rather than clinical outcomes. RCTs comparing brachytherapy versus radical prostatectomy are ongoing.

OPTION CRYOSURGERY

We found no RCTs about the effects of cryotherapy in men with clinically localised prostate cancer.

Benefits: We found no systematic review or RCTs.

Harms: Complications reported in case series include impotence (65%), transient scrotal oedema (10%), sloughed urethral tissue (3%), urethral stricture (1%), incontinence, urethrorectal fistula, and prostatic abscess (1%).[30]

Comment: One ongoing trial is comparing cryosurgery with radiation.

OPTION ANDROGEN SUPPRESSION

We found no RCTs assessing the effects of primary treatment with early androgen suppression in the absence of symptoms on length or quality of life in men with clinically localised prostate cancer. We found limited evidence from one RCT that androgen suppression with bicalutamide versus placebo significantly reduced disease progression after a median of 2.6 years, but interpreting the results is difficult because men with prostate cancer of different stages were included in the trial.

Benefits: We found no systematic reviews. We found one RCT (3603 men with prostate cancer stages T1 or T2 [65%], T3 [32%], or T4 [3%], any nodal status, and M0) of androgen suppression (see glossary, p 900) (with bicalutamide) versus placebo until disease progression.[31] About 45% of the men had received radical prostatectomy (see glossary, p 900), 20% had received radiotherapy, and 35% had received watchful waiting. The trial found bicalutamide significantly reduced disease progression (HR 0.57, 95% CI 0.48 to 0.69) after a median of 2.6 years. There were not enough events to assess the effect on mortality.

Harms: See harms of androgen suppression for the treatment of men with locally advanced prostate cancer, p 898. The most commonly reported adverse events were gynaecomastia and breast pain (gynaecomastia plus breast pain 47.5% with bicalutamide *v* 2.1% with placebo; $P < 0.05$), and hot flushes (9.3% with bicalutamide *v* 4.6% with placebo; $P < 0.05$).[32]

Comment: The RCT reported that results were consistent across clinical stages, but did not provide information to assess this.

QUESTION In men who have received primary treatment and remain asymptomatic, should androgen suppression be offered when raised concentrations of prostate specific antigens are detected?

We found no RCTs on the effects of initiating androgen suppression when prostate specific antigen rises or persists after primary treatment.

Benefits: We found one systematic review (search date 1998), that identified no RCTs.[33]

Harms: See harms of androgen suppression for the treatment of men with locally advanced prostate cancer, p 898.

Comment: In the USA, clinicians often monitor blood concentrations of prostate specific antigen and offer androgen suppression (see glossary, p 900) when these rise. Consequently, more men with persistent disease are considered for androgen suppression and treatment is initiated earlier in the natural course of the disease. RCTs are needed to evaluate the effectiveness of this approach and of intermittent treatment, in which androgen suppression is initiated when prostate specific antigen rises after primary treatment and discontinued when the antigen concentrations return to nadir.[33]

QUESTION **What are the effects of treatments for locally advanced prostate cancer?**

OPTION **ANDROGEN SUPPRESSION**

RCTs found limited evidence that, in men with locally advanced disease, androgen suppression initiated at diagnosis versus no initial treatment or versus deferred androgen suppression reduced complications and may improve survival.

Benefits: **Versus no initial treatment:** We found no recent RCTs. Three RCTs performed between 1960 and 1975 (about 4000 men with all stages of prostate cancer) compared androgen suppression (see glossary, p 900) (diethylstilbestrol [stilboestrol], orchiectomy, or oestrogens) versus no initial treatment. They found no difference in overall survival. Re-analysis of updated data from these RCTs provided tentative evidence of a modest survival advantage with androgen suppression.[34] **Immediate (initiated at diagnosis) versus deferred androgen suppression:** We found one systematic review (search date 1998, 3 RCTs, 2143 men).[33] Two of the RCTs were conducted in the 1960s. None had a uniform protocol for initiating deferred treatment, so deferred treatment in these RCTs reflects the varied practices of the treating clinicians. Men in the deferred hormonal treatment group were not closely monitored with prostate specific antigen testing. The systematic review found no significant survival difference at 5 years between immediate compared with deferred androgen suppression (HR 0.91, 95% CI 0.81 to 1.03).[34] A more recent trial, which included 938 men with stage C (locally advanced) and D (asymptomatic metastatic) disease, reported a survival benefit from immediate treatment in men with stage C disease (survival benefit measured by survival curve P = 0.02; CI not calculable).[35] In people with stage C disease, immediate androgen suppression was associated with a non-significantly lower risk of major complications, such as pathological fractures (3/256 [1.2%] *v* 6/244 [2.5%] with deferred treatment; RR 0.48, 95% CI 0.12 to 1.9 with deferred treatment), ureteric obstruction (22/256 [8.6%] *v* 28/244 [11.5%]; RR 0.75, 95% CI 0.44 to 1.3), and extraskeletal metastases (17/256 [6.6%] *v* 26/244 [10%]; RR 0.62, 95% CI 0.35 to 1.1). The trial did not make clear the time interval over which outcomes were recorded, although this seemed to be at least 10 years. The lower incidence of complications was more apparent in men presenting with stage C disease. One additional RCT in men with cancers of different stages found an improvement in disease free survival with bicalutamide versus placebo.[31] See benefits of androgen suppression under effects of treating clinically localised prostate cancer, p 897.

Harms: Adverse events were not well reported in the review. Earlier initiation of androgen suppression means longer exposure to adverse effects, which include osteoporosis, weight gain, hot flushes (10–60%), loss of muscle mass, gynaecomastia (5–10%), impotence (10–30%), and loss of libido (5–30%).[33] These adverse effects are particularly important in the treatment of men with long life expectancy or younger men with lower grade cancers. The review did not report on quality of life.

Comment: The RCTs conducted in the 1960s[33] included men who were older and had more advanced cancers than those in the more recent RCT.[35] RCTs are needed to evaluate the effectiveness of androgen suppression before surgery when disease extends beyond the capsule.

OPTION ANDROGEN SUPPRESSION IN ADDITION TO EXTERNAL BEAM RADIATION

One systematic review has found that early androgen suppression versus deferred androgen suppression significantly improves overall survival at 5 years in men with locally advanced disease treated with radiotherapy. One additional RCT found no difference in overall survival or local disease control after orchiectomy, whether or not it was combined with radiotherapy, but the results are difficult to interpret.

Benefits: We found one systematic review (search date 1998, 4 RCTs, 1565 men)[33] and one additional RCT.[36] The review compared early versus deferred androgen suppression in men receiving external beam radiation.[33] Early androgen suppression was initiated at the same time as radiation treatment for locally advanced, or asymptomatic but clinically evident, metastatic prostate cancer, and was continued until the development of hormone refractory disease. The deferred group received radiation treatment alone, with androgen suppression initiated only in those in whom the disease progressed. The systematic review found that early androgen suppression improved overall 5 year survival compared with deferred treatment (percentage surviving at 5 years 76.5% *v* 68.2%; ARR 8.3%; HR 0.63, 95% CI 0.48 to 0.83; NNT at 5 years 12).[33] Long term follow up of one of the RCTs (476 men, stages T2–T4, with or without pelvic lymph node involvement) included in the review found more people survived with androgen suppression at 8 years but the difference was not significant (53% with androgen suppression *v* 44% without androgen suppression; P = 0.10), but there was a significant improvement in disease free survival (33% *v* 21%; P = 0.004) and in the incidence of distant metastases (34% *v* 45%; P = 0.04).[31] The additional RCT (277 men with advanced localised prostate cancer; T2–T4, M0, with and without nodal disease) compared orchiectomy alone versus radiotherapy alone versus radiotherapy in addition to orchiectomy.[36] It found no significant difference in overall survival or need for further treatment for local disease progression between the three treatment groups (data presented as a diagram; no P value provided).

Harms: The review reported adverse effects of androgen suppression (see harms of androgen suppression for the treatment of men with locally advanced prostate cancer, p 898).[33] In the additional RCT, adverse effects attributable to radiotherapy included bowel symptoms (19%), urinary symptoms excluding transient frequency (8%), bowel and urinary complications (1%), rectal bleeding necessitating blood transfusion (2%), and radiation proctitis (1%), which was a contributory factor in the two peoples' deaths. After orchiectomy, hot flushes (15%) were the predominant adverse effect.[36]

Comment: We found no evidence from RCTs about the effectiveness of external beam radiation alone versus no treatment in men with locally advanced prostate cancer. The additional RCT may have been underpowered to detect a difference in mortality.[36]

OPTION **ANDROGEN SUPPRESSION AFTER RADICAL PROSTATECTOMY AND PELVIC LYMPHADENECTOMY**

One RCT in men with node positive prostate cancer found that immediate androgen suppression after radical prostatectomy and pelvic lymphadenectomy versus deferred androgen suppression significantly improved survival over a median 7.1 years and reduced the risk of recurrence.

Benefits: We found one RCT (98 men after radical prostatectomy and pelvic lymphadenectomy for nodal metastases) of immediate androgen suppression (with either goserelin or bilateral orchiectomy) versus androgen suppression deferred until disease progression.[37] It found that antiandrogens decreased mortality in the long term (median follow up 7.1 years; mortality 7/47 [14.9%] with antiandrogen *v* 18/51 [35.3%] with watchful waiting; ARR 20.4%; RR 0.42, 95% CI 0.19 to 0.92; NNT 4, 95% CI 3 to 33), and resulted in a higher proportion of men with undetectable prostate specific antigen ($P < 0.001$).

Harms: The RCT found that, compared with deferred androgen suppression, immediate androgen suppression caused more haematological effects (15% *v* 4%), gastrointestinal effects (25% *v* 6%), non-specific genitourinary effects (48% *v* 12%), hot flushes (56% *v* 0%), and weight gain (18% *v* 2%).[37]

Comment: None.

GLOSSARY

Androgen suppression Monotherapy uses a single drug or surgical procedure for androgen suppression. Methods include orchiectomy (removal of both testes), diethylstilbestrol, luteinising hormone releasing agonist injections, or non-steroidal antiandrogens. Combined androgen blockade uses the addition of a non-steroidal antiandrogen to standard androgen suppression monotherapy with orchiectomy, diethylstilbestrol, or luteinising hormone releasing agonist injection.

Brachytherapy Radiotherapy where the sources of ionising radiation are radioactive implants, many of which are permanently inserted directly into the prostate gland.

Conformal radiotherapy 3D radiotherapy planning systems and methods to match the radiation treatment to irregular tumour volumes.

Gleason score A number from 1–10 with 1 being the most well differentiated and 10 being the most poorly differentiated tumour or a histological examination.

Radical prostatectomy Surgical removal of the prostate with its capsule, seminal vesicles, ductus deferens, some pelvic fasciae, and sometimes pelvic lymph nodes; performed through either the retropubic or the perineal route.

REFERENCES

1. Middleton RG, Thompson IM, Austenfeld MS, et al. Prostate cancer clinical guidelines panel summary report on the management of clinically localized prostate cancer. *J Urol* 1995;154:2144–2148. Search date 1993; primary source Medline.
2. Landis SH, Murray T, Bolden S, et al. Cancer statistics. *CA Cancer J Clin* 2000;50:12–13.
3. Whitmore WF. Localized prostatic cancer: management and detection issues. *Lancet* 1994;343:1263–1267.
4. Stanford JL, Stephenson RA, Coyle LM, et al. Prostate Cancer Trends 1973–1995, SEER Program, National Cancer Institute. NIH Pub. No. 99–4543. Bethesda, MD, 1999.
5. Adolfsson J, Steineck G, Hedund P. Deferred treatment of clinically localized low-grade prostate cancer: actual 10-year and projected 15-year follow-up of the Karolinska series. *Urology* 1997;50:722–726.
6. Johansson J-E, Holmberg L, Johansson S, et al. Fifteen-year survival in prostate cancer: prospective, population-based study in Sweden. *JAMA* 1997;277:467–471.
7. Pound CR, Partin AW, Eisenberger MA, et al. Natural history of progression after PSA elevation following radical prostatectomy. *JAMA* 1999;281:1591–1597.
8. Brawley OW. Prostate carcinoma incidence and patient mortality. *Cancer* 1997;80:1857–1863.
9. Wingo PA, Ries LAG, Rosenberg HM, et al. Cancer incidence and mortality, 1973–1995. *Cancer* 1998;82:1197–1207.
10. Fleming C, Wasson J, Albertsen PC, et al. A decision analysis of alternative strategies for clinically localized prostate cancer. *JAMA* 1993;269:2650–2658.
11. Albertsen PC, Hanley JA, Gleason DF, Barry MJ. Competing risk analysis of men aged 55 to 74 years at diagnosis managed conservatively for clinically localized prostate cancer. *JAMA* 1998;280:975–980.
12. Lu-Yao GL, Yao S. Population-based study of long-term survival in patients with clinically localised prostate cancer. *Lancet* 1997;349:906–910.
13. Iversen P, Madsen PO, Corle DK. Radical prostatectomy versus expectant treatment for early carcinoma of the prostate: 23 year follow-up of a prospective randomized study. *Scand J Urol Nephrol Suppl* 1995;172(suppl):65–72.
14. Paulson DF, Lin GH, Hinshaw W, Stephani S, and the Uro-oncology Research Group. Radical surgery versus radiotherapy for adenocarcinoma of the prostate. *J Urol* 1982;128:502–504.
15. Lu-Yao GL, McLerran D, Wasson JH. An assessment of radical prostatectomy: time trends, geographic variation, and outcomes. *JAMA* 1993;269:2633–2636.
16. Anonymous. Screening for prostate cancer. *Ann Intern Med* 1997;126:480–484.
17. Fowler FJ, Barry MJ, Lu-Yao G, et al. Patient-reported complications and follow-up treatment after radical prostatectomy: the national Medicare experience 1988–1990 (updated June 1993). *Urology* 1993;42:622–629.
18. Bishoff JT, Motley G, Optenberg SA, et al. Incidence of fecal and urinary incontinence following radical perineal and retropubic prostatectomy in a national population. *J Urol* 1998;160:454–458.
19. Litwin MS, Hays RD, Fink A, et al. Quality-of-life outcomes in men treated for localized prostate cancer. *JAMA* 1995;273:129–135.
20. Wilt TJ, Brawer MK. The prostate cancer intervention versus observation trial. *Oncology* 1997;11:1133–1139.
21. Norlen BJ. Swedish randomized trial of radical prostatectomy versus watchful waiting. *Can J Oncol* 1994;4(suppl 1):38–42.
22. Dearnaley DP, Khoo VS, Norman AR, et al. Comparison of radiation side-effects of conformal and conventional radiotherapy in prostate cancer: a randomized trial. *Lancet* 1999;353:267–272.
23. Fowler FJ, Barry MJ, Lu-Yao G, et al. Outcomes of external beam radiation therapy for prostate cancer: a study of Medicare beneficiaries in three surveillance, epidemiology, and end results areas. *J Clin Oncol* 1996;14:2258–2265.
24. Crook J, Perry G, Robertson S, Esche B. Routine prostate biopsies: results for 225 patients. *Urology* 1995;45:624–632.
25. Shipley WU, Thames HD, Sandler HM, et al. Radiation therapy for clinically localized prostate cancer. A multi-institutional pooled analysis. *JAMA* 1999;281:1598–1604.
26. Brachytherapy for prostate cancer. Tec assessment program. *Blue Cross Blue Shield Assoc* 1997;12:1–27. Search date 1997; primary sources Medline, Current Contents, bibliographies, and abstracts of proceedings of scientific meetings.
27. Crook J, Lukka H, Klotz L, Bestic N, Johnston M, and the Genitourinary Cancer Disease Site Group of the Cancer Care Ontario Practice Guidelines Initiative. Systematic overview of the evidence for brachytherapy in clinically localized prostate cancer. *Can Med Assoc J* 2001;164:975–981. Search date 1999; primary sources Medline and Cancerlit.
28. Wills F, Hailey D. Brachytherapy for prostate cancer. *Edmonton, AB, Canada: The Alberta Heritage Foundation for Medical Research. Health Technology Assess* 1999:1–65. Search date 1999; primary sources The Cochrane Library, Medline, Healthstar, Cancerlit, Embase, Cinahl, hand search of reference lists, and internet searches.
29. Talcott JA, Clark JC, Stark P, Nadir B, Ragde N. Long term complications of brachytherapy for early prostate cancer. A survey of treated patients. *American Society of Clinical Oncology Annual Meeting* 1999; Abstract 1196.
30. Littrup PJ, Mody A, Sparschu RA. Prostate cryosurgery complications. *Semin Int Radiol* 1994;11:226–230.
31. Pilepich M, Winter M, Madhu J, et al. Phase III radiation therapy oncology group (RTOG) trial 86–10 of androgen deprivation adjuvant to definitive radiotherapy in locally advanced carcinoma of the prostate. *Int J Radiat Oncol Biol Phys* 2001;50:1243–1252.
32. Wirth M, Tyrrell C, Wallace M, et al. Bicalutamide (Casodex) 150 mg as immediate therapy in patients with localized or locally advanced prostate cancer significantly reduces the risk of disease progression. *Urology* 2001;58:146–150.
33. Agency for Health Care Policy and Research. Relative effectiveness and cost-effectiveness of methods of androgen suppression in the treatment of advanced prostatic cancer. Summary. Rockville, MD: Agency for Health Care Policy and Research, 1999. (Evidence Report/Technology Assessment: No 4.) http://www.ahcpr.gov/clinic/prossumm.htm. Search date 1998; primary sources Medline, Cancerlit, Embase, Current Contents, and Cochrane Library.
34. Byar DP, Corle DK. Hormone treatment for prostate cancer: results of the Veterans'

Administration cooperative urologic research group studies. *NCI Monograph* 1988;7:165–170.
35. The Medical Research Council Prostate Cancer Working Party Investigators Group. Immediate versus deferred treatment for advanced prostatic cancer: initial results of the Medical Research Council trial. *Br J Urol* 1997;79:235–246.
36. Fellows GJ, Clark PB, Beynon LL, et al. Treatment of advanced localised prostatic cancer by orchiectomy, radiotherapy, or combined treatment. *Br J Urol* 1992:70;304–309.
37. Messing EM, Manola J, Sarodsy M, Wilding G, Crawford ED, Trump D. Immediate hormonal therapy compared with observation after radical prostatectomy and pelvic lymphadenectomy in men with node-positive prostate cancer. *N Engl J Med* 1999;341:1781–1789.

Timothy Wilt
Professor of Medicine
VA Coordinating Center for the Cochrane Review Group in Prostate Diseases and Urologic Malignancies and the Center for Chronic Diseases Outcomes Research
Minneapolis VA Hospital, Minneapolis, USA

Competing interests: None declared.

TABLE 1 **Prostatic cancer staging systems (see text, p 892).**

Tumour, node, metastasis (TNM) classification system	
Tumour	
T0	Clinically unsuspected
T1	Clinically inapparent (not palpable or visible by imaging)
T2	Tumour confined within prostate
T3	Tumour outside capsule or extension into vesicle
T4	Tumour fixed to other tissue
Nodes	
N0	No evidence of involvement of regional nodes
N1	Involvement of regional nodes
Metastases	
M0	No evidence of distant metastases
M1	Evidence of distant metastases
American urologic staging system	
Stage A	No palpable tumour
Stage B	Tumour confined to the prostate gland
Stage C	Extracapsular extension
Stage D	Metastatic prostate cancer
Stage D1	Pelvic lymph node metastases
Stage D2	Distant metastases

Anorexia nervosa

Search date December 2001

Janet Treasure and Ulrike Schmidt

QUESTIONS

INTERVENTIONS

See glossary, p 912

Key Messages

- **Cisapride** One small RCT found no significant difference with cisapride versus placebo in weight gain at 8 weeks. Cisapride has now been withdrawn in many countries because of an increased risk of cardiac irregularities, including ventricular tachycardia, torsades de pointes, and sudden death.
- **Cyproheptadine** Three small RCTs found no significant difference with cyproheptadine versus placebo in weight gain.
- **Inpatient versus outpatient treatment setting (in people not so severely ill as to warrant emergency intervention)** Limited evidence from one small RCT found that outpatient treatment was as effective as inpatient treatment in increasing weight and improving Morgan Russell scale global scores at 1, 2, and 5 years in those individuals who do not warrant emergency intervention.
- **Neuroleptic drugs that increase the QT interval** We found no RCTs. The QT interval may be prolonged in people with anorexia nervosa, and many neuroleptic drugs (haloperidol, pimozide, sertindole, thioridazine, chlorpromazine, and others) also increase the QT interval. Prolongation of the QT interval may be associated with increased risk of ventricular tachycardia, torsades de pointes, and sudden death.
- **Oestrogen treatment (for prevention of fractures)** We found no good evidence about the effects of hormonal treatment on fracture rates. One small RCT found no effect of oestrogen versus no treatment on bone mineral density.
- **Psychotherapies** One small RCT found limited evidence that focal analytical therapy or family therapy versus treatment as usual significantly increased the number of people recovered or improved as assessed by the Morgan Russell scale at 1 year. One small RCT found no significant difference in outcomes

between psychotherapy and dietary counselling at 1 year. A second RCT comparing cognitive therapy versus dietary counselling found a 100% non-take up/withdrawal rate with dietary counselling. Six small RCTs found no significant difference between different psychotherapies. However, all the RCTs were small and were unlikely to have been powered to detect a clinically important difference between treatments.

- **Selective serotonin reuptake inhibitors (fluoxetine)** One small RCT found no significant difference with fluoxetine versus placebo in weight gain, eating symptoms, or depressive symptoms after 36 days of treatment, but another small RCT found limited evidence that fluoxetine reduced relapse in people discharged from hospital.
- **Tricyclic antidepressants** Two small RCTs found no evidence of beneficial effects from the use of amitriptyline, but amitriptyline was associated with more adverse events than placebo. Observational studies found the QT interval may be prolonged in people with anorexia nervosa, and tricyclic antidepressants (amitriptyline, protriptyline, nortriptyline, doxepin, and maprotiline) also increase the QT interval. Prolongation of the QT interval may be associated with increased risk of ventricular tachycardia, torsades de pointes, and sudden death.
- **Zinc** One small RCT in people admitted to an eating disorder unit found limited evidence of a significant improvement with zinc versus placebo in average daily body mass index gain.

DEFINITION Anorexia nervosa is characterised by a refusal to maintain weight at or above a minimally normal weight (< 85% of expected weight for age and height, or body mass index [see glossary, p 912] < 17.5 kg/m^2), or a failure to show the expected weight gain during growth. In association with this there is often an intense fear of gaining weight, preoccupation with weight, denial of the current low weight and its adverse impact on health, and amenorrhoea. Two subtypes of anorexia nervosa, binge–purge and restricting, have been defined.[1]

INCIDENCE/ PREVALENCE A mean incidence in the general population of 19/100 000 a year in females and 2/100 000 a year in males has been estimated from 12 cumulative studies.[2] The highest rate was in female teenagers (age 13–19 years), where there were 50.8 cases/100 000 a year. A large cohort study of Swedish school children (4291 people, aged 16 years) were screened by weighing and subsequent interview, and the prevalence of anorexia nervosa cases (defined using DSM-III and DSM-III-R criteria) was found to be 7/1000 for girls and 1/1000 for boys.[3] Little is known of the incidence or prevalence in Asia, South America, or Africa.

AETIOLOGY/ RISK FACTORS The aetiology of anorexia nervosa has been related to family, biological, social, and cultural factors.[4] Studies have found that anorexia nervosa is associated with a family history of anorexia nervosa (HR 11.4, 95% CI 1.1 to 89.0), of bulimia nervosa (adjusted HR 3.5, 955 CI 1.1 to 14.0),[5] depression, generalised anxiety disorder, obsessive compulsive disorder, or obsessive compulsive personality disorder (adjusted RR 3.6, 95% CI 1.6 to 8.0).[6] A twin study estimated the heritability to be 58% (95% CI 33% to 77%), with the remaining variance apparently due to non-shared environment. However, the study was unable to completely rule out a contribution of a non-shared environment. Specific aspects of childhood temperament thought to be related include perfectionism, negative self-evaluation, and extreme compliance.[7] Perinatal factors include prematurity (OR 3.2, 95% CI 1.6 to 6.2), particularly if the baby was small for gestational age (OR 5.7, 95% CI 1.4 to 4.1).

PROGNOSIS We found no good evidence on the prognosis of people with anorexia nervosa who do not access formal medical care. A summary of treatment studies (68 studies published between 1953 and 1989, 3104 people, length of follow up 1–33 years) found that 43% of people recover completely (range 7–86%), 36% improve (range 1–69%), 20% develop a chronic eating disorder (range 0–43%), and 5% die from anorexia nervosa (range 0–21%).[8] Favourable prognostic factors include an early age at onset and a short interval between onset of symptoms and the beginning of treatment. Unfavourable prognostic factors include vomiting, bulimia, profound weight loss, chronicity, and a history of premorbid developmental or clinical abnormalities. The all cause standardised mortality ratio of eating disorders (anorexia nervosa and bulimia nervosa) has been estimated at 538, about three times higher than other psychiatric illnesses.[9] The average annual risk of mortality was 0.59% a year in females in 10 eating disorder populations (1322 people) with a minimum follow up of 6 years.[10] The mortality risk was higher for people with lower weight and with older age at presentation. Young women with anorexia nervosa are at an increased risk of fractures later in life.[11]

AIMS To restore physical health (weight within the normal range and no sequelae of starvation, e.g. regular menstruation, normal bone mass), normal patterns of eating and attitudes towards weight and shape, and no additional psychiatric comorbidity (e.g. depression, anxiety, obsessive compulsive disorder); to reduce the impact of the illness on social functioning and quality of life.

OUTCOMES The most widely used measure of outcome is the Morgan Russell scale (see glossary, p 912),[12] which includes nutritional status, menstrual function, mental state, and sexual and social adjustment. Biological outcome criteria alone such as weight (body mass index or in relation to matched population weight) and menstrual function are used infrequently as outcome measures. RCTs do not usually have sufficient power or long enough follow up periods to address mortality. Other validated outcome measures used include eating symptom measures.[13–16] Bone mass density is included as a proxy outcome for the risk of fractures.

METHODS *Clinical Evidence* update search and appraisal December 2001, and hand search of reference lists of identified reviews. To be included, an RCT had to have at least 30 people and follow up greater than 75%. Results from each of the identified trials were extracted independently by the two reviewers. Any disagreements were discussed until a consensus was reached. A systematic review (in German) was identified through direct contact with the author.[17] This will be translated and may be included in future *Clinical Evidence* updates.

QUESTION What are the effects of treatments in anorexia nervosa?

OPTION PSYCHOTHERAPIES

One small RCT found limited evidence that focal analytical therapy or family therapy versus treatment as usual significantly increased the number of people recovered or improved as assessed by the Morgan Russell scale at 1 year. One small RCT found no significant difference in outcomes between psychotherapy and dietary advice at 1 year. A second RCT comparing cognitive therapy versus dietary counselling found a 100% non-take up/withdrawal rate with dietary counselling. Six small RCTs found no significant difference between different psychotherapies. However, all the RCTs were small and were unlikely to have been powered to detect a clinically important difference between treatments.

Benefits: We found no systematic review. We found eight small RCTs. Three small RCTs of limited quality compared different psychotherapies (see glossary, p 912) versus dietary counselling (see glossary, p 912) or treatment as usual (see web extra table A at www.clinicalevidence.com). All three RCTs were carried out in an outpatient setting in people with a late age of onset and long duration of illness.[18–20] The largest RCT found significant improvements in weight gain for some psychotherapies versus treatment as usual and for the number of people classified as recovered.[18] The second RCT found a significant improvement for cognitive therapy versus baseline.[20] All people treated with dietary counselling either did not take up or withdrew from treatment and refused release of their results, making it impossible to compare the two groups. The third RCT found no difference in outcomes between the groups.[19] Six small RCTs of limited quality compared different psychotherapies. Three of these were undertaken in an outpatient setting,[21–23] in people with an early age of onset and short illness duration. Two of the RCTs were carried out in an outpatient setting in people with a later age of onset and longer duration of illness.[18,24] One RCT included people with early and late onset anorexia nervosa and with long and short duration of illness (see web extra table A at www.clinincalevidence.com).[25,26] No RCT found an overall significant difference between different psychotherapies.

Harms: The acceptability of the treatment varied between RCTs. Failure to take up treatment ranged from 0–30% between RCTs (4/84 [5%];[18] 0/30 [0%];[19] 0/25 [0%] in cognitive therapy and 3/10 [30%] in dietary counselling group;[20] 3/43 [7%];[21] 15/56 [27%];[22] 7/33 [21%];[23] 1/31 [3%];[24] 3/57 [5%][25]) and withdrawal from treatment ranged from 0–70% between RCTs (25/84 [30%] 7 from focal psychotherapy; 5 from family therapy; 9 from cognitive analytical therapy; 4 from treatment as usual;[18] 1/15 [7%] from psychotherapy; 4/15 [27%] from dietary advice;[19] 2/25 [8%] from cognitive therapy; 7/10 [70%] from dietary counselling;[20] 11/40 [27.5%];[21] 4/41 [10%];[22] 0/26 [0%];[23] 10/30 [33%];[24] 16/57 [28%] 6 from family therapy; 10 from individual therapy[25]), but this may have been caused by different methods of case ascertainment. The number of people admitted for inpatient treatment (see glossary, p 912) also varied between RCTs, ranging from 0–36% (12/84

[14%];[18] 3/30 [10%];[19] 0/30 [0%];[24] 4/40 [10%];[21] 16/41 [36%];[22] 8/33 [24%][23]). One death was attributed to anorexia nervosa in the control group in one outpatient RCT with a 1 year follow up.[18] Three deaths attributed to anorexia nervosa occurred in the 5 year follow up period in one inpatient based RCT.[26]

Comment: All the RCTs were small and had limited power to detect clinically important differences if they existed. The amount of therapeutic input varied considerably between and within the RCTs. There was variation in methods of recruitment, reporting of key results (e.g. withdrawal rates), and the description of participants' characteristics and selection. The people in the inpatient RCT covered a broad range of severity.[25]

OPTION TRICYCLIC ANTIDEPRESSANTS

Two small RCTs found no evidence of beneficial effects from the use of amitriptyline, but amitriptyline was associated with more adverse events. Observational studies found that the QT interval may be prolonged in people with anorexia nervosa, and tricyclic antidepressants (amitriptyline, protriptyline, nortriptyline, doxepin, and maprotiline) also increase the QT interval. Prolongation of the QT interval may be associated with increased risk of ventricular tachycardia, torsades de pointes, and sudden death.

Benefits: We found no systematic review. We found two small RCTs.[27,28] The first RCT (43 people with early onset and short duration anorexia nervosa, mean age 16.6 years, mean 27% below average weight, mean duration of anorexia nervosa 1.5 years) in two units (5 outpatients) compared amitriptyline versus placebo.[28] Participants could also receive various kinds of psychotherapy (see glossary, p 912). Eighteen people refused to participate and were used as a third comparison group. The RCT found no significant difference between the groups on any of the outcome scales measured at 5 weeks (> 50% improvement in global response 1/11 [9%] with amitriptyline *v* 1/14 [7%] with placebo; RR 1.2, 95% CI 0.1 to 16.7). The second RCT (72 women, mean age 20.6 years, mean 2.9 years duration) compared amitriptyline, cyproheptadine, and placebo.[28] The drug treatment had no significant effect on treatment efficiency — that is, the reciprocal of days to reach target weight times 90 (a dummy figure of 120 days was used if people failed to reach target weight) (see benefits under cyproheptadine, p 909).[28]

Harms: Adverse events more common with amitriptyline included increased perspiration (2/11 [18%] with amitriptyline *v* 0/14 [0%] with placebo), drowsiness (6/11 [55%] *v* 0/14 [0%]), dry mouth (4/11 [36%] *v* 2/14 [14%]), blurred vision (1/11 [9%] *v* 0/14 [0%]), urinary retention (1/11 [9%] *v* 0/14 [0%] with placebo), hypotension (2/11 [18%] *v* 0/14 [0%]), and leukopenia (1/11 [9%] *v* 0/14 [0%]). Adverse events more common with placebo included palpitations (0/11 [0%] with amitriptyline *v* 1/14 [7%] with placebo), and dizziness (0/11 [0%] with amitriptyline *v* 2/14 [14%] with placebo). The QT interval may be prolonged in people with anorexia nervosa,[29] and tricyclic antidepressants (amitriptyline, protriptyline, nortriptyline, doxepin, and maprotiline) also increase the QT interval.[30–32] In an observational study (495 people with mental illness and 101 healthy controls), an increased risk of QTc was seen with tricyclic use, adjusting for age and other drug use (adjusted OR 2.6, 95% CI 1.2 to 5.6).[33] The RCT of amitriptyline versus placebo found more adverse effects with amitriptyline than placebo. General harms of tricyclic antidepressants are described in the section on depression (see depressive disorders, p 951).

Comment: The RCTs were both of short duration. Prolongation of the QT interval may be associated with increased risk of ventricular tachycardia, torsades de pointes, and sudden death.[31,32] It is not clear if people in the second amitriptyline RCT also received psychotherapy.[28]

OPTION SELECTIVE SEROTONIN REUPTAKE INHIBITORS

One small RCT found no significant difference with fluoxetine versus placebo in weight gain, eating symptoms, or depressive symptoms after 36 days of treatment, but another small RCT found limited evidence that fluoxetine reduced relapse in people discharged from hospital.

Benefits: We found two small RCTs.[34,35] The first RCT (33 women; mean age 26.2 years; mean body mass index (see glossary, p 912) 15.0 kg/m^2; mean duration of anorexia nervosa 8.0 years) compared fluoxetine (60 mg) versus placebo for the duration (mean 36 days) of inpatient treatment (which included individual and group psychotherapy [see glossary, p 912]).[34] There were two early withdrawals from the fluoxetine group. The RCT found no significant differences in weight gain, eating symptoms, or depressive symptoms between the groups. The second RCT (39 women with restricting or restricting purging type anorexia, mean age 22–23 years, mean duration of anorexia nervosa 4–7 years) compared fluoxetine (starting dosage 20 mg daily) versus placebo for 1 year. All women had been discharged from hospital after weight gain (minimum weight restoration was 75% of average body weight). Women were allowed additional psychotherapy. Women who had substantial and incapacitating symptoms were encouraged to withdraw from the study. It found significantly lower withdrawal rate with fluoxetine versus placebo (6/16 [37%] with fluoxetine *v* 16/19 [84%] with placebo; RR 0.45, 95% CI 0.23 to 0.86).[35]

Harms: General harms of selective serotonin reuptake inhibitors are described in the section on depression (see depressive disorders, p 951).

Comment: In the second RCT, four women were excluded from the analysis; three people on fluoxetine because the blinding was broken, and one person on placebo because they stopped taking mediation before the end of 30 days.[35]

OPTION NEUROLEPTIC MEDICATION

We found no good evidence.

Benefits: We found no systematic review and no RCTs.

Harms: General harms of neuroleptic drugs are described in the section on schizophrenia (see schizophrenia, p 1019). The QT interval may be prolonged in people with anorexia nervosa,[29,30] and many neuroleptic drugs (haloperidol, pimozide, sertindole, thioridazine, chlorpromazine, and others) may also increase the QT interval.[31,32] An observational study (495 people with mental illness and 101 healthy controls) found an increased risk of QTc with high and very high dose neuroleptic use after adjusting for age and other drug use (high dose: adjusted OR 3.4, 95% CI 1.2 to 10.1; very high dose: adjusted OR 5.6, 95% CI 1.6 to 19.3).[33]

Comment: Prolongation of the QT interval may be associated with increased risk of ventricular tachycardia, torsades de pointes, and sudden death.[31,32]

OPTION ZINC

One small RCT found limited evidence of an improvement in daily body mass index gain with the addition of zinc to an inpatient regime.

Benefits: We found no systematic review. We found one RCT (54 people aged > 15 years, mean body mass index (see glossary, p 912) 15.8 kg/m^2, mean duration of anorexia nervosa 3.7 years, admitted to 2 eating disorder units), which compared 100 mg zinc gluconate versus placebo.[36] All but three of the people had normal zinc levels at pretreatment. Treatment was continued until the individual had gained 10% of weight over the admission weight on two consecutive weeks. Ten people in the zinc group and nine in the placebo group did not complete the study. The RCT found a significant difference in rate of body mass index gain per day (0.079 kg/m^2/day with zinc *v* 0.039 kg/m^2/day with placebo; $P = 0.03$).

Harms: None reported.

Comment: The rationale for zinc supplements in people with normal zinc levels at pretreatment is unclear.

OPTION CYPROHEPTADINE

One RCT in outpatients and two RCTs in inpatients found no significant difference between cyproheptadine and placebo in weight gain.

Benefits: We found no systematic review. We found three small RCTs. The first RCT (24 women in an outpatient setting) compared cyproheptadine versus placebo.[37] The trial found no significant difference in response to treatment after 2 months. The second RCT (81 women in 3 specialised inpatient units) compared cyproheptadine versus placebo, and behaviour therapy versus no behaviour therapy.[38] The effect of behaviour therapy was not reported. There were no significant differences in weight gain between the cyproheptadine and placebo groups. The third RCT (72 women, mean age 20.6 years, mean 77% of target weight, mean duration of anorexia 2.9 years, at 2 specialised inpatient units) compared amitriptyline (up to a maximum of 160 mg) versus cyproheptadine (up to a maximum of 32 mg) versus placebo.[28] The drug treatment had no significant effect on treatment efficiency — that is, the reciprocal of days to reach target weight times 90 (a dummy figure of 120 days was used if people failed to reach target weight).

Harms: No harms were reported in the first two RCTs.[37,38] In the third RCT, on both day 7 and day 21, placebo exceeded the amitriptyline group in number of physical adverse events rated moderate or severe. Cyproheptadine had the lowest number of adverse effects. No one had to be withdrawn from the protocol because of adverse experiences.[28]

Comment: All three RCTs were brief.

OPTION INPATIENT VERSUS OUTPATIENT TREATMENT SETTING IN ANOREXIA NERVOSA

Limited evidence from one small RCT found that outpatient treatment was as effective as inpatient treatment in increasing weight and improving Morgan Russell scale global scores at 1, 2, and 5 years in those individuals who do not warrant emergency intervention.

Benefits: We found one systematic review (search date 1999)[39] comparing inpatient treatment (see glossary, p 912) with outpatient care. The review identified one RCT, which had a 5 year follow up.[40,41] Ninety people referred with anorexia nervosa (mean age 22 years, weight loss 26% of matched population mean weight, mean duration 3.2 years) were randomised to four treatment groups: inpatient treatment (see glossary, p 912), outpatient treatment (individual and family therapy (see glossary, p 912)), outpatient group therapy, and assessment interview only. Assessors were not blind to treatment allocation. Adherence to allocated treatment (defined as accepting allocation and at least 1 attendance at a treatment group or individual treatment session) differed significantly between groups: inpatient treatment 18/30 (60%); outpatient treatment (individual and family therapy) 18/20 (90%); outpatient group psychotherapy (see glossary, p 912) 17/20 (85%); and assessment interview only 20/20 (100%). Treatment adherence differed significantly between outpatient and inpatient treatment (RR 1.5, 95% CI 1.1 to 2.0). Average acceptance of therapeutic input also varied between groups (20 weeks inpatient treatment, 9 outpatient sessions, and 5 group sessions). In the assessment interview only group, six people had no treatment of any kind in the first year, and the others had treatment elsewhere (6 had inpatient treatment, 5 had outpatient hospital treatment, and 3 had at least weekly contact with their general practitioners). Six people in this group spent almost the entire year in treatment. There were no significant differences in mean weight or in the Morgan Russell scale (see glossary, p 912) global scores between any of the four groups at 1, 2, and 5 years. The proportion of people with a good outcome with inpatient treatment was 5/29 (17%) at 2 years and 9/27 (33%) at 5 years; with outpatient treatment (individual and family therapy) 4/20 (20%) at 2 years and 8/17 (47%) at 5 years; with outpatient group psychotherapy 5/19 (26%) at 2 years and 10/19 (53%) at 5 years; and with assessment interview only 2/20 (10%) at 2 years and 6/19 (32%) at 5 years.

Harms: One person died as a result of anorexia nervosa between the assessment and the start of outpatient group treatment, and one of the people allocated to inpatient treatment died as a result of anorexia nervosa by 5 years.[40,41]

Comment: The systematic review[39] was unable to draw meaningful conclusions from numerous case series as participant characteristics, treatments, mortality, and outcomes varied widely. Individuals admitted for inpatient treatment had a lower mean weight than those treated as outpatients. One subsequent observational study (355 people with anorexia nervosa; 169 with anorexia nervosa bulimic type; mean age 25 years; mean duration of illness 5.7 years; 75% available for 2.5 years' follow up) found that people with longer duration of illness had a higher likelihood of good outcome with longer than with briefer duration of inpatient treatment, and those with a shorter duration of illness had a higher likelihood of good outcome with briefer inpatient treatment.[42] Median duration of inpatient treatment was 11.6 weeks for anorexia nervosa and 10.6 weeks for anorexia nervosa bulimic type.

OPTION CISAPRIDE

One small RCT found no significant difference with cisapride versus placebo in weight gain at 8 weeks. Cisapride has now been withdrawn in many countries because of an increased risk of cardiac irregularities, including ventricular tachycardia, torsades de pointes, and sudden death.

Benefits: We found no systematic review. We found one small RCT (34 inpatients aged 18–40 years at 2 hospitals; mean duration 2.7 years; body mass index [see glossary, p 912] 15.1 kg/m^2) comparing cisapride (30 mg) versus placebo for 8 weeks.[43] The trial found no difference in weight gain (placebo 5.7 kg *v* cisapride 5.1 kg; $P > 0.05$).

Harms: No adverse events were noted in this RCT. The QT interval in anorexia nervosa is prolonged even in the absence of medication; therefore, cisapride is not recommended in anorexia nervosa. Cisapride has now been withdrawn in many countries because of an increased risk of cardiac irregularities, including ventricular tachycardia, torsades de pointes, and sudden death.[31,32]

Comment: Five people withdrew from the RCT and were not included in the analysis.

QUESTION What are the effects of interventions to prevent or treat complications of anorexia?

OPTION HORMONAL TREATMENT

We found no good evidence about the effects of hormonal treatment on fracture rates. One small RCT found no effect of oestrogen versus no treatment on bone mineral density.

Benefits: We found no systematic review. We found one RCT (48 women, mean age 23.7 years, mean duration of anorexia nervosa 4.0 years) of hormone replacement therapy (Premarin 0.625 mg on days 1–25 of each month plus Provera 5 mg on days 16–25) versus an oral contraceptive containing 35 μg ethinyl estradiol (oestradiol) versus no medication over 6 months.[44] All women maintained a calcium intake of 1500 mg using oral calcium carbonate. Spinal bone mineral density was measured at 6 monthly intervals. There was no significant difference in the final bone density at follow up of 0.5–3.0 years.

Harms: Three women withdrew from the oestrogen treatment; two because of adverse effects, and one because she had left the country. One woman who was in the control group was unwilling to return for further testing.

Anorexia nervosa

Comment: Improvements in bone mineral density would not necessarily lead to reductions in risk of fractures.

GLOSSARY

Body mass index Weight (kg) divided by height (m) squared.

Dietary counselling Dieticians with experience of eating disorders discuss diet, mood, and daily behaviours.

Family therapy Treatment that includes members of the family of origin or the constituted family, and that addresses the eating disorder as a problem of family life.

Inpatient treatment This has been regarded as the standard approach to the management of anorexia nervosa.[45] One of the key components of inpatient treatment is refeeding, which is achieved through structured, supervised meals. Psychotherapy (of a variety of different types) and pharmacotherapy are included in many programmes.

Morgan Russell scale A widely used measure of outcome for anorexia nervosa that consists of two scores: an average outcome score and a general outcome score. The average outcome score is based on the outcome in five areas: nutritional status, menstrual function, mental state, sexual adjustment, and socioeconomic status.

Psychotherapy Different types of psychological treatments given individually or in groups are included here. These use psychodynamic, cognitive behavioural, or supportive techniques, or combinations of these.

Substantive changes

Antidepressant medication: New RCT;[35] found limited evidence that fluoxetine reduces relapse.

REFERENCES

1. American Psychiatric Association. *Diagnostic and statistical manual of mental disorders (DSM-IV).* 4th ed. Washington DC: APA, 1994.
2. Pawluck DE, Gorey KM. Secular trends in the incidence of anorexia nervosa: integrative review of population-based studies. *Int J Eat Disord* 1998;23:347–352.
3. R stam M, Gillberg C, Garton M. Anorexia nervosa in a Swedish urban region. A population-based study. *Br J Psychiatry* 1989;155:642–646.
4. Strober M, Freeman R, Lampert C, et al. Controlled family study of anorexia nervosa and bulimia nervosa: evidence of shared liability and transmission of partial syndromes. *Am J Psychiatry* 2000;157;393–401.
5. Lilenfeld LR, Kaye WH, Greeno CG, et al. A controlled family study of anorexia nervosa and bulimia nervosa: psychiatric disorders in first-degree relatives and effects of proband comorbidity. *Arch Gen Psychiatry* 1998;55:603–610.
6. Wade TD, Bulik CM, Neale M, et al. Anorexia nervosa and major depression: shared genetic and environmental risk factors. *Am J Psychiatry* 2000;157:469–471.
7. Fairburn CG, Cooper Z, Doll HA, et al. Risk factors for anorexia nervosa: three integrated case-control comparisons. *Arch Gen Psychiatry* 1999;56:468–476.
8. Steinhausen, H-C. The course and outcome of anorexia nervosa. In: Brownell K, Fairburn CG, eds. *Eating disorders and obesity: a comprehensive handbook*. New York: Guilford Press, 1995:234–237.
9. Harri, EC, Barraclough B. Excess mortality of mental disorder. *Br J Psychiatry* 1998;173:11–53.
10. Nielsen S, Møller-Madsen S, Isager T, et al. Standardized mortality in eating disorders: a quantitative summary of previously published and new evidence. *J Psychosom Res* 1998;44:413–434.
11. Lucas A, Melton L, Crowson C, et al. Long term fracture risk among women with anorexia nervosa: a population-based cohort study. *Mayo Clin Proc* 1999;74:972–977.
12. Morgan HG, Russell GF. Value of family background and clinical features as predictors of long-term outcome in anorexia nervosa: four-year follow-up study of 41 patients. *Psychol Med* 1975;5:355–371.
13. Cooper Z, Fairburn CG. The Eating Disorders Examination. A semi-structured interview for the assessment of the specific psychopathology of eating disorders. *Int J Eat Disord* 1987;6:1–8.
14. Garner DM. *Eating Disorder Inventory-2 (EDI-2): professional manual*. Odessa FL: Psychological Assessment Resources Inc, 1991.
15. Garner DM, Garfinkel PE. The eating attitudes test: an index of the symptoms of anorexia nervosa. *Psychol Med* 1979;10:647–656.
16. Henderson M, Freeman CPL. A self-rating scale for bulimia: the 'BITE'. *Br J Psychiatry* 1987;150:18–24.
17. Herzog T. Stand der vergleichenden Therapieforschung bei Anorexia nervosa. Ergebnisse einer Systematischen Literaturübersicht. In: Gastpar M, Remschmidt HJ, Senf W, eds. *Forschungsperspektiven bei esstorungen*. Berlin: Verlag Wissenschaft und Praxis 2000.
18. Dare C, Eisler I, Russell G, et al. Psychological therapies for adult patients with anorexia nervosa:

a randomised controlled trial of outpatient treatments. *Br J Psychiatry* 2001;178:216–221.
19. Hall A, Crisp AH. Brief psychotherapy in the treatment of anorexia nervosa. Outcome at one year. *Br J Psychiatry* 1987;151:185–191.
20. Serfaty MA. Cognitive therapy versus dietary counselling in the outpatient treatment of anorexia nervosa: effects of the treatment phase. *Eur Eat Dis Rev* 1999;7:334–350.
21. Eisler I, Dare C, Hodes M, et al. Family therapy for adolescent anorexia nervosa: the results of a controlled comparison of two family interventions. *J Child Psychol Psychiatry* 2000;41:727–736.
22. Robin AL, Siegel PT, Moye AW, et al. A controlled comparison of family versus individual therapy for adolescents with anorexia nervosa. *J Am Acad Child Adolesc Psychiatry* 1999;38:1482–1489.
23. Wallin U, Kronvall P, Majewski ML. Body awareness therapy in teenage anorexia nervosa: outcome after 2 years. *Eur Eat Dis Rev* 2000;8:19–30.
24. Treasure JL, Todd G, Brolly M, et al. A pilot study of a randomized trial of cognitive analytical therapy vs educational behavioral therapy for adult anorexia nervosa. *Behav Res Ther* 1995;33:363–367.
25. Russell GFM, Szmukler G, Dare C, et al. An evaluation of family therapy in anorexia nervosa and bulimia nervosa. *Arch Gen Psychiatry* 1987;44:1047–1056.
26. Eisler I, Dare C, Russell GFM, et al. Family and individual therapy in anorexia nervosa. A 5-year follow-up. *Arch Gen Psychiatry* 1997;54:1025–1030.
27. Biederman J, Herzog DB, Rivinus TM, et al. Amitriptyline in the treatment of anorexia nervosa: a double-blind, placebo-controlled study. *J Clin Psychopharmacol* 1985;5:10–16.
28. Halmi KA, Eckert E, LaDu TJ, et al. Anorexia nervosa. Treatment efficacy of cyproheptadine and amitriptyline. *Arch Gen Psychiatry* 1986;43:177–181.
29. Ackerman MJ. The long QT syndrome: ion channel diseases of the heart. *Mayo Clin Proc* 1998;73:250–269.
30. Becker A, Grinspoon SK, Klibanski A, et al. Current concepts: eating disorders. *N Engl J Med* 1999;340:1092–1098.
31. Yap Y, Camm J. Risk of torsades de pointes with non-cardiac drugs: doctors need to be aware that many drugs can cause QT prolongation. *BMJ* 2000;320:1158–1159.
32. Sheridan DJ. Drug-induced proarrhythmic effects: assessment of changes in QT interval. *Br J Clin Pharmacol* 2000;50:297–302.
33. Reilly JG, Ayis SA, Ferrier IN, et al. QTc interval abnormalities and psychotropic drug therapy in psychiatric patients. *Lancet* 2000;355:1048–1052.
34. Attia E, Haiman C, Walsh BT, et al. Does fluoxetine augment the inpatient treatment of anorexia nervosa? *Am J Psychiatry* 1998;155:548–551.
35. Kaye WH, Nagata T, Weltzin TE, et al. Double-blind placebo-controlled administration of fluoxetine in restricting- and restricting-purging-type anorexia nervosa. *Soc Biol Psych* 2001;49:644–652.
36. Birmingham CL, Goldner EM, Bakan R. Controlled trial of zinc supplementation in anorexia nervosa. *Int J Eat Disord* 1994;15:251–255.
37. Vigersky RA, Loriaux L. The effect of cyproheptadine in anorexia nervosa: a double blind trial. In: Vigersky RA, ed. *Anorexia nervosa.* New York: Raven Press, 1977:349–356.
38. Goldberg SC, Halmi KA, Eckert RC, et al. Cyproheptadine in anorexia nervosa. *Br J Psychiatry* 1979;134:67–70.
39. West Midlands Development and Evaluation Service. *In-patient versus out-patient care for eating disorders.* DPHE 1999 Report No 17. Birmingham: University of Birmingham, 1999. Search date 1999; primary sources Medline, Psychlit, Cochrane Library, variety of internet sites, and hand searches of relevant editions of relevant journals and references from identified articles.
40. Crisp AH, Norton K, Gowers S, et al. A controlled study of the effect of therapies aimed at adolescent and family psychopathology in anorexia nervosa. *Br J Psychiatry* 1991;159:325–333.
41. Gowers S, Norton K, Halek C, et al. Outcome of outpatient psychotherapy in a random allocation treatment study of anorexia nervosa. *Int J Eat Disord* 1994;15:65–177.
42. Kächele H for the study group MZ-ESS. Eine multizentrische Studie zu Aufwand und Erfolg bei psychodynamischer Therapie von Eβstörungen. *Psychother Med Psychol (Stuttg)* 1999;49:100–108.
43. Szmukler GI, Young GP, Miller G, et al. A controlled trial of cisapride in anorexia nervosa. *Int J Eat Disord* 1995;17:347–357.
44. Klibanski A, Biller BMK, Schoenfeld DA, et al. The effects of estrogen administration on trabecular bone loss in young women with anorexia nervosa. *J Clin Endocrinol Metab* 1995;80:898–904.
45. American Psychiatric Association. Practice guideline for the treatment of patients with eating disorders (revision). *Am J Psychiatry* 2000;157(suppl 1):1–39.

Janet Treasure
Psychiatrist
Institute of Psychiatry
Kings College London
London, UK

Ulrike Schmidt
Psychiatrist
South London and Maudsley NHS Trust
London, UK

Competing interests: None declared.

Bulimia nervosa

Search date April 2002

Phillipa Hay and Josue Bacaltchuk

QUESTIONS

INTERVENTIONS

See glossary, p 923

Key Messages

Psychotherapy

- **Cognitive behavioural therapy** Systematic reviews have found that cognitive behavioural therapy versus remaining on a waiting list significantly reduces specific symptoms of bulimia nervosa (binge eating, purging, disturbed eating patterns), and improves non-specific symptoms such as depression. One review and subsequent RCTs found no clear benefit from cognitive behavioural therapy versus other psychotherapies.
- **Other psychotherapies** One systematic review and one subsequent RCT have found that non-cognitive behavioural psychotherapy versus being on a waiting list significantly improve the symptoms of bulimia nervosa.

Antidepressants

- **Antidepressant medication (tricyclic antidepressants and monoamine oxidase inhibitors, and fluoxetine)** Systematic reviews and one subsequent RCT have found short term reduction in bulimic symptoms (significant for vomiting only in the subsequent RCT) and a small reduction in depressive symptoms with tricyclic and monoamine oxidase inhibitor antidepressants. One systematic review and one subsequent have RCT found that fluoxetine versus placebo significantly reduces bulimic symptoms in the short term.
- **Antidepressants as maintenance** We found insufficient evidence to assess the effects of antidepresssants for maintenance.
- **Other antidepressants (venlafaxine, mirtazapine, and reboxetine)** We found no RCTs on the effects of venlafaxine, mirtazapine, and reboxetine.
- **Selective serotonin reuptake inhibitor (other than fluoxetine)** We found no good evidence on selective serotonin reuptake inhibitors other than fluoxetine.

Combinations of antidepressants and psychotherapy

- **Combination treatment with an antidepressant and psychotherapy** One systematic review has found that combination treatment (antidepressants plus psychotherapy) versus antidepressants alone reduces binge frequency and depressive symptoms but found no significant effect on remission rates. It has also found that combination treatment versus psychotherapy alone improves short term remission from binge eating and depressive symptoms but has no significant effect on binge eating frequency.

DEFINITION Bulimia nervosa (see glossary, p 923) is an intense preoccupation with body weight and shape, with regular episodes of uncontrolled overeating of large amounts of food (binge eating — see glossary, p 923) associated with use of extreme methods to counteract the feared effects of overeating. If a person also meets the diagnostic criteria for anorexia nervosa, then the diagnosis of anorexia nervosa takes precedence.[1] Bulimia nervosa can be difficult to identify because of extreme secrecy about binge eating and purgative behaviour. Weight may be normal but there is often a history of anorexia nervosa or restrictive dieting. Some people alternate between anorexia nervosa and bulimia nervosa.

INCIDENCE/ PREVALENCE In community based studies, the prevalence of bulimia nervosa is between 0.5% and 1.0% in young women, with an even social class distribution.[2–4] About 90% of people diagnosed with bulimia nervosa are women. The numbers presenting with bulimia nervosa in industrialised countries increased during the decade that followed its recognition in the late 1970s and "a cohort effect" is reported in community surveys,[2,5,6] implying an increase in incidence. The prevalence of eating disorders such as bulimia nervosa is lower in non-industrialised populations,[7] and varies across ethnic groups. African-American women have a lower rate of restrictive dieting than white American women, but have a similar rate of recurrent binge eating.[8]

AETIOLOGY/ RISK FACTORS Young women from the developed world who restrict their dietary intake are at greatest risk of developing bulimia nervosa and other eating disorders. One community based case control study compared 102 people with bulimia nervosa with 204 healthy controls and found higher rates of the following in people with the eating disorder: obesity, mood disorder, sexual and physical abuse, parental obesity, substance misuse, low self esteem, perfectionism, disturbed family dynamics, parental weight/shape concern, and early menarche.[9] Compared with a control group of 102 women who had other psychiatric disorders, women with bulimia nervosa had higher rates of parental problems and obesity.

PROGNOSIS A 10 year follow up study (50 people with bulimia nervosa from a former trial of mianserin treatment) found that 52% had fully recovered, and only 9% continued to experience full symptoms of bulimia nervosa.[10] A larger study (222 people from a trial of antidepressants and structured, intensive group psychotherapy, 101 of whom were from a controlled trial of imipramine and a structured, intensive cognitive behavioural group psychotherapy) found that, after a mean follow up of 11.5 years, 11% still met criteria for bulimia nervosa, whereas 70% were in full or partial remission.[11] For the people from the controlled trial, being in either the imipramine, psychotherapy plus imipramine, or psychotherapy plus placebo groups, versus the placebo only group, was associated with significantly better psychosocial adjustment, but not bulimic symptoms, at follow up. Short term studies found similar results: about 50% of people made a full recovery, 30% made a partial recovery, and 20% continued to be symptomatic.[12] There are few consistent predictors of longer term outcome. Good prognosis has been associated with shorter illness duration, a younger age of onset, higher social class, and a family history of alcohol abuse.[10] Poor prognosis has been associated with a history of substance misuse,[13] premorbid and paternal obesity,[14] and, in some studies, personality disorder.[15–18] One study (102 people) of the natural course of bulimia nervosa found that 31% still had the disorder at 15 months and 15% at 5 years.[19] Only 28% received treatment during the follow up period. In an evaluation of response to cognitive behavioural therapy (see glossary, p 923), early progress (by session 6) best predicted outcome.[20] A subsequent systematic review of the outcome literature found no consistent evidence to support early intervention and a better prognosis.[21]

AIMS To reduce symptoms of bulimia nervosa; to improve general psychiatric symptoms; to improve social functioning and quality of life.

OUTCOMES Frequency of binge eating, abstinence from binge eating, frequency of behaviours to reduce weight and counter the effects of binge eating, severity of extreme weight and shape preoccupation, severity of general psychiatric symptoms, severity of depression, improvement in social and adaptive functioning, remission rates, relapse rates, and withdrawal rates.

METHODS *Clinical Evidence* update search and appraisal April 2002 and hand search of reference lists from identified reviews. One systematic review was not included because it included uncontrolled studies.[22]

QUESTION What are the effects of treatments for bulimia nervosa in adults?

OPTION COGNITIVE BEHAVIOURAL THERAPY

Systematic reviews have found that cognitive behavioural therapy versus remaining on a waiting list reduces specific symptoms of bulimia nervosa and improves non-specific symptoms such as depression. One RCT in the review found that cognitive behavioural therapy versus interpersonal psychotherapy significantly reduced binge eating in the short term, but there was no significant difference in the longer term. One subsequent RCT found significantly higher abstinence rates for people receiving cognitive behavioural therapy versus those in a support group.

Benefits: We found three systematic reviews of psychotherapy,[23–25] three subsequent RCTs,[26–28] and two subsequent analyses.[29,30] The third systematic review is in German and may be included in a future *Clinical Evidence* update.[25] The first systematic review (search date 2000, 27 RCTs) included RCTs of other binge eating disorders (see glossary, p 923), although most studies were of people with bulimia nervosa (see glossary, p 923) (18 RCTs in people with bulimia nervosa characterised by purging behaviour).[23] The second review (search date 1998, 26 RCTs) used a broad definition of cognitive behavioural therapy (CBT) (see glossary, p 923), including exposure and response prevention, and included non-randomised trials.[24] **Versus waiting list controls:** One systematic review (search date 2000; individual analyses included a maximum of 10 RCTs and 668 people) found that CBT versus remaining on a waiting list increased the proportion of people abstaining from binge eating at the end of the trial (7 RCTs; RR 0.64, 95% CI 0.53 to 0.78) and reduced depression scores (4 RCTs, 159 people) (see table 1, p 926).[23] There was no significant difference between CBT and remaining on the waiting list in weight at the end of treatment (3 RCTs; 135 people). The review found insufficient evidence about other outcomes, such as social functioning. A second systematic review (search date 1998, 9 RCTs of specific CBT, 173 people) found a wide range of abstinence from binge eating at the end of treatment (mean 55%, range 33% to 92%).[24] Pooled effect sizes (weighted for sample size) ranged from 1.22–1.35 for reduction in binge eating frequency, purging frequency, depression, and disturbed eating attitudes. Tests for heterogeneity were not significant. In one of the included RCTs, the benefits of CBT were maintained for up to 5 years.[14] **Versus placebo medication:** One subsequent RCT (91 people) found no significant difference in efficacy with unguided manual based self help CBT versus placebo medication (see benefits of antidepressants, p 920).[28] **Versus other psychotherapies:** One systematic review (search date 2000) found that a higher percentage of people abstained from binge eating after CBT than after other psychotherapies, but the difference did not quite reach significance (7 RCTs; RR 0.80, 95% CI 0.61 to 1.04).[24] CBT in a full or less intensive form was not significantly superior to CBT in a pure self help form (see glossary, p 924) (4 RCTs; RR 0.90, 95% CI 0.74 to 1.10). CBT was associated with significantly lower depression scores at the end of treatment compared with other psychotherapies (8 RCTs, 273 people; SMD –0.52, 95% CI –0.76 to –0.27). CBT plus exposure therapy was not significantly more effective than CBT alone (3 RCTs; RR for abstinence from binge eating 0.87, 95% CI 0.65 to 1.16). Depression scores were significantly lower at the end of treatment with CBT plus exposure therapy versus CBT alone (3 RCTs, 122 people; SMD 0.54, 95% CI 0.17 to 0.91). One RCT included in the review (220 people) compared classic CBT versus interpersonal psychotherapy (see glossary, p 923) for bulimia nervosa that involved purging.[31] It found that CBT significantly improved abstinence from binge eating at the end of treatment (19 individual sessions conducted ≥ 20 wks; intention to treat analysis; 29% with CBT *v* 6% with interpersonal psychotherapy); however, the difference was not significant at 4, 8, and 12 months of follow up, although both groups improved from baseline. We found one subsequent RCT (125 people with bulimia nervosa), which compared four sessions of CBT versus motivational enhancement therapy (see glossary, p 923).[27] It found no significant differences between CBT and motivational enhancement therapy in engaging participants or the chance of achieving a clinically significant reduction in binge frequency (17/25 [68%] *v* 23/43 [53%]; RR 1.3, 95% CI 0.9 to 1.9). However, results were reported only on the first 4 weeks of treatment, which was prior to all people receiving a further 8 weeks of individual or group CBT.

Harms: One systematic review found that the RCTs did not report details of adverse effects, subsequent RCTs did not report details of adverse effects.[23,27,31] One systematic review (search date 2000) found no significant difference in completion rates between interventions,[23] suggesting no major difference in acceptability. However, neither review could exclude infrequent serious adverse effects.[23,24] An observational study found that group psychotherapy offered very soon after presentation was sometimes perceived as threatening.[10]

Comment: One systematic review (search date 2000) defined CBT as psychotherapy that uses the techniques and models specified by Wilson and Fairburn,[32] but it did not specify the number of sessions or specialist expertise (classical CBT for bulimia nervosa specifies 19 individual sessions over 20 wks conducted by trained therapists[32]). Effect sizes for CBT were large, but over 50% of people were still binge eating at the end of treatment.[23,24] Further research is needed to evaluate the specific and non-specific effects of CBT and other psychotherapies, to explore individual characteristics (such as readiness to change) that may predict response, and to explore the long term effects of treatment. In the first review, abstinence from binge eating was higher in all experimental groups, but the differences reached significance only when compared with those in a waiting list control.[23] However, waiting list or delayed treatment control groups are subject to bias because it is not possible to "blind" someone to the knowledge they are not in the active treatment group. It is difficult to interpret the clinical importance of the statistically significant changes in depression scores. It is also difficult to interpret directly the clinical importance of the benefits reported as effect sizes, where the individual RCTs used different outcomes. Further limitations are that the quality of trials was variable (e.g. 57% were not blinded).[23] Sample sizes were often small. None of the studies measured harms rigorously. Two further analyses[29,30] found limited observational evidence that motivation and compliance factors may influence outcomes. One study[29] performed additional analyses in an RCT of CBT versus interpersonal psychotherapy.[31] It found that "stage of change", or psychological motivation and greater readiness to change, was not related to non-completion, but was associated with a good outcome in those who completed interpersonal psychotherapy. The second RCT examined the effects of compliance on outcome in 62 people randomised to guided self help or to full CBT for 16 weeks.[30] At 6 months' follow up, but not the end of treatment, binge eating abstinence rates were greater in those who had completed two or more of the CBT exercises ($P = 0.04$; CI not provided). **Versus antidepressants:** See option, p 919.

OPTION OTHER PSYCHOTHERAPIES

One systematic review and one subsequent RCT have found that non-cognitive behavioural psychotherapy increases abstinence from binge eating compared with waiting list controls. The systematic review

found that three specific psychotherapies other than cognitive behavioural therapy significantly reduced bulimic symptoms compared with specified control psychotherapies, but the review included RCTs with weak methods.

Benefits: **Versus waiting list controls:** We found one systematic review (search date 2000)[23] and one subsequent RCT.[33] The review also included data from studies of other binge eating (see glossary, p 923) syndromes. It found that non-cognitive behavioural therapy (CBT) psychotherapies (e.g. hypnobehavioural therapy and interpersonal psychotherapy (see glossary, p 923)) versus waiting list control significantly increased abstinence from binge eating (3 RCTs, 131 people; RR 0.67, 95% CI 0.56 to 0.81) and reduced bulimia nervosa (see glossary, p 923) symptom severity measures (4 RCTs, 177 people; SMD –1.2, 95% CI –1.52 to –0.87). The additional small RCT (32 people) found that people randomised to dialectical behaviour therapy (see glossary, p 923) had significantly fewer binge eating episodes at the end of 20 sessions of treatment than did those on a waiting list ($P < 0.001$; CI not provided).[33] **Versus a control therapy:** The systematic review reported three RCTs in which psychotherapies other than CBT were compared with a control therapy.[23] One compared nutritional counselling and stress management, one compared guided imagery and self monitoring, and the third was a three-armed RCT comparing self psychology (see glossary, p 924) (the active treatment), cognitive orientation (see glossary, p 923), and a control nutritional counselling therapy. Meta-analysis favoured the active or experimental therapies over the control therapies for reduction in bulimic symptoms. **Versus CBT:** See benefits of cognitive behavioural therapy, p 916.

Harms: The RCTs did not report details of individual adverse events (see harms of CBT, p 918). Non-CBT psychotherapies include a large number of options, and it remains unclear which therapies are most effective.

Comment: The quality of trials was variable, few were blinded, sample sizes were small, and none of the studies measured harms rigorously (see comment under CBT, p 918). Waiting list or delayed treatment control groups are subject to bias because it is not possible to "blind" someone to the knowledge they are not in the active treatment group.

OPTION ANTIDEPRESSANTS

Two systematic reviews and one subsequent RCT have found short term reduction in bulimic symptoms (significant for vomiting only in the subsequent RCT) and a small reduction in depressive symptoms with tricyclic and monoamine oxidase inhibitor antidepressants, and with fluoxetine. We found no good evidence on other selective serotonin reuptake inhibitors. A further subsequent RCT found no significant benefit with moclobemide 600 mg daily versus placebo. One systematic review found no significant difference in symptoms or relapse rates with antidepressants versus cognitive behavioural therapy. We found insufficient evidence to assess the effects of antidepresssants for maintenance.

Benefits: We found two systematic reviews,[24,34] three additional RCTs of longer term maintenance (not primary treatment studies),[35–37] and three subsequent RCTS.[28,38,39] The second review included an RCT of fluoxetine in those who relapsed after psychotherapy.[38] **Versus placebo:** Both reviews found that antidepressants reduced bulimic symptoms.[24,34] The first review (search date 1998, 9 RCTs; antidepressants were imipramine [1 RCT], desipramine [3 RCTs], phenelzine [1 RCT], fluoxetine [2 RCTs], brofaromine [1 RCT], and isocarboxazid [1 RCT]) found that antidepressants versus placebo significantly reduced binge eating (see glossary, p 923) (5 RCTs; 1 imipramine, 3 desipramine, and 1 brofaromine RCT; 163 people; at the end of the RCTs 16% were not binge eating with antidepressants; effect size weighted for sample size 0.66, 95% CI 0.52 to 0.81).[24] Antidepressants versus placebo improved purging (6 RCTs; 2 desipramine, 2 fluoxetine, 1 isocarboxazid, and 1 brofaromine; effect size 0.39, 95% CI 0.24 to 0.54), depression (all 9 RCTs; effect size 0.73, 95% CI 0.58 to 0.88), and improved scales of eating attitudes. The second review (search date 1997, 8 RCTs; antidepressants were imipramine [5 RCTs], amitriptyline [1 RCT], desipramine [5 RCTs], phenelzine [2 RCTs], isocarboxazid [1 RCT], brofaromine [1 RCT], fluoxetine [5 RCTs], mianserin [1 RCT], bupropion [1 RCT], and trazodone [1 RCT]) found more frequent remission of bulimic episodes with antidepressants (19% *v* 8% with placebo; pooled RR 0.88, 95% CI 0.83 to 0.94; NNT 9, 95% CI 6 to 16).[34] The review found no significant difference in effect between different classes of antidepressants, but there were too few RCTs to exclude a clinically important difference (see table 2, p 926). Most RCTs were of tricyclic antidepressants or monoamine oxidase inhibitors, fluoxetine was the only selective serotonin reuptake inhibitor included in the reviews, and only one RCT reported remission rates.[34] One RCT (the first subsequent RCT; 22 people who relapsed following a RCT of psychotherapy) compared fluoxetine versus placebo.[38] It found that more people taking fluoxetine reported 1 month of abstinence from bingeing and purging (5/13 [39%] with antidepressants *v* 0/9 [0%] taking placebo; P = 0.05; CI not provided). The second subsequent, four-armed RCT compared fluoxetine 60 mg daily versus placebo versus a self help cognitive behavioural therapy manual (see benefits of cognitive behavioural therapy, p 916) versus fluoxetine plus a self help manual (see benefits of combination treatment, p 922).[28] It found a significantly greater reduction with fluoxetine versus placebo in vomiting and binge eating symptoms at week four. Small numbers (26 and 22 in each group, 91 people in total) might have prevented the trial from detecting a clinically relevant difference if one existed. Remission rates after a 16 week treatment period with fluoxetine were 16%, and were not reported for placebo. The third subsequent RCT (75 women with bulimia nervosa (see glossary, p 923)) compared moclobemide (a reversible monamine oxide inhibitor) 600 mg daily versus placebo.[39] Outcomes were reported for the 52 who completed the study, and active treatment was not found to be more efficacious. Remission rates were not reported. **Versus cognitive behavioural therapy:** See cognitive behavioural therapy, p 916. **Versus psychotherapy:** We found one systematic review (search date 1997, 5 RCTs) of antidepressants versus psychotherapy (all cognitive behavioural therapy RCTs), which found no significant difference in remission rates (39% with psychotherapies *v* 20% with antidepressants; effect size 1.28; P = 0.07; CI not provided), bulimic symptom severity (3 RCTs), or depression symptom severity at the end of the RCT (3 RCTs).[40] **Versus antidepressants plus psychotherapy:** See combination therapy, p 922. **Antidepressants as maintenance:** We found two small RCTs of maintenance treatment.[35,36] The first very small RCT (9 people who had responded well to despiramine over the previous 24 wks) compared continuation of desipramine versus placebo.[35] It found no significant difference between treatments (relapse: 1/5 [20%] with desipramine *v* 2/4 [50%] with placebo, RR 0.4, 95% CI 0.1 to 3.0). The second very small RCT (9 women who had responded well to imipramine over the previous 10 wks) compared continuation of imipramine versus placebo.[36] It found no significant difference in relapse (relapse: 2/3 [67%] with imipramine *v* 5/6 [83%] with placebo, RR 0.8, 95% CI 0.3 to 1.9).[36]

Harms: One systematic review found increased withdrawal with antidepressants compared with psychotherapy (4 RCTs, 189 people; AR 40% *v* 18%; RR 2.18, 95% CI 1.09 to 4.35).[40] The second systematic review found significantly increased withdrawal in people taking antidepressants compared with placebo (12 RCTs; 1123 people; 10.5% with any antidepressant *v* 5.1% with placebo, RR 1.83, 95% CI 1.13 to 2.95; NNH 7, 95% CI 4 to 18).[34] It found no significant difference in withdrawal due to adverse effects between and within classes of antidepressants. It found that withdrawal due to any cause was more likely with tricyclic antidepressants than with placebo (6 RCTs; 277 people; 29% with tricyclic *v* 14% with placebo; RR 1.93, 95% CI 1.15 to 3.25), but was more likely with placebo than with selective serotonin reuptake inhibitors (3 RCTs; 706 people; 37% with a selective serotonin re-uptake inhibitor *v* 40% with placebo; RR 0.83, 95% CI 0.68 to 0.99). We found two RCTs examining specific adverse effects. One found significant increases in reclining and standing blood pulse rate, lying systolic and diastolic blood pressure, and greater orthostatic effects on blood pressure with desipramine versus placebo.[41] Cardiovascular changes were well tolerated and few people withdrew because of these effects. Meta-analysis of two double blind RCTs of fluoxetine versus placebo found no significant difference in the incidence of suicidal acts or ideation in people treated with fluoxetine versus placebo.[42] However, the overall incidence of events was low (suicide attempts 1.2%, none fatal; emergent suicidal ideation 3.1%). The third subsequent RCT did not report on withdrawal or adverse events.[28]

Comment: We found no consistent predictors of response to treatment. Antidepressants included in the RCTs were imipramine, amitriptyline, desipramine, phenylzine, isocarboxazid, brofaramine, fluoxetine, mianserin, and buproprion. We found no good evidence for the efficacy of the "newer" antidepressants venlafaxine, reboxetine, and mirtazapine. Both reviews commented on the lack of follow up.[24,34] The fourth subsequent RCT found no differences between active and placebo groups in withdrawal rates because of adverse events, and no changes in blood pressure in those on moclobemide despite reports in food diaries of a high consumption of tyramine-containing foods.[39] The RCTs of maintenance both made multiple randomisations and compared a number of different groups. This meant that there were very few people in the groups for maintenance treatment

OPTION COMBINATION TREATMENT

One systematic review has found that combination treatment (antidepressants plus psychotherapy) versus antidepressants alone reduces binge frequency and depressive symptoms but found no significant effect on remission rates. It has also found that combination treatment versus psychotherapy alone improves short term remission and depressive symptoms but has no significant effect on binge frequency. Antidepressants in combination with psychotherapy are associated with higher withdrawal rates versus psychotherapy alone. One subsequent study of cognitive behavioural therapy in a self help form plus fluoxetine also found reduced bulimic symptoms with combination treatment.

Benefits: We found one systematic review (search date 1997, 7 RCTs, 343 people) comparing combination treatment (antidepressants plus psychotherapy) versus either treatment alone.[43] Meta-analysis found that combined treatment with antidepressants plus psychotherapy versus antidepressants alone significantly improved binge frequency and depressive symptoms (3 RCTs; effect size 0.47; P = 0.04; CI not provided), but found no significant difference in short term remission rates (4 RCTs; 141 people; 42% with combined treatment *v* 23% with antidepressants alone; RR 1.38; P = 0.06; CI not provided).[43] A second meta-analysis compared psychotherapy alone versus a combination of psychotherapy plus antidepressants.[43] Combination treatment was associated with significantly higher rates of short term remission (6 RCTs; 257 people; 49% *v* 36%; RR 1.21; P = 0.03; CI not provided) and greater improvement in depressive symptoms, but no significant difference in frequency of binge eating (see glossary, p 923) compared with psychotherapy alone. In the subsequent RCT (see benefits of antidepressants, p 920), people who received both the self help manual and fluoxetine (60 mg) daily had the greatest reduction in bulimic symptoms, compared with those in the placebo, fluoxetine, or self help only arms, but significance was not reported.[28] Remission rates did not differ significantly across the three active treatment arms.

Harms: Withdrawal rates were lower after psychotherapy plus antidepressants than with antidepressants alone, but the difference was not significant (4 RCTs; 196 people; 34% with psychotherapy plus antidepressant *v* 41% with antidepressants alone; RR 1.19, 95% CI 0.69 to 2.05).[43] Withdrawal rates were significantly higher with psychotherapy plus antidepressants than with psychotherapy alone (6 RCTs; 295 people; 30% *v* 16%; RR 0.57; P = 0.01; CI not provided).[43]

Comment: None.

GLOSSARY

Binge eating Modified from DSM-IV.[1] Eating, in a discrete period (e.g. hours), a large amount of food, accompanied by a lack of control over eating during the episode.

Bulimia nervosa The American Psychiatric Association DSM-IV[1] criteria include recurrent episodes of binge eating; recurrent inappropriate compensatory behaviour to prevent weight gain; frequency of binge eating and inappropriate compensatory behaviour both, on average, at least twice a week for 3 months; self evaluation unduly influenced by body shape and weight; and disturbance occurring not exclusively during episodes of anorexia nervosa. Types of bulimia nervosa, modified from DSM-IV[1], are purging: using self induced vomiting, laxatives, diuretics, or enemas; non-purging: fasting, exercise, but not vomiting or other abuse as for the purging type.

Cognitive behavioural therapy In bulimia nervosa this uses three overlapping phases. Phase one aims to educate the person about bulimia nervosa. People are helped to increase regularity of eating, and resist urge to binge or purge. Phase two introduces procedures to reduce dietary restraint (e.g. broadening food choices). In addition, cognitive procedures supplemented by behavioural experiments are used to identify and correct dysfunctional attitudes and beliefs, and avoidance behaviours. Phase three is the maintenance phase. Relapse prevention strategies are used to prepare for possible future set backs.[44]

Cognitive orientation therapy The cognitive orientation theory aims to generate a systematic procedure for exploring the meaning of a behaviour around themes, such as avoidance of certain emotions. Therapy for modifying behaviour focuses on systematically changing beliefs related to themes, not beliefs referring directly to eating behaviour. No attempt is made to persuade the people that their beliefs are incorrect or maladapative.[45]

Dialectical behaviour therapy A type of behavioural therapy that views emotional dysregulation as the core problem in bulimia nervosa, with binge eating and purging understood as attempts to influence, change, or control painful emotional states. Patients are taught a repertoire of skills to replace dysfunctional behaviours.[33]

Hypnobehavioural psychotherapy Uses a combination of behavioural techniques, such as self monitoring to change maladaptive eating disorders, and hypnotic techniques to reinforce and encourage behaviour change.

Interpersonal psychotherapy In bulimia nervosa this is a three phase treatment. Phase one analyses in detail the interpersonal context of the eating disorder. This leads to the formulation of an interpersonal problem area; this forms the focus of the second stage, which is aimed at helping the person make interpersonal changes. Phase three is devoted to the person's progress and an exploration of ways to handle future interpersonal difficulties. At no stage is attention paid to eating habits or body attitudes.[31]

Motivational enhancement therapy (MET) This is based on a model of change with focus on stages of change. Stages of change represent constellations of intentions and behaviours through which individuals pass as they move from having a problem to doing something to resolve it. People in "precontemplation" show no intention to change. People in "contemplation" acknowledge they have a problem and are thinking about change, but have not yet made a commitment to change. People in the third "action" stage are actively engaged in overcoming their problem, and people in "maintenance" work to prevent relapse. Transition from one stage to the next is sequential, but not linear. The aim of MET is to help people move from earlier stages into "action, utilising cognitive and emotional strategies". There is an emphasis on the therapeutic alliance. With precontemplators, the therapist explores perceived positive and negative aspects of their behaviours. Open-ended questions are used to elicit client expression, and reflective paraphrase is used to reinforce key points of motivation. During a session following structured assessment, most of the time is devoted to explaining feedback to the client. Later in MET, attention is devoted to developing and consolidating a change plan.[46]

Pure self help cognitive behavioural therapy A modified form of cognitive behavioural therapy, in which a treatment manual is provided for people to proceed with treatment on their own, or with support from a non-professional. "Guided self help" usually implies that the support person may or may not have some professional training, but is usually not a specialist in eating disorders.

Self psychology therapy This approaches bulimia nervosa as a specific case of the pathology of the self. The treated person cannot rely on people to fulfil their needs such as self esteem. They instead rely on a substance, food, to fulfill personal needs. Therapy progresses when the people move to rely on humans, starting with the therapist.[45]

REFERENCES

1. American Psychiatric Association. *Diagnostic and statistical manual of mental disorders* 4th ed. Washington DC: American Psychiatric Press, 1994.
2. Bushnell JA, Wells JE, Hornblow AR, et al. Prevalence of three bulimic syndromes in the general population. *Psychol Med* 1990;20:671–680.
3. Garfinkel PE, Lin B, Goering P, et al. Bulimia nervosa in a Canadian community sample: prevalence, co-morbidity, early experiences and psychosocial functioning. *Am J Psychiatry* 1995;152:1052–1058.
4. Gard MCE, Freeman CP. The dismantling of a myth: a review of eating disorders and socioeconomic status. *Int J Eat Disord* 1996;20:1–12.
5. Hall A, Hay PJ. Eating disorder patient referrals from a population region 1977–1986. *Psychol Med* 1991;21:697–701.
6. Kendler KS, Maclean C, Neale M, et al. The genetic epidemiology of bulimia nervosa. *Am J Psychiatry* 1991;148:1627–1637.
7. Choudry IY, Mumford DB. A pilot study of eating disorders in Mirpur (Pakistan) using an Urdu version of the Eating Attitude Test. *Int J Eat Disord* 1992;11:243–251.
8. Striegel-Moore RH, Wifley DE, Caldwell MB, et al. Weight-related attitudes and behaviors of women who diet to lose weight: a comparison for black dieters and white dieters. *Obes Res* 1996;4:109–116.
9. Fairburn CG, Welch SL, Doll HA, et al. Risk factors for bulimia nervosa: a community-based case-control study. *Arch Gen Psychiatry* 1997;54:509–517.
10. Collings S, King M. Ten year follow-up of 50 patients with bulimia nervosa. *Br J Psychiatry* 1994;164:80–87.
11. Keel PK, Mitchell JE, Davis TL, et al. Long-term impact of treatment in women diagnosed with bulimia nervosa *Int J Eat Disord* 2002;31:151–158.
12. Keel PK, Mitchell JE. Outcome in bulimia nervosa. *Am J Psychiatry* 1997;154:313–321.
13. Keel PK, Mitchell JE, Miller KB, et al. Long-term outcome of bulimia nervosa. *Arch Gen Psychiatry* 1999;56:63–69.
14. Fairburn CG, Norman PA, Welch SL, et al. A prospective study of outcome in bulimia nervosa and the long-term effects of three psychological treatments. *Arch Gen Psychiatry* 1995;52:304–312.
15. Coker S, Vize C, Wade T, et al. Patients with bulimia nervosa who fail to engage in cognitive behaviour therapy. *Int J Eat Disord* 1993;13:35–40.
16. Fahy TA, Russell GFM. Outcome and prognostic variables in bulimia. *Int J Eat Disord* 1993;14:135–146.
17. Rossiter EM, Agras WS, Telch CF, et al. Cluster B personality disorder characteristics predict outcome in the treatment of bulimia nervosa. *Int J Eat Disord* 1993;13:349–358.
18. Johnson C, Tobin DL, Dennis A. Differences in treatment outcome between borderline and nonborderline bulimics at 1-year follow-up. *Int J Eat Disord* 1990;9:617–627.
19. Fairburn C, Cooper Z, Doll H, et al. The natural course of bulimia nervosa and binge eating disorder in young women. *Arch Gen Psychiatry* 2000:57:659–665.
20. Agras WS, Crow SJ, Halmi KA, et al. Outcome predictors for the cognitive behavior treatment of bulimia nervosa: data from a multisite study. *Am J Psychiatry* 2000;157:1302–1308.
21. Reas DL, Schoemaker C, Zipfel S, et al. Prognostic value of duration of illness and early intervention in bulimia nervosa: a systematic review of the outcome literature. *Int J Eat Disord* 2001;30:1–10.
22. Lewandowski LM, Gebing TA, Anthony JL, et al. Meta-analysis of cognitive behavioural treatment studies for bulimia. *Clin Psychol Rev* 1997;17:703–718. Search date 1995; primary sources Psychinfo and hand searches of references lists.
23. Hay PJ, Bacaltchuk J. Psychotherapy for bulimia nervosa and binging (Cochrane Review). In: The Cochrane Library, Issue 2, 2002. Oxford: Update Software. Search date 2000; primary sources Medline, Extramed, Embase, Psychlit, Current Contents, Lilacs, Scisearch, The Cochrane Controlled Trials Register 1997, The Cochrane Collaboration Depression and Anxiety Trials Register, hand search of *Int J Eat Disord* since its first issue, citation lists in identified studies and reviews, and personal contacts.
24. Whittal ML, Agras WS, Gould RA. Bulimia nervosa: a meta-analysis of psychosocial and pharmacological treatments. *Behav Ther* 1999;30:117–135. Search date 1998; primary sources Psychlit, Medline, hand search of *Int J Eat Disord* 1990–1998, and hand search other relevant (not specified) journals and identified studies. This was reviewed in Waller G. *Evidence Based Medicine* (September/October 1999).
25. Jacobi C, Dahme B, Rustenbach S. Comparison of controlled pshco- and pharmacotherapy studies in

bulimia anorexia nervosa [German] *Psychother Psychosom Med Psychol* 1997;47:346–364. Search date not stated; primary sources Psychological Abstracts, Medline, Psychindex, and Psychinfo.

26. Hsu LKG, Rand W, Sullivan S, et al. Cognitive therapy, nutritional therapy and their combination in the treatment of bulimia nervosa. *Psychol Med* 2001;31:871–879.
27. Treasure JL, Katzman M, Schmidt U, et al. Engagement and outcome in the treatment of bulimia nervosa: first phase of a sequential design comparing motivation enhancement therapy and cognitive behavioural therapy. *Behav Res Ther* 1999;37:405–418.
28. Mitchell JE, Fletcher L, Hanson K, et al. The relative efficacy of fluoxetine and manual-based self-help in the treatment of outpatients with bulimia nervosa. *J Clin Psychopharmacol* 2001;21:298–304.
29. Wolk SL, Devlin MJ. Stage of change as a predictor of response to psychotherapy for bulimia nervosa. *Int J Eat Disord* 2001;30:96–100.
30. Thiels C, Schmidt U, Troop N, et al. Compliance with a self-care manual in guided self-change for bulimia nervosa. *Eur Eat Disord Rev* 2001;9:115–122.
31. Agras WS, Walsh BT, Fairburn CG, et al. A multicenter comparison of cognitive-behavioral therapy and interpersonal psychotherapy. *Arch Gen Psychiatry* 2000; 54:459–465.
32. Wilson GT, Fairburn CG. Treatments for eating disorders. In: Nathan PE, Gorman JM, eds. *A Guide to Treatments that Work*. New York: Oxford University Press, 1998:501–530.
33. Safer DL, Telch CF, Agras WS. Dialectical behavior therapy for bulimia nervosa. *Am J Psychiatry* 2001;158:632–634.
34. Bacaltchuk J, Hay P. Antidepressants versus placebo for people with bulimia nervosa. In: The Cochrane Library Issue 2, 2002. Oxford: Update Software. Search date 1997; primary sources Medline, Extramed, Embase, Psychlit, Current Contents, Lilacs, Scisearch, The Cochrane Controlled Trials Register, The Cochrane Collaboration Depression and Anxiety Trials Register, hand search of citation lists in identified studies and reviews, and personal contact.
35. Walsh BT, Hadigan CM, Devlin MJ, et al. Long-term outcome of antidepressant treatment for bulimia nervosa. *Am J Psychiatry* 1991;148:1206–1212.
36. Pyle RL, Mitchell JE, Eckert ED, et al. Maintenance treatment and 6-month outcome for bulimic patients who respond to initial treatment. *Am J Psychiatry* 1990;147:871–875.
37. Agras WS, Rossiter EM, Arnow B, et al. One-year follow-up of psychosocial and pharmacologic treatments for bulimia nervosa *J Clin Psychiatry* 1994;55:179–183.
38. Walsh BT, Agras WS, Devlin MJ, et al. Fluoxetine for bulimia nervosa following poor response to psychotherapy. *Am J Psychiatry* 2000;157:1332–1334.
39. Carruba MO, Cuzzolaro M, Riva L, et al. Efficacy and tolerability of moclobemide in bulimia nervosa: a placebo-controlled trial. *Int Clin Psychopharmacol* 2001;16:27–32.
40. Bacaltchuk J, Hay P, Trefiglio R. Antidepressants versus psychological treatments and their combination for bulimia nervosa (Cochrane Review). In: The Cochrane Library, Issue 2, 2002. Oxford: Update Software. Search date 1997; primary sources Medline, Extramed, Embase, Psychlit, Current Contents, Lilacs, Scisearch, Cochrane Controlled Trials Register, Cochrane Collaboration Depression and Anxiety Trials Register, hand search of *Int J Eat Disord* since its first issue, citation lists of identified studies and reviews, and personal contacts.
41. Agras WS, Rossiter EM, Arnow B, et al. Pharmacologic and cognitive-behavioral treatment for bulimia nervosa: a controlled comparison. *Am J Psychiatry* 1992;149:82–87.
42. Wheadon DE, Rampey AH, Thompson VL, et al. Lack of association between fluoxetine and suicidality in bulimia nervosa. *J Clin Psychiatry* 1992;53:235–241.
43. Bacaltchuk J, Trefiglio RP, Oliveira IR, et al. Combination of antidepressants and psychotherapy for bulimia nervosa: a systematic review. *Acta Psychiatr Scand* 2000;101:256–264. Search date 1997; primary sources handsearch of *Int J Eat Disord* since its first issue, Medline, Extramed, Embase, Psychlit, Current Contents, Lilacs, Scisearch, Cochrane Controlled Trials Register 1997 Internet version, Cochrane Collaboration Depression and Anxiety Trials Register, hand search of all citation lists in identified studies and reviews, and personal contact.
44. Fairburn CG, Marcus MD, Wilson GT. Cognitive-behavioral therapy for binge eating and bulimia nervosa: a comprehensive treatment manual. In :Fairburn CG, Wilson GT eds. *Binge eating: Nature, Assessment, and Treatment*. New York, NY: Guilford Press; 1993:361–404.
45. Bachar E, Latzer Y, Kreitler S, et al. Empirical comparison of two psychological therapies. Self psychology and cognitive orientation in the treatment of anorexia and bulimia. *J Psychother Pract Res* 1999;8:115–128.
46. Schmidt U, Treasure J. 1997 Clinician's guide to getting better bit(e) by bit(e) Hove: Psychology Press.

Phillipa Hay
Psychiatrist
University of Adelaide, Adelaide, Australia

Josue Bacaltchuk
Psychiatrist
Federal University of Sao Paulo, Sao Paulo, Brazil

Competing interests: PH has received reimbursement for attending symposia from Solvay Pharmaceuticals, Bristol-Myers Squibb, and Pfizer Pharmaceuticals, and for educational training of family doctors from Bristol-Myers Squibb, Pfizer Pharmaceuticals, and Lundbeck, and has been funded by Jansenn-Cilag to attend symposia. JB has received fees from Janssen-Cilag Farmaceutica.

TABLE 1 Comparison of remission rates between cognitive behaviour therapy or other active psychotherapy and comparison group (see text, p 916).[24]

Comparison	Number of RCTs	Number of people	Absolute remission rates	RR of not remitting (95% CI)
CBT *v* waiting list	7	300	42% *v* 6%	0.64 (0.53 to 0.78)
CBT *v* other psychotherapy	7	474	40% *v* 21%	0.80 (0.61 to 1.04)
CBT *v* pure self help CBT	4	223	46% *v* 36%	0.90 (0.74 to 1.10)
Other psychotherapy *v* waiting list	3	131	36% *v* 3%	0.67 (0.56 to 0.81)

CBT, cognitive behavioural therapy.

TABLE 2 Comparison of remission rates between active drug and placebo by class of antidepressant (see text, p 920).[34]

Class: drug(s)	Number of RCTs	Number of people	RR	95% CI
TCA: desipramine, imipramine	3	132	0.86	0.7 to 1.07
SSRI: fluoxetine	1	398	0.92	0.84 to 1.01
MAOI: phenylzine, brofaramine	2	98	0.81	0.68 to 0.96
Other: bupropion, trazodone	2	87	0.86	0.76 to 0.97

MAOI, monoamine oxidase inhibitor; SSRI, selective serotonin reuptake inhibitor; TCA, tricyclic antidepressant.

Dementia

Search date February 2002

James Warner, Rob Butler, and Elizabeth Jackson

QUESTIONS

INTERVENTIONS

See glossary, p 946

Key Messages

- People in dementia RCTs are often not representative of people in routine settings. Few RCTs are conducted in primary care.

- **Carbamazepine (for behavioural symptoms)** One RCT found that carbamazepine versus placebo significantly reduced agitation and aggression in people with unspecified dementia.
- **Cholinesterase inhibitors (for behavioural symptoms)** One RCT in people with Alzheimer's disease found no significant difference in psychiatric symptoms at 3 months with galantamine versus placebo, but another RCT found that galantamine versus placebo significantly improved psychiatric symptoms at 6 months. One RCT in people with Alzheimer's disease found that donepezil versus placebo significantly improved functional and behavioural symptoms at 24 weeks, and another RCT found no significant difference in psychiatric symptoms at 24 weeks with donepezil versus placebo.
- **Donepezil (cognitive benefit, Alzheimer's disease)** One systematic review has found that donepezil versus placebo significantly improves cognitive function at up to 52 weeks in people with mild to moderate Alzheimer's disease. One subsequent RCT in people with moderate to severe Alzheimer's disease has found that donepezil versus placebo significantly improves cognitive function and functional and behavioural symptoms at 24 weeks.
- **Galantamine (cognitive benefit, Alzheimer's disease)** One systematic review and one additonal RCT have found that galantamine versus placebo significantly improves functioning and cognition at 6 months.
- **Ginkgo biloba (cognitive benefit, Alzheimer's disease)** One systematic review has found that Ginkgo biloba versus placebo significantly improves cognitive function and is well tolerated.
- **Ginkgo biloba (for vascular and Lewy body dementia)** One systematic review and one subsequent RCT found no clear evidence of benefit with Ginkgo biloba versus placebo in people with vascular dementia. We found no RCTs in people with Lewy body dementia.
- **Haloperidol (for behavioural symptoms)** One systematic review in people with various types of dementia found no significant difference in agitation with haloperidol versus placebo, but found limited evidence that haloperidol may significantly reduce aggression.
- **Lecithin** One systematic review of small, poor quality RCTs in people with Alzheimer's disease found no significant difference between lecithin versus placebo in cognition, functional performance, quality of life, or global impression. We found insufficient evidence about lecithin versus placebo in people with vascular and Lewy body dementia.
- **Music therapy (for behavioural symptoms)** One systematic review of studies with weak methods found insufficient evidence about music therapy.
- **Nicotine** One systematic review found no RCTs of adequate quality on the effects of nicotine.
- **Non-steroidal anti-inflammatory drugs** One RCT in people with Alzheimer's disease found no significant difference in cognitive function after 25 weeks' treatment with diclofenac plus misoprostol versus placebo. Another RCT in people with Alzheimer's disease found that indometacin versus placebo significantly improved cognitive function after 6 months' treatment. We found no RCTs of non-steroidal anti-inflammatory drugs in people with vascular or Lewy body dementia.
- **Oestrogen (cognitive benefit, Alzheimer's disease)** One systematic review in women with established Alzheimer's disease has found that hormone replacement therapy versus no hormone replacement therapy significantly improves cognition.

- **Olanzapine (improved agitation, hallucinations, and delusions)** One RCT in people with Alzheimer's disease and behavioural and psychological symptoms found that olanzapine (5–10 mg daily) versus placebo reduced agitation, hallucinations, and delusions.
- **Physostigmine (for cognitive outcomes, Alzheimer's disease)** One systematic review found that slow release physostigmine versus placebo improved cognition, but adverse effects, including nausea, vomiting, diarrhoea, dizziness, and stomach pain, were common.
- **Reality orientation (cognitive and behavioural symptoms)** One systematic review in people with unspecified dementia found that reality orientation versus no treatment significantly improved cognitive function and behaviour.
- **Reminiscence therapy (for behavioural symptoms)** One systematic review found insufficient evidence on the effects of reminiscence therapy.
- **Risperidone (reduced psychotic symptoms and aggression)** One RCT in people with moderate to severe dementia including Alzheimer's disease and vascular dementia found that risperidone versus placebo significantly improved behavioural and psychological symptoms over 12 weeks (risperidone 2 mg, NNT 6, 95% CI 4 to 17), but another RCT in people with severe dementia and agitation found no significant difference in symptoms over 13 weeks.
- **Rivastigmine (for cognitive outcomes, Alzheimer's disease)** One systematic review has found that rivastigmine versus placebo significantly improves cognitive function, but increases the frequency of nausea, vomiting, anorexia, diarrhoea, and discontinuation of treatment.
- **Rivastigmine (for vascular and Lewy body dementia)** One RCT in people with Lewy body dementia found that rivastigmine versus placebo significantly improved cognitive function and behaviour after 20 weeks (NNT 3, 95% CI 2 to 6 for at least 30% improvement on Neuropsychiatric Inventory score). Discontinuation of treatment and adverse effects including nausea, vomiting, anorexia, and diarrhoea are common. We found insufficient evidence about the effects of rivastigmine in people with vascular dementia.
- **Selegiline (cognitive benefit, Alzheimer's disease)** One systematic review has found that in people with Alzheimer's disease, selegiline versus placebo significantly improves cognitive function, behavioural disturbance, and mood after about 3 months, but found no evidence of improved clinical global state.
- **Sodium valproate (for behavioural symptoms)** One RCT found that sodium valproate versus placebo significantly reduced agitation in unspecified dementia.
- **Tacrine** Systematic reviews found limited evidence that tacrine versus placebo significantly improved cognitive function and global state in Alzheimer's disease, but adverse effects, including nausea and vomiting, diarrhoea, anorexia, and abdominal pain, were common. We found no RCTs in people with vascular or Lewy body dementia.
- **Trazodone (for behavioural symptoms)** One RCT in people with Alzheimer's disease found no significant difference between trazodone versus haloperidol in reducing agitation. Another RCT in people with dementia plus agitated behaviour found no significant difference in agitation between trazodone, haloperidol, behavioural management techniques, and placebo. The RCTs may have been too small to exclude a clinically important difference.

- **Vitamin E (for cognitive outcomes)** One RCT in people with Alzheimer's disease found no significant difference in cognitive function after 2 years' treatment with vitamin E versus placebo, but found that vitamin E significantly reduced mortality, institutionalisation, loss of ability to perform activities of daily living, and the proportion of people who developed severe dementia. We found no RCTs about vitamin E in vascular or Lewy body dementia.
- **Donepezil (for vascular and Lewy body dementia); galantamine (for vascular and Lewy body dementia); oestrogen (for vascular and Lewy body dementia); physostigmine (for vascular and Lewy body dementia) selegiline (for vascular and Lewy body dementia)** We found no RCTs on the effects of donepezil, galantamine, oestrogen, physostigmine, and selegiline in vascular dementia or Lewy body dementia.

DEFINITION **Dementia** is characterised by chronic, global, non-reversible impairment of cerebral function. It usually results in loss of memory (initially of recent events), loss of executive function (such as the ability to make decisions or sequence complex tasks), and changes in personality. **Alzheimer's disease** is a type of dementia characterised by an insidious onset and slow deterioration, and involves speech, motor, personality, and executive function impairment. It should be diagnosed after other systemic, psychiatric, and neurological causes of dementia have been excluded clinically and by laboratory investigation. **Vascular dementia** (multi-infarct dementia) is a stepwise deterioration of executive function with or without language and motor dysfunction occurring as a result of cerebral arterial occlusion. It usually occurs in the presence of vascular risk factors (diabetes, hypertension, and smoking). Characteristically, it has a more sudden onset and stepwise progression than Alzheimer's disease. **Lewy body dementia** is an insidious impairment of executive functions with (1) Parkinsonism, (2) visual hallucinations, and (3) fluctuating cognitive abilities and increased risk of falls or autonomic failure.[1,2] Careful clinical examination of people with mild to moderate dementia, and the use of established diagnostic criteria, has an antemortem positive predictive value of 70–90% compared with the gold standard of postmortem diagnosis.[3,4]

INCIDENCE/ PREVALENCE About 6% of people aged over 65 years and 30% of people aged over 90 years have some form of dementia.[5] Dementia is rare before the age of 60 years. The most common types of dementia are Alzheimer's disease, vascular dementia, mixed vascular and Alzheimer's disease, and Lewy body dementia. Alzheimer's disease and vascular dementia (including mixed dementia) are each estimated to account for 35–50% of dementia, and Lewy body dementia is estimated to account for up to 20% of dementia in the elderly, varying with geographical, cultural, and racial factors.[1,5–10]

AETIOLOGY/ RISK FACTORS **Alzheimer's disease:** The cause of Alzheimer's disease is unclear. A key pathological process is deposition of abnormal amyloid in the central nervous system.[11] Most people with the relatively rare condition of early onset Alzheimer's disease (before age 60 years) show an autosomal dominant inheritance due to mutations on presenelin or amyloid precursor protein genes. Several genes (*APP*, *PS-1*, and *PS-2*) have been identified. Later onset dementia is sometimes clustered in families, but specific gene mutations have not been identified. Head injury, Down's syndrome, and lower premorbid intellect may be risk factors for Alzheimer's disease. **Vascular dementia** is related to cardiovascular risk factors, such as smoking, hypertension, and diabetes. **Lewy body dementia:** The aetiology of Lewy body dementia is unknown. Brain acetylcholine activity is reduced in many forms of dementia, and the level of reduction correlates with cognitive impairment. Many treatments for Alzheimer's disease enhance cholinergic activity.[1,6]

PROGNOSIS **Alzheimer's disease:** Alzheimer's disease usually has an insidious onset with progressive reduction in cerebral function. Diagnosis is difficult in the early stages. Average life expectancy after diagnosis is 7–10 years.[10] **Lewy body dementia:** People with Lewy body dementia have an average life expectancy of around 6 years after diagnosis.[5] Behavioural problems, depression, and psychotic symptoms are common in all types of dementia.[12,13] Eventually, most people with dementia find it difficult to perform simple tasks without help.

AIMS To improve cognitive function (memory, orientation, attention, and concentration); to reduce behavioural and psychological symptoms (wandering, aggression, anxiety, depression, and psychosis); to improve quality of life for both the individual and carer, with minimum adverse effects.

OUTCOMES Quality of life of the person with dementia and their carer (rarely used in clinical trials). Comprehensive scales of cognitive function (e.g. Alzheimer's Disease Assessment Scale cognitive subscale [ADAS-cog], 70-point scale, lower scores signify better function;[14] Mini Mental State Examination, 30-point scale, higher scores signify better function[15]). ADAS-cog is more sensitive than Mini Mental State Examination, but neither scale directly reflects outcomes important to people with dementia or their carers. A 7 point change in the ADAS-cog has been regarded as clinically important. Measures of global state (e.g. clinician interview-based impression of change with caregiver input scale, Clinician's Interview Based Impression of Change-Plus: 7 points). Measures of psychiatric symptoms (e.g. Neuropsychiatric Inventory, 12-item caregiver-rated, maximum score 144, higher scores indicate greater difficulties; Dementia Mood Assessment Scale, and Brief Psychiatric Rating Scale, which use lower scores to signify improved symptoms; Behave-AD scale, scores 0–75, lower scores indicate better function). Time to institutionalisation or death are rarely reported because of the short duration of most trials.[16] Functional measures include the Disability Assessment for Dementia, a 40-item scale assessing 10 domains of function[17] and the Instrumental Activities of Daily Living Scale, maximum score 14 (higher scores indicate better function).[18]

METHODS *Clinical Evidence* update search and appraisal February 2002. Dementia is often considered to have two domains of symptoms: cognitive impairment and non-cognitive symptoms (behavioural and psychological symptoms of dementia). We have separated the evidence into these two domains because they are often therapeutic targets at different stages of dementia and many RCTs focus on one or other domain of symptoms. In many RCTs, missing data were managed using "last observation carried forward", which does not account for the tendency of people with dementia to deteriorate with time; therefore, these studies may overestimate the benefit derived from interventions, especially when there are higher withdrawal rates in the intervention arm compared with controls.

QUESTION **What are the effects of treatments on cognitive symptoms of dementia?**

OPTION **DONEPEZIL**

One systematic review has found that donepezil versus placebo significantly improves cognitive function at up to 52 weeks in people with mild or moderate Alzheimer's disease. One subsequent RCT in people with moderate to severe Alzheimer's disease has found that donepezil versus placebo significantly improves cognitive function and functional and behavioural symptoms at 24 weeks. We found no RCTs assessing the effects of donepezil on quality of life. We found no RCTs of donepezil in vascular dementia or Lewy body dementia.

Benefits: **Alzheimer's disease:** We found one systematic review[19] and one subsequent RCT.[20] The systematic review (search date 2000) identified eight RCTs of 12, 24, and 52 weeks duration (2664 people with mild or moderate Alzheimer's disease) comparing donepezil versus placebo.[19] Five RCTs identified by the review reported results using the Alzheimer's Disease Assessment Scale cognitive subscale (ADAS-cog) or the Clinician's Interview Based Impression of Change-Plus (CIBIC-Plus); three of 12 weeks' duration and two of 24 weeks' duration. The review found that donepezil 5 mg or 10 mg daily versus placebo significantly improved cognitive function (measured by ADAS-cog scores) at 12 and 24 weeks (see table 1, p 949), and significantly improved global clinical state at 12 weeks (CIBIC-Plus score unchanged or worse; donepezil 5 mg: 1 RCT 104/153 [68%] *v* 123/150 [82%]; RR 0.83, 95% CI 0.73 to 0.95; donepezil 10 mg: 1 RCT; 302 people; 94/152 [60%] *v* 123/150 [82%]; RR 0.75, 95% CI 0.65 to 0.87) and 24 weeks (CIBIC-Plus score unchanged or worse: donepezil 5 mg; 2 RCTs; 812 people; 311/403 [77%] *v* 356/409 [87%]; RR 0.89, 95% CI 0.83 to 0.95; donepezil 10 mg: 799 people; 295/390 [76%] *v* 356/409 [87%]; RR 0.87, 95% CI 0.81 to 0.93), but did not significantly improve patient or carer rated quality of life.[19] One large RCT identified by the review (double blind, 473 people with mild to moderate Alzheimer's disease) comparing donepezil 10 mg daily versus placebo found that donepezil significantly improved cognitive function over 24 weeks (NNT 4, 95% CI 3 to 7 for a 4 point improvement in ADAS-cog; NNT 6, 95% CI 4 to 12 for a 7 point improvement).[23] A third RCT identified by the review (206 people living in a nursing home, mean age 85, mean Mini Mental State Examination [MMSE] 14) comparing donepezil versus placebo found that donepezil significantly improved cognitive function over 24 weeks (NNT for a 3 point improvement in MMSE score 7, 95% CI 4 to 50). Another RCT (286 people) identified by the review found that donepezil 10 mg daily versus placebo significantly improved cognitive function over 52 weeks (MMSE: WMD 1.7, 95% CI 0.8 to 2.6) and activities of daily living. An unblinded extension of one of the RCTs identified by the review observed 133 people on donepezil 3–10 mg daily for up to 240 weeks.[24] Improved cognitive function compared with baseline was present for 38 weeks, and throughout the period of observation cognitive function remained above the level estimated had people not been treated. One subsequent RCT (24 wks, 290 people with moderate to severe Alzheimer's disease aged 48–92 years, MMSE score 5 to 17) compared donepezil 5–10 mg daily versus placebo.[20] It found that donepezil versus placebo significantly improved CIBIC-Plus scores at 24 weeks (mean difference 0.54, no 95% CI provided, results presented graphically; NNT 5, 95% CI 4 to 10 for improved or no change on CIBIC-Plus).[20] **Vascular dementia:** We found no systematic review or RCTs relating to donepezil treatment and its effect on cognitive function in vascular dementia. **Lewy body dementia:** We found no systematic review and no RCTs relating to donepezil treatment and its effect on cognitive function in Lewy body dementia.

Harms: **Alzheimer's disease:** Adverse effects common to all cholinesterase inhibitors include anorexia, nausea, vomiting, and diarrhoea (see table 2, p 950). The RCTs identified by the review found that donepezil was associated with nausea, vomiting, and diarrhoea, which tended to be mild and transient.[19] Hepatotoxicity was reported as non-significant. The review found no difference in the proportion of people who withdrew for any cause (27% with 10 mg donepezil *v* 20% with 5 mg *v* 21% with placebo).[19] Long term follow up of people taking donepezil up to 10 mg (open label extension) found that 86% experienced at least one adverse effect, often occurring later in the study. Common adverse events included agitation (24%), pain (20%), insomnia (11%), and diarrhoea (9%).[24] The subsequent RCT found no significant difference with donepezil versus placebo in the proportion of people who experienced any adverse event over 24 weeks (120/144 [83%] *v* 117/146 [80%]; RR 1.04, 95% CI 0.93 to 1.16).[20] **Vascular or Lewy body dementia:** We found no RCTs assessing harms specifically in people with vascular or Lewy body dementia.

Comment: Donepezil appears relatively safe and confers some benefit for some individuals. However, more pragmatic trials in routine clinical settings are required. Quality of life of carers has not been assessed in existing trials.[19] Donepezil is taken once daily; this is a potential advantage over other cholinesterase inhibitors for people with dementia. Improvement usually starts within 2–4 months of starting donepezil. Open label studies should be interpreted with caution, but do suggest that the effect of continued treatment is sustained in the long term.[24] Many trials that found benefit from donepezil also found much higher withdrawal rates (30% or more) with donepezil than with placebo.

OPTION RIVASTIGMINE

One systematic review has found that rivastigmine improves cognitive function in people with Alzheimer's disease, but adverse effects such as nausea, vomiting, and anorexia are common. We found no RCTs about the effects of rivastigmine in people with vascular dementia. One RCT in people with Lewy body dementia found improvement of cognitive function and behaviour with rivastigmine versus placebo.

Benefits: **Alzheimer's disease:** We found one systematic review (search date 2000, 4 RCTs, 12 or 26 wks duration, 3370 people with mild to moderate Alzheimer's disease[21]) (see table 1, p 949). The review found that over 26 weeks, rivastigmine (6–12 mg twice daily) versus placebo produced small but significant improvements in cognitive function (Alzheimer's Disease Assessment Scale cognitive subscale [ADAS-cog]: 4 RCTs; 1917 people WMD –2.1, 95% CI –2.7 to –1.5; Mini Mental State Examination: WMD 0.8, 95% CI 0.5 to 1.1), and global clinical state (Clinician's Interview Based Impression of Change: OR 0.7, 95% CI 0.6 to 0.9). Quality of life results were not provided. **Vascular dementia:** We found no systematic review or RCTs of rivastigmine in people with vascular dementia. A subgroup analysis of an RCT (699 people with Alzheimer's disease but not vascular dementia) comparing rivastigmine (1–4 mg daily or 6–12 mg daily) versus placebo over 26 weeks found that people with vascular risk factors responded more than those without (mean ADAS-cog difference –2.3).[25] **Lewy body dementia:** We found no systematic review but found one RCT (120 people with Lewy body dementia), which found that rivastigmine (dose titrated to 6 mg twice daily) versus placebo for 20 weeks significantly improved a computerised psychometric measure of cognitive function (intention to treat analysis; P = 0.05; further exploration of effect size not possible) and a global measure of behavioural function (NNT for at least 30% improvement on Neuropsychiatric Inventory score 3, 95% CI 2 to 6).[26]

Harms: **Alzheimer's disease:** Adverse effects common to all cholinesterase inhibitors include anorexia, nausea, vomiting, and diarrhoea (see table 2, p 950). The systematic review found that rivastigmine versus placebo increased the proportion of people who discontinued treatment (35% with 6–12 mg rivastigmine *v* 18% with 1–4 mg rivastigmine *v* 17% with placebo).[21] **Lewy body dementia:** The RCT in people with Lewy body dementia found that rivastigmine versus placebo increased the proportion of people who had nausea (37% *v* 22%), vomiting (25% *v* 15%), anorexia (19% *v* 10%), and somnolence (9% *v* 5%; no further data provided).[26]

Comment: The rates of adverse effects seemed higher with rivastigmine than with other anticholinesterase drugs, but direct comparisons have not been performed.

OPTION GALANTAMINE

One systematic review and one additional RCT have found that galantamine versus placebo significantly improves cognition and functioning in older people with Alzheimer's disease. We found no RCTs of galantamine in people with vascular or Lewy body dementia.

Benefits: **Alzheimer's disease:** We found one systematic review (search date 2000, 7 RCTs)[22] and one additional RCT comparing galantamine versus placebo.[27] The review found that galantamine (8 mg, 12 mg, or 16 mg twice daily) versus placebo significantly improved cognitive function (measured by Alzheimer's Disease Assessment Scale cognitive subscale [ADAS-cog] score) over 6 months (see table 1, p 949), global status (Clinician's Interview Based Impression of Change: OR 1.8, 95% CI 1.5 to 2.3), and psychiatric symptoms (Neuropsychiatric Inventory score: WMD –2.3, 95% CI –4.0 to –0.6).[22] The additional RCT (653 people) found that galantamine (24 mg daily) versus placebo significantly improved cognitive function over 26 weeks (ADAS-cog mean difference: –3.1, 95% CI –4.5 to –1.7).[27] It also found that galantamine (32 mg daily) versus placebo significantly improved cognitive function (ADAS-cog mean difference: –4.1, 95% CI –5.6 to –2.7; NNT for 4 point difference 6, 95% CI 4 to 12) and disability (disability assessment scale, 100 point scale, higher score = better function: mean difference: 3.4, 95% CI 0.1 to 6.7).[27] **Vascular dementia:** We found no systematic review or RCTs of galantamine versus placebo in people with vascular dementia. **Lewy body dementia:** We found no systematic review or RCTs of galantamine versus placebo in people with Lewy body dementia.

Harms: **Alzheimer's disease:** Adverse effects common to all cholinesterase inhibitors include anorexia, nausea, vomiting, and diarrhoea (see table 2, p 950) The review found that adverse effects over 6 months were more frequent with larger doses of galantamine, including nausea (42% with galantamine 16 mg twice daily *v* 24% with placebo), vomiting (21% with galantamine *v* 7% with placebo). It also found that higher doses of galantamine increased the proportion of people who discontinued treatment because of adverse effects over 6 months (38% with galantamine 16 mg twice daily *v* 25% with galantamine 12 mg twice daily *v* 16% with placebo).[22]

Comment: None.

OPTION TACRINE

Two systematic reviews found limited evidence that tacrine versus placebo improved cognitive function and global state in Alzheimer's disease, but adverse effects, including nausea and vomiting, diarrhoea, anorexia, and abdominal pain were common. We found no RCTs assessing its use in people with vascular or Lewy body dementia.

Benefits: **Alzheimer's disease:** We found two systematic reviews of tacrine versus placebo in people with Alzheimer's disease (search date not stated, 12 RCTs, 1984 people;[28] search date 1997, 21 RCTs, including 12 RCTs identified by the first review, 3555 people[29]). Various doses of tacrine were used in the RCTs, and the duration of treatment varied from 3–36 weeks. The first review found that tacrine versus placebo significantly improved overall clinical improvement (OR 1.58, 95% CI 1.18 to 2.11), and cognition (Mini Mental State Examination at 12 wks: SMD 0.77, 95% CI 0.35 to 1.20; Alzheimer's Disease Assessment Scale cognitive subscale at

12 wks SMD −2.7, 95% CI −1.36 to −2.78).[28] A subsequent subgroup analysis indicated that the five non-industry sponsored studies found no significant effect with tacrine versus placebo, but most (6/7) manufacturer supported studies found clinical benefit (1 RCT was not located for the subgroup analysis).[30] **Vascular dementia:** We found no systematic review and no RCTs. **Lewy body dementia:** We found no systematic review and no RCTs.

Harms: One RCT identified by the review found that withdrawals because of adverse events were common (OR for withdrawal 3.6, 95% CI 2.8 to 4.7)[28] and were more likely with higher doses (265/479 [55%] with high dose tacrine *v* 20/184 [11%] with placebo; RR 5.1, 95% CI 3.3 to 7.7; NNH 3, 95% CI 2 to 3), and reversible elevation of liver enzymes was found in 133/265 (50%) of people taking tacrine.[31] Common adverse events included nausea and vomiting (35% with 160 mg daily), diarrhoea (18%), anorexia (12%), and abdominal pain (9%).

Comment: The quality of tacrine trials was generally poor.[28,29]

OPTION PHYSOSTIGMINE

One systematic review in people with Alzheimer's disease found that slow release physostigmine versus placebo improved cognition, but adverse effects including nausea, vomiting, diarrhoea, dizziness, and stomach pain were common. We found no evidence about its use in people with vascular or Lewy body dementia.

Benefits: **Alzheimer's disease:** We found one systematic review (search date 2000, 15 RCTs).[32] The RCTs differed widely in the preparations of physostigmine used, which makes it difficult to generalise results. Four RCTs were small trials of intravenous physostigmine, and seven were small trials (131 people) of standard oral preparation. Four RCTs (1456 people) used controlled release preparations. Two RCTs reported results only for people who responded to physostigmine in a prestudy titration phase. One RCT (170 people) found that physostigmine (27 mg daily) versus placebo improved cognition after 12 weeks (Alzheimer's Disease Assessment Scale cognitive subscale: −2.0, 95% CI −3.6 to −0.5), but did not significantly improve activities of daily living or clinician impression of change. **Vascular dementia:** We found no systematic review and no RCTs in people with vascular dementia. **Lewy body dementia:** We found no systematic review and no RCTs.

Harms: Common adverse effects include nausea, vomiting, diarrhoea, dizziness, and stomach pain. In RCTs that randomised all people with Alzheimer's disease rather than selecting those who tolerated and responded to physostigmine, withdrawals were more common with physostigmine (234/358 [65%] with physostigmine *v* 31/117 [26%] with placebo; OR 4.80, 95% CI 3.17 to 7.33).[32]

Comment: Physostigmine is a sympathomimetic drug and has a very short half life. We found only limited evidence that physostigmine improved cognition, and no evidence that it improved other domains of function. Adverse affects are common. Screening out non-responders before the trial is likely to overestimate the effectiveness of this drug.

OPTION NICOTINE

We found one systematic review, which found no RCTs of adequate quality.

Benefits: One systematic review (search date 2001) found no RCTs of adequate quality.[33]

Harms: We found no RCTs.

Comment: None.

OPTION LECITHIN

One systematic review in people with Alzheimer's disease found no significant benefit with lecithin versus placebo. We found insufficient evidence about lecithin versus placebo in people with vascular and Lewy body dementia.

Benefits: **Alzheimer's disease:** We found one systematic review (search date 2000, 10 RCTs, 256 people with mild to severe disease Alzheimer's disease) of lecithin, which found no significant improvement in cognition, functional performance, quality of life, or global impression (see comment below).[34] **Vascular dementia:** We found no systematic review or RCTs. **Lewy body dementia:** We found one systematic review[34] including one RCT (90 people with "Parkinsonian dementia", which may have included people with causes of dementia apart from Lewy body dementia). The RCT found no benefit from lecithin versus placebo.

Harms: The review found that adverse effects were more common with lecithin (41% with lecithin *v* 10% with placebo; OR 6.0, 95% CI 1.5 to 24).[34] The specific nature of the adverse effects was not stated.

Comment: One RCT (included in the systematic review[34]) of lecithin versus placebo in people with minimal cognitive impairment, found some components of cognition were significantly better in the placebo group. Most studies of lecithin are small and old. Meta-analysis in the systematic review was hampered by diverse outcome criteria.

OPTION NON-STEROIDAL ANTI-INFLAMMATORY DRUGS

One RCT in people with Alzheimer's disease found no significant difference in cognitive function after 25 weeks' treatment with diclofenac plus misoprostol versus placebo. Another RCT in people with Alzheimer's disease found that indometacin versus placebo significantly improved cognitive function after 6 months' treatment. We found no RCTs of non-steroidal anti-inflammatory drugs in people with vascular or Lewy body dementia.

Benefits: **Alzheimer's disease:** We found no systematic review but found two RCTs.[35,36] The first RCT (41 people) found no significant difference in cognitive function after 25 weeks' treatment with diclofenac plus misoprostol versus placebo (Alzheimer's Disease Assessment Scale cognitive subscale [ADAS-cog] score: mean difference +1.14, 95% CI –2.9 to +5.2) or global status (Clinician's Interview Based Impression of Change score: +0.24, 95% CI

–0.26 to +0.74).[35] The second RCT (44 people with mild to moderate Alzheimer's disease) found that indometacin (indomethacin) (up to 150 mg daily) versus placebo for 6 months significantly improved cognitive function (Mini Mental State Examination and ADAS-cog score; inadequately described results for only 28/44 completers).[36] **Vascular dementia:** We found one systematic review of aspirin for vascular dementia (search date 2000) that found no RCTs (see comment below).[37] **Lewy body dementia:** We found no systematic review and no RCTs.

Harms: See non-steroidal anti-inflammatory drugs, p 1203. In one RCT,[35] more people withdrew by week 25 with diclofenac plus misoprostol versus placebo (12 [50%] *v* 2 [12%]). No serious drug related adverse events were reported.[35] In the RCT of indometacin, 21% of people on indometacin withdrew because of gastrointestinal symptoms.[36]

Comment: Earlier versions of a systematic review of aspirin in vascular dementia included one RCT (70 people), which was subsequently removed because of inadequate quality, including a lack of placebo control.[37]

OPTION OESTROGEN

One systematic review in women with established Alzheimer's disease has found that oestrogen versus no oestrogen improves cognition. We found no evidence about its use in people with vascular or Lewy body dementia.

Benefits: **Alzheimer's disease:** We found one systematic review (search date 2000, 8 placebo controlled RCTs of oestrogen 0.625–1.25 mg daily, 313 people, 7 wks to 12 months' duration).[38] The review found that oestrogen versus no oestrogen improves cognitive function (5 RCTs, Mini Mental State Examination: WMD 2.3, 95% CI 1.7 to 3.4). The largest and longest RCT (120 women with mild to moderate Alzheimer's disease) found that conjugated equine oestrogen (0.625 mg daily) versus placebo for 52 weeks had no significant effect on the Clinical Global Impression of Change 7 point scale, on secondary outcome measures, or on Mini Mental State Examination score at 12 months.[39] **Vascular dementia:** We found no systematic review or RCTs. **Lewy body dementia:** We found no systematic review or RCTs.

Harms: There is concern that oestrogen treatment may increase the risk of developing breast cancer and cardiovascular events (see harms of hormone replacement therapy under secondary prevention of ischaemic cardiac events, p 129).

Comment: Most RCTs in the meta-analysis were small and heterogeneity may have distorted the results. A meta-analysis of 14 observational studies (5990 people, length of follow up not stated) found that hormone replacement therapy is associated with a lower risk of developing dementia (dementia in 13% with HRT *v* 21% with controls; RR 0.56, 95% CI 0.46 to 0.68). Observational studies provide only indirect evidence; the observed association may be explained by confounders (e.g. educational level, lifestyle factors).

OPTION VITAMIN E

One RCT in people with Alzheimer's disease found no significant difference in cognitive function after 2 years' treatment with vitamin E versus placebo, but found that vitamin E significantly reduced mortality, institutionalisation, loss of ability to perform activities of daily living, and the proportion of people who developed severe dementia. We found no RCTs about vitamin E in vascular or Lewy body dementia.

Benefits: **Alzheimer's disease:** We found one systematic review (search date 2000, 1 RCT, 169 people with moderate to severe Alzheimer's disease).[40] The multicentre RCT[41] compared high dose α-tocopherol (vitamin E, 2000 IU daily) versus placebo and compared selegiline versus placebo. It found that high dose α-tocopherol versus placebo for 2 years did not significantly affect cognitive function (measured by the cognitive portion of the Alzheimer's Disease Assessment Scale). It found that vitamin E versus placebo significantly increased event free survival (defined as death, or survival until institutionalisation, loss of ability to perform activities of daily living, or severe dementia [clinical dementia rating of 3]; OR 0.49, 95% CI 0.25 to 0.96). **Vascular dementia:** We found no systematic review or RCTs. **Lewy body dementia:** We found no systematic review or RCTs.

Harms: The RCT found no significant differences in adverse effects between placebo and α-tocopherol.[41] Other studies have found weak evidence of associations between high dose α-tocopherol and bowel irritation, headache, muscular weakness, visual complaints, vaginal bleeding, bruising, thrombophlebitis, deterioration of angina pectoris, worsening of diabetes, syncope, and dizziness.[42] A few case reports have created concern that vitamin E may increase the risk of haemorrhagic stroke.

Comment: The groups in the RCT[41] were not matched evenly at baseline: the placebo group had a higher mean Mini Mental State Examination score, and these baseline scores were a significant predictor of outcome. Attempts to correct for this imbalance suggested that α-tocopherol might increase mean survival, but the need for statistical adjustments weakens the strength of this conclusion.

OPTION SELEGILINE

One systematic review has found that in people with Alzheimer's disease, selegiline versus placebo improves cognitive function, behavioural disturbance, and mood, but found no evidence of improved clinical global state. Selegiline was well tolerated and no serious adverse events were reported. We found no evidence about its use in vascular or Lewy body dementia.

Benefits: **Alzheimer's disease:** We found one systematic review in people with Alzheimer's disease (search date not stated, 15 RCTs) comparing selegiline versus placebo (average number of people 50, typical duration of treatment 3 months).[43] Analysis of pooled results found that selegiline improved several outcome measures: cognitive function scores (measured by several parameters: SMD –0.56, 95% CI –0.88 to –0.24), mood score (Dementia Mood Assessment

Scale: SMD –1.14, 95% CI –2.11 to –0.18), and behavioural symptom score (Brief Psychiatric Rating Scale: SMD –0.53, 95% CI –0.94 to –0.12). The review found no evidence of an effect on global rating scales (SMD –0.11, 95% CI –0.49 to +0.27). **Vascular dementia:** We found no systematic review or RCTs. **Lewy body dementia:** We found no systematic review or RCTs.

Harms: The RCTs identified by the review found no difference in adverse effects (anxiety, agitation, dizziness, nausea, dyspepsia) with selegiline versus placebo.[43]

Comment: The trials used a variety of outcomes, making comparison with other treatments difficult.

OPTION GINKGO BILOBA

One systematic review has found that Ginkgo biloba versus placebo significantly improves cognitive function and is well tolerated in Alzheimer's disease. We found no clear evidence to support its use in vascular or Lewy body dementia.

Benefits: **Alzheimer's disease:** We found one systematic review[44] and one subsequent RCT.[45] The systematic review (search date 1998, 9 double blind RCTs, 1457 people with Alzheimer's disease, vascular dementia, or mixed Alzheimer's disease and vascular dementia)[44] found that in eight RCTs Ginkgo biloba was superior to placebo for a variety of outcomes. The largest and longest trial (52 wks, 309 people of which 236 had Alzheimer's disease) found that in people with Alzheimer's disease, Ginkgo biloba versus placebo significantly improved cognition (completer analysis for people with Alzheimer's disease or vascular dementia, change in Alzheimer's Disease Assessment Scale cognitive subscale score: –1.7, 95% CI –3.2 to –0.20; NNT for 4 point change in ADAS-cog: 8, 95% CI 5 to 50), care giver assessed improvement (change in Geriatric Evaluation by Relative's Rating Instrument score: –0.19, 95% CI –0.28 to –0.08), but did not significantly improve the mean Clinician's Global Impression of Change score (change in score: 0, 95% CI –0.2 to +0.2).[46] The RCT had a high withdrawal rate (137 people [44%] withdrew). The subsequent RCT (24 wks, 214 people in elderly people homes) compared Ginkgo biloba 240 mg daily versus Ginkgo biloba 160 mg daily versus placebo in people with dementia (30%) or mild cognitive impairment (70%).[45] People receiving active medication were rerandomised after 12 weeks to continuing active medication or placebo. Placebo included quinine to mimic the bitter taste of Ginkgo biloba. The study found no significant benefits for Ginkgo biloba. **Vascular dementia:** One systematic review[44] included a meta-analysis for people with vascular dementia, and one subsequent RCT[45] separately analysed results for people with vascular dementia. No benefits were found for Ginkgo biloba versus placebo. **Lewy body dementia:** We found no systematic review or RCTs.

Harms: The largest RCT found adverse events were equally likely with Ginkgo biloba versus placebo (31% *v* 31%).[46] No specific pattern of adverse events was reported.

Comment: Most of the RCTs were brief, with different entry criteria, outcomes, and doses. The effect size of Ginkgo biloba was minimal in the study that used a bitter tasting placebo.[45] Deblinding is common in dementia trials, and may account for some of the perceived treatment effect. However, 70% of the people in this study did not meet criteria for dementia, so the true effect size is uncertain. The high withdrawal rate in the largest RCT weakens its conclusions, although the authors did conduct both completer and intention to treat analyses.[46]

OPTION REMINISCENCE THERAPY

We found insufficient evidence on the effects of reminiscence therapy in people with unspecified dementia.

Benefits: We found one systematic review of reminiscence therapy (see glossary, p 946) (search date 2000, 2 RCTs, 42 people).[47] Analysis of pooled data was hindered by poor trial methods, diverse outcomes, and no separation of data for different types of dementia.

Harms: We found no evidence.

Comment: None.

OPTION REALITY ORIENTATION

One systematic review found that reality orientation improved cognitive function and behaviour compared with no treatment in people with unspecified dementia. We found no evidence about harms.

Benefits: We found one systematic review (search date 2000, 6 RCTs, 125 people).[48] The RCTs compared reality orientation (see glossary, p 946) versus no treatment and used different measures of cognition. The review found that reality orientation improved cognitive function score (SMD –0.59, 95% CI –0.95 to –0.22) and behavioural symptom score (SMD –0.66, 95% CI –1.27 to –0.05). No separate analysis was done for specific types of dementia.

Harms: The RCTs gave no information on adverse effects.[48]

Comment: The RCTs did not use standardised interventions or outcomes.[48]

OPTION MUSIC THERAPY

One systematic review of studies with weak methods found insufficient evidence about music therapy.

Benefits: We found one systematic review of music therapy (search date 1998, 21 studies, 336 people).[49] It included studies with weak methods and found in a meta-analysis that music therapy versus control interventions significantly improved cognitive and behavioural outcomes (mean effect size 0.79, 95% CI 0.62 to 0.95). Significant effects were noted with different types of music therapy (active *v* passive, taped *v* live).

Harms: The systematic review gave no information on harms.[49]

Comment: The primary studies lacked adequate controls, had potential for bias, used diverse interventions, and used inadequate outcome measures. Although one meta-analysis found significant benefits for music therapy on pooling the results of many studies, further high quality studies are needed to clarify whether the results are explained by a true effect or by bias. A previous Cochrane systematic review has been withdrawn.[50]

QUESTION What are the effects of treatments on behavioural and psychological symptoms of dementia?

OPTION ANTIPSYCHOTICS

One systematic review in people with various types of dementia found no significant difference in agitation with haloperidol versus placebo, but found limited evidence that haloperidol may significantly reduce aggression. One RCT in people with moderate to severe dementia including Alzheimer's disease and vascular dementia found that risperidone versus placebo significantly improved behavioural and psychological symptoms over 12 weeks, but another RCT in people with severe dementia and agitation found no significant difference in symptoms over 13 weeks. One RCT in people with Alzheimer's disease and behavioural and psychological symptoms found that olanzapine versus placebo reduced agitation, hallucinations, and delusions. RCTs have found no significant difference in efficacy between different antipsychotics.

Benefits: **Haloperidol versus placebo:** We found one systematic review (search date 2000, 5 RCTs, none of which were included in the older review) of haloperidol for agitation in various types of dementia including Alzheimer's disease and vascular dementia.[51] It found no significant difference in agitation at 6–16 weeks with haloperidol versus placebo (change in symptoms from baseline measured by the Cohen-Mansfield Agitation Inventory or the psychomotor score of the Behavioural Symptoms Scale for Dementia; WMD –0.48, 95% CI –1.43 to +0.53). However, it found limited evidence that haloperidol versus placebo significantly reduced aggression from baseline at 3–6 weeks (2 RCTs, 240 people: WMD –1.11, 95% CI –2.02 to –0.11).[51] **Risperidone versus placebo:** We found two RCTs.[52,53] The first RCT (double blind, 625 people with moderate to severe dementia plus behavioural and psychological symptoms, 73% with Alzheimer's disease, mean age 83 years, 68% women) compared risperidone versus placebo over 12 weeks.[52] A response was defined as a reduction of at least 50% in the Behave-AD scale. It found that risperidone 1 and 2 mg versus placebo significantly improved the chance of responding over 12 weeks (45% with risperidone 1 mg *v* 33% with placebo *v* 50% with risperidone 2 mg; for risperidone 1 mg *v* placebo NNT 9, 95% CI 5 to 100; for risperidone 2 mg *v* placebo NNT 6, 95% CI 4 to 17). Gender and the type of dementia did not significantly affect the results. The second RCT (344 people with agitation and severe dementia, 67% with Alzheimer's, 26% with vascular dementia, mean age 81 years, 56% women) identified by the later review compared adjusted doses of risperidone (mean dose 1.1 mg) versus placebo or versus haloperidol (mean dose 1.2 mg) over 13 weeks for the treatment of behavioural symptoms.[53] A response was defined as a reduction of at least 30% in the Behave-AD scale. It found no significant difference in the proportion of people who responded over 13 weeks with risperidone versus placebo (37/68 [54%] with risperidone *v* 35/74 [47%] with placebo; ARI +7%, 95% CI, −9% to +23%; see below for risperidone versus haloperidol). **Olanzapine versus placebo:** We found one RCT (double blind, 6 wks' duration, 206 elderly US nursing home residents with Alzheimer's disease plus psychotic or behavioural symptoms).[54] The RCT compared olanzapine (given as a fixed dose of 5, 10, or 15 mg daily) versus placebo. Agitation, hallucinations, and delusions were improved by the two lower doses but not by the highest dose of olanzapine when compared with placebo (subscale of the Neuropsychiatric Inventory [nursing home version]: −7.6 with olanzapine 5 mg *v* −6.1 with olanzapine 10 mg *v* −4.9 with olanzapine 15 mg *v* −3.7 with placebo). **Comparisons between antipsychotics:** The RCT comparing adjusted doses of risperidone versus haloperidol or versus placebo found no significant difference in the proportion of people who responded over 13 weeks with risperidone versus haloperidol.[53] A response was defined as a reduction of at least 30% in the Behave-AD scale.

Harms: **Antipsychotics versus placebo:** One study (2 year prospective, longitudinal, 71 people with dementia) found that the mean decline in cognitive scores in 16 people who took antipsychotics was twice that of people who did not (expanded Mini Mental State Examination 21 *v* 9; P = 0.002). See schizophrenia, p 1019.[55] **Risperidone versus placebo:** The first RCT of risperidone found discontinuation because of adverse events was more common with high dose risperidone (12% with placebo *v* 8% with 0.5 mg *v* 16% with 1 mg *v* 24% with 2 mg).[52] **Olanzapine versus placebo:** The RCT found that olanzapine versus placebo increased sedation (25% with 5 mg olanazapine *v* 26% with 10 mg *v* 36% with 15 mg *v* 6% with placebo), and gait disturbance (20% with 5 mg olanzapine *v* 14% with 10 mg *v* 17% with 15 mg *v* 2% with placebo).[54] **Comparisons between antipsychotics:** In the RCT comparing risperidone versus placebo or versus haloperidol, about 18% of people withdrew because of adverse effects from each of the three arms.[53] Extrapyramidal adverse effects were more common in people receiving haloperidol than placebo (22% with haloperidol *v* 15% with risperidone *v* 11% with placebo).

Comment: **Antipsychotics versus placebo:** We found one systematic review (search date 1995, 7 RCTs, 4–12 wks' duration, 294 people with unspecified dementia and behavioural problems).[56] It assessed a variety of antipsychotics, including haloperidol (2 RCTs). The other antipsychtics assessed (acetophenazine, loxapine, trifluoperazine, thiothixene) are no longer commonly used. It found that antipsychotics versus placebo increased the number of people who improved (61%, 95% CI 47% to 75% with antipsychotics *v* 34%, 95% CI 18% to 50% with placebo). It found that adverse effects were more common with antipsychotics than placebo (ARI 25%, 95% CI 13% to 37%), including sedation (21%), movement disorders (13%), and orthostatic hypotension (8%).[56] However, pooled withdrawal rates were not different between antipsychotics and placebo (ARI 4%, 95% CI −7% to 14%).[56] **Comparisons between antipsychotics:** The review (search date 1995) identified eleven RCTs comparing different antipsychotics.[56] It found no difference in efficacy between haloperidol, diazepam, thioridazene, loxapine or oxazepam.[56] Most studies suggest that antipsychotic medications are effective at reducing behavioural and psychiatric symptoms in people with dementia. However, high response rates with placebo indicate that many behavioural problems resolve spontaneously in the short term. Most people with dementia are sensitive to adverse effects from antipsychotics, especially sedation and extrapyramidal symptoms. People with Lewy body dementia are particularly sensitive to these adverse effects, suggesting that antipsychotics have a poor balance of benefits and harms in people with Lewy body dementia. More studies are needed to determine whether newer atypical antipsychotics have a better ratio of benefits to harms than older antipsychotics.

OPTION ANTIEPILEPTIC DRUGS

One RCT found that carbamazepine versus placebo significantly reduced agitation and aggression in people with agitation and unspecified dementia. Another RCT found that sodium valproate reduced agitation in unspecified dementia. We found no RCTs about other antiepileptic drugs.

Benefits: We found no systematic review but we found two RCTs.[57,58] The first RCT (single blind, 51 nursing home patients with agitation and Alzheimer's disease, vascular dementia or mixed Alzheimer's disease and vascular dementia, 6 wks' duration) compared carbamazepine (individualised doses; modal dose 300 mg; mean serum level 5.3 μg/mL versus placebo).[57] It found that carbamazepine versus placebo significantly improved a measure of agitation and aggression (mean total Brief Psychiatric Rating Scale score: 7.7 with carbamazepine *v* 0.9 with placebo) and a measure of global status (Clinical Global Impressions rating: 77% with carbamazepine *v* 21% with placebo). The second RCT (single blind, 56 people with Alzheimer's disease or vascular dementia in nursing homes, 6 wks' duration) compared sodium valproate with placebo.[58] It found that when several covariates were taken into account, sodium valproate improved agitation and aggression (measured by Brief Psychiatric Rating Scale score; P = 0.05 only after adjustment), and a measure of global status (Clinical Global Impressions rating: 68% with sodium valproate *v* 52% with placebo; P = 0.06).

Harms: Harms were significantly more common with carbamazepine than with placebo (16/27 [59%] *v* 7/24 [29%]; P = 0.003). These were considered clinically significant in two cases (1 person with tics, 1 with ataxia). Carbamazepine in the elderly may cause cardiac toxicity. Harms, which were generally rated as mild, were also more common with sodium valproate than with placebo (68% sodium valproate *v* 33% with placebo; P = 0.003).[58] See epilepsy, p 1313.

Comment: The need to perform adjustments for covariates in the second RCT weakens the strength of the findings.

OPTION ANTIDEPRESSANTS

One RCT in people with dementia plus agitated behaviour found no significant difference in agitation with trazodone versus haloperidol. Another RCT in people with Alzheimer's disease and agitated behaviours found no significant difference in outcomes between trazodone, haloperidol, behaviour management techniques, and placebo. The RCTs may have been too small to exclude a clinically important difference.

Benefits: We found no systematic review but found two RCTs.[59,60] The first small RCT (double blind, 28 elderly people Alzheimer's disease, vascular dementia or mixed Alzheimer's disease and vascular dementia and agitated behaviour, 9 wks' duration) compared trazodone (50–250 mg daily) versus haloperidol (1–5 mg daily).[59] It found no significant difference in agitation between the groups, but the trial was too small to exclude a clinically important difference. The second RCT (double blind, 149 people with Alzheimer's disease and agitated behaviours, 16 wks' duration) compared the reduction of agitation with haloperidol (mean dose 1.1 mg daily) versus trazodone (mean dose 200 mg daily) versus behaviour management techniques versus placebo.[60] It found no significant differences in outcome (Alzheimer's Disease Co-operative Study Clinical Global Impression of Change) between the four interventions, but may have been too small to exclude a clinically important difference.

Harms: In the first RCT, adverse effects were more common in the group treated with haloperidol than trazodone.[59] In the second RCT no significant differences in adverse events were seen between the trazodone group and the placebo group.[60] Priapism has been reported with trazodone, occurring in about 1/10 000 people.

Comment: The RCTs were too small to exclude clinically important differences between the interventions.[59,60]

OPTION CHOLINESTERASE INHIBITORS New

One RCT in people with Alzheimer's disease found no significant difference in psychiatric symptoms at 3 months with galantamine versus placebo, but another RCT found that galantamine versus placebo significantly improved psychiatric symptoms at 6 months. One RCT in people with Alzheimer's disease found that donepezil versus placebo significantly improved functional and behavioural symptoms at 24 weeks, and another RCT found no significant difference in psychiatric symptoms at 24 weeks with donepezil versus placebo.

Benefits: **Galantamine:** We found one systematic review (search date 2000, 2 RCTs).[22] It could not perform a meta-analysis because of differences in length of follow up between the trials. Both trials provided data using the Neuropsychiatric Inventory; scored 0–120, negative change indicates improvement. The first RCT (386 people with Alzheimer's disease) identified by the review found no significant difference in psychiatric symptoms at 3 months with galantamine (12–16 mg twice daily) versus placebo (mean change in NPI score: –0.30 with galantamine *v* +0.50 with placebo; WMD –0.80, 95% CI –2.67 to +1.07). The second RCT identified by the review (978 people with Alzheimer's disease) found that galantamine (16 mg daily) versus placebo significantly reduced psychiatric symptoms at 6 months (mean change in Neuropsychiatric Inventory scores –0.10 with galantamine *v* +2.00 with placebo; WMD –2.10, 95% CI –4.04 to –0.16), but found no significant difference with galantamine 8 mg daily or 24 mg daily.[22]

Donepezil: We found two RCTs.[20,61] The first RCT (290 people with moderate to severe Alzheimer's disease aged 48–92 years, Mini Mental State Examination score 5–17) compared donepezil (5–10 mg daily) versus placebo.[20] It found that donepezil versus placebo significantly improved functional and behavioural symptoms at 24 weeks (Disability Assessment for Dementia score; mean difference 8.23, no 95% CI provided; $P < 0.001$; Neuropsychiatric Inventory score; mean difference 5.64, no 95% CI provided; $P < 0.0001$). The second RCT (208 people with Alzheimer's disease, at least one symptom on the Neuropsychiatric Inventory Nursing Home version and living in a nursing home) found that donepezil versus placebo improved psychiatric symptoms after 24 weeks of treatment, but the difference was not significant (change in mean Neuropsychiatric Inventory Nursing Home version scores –4.9 with donepezil *v* –2.3 with placebo; reported as non-significant; no further data provided).[61]

Harms: See harms of donepezil, p 933 and galantamine, p 935 (see table 2, p 950).

Comment: Cholinesterase inhibitors improve cognitive function and are well tolerated in older people. Further studies are needed to show whether they also improve behavioural and psychological symptoms of dementia.

GLOSSARY

Reality orientation Involves presenting information that is designed to reorient a person in time, place, or person. It may range in intensity from a board giving details of the day, date, and season, to staff reorienting a patient at each contact.

Reminiscence therapy Involves encouraging people to talk about the past in order to enable past experiences to be brought into consciousness. It relies on remote memory, which is relatively well preserved in mild to moderate dementia.

Substantive changes

Donepezil One new RCT;[20] conclusions unchanged.

Antipsychotics One new systematic review in people with various types of dementia found no significant difference in agitation with haloperidol versus placebo, but found limited evidence that haloperidol may significantly reduce aggression.[51]

REFERENCES

1. van Duijn CM. Epidemiology of the dementia: recent developments and new approaches *J Neurol Neurosurg Psychiatry* 1996;60:478–488.
2. McKeith IG, Galasko D, Kosaka K, et al. Consensus guidelines for the clinical and pathological diagnosis of dementia with Lewy bodies (DLB): report of the consortium on DLB International workshop. *Neurology* 1996;47:1113–1124.
3. Rasmusson DX, Brandt J, Steele C, et al. Accuracy of clinical diagnosis of Alzheimer disease and clinical features of patients with non-Alzheimer's disease neuropathology. *Alzheimer Dis Assoc Disord* 1996;10:180–188.
4. Verghese J, Crystal HA, Dickson DW, et al. Validity of clinical criteria for the diagnosis of dementia with Lewy bodies. *Neurology* 1999;53:1974–1982.
5. Lobo A, Launer LJ, Fratiglioni L, et al. Prevalence of dementia and major subtypes in Europe: a collaborative study of population-based cohorts. *Neurology* 2000;54:S4–S9.
6. Farrer L. Intercontinental epidemiology of Alzheimer's disease: a global approach to bad gene hunting. *JAMA* 2001;285:796–798.
7. Skoog I. A population-based study of dementia in 85 year olds. *N Engl J Med* 1993;328:153–158.
8. McKeith IG. Clinical Lewy body syndromes. *Ann N Y Acad Sci* 2000;920:1–8.
9. Inkeda M, Hokoishi K, Maki N, et al. Increased prevalence of vascular dementia in Japan: a community-based epidemiological study. *Neurology* 2001;57:839–844.
10. McKeith I. The differential diagnosis of dementia. In: Burns A, Levy R, eds. *Dementia*. 1st ed. London: Chapman and Hall, 1994:39–57.

11. Hardy J. Molecular classification of Alzheimer's disease. *Lancet* 1991;1:1342–1343.
12. Eastwood R, Reisberg B. Mood and behaviour. In: Panisset M, Stern Y, Gauthier S, eds. *Clinical diagnosis and management of Alzheimer's disease*. 1st ed. London: Dunitz, 1996:175–189.
13. Absher JR, Cummings JL. Cognitive and noncognitive aspects of dementia syndromes. In: Burns A, Levy R, eds. *Dementia*. 1st ed. London: Chapman and Hall, 1994:59–76.
14. Rosen WG, Mohs RC, Davis KL. A new rating scale for Alzheimer's disease. *Am J Psychiatry* 1984;141:1356–1364.
15. Folstein MF, Folstein SE, McHugh PR. Mini Mental State: a practical method for grading the cognitive state of patients for the clinician. *J Psychiatr Res* 1975;12:189–198.
16. Burns A, Lawlor B, Craig S. Assessment scales in old age psychiatry. London: Martin Dunitz. 1998
17. Gelinas I, Gauthier L, McIntyre M, et al. Development of a functional measure for persons with Alzheimer's disease: the Disability Assessment of Dementia. *Am J Occupat Ther* 1999;53:471–481.
18. Lawton MP, Brody EM. Assessment of older people: self-maintaining and instrumental activities of daily living. *Gerontologist* 1969;9:179–186.
19. Birks JS, Melzer D, Beppu H. Donepezil for mild and moderate Alzheimer's disease. In: The Cochrane Library, Issue 1, 2002. Oxford: Update Software. Search date 2000; primary sources Cochrane Dementia and Cognitive Impairment Group Specialized Register of Clinical Trials, Medline, Psychlit, Embase, the Donepezil Study Group, and Eisai Inc.
20. Feldman H, Gauthier S, Hecker J, et al. A 24-week, randomized, double blind study of donepezil in moderate to severe Alzheimer's disease. *Neurology* 2001;57:613–620.
21. Birks J, Iakovidou V, Tsolaki M, et al. Rivastigmine for Alzheimer's disease (Cochrane Review). In: The Cochrane Library, Issue 1, 2002. Oxford: Update Software. Search date 2000; primary sources Cochrane Controlled Trials Register, Cochrane Dementia Group Specialized Register of Clinical Trials, Medline, Embase, Psychlit, Cinahl, and hand searches of geriatric and dementia journals and conference abstracts.
22. Olin J, Schneider L. Olin J, et al. Galantamine for Alzheimer's disease. In: The Cochrane Library, Issue 1, 2002. Oxford: Update Software. Search date 2000; primary sources Cochrane Dementia Group Specialized Register of Clinical Trials, Cochrane Controlled Trials Register, Embase, Medline, Psychlit, Combined Health Information Database, National Research Register, Alzheimer's Disease Education and Referral Centre Clinical Database, Biomed (Biomedicine and Health), GlaxoWellcome Clinical Trials Register, National Institutes of Health Clinical Trials Databases, Current Controlled Trials, Dissertation Abstracts, Index to UK Theses, hand searched reference lists, and additional information was collected from an unpublished investigational brochure for galantamine.
23. Rogers SL, Farlow MR, Doody RS, et al. A 24-week double blind placebo controlled trial of donepezil in patients with Alzheimer's disease. *Neurology* 1998;50:136–145.
24. Rogers SL, Doody RS, Pratt RD, et al. Long term efficacy and safety of donepezil in the treatment of Alzheimer's disease: final analysis of a US multicentre open-label study. *Eur Neuropsychopharmacol* 2000;10:195–203.
25. Kumar V, Anand R, Messina J, et al. An efficacy and safety analysis of Exelon in Alzheimer's disease patients with concurrent vascular risk factors. *Eur J Neurol* 2000;7:159–169.
26. McKeith I, Del Ser T, Spano P, et al. Efficacy of rivastigmine in dementia with Lewy bodies: a randomised, double-blind, placebo-controlled international study. *Lancet* 2000;356:2031–2036.
27. Wilcock G, Lilienfield S, Gaens E. Efficacy and safety of galantamine in patients with mild to moderate Alzheimer's disease: multicentre randomised controlled trial. *BMJ* 2000;321:1–7.
28. Qizilbash N, Whitehead A, Higgins J, et al. Cholinesterase inhibition for Alzheimer disease. *JAMA* 1998;280:1777–1782. Search date not stated; primary sources Cochrane Dementia Group Registry of Clinical Trials, trial investigators, and Parke-Davis Pharmaceuticals.
29. Arrieta JR, Artalejo FR. Methodology, results and quality of clinical trials of tacrine in the treatment of Alzheimer's disease: a systematic review of the literature. *Age ageing* 1998;27:161–179. Search date 1997; primary sources Cochrane Library and Medline.
30. Koepp R, Miles SH. Meta-analysis of tacrine for Alzheimer's disease: the influence of industry sponsors. *JAMA* 1999;281:2287–2288.
31. Knapp MJ, Knopman DS, Solomon PR, et al. A 30-week randomized controlled trial of high-dose tacrine in patients with Alzheimer's disease. The Tacrine Study Group. *JAMA* 1994;271:985–991.
32. Coelho F, Filho JM, Birks J. Physostigmine for Alzheimer's disease. In: The Cochrane Library, Issue 1, 2002. Oxford: Update Software. Search date 2000; primary sources the Cochrane Dementia Group Specialized Register of Clinical Trials and pharmaceutical companies.
33. López-Arrieta JM, Rodr guez JL, Sanz F. Efficacy and safety of nicotine on Alzheimer's disease patients. In: The Cochrane Library, Issue 1, 2002. Oxford: Update Software. Search date 2001; primary source Cochrane Dementia Group Specialized Register of Clinical Trials.
34. Higgins JPT, Flicker L. Lecithin for dementia and cognitive impairment. In: The Cochrane Library, Issue 1, 2002. Oxford: Update Software. Search date 2000; primary sources Cochrane Dementia and Cognitive Impairment Group Specialized Register of Clinical Trials, Medline, Embase, Psychlit, ISI, Current Contents, and hand searched reference lists and textbooks.
35. Scharf S, Mander A, Ugoni A, et al. A double-blind, placebo-controlled trial of diclofenac/misoprostol in Alzheimer's disease. *Neurology* 1999;53:197–201.
36. Rogers J, Kirby LC, Hempleman SR, et al. Clinical trial of indomethacin in Alzheimer's disease. *Neurology* 1993;43:1609–1611.
37. Williams PS, Spector A, Orrell M, et al. Aspirin for vascular dementia. In: The Cochrane Library, Issue 1, 2002. Oxford: Update Software. Search date 2000; primary sources Medline, Cochrane Library Trials Register, Embase, Cinahl, Psychlit, Amed, Sigle, National Research Register, hand searched reference lists, and contact with specialists.
38. Hogervorst E, Williams J, Budge M, et al. The nature of the effect of female gonadal hormone replacement therapy on cognitive function in post-menopausal women: a meta-analysis. *Neuroscience* 2000;101:485–512. Search date 2000, primary sources Medline, Embase, Psychlit, and hand searches of reference lists.
39. Mulnard RA, Cotman CW, Kawas C, et al. Estrogen replacement therapy for treatment of mild to moderate Alzheimer disease: a randomized controlled trial. Alzheimer's Disease Co-operative Study. *JAMA* 2000;283:1007–1015.
40. Tabet N, Birks J, Grimley Evans J. Vitamin E for Alzheimer's disease. In: The Cochrane Library, Issue 1, 2002. Oxford: Update Software. Search date

2000; primary sources Cochrane Dementia and Cognitive Impairment Group Specialized Register of Clinical Trials
41. Sano M, Ernesto C, Thomas RG, et al. A controlled trial of selegiline, α-tocopherol, or both as treatment for Alzheimer's disease. *N Engl J Med* 1997;336:1216–1222.
42. Myers DG, Maloley PA, Weeks D. Safety of antioxidant vitamins. *Arch Intern Med* 1996;156:925–935.
43. Birks J, Flicker L. Selegiline for Alzheimer's disease. In: The Cochrane Library, Issue 1, 2002. Oxford: Update Software. Search date not stated, review amended 1998; primary source Cochrane Dementia and Cognitive Impairment Group Register of Clinical Trials.
44. Ernst E, Pittler MH. Ginkgo biloba for dementia. *Clin Drug Invest* 1999;17:301–308. Search date 1998; primary sources Medline, Embase, Biosis, Cochrane Register of Controlled Clinical Trials, hand searches of bibliographies, and contact with manufacturers.
45. Van Dongen MC, van Rossum E, Kessels AG, et al. The efficacy of Ginkgo for elderly people with dementia and age-associated memory impairment: New results of a randomised controlled trial. *J Am Geriatr Soc* 2000;48:1183–1194.
46. Le Bars P, Katz MM, Berman N, et al. A placebo-controlled, double-blind, randomised trial of an extract of Ginkgo biloba for dementia. *JAMA* 1997;278:1327–1332.
47. Spector A, Orrell M. Reminiscence therapy for dementia. In: The Cochrane Library, Issue 1, 2002. Oxford: Update Software. Search date 2000; primary sources Cochrane Controlled Trials Register, Medline, Psychlit, Embase, Omni, Bids, Dissertation Abstracts International, Sigle, reference lists of relevant articles, internet sites, and hand searching of specialist journals.
48. Spector A, Orrell M, Davies S, et al. Reality orientation for dementia. In: The Cochrane Library, Issue 1, 2002. Oxford: Update Software. Search date 2000; primary sources Medline, Psychlit, Embase, Cochrane Database of Systematic Reviews, Omni, Bids, Dissertation Abstracts International, Sigle, plus internet searching of HealthWeb, Mental Health Infosources, American Psychiatric Association, Internet Mental Health, Mental Health Net, NHS Confederation, and hand searching of specialist journals.
49. Koger SM, Chaplin K, Brotons M. Is music therapy an effective intervention for dementia? A meta-analytic review of the literature. *J Music Ther* 1999;36:2–15. Search date 1998; primary sources Medline, Psychlit, and hand searched reference lists.
50. Koger SM, Brotons M. Music therapy for dementia symptoms. In: Cochrane Library, Issue 1, 2002. Oxford: Update Software. Search date 2000; primary sources Medline, Cochrane Dementia and Cognitive Improvement Group Trials Register, Embase, Cinahl, and Psychlit.
51. Lonergan E, Luxenberg J, Colford J. Haloperidol for agitation in dementia. In: The Cochrane Library, Issue 1, 2002. Oxford: Update Software. Search date 2000; primary sources Cochrane Controlled Trials Register, Cochrane Dementia Group Specialized Register of Clinical Trials, Medline, Embase, Psychlit, Cinahl, and Glaxo-Wellcome Trials database.
52. Katz IR, Jeste DV, Mintzer JE, et al. Comparison of risperidone and placebo for psychosis and behavioural disturbances associated with dementia: a randomized double-blind trial. *J Clin Psychiatry* 1999;60:107–115.
53. De Deyn PP, Rabheru K, Rasmussen A, et al. A randomized trial of risperidone, placebo, and haloperidol for behavioural symptoms of dementia. *Neurology* 1999;53:946–955.
54. Street JS, Clark WS, Gannon KS, et al. Olanzapine treatment of psychotic and behavioural symptoms in patients with Alzheimer's disease in nursing care facilities: a double-blind, randomised, placebo-controlled trial. *Arch Gen Psychiatry* 2000;57:968–976.
55. McShane R, Keene J, Gedling K, et al. Do neuroleptic drugs hasten cognitive decline in dementia? Prospective study with necropsy follow up. *BMJ* 1997;314:266–269.
56. Lanctot KL, Best TS, Mittmann N, et al. Efficacy and safety of neuroleptics in behavioural disorders associated with dementia. *J Clin Psychiatry* 1998;59:550–561. Search date 1995; primary sources Medline and hand search of references.
57. Tariot PN, Erb R, Podgorski CA, et al. Efficacy and tolerability of carbamazepine for agitation and aggression in dementia. *Am J Psychiatry* 1998;155:54–61.
58. Porsteinsson AOP, Tariot PN, Erb R, et al. Placebo-controlled study of divalproex sodium for agitation in dementia. *Am J Geriatr Psychiatry* 2001;9:58–66.
59. Sultzer DL, Gray KF, Gunay I, et al. A double-blind comparison of trazodone and haloperidol for treatment of agitation in patients with dementia. *Am J Geriatr Psychiatry* 1997;5:60–69.
60. Teri L, Logsdon RG, Peskind E, et al. Treatment of agitation in AD: a randomised, placebo-controlled clinical trial. *Neurology* 2000;55:1271–1278.
61. Taroit PN, Cummings JL, Katz IR, et al. A randomized double blind placebo controlled study of the efficacy and safety of donepezil in patients with Alzheimer's disease in the nursing home setting. *J Am Geriatr Soc* 2001;49:1590–1599.

James Warner
Senior Lecturer/Consultant in Old Age Psychiatry
Imperial College, London, UK

Rob Butler
Honorary Senior Lecturer in Psychiatry and Consultant in Old Age Psychiatry
University of Auckland and Waitemata Health, Auckland, New Zealand

Elizabeth Jackson
Specialist Registrar
CNWL Mental Health Trust, London, UK

Competing interests: JW has been reimbursed by Novartis, the manufacturer of rivastigmine, for conference attendance and has received speaker fees from Janssen Pharmaceuticals for educational events. RB, none declared. EJ none declared.

TABLE 1 Effects of donepezil, rivastigmine, and galantamine on Alzheimer's Disease Assessment Scale cognitive subscale (ADAS-cog) scores (see text, p 932).

Drug	Dose (mg)	Duration (wk)	Number randomised	Effect size (difference in ADAS-cog between treatment and placebo arms) (95% CI)	NNT (95% CI) 4 point change in ADAS-cog	OR (95% CI) for treatment withdrawal	Ref
Donepezil	5 od	12	488	−2.3 (−3.2 to −1.5)	N/A	2.3 (1.0 to 5.3)	19
		24	831	−1.9 (−2.6 to −1.1)	N/A	0.9 (0.5 to 1.4)	19
	10 od	12	301	−3.1 (−4.2 to −1.9)	N/A	4.1 (1.6 to 10.4)	19
		24	821	−2.9 (−3.7 to −2.2)	N/A	1.6 (1.1 to 2.3)	19
Rivastigmine	1–4 bd	12	1293	−0.3 (−0.9 to +0.3)	+50 (+25 to −50)	2.7 (1.1 to 6.8)	21
		26	1293	− 0.8 (−15 to −0.2)	+100 (+15 to −20)	1.0 (0.7 to 1.5)	21
	6–12 bd	12	1917	−1.5 (−2.0 to −1.0)	15 (10 to 25)	3.1 (1.3 to 7.6)	21
		26	1917	−2.1 (−2.7 to −1.5)	17 (12 to 34)	3.0 (2.3 to 3.8)	21
Galantamine	8 bd	24	565	−3.3 (−4.5 to −2.2)	7 (5 to 13)	1.0 (0.51 to 1.9)	22
	12 bd	24	1352	−3.3 (−3.9 to −2.7)	7 (5 to 12)	1.5 (0.8 to 2.6)	22
	16 bd	24	825	−3.3 (−4.1 to −2.4)	5 (4 to 10)	4.7 (2.9 to 7.5)	22

bd, twice daily; od, once daily; N/A, not applicable; ref, reference.

TABLE 2 **Common adverse effects of cholinesterase inhibitors (see text, p 933).**

	Nausea		Vomiting		Diarrhoea		
	% in treatment group	OR	% in treatment group	OR	% in treatment group	OR	Ref
Donepezil 10 mg od	19	3.6 (2.1 to 6.4)	14	2.8 (1.8 to 4.2)	16	2.9 (2.0 to 4.2)	19
Rivastigmine 6–12 mg bd	47	5.4 (4.4 to 6.6)	31	5.3 (4.2 to 6.7)	19	1.7 (1.4 to 2.3)	21
Galantamine 12 mg bd	30	3.7 (2.8 to 4.8)	16	3.0 (2.1 to 4.2)	8	1.4 (0.9 to 2.1)	22

bd, twice daily; od, once daily.

Depressive disorders

Search date November 2001

John Geddes, Rob Butler, and Simon Hatcher

QUESTIONS

INTERVENTIONS

See glossary, p 968

Key Messages

- We found no reliable direct evidence that one type of treatment (drug or non-drug) is superior to another in improving symptoms of depression. However, we found strong evidence that some treatments are effective, whilst the effectiveness of others remains uncertain. Of the interventions examined, prescription antidepressant drugs and electroconvulsive therapy are the only treatment for which there is good evidence of effectiveness in severe and psychotic depressive disorders. We found no RCTs comparing drug and non-drug treatments in severe depressive disorders.

- **Prescription antidepressant drugs (in mild, moderate, and severe depression)** Systematic reviews in people aged 16 years or over have found that antidepressant drugs are effective in acute treatment of all grades of depressive disorders. Systematic reviews have found no clinically significant difference in outcomes with different kinds of antidepressant drug. One systematic review in people aged 55 years or over with all grades of depressive disorder has found that tricyclic antidepressants, selective serotonin reuptake inhibitors, or monoamine oxidase inhibitors versus placebo significantly reduce the proportion of people who fail to recover over 26–49 days. We found no specific evidence on adverse effects in older adults. However, the drugs differ in their adverse event profiles.
  - **Monoamine oxidase inhibitors** One systematic review found that monoamine oxidase inhibitors were less effective than tricyclic antidepressants in people with severe depressive disorders, but may be more effective in atypical depressive disorders, for example, increased sleep, increased appetite, mood reactivity, and rejection sensitivity.
  - **Selective serotonin reuptake inhibitors and related drugs** One systematic review found that, on average, people seem to tolerate selective serotonin reuptake inhibitors a little better than tricyclic antidepressants, but the difference was small. Another systematic review and one retrospective cohort study found no strong evidence that fluoxetine was associated with increased risk of suicide. One RCT and observational data suggest that abrupt withdrawal of selective serotonin reuptake inhibitors is associated with symptoms including dizziness and rhinitis, and that these symptoms are more likely with drugs with a short half life, such as paroxetine.
  - **Tricyclic and heterocyclic antidepressants** One systematic review found that, on average, people seem to tolerate tricyclic antidepressants a little less well than selective serotonin reuptake inhibitors but the difference was small.
- **Befriending (in mild to moderate depression)** One small RCT found limited evidence that befriending versus waiting list control reduced symptoms of depression.
- **Bibliotherapy (in mild to moderate depression)** One systematic review in younger and older adults found limited evidence that bibliotherapy versus waiting list control or standard care may reduce mild depressive symptoms. Another systematic review found limited evidence in people with anxiety, chronic fatigue, or combined anxiety and depression that bibliotherapy versus standard care may improve symptoms over 2–6 months.
- **Care pathways (in mild to moderate depression)** Five RCTs in people aged over 18 years found that the effectiveness of antidepressant treatment may be improved by several approaches, including collaborative working between primary care clinicians and psychiatrists plus intensive patient education, case management, telephone support, and relapse prevention programmes. One RCT found that a clinical practice guideline and practice based education versus usual care did not improve either detection or outcome of depression.
- **Care pathways versus usual care for long term outcomes (in mild to moderate depression)** One RCT found that a multifaceted quality improvement programme versus usual care significantly improved symptoms over 1 year, but found no significant difference in outcomes at 2 years.
- **Cognitive therapy (in mild to moderate depression)** One systematic review in younger and older adults has found that cognitive therapy versus placebo significantly improves the symptoms of depression.

- **Cognitive therapy versus antidepressants for long term outcomes (in mild to moderate depression)** One systematic review and one additional RCT found limited evidence that cognitive therapy versus antidepressants may reduce the risk of relapse over 2 years.
- **Combining drug and psychological treatment (in mild to moderate and severe depression)** One meta-analysis of RCTs in people aged 18–80 years has found that in people with severe depression, adding drug treatment to interpersonal psychotherapy or to cognitive therapy versus either psychological treatment alone improves symptoms, but has found no significant difference in symptoms in people with mild to moderate depression. Subsequent RCTs in younger and older adults with mild to moderate depression have found that antidepressants plus psychotherapy improve symptoms significantly more than either antidepressants or psychotherapy alone. One RCT in older adults with mild to moderate depression found that cognitive behavioural therapy plus desipramine improved symptoms significantly more than desipramine alone.
- **Continuation drug treatment in mild to moderate depression (reduces risk of relapse)** One systematic review and subsequent RCTs in younger and older adults have found that continuation treatment with antidepressant drugs versus placebo for 4–6 months after recovery significantly reduces the risk of relapse. One RCT in people aged over 60 years has found that continuation treatment with dosulepin versus placebo significantly reduces the risk of relapse over 2 years.
- **Electroconvulsive therapy (in severe depression)** Systematic reviews and additional RCTs have found that electroconvulsive therapy versus sham electroconvulsive therapy improves symptoms in the acute treatment of severe depression.
- **Exercise (in mild to moderate depression)** One systematic review found limited evidence from poor quality RCTs that exercise versus placebo may improve symptoms, and that exercise may be as effective as cognitive therapy.
- **Interpersonal psychotherapy (in mild to moderate depression)** One large RCT has found that interpersonal psychotherapy versus antidepressants or versus standard care significantly improves rates of recovery from depression after 16 weeks (NNT 5, 95% CI 3 to 22).
- **Non-directive counselling (in mild to moderate depression)** One systematic review in people aged over 18 years with recent onset psychological problems, including depression, found that brief, non-directive counselling versus usual care by a physician significantly reduced symptom scores in the short term (< 6 months), but found no significant difference in scores in the long term (> 6 months).
- **Problem solving treatment (in mild to moderate depression)** RCTs have found that problem solving treatment versus placebo or versus control significantly improves symptoms over 3–6 months, and have found no significant difference in symptoms with problem solving treatment versus drug treatment.
- **Psychological treatments (cognitive therapy, interpersonal psychotherapy, and problem solving treatment) in severe depression** RCTs found limited evidence about the effects of psychological treatments in severe depression.
- **St John's Wort (in mild to moderate depression)** Systematic reviews in people with mild to moderate depressive disorders have found that St John's Wort (*Hypericum perforatum*) versus placebo significantly improves depressive symptoms over 4–12 weeks, and have found no significant difference in symptoms with St John's Wort versus prescription antidepressant drugs.

DEFINITION **Depressive disorders** are characterised by persistent low mood, loss of interest and enjoyment, and reduced energy. They often impair day to day functioning. Most of the RCTs assessed in this review classify depression using the *Diagnostic and statistical manual of mental disorders* (DSM IV)[1] or the *ICD-10 classification of mental and behavioural disorders* (ICD-10).[2] DSM IV divides depression into major depressive disorder or dysthymic disorder. **Major depressive disorder** is characterised by one or more major depressive episodes (that is, at least 2 wks of depressed mood or loss of interest accompanied by at least 4 additional symptoms of depression). **Dysthymic disorder** is characterised by at least 2 years of depressed mood for more days than not, accompanied by additional symptoms that do not reach the criteria for major depressive disorder.[1] ICD-10 divides depression into mild to moderate or severe depressive episodes.[2] **Mild to moderate depression** is characterised by depressive symptoms and some functional impairment. **Severe depression** is characterised by additional agitation or psychomotor retardation with marked somatic symptoms.[2] In this review, we use both DSM IV and ICD-10 classifications, but treatments are considered to have been assessed in severe depression if the RCT included inpatients. **Older adults:** Older adults are generally defined as people aged 65 years or older. However, some of the RCTs of older people in this review included people aged 55 years or over. The presentation of depression in older adults may be atypical: low mood may be masked and anxiety or memory impairment may be the principal presenting symptoms. Dementia should be considered in the differential diagnosis of depression in older adults.[3]

INCIDENCE/ PREVALENCE Depressive disorders are common, with a prevalence of major depression between 5% and 10% of people seen in primary care settings.[4] Two to three times as many people may have depressive symptoms but do not meet DSM IV criteria for major depression. Women are affected twice as often as men. Depressive disorders are the fourth most important cause of disability worldwide and they are expected to become the second most important cause by the year 2020.[5,6] **Older adults:** Between 10% and 15% of older people have depressive symptoms, although major depression is relatively rare in older adults.[7]

AETIOLOGY/ RISK FACTORS The causes are uncertain but include both childhood events and current psychosocial adversity.

PROGNOSIS About half of people suffering a first episode of major depressive disorder experience further symptoms in the next 10 years.[8] **Older adults:** One systematic review (search date 1996, 12 prospective cohort studies, 1268 people, mean age 60 years) found that the prognosis may be especially poor in elderly people with a chronic or relapsing course of depression.[9] Another systematic review (search date 1999, 23 prospective cohort studies in people aged ≥65 years, including 5 identified by the first review) found that depression in older people was associated with increased mortality (15 studies; pooled OR 1.73, 95% CI 1.53 to 1.95).[10]

AIMS To improve mood, social and occupational functioning, and quality of life; to reduce morbidity and mortality; to prevent recurrence of depressive disorder; and to minimise adverse effects of treatment.

OUTCOMES Depressive symptoms rated by the depressed person and clinician, social functioning, occupational functioning, quality of life, admission to hospital, rates of self harm, relapse of depressive symptoms, rates of adverse events. Trials often use continuous scales to measure depressive symptoms (such as the Hamilton Depression Rating Scale and the Beck Depression Inventory). Clinician reports and self reported global outcome measures are also used. Changes in continuous measures can be dealt with in two ways. They can be dichotomised in an arbitrary but clinically helpful manner (e.g. taking a reduction in depressive symptoms of more than 50% as an end point), which allows results to be expressed as relative risks and numbers needed to treat. Alternatively, they can be treated as continuous variables, as is done for systematic analysis. In this case, the pooled estimate of effect (the effect size) expresses the degree of overlap between the range of scores in the control and experimental groups. The effect size can be used to estimate the proportion of people in the control group who had a poorer outcome than the average person in the experimental group; a proportion of 50% indicates that the treatment has no effect. **Older adults:** The Hamilton Depression Rating Scale is not ideal for older people because it includes several somatic items that may be positive in older people who are not depressed. It has been the most widely used scale, although specific scales for elderly people (such as the Geriatric Depression Scale) avoid somatic items.

METHODS The contributors conducted a validated search for systematic reviews and RCTs between May and September 1998 from the Cochrane Database of Systematic Reviews and the Database of Abstract of Reviews of Effectiveness, *Best Evidence* and *Evidence-Based Mental Health*, Medline, Psychlit, and Embase. Studies were included by using epidemiological criteria and relevance to the clinical question. A *Clinical Evidence* update search and appraisal was conducted in November 2001, including a search for data on depression in older adults. To date, few studies have concentrated on older adults as a separate subgroup. Most published evidence for the efficacy of antidepressants includes all ages over 16 years or is limited to people aged under 65 years. Studies including those aged over 16 years sometimes include few older people and caution should be applied in generalising the results to older people. In this review, studies are included under the heading **Older adults** if they specifically included people aged over 55 years.

QUESTION What are the effects of treatments?

OPTION PRESCRIPTION ANTIDEPRESSANT DRUGS

Systematic reviews in people aged 16 years or over have found that antidepressant drugs (monoamine oxidase inhibitors, selective serotonin reuptake inhibitors, or tricyclic antidepressants) versus placebo improve symptoms in acute treatment of all grades of depressive disorder. Two

systematic reviews have found no clinically significant difference in outcomes with different kinds of antidepressant drug, although one systematic review found that monoamine oxidase inhibitors were less effective than tricyclic antidepressants in people with severe depressive disorders, but may be more effective in atypical depressive disorders, for example increased sleep, increased appetite, mood reactivity, and rejection sensitivity. Systematic reviews have found that antidepressant drugs differ in their adverse event profiles. One systematic review has found that, on average, people seem to tolerate selective serotonin reuptake inhibitors a little better than tricyclic antidepressants, but the difference was small. Another systematic review and one retrospective cohort study found no strong evidence that fluoxetine was associated with increased risk of suicide. One RCT and observational data suggest that abrupt withdrawal of selective serotonin reuptake inhibitors is associated with symptoms including dizziness and rhinitis, and that these symptoms are more likely with drugs with a short half life, such as paroxetine. One systematic review in people aged 55 years or over with all grades of depressive disorder has found that tricyclic antidepressants, selective serotonin reuptake inhibitors, or monoamine oxidase inhibitors versus placebo significantly reduce the proportion of people who fail to recover over 26–49 days. We found no specific evidence on adverse effects in older adults.

Benefits: **Antidepressants versus placebo:** We found two systematic reviews.[11,12] The first review (search date 1995, 49 RCTs in people aged 18–70 years with mild to moderate or severe depressive disorders) included five RCTs in people admitted to hospital (probably with severe depressive disorders), 40 RCTs in a setting outside hospital, one in both settings, and three that did not specify the setting.[11] All of the RCTs identified by the review included three way comparisons: two antidepressant drugs (monoamine oxidase inhibitors [MAOIs], selective serotonin reuptake inhibitors [SSRIs], or tricyclic antidepressants [TCAs] and placebo and were of least 4 weeks' duration). The review only included RCTs that measured improvement in depressive symptoms using scales such as the Hamilton Depression Rating Scale and Montgomery-Asberg Depression Rating Scale. It found that the mean effect size for change in score with antidepressants versus placebo was 0.5, which means that 69% of people taking placebo had worse outcomes than the average person taking antidepressants. Antidepressants were more effective in those with depressive disorders diagnosed according to standard criteria (mainly *Diagnostic and Statistical Manual of Mental Disorders*, 3rd edition, revised [DSM-III-R]).[11] The second systematic review (search date 1997, 15 RCTs, 1871 people aged ≥ 18 years) compared antidepressants (SSRIs; TCAs; MAOIs; or amisulpride, amineptine or ritanserin) versus placebo in people with dysthymia (chronic mild depressive disorders).[12] It found that antidepressants versus placebo significantly increased the proportion of people who responded to treatment at 4–12 weeks (response defined as a 50% decrease in Hamilton Rating Score for Depression or scoring 1 or 2 on item 2 of the Clinical Global Impression Score; RR 1.9, 95% CI 1.6 to 2.3; NNT 4, 95% CI 3 to 5). **In older adults; antidepressants versus placebo:** We found one systematic review (search date 2000, 17 RCTs, 1326 people aged ≥ 55 years with mild to moderate or severe depression) comparing antidepressants versus placebo.[13] It found that TCAs, SSRIs, or MAOIs versus placebo significantly reduced the proportion of people who failed to recover over 26–49 days (125/245 [51%] with TCAs v 167/223 [75%] with placebo: RR 0.68, 95% CI 0.59 to 0.68, NNT 4, 95% CI 4 to 5; 261/365 [72%] with SSRIs v 310/372 [83%] with placebo: RR 0.86, 95% CI 0.79 to 0.93, NNT 9, 95% CI 9 to 10; 34/58 [59%] with MAOIs v 57/63 [90%] with placebo: RR 0.64, 95% CI 0.50 to 0.81, NNT 4, 95% CI 3 to 4).[13] **In people with depression plus a physical illness; antidepressants versus placebo:** One systematic review (search date 1998, 18 RCTs, 838 people aged > 18 years with depression and a physical illness) found that antidepressants versus placebo significantly reduced the proportion of people who failed to recover over 4–12 weeks (177/366 [48%] with antidepressant v 229/325 [70%] with placebo; RR 0.68, 95% CI 0.60 to 0.77; NNT 4, 95% CI 3 to 7).[14] People allocated to antidepressants were more likely to withdraw from the study than those on placebo (NNH 10, 95% CI 5 to 43).[14] **TCAs versus SSRIs:** We found three systematic reviews (search dates 1999,[15] 1997,[16] and 1998[17]) and one subsequent RCT[18] in people with mild to moderate or severe depression comparing SSRIs versus TCAs. The reviews found no significant difference in overall effectiveness. The second review (search date 1997, 95 RCTs, 10 533 people aged 18–80 years) found that SSRIs may be slightly more acceptable overall, as measured by the number of people who withdrew from clinical trials (RR 0.88, 95% CI 0.83 to 0.93; NNH 26).[15] The third systematic review (search date 1998, 28 RCTs, 5940 people aged ≥ 18 years) compared the efficacy of newer antidepressants versus placebo or versus older antidepressants in primary care.[17] The average response rate was 63% for newer agents, 35% for placebo, and 60% for TCAs (RR for SSRIs versus placebo 1.6, 95% CI 1.2 to 2.1). One subsequent small RCT (152 people with major depression) compared adherence on dosulepin (dothiepin) with fluoxetine over 12 weeks and found no significant difference between the drugs. However, the study was probably underpowered.[18] **MAOIs versus TCAs:** We found one systematic review (search date not stated, 55 RCTs comparing MAOIs v TCAs in several subgroups of people with depression aged 18–80 years).[19] It found that MAOIs were less effective than TCAs in people with severe depressive disorders but may be more effective in atypical depressive disorders (depressive disorders with reversed biological features, e.g. increased sleep, increased appetite, mood reactivity, and rejection sensitivity). **Antidepressants plus benzodiazepines versus antidepressants alone:** We found one systematic review (search date 1999, 8 RCTs, 679 people aged 18–65 years, 1 RCT in people aged 20–73 years with major depression) comparing combination treatment with antidepressants plus benzodiazepines versus antidepressants alone.[20] It found that combination treatment versus antidepressants alone was significantly more likely to produce a response within 1 week (RR of > 50% reduction on symptom rating scale 1.64, 95% CI 1.19 to 2.27), although this difference was not apparent at 6 weeks.

Harms: **Common adverse events with TCAs versus SSRIs:** One systematic review (search date 1996) compared adverse events with TCAs versus SSRIs in people aged 18 years or over with all severities of depression (see table 1, p 972).[21] **Adverse effects with different SSRIs:** One large cohort study of people receiving four different SSRIs (fluvoxamine [983 people], fluoxetine [692 people], sertraline [734 people], and paroxetine [13 741 people]) in UK primary care found that reports of common adverse events (nausea/vomiting, malaise/lassitude, dizziness, and headache/migraine) varied between SSRIs (fluvoxamine 78/1000 participant months; fluoxetine 23/1000 participant months; RR v fluvoxamine 0.29; 95% CI 0.27 to 0.32; paroxetine 28/1000 participant months; RR 0.35, 95% CI 0.33 to 0.37; sertraline 21/1000 participant months; RR 0.26, 95% CI 0.25 to 0.28).[22] Only 52% of people responded to the questionnaire, although this response rate was similar for all four drugs. A study of spontaneous reports to the UK Committee on Safety of Medicines found no difference in safety profiles between the same four SSRIs.[23] **Suicide with TCAs versus SSRIs:** One systematic review (search date not stated, which included RCTs completed by December 1989) pooled data from 17 double blind RCTs in people with depressive disorders aged 12–90 years comparing a TCA (731 people) versus fluoxetine (1765 people) or versus placebo (569 people).[24] It found no significant difference in the rate of suicidal acts between the groups (TCAs 0.4%, fluoxetine 0.3%, and placebo 0.2%), but development of suicidal ideation was less frequent in the fluoxetine group (1% fluoxetine *v* 3% placebo, P = 0.04; and *v* 4% TCAs, P = 0.001). One historical cohort study followed 172 598 people who had at least one prescription for 1/10 antidepressants during the study period in general practice in the UK. The risk of suicide was higher in people who received fluoxetine (19/10 000 person years, 95% CI 9 to 34) than those receiving dosulepin (RR of suicide *v* dosulepin 2.1, 95% CI 1.1 to 4.1).[25] In a nested case controlled subanalysis in people with no history of suicidal behaviour or previous antidepressant prescription, the risk remained the same, although the confidence interval broadened to make the result non-significant (RR 2.1, 95% CI 0.6 to 7.9). Although the apparent association may be because of residual confounding, there remains uncertainty about the possible association between fluoxetine and suicide. However, any absolute increase in risk is unlikely to be large. **Withdrawal effects with SSRIs:** We found one RCT in people aged 18 years or over (average age 30–40 years) comparing abrupt discontinuation of fluoxetine (96 people) versus continued treatment (299 people) in people who had been taking the drug for 12 weeks. Abrupt discontinuation was associated with increased dizziness (7% *v* 1%), dysmenorrhoea (3% *v* 0%), rhinitis (10% *v* 3%), and somnolence (4% *v* 0%). However, there was a high withdrawal rate in this study because of the return of symptoms of depression (39%), so these may be underestimates of the true rate of withdrawal symptoms.[26] Between 1987 and 1995 the rate of spontaneous reports of suspected withdrawal reactions per million defined daily doses to the World Health Organization Collaborating Centre for International Drug Monitoring was higher for paroxetine than for sertraline and fluoxetine.[27] The most common withdrawal effects were dizziness, nausea, paraesthesia, headache, and vertigo. **During pregnancy:** One systematic review (search date 1999) assessing the risk of fetal harm of antidepressants in pregnancy found four small prospective studies published since 1993.[28] No evidence of increased risk was found, although the chances of adverse effects with a low incidence cannot be excluded. Decreased birth weights of infants exposed to fluoxetine in the third trimester were identified in one study and direct drug effects and withdrawal syndromes were identified in some neonates. **In older adults:** We found no specific evidence on adverse effects in older adults.

Comment: The systematic review of antidepressants versus placebo in older people[13] was limited by the diversity of populations included, and the brevity of the studies. The reviewers recommended at least 6 weeks of antidepressant treatment in elderly people to achieve optimal effect. A systematic review is under way to examine adverse effects in elderly people.[13] Metabolic and physical changes with age mean that older people may be more prone to adverse effects such as falls. As older people take more medications, they are at more risk of drug interactions. Suicide is a risk in elderly people.

OPTION CARE PATHWAYS

Five RCTs in people aged over 18 years found that the effectiveness of antidepressant treatment may be improved by several approaches, including collaborative working between primary care clinicians and psychiatrists plus intensive patient education, case management, telephone support, and relapse prevention programmes. One RCT found that a clinical practice guideline and practice based education versus usual care did not improve either detection or outcome of depression.

Benefits: We found no systematic review but found six RCTs.[29–34] **Collaborative working between primary care clinicians and psychiatrists plus intensive patient education:** The first RCT (217 people aged 19–76 years with mild to moderate or major depression in primary care in the USA) found that compared to standard treatment (including antidepressants), the addition of a multifaceted programme, including collaborative working between primary care physician and psychiatrist plus intensive patient education, improved outcomes over 12 months.[29] Improvement in depressive symptoms assessed by Symptom Checklist-90 was significant only in the subgroup of people with major depressive disorder (91 people; AR of clinical response of > 50% reduction on symptom checklist 74% *v* 44% with standard treatment; NNT 4, 95% CI 3 to 10).[29] **Care management:** The second RCT (613 people, mean age 46 years) in a Health Maintenance Organization in Seattle (USA) compared three interventions: usual care (antidepressants), usual care plus feedback (in which doctors received a detailed report on each person at 8 and 16 weeks after randomisation), or usual care plus feedback plus care management (in which the care manager assessed people with depression by telephone at 8 and 16 weeks, doctors received a detailed report, and care managers facilitated the follow up). It found that feedback plus care management versus usual care significantly increased the proportion of people with a clinically important reduction in depressive symptoms at 6 months after randomisation (about 56% of people with care management *v* 40% with usual care [results presented graphically]; OR 2.22, 95% CI 1.31 to 3.75).[30] **Clinical practice guideline and practice based education:** The third RCT (cluster randomised, based in UK primary care, people aged over 16 years) compared the effects of a clinical practice guideline and practice based education versus usual care and found that the intervention did not improve either detection or outcome of depression.[31] **Telephone support:** The fourth RCT (302 people with major depressive disorder or dysthymia aged 19–90 years) compared usual physician care (selective serotonin reuptake inhibitor [SSRI]; 117 people), usual care plus nurse telehealth (SSRI plus 12–14 telephone support calls during 16 wks of treatment; 62 people), or usual care plus telehealth plus peer support (123 people).[31] Nurse telehealth versus usual clinician care significantly increased the proportion of people with a 50% reduction in symptoms at 6 months (57% with nurse telehealth *v* 38% with usual care; NNT 6, 95% CI 4 to 18). **Relapse prevention programme:** The fifth RCT (386 people aged > 18 with recurrent major depression or dysthymia who had largely recovered after 8 weeks of antidepressant treatment) compared a relapse prevention programme (2 primary care visits and 3 telephone calls) versus usual care for 1 year. It found that relapse prevention versus usual care significantly improved depressive symptoms over 1 year (results presented graphically; P = 0.04), but found no significant difference in relapse rates (35% in both groups).[33] **Multifaceted quality improvement programme:** The sixth RCT compared a multifaceted quality improvement programme (including antidepressants plus psychotherapy or plus [cognitive behavioural therapy (see glossary, p 968)]) versus usual care and assessed outcomes at 1 and 2 years (see which treatments are most effective at improving long term outcome, p 967) **Older adults:** We found no systematic review or RCTs specifically in older adults.

Harms: The RCTs gave no information about adverse effects.[29–34]

Comment: None.

OPTION ST JOHN'S WORT (*HYPERICUM PERFORATUM*)

Two systematic reviews in people with mild to moderate depressive disorders have found that St John's Wort (*H perforatum*) versus placebo significantly improves depressive symptoms over 4–12 weeks, and have found no significant difference in symptoms with St John's Wort versus prescription antidepressant drugs. However, these findings have not yet been repeated in people with all grades of depression using standardised preparations of St John's Wort.

Benefits: We found two systematic reviews.[35,36] The first review (search date 1998, 2291 people aged > 18 years with mild to moderate depression) identified 17 RCTs comparing St John's Wort versus placebo (1168 people) and 10 RCTs (1123 people) comparing St John's Wort (8 RCTs using single preparations of hypericum, and 2 using combinations of hypericum and valeriana) versus other antidepressant or sedative drugs. It found that *H perforatum* preparations versus placebo significantly increased the proportion of people who responded over 4–12 weeks (response defined as a

Hamilton Depression Rating Score of < 10 or < 50% of baseline score; 267/465 [57%] with hypericum v 122/485 [25%] with placebo; RR 2.47, 95% CI 1.69 to 3.61), but found no significant difference in the proportion of people who responded with St John's Wort versus antidepressants (177/352 [50%] with single preparations of hypericum v 176/339 [52%] with placebo; 88/130 [68%] v 66/132 [50%]; RR 1.01, 95% CI 0.87 to 1.16; combinations RR 1.52, 95% CI 0.78 to 2.94).[35] The second systematic review (search date 2000, 23 RCTs, 2776 people with mild to moderate depression) included 14 RCTs identified by the first review, but applied different inclusion criteria for RCTs and excluded 13 of the RCTs included in the first review.[36] It identified 14 RCTs (1336 people) comparing St John's Wort versus placebo and nine RCTs (1394 people) comparing St John's Wort versus other antidepressants. It found that St John's Wort versus placebo significantly increased the proportion of people who responded over 4–8 weeks (390/690 [57%] v 184/646 [28%]; RR 1.98, 95% CI 1.49 to 2.62), but found no significant difference in depressive symptoms over 4–6 weeks with St John's Wort versus other antidepressants (422/694 [61%] v 423/700 [60%]; RR 1.00, 95% CI 0.91 to 1.11). These results did not change when only RCTs which met stricter methodological treatment were combined (6 RCTs; St John's Wort v placebo: 153/257 [60%] v 79/232 [34%]; RR 1.77, 95% CI 1.16 to 2.70; St John's Wort v other antidepressants: 260/440 [59%] v 261/468 [56%]; RR 1.04, 95% CI 0.94 to 1.15).[36] **Older adults:** We found no systematic review or RCTs specifically in older adults.

Harms: We found three systematic reviews (two already cited [see benefits above][35,36] and one other, search date 1997[37]). The first review[35] found that adverse events were poorly reported in the trials. Adverse effects were reported by 26% of people taking St John's Wort versus 45% of people taking standard antidepressants (RR 0.57, 95% CI 0.47 to 0.69), and by 15% of people taking combinations of hypericum and valeriana versus 27% taking amitriptyline or desipramine (RR 0.49, 95% CI 0.23 to 1.04).[35] The second systematic review[36] found no significant difference in the proportion of people who had adverse effects (including gastrointestinal effects, headaches, restlessness, and fatigue) with St John's Wort versus placebo (43/236 [18%] v 29/177 [16%]; RR 1.04, 95% CI 0.68 to 1.58), and found that St John's Wort versus antidepressants significantly reduced the proportion of people with adverse effects (260/440 [59%] v 261/448 [58%]; RR 0.59, 95% CI 0.52 to 0.71). The third systematic review included RCTs and observational surveillance studies after marketing of St John's Wort.[37] It found that the most common adverse effects of St John's Wort in the included studies were gastrointestinal symptoms, dizziness/confusion, tiredness/sedation, and dry mouth, although all occurred less frequently than on conventional drugs. Findings from observational studies were consistent with these results. Photosensitivity is theoretically possible; however, only two cases have been reported.

Comment: The evidence cited (see benefits above) must be interpreted cautiously because it is unclear how closely people in these trials match people in clinical practice, and the preparations and doses of

H perforatum and types and doses of standard antidepressants varied. More studies are needed on clearly defined, clinically representative people using standardised preparations. Interactions with other drugs are possible and should be considered.

OPTION ELECTROCONVULSIVE THERAPY

Two systematic reviews and additional RCTs in people aged over 16 years have found that electroconvulsive therapy versus simulated electroconvulsive therapy improves symptoms in the acute treatment of severe depressive illness.

Benefits: We found two systematic reviews,[38,39] three additional RCTs,[40–42] and two subsequent RCTs.[43,44] The first review (search date not stated, 6 RCTs published between 1960 and 1978, 205 people with severe depressive disorder, aged range not stated) compared electroconvulsive therapy (ECT) versus simulated ECT (in which people received everything but electric stimulation).[38] People treated with real ECT were more likely to respond to treatment (pooled OR 3.7, 95% CI 2.1 to 6.5; NNT 3, 95% CI 2 to 5; calculated from data in the article). The second review (search date 1998, which included 11 additional RCTs published between 1987 and 1998) also found good evidence for the beneficial effects of ECT, but did not quantify its conclusions.[39] The results of the additional and subsequent RCTs are consistent with the findings of the review.[40–44] **Older adults:** We found no systematic review or RCTs specifically in older adults.

Harms: The systematic reviews gave no information on adverse effects,[38,39] and we found no good evidence about possible adverse cognitive effects of ECT. However, people often complain of memory impairment after ECT. One of the main difficulties in studying the association between memory impairment and ECT is that depressive disorders also lead to cognitive impairment that usually improve during the course of treatment. For this reason, most of the small studies in this area find an average improvement in memory in people treated with ECT. This does not rule out the possibility of more subtle, subjective memory impairment secondary to ECT. Adverse memory effects would probably vary according to the dose and electrode location.

Comment: A further systematic review is in progress.[45] As ECT may be unacceptable to some people and, because it is a short term treatment, there is consensus that it should normally be reserved for people who cannot tolerate or have not responded to drug treatment, although it may be useful when a rapid response is required.

OPTION PSYCHOLOGICAL TREATMENTS

One systematic review in younger and older adults with mild to moderate depression has found that cognitive therapy versus placebo significantly improves symptoms. One systematic review in people aged over 18 years with recent onset psychological problems, including depression, found that brief, non-directive counselling versus usual care by a physician significantly reduced symptom scores in the short term (< 6 months), but

found no significant difference in scores in the long term (> 6 months). RCTs in younger and older adults with mild to moderate depression found that problem solving treatment or interpersonal psychotherapy versus placebo significantly improved depressive symptoms in the short term, and have found no significant difference in symptoms with problem solving treatment or interpersonal psychotherapy versus antidepressant treatment. RCTs found limited evidence on the relative efficacy of drug and non-drug treatment in severe depression. One systematic review in people aged over 55 years with mild to moderate depression has found no significant difference in symptoms with psychological treatments (such as cognitive therapy or cognitive behaviour therapy), versus no treatment. However, it also found no significant difference in symptoms with psychological treatments versus similar but non-specific attention. This review was based on a small number of studies, the populations varied (although most were community samples), and many of the studies were short term. RCTs found limited evidence about the effects of psychological treatments in severe depression.

Benefits: The evidence comparing psychological treatments versus drug or no treatment is summarised in table 2 (see, p 973).[46–50] We found limited evidence on the relative efficacy of drug and non-drug treatment in severe depression (see comment below). **Older adults:** We found one systematic review (search date 1995, 14 small RCTs, < 24 people, age > 55 years in an outpatient or community setting) of pharmacological and psychological treatments.[51] It found four RCTs in older adults that compared psychological treatments versus no treatment. None of the RCTs found a significant difference between treatment and no treatment, measured on the Hamilton Depression Rating Scale. It also found six RCTs comparing different psychological treatments. Five of six comparisons of "rational" treatments (such as cognitive therapy or cognitive behaviour therapy [see glossary, p 968]), versus no treatment in older adults found significant benefit with treatment. Combined, the "rational" treatments performed significantly better than no treatment (mean difference in the Hamilton Depression Rating Score −7.3 95% CI −10.1 to −4.4), but were not significantly different from the "non-specific attention" control. None of the RCTs found significant differences in effectiveness between psychological treatments.

Harms: The systematic review and RCTs gave no information on adverse effects.[46–50]

Comment: Large RCTs are needed in more representative people in a range of clinical settings, including primary care. Because of varying exclusion criteria, the generalisability of the studies is questionable (see table 2, p 973). Other factors to be considered when psychological treatments are compared with drug treatment include whether serum concentrations of drugs reach therapeutic concentrations, whether changes in medication are allowed (reflecting standard clinical practice), and whether studies reflect the natural course of depressive disorders. It is difficult to conduct studies of psychological treatments for severe depression because of the ethics surrounding withholding a proved treatment (antidepressant drugs) in a group of people at risk of self harm or neglect.[52]

OPTION **PSYCHOLOGICAL TREATMENTS PLUS DRUG TREATMENT**

One non-systematic review of RCTs in people aged 18–80 years has found that, in people with severe depression, adding drug treatment to interpersonal psychotherapy or to cognitive therapy versus either psychological treatment alone improves symptoms, but has found no significant difference in symptoms in people with mild to moderate depression. Subsequent RCTs in younger and older adults with mild to moderate depression have found that antidepressants plus psychotherapy improve symptoms significantly more than either antidepressants or psychotherapy alone. One RCT in older adults with mild to moderate depression found that cognitive behavioural therapy plus desipramine improved symptoms significantly more than desipramine alone.

Benefits: We found no systematic review, but found one non-systematic review of RCTs[52] and two subsequent RCTs.[53,54] The non-systematic review of six RCTs (595 people aged 18–80 years with major depression) found no advantage in combining drug and specific psychological treatments in mild to moderate depressive disorders, but found that in more severe depressive disorders combining drug and interpersonal psychotherapy or cognitive therapy (see glossary, p 968) was more effective than interpersonal psychotherapy or cognitive therapy alone.[52] The first subsequent RCT (681 adults with chronic depressive disorder, mean age 43 years) compared three interventions: nefazodone alone, cognitive behavioural therapy (see glossary, p 968) alone, or nefazodone plus cognitive behavioural therapy.[53] It found that combined treatment versus either treatment alone significantly improved the proportion of people with a clinical response (defined as at least 50% reduction on the Hamilton Depression Rating Scale and a score of ≤ 15; 152/226 [67%] with combined treatment *v* 92/220 [42%] with nefazodone alone *v* 90/226 [40%] with psychotherapy alone; combined treatment *v* either single intervention; P < 0.001; NNT 5, 95% CI 3 to 6). The second subsequent RCT (167 people with a major depressive episode) compared antidepressants (fluoxetine, amitriptyline, or moclobemide) plus short term psychodynamic supportive psychotherapy (see glossary, p 969) versus antidepressants alone (see comment below).[54] It found that combined treatment versus antidepressants significantly increased the proportion of people who had improved after 24 weeks (improvement defined as Hamilton Depression Rating Score of ≤ 7, Clinical Global Impression score of 1 or 2, SCL-90 or Quality of Life Depression Scale score of a least 1 standard deviation from baseline; mean success rate 41% *v* 59%; NNT 5, 95% CI 3 to 11).[54] **Older adults:** We found one RCT (102 people aged > 60 years with major depressive disorder) that compared three interventions: desipramine plus cognitive behavioural therapy; desipramine alone; or cognitive behavioural therapy alone.[55] It found that all three groups showed a significant reduction in symptoms from baseline assessed by the Hamilton Depression Rating Scale after 16–20 weeks of treatment (desipramine 0.20, cognitive behavioural therapy 0.36, and combined treatments 0.41). It found that combined treatments versus desipramine alone significantly improved symptoms over 16–20 weeks ($P < 0.05$). It found no significant difference between the three groups in the proportion of people who withdrew for any cause (desipramine 34%, cognitive behavioural therapy 23%, and combined treatments 33%).[55]

Harms: The non-systematic review and RCTs gave no information on adverse effects.[52–55]

Comment: A systematic review is needed to address this question. In the second subsequent RCT, 38/167 people initially randomised refused the proposed treatment: 27/84 (32%) of people offered antidepressants and 11/83 (13%) of people offered combined treatment.[54] This makes the results of the RCT very difficult to interpret.

OPTION EXERCISE

One systematic review found limited evidence from poor quality RCTs that exercise versus placebo may improve symptoms, and that exercise may be as effective as cognitive therapy. One poor quality RCT in older adults identified by the review found limited evidence that exercise may be as effective as antidepressants in improving symptoms and may reduce relapse over 10 months.

Benefits: We found one systematic review (search date 1999, 14 RCTs, 851 people).[56] It found limited evidence that exercise versus no treatment may improve symptoms and found that exercise may be as effective as cognitive therapy (see glossary, p 968). However, it suggested that these results were inconclusive because of methodological problems in all the RCTs; randomisation was adequately concealed in only three of the RCTs, intention to treat analysis was undertaken in only two, and assessment of outcome was blinded in only one of the RCTs. **Older adults:** The systematic review[56] identified one RCT (156 people with major depression, mean age 57 years) comparing aerobic exercise, sertraline hydrochloride (a selective serotonin reuptake inhibitors), and combined treatment for 16 weeks. It found that the proportion of people who recovered (those no longer meeting criteria for depression or with a Hamilton Depression Rating Scale < 8) was not significantly different across the treatment groups (60% with exercise *v* 69% with sertraline *v* 66% with combined treatments).[57] A 10 month follow up of this RCT found lower rates of relapse with exercise versus medication (30% with exercise *v* 52% with sertraline *v* 55% with combined treatment).[58] However, about half of the people in the medication group engaged in exercise during follow up, making it difficult to draw firm conclusions about specific effects of exercise treatment. The clinical importance of the observed difference at 10 months remains unclear.[58]

Harms: The review gave no information about adverse effects.[56]

Comment: There is a need for a well designed RCT of the effects of exercise in people with all grades of depression assessing clinical outcomes over an adequate time period.

OPTION BIBLIOTHERAPY

One systematic review in younger and older adults found limited evidence that bibliotherapy versus waiting list control or standard care may reduce mild depressive symptoms. Another systematic review found limited evidence in people with anxiety, chronic fatigue, or combined anxiety and depression that bibliotherapy versus standard care may improve symptoms over 2–6 months.

Benefits: **Younger and older adults:** We found two systematic reviews (search date not stated[59] and search date 1999[60]). The first review identified six small short term RCTs of bibliotherapy (see glossary, p 968) versus waiting list control in 273 people (described as adults in 4 RCTs and elderly in 2 RCTs; no age range provided) recruited by advertisement through the media and probably with only mild depression (see comment below).[59] The mean effect size of bibliotherapy was 0.82 (95% CI 0.50 to 1.15). This means that 79% of people in the waiting list control group had a worse outcome than the average person in the bibliotherapy group. The second systematic review identified eight randomised and non-randomised trials in younger and older people, but only one of them included people with depression.[60] It found limited evidence in people with anxiety, chronic fatigue, or combined anxiety and depression that bibliotherapy versus standard care may improve symptoms over 2–6 months. The RCT that included people with depression found that bibliotherapy versus standard care significantly improved symptoms of anxiety over 4 weeks assessed by the Hamilton Depression Rating Scale, but found no significant difference in symptoms of depression at 4 or 12 weeks. **Older adults:** We found no systematic review or RCTs specifically in older adults.

Harms: None reported.

Comment: The review did not clearly describe the characteristics of the people in the RCTs it identified, and it is unclear whether people were receiving interventions in addition to bibliotherapy.[59] Further studies are needed in clinically representative groups.

OPTION BEFRIENDING

One small RCT found limited evidence that befriending versus waiting list control reduced symptoms of depression.

Benefits: We found one small RCT (86 women with chronic depression, aged > 18 years, primarily aged 25–40 years, based in London, UK) of befriending (see glossary, p 968) versus waiting list control.[61] Initial identification was by postal screening of women registered with, but not attending, primary care. It found that befriending versus waiting list control significantly increased the proportion of women with remission of symptoms at 13 months (65% with befriending *v* 39% with control; $P < 0.05$; NNT 4, 95% CI 2 to 18). **Older adults:** We found no systematic review or RCTs specifically in older adults.

Harms: The RCT gave no information on harms.[61]

Comment: In the RCT, 14% of women in the befriending group were taking antidepressants and 12% of women in the waiting list control group.[61] Fewer than half of the women screened by post were interested in befriending as a treatment option.

QUESTION What are the effects of continuation treatment with antidepressant drugs?

One systematic review and subsequent RCTs in younger and older adults have found that continuation treatment with antidepressant drugs versus placebo for 4–6 months after recovery significantly reduces the risk of relapse. One RCT in people aged over 60 years has found that continuation treatment with dosulepin versus placebo significantly reduces the risk of relapse over 2 years.

Benefits: We found one systematic review (search date not stated, 6 RCTs, 312 people, age range not stated).[62] It found that continuation of antidepressant medication versus placebo for 4–6 months after acute treatment reduced the relapse rate by nearly half (RR 0.6, 95% CI 0.4 to 0.7). Several more recent RCTs confirm this reduction in risk of early relapse with continuing antidepressant treatment for 6–12 months after acute treatment. **Older adults:** We found one RCT (69 people aged > 60 years with mild to moderate or severe depression who had recovered sufficiently and consented to enter a 2 year trial of [continuation treatment (see glossary, p 969)]), which compared dosulepin versus placebo.[63] It found that dosulepin versus placebo reduced the risk of relapse over 2 years by 55% (RR 0.45, 95% CI 0.22 to 0.96).

Harms: Adverse effects seem to be similar to those reported in trials of acute treatment.

Comment: We found no adequate systematic review of maintenance treatment (see glossary, p 969), but several RCTs have found that maintenance treatment reduced recurrence compared with placebo in recurrent depressive disorder. However, they all have problems with their methods (e.g. high withdrawal rates)[64] and will be considered in future *Clinical Evidence* updates. A systematic review of antidepressant treatment duration is in progress.[65]

QUESTION Which treatments are most effective at improving long term outcome (≥ 1 year)

One systematic review and one additional RCT in younger and older adults found limited evidence that cognitive therapy versus antidepressants may reduce the risk of relapse over 2 years. One RCT found that a multifaceted quality improvement programme versus usual care significantly improved symptoms over 1 year, but found no significant difference in outcomes at 2 years.

Benefits: **Cognitive therapy versus antidepressants:** We found one systematic review (search date not stated) comparing cognitive therapy (see glossary, p 968) versus antidepressants in people with mainly mild to moderate depressive disorders.[46] The review identified eight small RCTs (261 people, mean age 39.3 years) that assessed long term (1–2 year) recovery or relapse rates after treatment had stopped. It found limited evidence by combining relapse rates across different RCTs that overall, 30% of people treated with cognitive therapy relapsed compared with 60% of those treated with either antidepressants or antidepressants plus cognitive therapy.[46] We found one small additional RCT (40 people) comparing cognitive therapy versus normal clinical management (antidepressants) for residual depressive symptoms in people who had responded to antidepressants. It also found that at 2 years, fewer people relapsed with cognitive therapy than with antidepressants.[66] **Care pathways versus usual care:** One RCT (1356 people aged > 18 years with mild to moderate or major depression in 46 primary care clinics in US Health Maintenance Organisations) compared a multifaceted quality improvement programme (including antidepressants plus psychotherapy or plus [cognitive behavioural therapy (see glossary, p 968)]) versus usual care (including mailed practice guidelines).[34] It found that the quality improvement programme versus usual care significantly increased the proportion of people who improved on continuous depression rating scales over 1 year. It found that among people initially employed, 90% of people in the quality improvement programme worked at 12 months *v* 85% of the people receiving usual care (P = 0.05). For people initially not working, there was no difference in employment rates at 12 months with quality improvement versus usual care (17% *v* 18%).[34] A 2 year follow up of this RCT found no significant difference in outcomes with quality improvement versus usual care.[67] **Older adults:** We found no systematic review or RCTs specifically in older adults.

Harms: See harms of prescription antidepressant drugs, p 957.

Comment: The review did not present information on the proportion of people who recovered and continued to remain well after 2 years.[46] The largest RCT identified by the review found that only a fifth of people remained well over 18 months' follow up, and that there were no significant differences between interpersonal psychotherapy (see glossary, p 969), cognitive therapy, or drug treatment.[46] It is possible that different people respond to different treatments. Further large scale comparative studies are needed of the long term effectiveness of treatments in people with all severities of depressive disorders.

GLOSSARY

Befriending Consists of a befriender meeting the person to talk and socialise for at least 1 hour a week, acting as a friend.

Bibliotherapy Advising people to read written material such as *Feeling good: the new mood therapy* by David Burns (New York: New American Library, 1980).

Brief, non-directive counselling Helping people to express feelings and clarify thoughts and difficulties; therapists suggest alternative understandings and do not give direct advice but try to encourage people to solve their own problems.

Cognitive behavioural therapy Brief (20 sessions over 12–16 wks) structured treatment incorporating elements of cognitive therapy and behavioural therapy. Behavioural therapy is based on learning theory and concentrates on changing behaviour.

Cognitive therapy Brief (20 sessions over 12–16 wks) structured treatment aimed at changing the dysfunctional beliefs and negative automatic thoughts that characterise depressive disorders. It requires a highly trained therapist.[68]

Continuation treatment Continuation of treatment after successful resolution of a depressive episode to prevent relapse.

Interpersonal psychotherapy Standardised form of brief psychotherapy (usually 12–16 weekly sessions) primarily intended for outpatients with unipolar non-psychotic depressive disorders. It focuses on improving the person's interpersonal functioning and identifying the problems associated with the onset of the depressive episode.[69]

Maintenance treatment Long term treatment of recurrent depressive disorder to prevent the recurrence of further depressive episodes.

Problem solving treatment Consists of three stages: (1) identifying the main problems for the person; (2) generating solutions; and (3) trying out the solutions. Potentially briefer and simpler than cognitive therapy and may be feasible in primary care.[48]

Psychodynamic supportive psychotherapy Aims to facilitate change by detecting and resolving underlying psychological conflicts. The treatment aims to be less challenging by incorporating supportive elements.

Substantive changes

Prescription antidepressant drugs One new systematic review in older people;[13] conclusions unchanged.

Care pathways One new systematic review in younger and older adults;[33] recatagorised as likely to be beneficial.

St John's Wort (*H perforatum*) One new RCT in younger and older adults;[36] conclusions unchanged.

Psychological treatments One new RCT[49] and one new systematic review[50] comparing psychological treatments versus drug or no treatment; conclusions unchanged.

Psychological treatments plus drug treatment One new RCT in younger and older adults;[54] conclusions unchanged.

Psychological treatments plus drug treatment One new RCT in older adults found that cognitive behavioural therapy plus desipramine improved symptoms significantly more than desipramine alone.[55]

Exercise One new systematic review in younger and older adults;[56] conclusions unchanged.

Bibliotherapy One new systematic review;[60] conclusions unchanged.

REFERENCES

1. American Psychiatric Association. *Diagnostic and statistical manual of mental disorders*, 4th ed. Washington, DC: American Psychiatric Association, 1994.
2. World Health Organization. *The ICD-10 classification of mental and behavioural disorders*. Geneva: World Health Organization, 1992.
3. Rosenstein, Leslie D. Differential diagnosis of the major progressive dementias and depression in middle and late adulthood: a summary of the literature of the early 1990s. *Neuropsychol Rev* 1998;8:109–167.
4. Katon W, Schulberg H. Epidemiology of depression in primary care. *Gen Hosp Psychiatry* 1992;14:237–247.
5. Murray CJ, Lopez AD. Regional patterns of disability-free life expectancy and disability-adjusted life expectancy: global burden of disease study. *Lancet* 1997;349:1347–1352.
6. Murray CJ, Lopez AD. Alternative projections of mortality and disability by cause 1990–2020: global burden of disease study. *Lancet* 1997;349:1498–1504.
7. Beekman ATF, Copeland JRM, Prince MJ. Review of community prevalence of depression in later life. *Br J Psychiatry* 1999;174:307–311.
8. Judd LL, Akiskal HS, Maser JD, et al. A prospective 12 year study of subsyndromal and syndromal depressive symptoms in unipolar major depressive disorders. *Arch Gen Psychiatry* 1988;55:694–700.
9. Cole MG, Bellavance F, Mansour A. Prognosis of depression in elderly community and primary care populations: a systematic review and meta-analysis. *Am J Psychiatry* 1999;156:1182–1189. Search date 1996; primary sources Medline 1981–1996, Psychinfo 1984–1996, and hand searches of the bibliographies of relevant articles.
10. Saz P, Dewey ME. Depression, depressive symptoms and mortality in persons aged 65 and older living in the community: a systematic review of the literature. *Int J Geriatr Psychiatry* 2001;16:622–630. Search date 1999; primary sources Embase, Medline, personal files, and hand searches of reference lists.

11. Joffe R, Sokolov S, Streiner D. Antidepressant treatment of depression: a meta-analysis. *Can J Psychiatry* 1996;41:613–616. Search date 1995; primary source Medline.
12. Lima MS, Moncrieff J. Drugs versus placebo for dysthymia. In: Cochrane Library, Issue 4, 2001. Oxford: Update Software. Search date 1997; primary sources Biological Abstracts, Medline, Psychlit, Embase, Lilacs, Cochrane Library, personal communication, conference abstracts, unpublished trials from the pharmaceutical industry, and book chapters on the treatment of depression.
13. Wilson K, Mottram P, Sivanranthan A, et al. Antidepressant versus placebo for the depressed elderly. In: The Cochrane Library, Issue 4, 2001. Oxford: Update Software. Search date 2000; primary sources Psychlit, Medline, Embase, Cinahl, Cochrane Controlled Trials register, CCDAN trials register, and hand searches.
14. Gill D, Hatcher S. Antidepressants for depression in medical illness. In: The Cochrane Library, Issue 4, 2001. Oxford: Update Software. Search date 1998; primary sources Medline, Cochrane Library Trials Register, Cochrane Depression and Neurosis Group Trials Register, and hand searches of two journals and reference lists.
15. Geddes JR, Freemantle N, Mason J, et al. Selective serotonin reuptake inhibitors (SSRIs) for depression. In: The Cochrane Library, Issue 4, 2001. Oxford: Update Software. Search date 1999; primary sources Medline, Embase, Cochrane Group Register of Controlled Trials, hand searches of reference lists of all located studies, and contact with manufacturers.
16. Anderson IM. Selective serotonin reuptake inhibitors versus tricyclic antidepressants: a meta-analysis of efficacy and tolerability. *J Affect Disord* 2000;58:19–36. Search date 1997; primary sources Medline, and hand searches of reference lists of meta-analyses and reviews.
17. Mulrow CD, Williams JW, Chiqueete E, et al. Efficacy of newer medications for treating depression in primary care people. *Am Med J* 2000;108:54–64. Search date 1998; primary sources Cochrane Depression Anxiety and Neurosis Group Specialised Register of Clinical Trials, hand searches of trials and 46 pertinent meta-analyses, and consultation with experts.
18. Thompson C, Peveler RC, Stephenson D, et al. Compliance with antidepressant medication in the treatment of major depressive disorder in primary care: a randomized comparison of fluoxetine and a tricyclic antidepressant. *Am J Psychiatry* 2000;157:338–343.
19. Thase ME, Trivedi MH, Rush AJ. MAOIs in the contemporary treatment of depression. *Neuropsychopharmacology* 1995;12:185–219. Search date not stated; primary sources Medline and Psychological Abstracts.
20. Furukawa TA, Streiner DL, Young LT. Antidepressant and benzodiazepine for major depression. In: The Cochrane Library, Issue 4, 2001. Oxford: Update Software. Search date 1999; primary sources Medline, Embase, International Pharmaceutical Abstracts, Biological Abstracts, LILACS, Psychlit, Cochrane Library, Cochrane Depression, Anxiety and Neurosis Group Trial Register, SciSearch, hand searches of reference lists, and personal contacts.
21. Trindade E, Menon D. *Selective serotonin reuptake inhibitors (SSRIs) for major depression. Part I. Evaluation of the clinical literature*. Ottawa: Canadian Coordinating Office for Health Technology Assessment, 1997 August Report 3E. *Evidence-Based Mental Health* 1998;1:50. Search date 1996; primary sources Medline, Embase, Psychinfo, International Pharmaceutical Abstracts, Pascal, Health Planning and Administration, Mental Health Abstracts, Pharmacoeconomics and Outcomes News, Current Contents databases, scanning bibliographies of retrieved articles, hand searching of journals, and consulting researchers.
22. Mackay FJ, Dunn NR, Wilton LV, et al. A comparison of fluvoxamine, fluoxetine, sertraline and paroxetine examined by observational cohort studies. *Pharmacoepidemiol Drug Safety* 1997;6:235–246.
23. Price JS, Waller PC, Wood SM, et al. A comparison of the post marketing safety of four selective serotonin reuptake inhibitors including the investigation of symptoms occurring on withdrawal. *Br J Clin Pharmacol* 1996;42:757–763.
24. Beasley CM Jr, Dornseif BE, Bosomworth JC, et al. Fluoxetine and suicide: a meta-analysis of controlled trials of treatment for depression. *BMJ* 1991;303:685–692. Search date not stated, but included trials that had been completed/analysed by December 1989; primary sources not given in detail but based on clinical report form data from trials and data from the Drug Experience Network Database.
25. Jick SS, Dean AD, Jick H. Antidepressants and suicide. *BMJ* 1995;310:215–218.
26. Zajecka J, Fawcett J, Amsterdam J, et al. Safety of abrupt discontinuation of fluoxetine: a randomised, placebo controlled study. *J Clin Psychopharmacol* 1998;18:193–197.
27. Stahl MM, Lindquist M, Pettersson M, et al. Withdrawal reactions with selective serotonin reuptake inhibitors as reported to the WHO system. *Eur J Clin Pharmacol* 1997;53:163–169.
28. Wisner KL, Gelenberg AJ, Leonard H, et al. Pharmacologic treatment of depression during pregnancy. *JAMA* 1999;282:1264–1269. Search date 1999; primary sources Medline, Healthstar, hand searches of bibliographies of review articles, and discussions with investigators in the field.
29. Katon W, Von Korff M, Lin E, et al. Collaborative management to achieve treatment guidelines: impact on depression in primary care. *JAMA* 1995;273:1026–1031.
30. Simon GE, Vonkorff M, Rutter C, et al. Randomised trial of monitoring, feedback, and management of care by telephone to improve treatment of depression in primary care. *BMJ* 2000;320:550–554.
31. Thompson C, Kinmonth AL, Stevens L, et al. Effects of a clinical-practice guideline and practice-based education on detection and outcome of depression in primary care: Hampshire Depression Project randomised controlled trial. *Lancet* 2000;355:185–191.
32. Hunkeler EM, Meresman JF, Hargreaves WA, et al. Efficacy of nurse telehealth care and peer support in augmenting treatment of depression in primary care. *Arch Fam Med* 2000;9:700–708.
33. Katon W, Rutter C, Ludman EJ, et al. A randomized trial of relapse prevention of depression in primary care. *Arch Gen Psychiatry* 2001;58:241–247.
34. Wells KB, Sherbourne C, Schoenbaum M, et al. Impact of disseminating quality improvement programs for depression in managed primary care: a randomized controlled trial. *JAMA* 2000;283:212–220.
35. Linde K, Mulrow CD. St John's Wort for depression. In: The Cochrane Library, Issue 4, 2001. Oxford: Update Software. Search date 1998; primary sources Medline, Embase, Psychlit, Psychindex, specialised databases: Cochrane Complementary Medicine Field, Cochrane

Depression and Neurosis CRG, Phytodok, hand searches of references of pertinent articles, and contact with manufacturers, and researchers.
36. Whiskey A, Werneke U, Taylor D. A systematic review and meta-analysis of *Hypericum perforatum* in depression: a comprehensive clinical review. *Int Clin Psychopharmacol* 2001;16:239–252. Search date 2000; primary sources (in English or German) Medline, Embase, and hand searched references of primary studies.
37. Ernst E, Rand JI, Barnes J, et al. Adverse effects profile of the herbal antidepressant St John Wort (*Hypericum perforatum L*). *Eur J Clin Pharmacol* 1998;54:589–594. Search date 1997; primary sources AMED, Cochrane Library 1997 Issue 2, Embase, Medline, hand searched reference lists, contacted WHO Collaborating Centre for International Drug Monitoring, UK Committee on Safety of Medicines, and German Bundesinstitut für Arzneimittel und Medizinproducte plus 12 German manufacturers of hypericum products.
38. Janicak PG, Davis JM, Gibbons RD, et al. Efficacy of ECT: a meta-analysis. *Am J Psychiatry* 1985;142:297–302. Search date not stated; primary source Medline.
39. Wijeratne C, Halliday GS, Lyndon RW. The present status of electroconvulsive therapy: a systematic review. *Med J Austr* 1999;171:250–254. Search date 1998; primary source Medline.
40. Johnstone EC, Deakin JF, Lawler P, et al. The Northwick Park electroconvulsive therapy trial. *Lancet* 1980;1:1317–1320.
41. Brandon S, Cowley P, McDonald C, et al. Electroconvulsive therapy: results in depressive illness from the Leicestershire trial. *BMJ* 1984;288:22–25.
42. Gregory S, Shawcross CR, Gill D. The Nottingham ECT study. A double-blind comparison of bilateral, unilateral and simulated ECT in depressive illness. *Br J Psychiatry* 1985;146:520–524.
43. Vaughan McCall W, Reboussin DM, Weiner RD, et al. Titrated moderately suprathreshold vs fixed high-dose right unilateral electroconvulsive therapy. *Arch Gen Psychiatry* 2000;57:438–444.
44. Sackeim HA, Prudic J, Devanand DP, et al. A prospective, randomized, double-blind comparison of bilateral and right unilateral electroconvulsive therapy at different stimulus intensities. *Arch Gen Psychiatry* 2000;57:425–434.
45. Scott AIF, Doris AB. Electroconvulsive therapy for depression (protocol). In: The Cochrane Library, Issue 4, 2001. Oxford: Update Software.
46. Gloaguen V, Cottraux J, Cucherat M, et al. A meta-analysis of the effects of cognitive therapy in depressed people 1998. *J Affect Disord* 1998;49:59–72. Search date not stated; primary sources Medline, Embase, references in books and papers, previous reviews and meta-analyses, abstracts from congress presentations, and preprints sent by authors.
47. Elkin I, Shea MT, Watkins JT, et al. National Institute of Mental Health treatment of depression collaborative research program: general effectiveness of treatments. *Arch Gen Psychiatry* 1989;46:971–982.
48. Mynors-Wallis LM, Gath DH, Lloyd-Thomas, AR, et al. Randomised controlled trial comparing problem solving treatment with amitriptyline and placebo for major depression in primary care. *BMJ* 1995;310:441–445.
49. Dowrick C, Dunn G, Ayuso-Mateos JL, et al. Problem solving treatment and group psychoeducation for depression: multicentre randomised controlled trial. *BMJ* 2000;321:1450–1454.
50. Bower P, Rowland N, Mellor Clark J, et al. Effectiveness and cost effectiveness of counselling in primary care. In: The Cochrane Library, Issue 4, 2001. Oxford: Update Software. Search date 2001; primary sources Medline, Embase, Psychlit, Cinahl, Cochrane Controlled Trials Register, CCDAN trials register, personal contact with experts and CCDAN members, search of unpublished sources (clinical trials, books, dissertations, agency reports, etc.), and hand searches of one journal and reference lists.
51. McCusker J, Cole M, Keller E, et al. Effectiveness of treatments of depression in older ambulatory people. *Arch Intern Med* 1998;158:705–712. Search date 1995; primary sources Medline, Psychinfo, and hand searches of references.
52. Thase ME, Greenhouse JB, Frank E, et al. Treatment of major depression with psychotherapy or psychotherapy — pharmacotherapy combinations. *Arch Gen Psychiatry* 1997;54:1009–1015. Pooled results of six research protocols conducted 1982 to 1992 at the Mental Health Clinical Research Center, University of Pittsburgh School of Medicine.
53. Keller MB, McCullough JP, Klein DN, et al. A comparison of nefazodone, the cognitive behavioral-analysis system of psychotherapy, and their combination for the treatment of chronic depression. *N Engl J Med* 2000;342:1462–1470.
54. De Jonghe F, Kool S, van Aalst G, Dekker J, Peen J. Combining psychotherapy and antidepressants in the treatment of depression. *J Affect Disord* 2001;64:217–229.
55. Thompson LW, Coon DW, Gallagher-Thompson D, Sommer BR, Koin D. Comparison of desipramine and cognitive behavioural therapy in the treatment of elderly outpatients with mild-to-moderate depression. *Am J Geriatr Psychiatry* 2001;9:225–240.
56. Lawlor DA, Hopker SW. The effectiveness of exercise as an intervention in the management of depression: systematic review and meta-regression analysis of randomised controlled trials. *BMJ* 2001;322:763–767. Search date 1999; primary sources Medline, Embase, Sports Discus, Psychlit, Cochrane Library, and hand searches of reference lists and nine journals.
57. Blumenthal JA, Babyak MA, Moore KA, et al. Effects of exercise training on older people with major depression. *Arch Intern Med* 1999;159:2349–2356.
58. Babyak M, Blumenthal JA, Herman S, et al. Exercise treatment for major depression: maintenance of therapeutic benefit at 10 months. *Psychosom Med* 2000;62:633–638.
59. Cuijpers P. Bibliotherapy in unipolar depression: a meta-analysis. *J Behav Ther Exp Psychiatry* 1997;28:139–147. Search date not stated; primary sources Psychlit, Psychinfo, and Medline.
60. Bower P, Richards D, Lovell K. The clinical and cost-effectiveness of self-help treatments for anxiety and depressive disorders in primary care: a systematic review. *Br J Gen Pract* 2001;51:838–845. Search date 1999; primary sources Psychinfo, Medline, Embase, Cinahl, Cochrane Library, Counselling in Primary Care Counsel.lit database, National Research Register, personal contact with researchers, hand searches of reference lists and two journals.
61. Harris T, Brown GW, Robinson R. Befriending as an intervention for chronic depression among women in an inner city: randomised controlled trial. *Br J Psychiatry* 1999;174:219–224.
62. Loonen AJ, Peer PG, Zwanikken GJ. Continuation and maintenance therapy with antidepressive agents: meta-analysis of research. *Pharm Week Sci* 1991;13:167–175. Search date not stated;

primary sources references of textbooks and review articles, Medline, Embase, and review of reference lists of primary studies.

63. Old age depression interest group. How long should the elderly take antidepressants? A double-blind placebo-controlled study of continuation/prophylaxis therapy with dothiepin. *Br J Psychiatry* 1993;162:175–182.
64. Keller MB, Kocsis JH, Thase ME, et al. Maintenance phase efficacy of sertraline for chronic depression: a randomized controlled trial. *JAMA* 1998;280:1665–1672.
65. Carney S, Geddes J, Davies D, et al. Antidepressants treatment duration for depressive disorder (protocol). In: The Cochrane Library, Issue 4, 2001. Oxford: Update Software.
66. Fava GA, Rafanelli C, Grandi S, et al. Prevention of recurrent depression with cognitive behavioral therapy: preliminary findings. *Arch Gen Psychiatry* 1998;55:816–820.
67. Sherbourne CD, Wells KB, Duan N, et al. Long term effectiveness of disseminating quality improvement for depression in primary care. *Arch Gen Psychiatry* 2001;58:696–703.
68. Haaga DAF, Beck AT. Cognitive therapy. In: Paykel ES, ed. *Handbook of affective disorders.* Edinburgh: Churchill Livingstone, 1992:511–523.
69. Klerman GL, Weissman H. Interpersonal psychotherapy. In: Paykel ES, ed. *Handbook of affective disorders.* Edinburgh: Churchill Livingstone, 1992:501–510.

John Geddes
Senior Clinical Research Fellow/Honorary Consultant Psychiatrist
University of Oxford
Oxford
UK

Rob Butler
Honorary Senior Lecturer in Psychiatry/Consultant in Old Age Psychiatry
University of Auckland and Waitemata Health
Auckland
New Zealand

Simon Hatcher
Senior Lecturer in Psychiatry/Honorary Consultant in Liaison Psychiatry
University of Auckland
Auckland
New Zealand

Competing interests: RB has been reimbursed by Novartis for attending a conference.

TABLE 1 **Adverse events (% of people) with selective serotonin reuptake inhibitors versus tricyclic antidepressants (see text, p 957).[21]**

Adverse effects	SSRI event rates (%)	TCA event rates (%)
Dry mouth	21	55
Constipation	10	22
Dizziness	13	23
Nausea	22	12
Diarrhoea	13	5
Anxiety	13	7
Agitation	14	8
Insomnia	12	7
Nervousness	15	11
Headache	17	14

SSRI, selective serotonin reuptake inhibitors; TCA, tricyclic antidepressants.

TABLE 2 **Effects of specific psychological treatments for depressive disorders (see text, p 963).**

Intervention	Evidence	Benefits	Harms	Disadvantages
Cognitive therapy	1 SR (48 RCTs of psychological therapies [2765 people, mean age 39.3 y] mainly outpatients in secondary care; therefore, probably with mild to moderate depression; people with psychotic or bipolar symptoms were excluded); 20 RCTs compared CT with waiting list or placebo and 17 compared it with drug treatment.[46]	79% of people receiving placebo were more symptomatic than the average person receiving CT ($P < 0.0001$).[43] 65% of people receiving CT were less symptomatic than the average person treated with antidepressant drugs ($P < 0.0001$).[46]	No harms reported.	Requires extensive training. Limited availability. RCTs in primary care suggest limited acceptability to some people.
Interpersonal psychotherapy	No SR. 1 large RCT (people with mild to moderate depression, mean age 35 y) compared interpersonal psychotherapy *v* either drug treatment, CT, or placebo plus clinical management for 16 wks.[47]	Rates of recovery from depression: interpersonal psychotherapy (43%; NNT 5, 95% CI 3 to 19), imipramine (42%; NNT 5, 95% CI 3 to 22), placebo clinical management (21%).[47]	No harms reported.	Requires extensive training. Limited availability.
Problem solving therapy	No SR. 1 large RCT (452 people aged 18–65 y with mild to moderate depression or adjustment disorders) compared PS, group treatment, and control.[49] 1 RCT (91 people aged 18–65 y with mild to moderate depression) compared problem solving, placebo, and amitriptyline.[48]	PS *v* control significantly increased the proportion of people who were not depressed at 6 mo, but no significant difference at 1 y.[49] PS *v* placebo significantly improved symptoms at 12 wks, and no significant difference in symptoms with PS *v* amitriptyline.[48]	No harms reported.	Requires some training. Limited availability.
Non-directive counselling	1 SR (7 RCTs, 772 people aged over 18 y with recent onset psychological problems, including depression in UK primary care) compared counselling *v* standard physician care.[50]	Counselling *v* standard care significantly improved symptoms in the short term (1–6 mo; WMD –2.03, 95% CI –3.82 to –0.24), but no significant difference in the long term (> 6 mo; WMD –0.03, 95% CI –0.39 to +0.32).[50]	No harms reported.	Requires some training. Limited availability.

CT, cognitive therapy; mo, month; PS, problem solving; SR, systematic review; y, year.

Generalised anxiety disorder

Search date February 2002

Christopher Gale and Mark Oakley-Browne

QUESTIONS

INTERVENTIONS

See glossary, p 988

Key Messages

- **Abecarnil** RCTs found conflicting evidence of the effects of abecarnil versus placebo in improving symptoms.
- **Antipsychotic drugs** One RCT found that trifluoperazine versus placebo significantly reduced anxiety after 4 weeks, but caused more drowsiness, extrapyramidal reactions, and other movement disorders.
- **Applied relaxation** We found no RCTs of applied relaxation versus placebo or no treatment. One systematic review found limited evidence, by making indirect comparisons of treatments across different RCTs, that more people given applied relaxation maintained recovery after 6 months than those given individual cognitive therapy, non-directive treatment, group cognitive, group behaviour therapy, individual behaviour therapy, or analytical psychotherapy. One subsequent RCT found no significant difference in symptoms at 13 weeks with applied relaxation versus cognitive behaviour therapy.
- **Benzodiazepines** One systematic review and one subsequent RCT found limited evidence that benzodiazepines versus placebo reduced symptoms over 2–9 weeks. However, RCTs and observational studies found that benzodiazepines increased the risk of dependence, sedation, industrial accidents, and road traffic accidents. One systematic review found that, if used in late pregnancy or while breast feeding, benzodiazepines may cause adverse effects in neonates. Limited evidence from RCTs found no significant difference in symptoms over 6–8 weeks with benzodiazepines versus buspirone, abecarnil, or antidepressants. One systematic review of poor quality RCTs found insufficient evidence about the effects of long term treatment with benzodiazepines.

- **β Blockers** We found no RCTs on the effects of β blockers.
- **Buspirone** RCTs have found that buspirone versus placebo significantly improves symptoms over 4–9 weeks. Limited evidence from RCTs found no significant difference in symptoms over 6–8 weeks with buspirone versus antidepressants or hydroxyzine.
- **Certain antidepressants (imipramine, opipramol, paroxetine, trazodone, venlafaxine)** RCTs have found that imipramine, opipramol, paroxetine, trazodone, or venlafaxine versus placebo significantly improve symptoms over 4–8 weeks, and that they are not significantly different from each other. RCTs and observational studies have found that antidepressants are associated with sedation, dizziness, nausea, falls, and sexual dysfunction. Limited evidence from RCTs found no significant difference in symptoms over 8 weeks with antidepressants versus benzodiazepines or buspirone.
- **Cognitive therapy** Systematic reviews have found that cognitive behaviour therapy, using a combination of interventions such as exposure, relaxation, and cognitive restructuring, improves anxiety and depression more over 4–12 weeks than remaining on a waiting list (no treatment), anxiety management training alone, relaxation training alone, or non-directive psychotherapy. One systematic review found limited evidence, by making indirect comparisons of treatments across different RCTs, that more people given individual cognitive therapy maintained recovery after 6 months than those given non-directive treatment, group cognitive, group behaviour therapy, individual behaviour therapy, or analytical psychotherapy. The review found that fewer people maintained recovery after 6 months with cognitive therapy versus applied relaxation. One subsequent RCT found no significant difference in symptoms at 13 weeks with cognitive therapy versus applied relaxation. Another subsequent RCT in people aged over 55 years with a variety of anxiety disorders found that cognitive behavioural therapy versus supportive counselling significantly improved symptoms of anxiety over 12 months NNT 3, 95% CI 2 to 49, but found no significant difference in symptoms of depression.
- **Hydroxyzine** One RCT found that hydroxyzine versus placebo significantly improved symptoms of anxiety after 4 weeks. Another RCT found no significant difference between hydroxyzine versus placebo or buspirone in the proportion of people with improved symptoms of anxiety at 35 days.
- **Kava** One systematic review in people with anxiety, including generalised anxiety disorder, found that kava versus placebo significantly reduced symptoms of anxiety over 4 weeks. Observational evidence suggests that kava may be associated with hepatotoxicity.

DEFINITION Generalised anxiety disorder (GAD) is defined as excessive worry and tension about every day events and problems, on most days, for at least 6 months to the point where the person experiences distress or has marked difficulty in performing day-to-day tasks.[1] It may be characterised by the following symptoms and signs: increased motor tension (fatigability, trembling, restlessness, and muscle tension); autonomic hyperactivity (shortness of breath, rapid heart rate, dry mouth, cold hands, and dizziness); and increased vigilance and scanning (feeling keyed up, increased startling, and impaired concentration), but not panic attacks.[1] One non-systematic review of epidemiological and clinical studies found marked reduction of quality of life and psychosocial functioning in people with anxiety disorders (including GAD).[2] It also found that (using the Composite Diagnostic International Instrument) people with GAD have low overall life satisfaction and some impairment in ability to fulfil roles, social tasks, or both.[2]

INCIDENCE/ PREVALENCE Assessment of the incidence and prevalence of GAD is difficult as a large proportion of people with GAD have a co-morbid diagnosis. One non-systematic review identified the US National Comorbidity Survey, which found that over 90% of people diagnosed with GAD had a co-morbid diagnosis, including dysthymia (22%), depression (39–69%), somatisation, other anxiety disorders, bipolar disorder, or substance abuse.[3] The reliability of the measures used to diagnose GAD in epidemiological studies is unsatisfactory.[4,5] One US study, with explicit diagnostic criteria (DSM-III-R), estimated that 5% of people will develop GAD at some time during their lives.[5] A recent cohort study of people with depressive and anxiety disorders found that 49% of people initially diagnosed with GAD retained this diagnosis over 2 years.[6] One non-systematic review found that the incidence of GAD in men is only half the incidence in women.[7] One non-systematic review of seven epidemiological studies found reduced prevalence of anxiety disorders in older people.[8] Another non-systematic review of 20 observational studies in younger and older adults suggested that the autonomic arousal to stressful tasks is decreased in older people, and that older people become accustomed to stressful tasks more quickly than younger people.[9]

AETIOLOGY/ RISK FACTORS One community study and a clinical study have found that GAD is associated with an increase in the number of minor stressors, independent of demographic factors,[10] but this finding was common in people with other diagnoses in the clinical population.[6] One non-systematic review (5 case control studies) of psychological sequelae to civilian trauma found that rates of GAD reported in four of the five studies were increased significantly compared with a control population (rate ratio 3.3, 95% CI 2.0 to 5.5).[11] One systematic review of cross-sectional studies found that bullying (or peer victimisation) was associated with a significant increase in the incidence of GAD (effect size 0.21).[12] One systematic review (search date not stated) of the genetic epidemiology of anxiety disorders (including GAD) identified two family studies and three twin studies.[13] The family studies (45 index cases, 225 first degree relatives) found a significant association between GAD in the index cases and in their first degree relatives (OR 6.1, 95% CI 2.5 to 14.9). The twin studies (13 305 people) estimated that 31.6% (95% CI 24% to 39%) of the variance to liability to GAD was explained by genetic factors.[13]

PROGNOSIS GAD often begins before or during young adulthood and can be a lifelong problem.[14] Spontaneous remission is rare.

AIMS To reduce anxiety; to minimise disruption of day-to-day functioning; and to improve quality of life, with minimum adverse effects.

OUTCOMES Severity of symptoms and effects on quality of life, as measured by symptom scores: usually the HAM-A, State-Trait Anxiety Inventory, or Clinical Global Impression Symptom Scores. Where numbers needed to treat are given, these represent the number of people requiring treatment within a given time period (usually 6–12 wks) for one additional person to achieve a certain improvement in symptom score. The method for obtaining numbers needed to treat was not standardised across studies. Some used a reduction by, for example, 20 points in the HAM-A as a response, others defined a response as a reduction, for example, by 50% of the premorbid score. We have not attempted to standardise methods, but instead have used the response rates reported in each study to calculate numbers needed to treat. Similarly, we have calculated numbers needed to harm from original trial data.

METHODS *Clinical Evidence* update search and appraisal February 2002. Recent changes in diagnostic classification make it hard to compare older studies with more recent ones. In the earlier classification system (DSM-III-R) the diagnosis was made only in the absence of other psychiatric disorders. In current systems (DSM-IV and ICD-10), GAD can be diagnosed in the presence of any comorbid condition. All drug studies were short term — at most 12 weeks.

QUESTION What are the effects of treatments?

OPTION COGNITIVE THERAPY

Two systematic reviews and one non-systematic review have found that cognitive behavioural therapy, using a combination of interventions such as exposure, relaxation, and cognitive restructuring, improves anxiety and depression over 4–12 weeks more than remaining on a waiting list (no treatment), anxiety management training alone, relaxation training alone, or non-directive psychotherapy. One systematic review found limited evidence (by making indirect comparisons of treatments across different RCTs) that more people given individual cognitive therapy maintained recovery after 6 months than those given non-directive treatment, group cognitive, group behaviour therapy, individual behaviour therapy, or analytical psychotherapy, but that fewer people maintained recovery after 6 months with cognitive therapy versus applied relaxation. One subsequent RCT found no significant difference in symptoms at 13 weeks with cognitive therapy versus applied relaxation. Another subsequent RCT in people aged over 55 years with a variety of anxiety disorders found that cognitive behavioural therapy versus supportive counselling significantly improved symptoms of anxiety over 12 months, but found no significant difference in symptoms of depression.

Benefits: We found three systematic reviews,[15–17] one non-systematic review,[18] and two subsequent RCTs[19,20] comparing cognitive therapy (see glossary, p 988) versus waiting list control (no treatment) or versus other psychotherapies. The first systematic review (search date 1996) identified 13 RCTs (722 people, 60% women) comparing 22 cognitive behavioural therapies (see glossary, p 988), which involved (alone or in combination) cognitive restructuring, relaxation training, exposure, and systematic desensitisation versus control.[15] Controls included remaining on a waiting list, anxiety management training, relaxation training, and non-directive psychotherapy. The review found that cognitive behavioural therapies versus control significantly improved symptoms over 4–12 weeks (effect size for anxiety 0.70, 95% CI 0.57 to 0.83 and for depression 0.77, 95% CI 0.64 to 0.90; dichotomous data not available). The second systematic review (search date 1998, 6 RCTs, 404 people) included four RCTs identified by the first review.[16] It indirectly compared treatment arms across RCTs and reanalysed the raw data from individual RCTs to calculate the proportion of people who experienced a clinically significant improvement in symptoms after treatment and maintained that improvement for 6 months (see comment below). It found limited evidence that more people given individual cognitive therapy maintained recovery after 6 months than those given psychotherapies other than applied relaxation (see glossary, p 988) (individual cognitive therapy 41%; applied relaxation 52%; non-directive treatment 19%; group cognitive therapy 18%; group behaviour therapy 12%; individual behaviour therapy 18%; and analytical psychotherapy 0%; P values not provided).[16] One year follow up of one of the RCTs found that cognitive therapy was associated with better outcomes than analytical psychotherapy and anxiety management training.[21] The third systematic review (search date not stated, 5 RCTs, 313 people) included three RCTs identified by the first review and one RCT identified by the second review.[17] It found that cognitive behavioural therapies (including relaxation, cognitive therapy, cognitive behavioural therapy, analytical psychotherapy, and anxiety management training [alone or in combination]) versus waiting list control were associated with an improvement in symptoms (median effect size 0.9; CI not provided).[17] The non-systematic review (13 RCTs, including 9 RCTs identified by the first systematic review and 1 RCT identified by the second systematic review) found that cognitive behavioural therapy versus cognitive therapy or behavioural therapy alone, or versus placebo, alternative treatment, waiting list control, or no treatment was associated with an improvement in symptoms of anxiety and depression.[18] Many of the RCTs identified by the reviews used the State-Trait Anxiety Inventory (see comment below).[15–18] The first subsequent RCT (36 people aged 18–60 years with generalised anxiety disorder) compared weekly sessions of cognitive therapy versus applied relaxation for 12 weeks.[19] It found no significant difference in the proportion of people who responded after 13 weeks with cognitive therapy versus applied relaxation (response defined as improvement to score 3 or 4 on Cognitive Global Impression Scale, 10/18 [56%] with cognitive therapy *v* 8/15 [53%] with applied relaxation; ARR –2%, 95% CI –33% to +29%; RR 1.04, 95% CI 0.55 to 1.95).[19] The second subsequent RCT (40 people aged ≥ 55 years with a variety of anxiety disorders, 19% of whom had generalised anxiety disorder) compared cognitive behavioural therapy versus supportive counselling.[20] It found that cognitive behavioural therapy versus supportive counselling significantly improved symptoms of anxiety at 12 months (response defined as > 20% improvement in anxiety symptoms on the Beck Anxiety Inventory or the Hamilton Anxiety Inventory; 12/17 [71%] of people responded with cognitive behavioural therapy *v* 9/23 [39%] of people with supportive counselling; RR 1.80, 95% CI 1.15 to 2.10; NNT 3, 95% CI 2 to 49), but found no significant difference in symptoms of depression at 12 months (response defined as > 20% improvement in depressive symptoms on the Beck Depression Inventory or the Geriatric Depression Scale; 10/17 [59%] people responded with cognitive behavioural therapy *v* 9/23 [39%] with supportive counselling; RR 1.50, 95% CI 0.79 to 2.87).[20]

Harms: The reviews and subsequent RCTs gave no information on harms.[15–20]

Comment: The second systematic review made indirect comparisons of treatments from different RCTs.[16] This loses the benefits of randomisation as the populations compared may not be equivalent. The figures presented in the systematic review produce estimates of relative effectiveness with wide confidence intervals: a clinically important difference between applied relaxation and cognitive therapy has not been established or excluded.[16] The State-Trait Anxiety Inventory covers a restricted range of symptoms, and may not satisfactorily reflect treatment outcomes in generalised anxiety disorder.[15–18]

OPTION APPLIED RELAXATION

We found no RCTs of applied relaxation (see glossary, p 988) versus placebo or no treatment. One systematic review found limited evidence, by making indirect comparisons of treatments across different RCTs, that more people given applied relaxation maintained recovery after 6 months than those given individual cognitive therapy (see glossary, p 988), non-directive treatment, group cognitive therapy, group behaviour therapy, individual behaviour therapy, or analytical psychotherapy. One subsequent RCT found no significant difference in symptoms at 13 weeks with applied relaxation versus cognitive behaviour therapy (see glossary, p 988).

Benefits: **Versus placebo or no treatment:** We found no systematic review or RCTs. **Versus other psychological treatments:** We found one systematic review (search date 1998)[16] and one subsequent RCT[19] (see benefits of cognitive therapy, p 977).

Harms: The systematic review and subsequent RCT gave no information on harms.[16,19]

Comment: None.

OPTION BENZODIAZEPINES

One systematic review and one subsequent RCT found limited evidence that benzodiazepines versus placebo reduced symptoms over 2–9 weeks. However, RCTs and observational studies found that benzodiazepines increased the risk of dependence, sedation, industrial accidents, and road traffic accidents. One non-systematic review found that, if used in late pregnancy or while breast feeding, benzodiazepines may cause adverse effects in neonates. One subsequent RCT found no significant difference in symptoms of anxiety with sustained release alprazolam versus bromazepam, and another subsequent RCT found no significant difference in overall symptoms with mexazolam versus alprazolam. Limited evidence from RCTs found no significant difference in symptoms

over 6–8 weeks with benzodiazepines versus buspirone, abecarnil, or antidepressants. One systematic review of poor quality RCTs found insufficient evidence about the effects of long term treatment with benzodiazepines.

Benefits: **Versus placebo:** We found one systematic review (search date 1996, 17 RCTs, 2044 people)[15] and one subsequent RCT.[22] The review found that benzodiazepines versus placebo were associated with a better response over 2–9 weeks (pooled mean effect size 0.70; CI not provided). The subsequent RCT (310 people) compared three interventions: diazepam (15–35 mg daily), abecarnil (7.5–17.5 mg daily), and placebo.[22] It found that diazepam versus placebo significantly increased the proportion of people with moderate improvement on the Clinical Global Impression scores at 6 weeks (73% with diazepam *v* 56% with placebo; $P < 0.01$).[22] **Versus each other:** The systematic review did not directly compare different benzodiazepines.[15] One subsequent RCT (121 people) compared sustained release alprazolam versus bromazepam and found no significant difference in Hamilton Anxiety Scale scores or Clinical Global Impression scores over 5 weeks (results presented graphically).[23] A second subsequent RCT (64 people) comparing mexazolam versus alprazolam found no significant difference in the proportion of people who had "highly improved" or "moderately improved" Clinical Global Impression scores at 3 weeks (98% *v* 87%; $P > 0.05$; results presented graphically).[24] **Long term treatment:** We found one systematic review (search date 1998, 8 RCTs, any benzodiazepine medication, > 2 months' duration).[25] It found that the weak methods of the RCTs identified prevent firm conclusions being made.[25] **Versus buspirone:** See benefits of buspirone, p 981. **Versus abecarnil:** See benefits of abecarnil, p 983. **Versus antidepressants:** See benefits of antidepressants, p 984.

Harms: **Sedation and dependence:** Benzodiazepines have been found to cause impairment in attention, concentration, and short term memory. One RCT identified by the review found an increased rate of drowsiness (71% with diazepam *v* 13% with placebo; $P = 0.001$) and dizziness (29% *v* 11%; $P = 0.001$).[15] Sedation can interfere with concomitant psychotherapy. One non-systematic review of the harms of benzodiazepines found that rebound anxiety on withdrawal has been reported in 15–30% of participants.[26] It also found that there is a high risk of substance abuse and dependence with benzodiazepines. **Memory:** Thirty one people with agoraphobia/panic disorder from an RCT of 8 weeks' alprazolam versus placebo were reviewed after 3.5 years.[27] Five people were still taking benzodiazepines and had significant impairment in memory tasks.[27] There was no difference in memory performance between those who had been in the placebo group and those who had been given alprazolam but were no longer taking the drug. **Road traffic accidents:** We found one systematic review (search date 1997) examining the relation between benzodiazepines and road traffic accidents.[28] In the case control studies, the odds ratio for death or emergency medical treatment in those who had taken benzodiazepines compared with those who had not taken them ranged from 1.45 to 2.40. The odds ratio increased with higher doses and more recent intake. In the police and emergency ward studies, benzodiazepine use was a factor in 1–65% of accidents (usually 5–10%). In two studies in which participants had blood alcohol concentrations under the legal limit, benzodiazepines were found in 43% and 65% of people. For drivers over 65 years of age, the risk of being involved in reported road traffic accidents was higher if they had taken longer acting and larger quantities of benzodiazepines. These results are from case control studies and, therefore, are subject to confounding factors. **Pregnancy and breast feeding:** One systematic review (search date 1997) of 23 case series and reports found no association between cleft lip and palate and use of benzodiazepines in the first trimester of pregnancy.[29] However, one non-systematic review found that the use of benzodiazepines in late pregnancy is associated with neonatal hypotonia and withdrawal syndrome.[30] Benzodiazepines are secreted in breast milk, and there have been reports of sedation and hypothermia in infants.[31] **Other:** One non-systematic industry funded review of eight RCTs of benzodiazepines versus placebo or buspirone found consistent improvement with benzodiazepines.[31] However, it found that recent use of benzodiazepines limited the effectiveness of buspirone (see benefits of buspirone, p 981).[31]

Comment: All of the RCTs assessing benzodiazepines were short term (at most 12 wks).[15,23,24] There was usually a significant improvement in symptoms at 6 weeks, but response rates were given at the end of the RCTs.

OPTION BUSPIRONE

RCTs have found that buspirone versus placebo significantly improves symptoms over 4–9 weeks. Limited evidence from RCTs found no significant difference in symptoms over 6–8 weeks with buspirone versus antidepressants or hydroxyzine.

Benefits: **Versus placebo:** We found one systematic review (search date 1996, 8 RCTs, 1 non-systematic review, 1884 people),[15] two subsequent RCTs,[32,33] and one non-systematic review.[31] The systematic review found that buspirone versus placebo was associated with a greater response over 4–9 weeks (pooled mean effect size 0.39; CI not provided).[15] One of the studies included in the review[15] was a non-systematic review (8 RCTs, 520 people; see comment below).[34] It found that buspirone versus placebo significantly increased the proportion of people "much or very much improved" as rated by their physician (54% with buspirone *v* 28% with placebo; $P \leq 0.001$).[34] The first subsequent RCT (162 people) of buspirone versus placebo found similar results (55% with buspirone *v* 35% with placebo; $P < 0.05$).[32] The second subsequent RCT (365 people) compared four interventions: buspirone (30 mg/day), venlafaxine (75 mg/day), venlafaxine (150 mg/day), and placebo over 8 weeks (see benefits of antidepressants, p 984).[33] It found that buspirone versus placebo significantly increased the proportion of people who responded after 8 weeks of treatment (response defined as score of 1 or 2 on the Clinical Global Impression Scale; 52/95 [55%] with buspirone *v* 38/98 [39%] with placebo; $P = 0.03$).[33] A non-systematic reanalysis by the manufacturer of pooled data from eight RCTs (735 people) compared buspirone versus placebo or versus benzodiazepines (see benefits of antidepressants, p 984). It found limited evidence from indirect comparisons across RCTs of a differential response to buspirone depending on whether the participant had been exposed to benzodiazepines (response defined "much or very much improved" on the Clinical Global Impression Scale: no previous exposure to benzodiazepines; response rate 59% with buspirone *v* 31% with placebo, P = 0.01; recent benzodiazepine use; response rate 41% with buspirone *v* 26% with placebo, P = 0.07). It did not assess whether this difference in response rates to buspirone was significant.[31] **Versus benzodiazepines:** The systematic review did not directly compare buspirone versus benzodiazepines.[15] One large RCT (240 people) identified by the review[15] compared buspirone versus diazepam versus placebo.[35] It found no difference in the proportion of people who responded over 6 weeks with buspirone versus diazepam (response defined as ≥ 40% reduction in Hamilton Anxiety Scale score; 61% with diazepam *v* 54% with buspirone; P values not provided).[35] A non-systematic reanalysis by the manufacturer of pooled data from eight RCTs (735 people) comparing buspirone versus placebo or versus benzodiazepines found limited evidence of a differential response to buspirone depending on whether the participant had been exposed to benzodiazepines (response defined "much or very much improved" on the Clinical Global Impression Scale: no previous exposure to benzodiazepines; response rate 59% with buspirone *v* 61% with benzodiazepines; recent benzodiazepine use: response rate 41% with buspirone *v* 69% with benzodiazepines; P values not provided). It did not assess whether this difference in response rates to buspirone was significant.[31] **Versus antidepressants:** See benefits of antidepressants, p 984. **Versus hydroxyzine:** See benefits of hydroxyzine, p 983.

Harms: **Sedation and dependence:** The subsequent RCT found that buspirone significantly increased the proportion of people with nausea (27/80 [34%] with buspirone *v* 11/82 [13%] with placebo; RR 2.5, 95% CI 1.3 to 4.7; NNH 5, 95% CI 4 to 14), dizziness (51/80 [64%] with buspirone *v* 10/82 [12%] with placebo; RR 5.2, 95% CI 2.9 to 9.6; NNH 2, 95% CI 2 to 3), and somnolence (15/80 [19%] with buspirone *v* 6/82 [7%] with placebo; RR 2.6, 95% CI 1.0 to 6.3; NNH 9, 95% CI 5 to 104).[32] The RCT found no significant difference in the number of people reporting any adverse effect with buspirone versus diazepam (49% with buspirone *v* 63% with diazepam). Diazepam was associated with more fatigue and weakness compared with buspirone but less headache and dizziness. The non-systematic review did not report on the comparative adverse effects of buspirone versus benzodiazepines.[31] **Pregnancy and breast feeding:** We found no evidence.

Comment: All of the RCTs in the non-systematic review were sponsored by pharmaceutical companies and had been included in regulatory submissions for buspirone.[34]

OPTION HYDROXYZINE

One RCT identified by a non-systematic review found that hydroxyzine versus placebo significantly improved symptoms of anxiety after 4 weeks. Another RCT identified by the review found no significant difference in the proportion of people with improved symptoms of anxiety at 35 days with hydroxyzine versus placebo or buspirone.

Benefits: **Versus placebo:** We found one non-systematic review (2 RCTs, 354 people).[36] The first RCT (110 people) identified by the review found a significantly greater improvement in Hamilton Anxiety Scale scores after 4 weeks with hydroxyzine (50 mg/day) versus placebo (results presented graphically). The second RCT (244 people) identified by the review compared hydroxyzine versus buspirone versus placebo for 28 days (followed by placebo in all groups for 7 days). It found no significant difference in the proportion of people with a Hamilton Anxiety Scale reduction of 50% or greater at 35 days with hydroxyzine (50 mg/day) versus placebo (30/71 [42%] with hydroxyzine *v* 20/70 [29%] with placebo; ARR 14%, 95% CI –2% to +29%; RR 1.50, 95% CI 0.93 to 2.23; not intention to treat).[36] **Versus buspirone:** The second RCT identified by the non-systematic review also found no significant difference with hydroxyzine versus buspirone on the number of people with a Hamilton Anxiety Scale reduction of 50% or greater after 28 days (30/71 [42%] with hydroxyzine *v* 26/72 [36%] with buspirone; RR 1.20, 95% CI 0.78 to 1.80; ARR 5%, 95% CI –11% to +21%).[36]

Harms: The second RCT (244 people) identified by the review found that hydroxyzine versus placebo increased the proportion of people with somnolence (10% *v* 0%) and headaches (6% *v* 1%).[36] Overall adverse effects were reported in 40% of people taking hydroxyzine versus 38% taking buspirone versus 28% taking placebo.

Comment: None.

OPTION ABECARNIL

One RCT found no significant difference in symptoms at 6 weeks with abecarnil versus placebo or versus diazepam. One smaller RCT found limited evidence that low dose abecarnil versus placebo significantly improved symptoms.

Benefits: We found no systematic review, but found two multicentre RCTs.[22,37] The first RCT (310 people) compared three interventions: abecarnil (7.5–17.5 mg/day), diazepam (15–35 mg/day), and placebo.[22] It found no significant difference with abecarnil versus placebo or versus diazepam in the proportion of people with moderate improvement on the Clinical Global Impression scores at 6 weeks (62% with abecarnil *v* 56% with placebo; $P < 0.031$; 62% with abecarnil *v* 73% with diazepam; P value not provided).[22] A second RCT (129 people) compared 3 weeks of treatment with abecarnil (3–9 mg, 7.5–15 mg, and 15–30 mg/day) versus placebo.[37] Within each group the dose was escalated from the minimum to the maximum over the length of the trial. It found that abecarnil (3–9 mg) versus placebo significantly improved symptoms (outcome 50% reduction in Hamilton Anxiety Scale score; 19/31 [61%] with abecarnil v 8/26 [31%] with placebo; P = 0.05), but found no significant difference in symptoms with higher doses of abecarnil versus placebo.[37] Results were not intention to treat (12/34 [35%] people withdrew with abecarnil 15–30 mg v 4/35 [11%] with abecarnil 7.5–15 mg v 1/32 [3%] with abecarnil 3–9 mg v 2/28 [7%] with placebo).

Harms: The second RCT found that abecarnil (3–9 mg/day) versus placebo significantly increased fatigue (4/32 [13%] with abecarnil v 0/28 [0%] with placebo; NNH 3, 95% CI 3 to 7) and equilibrium loss (2/32 [6%] with abecarnil v 0/28 [0%] with placebo; NNH 7, 95% CI 4 to 14).[37] Abercarnil versus placebo was also associated with more drowsiness (10/32 [31%] with abecarnil v 4/28 [14%] with placebo; RR 2.12, 95% CI 0.77 to 6.21). Higher doses were associated with more adverse effects (62% of people taking abecarnil 15–30 mg experienced at least 1 adverse effect v 51% of people taking abecarnil 7.5–15 mg v 22% of people taking abecarnil 3–9 mg v 21% of people taking placebo).[37]

Comment: None.

OPTION ANTIDEPRESSANTS

RCTs have found that imipramine, opipramol, paroxetine, trazodone, or venlafaxine versus placebo significantly improve symptoms over 4–8 weeks, and that they are not significantly different from each other. RCTs and observational studies have found that antidepressants are associated with sedation, dizziness, nausea, falls, and sexual dysfunction. Limited evidence from RCTs found no significant difference in symptoms over 8 weeks with antidepressants versus benzodiazepines or buspirone. We found no systematic review or RCTs assessing sedating tricyclic antidepressants in people with generalised anxiety disorder.

Benefits: **Versus placebo or versus each other:** We found one systematic review (search date 1996, 3 RCTs)[15] and seven subsequent RCTs.[33,38–43] The systematic review found that trazodone, imipramine, or ritanserin versus placebo were associated with a significantly greater response (pooled mean effect size 0.57; CI not provided).[15] The first subsequent RCT (230 people) compared four interventions: imipramine, trazodone, placebo, and diazepam.[38] It found that both antidepressants versus placebo significantly increased the proportion of people with patient assessed global improvement at the end of 8 weeks of treatment, but imipramine and trazodone were not significantly different from each other (73% with imipramine v 67% with trazodone v 39% with placebo). The results were not intention to treat (18/58 [31%] people withdrew with imipramine, 22/61 [36%] with trazodone, 18/56 [32%] with diazepam, and 20/55 [36%] with placebo).[38] The second subsequent RCT (318 people) compared opipramol (a tricyclic antidepressant with minimal serotonin reuptake blocking properties) versus placebo or versus alprazolam over 28 days. It found that opipramol versus placebo significantly increased the proportion of people who responded after 28 days (response defined as Clinical Global Impression score of < 2; 63/100 [63%] with opipramol v

50/107 [47%] with placebo; RR 1.35, 95% CI 1.05 to 1.69; NNT 7; 95% CI 1 to 26), but found no significant difference in the proportion of people who responded with opipramol versus alprazolam (63/100 [63%] with opipramol *v* 67/105 [64%] with alprazolam; RR 1.01, 95% CI 0.79 to 1.25).[39] The third subsequent RCT (324 people) found that paroxetine versus placebo significantly increased the proportion of people who responded after 8 weeks (response defined as a score of 1 or 2 on the Clinical Global Impression Scale; 100/161 [62%] with paroxetine *v* 77/163 [47%] with placebo; RR 1.31, 95% CI 1.07 to 1.61; NNT 6, 95% CI 4 to 24).[42] The fourth subsequent RCT (365 people) compared venlafaxine at two different doses (75 or 150 mg/day), buspirone (30 mg/day) versus placebo over 8 weeks.[33] It found that both doses of venlafaxine versus placebo significantly increased the proportion of people who responded after 8 weeks of treatment (response defined as a score of 1 or 2 on the Clinical Global Impression Scale; 54/87 [62%] with venlafaxine 75 mg *v* 38/98 [39%] with placebo; P = 0.002; 44/89 [49%] with 150 mg venlafaxine *v* 38/98 [39%] with placebo; P = 0.05).[33] The fifth subsequent RCT compared three venlafaxine regimens (75 mg, 150 mg, and 225 mg/day) versus placebo over 8 weeks. It found that all doses of venlafaxine versus placebo significantly improved Hamilton Anxiety Scale and Hospital Anxiety and Depression scale scores, and were not significantly different from each other at 8 weeks (results presented graphically).[40] The sixth subsequent RCT (261 people) compared venlafaxine (75–225 mg/day) versus placebo for 6 months.[41] Intention to treat analysis (last observation carried forward, 44/127 [35%] taking placebo and 60/124 [48%] taking venlafaxine completed) found that venlafaxine versus placebo significantly increased the proportion of people with a reduction of 40% on baseline Hamilton Anxiety score in both Hamilton Anxiety Scale and Clinical Global Impression Scale over 6 months (42% response with venlafaxine *v* 21% with placebo). We were unable, because of the nature of the analysis and reporting, to calculate relative risk or number needed to treat with meaningful confidence intervals.[41] The seventh subsequent RCT (541 people) compared venlafaxine at three different doses (35, 75, or 150 mg/day) versus placebo.[43] It found that venlafaxine (75 mg or 150 mg) versus placebo significantly increased the proportion of people who responded to treatment at week 24 (response defined as 50% reduction in Hamilton Anxiety Scale score or Clinical Global Impression score of 1 or 2; results presented graphically; P < 0.001 for both doses). **Versus benzodiazepines:** We found no systematic review, but found two RCTs.[38,44] The first RCT (230 people) compared four interventions: flexible doses of imipramine, trazodone, placebo, and diazepam.[38] It found no significant difference in the proportion of people with patient assessed global improvement at the end of 8 weeks of treatment with antidepressants versus diazepam (73% of people improved with imipramine *v* 67% with trazodone *v* 66% with diazepam). The results were not intention to treat (18/58 [31%] people withdrew with imipramine, 22/61[36%] with trazodone, 18/56 [32%] with diazepam, and 20/55 [36%] with placebo).[38] The second RCT (81 people) compared paroxetine, imipramine, and 2'-chlordesmethyldiazepam for 8 weeks.[44] Paroxetine and imipramine were significantly more effective than 2'-chlordesmethyldiazepam in improving anxiety scores (mean Hamilton Anxiety Scale after 8 wks: 11.1 for paroxetine, 10.8 for imipramine, 12.9 for 2'-chlordesmethyldiazepam; P = 0.05). **Versus buspirone:** We found no systematic review. One RCT (365 people) compared venlafaxine at two different doses (75 or 150 mg/day) versus buspirone (30 mg/day) versus placebo over 8 weeks. It found no significant difference in the proportion of people who responded after 8 weeks of treatment with venlafaxine versus buspirone (response defined as score of 1 or 2 on the Clinical Global Impression Scale; 54/87 [62%] with venlafaxine 75 mg *v* 44/89 [49%] with 150 mg venlafaxine *v* 52/95 [55%] with buspirone; P values not provided).[33] **Sedating tricyclic antidepressants:** We found no systematic review or RCTs assessing sedating tricyclic antidepressants in people with generalised anxiety disorder.

Harms: **Common adverse effects:** One RCT found sedation, confusion, dry mouth, and constipation with both imipramine and trazodone.[38] RCTs reported nausea, somnolence, dry mouth, sweating, constipation, anorexia, and sexual dysfunction with venlafaxine. One of the RCTs found that 26% of people taking venlafaxine and 17% of people taking placebo withdrew because of adverse effects.[41] Most of the adverse effects (apart from dizziness and sexual dysfunction) decreased over 6 months in those who continued to take the medication.[41] There have been case reports of nausea in people taking paroxetine.[45] **Overdose:** In a series of 239 coroner directed necropsies from 1970–1989, tricyclic antidepressants were considered to be a causal factor in 12% of deaths and hypnosedatives (primarily benzodiazepines and excluding barbiturates) in 8% of deaths.[44] **Accidental poisoning:** Tricyclic antidepressants are a major cause of accidental poisoning.[46] A study estimated that there was one death for every 44 children admitted to hospital after ingestion of tricyclic antidepressants.[47] **Hyponatraemia:** One case series reported 736 incidents of hyponatraemia in people taking selective serotonin reuptake inhibitors; 83% of episodes were in hospital inpatients aged over 65 years.[48] It is not possible to establish causation from this type of data. **Falls:** One retrospective cohort study (2428 elderly residents of nursing homes) found an increased risk of falls in new users of antidepressants (665 people taking tricyclic antidepressants; adjusted RR 2.0, 95% CI 1.8 to 2.2; 612 people taking selective serotonin reuptake inhibitors; adjusted RR 1.8, 95% CI 1.6 to 2.0; and 304 people taking trazodone; adjusted RR 1.2, 95% CI 1.0 to 1.4).[49] The increased rate of falls persisted through the first 180 days of treatment and beyond. One case control study (8239 people aged ≥66 years, treated in hospital for hip fracture) found an increased risk of hip fracture in those taking antidepressants (adjusted OR, selective serotonin reuptake inhibitors 2.4, 95% CI 2.0 to 2.7; secondary amine tricyclic antidepressants such as nortriptyline 2.2, 95% CI 1.8 to 2.8; and tertiary amine tricyclic antidepressants such as amitriptyline 1.5, 95% CI 1.3 to 1.7).[50] This study could not control for confounding factors; people taking antidepressants may be at increased risk of hip fracture for other reasons. **In pregnancy:** We found no reports of harmful effects in pregnancy. One case controlled study found no evidence that imipramine or fluoxetine increased the rate of malformations in pregnancy.[51] **Sexual dysfunction:** A survey (1022 people mostly suffering from depression; 610 women) of people using antidepressants with previously acceptable sexual function has reported the incidence of sexual dysfunction to be 71% for paroxetine, 67% for venlafaxine, and 63% for fluvaxamine.[52]

Comment: None.

OPTION ANTIPSYCHOTIC DRUGS

One RCT found that trifluoperazine versus placebo significantly reduced anxiety after 4 weeks, but caused more drowsiness, extrapyramidal reactions, and other movement disorders.

Benefits: We found no systematic review. We found one RCT (415 people) comparing 4 weeks of trifluoperazine treatment (2–6 mg/day) versus placebo.[53] It found that trifluoperazine versus placebo significantly reduced the total score on the Hamilton Anxiety Scale (difference 14 points; $P < 0.001$).

Harms: The RCT reported more cases of drowsiness (43% with trifluoperazine *v* 25% with placebo) and extrapyramidal reactions and movement disorders (17% with trifluoperazine *v* 8% with placebo) with trifluoperazine versus placebo.[53] A cohort study found that in the longer term, rates of tardive dyskinesia are increased the more often treatment is interrupted.[54]

Comment: None.

OPTION β BLOCKERS

We found no RCTs assessing β blockers in people with generalised anxiety disorder.

Benefits: We found no systematic review or RCTs.

Harms: We found no good evidence.

Comment: None.

OPTION KAVA New

One systematic review in people with anxiety disorders, including generalised anxiety disorder, found that kava versus placebo significantly reduced symptoms of anxiety over 4 weeks. Observational evidence suggests that kava may be associated with hepatotoxicity.

Benefits: We found one systematic review (search date 1998, 7 RCTs, 377 people with anxiety disorders, proportion of people with generalised anxiety disorder not specified) comparing kava versus placebo.[55] It found that kava versus placebo significantly reduced Hamilton Anxiety Scores over 4 weeks (3 RCTs; 198 people; WMD 9.69, 95% CI 3.54 to 15.83).

Harms: The systematic review found that people taking kava experienced stomach complaints, restlessness, drowsiness, tremor, headache, and tiredness,[55] but provided no comparative information about adverse effects in people taking placebo. One RCT (38 people with generalised anxiety disorder) assessing adverse effects of kava found no difference in adverse effects or withdrawal symptoms with kava versus placebo, but one person had a mild increase in alanine aminotransferase.[56] One overview assessing the harms of a variety of herbal preparations reported that kava has been associated with several cases of toxic liver damage, and that long term use (not specified) at high doses (over 330 mg/day) may be associated with alopecia and yellow, dry skin.[57] Case reports also suggest that kava may be associated with fulminant hepatitis.[58] The United States National Center of Complementary and Alternative Medicine has suggested that kava may be associated with liver disease.[59]

Comment: None.

GLOSSARY

Applied relaxation A technique involving training in relaxation techniques and self monitoring of symptoms without challenging beliefs.

Cognitive behavioural therapy Brief (20 sessions over 12–16 wks) structured treatment incorporating elements of cognitive therapy and behavioural therapy. Behavioural therapy is based on learning theory and concentrates on changing behaviour.

Cognitive therapy Brief (20 sessions over 12–16 wks) structured treatment aimed at identifying anxiety associated thoughts and beliefs, changing over monitoring of physical symptoms, and minimising the catastophising that characterises generalised anxiety disorder. This is combined with relaxation, exercise, and testing the validity of beliefs in real life situations. It requires a highly trained therapist.

Substantive changes

Cognitive therapy: One new systematic review,[17] one new non-systematic review,[18] and one new subsequent RCT;[20] conclusions unchanged.

Benzodiazepines: One new RCT;[24] conclusions unchanged.

Antidepressants: Two new RCTs;[42,43] conclusions unchanged.

REFERENCES

1. American Psychiatric Association. *Diagnostic and statistical manual of mental disorders*, 4th ed. Washington, DC: American Psychiatric Association, 1994.
2. Mendlowicz MV, Stein MB. Quality of life in individuals with anxiety disorders. *Am J Psychiatry* 2000;157:669–682.
3. Stein D. Comorbidity in generalised anxiety disorder: impact and implications. *J Clin Psychiatry* 2001;62(suppl 11):29–34.(review).
4. Judd LL, Kessler RC, Paulus MP, et al. Comorbidity as a fundamental feature of generalised anxiety disorders: results from the national comorbidity study (NCS). *Acta Psychiatry Scand* 1998;98(suppl 393):6–11.
5. Andrews G, Peters L, Guzman AM, et al. A comparison of two structured diagnostic interviews: CIDI and SCAN. *Aust N Z J Psychiatry* 1995;29:124–132.
6. Kessler RC, McGonagle KA, Zhao S, et al. Lifetime and 12-month prevalence of DSM-III-R psychiatric disorders in the United States: results from the national comorbidity survey. *Arch Gen Psychiatry* 1994;51:8–19.
7. Seivewright N, Tyrer P, Ferguson B, et al. Longitudinal study of the influence of life events and personality status on diagnostic change in three neurotic disorders. *Depression Anx* 2000;11:105–113.
8. Pigott T. Gender differences in the epidemiology and treatment of anxiety disorders. *J Clin Psychiatry* 1999;60(suppl 18):15–18.
9. Jorm AF. Does old age reduce the risk of anxiety and depression? A review of epidemiological studies across the adult life span. *Psychol Med* 2000;30:11–22.
10. Lau AW, Edelstein BA, Larkin KT. Psychophysiological arousal in older adults: a critical review. *Clin Psychol Rev* 2001;21:609–630 (review).
11. Brantley PJ, Mehan DJ Jr, Ames SC, et al. Minor stressors and generalised anxiety disorders among low income patients attending primary care clinics. *J Nerv Ment Dis* 1999;187:435–440.

12. Brown ES, Fulton MK, Wilkeson A, Petty F. The psychiatric sequelae of civilian trauma. *Comp Psychiatry* 2000;41:19–23.
13. Hawker DSJ, Boulton MJ. Twenty years' research on peer victimisation and psychosocial maladjustment: a meta-analytic review of cross-sectional studies. *J Child Psychol Psychiatr* 2000;41:441–445.
14. Hettema JM, Neale MC, Kendler KS. A review and meta-analysis of the genetic epidemiology of anxiety disorders. *Am J Psychiatry* 2001;158:1568–1578. Search date not stated; primary source Medline.
15. Gould RA, Otto MW, Pollack MH, et al. Cognitive behavioural and pharmacological treatment of generalised anxiety disorder: a preliminary meta-analysis. *Behav Res Ther* 1997;28:285–305. Search date 1996; primary sources Psychlit, Medline, examination of reference lists, and unpublished articles presented at national conferences.
16. Fisher PL, Durham RC. Recovery rates in generalized anxiety disorder following psychological therapy: an analysis of clinically significant change in the STAI-T across outcome studies since 1990. *Psychol Med* 1999;29:1425–1434. Search date: 1998; primary sources Medline, Psychlit, and Cochrane Controlled Trials Register.
17. Western D, Morrison K. A multidimensional meta-analysis of treatments for depression, panic and generalized anxiety disorder: an empirical examination of the status of empirically supported therapies. *J Consult Clin Psychol* 2001;69:875–889. Search date not stated but only included studies published 1990–1999; primary sources hand searches of 10 journals and psychological abstracts.
18. Borkovec TD, Ruscio AM. Psychotherapy for generalized anxiety disorder. *J Clin Psychiatry* 2001;61(suppl 11):37–42.
19. Ost L, Breitholts E. Applied relaxation vs. cognitive therapy in the treatment of generalized anxiety disorder. *Behav Res Ther* 2000;38:777–790.
20. Barrowclough C, King P, Russell E, et al. A randomized trial of effectiveness of cognitive-behavioural therapy and supportive counselling for anxiety disorders in older adults. *J Consult Clin Psychol* 2001:69;756–762.
21. Durham RC, Fisher PL, Trevling LR, et al. One year follow-up of cognitive therapy, analytic psychotherapy and anxiety management training for generalised anxiety disorder: symptom change, medication usage and attitudes to treatment. *Behav Cogn Psychother* 1999;27:19–35.
22. Rickels K, DeMartinis N, Aufdembrinke B. A double-blind, placebo controlled trial of abecarnil and diazepam in the treatment of patients with generalized anxiety disorder. *J Clin Psychopharmacol* 2000:20:12–18.
23. Figueira ML. Alprazolam SR in the treatment of generalised anxiety: a multicentre controlled study with bromazepam. *Hum Psychother* 1999;14:171–177.
24. Vaz-Serra A, Figuerra L, Bessa-Peixoto A, et al. Mexazolam and alprazolam in the treatment of generalized anxiety disorder. *Clin Drug Invest* 2001;21:257–263.
25. Mahe V, Balogh A. Long-term pharmacological treatment of generalized anxiety disorder. *Int Clin Psychopharmacol* 2000;15:99–105. Search date 1998; primary sources Medline, Biosis, and Embase.
26. Tyrer P. Current problems with the benzodiazepines. In: Wheatly D, ed. *The anxiolytic jungle: where next?* Chichester: J Wiley and Sons, 1990:23–47.
27. Kilic C, Curran HV, Noshirvani H, et al. Long-term effects of alprazolam on memory: a 3.5 year follow-up of agoraphobia/panic patients. *Psychol Med* 1999;29:225–231.
28. Thomas RE. Benzodiazepine use and motor vehicle accidents. Systematic review of reported association. *Can Fam Physician* 1998;44:799–808. Search date 1997; primary source Medline.
29. Dolovich LR, Addis A, Regis Vaillancourt JD, et al. Benzodiazepine use in pregnancy and major malformations of oral cleft: meta-analysis of cohort and case-control studies. *BMJ* 1998;317:839–843. Search date 1997; primary sources Medline, Embase, Reprotox, and references of included studies and review articles.
30. Bernstein JG. *Handbook of drug therapy in psychiatry*, 3rd ed. St Louis, Missouri: Mosby Year Book, 1995:401.
31. DeMartinis N, Rynn M, Rickels K, et al. Prior benzodiazepine use and buspirone response in the treatment of generalized anxiety disorder. *J Clin Psychiatry* 2000;61:91–94.
32. Sramek JJ, Transman M, Suri A, et al. Efficacy of buspirone in generalized anxiety disorder with coexisting mild depressive symptoms. *J Clin Psychiatry* 1996;57:287–291.
33. Davidson JR, DuPont RL, Hedges D, et al. Efficacy, safety and tolerability of venlafaxine extended release and buspirone in outpatients with generalised anxiety disorder. *J Clin Psychiatry* 1999;60:528–535.
34. Gammans RE, Stringfellow JC, Hvisdos AJ, et al. Use of buspirone in patients with generalized anxiety disorder and coexisting depressive symptoms: a meta-analysis of eight randomized, controlled trials. *Pharmacopsychiatry* 1992;25:193–201.
35. Rickels K, Weisman K, Norstad N, et al. Buspirone and diazepam in anxiety: a controlled study. *J Clin Psychiatry* 1982;12:81–86.
36. Lader M, Anxiolytic effect of hydroxyzine: A double-blind trial versus placebo and buspirone. *Hum Psychopharmacol Clin Exp* 1999:14;S94–102.
37. Ballenger JC, McDonald S, Noyes R, et al. The first double-blind, placebo-controlled trial of a partial benzodiazepine agonist, abecarnil (ZK 112–119) in generalised anxiety disorder. *Adv Biochem Psychopharmacol* 1992;47:431–447.
38. Rickels K, Downing R, Schweizer E, et al. Antidepressants for the treatment of generalised anxiety disorder: a placebo-controlled comparison of imipramine, trazodone and diazepam. *Arch Gen Psychiatry* 1993;50:884–895.
39. Moller HJ, Volz HP, Reimann IW, et al. Opipramol for the treatment of generalised anxiety disorder: A placebo-controlled trial including an alprazolam-treated group. *J Clin Psychopharmacol* 2001;21:51–65.
40. Rickels K, Pollack MH, Sheehan D, et al. Efficacy of extended-release venlafaxine in nondepressed outpatients with generalized anxiety disorder. *Am J Psychiatry* 2000;157:968–974.
41. Gelenberg A, Lydiard R, Rudolph R, et al. Efficacy of venlafaxine extended releases capsules in nondepressed outpatients with generalized anxiety disorder: a 6-month randomized controlled trial. *JAMA* 2000;283:3082–3088.
42. Pollack MH, Zaninelli R, Goddard A, et al. Paroxetine in the treatment of generalized anxiety disorder: results of a placebo-controlled, flexible-dosage trial. *J Clin Psychiatry* 2001;62:350–357.
43. Allgulander C, Hackett D, Salinas E. Venlafaxine extended release (ER) in the treatment of

generalised anxiety disorder: twenty-four week placebo-controlled dose-ranging study. *Br J Psychiatry* 2001;179:15–22.
44. Dukes PD, Robinson GM, Thomson KJ, et al. Wellington coroner autopsy cases 1970–89: acute deaths due to drugs, alcohol and poisons. *N Z Med J* 1992;105:25–27. (Published erratum appears in *N Z Med J* 1992;105:135.)
45. Rocca P, Fonzo V, Scotta M, et al. Paroxetine efficacy in the treatment of generalized anxiety disorder. *Acta Psychiatr Scand* 1997:95:444–450.
46. Kerr GW, McGuffie AC, Wilkie S. Tricyclic antidepressant overdose: a review. *Emerg Med J* 2001;18:236–241.
47. Pearn J, Nixon J, Ansford A, et al. Accidental poisoning in childhood: five year urban population study with 15 year analysis of fatality. *BMJ* 1984;288:44–46.
48. Lui BA, Mitmann N, Knowles SR, et al. Hyponatremia and the syndrome of inappropriate secretion of antidiuretic hormone associated with the use of selective serotonin reuptake inhibitors: a review of spontaneous reports. *Can Med Assoc J* 1995;155:519–527.
49. Thapa PB, Gideon P, Cost TW, et al. Antidepressants and the risk of falls among nursing home residents. *N Engl J Med* 1998;339:875–882.
50. Liu B, Anderson G, Mittmann N, et al. Use of selective serotonin-reuptake inhibitors of tricyclic antidepressants and risk of hip fractures in elderly people. *Lancet* 1998;351:1303–1307.
51. Kulin NA, Pastuszak A, Koren G. Are the new SSRIs safe for pregnant women? *Can Fam Physician* 1998;44;2081–2083.
52. Montejo AL, Llorca G, Izquierdo JA, et al. Incidence of sexual dysfunction associated with antidepressant agents: A prospective multicentre study of 1022 outpatients. *J Clin Psychiatry* 2000;62(suppl 3):10–21.
53. Mendels J, Krajewski TF, Huffer V, et al. Effective short-term treatment of generalized anxiety with trifluoperazine. *J Clin Psychiatry* 1986;47:170–174.
54. Van Harten PN, Hoek HW, Matroos GE, et al. Intermittent neuroleptic treatment and risk of tardive dyskinesia: Curacao extrapyramidal syndromes study III. *Am J Psychiatry* 1998;155:565–567.
55. Pittler MH, Ernst E. Kava extract for treating anxiety. In: The Cochrane Library, Issue 1, 2002. Oxford: Update Software. Search date 1998; primary sources Medline, Embase, Biosis, Amed, Ciscom, Cochrane Library, hand searches of references, personal files, and contact with manufacturers of kava preparations and experts.
56. Conner KM, Davidson JRT, Churchill LE. Adverse-effect profile of Kava. *CNS Spectrums* 2001;6:848–853.
57. Ernst E. The risk–benefit profile of commonly used herbal therapies: Ginkgo, St. John's Wort, Ginseng, Echinacea, Saw Palmetto, and Kava. *Ann Intern Med* 2002;136:42–53. Search date 2000; primary sources Medline, Embase, Ciscom, Amed, and the Cochrane Library and personal contact with nine experts.
58. Escher M, Desmueles J. Hepatitis associated with kava, a herbal remedy for anxiety. *BMJ* 2001;322:139.
59. National Center for Complimentary and Alternative Medicine. Consumer Advisory. Kava linked to liver damage. Internet 2002 [cited March26]; http://nccam.nih.gov/fcp/kava/kava.htm.

Christopher Gale
Consultant Psychiatrist, Clinical Senior Lecturer
Faculty of Medicine and Health Sciences
University of Auckland
Auckland
New Zealand

Mark Oakley-Browne
Professor of Rural Psychiatry
University of Monash
Victoria
Australia

Competing interests: CG has been paid by Eli Lilly, the manufacturer of Prozac, to attend symposia. MOB has been reimbursed by Eli Lilly for attending a conference and for running an educational programme.

Obsessive compulsive disorder

Search date May 2002

G Mustafa Soomro

QUESTIONS

INTERVENTIONS

INITIAL TREATMENT

Beneficial

IN PEOPLE WHO DO NOT RESPOND TO SEROTONIN REUPTAKE INHIBITORS

Likely to be beneficial

To be covered in future updates

Other forms of psychotherapy
Other drug monotherapies
Other adjuvant/augmentation drug treatment
Psychosurgery
Electroconvulsive treatment
Treatment in children and adolescents

See glossary, p 999

Key Messages

- **Behavioural therapy** One systematic review and one subsequent RCT have found that behavioural therapy improves symptoms compared with relaxation. Two observational studies found that improvement was maintained for up to 2 years. Another systematic review found no significant difference in symptoms with behavioural therapy versus cognitive therapy. One additional RCT found limited evidence that group behavioural therapy versus group cognitive therapy improved symptoms after 3 months (NNT 3, 95% CI 2 to 9).
- **Cognitive therapy** One systematic review has found no significant difference in symptoms with cognitive therapy versus behavioural therapy. One subsequent RCT found limited evidence that group cognitive therapy improved symptoms less than group behavioural therapy after 12 weeks.
- **Drug treatment (fluvoxamine) plus behavioural therapy** Systematic reviews have found that monotherapy with drug therapy (serotonin reuptake inhibitors) or behavioural therapy improve symptoms. But RCTs have found only limited evidence that behavioural therapy plus fluvoxamine reduces symptoms more than behavioural therapy alone.
- **Selective and non-selective serotonin reuptake inhibitors** Systematic reviews and subsequent RCTs have found that serotonin reuptake inhibitors versus placebo significantly improve symptoms after 12 weeks. One observational study found that most people relapsed within 7 weeks of stopping treatment with clomipramine (a non-selective serotonin reuptake inhibitor). RCTs have found no consistent

evidence of different efficacy among serotonin reuptake inhibitors. One systematic review and two subsequent RCTs have found that serotonin reuptake inhibitors reduce symptoms significantly more than other types of antidepressants. RCTs have found that clomipramine is associated with more adverse effects than selective serotonin reuptake inhibitors.

- **Addition of antipsychotics in people who have not responded to serotonin reuptake inhibitors** Two small RCTs in people unresponsive to serotonin reuptake inhibitors found that the addition of antipsychotics versus placebo significantly improved symptoms (NNT 2, 95% CI 2 to 3).

DEFINITION Obsessive compulsive disorder involves obsessions or compulsions (or both) that are not caused by drugs or a physical disorder, and which cause significant personal distress or social dysfunction. **Obsessions** are recurrent and persistent ideas, images, or impulses that cause pronounced anxiety and that the person perceives to be self produced. **Compulsions** are intentional repetitive behaviours or mental acts performed in response to obsessions or according to certain rules, and are aimed at reducing distress or preventing certain imagined dreaded events. Obsessions and compulsions are usually recognised as pointless and are resisted by the person. (There are minor differences in the criteria for obsessive compulsive disorder between the third, revised third, and fourth editions of the *Diagnostic and Statistical Manual:* DSM-III, DSM-III-R, and DSM-IV.)[1]

INCIDENCE/ PREVALENCE One national, community based survey of obsessive compulsive disorder in the UK (1993, 10 000 people) found a prevalence of 1% in men and 1.5% in women.[2] A survey in the USA (18 500 people) found a lifetime prevalence of obsessive compulsive disorder of between 1.9 and 3.3% in 1984.[3] An international study found a lifetime prevalence of 3% in Canada, 3.1% in Puerto Rico, 0.3–0.9% in Taiwan, and 2.2% in New Zealand.[2]

AETIOLOGY/ RISK FACTORS Behavioural, cognitive, genetic, and neurobiological factors are implicated in obsessive compulsive disorder.[4–10]

PROGNOSIS One study (144 people followed for a mean of 47 years) found that an episodic (see glossary, p 1000) course of obsessive compulsive disorder was more common during the initial years (about 1–9 years), but a chronic (see glossary, p 999) course was more common afterwards.[11] Over time, the study found that 39–48% of people had symptomatic improvement. A 1 year prospective cohort study found 46% of people had an episodic course and 54% had a chronic course.[12]

AIMS To improve symptoms, and to reduce impact of illness on social functioning and quality of life.

OUTCOMES Severity of symptoms; adverse effects of treatment; and social functioning. Commonly used instruments for measuring symptoms include the Hamilton Anxiety Rating scale, the Hamilton Depression Rating scale, and the Yale–Brown obsessive compulsive scale, which is observer rated and well validated.[13–16] Most trials use a 25% reduction in Yale–Brown scale scores from baseline as indicative of clinically important improvement, but some studies use a 35% reduction.[16]

METHODS *Clinical Evidence* update search and appraisal May 2002.

QUESTION What are the effects of treatments in adults?

OPTION SEROTONIN REUPTAKE INHIBITORS

Systematic reviews and subsequent RCTs have found that serotonin reuptake inhibitors versus placebo significantly reduce symptoms. One observational study found that most people relapsed within 7 weeks of stopping treatment with clomipramine (a non-selective serotonin reuptake inhibitor). RCTs have found no consistent evidence of different efficacy among serotonin reuptake inhibitors. One systematic review and two subsequent RCTs have found that serotonin reuptake inhibitors reduce symptoms significantly more than other types of antidepressants. RCTs have found that clomipramine is associated with more adverse effects than selective serotonin reuptake inhibitors. One RCT in people who had responded to 20 weeks of treatment with fluoxetine (selective serotonin reuptake inhibitor) found that maintenance of fluoxetine versus replacement by placebo did not significantly reduce relapse rate over 1 year. One RCT in people who had previously responded to 1 years' treatment with sertraline found that the maintenance of sertraline versus placebo significantly reduced the proportion of people who had worsening of symptoms, or who withdrew because of relapse or insufficient clinical response, but found no significant difference in the proportion of people who relapsed over 24 weeks.

Benefits: **Versus placebo:** We found three systematic reviews[17–19] and three subsequent RCTs.[20–22] The first review (search date 1994, mean treatment duration 12 wks) compared clomipramine (a non-selective serotonin reuptake inhibitor [see glossary, p 1000]), fluoxetine, fluvoxamine, and sertraline (selective serotonin reuptake inhibitors [see glossary, p 1000]) versus placebo.[17] Two RCTs of clomipramine versus placebo included 73 children, but the review did not analyse these RCTs separately. It found that clomipramine versus placebo significantly reduced symptoms (9 RCTs, 668 people, SMD 1.31, 95% CI 1.15 to 1.47). It also found significantly reduced symptoms with fluoxetine versus placebo (1 RCT, 287 people, change in Yale–Brown scale SMD 0.57, 95% CI 0.33 to 0.81), fluvoxamine versus placebo (3 RCTs, 395 people, SMD 0.57, 95% CI 0.37 to 0.77) and sertraline versus placebo (3 RCTs, 270 people, SMD 0.52, 95% CI 0.27 to 0.77).[17] The second review (search date not stated, 8 RCTs including 4 from the first review, 1131 people) found that clomipramine was significantly more effective than placebo (SMD 1.31; $P < 0.01$; CI not provided).[18] The third review (search date 1997, 1 study, 338 people) found that paroxetine (a selective serotonin reuptake inhibitor) versus placebo significantly reduced symptoms over 12 weeks (SMD after adjustment for method variables 0.48, 95% CI 0.24 to 0.72).[19] The first subsequent RCT (350 people) compared fluoxetine 20 mg daily versus 40 mg daily versus 60 mg daily versus placebo.[20] It found significant improvement of symptoms with all doses of fluoxetine versus placebo (improvement of Yale–Brown scale, fluoxetine 20 mg 19.5%; 40 mg 22.1%; 60 mg 26.6%; placebo 3.3%; CI not provided; all P values *v* placebo < 0.001). Larger doses produced a significantly greater response ($P < 0.001$). The second subsequent RCT (164 people) found that sertraline versus placebo significantly reduced symptoms (mean reduction of Yale–Brown scale 9 points with sertraline *v* 4 points with placebo; CI not stated; $P < 0.01$).[21] The third subsequent RCT (401 people) compared three doses of citalopram (selective serotonin reuptake inhibitor) (20 mg, 40 mg, 60 mg) versus placebo over 12 weeks.[22] It found that citalopram versus placebo significantly improved symptoms (AR for > 25% reduction in Yale–Brown scale: 57.4% with citalopram 20 mg *v* 52% with 40 mg *v* 65% with 60 mg *v* 36.6% with placebo; NNT for 20 mg citalopram *v* placebo 5, 95% CI 3 to 14). There was no significant difference between the three doses of citalopram. **Versus each other:** We found one systematic review[17] and five subsequent RCTs.[23–27] The review (search date 1994, 85 people, 3 RCTs) found no significant difference in symptoms with clomipramine versus fluoxetine or fluvoxamine (SMD –0.04, 95% CI –0.43 to +0.35).[17] The first subsequent RCT (170 people) found that sertraline versus clomipramine significantly reduced symptoms (8% greater mean reduction in Yale–Brown scale, $P = 0.036$).[23] The second subsequent RCT (133 people) found that clomipramine versus fluvoxamine did not significantly improve symptoms (change in Yale–Brown scale, 50.2% with clomipramine *v* 45.6% with fluvoxamine; CI and P value not stated).[24] The third subsequent RCT (227 people, double blind) found no significant difference with fluvoxamine (150–300 mg) versus clomipramine (150–300 mg) in severity of symptoms after 10 weeks (reduction in Yale–Brown score about 46% in both groups; P value not stated; proportion of people achieving at least 35% reduction in Yale–Brown score 62% with fluvoxamine *v* 65% with clomipramine, reported as non-significant).[25] The fourth subsequent RCT (150 people double blind) compared sertraline (50–200 mg) versus fluoxetine (20–80 mg). It found no significant difference in symptom severity at 24 weeks with sertraline versus fluoxetine (reduction in Yale–Brown score 9.6 points with sertraline *v* 9.7 points with fluoxetine, P value not stated).[26] The fifth subsequent RCT (30 people, observer blinded) compared three treatments: fluvoxamine, paroxetine, and citalopram. It found no significant difference in the effects of these drugs, but was too small to exclude a clinically important difference.[27] **Versus other antidepressants:** We found one systematic review[17] and two subsequent RCTs.[28,29] The systematic review (search date 1997, 7 RCTs, 147 people with obsessive compulsive disorder, including 67 children/adolescents) found clomipramine versus other antidepressants (desipramine, imipramine, nortripytyline, clorgyline, phenelzine) significantly reduced symptoms (SMD 0.65, 95% CI 0.36 to 0.92).[17] One subsequent RCT (54 people) of fluoxetine versus phenelzine (a monoamine-oxidase inhibitor) versus placebo found the largest symptom reduction over 10 weeks with fluoxetine (mean relative reduction in Yale–Brown scale 15% fluoxetine, 9% phenelzine, and 1% placebo).[28] The second subsequent RCT (164 people with concurrent obsessive compulsive disorder and major depressive disorder) found that sertraline versus desipramine (non-selective serotonin reuptake inhibitor) significantly reduced obsessive compulsive symptoms (> 40% improvement on Yale–Brown scale 48% with sertraline *v* 31% with desipramine, $P = 0.01$) and significantly increased the number of people with remission of depressive symptoms (< 7 on Hamilton Depression Rating Scale 49% with sertraline *v* 35% with desipramine, P = 0.04).[29] **Versus behavioural therapy:** We found one systematic review (search date 1997, number of studies and people not stated).[19] It found no significant difference in symptoms with serotonin reuptake inhibitors versus placebo or behavioural therapy versus placebo, but these conclusions must be treated with caution as the review made indirect comparisons of effect sizes.[19]

Harms: **Versus placebo:** One systematic review (search date not stated, 16 RCTs) found a greater incidence of adverse effects with serotonin reuptake inhibitors versus placebo (RRI 54% for clomipramine, 11% for fluoxetine, 19% for fluvoxamine, and 27% for sertraline).[18] An RCT that compared citalopram versus placebo found that nausea, insomnia, fatigue, sweating, dry mouth, and ejaculatory failure were significantly more common with citalopram.[22] **Versus each other:** One systematic review (search date 1997) of controlled and uncontrolled studies found the withdrawal rate because of adverse effects to be 11% for clomipramine, 10% for fluoxetine, 13% for fluvoxamine, 9% for sertraline, and 11% for paroxetine.[19] Anti cholinergic adverse effects (dry mouth, blurred vision, constipation, and urinary retention), cardiac adverse effects, drowsiness, dizziness, and convulsions (convulsions usually at doses > 250 mg/day) have been reported to be most common with the non-selective serotonin inhibitor clomipramine,[30–32] whereas selective serotonin reuptake inhibitors were associated with fewer adverse effects but more nausea, diarrhoea, anxiety, agitation, insomnia, and headache.[30] Both clomipramine and selective serotonin reuptake inhibitors were associated with weight change and sexual dysfunction.[30,32] One RCT comparing clomipramine versus fluvoxamine (227 people) found that more people stopped clomipramine prematurely (16% withdrew with clomipramaine *v* 8% with fluvoxamine; CI and P value not reported), and found that clomipramine versus fluvoxamine significantly increased the proportion of people who had anticholinergic adverse effects (dry mouth 43% with clomipramine *v* 10% with fluvoxamine; constipation 25% *v* 9%; tremor 22% *v* 9%; and dizziness 18% *v* 7%; P = 0.05 for frequency of all anticholenergic adverse effects).[25] One non-systematic review of three prospective cohort studies and five surveys found that fluoxetine during pregnancy did not significantly increase the risk of spontaneous abortion or major malformation (figures not provided).[33] The review included one prospective cohort study (174 people) and three surveys that found similar outcomes with other selective serotonin reuptake inhibitors (sertraline, paroxetine, and fluvoxamine). One prospective cohort study of 55 preschool children exposed to fluoxetine *in utero* found no significant difference from unexposed children in global IQ, language, or behaviour. It included no information on long term harms for the other selective serotonin reuptake inhibitors. The non-systematic review of effects in pregnancy did not make explicit how articles were selected.[33] **Versus other antidepressants:** One RCT (164 people) found that more people discontinued treatment because of adverse effects with desipramine than with sertraline (26% *v* 10%; P = 0.009).[29]

Comment: **Duration and discontinuation of treatment:** We found insufficient evidence to define the optimum duration of treatment. Most RCTs lasted only 10–12 weeks.[32,34] A prospective, 1 year study found further significant improvement after a 40 week open label extension of the study, with continuing adverse effects.[35] One observational study found that 16/18 (89%) people relapsed within 7 weeks of replacing clomipramine with placebo treatment.[36] One RCT (70 people who had responded to a 20 wk course of fluoxetine) found maintenance of fluoxetine versus replacement by placebo for 1 year did not significantly change the 1 year relapse rate or adverse event rate.[37] A subgroup analysis found that the risk of relapse was lower among people taking 60 mg fluoxetine at randomisation compared to people taking 40 mg, 20 mg, or placebo. But the dose of fluoxetine was not itself randomly allocated, and so this evidence does not establish that the difference in relapse was an effect of high dose fluoxetine. We found one RCT that compared continued sertraline versus placebo in 223 people with obsessive compulsive disorder, who had all previously responded to 1 years' treatment with sertraline (response defined as at least 25% reduction in Yale–Brown score from baseline).[38] People continuing on sertraline were prescribed their previous dose (mean 183 mg). It found that sertraline versus placebo significantly reduced the proportion of people who withdrew because of relapse or insufficient clinical response over 24 weeks (9% with sertraline *v* 24% with placebo; P = 0.006; CI not stated). It found that sertraline versus placebo reduced the proportion of people who had worsening of symptoms (12% with sertraline *v* 35% with placebo; P = 0.001; CI not reported), but found no significant difference in relapse rate over 24 weeks (2.7% with sertraline *v* 4.4% with placebo; P = 0.34).[38] **Effects on people without depression:** The first systematic review found that serotonin reuptake inhibitors reduced symptoms of obsessive compulsive disorder in people without depression (5 RCTs, 594 people, SMD 1.37, 95% CI 1.19 to 1.55).[17] **Factors predicting outcome:** Four RCTs found that people who did not respond to serotonin reuptake inhibitors had younger age of onset, longer duration of the condition, higher frequency of symptoms, coexisting personality disorders, and a greater likelihood of previous hospital admission. Predictors of good response were older age of onset, history of remissions, no previous drug treatment, more severe obsessive compulsive disorder, and either high or low score on the Hamilton Depression Rating Scale.[39–42] Two cohort studies of people with obsessive compulsive disorder found that poor response to serotonin reuptake inhibitors was predicted by concomitant schizotypal personality disorder (see glossary, p 1000), by tic disorder (see glossary, p 1000), and also by severe obsessive compulsive disorder with cleaning rituals (OR 4.9, 95% CI 1.1 to 21.2).[43,44]

OPTION BEHAVIOURAL THERAPY OR COGNITIVE THERAPY

We found no studies of behavioural treatment versus no treatment. One systematic review and one subsequent RCT found that behavioural therapy versus relaxation significantly reduced symptoms. The review and one subsequent RCT found no significant difference in symptoms with

behavioural therapy versus cognitive therapy. Another subsequent RCT found limited evidence that group behavioural therapy versus group cognitive therapy significantly reduced symptoms over 12 weeks. One systematic review found limited evidence from indirect comparisons of similar reductions in symptoms with behavioural therapy versus placebo, behavioural therapy plus serotonin reuptake inhibitors versus placebo, and serotonin reuptake inhibitors versus placebo. One subsequent RCT found no significant difference in symptoms with behavioural therapy, cognitive therapy, behavioural therapy plus fluvoxamine, or cognitive therapy plus fluvoxamine. Another subsequent RCT found that behavioural therapy plus fluvoxamine versus behavioural therapy alone significantly increased the proportion of people with improved symptoms after 9 weeks' treatment. Two follow up studies found significant improvement maintained for up to 2 years after behavioural treatment, although some people required additional behavioural treatment.

Benefits: **Behavioural therapy or cognitive therapy versus no treatment:** We found no systematic review or RCTs. **Behavioural therapy versus relaxation:** We found one systematic review (search date not stated, 2 RCTs, 121 people) that found that behavioural therapy (see glossary, p 999) versus relaxation significantly reduced symptoms (SMD 1.18; $P < 0.01$; CI not provided).[18] One subsequent RCT (218 people with DSM-IV obsessive compulsive disorder, 49% of whom were also taking a serotonin reuptake inhibitor that was continued after randomisation) compared three treatments: behavioural therapy guided by a computer, behavioural therapy guided by clinician, and relaxation.[45] It found limited evidence that either type of behavioural therapy versus relaxation significantly improved Yale–Brown score after 10 weeks' treatment (reduction of score 5.6 points with computer guided behavioural therapy, 8.0 points with clinician guided behavioural therapy and 1.7 points with relaxation; $P = 0.001$ for relaxation *v* either type of behavioural therapy; $P = 0.035$ for clinician guided *v* computer guided behavioural therapy; analysis not by intention to treat). **Behavioural therapy versus cognitive therapy:** We found one systematic review[18] and two subsequent RCTs.[46,47] The systematic review (search date not stated, 4 RCTs, 92 people) found no significant difference in symptoms with behavioural therapy versus cognitive therapy (see glossary, p 1000) (SMD –0.19; $P > 0.05$; CI not available).[18] The first subsequent RCT (76 people) found that group behavioural therapy (exposure with response prevention) versus group cognitive behavioural therapy improved symptoms over 12 weeks and the difference had borderline significance (mean final Yale–Brown score 13.6 with behavioural therapy *v* 16.3 with cognitive therapy; CI not stated; $P = 0.049$; 13 people lost to follow up; analysis not by intention to treat).[46] Recovery (defined as ≥6 point Yale Brown scale reduction and score ≤12) was not significantly increased immediately after treatment (AR 38% with behavioural therapy *v* 16% with cognitive therapy; $P = 0.09$), but was significantly improved after 3 months follow up (AR 45% with behavioural therapy *v* 13% with cognitive therapy; NNT 3, 95% CI 2 to 9; $P = 0.01$). The second RCT (63 people) found no significant difference with behavioural therapy versus cognitive therapy in the proportion of people achieving at least 25% improvement in Yale–Brown score after 16 weeks (OR 0.7, 95% CI 0.2 to 2.0).[47]

Behavioural therapy or cognitive therapy plus serotonin reuptake inhibitors: We found one systematic review[19] and two subsequent RCTs.[48,49] The systematic review (search date 1997, number of studies and people not stated) did not make direct comparisons between treatments.[19] In indirect comparisons, it found similar reductions in symptoms with behavioural therapy alone versus placebo, behavioural therapy plus serotonin reuptake inhibitors versus placebo, and serotonin reuptake inhibitors alone versus placebo. One subsequent RCT (99 people in an outpatient setting) compared four treatments: behavioural therapy, cognitive therapy, behavioural therapy plus fluvoxamine, and cognitive therapy plus fluvoxamine. It found no significant differences in symptoms (mean change in Yale–Brown scale 32% with behavioural therapy *v* 47% with cognitive therapy *v* 49% with behavioural therapy plus fluvoxamine *v* 43% with cognitive therapy plus fluvoxamine).[48] Another subsequent RCT (49 people in a hospital setting) found that behavioural therapy plus fluvoxamine versus behavioural therapy plus pill placebo significantly increased the proportion of people with improved symptoms after 9 weeks' treatment (number of people with > 35% reduction of Yale–Brown score 21/24 [88%] *v* 15/25 [60%]; RR 1.46, 95% CI 1.02 to 2.08).[49]

Harms: We found no evidence from RCTs or cohort studies of adverse effects from behavioural or cognitive therapy. Case reports have described unbearable and unacceptable anxiety in some people receiving behavioural therapy (see glossary, p 999).

Comment: **Factors predicting outcome:** We found two RCTs of behavioural therapy (total 96 people, duration 2.5 months and 32 wks) and two retrospective cohort studies (total 346 people, duration 1 year and 11 wks).[50–53] These found poorer outcome to be predicted by initial severity, depression, longer duration, poorer motivation, and dissatisfaction with the therapeutic relationship. Good outcome was predicted by early adherence to "exposure homework" (that is, tasks to be carried out outside regular therapy sessions involving contact with anxiety provoking situations), employment, living with one's family, no previous treatment, having fear of contamination, overt ritualistic behaviour, and absence of depression.[50–52] Good outcome for women was predicted by having a co-therapist (someone, usually related to her, who is enlisted to help with treatment outside regular treatment sessions; OR 19.5, 95% CI 2.7 to 139).[53] Two systematic reviews of drug, behavioural, cognitive, and combination treatments for obsessive compulsive disorder are being prepared. **Maintenance of improvement:** A prospective follow up (20 people with obsessive compulsive disorder, specific diagnostic criteria not provided) after a 6 month RCT of behavioural therapy found that 79% maintained improvement in obsessive compulsive symptoms at 2 years' follow up.[54] A prospective non-inception cohort study of behavioural therapy in 21 people with obsessive compulsive disorder (specific diagnostic criteria not provided) found that, after 2 weeks of treatment, 68–79% maintained complete or much improvement in symptoms at 3 months' follow up.[55] In both studies, some people received additional behavioural therapy during follow up.

QUESTION **What are the effects of treatments in adults who have not responded to initial serotonin reuptake inhibitors?**

OPTION **COMBINED ANTIPSYCHOTICS AND SEROTONIN REUPTAKE INHIBITORS**

In people who have not responded to serotonin reuptake inhibitors alone, two small RCTs found that antipsychotics combined with serotonin reuptake inhibitors reduced symptoms.

Benefits: We found no systematic review, but found two small RCTs that assessed combined antipsychotics and serotonin reuptake inhibitors in people who did not respond to serotonin treatment alone.[56,57] The first RCT (34 people with obsessive compulsive disorder who had not responded to 8 wks' treatment with fluvoxamine) compared fluvoxamine (a selective serotonin reuptake inhibitor) plus haloperidol (an antipsychotic) maximum dose of haloperidol 10 mg/day versus fluvoxamine plus placebo.[56] It found that those in the combined haloperidol plus fluvoxamine arm were significantly more likely to have met two out of three different response criteria (11/17 [65%] with combined haloperidol plus fluvoxamine *v* 0/17 [0%] with fluvoxamine plus placebo; NNT 2, 95% CI 2 to 3; P < 0.0002). The second RCT (36 people with obsessive compulsive disorder who did not respond to 12 wks of serotonin reuptake inhibitor) found that 6 weeks of risperidone (an antipsychotic) versus placebo added to the prior serotonin reuptake inhibitor significantly reduced symptoms of obsessive compulsive disorder (reduction in the Yale–Brown scale 36% *v* 9%; P = 0.001), depression (reduction in the Hamilton Depression Rating Scale 35% *v* 20%; P = 0.002), and anxiety (reduction in the Hamilton Anxiety Rating Scale 31% *v* 12%; P = 0.007).[57] People in the combined risperidone arm were more likely to have met two of the response criteria (8/18 [44%] with risperidone plus serotonin reuptake inhibitor *v* 0/15 [0%] with placebo plus serotonin reuptake inhibitor; NNT 2, 95% CI 2 to 3; P < 0.005).

Harms: One RCT of serotonin reuptake inhibitors with risperidone found that adverse effects (sedation, restlessness, increased appetite, dry mouth, or tinnitus) were experienced by at least 10% of people.[57] Risperidone is commonly associated with hypotension and prolactinaemia. Extrapyramidal adverse effects are more common with haloperidol, which can also cause prolactinaemia.

Comment: None.

GLOSSARY

Behavioural therapy Consists of exposure to the anxiety provoking stimuli and prevention of ritualistic behaviour (engaging in compulsions).

Chronic Continuous course of obsessive compulsive disorder without periods of remission since first onset.

Obsessive compulsive disorder

Cognitive therapy Aims to correct distorted thoughts (such as exaggerated sense of harm and personal responsibility) by Socratic questioning, logical reasoning, and hypothesis testing.
Episodic Episodic course of obsessive compulsive disorder with periods of remission since first onset.
Non-selective serotonin reuptake inhibitors Clomipramine, desipramine. In one systematic review, desipramine is classed as a triycyclic antidepressant.[17]
Selective serotonin reuptake inhibitors Citalopram, fluoxetine, fluvoxamine, paroxetine, and sertraline.
Schizotypal personality disorder Characterised by discomfort in close relationships, cognitive and perceptual distortions, and eccentric behaviour.
Tic disorder Characterised by motor tics, vocal tics, or both.

Substantive changes

Serotonin reuptake inhibitors Two additional RCTs comparing different serotonin reuptake inhibitors;[25,26] conclusions unchanged.
Behavioural therapy or cognitive therapy One additional RCT comparing behavioural therapies versus relaxation therapy;[45] conclusions unchanged.
Behavioural therapy or cognitive therapy One additional RCT comparing cognitive and behavioural therapies;[47] conclusions unchanged.

REFERENCES

1. American Psychiatric Association. *Diagnostic and statistical manual of mental disorders*, 4th ed. Washington, DC: APA, 1994.669–673.
2. Bebbington PE. Epidemiology of obsessive–compulsive disorder. *Br J Psychiatry* 1998;35(suppl.):2–6.
3. Karno M, Golding JM, Sorenson SB, et al. The epidemiology of obsessive–compulsive disorder in five US communities. *Arch Gen Psychiatry* 1988;45:1094–1099.
4. Baer L, Minichiello WE. Behavior therapy for obsessive–compulsive disorder. In: Jenike MA, Baer L, Minichiello WE, eds. *Obsessive–compulsive disorders*. St Louis: Mosby, 1998: 337–367.
5. Steketee GS, Frost RO, Rheaume J, et al. Cognitive theory and treatment of obsessive–compulsive disorder. In: Jenike MA, Baer L, Minichiello WE, eds. *Obsessive–compulsive disorders*. St Louis: Mosby, 1998: 368–399.
6. Alsobrook JP, Pauls DL. The genetics of obsessive–compulsive disorder. In: Jenike MA, Baer L, Minichiello WE, eds. *Obsessive–compulsive disorders*. St Louis: Mosby, 1998: 276–288.
7. Rauch SL, Whalen PJ, Dougherty D, et al. Neurobiologic models of obsessive compulsive disorder. In: Jenike MA, Baer L, Minichiello WE, eds. *Obsessive–compulsive disorders*. St Louis: Mosby, 1998: 222–253.
8. Delgado PL, Moreno FA. Different roles for serotonin in anti-obsessional drug action and the pathophysiology of obsessive–compulsive disorder. *Br J Psychiatry* 1998;35(suppl.):21–25.
9. Saxena S, Brody AL, Schwartz JM, et al. Neuroimaging and frontal–subcortical circuitry in obsessive–compulsive disorder. *Br J Psychiatry* 1998;35(suppl.):26–37.
10. Rauch SL, Baxter LR Jr. Neuroimaging in obsessive–compulsive disorder and related disorders. In: Jenike MA, Baer L, Minichiello WE, eds. *Obsessive–compulsive disorders*. St Louis: Mosby, 1998: 289–317.
11. Skoog G, Skoog I. A 40-year follow up of patients with obsessive–compulsive disorder. *Arch Gen Psychiatry* 1999;56:121–127.
12. Ravizza L, Maina G, Bogetto F. Episodic and chronic obsessive–compulsive disorder. *Depress Anxiety* 1997;6:154–158.
13. Goodman WK, Price LH, Rasmussen SA, et al. The Yale–Brown obsessive compulsive scale. I. Development, use, and reliability. *Arch Gen Psychiatry* 1989;46:1006–1011.
14. Insel TR, Murphy DL, Cohen RM, et al. Obsessive–compulsive disorder. A double-blind trial of clomipramine and clorgyline. *Arch Gen Psychiatry* 1983;40:605–612.
15. Goodman WK, Price LH, Rasmussen SA, et al. The Yale–Brown obsessive compulsive scale. II. Validity. *Arch Gen Psychiatry* 1989;46:1012–1016.
16. Goodman WK, Price LH. Rating scales for obsessive–compulsive disorder. In: Jenike MA, Baer L, Minichiello WE, eds. *Obsessive–compulsive disorders*. St Louis: Mosby, 1998: 97–117.
17. Piccinelli M, Pini S, Bellantuono C, et al. Efficacy of drug treatment in obsessive–compulsive disorder. A meta-analytic review. *Br J Psychiatry* 1995;166:424–443. Search dates 1994; primary sources Medline and Excerpta Medica-Psychiatry.
18. Abramowitz JS. Effectiveness of psychological and pharmacological treatments for obsessive–compulsive disorder: a quantitative review. *J Consult Clin Psychol* 1997;65:44–52. Search date not stated; primary sources Medline and PsycLIT.
19. Kobak KA, Greist JH, Jefferson JW, et al. Behavioral versus pharmacological treatments of obsessive compulsive disorder: a meta-analysis. *Psychopharmacology (Berl)* 1998;136:205–216. Search date 1997; primary sources Medline, PsycINFO, Dissertations, and Abstracts International databases.
20. Tollefson GD, Rampey AH, Potvin JH, et al. A multicenter investigation of fixed-dose fluoxetine in the treatment of obsessive–compulsive disorder. *Arch Gen Psychiatry* 1994;51:559–567.
21. Kronig MH, Apter J, Asnis G, et al. Placebo controlled multicentre study of sertraline treatment for obsessive–compulsive disorder. *J Clin Psychopharmacol* 1999;19:172–176.

22. Montgomery SA, Kasper S, Stein DJ, et al. Citalopram 20 mg, 40 mg and 60 mg are all effective and well tolerated compared with placebo in obsessive-compulsive disorder. *Int Clin Psychopharmacol* 2001;16:75–86.
23. Bisserbe JC, Lane RM, Flament MF. A double blind comparison of sertraline and clomipramine in outpatients with obsessive–compulsive disorder. *Eur Psychiatry* 1997;12:82–93.
24. Mundo E, Maina G, Uslenghi C. Multicentre, double-blind, comparison of fluvoxamine and clomipramine in the treatment of obsessive–compulsive disorder. *Int Clin Psychopharmacol* 2000;15:69–76.
25. Mundo E, Rouillon F, Figuera L, et al. Fluvoxamine in obsessive-compulsive disorder: Similar efficacy but superior tolerability in comparison with clomipramine. *Hum Psychopharmacol* 2001;16:461–468.
26. Bergeron R, Ravindran AV, Chaput Y, et al. Sertraline and fluoxetine treatment of obsessive-compulsive disorder: Results of a double-blind, 6-month treatment study. *J Clin Psychopharmacol* 2002;22:148–154.
27. Mundo E, Bianchi L, Bellodi L. Efficacy of fluvoxamine, paroxetine, and citalopram in the treatment of obsessive–compulsive disorder: a single-blind study. *J Clin Psychopharmacol* 1997;17:267–271.
28. Jenike MA, Baer L, Minichiello WE, et al. Placebo-controlled trial of fluoxetine and phenelzine for obsessive–compulsive disorder. *Am J Psychiatry* 1997;154:1261–1264.
29. Hoehn-Saric R, Ninan P, Black DW, et al. Multicenter double-blind comparison of sertraline and desipramine for concurrent obsessive–compulsive and major depressive disorders. *Arch Gen Psychiatry* 2000;57:76–82.
30. BMJ Books and Pharmaceutical Press. *British national formulary*. London: British Medical Association and Royal Pharmaceutical Society of Great Britain, 2002.
31. Trindade E, Menon D. Selective serotonin reuptake inhibitors differ from tricyclic antidepressants in adverse events (Abstract). Selective serotonin reuptake inhibitors for major depression. Part 1. Evaluation of clinical literature. Ottawa: Canadian Coordinating Office for Health Technology Assessment, August 1997 Report 3E. *Evid Based Ment Health* 1998;1:50.
32. Jenike MA. Drug treatment of obsessive–compulsive disorders. In: Jenike MA, Baer L, Minichiello WE, eds. *Obsessive–compulsive disorders*. St Louis: Mosby, 1998:469–532.
33. Goldstein DJ, Sundell K. A review of safety of selective serotonin reuptake inhibitors during pregnancy. *Hum Psychopharmacol Clin Exp* 1999;14:319–324.
34. Rauch SL, Jenike MA. Pharmacological treatment of obsessive compulsive disorder. In: Nathan PE, Gorman JM, eds. *Treatments that work*. New York: Oxford University Press, 1998:359–376.
35. Rasmussen S, Hackett E, DuBoff E, et al. A 2-year study of sertraline in the treatment of obsessive–compulsive disorder. *Int Clin Psychopharmacol* 1997;12:309–316.
36. Pato MT, Zohar-Kadouch R, Zohar J, et al. Return of symptoms after discontinuation of clomipramine in patients with obsessive–compulsive disorder. *Am J Psychiatry* 1988;145:1521–1525.
37. Romano S, Goodman W, Tamura R, et al. Long-term treatment of obsessive-compulsive disorder after an acute response: a comparison of fluoxetine versus placebo. *J Clin Psychopharmacol* 2001;21:46–52.
38. Koran LM, Hackett E, Rubin A, et al. Efficacy of sertraline in the long-term treatment of obsessive-compulsive disorder. *Am J Psychiatry* 2002;159:88–95.
39. Ravizza L, Barzega G, Bellino S, et al. Predictors of drug treatment response in obsessive–compulsive disorder. *J Clin Psychiatry* 1995;56:368–373.
40. Cavedini P, Erzegovesi S, Ronchi P, et al. Predictive value of obsessive–compulsive personality disorder in antiobsessional pharmacological treatment. *Eur Neuropsychopharmacol* 1997;7:45–49.
41. Ackerman DL, Greenland S, Bystritsky A. Clinical characteristics of response to fluoxetine treatment of obsessive–compulsive disorder. *J Clin Psychopharmacol* 1998;18:185–192.
42. Ackerman DL, Greenland S, Bystritsky A, et al. Predictors of treatment response in obsessive–compulsive disorder: multivariate analyses from a multicenter trial of clomipramine. *J Clin Psychopharmacol* 1994;14:247–254.
43. Mundo E, Erzegovesi S, Bellodi L. Follow up of obsessive–compulsive patients treated with proserotonergic agents (letter). *J Clin Psychopharmacol* 1995;15:288–289.
44. Alarcon RD, Libb JW, Spitler D. A predictive study of obsessive–compulsive disorder response to clomipramine. *J Clin Psychopharmacol* 1993;13:210–213.
45. Greist JH, Marks IM, Baer L, et al. Behavior therapy for obsessive-compulsive disorder guided by a computer or by a clinician compared with relaxation as a control. *J Clin Psychiatry* 2002;63:138–145.
46. McLean PD, Whittal ML, Thordarson DS, et al. Cognitive versus behavior therapy in the group treatment of obsessive-compulsive disorder. *J Consult Clin Psychol* 2001;69:205–214.
47. Cottraux J, Note I, Yao SN, et al. A randomized controlled trial of cognitive therapy versus intensive behavior therapy in obsessive compulsive disorder. *Psychother Psychosom* 2001;70:288–297.
48. van Balkom AJ, de Haan E, van Oppen P, et al. Cognitive and behavioral therapies alone versus in combination with fluvoxamine in the treatment of obsessive compulsive disorder. *J Nerv Ment Dis* 1998;186:492–499.
49. Hohagen F, Winkelmann G, Rasche-Ruchle H, et al. Combination of behaviour therapy with fluvoxamine in comparison with behaviour therapy and placebo. Results of a multicentre study. *Br J Psychiatry* 1998;35(suppl.):71–78.
50. Keijsers GP, Hoogduin CA, Schaap CP. Predictors of treatment outcome in the behavioural treatment of obsessive–compulsive disorder. *Br J Psychiatry* 1994;165:781–786.
51. De Araujo LA, Ito LM, Marks IM. Early compliance and other factors predicting outcome of exposure for obsessive–compulsive disorder. *Br J Psychiatry* 1996;169:747–752.
52. Buchanan AW, Meng KS, Marks IM. What predicts improvement and compliance during the behavioral treatment of obsessive compulsive disorder? *Anxiety* 1996;2:22–27.
53. Castle DJ, Deale A, Marks IM, et al. Obsessive–compulsive disorder: prediction of outcome from behavioural psychotherapy. *Acta Psychiatr Scand* 1994;89:393–398.
54. Marks IM, Hodgson R, Rachman S. Treatment of chronic obsessive–compulsive neurosis by in-vivo exposure. A two-year follow up and issues in treatment. *Br J Psychiatry* 1975;127:349–364.
55. Foa EB, Goldstein A. Continuous exposure and complete response prevention in obsessive–compulsive neurosis. *Behav Ther* 1978;9:821–829.

56. McDougle CJ, Goodman WK, Leckman JF, et al. Haloperidol addition in fluvoxamine-refractory obsessive-compulsive disorder. A double-blind, placebo-controlled study in patients with and without tics. *Arch Gen Psychiatry* 1994;51:302–308.

57. McDougle CJ, Epperson CN, Pelton GH, et al. A double-blind, placebo-controlled study of risperidone addition in serotonin reuptake inhibitor-refractory obsessive-compulsive disorder. *Arch Gen Psychiatry* 2000;57:794–801.

G Mustafa Soomro
Honorary Research Fellow
Section of Community Psychiatry
St George's Hospital Medical School
London, UK

Competing interests: None declared.

Panic disorder

Search date May 2002

Shailesh Kumar and Mark Oakley-Browne

QUESTIONS

INTERVENTIONS

See glossary, p 1008

Key Messages

- **Benzodiazepines** One systematic review and one additional RCT have found that alprazolam versus placebo significantly reduces the number of panic attacks and improves symptoms. However, benzodiazepines are associated with a wide range of adverse effects both during their use and after treatment has been withdrawn.
- **Buspirone** RCTs found insufficient evidence on the effects of buspirone versus placebo.
- **Monoamine oxidase inhibitors** We found no RCTs on the effects of monoamine oxidase inhibitors.
- **Selective serotonin reuptake inhibitors** Systematic reviews and one additional RCT have found that selective serotonin reuptake inhibitors versus placebo improve symptoms in panic disorder. One RCT found that discontinuation of sertraline in people with a good response significantly increased exacerbation of symptoms.
- **Tricyclic antidepressants (imipramine)** One systematic review and subsequent RCTs have found that imipramine versus placebo significantly improves symptoms. One RCT found that imipramine significantly reduced relapse rates over 12 months (NNT 5, 95% CI 3 to 14).

Panic disorder

DEFINITION A panic attack is a period in which there is sudden onset of intense apprehension, fearfulness, or terror often associated with feelings of impending doom. Panic disorder occurs when there are recurrent, unpredictable attacks followed by at least 1 month of persistent concern about having another panic attack, worry about the possible implications or consequences of the panic attacks, or a significant behavioural change related to the attacks.[1] The term panic disorder excludes panic attacks attributable to the direct physiological effects of a general medical condition, substance, or another mental disorder. Panic disorder is sometimes categorised as with or without agoraphobia.[1] Alternative categorisations focus on phobic anxiety disorders and specify agoraphobia with or without panic disorder.[2]

INCIDENCE/ PREVALENCE Panic disorder often starts around 20 years of age (between late adolescence and the mid-30s).[3] Lifetime prevalence is 1–3%, and panic disorder is more common in women than in men.[4] An Australian community study found 1 month prevalence rates for panic disorder (with or without agoraphobia) of 0.4% using International Classification of Diseases (ICD)-10 diagnostic criteria and of 0.5% using Diagnostic and Statistical Manual (DSM)-IV diagnostic criteria.[5]

AETIOLOGY/ RISK FACTORS Stressful life events tend to precede the onset of panic disorder,[6,7] although a negative interpretation of these events in addition to their occurrence has been suggested as an important causal factor.[8] Panic disorder is associated with major depression,[9] social phobia, generalised anxiety disorder, obsessive compulsive disorder,[10] and a substantial risk of drug and alcohol abuse.[11] It is also associated with avoidant, histrionic, and dependent personality disorders.[10]

PROGNOSIS The severity of symptoms in people with panic disorder fluctuates considerably, with periods of no attacks, or only mild attacks with few symptoms, being common. There is often a long delay between the initial onset of symptoms and presentation for treatment. Recurrent attacks may continue for several years, especially if associated with agoraphobia. Reduced social or occupational functioning varies among people with panic disorder and is worse in people with associated agoraphobia. Panic disorder is also associated with an increased rate of attempted but unsuccessful suicide.[12]

AIMS To reduce the severity and frequency of panic attacks, phobic avoidance, and anticipatory anxiety; to improve social and occupational functioning, with minimal adverse effects of treatment.

OUTCOMES Measures of panic attacks, agoraphobia, and associated disability (self reported and clinician rated, before and after treatment, and longer term) using general scales or specific scales for panic disorder (e.g. the panic and agoraphobia scale, the mobility inventory for agoraphobia).

METHODS *Clinical Evidence* search and appraisal May 2002. Studies with follow up periods of less than 6 months were excluded.

QUESTION **What are the effects of drug treatments for panic disorder?**

OPTION **TRICYCLIC ANTIDEPRESSANTS**

One systematic review and subsequent RCTs have found that imipramine versus placebo improves symptoms in people with panic disorder. One RCT found that imipramine reduced relapse rates in people with panic disorder.

Benefits: We found one systematic review,[13] one additional RCT,[14] and two subsequent RCTs.[15,16] The systematic review (search date not stated, 27 RCTs, 2348 people) compared imipramine, selective serotonin reuptake inhibitors (paroxetine, fluvoxamine, zimelidine, and clomipramine; see comment below) and alprazolam versus placebo and versus each other (see benefits of selective serotonin reuptake inhibitors, p 1006 and benzodiazepines, p 1008).[13] It found that imipramine versus placebo significantly increased the number of people judged to have improved ($P < 0.0001$; see comment below). The additional RCT (181 people with panic disorder with or without agoraphobia) compared three treatments: oral imipramine (maximum dose 225 mg; see comment below); oral alprazolam (maximum dose 10 mg; see comment below); and placebo (see benefits of benzodiazepines, p 1008).[14] It found that imipramine versus placebo reduced the number of panic attacks after 8 months (results presented graphically, significance not calculated). The first subsequent RCT (56 adults with panic disorder and agoraphobia in stable remission after 24 wks' treatment with oral imipramine) comparing oral imipramine (2.25 mg/kg daily) versus placebo found that significantly fewer people taking imipramine relapsed after 12 months (see comment below; 1/29 [3%] with imipramine *v* 10/27 [37%] with placebo; RR 0.09, 95% CI 0.01 to 0.68; NNT 5, 95% CI 3 to 14).[16] The second subsequent RCT (312 people) compared five groups: oral imipramine (maximum dose 300 mg daily; see comment below); cognitive behavioural therapy (see glossary, p 1008); placebo; cognitive behavioural therapy plus oral imipramine (maximum dose 300 mg daily; see comment below); and cognitive behavioural therapy plus placebo.[15] It found that imipramine versus placebo significantly increased the number of people judged to have responded using the panic disorder severity scale after 6 months (38% response rate with imipramine *v* 13% response rate with placebo; absolute numbers not provided; $P = 0.02$).

Harms: Adverse effects associated with imipramine treatment included blurred vision, tachycardia, palpitations, blood pressure changes, insomnia, nervousness, malaise, dizziness, headache, nausea, vomiting, and reduced appetite (see harms of prescription antidepressant drugs under depressive disorders, p 951).[14,17]

Comment: The review included clomipramine as a serotonin reuptake inhibitor. This drug is also often described as a tricyclic antidepressant.[13] The review used improvement as an outcome measure without a clear definition of this term. In the additional RCT and the second subsequent RCT, flexible dosing was used according to tolerance and therapeutic need.[14,15] In the subsequent RCT comparing imipramine versus placebo, relapse rate was not clearly defined.[16]

OPTION SELECTIVE SEROTONIN REUPTAKE INHIBITORS

Systematic reviews and one additional RCT have found that selective serotonin reuptake inhibitors versus placebo improve symptoms in panic disorder. One RCT found that discontinuation of sertraline in people with a good response significantly increased exacerbation of symptoms.

Benefits: We found two systematic reviews (see benefits of tricyclic antidepressants, p 1005 and benzodiazepines, p 1008),[13,18] one additional RCT,[20] and one subsequent RCT.[19] The first systematic review (search date not stated, 27 RCTs, 2348 people) found that selective serotonin reuptake inhibitors (paroxetine, fluvoxamine, zimelidine, and clomipramine; see comment below) versus placebo significantly increased the number of people who improved ($P < 0.0001$; see comment below).[13] The second systematic review (search date not stated, 12 RCTs, 1741 people) only reported combined results as an effect size against placebo (effect size 0.55), and did not report statistical significance.[18] The additional RCT (279 people) compared five groups: oral citalopram (10 or 15 mg daily); oral citalopram (20 or 30 mg daily); oral citalopram (40 or 60 mg daily); oral clomipramine (60 or 90 mg daily); and placebo.[20] It found that citalopram (at all doses) versus placebo significantly increased the number of people who responded (defined as no panic attacks and either no episodic increases in anxiety or only slight increases in anxiety precipitated by definite events or activities) after 12 months (citalopram 10 or 15 mg daily *v* placebo; $P = 0.05$; citalopram 20 or 30 mg daily *v* placebo; $P = 0.001$; citalopram 40 or 60 mg daily *v* placebo; $P = 0.003$; results presented graphically). The subsequent RCT (182 people who had responded to open label sertraline for 52 wks) compared double blind placebo (discontinuation of sertraline) versus sertraline for 28 weeks.[19] It found significantly more people on placebo had exacerbation of symptoms (33% with placebo *v* 13% with sertraline; $P = 0.005$; CI not available).

Harms: The additional RCT reported that harms associated with citalopram included headache, tremor, dry mouth, and somnolence (see harms of prescription antidepressant drugs under depressive disorders, p 951).[20]

Comment: The first review included clomipramine as a selective serotonin reuptake inhibitor, although this drug is often described as a tricyclic antidepressant.[13] In addition, the review used improvement as an outcome measure without clearly defining this term. In the additional RCT, only just over half of people (28/54 [52%]) completed the trial; analysis was by intention to treat and people who withdrew from the trial were counted as treatment failures.[20] The RCT used flexible dosing according to tolerance and therapeutic need. Selective serotonin reuptake inhibitors can cause initial increased anxiety, which can exacerbate a tendency to focus on internal sensations and to avoid situations that trigger these sensations (catastrophise somatic sensations). Education about this event is likely to improve adherence with medication. The second systematic review found smaller RCTs were associated with larger effect sizes suggesting the possibility of publication bias.[18]

OPTION MONOAMINE OXIDASE INHIBITORS

We found no evidence on the effects of monoamine oxidase inhibitors in panic disorder.

Benefits: We found no systematic review and no RCTs.

Harms: We found no evidence of harms associated specifically with the use of monoamine oxidase inhibitors in the long term treatment of panic disorder.

Comment: Our search strategy excluded studies with follow up of less than 6 months.

OPTION BUSPIRONE

Two RCTs found insufficient evidence on the effects of buspirone in people with panic disorder.

Benefits: We found no systematic review but found two RCTs.[21,22] The first RCT (48 people) compared oral buspirone (maximum 60 mg daily) plus cognitive behavioural therapy (see glossary, p 1008) versus placebo plus cognitive behavioural therapy for 16 weeks.[21] It found that oral buspirone plus cognitive behavioural therapy significantly improved self rated panic and agoraphobia scores after 1 year (using a 90 point symptom scale where each symptom was graded from 0 = not present to 4 = severe; P = 0.03; absolute numbers not provided). The second RCT (41 people with panic disorder and agoraphobia) compared 16 weeks of oral buspirone (30 mg daily) plus cognitive behavioural therapy versus 16 weeks of placebo plus cognitive behavioural therapy.[22] It found no significant difference in the number of people who had a reduction of at least 50% in their agoraphobic symptoms after 68 weeks (44% with buspirone plus cognitive behavioural therapy *v* 68% with placebo plus cognitive behavioural therapy; absolute numbers of people not provided).

Harms: The RCTs did not report harms (see harms of buspirone under generalised anxiety disorder, p 974).

Comment: The first RCT used a flexible dosing regimen with maximum dose adjustment according to tolerance and therapeutic need.[21]

OPTION BENZODIAZEPINES

One systematic review and one additional RCT have found that alprazolam reduces the numbers of panic attacks and improves symptoms in people with panic disorder. Benzodiazepines are associated with a wide range of adverse effects both during their use and after treatment has been withdrawn.

Benefits: We found one systematic review (search date not stated, 27 RCTs, 2348 people; see benefits of tricyclic antidepressants, p 1005 and see benefits of selective serotonin reuptake inhibitors, p 1006),[13] and one additional RCT.[14] The review found that alprazolam versus placebo significantly increased the number of people judged to have improved ($P < 0.0001$; see comment below).[13] The additional RCT (181 people with panic disorder with or without agoraphobia) compared three treatments: oral alprazolam (maximum 10 mg daily; see comment below), oral imipramine (maximum 225 mg daily; see comment below), and placebo (see benefits of tricyclic antidepressants, p 1005 and selective serotonin reuptake inhibitors, p 1006).[14] It found that alprazolam versus placebo was associated with fewer panic attacks after 8 months (results presented graphically; significance not calculated).

Harms: The systematic review did not report harms.[13] Adverse effects associated with alprazolam include sedation, insomnia, memory lapses, nervousness, irritability, dry mouth, tremor, impaired coordination, constipation, urinary retention, altered libido, and altered appetite (see harms of benzodiazepines under generalised anxiety disorder, p 974).[14] We found one non-systematic review of the effects of benzodiazepines in anxiety disorder in people with a history of substance abuse or dependence.[23] The review reported that the mortality of long term benzodiazepine users was no higher than matched controls. It reported that the most pronounced adverse effects followed sudden withdrawal and included tinnitus, paraesthesia, vision disturbance, depersonalisation, seizures, withdrawal psychosis, and persistent discontinuation syndrome.

Comment: The review used improvement as an outcome measure without clearly defining this term.[13] The additional RCT used flexible dosing according to tolerance and therapeutic need.[14] Many RCTs of psychological and pharmacological treatments (even those not involving benzodiazepines) allowed people to receive small amounts of anxiolytic drugs during the study because benzodiazepine abuse is quite prevalent in people who suffer from panic disorder.

GLOSSARY

Cognitive behavioural therapy Brief structured treatment using relaxation and exposure procedures, and aimed at changing dysfunctional beliefs and negative automatic thoughts (typically 20 sessions over 12–16 wks).

Substantive changes

Selective serotonin reuptake inhibitors One new systematic review[18] and one new RCT.[19] The RCT found that discontinuation of sertraline in people with a good response significantly increased symptom exacerbation.

REFERENCES

1. American Psychiatric Association. *Diagnostic and statistical manual of mental disorders*, 4th ed. Washington, DC: American Psychiatric Association, 1994.
2. World Health Organization. *The ICD-10 classification of mental and behavioural disorders*. Geneva: World Health Organization, 1992.
3. Robins LN, Regier DA, eds. *Psychiatric disorders in America: the epidemiologic catchment area study*. New York, NY: Free Press, 1991.
4. Weissman MM, Bland MB, Canino GJ, et al. The cross-national epidemiology of panic disorder. *Arch Gen Psychiatry* 1997;54:305–309.
5. Andrews G, Henderson S, Hall W. Prevalence, comorbidity, disability and service utilisation. Overview of the Australian National Mental Health Survey. *Br J Psychiatry* 2001;178:145–153.
6. Last CG, Barlow DH, O'Brien GT. Precipitants of agoraphobia: role of stressful life events. *Psychol Rep* 1984;54:567–570.

7. De Loof C, Zandbergen H, Lousberg T, et al. The role of life events in the onset of panic disorder. *Behav Res Ther* 1989;27:461–463.
8. Rapee RM, Mattick RP, Murrell E. Impact of life events on subjects with panic disorder and on comparison subjects. *Am J Psychiatry* 1990;147:640–644.
9. Hirschfield RMA. Panic disorder: diagnosis, epidemiology and clinical course. *J Clin Psychiatry* 1996;57:3–8.
10. Andrews G, Creamer M, Crino R, et al. *The treatment of anxiety disorders*. Cambridge: Cambridge University Press, 1994.
11. Page AC, Andrews G. Do specific anxiety disorders show specific drug problems? *Aust N Z J Psychiatry* 1996;30:410–414.
12. Gorman JM, Coplan JD. Comorbidity of depression and panic disorder. *J Clin Psychiatry* 1996;57:34–41.
13. Boyer W. Serotonin uptake inhibitors are superior to imipramine and alprazolam in alleviating panic attacks: a meta-analysis. *Int Clin Psychopharmacol* 1995;10:45–49. Search date not stated; primary sources Medline, Embase, Psychlit, and sponsoring agencies of two trials contacted for supplementary statistical information.
14. Curtis GC, Massana J, Udina C, et al. Maintenance drug therapy of panic disorder. *J Psychiatr Res* 1993;27:127–142.
15. Barlow DH, Gorman J, Shear MK, et al. Cognitive-behavioral therapy, imipramine, or their combination for panic disorder: a randomized controlled trial. *JAMA* 2000;283:2529–2536.
16. Mavissakalian MR, Perel JM. Long-term maintenance and discontinuation of imipramine therapy in panic disorder with agoraphobia. *Arch Gen Psychiatry* 1999;56:821–827.
17. Cassano GB, Toni C, Petracca A, et al. Adverse effects associated with the short-term treatment of panic disorder with imipramine, alprazolam or placebo. *Eur Neuropsychopharmacol* 1994;4:47–53.
18. Otto M, Tuby K, Gould R, et al. An effect-size analysis of the relative efficacy and tolerability of serotonin selective reuptake inhibitors for panic disorder. *Am J Psychiatry* 2001;158:1989–1992. Search date not stated; primary sources Medline, Psychlit, and hand searched references.
19. Rapaport M, Wolkow R, Rubin A, et al. Sertraline treatment of panic disorder: results of a long term study. *Acta Psych Scand* 2001;104:289–298.
20. Lepola UM, Wade AG, Leinonen EV, et al. A controlled, prospective, 1-year trial of citalopram in the treatment of panic disorder. *J Clin Psychiatry* 1998;59:528–534.
21. Bouvard M, Mollard E, Guerin J, et al. Study and course of the psychological profile in 77 patients expressing panic disorder with agoraphobia after cognitive behaviour therapy with or without buspirone. *Psychother Psychosom* 1997;66:27–32.
22. Cottraux J, Note ID, Cungi C, et al. A controlled study of cognitive behaviour therapy with buspirone or placebo in panic disorder with agoraphobia. *Br J Psychiatry* 1995;167:635–641.
23. Posternak M, Mueller T. Assessing the risks and benefits of benzodiazepines for anxiety disorders in patients with a history of substance abuse or dependence. *Am J Addict* 2001;10:48–68.

Shailesh Kumar
Division of Psychiatry
Auckland Medical School
Auckland
New Zealand

Mark Oakley Browne
Professor of Rural Psychiatry
Monash University
Gippsland, Victoria
Australia

Competing interests: SK was reimbursed by Eli-Lilly, the manufacturers of Prozac (fluoxetine), to attend two psychiatric symposia. MOB has been paid by GlaxoSmithKline, the manufacturer of Aropax (paroxetine), for contributing to educational sessions for general practitioners. The programme topic was “The recognition and management of generalized anxiety disorder”.

Post-traumatic stress disorder

Search date January 2002

Jonathan Bisson

QUESTIONS

INTERVENTIONS

PREVENTION

Likely to be beneficial

Multiple episode cognitive behavioural therapy or prolonged exposure therapy versus supportive counselling in people with acute stress disorder. .1012

Unknown effectiveness

Multiple episode cognitive behavioural therapy or prolonged exposure therapy versus no treatment or versus standard care in all people exposed to a traumatic event 1012

Unlikely to be beneficial

Single episode psychological interventions ("debriefing") .1012

TREATMENT

Beneficial

Cognitive behavioural therapies/exposure therapies..............1014

Eye movement desensitisation and reprocessing........1014

Sertraline................1015

Paroxetine New 1015

Unknown effectiveness

Supportive counselling......1014

Inpatient programmes......1014

Affect management........1014

Psychodynamic psychotherapy..........1014

Hypnotherapy............1014

Drama therapy 1014

Other drug treatments (fluoxetine, brofaromine, amitriptyline, lamotrigine, benzodiazepines, antipsychotics, carbamazepine, imipramine, or phenelzine) .1015

See glossary, p 1016

Key Messages

Prevention

- **Multiple episode cognitive behavioural therapy or prolonged exposure therapy versus supportive counselling** Two small RCTs in people with acute stress disorder after a traumatic event (accident or non-sexual assault) found that five sessions of either cognitive behavioural therapy or prolonged exposure versus supportive counselling significantly reduced the number of people with post-traumatic stress disorder after 6 months.
- **Multiple episode cognitive behavioural therapy versus no treatment or standard care** One RCT found that 1–6 sessions of cognitive behavioural therapy versus standard care improved anxiety and intrusive symptoms measures, but there were no significant differences in depression or avoidance symptom measures at 6 months.

- **Single episode psychological interventions (debriefing)** One systematic review in people who had been exposed to a traumatic event in the previous month found no significant difference between debriefing versus no debriefing in the incidence of post-traumatic stress disorder at 3 months or 1 year.

Treatment

- **Cognitive behavioural therapies** RCTs have found that cognitive behavioural therapies versus no treatment or supportive counselling significantly improve post-traumatic stress disorder symptoms, anxiety, and depression.
- **Eye movement desensitisation and reprocessing** RCTs have found that eye movement desensitisation and reprocessing versus waiting list control or relaxation treatment improves symptoms. Two RCTs found no significant difference between eye movement desensitisation and reprocessing versus exposure therapy in improving symptoms.
- **Paroxetine** One systematic review and subsequent RCTs found evidence that paroxetine versus placebo reduced symptoms at 3 months.
- **Sertraline** One systematic review found evidence that sertraline versus placebo significantly reduced symptoms at up to 6 months.
- **Affect management; drama therapy; hypnotherapy; inpatient programmes; other drug treatments (fluoxetine, brofaromine, amitriptyline, lamotrigine, benzodiazepines, antipsychotics, carbamazepine, imipramine, or phenelzine); psychodynamic psychotherapy; and supportive counselling** We found insufficient evidence of the effects of these interventions in improving symptoms.

DEFINITION Post-traumatic stress disorder (PTSD) can occur after a major traumatic event. Symptoms include upsetting thoughts and nightmares about the traumatic event, avoidance behaviour, numbing of general responsiveness, increased irritability, and hypervigilance.[1]

INCIDENCE/ PREVALENCE One large cross sectional study in the USA found that 1/10 (10%) women and 1/20 (5%) men experience PTSD at some stage in their lives.[2]

AETIOLOGY/ RISK FACTORS Risk factors include major trauma such as rape, a history of psychiatric disorders, acute distress and depression after the trauma, lack of social support, and personality factors (such as neuroticism).[3]

PROGNOSIS One large cross sectional study in the USA found that over a third of sufferers continued to satisfy the criteria for a diagnosis of PTSD 6 years after diagnosis.[2] Cross sectional studies provide weak evidence about prognosis.

AIMS To reduce initial distress after a traumatic event; to prevent PTSD and other psychiatric disorders; to reduce levels of distress in the long term; and to improve function and quality of life.

OUTCOMES Presence or absence of PTSD and severity of symptoms. Scoring systems include impact of event scale and clinician administered PTSD scale.

METHODS *Clinical Evidence* update search and appraisal January 2002.

QUESTION **What are the effects of preventive psychological interventions?**

One systematic review in people who had been exposed to a traumatic event in the previous month found no significant difference between debriefing versus no debriefing in the incidence of post-traumatic stress disorder at 3 months or 1 year. Two small RCTs in people with acute stress disorder after a traumatic event (accident or non-sexual assault) found that five sessions of either cognitive behavioural therapy or prolonged exposure versus supportive counselling significantly reduced the number of people with post-traumatic stress disorder after 6 months. One RCT found that 1–6 sessions of cognitive behavioural therapy versus standard care improved anxiety and intrusive symptoms measures, but there were no significant differences in depression or avoidance symptom measures at 6 months. One RCT found that a social work intervention improved outcome more than an immediate debriefing or no intervention. One RCT found no significant difference between collaborative care and no intervention for preventing post-traumatic stress disorder at 4 months, although it may have lacked power to exclude a clinically important effect.

Benefits: **Single episode intervention:** We found one systematic review (search date 2001, 11 RCTs, 1759 people) comparing early (within 1 month) single episode interventions ("debriefing") versus no intervention,[4] and one subsequent RCT.[5] The RCTs in the review used psychological debriefing (see glossary, p 1017) or similar techniques after traumatic events. The review found that debriefing was associated with a non-significant increase in the risk of post-traumatic stress disorder (PTSD) at 3 months and 1 year (OR at 3 months 1.1, 95% CI 0.6 to 2.5; OR at 12 months 2.0, 95% CI 0.9 to 4.5). One subsequent RCT (77 people who had been robbed) compared early group debriefing (within 10 h) versus delayed group debriefing (after > 48 h). Early debriefing reduced symptom severity measured on the Post-traumatic Stress Diagnostic Scale at 2 weeks compared with delayed debriefing (early debriefing: mean score 6.94, delayed debriefing: mean 33.10, $P < 0.001$).[5]
Multiple episode intervention: We found no systematic review. We found six RCTs. The first RCT (70 people) compared three treatments: social work intervention (emotional, practical, and social support for 2–10 h in the first 3 months); immediate review (a single debriefing type intervention), and no intervention after a road traffic accident.[6] The social work intervention reduced the risk of a poor outcome (based on traumatic neurosis symptoms) compared with immediate review, although both interventions reduced the risk of a poor outcome compared with no intervention (AR for poor outcome 87% with no intervention *v* 60% with immediate review *v* 30% with social work; ARR for social work *v* no intervention 57%, NNT 2; ARR for immediate review *v* no intervention 27%, NNT 4; CI not provided; $P < 0.001$ for either intervention group *v* no intervention; $P < 0.05$ for comparison between the intervention groups). The second RCT (151 people) compared 3–6 sessions of educational and cognitive behavioural therapy (see glossary, p 1016) techniques versus no psychological intervention.[7] People were randomised before being offered the intervention, resulting in a much higher take up rate for the monitoring group and a higher level

of symptoms at baseline in the treatment group. This makes the results difficult to interpret. Intervention began at least 1 month after a road traffic accident. It found no significant differences in rates of development of PTSD between groups at 6 months. The third RCT (24 people with acute stress disorder) compared five sessions of cognitive behavioural therapy versus five sessions of supportive counselling (see glossary, p 1017) within 2 weeks of a road traffic accident or industrial accident.[8] Cognitive behavioural therapy was associated with a large reduction in the number of people who met PTSD diagnostic criteria immediately after treatment (8% *v* 83% with supportive counselling; $P < 0.001$) and at 6 months (17% *v* 67% with supportive counselling; $P < 0.05$).[9] The fourth RCT (66 survivors of road traffic accidents or non-sexual assault with acute stress disorder) evaluated five 90 minute sessions of prolonged exposure therapy (see glossary, p 1017) versus supportive counselling versus prolonged exposure therapy plus anxiety management. Immediately after completion of treatment, significantly lower rates of PTSD were found in the prolonged exposure group (2/14 [14%]) and in the prolonged exposure plus anxiety management group (3/15 [20%]) compared with the supportive counselling group (9/16 [56%]; $P < 0.05$ for each group *v* supportive counselling). The differences were still significant at 6 months' follow up (2/13 [15%] with prolonged exposure *v* 3/13 [23%] with anxiety management *v* 10/15 [67%] with supportive counselling; $P < 0.05$ for each group *v* supportive counselling).[10] The fifth RCT (132 French bus drivers who had been attacked) compared 1–6 sessions of cognitive behavioural therapy versus standard care.[11] At 6 months' follow up, the reductions in anxiety and intrusive symptoms measures were significantly greater in the treatment group, but there were no significant differences in depression or avoidance symptom measures between the groups. The sixth RCT (34 people) compared a 4 month collaborative care (see glossary, p 1016) input intervention with no intervention.[12] After 4 months, the risk of developing PTSD was lower with collaborative care versus no intervention, but the difference was not significant (AR for PTSD 43% with no intervention *v* 17% with collaborative care; CI not provided; $P > 0.1$). The trial may have lacked power to exclude a clinically important difference between treatments.

Harms: Two RCTs of single episode intervention included in the systematic review found an increased risk of subsequent psychological problems in people receiving the intervention. However, initial traumatic exposure had been higher in these people.[4]

Comment: The systematic review found that the overall quality of the RCTs was poor.[4] Problems included lack of blinding, failure to state loss to follow up, and lack of intention to treat analysis despite high withdrawal rates. These method problems are also apparent in the multiple episode intervention RCTs. The first multiple episode psychological treatment RCT included multiple types of intervention (help, information, support, and reality testing/confrontation) in the treatment group.[7]

QUESTION What are the effects of psychological treatments?

Mainly small RCTs have found evidence of benefit from specific psychological treatments compared with supportive counselling, relaxation treatment, or no treatment.

Benefits: We found one systematic review of psychological treatments for post-traumatic stress disorder (PTSD) (search date not stated, 17 RCTs, 690 people).[9] The RCTs compared a range of specific psychological treatments versus supportive counselling (see glossary, p 1017) or no intervention. All trials found that psychological treatment was associated with a greater improvement in immediate outcome (using a composite score of PTSD symptoms, anxiety, and depression) compared with supportive counselling or no treatment (overall effect size immediately after treatment 0.54; CI not provided). The difference was still evident at 1 year (overall effect size from 12 RCTs with long term follow up 0.53; CI not provided). **Cognitive behavioural therapy:** We found one systematic review (search date not stated, 17 RCTs, 690 people)[9] and three subsequent RCTs.[13–15] The review identified 14 RCTs of cognitive behavioural therapy (see glossary, p 1016) in people with PTSD. Although many were of poor quality, all described a positive effect compared with no treatment. One RCT (45 people) in the review evaluated three types of cognitive therapy and found that all were better than no treatment at 3 months (effect sizes compared with no treatment: stress inoculation 1.1, 95% CI 0.7 to 1.5; supportive counselling 0.6, 95% CI 0.2 to 0.9; prolonged exposure 1.7, 95% CI 1.2 to 2.1).[16] One subsequent RCT (87 people) compared exposure, cognitive therapy, or both, with relaxation treatment (see glossary, p 1017).[13] The trial found that all cognitive behavioural therapies reduced symptoms of PTSD more than relaxation treatment, immediately and at 3 months (53 people evaluated; no intention to treat analysis performed).[13] The second subsequent RCT (54 people) found that 39% of people continued to suffer from PTSD 1 year after 16 1-hour sessions of imaginal exposure therapy or cognitive therapy. There was no difference in the prevalence of PTSD between the two treatment groups.[14] The third subsequent RCT (168 people with PTSD and chronic nightmares) compared three sessions of imagery rehearsal therapy (see glossary, p 1017) versus no treatment. It found that imagery rehearsal therapy improved PTSD symptoms (AR for symptoms improving by at least one level of clinical severity 65% with imagery rehearsal *v* 31% with no treatment; ARR 34%; NNT 3, CI not provided, $P < 0.001$).[15] **Eye movement desensitisation and reprocessing:** We found one systematic review (search date 2000, 33 RCTs and 1 controlled study, number of people not stated).[17] It found that eye movement desensitisation and reprocessing (EMDR) (see glossary, p 1017) was more effective than no treatment in people with PTSD (effect size 0.44, 95% CI 0.31 to 0.55). However, it found no significant difference between EMDR and cognitive behavioural therapy/exposure therapy (effect size for EMDR *v* cognitive behavioural therapy/exposure therapy –0.28, 95% CI –0.54 to +0.02) or between EMDR with eye movements and EMDR without eye movements (effect size +0.10, 95% CI –0.08 to +0.27). **Affect management:** We found one RCT (48 women) comparing

15 weeks of affect management (see glossary, p 1016) treatment (as adjunctive therapy to drug treatment) versus waiting list control.[18] The RCT found that control of PTSD and dissociative symptoms were greater with affect management. **Other psychological treatments:** We found one RCT (112 people), which found no significant difference between psychodynamic psychotherapy (see glossary, p 1017), exposure therapy, and hypnotherapy (see glossary, p 1017). However, it reported that symptoms were improved more in all active groups than remaining on the waiting list (no treatment control). However, the trial did not test the significance of comparative results.[19] One RCT (42 police officers)[20] evaluated brief eclectic psychotherapy (which combines components of cognitive behavioural therapy and psychodynamic psychotherapy) over 16 sessions of treatment. The treatment group improved more than a waiting list control after treatment (9% *v* 50% remained PTSD positive, $P < 0.01$; CI not available) and at 3 months' follow up (4% *v* 65% remained PTSD positive). **Inpatient treatment programme:** We found no RCTs. **Drama therapy:** See glossary, p 1016. We found no RCTs.

Harms: The RCTs gave no information of harms. Overall, cognitive behavioural therapy seems well tolerated. However, there have been case reports in some people of "imaginal flooding" (a form of cognitive behavioural therapy) worsening symptoms, leading to calls for caution when evaluating people for treatment.[21] The RCT of affect management treatment had a high withdrawal rate (31%), specific drug treatments were not stated, and the analysis was not by intention to treat.

Comment: None.

QUESTION What are the effects of drug treatments?

One systematic review and subsequent RCTs have found that sertraline reduces symptoms more than placebo. We found more limited evidence from the systematic review and subsequent RCTs that paroxetine also reduced symptoms more than placebo. We found insufficient evidence on the effects of fluoxetine, brofaromine, amitriptyline, lamotrigine, benzodiazepines, antipsychotics, carbamazepine, imipramine, or phenelzine.

Benefits: We found one systematic review (search date 1999,[22] 15 RCTs, 9 with sufficient data for inclusion in the analysis, 868 people) of pharmacotherapy for post-traumatic stress disorder (PTSD), which used the Clinical Global Impressions scale change item or close equivalent as the primary outcome measure. The proportion of non-responders was lower in the pharmacotherapy group than the control group (RR 0.72, 95% CI 0.64 to 0.83). Two studies considered sertraline (42 people: OR 0.44, 95% CI 0.12 to 1.60; 183 people: OR 0.44, 95% CI 0.24 to 0.78), one paroxetine (280 people: OR 0.64, 95% CI 0.40 to 1.02), one fluoxetine (53 people: OR 0.30, 95% CI 0.09 to 1.02), two brofaromine (114 people: OR 0.94, 95% CI 0.45 to 1.99; 64 people: OR 0.40, 95% CI 0.15 to 1.08), one amitriptyline (40 people: OR 0.41, 95% CI 0.12 to 1.42), one lamotrigine (14 people: OR 0.39, 95% CI 0.04 to 3.71), one imipramine (41 people: OR 0.23, 95% CI 0.07 to 0.78), and one phenelzine (37 people: OR 0.21, 95% CI 0.06 to 0.73). We found four subsequent RCTs; two comparing sertraline versus placebo[23,24] and two comparing paroxetine versus placebo[25,26] in people with PTSD. The first RCT (208 people) found that sertraline (50–200 mg daily) reduced symptoms compared with placebo at 12 weeks (mean change in PTSD symptom score on the Clinical Administered PTSD scale total score −33.0 with sertraline *v* −26.2 with placebo; $P = 0.04$).[23] The second RCT (96 people) found that sertraline reduced PTSD relapse compared with placebo after 28 weeks (AR for relapse 5% with sertraline *v* 26% with placebo; ARR 21%; NNT 5; CI not provided; $P < 0.02$).[24] The third RCT (307 people) found that paroxetine (20–50 mg daily) versus placebo increased response rate (defined as "very much improved" or "much improved" on the Clinical Global Impressions–Global Improvement scale) versus placebo at 12 weeks (AR for response 59% with paroxetine *v* 38% with control; ARR 21%; NNT 5; CI not provided; $P = 0.008$).[25] The final RCT (551 people) similarly found that paroxetine (20 or 40 mg daily) improved response rate (using same definition) compared with placebo at 12 weeks (AR for response 62% with 20 mg paroxetine *v* 54% with 40 mg paroxetine *v* 37% with placebo; CI not provided; $P < 0.001$ for both paroxetine groups compared with placebo).[26] **Antipsychotic drugs:** We found no systematic review and no RCTs. **Carbamazepine:** We found no systematic review and no RCTs. **Benzodiazepines:** We found no systematic review. One RCT was not included in the systematic review above because of insufficient data.

Harms: Known adverse effects include possible hypertensive crisis with monoamine oxidase inhibitors (and also the need for dietary restriction), anticholinergic effects with tricyclic antidepressants, nausea and headache with selective serotonin reuptake inhibitors (see harms of prescription antidepressant drugs under depressive disorders, p 951) and dependency with benzodiazepines (see harms of benzodiazepines under generalised anxiety disorder, p 974).

Comment: Small trial sizes and different populations make it difficult to compare results. Other treatments or combinations of drug and psychological treatment await evaluation. It is difficult to interpret effect sizes in terms of clinical importance rather than statistical significance. Some categorise effect sizes of less than 0.5 as small; 0.5–0.8 as medium; and greater than 0.8 as large.

GLOSSARY

Affect management A type of group treatment focusing on regulation of mood.

Cognitive behavioural therapy Covers a variety of techniques. *Imaginal exposure* entails exposure to a detailed account or image of what happened. *Real life exposure* involves confronting real life situations that have become associated with the trauma and cause fear and distress. *Cognitive therapy* entails challenging distorted thoughts about the trauma, the self, and the world. *Stress inoculation* entails instruction in coping skills and some cognitive techniques such as restructuring.

Collaborative care Entails counselling, liaison, and co-ordination of care after discharge.

Drama therapy Entails using drama as a form of expression and communication.

Eye movement desensitisation and reprocessing (EMDR) Entails asking the person to focus on the traumatic event, a negative cognition associated with it, and the associated emotions.[27] The person is then asked to follow the therapist's finger as it moves from side to side.

Hypnotherapy Entails hypnosis to allow people to work through the traumatic event.

Imagery rehearsal therapy Involves encouraging participants to practice pleasant imagery exercises and employ cognitive behavioural tools to deal with unpleasant images.

Prolonged exposure A type of cognitive behavioural therapy that includes repeated exposure to memories of the trauma, and to non-dangerous real life situations that are avoided because of trauma related fear.

Psychodynamic psychotherapy Entails analysis of defence mechanisms, interpretations, and pre-trauma experiences.

Psychological debriefing A technique that entails detailed consideration of the traumatic event and the normalisation of psychological reactions.

Relaxation treatment A technique involving imagination of relaxing situations to induce muscular and mental relaxation.

Supportive counselling A non-directive intervention dealing with current issues rather than the trauma itself.

Substantive changes

Single episode intervention Systematic review updated[4] and one subsequent RCT found;[5] conclusion unchanged.

Multiple episode intervention Two new RCTs;[6,12] conclusion unchanged.

Treatments: Cognitive behavioural therapy New RCT;[15] conclusion unchanged.

Eye movement desensitisation and reprocessing New systematic review;[17] conclusion amended and intervention re-categorised as beneficial.

Drug treatments Four new RCTs;[23–26] conclusion amended. Sertraline recategorised as beneficial.

REFERENCES

1. American Psychiatric Association. *Diagnostic and statistical manual of mental disorders*. 4th ed. Washington: APA, 1994.
2. Kessler RC, Sonnega A, Bromet E, et al. Posttraumatic stress disorder in the national comorbidity survey. *Arch Gen Psychiatry* 1995;52:1048–1060.
3. O'Brien S. *Traumatic events and mental health*. Cambridge: Cambridge University Press, 1998.
4. Rose S, Bisson J, Wessely S. Psychological debriefing for preventing post traumatic stress disorder (PTSD) (Cochrane Review). In: The Cochrane Library, Issue 4, 2001. Oxford: Update Software. Search date 2001; primary sources Medline, Embase, PsychLit, Pilots, Biosis, Pascal, Occupational Safety and Health, Sociofile, Cinahl, Psycinfo, Psyndex, Sigle, Lilacs, Cochrane Controlled Clinical Trials, National Research Register, hand search of Journal of Traumatic Stress and contact with leading researchers.
5. Campfield KM, Hills AM. Effect of timing of critical incident stress debriefing (CISD) on posttraumatic symptoms. *J Traum Stress* 2001;14:327–340.
6. Bordow S, Porritt D. An experimental evaluation of crisis intervention. *Soc Sci Med* 1979;13A:251–256.
7. Brom D, Kleber RJ, Hofman MC. Victims of traffic accidents: incidence and prevention of post-traumatic stress disorder. *J Clin Psychol* 1993;49:131–140.
8. Bryant RA, Harvey AG, Basten C, et al. Treatment of acute stress disorder: a comparison of cognitive behavioural therapy and supportive counselling. *J Consult Clin Psychol* 1998;66:862–866.
9. Sherman JJ. Effects of psychotherapeutic treatments for PTSD: a meta-analysis of controlled clinical trials. *J Trauma Stress* 1998;11:413–436. Search date not stated; primary sources Psychlit, Eric, Medline, Cinahl, Dissertation Abstracts, and Pilots Traumatic Stress Database.
10. Bryant RA, Sackville T, Dang ST, et al. Treating acute stress disorder: an evaluation of cognitive behavior therapy and supportive counselling techniques. *Am J Psychiatry* 1999;156:1780–1786.
11. Andre C, Lelord F, Legeron P, et al. Controlled study of outcomes after 6 months to early intervention of bus driver victims of aggression [in French]. *Encephale* 1997;23:65–71.
12. Zatzick DF, Roy-Byrne P, Russo JE, et al. Collaborative interventions for physically injured trauma survivors: a pilot randomized effectiveness trial. *Gen Hosp Psychiatry* 2001;23:114–123.
13. Marks I, Lovell K, Noshirvani H, et al. Treatment of posttraumatic stress disorder by exposure and/or cognitive restructuring: a controlled study. *Arch Gen Psychiatry* 1998;55:317–325.
14. Tarrier N, Sommerfield C, Pilgrim H, et al. Cognitive therapy or imaginal exposure in the treatment of post-traumatic stress disorder. *Br J Psychiatry* 1999;175:571–575.
15. Krakow B, Hollifield M, Johnston L, et al. Imagery rehearsal therapy for chronic nightmares in sexual

assault survivors with posttraumatic stress disorder: a randomized controlled trial. *JAMA* 2001;286:537–545.
16. Foa Ebv , Rothbaum BO, Riggs DS, et al. Treatment of posttraumatic stress disorder in rape victims: a comparison between cognitive-behavioural procedures and counselling. *J Consult Clin Psychol* 1992;59:715–723.
17. Davidson PR, Parker KC. Eye movement desensitisation and reprocessing (EMDR): a meta-analysis. *J Consult Clin Psychol* 2001;69:305–316. Medline and Psychinfo searched between 1988 and April 2000, and Current Contents searched from 1997 to March 2000, plus reference lists from articles found in these searches.
18. Zlotnick C, Shea T, Rosen K, et al. An affect-management group for women with posttraumatic stress disorder and histories of childhood sexual abuse. *J Trauma Stress* 1997;10:425–436.
19. Brom D, Kleber RJ, Defares PB. Brief psychotherapy of posttraumatic stress disorders. *J Consult Clin Psychol* 1989;57:607–612.
20. Gersons BPR, Carlier IVE, Lamberts RD, et al. Randomised clinical trial of brief eclectic psychotherapy for police officers with posttraumatic stress disorder. *J Trauma Stress* 2000;13:333–348.
21. Pitman RK, Altman B, Greenwald E, et al. Psychiatric complications during flooding therapy for posttraumatic stress disorder. *J Clin Psychiatry* 1991;52:17–20.
22. Stein DJ, Zungu-Dirwayi N, Van der Linden GJ, et al. Pharmacotherapy for posttraumatic stress disorder (Cochrane Review). In: The Cochrane Library, Issue 4, 2001. Oxford: Update Software. Search date 1999; primary sources Medline, Psychlit, Pilots Traumatic Stress Database, Dissertation Abstracts, trials register of the Cochrane Depression, Anxiety and Neurosis Controlled Group, hand searches of reference lists, and personal contact with PTSD researchers and pharmaceutical companies.
23. Davidson JR, Rothbaum BO, van der Kolk BA, et al. Multicenter, double blind comparison of sertraline and placebo in the treatment of posttraumatic stress disorder. *Arch Gen Psychiatry* 2001;58:485–492.
24. Davidson J, Pearlstein T, Londborg P, et al. Efficacy of sertraline in preventing relapse of posttraumatic stress disorder: results of a 28-week double-blind, placebo-controlled study. *Am J Psychiatry* 2001;158:1974–1981.
25. Tucker P, Zaninelli R, Yehuda R, et al. Paroxetine in the treatment of chronic posttraumatic stress disorder: results of a placebo-controlled, flexible-dosage trial. *J Clin Psychiatry* 2001;62:860–868.
26. Marshall RD, Beebe KL, Oldham M, et al. Efficacy and safety of paroxetine treatment for chronic PTSD: a fixed-dose, placebo-controlled study. *Am J Psychiatry* 2001;158:1982–1988.
27. Shapiro F. Eye movement desensitisation: a new treatment for post-traumatic stress disorder. *J Behav Ther Exp Psychiatry* 1989;20:211–217.

Jonathan Bisson
Consultant Liaison Psychiatrist
Cardiff and Vale NHS Trust
Cardiff
UK

Competing interests: None declared.

Schizophrenia

Search date April 2002

Zia Nadeem, Andrew McIntosh, and Stephen Lawrie

QUESTIONS

INTERVENTIONS

See glossary, p 1045

Key Messages

- Most evidence is from systematic reviews of RCTs that report different outcomes. There is a need for larger RCTs, over longer periods, with well designed end points, including standardised, validated symptom scales. No intervention has been consistently found to reduce negative symptoms.

Clin Evid 2002;8:1019–1049.

- **Behavioural therapy for improving adherence** One RCT found that behavioural interventions versus usual treatment improved adherence to antipsychotic medication over 3 months. Two RCTs found that behavioural interventions versus psychoeducational therapy improved adherence.
- **Chlorpromazine** One systematic review has found that chlorpromazine versus placebo significantly reduces the proportion of people who have no improvement (NNT 7, 95% CI 5 to 10), or have marked/worse severity of illness at 6 months (NNT 5, 95% CI 4 to 8) on a psychiatrist rated scale. The review found that chlorpromazine versus placebo caused significantly more adverse effects, such as sedation, acute dystonia, and parkinsonism.
- **Clozapine** Two systematic reviews found that clozapine versus standard antipsychotic drugs improved symptoms over 4–10 weeks, and may improve symptoms in the longer term. However, RCTs found that clozapine may be associated with blood dyscrasias. Three systematic reviews found no strong evidence about the effectiveness or safety of clozapine versus new antipsychotic drugs. One systematic review in people resistant to standard treatment has found that clozapine versus standard treatment improves symptoms after 12 weeks and after 2 years.
- **Cognitive behavioural therapy to reduce relapse rates** Limited evidence from RCTs found no significant difference in relapse rates with the addition of cognitive behavioural therapy to standard care.
- **"Compliance" therapy** One RCT found limited evidence that compliance therapy versus non-specific counselling may increase adherence to antipsychotic medication at 6 and 18 months.
- **Continuation of medication for 6–9 months after an acute episode** Systematic reviews have found that continuing antipsychotic medication for at least 6 months after an acute episode significantly reduces relapse rates, and that some benefit of continuing medication is apparent for up to 2 years.
- **Depot bromperidol decanoate** One systematic review found no significant difference in the proportion of people who needed additional medication or left the study early over 6–12 months with bromperidol versus haloperidol or fluphenazine decanoate. One RCT found no significant difference in anticholinergic adverse effects at 12 months with depot bromperidol decanoate versus fluphenazine, and two RCTs found no significant difference in movement disorders over 6–12 months with bromperidol versus haloperidol or fluphenazine.
- **Depot haloperidol decanoate** One RCT found that depot haloperidol decanoate versus placebo reduced the need for additional medication at 4 months (NNT 2, 95% CI 1 to 2 with 4 months' treatment). One systematic review has found that haloperidol versus placebo is associated with with acute dystonia (NNH 5, 95% CI 3 to 9), akathisia (NNH 6, 95 % CI 4 to 14), and parkinsonism (NNH 3, 95% CI 2 to 5)
- **Depot pipotiazine palmitate** One RCT found no significant difference with depot pipotiazine palmitate versus standard antipsychotic drugs in symptoms or in the proportion of people requiring anticholinergic drugs at 18 months. RCTs found no significant difference with depot pipotiazine versus antipsychotic drugs in the proportion of people who left the trial early.
- **Family interventions to improve adherence** One systematic review has found that family therapy versus usual care is unlikely to improve adherence to antipsychotic medication.

- **Family interventions to reduce relapse rates** One systematic review has found that family intervention versus usual care significantly reduces relapse rates at 12 and 24 months. Seven families would have to be treated to avoid one additional relapse (and likely hospitalisation) in the family member with schizophrenia (NNT 7, 95% CI 4 to 14). One RCT found that fewer people receiving a multiple family versus single family intervention relapsed over 2 years, but the difference did not quite reach significance.
- **Haloperidol** One systematic review has found that haloperidol versus placebo significantly increases physician rated global improvement for up to 2 years (NNT 3, 95% CI 3 to 5), but is associated with acute dystonia (NNH 5, 95% CI 3 to 9), akathisia (NNH 6, 95 % CI 4 to 14), and parkinsonism (NNH 3, 95% CI 2 to 5).
- **Polyunsaturated fatty acids** One small RCT found limited evidence that polyunsaturated fatty acids versus placebo reduced the subsequent use of antipsychotic medication after 12 weeks.
- **Psychoeducational interventions to improve adherence** One systematic review found limited evidence that psychoeducation versus usual care improved adherence with antipsychotic medication. Two RCTs found that psychoeducational therapy improved adherence less than behavioural therapy.
- **Psychoeducational interventions to reduce relapse rates** One systematic review has found that psychoeducation versus control intervention significantly reduces relapse rates at 9–18 months.
- **Social skills training to reduce relapse rates** Limited evidence from a systematic reviews of RCTs and observational studies suggests that social skills training versus usual care may reduce relapse rates.
- **Amisulpride; loxapine; molindone; olanzapine; pimozide; quetiapine; risperidone; sulpiride; thioridazine; ziprasidone; zotepine** Systematic reviews have found that these antipsychotic drugs are as effective as standard antipsychotic drugs, and have different profiles of adverse effects.
- **Benperidol; perazine** Systematic reviews of poor quality RCTs found insufficient evidence about the effects of these interventions.

DEFINITION Schizophrenia is characterised by the positive symptoms (see glossary, p 1045) of auditory hallucinations, delusions, and thought disorder, and by the negative symptoms (see glossary, p 1045) of demotivation, self neglect, and reduced emotion.[1]

INCIDENCE/ PREVALENCE Onset of symptoms typically occurs in early adult life (average age 25 years) and is earlier in men than women. Prevalence worldwide is 2–4/1000. One in 100 people will develop schizophrenia in their lifetime.[2,3]

AETIOLOGY/ RISK FACTORS Risk factors include a family history (although no major genes have been identified); obstetric complications; developmental difficulties; central nervous system infections in childhood; cannabis use; and acute life events.[2] The precise contributions of these factors and ways in which they may interact are unclear.

PROGNOSIS About three quarters of people suffer recurrent relapse and continued disability, although the proportion of people who improved significantly increased after the mid 1950s (mean 48.5% from 1956–1985 *v* 35.4% from 1895–1956).[4] Outcome may be worse in people with insidious onset and delayed initial treatment, social isolation, or a strong family history; in people living in industrialised countries; in men; and in people who misuse drugs.[3] Drug treatment is generally successful in treating positive symptoms, but up to a third of people derive little benefit and negative symptoms are notoriously difficult to treat. About half of people with schizophrenia do not adhere to treatment in the short term. The figure is even higher in the longer term.[5]

AIMS To relieve symptoms and to improve quality of life, with minimal adverse effects of treatment.

OUTCOMES Severity of positive and negative symptoms; global clinical improvement; global clinical impression (a composite measure of symptoms and everyday functioning); rate of relapse; adherence to treatment; adverse effects of treatment.

METHODS *Clinical Evidence* update search and appraisal April 2002. Most of the RCTs we found were small, short term, with high withdrawal rates, and many different outcome measures.[6] There were a large number of high quality recent systematic reviews. Therefore, if possible, we focused primarily on systematic reviews and included only the outcomes we thought were the most clinically relevant (because each treatment is associated with different benefits and harms, we used estimates of global effectiveness if they were available). We searched for placebo controlled studies for standard antipsychotic medication and comparative studies for newer antipsychotic drugs.

QUESTION What are the effects of drug treatments?

OPTION CHLORPROMAZINE

One systematic review has found that chlorpromazine versus placebo significantly reduces the proportion of people who have no improvement, or marked/worse severity of illness at 6 months on a psychiatrist rated scale. The review found that chlorpromazine versus placebo caused significantly more adverse effects, such as sedation, acute dystonia, and parkinsonism.

Benefits: **Versus placebo:** We found one systematic review (search date 1999, 45 RCTs, 3116 people, mean dose 511 mg daily, range 25–2000 mg daily).[7] It found that chlorpromazine versus placebo significantly reduced the proportion of people who had no improvement on a psychiatrist rated global impression scale at 6 months (583/921 [63%] with chlorpromazine *v* 609/790 [77%] with placebo; RR 0.76, 95% CI 0.71 to 0.80; NNT 7, 95% CI 5 to 10) and significantly reduced the proportion of people who had marked or worse severity of illness on a psychiatrist rated scale at 6 months (323/493 [66%] with chlorpromazine *v* 231/285 [81%] with placebo; RR 0.77, 95% CI 0.71 to 0.84; NNT 5, 95% CI 4 to 8).[7]

Harms: **Versus placebo:** The systematic review found that chlorpromazine versus placebo caused significantly higher rates of sedation (RR 2.4, 95% CI 1.7 to 3.3; NNH 6, 95% CI 4 to 8), acute dystonia (RR 3.1, 95% CI 1.3 to 7.6; NNH 24, 95% CI 14 to 77), parkinsonism (RR 2.6, 95% CI 1.2 to 5.4; NNH 10, 95% CI 8 to 16), weight gain (RR 4.4, 95% CI 2.1 to 9; NNH 3, 95% CI 2 to 5), skin photosensitivity (RR 5.2, 95% CI 3 to 10; NNH 7, 95% CI 6 to 10), dizziness caused by hypotension (RR 1.9, 95% CI 1.3 to 2.6; NNH 12, 95% CI 8 to 20), and dry mouth (RR 4, 95% CI 1.6 to 10; NNH 19, 95% CI 12 to 37).[7] Chlorpromazine versus placebo was also associated with a non-significantly higher rate of seizures (RR 2.4, 95% CI 0.4 to 16) and blood dyscrasias (RR 2.0, 95% CI 0.7 to 6). We found no long term data on the risk of tardive dyskinesia or the rare but potentially fatal neuroleptic malignant syndrome. Despite the frequent adverse effects, the review found that people receiving chlorpromazine versus placebo were more likely to stay in RCTs in both the short and the medium term.

Comment: The review did not categorise symptoms as positive or negative as this information was rarely available from included RCTs.[7] Relative risks and numbers needed to treat were based on 6 months' data. There was significant heterogeneity of the benefits results from the RCTs, but the analyses remained significant after removal of the heterogenous RCTs.[7]

OPTION HALOPERIDOL

One systematic review has found that haloperidol versus placebo significantly increases the proportion of people with psychiatrist rated global improvement after 6 weeks and 2 years, but is associated with acute dystonia, akathisia, and parkinsonism.

Benefits: **Versus placebo:** We found one systematic review (search date 1998, 20 RCTs, 1001 people).[8] It found that haloperidol (over a wide range of doses) versus placebo significantly increased psychiatrist rated global improvement after 6 weeks (3 RCTs: RR for global improvement with haloperidol *v* placebo 2.3, 95% CI 1.7 to 3.3; NNT 3, 95% CI 2 to 5), and after 24 months (8 RCTs: RR 1.5, 95% CI 1.2 to 1.7; NNT 3, 95% CI 3 to 5).

Harms: **Versus placebo:** The systematic review found that haloperidol versus placebo significantly increased the risk of acute dystonia (2 RCTs: RR 4.7, 95% CI 1.7 to 44; NNH 5, 95% CI 3 to 9), akathisia (3 RCTs: RR 6.5, 95% CI 1.5 to 28; NNH 6, 95%CI 4 to 14), and parkinsonism (4 RCTs: RR 8.9, 95% CI 2.6 to 31; NNH 3, 95% CI 2 to 5).[8] People taking haloperidol were more likely to be treated with anticholinergic drugs than those taking placebo (4 RCTs: R 4.9, 95% CI 1.01 to 24; NNH 2, 95% CI 1 to 3).

Comment: The median size of RCTs in the review was 38 people, but the quality of the RCTs was higher than average for schizophrenia trials.[8] Although the dose range was very wide, most RCTs used 4–20 mg daily and adjusted dose according to need. The review found evidence of publication bias for the 6–24 months global outcome ratings.[8]

OPTION THIORIDAZINE

One systematic review has found that thioridazine versus placebo significantly improves global mental state over 3–12 months. It has found no significant difference with thioridazine versus standard antipsychotic

drugs in global clinical impression or improvement in mental state at 3–12 months, and has found that thioridazine versus standard antipsychotic medication causes fewer extrapyramidal adverse events and parkinsonism at 3 months.

Benefits: We found one systematic review (search date 1999, 11 RCTs, 560 people).[9] **Versus placebo:** The review found that thioridazine versus placebo significantly reduced the proportion of people who were "no better or worse" on global clinical impression at 3–12 months (5 RCTs; RR of 27/84 [32%] *v* 57/81 [70%]; RR 0.5, 95% CI 0.37 to 0.68, NNT 3 95% CI 3 to 5). **Versus standard antipsychotic drugs:** The review found no significant difference between thioridazine versus standard antipsychotic medication in the risk of "being no better or worse" on clinical global impression at 3 months (11 RCTs, 137/372 [37%] *v* 157/399 [39%]; RR 0.98, 95% CI 0.84 to 1.14) or at 6–11 months (2 RCTs 7/43 [16%] *v* 15/39 [38%], RR 1.03, 95% CI 0.59 to 1.79) or in improvement in mental state.[9]

Harms: **Versus placebo:** The review found no significant difference in adverse events.[9] **Versus standard antipsychotic drugs:** The review identified one RCT (74 people) comparing thioridazine versus chlorpromazine, which found that thioridazine caused more cardiovascular adverse events at 3 months (RR 3.2, 95% CI 1.4 to 7.0; NNH 3, 95% CI 2 to 7), although by 6 months the difference was not significant. The review found that thioridazine versus standard antipsychotic drugs caused fewer extrapyramidal adverse events or use of antiparkinsonian medication over 3 months (7 RCTs, 1082 people, 108/426 [25%] *v* 306/656 [47%]; RR 0.50, 95% CI 0.42 to 0.60) and reduced parkinsonism (2 RCTs, 340 people, 5/119 [4%] with thioridazine *v* 35/221 [16%] with standard antipsychotics; RR 0.29, 95% CI 0.12 to 0.70).[9]

Comment: None.

OPTION DEPOT HALOPERIDOL DECANOATE

One systematic review found limited evidence that depot haloperidol decanoate versus placebo reduced the need for additional medication at 4 months and reduced the proportion of people who withdrew from the trial. One systematic review has found that haloperidol versus placebo is associated with acute dystonia, akathisia, and parkinsonism.

Benefits: **Versus placebo:** We found one systematic review (search date 1998, 2 RCTs, 78 people).[10] Both RCTs found that people taking depot haloperidol versus placebo were more likely to stay in the RCT (RR 0.2, 95% CI 0.1 to 0.4; NNT 2, 95% CI 1 to 3).[10] One of the RCTs (22 people) identified by the review comparing intramuscular depot haloperidol decanoate (mean dose 150 mg monthly) versus placebo found that haloperidol decanoate was more likely to result in a "reduced need for additional medication" at 4 months (RR 2.6, 95% CI 1.1 to 5.6; NNT with 4 months' treatment 2, 95% CI 1 to 2; see comment below).

Harms: The systematic review gave no information on harms.[10] See harms of haloperidol, p 1023.

Comment: The RCT (22 people) identified by the review did not report how "reduced need for medication" was measured.[10] Depot injection is believed to ensure adherence, but we found no evidence from RCTs to support this belief.

OPTION DEPOT PIPOTIAZINE PALMITATE

One RCT found no significant difference with depot pipotiazine palmitate versus standard antipsychotic drugs in symptoms or in the proportion of people requiring anticholinergic drugs at 18 months. Two RCTs found no significant difference with depot pipotiazine versus standard antipsychotic drugs in the proportion of people who left the trial early.

Benefits: **Versus standard antipsychotic drugs:** We found one systematic review (search date 1998), which identified two RCTs comparing intramuscular depot pipotiazine (pipothiazine) palmitate versus standard antipsychotic drugs, chosen by physicians.[11] The first RCT (124 people) identified by the review found no significant difference in brief psychiatric rating scores with depot pipotiazine (mean dose 90 mg monthly) versus standard antipsychotic drugs at 18 months (WMD –3.1, 95% CI –7.3 to +1.2). The other RCT identified by the review gave no information on the effects of depot pipotiazine versus standard antipsychotic drugs on symptoms or the need for additional medication.

Harms: **Versus standard antipsychotic drugs:** The first RCT identified by the review found no significant difference in the proportion of people who needed to take anticholinergic drugs for unspecified reasons with depot pipotiazine palmitate versus standard antipsychotic drugs (42/61 [69%] *v* 49/63 [78%]; RR 0.89, 95% CI 0.71 to 1.10)[11] The review found no significant difference in the proportion of people who left the trial early with thioridazine (mean dose 113 mg a month for 6 months) versus standard antipsychotic drugs (2 RCTs, 25% in both groups, RR 1.0, 95% CI 0.5 to 1.9).

Comment: None.

OPTION BENPERIDOL New

We found no RCTs comparing benperidol versus placebo. One RCT found that benperidol was significantly less likely than perphenazine to improve global mental state over 30 days.

Benefits: **Versus placebo:** We found no RCTs. **Versus standard antipsychotic drugs:** We found one systematic review (search date 2001, 1 RCT, 40 people) which found that benperidol was significantly less likely than perphenazine to improve global mental state over 30 days (RR of failure to improve 8.00, 95% CI 2.11 to 30; NNT 1.4, 95% CI 1 to 2).[12]

Harms: The RCT gave no information on adverse effects.[12]

Comment: None.

OPTION PERAZINE New

Two poor quality RCTs found no significant difference in global clinical impression over 28 days with perazine versus haloperidol. Two RCTs found insufficient evidence of the effects of perazine versus zotepine, and one

RCT found no significant difference in mental state at 28 days with perazine versus amisulpride. Three RCTs found no significant difference in the risk of extrapyramidal effects over 28 days with perazine versus zotepine or amisulpride.

Benefits: **Versus placebo:** We found no RCTs. **Versus standard antipsychotic drugs:** We found one systematic review (search date 2001) which identified two RCTs (71 people) comparing perazine versus haloperidol.[13] It could not perform a meta-analysis because of poor reporting in one of the RCTs. It found no significant difference in the proportion of people who were "no better or worse" for global clinical impression with perazine versus halpoperiodol at 28 days (1 RCT, 32 people, 8/17 [47%] with perazine *v* 6/15 [60%] with haloperidol; RR 1.18, 95% CI 0.53 to 2.62). **Versus new antipsychotic drugs:** The review identified two RCTs comparing perazine versus zotepine.[13] It could not perform a meta-analysis because of methodological differences between the trials. The first RCT (34 people) found that perazine was significantly less effective than zotepine in improving symptoms assessed by mean Brief Psychiatric Rating Scale score at 28 days (WMD 7.9, 95% CI 1.1 to 14.7). The second RCT (40 people), which used a different method to calculate mean Brief Psychiatric Rating Scale score, found that perazine was significantly more effective than zotepine in improving symptoms at the end of the trial, which was not specified (WMD –0.4, 95% –0.7 to –0.1). One RCT identified by the review found no significant difference between perazine versus amisulpride in the proportion of people whose mental state was "no better or worse" at 28 days (4/15 [27%] *v* 3/15 [20%]; RR 1.33, 95% CI 0.36 to 4.97).[13]

Harms: **Versus standard antipsychotic drugs:** The review gave no information about the adverse effects of perazine versus haloperidol.[13] **Versus new antipsychotic drugs:** The review (3 RCTs) found no significant difference with perazine versus zotepine or versus amisulpride in the risk of akathesia over 28 days (3/56 [5%] with perazine *v* 10/55 [18%] with zotepine or amisulpride; RR 0.30, 95% CI 0.09 to 1.00; dyskinesia (1/56 [2%] *v* 3/55 [5%] ; RR 0.42, 95% CI 0.06 to 2.74) or parkinsonism over 28 days (10/41 [24%] with perazine *v* 8/40 [24%] with zotepine or amisulpride; RR 1.22, 95% CI 0.54 to 2.78).[13]

Comment: None.

OPTION DEPOT BROMPERIDOL DECANOATE New

One RCT found no significant difference in global mental state or in anticholinergic adverse effects with depot bromperidol deconoate versus placebo at 6 months, but may have been too small to exclude a clinically important difference. One systematic review found no significant difference in the proportion of people who needed additional medication or left the study early over 6–12 months with bromperidol versus haloperidol or fluphenazine decanoate. One RCT found no significant difference in anticholinergic adverse effects at 12 months with depot bromperidol decanoate versus fluphenazine, and two RCTs found no significant difference in movement disorders over 6–12 months with bromperidol versus haloperidol or fluphenazine.

Benefits: We found one systematic review (search date 1999, 4 RCTs, 117 people).[14] **Versus placebo:** One small RCT (20 people) identified by the review found no significant difference in global mental state at 6 months with depot bromperidol deconoate versus placebo (no raw data available). The RCT may have been too small to exclude a clinically important difference. **Versus standard antipsychotic drugs:** The review (3 RCTs, 97 people) found no significant difference with bromperidol versus haloperidol or versus fluphenazine decanoate in the proportion of people who needed additional antipsychotics or benzodiazepines over 6–12 months (19/48 [39.5%] with bromperidol *v* 18/49 [37%] with haloperidol or fluphenazine; RR 1.08, 95% CI 0.68 to 1.70 and who left the RCT early (10/48 [21%] with bromperidol *v* 5/49 [10%] with haloperidol or fluphenazine; RR 1.92, 95% CI 0.80 to 4.60).[14]

Harms: **Versus placebo:** The RCT found no significant difference in anticholinergic adverse effects and movement disorders at 6 months with bromperidol versus placebo, but may have been too small to detect a clinically important difference.[14] **Versus standard antipsychotic drugs:** One RCT (47 people) found no significant differcnce in the frequency of anticholinergic adverse effects at 12 months with bromperidol versus fluphenazine (6/23 [26%] *v* 2/24 [8%]; RR 3.13, 95% CI 0.70 to 13.95), but may have been too small to exclude a clinically important difference. Two RCTs (77 people) found no significant difference in movement disorders over 6–12 months with bromperidol versus haloperidol or fluphenazine (16/38 [42%] *v* 22/39 [56%]; RR 0.74, 95% CI 0.47 to 1.17).[14]

Comment: None.

OPTION LOXAPINE

One systematic review comparing loxapine versus standard antipsychotic drugs found no significant difference in global improvement or adverse effects.

Benefits: **Versus standard antipsychotic drugs:** We found one systematic review (search date 1999, 22 RCTs, 1073 peoplc), which compared loxapine (dose range 25–250 mg daily) versus standard antipsychotic drugs, usually chlorpromazine.[15] It found no significant difference in global improvement with loxapine versus standard antipsychotic drugs (9 RCTs, 411 people: RR of no improvement 0.9, 95% CI 0.7 to 1.2).

Harms: The review found no significant difference in adverse effects with loxapine versus standard antipsychotic drugs.[15]

Comment: All of the RCTs identified by the review were conducted in the USA or India and none lasted longer than 12 weeks.[15]

OPTION MOLINDONE

One systematic review found no significant difference in global clinical improvement or total number of adverse events over 4–12 weeks with molindone versus standard antipsychotic drugs.

Benefits: **Versus placebo:** We found no RCTs. **Versus standard antipsychotic drugs:** We found one systematic review (search date 1999, 4 RCTs, 150 people) of molindone versus standard antipsychotic drugs.[16] It found no significant difference between molindone and standard antipsychotic drugs in global clinical improvement over 4–12 weeks as assessed by a physician (4 RCTs; 25/84 [29.8%] *v* 20/66 [30.3%]; RR of no improvement 1.1, 95% CI 0.7 to 1.8).

Harms: The review found no significant difference with molindone versus standard antipsychotic drugs in movement disorders (rigidity, tremor, akasthesia, use of antiparkinsonian medication) or total number of adverse events (2 RCTs, 1 controlled trial; 24/42 [57%] *v* 25/42 [59%]; RR 0.96, 95% CI 0.73 to 1.27).[16] One RCT identified by the review found that the rate of confusion was significantly higher in people taking molindone versus standard antipsychotic drugs (9/14 [64%] with molindone *v* 6/30 [20%] with standard antipsychotic drugs; RR 3.2, 95% CI 1.4 to 7.3). The review found that weight loss was more frequent in those taking molindone versus standard antipsychotic drugs (2 RCTs, 12/30 [40%] *v* 4/30 [13%]; RR 2.8, 95% CI 1.1 to 7.0), and that molindone was associated with less frequent weight gain than standard antipsychotic drugs (2 RCTs, 4/30 [13%] *v* 11/30 [37%]; RR 0.4, 95% CI 0.1 to 1.0).[16]

Comment: None.

OPTION PIMOZIDE

We found insufficient evidence from RCTs comparing pimozide versus placebo. One systematic review comparing pimozide versus standard antipsychotic drugs found no significant difference in global clinical impression, and found that pimozide versus standard antipsychotic drugs significantly decreased sedation but increased tremor. It found no overall difference in cardiovascular adverse effects such as rise or fall in blood pressure or dizziness with pimozide versus standard antipsychotic drugs.

Benefits: **Versus placebo:** We found one systematic review (search date 1999, 3 RCTs, 86 people) of pimozide versus placebo.[17] One RCT (20 people) found no significant difference in clinical global impression at 3 months. Two further small RCTs (66 people) found greater improvement at 6 months with pimozide, the significance of which depend on the statistical method used. **Versus standard antipsychotic drugs:** We found one systematic review (search date 1999) of pimozide (mean dose 7.5 mg daily, range 1–75 mg daily) versus standard antipsychotic drugs.[17] It found no significant difference in global clinical impression (3 RCTs, 206 people: RR 0.9, 95% CI 0.8 to 1.1).

Harms: **Versus placebo:** One small short RCT identified by the review found significantly more electrocardiogram (ECG) changes with pimozide versus placebo (T wave changes RR 5, 95% CI 0.3 to 93).[17] Doses used were on a sliding scale up to 40 mg daily. **Versus standard antipsychotic drugs:** The review found that pimozide caused significantly less sedation than standard antipsychotic drugs (RR 0.4, 95% CI 0.2 to 0.7; NNT 6, 95% CI 4 to 16), but was more likely to cause tremor (RR 1.6, 95 CI 1.1 to 2.3; NNH 6, 95% CI 3 to 44).[17] It found no difference in cardiovascular symptoms such as rise or fall in blood pressure and dizziness between pimozide and standard antipsychotic drugs. There was little usable ECG data. One RCT in the review found no significant difference in ECG changes with pimozide versus standard antipsychotic drugs (RR 0.67, 95% CI 0.1 to 3.7).

Comment: Sudden death has been reported in a number of people taking pimozide at doses over 20 mg daily, but we found no evidence from RCTs that pimozide is more likely to cause sudden death than other antipsychotic drugs.[17] The manufacturer recommends periodic ECG monitoring in all people taking more than 16 mg daily of pimozide and avoidance of other drugs known to prolong the QT interval on an ECG or cause electrolyte disturbances (other antipsychotic drugs, antihistamines, antidepressants, and diuretics). The RCTs comparing pimozide versus placebo may be too small to detect a clinically significant difference.

OPTION POLYUNSATURATED FATTY ACIDS

One small RCT found limited evidence that polyunsaturated fatty acids versus placebo reduced the subsequent use of antipsychotic medication after 12 weeks.

Benefits: **Versus placebo:** We found one systematic review (search date 2000, 1 RCT, 30 people) of fatty acid supplementation versus placebo.[18] It found that fish oil versus placebo significantly reduced the proportion of people who needed subsequent antipsychotic medication after 12 weeks (RR 0.6, 95% CI 0.4 to 0.9).The review also found a slight difference in average symptom severity scores favouring fish oil (26 people: WMD –13, 95% CI –22 to –3).

Harms: The RCT did not find significant adverse events.[18]

Comment: The RCT identified by the systematic review is an unpublished conference proceeding.[18]

OPTION SULPIRIDE

One systematic review found that sulpiride versus placebo significantly improved global clinical impression over 10 weeks, and found no significant difference in global clinical impression over 4–10 weeks with sulpiride versus standard antipsychotic drugs. The review found that the use of antiparkinson drugs over 4–10 weeks was significantly less frequent with sulpiride versus standard antipsychotic drugs.

Benefits: We found one systematic review (search date 1998) comparing sulpiride versus placebo or versus standard antipsychotic drugs.[19] **Versus placebo:** The review identified three RCTs (see comment below). One RCT (28 people) found that sulpiride versus placebo significantly reduced the proportion of people who had no improvement in global clinical impression over 10 weeks (8/16 [50%] with sulpiride *v* 11/12 [92%] with placebo; RR 0.55, 95% CI 0.32 to 0.92). **Versus standard antipsychotic drugs:** The review (7 RCTs,

366 people) found no significant difference in the proportion of people who had no improvement in global clinical impression with sulpiride versus standard antipsychotic drugs over 4–10 weeks (172/196 [88%] with sulpiride v 194/212 [91%] with placebo; RR 0.96, 95% CI 0.90 to 1.02).[19]

Harms: **Versus placebo:** The review found no difference with sulpiride versus placebo in involuntary movements or hypersalivation.[19] **Versus standard antipsychotic drugs:** The review found that the use of antiparkinson drugs over 4–10 weeks was significantly less frequent with sulpiride versus standard antipsychotic drugs (RR 0.73, 95% CI 0.59 to 0.90).[19]

Comment: The review stated that the other two RCTs it identified reported improvement in mental state with sulpiride versus placebo, but that no raw data could be obtained because of poor reporting in the RCTs.[19] Observational evidence and clinical experience suggest sulpiride may be associated with galactorrhoea, but RCT data did not quantify the risk of occurrence.[20]

OPTION AMISULPRIDE

One RCT found that amisulpride versus placebo significantly increased the proportion of people who were "much improved" in global clinical impression. Three systematic reviews found limited evidence that amisulpride may improve symptoms more than standard antipsychotic drugs, although one of the reviews suggested that effects may be attributable to differences in dose. One RCT found no significant difference in symptoms with amisulpride versus risperidone. The systematic reviews found that extrapyramidal adverse effects were less likely with amisulpride versus standard antipsychotic drugs.

Benefits: **Versus placebo:** We found two systematic reviews.[21,22] The first review (search date 2000) identified one RCT comparing amisulpride versus placebo that assessed symptoms using the Clinical Global Assessment scale.[21] It found that amisulpride versus placebo significantly reduced the proportion of people who were less than "much improved" in global clinical impression (79/159 [50%] with amisulpride v 66/83 [79%] with placebo; RR 0.62, 95% CI 0.52 to 0.76; NNT 4, 95% CI 3 to 6). The second review (search date 2000) identified no RCTs comparing amisulpride versus placebo in people with both positive and negative symptoms.[22] **Versus standard antipsychotic drugs**: We found three systematic reviews.[21–23] The first systematic review (search date 2000) identified four RCTs (651 people) comparing amisulpride versus a standard antipsychotic that used the Clinical Global Impression scale to assess outcomes.[21] It found that amisulpride versus standard antipsychotic drugs significantly reduced the proportion of people who were less than "much improved" in global clinical impression (107/324 [33%] with amisulpride v 163/327 [50%] with standard antipsychotic drugs; RR 0.66, 95% CI 0.55 to 0.80; NNT 6, 95% CI 5 to 11).[21] The second systematic review (search date 1998, 4 RCTs, including 2 RCTs identified by the first review, duration 4–6 weeks, 683 people) compared amisulpride versus standard antipsychotic drugs, usually haloperidol.[23] Allocation concealment was unclear in all included RCTs. It found that symptom reduction was greater with amisulpride versus standard antipsychotic drugs (standardised effect size –0.35, 95% CI –0.52 to –0.18, indicating that about 64% [95% CI 57% to 70%] of people do worse with standard antipsychotic drugs compared with amisulpride). The third systematic review (11 RCTs, 6 of which were included in the first or second reviews) found that amisulpride versus standard antipsychotic drugs improved Brief Psychiatric Rating scale scores (mean effect size 0.11; CI not stated; no further data provided).[22] **Versus risperidone:** The first review identified one RCT (228 people) which found no significant difference with amisulpride versus risperidone in brief psychiatric rating scale total symptom scores.[21]

Harms: **Versus placebo:** The first review found that extrapyramidal symptoms were significantly more common in people taking amisulpride than those treated with placebo, (2 RCTs; 20/173 [12%] *v* 7/96 [7%]; RR 2.18, 95% CI 1.09 to 4.38).[21] The second review comparing amisulpride (50–300 mg/daily) versus placebo in people with predominately negative symptoms found no significant difference in the use of antiparkinsonian medication. **Versus standard antipsychotic drugs:** The first review found that amisulpride versus standard antipsychotic drugs significantly reduced the proportion of people who had at least one adverse effect (6 RCTs; 261/373 [70%] *v* 308/378 [81%]; RR 0.85, 95% CI 0.79 to 0.92; NNT 9, 95% 5% CI 6 to 17).[21] It also found that people taking amisulpride versus standard antipsychotic drugs were significantly less likely to experience at least one extrapyramidal symptom (7 RCTs; 161/383 [42%] *v* 234/388 [60%]; RR 0.68, 95% CI 0.60 to 0.79; NNT 5, 95% CI 4 to 8). It also found that amisulpride versus standard antipsychotic drugs significantly reduced the proportion of people who left the study early (14 RCTs; 282/881 [32%] *v* 242/631 [38%]; RR 0.72, 95% CI 0.62 to 0.83; NNT 9, 95% CI 7 to 16). The second review found that amisulpride versus standard antipsychotic drugs significantly reduced the proportion of people who withdrew from the trial (NNH 9, 95% CI 5 to 22).[23] It also found that movement disorders, measured by the Simpson Angus scale, were significantly less frequent with amisulpride versus standard antipsychotic drugs (SMD –0.44, 95% CI –0.26 to –0.61).[23] The third systematic review found that people taking amisulpride versus standard antipsychotic drugs were less likely to withdraw from the study early and experienced fewer movement disorders.[22] It found that amisulpride versus standard antipsychotic drugs significantly reduced the use of antiparkinsonian medication (effect size 0.25, 95% CI 0.17 to 0.32). **Versus risperidone:** The RCT identified by the first review found no significant difference in adverse effects, extrapyramidal symptoms, or withdrawal rate with amisulpride versus risperidone.[21]

Comment: All four short term RCTs identified by the second review included people randomised to relatively high doses of amisulpride (estimated equivalent to 20 mg haloperidol), which may have exaggerated results in favour of amisulpride.[23] Meta-regression analysis found that, after adjustment for dose differences, new antipsychotic drugs lose their therapeutic advantage over standard antipsychotic drugs, but remain superior for extrapyramidal adverse effects. Meta-regression was not available for amisulpride alone.

OPTION OLANZAPINE

Four systematic reviews found limited evidence that olanzapine may improve symptoms more than standard antipsychotic drugs and good evidence that olanzapine has fewer adverse effects, although one of the reviews suggested that effects may be attributable to differences in dose. Four systematic reviews found no clear difference in symptoms or adverse effects with olanzapine versus risperidone or clozapine.

Benefits: We found six systematic reviews[23–28] and one subsequent RCT.[29] comparing olanzapine versus standard antipsychotic drugs or versus other new antipsychotic drugs. **Versus standard antipsychotic drugs:** The first systematic review (search date 1999, 15 RCTs, 3282 people) compared olanzapine versus standard antipsychotic drugs, usually haloperidol.[24] It found that olanzapine (2.5–25 mg daily) did not significantly reduce psychotic symptoms over 6–8 weeks compared with standard antipsychotic drugs (2778 people: RR for no important response, defined as a 40% reduction on any scale 0.9, 95% CI 0.76 to 1.06). The second systematic review (search date 1999, 4 RCTs, 2914 people) found that olanzapine was associated with slightly greater treatment success than haloperidol on a composite measure of positive and negative symptoms.[25] The third systematic review (search date 1998, 4 RCTs) similarly found that olanzapine improved symptoms compared with standard antipsychotic drugs (WMD –0.22, 95% CI –0.30 to –0.14) indicating that 59% of people taking standard antipsychotics had poorer symptom score than people taking olanzapine. However, after adjustment for treatment doses, no significant benefit was found (see comment on amisulpride, p 1031).[23] The fourth systematic review (search date 1998, 3 RCTs, 2606) compared olanzapine versus standard antipsychotic medication.[26] It found no significant difference in the mean change on a combined rating of positive and negative symptoms (PANSS) with olanzapine versus standard antipsychotic drugs. A subsequent meta-regression analysis was conducted to control for confounding variables (age, duration of illness, etc.) and found that the mean improvement in the PANSS rating scale was significantly greater in people treated with olanzapine (WMD –5.9, 95% CI –11.1 to –0.6). The meta-regression analysis did not appear to take account of the dose of standard antipsychotic (usually haloperidol).[26] **Versus risperidone:** Two systematic reviews (search date 1999, 1 RCT;[25] search date 1998, 2 RCTs[23]) and one subsequent RCT[29] found no significant difference between olanzapine and risperidone (results from first systematic review; RR for no clinically important response after 8 wks 0.93, 95% CI 0.85 to 1.01).[25] However, one further systematic review (search date 1999, 3 RCTs) found that olanzapine reduced symptom severity in the medium term, although it found no significant difference in the long term (at medium term follow up in 392 participants, composite symptom scores improved by 7.5 points with olanzapine *v* risperidone on a 210 point scale, 95% CI 2.9 to 12.0).[27] **Versus clozapine:** One systematic review (search date 1998, 1 RCT, 180 people) comparing olanzapine versus clozapine found no significant difference for clinical response rates (RR for no important clinical response 0.7, 95% CI 0.5 to 1.1).[28]

Harms: **Versus standard antipsychotic drugs:** Olanzapine versus standard antipsychotic drugs did not significantly reduce the number of people who withdrew from the trials at 6–8 weeks (36% *v* 49%; RR 0.9, 95% CI 0.7 to 1.1) or at one year (83% *v* 90%; OR 0.9, 95% CI 0.86 to 1.02).[24] Olanzapine versus standard antipsychotic drugs caused fewer extrapyramidal adverse effects (in heterogeneous data prone to bias), less nausea (2347 people; RR 0.7, 95% CI 0.6 to 0.9; NNT 25, 95% CI 14 to 85), vomiting (1996 people: RR 0.6, 95% CI 0.4 to 0.8; NNT 20, 95% CI 12 to 46), or drowsiness (2347 people: RR 0.8, 95% CI 0.7 to 0.9) than standard antipsychotic drugs.[24] Olanzapine was associated with a greater increase in appetite (1996 people: RR 1.7, 95% CI 1.4 to 2.0; NNH 10, 95% CI 7 to 15), and weight gain (heterogeneous data) than standard antipsychotic drugs.[24] The third systematic review found that drop out rate was lower with olanzapine than with haloperidol, but the difference did not persist after adjustment for dose.[23] Dystonia and akathisia were less frequent with olanzapine than haloperidol, even after adjustment for dose (ARR for dystonia with olanzapine *v* haloperidol 14%, 95% CI 11% to 17%; ARR for akathisia with olanzapine *v* haloperidol 4.8%, 95% CI 3.1% to 6.5%). Olanzapine was associated with a 12% (95% CI 8% to 15%) increase in excessive appetite compared with haloperidol.[23] **Versus risperidone:** The first systematic review (search date 1999, 1 RCT, 84 people) found that olanzapine compared with risperidone was associated with fewer extrapyramidal adverse effects (NNT to avoid causing 1 adverse effect 8), less parkinsonism (NNT 11), and less need for anticholinergic medication (NNT 8), but olanzapine caused more dry mouth (NNH 9), and greater weight gain (NNH 11).[24] One additional review found that risperidone was associated with a higher drop out rate than olanzapine (RR for drop out with risperidone *v* olanzapine 1.3, 95% CI 1.1 to 1.6).[27] One subsequent RCT (377 people) comparing olanzapine and risperidone found no significant difference for severity of extrapyramidal adverse effects, need for anticholinergics, or for drop out rate. Fewer people on risperidone experienced weight gain (AR for ≥ 7% weight gain 27.3% with olanzapine, 11.6% with risperidone).[29] **Versus clozapine:** One RCT (search date 1999, 180 people) found that olanzapine was associated with significantly less nausea than clozapine (RR 0.1, 95% CI 0.01 to 0.8), but found no significant difference for movement disorders (RR for self reported symptoms of movement disorder 0.4, 95% CI 0.1 to 1.4).[28]

Comment: The results of the reviews are dominated by one large multicentre RCT reported by drug company employees. [23–28] Benefits seem to be maximal at a dose of 15 mg daily, and higher doses may be associated with more harms. Results depended on the precise statistical test used. Reliability of results may be compromised by heterogeneity.

OPTION QUETIAPINE

Three systematic reviews comparing quetiapine with standard antipsychotic drugs found no significant difference in symptoms, but two of the reviews found that quietiapine significantly reduced akathisia, parkinsonism, and the proportion of people who left the trial early.

Benefits: **Versus standard antipsychotic drugs:** We found three systematic reviews.[23,25,30] The first review (search date 1999, 6 RCTs, 1414 people) identified two RCTs (809 people) comparing quetiapine versus haloperidol and found no evidence of a difference in effectiveness on a composite measure of positive and negative symptoms.[25] The second review (search date 2000, 7 RCTs) of quetiapine (50–800 mg daily) versus standard antipsychotic drugs (usually haloperidol) found no significant difference in global improvement (1247 people: RR no important improvement in mental state 0.93, 95% CI 0.83 to 1.04).[30] The third review (search date 1998, 2 RCTs) also found no difference in overall symptom score (WMD –0.03, 95% CI –0.23 to +0.18).[23]

Harms: **Versus standard antipsychotic drugs:** The second review found that quetiapine versus standard antipsychotic drugs was associated with significantly fewer people leaving trials early (RR 0.87, 95% CI 0.76 to 0.99), less dystonia (RR 0.14, 95% CI 0.04 to 0.49), less akathisia (RR 0.24, 95% CI 0.15 to 0.38), and less parkinsonism (RR 0.22, 95% CI 0.15 to 0.33), but more dry mouth (RR 2.85, 95% CI 1.46 to 5.57).[30] The third systematic review found no difference in withdrawal rate with quetiapine versus standard antipsychotic drugs (OR 0.70, 95% CI 0.46 to 1.06).[23] Meta-regression analysis, which controlled for dose differences, found that as a group, new antipsychotic drugs reduced extrapyramidal adverse effects compared with standard drugs (see comment on amisulpiride, p 1031).

Comment: The evidence comes from a small number of short term RCTs that had substantial withdrawal rates and did not conduct intention to treat analyses.

OPTION RISPERIDONE

Four systematic reviews found limited evidence that risperidone may be more effective than standard antipsychotic drugs (mainly haloperidol), and good evidence that, at lower doses, risperidone has fewer adverse effects, although one of the reviews suggested that effects may be attributable to differences in dose. Three systematic reviews found no significant difference between risperidone versus new antipsychotic drugs.

Benefits: **Versus standard antipsychotic drugs:** We found four systematic reviews[24–26,31] and one additional RCT.[32] The first systematic review (search date 1997, 14 RCTs, 3401 people) found that, at 12 weeks, risperidone (mean daily dose range 6.1–12 mg) was significantly more effective in improving outcome than standard antipsychotic drugs, usually haloperidol.[31] Outcome was "clinical improvement", variably defined but usually defined as a 20% reduction in general symptoms (2171 people: 11 RCTs; RR no improvement 0.8, 95% CI 0.7 to 0.9; NNT 10, 95% CI 7 to 16). No benefit was observed for the outcome of global clinical impression. The second systematic review (search date 1999, 9 RCTs, 2215 people) found that risperidone was associated with slightly greater success than haloperidol on a composite measure of positive and negative symptoms.[25] The third systematic review (search date 1998,

8 RCTs) found significant heterogeneity among six short term RCTs. Two long term RCTs found that risperidone improved symptom scores compared with standard antipsychotic drugs (WMD –0.40, 95% CI –0.27 to –0.54 indicating that about 66% of people taking standard antipsychotics had worse composite symptom scores than with risperidone). However, this difference did not persist after controlling for dose of standard drug (see benefits of amisulpride, p 1030).[23] The fourth systematic review (search date 1998, 7 RCTs, 1036 people) found that risperidone versus haloperidol significantly improved negative and positive symptoms as measured by the PANSS (WMD –8.3 95%CI –13.8 to –2.7).[26] The additional RCT (99 people) comparing a range of doses of risperidone with haloperidol found no overall significant difference in global outcome.[32] **Versus new antipsychotic drugs:** See benefits of olanzapine, p 1032. We found three systematic reviews,[23,27,28] which found no significant difference between risperidone versus clozapine (5 RCTs) or versus amisulpride (1 RCT) for outcomes including improvement in mental state. However, the RCTs were small and short, with high withdrawal rates. The third review (2 RCTs) found no difference in efficacy with risperidone versus clozapine.[23]

Harms: **Versus standard antipsychotic drugs:** The first systematic review found no significant difference with risperidone versus standard antipsychotic drugs in the proportion of people who withdrew from treatment (2166 people: RR 0.8, 95% CI 0.6 to 1.1). People taking risperidone versus standard antipsychotic drugs developed significantly fewer extrapyramidal effects (2279 people: RR 0.6, 95% CI 0.5 to 0.7; NNT 5, 95% CI 5 to 10), required less antiparkinsonian medication (2436 people: RR 0.6, 95% CI 0.5 to 0.7; NNT 7, 95% CI 5 to 10), and were less likely to develop daytime somnolence (2098 people: RR 0.9, 95% CI 0.7 to 0.99; NNT 22, 95% CI 11 to 500). Risperidone versus standard antipsychotic drugs was associated with significantly more weight gain (1652 people: RR 1.4, 95% CI 1.1 to 1.7; NNH 13, 95% CI 8 to 36).[31] The additional RCT found no significant difference in the rate of overall adverse effects between risperidone and haloperidol.[32] The third systematic review found no significant difference in the proportion of people who withdrew from treatment with risperidone versus haloperidol, but found that risperidone reduced symptoms of dystonia (WMD –0.26, 95% CI –0.39 to –0.12), parkinsonism (WMD –0.39, 95% CI –0.51 to –0.27), and dyskinesia (WMD –0.16, 95% CI –0.28 to –0.04) compared with haloperidol. Differences persisted after controlling for dose.[23] The fourth systematic review found that risperidone versus haloperidol significantly reduced the proportion of people who required medication for extrapyramidal side effects (OR 0.42, 95% CI 0.19 to 0.96).[26] **Versus new antipsychotic drugs:** See harms of olanzapine, p 1033. We found three systematic reviews,[23,27,28] which found no significant difference between risperidone and clozapine. The second systematic review (search date 1999, 1 RCT, 228 people) found amisulpride versus risperidone caused less agitation (RR 0.29, 95% CI 0.1 to 0.86), and less constipation (RR 0.13, 95% CI 0.2 to 1.0).[27]

Comment: The reported benefits in the first review over standard antipsychotic drugs were marginal, and it found evidence of publication bias.[31] Sensitivity analyses found that benefits in clinical improvement and continuing treatment of risperidone compared with standard antipsychotic drugs were no longer significant if RCTs using more than 10 mg haloperidol daily were excluded.[31] This loss of significance could be because of loss of power when RCTs were excluded. Exclusion of the higher dosage RCTs did not remove the difference in rate of extrapyramidal adverse effects.[31]

OPTION ZIPRASIDONE

One systematic review found no significant difference in mental state improvement with ziprasidone versus haloperidol, and found that ziprasidone versus haloperidol significantly reduced akathisia and acute dystonia, but increased nausea and vomiting.

Benefits: **Versus standard antipsychotic drugs:** We found one systematic review (search date 1999) that identified one RCT (301 people) that assessed improvement in mental state.[33] It found no significant difference in mental state improvement with ziprasidone versus haloperidol (RR no important improvement in mental state 0.9, 95% CI 0.7 to 1.0).[33]

Harms: **Versus standard antipsychotic drugs:** The review found no clear difference in total adverse events between ziprasidone and haloperidol.[33] Ziprasidone versus haloperidol was significantly less likely to cause akathisia in the short term (2 RCTs, 438 people: RR 0.3, 95% CI 0.2 to 0.6; NNT 8, 95% CI 5 to 18), and in the long term (1 RCT, 301 people: RR 0.3, 95% CI 0.1 to 0.7; NNT 9, 95% CI 5 to 21), and less likely to cause acute dystonia in the short term (2 RCTs, 438 people: RR 0.4, 95% CI 0.2 to 0.9; NNT 16, 95% CI 9 to 166). Ziprasidone versus haloperidol was more likely to produce nausea and vomiting in both the short term (1 RCT, 306 people: RR 3.6, 95% CI 1.8 to 7; NNT 5, 95% CI 4 to 8), and in the long term (1 RCT, 301 people: RR 2.1, 95% CI 1 to 4; NNT 9, 95% CI 5 to 33). Intramuscular ziprasidone was significantly more likely to be associated with injection site pain than haloperidol (1 RCT, 306 people: RR 5.3, 95% CI 1.3 to 22; NNT 12, 95% CI 7 to 27).

Comment: The duration of RCTs in the review was less than 6 weeks.[33] Most reported a withdrawal rate of over 20% and no RCT clearly described adequate precautions for the blinding of treatment allocation. We found no evidence comparing ziprasidone with other new antipsychotic drugs.

OPTION ZOTEPINE

One systematic review found weak evidence that zotepine versus standard antipsychotic drugs significantly increased the proportion of people with a clinically important improvement in symptoms, and reduced akasthesia, dystonia and rigidity. This finding was not robust as removal of a single RCT from the analysis meant that the difference between zotepine and standard antipsychotics was no longer significant.

Benefits: **Versus standard antipsychotic drugs:** We found one systematic review (search date 1999, 8 RCTs, 356 people) comparing zotepine (75–450 mg daily) versus a variety of standard antipsychotic drugs.[34] It found that zotepine was significantly more likely than standard antipsychotic drugs to bring about "clinically important improvement" as defined by a pre-stated cut off point on the brief psychiatric rating scale (RR 1.25, 95% CI 1.1 to 1.4; NNT 7, 95% CI 4 to 22; see comment below).

Harms: The review found zotepine caused significantly less akathisia (396 people: RR 0.7, 95% CI 0.6 to 0.9; NNT 8, 95% CI 5 to 34), dystonia (70 people: RR 0.5, 95% CI 0.2 to 0.9; NNT 4, 95% CI 2 to 56), and rigidity (164 people: RR 0.6, 95% CI 0.4 to 0.9; NNT 7, 95% CI 4 to 360) than standard antipsychotic drugs.[34]

Comment: All but one RCT identified by the review were of 12 weeks or less duration and all were conducted in Europe.[23] Only one RCT favoured zotepine over standard antipsychotic drugs, and removal of this RCT from the analysis changed the result from a significant to a non-significant effect. Two RCTs found abnormal electrocardiogram results in people taking zotepine, but few additional details were given. We found too few RCTs to compare zotepine reliably with other new antipsychotic drugs.

OPTION CLOZAPINE

Two systematic reviews found that clozapine versus standard antipsychotic drugs improved symptoms over 4–10 weeks, and may improve symptoms in the longer term. However, RCTs found that clozapine may be associated with blood dyscrasias. Three systematic reviews found no strong evidence about the effectiveness or safety of clozapine versus new antipsychotic drugs.

Benefits: We found four systematic reviews.[23,27,28,35] **Versus standard antipsychotic drugs:** One systematic review (search date 1999, 31 RCTs, 2530 people, 73% men) compared clozapine versus standard antipsychotic drugs, such as chlorpromazine and haloperidol. It found that clozapine was associated with greater clinical improvement both in the short term (4–10 wks, 14 RCTs, 1131 people: RR no important improvement 0.7, 95% CI 0.7 to 0.8; NNT 6, 95% CI 5 to 7) and the long term (heterogeneous data).[35] A second review (search date 1998, 12 RCTs) also found that clozapine improved symptoms compared with standard antipsychotic drugs (WMD –0.68, 95% CI –0.82 to –0.55, indicating that 75% of people taking standard antipsychotic drugs had worse composite symptom scores than those taking clozapine). However, the two long term RCTs included in the review were heterogeneous and the short term benefit was not observed after controlling for the dose of standard drug (see benefits of amisulpride, p 1030).[23] **Versus new antipsychotic drugs:** We found one systematic review (search date 1999, 8 RCTs), which compared clozapine versus new antipsychotic drugs, including olanzapine and risperidone,[28] and two systematic reviews, which included comparisons of clozapine versus risperidone (search date 1999, 5 RCTs;[27] search date 1998, 2 RCTs[23]). All three systematic reviews found no significant difference in efficacy, but the number of people studied was too small to rule out a clinically important difference.

Harms: **Versus standard antipsychotic drugs:** Clozapine versus standard antipsychotic drugs was more likely to cause hypersalivation (1419 people: RR 3.0, 95% CI 1.8 to 4.7; NNH 3), temperature increases (1147 people: RR 1.8, 95% CI 1.2 to 2.7; NNH 11), and sedation (1527 people: RR 1.2, 95% CI 1.1 to 1.4; NNH 10), but less likely to cause dry mouth (799 people: RR 0.4, 95% CI 0.3 to 0.6; NNT 6), and extrapyramidal adverse effects (1235 people: RR 0.7, 95% CI 0.5 to 0.9; NNT 6).[23] One systematic review found that blood problems occurred more frequently with clozapine than with standard antipsychotic drugs (1293 people: AR 3.6% *v* 1.9%; NNH 58, 95% CI 31 to 111).[35] In a large observational case series, leucopenia was reported in 3% of 99 502 people over 5 years. However, it found monitoring white cell (neutrophil) counts was associated with a lower than expected rate of cases of agranulocytosis (382 *v* 995; AR 0.38% *v* 1%) and deaths (12 *v* 149).[36] Dyscrasias were significantly more common with clozapine versus standard antipsychotic drugs in younger people in a single RCT included in the first systematic review (21 people: RR 5.4, 95% CI 10 to 162; NNH 2.5).[35,37] One review found that, despite the requirement for regular blood tests, fewer people withdrew from treatment with clozapine in the long term (1513 people: RR 0.8, 95% CI 0.6 to 0.9; NNH 3).[35] However, another review found that long term drop out rate was only lower on fixed effects but not on random effects analyses. The difference in drop out rates did not persist after controlling for dose of haloperidol in an meta-regression analysis of all new antipsychotic drugs considered together.[23] **Versus new antipsychotic drugs:** Compared with new antipsychotic drugs (mainly risperidone), clozapine was less likely to cause extrapyramidal adverse effects (305 people: RR 0.3, 95% CI 0.1 to 0.6; NNT 6, 95% CI 4 to 9). Clozapine versus new antipsychotic drugs may also be less likely to cause dry mouth and more likely to cause fatigue, nausea, dizziness, hypersalivation, and hypersomnia, but these findings were from one or at most two RCTs.[28] Compared with new antipsychotic drugs, people on clozapine tended to be more satisfied with their treatment, but also tended to withdraw from RCTs more often.[28] Two reviews found no difference in rates of blood dyscrasias between clozapine and the new antipsychotic drugs, but the number of people studied was too small (558) to rule out a clinically important difference.[27,28]

Comment: Some of the benefits of clozapine were more apparent in the long term, depending on which drug was used for comparison in the RCTs.

QUESTION Which interventions reduce relapse rates?

OPTION CONTINUED TREATMENT WITH ANTIPSYCHOTIC DRUGS

Systematic reviews have found that continuing antipsychotic medication for at least 6 months after an acute episode significantly reduces relapse rates, and that some benefit of continuing medication is apparent for up to 2 years. We found no evidence of a difference in relapse rates among standard antipsychotic drugs, but one systematic review has found that clozapine versus standard antipsychotic drugs reduces relapse rates over

12 weeks and another review found that bromperidol versus haloperidol or fluphenazine significantly increased the proportion of people who relapsed. One additional RCT found that risperidone versus haloperidol reduced relapse over 2.2 years.

Benefits: **Versus no treatment or placebo:** We found three systematic reviews.[6,8,38] One review (search date not stated, 66 studies, 4365 people taking antipsychotic drugs, mean dose 630 mg chlorpromazine equivalents daily, mean follow up of 6.3 months) included 29 controlled trials with a mean follow up of 9.7 months.[38] It found significantly lower relapse in 1224 people maintained on treatment compared with 1224 withdrawn from treatment (16.2% *v* 51.5%; ARR 35%, 95% CI 33% to 38%; NNT 3, 95% CI 2.6 to 3.1). Over time, the relapse rate in people maintained on antipsychotic treatment approached that in those withdrawn from treatment, but was still lower in those on treatment at 2 years (ARR 22%; NNT 5). The second review (search date 1997) found that relapse rates over 6–24 months were significantly lower on chlorpromazine than placebo (3 RCTs; RR 0.7, 95% CI 0.5 to 0.9; NNT 3, 95% CI 2.5 to 4).[6] One subsequent systematic review (search date 1998, 20 RCTs) comparing haloperidol versus placebo included two RCTs (70 people currently in remission; duration 1 year). Haloperidol was more effective than placebo for preventing relapse (ARR 33%, 95% CI 16% to 50%; NNT 4, 95% CI 2 to 7).[8] **Choice of drug:** We found 11 systematic reviews [10,11,14,17,24,35,39–43] and one additional RCT (see table 1, p 1049).[44] The first systematic review (search date 1995) identified six RCTs comparing oral with depot fluphenazine.[39] A second systematic review (search date 1998) identified seven RCTs comparing haloperidol decanoate versus other depot antipsychotic drugs.[10] A third systematic review (search date 1998) identified eight RCTs comparing flupentixol (flupenthixol) decanoate versus other depot antipsychotic drugs.[40] A fourth systematic review (search date 1998, 14 RCTs) identified seven RCTs (417 people) comparing pipotiazine palmitate versus other depots, and one RCT (124 people) comparing pipotiazine palmitate with oral antipsychotic drugs.[11] A fifth systematic review (search date 1998) identified one RCT comparing fluspirilene decanoate versus oral chlorpromazine, and three RCTs comparing fluspirilene decanoate with other depot preparations.[41] A sixth systematic review (search date 1998) found one RCT comparing perphenazine enanthate versus clopenthixol decanoate.[42] Two reviews comparing pimozide and olanzapine versus typical antipsychotic drugs also found no significant difference in relapse rates.[17,24] The number of people studied was too small to rule out a clinically important difference. A ninth review (search date 1998) comparing clozapine with standard antipsychotic drugs found that relapse rates up to 12 weeks were significantly lower with clozapine (19 RCTs; RR 0.6, 95% CI 0.5 to 0.8; NNT 20).[35] A tenth review (search date 1998) found that significantly fewer people taking depot zuclopenthixol decanoate relapsed over 12 weeks to 1 year compared with people taking other depot preparations (3 RCTs, 296 people: RR 0.7, 95% CI 0.6 to 1.0; NNT 9, 95% CI 5 to 53).[43] An eleventh review (search date 1999) found that bromperidol versus haloperidol or fluphenazine significantly increased the proportion of people who relapsed (2 RCTs; RR 3.92 95% CI 1.05 to 14.6 NNH 5, 95% CI 3 to 28).[14] One additional RCT (365 people) found that risperidone versus haloperidol significantly reduced relapse over 2.2 years (NNT 5, 95% CI 4 to 10).[44]

Harms: Mild transient nausea, malaise, sweating, vomiting, insomnia, and dyskinesia were reported in an unspecified number of people after sudden drug cessation, but were usually acceptable with gradual dose reduction.[45] Annual incidence of tardive dyskinesia was 5%.[43]

Comment: In the systematic review of continued treatment versus withdrawal of treatment, meta-analysis of the 29 controlled trials gave similar results to those obtained when all 66 studies were included (ARR 37%, NNT 3).[43] The review was weakened because all RCT results were used rather than weighted comparisons, no length of time was given since the last acute episode, and no distinction was made between people experiencing a first episode and those with chronic illness.[43] Some clinicians use depot antipsychotic medication in selected people to ensure adherence to medication. We found no evidence from RCTs to support this practice.

OPTION FAMILY INTERVENTIONS

One systematic review has found that family intervention versus usual care significantly reduces relapse rates at 12 and 24 months. Seven families would have to be treated to avoid one additional relapse (and likely hospitalisation) in the family member with schizophrenia. One RCT found that fewer people receiving a multiple family versus single family intervention relapsed over 2 years, but the difference did not quite reach significance.

Benefits: **Versus usual care:** We found one systematic review (search date 1998, 13 RCTs).[46] Family interventions consisted mainly of education about the illness and training in problem solving over at least six weekly sessions. Three of the RCTs identified by the review included substantial proportions of people experiencing their first episode. The review found that family interventions versus usual care significantly reduced relapse rates at 12 and 24 months. At 12 months, the risk of relapse was significantly reduced (6 RCTs, 516 people: RR 0.7, 95% CI 0.5 to 1.0), such that seven families would have to be treated to avoid one additional relapse (and likely hospitalisation) in the family member with schizophrenia (NNT 7, 95% CI 4 to 14). **Multiple family psychoeducational intervention versus single family psychoeducational intervention:** We found one RCT (172 people aged 18–45 years with schizophrenia, and their families) that compared multiple family psychoeducational therapy versus single family psychoeducational therapy.[47] Psychoeducational therapy involved promoting family interactions to support recovery from an acute episode over one year and aiding vocational and social functioning over a second year, either in sessions with three families (multiple) or a single family. The RCT found that fewer people receiving multiple versus single family therapy relapsed over two years, but the difference did not quite reach significance (23/83 [28%] with multiple therapy *v* 37/89 [42%] with single family; RR 0.67, 95% CI 0.43 to 1.02).[40]

Harms: No harms were reported in the review or RCT.[46,47]

Comment: These results may overestimate treatment effect because of the difficulty of blinding people and investigators.[46] Although no harms were reported, illness education could possibly have adverse consequences on morale and outlook. The mechanism for the effects of family intervention remains unclear. It is thought to work by reducing "expressed emotion" (hostility and criticism) in relatives of people with schizophrenia. The time consuming nature of this intervention, which must normally take place at evenings or weekends, can limit its availability. It cannot be applied to people who have little contact with home based carers.

OPTION SOCIAL SKILLS TRAINING

Limited evidence from a systematic reviews of RCTs and observational studies suggests that social skills training versus usual care may reduce relapse rates.

Benefits: We found one systematic review (search date not stated 27 studies, number of RCTs not specified) comparing social skills training versus usual care.[48] The RCTs were mainly in men admitted to hospital, not all of whom had schizophrenia, using different techniques that generally included instruction in social interaction. Four studies provided quantitative information, of which three defined relapse as rehospitalisation. The review found that social skills training versus usual care significantly reduced relapse rates (WMD 0.47). However, sensitivity analysis indicated that five negative results (in studies not identified by a search) would render the difference non-significant. One systematic review (search date 1988) identified 73 trials in people with a variety of psychiatric disorders and found similar results, but suggested that motivation was an important predictor of benefit from treatment.[49]

Harms: None reported.

Comment: Many of the RCTs simultaneously compared the effects of other interventions (medication, education), so the effects of individual interventions are difficult to assess. Overall, it remains uncertain whether people at different stages of illness and function require different approaches. Selected people may benefit even from interventions of short duration.

OPTION COGNITIVE BEHAVIOURAL THERAPY

Limited evidence from RCTs found no significant difference in relapse rates with cognitive behavioural therapy plus standard care versus standard care alone.

Benefits: We found one systematic review (search date 2001, 2 RCTs, 123 people) comparing cognitive behavioural therapy plus standard care versus standard care alone.[50] Both RCTs incorporated the challenging of key beliefs, problem solving, and enhancement of coping. It found no significant difference with cognitive behavioural therapy versus standard care in relapse or readmission to hospital in the medium term (1 RCT, 0/33 [0%] *v* 4/28 [14%]; RR 0.09, 95% CI 0.01 to 1.69) or the long term (2 RCTs; 36/63 [57%] *v* 31/60 [52%]; RR 1.13, 95% CI 0.82 to 1.56; see comment below).[50]

Harms: The systematic review gave no information on harms.[50]

Comment: Neither of the RCTs contributing long term results was blinded, and each concentrated on different clinical issues — symptoms, adherence to treatment, or general rehabilitation. The results are sensitive to the method of statistical calculation used; peto odds ratios found a significant benefit with cognitive behavioural therapy in the medium term (1 RCT, 61 people), but absolute risk reductions and relative risks found no significant difference.[50]

OPTION PSYCHOEDUCATIONAL INTERVENTIONS

One systematic review has found that psychoeducation versus control intervention significantly reduces relapse rates at 9–18 months.

Benefits: **Versus usual treatment:** We found one systematic review (search date 2002, 10 RCTs, 1128 people, 53% male).[51] The systematic review included one RCT of a brief individual intervention (10 sessions or less), but no standard length individual psychoeducational interventions (11 sessions or more). It included six RCTs of brief group psychoeducational interventions and four of standard length. Standard length interventions were significantly more effective than treatment as usual in preventing relapse during 9–18 months (6 RCTs, 720 people: RR 0.80, 95% CI 0.70 to 0.92; NNT 6, 95% CI 3 to 83). Brief group psychoeducational interventions were also more effective than treatment as usual in preventing relapse or re admission by 1 year (RR 0.85, 95% CI 0.74 to 0.98; NNT 12, CI 6 to 83). When all RCTs were pooled, relapse rates at 9–18 months' follow up were significantly lower in the psychoeducation group than in the control intervention group (6 RCTs; RR 0.80, 95% CI 0.70 to 0.92; NNT 9, 95% CI 6 to 22).

Harms: None reported.

Comment: The systematic review found few good RCTs. There was significant heterogeneity of both interventions and outcomes.

QUESTION Which interventions are effective in people resistant to standard treatment?

One systematic review in people resistant to standard treatment has found that clozapine versus standard treatment improves symptoms after 12 weeks and after 2 years.

Benefits: **Clozapine:** We found one systematic review (search date 1999, 6 RCTs) comparing clozapine versus standard antipsychotic drugs in people who were resistant to standard treatment.[35] Clozapine achieved improvement both in the short term (6–12 wks, 4 RCTs, 370 people: RR for no improvement compared with standard antipsychotic drugs 0.7, 95% CI 0.6 to 0.8; NNT 5), and in the longer term (12–24 months: 2 RCTs, 648 people: RR 0.8, 95% CI 0.6 to 1.0). There was no difference in relapse rates in the short term. **Other interventions:** We found no good evidence on the effects of other interventions in people resistant to standard treatment.

Harms: See harms of clozapine, p 1038.

Comment: RCTs are under way to clarify the mode of action of cognitive behavioural therapy and establish its effects in people who are resistant to standard treatments.

QUESTION Which interventions improve adherence to antipsychotic medication?

OPTION COMPLIANCE THERAPY

One RCT found limited evidence that compliance therapy versus non-specific counselling may increase adherence to antipsychotic medication at 6 and 18 months.

Benefits: We found no systematic review. We found one RCT (47 people with acute psychoses, most of whom fulfilled criteria for schizophrenia or had been admitted with the first episode of a psychotic illness) of compliance therapy (see glossary, p 1045) versus supportive counselling, that assessed outcomes immediately after treatment, at 6 months[52], and at 18 months.[53] It found that people treated with compliance therapy were significantly more likely to attain at least passive acceptance of antipsychotic medication versus people who received non-specific counselling, both immediately after the intervention (OR 6.3, 95% CI 1.6 to 24.6) and at 6 months' follow up (OR 5.2, 95% CI 1.5 to 18.3).[52] At 18 months (for an extended sample of 74 people), it found a significant improvement on a seven point scale of medication adherence was found for people treated with compliance therapy (mean difference 1.4, 95% CI 0.9 to 1.6).[52]

Harms: None reported.[52,53]

Comment: Other trials have examined the potential benefits of compliance therapy, but either did not employ a standardised measure of adherence or adherence was not rated in a blind fashion. The RCT above requires independent replication. About a third of each group did not complete the RCTs, and missing data are estimated from the mean scores in each group. Calculation of numbers needed to treat was not possible because of missing data.

OPTION FAMILY INTERVENTIONS

One systematic review has found that family interventions versus usual care are unlikely to improve adherence to antipsychotic medication.

Benefits: We found one systematic review (search date 1998) comparing family interventions versus usual care.[46] Family interventions consisted mainly of education about the illness and training in problem solving over at least six weekly sessions. "Poor compliance with medication" (5 RCTs, 257 people, 9 months' to 2 years' duration) and "poor compliance with treatment protocol" (12 RCTs, 745 people) were not altered by family therapy compared with usual care (OR for poor compliance with medication: family therapy *v* control 0.63, 95% CI 0.38 to 1.03; OR for poor compliance with treatment protocol: family therapy *v* control 1.10, 95% CI 0.72 to 1.66).

Harms: No harms were reported, although illness education could possibly have adverse consequences on morale and outlook.[46]

Comment: None.

OPTION PSYCHOEDUCATIONAL INTERVENTIONS

One systematic review found limited evidence that psychoeducation versus usual care improved adherence with antipsychotic medication. Two RCTs found that psychoeducational therapy improved adherence less than behavioural therapy.

Benefits: **Versus usual treatment:** We found one systematic review (search date 2002, 10 RCTs, 1128 people, 53% male).[51] The systematic review considered individual and group psychoeducation of either standard length (11 sessions or more) or brief interventional types (10 sessions or less). One RCT (67 people with DSM-III-R schizophrenia) measured the effect of individual psychoeducation on compliance. It found no significant difference between the brief individual psychoeducation and treatment as usual on the compliance subscale of the schedule for assessment of insight. Two RCTs compared brief group psychoeducational interventions versus control group. Both suggest psychoeducation to be more effective than the comparison treatment. The first RCT (236 people) found a significant advantage group of psychoeducational intervention versus usual treatment on a continuous scale of medication concordance (WMD –0.4, 95% CI –0.6 to –0.2). The second RCT (46 people) of a brief psychoeducational intervention versus usual treatment reported compliance episodes at 1 year follow up. Skewed data suggested an advantage of psychoeducational interventions (treatment group: 24 people, mean number of non-compliant episodes at 1 year 0.38; control group: 22 people, mean 1.14). One RCT (82 people, 18 months' duration) compared standard length group interventions versus treatment as usual and found no significant difference in compliance. **Versus behavioural therapy:** We found two RCTs.[54,55] One RCT (36 men) compared behavioural therapy versus psychoeducation versus usual treatment.[54] The behavioural training method comprised being told the importance of complying with antipsychotic medication and instructions on how to take medication. Each participant was given a self monitoring spiral calendar, which featured a dated slip of paper for each dose of antipsychotic. Adherence was estimated by pill counts. After 3 months, fewer people had high pill adherence after psychoeducation compared with behaviour therapy (3/11 *v* 8/11 had pill adherence scores of 80% measured by pill counts). The second RCT (39 people) compared a behavioural intervention given individually, a behavioural intervention involving the person with schizophrenia and their family, and a psychoeducational intervention.[55] The behavioural intervention consisted of specific written guidelines, and oral instructions, given to people to use a pill box consisting of 28 compartments for every medication occasion during a week. The behavioural intervention, when given to the individual and their family, also consisted of instructions for the family member to compliment the person with schizophrenia for taking their prescribed medication. The primary outcome measure was pill count at 2 months. Medication adherence was more likely with behavioural interventions than with psychoeducation (> 90% adherence at 2 months, 25/26 [96%] with behavioural methods *v* 6/13 [46%] with psychoeducation; ARR 0.5; RR 2.1; NNT 2 95% CI 2 to 5).

Harms: None reported.

Comment: There are few RCTs of psychoeducational interventions and most do not measure medication adherence. Each psychoeducational intervention varied in the protocol used and few employed the same outcome ratings.

OPTION BEHAVIOURAL THERAPY

One RCT found that behavioural interventions improved adherence to antipsychotic medication compared with usual treatment. Two RCTs found that behavioural interventions improved adherence compared with psychoeducational therapy.

Benefits: We found no systematic review. **Versus usual treatment:** We found one RCT (36 men).[54] The behavioural training method comprised being told the importance of complying with antipsychotic medication and instructions on how to take medication. Each participant was given a self monitoring spiral calendar, which featured a dated slip of paper for each dose of antipsychotic. Adherence was estimated by pill counts. After 3 months fewer people had high pill adherence after usual treatment compared with behaviour therapy (figures not provided). **Versus psychoeducational therapy:** See benefits of psychoeducational therapy, p 1044.

Harms: None reported.

Comment: None.

GLOSSARY

Compliance therapy A treatment based on cognitive behavioural therapy and motivational interviewing techniques with a view to improving concordance to medication.

Negative symptoms This generally refers to qualities abnormal by their absence (e.g. loss of drive, motivation, and self care).

Positive symptoms This refers to symptoms that characterise the onset or relapse of schizophrenia, usually hallucinations and delusions, but sometimes including thought disorder.

Substantive changes

Amisulpride Two new systematic reviews;[21,22] conclusions unchanged.

Olanzapine One new systematic review;[26] conclusions unchanged.

Risperidone One new systematic review;[26] conclusions unchanged.

Preventing relapse, continued treatment with antipsychotic drugs, choice of drug One new systematic review found that bromperidol versus haloperidol or flupehenazine significantly increased the proportion of people who relapsed.[14] One new RCT found that risperidone versus haloperidol reduced relapse over 2.2 years.[44]

Cognitive behavioural therapy to reduce relapse rates Limited evidence from one new systematic review of two RCTs found no significant difference in relapse rates with cognitive behavioural therapy plus standard care versus standard care alone.[50] Recategorised as unknown effectiveness.

REFERENCES

1. Andreasen NC. Symptoms, signs and diagnosis of schizophrenia. *Lancet* 1995;346:477–481.
2. Cannon M, Jones P. Neuroepidemiology: schizophrenia. *J Neurol Neurosurg Psychiatry* 1996;61:604–613.
3. Jablensky A, Sartorius N, Ernberg G, et al. Schizophrenia: manifestations, incidence and course in different cultures. A World Health Organisation ten-country study. *Psychol Med* 1992;monograph supplement 20:1–97.
4. Hegarty JD, Baldessarini RJ, Tohen M, et al. One hundred years of schizophrenia: a meta-analysis of the outcome literature. *Am J Psychiatry* 1994;151:1409–1416.
5. Johnstone EC. Schizophrenia: problems in clinical practice. *Lancet* 1993; 341:536–538.
6. Thornley B, Adams C. Content and quality of 2000 controlled trials in schizophrenia over 50 years. *BMJ* 1998;317:1181–1184. Search date 1997; primary sources hand searching of conference proceedings, Biological Abstracts, Cinahl, The Cochrane Library, Embase, Lilacs, Psychlit, Pstndex, Medline, and Sociofile.
7. Thornley B, Adams CE, Awad G. Chlorpromazine versus placebo for those with schizophrenia. In: The Cochrane Library, Issue 2, 2002. Oxford: Update Software. Search date 1999; primary sources Biological Abstracts, Embase, Medline, Psychlit, SciSearch, Cochrane Library, Cochrane Schizophrenia Group's Register, hand searches of reference lists, and personal contact with pharmaceutical companies and authors of trials.
8. Joy CB, Adams CE, Lawrie SM. Haloperidol versus placebo for schizophrenia. In: The Cochrane Library, Issue 2, 2002. Oxford: Update Software. Search date 1998; primary sources Biological Abstracts, Cinahl, The Cochrane Schizophrenia Group's Register, Embase, Medline, Psychlit, SciSearch, hand searches of references, and contact with authors of trials and pharmaceutical companies.
9. Sultana A, Reilly J, Fenton M. Thioridazine for schizophrenia. In: The Cochrane Library, Issue 2, 2002. Oxford: Update Software. Search date 1999; primary sources Biological Abstracts, Cinahl, The Cochrane Library, The Cochrane Schizophrenia Group's Register, Embase, Medline, Psychlit, Sociofile, reference lists, pharmaceutical companies, and authors of trials.
10. Quraishi S, David A. Depot haloperidol decanoate for schizophrenia. In: The Cochrane Library, Issue 2, 2002. Oxford: Update Software. Search date 1998; primary sources Biological Abstracts, Embase, Medline, Psychlit, SciSearch, The Cochrane Library, reference lists, authors of studies, and pharmaceutical companies.
11. Quraishi S, David A. Depot pipothiazine palmitate and undeclynate for schizophrenia. In: The Cochrane Library, Issue 2, 2002. Oxford: Update Software. Search date 1998; primary sources Biological Abstracts, Cochrane Library, Cochrane Schizophrenia Group's Register, Embase, Medline, Psychlit, hand searches of reference lists, and personal communication with pharmaceutical companies.
12. Leucht S, Hartung B. Benperidol for schizophrenia. In: The Cochrane Library, Issue 2, 2002. Search date 2001; primary sources Cochrane Schizophrenia Group's register (January 2001), Biological Abstracts, CINAHL, The Cochrane Library, Embase, Medline, Psyclit, Lilacs, Psyndex, Sociological Abstracts, Sociofile, hand searches of reference lists and personal contact with pharmaceutical companies and authors.
13. Leucht S, Hartung B. Perazine for schizophrenia. In: The Cochrane Library, Issue 2, 2002. Search date 2001; primary sources Cochrane Schizophrenia Group's register (January 2001) , Biological Abstracts, CINAHL, The Cochrane Library, Embase, Medline, Psyclit, Lilacs, Psyndex, Sociological Abstracts, Sociofile, hand searches of reference lists and personal contact with pharmaceutical companies and authors.
14. Quraishi S, David A, Adams, CE. Depot bromperidol decanoate for schizophrenia. In: The Cochrane Library, Issue 2, 2002. Search date 1999; primary sources Biological Abstracts, Cochrane Library, Cochrane Schizophrenia Group's Register, Embase, Medline, PsycLIT, hand searches of reference lists and personal contact with Janssen Cilag.
15. Fenton M, Murphy B, Wood J, et al. Loxapine for schizophrenia. In: The Cochrane Library, Issue 2, 2002. Oxford: Update Software. Search date 1999; primary sources Biological Abstracts, The Cochrane Library, The Cochrane Schizophrenia Group's Register, Embase, Lilacs, Psyndex, Psychlit, and hand searches of reference lists.
16. Bagnall AM, Fenton M, Lewis R, et al. Molindone for schizophrenia and severe mental illness. In: The Cochrane Library, Issue 2, 2002. Oxford: Update Software. Search date 1999; primary sources Biological Abstracts, The Cochrane Library, The Cochrane Schizophrenia Group's Register, Cinahl, Embase, Psychlit, pharmaceutical databases, hand searches of reference lists, and personal contact with authors of trials.
17. Sultana A, McMonagle T. Pimozide for schizophrenia or related psychoses. In: The Cochrane Library, Issue 2, 2002. Oxford: Update Software. Search date 1999; primary sources Biological Abstracts, The Cochrane Schizophrenia Group's Register, Embase, Janssen-Cilag UK's register of studies, Medline, hand searches of reference lists, and personal contact with pharmaceutical companies.
18. Joy CB, Mumby-Croft R, Joy LA. Polyunsaturated fatty acid (fish or evening primrose oil) for schizophrenia. In: The Cochrane Library, Issue 2, 2002. Oxford: Update Software. Search date 2000; primary sources Biological Abstracts, Cinahl, The Cochrane Library, The Cochrane Schizophrenia Group's Register, Embase, Psychlit, hand searches of reference lists and personal contact with the authors.
19. Soares BGO, Fenton M, Chue P. Sulpiride for schizophrenia. In: The Cochrane Library, Issue 2, 2002. Oxford: Update Software. Search date 1998; primary sources Biological Abstracts, Cinahl, Cochrane Schizophrenia Group's Register, The Cochrane Library, Embase, Medline, Psychlit, Sigle, and Sociofile.
20. Harnryd C, Bjerkenstedt L, Bjork K, et al. Clinical evaluation of sulpiride in schizophrenic patients — a double-blind comparison with chlorpromazine. *Acta Psych Scand.* 1984;311:7–30.

21. Mota Neto JIS, Lima MS, Soares BGO. Amisulpride for schizophrenia. In: The Cochrane Library, Issue 2, 2002. Oxford: Update Software. Search date 2000, Biological Abstracts Cinahl, Cochrane Library, Cochrane Schizophrenia Group's Register, Embase, Lilacs, Medline, Psyclit, Science Citation Index, hand searches of reference lists and personal contact with the manufacturer of amisulpride.
22. Leucht S, Pitschel-Walz G, Engel RR, et al. Amisulpride, an unusual "atypical" antipsychotic: a meta-analysis of randomized controlled trials. *Am J Psychiatry* 2002;159:177–179. Search date 2000; primary sources Medline, Current Contents, hand searches of reference lists and personal contact with the manufacturer of amisupride.
23. Geddes J, Freemantle N, Harrison P, et al, for the National Schizophrenia Development Group. Atypical antipsychotics in the treatment of schizophrenia: systematic review and meta-regression analysis. *BMJ* 2000;321:1371–1377. Search date 1998; primary sources Medline, Embase, Psychlit, and Cochrane Controlled Trials Register.
24. Duggan L, Fenton M, Dardennes RM, et al. Olanzapine for schizophrenia. In: The Cochrane Library, Issue 2, 2002. Oxford: Update Software. Search date 1999; primary sources Biological Abstracts, Embase, Medline, Psychlit, Cochrane Library, hand searches of reference lists and conference abstracts, and personal communication with authors of trials and pharmaceutical companies.
25. Leucht S, Pitschel Walx G, Abraham D, et al. Efficacy and extrapyramidal side-effects of the new antipsychotics olanzapine, quetiapine, risperidone and sertindole compared to conventional antipsychotics and placebo. A meta-analysis of randomised controlled trials. *Schizophr Res* 1999;35:51–68. Search date 1999; primary sources Medline, Current Contents, hand searches of reference lists, and personal communication with pharmaceutical companies.
26. Peuskens J, de Hert M, Jones, M. The clinical value of risperidone and olanzapine: a meta-analysis of efficacy and safety. *Int J Psych Clin Prac* 2001;5:170–187. Search date 1998, primary sources Medline, Embase, Psychlit 1991–1998.
27. Gilbody SM, Bagnall AM, Duggan L, et al. Risperidone versus other atypical antipsychotic medication for schizophrenia. In: The Cochrane Library, Issue 2, 2002. Oxford: Update Software. Search date 1999; primary sources Biological Abstracts, Cochrane Library, Cochrane Schizophrenia Group's Register, Embase, Medline, Lilacs, Psyindex, Psychlit, pharmaceutical databases on the Dialog Corporation Datastar and Dialog services, hand search of reference lists, and contact with pharmaceutical companies and authors of trials.
28. Tuunainen A, Gilbody SM. Newer atypical antipsychotic medication versus clozapine for schizophrenia. In: The Cochrane Library, Issue 2, 2002. Oxford: Update Software. Search date 1998; primary sources Biological Abstracts, Cochrane Schizophrenia Group's Register, Cochrane Library, Embase, Lilacs, Medline, Psychlit, hand searches of reference lists, and personal contact with authors of trials and pharmaceutical companies.
29. Conley RR, Mahmoud R. A randomized double-blind study of risperidone and olanzapine in the treatment of schizophrenia or schizoaffective disorder. *Am J Psychiatry* 2001;158:765–774.
30. Srisurapanont M, Disayavanish C, Taimkaew K. Quetiapine for schizophrenia. In: The Cochrane Library, Issue 2, 2002. Oxford: Update Software. Search date 2000; primary sources Biological Abstracts, Embase, Medline, Psychlit, The Cochrane Library, Cinahl, Sigle, Sociofile, hand searches of journals, and personal communication with authors of studies and pharmaceutical companies.
31. Kennedy E, Song F, Hunter R, et al. Risperidone versus typical antipsychotic medication for schizophrenia. In: The Cochrane Library, Issue 2, 2002. Oxford: Update Software. Search date 1997; primary sources Biological Abstracts, The Cochrane Trials Register, Embase, Medline, Psychlit, hand searches of reference lists, and personal communication with pharmaceutical companies.
32. Lopez Ibor JJ, Ayuso JL, Gutierrez M, et al. Risperidone in the treatment of chronic schizophrenia: multicenter study comparative to haloperidol. *Actas Luso Esp Neurol Psiquiatr Cienc Afines* 1996;24:165–172.
33. Bagnall AM, Lewis RA, Leitner ML, et al. Ziprasidone for schizophrenia and severe mental illness. In: The Cochrane Library, Issue 2, 2002. Oxford: Update Software. Search date 1999; primary sources Biological Abstracts, The Cochrane Library, The Cochrane Schizophrenia Group's Register, Embase, Lilacs, Psyndex, Psychlit, pharmaceutical databases, hand searches of reference lists, and personal contact with authors of trials.
34. Fenton M, Morris F, De Silva P, et al. Zotepine for schizophrenia. In: The Cochrane Library, Issue 2, 2002. Oxford: Update Software. Search date 1999; primary sources Biological Abstracts, The Cochrane Library, The Cochrane Schizophrenia Group's Register, Embase, Dialog Corporation Datastar service, Medline, Psychlit, hand searches of reference lists, and personal contact with authors of trials and pharmaceutical companies.
35. Wahlbeck K, Cheine M, Essali MA. Clozapine versus typical neuroleptic medication for schizophrenia. In: The Cochrane Library, Issue 2, 2002. Oxford: Update Software. Search date 1999; primary sources Biological Abstracts, Cochrane Schizophrenia Group's Register, Cochrane Library, Embase, Lilacs, Medline, Psychlit, SciSearch Science Citation Index, hand searches of reference lists, and personal communication with pharmaceutical companies.
36. Honigfeld G, Arellano F, Sethi J, et al. Reducing clozapine-related morbidity and mortality: five years experience of the clozaril national registry. *J Clin Psychiatry* 1998;59(suppl 3):3–7.
37. Kumra S, Frazier JA, Jacobsen LK, et al. Childhood-onset schizophrenia. A double-blind clozapine-haloperidol comparison. *Arch Gen Psychiatry* 1996;53:1090–1097.
38. Gilbert PL, Harris MJ, McAdams LA, et al. Neuroleptic withdrawal in schizophrenic people: a review of the literature. *Arch Gen Psychiatry* 1995;52:173–188. Search date not stated; primary source Medline.
39. Adams CE, Eisenbruch M. Depot fluphenazine versus oral fluphenazine for those with schizophrenia. In: The Cochrane Library, Issue 2, 2002. Oxford: Update Software. Search date 1995; primary sources Biological Abstracts, The Cochrane Library, Cochrane Schizophrenia Group's Register, Embase, Medline, Psychlit, Science Citation Index, hand searches of reference lists, and personal communication with pharmaceutical companies.
40. Quraishi S, David A. Depot flupenthixol decanoate for schizophrenia or similar psychotic disorders. In:

The Cochrane Library, Issue 2, 2002. Oxford: Update Software. Search date 1998; primary sources Biological Abstracts, The Cochrane Library, Cochrane Schizophrenia Group's Register, Embase, Medline, Psychlit, SciSearch, references, and personal communication with authors of trials and pharmaceutical companies.

41. Quraishi S, David A. Depot fluspirilene for schizophrenia. In: The Cochrane Library, Issue 2, 2002. Oxford: Update Software. Search date 1998; primary sources Biological Abstracts, The Cochrane Library, The Cochrane Schizophrenia Group's Register, Embase, Medline, Psychlit, and hand searches of reference lists.
42. Quraishi S, David A. Depot perphenazine decanoate and enanthate for schizophrenia. In: The Cochrane Library, Issue 2, 2002. Oxford: Update Software. Search date 1998; primary sources Biological Abstracts, The Cochrane Library, The Cochrane Schizophrenia Group's Register, Embase, Medline, Psychlit, hand searches of reference lists, and personal communication with pharmaceutical companies.
43. Coutinho E, Fenton M, Quraishi S. Zuclopenthixol decanoate for schizophrenia and other serious mental illnesses. In: The Cochrane Library, Issue 2, 2002. Oxford: Update Software. Search date 1998; primary sources Biological Abstracts, Cinhal, The Cochrane Library, The Cochrane Schizophrenia Group's Register, Embase, Medline, and Psychlit. References of all eligible studies were searched for further trials. The manufacturer of zuclopenthixol was contacted.
44. Csernansky JG, Mahmoud R, Brenner R; The Risperidone-USA-79 Study Group. A comparison of risperidone and haloperidol for the prevention of relapse in patients with schizophrenia. *New Engl J Med* 2002;346:1:16–22.
45. Jeste D, Gilbert P, McAdams L, et al. Considering neuroleptic maintenance and taper on a continuum: need for an individual rather than dogmatic approach. *Arch Gen Psychiatry* 1995;52:209–212.
46. Pharaoh FM, Mari JJ, Streiner D. Family intervention for schizophrenia. In: The Cochrane Library, Issue 2, 2002. Oxford: Update Software. Search date 1998; primary sources Medline, Embase, The Cochrane Library, Cochrane Schizophrenia Group's Register, and reference lists of articles.
47. McFarlane WR, Lukens E, Link B, et al. Multiple-family groups and psychoeducation in the treatment of schizophrenia. *Arch Gen Psychiatry* 1995;52:679–687.
48. Benton MK, Schroeder HE. Social skills training with schizophrenics: a meta-analytic evaluation. *J Consult Clin Psychol* 1990;58:741–747. Search date not stated; primary sources computerised databases and manual search but sources not specified.
49. Corrigan PW. Social skills training in adult psychiatric populations: a meta-analysis. *J Behav Ther Exp Psychiatry* 1991;22:203–210. Search date 1988; primary source Psychological Abstracts.
50. Cormac I, Jones C, Campbell C. Cognitive behavioural therapy for schizophrenia. In: The Cochrane Library, Issue 2, 2002. Oxford: Update Software. Search date 2001, primary sources Biological Abstracts, Cochrane Schizophrenia Group's Register, Cinahl, The Cochrane Library, Medline, Embase, Psychlit, Sigle, Sociofile, reference lists of articles, and personal communication with authors of trials.
51. Pekkala E, Merinder L. Psychoeducation for schizophrenia. In: The Cochrane Library, Issue 2, 2002. Oxford: Update Software. Search date 2002; primary sources Cinahl, The Cochrane Library, Cochrane Schizophrenia Group's Register, Embase, Medline, Psychlit, Sociofile, hand searched reference lists, and personal contact with authors.
52. Kemp R, Kirov G, Everitt B, et al. Randomised controlled trial of compliance therapy. 18-month follow-up. *Br J Psychiatry* 1998;172:413–419.
53. Kemp R, Hayward P, Applewhaite G, et al. Compliance therapy in psychotic people: randomised controlled trial. *BMJ* 1996;312:345–349.
54. Boczkowski JA, Zeichner A, DeSanto N. Neuroleptic compliance among chronic schizophrenic outpeople: an intervention outcome report. *J Consult Clin Psychol* 1985;53:666–671.
55. Azrin NH, Teichner G. Evaluation of an instructional program for improving medication compliance for chronically mentally ill outpatients. *Behaviour Res Ther* 1998;36:849–861.

Zia Nadeem
Research Fellow
Department of Psychiatry

Andrew McIntosh
Lecturer in Psychiatry
Department of Psychiatry

Stephen Lawrie
Senior Clinical Research Fellow and
Honorary Consultant Psychiatrist
University of Edinburgh
UK

Competing interests: SML has been paid for speaking about critical appraisal by employees of the manufacturers of olanzapine, quetiapine, risperidone, and ziprasidone, and has been paid to speak about the management of schizophrenia by employees of the manufacturers of amisulpiride, olanzapine, risperidone, and clozapine. AM none declared. ZN none declared.

TABLE 1 **Continued treatment with antipsychotic drugs: choice of drugs** **(see text, p 1039).**

Ref	Search Date	Number of RCTs	Comparisons	Main conclusion
39	1995	6	Oral *v* depot fluphenazine	No significant difference
10	1998	7	Haloperidol decanoate *v* other depots	No significant difference
40	1999	8	Flupenthixol decanoate *v* other depots	No significant difference
11	1999	7	Pipotiazine (pipothiazine) palmitate *v* other depots	No significant difference
11	1999	2	Pipotiazine (pipothiazine) palmitate *v* oral antipsychotics	No significant difference
41	1999	1	Fluspirilene decanoate *v* oral chlorpromazine	No significant difference
41	1999	3	Fluspirilene decanoate *v* other depots	No significant difference
42	1999	1	Perphenazine enanthate *v* clopenthixol decanoate	No significant difference
17	2000	11	Pimozide *v* standard antipsychotics	No significant difference
24	1999	1	Olanzapine *v* standard antipsychotics	No significant difference
43	1998	3	Zuclopenthixol decanoate *v* other depots	People taking zuclopenthixol had lower relapse rates over 12 weeks to 1 year
35	1999	19	Clozapine *v* standard antipsychotics	Relapse rates up to 12 weeks were lower with clozapine
14	1999	2	Bromperidol *v* haloperidol or fluphenazine	Relapse rates over 6–12 months were lower with haloperidol or fluphenazine

Ankle sprain

Search date March 2002

Peter Struijs and Gino Kerkhoffs

QUESTIONS

INTERVENTIONS

See glossary, p 1057

Key Messages

- **Cold pack compression** Two RCTs found no significant difference in symptoms with cold pack placement versus placebo or control. One RCT found significantly less oedema with cold pack placement versus heat or a contrast bath at 3–5 days post injury.
- **Diathermy** One systematic review found insufficient evidence on the effects of diathermy versus placebo in walking ability and reduction in swelling.
- **Functional treatment** One systematic review and one subsequent RCT found limited evidence that functional treatment versus minimal treatment significantly reduced the risk of the ankle giving way. One systematic review and two RCTs comparing functional treatment versus surgery found conflicting evidence. One systematic review found that functional treatment versus immobilisation significantly improved six outcome measures at either short (up to 6 weeks), intermediate (6 weeks to 1 year), or long term (over 1 year) follow up. Effects were less marked at long term follow up. Another systematic review found that functional treatment versus immobilisation resulted in significantly less persistent subjective instability but no significant difference in pain. We found insufficient evidence comparing different functional treatments.
- **Homeopathic ointment** One systematic review of one RCT found limited evidence that homeopathic ointment versus placebo significantly improved outcome on a "composite criteria" of treatment success.
- **Immobilisation** One systematic review found that immobilisation versus functional treatment was associated with significantly less improvement in six outcome measures at either short (up to 6 weeks), intermediate (6 weeks to 1 year), or long term (over 1 year) follow up. Effects were less marked at long term follow up. One other systematic review found that immobilisation versus functional treatment resulted in significantly more persistent subjective instability but no significant difference in pain. One systematic review has found no significant difference with immobilisation versus surgery in pain or subjective instability.

- **Surgery** One systematic review has found no significant difference with surgery versus immobilisation in pain or subjective instability. One systematic review and two RCTs comparing surgery versus functional treatment found conflicting evidence.
- **Ultrasound** One systematic review found no significant difference with ultrasound versus sham ultrasound in the general improvement of symptoms or the ability to walk or bear weight at 7 days. Three RCTs found conflicting evidence with ultrasound versus other treatments.

DEFINITION Ankle sprain is an injury of the lateral ligament complex of the ankle joint. Such injury can range from mild to severe and is graded on the basis of severity.[1–5] Grade I is a mild stretching of the ligament complex without joint instability; Grade II is a partial rupture of the ligament complex with mild instability of the joint (such as isolated rupture of the anterior talofibular ligament); Grade III involves complete rupture of the ligament complex with instability of the joint.

INCIDENCE/ PREVALENCE Ankle sprain is a common problem in acute medical care occurring at a rate of about one injury/10 000 population a day.[6] Injuries of the lateral ligament complex of the ankle form a quarter of all sports injuries.[6]

AETIOLOGY/ RISK FACTORS The usual mechanism of injury is inversion and adduction (usually referred to as supination) of the plantar-flexed foot. Predisposing factors are a history of ankle sprains and specific malalignment, like crus varum and pes cavo-varus.

PROGNOSIS Some sports (e.g. basketball, football [soccer], and volleyball) have a particularly high incidence of ankle injuries. Pain is the most frequent residual problem, often localised on the medial side of the ankle.[4] Other residual complaints include mechanical instability, intermittent swelling, and stiffness. People with more extensive cartilage damage have a higher incidence of residual complaints.[4] Long term cartilage damage can lead to degenerative changes and this is especially true if there is persistent or recurrent instability. Every further sprain has the potential to add new damage.

AIMS Reduction of swelling and pain, and the restoration of the stability of the ankle joint.

OUTCOMES Return to pre-injury level of sports; return to pre-injury level of work; pain; swelling; subjective instability; objective instability; recurrent injury; ankle mobility; complications; patient satisfaction.

METHODS *Clinical Evidence* search and appraisal March 2002

QUESTION **What are the effects of treatment strategies for acute ankle ligament ruptures?**

OPTION **IMMOBILISATION**

One systematic review found that immobilisation versus functional treatment was associated with significantly less improvement in six outcome measures at either short (up to 6 weeks), intermediate (6 weeks to 1 year), or long term (over 1 year) follow up. Effects were less marked at long term follow up. One other systematic review found that

immobilisation versus functional treatment resulted in significantly more persistent subjective instability but no significant difference in pain. One systematic review has found no significant difference with immobilisation versus surgery in pain or subjective instability.

Benefits: We found four systematic reviews (search dates 1993,[7] 1994,[8] 1998,[9] 1999[10]) describing 30 RCTs. **Versus functional treatment:** We found four systematic reviews describing 21 RCTs (2719 people).[7–10] The most recent review[10] included any inpatient, outpatient, or home based intervention program that comprised immobilisation (see glossary, p 1057) with or without a plaster cast. The systematic review reported outcomes at short, intermediate, or long term follow up (see comment). It found significant differences in six outcomes measured at different times. At short term follow up it found that functional treatment (see glossary, p 1057) versus immobilisation significantly increased the number of people satisfied with treatment (6 RCTs; RR 6.50, 95% CI 1.8 to 24.0) and significantly reduced the number of people with persistent swelling (7 RCTs; RR 1.44, 95% CI 1.1 to 2.0) or an impaired range of motion (3 RCTs; RR 1.64, 95% CI 1.1 to 2.6). At intermediate term follow up with functional treatment versus immobilisation it found that significantly more people were satisfied with treatment (6 RCTs; RR 4.25, 95% CI 1.1 to 16). At intermediate term follow up with immobilisation versus functional treatment it found significantly increased objective instability with stress x ray (1 RCT; weighted mean difference [WMD] 2.48°, 95% CI 1.3° to 3.6°). At long term follow up with functional treatment versus immobilisation it found that significantly more people returned to sports (5 RCTs; RR 1.85, 95% CI 1.2 to 2.8). It also found that functional treatment versus immobilisation significantly reduced the time taken to return to work (7 RCTs; WMD 7.1 days, 95% CI 5.6 to 8.7). At long-term follow up, differences in outcomes for persistent swelling, objective instability, range of motion, and patient satisfaction, were no longer statistically significant (results presented graphically). The review included a variety of different forms of functional treatment, including strapping, bracing, use of an orthosis, and special shoes for at least 5 weeks. The second most recent review found significantly less persistent subjective instability with functional treatment (5 RCTs; RR 0.6, 95% CI 0.4 to 0.8; absolute risks not provided; timescale not provided), but no significant difference in pain (5 RCTs; RR 0.8, 95% CI 0.5 to 1.2; absolute risks not provided).[9] The review included a variety of different forms of functional treatment including strapping, bracing, use of an orthosis, elastic wrapping, special shoes for at least 5 weeks, and short term (up to 3 weeks) cast immobilisation. The two oldest reviews were narrative in character and no data were pooled.[7,8] **Versus surgery:** We found one systematic review (search date 1998, 9 RCTs, 694 people) that compared operative treatment followed by 6 weeks of cast treatment versus 6 weeks of cast treatment alone.[9] It found no significant differences for either pain (5 RCTs; RR 1.1, 95% CI 0.6 to 2.1; absolute risks not provided) or subjective instability (5 RCTs; RR 1.0, 95% CI 0.7 to 1.4; absolute risks not provided). One of the RCTs (150 people) found immobilisation to be less effective than surgery for subjective instability at long term follow up (minimum 2 years' follow up; RR 3.6, 95% CI 1.1 to 11.5).[11] The RCT identified no significant differences for recurrent sprains, return to sports, and objective instability.

Harms: One RCT found fewer cases of deep venous thrombosis after cast immobilisation than with surgery (deep venous thrombosis: 2/47 [4%] after cast immobilisation *v* 3/34 [9%] after surgery; RR 0.48, 95% CI 0.09 to 2.7).[11] Other RCTs did not specifically address harms. Other known harms of immobilisation include pain and impairment in activities of daily living.[11]

Comment: The most recent systematic review did not provide absolute figures, only summary risk estimations.[10] Follow up periods for outcome measures were categorised as short term (within 6 wks of randomisation), intermediate term (6 wks to 1 year), or long term (more than 1 year follow up). The different treatment modalities included as functional treatment in the reviews makes it difficult to draw definitive conclusions on individual forms of functional treatment versus immobilisation.

OPTION FUNCTIONAL TREATMENT

One systematic review and one subsequent RCT found limited evidence that functional treatment versus minimal treatment significantly reduced the risk of the ankle giving way. One systematic review and two RCTs comparing functional treatment versus surgery found conflicting evidence. One systematic review found that functional treatment versus immobilisation significantly improved six outcome measures at either short (up to 6 wks) intermediate (6 wks to 1 year) or long term (over 1 year) follow up. Effects were less marked at long term follow up. One other systematic review found that functional treatment versus immobilisation significantly reduced persistent subjective instability but no significant difference in pain. We found insufficient evidence comparing different functional treatments.

Benefits: We found four systematic reviews (search dates 1993,[7] 1994,[8] 1998,[9] and 1999,[10] describing 30 RCTs and eight additional RCTs[12–19]) comparing functional treatment (see glossary, p 1057) as a treatment strategy. **Versus minimal treatment:** We found two systematic reviews and one subsequent RCT.[8,9,12] The most recent systematic review (search date 1998, 3 RCTs, 214 people) compared functional treatment versus a minimal treatment policy.[9] It found that functional treatment significantly reduced the risk of the ankle giving way (RR 0.34, 95% CI 0.17 to 0.71). Although pain scores were better with functional treatment the difference was not significant (RR 0.53, 95% CI 0.27 to 1.02). The older systematic review was narrative in character and no data were pooled.[8] The subsequent RCT (30 people with subacute or chronic ankle sprain without gross mechanical instability) compared the mortise separation adjustment (see glossary, p 1057) versus detuned ultrasound.[12] It found mobilisation significantly reduced pain, increased ankle range of motion, and improved ankle function at 1 month (results presented graphically). **Versus immobilisation:** See immobilisation option, p 1051. **Versus surgery:** We found three systematic reviews (search dates 1993,[7] 1994,[8] and 1998[9]) including 15 RCTs and two additional RCTs.[15,16] The most recent systematic review (search date 1998, 7 RCTs, 914 people) included only people with rupture of the lateral ankle ligament.[9] It did not specify the kinds of surgery included within the RCTs. It found that surgery versus functional treatment significantly reduced long term subjective instability (7 RCTs; RR 0.2, 95% CI 0.2 to 0.3; absolute risks not provided), but had no significant effect on long term pain (6 RCTs; RR 0.5, 95% CI 0.2 to 1.5; absolute risks not provided). One RCT in the review (116 people) found that surgery increased the proportion of people with impaired range of movement in the short term compared to those treated with a semi-rigid device (RR 60, 95% CI 3.8 to 946).[13] The two oldest reviews were narrative in character and no data were pooled.[7,8] The two additional RCTs did not describe significant differences between functional treatment and surgery.[15,16] **Versus functional treatment:** We found five RCTs comparing different functional treatment strategies.[13,14,17–19] One RCT (61 people without previous fractures in the ankle joint or clinically demonstrable ankle instability; mean follow up of 230 days) found a reduced risk of recurrent sprains after elastic bandage plus propriocepsis training versus elastic bandage only (RR 0.46, 95% CI 0.2 to 1.0).[17] Thirteen people withdrew from the RCT and were not included in the analysis. The second RCT (73 people with time from injury to treatment of < 24 h) identified a faster return to work for the semi-rigid device group compared with treatment with an elastic bandage (up to 10 weeks' follow up; 9.1 *v* 5.3 days; mean difference 3.8 days, 95% CI 1.1 to 6.5).[14] Fifteen people did not complete 10 weeks' follow up, and it was not reported if results were intention to treat. The third RCT (41 people within 72 h of injury and requiring assisted ambulation but without previous injury, presence of severe vascular disease, or use of anticoagulant or anti-inflammatory medications) compared anteroposterior mobilisation plus rest, ice, compression, and elevation versus rest, ice, compression, and elevation alone.[19] People treated with anteroposterior mobilisation required fewer treatment sessions, had greater improvement in range of motion (after 2 treatment sessions 10.5° with added mobilisation *v* 5.8°; $P < 0.05$), and greater increases in stride speed. Three people withdrew from the mobilisation group and analysis was not intention to treat. The remaining two RCTs found no significant differences. The first RCT (116 people with all grades of ankle sprain) compared a semi-rigid device with tape (recurrent sprains were found in 4% *v* 0%).[13] The second RCT (119 people not requiring surgery treated within 24 h of injury) compared two types of tape treatment with follow up of 5–7 days (short term pain 8% *v* 5%; swelling 58% *v* 47%; limited range of movement 36% *v* 47%).[18]

Harms: Allergic reactions and skin problems have been recorded with tape;[20] however, none of the RCTs reported this.

Comment: The more recent systematic review of functional treatment versus surgery presented results only as relative risks, which does not allow assessment of the number of people who benefited.[9] It also categorised short term cast use as a functional treatment. The older systematic reviews did not perform meta-analysis and included people with different severity of ankle sprain.[7,8]

OPTION SURGERY

One systematic review has found no significant difference with surgery versus immobilisation in pain or subjective instability. One systematic review and two RCTs comparing surgery versus functional treatment found conflicting evidence.

Benefits: We found three systematic reviews (search dates 1993,[7] 1994,[8] and 1998[9]) describing 19 RCTs and three additional RCTs.[15,16,21] **Versus immobilisation:** See immobilisation option, p 1051. **Versus functional treatment:** See functional treatment option, p 1053.

Harms: Neurological injuries, infections, bleeding, osteoarthritis, and death are known harms of surgery.[11,21,22] One RCT found fewer cases of deep venous thrombosis after cast immobilisation than with surgery (deep venous thrombosis: 2/47 [4%] after cast immobilisation *v* 3/34 [9%] after surgery; RR 0.48, 95% CI 0.09 to 2.7).[11] Another RCT found dysaesthesia (see glossary, p 1057) in 6/102 (6%) after surgery.[23]

Comment: None.

OPTION ULTRASOUND

One systematic review found no significant difference with ultrasound versus sham ultrasound in the general improvement of symptoms or the ability to walk or bear weight at 7 days. Three RCTs found conflicting evidence with ultrasound versus other treatments.

Benefits: We found one systematic review (search date 2001, 5 RCTs, 572 people; see comment).[24] **Versus placebo:** Four RCTs in the review compared ultrasound with a sham ultrasound treatment.[24] None of the RCTs demonstrated a significant difference for any outcome measure. There was no significant difference in the pooled risk for general improvement with ultrasound versus sham ultrasound at 7 days (3 RCTs; 121/169 [72%] with ultrasound *v* 116/172 [68%] with sham ultrasound; RR 1.04, 95% CI 0.92 to 1.17). There was no significant difference in the pooled risk for functional disability (the ability to walk or bear weight) with ultrasound versus sham ultrasound at 7 days (2 RCTs; 69/95 [73%] with ultrasound *v* 61/92 [66%] with sham ultrasound; RR 1.09, 95% CI 0.92 to 1.30). **Versus other treatments:** Three RCTs in the review compared the effectiveness of ultrasound versus other treatment modalities.[24] The largest RCT (72 people in the smallest group) compared ultrasound plus placebo gel versus ultrasound plus felbinac gel versus sham ultrasound plus felbinac gel over about 7 days. The comparison between ultrasound and felbinac gel resulted in small and non significant differences. The second RCT (20 people in the smallest group) compared ultrasound versus electrotherapy. It found no significant difference in swelling, ability to walk, and recovery. The third low quality RCT (40 people in the smallest group) compared ultrasound versus immobilisation (see glossary, p 1057) with elastoplast over 2 weeks' follow up. It found no significant improvement in the number of people who recovered with ultrasound versus immobilisation after 7 days (46% ultrasound *v* 27% immobilisation; ARR 19%, 95% CI –2% to +40%) but found a significant difference after 14 days (86% ultrasound *v* 59% immobilisation; ARR 27%, 95% CI 8% to 46%).

Harms: Two included RCTs addressed adverse reactions. One RCT found none.[25] The systematic review reported that in the other RCT, 8/73 (11%) people in the ultrasound group (plus placebo gel) reported 11 non-serious adverse reactions, including gastrointestinal events and skin reactions, and in one person treatment was discontinued due to skin reactions and the person was withdrawn from the RCT.[26]

Comment: In the review, the quality of four of the included RCTs was described as "modest" and one as "good".[24] The review reported RCTs in which pain, swelling, and/or functional disability due to an acute ankle sprain was present, and in which at least one group was treated with active ultrasound therapy. All the RCTs included followed people for less than 4 weeks.

OPTION COLD PACK COMPRESSION

Two RCTs found no significant difference in symptoms with cold pack placement versus placebo or control. One RCT found significantly less oedema with cold pack placement versus heat or a contrast bath at 3–5 days post injury.

Benefits: We found one systematic review (search date 1994, 3 RCTs, 203 people).[8] The first RCT (143 people) identified by the review compared cryotherapy versus placebo (simulated) therapy.[27] The second RCT (30 people) identified by the review compared ice treatment plus physiotherapy versus no ice plus physiotherapy.[28] In both RCTs, no significant differences were found. The third RCT (30 people) identified by the review found significantly less oedema with cold versus heat or a contrast bath at 3–5 days post injury ($P < 0.05$).[29]

Harms: None of the RCTs addressed harms from cold pack placement.

Comment: The systematic review was narrative in character and no data were pooled.[8] The systematic review did not report the grade of injuries.

OPTION DIATHERMY

One systematic review found insufficient evidence on the effects of diathermy versus placebo in walking ability and reduction in swelling.

Benefits: We found one systematic review (search date 1994, 5 RCTs, 490 people).[8] The review included a range of severity of ankle sprains but excluded the most severe injuries (avulsion and osteochondral fractures). The largest high quality RCT (300 people with time from injury to treatment of 4 days or less) compared two forms of pulsating shortwave treatment versus placebo.[30] The RCT found that walking ability improved significantly more quickly with high frequency electromagnetic pulsing than with placebo ($P < 0.01$). The difference was not significant with low frequency electromagnetic pulsing. However, reduction of swelling was significantly better for the low frequency group versus placebo but not for high frequency versus placebo (change in circumference of ankle with high frequency 4.5 mm *v* low frequency 5.0 mm *v* placebo 2.6 mm; $P < 0.01$ for low frequency *v* placebo). A second RCT (50 people) found significantly reduced oedema with pulsating shortwave diathermy compared with placebo ($P < 0.01$).[31] The other RCTs (73, 37, and 30 people) found no significant differences for pain, oedema, or range of motion compared with placebo.[32–34] The first of these presented results as graphs.[32] From these RCTs the grades of injuries were not clear. No other outcome measures were reported and no results were pooled.

Harms: No evidence of any harm was reported.

Comment: None.

OPTION HOMEOPATHIC OINTMENT

One systematic review of one RCT found limited evidence that homeopathic ointment versus placebo significantly improved outcome based on a "composite criteria" of treatment success.

Benefits: We found one systematic review (search date 1998)[35] which included one RCT in German (69 people with acute ankle sprains).[36] The review found that people treated with Traumeel ointment had a significantly better outcome based on a "composite criteria of treatment success" versus placebo. The review did not provide specific numeric results or timescale of outcome measurement but described a P value of 0.028.[35] People initially randomised in the RCT and losses to follow up were not reported.

Harms: Harms were not addressed in the review.

Comment: The RCT included in the systematic review will be translated and further details included in future *Clinical Evidence* updates.

GLOSSARY

Dysaesthesia Decreased sensitivity of the skin for stimuli.

Functional treatment Diverse functional treatments have been used. The main differences are the type of external device applied for treatment. The supports can be divided according to rigidity into elastic bandage; tape; lace-up ankle support; and semi-rigid ankle support. Propriocepsis training (to enhance joint stability) has also been used.

Immobilisation Limiting the mobility of a joint complex to zero degrees.

Mortise separation adjustment An adjustment technique involving special manual manipulation of the foot and ankle.[12]

Substantive changes

Immobilisation One new systematic review of immobilisation including a comparison of immobilisation versus functional treatment;[10] functional treatment recategorised as beneficial.

Surgery One new RCT;[16] conclusions unchanged.

Ultrasound Updated systematic review;[24] conclusions unchanged.
Homeopathic ointment One new systematic review;[35] conclusions unchanged.

REFERENCES

1. Bernett P, Schirmann A. Sportverletzungen des sprunggelenkes. *Unfallheilkunde* 1979;82:155–160.
2. Lassiter TE, Malone TR, Garret WE. Injuries to the lateral ligaments of the ankle. *Orthop Clin North Am* 1989;20:629–640.
3. Marti RK. Bagatelletsels van de voet. 56–61. 1982. Capita selecta, Reuma Wereldwijd.
4. Van Dijk CN, Bossuyt PM, Marti RK. Medial ankle pain after lateral ligament rupture. *J Bone Joint Surg (Br)* 1996;78:562–567.
5. Watson-Jones R. *Fractures and joint injuries*. London: Churchill Livingstone, 1976.
6. Katcherian DA. Treatment of Freiberg's disease. *Orthop Clin North Am* 1994;25:69–81.
7. Shrier I. Treatment of lateral collateral ligament sprains of the ankle: A critical appraisal of the literature. *Clin J Sport Med* 1995;5:187–195. Search date 1993; primary sources hand searches of bibliographies and reference lists.
8. Ogilvie-Harris DJ, Gilbart M. Treatment modalities for soft tissue injuries of the ankle: A critical review. *Clin J Sport Med* 1995;5:175–186. Search date 1994; primary sources Medline, and Excerpta Medica.
9. Pijnenburg AC, Van Dijk CN, Bossuyt PM, et al. Treatment of ruptures of the lateral ankle ligaments: a meta-analysis. *J Bone Joint Surg (Am)* 2000;82:761–773. Search date 1998; primary sources Cochrane, Medline, Embase, hand searches of references from the published reviews, and personal contact with authors.
10. Kerkhoffs GMMJ, Rowe BH, Assendelft WJJ, et al. Immobilisation for acute ankle sprain: a systematic review. *Arch Orthop Trauma Surg* 2001;121:462–471. Search date 1999; primary sources Medline, Embase, Biosis, Cochrane Controlled Trials Register, Current Contents and hand searches of reference lists of all papers, and personal contact with authors and relevant organisations.
11. Korkala O, Rusanen M, Jokipii P, et al. A prospective study of the treatment of severe tears of the lateral ligament of the ankle. *Int Orthop* 1987;11:13–17.
12. Pellow JE, Brantingham JW. The efficacy of adjusting the ankle in the treatment of subacute and chronic grade I and Grade II ankle inversion sprains. *J Manipulative Physiol Ther* 2001;24:17–24.
13. Johannes EJ, Sukul DM, Spruit PJ, Putters JL. Controlled trial of a semi-rigid bandage ('Scotchrap') in patients with ankle ligament lesions. *Curr Med Res Opin* 1993;13:154–162.
14. Leanderson J, Wredmark T. Treatment of acute ankle sprain. Comparison of a semi-rigid ankle brace and compression bandage in 73 patients. *Acta Orthop Scand* 1995;66:529–531.
15. Otto M, Novak L, Fekecs G. Functional conservative versus operative treatment of outer ankle ligament ruptures. *J Bone Joint Surg (Br)* 1997;(suppl II):250.
16. Specchiulli F, Cofano RE. A comparison of surgical and conservative treatment in ankle ligament tears. *Sports Med* 2001;24:686–688.
17. Wester JU, Jespersen SM, Nielsen KD, et al. Wobble board training after partial sprains of the lateral ligaments of the ankle: a prospective randomized study. *J Orthop Sports Phys Ther* 1996;23:332–336.
18. Viljakka T, Rokkanen P. The treatment of ankle sprain by bandaging and antiphlogistic drugs. *Ann Chir Gynaecol* 1983;72:66–70.
19. Green T, Refshauge K, Crosbie J, et al. A randomized controlled trial of a passive accessory joint mobilization on acute ankle inversion sprains. *Phys Ther* 2001;81:984–994.
20. Zeegers AVCM. Supination injury of the ankle joint. University of Utrecht, The Netherlands, Thesis, 1995.
21. Biegler M, Lang A, Ritter J. Comparative study on the effectiveness of early functional treatment using special shoes following surgery of ruptures of fibular ligaments [German]. *Unfallchirurg* 1985;88:113–117.
22. Sommer HM, Schreiber H. Early functional conservative therapy of fresh fibular capsular ligament rupture from the socioeconomic viewpoint. *Sportverletz Sportschaden* 1993;7:40–46.
23. Zwipp H, Hoffmann R, Thermann H, et al. Rupture of the ankle ligaments. *Int Orthop* 1991;15:245–249.
24. Van der Windt DAWM, Van der Heijden GJMG, Van den Berg SGM, et al. Ultrasound therapy for acute ankle sprains (Cochrane Review). In: The Cochrane Library, Issue 1, 2002. Oxford: Update Software. Search date 2001; primary sources Cochrane Musculoskeletal Injuries Group specialised register, Cochrane Controlled Trials Register, Cochrane Rehabilitation and Related Therapies Field database, Medline, Embase, Cinahl, PEDro — the Physiotherapy Evidence Database, and hand searches of reference lists of articles and personal contact with colleagues.
25. Nyanzi CS, Langridge J, Heyworth JR, et al. Randomized controlled study of ultrasound therapy in the management of acute lateral ligament sprains of the ankle joint. *Clin Rehabil* 1999;13:16–22.
26. Oakland C. A comparison of the efficacy of the topical NSAID felbinac and ultrasound in the treatment of acute ankle injuries. *Br J Clin Res* 1993 ;4 :89–96.
27. Sloan JP, Hain R, Pownall R. Clinical benefits of early cold therapy in accident and emergency following ankle sprain. *Arch Emerg Med* 1989;6:1–6.
28. Laba E, Roestenburg M. Clinical evaluation of ice therapy for acute ankle sprain injuries. *New Zeal J Physiother* 1989;17:7–9.
29. Cote DJ, Prentice WEJ, Hooker DN, et al. Comparison of three treatment procedures for minimizing ankle sprain swelling. *Physical Ther* 1988;68:1072–1076.
30. Pasila M, Visuri T, Sundholm A. Pulsating shortwave diathermy: value in treatment of recent ankle and foot sprains. *Arch Phys Med Rehabil* 1978;59:383–386.
31. Pennington GM, Danley DL, Sumko MH, et al. Pulsed, non-thermal, high-frequency electromagnetic energy (DIAPULSE) in the treatment of grade I and grade II ankle sprains. *Mil Med* 1993;158:101–404.
32. Barker AT, Barlow PS, Porter J, et al. A double-blind clinical trial of low power pulsed shortwave therapy in the treatment of a soft tissue injury. *Physiotherapy* 1985;71:500–504.
33. McGill SN. The effects of pulsed shortwave therapy on lateral ligament sprain of the ankle. *New Zeal J Physiother* 1988;16:21–24.

34. Michlovitz S, Smith W, Watkins M. Ice and high voltage pulsed stimulation in treatment of acute lateral ankle sprains. *J Orthop Sports Phys Ther* 1988;9:301–304.
35. Cucherat M, Haugh MC, Gooch M, et al. Evidence of clinical efficacy of homeopathy: a meta-analysis of clinical trials. *European Journal of Clinical Pharmacology* 2000;56:27–33. Search date 1998; primary sources Medline, Embase, Biosis, PsychInfo, Cinahl, British Library Stock Alert Service, SIGLE, AMED and hand searches of homeopathy journals, conference abstracts, references provided by colleagues, reference lists of selected papers, and personal contact with pharmaceutical companies.
36. Zell R, Connert WD, Mau J, et al. Treatment of acute sprains of the ankle joint. Double-blind study assessing the effectiveness of a homeopathic ointment preparation [German]. *Fortschr Med* 1988;106:96–100.

Peter Struijs

Gino Kerkhoffs

Academic Medical Center
Amsterdam
The Netherlands

Competing interests: None declared.

Carpal tunnel syndrome

Search date January 2002

Shawn Marshall

QUESTIONS

INTERVENTIONS

See glossary, p 1072

Key Messages

- **Diuretics** One small RCT found no significant difference with trichlormethiazide versus placebo in mean Global Symptom Score after 2 weeks or 4 weeks.
- **Endoscopic carpal tunnel release** We found no RCTs on the effects of surgery versus placebo. One systematic review found no significant difference with endoscopic versus open carpal tunnel release surgery in symptoms after 3–12 months. One subsequent small RCT found no significant difference between endoscopic versus open carpal tunnel release in tingling sensations or severity of night time numbness after 4 weeks, but found that endoscopic versus open carpal tunnel release significantly improved the severity of night time hand or wrist pain after 4 weeks. RCTs found conflicting evidence on difference in the time taken to return to work between endoscopic versus open carpal tunnel release. Harms resulting from endoscopic carpal tunnel release vary between RCTs. One systematic review comparing the two interventions suggested that endoscopic carpal tunnel release may cause more transient nerve problems whereas open carpal tunnel release may cause more wound problems.

Clin Evid 2002;8:1060–1074.

- **Internal neurolysis in conjunction with open carpal tunnel release** Three RCTs found no significant difference with open carpal tunnel release alone versus open carpal tunnel release plus internal neurolysis in symptoms.
- **Local corticosteroid injection (short term)** One systematic review has found that local corticosteroid injections versus placebo injection significantly improve symptoms after 1 month (NNT 3, 95% CI 2 to 4). One subsequent RCT found that hydrocortisone injection versus no injection significantly improved symptoms after 6 weeks (NNT 2, 95% CI 2 to 3). One RCT found that local methylprednisolone injection versus oral prednisolone significantly improved symptoms after 8 weeks and 12 weeks.
- **Non-steroidal anti-inflammatory drugs** One small RCT found no significant difference with tenoxicam versus placebo in mean global symptom score after 2 weeks or 4 weeks. One RCT found no significant difference in symptom severity scores with ibuprofen plus nocturnal wrist splint versus chiropractic manipulation plus ultrasound plus nocturnal wrist splint after 9 weeks.
- **Open carpal tunnel release** We found no RCTs on the effects of surgery versus placebo. One systematic review found no significant difference with endoscopic versus open carpal tunnel release surgery in symptoms after 3–12 months. One subsequent small RCT found no significant difference between endoscopic versus open carpal tunnel release in tingling sensations or severity of night time numbness after 4 weeks, but found that endoscopic versus open carpal tunnel release significantly improved the severity of night time hand or wrist pain after 4 weeks. RCTs found conflicting evidence on difference in the time taken to return to work between open versus endoscopic carpal tunnel release. Harms resulting from open carpal tunnel release vary between RCTs. One systematic review comparing the two interventions suggested that open carpal tunnel release may cause more wound problems whereas endoscopic carpal tunnel release may cause more transient nerve problems.
- **Oral corticosteroids (short term)** Three RCTs have found that oral corticosteroids (prednisone or prednisolone) versus placebo significantly improve symptoms after 2 weeks. One RCT found that local methylprednisolone injection versus oral prednisolone significantly improved symptoms after 8 weeks and 12 weeks.
- **Wrist splints** One RCT found a significant improvement with a nocturnal hand brace versus no treatment in symptoms after 2 weeks and 4 weeks. RCTs found no significant difference in symptoms with neutral angle versus 20° extension wrist splinting, or with full time versus night time only neutral angle wrist splinting.
- **Wrist splints after carpal tunnel release surgery** Two RCTs in people after carpal tunnel release surgery found no significant difference with wrist splinting versus no splinting in median grip strength or in the number of people who considered themselves "cured". Another RCT found that splinting versus no splinting significantly increased pain at 1 month and the number of days taken to return to work.
- **Local corticosteroid injection (long term); nerve and tendon gliding exercises; oral corticosteroids (long term); surgery versus no surgery** We found no RCTs on the effects of these interventions.
- **Pyridoxine; therapeutic ultrasound** RCTs found conflicting results on the effects of these interventions.

Carpal tunnel syndrome

DEFINITION Carpal tunnel syndrome is a neuropathy caused by compression of the median nerve within the carpal tunnel.[1] Classical symptoms of carpal tunnel syndrome include numbness, tingling, burning, or pain in at least two of the three digits supplied by the median nerve (i.e. the thumb, index, and middle fingers).[2] The American Academy of Neurology has described diagnostic criteria (see glossary, p 1072) that rely on a combination of symptoms and physical examination findings.[3] Other diagnostic criteria include results from electrophysiological studies.[2]

INCIDENCE/ PREVALENCE A general population survey in Rochester, Minnesota, found the age adjusted incidence of carpal tunnel syndrome to be 105 (95% CI 99 to 112) cases per 100 000 person years.[4,5] Age adjusted incidence rates were 52 (95% CI 45 to 59) cases for men and 149 (95% CI 138 to 159) cases for women per 100 000 person years. The study found incidence rates increased from 88 (95% CI 75 to 101) cases per 100 000 person years in 1961–1965 to 125 (95% CI 112 to 138) cases per 100 000 person years in 1976–1980. Incidence rates of carpal tunnel syndrome increased with age for men, whereas for women they peaked between the ages of 45–54 years. A general population survey in the Netherlands found prevalence to be 1% for men and 7% for women.[6] A more comprehensive study in southern Sweden found the general population prevalence for carpal tunnel syndrome was 3% (95% CI 2 to 3%).[7] As in other studies, the overall prevalence in women was higher than in men (male to female ratio 1 : 1.4); however, among older people, the prevalence in women was almost four times that in men (age group 65–74 years: men 1%, 95% CI 0 to 4%; women 5%, 95% CI 3 to 8%).

AETIOLOGY/ RISK FACTORS Most cases of carpal tunnel syndrome have no easily identifiable cause (idiopathic). Non-specific tenosynovitis is believed to contribute to compression of the median nerve within the carpal tunnel.[4] Secondary causes of carpal tunnel syndrome include the following: space occupying lesions (tumours, hypertrophic synovial tissue, fracture callus, and osteophytes); metabolic and physiological (pregnancy, hypothyroidism, rheumatoid arthritis); infections; neuropathies (associated with diabetes mellitus or alcoholism); and familial disorders. One case control study found that risk factors in the general population included repetitive activities requiring wrist extension or flexion, obesity, very rapid dieting, shorter height, hysterectomy without oopherectomy, and recent menopause.[8]

PROGNOSIS We found little good evidence. One observational study (carpal tunnel syndrome defined by symptoms and electrophysiological study results) found that 34% of people with idiopathic carpal tunnel syndrome without treatment had complete resolution of symptoms (remission) within 6 months of diagnosis.[9] Remission rates were higher for younger age groups, for women versus men, and for pregnant versus non-pregnant women.

AIMS To improve symptoms and reduce the physical signs of carpal tunnel syndrome; to prevent progression and loss of hand function secondary to carpal tunnel syndrome; to minimise loss of time from work.

OUTCOMES Clinical improvement of symptoms and reduction in physical signs; hand function; time to return to work.

METHODS *Clinical Evidence* search and appraisal January 2002.

QUESTION What are the effects of drug treatment?

OPTION ORAL CORTICOSTEROIDS

Three RCTs have found that oral corticosteroids (prednisone or prednisolone) versus placebo significantly improve symptoms after 2 weeks. One RCT found that local methylprednisolone injection versus oral prednisolone significantly improved symptoms after 8 weeks and 12 weeks.

Benefits: We found no systematic review. **Versus placebo:** We found three RCTs.[10–12] The first RCT (15 people) compared oral prednisone (20 mg daily for the first wk followed by 10 mg daily for the second wk) versus placebo.[10] The RCT found that prednisone significantly improved symptoms based on the Global Symptom Score (GSS) (see glossary, p 1072) at 2 weeks' follow up, but significance was not maintained at 4 or 8 weeks' follow up (results presented graphically; CI not provided). The second RCT (91 people) compared four treatments: oral prednisolone (prednisolone 20 mg daily for 2 wks followed by 10 mg daily for another 2 wks); an oral slow release non-steroidal anti-inflammatory drug (tenoxicam 20 mg daily); an oral diuretic (trichlormethiazide 2 mg daily) and placebo (see comment below).[11] The RCT found that prednisolone (26 people) versus placebo (23 people) significantly reduced the mean GSS after 2 weeks (difference in mean GSS –6.6, 95% CI –10.4 to –2.8) and after 4 weeks (–10.8, 95% CI –15.0 to –6.7). The third RCT (36 people) compared oral prednisolone (25 mg daily for 10 days) versus placebo.[12] The RCT found that prednisolone (18 people) versus placebo (18 people) significantly reduced the median GSS after 2 weeks (difference in median GSS –6, 95% CI –11 to –1) and after 8 weeks (difference in median GSS –6, 95% CI –11 to 0). **Versus injected corticosteroids:** One RCT (60 people) compared a single local corticosteroid injection (methylprednisolone acetate 15 mg into the carpal tunnel) plus oral placebo versus oral corticosteroid (prednisolone 25 mg daily for 10 days) plus placebo injection.[13] The RCT found no significant difference in the mean GSS with local methylprednisolone injection (30 people) versus oral prednisolone (30 people) after 2 weeks (difference in mean GSS –4.2, 95% CI –8.7 to +0.3), but found a significant improvement with local methylprednisolone injection versus oral prednisolone after 8 weeks (difference in mean GSS –7.1, 95% CI –11.4 to –2.8) and 12 weeks (difference in mean GSS –7.1, 95% CI –11.7 to –2.5).[13]

Harms: In the first RCT (15 people), three people in each group reported adverse effects, although none of these people discontinued their treatment.[10] In the prednisone group, one person with diabetes reported mild hyperglycaemia, whereas other reported symptoms included nausea, abdominal discomfort, constipation, and altered taste sensation. Symptoms in the placebo group included nausea, abdominal discomfort, constipation, insomnia, headache, dysuria, and burning nostrils. The second RCT did not report harms.[11] The third RCT did not report adverse events.[12] The RCT comparing local corticosteroid injection versus oral corticosteroid reported nine side effects in the oral prednisolone and placebo injection group:[13] bloating (2 people), insomnia (2 people), polyphagia (3 people), and injection pain (2 people). The RCT reported two people had injection pain in the local corticosteroid injection group. Common adverse reactions to oral corticosteroids include nausea, anxiety, acne, menstrual irregularities, insomnia, headaches, and mood swings. More serious adverse reactions include peptic ulcer, steroid psychosis, osteoporosis, and adrenal insufficiency.[14]

Comment: The second RCT reported that 18/91 (20%) people did not complete the trial, although analysis of data was not by intention to treat.[11]

OPTION NON-STEROIDAL ANTI-INFLAMMATORY DRUGS

One small RCT found no significant difference with tenoxicam versus placebo in mean global symptom score after 2 weeks or 4 weeks. One RCT found no significant difference in symptom severity scores with ibuprofen plus nocturnal wrist splint versus chiropractic manipulation plus ultrasound plus nocturnal wrist splint after 9 weeks.

Benefits: We found no systematic review. We found two RCTs.[11,15] **Versus placebo:** One RCT (91 people) compared four treatments: prednisolone; an oral slow release non-steroidal anti-inflammatory drug (NSAID) (tenoxicam 20 mg daily for 4 wks); a diuretic; and placebo (see the benefits and comment under oral corticosteroids, p 1063).[11] It found that tenoxicam (18 people) versus placebo (16 people) did not significantly alter mean Global Symptom Score (see glossary, p 1072) after 2 weeks (difference in mean Global Symptom Score +3.1, 95% CI –1.4 to +7.6) or after 4 weeks (+3.2, 95% CI –1.7 to +8.1). **Versus other treatments:** The second RCT (91 people, age 21–45 years) compared an oral NSAID (ibuprofen 800 mg 3 times daily for 1 wk, then twice daily for 1 wk, and then as needed for 7 wks) plus nocturnal wrist splints versus chiropractic manipulation plus ultrasound treatments plus nocturnal wrist splints.[15] The RCT found no significant difference between treatments in symptom severity after 9 weeks (see comment below; difference in mean symptom severity score for NSAID group *v* non-NSAID group –2.4, 95% CI –7.5 to +2.7).

Harms: The first RCT did not report harms.[11] In the second RCT, 10/46 (22%) people taking ibuprofen reported acute gastrointestinal intolerance, headache, and nausea.[15] Of these 10 people, 5/46 (11%) withdrew from the medication and 5/46 (11%) continued to take ibuprofen with an additional liquid antacid (see NSAIDs topic, p 1203).

Comment: The second RCT used a numerical scoring system to grade symptom severity (0 = no symptoms; 16 = severe symptoms).[15]

OPTION DIURETICS

One small RCT found no significant difference with trichlormethiazide versus placebo in mean Global Symptom Score after 2 weeks or 4 weeks.

Benefits: We found no systematic review but found one RCT (91 people), which compared four treatments: prednisolone; a non-steroidal anti-inflammatory drug; an oral diuretic (trichlormethiazide 2 mg daily for 4 wks); and placebo (see the benefits and comment under oral corticosteroids, p 1063).[11] It found that trichlormethiazide (16 people) versus placebo (16 people) did not significantly alter mean Global Symptom Score (see glossary, p 1072) after either 2 weeks (difference in mean Global Symptom Score +0.7, 95% CI –3.0 to +4.4) or after 4 weeks (+0.8, –3.2 to +4.8).

Harms: This RCT did not report harms.

Comment: None.

OPTION **PYRIDOXINE**

Two small RCTs found conflicting results on the effects of pyridoxine (vitamin B6) versus placebo in carpal tunnel syndrome.

Benefits: We found no systematic review. We found two small RCTs.[16,17] The first RCT (11 people) compared oral pyridoxine (200 mg daily) versus placebo.[17] It found no significant difference between treatments in the number of people who reported symptomatic improvement at 10 weeks (see comment below; 3/6 [50%] improved with pyridoxine *v* 4/5 [80%] with placebo; RR 1.6, 95% CI 0.6 to 4). The second RCT (35 people) compared oral pyridoxine (200 mg daily) versus placebo.[16] It found after 12 weeks that pyridoxine significantly reduced mean symptom severity score for finger discomfort after repetitive movement (see comment below; difference –1.0, 95% CI –2.0 to –0.1), but did not significantly reduce mean symptom severity score for night time discomfort (difference –0.5, 95% CI –1.4 to +0.4).

Harms: Neither RCT reported harms. Common adverse reactions associated with pyridoxine include numbness, paraesthesia, and an unsteady gait.[14]

Comment: The first RCT did not specify which symptoms were assessed nor how changes were scored.[17] The second RCT used an unvalidated 4-point questionnaire with discrete numerical scoring of symptom severity (0 = no symptoms; 4 = severe symptoms).[16]

OPTION **LOCAL CORTICOSTEROID INJECTION**

One systematic review has found that local corticosteroid injections versus placebo injection significantly improve symptoms after 1 month. One subsequent RCT found that hydrocortisone injection versus no injection significantly improved symptoms after 6 weeks. One RCT found that local methylprednisolone injection versus oral prednisolone significantly improved symptoms after 8 weeks and 12 weeks.

Benefits: **Versus placebo or no treatment:** We found one systematic review (search date not stated, 2 RCTs, 97 people)[18] and one subsequent RCT (84 people).[19] The first RCT included in the systematic review compared local injection of methylprednisolone (40 mg) versus local placebo injection,[20] whereas the second RCT compared local injection of betamethasone (1.5 mg) plus placebo injection into the deltoid muscle versus local placebo injection plus betamethasone (1.5 mg) injection into the deltoid muscle.[21] Meta-analysis of data from both RCTs found significantly more people with symptom improvement at 1 month with corticosteroid (methylprednisolone or betamethasone) injection (see comment below; 32/48 [67%] people with corticosteroid injection *v* 9/49 [18%] people with placebo injection; RR 3.6, 95% CI 1.9 to 6.8; NNT 3, 95% CI 2 to 4).[18] The subsequent RCT compared three treatments: local injection of low dose hydrocortisone (25 mg); local injection of high dose hydrocortisone (100 mg); and no injection.[19] It found significant improvement after 6 weeks in the number of people with improved symptoms with both doses of hydrocortisone versus no injection (see comment below; 21/32 [66%] with low dose hydrocortisone *v* 1/20 [5%] with no injection; RR 13.1, 95% CI 1.9 to 90.1; NNT 2, 95% CI 2 to 3; 20/32 [63%] with high dose hydrocortisone *v* 1/20 [5%] with no injection; RR 12.5, 95% CI 1.8 to 86.0; NNT 2, 95% CI 2 to 4). The RCT found no significant difference after 6 weeks in the number of people with improvement with low dose versus high dose hydrocortisone (21/32 [66%] with low dose hydrocortisone *v* 20/32 [63%] with high dose hydrocortisone; RR 1.0, 95% CI 0.7 to 1.5). **Versus oral corticosteroids:** We found one RCT, which compared a single local corticosteroid injection plus oral placebo versus oral corticosteroid plus placebo injection.[13] See benefits of oral corticosteroids, p 1063.

Harms: The RCTs in the systematic review and subsequent RCT did not report adverse events.[18,19] The RCT comparing local corticosteroid injection versus oral corticosteroid reported nine side effects in the oral prednisolone plus placebo injection group:[13] bloating (2 people), insomnia (2 people), polyphagia (3 people), and injection pain (2 people). The RCT reported two people had injection pain in the local corticosteroid injection group. Known serious adverse effects of local corticosteroid injection into the carpal tunnel include tendon rupture and injection into the median nerve.[22]

Comment: The two RCTs included in the systematic review only defined clinical outcomes loosely using a subjective ordinal ranking scale and neither RCT specified the magnitude of symptomatic improvement or the changes in specific symptoms.[18] The subsequent RCT reported the number of people who scored their symptoms as "better" or "much better", but these terms were not quantified and changes in individual symptoms were not described.[19]

QUESTION What are the effects of non-drug treatment?

OPTION WRIST SPLINTS

One RCT found a significant improvement with a nocturnal hand brace versus no treatment in symptoms after 2 weeks and 4 weeks. RCTs found no significant difference in symptoms with neutral angle versus 20° extension wrist splinting, or with full time versus night time only neutral angle wrist splinting.

Benefits: **Versus no treatment:** We found one RCT (83 people) that compared a new style of nocturnal hand brace worn for 4 weeks versus no treatment.[23] The RCT found a significant improvement with nocturnal hand brace versus no treatment in symptoms measured by the Boston Carpal Tunnel Symptom Questionnaire at 2 weeks

(−1.03, 95% CI −1.98 to −0.08) and 4 weeks (−1.07, 95% CI −2.01 to −0.13). **Versus other treatments:** We found no RCTs. **Versus different splinting regimens:** We found one systematic review (search date 1997, 1 RCT)[24] and one subsequent RCT.[25] The RCT in the review (59 people, 90 wrists) compared neutral angle wrist splinting versus wrist splinting in 20° extension (see comment below).[26] It found no significant difference after 2 weeks' follow up in the number of people who reported some degree of improvement in their symptoms (40/45 [89%] with neutral angle splinting *v* 38/45 [84%] with extension splinting; RR 1.1, 95% CI 0.9 to 1.2). The subsequent RCT (24 people) compared full time (day and night) wear of neutral angle wrist splints versus night time only wear. It found no significant difference after 6 weeks in mean symptom severity score (see comment below; difference in mean symptom severity score +0.1, 95% CI −0.3 to +0.5).[25]

Harms: In the RCT comparing nocturnal hand brace to no treatment, four people in the hand brace group experienced transient paraesthesias after the hand brace was removed.[23] Harms were not reported by the other RCTs.

Comment: The RCT in the systematic review graded improvement in symptoms as "none", "some", "a lot", or "complete"; however, individual symptoms and the method for grading changes in symptoms were not described.[26] The subsequent RCT used a validated numerical scale to assess changes in symptom severity.[25] The use of a night time splint was complete or nearly complete in 85% of people allocated to night time splinting only, but 23% of the people reported limited additional daytime use. Complete or nearly complete daytime wear was reported by only 27% of people allocated to full time wear. More men than women were included in the trial than would have been expected from the usual sex distribution of carpal tunnel syndrome.

OPTION NERVE AND TENDON GLIDING EXERCISES

We found no RCTs on the effects of nerve gliding or tendon gliding exercises (see glossary, p 1072).

Benefits: We found no RCTs.

Harms: We found no RCTs.

Comment: None.

OPTION THERAPEUTIC ULTRASOUND

Three RCTs found conflicting results on the effects of ultrasound therapy.

Benefits: We found no systematic review but found three RCTs.[15,27,28] The first RCT (45 people, 90 wrists) compared ultrasound (15 mins, 5 times weekly for 2 wks followed by twice weekly for 5 wks at an intensity of 1.0 W/cm^2) versus placebo.[28] The dominant wrist was randomly allocated to ultrasound or placebo and the contralateral wrist was allocated to the other treatment. The RCT found at 6 months that significantly more wrists receiving ultrasound treatment had satisfactory improvement or complete remission (see comment below; 22/30 [73%] wrists with ultrasound v 6/30 [20%] wrists with placebo; RR 3.7, 95% CI 1.7 to 7.7; NNT 2, 95% CI 2 to 4). The second RCT (18 women, 30 wrists) compared three groups: low intensity ultrasound (0.8 W/cm^2); high intensity ultrasound (1.5 W/cm^2); and placebo.[27] Each treatment was performed for 5 minutes, five times a week for 2 weeks. The RCT found no significant difference between low and high intensity ultrasound treatments or between either ultrasound treatment and placebo in mean symptom severity graded on a visual analogue scale at 2 weeks (mean difference with high intensity ultrasound v placebo –1.1, 95% CI –3.0 to +0.9; mean difference with low intensity ultrasound v placebo –0.4, 95% CI –2.5 to +1.6; mean difference with high intensity ultrasound v low intensity ultrasound –0.7, 95% CI –2.4 to +0.9). The third RCT (91 people) compared ultrasound (1.0–1.5 W/cm^2 for 5 mins) plus nocturnal wrist splints plus chiropractic manipulation (3 sessions/wk for 2 wks, then 2 sessions/wk for 3 wks, then 1 session/wk for 4 wks) versus nocturnal wrist splints plus a non-steroidal anti-inflammatory drug (see non-steroidal anti-inflammatory drugs topic, p 1203).[15] The RCT found no significant difference between treatments in symptom severity scores at 9 weeks (see comment below; non-ultrasound group v ultrasound group –2.4, 95% CI –7.5 to +2.7).

Harms: In the third RCT, one person reported a sore neck after chiropractic manipulation.[15]

Comment: In the first RCT, 15/45 (33%) people did not complete the trial and analysis of data was not by intention to treat.[28] The RCT used "satisfactory improvement" and "complete remission" as outcome measures, although these terms were not clearly defined. The third RCT used numerical scoring system to grade symptom severity (0 = no symptoms; 16 = severe symptoms).[15]

QUESTION What are the effects of surgical treatment?

OPTION SURGERY

We found no RCTs on the effects of surgery versus placebo. One systematic review found no significant difference with endoscopic versus open carpal tunnel release surgery in symptoms after 3–12 months. One subsequent small RCT found no significant difference between endoscopic versus open carpal tunnel release in tingling sensations or severity of night time numbness after 4 weeks, but found that endoscopic versus open carpal tunnel release significantly improved the severity of night time hand or wrist pain after 4 weeks. RCTs found conflicting evidence on differences in the time taken to return to work between the two procedures. Harms resulting from endoscopic and open carpal tunnel release vary between RCTs. One systematic review comparing the two interventions suggests that endoscopic carpal tunnel release may cause more transient nerve problems whereas open carpal tunnel release may cause more wound problems.

Benefits: **Surgery versus placebo:** We found one systematic review (search date 2000, 14 RCTS, 1179 people)[29] and one non-systematic review (search date 1997, 4 RCTs, 1394 people).[30] Neither review found RCTs comparing surgery versus placebo or no treatment. **Endoscopic versus open carpal tunnel release:** We found one systematic review (search date 2000, 7 RCTS, 739 people; see comment below)[29] and one subsequent small RCT (26 men).[31] The systematic review included three "high quality" RCTs and four "low quality" RCTs comparing endoscopic carpal tunnel release versus open carpal tunnel release.[29] The systematic review included three RCTs that assessed effects on symptoms after 3 months.[29] It found no significant difference in symptoms after 3 months with endoscopic versus open carpal tunnel release (reported as improvement in paraesthesia, numbness in 99% with endoscopic carpal tunnel release *v* 98% with open carpal tunnel release after 12 wks, difference 1%, 95% CI −3 to +5% in 1 RCT; reported as "no significant difference" in pain after 3 months in 1 RCT; reported as "no significant difference" in symptom severity score after 3 months in 1 RCT; P values not provided).[29] The systematic review included one RCT that evaluated effects on symptoms after 6 months and 12 months. It found no significant difference in pain with endoscopic versus open carpal tunnel release after 6 months and 12 months (reported as "no significant difference"; P value not provided).[29] One subsequent small RCT found that tingling sensations and severity of night time numbness were improved in the endoscopic versus the open carpal tunnel release group at 2 weeks, but were no longer significantly different by 4 weeks (P values not provided).[31] It found endoscopic versus open carpal tunnel release significantly improved the severity of night time hand or wrist pain after 4 weeks (P value not provided).[31] Four RCTs included in the review found a significant decrease in the time taken to return to work and/or activities of daily living with endoscopic carpal tunnel release versus open carpal tunnel release (endoscopic carpal tunnel release *v* open carpal tunnel release: reported as median 14 days *v* 28 days, $P < 0.05$ in 1 RCT; mean 24 days *v* 42 days, $P < 0.05$ in 1 RCT; mean 14 days *v* 39 days, $P < 0.05$ in 1 RCT; mean 20 days *v* 30 days, $P < 0.05$ in 1 RCT), whereas three RCTs included in the review found no significant difference (endoscopic carpal tunnel release *v* open carpal tunnel release: reported as mean 17 days *v* 19 days, "no significant difference" in 1 RCT; reported as more than 4 wks absence from work 16% *v* 13%, difference 3%, 95% CI −7 to + 14% in 1 RCT; reported as time to return to work 17 days *v* 17 days, "no significant difference" in 1 RCT; P value not provided).[29]

Harms: **Endoscopic versus open carpal tunnel release:** All seven RCTs included in the systematic review reported complications.[29] For endoscopic carpal tunnel release complications reported included partial transection of superficial palmar arch, digital nerve contusion, ulnar nerve neurapraxia (see glossary, p 1072), wound haematoma, four conversion to the open procedure, transient neurapraxia, three transient numbness on radial side of ring finger, ulnar nerve paraesthesia, incomplete release, increased numbness in fingertips, subcutaneous heamatoma, loss of strength and mobility in wrist, and algodystrophy. For open carpal tunnel release, complications reported included painful hypertrophic scar, reflex sympathetic dystrophy, prolonged wound secretion, wound infection, scar tethering, five scar hypertrophy, two loss of strength, and swollen/stiff fingers. The systematic review stated "it seems that endoscopic carpal tunnel release gives more transient nerve problems (e.g. neurapraxia, numbness, paraesthesia) and open carpal tunnel release more wound problems (e.g. infection, hypertrophic scar, scar tenderness)".[29] Harms resulting from endoscopic and open carpal tunnel release vary between RCTs, although rates of complications for both procedures are generally low.[31–38]

Comment: Meta-analysis in the systematic review was not undertaken as the data could not be pooled. Endoscopic release techniques vary between RCTs, which may account for some of the variation in complication rates.[30]

OPTION INTERNAL NEUROLYSIS IN CONJUNCTION WITH OPEN CARPAL TUNNEL RELEASE

Three RCTs found no significant difference with open carpal tunnel release alone versus open carpal tunnel release plus internal neurolysis in symptoms.

Benefits: We found one systematic review (search date 2000, 3 RCTs, 148 people; see comment below),[29] which included three RCTs comparing open carpal tunnel release alone versus open carpal tunnel release plus internal neurolysis (see glossary, p 1072).[39–41] The first RCT (59 people, 63 wrists) found no significant difference between treatments in the number of people reporting relief from all or the majority of their symptoms after 12 months (28/32 [88%] with open carpal tunnel release alone *v* 25/31 [81%] with open carpal tunnel release plus internal neurolysis; RR 1.1, 95% CI 0.9 to 1.3).[39] The second RCT (48 people, 48 wrists) found no significant difference between treatments in the number of people who reported complete relief of symptoms after 6 months (23/24 [96%] with open carpal tunnel release alone *v* 23/24 [96%] with open carpal tunnel release plus internal neurolysis; RR 1.0, 95% CI 0.9 to 1.1).[41] The third RCT (41 people, 47 wrists with severe carpal tunnel syndrome; see comment below) found no significant difference between treatments in the number of wrists with a good (resolution of pain, improvement in sensory deficit, and no surgical complications) or excellent (resolution of pain, resolution of sensory deficit, and no surgical complications) clinical response (15/23 [65%] wrists with open carpal tunnel release alone *v* 16/24 [67%] wrists with open carpal tunnel release plus internal neurolysis; RR 1.0, 95% CI 0.6 to 1.5).[40]

Harms: The first and second RCTs did not report harms.[39,41] The third RCT (41 people, 47 wrists) found no significant difference between treatments in the number of wrists with persistent incisional pain, which was the most common complication reported in the trial (3/23 [13%] of wrists with open carpal tunnel release alone *v* 4/24 [17%] of wrists with open carpal tunnel release plus internal neurolysis; RR 0.8, 95% CI 0.2 to 3.1).[40] Other complications included 4% (1/24) wrists with hand swelling, 4% (1/24) wrists with adhesive capsulitis (see glossary, p 1072) in the open carpal tunnel release plus internal neurolysis group, and 4% (1/23) wrists with causalgia in the open carpal tunnel release alone group.

Comment: Meta-analysis in the systematic review was not undertaken as the data could not be pooled. The third RCT defined severe carpal tunnel syndrome as including thenar atrophy, a fixed sensory deficit, or both, in addition to the more common symptoms and signs associated with the syndrome.[39]

QUESTION What are the effects of postoperative treatment?

OPTION WRIST SPLINTS AFTER CARPAL TUNNEL RELEASE SURGERY

Two RCTs in people after carpal tunnel release surgery found no significant difference with wrist splinting versus no splinting in median grip strength or in the number of people who considered themselves "cured". Another RCT found that splinting versus no splinting significantly increased pain at 1 month and the number of days taken to return to work.

Benefits: **Versus unrestricted range of motion:** We found no systematic review. We found three RCTs.[42–44] The first RCT (74 people, 82 wrists) compared rigid wrist splinting for 4 weeks after surgery versus no splinting plus advice to mobilise the affected wrist or wrists.[42] It found no significant difference between treatments in median grip strength (as a percentage of median preoperative grip strength: unsplinted 78%, 95% CI 70% to 86% *v* splinted 76%, 95% CI, 71% to 85%). The second RCT (47 people, 51 wrists) compared rigid wrist splinting for 2 weeks after surgery versus no splinting.[43] It found no significant difference in the number of people who considered themselves "cured" at follow up (see comment below; 12/26 [46%] with splinting *v* 8/17 [47%] with no splinting; RR 1.0, 95% CI 0.5 to 1.9). The third RCT (50 people, 50 wrists) compared rigid wrist splinting for 2 weeks after surgery versus no splinting.[44] It found that the average number of days taken to return to work was significantly lower in the unsplinted group (17 days with no splinting *v* 27 days with splinting; P = 0.005; RR and CI not provided). **Versus bulky dressings:** We found one systematic review (search date 1997) comparing wrist splinting versus bulky dressings after carpal tunnel decompression.[24] It found no RCTs.

Harms: The first RCT found no significant difference between treatments in the number of people reporting scar pain after 6 months (6/37 [16%] with splinting *v* 6/44 [14%] with no splinting; RR 1.2, 95% CI 0.4 to 3.4).[42] The second RCT reported complications for one person in the unsplinted group who had persistent symptoms and required reoperation.[43] The third RCT reported that pillar pain (see glossary, p 1072) was increased at 1 months' follow up for the splinted group (P = 0.02), as was scar tenderness (P = 0.04), although subjective scores for pain were not significantly different between treatments at 3 or 6 months after surgery (data not available).[44]

Comment: In the second RCT, although the term "cured" was used as an outcome measure, its meaning was not defined in the context of the trial and the length of follow up was not specified.[42] The RCT found that 7/47 (15%) people were lost to follow up. Analysis of data was not by intention to treat. The RCTs were too small to exclude the possibility of a clinically important increase in the risk of some complications (e.g. transient ulnar nerve injury) with splinting compared with no splinting.

GLOSSARY

Adhesive capsulitis A condition in which the joint capsule becomes contracted and thickened causing restriction in the range of movement.

American Academy of Neurology diagnostic criteria[3] The likelihood of carpal tunnel syndrome increases with the number of standard symptoms and provocative factors. Symptoms include dull aching discomfort in the hand, forearm or upper arm; paraesthesia in the hand; weakness or clumsiness of the hand; dry skin, swelling, or colour changes in the hand; or occurrence of any of these symptoms in the distribution of the median nerve. Provocative factors include sleep, sustained arm or hand positions, or repetitive actions of the hand or wrist. Relieving factors include changes in hand posture and shaking the hand. Physical examination may be normal, or symptoms may be elicited by tapping or direct pressure over the median nerve at the wrist or with forced flexion or extension of the wrist. Physical signs include sensory loss in the median nerve distribution; weakness or atrophy in the thenar muscles; and dry skin on the thumb, index, or middle fingers. Electromyography and nerve conduction studies can confirm, but not exclude, the diagnosis of carpal tunnel syndrome.

Global Symptom Score (GSS) The numerical sum of five common carpal tunnel syndrome symptoms (pain, numbness, paresthesia, weakness/clumsiness, and nocturnal wakening), which are each rated from 0 (no symptoms) to 10 (severe symptoms).[10,11]

Internal neurolysis Decompression within the nerve accomplished by performing an epineurotomy and then dividing the nerve into multiple fascicular groups.[40]

Nerve gliding exercises Exercise therapy directed at restoring and maximising excursion of the median nerve through the carpal tunnel.[45]

Pillar pain Pain at the radial or ulnar border of the carpal tunnel.

Tendon gliding exercises Exercise therapy directed at restoring and maximising excursion of the finger flexor tendons through the carpal tunnel.[45]

Ulnar neurapraxia Failure of nerve conduction of the ulnar nerve, usually reversible, due to metabolic or microstructural abnormalities without disruption of the axon.

Substantive changes

Oral corticosteroids Two new RCTs;[12,13] conclusions unchanged.

Local corticosteroid injection One new RCT;[13] conclusions unchanged.

Wrist splints One new RCT;[23] conclusions unchanged.

Surgery One new systematic review;[29] conclusions unchanged.

Internal neurolysis plus open carpal tunnel release One new systematic review;[29] conclusions unchanged.

REFERENCES

1. Rozmaryn LM. Carpal tunnel syndrome: a comprehensive review. *Curr Opin Orthop* 1997;8:33–43.
2. Rempel D, Evanoff B, Amadio PC, et al. Consensus criteria for the classification of carpal tunnel syndrome in epidemiologic studies. *Am J Public Health* 1998;88:1447–1451.
3. Anonymous. Practice parameter for carpal tunnel syndrome (summary statement). Report of the Quality Standards Subcommittee of the American Academy of Neurology. *Neurology* 1993;43:2406–2409.
4. von Schroeder H, Botte MJ. Carpal tunnel syndrome. *Hand Clin* 1996;12:643–655.
5. Stevens JC, Sun S, Beard CM, et al. Carpal tunnel syndrome in Rochester, Minnesota, 1961 to 1980. *Neurology* 1988;38:134–138.
6. Dumitru D. *Textbook of Electrodiagnostic Medicine*. Hanley and Belfus, eds. Philadelphia: Mosby Publications, 1995.

7. Atroshi I, Gummesson C, Johnsson R, et al. Prevalence of carpal tunnel syndrome in a general population. *JAMA* 1999;282:153–158.
8. De Krom MCTF, Kester A, Knipschild P, et al. Risk factors for carpal tunnel syndrome. *Am J Epidemiol* 1990;132:1102–1110.
9. Fatami T, Kobayashi A, Utika T, et al. Carpal tunnel syndrome; its natural history. *Hand Surgery* 1997;2:129–130.
10. Herskovitz S, Berger AR, Lipton RB. Low-dose, short-term oral prednisone in the treatment of carpal tunnel syndrome. *Neurology* 1995;45:1923–1925.
11. Chang MH, Chiang HT, Lee SS, et al. Oral drug of choice in carpal tunnel syndrome. *Neurology* 1998;51:390–393.
12. Hiu ACF, Wong SM, Wong KS, et al. Oral steroid in the treatment of carpal tunnel syndrome. *Ann Rheum Dis* 2001;60(8):813–814.
13. Wong SM, Hui ACF, Tang A, et al. Local vs systemic corticosteroids in the treatment of carpal tunnel syndrome. Neurology 2001; 56(11):1565–1567.
14. Canadian Pharmacists Association. *Compendium of pharmaceuticals and specialties 2000.* Ottawa: Canadian Pharmacists Association, 2000.
15. Thomas P, James D, Hulbert R, et al. Comparative efficacy of conservative medical and chiropractic treatments for carpal tunnel syndrome: a randomized clinical trial. *J Manipulative Physiol Ther* 1998;21:317–326.
16. Spooner GR, Desai HB, Angel JF, et al. Using pyridoxine to treat carpal tunnel syndrome. Randomized control trial. *Can Fam Physician* 1993;39:2122–2127.
17. Stransky M, Rubin A, Lava NS, et al. Treatment of carpal tunnel syndrome with vitamin B6: a double-blind study. *South Med J* 1989;82:841–842.
18. Marshall S, Tardif G, Ashworth N. Local corticosteroid injection for carpal tunnel syndrome. In: The Cochrane Library, Issue 4, 2001. Oxford: Update Software. Search date not stated; primary sources Cochrane Neuromuscular Disease Group Register, Medline, Embase, and Cinahl. No company sponsorship declared.
19. O'Gradaigh D, Merry P. Corticosteroid injection for the treatment of carpal tunnel syndrome *Ann Rheum Dis* 2000;59:918–919.
20. Dammers JW, Veering MM, Vermeulen M, et al. Injection with methylprednisolone proximal to the carpal tunnel: randomized double blind trial. *BMJ* 1999;319:884–886.
21. Ozdogan H, Yazici H. The efficacy of local steroid injections in idiopathic carpal tunnel syndrome: a double-blind study. *Br J Rheumatol* 1984;23:272–275.
22. Babu SR, Britton JM. The role of steroid injection in the management of carpal tunnel syndrome. *J Orthop Rheumatol* 1994;7:59–60.
23. Manente G, Torrieri F, Di Blasio F, et al. An innovative hand brace for carpal tunnel syndrome: a randomised controlled trial. *Muscle Nerve* 2001;24(8):1020–1025.
24. Feuerstein M, Burrell LM, Miller VI, et al. Clinical management of carpal tunnel syndrome: a 12-year review of outcomes. *Am J Ind Med* 1999;35:232–245. Search date 1997; primary sources Medline, Cinahl, Psychlit, and Nioshtic. No company sponsorship declared.
25. Walker WC, Metzler M, Cifu DX, et al. Neutral wrist splinting in carpal tunnel syndrome: a comparison of night-only versus full-time wear instructions. *Arch Phys Med Rehabil* 2000;81:424–429.
26. Burke TD, Burke MM, Stewart GW, et al. Splinting for carpal tunnel syndrome: In search of the optimal angle. *Arch Phys Med Rehabil* 1994;75:1241–1244.
27. Oztas O, Turan B, Bora I, et al. Ultrasound therapy effect in carpal tunnel syndrome. *Arch Phys Med Rehabil* 1998;79:1540–1544.
28. Ebenbichler GR, Resch KL, Nicolakis P, et al. Ultrasound treatment for treating the carpal tunnel syndrome: randomised "sham" controlled trial. *BMJ* 1998;316:730–735.
29. Gerritsen AA, Uitdehaag BMJ, van Geldere D, et al. Systematic review of randomised clinical trials of surgical treatment for carpal tunnel syndrome. *Br J Surg* 2001;88(10):1285–1295. Search date 2000; primary sources Medline, Embase, the Cochrane Controlled Trials Register, reference lists of retrieved studies.
30. Jimenez DF, Gibbs SR, Clapper AT. Endoscopic treatment of carpal tunnel syndrome: a critical review [see comments]. *J Neurosurg* 1998;88:817–826. Search date 1997; primary sources not stated.
31. Mackenzie DJ, Hainer R, Wheatley MJ. Early recovery after endoscopic vs. short-incision open carpal tunnel release. *Ann Plastic Surg* 2000;44:601–604.
32. Hoefnagels WAJ, Van Kleef JGF, Mastenbroek GGA, et al. Surgical treatment of the carpal tunnel syndrome: Endoscopic or classical (open) surgery? A prospective randomised study. *Ned Tijdschr Geneeskd* 1997;141:878–882.
33. Benedetti RB, Sennwald G. Endoscopic decompression of the median nerve by the technique of Agee: A prospective study in comparison with the open decompression. *Handchir Mikrochir Plast Chir* 1996;28:151–155.
34. Stark B, Engkvist-Lofmark C. Carpal tunnel syndrome. Endoscopic release or conventional surgery. *Handchir Mikrochir Plast Chir* 1996;28:128–132.
35. Herren DB. Complications after endoscopic carpal tunnel decompression. *Z Unfallchir Versicherungsmed* 1994;87:120–127.
36. Brown RA, Gelberman RH, Seiler III, et al. Carpal tunnel release. A prospective, randomized assessment of open and endoscopic methods. *J Bone Joint Surg Am* 1993;75:1265–1275.
37. Erdmann MWH. Endoscopic carpal tunnel decompression. *J Hand Surg* 1994;19:5–13.
38. Agee JM, McCarroll J, Tortosa RD, et al. Endoscopic release of the carpal tunnel: a randomized prospective multicenter study. *J Hand Surg* 1992;17:987–995.
39. Mackinnon SE, McCabe S, Murray JF, et al. Internal neurolysis fails to improve the results of primary carpal tunnel decompression. *J Hand Surg Am* 1991;16:211–218.
40. Lowry WE Jr, Follender AB. Interfascicular neurolysis in the severe carpal tunnel syndrome. A prospective, randomized, double-blind, controlled study. *Clin Orthop* 1988;227:251–254.
41. Holmgren-Larsson H, Leszniewski W, Linden U et al. Internal neurolysis or ligament division only in carpal tunnel syndrome — results of a randomized study. *Acta Neurochir (Wien)* 1985;74:118–121.
42. Finsen V, Andersen K, Russwurm H. No advantage from splinting the wrist after open carpal tunnel release. A randomized study of 82 wrists. *Acta Orthop Scand* 1999;70:288–292.
43. Bury TF, Akelman E, Weiss AP. Prospective, randomized trial of splinting after carpal tunnel release. *Ann Plastic Surg* 1995;35:19–22.

44. Cook AC, Szabo RM, Birkholz SW, et al. Early mobilization following carpal tunnel release. A prospective randomized study. *J Hand Surg Br* 1995;20:228–230.

45. Rozmaryn LM, Dovelle S, Rothman ER, et al. Nerve and tendon gliding exercises and the conservative management of carpal tunnel syndrome. *J Hand Ther* 1998;11:171–179.

Shawn Marshall
Assistant Professor
University of Ottawa
Ottawa
Canada

Competing interests: None declared.

Chronic fatigue syndrome

Search date July 2002

Steven Reid, Trudie Chalder, Anthony Cleare, Matthew Hotopf, and Simon Wessely

QUESTIONS

INTERVENTIONS

Key Messages

- **Cognitive behavioural therapy** One systematic review has found that cognitive behavioural therapy versus standard care or relaxation therapy administered by highly skilled therapists in specialist centres improves quality of life and physical functioning. One additional multicentre RCT has found that cognitive behavioural therapy administered by less experienced therapists compared with guided support groups or no intervention may also be effective.
- **Evening primrose oil** One small RCT found no significant difference with evening primrose oil versus placebo in depression scores at 3 months.
- **Graded aerobic exercise** RCTs have found that a graded aerobic exercise programme versus flexibity and relaxation training or general advice significantly improves measures of fatigue and physical functioning. One RCT has found a significant improvement in measures of physical functioning, fatigue, mood, and sleep at 1 year with an educational package to encourage graded exercise versus written information only.
- **Immunotherapy** Small RCTs found that immunoglobulin G versus placebo modestly improved physical functioning and fatigue at 3–6 months, but was associated with considerable adverse effects. Small RCTs found insufficient evidence on the effects of interferon alfa versus placebo.
- **Magnesium (intramuscular)** One small RCT found that magnesium injections versus placebo significantly improved symptoms at 6 weeks (NNT 2, 95% 2 to 4).
- **Prolonged rest** We found no RCTs on the effects of prolonged rest. Indirect observational evidence in healthy volunteers and in people recovering from a viral illness suggests that prolonged rest may perpetuate or worsen fatigue and symptoms.
- **Antidepressants; corticosteroids; oral nicotinamide adenine dinucleotide** RCTs found insufficient evidence on the effects of these interventions.

Chronic fatigue syndrome

DEFINITION Chronic fatigue syndrome (CFS) is characterised by severe, disabling fatigue and other symptoms, including musculoskeletal pain, sleep disturbance, impaired concentration, and headaches. Two widely used definitions of CFS, from the US Centers for Disease Control and Prevention[1] and from Oxford, UK,[2] were developed as operational criteria for research (see table 1, p 1088). There are two important differences between these definitions. The UK criteria insist upon the presence of mental fatigue, whereas the US criteria include a requirement for several physical symptoms, reflecting the belief that CFS has an underlying immunological or infective pathology.

INCIDENCE/ PREVALENCE Community and primary care based studies have reported the prevalence of CFS to be 0–3%, depending on the criteria used.[3,4] Systematic population surveys have found similar prevalence of CFS in people of different socioeconomic status, and in all ethnic groups.[4,5]

AETIOLOGY/ RISK FACTORS The cause of CFS is poorly understood. Women are at higher risk than men (RR 1.3–1.7 depending on diagnostic criteria used).[6]

PROGNOSIS Studies have focused on people attending specialist clinics. A systematic review of studies of prognosis (search date 1996) found that children with CFS had better outcomes than adults: 54–94% of children showed definite improvement (after up to 6 years' follow up), whereas 20–50% of adults showed some improvement in the medium term and only 6% returned to premorbid levels of functioning.[7] Despite the considerable burden of morbidity associated with CFS, we found no evidence of increased mortality. The systematic review found that outcome was influenced by the presence of psychiatric disorders (depression and anxiety), and beliefs about causation and treatment.[7]

AIMS To reduce levels of fatigue and associated symptoms; to increase levels of activity; to improve quality of life.

OUTCOMES Severity of symptoms and their effects on physical function and quality of life. These outcomes are measured in several different ways: the medical outcomes survey short form general health survey (SF-36),[8] a rating scale measuring limitation of physical functioning caused by ill health (score range 0–100, where 0 = limited in all activities and 100 = able to carry out vigorous activities); the Karnofsky scale,[9] a modified questionnaire originally developed for the rating of quality of life in people undergoing chemotherapy for malignancy; the Beck Depression Inventory,[10] a checklist for quantifying depressive symptoms; the sickness impact profile,[11] a measure of the influence of symptoms on social and physical functioning; the Chalder fatigue scale,[12] a rating scale measuring subjective fatigue (score range 0–11, where scores ≥ 4 = excessive fatigue); the clinical global impression scale,[13] a validated measure of overall change compared with baseline at study onset, with seven possible scores from "very much worse" (score 7) to "very much better" (score 1); and self reported severity of symptoms and levels of activity, the Nottingham health profile[14] contains questions in

6 categories — energy, pain perception, sleep patterns, sense of social isolation, emotional reactions, physical mobility (weighted scores give maximum 100 for answer yes to all questions, and minimum 0 for someone with no complaints).

METHODS *Clinical Evidence* update search and appraisal July 2002.

QUESTION What are the effects of treatments?

OPTION ANTIDEPRESSANTS

RCTs found insufficient evidence about the effects of antidepressants in people with chronic fatigue syndrome.

Benefits: We found one systematic review (search date 2000), which did not report quantified results.[15] **Fluoxetine:** The review identified two RCTs.[16,17] The first RCT (107 depressed and non-depressed people with chronic fatigue syndrome [CFS]) compared fluoxetine versus placebo for 8 weeks.[16] It found that fluoxetine versus placebo significantly improved the Beck Depression Inventory (mean difference between fluoxetine and placebo in improvement in Beck Depression Inventory –0.19, 95% CI –0.35 to –0.02), but the difference may not be clinically important. It found no significant difference with fluoxetine versus placebo in the sickness impact profile (mean difference between fluoxetine and placebo measured by fatigue subscale of Checklist Individual Strength –0.16, 95% CI –0.64 to +0.31).[18] The second RCT (136 people with CFS) compared four groups: fluoxetine plus graded exercise; drug placebo plus graded exercise; fluoxetine plus general advice to exercise; and drug placebo plus general advice to exercise. It found no significant difference in the level of fatigue, although there were modest improvements in measures of depression at 12 weeks (Hospital Anxiety and Depression scale, mean change 1.1, 95% CI 0.03 to 2.2).[17,19] **Phenelzine:** The review identified one RCT.[15,20] The RCT (30 people with CFS) compared phenelzine versus placebo, using a modified Karnofsky scale and other outcome measures (including functional status questionnaire, profile of mood states, Centres for Epidemiological Study of Depression fatigue severity scale, and symptom severity checklist).[19] This study concluded that there was a pattern of improvement across several measures (significance tests for individual measures not carried out). **Moclobemide:** The review identified one RCT but did not report quantified results.[15,21] The RCT (90 people with CFS) compared moclobemide (450–600 mg daily) versus placebo.[21] It found that moclobemide was associated with a non-significant increase in subjectively reported global improvement (moclobemide 24/47 [51%] *v* placebo 14/43 [33%]; OR 2.16, 95% CI 0.9 to 5.1), and a non-significant improvement in the clinician rated Karnofsky scale. **Sertraline versus clomipramine:** We found one RCT comparing sertraline versus clomipramine in people with CFS.[22] It found no significant difference between sertraline and clomipramine. There was no placebo group, making it difficult to draw useful conclusions.

Harms: **Fluoxetine:** One RCT assessed separately the symptoms (which could be attributed to either CFS or to known adverse effects of fluoxetine) before starting treatment, after 2 weeks, after 6 weeks, and at the end of treatment (wk 8). It found that more people taking fluoxetine complained of tremor and perspiration compared with placebo at 8 weeks (tremor: P = 0.006; perspiration: P = 0.008).[16] It found no significant difference between fluoxetine and placebo at 2 and 6 weeks. More people taking fluoxetine withdrew from the trial because of adverse effects (9/54 [17%] *v* 2/53 [4%]).[16] The second RCT also found more people taking fluoxetine withdrew from the trial (24/68 people [36%] with fluoxetine withdrew *v* 16/69 people [24%] with placebo).[17] **Phenelzine:** Three of 15 people (20%) taking phenelzine withdrew because of adverse effects compared with none taking placebo.[20] **Sertraline versus clomipramine:** The RCT provided no information on adverse effects.[22]

Comment: Clinical trials were performed in specialist clinics. **Fluoxetine:** The first RCT[16] used a shorter duration of treatment and studied people with a longer duration of illness compared with the second RCT.[17]

OPTION CORTICOSTEROIDS

Four RCTs found insufficient evidence about the effects of corticosteroids versus placebo in people with chronic fatigue syndrome.

Benefits: We found one systematic review (search date 2000), which did not report quantified results.[15] **Fludrocortisone:** The systematic review[15] identified two RCTs.[23,24] The first large RCT (100 people with chronic fatigue syndrome [CFS] and neurally mediated hypotension) compared fludrocortisone (titrated to 0.1 mg daily) versus placebo for 9 weeks. It found no significant difference on a self rated global scale of "wellness" (recorded improvement of ≥ 15 points: fludrocortisone 14% *v* placebo 10%; P = 0.76; raw data not provided).[23] The second randomised crossover trial (20 people), which measured change in symptom severity (visual analogue scale of symptoms from 0–10 corresponding to "no problem" to "could not be worse") and functional status (using the SF-36) for 6 weeks. It found no significant difference between fludrocortisone and placebo.[24] **Hydrocortisone:** The review identified two RCTs.[15,25,26] The first RCT (65 people) compared hydrocortisone (25–35 mg daily) versus placebo for 12 weeks. It found that people taking hydrocortisone had a greater improvement in a self rated scale of "wellness" (recorded improvement of ≥ 5 points: hydrocortisone 53% *v* placebo 29%; P = 0.04). Other self rating scales did not show significant benefit (Beck Depression Inventory: hydrocortisone –2.1 *v* placebo –0.4, P = 0.17; activity scale: hydrocortisone 0.3 *v* placebo 0.7, P = 0.32; sickness impact profile: hydrocortisone –2.5 *v* placebo –2.2; P = 0.85).[25] The second randomised crossover trial (32 people) compared a lower dose of hydrocortisone (5 or 10 mg daily) versus placebo for 1 month. It found that more people taking hydrocortisone had short term improvement in fatigue (self report fatigue scale: hydrocortisone 28% *v* placebo 9%; results before crossover not provided).[26]

Harms: **Fludrocortisone:** In the first RCT, more people on fludrocortisone withdrew because of adverse events (12/50 [24%] *v* 4/50 [8%]; RR 3, 95% CI 1.04 to 8.67; NNT 6, 95% CI 3 to 8).[23] Four people withdrew from the trial because of worsening symptoms.[24] **Hydrocortisone:** One RCT (using 25–35 mg daily doses of hydrocortisone) found that 12 people (40%) experienced adrenal suppression (assessed by measuring cortisol levels).[25] Another RCT (using 5 or 10 mg daily doses of hydrocortisone) reported minor adverse effects in up to 10% of participants. Three people on hydrocortisone had exacerbation of acne and nervousness, and one person on placebo had an episode of fainting.[26]

Comment: The RCTs used different reasons for their choice of active treatment. The use of fludrocortisone, a mineralocorticoid, was based on the hypothesis that CFS is associated with neurally mediated hypotension.[27] The use of hydrocortisone, a glucocorticoid, in the other RCTs was based on evidence of underactivity of the hypothalamic–pituitary–adrenocortical axis in some people with CFS.[28] Any benefit from low dose glucocorticoids seems to be short lived, and higher doses are associated with adverse effects.

OPTION ORAL NICOTINAMIDE ADENINE DINUCLEOTIDE

One small RCT found insufficient evidence about the effects of oral nicotinamide adenine dinucleotide versus placebo in people with chronic fatigue syndrome.

Benefits: We found one systematic review (search date 2000), which did not report quantified results.[15] It identified one poor quality randomised crossover trial (35 people) comparing nicotinamide adenine dinucleotide (10 mg daily) versus placebo for 4 weeks.[29] Of the 35 people, two were excluded for non-compliance and seven were excluded for using psychotropic drugs. It found a significant improvement on a self devised 50 item symptom rating scale with nicotinamide adenine dinucleotide (8/26 people [30%] attained a 10% improvement with nicotinamide adenine dinucleotide *v* 2/26 people [8%] with placebo; $P < 0.05$, calculated by authors).

Harms: Minor adverse effects (loss of appetite, dyspepsia, flatulence) were reported on active treatment but did not lead to cessation of treatment.[29]

Comment: The RCT had a number of problems with its methods, including the use of inappropriate statistical analyses, the inappropriate exclusion of people from the analysis, and lack of numerical data preventing independent re-analysis of the published results.[30]

OPTION EXERCISE

RCTs have found that a graded aerobic exercise programme versus flexibity and relaxation training or general advice significantly improves measures of fatigue and physical functioning. One RCT has found a significant improvement in measures of physical functioning, fatigue, mood, and sleep at 1 year with an educational package to encourage graded exercise versus written information only.

Benefits: We found one systematic review (search date 2000), which did not report quantified results.[15] **Graded aerobic exercise:** The review identified two RCTs.[15,17,31] One RCT (66 people) compared graded aerobic exercise (active intervention) versus flexibility and relaxation training (control intervention) over 12 weeks.[31] All participants undertook individual weekly sessions supervised by an exercise physiologist. The aerobic exercise group built up their level of activity to 30 minutes of exercise a day (walking, cycling, swimming up to a maximum oxygen consumption of VO_2max 60%). People in the flexibility and relaxation training group were taught stretching and relaxation techniques (maximum 30 min daily, 5 days/wk) and were specifically told to avoid any extra physical activities. It found that more people from the aerobic exercise group reported feeling "better" or "very much better", and an improvement in physical fatigue and physical functioning versus the control group (clinical global impression scale: 52% *v* 27%, $P = 0.04$; Chalder fatigue scale: –8.4 *v* –3.1, $P = 0.004$; SF-36 scale: 20.5 *v* 8.0, $P = 0.01$). The flexibility training group crossed over to aerobic exercise at the end of the trial and significant improvements from baseline were found (peak oxygen consumption; $P < 0.0001$: physical function; $P = 0.002$ compared with baseline). The second RCT (136 people) compared four groups (graded aerobic exercise plus fluoxetine; graded aerobic exercise plus drug placebo; general advice plus fluoxetine; general advice plus drug placebo) over 24 weeks.[17] The graded exercise groups were given specific advice to undertake preferred aerobic exercise (such as walking, jogging, swimming, or cycling) for 20 minutes three times a week up to an energy expenditure of 75% of VO_2max. The general advice (exercise placebo) groups were not given any specific advice on frequency, intensity, or duration of aerobic activity they should be undertaking. It found that, at week 26, there were fewer cases of fatigue in the graded exercise groups versus people receiving general advice (Chalder fatigue scale < 4: 12/67 [18%] *v* 4/69 [6%]; RR 3.1, 95% CI 1.05 to 9.10; NNT 9, 95% CI 5 to 91). **Educational intervention:** The review identified one RCT (148 people) but did not report quantified results.[15,32] The RCT compared three types of educational interventions to encourage graded exercise versus only providing written information (control group).[32] The participants in the three educational intervention groups received two treatment sessions, two telephone follow ups, and an educational package that provided an explanation of symptoms and encouraged home based exercise. One group received seven additional follow up telephone calls and another received seven additional face to face sessions over 4 months. People in the written information group received advice and an information booklet that encouraged graded activity but gave no explanation for the symptoms. The RCT found that, in people who had received an educational intervention, there was improvement in physical functioning, fatigue, mood, sleep, and disability (self reported) compared with the people who had only received written information. No significant differences were found between the educational intervention groups (mean for 3 educational intervention groups versus written information, SF-36 subscale: ≥25 or an increase of ≥10, 1 year after randomisation, 69% *v* 6%, P < 0.001; Chalder fatigue scale: 3 *v* 10, P < 0.001; Hospital Anxiety and Depression scale: depression 4 *v* 10, P < 0.001; anxiety 7 *v* 10, P < 0.01).

Harms: None of the RCTs reported data on adverse effects, and we found no evidence that exercise is harmful in people with chronic fatigue syndrome. In the second aerobic exercise RCT, more people withdrew with exercise than without exercise but the difference was not significant (25/68 [37%] with exercise *v* 15/69 [22%] without exercise; RR 1.7, 95% CI 0.98 to 2.9).[17] The reasons for the withdrawals from the graded exercise groups were not stated.

Comment: Experience suggests that symptoms of chronic fatigue syndrome may be exacerbated by overly ambitious or overly hasty attempts at exercise.

OPTION PROLONGED REST

We found no RCTs on the effects of prolonged rest. Indirect observational evidence in healthy volunteers and in people recovering from a viral illness suggests that prolonged rest may perpetuate or worsen fatigue and symptoms.

Benefits: We found no systematic review or RCTs of prolonged rest in people with chronic fatigue syndrome.

Harms: We found no direct evidence of harmful effects of rest in people with chronic fatigue syndrome. We found observational evidence suggesting that prolonged inactivity may perpetuate or worsen fatigue and is associated with symptoms in both healthy volunteers[33] and in people recovering from viral illness.[34]

Comment: It is not clear that evidence from people recovering from viral illness can be extrapolated to people with chronic fatigue syndrome.

OPTION MAGNESIUM

One small RCT found that intramuscular magnesium injections versus placebo significantly improved symptoms at 6 weeks.

Benefits: We found one systematic review (search date 2000), which did not report quantified results.[15] The review identified one RCT (32 people with chronic fatigue syndrome), which compared weekly intramuscular injections of magnesium sulphate 50% versus placebo (water for injection) for 6 weeks.[35] It found that magnesium improved overall benefit (12/15 [80%] *v* 3/17 [18%]; RR 4.5, 95% CI 1.6 to 13.1; NNT 2, 95% CI 2 to 4), energy (P = 0.002), pain (P = 0.001), and emotional reactions (P = 0.013).

Harms: The RCT reported no adverse effects.

Comment: Subsequent studies have not found a deficiency of magnesium in people with chronic fatigue syndrome.[36–38] In the RCT, only red blood cell magnesium was slightly lower than the normal range. In the three subsequent studies, magnesium was in the normal range and no different from controls. However, none of the studies state where the normal range comes from so it is difficult to say if they are equivalent.

OPTION EVENING PRIMROSE OIL

One small RCT found no significant difference with evening primrose oil versus placebo in depression scores at 3 months.

Benefits: We found one systematic review (search date 2000), which did not report quantified results.[15] The review identified one RCT (50 people with chronic fatigue syndrome according to Oxford, UK, diagnostic criteria), which compared evening primrose oil (4 g daily) versus placebo for 3 months.[39] It found no significant difference between groups in depression scores (Beck Depression Inventory), physical symptoms, or participant assessment (at 3 months 46% were improved with placebo *v* 29% with evening primrose oil; $P = 0.09$; figures were not presented in a manner that allowed RR with CI to be calculated).

Harms: The RCT reported no adverse effects.

Comment: One RCT (63 people) compared evening primrose oil (4 g daily) versus placebo in people with a diagnosis of postviral fatigue syndrome.[40] This diagnosis was made on the basis of overwhelming fatigue, myalgia, and depression, which had been present for at least 1 year and all had been preceded by a febrile illness. At 3 months, 33/39 (85%) of the people on active treatment had improved compared with 4/24 (17%) on placebo — a significant benefit ($P < 0.0001$). The difference in outcome may be partly explained by participant selection; the study in people with chronic fatigue syndrome used currently accepted diagnostic criteria.[39] Also, whereas this RCT used liquid paraffin as a placebo,[40] the chronic fatigue syndrome RCT used sunflower oil, which is better tolerated and less likely to affect the placebo response adversely.[39]

OPTION IMMUNOTHERAPY

Small RCTs found that immunoglobulin G versus placebo modestly improved physical functioning and fatigue at 3–6 months, but was associated with considerable adverse effects. Small RCTs found insufficient evidence on the effects of interferon alfa versus placebo.

Benefits: We found one systematic review (search date 2000), which did not report quantified results.[15] **Immunoglobulin G:** The review identified four relevant RCTs comparing immunoglobulin G versus placebo for 6 months.[41–44] The first RCT (30 people) compared monthly intravenous injections of immunoglobulin G (1 g/kg) versus placebo (albumin).[41] After 6 months, no large differences were found in measures of fatigue (self reported symptom severity) or in physical and social functioning (SF-36). There was a significant improvement in social function with placebo versus immunoglobulin G (dichotomous figures not provided). The second RCT (49 people) compared monthly intravenous immunoglobulin G (2 g/kg) versus intravenous placebo (a maltose solution) for 3 months.[42] More people receiving immunoglobulin G versus placebo improved in terms of a physician rated assessment of symptoms and disability (10/23 [44%] v 3/26 [11%]; P = 0.03). The third RCT (99 adults) compared placebo versus three doses of immunoglobulin G (0.5, 1, or 2 g/kg).[43] It found no significant difference in quality of life, scores on visual analogue scales, or in changes in hours spent in non-sedentary activities. The fourth RCT (71 adolescents aged 11–18 years) compared immunoglobulin G (1 g/kg) versus placebo.[44] Three infusions were given 1 month apart. There was a significant difference between the active treatment and control groups in mean functional outcome, which was determined by taking the mean of clinician ratings from four areas of the participants' activities (number of people achieving improvement of ≥25% at 6 months: 26/36 [52%] with immunoglobin v 15/34 [31%] with placebo, RR 1.6, 95% CI 1.1 to 2.5). However, both groups showed significant improvements from baseline, continuing to the 6 month assessment after treatment. **Other treatments:** The review identified two RCTs (30 people) comparing interferon alfa versus placebo.[45,46] The first RCT only found treatment benefit on subgroup analysis of people with isolated natural killer cell dysfunction.[45] The second randomised crossover trial did not present results in a manner that allowed clear interpretation of treatment effect.[46] Other RCTs found no significant advantage over placebo from aciclovir,[47] dialysable leucocyte extract (in a factorial design with cognitive behavioural therapy),[48] or terfenadine.[49]

Harms: **Immunoglobulin G:** In the first RCT, adverse effects judged to be worse than pretreatment symptoms in either group included gastrointestinal complaints (18 people), headaches (23 people), arthralgia (6 people), and worsening fatigue. Of these symptoms, only headaches differed significantly between the groups (immunoglobulin G 14/15 [93%] v placebo 9/15 [60%]). Six participants (3 immunoglobulin G, 3 placebo) were considered to have major adverse effects. Adverse events by treatment group were only reported for headache.[41] **Other treatments:** In the RCT comparing interferon alfa 2/13 (15%) people taking active treatment developed neutropenia.[45]

Comment: **Immunoglobulin G:** The first two RCTs differed in that the second used twice the dose of immunoglobulin G, did not require that participants fulfil the operational criteria (similar but not identical to US Centers for Disease Control and Prevention criteria) for chronic fatigue syndrome, and made no assessments of them during the study, waiting until 3 months after completion.[42] **Other treatments:** Terfenadine, particularly at high blood concentrations, is associated with rare hazardous cardiac arrhythmias.[50]

OPTION COGNITIVE BEHAVIOURAL THERAPY

One systematic review has found that cognitive behavioural therapy versus standard medical care or relaxation therapy administered by highly skilled therapists in specialist centres improves quality of life and

physical functioning. One additional multicentre RCT has found that cognitive behavioural therapy administered by less experienced therapists versus guided support groups or no interventions may also be effective.

Benefits: We found two systematic reviews (search dates 1998[51] and 2000[15]). The first review[51] identified three RCTs that met the reviewers' inclusion criteria (all participants fulfilled accepted diagnostic criteria for chronic fatigue syndrome [CFS], use of adequate randomisation, and use of controls).[48,52,53] The second review identified one additional RCT that met inclusion criteria but the review did not report quantified results.[16,54] The first RCT (90 people with CFS according to Australian diagnostic criteria that are similar to US Centers for Disease Control and Prevention [CDC] criteria) identified by the reviews evaluated cognitive behavioural therapy (CBT) and immunological therapy (dialysable leucocyte extract) using a factorial design.[48] The comparison group received standard medical care. It found no significant difference in quality of life measures (Karnofsky scale and symptom report on a visual analogue scale) between CBT and standard medical care. CBT was given every 2 weeks for six sessions lasting 30–60 minutes each. Treatment involved encouraging participants to exercise at home and feel less helpless. The second RCT (60 people with CFS according to Oxford, UK, diagnostic criteria) identified by the reviews compared CBT versus normal general practice care in people attending a secondary care centre.[53] It found that, at 12 months, CBT improved quality of life (Karnofsky scale) compared with those receiving standard medical care (final score > 80: 22/30 [73%] with CBT *v* 8/30 [27%] with placebo; RR 2.75, 95% CI 1.54 to 5.32; NNT 3, 95% CI 2 to 5). The active treatment consisted of a cognitive behavioural assessment, followed by 16 weekly sessions of behavioural experiments, problem solving activity, and re-evaluation of thoughts and beliefs inhibiting return to normal functioning. The third RCT (60 people with CFS according to CDC diagnostic criteria in people attending a secondary care centre) identified by the reviews compared CBT with relaxation therapy.[52] It found substantial improvement in physical functioning (based on predefined absolute or relative increases in the SF-36 score) with CBT compared with relaxation therapy (19/30 [63%] with CBT *v* 5/30 [17%] with relaxation; RR 3.7, 95% CI 2.37 to 6.31; NNT 3, 95% CI 1 to 7). Improvement continued over 6–12 months' follow up. CBT was given in 13 weekly sessions. A 5 year follow up study of 53 (88%) of the original participants found that more people rated themselves as "much improved" or "very much improved" with CBT compared with relaxation therapy (17/25 [68%] with CBT *v* 10/28 [36%] with relaxation therapy; RR 1.9, 95% CI 1.1 to 3.4; NNT 4, 95% CI 2 to 19).[55] More people treated with CBT met the authors' criteria for complete recovery at 5 years but the difference was not significant (17/31 [55%] with CBT *v* 7/22 [32%] with relaxation therapy; RR 1.7, 95% CI 0.9 to 3.4). The additional multicentre RCT identified by the second review (278 people with CFS according to CDC criteria) compared CBT, guided support groups, or no intervention.[54] The CBT consisted of 16 sessions over 8 months administered by 13 therapists with no previous experience of treating CFS. The guided support groups were similar to CBT in terms of treatment schedule, with the participants receiving non-directive support from a social worker. At 8 months' follow up it found that more people in the CBT group met the criteria for clinical improvement for fatigue severity (checklist individual strength) and self reported improvement in fatigue compared with the guided support and no treatment groups (fatigue severity: CBT *v* support group, 27/83 [33%] *v* 10/80 [13%], RR 2.6, 95% CI 1.3 to 5.0; CBT *v* no intervention 27/83 [33%] *v* 8/62 [13%], RR 2.5, 95% CI 1.2 to 5.2; self reported improvement: CBT *v* support group 42/74 [57%] *v* 12/71 [17%], RR 3.4, 95% CI 1.9 to 5.8; CBT *v* no intervention 42/74 [57%] *v* 23/78 [30%], RR 1.9, 95% CI 1.3 to 2.9). The results were not corrected for multiple comparisons.

Harms: No harmful effects were reported.

Comment: The effectiveness of CBT for CFS outside of specialist settings has been questioned. The results of the multicentre RCT suggest that cognitive behavioural therapy may be effective when administered by less experienced therapists given adequate supervision. The trial had a high withdrawal rate (25% after 8 months), especially in the CBT and guided support groups. Although the presented confidence intervals are not adjusted for multiple comparisons the results would remain significant after any reasonable adjustment. The authors comment that the results were similar following intention to treat analysis but these results were not presented.[54] A randomised trial comparing CBT and non-directive counselling found that both interventions were of benefit in the management of people consulting their family doctor because of fatigue symptoms. In this study, 28% of the sample conformed to CDC criteria for CFS.[56]

REFERENCES

1. Fukuda K, Straus S, Hickie I, et al. The chronic fatigue syndrome: a comprehensive approach to its definition and study. *Ann Intern Med* 1994;121:953–959.
2. Sharpe M, Archard LC, Banatvala JE. A report — chronic fatigue syndrome: guidelines for research. *J R Soc Med* 1991;84:118–121.
3. Wessely S, Chalder T, Hirsch S, et al. The prevalence and morbidity of chronic fatigue and chronic fatigue syndrome: a prospective primary care study. *Am J Public Health* 1997;87:1449–1455.
4. Steele L, Dobbins JG, Fukuda K, et al. The epidemiology of chronic fatigue in San Francisco. *Am J Med* 1998;105(suppl 3A):83–90.
5. Lawrie SM, Pelosi AJ. Chronic fatigue syndrome in the community: prevalence and associations. *Br J Psychiatry* 1995;166:793–797.
6. Wessely S. The epidemiology of chronic fatigue syndrome. *Epidemiol Rev* 1995;17:139–151.
7. Joyce J, Hotopf M, Wessely S. The prognosis of chronic fatigue and chronic fatigue syndrome: a systematic review. *QJM* 1997;90:223–133. Search date 1996; primary sources Medline, Embase, Current Contents, and Psychlit.
8. Stewart AD, Hays RD, Ware JE. The MOS short-form general health survey. *Med Care* 1988;26:724–732.
9. Karnofsky DA, Burchenal JH, MacLeod CM. *The clinical evaluation of chemotherapeutic agents in cancer.* New York Academy of Medicine, New York: Columbia University Press; 1949:191–206.
10. Beck AT, Ward CH, Mendelson M, et al. An inventory for measuring depression. *Arch Gen Psychiatry* 1961;4:561–571.
11. Bergner M, Bobbit RA, Carter WB, et al. The sickness impact profile: development and final revision of a health status measure. *Med Care* 1981;19:787–805.
12. Chalder T, Berelowitz C, Pawlikowska I. Development of a fatigue scale. *J Psychosom Res* 1993;37:147–154.
13. Guy W. *ECDEU assessment manual for psychopharmacology*. Rockville, MD: National Institute of Mental Health, 1976:218–222.
14. Hunt SM, McEwen J, McKenna SP. Measuring health status: a new tool for clinicians and epidemiologists. *J Roy Coll Gen Prac* 1985,35:185–188.
15. Whiting P, Bagnall A-M, Sowden A, et al. Interventions for the treatment and management of chronic fatigue syndrome: A systematic review. *JAMA* 2001;286:1360–1368. Search date 2000; primary sources Medline, Embase, Psychlit, ERIC, Current Contents, Internet searches, bibliographies from the retrieved references, individuals and organisations through a web site dedicated to the review, and members of advisory panels.

16. Vercoulen J, Swanink C, Zitman F. Randomised, double-blind, placebo-controlled study of fluoxetine in chronic fatigue syndrome. *Lancet* 1996;347:858–861.
17. Wearden AJ, Morriss RK, Mullis R, et al. Randomised, double-blind, placebo controlled treatment trial of fluoxetine and a graded exercise programme for chronic fatigue syndrome. *Br J Psychiatry* 1998;172:485–490.
18. Vercoulen JHMM, Swanink CMA, Galama JMD, et al. Dimensional assessment of chronic fatigue syndrome. *J Psychosom Res* 1994;38:383–392.
19. Zigmond AS, Snaith RP. The Hospital Anxiety and Depression Scale (HAD). *Acta Psychiatr Scand* 1983;67:361–370.
20. Natelson BH, Cheu J, Pareja J, et al. Randomised, double blind, controlled placebo-phase in trial of low dose phenelzine in the chronic fatigue syndrome. *Psychopharmacology* 1996;124:226–230.
21. Hickie IB, Wilson AJ, Murray Wright J, et al. A randomized, double-blind, placebo-controlled trial of moclobemide in patients with chronic fatigue syndrome. *J Clin Psychiatry* 2000;61:643–648.
22. Behan PO, Hannifah H. 5-HT reuptake inhibitors in CFS. *J Immunol Immunopharmacol* 1995;15:66–69.
23. Rowe PC, Calkins H, DeBusk K, et al. Fludrocortisone acetate to treat neurally mediated hypotension in chronic fatigue syndrome. *JAMA* 2001;285:52–59.
24. Peterson PK, Pheley A, Schroeppel J, et al. A preliminary placebo-controlled crossover trial of fludrocortisone for chronic fatigue syndrome. *Arch Intern Med* 1998;158:908–914.
25. McKenzie R, O'Fallon A, Dale J, et al. Low-dose hydrocortisone for treatment of chronic fatigue syndrome. *JAMA* 1998;280:1061–1066.
26. Cleare AJ, Heap E, Malhi G, et al. Low-dose hydrocortisone in chronic fatigue syndrome: a randomised crossover trial. *Lancet* 1999;353:455–458.
27. Bou-Holaigah I, Rowe P, Kan J, et al. The relationship between neurally mediated hypotension and the chronic fatigue syndrome. *JAMA* 1995;274:961–967.
28. Demitrack M, Dale J, Straus S, et al. Evidence for impaired activation of the hypothalamic-pituitary-adrenal axis in patients with chronic fatigue syndrome. *J Clin Endocrinol Metab* 1991;73:1224–1234.
29. Forsyth LM, Preuss HG, MacDowell AL, et al. Therapeutic effects of oral NADH on the symptoms of patients with chronic fatigue syndrome. *Ann Allergy Asthma Immunol* 1999;82:185–191.
30. Colquhoun D, Senn S. Re: Therapeutic effects of oral NADH on the symptoms of patients with chronic fatigue syndrome. *Ann Allergy Asthma Immunol* 2000;84:639–640.
31. Fulcher KY, White PD. A randomised controlled trial of graded exercise therapy in patients with the chronic fatigue syndrome. *BMJ* 1997;314:1647–1652.
32. Powell P, Bentall RP, Nye FJ, et al. Randomised controlled trial of patient education to encourage graded exercise in chronic fatigue syndrome. *BMJ* 2001;322:387–390.
33. Sandler H, Vernikos J. *Inactivity: physiological effects*. London: Academic Press, 1986.
34. Dalrymple W. Infectious mononucleosis: 2. Relation of bed rest and activity to prognosis. *Postgrad Med* 1961;35:345–349.
35. Cox IM, Campbell MJ, Dowson D. Red blood cell magnesium and chronic fatigue syndrome. *Lancet* 1991;337:757–760.
36. Clague JE, Edwards RHT, Jackson MJ. Intravenous magnesium loading in chronic fatigue syndrome. *Lancet* 1992;340:124–125.
37. Hinds G, Bell NP, McMaster D, et al. Normal red cell magnesium concentrations and magnesium loading tests in patients with chronic fatigue syndrome. *Ann Clin Biochem* 1994;31:459–461.
38. Swanink CM, Vercoulen JH, Bleijenberg G, et al. Chronic fatigue syndrome: a clinical and laboratory study with a well matched control group. *J Intern Med* 1995;237:499–506.
39. Warren G, McKendrick M, Peet M. The role of essential fatty acids in chronic fatigue syndrome. *Acta Neurol Scand* 1999;99:112–116.
40. Behan PO, Behan WMH, Horrobin D. Effect of high doses of essential fatty acids on the postviral fatigue syndrome. *Acta Neurol Scand* 1990;82:209–216.
41. Peterson PK, Shepard J, Macres M, et al. A controlled trial of intravenous immunoglobulin G in chronic fatigue syndrome. *Am J Med* 1990;89:554–560.
42. Lloyd A, Hickie I, Wakefield D, et al. A double-blind, placebo-controlled trial of intravenous immunoglobulin therapy in patients with chronic fatigue syndrome. *Am J Med* 1990;89:561–568.
43. Vollmer-Conna U, Hickie I, Hadzi-Pavlovic D, et al. Intravenous immunoglobulin is ineffective in the treatment of patients with chronic fatigue syndrome. *Am J Med* 1997;103:38–43.
44. Rowe KS. Double-blind randomized controlled trial to assess the efficacy of intravenous gammaglobulin for the management of chronic fatigue syndrome in adolescents. *J Psychiatr Res* 1997;31:133–147.
45. See DM, Tilles JG. Alpha interferon treatment of patients with chronic fatigue syndrome. *Immunol Invest* 1996;25:153–164.
46. Brook M, Bannister B, Weir W. Interferon-alpha therapy for patients with chronic fatigue syndrome. *J Infect Dis* 1993;168:791–792.
47. Straus SE, Dale JK, Tobi M, et al. Acyclovir treatment of the chronic fatigue syndrome. Lack of efficacy in a placebo-controlled trial. *N Engl J Med* 1988;319:1692–1698.
48. Lloyd A, Hickie I, Boughton R, et al. Immunologic and psychological therapy for patients with chronic fatigue syndrome. *Am J Med* 1993;94:197–203.
49. Steinberg P, McNutt BE, Marshall P, et al. Double-blind placebo-controlled study of efficacy of oral terfenadine in the treatment of chronic fatigue syndrome. *J Allergy Clin Immunol* 1996;97:119–126.
50. Medicines Control Agency (UK). *Current Problems in Pharmacovigilance*, Volume 23, September 1997.
51. Price JR, Couper J. Cognitive behaviour therapy for CFS. In: The Cochrane Library, Issue 2, 2002. Oxford: Update Software. Search date 1998; primary sources Medline, Embase, Biological Abstracts, Sigle, Index to Theses of Great Britain and Ireland, Index to Scientific and Technical Proceedings, Science Citation Index, Trials Register of the Depression, Anxiety and Neurosis Group, citation lists, and personal contacts.
52. Deale A, Chalder T, Marks I, et al. Cognitive behaviour therapy for chronic fatigue syndrome: a randomized controlled trial. *Am J Psychiatry* 1997;154:408–414.
53. Sharpe M, Hawton K, Simkin S, et al. Cognitive behaviour therapy for chronic fatigue syndrome: a randomized controlled trial. *BMJ* 1996;312:22–26.

54. Prins JB, Bleijenberg G, Bazelmans E, et al. Cognitive behaviour therapy for chronic fatigue syndrome: a multicentre randomised controlled trial. *Lancet* 2001;357:841–847.

55. Deale A, Husain K, Chalder T, et al. Long-term outcome of cognitive behaviour therapy versus relaxation therapy for chronic fatigue syndrome: a 5-year follow-up study. *Am J Psychiatry* 2001;158:2038–2042.

56. Ridsdale L, Godfrey E, Chalder T, et al. Chronic fatigue in general practice: is counselling as good as cognitive behaviour therapy? A UK randomised trial. *Br J Gen Pract* 2001;51:19–24.

Steven Reid
Consultant Liaison Psychiatrist
St Mary's Hospital
London
UK

Trudie Chalder
Reader

Anthony Cleare
Senior Lecturer

Matthew Hotopf
Reader

Simon Wessely
Professor of Epidemiological and Liaison Psychiatry

Guy's, King's and St Thomas' School of Medicine and Institute of Psychiatry
London
UK

Competing interests: None declared.

TABLE 1 Diagnostic criteria for chronic fatigue syndrome (see text, p 1076).

CDC 1994[1]	Oxford, UK[2]
Clinically evaluated, medically unexplained fatigue of at least 6 months' duration that is:	Severe, disabling fatigue of at least 6 months' duration that:
• of new onset	• affects both physical and mental functioning
• not a result of ongoing exertion	• was present for more than 50% of the time
• not substantially alleviated by rest	
• a substantial reduction in previous levels of activity	
The occurrence of four or more of the following symptoms:	Other symptoms, particularly myalgia, sleep, and mood disturbance, may be present.
• subjective memory impairment	
• tender lymph nodes	
• muscle pain	
• joint pain	
• headache	
• unrefreshing sleep	
• postexertional malaise (> 24 h)	
Exclusion criteria	
• Active, unresolved, or suspected disease likely to cause fatigue	• Active, unresolved, or suspect disease likely to cause fatigue
• Psychotic, melancholic, or bipolar depression (but not uncomplicated major depression)	• Psychotic, melacholic, or bipolar depression (but not uncomplicated major depression)
• Psychotic disorders	• Psychotic disorders
• Dementia	• Dementia
• Anorexia or bulimia nervosa	• Anorexia or bulimia nervosa
• Alcohol or other substance misuse	
• Severe obesity	

CDC, US Centers for Disease Control and Prevention

Fracture prevention in postmenopausal women

Search date January 2002

Olivier Bruyere, John Edwards, and Jean-Yves Reginster

QUESTIONS

INTERVENTIONS

See glossary, p 1101

Key Messages

- **Alendronate** One systematic review and one subsequent RCT have found that alendronate versus placebo significantly reduces vertebral and non-vertebral fractures over 1–4 years.
- **Calcitonin** One large RCT found that calcitonin versus placebo significantly reduced the incidence of new vertebral fractures over 5 years. One systematic review found limited evidence about the effects of calcitonin versus placebo, no treatment, calcium, or calcium plus vitamin D.
- **Calcium alone** One RCT found that in women with existing fractures calcium versus placebo significantly reduced the incidence of new vertebral or non-vertebral fractures over 3 years, but found no significant difference in new fractures in women without existing fractures. Another RCT found no significant difference with calcium versus placebo in the proportion of women who had one or more new fractures over 2–4 years.
- **Calcium plus vitamin D** One RCT in elderly women in nursing homes has found that calcium plus vitamin D3 versus placebo significantly reduced the incidence of non-vertebral fractures over 18 months to 3 years. Another RCT found no significant difference in the incidence of vertebral fractures over 3 years with calcium plus vitamin D3 versus placebo, but it may have been underpowered to exclude a clinically important difference.

Clin Evid 2002;8:1089–1102.

Fracture prevention in postmenopausal women

- **Etidronate** One systematic review has found that etidronate versus placebo, calcium, or calcium plus vitamin D significantly reduces vertebral fractures over 2 years. One systematic review has found no significant difference in non-vertebral fractures over 2 years with etidronate versus placebo, versus calcium, or versus calcium plus vitamin D.
- **Hip protectors** RCTs in elderly nursing home residents found that hip protectors versus no hip protectors significantly reduced the incidence of hip fracture over 9–19 months, but found no significant difference in the incidence of pelvic fracture.
- **Hormone replacement therapy** RCTs found no significant difference with hormone replacement therapy versus placebo in the proportion of women who sustained vertebral fractures. One systematic review found that hormone replacement therapy versus placebo significantly reduced the proportion of women with non-vertebral fractures. Pooled estimates from observational studies found an increased risk of endometrial cancer and breast cancer when oestrogen was used for over 8 years, and found that hormone replacement therapy increased the risk of venous thromboembolism.
- **Risedronate** One large RCT in women with one or more existing fractures found that risedronate versus placebo reduced non-vertebral fractures over 3 years, but another large RCT found no significant difference. One large RCT in women aged over 70 years has found that risedronate versus placebo significantly reduces the incidence of hip fracture over 3 years. Two large RCTs in women with one or more existing fractures have found that risedronate versus placebo significantly reduces the incidence of vertebral fracture over 3 years. Observational evidence suggests that risedronate may be associated with significant increase in the occurrence of pulmonary cancer.
- **Tiludronate** One large RCT in women with low bone mineral density with and without one or more existing fracture found no significant difference with tiludronate versus placebo in the incidence of vertebral fractures over 3 years.
- **Vitamin D alone** One large RCT found no significant difference with vitamin D3 versus placebo in the incidence of non-vertebral fracture over 3 years. One systematic review found that calcitriol versus placebo significantly reduced the incidence of vertebral fractures during the third year of treatment.
- **Environmental manipulation; exercise; pamidronate** RCTs found insufficient evidence about the effects of these interventions in preventing vertebral and non-vertebral fractures.

DEFINITION A fracture is a break or disruption of bone or cartilage. Symptoms and signs may include immobility, pain, tenderness, numbness, bruising, joint deformity, joint swelling, limb deformity, and limb shortening. Diagnosis is usually based on a typical clinical picture combined with results from an appropriate imaging technique.

INCIDENCE/ PREVALENCE The lifetime risk of fracture in white women is 20% for the spine, 15% for the wrist, and 18% for the hip.[1]

AETIOLOGY/ RISK FACTORS Fractures usually arise from trauma. Risk factors include those associated with an increased tendency to fall (such as ataxia, drug and alcohol intake, loose carpets), age, osteoporosis, bony metastases, and other disorders of bone.

PROGNOSIS Fractures may result in pain, short or long term disability, haemorrhage, thromboembolic disease (see thromboembolism, p 209), shock, and death. Vertebral fractures are associated with pain, physical impairment, muscular atrophy, changes in body shape, loss of physical function, and lower quality of life. About 20% of women die in the first year after a hip fracture, representing an increase in mortality of 12–20% compared with women of similar age and no hip fracture. Half of elderly women who had been independent become partly dependent after hip fracture. One third become totally dependent.

AIMS To prevent fractures, with minimal adverse effects from treatment.

OUTCOMES Incidence of hip, wrist, and vertebral fractures.

METHODS *Clinical Evidence* update search and appraisal January 2002. We also hand searched journals of bone diseases and carried out manual searches using the bibliographies of review articles published after 1985. Some of the RCTs identified provide results generalised to fracture per person/year or overall fractures. These results provide an idea of the group effect of an intervention, but not of its effects on the incidence of fracture in an individual. Data on multiple fractures in one person clearly differ from data on multiple people experiencing a single fracture. Regulatory authorities and scientific groups have recommended that the results of studies evaluating new chemical entities are expressed in terms of the proportion of people experiencing new fractures.[2]

QUESTION **What are the effects of treatments to prevent fractures in postmenopausal women?**

OPTION **BISPHOSPHONATES** New

Olivier Bruyere and Jean-Yves Reginster

One systematic review and one subsequent RCT have found that alendronate versus placebo significantly reduces vertebral and non-vertebral fractures over 1–4 years. One systematic review has found that etidronate versus placebo, calcium, or calcium plus vitamin D significantly reduces vertebral fractures over 2 years, but has found no significant difference in non-vertebral fractures. Two large RCTs in women with one or more existing fracture have found that risedronate versus placebo significantly reduces the incidence of new vertebral fracture over 3 years. One of the RCTs found that risedronate versus placebo reduced non-vertebral fractures over 3 years, but the other found no significant difference. One large RCT in women aged over 70 years has found that risedronate versus placebo significantly reduces the incidence of hip fracture over 3 years. Observational evidence suggests that risedronate may be associated with significant increase in the occurrence of pulmonary cancer. One large RCT in women with low bone mineral density with and without one or more existing fractures found that tiludronate versus placebo significantly reduced the incidence of non-vertebral fractures. It found no significant difference with tiludronate versus placebo in the incidence of vertebral fractures over 3 years, but may have been too small to detect a clinically important difference. One small RCT found no significant difference with pamidronate versus placebo in the incidence of vertebral fracture per patient year.

Benefits: **Alendronate:** We found one systematic review[3] and one subsequent RCT.[4] The systematic review (search date 1998, 7 RCTs, 10 287 postmenopausal women aged 39–85 years) found that alendronate versus placebo significantly reduced vertebral fractures (RR 0.54, 95% CI 0.45 to 0.66) and non-vertebral fractures (RR 0.81, 95% CI 0.72 to 0.92). It found a non-significant reduction of hip fractures over 1–4 years (RR 0.64, 95% CI 0.40 to 1.01; results presented graphically).[3] One large subsequent RCT (3658 women with vertebral fracture or osteoporosis) compared alendronate (5–10 mg/day) versus placebo for 3–4 years.[4] It found that alendronate versus placebo significantly reduced non-vertebral fractures, including hip fractures, over 3 years (all non-vertebral: RR 0.73, 95% CI 0.61 to 0.87; hip: RR 0.47, 95% CI 0.2 to 0.79; no further data provided) and both clinical and radiologic vertebral fractures over 3 years (radiologic vertebral: RR 0.52, 95% CI 0.42 to 0.66; no further data provided).[4] **Etidronate:** We found one systematic review (search date 1998, 13 RCTs, 1010 women) comparing etidronate versus placebo, calcium, or calcium plus vitamin D.[5] It found that etidronate versus placebo significantly reduced vertebral fractures over 2 years (9 RCTs: 32/538 [6%] *v* 54/538 [10%]; RR 0.60, 95% CI 0.41 to 0.88), but found no significant difference in non-vertebral fractures (7 RCTs: 48/433 [11%] *v* 49/434 [11%]; RR 0.98, 95% CI 0.68 to 1.42).[5] **Pamidronate:** We found no systematic review but found one RCT (48 women with osteoporosis) comparing pamidronate (150 mg/day) versus placebo for 2 years.[6] It found no significant difference with pamidronate versus placebo in the incidence of vertebral fracture per patient year (13/100 *v* 24/100; P = 0.07; see methods, p 1091). **Risedronate:** We found no systematic review but found three RCTs.[7–9] The first RCT (2458 women < 85 years with at least 1 vertebral fracture) compared oral risedronate (2.5 mg/day or 5 mg/day) versus placebo for 3 years.[7] After 1 year the 2.5 mg dose of risedronate was discontinued as 5 mg was found to be more effective. It found that risedronate 5 mg versus placebo significantly reduced the incidence of new vertebral fractures over 3 years (Kaplen-Meier survival data 11% with risedronate *v* 16% with placebo; RR 0.59, 95% CI 0.43 to 0.82) and non-vertebral fractures (Kaplen-Meier survival data 5% with risedronate *v* 8% with placebo; RR 0.6, 95% CI 0.39 to 0.94).[7] The second RCT (1226 women with 2 or more existing vertebral fractures) compared risedronate 2.5 mg or 5 mg daily versus placebo for 3 years.[8] After 2 years the 2.5 mg dose of risedronate was discontinued as 5 mg was found to be more effective. It found that risedronate 5 mg versus placebo significantly reduced the proportion of women with new vertebral fractures over 3 years (Kaplan-Meier survival data 18% *v* 29%; RR 0.51, 95% CI 0.36 to 0.73), but found no significant difference in the proportion of women with osteoporosis related non-vertebral fractures (Kaplan-Meier survival data 8.9% with risedronate *v* 16% with placebo; RR 0.67, 95% CI 0.44 to 1.04).[8] The third RCT (9331 women > 70 years) compared risedronate 2.5 mg or 5 mg versus placebo.[9] It found that risedronate significantly reduced the proportion of women who had hip fracture over 3 years (Kaplan-Meier survival data 3% with risedronate *v* 4% with placebo; RR 0.7, 95% CI 0.6 to 0.9; see comment below). **Tiludronate:** We found no systematic review. We found one RCT (1805 women with low vertebral bone mineral density and at least 1 existing vertebral fracture and 488 women with low bone mineral density and no existing fracture) comparing tiludronate 50 mg or 200 mg daily versus placebo for the first 7 days of each month for 3 years.[10] It found no significant difference with tiludronate versus placebo in the incidence of vertebral fractures over 3 years, but may have been too small to detect a clinically important difference (20% with tiludronate 50 mg *v* 19% with placebo; RRR –8%, 95% CI –35 to +19%; 19.2% with tiludronate 200 mg *v* 18.9% with placebo; RRR –1.4%, 95% CI –27 to +25%; no raw data provided). It found that tiludronate 200 mg/day versus tiludronate 50 mg/day or versus placebo reduced the incidence of non-vertebral fractures (6% with tiludronate 200 mg/day *v* 9% with tiludronate 50 mg *v* 12% with placebo; no further data provided).

Harms: **Alendronate:** Observational evidence suggests that oral alendronate is associated with oesophageal erosions and ulcerative oesophagitis. However, one RCT[11] identified by the review[3] (where people took alendronate with 180–240 mL water on arising in the morning and remained upright for at least 30 min after swallowing the tablet and until the first food of the day had been ingested) found no significant difference in oesophagitis with alendronate versus placebo. **Risedronate:** One observational study found limited evidence suggesting that the gastrointestinal safety of risedronate appears to be in the same range as alendronate.[12] One non-systematic review (10 phase III studies) found limited evidence that risedronate versus placebo may be associated with a significant increase in the occurrence of pulmonary cancer (3.9/1000 people/year of exposure with risedronate 2.5 mg/day *v* 1.9/1000 patients/year of exposure with risedronate 5 mg/day *v* 1.2/1000 patients/year of exposure with placebo; significance not stated; see comment below).[13]

Comment: **Risedronate:** In the third RCT, risedronate versus placebo reduced the risk of hip fracture by 60% in women aged 70–79 years with osteoporosis and baseline vertebral fractures.[9] However, this subgroup included only 1128/6197 women in the trial and, although the RCT found an overall 30% reduction in the relative risk of hip fracture, this reduction was not significant either in women aged 70–79 years without existing vertebral fracture, or in women over the age of 80 with at least one clinical risk factor for hip fracture.[9] The non-systematic review assessing the harms of risedronate[13] did not provide a source of reference and the methods of the phase III studies identified are unclear.

OPTION CALCIUM AND VITAMIN D ALONE OR IN COMBINATION

New

Olivier Bruyere and Jean-Yves Reginster

One RCT found that in women with existing fractures calcium versus placebo significantly reduced the incidence of new vertebral or non-vertebral fractures over 3 years, but found no significant difference in new fractures in women without existing fractures. Another RCT found no significant difference with calcium versus placebo in the proportion of women who had one or more new fracture over 2–4 years. One large RCT identified by a systematic review found no significant difference with vitamin D3 versus placebo in the incidence of non-vertebral fracture over 3 years. One systematic review found that calcitriol versus placebo

significantly reduced the incidence of vertebral fractures during the third year of treatment. One RCT has found that calcium plus vitamin D3 versus placebo significantly reduces the incidence of non-vertebral fractures over 18 months to 3 years. Another RCT found no significant difference in the incidence of vertebral fractures over 3 years with calcium plus vitamin D3 versus placebo, but it may have been underpowered to exclude a clinically important difference.

Benefits: **Calcium versus placebo:** We found no systematic review but found two RCTs.[14,15] The first RCT (78 women) comparing elemental calcium (calcium lactate–gluconate plus calcium carbonate) 1 g/day versus placebo found no significant difference in the proportion of women who had one or more new fractures over 2–4 years, but may have been too small to exclude a clinically important difference (2/38 [5%] *v* 7/40 [17%]; RR 0.30, 95% CI 0.06 to 1.36).[14] The second RCT (197 women) compared oral calcium carbonate (1.2 g/day) versus placebo for a mean 3 years in women aged over 60 years with or without existing fractures (see comment below).[15] It found that in women with existing fractures (94 women, mean age 74.9 years) calcium versus placebo significantly reduced the proportion of women who had vertebral and non-vertebral fractures over a mean 3 years (15/53 [28%] *v* 21/41 [51%]; RR 0.55, 95% CI 0.33 to 0.93), but found no significant difference in the incidence of vertebral and non-vertebral fractures in women without existing fractures (103 women, mean age 72.4; 12/42 [28%] with calcium *v* 13/61 [21%] with placebo; RR 1.34, 95% CI 0.68 to 2.64).[15] **Vitamin D or vitamin D analogue versus placebo:** We found one systematic review (search date 2000, 3 RCTs).[16] The first RCT (2578 people; 1916 women, 662 men, mean age 80 years, living at home; see comment) found no significant difference with vitamin D3 versus placebo in the incidence of hip fracture (58/1284 [4.5%] *v* 48/1280 [3.7%]; RR 1.20, 95% CI 0.83 to 1.75) or any non-vertebral fracture over 3 years (135/1284 [10%] *v* 122/1280 [9%]; RR 1.10 95% CI 0.87 to 1.39). The review identified two small RCTs (68 women aged ≥ 54 years) comparing calcitriol (1,25 dihydroxy vitamin D) versus placebo. It found that calcitriol versus placebo significantly reduced the incidence of new vertebral fractures over 3 years (8/34 [23%] *v* 17/34 [50%]; RR 0.49, 95% CI 0.25 to 0.95). **Vitamin D or vitamin D analogue versus calcium:** We found one systematic review[16] that identified one RCT (622 women)[17] comparing calcitriol versus calcium (see comment below). It found that calcitriol significantly reduced the frequency of new vertebral fractures during the third year of treatment (12/213[6%] *v* 44/219 [20%]; RR 0.28, 95% CI 0.15 to 0.52; see comment below). **Calcium plus vitamin D versus placebo:** We found one systematic review (search date 2002, 2 RCTs, 3715 people).[16] One of the RCTs (3270 mobile elderly women, age range 69–106 years, living in 180 nursing homes) found that calcium plus vitamin D3 versus placebo significantly reduced the incidence of hip fractures (80/1387 [6%] *v* 110/1403 [8%]; RR 0.74, 95% CI 0.60 to 0.91) and all non-vertebral fractures (160/1387 [11%] *v* 215/1403 [15%]; RR 0.75, 95% CI 0.62 to 0.91) over 18 months. This difference remained significant after 3 years' treatment (hip fracture: 137/1176 [12%] *v* 178/1127 [16%]; RR 0.74, 95% CI 0.60 to 0.91; all non-vertebral fracture: 255/1176 [22%] *v* 308/1127 [27%]; RR 0.72, 95% CI 0.60 to 0.84). The other RCT (246 women, 199 men, mean age 71 years, living at home; see comment) found no significant difference with calcium plus vitamin D versus placebo in the incidence of hip fractures over 3 years (0/187 [0%] *v* 1/202 [0.5%]; RR 0.36, 95% CI 0.01 to 8.78), but may have been underpowered to exclude a clinically important difference. It found that calcium plus vitamin D significantly reduced overall non-vertebral fractures (11/187 [6%] *v* 26/202 [13%]; RR 0.46, 95% CI 0.23 to 0.90).[16]

Harms: The systematic review found that vitamin D or vitamin D analogues versus placebo or calcium significantly increased hypercalcaemia (5 RCTs, 1009 people; 22/498 [4.4%] *v* 18/511 [3.5%]; RR 1.71, 95% CI 1.01 to 2.89).[16]

Comment: In the RCT comparing calcium versus placebo in subgroups of women with and without existing fractures, randomisation was not stratified according to existing fracture status and there was an unequal number of women taking calcium or placebo in each subgroup.[15] In the RCT[17] comparing calcitriol versus placebo, identified by the review,[16] the rate of vertebral fractures in the calcitriol group did not change over time. The statistical difference in fracture rates observed between the groups may have occurred because people taking calcium had an increase in fracture incidence during the third year of the trial.[17] The results of the RCT should be interpreted with caution as they are not intention to treat, and there was a high withdrawal rate, particularly in the third year. This RCT did not have a central x ray reading facility for the assessment of vertebral fractures.[17] Although some RCTs included both men and women at risk of hip fracture,[16] it is likely that the results are generalisable to postmenopausal women.

OPTION CALCITONIN New

Olivier Bruyere and Jean-Yves Reginster

One large RCT found that calcitonin versus placebo significantly reduced the incidence of new vertebral fractures over 5 years. One systematic review found limited evidence about the effects of calcitonin versus placebo, no treatment, calcium, or calcium plus vitamin D.

Benefits: We found one systematic review[18] and one subsequent RCT.[19] The systematic review (search date 1997, 14 RCTs, 7 RCTs in perimenopausal women with crush fractures or osteoporosis, 7 RCTs in men and women with osteoporosis or taking corticosteroids, 1309 people, exact proportions of women and men not specified; see comment) compared calcitonin (salcatonin) versus placebo, no treatment, calcium, or calcium plus vitamin D (see comment below).[18] It found that fewer people developed vertebral or non-vertebral fractures with calcitonin versus no calcitonin, but the difference was not significant (vertebral fractures: 166/1190 [14%] people with calcitonin *v* 96/554 [17%] with no calcitonin; RR 0.80, 95% CI 0.64 to 1.01; non-vertebral fractures; RR 0.48, 95% CI 0.20 to 1.15; no raw data provided).[18] One subsequent RCT (1108 postmenopausal women with osteoporosis receiving calcium

1000 mg/day and vitamin D 400 IU/day) compared salmon calcitonin nasal spray (100, 200, or 400 IU) daily versus placebo for 5 years.[19] It found that calcitonin 200 IU versus placebo significantly reduced the proportion of women with new vertebral fractures over 5 years (51/287 [18%] with calcitonin 200 IU *v* 70/270 [26%] with placebo; RR 0.67, 95% CI 0.47 to 0.97). The difference remained significant in women with one to five existing vertebral fractures at baseline (60/203 [30%] *v* 40/207 [19%]; RR 0.64, 95% CI 0.43 to 0.96). It found no significant difference in the risk of vertebral fractures with calcitonin 100 IU or 400 IU versus placebo.[19]

Harms: The systematic review gave no information on harms.[18] The subsequent RCT found that nasal spray calcitonin versus placebo significantly increased nasal congestion, nasal discharge, or sneezing (22% *v* 15%: $P < 0.01$; no raw data provided).[19]

Comment: The systematic review commented that its conclusions are limited because many of the RCTs identified did not report the occurrence of fractures, were not double blinded, and only two of the RCTs identified were of over 2 years duration.[18] Although the review included some RCTs in both men and women at risk of hip fracture, it is likely that the results are generalisable to postmenopausal women.[18]

OPTION ENVIRONMENTAL MANIPULATION *New*

John Edwards

We found no RCTs assessing environmental manipulation alone. One RCT in men and women aged over 70 years found no significant difference in the fracture rate over 4 years with health visitor care versus control.

Benefits: We found no systematic review and no RCTs assessing environmental manipulation alone (see glossary, p 1101). We found one RCT (674 men and women > 70 years; similar proportions of women and men; see comment) comparing health visitor care (aimed at assessing nutritional deficiencies, reducing smoking and alcohol intake, improving muscle tone and fitness, assessing medical conditions and use of medication, and improving home environment, such as lighting) versus control (not specified).[20] It found no significant difference with health visitor versus control in the incidence of new fractures over 4 years (16/350 [5%] *v* 14/324 [4%]; RR 1.06, 95% CI 0.52 to 2.13).

Harms: The RCT gave no information on harms.[20]

Comment: Although the RCT included both men and women at risk of hip fracture, it is likely that the results are generalisable to postmenopausal women.[20]

OPTION EXERCISE New

John Edwards

Three RCTs found no significant difference in the incidence of falls resulting in fracture over 1 year with exercise versus control.

Benefits: We found one systematic review (search date 2001) that identified three RCTs comparing the effects of exercise versus control in preventing falls resulting in fracture.[21] The review did not perform a meta-analysis because of heterogeneity of methods and interventions between the trials. The first RCT identified by the review (165 postmenopausal women living in the community who had fractured an upper limb in the previous 2 years) compared advice to walk briskly for up to 40 minutes three times weekly versus advice to carry out upper limb exercises. It found no significant difference in the incidence of falls resulting in fracture after 1 year (2/81 [2%] with brisk walking *v* 3/84 [4%] with upper limb exercises; RR 0.69, 95% CI 0.12 to 4.03). The second RCT identified by the review (77 women and 22 men, aged > 65 years, living in the community; see comment) compared a home based exercise programme (balance and strength exercises plus walking) versus no exercise programme for 14 weeks. It found no significant difference in the incidence of falls resulting in fracture over 44 weeks (1/45 [2%] with exercise *v* 0/48 [0%] with no exercise; RR 3.20, 95% CI 0.13 to 76.48). The third RCT (162 women, 78 men, aged > 75 years; see comment) found no significant difference with a home exercise programme (balance and strength exercises plus walking) versus usual care over 1 year (2/121 [2%] with home exercise *v* 7/119 [6%] with usual care; RR 0.28, 95% CI 0.06 to 1.33).[21]

Harms: One of the RCTs found that brisk walking versus control increased the number of falls (15/100 person/years, 95% CI 1.4 to 29) (see methods of fracture prevention in postmenopausal women, p 1091).[21] This result should be interpreted with caution as falls are subject to memory bias.

Comment: Most of the RCTs identified by the review examined falls rather than fractures as the main outcome of interest.[21] Although two of the RCTs included both men and women at risk of hip fracture, it is likely that the results are generalisable to postmenopausal women.

OPTION HIP PROTECTORS New

John Edwards

RCTs in elderly nursing home residents found that hip protectors versus no hip protectors significantly reduced the incidence of hip fracture over 9–19 months, but found no significant difference in the incidence of pelvic fracture.

Benefits: **Non-vertebral fractures:** We found one systematic review[22] and two subsequent RCTs.[23,24] The systematic review (search date 2000) identified six RCTs (3412 people, predominantly women, see comment) assessing the effects of hip protectors versus no hip protectors on hip fractures.[22] It could not perform a meta-analysis of all of the RCTs because some of the RCTs used cluster randomisation and others randomised individuals. In the RCTs that randomised individuals, it found that hip protectors versus no hip protectors significantly reduced the incidence of hip fractures over 9–19 months (3 RCTs, 202 people, 90–100% women in 2 RCTs, proportion of women and men not stated in 1 RCT; 4/111 [4%] *v* 15/91 [16%]; RR 0.22, 95% CI 0.09 to 0.57).[22] The first subsequent RCT (164 elderly women) found that hip protectors versus control significantly reduced hip fractures over a mean 377 days (1/88 [1%] *v* 8/76 [10%]; RR 0.11, 95% CI 0.01 to 0.84).[23] The second subsequent RCT (64 women and 8 men in a nursing home) found no significant difference with hip protectors versus no hip protectors in hip fractures over 1 year (1/36 [3%] *v* 7/36 [19%]; RR 0.14, 95% CI 0.02 to 1.10), but it may have been too small to exclude a clinically important difference (see comment).[24] **Pelvic fractures:** The review identified three RCTs.[22] It could not perform a meta-analysis because of methodological differences between the trials. All three RCTs included men and women (see comment). The first RCT (1801 people aged > 75 years, 77–79% women) identified by the review found no significant difference in the incidence of pelvic fractures over a mean 11–15 months with hip protectors versus no hip protectors (2/653 [0.3%] *v* 12/1148 [1%]; RR 0.29, 95% CI 0.07 to 1.31). The second RCT identified by the review (665 people aged > 69 years living in a nursing home, 70% women) found no significant difference in the incidence of pelvic fractures over 11 months (0/247 [0%] *v* 2/418 [0.5%]; RR 0.34, 95% CI 0.02 to 7.01). The third RCT identified by the review (64 men and 8 women, aged 71–96 years living in a nursing home) found no significant difference with hip protectors versus no hip protectors in pelvic fractures over 12 months, but may have been too small to exclude a clinically important difference (0/36 [0%] hip protector *v* 2/36 [5%]; RR 0.20, 95% CI 0.01 to 4.03).[22]

Harms: **Non-hip or non-pelvic fractures and injuries:** One of the RCTs identified by the review (665 people) found that more people had non-hip fractures over 11 months with hip protectors versus no hip protectors, but the difference was not significant (15/247 [6.1%] *v* 25/418 [6.0%]; RR 1.02, 95% CI 0.55 to 1.89). Another small RCT identified by the review found no significant difference in the incidence of non-hip fractures with hip protectors versus no hip protectors (2/35 [5.7%] *v* 0/24 [0%]; RR 3.47, 95% CI 0.17 to 69.27). A third RCT identified by the review (1801 people) also found no significant difference in the proportion of people with lower limb or other non-hip fractures over a mean 11–15 months with hip protectors versus no hip protectors (23/653 [3.5%] *v* 59/1148 [5%]; RR 0.69, 95% CI 0.43 to 1.10). The first subsequent RCT found no significant difference in the incidence of non-hip fractures over a mean 377 days with hip protectors versus no hip protectors (2/88 [2.3%] *v* 0/76 [0%]).[23] **Falls:** One of the RCTs identified by the review found that more people fell on the hip with hip protectors versus no hip protectors, but the difference was not significant (8/101 [7.9%] *v* 1/40 [2.5%]; RR 3.17, 95% CI 0.41 to 24.5). The first subsequent RCT found no significant difference in the proportion of people sustaining one or more falls over a mean 377 days (40/88 [45%] *v* 28/76 [37%]; RR 1.23, 95% CI 0.85 to 1.79). The other five RCTs identified by the review and the second subsequent RCT found no difference in the incidence of falls with hip protectors versus no hip protectors, but gave no information on the proportion of people who fell.[22,24] These results should be interpreted with caution as falls are subject to memory bias. **Mortality:** One RCT identified by the review found no significant difference in mortality over 12 months with hip protectors versus no hip protectors (6/36 [17%] *v* 8/36 [22%]; RR 0.75, 95% CI 0.29 to 1.94). The first subsequent RCT also found no significant difference in mortality with hip protectors versus no hip protectors but may have been too small to exclude a clinically important difference (6/88 [7%] *v* 8/76 [10%]; RR 0.65, 95% CI 0.23 to 1.78).[23] **Hospitalisation:** One of the RCTs identified by the review found no significant difference with hip protectors versus no hip protectors in the proportion of people permanently hospitalised over 12 months (10/36 [28%] *v* 9/36 [25%]; RR 1.11, 95% CI 0.51 to 2.41). The first subsequent RCT found no significant difference in the proportion of people who were hospitalised for reasons other than fracture over a mean 377 days, but may have been too small to exclude a clinically important difference (10/88 [11%] *v* 9/76 [12%]; RR 0.96, 95% CI 0.41 to 2.24).[23]

Comment: Much of the evidence is taken from RCTs that included both men and women at risk of hip fracture, however, it is likely that the results are generaliseable to postmenopuasal women.[22] The results of the second subsequent RCT should be interpreted with caution as 60% of people who entered the trial were lost to follow up.[24] The RCT had protocol violations as three people were allocated to the hip protector group after randomisation when people initially randomised to hip protectors refused to wear them.[24]

OPTION HORMONE REPLACEMENT THERAPY

RCTs found no significant difference with hormone replacement therapy versus placebo in the proportion of women who sustained vertebral fractures. One systematic review and one subsequent RCT found that hormone replacement therapy versus placebo significantly reduced the proportion of women with non-vertebral fractures. Pooled estimates from observational studies found an increased risk of endometrial cancer and breast cancer when oestrogen was used for over 8 years, and found that hormone replacement therapy versus no hormone replacement therapy increased the risk of venous thromboembolism, including pulmonary embolism and deep vein thrombosis.

Benefits: **Vertebral fractures:** We found no systematic review. We found four RCTs.[25–28] The first RCT (75 postmenopausal women aged 47–75 years with 1 or more vertebral fractures) compared transdermal hormone replacement therapy (HRT) (17β estradiol [oestradiol] and oral medroxyprogesterone acetate) versus placebo.[25] It found no significant difference with HRT versus placebo in the proportion of women with at least one vertebral fracture after 12 months, but may have been too small to exclude a clinically important difference (7/34 [21%] *v* 12/34 [35%]; RR 0.58, 95% CI 0.26 to 1.30). The second RCT (100 postmenopausal women) compared transdermal oestrogen versus placebo.[26] It found that over a median 9 years (range 6–12 years) oestrogen versus placebo significantly reduced total spine score, an indirect measurement of vertebral fracture rate ($P < 0.01$), but had no significant effect on the number of women with a vertebral crush fracture (1/57 [2%] women with oestrogen treatment *v* 5/42 [12%] with placebo; RR 0.15, 95% CI 0.02 to 1.22). The third RCT (1006 women 3–24 months past their last menstrual bleeding aged 45–58 years) compared oral HRT versus placebo.[27] It found no significant difference with HRT versus placebo in the proportion of women who had vertebral fractures at 5 years' follow up (8/502 [1.6%] *v* 4/504 [0.8%]; RR 2.00, 95% CI 0.62 to 6.49). The fourth RCT (2763 postmenopausal women aged < 80 years) comparing oral HRT versus placebo for a mean 4.1 years found no significant difference in the incidence of spine fracture, but it may have been too small to exclude a clinically important difference (RR 0.7, 95% CI 0.3 to 1.4).[28] **Non-vertebral fractures:** We found one systematic review[29] and one subsequent RCT[28] comparing HRT versus placebo, no treatment, calcium, or calcium plus vitamin D. The review (search date 2000, 22 RCTs, 8774 women) found that HRT versus placebo significantly reduced the proportion of women with non-vertebral fractures at the end of the study, which ranged from 1–10 years (258/4929 [5%] *v* 307/3845 [8%]; RR 0.73, 95% CI 0.56 to 0.94).[29] This reduction remained significant in women taking HRT who had a mean age younger than 60 years (14 RCTs: RR 0.67, 95% CI 0.46 to 0.98; no further data provided). When RCTs in women with a mean age of 60 years or older were analysed, it found no significant difference in the incidence of non-vertebral fractures with HRT versus placebo (8 RCTs: RR 0.88, 95% CI 0.71 to 1.08; no further data provided).[29] One large subsequent RCT (2763 postmenopausal women aged < 80 years) found no significant difference with HRT versus placebo in the incidence of hip fracture (RR 1.1, 95% CI 0.5 to 2.3) or wrist fracture (RR 1.0, 95% CI 0.6 to 1.7), but may have been too small to exclude a clinically important difference.[28]

Harms: See HRT under secondary prevention of ischaemic cardiac events, p 129. In one of the RCTs identified by the review assessing non-vertebral fractures, 96/464 women (21%) withdrew from the trial, and significantly more women withdrew from the HRT groups versus non-HRT groups (72/232 [31%] women *v* 24/232 [10%]; RR 3.0, 95% CI 2.0 to 4.6).[30] The most common reasons cited for withdrawal were menstrual disorders and headache.

Comment: In the second RCT identified by the review assessing non-vertebral fractures, the use of multiple treatment groups without the correct statistical analyses limit the validity of the study results.[30] In the subsequent large RCT (2763 postmenopausal women aged < 80 years), prevention of fractures was a secondary outcome, the primary outcome was the secondary prevention of coronary heart disease.[28] In addition to the RCTs described, we found many observational studies with conflicting results.[1,31–37] One non-systematic review of 11 observational studies found a reduced risk of hip fracture in women taking oestrogen compared with non-users.[1] A prospective cohort study (9704 women, ≥ 65 years) found a significant reduction in the risk of hip fracture with oral oestrogen only in women who started HRT within 5 years of menopause and who used it continuously thereafter.[34] Other observational studies found no differences in fracture rates with HRT use.[38] We found no observational studies that detected an increased risk of fracture with HRT. Several observational studies found that only 8–20% of women continued HRT for at least 3 years.[39,40]

GLOSSARY

Environmental manipulation Involves the restructuring of a person's environment to remove hazards and reduce the risk of falling or of a fall resulting in fracture.

Substantive changes

Hormone replacement therapy; non vertebral fractures One new systematic review and one new subsequent RCT;[28,29] recategorised as likely to be ineffective or harmful.

REFERENCES

1. Grady D, Rubin S, Petitti D, et al. Hormone therapy to prevent disease and prolong life in postmenopausal women. *Ann Intern Med* 1992;117:1016–1037.
2. Reginster JY, Jones EA, Kaufman JM, et al (on behalf of the GREES). Recommendations for the registration of new chemical entities used in the prevention and treatment of osteoporosis. *Calcif Tissue Int* 1995;57:247–250.
3. Arboleya LR, Morales A, Fitcr J. Effect of alendronate on bone mineral density and incidence of fractures in postmenopausal women with osteoporosis. A meta-analysis of published studies. *Med Clin* 2000;114(Suppl. 2):79–84. Search date 1998; primary sources: Medline and Embase.
4. Black DM, Thompson DE, Bauer DC, et al. Fracture risk reduction with alendronate in women with osteoporosis: the fracture intervention trial. *J Clin Endocrinol Metab* 2000;85:4118–4124.
5. Crannney A, Welch V, Adachi JD, et al. Etidronate for treating and preventing postmenopausal osteoporosis. In: The Cochrane Library, Issue 4, 2001. Oxford: Update Software. Search date 1998; primary sources: Medline, HealthSTAR, Embase, Current Contents, hand searching of conference abstracts, citations of relevant articles, the proceedings of international osteoporosis meetings, and contact with osteoporosis investigators to identify additional studies, primary authors, and pharmaceutical industry sources for unpublished data.
6. Reid IR, Wattie DJ, Evans MC, et al. Continuous therapy with pamidronate, a potent bisphosphonate, in postmenopausal osteoporosis. *J Clin Endocrinol Metab* 1994;79:1595–1599.
7. Harris ST, Watts NB, Genant HK, et al. Effects of risedronate treatment on vertebral and nonvertebral fractures in women with postmenopausal osteoporosis. A randomized controlled trial. *JAMA* 1999;282:1344–1352.
8. Reginster J-Y, Minne HW, Sorensen OH, et al. Randomized trial of the effects of risedronate on vertebral fractures in women with established postmenopausal osteoporosis. *Osteoporos Int* 2000;11:83–91.
9. McClung MR, Geusens P, Miller PD, et al. Effect of risedronate on the risk of hip fracture in elderly women. *N Engl J Med* 2001;344:333–340.
10. Reginster J-Y, Christiansen C, Roux C, et al. Intermittent cyclic tiludronate in the treatment of osteoporosis. *Osteoporos Int* 2001;12:169–177.
11. Black DM, Cummings SR, Karpf DB, et al, for the Fracture Intervention Trial Research Group. Randomised trial of the effect of alendronate on the risk of fracture in women with existing vertebral fractures. *Lancet* 1996;348:1535–1541.
12. Lanza F, Schwartz H, Sahba B, et al. An endoscopic comparison of the effects of alendronate and risedronate on upper gastrointestinal mucosae. *Am J Gastroenterol* 2000;95:3112–3117.
13. Reginster JY, Biermans A, Monville JF. Bisphosphonates in the prevention and treatment of osteoporosis: state of the art. In: Aso T, Yanaihara T, Fujimito S, eds. *Menopause at the millennium*. Yokohama, Japan: Parthenon Publishing, 1999:323–332.
14. Reid IR, Ames RW, Evans MC, et al. Long-term effects of calcium supplementation on bone loss and fractures in post-menopausal women: a randomized controlled trial. *Am J Med* 1995;98:331–335.
15. Recker RR, Hinders S, Davies KM, et al. Correcting calcium nutritional deficiency prevents spine fractures in elderly women. *J Bone Miner Res* 1996;11:1961–1966.
16. Gillespie WJ, Avenell A, Henry DA, et al. Vitamin D and vitamin D analogues for preventing fractures associated with involutional and post-menopausal osteoporosis. In: The Cochrane Library, Issue 4, 2001. Oxford: Update Software. Search date 2000; primary sources Medline, Embase, Cinahl, Lilacs, Cabnar, Biosis, Healthstar, Current Contents, The Cochrane Database of Systematic Reviews, the Cochrane Musculoskeletal Injuries Group trials register, and bibliographies of identified trials and reviews.
17. Tilyard MW, Spears GFS, Thomson J, et al. Treatment of postmenopausal osteoporosis with calcitriol or calcium. *N Engl J Med* 1992;326:357–362.
18. Kanis JA, McCloskey EV. Effect of calcitonin on vertebral and other fractures. *QJM* 1999;92:143–149. Search date 1997; primary sources Medline, conference proceedings, and reference lists of various review articles and books.
19. Chesnut CH, Silverman S, Andriano K, et al. A randomized trial of nasal spray salmon calcitonin in postmenopausal women with established osteoporosis: the prevent recurrence of osteoporotic fractures study. *Am J Med* 2000;109:267–276.
20. Vetter NJ, Lewis PA, Ford D. Can health visitors prevent fractures in elderly people? *BMJ* 1992;304:888–890.
21. Gillespie LD, Gillespie WJ, Robertson MC, et al. Interventions for preventing falls in elderly people. In: The Cochrane Library, Issue 4, 2001. Oxford: Update Software. Search date 2001; primary sources Cochrane Musculoskeletal Group specialised register, Cochrane Controlled Trials Register, Medline, Embase, Cinahl, The National Research Register, Current Controlled Trials, reference lists of articles, and contact with researchers in the field.
22. Parker MJ, Gillespie LD, Gillespie WJ. Hip protectors for preventing hip fractures in the elderly. In: The Cochrane Library, Issue 4, 2001. Oxford: Update Software. Search date 2000; primary sources the Cochrane Musculoskeletal Injuries Group specialised register, Cochrane Controlled Trials Register, Medline, Embase, Cinahl, and reference lists of relevant articles.

23. Harada A, Mizuno M, Takemura M, et al. Hip fracture prevention trial using hip protectors in Japanese nursing homes. *Osteoporos Int* 2001;12:215–221.
24. Jäntti P, Aho H, Mäki-Jokela P. Turvahousut lonkanseudun murtumien ehkäisyssä. [Protector pants in the prevention of hip fractures.] *Suomen Lääkärilehti* 1996;51:3387–3389.
25. Lufkin E, Wahner H, O'Fallon W, et al. Treatment of postmenopausal osteoporosis with transdermal estrogen. *Ann Intern Med* 1992;117:1–9.
26. Lindsay R. Prevention of spinal osteoporosis in oophorectomised women. *Lancet* 1980;1:1152–1154.
27. Mosekilde L, Beck-Nielsen H, Sorensen OH, et al. Hormonal replacement therapy reduces forearm fracture incidence in recent postmenopausal women–results of the Danish Osteoporosis Prevention Study. *Maturitas* 2000;36:181–193.
28. Cauley JA, Black DM, Barrett-Connor, et al. Effects of hormone replacement therapy on clinical fractures and height loss: the heart and estrogen/progestin replacement study (HERS). *Am J Med* 2001;110:442–450.
29. Torgerson DJ, Bell-Syer SEM. Hormone replacement therapy and prevention of nonvertebral fractures. A meta-analysis of randomized trials. *JAMA* 2001;285:2891–2897. Search date 2000; primary sources Medline, Embase, Science Citation Index, Cochrane Controlled Trials Register, reference lists of systematic reviews, and contact with authors, researchers in the field, and pharmaceutical companies.
30. Komulainen M, Kröger H, Tuppurainen M, et al. HRT and vitamin D in prevention of non-vertebral fractures in postmenopausal women; a 5 year randomized trial. *Maturitas* 1998;31:45–54.
31. Ettinger B, Genant H, Cann C. Long-term estrogen replacement therapy prevents bone loss and fractures. *Ann Intern Med* 1985;102:319–324.
32. Maxim P, Ettinger B, Spitalny M. Fracture protection provided by long-term estrogen treatment. *Osteoporos Int* 1995;5:23–29.
33. Kanis J, Johnell O, Gullberg B, et al. Evidence for efficacy of drugs affecting bone metabolism in preventing hip fracture. *BMJ* 1992;305:1124–1128.
34. Cauley J, Seeley D, Ensrud K, et al. Estrogen replacement therapy and fractures in older women. *Ann Intern Med* 1995;122:9–16.
35. Michaëlsson K, Varon J, Farahmand B, et al, on behalf of the Swedish Hip Fracture Study Group. Hormone replacement therapy and risk of hip fracture: population based case-control study. *BMJ* 1998;316:1858–1863.
36. Michaëlsson K, Baron J, Johnell O, et al, for the Swedish Hip Fracture Study Group. Variation in the efficacy of hormone replacement therapy in the prevention of hip fracture. *Osteoporos Int* 1998;8:540–546.
37. Nguyen T, Jones G, Sambrook N, et al. Effects of estrogen exposure and reproductive factors on bone mineral density and osteoporotic fractures. *J Clin Endocrin Metab* 1995;80:2709–2714.
38. Kiel D, Baron J, Anderson J, et al. Smoking eliminates the protective effect of oral estrogens on the risk for hip fracture among women. *Ann Intern Med* 1992;116:716–721.
39. Ettinger B, Li D, Lein R. Continuation of postmenopausal hormone replacement therapy: comparison of cyclic versus continuous combined schedules. *Menopause* 1996;3:185–189.
40. Groeneveld F, Bareman F, Barentsen R, et al. Duration of hormonal replacement therapy in general practice: a follow up study. *Maturitas* 1998;29:125–131.

Olivier Bruyere
Research Fellow
WHO Collaborating Center for Public Health Aspects of Osteoarticular Disease
Liege
Belgium

John Edwards
General Practioner
Wolstanton Medical Centre
Newcastle-under-Lyme
UK

Jean-Yves Reginster
Professor of Epidemiology and Public Health
Bone and Cartilage Metabolism Unit
University of Liege
Liege
Belgium

Competing interests: OB, none declared. JR has participated in several pre-clinical and clinical trials, reviewed and consulted scientific documentation, has been an author of publications, and has chaired and spoken at scientific meetings for the following companies: Asahi, Bayer, Boehringer Ingelheim, Chiesi, Eli Lilly, Hoechst-Marion-Roussel, Hologic, Hybritech, Igea, Johnson & Johnson, Merck Sharp & Dohme, Negma, Organon, Pfizer, Pharmascience, Procter & Gamble Pharmaceuticals, Rotta research, Sanofi, Servier, SmithKline Beecham, Teva, Therabel, Tosse, Byk, UCB, and Will Pharma.

Hallux valgus (bunions)

Search date May 2002

Jill Ferrari

QUESTIONS

INTERVENTIONS

See glossary, p 1111

Key Messages

- **Antipronatory orthoses in children** One RCT in children aged 9–10 years found limited evidence that antipronatory orthoses versus no treatment may increase deterioration in metatarsophalangeal joint angles after 3 years.
- **Chevron osteotomy (compared with no treatment or with orthoses)** One RCT found that chevron osteotomy versus no treatment or orthoses significantly reduced pain intensity, and significantly improved cosmetic appearance, functional status, and footwear problems, but found no significant difference in ability to return to work after 1 year.
- **Chevron osteotomy (compared with proximal osteotomy)** RCTs identified by a systematic review comparing chevron osteotomy versus proximal osteotomy found conflicting results on hallux abductus angle, and found no significant difference in problems with footwear or mobility after a maximum of 38 months.
- **Chevron osteotomy plus Akin osteotomy** One small RCT found that chevron osteotomy plus Akin osteotomy versus Akin osteotomy plus distal soft tissue reconstruction significantly improved the hallux abductus angle, intermetatarsal angle, and tibial sesamoid position, but found no significant difference in patient satisfaction, cosmetic appearance, or motion at the toe after a minimum of 1 year.

Clin Evid 2002;8:1103–1112.

- **Chevron osteotomy plus adductor tenotomy** One RCT found no significant difference with chevron osteotomy plus adductor tenotomy versus chevron osteotomy alone in hallux abductus angle, range of motion, pain, satisfaction, problems with footwear, or mobility.
- **Continuous passive motion** One systematic review found no significant difference between continuous passive motion plus physiotherapy versus physiotherapy alone on joint range of motion or return to normal footwear after 3 months treatment, but was too small to rule out a clinically important effect.
- **Different methods of bone fixation** One RCT found no significant difference with a standard method of fixation versus absorbable pin fixation in clinical or radiological outcomes after a mean follow up of 11 months. One RCT found that screw fixation followed by early weight bearing in a plaster shoe versus vicryl suture fixation followed by 6 weeks non-weight bearing in a plaster boot significantly reduced both time taken to return to social activities and time taken to return to work but found no significant difference in clinical and radiological outcomes after 6 months.
- **Early weightbearing** One systematic review has found no significant difference with early versus late weight bearing in numbers of people with non-union at the site of arthrodesis.
- **Keller's arthroplasty** One systematic review found little good evidence on the effects of Keller's arthroplasty versus other types of operation.
- **Night splints** We found no RCTs examining the use of night splints in the treatment of hallux valgus.
- **Orthoses to prevent hallux valgus in high risk adults** One RCT in men with rheumatoid arthritis found no significant difference with orthoses versus no treatment in the number of people who developed hallux valgus after 3 years.
- **Orthoses to treat hallux valgus in adults** One RCT in adults found that orthoses versus no treatment significantly improved pain intensity after 6 months, but found no significant difference in pain after 12 months.
- **Slipper casts** One RCT of crepe bandage versus plaster cast slippers after Wilson osteotomy found no significant difference in hallux valgus angle, pain, overall assessment, joint range of movement, or return to normal activities, but was too small to rule out a clinically important effect.

DEFINITION **Hallux valgus** is a deformity of the great toe whereby the hallux (great toe) moves towards the second toe, overlying it in severe cases. This movement of the hallux is described as abduction (movement away from the midline of the body) and it is usually accompanied by some rotation of the toe so that the nail is facing the midline of the body (valgus rotation). With the deformity, the metatarsal head becomes more prominent and the metatarsal is said to be in an adducted position as it moves towards the midline of the body.[1] Radiological criteria for hallux valgus vary, but a commonly accepted criterion is to measure the angle formed between the metatarsal and the abducted hallux. This is called the metatarsophalangeal joint angle or hallux abductus angle and it is considered abnormal when it is greater than 14.5°.[2] **Bunion** is the lay term used to describe a prominent and often inflamed metatarsal head and overlying bursa. Symptoms include pain, limitation in walking, and problems with wearing normal shoes.

INCIDENCE/ PREVALENCE The prevalence of hallux valgus varies in different populations. In a recent study of 6000 UK school children aged 9–10 years, 2.5% had clinical evidence of hallux valgus, and 2% met both clinical and radiological criteria for hallux valgus. An earlier study found hallux valgus in 48% of adults.[2] Differences in prevalence may result from different methods of measurement, varying age groups, or different diagnostic criteria (e.g. metatarsal joint angle > 10° or > 15°).[3]

AETIOLOGY/ RISK FACTORS Nearly all population studies have found that hallux valgus is more common in women. Footwear may contribute to the deformity, but studies comparing people who wear shoes with those who do not have found contradictory results. Hypermobility of the first ray (see glossary, p 1112) and excessive foot pronation are associated with hallux valgus.[4]

PROGNOSIS We found no studies that looked at progression of hallux valgus. Progression of deformity and symptoms is rapid in some people, others remain asymptomatic. One study found that hallux valgus is often unilateral initially, but usually progresses to bilateral deformity.[2]

AIMS To reduce symptoms and deformity, with minimum adverse effects.

OUTCOMES **Hallux abductus/metatarsophalangeal joint angle**. Range of motion of the first metatarsophalangeal joint (the total range of both dorsiflexion and plantarflexion). Incidence of complications such as infection; re-operation; non-union; avascular necrosis; pain; general satisfaction and satisfaction with appearance; requirement for specialist or extra-width footwear; proportion of people with mobility problems; time to healing; development of transfer lesions (see glossary, p 1112); and adverse effects of treatment.

METHODS *Clinical Evidence* update search and appraisal May 2002. An earlier search (October 1998) was also made using a strategy developed by the Cochrane Musculoskeletal Injuries Group. We also hand searched podiatry journals up to July 2002.

QUESTION What are the effects of conservative treatments?

OPTION ORTHOSES

One RCT in children found limited evidence that antipronatory orthoses versus no treatment may increase deterioration in metatarsophalangeal joint angles after 3 years. One RCT in men with rheumatoid arthritis found no significant difference with orthoses versus no treatment in the number of people who developed of hallux valgus after 3 years. One RCT in adults found that orthoses versus no treatment significantly improved pain intensity after 6 months, but found no significant difference in pain after 12 months.

Benefits: We found no systematic review. We found three RCTs. **In children:** One RCT comparing antipronatory orthoses (see glossary, p 1111) versus no treatment screened 6000 UK school children aged 9–10 years.[2] On the basis of a clinical examination, 150 children were selected for x ray examination and 122 of these children (13% of whom were boys) found to have metatarsophalangeal joint angles greater than 14.5° in one or both feet were subsequently included in the trial (see comment). The RCT found that the metatarsophalangeal joint angles deteriorated both with orthoses and with no treatment, and found that the deterioration was greater in children treated with orthoses although this difference was not significant after 3 years (no direct statistical comparisons provided). **In adults:** We found no RCTs examining the use of orthoses in adults who already had hallux valgus. We found one RCT (102 men with rheumatoid arthritis, but without hallux valgus; see comment below) that compared the use of orthoses versus no treatment to prevent the development of hallux valgus.[5] The RCT found no significant difference between treatments in the number of people who developed hallux valgus after 3 years (5/50 [10%] for adults with orthoses *v* 12/48 [25%] no treatment; RR 0.4, 95% CI 0.2 to 1.1). We found one RCT (209 adults) which compared three treatments: chevron osteotomy (see glossary, p 1111); orthoses; and no treatment (see benefits of chevron osteotomy, p 1108).[6] The RCT found that orthoses versus no treatment significantly reduced pain intensity after 6 months (WMD −14, 95% CI −22 to −6), but found no significant difference in pain intensity after 12 months (WMD −6, 95% CI −15 to +3). The RCT also found that orthoses versus no treatment improved global assessment and satisfaction after 12 months (46% with orthoses versus 24% with no treatment; absolute numbers and significance not provided) but found no significant difference in duration of the pain, ability to work, and cosmetic disturbance.

Harms: The RCT in children did not report on harms.[2] The RCT in men with rheumatoid arthritis reported that orthoses caused mild discomfort in a small number of cases.[5]

Comment: The use of antipronatory orthoses in children is questionable because earlier studies have found that hallux valgus in children is not related to pronation but arises from positional changes in the first ray (see glossary, p 1112).[7] The first RCT reported that 29/122 (25%) children (mainly from the control group) were lost to follow up.[2] The RCT in people with rheumatoid arthritis included only men, although both rheumatoid arthritis and hallux valgus are more common in women.[5] This may limit the applicability of the results.

OPTION NIGHT SPLINTS

We found no RCTs examining the use of night splints in the treatment of hallux valgus.

Benefits: We found no systematic review and no RCTs.

Harms: We found no evidence of harms associated with night splints.

Comment: None.

QUESTION What are the effects of surgery?

OPTION KELLER'S ARTHROPLASTY

One systematic review found little good evidence on the effects of Keller's arthroplasty versus other types of operation.

Benefits: **Versus no treatment:** We found no RCTs. **Versus distal osteotomy:** We found one systematic review (search date 1998, 3 RCTs; see comment below)[8] that included one RCT (29 people) comparing distal metatarsal osteotomy (see glossary, p 1111) versus Keller's arthroplasty (see glossary, p 1112). The review found that osteotomy versus Keller's arthroplasty significantly improved both intermetatarsal angle (WMD −7.0°, 95% CI −8.9° to −1.1°) and range of movement (WMD 13°, 95% CI 5.0° to 21.1°), but found no significant difference in the number of people remaining in pain (OR 0.91, 95% CI 0.18 to 4.64) or in the number of people remaining dissatisfied (OR 0.91, 95% CI 0.18 to 4.64) after 3 years. **Versus arthrodesis:** The second RCT included in the review (81 people) found that Keller's arthroplasty versus arthrodesis significantly reduced the number of people with reduced mobility (OR 4.23, 95% CI 1.22 to 14.71), but found no significant difference in the number of people remaining in pain (OR 0.95, 95% CI 0.23 to 3.81) or in the number of people remaining dissatisfied (OR 1.11, 95% CI 0.41 to 3.01) after a minimum of 2 years.[8] **Plus joint distraction:** The third RCT included in the review found that the use of a Kirschner wire (see glossary, p 1112) to distract the joint during healing after Keller's arthroplasty versus no wire use significantly improved subjective assessment scores for symptoms ($P < 0.05$), but found no significant difference in the hallux abductus angle or intermetatarsal angle, pain, or movement after a minimum of 1 year.

Harms: The review did not report any specific complications associated with any of the procedures. Reduced toe function has been described after Keller's procedure.[8] The systematic review reported high levels of patient dissatisfaction (up to 33%) in most trials.[8]

Comment: Most of the people included in the review having surgery were under 50 years of age and were followed up for no more than 3 years.[8] Longer term outcomes remain unclear. Many of the RCTs reported results for numbers of feet, and did not always report standard deviations of the results. The systematic review analysed the results by numbers of people.[8]

OPTION CHEVRON OSTEOTOMY

One RCT found that chevron osteotomy versus no treatment or orthoses significantly reduced pain intensity, significantly improved cosmetic appearance, functional status and footwear problems, but found no significant difference in ability to return to work after 1 year. RCTs identified by a systematic review comparing chevron osteotomy versus proximal osteotomy found conflicting results on hallux abductus angle, and found no significant difference in problems with footwear or mobility after a maximum of 38 months. One RCT identified by the review found no

significant difference with chevron osteotomy plus adductor tenotomy versus chevron osteotomy alone in hallux abductus angle, range of motion, pain, satisfaction, problems with footwear, or mobility. One small RCT found that Akin osteotomy plus chevron osteotomy versus Akin osteotomy plus distal soft tissue reconstruction significantly improved the hallux abductus angle, intermetatarsal angle, and tibial sesamoid position, but found no significant difference in patient satisfaction, cosmetic appearance, or motion at the toe after a minimum of 1 year.

Benefits: **Versus no treatment or versus use of orthoses:** We found one RCT (209 adults) which compared three treatments: chevron osteotomy (see glossary, p 1111); orthoses; and no treatment (see benefits of orthoses, p 1105).[6] The RCT found that chevron osteotomy versus no treatment significantly reduced pain intensity (WMD −19, 95% CI −28 to −10), and significantly improved cosmetic appearance (WMD −1.2, 95% CI −1.8 to −0.6), functional status (WMD 11, 95% CI 7 to 16), and footwear problems (absolute numbers not provided; $p < 0.01$), but found no significant difference in the ability to work (WMD 4, 95% CI −3 to +11) after 1 year. The RCT found that chevron osteotomy versus orthoses significantly reduced pain intensity (WMD −14, 95% CI −22 to −5), and significantly improved cosmetic appearance (WMD −1.4, 95% CI −2.1 to −0.8), functional status (WMD 11, 95% CI 7 to 15), and footwear problems (absolute numbers not provided; $P < 0.001$), but found no significant difference in the ability to work (WMD 6, 95% CI 0 to 13) after 1 year. **Versus proximal osteotomy:** We found one systematic review (search date 1998, 3 RCTs, 205 people).[8] The first RCT (66 people) included in the review found no significant difference with proximal chevron osteotomy versus proximal crescentic osteotomy (see glossary, p 1112) in the hallux abductus angle, intermetatarsal angle or in transfer lesions (see glossary, p 1112) after 22 months.[8] The RCT found that proximal chevron osteotomy versus proximal crescentic osteotomy significantly reduced healing time ($P < 0.001$) and significantly reduced postoperative dorsiflexion at the healed site ($P = 0.005$). The second RCT (79 people) included in the review found that chevron osteotomy versus proximal osteotomy significantly improved the hallux abductus angle (WMD −5.0°, 95% CI −0.5° to −9.5°) and intermetatarsal angle (WMD −3.0°, 95% CI −1.0° to −5.0°), but found no significant difference in pain, satisfaction, problems with footwear, or mobility after 2 years. The third RCT (46 people) included in the review found that Wilson osteotomy (see glossary, p 1112) versus chevron osteotomy significantly improved the hallux abductus angle (WMD −12.4°, 95% CI −17.5° to −7.5°), but found no significant difference in problems with footwear or mobility after 38 months. **Plus adductor tenotomy:** We found one systematic review (search date 1998, 1 RCT, 84 people).[8] The RCT included in the review found no significant difference with chevron osteotomy plus adductor tenotomy versus chevron osteotomy alone in hallux abductus angle, range of motion, pain, satisfaction, problems with footwear, or mobility. **Plus Akin osteotomy:** One small RCT (23 people; see comment below) compared Akin osteotomy (see glossary, p 1111) plus chevron osteotomy versus Akin osteotomy plus distal soft tissue reconstruction (see glossary, p 1112).[9] It found that Akin osteotomy plus chevron osteotomy significantly improved the hallux abductus angle ($P < 0.01$), intermetatarsal angle ($P < 0.01$), and tibial sesamoid position ($P < 0.01$), but found no significant difference in patient satisfaction, cosmetic appearance, or motion at the toe after a minimum of 1 year.

Harms: Complications were reported by most of the RCTs. The RCT comparing chevron osteotomy, orthoses, and no treatment reported complications in 4/71 (6%) people undergoing chevron osteotomy (complications comprised one wound infection, one stress fracture, one episode of nerve damage, and one recurrence of deformity).[6] The RCT reported no complications associated with orthoses. The RCT comparing proximal crescentic osteotomy versus proximal chevron osteotomy found no significant difference in numbers of complications.[8] The RCT comparing proximal osteotomy versus chevron osteotomy reported one wound infection and two stress fractures in people undergoing chevron osteotomy and 11 complications in people undergoing proximal osteotomy, consisting mostly of pain in other areas of the forefoot (metatarsalgia).[8] The RCT comparing Wilson osteotomy versus chevron osteotomy, found no significant difference in the number of complications (11/26 [42%] with Wilson osteotomy *v* 9/24 [38%] with chevron osteotomy; RR 1.3, 95% CI 0.57 to 2.24).[8] Complications included swelling, over correction, slow healing, and recurrence of bunion. Transfer pain (see glossary, p 1112) and lesions were recurring problems in both groups. The RCT found that although Wilson osteotomy versus chevron osteotomy resulted in a significantly shortened metatarsal ($P = 0.02$), with metatarsal dorsiflexion in 20% of people, this change in position did not correlate with development of new corns, callous or pain. In the RCT of chevron osteotomy plus adductor tenotomy versus chevron osteotomy alone, about 25% of both groups remained dissatisfied during follow up.[8] This may be related to greater postoperative reduction in the circumference of the ball of the foot; the RCT found that the ball circumference of dissatisfied people was significantly greater than that of satisfied people ($P = 0.005$). The RCT comparing Akin osteotomy plus chevron osteotomy versus Akin osteotomy plus distal soft tissue reconstruction reported two complications with Akin osteotomy plus chevron osteotomy (one non-union and one where a transfer lesion developed resulting in further surgery), one complication with Akin osteotomy plus distal soft tissue reconstruction (nerve damage in the great toe).[9]

Comment: None of the RCTs included long term follow up. The RCT comparing chevron plus Akin osteotomy versus Akin osteotomy plus distal soft tissue reconstruction was poorly randomised and appears to be a subset of data from a larger RCT.[9]

OPTION DIFFERENT METHODS OF BONE FIXATION

One RCT found no significant difference with a standard method of fixation versus absorbable pin fixation in clinical outcomes or radiological outcomes after a mean follow up of 11 months. One RCT found that screw fixation followed by early weightbearing in a plaster shoe versus

vicryl suture fixation followed by 6 weeks non-weight bearing in a plaster boot significantly reduced both time taken to return to social activities and time taken to return to work but found no significant difference in clinical and radiological outcomes after 6 months.

Benefits: We found no systematic review. We found two RCTs comparing different methods of bone fixation following Mitchell's osteotomy (see glossary, p 1112).[10,11] The first RCT (28 people, 39 feet; see comment below) found no significant difference with a standard method of fixation versus absorbable pin fixation in clinical outcomes (range of movement, pain, metatarsalgia, walking ability, and cosmetic appearance) or radiological outcomes (hallux abductus angle, intermetatarsal angle, and the ratio of the first to second metatarsal length) after a mean follow up of 11 months (range 2–24 months). The second RCT (30 people) compared screw fixation followed by early weight bearing in a plaster shoe versus vicryl suture fixation followed by 6 weeks non-weight bearing in a plaster boot.[11] It found that screw fixation followed by early weight bearing in a plaster shoe significantly reduced time taken to return to social activities (mean 2.9 *v* 5.7 wks; $P < 0.001$) and time taken to return to work (mean 4.9 *v* 8.7 wks; $P < 0.001$), but found no significant difference in clinical and radiological outcomes after 6 months.[11]

Harms: The first RCT (28 people, 39 feet) reported more complications in people receiving standard versus pin fixation, although the difference was not significant (14/17 [82%] feet *v* 16/22 [73%] feet; RR 1.13, 95% CI 0.81 to 1.59).[10] These included recurrence of deformity (3/17 feet *v* 2/22 feet), problems primarily resulting in pain (5/17 feet *v* 6/22 feet), and continued swelling (3/17 feet *v* 0/22 feet). In the RCT (30 people) of screw versus suture fixation, 2/15 (13%) people had the screw removed because of pain.[11] The RCT reported that superficial infection occurred in three people overall (2 *v* 1) and also found that fixation followed by early weightbearing in a plaster shoe significantly increased metatarsophalangeal joint stiffness after both 3 and 6 months.

Comment: Applicability of the results from the first RCT may be limited as people were used as the unit of randomisation and feet as the unit of statistical analysis.[10]

QUESTION What are the effects of postoperative care?

OPTION CONTINUOUS PASSIVE MOTION

One systematic review found no significant difference between continuous passive motion plus physiotherapy versus physiotherapy alone on joint range of motion or return to normal footwear after 3 months' treatment, but was too small to rule out a clinically important effect.

Benefits: We found one systematic review (search date 1998, 1 RCT, 39 people).[8] The RCT included in the review found no significant difference in continuous passive motion plus physiotherapy versus physiotherapy alone in the range of motion (WMD –6.7°, 95% CI –13.6° to +0.3°) or in the number of people who returned to normal footwear after 3 months treatment.

Harms: No complications were reported by the RCT.[8]

Comment: None.

OPTION EARLY WEIGHTBEARING

One systematic review has found no significant difference with early weightbearing versus late weightbearing in numbers of people with non-union at the site of arthrodesis.

Benefits: We found one systematic review (search date 1998, 1 RCT).[8] The RCT (56 people; see comment below) compared early weightbearing (initial weightbearing in a cast from 2–4 wks postoperatively) versus late weightbearing (initial weightbearing 4 wks postoperatively).[8] It found no significant difference in numbers of people with non-union at the site of arthrodesis (1/29 [3%] with early weigthbearing versus 2/27 [7%] with late weightbearing; RR 0.46, 95% CI 0.05 to 4.85).

Harms: See benefits above.

Comment: The only outcome assessed by the RCT was non-union at the site of arthrodesis.[8]

OPTION SLIPPER CAST

One RCT of crepe bandage versus plaster cast slippers after Wilson osteotomy found no significant difference in hallux valgus angle, pain, overall assessment, joint range of movement, or return to normal activities, but was too small to rule out a clinically important effect.

Benefits: We found no systematic review, but found one RCT (54 feet), which compared the use of plaster slipper cast versus crepe bandage following a Wilson osteotomy (see glossary, p 1112).[12] Cast and dressings were changed 12 days after surgery and then kept on for a further 4 weeks. The RCT found no significant difference in hallux valgus angle, pain, overall assessment, joint range of movement, or return to normal activities.

Harms: The RCT reported that one failed union occurred with crepe bandaging versus none plaster slipper cast treatment, and that two people receiving plaster slipper cast treatment developed superficial wound infections.[12]

Comment: The RCT was small and could not exclude clinically important differences between the groups.[12]

GLOSSARY

Akin osteotomy A procedure involving resection of the medial prominence of the first metatarsal head and a medial wedge osteotomy of the proximal phalanx of the great toe.

Antipronatory orthoses Insoles designed to reduce the amount of in-roll or flattening of the foot during gait.

Chevron osteotomy A v-shaped wedge of bone is removed from the distal end of the metatarsal shaft, allowing the metatarsal head to be realigned on the shaft.

Distal osteotomy A cut is made in the neck of the metatarsal so that the head of the metatarsal can be realigned on the shaft.

Distal soft tissue reconstruction A procedure involving the release of various ligaments, the capsule, and tendons around the first metatarsophalangeal joint.
First ray The first metatarsal and medial cuneiform function as a single unit called the first ray.
Keller's arthroplasty A procedure involving removal of the medial side of the metatarsal head and straight resection of the base of the proximal phalanx.
Kirschner wire A thin but rigid wire that is used to fix bone fragments. It is passed through drilled channels in the bone (sometimes called K-wire).
Mitchell's osteotomy A distal metatarsal osteotomy whereby an incomplete osteotomy is performed perpendicular to the long axis of the bone. The distal portion is moved laterally and fixed in position. This results in shortening of the bone.
Proximal chevron osteotomy Removal of a v-shaped wedge of bone from the base of the metatarsal shaft followed by displacement and fixation of the distal portion of bone.
Proximal crescentic osteotomy A curved cut is made across the base of the metatarsal shaft. The distal portion of bone is slid across the proximal end of bone and fixed in a corrected position.
Transfer lesions Areas of corns or callus that develop when the weightbearing forces are transferred from one area of the foot to another.
Transfer pain Refers to pain that occurs in another area of the foot after surgery. It usually occurs in the second/third metatarsal heads after the surgeon has altered the first metatarsal head.
Wilson osteotomy A double oblique cut is made in the distal portion of the metatarsal shaft and the metatarsal head is slid into a corrected position.

REFERENCES

1. Dykyj D. Pathological anatomy of hallux abducto valgus. *Clin Podiatr Med Surg* 1989;6:1–15.
2. Kilmartin TE, Barrington RL, Wallace WA. A controlled prospective trial of a foot orthosis for juvenile hallux valgus. *J Bone Joint Surg Br* 1994;76:210–214.
3. Morris JB, Brash LF, Hird MD. Chiropodial survey of geriatric and psychiatric hospital in-patients – Angus District. *Chiropodist* 1980;April:128–139.
4. LaPorta G, Melillo T, Olinsky D. X-ray evaluation of hallux abducto valgus deformity. *J Am Podiatr Med Assoc* 1974;64:544–566.
5. Budiman-Mak E, Conrad KJ, Roach KE, et al. Can orthoses prevent hallux valgus deformity in rheumatoid arthritis? A randomised clinical trial. *J Clin Rheumatol* 1995;1:313–321.
6. Torkki M, Malmivaara A, Seitsalo S, et al. Surgery vs orthosis vs watchful waiting for hallux valgus. A randomised control trial. *JAMA* 2001;285:2474–2480.
7. Juriansz AM. Conservative treatment of hallux valgus: a randomised controlled trial of a hallux valgus night splint. MSc Thesis 1996: Faculty of Science, King's College London.
8. Ferrari J, Higgins JPT, William RL. Interventions for treating hallux valgus (abductovalgus) and bunions. In: The Cochrane Library, Issue 3, 2001. Oxford: Update Software. Search date 1998; primary sources Medline, Embase, Cinahl, Amed, Cochrane Controlled Trials Register, Cochrane Musculoskeletal Injuries Trials Register, bibliographies of identified trials, and hand searching of podiatry journals.
9. Basile A, Battaglia A, Campi A. Comparison of chevron-Akin osteotomy and distal soft tissue reconstruction-Akin osteotomy for correction of mild hallux valgus. *Foot Ankle Surg* 2000;6:155–163.
10. Prior TD, Grace DL, MacLean JB, et al. Correction of hallux abductovalgus by Mitchell's osteotomy: comparing standard fixation methods with absorbable polydioxanone pins. *Foot* 1997;7:121–125.
11. Calder JDF, Hollingdale JP, Pearse MF. Screw versus suture fixation of Mitchell's osteotomy. A prospective randomised study. *J Bone Joint Surg Br* 1999;81:621–624.
12. Meek RMD, Anderson EG. Plaster slipper versus crepe bandage after Wilson's osteotomy for hallux valgus. *Foot* 1999;9:138–141.

Jill Ferrari
Department of Podiatry
University College London
London
UK

Competing interests: None declared.

Herniated lumbar disc

Search date April 2002

Jo Jordan, Tamara Shawver Morgan, and James Weinstein

QUESTIONS

INTERVENTIONS

Covered elsewhere in *Clinical Evidence*

Non-specific acute low back pain (see low back pain and sciatica: acute, p 1156) and chronic low back pain (see low back pain and sciatica: chronic, p 1171).

See glossary, p 1123

Key Messages

- **Advice to stay active** One systematic review of conservative treatments found no RCTs on giving advice to stay active.
- **Automated percutaneous discectomy** We found no RCTs comparing automated percutaneous discectomy versus either conservative treatment or standard discectomy. We found conflicting evidence on the effects of automated percutaneous discectomy versus microdiscectomy. One RCT found that automated percutaneous discectomy versus microdiscectomy was associated with significantly lower success rates at interim analysis at 6 months, and was terminated prematurely. Another RCT comparing the same interventions found similar investigator rated clinical scores, although participant rated improvement was higher with automated percutaneous discectomy than with microdiscectomy after 2 years. One systematic review found that reoperation rates were higher with automated percutaneous discectomy than with either microdiscectomy or standard discectomy. One RCT in the review found that postoperative recovery was about three times shorter with automated percutaneous discectomy than with microdiscectomy.
- **Bed rest** One systematic review of conservative treatment found no RCTs on bed rest for symptomatic herniated discs.

- **Epidural corticosteroid injections** One systematic review found limited evidence that epidural steroid injections versus placebo may increase participant perception of global improvement. One subsequent RCT found no significant difference with the addition of epidural steroid injections to conservative treatment in pain, mobility, or return to work at 6 months.
- **Heat or ice** One systematic review identified no RCTs of heat or ice for sciatica caused by lumbar disc herniation.
- **Massage** One systematic review identified no RCTs of massage in symptomatic lumbar disc herniation.
- **Microdiscectomy (as effective as standard discectomy)** We found no RCTs comparing microdiscectomy versus conservative treatment. Three RCTs found no significant difference in clinical outcomes with microdiscectomy versus standard discectomy. One RCT found no significant difference with video-assisted arthroscopic microdiscectomy versus standard discectomy in self reported satisfaction or pain score after about 31 months. The duration of postoperative recovery with standard discectomy was almost twice that with arthroscopic discectomy. We found conflicting evidence on the effects of microdiscectomy versus automated percutaneous discectomy.
- **Non-steroidal anti-inflammatory drugs** One systematic review found no significant difference between non-steroidal anti-inflammatory drugs versus placebo in participant perception of overall improvement.
- **Spinal manipulation** One RCT in people with sciatica caused by disc herniation found that spinal manipulation versus a placebo of infrared heat increased self perceived improvement after 2 weeks (NNT 8, 95% CI 5 to 109). A second RCT found no significant difference in improvement between spinal manipulation, manual traction, exercise, and corsets after 1 month. A third RCT found that spinal manipulation versus traction significantly increased the number of people with improved symptoms.
- **Standard discectomy** One RCT found that standard discectomy versus conservative treatment (physiotherapy) significantly increased self reported improvement at 1 year (NNT 3, 95% CI 2 to 9), but not at 4 and 10 years. Three RCTs found no significant difference in clinical outcomes with standard discectomy versus microdiscectomy.
- **Analgesics; antidepressants; laser discectomy; muscle relaxants** We found no systematic review or RCTs on these interventions for treatment of symptomatic herniated lumbar disc.

DEFINITION Herniated lumbar disc is a displacement of disc material (nucleus pulposus or annulus fibrosis) beyond the intervertebral disc space.[1] The diagnosis can be confirmed by radiological examination; however, magnetic resonance imaging findings of herniated disc are not always accompanied by clinical symptoms.[2,3] This review covers treatment of people who have clinical symptoms relating to confirmed or suspected disc herniation. It does not include treatment of people with spinal cord compression or people with cauda equina syndrome (see glossary, p 1123), which often requires emergency intervention. The management of non-specific acute low back pain (see low back pain and sciatica: acute, p 1156) and chronic low back pain (see low back pain and sciatica: chronic, p 1171) are covered elsewhere.

INCIDENCE/ PREVALENCE The prevalence of symptomatic herniated lumbar disc is around 1–3% in Finland and Italy, depending on age and sex.[4] The highest prevalence is among people aged 30–50 years,[5] with a male : female ratio of 2 : 1.[6] In people aged between 25 and 55 years, about 95% of herniated discs occur at the L4–L5 level; in people over 55 years of age, disc herniation is more common above the L4–L5 level.[7,8]

AETIOLOGY/ RISK FACTORS Radiographical evidence of disc herniation does not necessarily predict low back pain in the future or indicate physical symptoms, because 19–27% of people without symptoms have disc herniation on imaging.[2,9] Risk factors for disc herniation include smoking (OR 1.7, 95% CI 1.0 to 2.5), weight bearing sports, and certain work activities such as repeated lifting (lifting objects < 11.3 kg, < 25 times daily while twisting body, knees not bent, OR 7.2, 95% CI 2.0 to 25.8; lifting objects < 11.3 kg, < 25 times daily while twisting body, knees bent, OR 1.9, 95% CI 0.8 to 4.8). Driving motor vehicles (possibly because of the resonant frequency of the spine being similar to that of certain vehicles) is also associated with increased risk (OR 1.7, 95% CI 0.2 to 2.7, depending on the vehicle model).[6,10,11]

PROGNOSIS The natural history of disc herniation is difficult to determine because most people take some form of treatment for their back pain, and a formal diagnosis is not always made.[6] Clinical improvement is usual in the majority of people, and only about 10% of people still have sufficient pain after 6 weeks to consider surgery. Sequential magnetic resonance images have shown that the herniated portion of the disc tends to regress over time, with partial to complete resolution after 6 months in two thirds of people.[12]

AIMS To relieve pain; increase mobility and function; and improve quality of life.

OUTCOMES **Primary outcomes:** pain, function, or mobility; individuals perceived overall improvement; quality of life; and adverse effects of treatment. **Secondary outcomes:** return to work; use of analgesia; and duration of hospitalisation.

METHODS *Clinical Evidence* search and appraisal April 2002.

QUESTION What are the effects of oral drug treatments? New

OPTION NON-STEROIDAL ANTI-INFLAMMATORY DRUGS

One systematic review of non-steroidal anti-inflammatory drugs versus placebo in people with sciatica caused by disc herniation found no significant difference in participant perception of overall improvement.

Benefits: We found one systematic review of medical treatments for sciatica caused by disc herniation (search date 1998, 3 RCTs, 321 people).[13] The RCTs compared non-steroidal anti-inflammatory drugs (NSAIDs) (piroxicam 40 mg daily for 2 days or 20 mg daily for 12 days; indometacin [indomethacin] 75–100 mg 3 times daily; phenylbutazone 1200 mg daily for 3 days or 600 mg daily for 2 days) versus placebo (tablet) after 5, 14, and 30 days of follow up.

The review found no significant difference between NSAIDs versus placebo in the number of people who improved (80/172 [46.5%] *v* 57/149 [38.3%] for number of people with improvement in pain or in the time taken to return to work; OR for global improvement 0.99, 95% CI 0.6 to 1.7; see comment below).

Harms: The systematic review did not report the adverse effects of NSAIDs. NSAIDs may cause gastrointestinal complications (see NSAIDs topic, p 1203).

Comment: The absolute numbers in the RCTs relate to the outcomes of improvement in pain (3 RCTs) and return to work (1 RCT).[13] However, the meta-analysis used the outcome measure of global improvement. The relationship between these measures is unclear.

OPTION ANALGESICS

We found no systematic review or RCTs of any analgesic to treat symptomatic herniated lumbar disc.

Benefits: We found no systematic review or RCTs.

Harms: We found no systematic review or RCTs.

Comment: None.

OPTION ANTIDEPRESSANTS

We found no systematic review or RCTs of antidepressants to treat symptomatic herniated lumbar disc.

Benefits: We found no systematic review or RCTs.

Harms: We found no systematic review or RCTs.

Comment: None.

OPTION MUSCLE RELAXANTS

We found no systematic review or RCTs of muscle relaxants to treat for herniated lumbar disc.

Benefits: We found no systematic review or RCTs that assessed the effectiveness of muscle relaxants in people with herniated lumbar disc.

Harms: We found no systematic review or RCTs.

Comment: None.

OPTION EPIDURAL CORTICOSTEROID INJECTIONS

One systematic review found limited evidence that epidural steroid injections versus placebo may increase participant perception of global improvement. One subsequent RCT found no significant difference with the addition of epidural steroid injections to conservative treatment in pain, mobility, or return to work at 6 months.

Benefits: We found one systematic review of medical treatments for sciatica caused by disc herniation (search date 1998, 4 RCTs of epidural steroids, 265 people)[13] and one subsequent RCT.[14] The review compared four different doses of epidural steroid injections (8 mL methylprednisolone 80 mg, 2 mL methylprednisolone 80 mg, 10 mL methylprednisolone 80 mg , and 2 mL methylprednisolone acetate 80 mg) versus placebo (saline or lidocaine [lignocaine] 2 mL) after follow up periods of 2, 21, and 30 days.[13] The review found limited evidence that epidural steroids versus placebo increased participant perceived global improvement (which was not defined). The result was of borderline significance (73/160 [45.6%] with steroid *v* 56/172 [32.5%] with placebo; OR 2.2, 95% CI 1.0 to 4.7). The subsequent RCT (36 people with disc herniation confirmed by magnetic resonance imaging) compared epidural steroids (3 injections of methylprednisolone 100 mg in 10 mL bupivacaine 0.25% during the first 14 days of hospitalisation) plus conservative non-operative treatment versus conservative treatment alone.[14] Conservative treatment involved initial bed rest and analgesia followed by graded rehabilitation (hydrotherapy, electroanalgesia, postural exercise classes) followed by physiotherapy. It found no significant difference in mean pain scores at 6 weeks and 6 months measured on a visual analogue scale (at 6 months, 32.9 [range 0–85] with steroids *v* 39.2 [range 0–100] with conservative treatment). There were no significant differences in mean mobility scores (Hannover Functional Ability Questionnaire: 61.8 [range 25–88] in with steroids *v* 57.2 [range 13–100]), in the number of people who had back surgery (2/17 [12%] with steroids *v* 4/19 [21%]; RR 0.56, 95% CI 0.09 to 2.17), or in people returning to work within 6 months (15/17 [88%] with steroids *v* 14/19 [74%]; RR 1.19, 95% CI 0.75 to 1.33).

Harms: No serious adverse effects were reported in the RCTs included in the systematic review, although 26 people complained of transient headache or transient increase in sciatic pain.[13] The subsequent RCT did not report adverse effects of epidural injections.[14]

Comment: None.

QUESTION What are the effects of non-drug treatments? New

OPTION BED REST

One systematic review of conservative treatment found no RCTs of bed rest for symptomatic herniated discs.

Benefits: We found one systematic review (search date 1998) of conservative treatments for sciatica caused by disc herniation, which identified no RCTs of bed rest for treatment of symptomatic herniated discs.[13] We found no subsequent RCTs.

Harms: We found no systematic review or RCTs.

Comment: None.

OPTION ADVICE TO STAY ACTIVE

One systematic review of conservative treatments for sciatica caused by lumbar disc herniation found no RCTs of giving advice to stay active.

Benefits: We found one systematic review (search date 1998) of conservative treatments for sciatica caused by disc herniation, which found no RCTs of giving advice to stay active.[13] We found no subsequent RCTs.

Harms: We found no RCTs.

Comment: None.

OPTION MASSAGE

One systematic review identified no RCTs of massage in symptomatic lumbar disc herniation.

Benefits: We found one systematic review (search date 1998) of conservative treatments for sciatica caused by disc herniation, which found no RCTs of massage.[13] We found no subsequent RCTs.

Harms: We found no systematic review or RCTs.

Comment: None.

OPTION HEAT AND ICE

One systematic review identified no RCTs of heat or ice for sciatica caused by lumbar disc herniation.

Benefits: We found one systematic review (search date 1998) of conservative treatments for sciatica caused by disc herniation, which identified no RCTs on the use of heat or ice for herniated lumbar discs.[13] We found no subsequent RCTs.

Harms: We found no systematic review or RCTs.

Comment: None.

OPTION SPINAL MANIPULATION

One RCT in people with sciatica caused by disc herniation found that spinal manipulation versus a placebo of infrared heat increased self perceived improvement after 2 weeks. A second RCT found no significant difference in improvement between spinal manipulation, manual traction, exercise, and corsets after 1 month. A third RCT found that spinal manipulation versus traction significantly increased the number of people with improved symptoms.

Benefits: We found two systematic reviews[13,15] and one subsequent RCT.[16] The first systematic review (search date 1998), which did not perform meta-analysis, identified two RCTs of spinal manipulation for sciatica caused by disc herniation.[13] The second systematic review (search date not stated) identified no RCTs.[15] **Versus placebo:** The first RCT (207 people) compared spinal manipulation (every day if necessary) versus placebo (infrared heat 3 times weekly).[13] It found that spinal manipulation versus placebo increased the number of people who perceived an overall improvement at 2 weeks (98/123 [80%] *v* 56/84 [67%]; RR 1.19, 95% CI 1.01 to 1.32; NNT 8, 95% CI 5 to 109).[13] **Versus other treatments:** The second RCT (322 people) compared four interventions: spinal manipulation, manual traction, exercise, and corsets, in a factorial design.[13] It found no significant difference between treatments in overall self perceived improvement after 28 days (quantified results not available). The subsequent RCT (112 people with symptomatic herniated lumbar disc) compared pulling and turning manipulation versus traction.[16] It found that significantly more people receiving spinal manipulation versus traction were "improved" (absence of lumbar pain, improvement in lumbar functional movement) or "cured" (absence of lumbar pain, straight leg raising of > 70°, ability to return to work) after treatment (54/62 [87.1%] *v* 33/50 [66%]; RR 1.32, 95% CI 1.06 to 1.65; NNT 5, 95% CI 4 to 16; timescale not stated).

Harms: The first systematic review did not report adverse effects.[13] The second systematic review identified one review of 135 case reports of serious complications following spinal manipulation published between 1950 and 1980.[15] The case review attributed these complications to cervical manipulation, misdiagnosis, presence of coagulation dyscrasias, presence of herniated nucleus pulposus, and/or improper techniques. The subsequent RCT found that 2/60 people receiving traction had syncope; no adverse effects were reported in people receiving manipulation.[16]

Comment: None.

QUESTION What are the effects of surgery? New

OPTION STANDARD DISCECTOMY

One RCT found that standard discectomy versus conservative treatment (physiotherapy) increased self reported improvement at 1 year, but not at 4 and 10 years. Three RCTs found no significant differences in clinical outcomes with standard discectomy versus microdiscectomy. Adverse effects were similar with both procedures.

Benefits: **Versus conservative treatment:** Two systematic reviews (search dates 1997[17] and not stated[18]) included the same RCT (126 people with symptomatic L5/S1 disc herniation), which compared standard discectomy (see glossary, p 1123) versus conservative treatment (6 wks of physiotherapy).[19] Each participant assessed and graded their improvement in terms of pain and function into four categories: "good" (completely satisfied), "fair", "poor", and "bad" (completely incapacitated for work because of pain). The RCT found that discectomy versus conservative treatment significantly increased the number of people reporting their improvement as "good" after 1 year (intention to treat analysis: 39/60 [65%] with surgery *v* 24/66 [36.4%] with conservative treatment; RR 1.79, 95% CI 1.30 to 2.18; NNT 3, 95% CI 2 to 9). However, at 4 and 10 years there was no significant difference in the same outcome (at 4 years: 40/60 [66.7%] with surgery *v* 34/66 [51.5%] with conservative treatment; RR 1.29, 95% CI 0.96 to 1.56; at 10 years: 35/60 [58.3%] *v* 37/66 [56.1%]; RR 1.04, 95% CI 0.73 to 1.32). **Versus microdiscectomy:** One systematic review (search date 1997) identified three RCTs (219 people) comparing standard discectomy versus microdiscectomy (see glossary, p 1123).[17] Meta-analysis was not performed because outcomes were not comparable. The first RCT in the review (60 people with lumbar disc herniation) found no significant difference between standard discectomy versus microdiscectomy in the number of people who rated their operative outcome as "good", "almost recovered", or "totally recovered" at 1 year (intention to treat analysis: 26/30 [87%] with standard discectomy *v* 24/30 [80%] with microdiscectomy; RR 1.08, 95% CI 0.78 to 1.20).[20] There was also no difference between treatments in the change in preoperative and postoperative pain scores (visual analogue scale; P value not provided) or in the duration of time taken to return to work (both 10 wks). The second RCT in the review (79 people with lumbar disc herniation) also found no significant differences between microdiscectomy versus standard discectomy in pain in the legs or back (visual analogue scale, not specified) or in analgesia use at any point during the 6 week follow up (absolute numbers not provided).[21] The third RCT (80 people; in French) also found that clinical outcomes and duration of sick leave were similar at 15 months, but the review did not provide further details.[17]

Harms: **Versus conservative treatment:** The RCT included in both systematic reviews did not report the complications of standard discectomy.[19] **Versus microdiscectomy:** One systematic review reported that there was no significant difference between standard discectomy versus microdiscectomy in perioperative bleeding, duration of stay, or scar tissue (numbers not provided).[17] The first RCT included in the review reported one person in each group with a nerve root tear and, of the people undergoing microdiscectomy, one had a dural leak and one had suspected discitis.[20] The second RCT included in the review did not report on the complications of either procedure.[21] Complication rates were reported inconsistently in studies, making it difficult to combine results to produce overall rates. Rates of complications for all types of discectomy have been compiled (see table 1, p 1125).[18]

Comment: The RCT of standard discectomy versus conservative treatment had considerable crossover between the two treatment groups. Of 66 people randomised to receive conservative treatment, 17 received surgery; of 60 people randomised to receive surgery, one refused the operation.[19] The results presented above are based on an intention to treat analysis.

OPTION MICRODISCECTOMY

We found no RCTs comparing microdiscectomy versus conservative treatment. Three RCTs found no significant difference in clinical outcomes with microdiscectomy versus standard discectomy. One RCT found no significant difference with video-assisted arthroscopic microdiscectomy versus standard discectomy in self reported satisfaction

or pain score after about 31 months. The duration of postoperative recovery with standard discectomy was almost twice that with arthroscopic discectomy. We found conflicting evidence on the effects of automated percutaneous discectomy versus microdiscectomy.

Benefits: We found no systematic review. **Versus conservative treatment:** We found no RCTs. **Versus standard discectomy:** See glossary, p 1123. See benefits of standard discectomy, p 1119. **Video-assisted arthroscopic microdiscectomy versus standard discectomy:** We found one RCT (60 people with proven lumbar disc herniation and associated radiculopathy after failed conservative treatment).[22] It found no significant difference between video-assisted arthroscopic discectomy versus standard discectomy in the number of people who were "very satisfied" on a 4-point satisfaction scale after about 31 months (22/30 [73%] with microdiscectomy [see glossary, p 1123] *v* 20/30 [67%] with standard discectomy ; RR 1.10, 95% CI 0.71 to 1.34). There was also no significant difference in mean pain score (visual analogue scale from 0 [no pain] to 10 [severe and incapacitating pain]: 1.9 with standard discectomy *v* 1.2 with microdiscectomy). However, the mean duration of postoperative recovery was almost twice as long with open surgery versus microdiscectomy (49 days *v* 27 days; P value not stated). **Versus automated percutaneous discectomy:** See glossary, p 1123. See benefits of automated percutaneous discectomy, p 1122.

Harms: **Video-assisted arthroscopic microdiscectomy versus open discectomy:** The RCT reported that one person undergoing open discectomy had leakage of spinal fluid from the dural sac 2 weeks postoperatively.[22] No other postoperative complications or neurovascular injuries were observed in either the standard discectomy or the microdiscectomy groups. Complication rates were reported inconsistently in studies, making it difficult to combine results to produce overall rates. Rates of complications for all types of discectomy have been compiled (see table 1, p 1125).[18]

Comment: None.

OPTION AUTOMATED PERCUTANEOUS DISCECTOMY

We found no RCTs comparing automated percutaneous discectomy versus either conservative treatment or standard discectomy. We found conflicting evidence on the effects of automated percutaneous discectomy versus microdiscectomy. One RCT found that automated percutaneous discectomy versus microdiscectomy was associated with significantly worse outcomes at interim analysis at 6 months, and was terminated prematurely. Another RCT comparing automated percutaneous discectomy versus microdiscectomy found similar investigator rated clinical scores, although participant rated improvement was higher with automated percutaneous discectomy after 2 years. One systematic review found that reoperation rates were higher with automated percutaneous discectomy than with either microdiscectomy or standard discectomy. One RCT in the review found that postoperative recovery was about three times shorter with automated percutaneous discectomy versus microdiscectomy.

Benefits: **Versus conservative treatment:** We found no systematic review or RCTs. **Versus standard discectomy:** One systematic review (search date not stated) identified no RCTs comparing automated percutaneous discectomy (APD) (see glossary, p 1123) versus standard discectomy (see glossary, p 1123).[18] **Versus microdiscectomy:** One systematic review (search date 1997) identified two RCTs that were not directly comparable because there were differences in the equipment used.[17] One RCT (71 people with radiographical confirmation of disc herniation) was stopped prematurely after an interim analysis at 6 months found that APD versus microdiscectomy (see glossary, p 1123) was associated with significantly lower success rate (overall outcome was classified as "success" or "failure" by the clinician and a masked observer [details not stated]: 9/31 [29%] with APD *v* 32/40 [80%] with microdisectomy; P < 0.001; CI not provided).[23] However, the other RCT (40 people with radiographical confirmation of disc herniation) reported similar improvements in the composite clinical score with APD versus microdiscectomy (scale 0–10, including back and leg pain, and sensory and motor deficit) at 2 years (preoperative scores: 4.55 with APD *v* 4.2 in microdiscectomy group; scores at 2 years: 8.23 with APD *v* 7.67 with microdiscectomy).[24] More people in the APD group rated their surgical outcomes as "excellent" or "good" than did those in the microdiscectomy group 2 years after surgery (14/20 [70%] with APD *v* 11/20 [55%] with microdiscectomy; P = 0.33).

Harms: The systematic review found that reoperations for recurrent or persistent disc herniations at the same level as the initial operations were reported more frequently in those who had APD versus either microdiscectomy or standard discectomy (APD 83%, 95% CI 76% to 88% *v* microdiscectomy 64%, 95% CI 48% to 78% *v* standard discectomy 49%, 95% CI 38% to 60%).[18] The first RCT did not report adverse effects.[23] The second RCT reported that no complications had occurred with APD, but did not comment on whether there had been any complications in the microdiscectomy group.[24] The mean duration of postoperative recovery was longer in people who had microdiscectomy compared with those who underwent APD (mean weeks of postoperative recovery [range]: 22.9 wks [4 wks to 1 year] for the microdiscectomy group *v* 7.7 wks [1–26 wks] for APD). Complication rates were reported inconsistently in studies, making it difficult to combine results to produce overall rates. Rates of complications for all types of discectomy have been compiled (see table 1, p 1125).[18]

Comment: None.

OPTION LASER DISCECTOMY

Systematic reviews found no RCTs on the effects of laser discectomy on disc herniations.

Benefits: Three systematic reviews (search dates 1997,[17] not stated,[18] and 2000[25]) found no RCTs on the effectiveness of laser discectomy.

Harms: We found no RCTs.

Comment: None.

GLOSSARY

Automated percutaneous discectomy Techniques using minimal skin incisions (generally several, all less than 3–5 mm) to allow small instruments to be inserted, using radiography to visualise these instruments, and using extensions for the surgeon to reach the operative site without having to dissect tissues.
Cauda equina A collection of spinal roots descending from the lower part of the spinal cord, which occupy the vertebral canal below the spinal cord.
Cauda equina syndrome Compression of the cauda equina causing symptoms, including changes in perineal sensation (saddle anaesthesia), and loss of sphincter control.
Laser discectomy The surgeon places a laser through a delivery device that has been directed under radiographic control to the disc, and removes the disc material using the laser. It uses many of the same techniques employed in automated percutaneous discectomy.
Microdiscectomy Removal of protruding disc material using various magnification techniques (i.e. an operating microscope).
Standard discectomy Surgical removal, in part or whole, of an intervertebral disc, generally with loop magnification (i.e. eyepieces).

REFERENCES

1. Fardon DF, Milette PC. Nomenclature and classification of lumbar disc pathology: recommendations of the Combined Task Forces of the North American Spine Society, American Society of Spine Radiology, and American Society of Neuroradiology. *Spine* 2001;26:E93–E113.
2. Boden SD. The use of radiographic imaging studies in the evaluation of patients who have degenerative disorders of the lumbar spine. *J Bone Joint Surg Am* 1996; 78:114–125.
3. Borenstein DG, O'Mara JW Jr, Boden SD, et al. The value of magnetic resonance imaging of the lumbar spine to predict low-back pain in asymptomatic subjects. *J Bone Joint Surg Am* 2001;83-A(9):1306–1311.
4. Andersson G. Epidemiology of spinal disorders. In: Frymoyer JW, Ducker TB, Hadler NM, et al. eds. *The adult spine: principles and practice*. New York, NY: Raven Press, 1997:93–141.
5. Heliovaara M. *Epidemiology of sciatica and herniated lumbar intervertebral disc*. Helsinki, Finland: The Social Insurance Institution, 1988.
6. Postacchini F, Cinotti G. Etiopathogenesis. In: Postacchini F, ed. *Lumbar disc herniation*. New York: Spring-Verlag/Wien, 1999
7. Friberg S, Hirsch C. Anatomical and clinical studies on lumbar disc degeneration. *Acta Orthop Scand* 1949;19:222–242.
8. Schultz A, Andersson G, Ortengren R, et al. Loads on the lumbar spine. *J Bone Joint Surg Am* 1982;64:713–720.
9. Jensen MC, Brant-Zawadzki MN, Obuchowski N, et al. Magnetic resonance imaging of the lumbar spine in people without back pain. *N Engl J Med* 1994;331:69–73.
10. Kelsey JL, Githens P, O'Connor T, et al. Acute prolapsed lumbar intervertebral disc: an epidemiologic study with special reference to driving automobiles and cigarette smoking. *Spine* 1984; 9:608–613.
11. Pedrini-Mille A, Weinstein JN, Found ME, et al. Stimulation of dorsal root ganglia and degradation of rabbit annulus fibrosus. *Spine* 1990;15:1252–1256.
12. Deyo RA, Weinstein JN. Low back pain. *N Engl J Med* 2001;344:365–370.
13. Vroomen PC, de Krom MC, Slofstra PD, et al. Conservative treatment of sciatica: a systematic review. *J Spinal Disord* 2000;13:463–469. Search date 1998; primary sources Medline and Embase/Excerpta Medica.
14. Buchner M, Zeifang F, Brocai DR, et al. Epidural corticosteroid injection in the conservative management of sciatica. *Clin Orthop* 2000;375:149–156.
15. Shekelle PG, Adams AH, Chassin MR, et al. Spinal manipulation for low-back pain. *Ann Intern Med* 1992;117:590–598. Search date not stated; primary sources Medline and Index Medicus 1952 onwards, reference lists, and consulted experts.
16. Liu J, Zhang S. Treatment of protrusion of lumbar intervertebral disc by pulling and turning manipulations. *J Tradit Chin Med* 2000;20:195–197.
17. Gibson JN, Grant IC, Waddell G. Surgery for lumbar disc prolapse (Cochrane Review). In: The Cochrane Library, Issue 1, 2002. Oxford: Update Software. Search date 1997; primary sources Medline, Embase, Biosis, dissertation abstracts, Index to UK Theses, Cochrane Controlled Trials Register, reference lists, personal bibliographies, and hand searched *Spine* 1975–1997.
18. Hoffman RM, Wheeler KJ, Deyo RA. Surgery for herniated lumbar discs: a literature synthesis. *J Gen Intern Med* 1993;8:487–496. Search date not stated; primary sources Medline, reference lists, book bibliographies, and colleagues' files.
19. Weber H. Lumbar disc herniation: a controlled, prospective study with ten years of observation. *Spine* 1983;8:131–140.
20. Tullberg T, Isacson J, Weidenhielm L. Does microscopic removal of lumber disc herniation lead to better results than the standard procedure? Results of a one-year randomized study. *Spine* 1993;18:24–27.
21. Henriksen L, Schmidt V, Eskesen V, et al. A controlled study of microsurgery versus standard lumbar discectomy. *Br J Neurosurg* 1996;10:289–293.
22. Hermantin FU, Peters T, Quartararo L, et al. A prospective, randomized study comparing the results of open discectomy with those of video-assisted arthroscopic microdiscectomy. *J Bone Joint Surg Am* 1999;81:958–965.
23. Chatterjee S, Foy PM, Findlay GF. Report of a controlled clinical trial comparing automated percutaneous lumbar discectomy and

microdiscectomy in the treatment of contained lumbar disc herniation. *Spine* 1995;20:734–738.
24. Mayer HM, Brock M. Percutaneous endoscopic discectomy: surgical technique and preliminary results compared to microdiscectomy. *J Neurosurg* 1993;78:216–225.
25. Boult M, Fraser RD, Jones N, et al. Percutaneous endoscopic laser discectomy. *Aust N Z J Surg* 2000;70:475–479. Search date 2000; primary sources Medline, Current Contents, Embase, and The Cochrane Library.

Jo Jordan
Systematic Reviewer
The Chartered Society of Physiotherapy
London
UK

Tamara Shawver Morgan
Chair, Orthopaedics, Dartmouth Medical School; Director, The Spine Center and the Center for Shared Decision-Making, Dartmouth-Hitchcock Medical Center; Co-Director, Dartmouth Clinical Trials Center, Dartmouth Medical School

James Weinstein
Dartmouth Medical School
Hanover, NH
USA

Competing interests: None declared.

TABLE 1 Reported complications from surgical procedures (see text, p 1120–1122).[18]

	Standard discectomy		Microdiscectomy		Percutaneous discectomy	
Complications	**Mean (% [95% CI])**	**Studies (n)***	**Mean (% [95% CI])**	**Studies (n)***	**Mean (% [95% CI])**	**Studies (n)***
Operative mortality	0.15 (0.09–0.24)	25	0.06 (0.01–0.42)	8	–	3
Total wound infections	1.97 (1.97–2.93)	25	1.77 (0.92–3.37)	16	–	2
Deep wound infections	0.34 (0.23–0.50)	17	0.06 (0.01–0.23)	8	–	2
Discitis	1.39 (0.97–2.01)	25	0.67 (0.44–1.02)	20	1.43 (0.42–4.78)	8
Dural tear	3.65 (1.99–6.65)	17	3.67 (2.03–6.58)	16	0.00	2
Total nerve root injuries	3.45 (2.21–5.36)	8	0.84 (0.24–2.92)	12	0.30 (0.11–0.79)	6
Permanent nerve root injuries	0.78 (0.42–1.45)	10	0.06 (0.00–0.26)	8	–	6
Thrombophlebitis	1.55 (0.78–1.30)	13	0.82 (0.49–1.35)	4	Not reported	0
Pulmonary emboli	0.56 (0.29–1.07)	14	0.44 (0.20–0.98)	5	Not reported	0
Meningitis	0.30 (0.15–0.60)	5	Not reported	0	Not reported	0
Cauda equina syndrome	0.22 (0.13–0.39)	3	Not reported	0	Not reported	0
Psoas haematoma	Not reported	0	Not reported	0	4.65 (1.17–15.5)	5
Transfusions	0.70 (0.19–2.58)	6	0.17 (0.08–0.39)	11	Not reported	0

*81 studies were included; 2 RCTs, 7 non-randomised controlled trials, 10 case control studies and 62 case series.

Hip fracture

Search date April 2002

William Gillespie

QUESTIONS

INTERVENTIONS

Covered elsewhere in *Clinical Evidence*

Fracture prevention, p 1089

Pressure sores, p 2021

See glossary, p 1145

Clin Evid 2002;8:1126–1148.

Key Messages

Surgical treatment

- **Arthroplasty for extracapsular fracture** One systematic review in people with unstable extracapsular hip fractures found limited evidence that arthroplasty versus internal fixation using a sliding hip screw did not significantly affect operating times, local wound complications, mortality, or mobility. Arthroplasty significantly increased the number of people who received a blood transfusion.
- **Arthroplasty for intracapsular fracture** One systematic review of randomised and observational studies, and five subsequent RCTs in people with displaced intracapsular fractures, found limited evidence that arthroplasty versus internal fixation significantly reduced the need for re-operation at 12–15 or 24 months after surgery, but significantly increased the number of deep infections and operative blood loss. Two of the subsequent RCTs found that arthroplasty versus internal fixation increased mortality.
- **Conservative (non-surgical) treatment of extracapsular fractures** One systematic review of people with extracapsular hip fractures comparing conservative versus operative treatment found limited evidence that operative treatment significantly reduced the number of people remaining in hospital after 12 weeks. The review found that conservative treatment significantly increased both leg shortening and varus deformity, but found insufficient evidence to determine whether any significant difference exists between treatments in medical complications, mortality, or long term pain.
- **Different types of implant for intracapsular fracture** One systematic review found insufficient evidence to determine the best implant for internal fixation of intracapsular fractures.
- **Intramedullary fixation with cephalocondylic nail versus extramedullary fixation for extracapsular fracture** One systematic review has found that cephalocondylic nails versus extramedullary fixation significantly reduce length of surgery, the incidence of deep wound sepsis, and operative blood loss. However, the review has also found that cephalocondylic nails significantly increase re-operation rates and the incidence of leg shortening and of external rotation deformity compared with extramedullary fixation.
- **Regional (versus general) anaesthesia for surgery** One systematic review of people after hip fracture surgery found limited evidence that regional versus general anaesthesia significantly reduced the risk of deep venous thrombosis, but had no significant effect on short term mortality.
- **Short cephalocondylic nail versus sliding hip screw for extracapsular fracture** One systematic review found no significant difference between intramedullary fixation with short cephalocondylic nail versus extramedullary fixation with sliding hip screw for pain at follow up, ability to return to a previous residence, and ability to walk after 3–12 months. The review also found no significant difference between treatments in mortality, wound infection, or fracture non-union, but found that cephalocondylic intramedullary fixation significantly increased intraoperative femoral fractures and re-operation rates.
- **Sliding hip screw device for internal fixation of extracapsular fracture** One systematic review found no significant difference with sliding hip screws versus fixed nail plates in mortality, pain at follow up, or impairment of mobility, but found that sliding hip screws significantly reduced the risk of fixation failure. It found limited evidence that a sliding hip screw versus the RAB fixed nail plate significantly increased the risk of leg shortening.

Hip fracture

Perioperative medical treatment

- **Cyclical compression of the foot or calf to reduce venous thromboembolism** One systematic review has found that cyclical compression devices (foot or calf pumps) significantly reduce deep venous thrombosis, but are associated with non-compliance and skin abrasion.
- **Graduated elastic compression to prevent venous thromboembolism** We found no RCTs in elderly people with hip fracture involving thromboembolism stockings for prevention of thrombotic complications. One systematic review in people undergoing elective total hip replacement has found that graduated elastic compression versus placebo significantly reduces the risk of deep venous thrombosis.
- **High specification versus standard hospital mattress on operating tables to prevent pressure sores** One systematic review has found that high specification foam mattresses and pressure relieving mattresses on operating tables versus standard hospital mattresses significantly reduce the number of pressure sores.
- **Nerve blocks for pain control before and after hip fracture** One systematic review of small RCTs and quasi-randomised trials found that nerve blocks significantly reduced total analgesic intake compared with no nerve block.
- **Nutritional supplementation after fracture** One systematic review in people who had undergone surgery for hip fracture found limited evidence that nutritional supplementation (oral protein and energy feeds) versus control significantly reduced postoperative complications.
- **Perioperative antibiotic prophylaxis** One systematic review has found that multiple dose perioperative and single dose preoperative antibiotic prophylaxis regimens versus control or no antibiotics significantly reduce infection after hip surgery.
- **Perioperative prophylaxis with antiplatelet agents** One systematic review has found that perioperative antiplatelet prophylaxis versus placebo or no prophylaxis significantly reduces the incidence of pulmonary embolism, but has no significant effect on the incidence of deep venous thrombosis. One subsequent RCT has found that aspirin versus placebo significantly reduces the incidence of both deep venous thrombosis and pulmonary embolism. The systematic review and subsequent RCT both found that antiplatelet treatment versus control significantly increases the risk of bleeding complications.
- **Perioperative prophylaxis with heparin to reduce venous thromboembolism** One systematic review has found that perioperative prophylaxis with either unfractionated heparin or low molecular weight heparin versus placebo or no treatment significantly reduces the incidence of deep venous thrombosis confirmed by imaging. The systematic review has also found that low molecular weight heparin versus unfractionated heparin significantly reduces deep venous thrombosis confirmed by imaging.
- **Preoperative bed traction to the injured limb** One systematic review found no significant difference in analgesic use or ease of fracture reduction with routine preoperative traction versus control. One RCT identified by the review found that skeletal versus skin traction significantly reduced analgesic use.

Rehabilitation programmes

- **Early supported discharge programmes** One systematic review of RCTs and observational studies has found that early supported discharge versus control significantly increases the number of people returning to their previous residence and reduces length of hospital stay, but significantly increases the frequency of readmission to hospital.

- **Geriatric hip fracture programmes in acute orthopaedic units** One systematic review of RCTs and observational studies, and one subsequent RCT in elderly people who have suffered hip fracture, found that geriatric hip fracture programmes versus control programmes significantly increased the number of people able to return to their previous residence, and significantly reduced morbidity whilst in hospital, but had no significant effect on mortality. The systematic review found that geriatric hip fracture programmes also reduced the length of hospital stay. Two additional RCTs found that a geriatrician led geriatric hip fracture programme versus control significantly reduced the incidence of severe delirium.
- **Specialised orthopaedic rehabilitation units for elderly people** One systematic review and one subsequent RCT found that rehabilitation in a geriatric outpatient rehabilitation unit versus control significantly increased the number of people able to return to their previous residence, although they found conflicting results on length of hospital stay. The systematic review found that geriatric outpatient rehabilitation units significantly reduced rates of readmission for acute care, but did not significantly reduce mortality or increase quality of life scores.
- **Systematic home based rehabilitation** One RCT comparing a systematic home based rehabilitation programme versus existing services found no significant difference in recovery to prefracture levels of self care, home management, social activity, balance, or lower extremity strength after 12 months.

DEFINITION Hip fracture is a fracture of the femur above a point 5 cm below the distal part of the lesser trochanter.[1] **Intracapsular fractures** occur proximal to the point at which the hip joint capsule attaches to the femur, and can be subdivided into displaced and undisplaced fractures. Undisplaced fractures include impacted or adduction fractures. Displaced intracapsular fractures may be associated with disruption of the blood supply to the head of the femur. Numerous subdivisions and classification methods exist for these fractures. In the most distal part of the proximal femoral segment (below the lesser trochanter), the term "subtrochanteric" is used. **Extracapsular fractures** occur distal to the hip joint capsule.

INCIDENCE/ PREVALENCE Hip fractures may occur at any age but are most common in elderly people. In industrialised societies, the lifetime risk of hip fracture is about 18% in women and 6% in men.[2] A recent study reported that prevalence increases from about 3/100 women aged 65–74 years to 12.6/100 women aged 85 years and above.[3] The age stratified incidence has also increased in some societies during the past 25 years; not only are people living longer, but the incidence of fracture in each age group may have increased.[4]

AETIOLOGY/ RISK FACTORS Hip fractures are usually sustained through a fall from standing height or less. The pattern of incidence is consistent with two main risk factors: increased risk of falling and loss of skeletal strength from osteoporosis. Both are associated with aging.

PROGNOSIS One in five people die in the first year after a hip fracture,[5] and one in four elderly people require a higher level of long term care after a fracture.[5,6] Those who do return to live in the community after a hip fracture have greater difficulty with activities of daily living than age and sex matched controls.[3]

AIMS To improve survival and quality of life; and to minimise complications and disability associated with hip fracture.

OUTCOMES Incidence of preoperative, operative, and postoperative complications (infection, venous thromboembolism, re-fracture, fixation failure, pressure sores, medical complications); proportion of people returning to previous residential and mobility status; rates of readmission to hospital and re-operation; measures of mobility and competence in activities of daily living; health related quality of life measures.

METHODS *Clinical Evidence* search and appraisal April 2002. We also scanned the bibliographies of included studies for additional references, contacted known trialists for up-to-date information, and included relevant results from Cochrane Library 2002, issue 2.

QUESTION **What are the effects of surgical interventions in the treatment of hip fracture?**

OPTION **REGIONAL VERSUS GENERAL ANAESTHESIA FOR HIP FRACTURE SURGERY**

One systematic review of people after hip fracture surgery found limited evidence that general versus regional anaesthesia significantly reduced the risk of deep venous thrombosis, but had no significant effect on short term mortality.

Benefits: We found one systematic review (search date 2000, 17 RCTs, 2305 people) comparing regional versus general anaesthesia.[7] The review found that regional anaesthesia significantly reduced the risk of deep venous thrombosis (3 RCTs; 39/129 [30%] with regional anaesthesia *v* 61/130 [47%] with general anaesthesia; RR 0.64, 95% CI 0.48 to 0.86; NNT 6, 95% CI 4 to 19; see comment below), although regional anaesthesia had no significant effect on mortality at 1 month (53/781 [7%] with regional anaesthesia *v* 78/826 [9%] with general anaesthesia; RR 0.72, 95% CI 0.51 to 1.00). Too few people were seen at 1 year follow up to confirm any long term benefit.

Harms: Regional anaesthesia was associated with marginally longer operation time (WMD 4.8 min, 95% CI 1.1 min to 8.6 min).[7]

Comment: Although the review indicated a significant reduction in risk of deep venous thrombosis, the three contributing RCTs had methodological limitations (probable selection and performance biases).[7] Therefore, this association may be insecure.

OPTION CHOICE OF IMPLANT FOR INTERNAL FIXATION OF INTRACAPSULAR HIP FRACTURES

One systematic review found insufficient evidence to determine the best implant for internal fixation of intracapsular fractures.

Benefits: We found one systematic review (search date 2000, 27 RCTs, 5269 people with intracapsular hip fractures) comparing different types of internal fixation (see glossary, p 1145) implants versus each other.[8] The authors grouped data to assess 18 comparisons; the numbers of participants in each comparison was insufficient to let a confident conclusion on the relative performance of individual implants.

Harms: The review found no evidence on harms associated with different types of internal fixation implant.[8]

Comment: None.

OPTION ARTHROPLASTY VERSUS INTERNAL FIXATION FOR INTRACAPSULAR HIP FRACTURES

One systematic review of randomised and observational studies and five subsequent RCTs in people with displaced intracapsular fractures found limited evidence that arthroplasty versus internal fixation significantly reduced the need for re-operation, but significantly increased the number of deep infections and blood loss. Two of the subsequent RCTs found that arthroplasty versus internal fixation increased mortality. Two RCTs comparing unipolar hemiarthroplasty versus bipolar hemiarthroplasty found conflicting results for mobility.

Benefits: **Arthroplasty versus internal fixation:** We found one systematic review (search date 1997, 1 RCT, 105 non-randomised studies in people aged > 65 years with a displaced intracapsular fracture),[9] and five subsequent RCTs[10–14] comparing arthroplasty (see glossary, p 1145) versus internal fixation (see glossary, p 1145). The review found that internal fixation versus arthroplasty significantly reduced the need for re-operation when assessed 12–15 months after surgery (1 RCT, 2 non-randomised studies; 36/285 [12.6%] with arthroplasty *v* 75/170 [44%] with internal fixation; RR 0.29, 95% CI 0.20 to 0.45) and 24 months after surgery (2 non-randomised studies; 26/144 [18%] with arthroplasty *v* 61/194 [31%] with internal fixation; RR 0.57, 95% CI 0.38 to 0.86), but significantly increased the number of deep infections (absolute numbers not provided).[9] The review also found no significant differences between treatments in mortality, mobility, deep vein thrombosis, or pulmonary embolism.[9] No health related quality of life results were available. Of the five subsequent RCTs, four reported comparisons between internal fixation and hemiarthroplasty,[10,12–14] and three reported comparisons between internal fixation and total hip arthroplasty.[10,11,13] All four RCTs found that arthroplasty versus internal fixation significantly reduced re-operation rates, but that arthroplasty versus internal fixation significantly increased blood loss. Two of the subsequent RCTs found that arthroplasty versus internal fixation increased mortality.[10,12] **Unipolar versus bipolar hemiarthroplasty:** We found no systematic review but found two RCTs comparing unipolar (see glossary, p 1146) versus bipolar hemiarthroplasty (see glossary, p 1145).[15,16] The first RCT (250 people aged > 80 years) found that unipolar hemiarthroplasty significantly increased the number of people who returned to preinjury residential status after 2 years (absolute numbers not provided; OR 1.94, 95% CI 1.03 to 3.67).[15] The second RCT (48 people, mean age 77 years) found that bipolar hemiarthroplasty improved performance in a 6 m walk after 6 months (unipolar 1.93 feet/s, range 1.16–3.30 *v* bipolar 2.67 feet/s, range 0.77–4.86; significance testing not possible).[16]

Harms: See benefits of arthroplasty above

Comment: None.

OPTION CONSERVATIVE VERSUS OPERATIVE TREATMENT FOR EXTRACAPSULAR HIP FRACTURES

One systematic review of people with extracapsular hip fractures comparing conservative versus operative treatment found limited evidence that operative treatment reduced time spent in hospital. The review found that conservative versus operative treatment significantly increased both leg shortening and varus deformity, but found insufficient evidence to determine whether any significant difference exists between treatments in medical complications, mortality, or long term pain.

Benefits: We found one systematic review (search date 2001, 5 RCTs).[17] Only one RCT (106 people) included in the review used a fixation device with the dynamic features used in contemporary practice (sliding nail plate). This RCT found that operative versus conservative treatment significantly reduced the number of people remaining in hospital after 12 weeks (11/55 [20%] with operative treatment *v* 20/51 [39%] with conservative treatment; RR 0.51, 95% CI 0.27 to 0.96).[17]

Harms: The RCT identified by the review found that conservative versus operative treatment significantly increased the number of people with leg shortening (29/39 [74%] with conservative treatment *v* 11/37 [30%] with operative treatment; RR 2.5, 95% CI 1.47 to 4.24; NNH 2, 95% CI 1 to 3) and varus deformity (see glossary, p 1146) (19/39 [49%] with conservative treatment *v* 3/35 [9%] with operative treatment; RR 5.7, 95% CI 1.8 to 17.6; NNH 2, 95% CI 1 to 4).[17] The review found insufficient evidence to determine whether any significant difference exists between treatments in medical complications, mortality, or long term pain.

Comment: Operative treatment was introduced in the 1950s with the expectation of improved functional outcome and reduced incidence of complications of immobilisation and prolonged bed rest. Although we found only limited evidence from RCTs about short term benefits of operation, the additional benefits of early mobilisation and early supported discharge (see benefits of early supported discharge programmes, p 1144) can be realised only after surgery.

OPTION ARTHROPLASTY VERSUS INTERNAL FIXATION FOR EXTRACAPSULAR FRACTURES

One systematic review in people with unstable extracapsular hip fractures found limited evidence that arthroplasty versus internal fixation using a sliding hip screw did not significantly affect operating times, local wound complications, mortality, or mobility, but that arthroplasty significantly increased the number of people who received a blood transfusion.

Benefits: We found one systematic review (search date 2001, 1 RCT, 90 people with unstable extracapsular hip fractures), which compared arthroplasty versus internal fixation using a sliding hip screw (see glossary, p 1146).[18] The review found no significant difference in operating times (inadequate data reported), local wound complications (3/41 [7%] with arthroplasty *v* 5/43 [12%] with internal fixation; RR 0.63, 95% CI 0.16 to 2.47), or mortality (12/43 [28%] with arthroplasty *v* 11/47 [23%] with internal fixation; RR 1.19, 95% CI 0.59 to 2.42) after 12 months. It also found no significant difference in the number of previously independent people who had lost ambulatory independence at discharge from hospital (12/30 [40%] with arthroplasty *v* 14/28 [50%] with internal fixation; RR 0.80, 95% CI 0.45 to 1.42).

Harms: The review found that arthroplasty versus internal fixation using a sliding hip screw significantly increased the number of people who received a blood transfusion (34/43 [79%] with arthroplasty *v* 27/47 [57%] with internal fixation; RR 1.38, 95% CI 1.03 to 1.84; NNH 4, 95% CI 2 to 21).[18]

Comment: The RCT identified by the review had limited methods (the method of randomisation was not specified, there was no blinding, analysis was not by intention to treat, and the outcome measures were not defined clearly), which may affect the generalisability of the results.[18]

OPTION DYNAMIC (SLIDING) VERSUS FIXED EXTRAMEDULLARY FIXATION FOR EXTRACAPSULAR HIP FRACTURE

One systematic review in people with extracapsular hip fractures found no significant difference with sliding hip screws versus fixed nail plates in mortality, pain at follow up, or impairment of mobility and found limited evidence that a sliding hip screw versus the RAB fixed nail plate significantly increased the risk of leg shortening. The review also found that sliding hip screws versus fixed nail plates significantly increased the risk of fixation failure.

Benefits: We found one systematic review (search date 2001).[19] Three RCTs (355 people) identified by the review compared a sliding hip screw (see glossary, p 1146) versus Jewett or McLaughlin fixed nail plate (see glossary, p 1145). One RCT (100 people) identified by the review compared a sliding hip screw versus the Pugh nail plate. The review found no significant difference in mortality (1 RCT: 9/51 [18%] with a sliding hip screw *v* 11/47 [23%] with a fixed nail plate; RR 0.75, 95% CI 0.34 to 1.66), pain at follow up (1 RCT: 4/42 [9%] with a sliding hip screw *v* 7/36 [19%] with a fixed nail plate; RR 0.49, 95% CI 0.16 to 1.54), or impairment of mobility (1 RCT:

11/42 [26%] with a sliding hip screw *v* 15/36 [42%] with a fixed nail plate; RR 0.63, 95% CI 0.33 to 1.20).[19] Two RCTs (433 people) identified by the review compared a sliding hip screw versus a RAB fixed nail plate (see glossary, p 1145) (see comment below). The review found that fixation with the RAB plate significantly decreased the risk of leg shortening (1 RCT: 186 people; RR for shortening 0.20, 95% CI 0.7 to 0.53).[14] The review also reported that a sliding hip screw significantly reduced operative blood loss compared with the Medoff fixed nail plate (1 RCT: 178 people; figures not stated). However, the Medoff sliding plate reduced fixation failure compared with the sliding hip screw (2 RCTs: 274 people; AR for fixation failure 2% with fixed nail plate *v* 9% with sliding hip screw, RR 0.23, 95% CI 0.08 to 0.64).

Harms: The review found that the use of a sliding hip screw versus Jewett or McLaughlin fixed nail plates significantly reduced the risk of fixation failure (12/83 [14%] with sliding hip screw *v* 38/62 [61%] with fixed nail plate; RR 0.24 95% CI 0.14 to 0.41).[19] The review also found that a sliding hip screw versus the Medoff fixed nail plate (1 RCT, 178 people) was reported to be associated with significantly lower operative blood loss, but statistical analysis was not available.

Comment: The two RCTs identified by the review comparing a sliding hip screw versus the RAB fixed nail plate found contrasting results in terms of operative complications and fixation failure.[19] This device remains of unproved value.

OPTION SHORT CEPHALOCONDYLIC NAILS VERSUS SLIDING HIP SCREW FOR EXTRACAPSULAR HIP FRACTURE

One systematic review has found no significant difference with short cephalocondylic intramedullary fixation versus sliding hip screw in pain at follow up, ability to return to a previous residence, and ability to walk. The review also found no significant difference between treatments in mortality, wound infection, or fracture non-union, but found that cephalocondylic intramedullary fixation significantly increases intraoperative femoral fractures and re-operation rates.

Benefits: We found one systematic review (search date 2001, 26 RCTs, 3610 people)[20] The review compared short cephalocondylic nails (see glossary, p 1145) (from different manufacturers) versus sliding hip screws (see glossary, p 1146) and found no significant difference in the number of people reporting pain at follow up (7 RCTs: 113/364 [31%] with nail *v* 106/307 [34%] with a sliding hip screw; RR 0.9, 95% CI 0.72 to 1.12), failing to return to previous residence (8 RCTs: 198/458 [43%] with nail *v* 207/488 [42%] with a sliding hip screw; RR 1.02, 95% CI 0.88 to 1.18), or impaired walking (6 RCTs: 180/377 [48%] with nail *v* 193/388 [50%] with a sliding hip screw; RR 0.96, 95% CI 0.83 to 1.11) after 3–12 months.[20] The review also found that the use of a short cephalocondylic intramedullary nail versus a sliding hip screw significantly reduced radiological screening time (a measure of radiation exposure; WMD nail *v* sliding hop screw –22.6 s, 95% CI –25.7 s to –19.5 s).

Harms: The review compared short cephalocondylic nails versus sliding hip screws and found no significant difference in mortality (18 RCTs: 240/1227 [20%] with nail *v* 251/1249 [20%] with a sliding hip screw; RR 0.97, 95% CI 0.83 to 1.13), incidence of deep wound infection (12 RCTs: 11/910 [1.2%] with nail *v* 9/912 [0.98%] with a sliding hip screw; RR 1.20, 95% CI 0.54 to 2.64), or fracture non-union (11 RCTs; 5/687 [0.7%] with nail *v* 5/698 [0.7%] with sliding hip screw; RR 1.01, 95% CI 0.36 to 2.84).[20] However, it found that the short cephalocondylic nail was associated with an increased risk of fracture of the femur during the operative procedure (18 RCTs, 27/1359 [2%] with nail *v* 4/1370 [0.3%] with sliding hip screw; RR 6.8, 95% CI 2.39 to 19.4) or later (19 RCTs, 36/1285 [2.8%] with nail *v* 2/1289 [0.16%] with sliding hip screw; RR 18, 95% CI 4.36 to 74.8), and an increased re-operation rate (74/1275 [5.8%] with nail *v* 43/1297 [3.3%] with sliding hip screw; RR 1.71, 95% CI 1.20 to 2.45).

Comment: We found no evidence that the theoretical mechanical advantages of intramedullary cephalocondylic devices for operative fixation of extracapsular hip fractures have so far been confirmed or rejected. The designs tested have been associated with higher risk of fracture fixation complications than alternative devices. The evidence refers to extracapsular hip fractures in the trochanteric region and may not apply to people with subtrochanteric fractures.

OPTION CEPHALOCONDYLIC NAILS VERSUS EXTRAMEDULLARY FIXATION FOR EXTRACAPSULAR HIP FRACTURE

One systematic review has found that cephalocondylic nails versus extramedullary fixation significantly reduce length of surgery, the incidence of deep wound sepsis, and operative blood loss. The review has also found that cephalocondylic nails significantly increase re-operation rates, the incidence of leg shortening, and of external rotation deformity.

Benefits: We found one systematic review (search date 1999, 11 RCTs, 1667 people), which compared cephalocondylic nails (see glossary, p 1145) versus extramedullary fixation.[21] It found that cephalocondylic nails significantly reduced the length of surgery (326 people: WMD –22.8 min, 95% CI –27.7 min to –17.8 min).

Harms: The review found that cephalocondylic nails versus extramedullary fixation significantly increased the risk of re-operation for fixation failure (8 RCTs: 118/564 [21%] with cephalocondylic nails *v* 31/566 [5%] with extramedullary fixation; RR 3.72, 95% CI 2.54 to 5.44), the incidence of leg shortening (7 RCTs: 44/401 [11%] with cephalocondylic nails *v* 19/442 [4%] extramedullary fixation; RR 2.71, 95% CI 1.65 to 4.59), and the incidence of external rotation deformity (5 RCTs: 86/345 [25%] with cephalocondylic nails *v* 28/396 [7%] with extramedullary fixation; RR 3.73, 95% CI 2.47 to 5.64).[21] However, the review also found that cephalocondylic nails significantly reduced the incidence of deep wound sepsis (5/554 [< 1%] with cephalocondylic nails *v* 23/549 [4%] with extramedullary fixation; RR 0.26, 95% CI 0.11 to 0.62) and significantly reduced operative blood loss (326 people: WMD –208 mL, 95% CI –262 to –154 mL).

Comment: None.

QUESTION What are the effects of perisurgical medical interventions on surgical outcome and prevention of complications?

OPTION TEMPORARY TRACTION BEFORE SURGERY FOR HIP FRACTURE

One systematic review has found no significant difference between routine preoperative traction versus control in analgesic use or ease of fracture reduction. One RCT identified by the review found that skeletal versus skin traction significantly reduced analgesic use.

Benefits: We found one systematic review (search date 2001, 7 RCTs, 1038 people with recent hip fracture), which compared traction versus control.[6] It found no significant difference in the number of people requiring analgesia in the 24 hours after admission (1 RCT: 54/101 [53%] with traction *v* 71/151 [47%] with control; RR 1.14, 95% CI 0.89 to 1.46), in the number of people requiring analgesia before surgery (1 RCT: 45/50 [90%] with traction *v* 39/50 [78%] with control; RR 2.42, 95% CI 0.84 to 7.01), or the difficulty of fracture reduction at time of surgery (1 RCT: 5/45 [11%] with traction *v* 7/64 [11%] with control; RR 1.02, 95% CI 0.34 to 3.00).[6] One RCT identified by the review comparing skeletal versus skin traction found that skeletal traction significantly reduced the mean number of analgesic doses required (1 RCT: skin traction 40 people, mean 2.5 doses, standard deviation 1.6 *v* skeletal traction 38 people, mean 1.7, standard deviation 1.4; WMD 0.80, 95% CI 0.13 to 1.46).

Harms: Two of the RCTs identified by the review compared skeletal traction versus skin traction. Although no important difference was identified between these two methods, initial skeletal traction was more painful.[6]

Comment: None.

OPTION NERVE BLOCKS FOR PAIN CONTROL BEFORE AND AFTER HIP FRACTURE

One systematic review found limited evidence that nerve blocks reduced total analgesic intake compared with no nerve block. One small RCT identified by the review found that femoral nerve block versus control significantly reduced the incidence of respiratory infections.

Benefits: We found one systematic review (search date 2001, 8 RCTs or quasi-randomised trials, 328 people with recent hip fracture; see comment below).[22] Two small RCTs identified by the review compared nerve block versus no nerve block at hospital admission, and the remaining five trials compared perioperative nerve block versus no nerve block. Nerve block was associated with reduced use of parenteral or oral analgesia to control pain from the fracture, operation, or during surgery. The review found that nerve block versus control significantly reduced the number of people requiring analgesia (lateral cutaneous nerve block with subcostal block, 2 trials: 19/26 [73%] with block *v* 25/25 [100%] with control; RR 0.73, 95% CI 0.58 to 0.92; lateral cutaneous nerve block alone, 1 trial: 7/17 [41%] with block v 16/16 [100%] without block; RR 0.41, 95% CI 0.23 to 0.73; triple nerve block, 1 trial: 13/25 [52%] with block v 22/24 [92%] with control; RR 0.57, 95% CI 0.38 to 0.84). It is not clear whether this reduction in analgesia was associated with clinical benefit. Administration of a psoas nerve block at time of admission to hospital significantly reduced complaints of unsatisfactory pain control, measured on a visual analogue scale both preoperatively (RR 0.25, 95% CI 0.08 to 0.75) and postoperatively (RR 0.10, 95% CI 0.01 to 0.71). A single small RCT identified by the review found that femoral nerve block at time of admission to hospital versus control significantly reduced the incidence of respiratory infections (2/25 [8%] with nerve block v 11/25 [44%] with control; RR 0.18, 95% CI 0.04 to 0.74).

Harms: None reported.

Comment: The trials were small, used different types of nerve blocks, and had varying times of insertion. It is unclear whether nerve blocks confer any benefit compared with other methods of analgesia in hip fracture. The possible reduction of respiratory infection is worthy of further study.

OPTION PERIOPERATIVE ANTIBIOTICS

One systematic review has found that multiple dose perioperative and single dose preoperative antibiotic prophylaxis regimens versus control or no antibiotics significantly reduce infection after hip surgery.

Benefits: **Multiple dose perioperative antibiotic regimens:** We found one systematic review (search date 2000, 11 RCTs, 1896 people with recent hip fracture), which compared multiple dose antibiotic regimens versus control or no prophylaxis.[23] The review found that antibiotics significantly reduced the incidence of deep wound infection (12/961 [1%] with antibiotic v 40/935 [4%] with control; RR 0.29, 95% CI 0.15 to 0.55), superficial wound infection (22/705 [3%] with antibiotic v 38/661 [6%] with control; RR 0.48, 95% CI 0.28 to 0.81), and urinary tract infection (31/259 [12%] with antibiotic v 44/241 [18%] with control; RR 0.66, 95% CI 0.43 to 1.00).[23] The review found that multiple dose perioperative antibiotic regimens did not significantly reduce the incidence of respiratory tract infections (14/259 [5%] with antibiotic v 16/241 [7%] with control; RR 0.81, 95% CI 0.41 to 1.63). **Single dose preoperative antibiotic regimens:** We found one systematic review (search date 2000, 7 RCTs, 3500 people with recent hip fracture, including 2195 people from one multicentre trial).[23] It found that single dose preoperative prophylaxis versus placebo or no treatment significantly reduced deep wound infection (20/1745 [1%] with antibiotic v 51/1755 [< 1%] with control; RR 0.41, 95% CI 0.25 to 0.65), superficial wound infection (59/1745 [3%] with antibiotic v 87/1755 [5%] with control; RR 0.69, 95% CI 0.50 to 0.95), urinary tract infection (131/1493 [9%] with antibiotic v 212/1482 [14%] with control; RR 0.63, 95% CI 0.53 to 0.76), and respiratory infection (41/1493 [3%] with antibiotic v 92/1482 [6%] with control; RR 0.46, 95% CI 0.33 to 0.65).

Harms: The systematic review found that adverse effects (allergy, rashes, gastrointestinal complaints) were rarely reported but were more common in people given multiple dose perioperative antibiotics, although the difference was not significant (24/520 [5%] with antibiotic *v* 12/362 [3%] with control; RR 1.83, 95% CI 0.96 to 3.50).[23]

Comment: Many different antimicrobials were studied (all active against *Staphylococcus aureus*). The absolute risk reduction with single dose regimens was not significantly less than with multiple dose regimens.

OPTION UNFRACTIONATED HEPARIN AND LOW MOLECULAR WEIGHT HEPARIN

One systematic review has found that perioperative prophylaxis with either unfractionated heparin or low molecular weight heparin versus placebo or no treatment significantly reduces the incidence of deep venous thrombosis confirmed by imaging. The review has also found that low molecular weight heparin versus unfractionated heparin significantly reduces deep venous thrombosis. We found insufficient evidence to confirm the effect on pulmonary thromboembolism or postphlebitic leg.

Benefits: We found one systematic review (search date 2000, 22 RCTs in elderly people undergoing surgery for hip fracture).[24] Overall, trial quality was poor. **Heparin versus placebo or no treatment:** The review identified 10 RCTs that compared unfractionated heparin versus placebo or no treatment and four RCTs that compared low molecular weight heparin (LMWH) versus placebo or no treatment.[24] The review found significantly fewer lower limb deep vein thromboses (identified by imaging) with unfractionated heparin (103/407 [25%] with unfractionated heparin *v* 166/409 [41%] with control; RR 0.59, 95% CI 0.49 to 0.72; NNT 7, 95% CI 5 to 12) and with LMWH (18/104 [17%] with heparin *v* 37/110 [34%] with control; RR 0.55, 95% CI 0.34 to 0.88; NNT 7, 95% CI 4 to 19). **Unfractionated heparin versus LMWH:** The review identified five RCTs that compared unfractionated heparin versus LMWH. It found that LMWH significantly reduced deep venous thrombosis confirmed by imaging (47/252 [19%] with LMWH *v* 64/227 [28%] with unfractionated heparin; RR 0.67, 95% CI 0.48 to 0.94; NNT 11, 95% CI 6 to 50).[24]

Harms: The review found a non-significant increase in overall mortality after hip fracture in the group receiving heparin (46/420 [11%] with heparin *v* 35/423 [8%] with control; RR 1.31, 95% CI 0.88 to 1.97).[24] One systematic review (search date not stated) summarised the risk of bleeding or transfusion in all RCTs of prophylactic subcutaneous unfractionated heparin in general, orthopaedic, and urological surgery.[25] Overall, excessive bleeding or need for transfusion was significantly increased with heparin (419/7027 [6%] with heparin *v* 244/6504 [< 1%] with control; OR 1.66). Another systematic review (search date 1991) included comparisons of unfractionated heparin and LMWH in general and orthopaedic surgery, and found insufficient evidence from published RCTs to confirm a difference in the rate of bleeding complications.[26]

Comment: We found no RCTs that reported the incidence of postphlebitic leg or wound complications.

OPTION ANTIPLATELET AGENTS

One systematic review has found that antiplatelet prophylaxis versus placebo or no prophylaxis significantly reduces the incidence of pulmonary embolism, but does not significantly affect the incidence of deep venous thrombosis. One subsequent RCT has found that aspirin versus placebo significantly reduces the incidence of both deep venous thrombosis and pulmonary embolism. The review and subsequent RCT have both found that antiplatelet treatment versus control significantly increases the risk of bleeding complications.

Benefits: We found one systematic review (search date 1990, 898 people)[27] and one subsequent large multicentre RCT (13 356 people having surgery for hip fracture).[28] The review compared prophylaxis with an antiplatelet agent versus placebo or no prophylaxis after fracture.[27] Most people in the review had a hip fracture. It found that antiplatelet prophylaxis had no significant effect on the incidence of deep venous thrombosis (163/454 [36%] with antiplatelet prophylaxis *v* 186/444 [42%] with control; RR 0.9, 95% CI 0.73 to 1.01), but significantly reduced the incidence of pulmonary embolism (14/504 [3%] with antiplatelet prophylaxis *v* 34/494 [7%] with control; RR 0.40, 95% CI 0.22 to 0.74; NNT 25, 95% CI 15 to 78).[27] The subsequent RCT compared antiplatelet treatment using aspirin versus placebo. Treatment was started preoperatively and continued for 35 days.[28] The RCT found that aspirin significantly reduced the incidence of symptomatic deep vein thrombosis (69/6679 [1.0%] with aspirin *v* 97/6677 [1.5%] with placebo; RR 0.71, 95% CI 0.52 to 0.97), of venous thromboembolism (symptomatic deep vein thrombosis or non-fatal pulmonary embolism, 87/6679 [1.3%] with aspirin *v* 122/6677 [1.8%] with control; RR 0.71, 95% CI 0.54 to 0.94), and of fatal pulmonary embolism (18/6679 [< 1%] with aspirin *v* 43/6677 [< 1%] with control; RR 0.42, 95% CI 0.24 to 0.73).[28]

Harms: The systematic review summarised the bleeding complications reported across all surgical procedures.[27] Fatal bleeds were rare (2/4441 [< 1%] with antiplatelet treatment *v* 0/4450 [0%] with control). The review found that antiplatelet treatment versus control or no antiplatelet treatment significantly increased the number of blood transfusions (28/2798 [1%] with antiplatelet treatment *v* 15/3808 [< 1%] with control; RR 2.5, 95% CI 1.36 to 4.75) and other bleeding related complications (re-operation, haematoma, or infection because of a bleed; 177/2269 [8%] with antiplatelet treatment *v* 129/2306 [6%] with control; RR 1.20, 95% CI 1.12 to 1.74). The subsequent RCT found that fatal bleeds were also rare (13/6679 [< 1%] with aspirin *v* 15/6677 [< 1%] with control), but that aspirin versus placebo significantly increased the number of non-fatal gastrointestinal bleeds (182/6679 [3%] with aspirin *v* 122/6677 [2%] with control; RR 1.50, 95% CI 1.19 to 1.87).[28]

Comment: None.

OPTION **GRADUATED ELASTIC COMPRESSION (THROMBOEMBOLISM STOCKINGS)**

We found no RCTs in elderly people with hip fracture involving thromboembolism stockings for prevention of thrombotic complications. One systematic review in people undergoing elective total hip replacement has found that graduated elastic compression versus placebo significantly reduces the risk of deep venous thrombosis.

Benefits: We found one systematic review (search date 1998), which found no RCTs in people with hip fracture.[29] The review pooled data from four RCTs in people undergoing elective total hip replacement.[29] The review found that graduated elastic compression versus control significantly reduced deep venous thrombosis (32/125 [26%] with stockings *v* 61/111 [55%] with control; RR 0.43, 95% CI 0.30 to 0.61; NNT 4, 95% CI 3 to 6). A second systematic review (search date 1999) included two of the four RCTs reported in the earlier review but did not present a separate analysis for lower limb surgery.[30]

Harms: The first review reported that manufacturers of stockings advise against their use in people with an ankle : brachial pressure of less than 0.7. People with peripheral arterial disease or with diabetes and neuropathy were stated to be at higher risk of worsening ischaemia, but we found no evidence in RCTs to measure this risk.

Comment: It is unclear whether extrapolation from elective hip replacement studies is appropriate for hip fracture.

OPTION **CYCLICAL COMPRESSION OF THE FOOT OR CALF**

One systematic review has found that cyclical compression devices (foot or calf pumps) significantly reduce deep venous thrombosis in people with hip fracture. Problems with skin abrasion and compliance have been reported.

Benefits: We found one systematic review (search date 2000, 4 RCTs, 442 people) comparing cyclical compression of the calf or foot using mechanical pumping devices versus no compression.[24] The review found that cyclical compression versus no compression significantly reduced the risk of deep venous thrombosis (12/202 [6%] with compression *v* 42/212 [20%] with control; RR 0.30, 95% CI 0.17 to 0.53). We found no adequate evidence about any effect on the incidence of pulmonary embolism or overall mortality.

Harms: Problems with skin abrasion and compliance were reported in all four RCTs of cyclical compression devices.

Comment: None.

OPTION **BEDS, MATTRESSES, AND CUSHIONS FOR PREVENTING PRESSURE SORES**

One systematic review has found that high specification foam mattresses and pressure relieving mattresses on operating tables versus standard hospital mattresses significantly reduce the number of pressure sores.

Benefits: We found one systematic review (search date 2000), which found that high specification foam mattresses versus "standard hospital" mattresses significantly reduced the number of pressure sores (4 RCTs, 52/678 [8%] with high specification *v* 57/172 [33%] with standard; RR 0.29, 95% CI 0.19 to 0.43).[31] The review identified three RCTs that compared different methods of pressure relief for people on the operating table.[31] It found that viscoelastic polymer (gel) pad versus a standard operating table significantly reduced the number of postoperative pressure sores (22/205 [11%] with gel pad *v* 43/211 [20%] with standard table; RR 0.53, 95% CI 0.33 to 0.85; ARR 9.6%; NNT 11, 95% CI 7 to 37). The review also identified two RCTs that compared an alternating pressure system (applied during and after surgery) versus control (a gel pad used during surgery plus standard mattress after surgery).[31] It found that the use of alternating pressure significantly reduced the number of pressure sores (3/188 [2%] with alternating pressure *v* 14/180 [8%] with control; RR 0.21, 95% CI 0.06 to 0.7; ARR 6.2%; NNT 17, 95% CI 10 to 83).

Harms: None identified.

Comment: None.

OPTION **NUTRITIONAL SUPPLEMENTATION AFTER HIP FRACTURE**

One systematic review in people who had undergone surgery for hip fracture found limited evidence that nutritional supplementation (oral protein and energy feeds) versus control significantly reduces complications after surgery for hip fracture.

Benefits: We found one systematic review (search date 2000, 15 RCTs, 1054 people).[32] Six RCTs identified by the review found that oral multinutrient feeds (providing non-protein energy, protein, some vitamins and minerals) versus control significantly reduced the overall incidence of complications by the end of the study (14/66 [21%] with multinutrient feeds *v* 26/73 [36%] with control; RR 0.52, 95% CI 0.32 to 0.84), but did not significantly affect mortality (12/91 [13%] with multinutrient feeds *v* 14/97 [14%] with control; RR 0.85, 95% CI 0.42 to 1.70). Three RCTs identified by the review found that nasogastric multinutrient feeding versus control had no significant effect on mortality (RR 0.99, 95% CI 0.50 to 1.97), but the studies included people with differing characteristics. Three RCTs identified by the review found that protein versus no protein in an oral feed significantly reduced unfavourable outcomes (complications or mortality combined; 66/113 [58%] with protein *v* 82/110 [75%] with no protein; RR 0.78, 95% CI 0.65 to 0.95), but had no significant effect on mortality alone. Two RCTs identified by the review (one testing intravenous thiamine and other water soluble vitamins and the other testing alfacalcidol) found no evidence of benefit for either vitamin supplement.

Harms: We found little evidence about harms. Nasogastric feeds were sometimes tolerated poorly. Complications, described in only one RCT identified by the review, included bloating and anorexia. We found no reports of feed induced diarrhoea or aspiration pneumonia.

Comment: The quality of trials reported in the review was poor. Defects included inadequate numbers of people, methodological problems (inadequate allocation concealment, assessor blinding, and intention to treat analysis), and limited outcome assessment.

QUESTION **What are the effects of rehabilitation programmes and treatment protocols after hip fracture?**

OPTION **INPATIENT REHABILITATION IN A GERIATRIC ORTHOPAEDIC REHABILITATION UNIT**

One systematic review and one subsequent RCT has found that geriatric outpatient rehabilitation units versus control significantly increase the number of people able to return to their previous residence, although they found conflicting results on length of hospital stay. The systematic review has found that geriatric outpatient rehabilitation units versus control significantly reduce rates of readmission for acute care but did not significantly reduce mortality or increase quality of life scores. Limited evidence from observational studies suggests that geriatric outpatient rehabilitation units may reduce the frequency of readmission for acute care, improve the rate of return to previous residence, and provide improved mobility and activities of daily living.

Benefits: We found one systematic review (search date 1998, 4 RCTs, 3 cohort studies)[33] and one subsequent RCT (243 elderly people with moderate dementia)[34] comparing geriatric outpatient rehabilitation units (GORU) versus control. **Length of hospital stay:** Significant heterogeneity was present between RCT results.[33] The review found no significant difference between programmes with GORU versus those without in total hospital stay (333 people with GORU *v* 375 people with control; WMD +1.6 days, 95% CI –28.0 days to +31 days). The subsequent RCT found that GORU versus control also reduced the median number of days spent in hospital (47 days, range 10–365 days with GORU *v* 147 days, range 18–365 days with control).[34] **Readmission for acute care:** The review found that GORU significantly reduced rates of readmission for acute care (36/182 [20%] with GORU *v* 57/196 [29%] with control; RR 0.68, 95% CI 0.47 to 0.97).[33] **Return to previous residence after discharge:** The review found that GORU significantly increased the number of people able to return to their previous residence (4 RCTs, 254/343 [74%] with GORU *v* 255/380 [67%] with control; RR 1.11, 95% CI 1.01 to 1.22). The subsequent RCT found that GORU versus control significantly reduced the number of people unable to return to their previous residence (RR 0.27, 95% CI 0.11 to 0.69).[34] **Mortality:** The review found that GORU versus control did not significantly reduce mortality (79/383 [21%] with GORU *v* 90/433 [21%] with control; RR 0.98, 95% CI 0.75 to 1.28).[33] **Health related quality of life:** The systematic review included one RCT (108 people) and one cohort study (723 people) comparing health related quality of life scores for GORU versus control. They both found no significant difference.

Harms: The review found that GORU versus control significantly increased the number of pressure sores (1 study: 17/142 [12%] with GORU *v* 8/193 [4%] with control; RR 2.89, 95% CI 1.28 to 6.50).[33]

Comment: **Hospital morbidity:** The review identified two cohort studies, which found no significant difference with GORU versus control in postoperative complications as a whole (1 study, 102 events from 521 admissions with GORU *v* 95 events from 202 admissions with control).[28] **Mobility and activities of daily living:** The review identified one cohort study, which found that GORU versus control significantly increased the number of people independently mobile at 6 months (221/336 [66%] with GORU *v* 104/127 [82%] with control; RR 1.25, 95% CI 1.11 to 1.39). The review also found that rehabilitation with GORU significantly reduced loss of daily living ability score at 12 months (22/44 [50%] with GORU *v* 28/36 [78%] with control; RR 0.64, 95% CI 0.46 to 0.91).

OPTION GERIATRIC HIP FRACTURE PROGRAMME WITHIN AN ACUTE ORTHOPAEDIC UNIT

One systematic review and one subsequent RCT in elderly people who have suffered hip fracture have found that geriatric hip fracture programmes versus control programmes significantly increase the number of people able to return to their previous residence, and significantly reduce morbidity whilst in hospital, but had no significant effect on mortality. The review has found that geriatric hip fracture programmes also reduce the length of hospital stay. Two additional RCTs have found that a geriatrician led geriatric hip fracture programme versus control significantly reduces the incidence of severe delirium.

Benefits: We found one systematic review (search date 1998, 5 studies),[33] two additional RCTs,[35,36] and one subsequent RCT[37] of geriatric hip fracture programmes (GHFP) versus control programmes. **Length of hospital stay:** Introduction of GHFP was associated with a reduction in length of hospital stay in four of the five included studies (crude average reduction of 9 days). **Readmission for acute care:** One RCT identified by the review found no significant difference in readmission rates after 4 months (16/127 [13%] with GHFP *v* 11/125 [9%] with control; RR 1.43, 95% CI 0.69 to 2.96). **Return to previous residence after discharge:** The review found that GHFP significantly increased the number of people able to return home (2 RCTs: 121/139 [87%] with GHFP *v* 100/131 [76%] with control; RR 1.14, 95% CI 1.02 to 1.28). **Mortality:** The review found no significant reduction in mortality with GHFP (2 RCTs: 27/165 [16%] with GHFP *v* 30/158 [19%] with control; RR 0.87, 95% CI 0.54 to 1.39). **Morbidity:** The review found that GHFP significantly reduced the number of people sustaining one or more complications whilst in hospital GHFP (162/431 [38%] with GHFP *v* 39/60 [65%] with control; RR 0.58, 95% CI 0.46 to 0.72). Two additional RCTs (246 people)[35,36] found that a geriatrician led GHFP versus control significantly reduced the incidence of severe delirium (7/60 [12%] with geriatrician GHFP *v* 18/62 [29%] with control; RR 0.40, 95% CI 0.18 to 0.89), but that a nurse led programme showed no significant effect on the incidence of delirium, but duration was significantly shorter and severity of the delirium significantly less. **Mobility and activities of daily living:** The review found that GHFP did not significantly reduce the number of people failing to walk independently by discharge (1 RCT: 63/127 [50%] GHFP *v* 51/125 [41%] with control; RR 1.22, 95% CI 0.9 to 1.6), that GHFP reduced the mean time taken to walk 20 m (1 RCT: 45 s with GHFP *v* 59 s with control; no standard deviation provided), and that GHFP increased mean modified Barthel Index (see glossary, p 1145) scores (1 RCT: 92.8, 95% CI 90.0 to 95.6 with GHFP *v* 85.6, 95% CI 81.3 to 89.8 with control). **Health related quality of life:** The review found no studies of this outcome. We found one subsequent RCT comparing GHFP with control programmes.[37] It found that GHFP significantly reduced hospital stay, but did not reduce complication or readmission rates.

Harms: We found no evidence of harms.

Comment: None.

OPTION EARLY SUPPORTED DISCHARGE PROGRAMMES

One systematic review in people after hip fracture has found that early supported discharge versus control significantly increases the number of people returning to their previous residence and reduces length of hospital stay, but significantly increases the frequency of readmission to hospital.

Benefits: We found one systematic review (search date 1998, 41 comparative studies, including 14 RCTs), which included six studies comparing early supported discharge (ESD) versus control.[33] **Length of hospital stay:** The review found that the introduction of ESD was associated with reduced length of both acute hospital stay and total number of days in hospital. The crude average reduction (no standard deviations provided) was 6.9 days in acute hospital stay and 2.0 days in total duration of care. **Mortality:** The review found that ESD had no significant effect on mortality (1 RCT: 12/160 [8%] with ESD *v* 6/81 [7%] with control; RR 1.01, 95% CI 0.39 to 2.60). **Mobility and activities of daily living:** One RCT identified by the review found no significant difference in Barthel Index (see glossary, p 1145) scores after 3 months (ESD 160 people, mean change 1.9, standard deviation 3.22 *v* control 81 people, mean change 1.7, standard deviation 2.68). **Health related quality of life:** One RCT found no significant difference in European quality of life (scale) score after 3 months (mean difference –0.04, 95% CI –0.13 to +0.06).

Harms: The review found that ESD versus control significantly increased the frequency of readmission to hospital (3 cohort studies: 69/922 [7%] with ESD *v* 17/406 [4%] with control; RR 1.91, 95% CI 1.11 to 3.29).[33]

Comment: **Return to previous residence after discharge:** The systematic review found that ESD versus control significantly increased rate of return to previous residence (3 cohort studies: 203/247 [82%] with

ESD v 129/197 [65%] with control; RR 1.25, 95% CI 1.11 to 1.41).[28] **Morbidity:** One cohort study identified by the review compared ESD versus control and found no significant difference in the incidence of one or more hospital complications (17/63 [27%] with ESD v 15/66 [23%] with control; RR 1.19, 95% CI 0.65 to 2.17). **Mobility and activities of daily living:** One cohort study identified by the review found no evidence of difference in Nottingham Health Profile mobility dimension mean score (48 with ESD v 50 with control; no standard deviation provided). **Health related quality of life:** The review found no significant difference in mean Nottingham Health Profile dimension score (1 cohort study: 110 people).

OPTION **SYSTEMATIC MULTICOMPONENT HOME REHABILITATION AFTER HIP FRACTURE**

One RCT comparing a systematic home based rehabilitation programme versus existing services found no significant difference in recovery to prefracture levels of self care, home management, social activity, balance, or lower extremity strength.

Benefits: We found no systematic review but found one RCT (304 people who had surgery for hip fracture and returned home within 100 days, 12 months' follow up),[38] which compared systematic home based multicomponent rehabilitation addressing physical impairments and activities of daily living versus "usual care". It found no significant difference between groups in recovery to prefracture levels of self care, home management, social activity, balance, or lower extremity strength. The systematic programme was associated with slightly greater upper arm strength and marginally better walking.

Harms: None reported.

Comment: The RCT examined whether systematising home assessment and treatment according to a protocol made a difference versus "usual care". The failure of this trial to find a difference between the systematic programme and "usual care" may be contextual, indicating that "usual care" was already being delivered competently.

GLOSSARY

Arthroplasty The use of a surgically inserted device to replace one or both sides of a joint after fracture or because of the consequences of chronic arthritis.

Bipolar hemiarthroplasty A type of hip arthroplasty, which replaces the femoral head with an artificial femoral head containing an internal articulation.

Cephalocondylic nail A device used for internal fixation of hip fractures, consisting of a nail inserted into the interior (medulla) of the femur from its upper end and driven through the fracture site towards the knee.

Fixed nail plate A device used for internal fixation of hip fractures, which consists of a rigid nail driven through the fracture site and attached to a plate on the outside (extramedullary) lateral surface of the femur.

Internal fixation The use of devices (usually metal) to immobilise fractures by open surgery.

Modified Barthel Index A scoring system for assessing a person's ability in activities of daily living.

RAB fixed nail plate A type of fixed nail plate, which has an additional oblique strut connecting the nail and the plate.

Hip fracture

Sliding hip screw A device used for internal fixation of hip fractures, consisting of a lag screw that is passed across the fracture site and then attached to a plate on the outside (extramedullary) lateral surface of the femur. The design allows the lag screw to slide into a sleeve on the plate to accommodate shortening at the fracture site. This sliding capability is referred to as dynamic fixation.
Unipolar hemiarthroplasty A type of hip arthroplasty, which replaces the femoral head with a monoblock metallic femoral head.
Varus deformity A deformity occurring in a limb, for any reason, in which the segment of the limb below the site of deformity is adducted towards the midline.

Substantive changes

Conservative versus operative treatment for extracapsular hip fractures Updated systematic review;[17] conclusions unchanged.
Arthroplasty versus internal fixation for extracapsular fracture Updated systematic review;[18] conclusions unchanged.
Dynamic (sliding) versus fixed extramedullary fixation for extracapsular hip fracture Updated systematic review;[19] conclusions unchanged.
Short cephalocondylic nail versus sliding hip screw Updated systematic review, which identified further RCTs;[20] conclusions unchanged.
Cephalocondylic nails versus extramedullary fixation for extracapsular fracture Updated systematic review;[21] conclusions unchanged.
Nerve blocks for pain control before and after hip fracture Updated systematic review;[22] conclusions unchanged.

REFERENCES

1. Parker MJ, Pryor GA. *Hip fracture management*. Oxford: Blackwell Scientific Publications, 1993.
2. Meunier PJ. Prevention of hip fractures. *Am J Med* 1993;95(suppl):75–78.
3. Hochberg MC, Williamson J, Skinner EA, et al. The prevalence and impact of self-reported hip fracture in elderly community-dwelling women: The Women's Health and Aging Study. *Osteoporos Int* 1998;8:385–389.
4. Boyce WJ, Vessey MP. Rising incidence of fracture of the proximal femur. *Lancet* 1985;1:150–151.
5. Schurch M-A, Rizzoli R, Mermillod B, et al. A prospective study on the socio-economic aspects of fracture of the proximal femur. *J Bone Miner Res* 1996;11:1935–1942.
6. Parker MJ, Handoll HHG. Pre-operative traction for fractures of the proximal femur. In: The Cochrane Library, Issue 2, 2002. Oxford: Update Software. Search date 2001; primary sources Cochrane Musculoskeletal Injuries Group specialised register (April 2001), the Cochrane Controlled Trials Register, Medline, Embase, Cinahl, the National Research Register, and reference lists of articles.
7. Parker MJ, Urwin SC, Handoll HHG, et al. General versus spinal/epidural anaesthesia for surgery for hip fractures in adults. In: The Cochrane Library, Issue 2, 2002. Oxford: Update Software. Search date 2000; primary sources Cochrane Musculoskeletal Injuries Group Trials Register, Medline, and hand searching of selected orthopaedic and anaesthetic journals, conference proceedings, and reference lists of relevant articles.
8. Parker MJ, Stockton G. Internal fixation implants for intracapsular proximal femoral fractures in adults. In: The Cochrane Library, Issue 2, 2002. Oxford: Update Software. Search date 2000; primary sources Cochrane Musculoskeletal Injuries Group specialised register, reference lists of articles, conference proceedings, and personal contact with trialists.
9. Parker MJ, Blundell C. Choice of implant for internal fixation of femoral neck fractures: meta-analysis of 25 randomised trials including 4925 patients. *Acta Orthop Scand* 1998;69:138–143. Search date 1997; primary sources Cochrane, Medline, and hand searches of six orthopaedic journals.
10. Davison JN, Calder SJ, Anderson GH, et al. Treatment for displaced intracapsular fracture of the proximal femur. A prospective, randomised trial in patients aged 65 to 79 years. *J Bone Joint Surg Br* 2001;83:206–212.
11. Johansson T, Jacobsson SA, Ivarsson I, et al. Internal fixation versus total hip arthroplasty in the treatment of displaced femoral neck fractures: a prospective randomized study of 100 hips. *Acta Orthop Scand* 2000;71:597–602.
12. Parker MJ, Pryor GA. Internal fixation or arthroplasty for displaced cervical hip fractures in the elderly: a randomised controlled trial of 208 patients. *Acta Orthop Scand* 2000;71:440–446.
13. Ravikumar KJ, Marsh G. Internal fixation versus hemiarthroplasty versus total hip arthroplasty for displaced subcapital fractures of femur — 13 year results of a prospective randomised study. *Injury* 2000;31:793–797.
14. Van Dortmont LM, Douw CM, Van Breukelen AM, et al. Cannulated screws versus hemiarthroplasty for displaced intracapsular femoral neck fractures in demented patients. *Ann Chir Gynaecol* 2000;89:132–137.
15. Calder SJ, Anderson GH, Jagger C, et al. Unipolar or bipolar prosthesis for displaced intracapsular hip fracture in octogenarians: a randomised prospective study. *J Bone Joint Surg Br* 1996;78:391–394.

16. Cornell CN, Levine D, O'Doherty J, et al. Unipolar versus bipolar arthroplasty for the treatment of femoral neck fractures in the elderly. *Clin Orthop* 1998;348;67–71.
17. Parker MJ, Handoll HHG. Conservative versus operative treatment for extracapsular hip fractures. In: The Cochrane Library, Issue 2, 2002. Oxford: Update Software. Search date 2001; primary sources Cochrane Musculoskeletal Injuries Group Trials Register, hand searches of reference bibliographies, and personal contact with trialists.
18. Parker MJ, Handoll HHG. Replacement arthroplasty versus internal fixation for extracapsular hip fractures. In: The Cochrane Library, Issue 2, 2002. Oxford: Update Software. Search date 2001; primary sources Cochrane Musculoskeletal Injuries Group Trials Register, hand searches of reference bibliographies, and personal contact with colleagues.
19. Parker MJ, Handoll HHG, Chinoy MA. Extramedullary fixation implants for extracapsular hip fractures. In: The Cochrane Library, Issue 2, 2002. Oxford: Update Software. Search date 2001; primary sources Cochrane Musculoskeletal Injuries Group Trials Register and hand searches of reference lists of relevant articles.
20. Parker MJ, Handoll HHG. Gamma and other cephalocondylic intramedullary nails versus extramedullary implants for extracapsular hip fractures. In: The Cochrane Library, Issue 2, 2002. Oxford: Update Software. Search date 2001; primary sources Cochrane Musculoskeletal Injuries Group Trials Register, Medline, hand searching of selected orthopaedic journals, conference proceedings, reference lists of relevant articles, and personal contact with trialists, colleagues, and implant manufacturers.
21. Parker MJ, Handoll HHG, Bhonsle S, et al. Cephalocondylic nails versus extramedullary implants for extracapsular hip fractures. In: The Cochrane Library, Issue 2, 2002. Oxford: Update Software. Search date 1999; primary sources Cochrane Musculoskeletal Injuries Group Trials Register, Medline, and hand searches of reference lists of relevant articles.
22. Parker MJ, Griffiths R, Appadu BN. Nerve blocks (subcostal, lateral cutaneous, femoral, triple, psoas) for hip fractures. In: The Cochrane Library, Issue 2, 2002. Oxford: Update Software. Search date 2001; primary sources Cochrane Musculoskeletal Injuries Group Trials Register, Medline, and hand searches of trial bibliographies.
23. Gillespie WJ, Walenkamp G. Antibiotic prophylaxis for surgery for proximal femoral and other closed long bone fractures. In: The Cochrane Library, Issue 2, 2002. Oxford: Update Software. Search date 2000; primary sources Medline, Embase, Current Contents, Dissertation Abstracts, Index to UK theses, and hand searches of bibliographies of identified articles.
24. Handoll HHG, Farrar MJ, McBirnie J, et al. Heparin, low molecular weight heparin and physical methods for preventing deep vein thrombosis and pulmonary embolism following surgery for hip fractures. In: The Cochrane Library, Issue 2, 2002. Oxford: Update Software. Search date 2000; primary sources Cochrane Musculoskeletal Injuries Group Trials Register, Medline, Embase, hand searches of published papers and books, and personal contact with trialists and other workers in the field.
25. Collins R, Scrimgeour A, Yusuf S, et al. Reduction in fatal pulmonary embolism and venous thrombosis by perioperative administration of subcutaneous heparin. *N Engl J Med* 1988;318:1162–1173. Search date not stated; primary sources Medline, hand searches of reference lists, and personal contact with colleagues, investigators, and manufacturers of heparin.
26. Jorgensen LN, Wille-Jorgensen P, Hauch O. Prophylaxis of postoperative thromboembolism with low molecular weight heparins. *Br J Surg* 1993;80:689–704. Search date 1991; primary sources Medline, Current Contents, hand searches of reference lists, and personal contact with authors of trials.
27. Antiplatelet Trialists' Collaboration. Collaborative review of randomized trials of antiplatelet therapy. III: reduction in venous thrombosis and pulmonary embolism by antiplatelet prophylaxis among surgical and medical patients. *BMJ* 1994;308:235–246. Search date 1990; primary sources Medline, Current Contents, hand searches of journals, reference lists, abstracts, conference proceedings, and personal contact with the International Committee on Thrombosis and Haemostastis, colleagues, and manufacturers.
28. Anonymous. Prevention of pulmonary embolism and deep vein thrombosis with low dose aspirin: Pulmonary Embolism Prevention (PEP) trial. *Lancet* 2000;355:1295–1302.
29. Agu O, Hamilton G, Baker D. Graduated compression stockings in the prevention of venous thromboembolism. *Br J Surg* 1999;86:992–1004. Search date 1998; primary sources Medline, Cochrane, and hand searches of reference lists.
30. Amarigiri SV, Lees TA. Elastic compression stockings for prevention of deep venous thrombosis. In: The Cochrane Library, Issue 2, 2002. Oxford: Update Software. Search date 1999; primary sources Cochrane Peripheral Vascular Disease Group Trials Register, Medline, Embase, hand searches of Index Medicus, and personal contact with manufacturers and trialists in ongoing trials.
31. Cullum N, Deeks J, Sheldon TA, et al. Beds, mattresses and cushions for pressure sore prevention and treatment. In: The Cochrane Library, Issue 2, 2002. Oxford: Update Software. Search date 2000; primary sources Cochrane Wounds Group Specialist Trials Register, hand searching of wound care journals, and relevant conference proceedings.
32. Avenell A, Handoll HHG. Nutritional supplementation for hip fracture aftercare in the elderly. In: The Cochrane Library, Issue 2, 2002. Oxford: Update Software. Search date 2000; primary sources Cochrane Musculoskeletal Injuries Group Trials Register, Cochrane Controlled Trials Register, Medline, Nutrition Abstracts and Reviews, Healthstar, Embase, Biosis, Cinahl, and hand searching of reference lists of selected nutrition journals.
33. Cameron I, Crotty M, Currie C, et al. Geriatric rehabilitation following fractures in older people: a systematic review. *Health Technol Assess* 2000;4. Search date 1998; primary sources Cochrane Musculoskeletal Injuries Group Trials Register, Cochrane Controlled Trials Register, Medline, Cinahl, and hand searches of reference lists.
34. Huusko TM, Karppi P, Avikainen V, et al. Randomised, clinically controlled trial of intensive geriatric rehabilitation in patients with hip fracture: subgroup analysis of patients with dementia. *BMJ* 2000;321:1107–1111.
35. Marcantonio ER, Flacker JM, Wright RJ, et al. Reducing delirium after hip fracture: a randomized trial. *J Am Geriatr Soc* 2001;49:516–522.
36. Milisen K, Foreman MD, Abraham IL, et al. A nurse-led interdisciplinary intervention program for delirium in elderly hip-fracture patients. *J Am Geriatr Soc* 2001;49:523–532.

37. Choong PFM, Langford AK, Dowsey MM, et al. Clinical pathway for fractured neck of femur: a prospective, controlled study. *Med J Aust* 2000;172:423–426.

38. Tinetti ME, Baker DI, Gottschalk M, et al. Home-based multi-component rehabilitation program for older persons after hip fracture: a randomized trial. *Arch Phys Med Rehab* 1999;80:916–922.

William Gillespie
Dean
Hull York Medical School
Universities of Hull and York
UK

Competing interests: The author has received grant funding from contestable public funds (as one member of a group of applicants) for randomised trial in fracture prevention. He is co-ordinating editor of the Cochrane Musculoskeletal Injuries Group.

Leg cramps

Search date February 2002

Gavin Young

QUESTIONS

INTERVENTIONS

To be covered in future updates

Treatments for leg cramps associated with venous insufficiency
Treatments for leg cramps associated with dialysis

Covered elsewhere in *Clinical Evidence*

Compression hosiery for venous leg ulcers, p 2032

See glossary, p 1154

Key Messages

In idiopathic leg cramps

- **Quinine** One systematic review has found that quinine versus placebo significantly reduces the frequency of nocturnal leg cramp attacks over 4 weeks.
- **Quinine plus theophylline** One small RCT found limited evidence that quinine plus theophylline versus quinine alone significantly reduced the number of nights affected by leg cramp over 2 weeks.
- **Vitamin E** One small RCT comparing vitamin E versus placebo found no significant difference in the number of nights disturbed by leg cramps.
- **Analgesics; antiepileptic drugs; compression hosiery** We found no RCTs on the effects of these interventions on idiopathic leg cramps.

In leg cramps in pregnancy

- **Calcium salts** Two RCTs identified by a systematic review comparing calcium versus placebo or no treatment found conflicting results.

Clin Evid 2002;8:1149–1155.

- **Magnesium salts** One systematic review of one small RCT found that magnesium tablets (primarily magnesium lactate, magnesium citrate) versus placebo significantly reduced the number of pregnant women with leg cramps after 3 weeks.
- **Multivitamins and mineral supplements** One systematic review of one small RCT found no significant difference with a multivitamin plus mineral tablet versus placebo in the number of pregnant women with cramps in the ninth month of pregnancy.
- **Sodium chloride** One systematic review found insufficient evidence about the effects of sodium chloride on leg cramps in pregnancy.

DEFINITION Leg cramps are involuntary, localised, and usually painful skeletal muscle contractions, which commonly affect calf muscles. Leg cramps typically occur at night and usually last only seconds to minutes. Leg cramps may be idiopathic (see glossary, p 1154) or related to a definable process or disease such as pregnancy, renal dialysis, or venous insufficiency.

INCIDENCE/ PREVALENCE Leg cramps are common and their incidence increases with age. About half of the people attending a general medicine clinic have had leg cramps within 1 month of their visit, and over two thirds of people over 50 years of age have experienced leg cramps.[1]

AETIOLOGY/ RISK FACTORS Very little is known about the causes of leg cramps. Risk factors include pregnancy, exercise, salt depletion, renal dialysis, electrolyte imbalances, peripheral vascular disease (both venous and arterial), peripheral nerve injury, polyneuropathies, motor neuron disease, muscle diseases, and the use of certain drugs. Other causes of calf pain include trauma, deep venous thrombosis (see thromboembolism, p 209), and ruptured Baker's cyst (see glossary, p 1154).

PROGNOSIS Leg cramps may cause severe pain and sleep disturbance, both of which are distressing.

AIMS To reduce the number and the severity of attacks of cramp, with minimal adverse effects of treatment.

OUTCOMES Number of attacks; severity of attacks; number of disturbed nights.

METHODS *Clinical Evidence* search and appraisal February 2002.

QUESTION What are the effects of treatments for idiopathic leg cramps?

OPTION COMPRESSION HOSIERY

We found no RCTs on the effects of compression hosiery on idiopathic leg cramps.

Benefits: We found no systematic review or RCTs.

Harms: We found no evidence on harms related to the use of compression hosiery in patients with idiopathic leg cramps (see compression under prevention and treatment of venous leg ulcers, p 2032).

Comment: None.

OPTION QUINININE

One systematic review has found that quinine versus placebo significantly reduces the frequency of nocturnal leg cramp attacks over 4 weeks.

Benefits: We found one systematic review (search date 1997, 8 RCTs, 659 people).[2] A meta-analysis of eight RCTs in the review found that quinine versus placebo significantly reduced the frequency of nocturnal leg cramps over a 4 week period (an absolute reduction of 2.9 cramps while taking quinine *v* placebo, 95% CI 0.2 to 5.54; RR not available).

Harms: Adverse effects of quinine include headache, digestive disorders, tinnitus, fever, blurred vision, dizziness, and pruritus.[2] In the systematic review, tinnitus was significantly more common in people taking quinine versus placebo (20/659 [3.0%] with quinine *v* 7/659 [1.1%] with placebo; RR 2.86, 95% CI 1.22 to 6.71; NNH 50, 95% CI 27 to 230). Elevated quinine levels may cause cinchonism (see glossary, p 1154): a syndrome that includes nausea, vomiting, tinnitus, and deafness.[3]

Comment: The systematic review excluded two RCTs because of a lack of individual patient data. Both these RCTs found a reduction in the number of leg cramps with quinine versus placebo. We found no evidence about the optimal dose of quinine or length of treatment.

OPTION QUININE PLUS THEOPHYLLINE

One small RCT found limited evidence that quinine plus theophylline versus quinine alone significantly reduced the number of nights affected by leg cramp over 2 weeks.

Benefits: We found no systematic review. We found one RCT (164 people), which compared quinine plus theophylline versus quinine alone for 2 weeks.[4] Baseline rates of leg cramp were measured for 1 week prior to randomisation, when all people received placebo (single blind). Pooled results for 126 people who completed at least 4 days treatment in the 2 week period found quinine plus theophylline to be rated significantly more often as "good" or "very good" compared with quinine alone or placebo (87% with quinine plus theophylline *v* 64% with quinine *v* 40% with placebo; see comment below). After 2 weeks of treatment, theophylline plus quinine versus quinine alone significantly reduced the mean number of nights affected by cramp (from 4.7 nights to 1.1 nights with theophylline plus quinine *v* 4.8 nights to 2.2 nights with quinine alone; P = 0.009).

Harms: During the placebo week, six people reported side effects (nausea to vomiting in 2 people, nausea, heartburn, depression, bitter after taste). When using quinine, three people reported adverse effects (bloating and tenesmus, nausea to vomiting and nausea) resulting in early withdrawal from the study in two people. When using quinine plus theophylline, four people had adverse effects (fall in blood pressure and dizziness, nausea in 2 cases, palpitations and tinnitus) resulting in the four people discontinuing the study.

Comment: The results of the RCT should be treated with caution as it did not specify criteria to categorise outcomes as "good" or "very good" and pooled the results only for people who received treatment for at least 4 out of 14 days (126 people out of 164 enrolled) without using an intention to treat analysis.

OPTION VITAMIN E

One small RCT comparing vitamin E versus placebo found no significant difference in the number of nights disturbed by leg cramps.

Benefits: We found no systematic review. We found one crossover RCT (27 men), which compared vitamin E versus placebo.[5] It found that vitamin E versus placebo did not significantly reduce the median number of nights with leg cramps (15 nights *v* 13 nights; $P > 0.05$).

Harms: Adverse effects were reported as similar in the vitamin E and placebo groups, but no details were provided.[5]

Comment: None.

OPTION ANALGESICS

We found no RCTs on the effects of analgesics on idiopathic leg cramps.

Benefits: We found no systematic review or RCTs.

Harms: We found no RCTs.

Comment: None.

OPTION ANTIEPILEPTIC DRUGS

We found no RCTs on the effects of antiepileptic drugs on idiopathic leg cramps.

Benefits: We found no systematic review or RCTs.

Harms: Harms associated with the use of antiepileptic drugs are well described (see epilepsy, p 1313).

Comment: None.

QUESTION What are the effects of treatments for leg cramps in pregnancy? New

OPTION MAGNESIUM SALTS

One systematic review of one small RCT found that magnesium tablets (primarily magnesium lactate, magnesium citrate) versus placebo significantly reduced the number of pregnant women with leg cramps after 3 weeks.

Benefits: We found one systematic review (search date 2001,[6] 1 RCT,[7] 73 pregnant women 22–36 wks gestation), which compared chewable magnesium tablets (primarily magnesium lactate, magnesium citrate) versus chewable placebo tablets (primarily sorbitol, fructose–dextrose) given for 3 weeks. The review found that magnesium versus placebo significantly reduced the number of pregnant women who still had cramps at the end of 3 weeks' treatment (23/34 [68%] with magnesium v 33/35 [94%] with placebo; OR 0.18, 95% CI 0.05 to 0.60; see comment below).[6] The RCT found that magnesium versus placebo decreased the proportion of women who rated themselves "unchanged" or "worse" ("unchanged": 7/34 [21%] with magnesium v 16/35 [46%] with placebo; "worse": 0/34 [0%] with magnesium v 5/35 [14%] with placebo).[7]

Harms: Side effects were described as infrequent in both groups, mainly slight nausea.[6] One woman in the placebo group discontinued treatment because of severe nausea.[6]

Comment: The RCT did not describe the method of randomisation used, and symptoms were assessed after 3 weeks of treatment with no further follow up.[6]

OPTION MULTIVITAMINS AND MINERAL SUPPLEMENTS

One systematic review of one small RCT found no significant difference with a multivitamin plus mineral tablet versus placebo in the number of pregnant women with cramps in the ninth month of pregnancy.

Benefits: We found one systematic review (search date 2001,[6] 1 RCT,[8] 62 pregnant women), which compared a multivitamin plus mineral tablet (containing 12 different ingredients; see comment below) versus placebo (no details provided). Supplements were given from 3 months' gestation. The review found no significant difference with multivitamin plus mineral versus placebo in the number of women still having cramps in the ninth month of pregnancy (2/11 [18%] with multivitamin plus mineral v 10/18 [56%] with placebo; OR 0.23, 95% CI 0.05 to 1.01).[6]

Harms: The RCT found that 4% of women had adverse effects (nausea, vomiting, diarrhoea). It is not clear which treatment these women were taking.[8]

Comment: This small RCT was primarily undertaken to examine the effects of a multivitamin mineral supplement on zinc and copper levels during pregnancy.[8] In total, 29/62 (48%) of women were assessed for cramp at 9 months' gestation.[6] The high drop out rate is not explained. The supplement contained: zinc gluconate, copper gluconate, iron gluconate, magnesium lactate, chromium chloride, ascorbic acid, thiamin nitrate, riboflavin (riboflavine), pyridoxal chlorhydrate, folic acid, cyanocobalamin, and α-tocopheral acetate.[6]

OPTION SODIUM CHLORIDE

One systematic review found insufficient evidence about the effects of sodium chloride on leg cramps in pregnancy.

Benefits: We found one systematic review (search date 2001),[6] which included one controlled clinical trial[9] published in 1947 (see comment below).

Harms: We found no RCTs.

Comment: The controlled clinical trial was of poor quality. Initially, sodium chloride and calcium lactate were given to alternate participants.[9] It was then decided, based on the difference between the results of the two treatments, to also use two further control groups (saccharin and no treatment).[9] The dose of sodium chloride changed during the course of the study.[6]

OPTION CALCIUM SALTS

Two RCTs identified by a systematic review comparing calcium versus placebo or no treatment found conflicting results.

Benefits: We found one systematic review (search date 2001),[6] which included two RCTs[10,11] and one controlled clinical trial (see comment below). The first RCT (42 pregnant women) included in the review found that calcium (calcium gluconate, lactate, and carbonate) versus no treatment significantly reduced the number of women with no improvement of cramps (2/21 [10%] with calcium *v* 18/21 [86%] with no treatment; OR 0.05, 95% CI 0.02 to 0.17).[6] The second RCT (60 pregnant women) included in the review found no significant difference with calcium (calcium gluconate, lactate, and carbonate) versus placebo (vitamin C) in the number of pregnant women with no improvement of cramps (11/30 [37%] with calcium *v* 8/30 [27%] with placebo; OR 1.58, 95% CI 0.54 to 4.63; see comment below).[6]

Harms: The RCTs did not report harms.[6]

Comment: The controlled clinical trial identified by the review was of poor quality (see comment under sodium chloride, p 1154). There was a marked difference in the response of the control group in the two included RCTs. In the first RCT using no treatment as control, 18/21 (86%) women with no treatment had no improvement in cramps.[10] In the second RCT using placebo (vitamin C) as control, 8/30 (27%) women with placebo had no improvement.[11]

GLOSSARY

Baker's cyst A cyst or out pouching that occurs in the lining of the knee joint. Rupture of the cyst may be associated with calf pain.

Cinchonism Adverse effects caused by quinine and other derivatives of cinchona bark. It usually presents with nausea, vomiting, headache, tinnitus, deafness, vertigo, and visual disturbances.

Idiopathic leg cramps A phrase indicating that the underlying cause of the leg cramps is currently unknown. It is used in this review to distinguish the commonest type of leg cramps from leg cramps in people who are receiving dialysis, have venous insufficiency, or are pregnant.

REFERENCES

1. Hall AJ. Cramp and salt balance in ordinary life. *Lancet* 1947;3:231–233.
2. Man-Son-Hing M, Wells G, Lau A. Quinine for nocturnal leg cramps: a meta-analysis including unpublished data. *J Gen Intern Med* 1998;13:600–606. Search date 1997; primary sources Medline, Embase, Current Contents, and contact with authorities.
3. McGee SR. Muscle cramps. *Arch Intern Med* 1990;150:511–518.
4. Gorlich HD, Gablez VE, Steinberg HW. Treatment of recurrent nocturnal leg cramps. A multicentric double blind, placebo controlled comparison between the combination of quinine and theophylline ethylene diamine and quinine. *Arzneimittelforschung* 1991;41:167–175.

5. Connolly PS, Shirley EA, Wasson JH, et al. Treatment of nocturnal leg cramps: A crossover trial of quinine vs vitamin E. *Arch Intern Med* 1992;152:1877–1880.
6. Young GL, Jewell D. Interventions for leg cramps in pregnancy (Cochrane Review). In: The Cochrane Library, Issue 1, 2002. Oxford: Update Software. Search date 2001; primary sources Cochrane Pregnancy and Childbirth Group trials register.
7. Dahle LO, Berg G, Hammar M, et al. The effect of oral magnesium substitution on pregnancy-induced leg cramps. *Am J Obstet Gynecol* 1995;173(1):175–180.
8. Thauvin E, Fusselier M, Arnaud J, et al. Effects of a multivitamin mineral supplement on zinc and copper status during pregnancy. *Biol Trace Elem Res* 1992;32:405–414.
9. Robinson M. Cramps in pregnancy. *Journal of Obstetrics and Gynaecology for the British Commonwealth* 1947;54:826–829.
10. Hammar M, Larsson L, Tegler L. Calcium treatment of leg cramps in pregnancy. *Acta Obstet Gynecol Scand* 1981;60:345–347.
11. Hammar M, Berg G, Solheim F, et al. Calcium and magnesium status in pregnant women. A comparison between treatment with calcium and vitamin C in pregnant women with leg cramps. *Int J Vitam Nutr Res* 1987;57:179–183.

Gavin Young
General Practitioner
Temple Sowerby Surgery
Penrith
UK

Competing interests: None declared.

Low back pain and sciatica: acute

Search date October 2001

Maurits van Tulder and Bart Koes

QUESTIONS

INTERVENTIONS

See glossary, p 1168

Key Messages

- **Acupuncture** We found no systematic review and no RCTs of acupuncture specifically in people with acute low back pain.
- **Advice to stay active** Two systematic reviews and one subsequent RCT have found that advice to stay active versus no advice significantly increases the rate of recovery and reduces pain, disability, and time spent off work.
- **Analgesics (paracatemol, opioids)** Systematic reviews have found no consistent difference with analgesics versus non-steroidal anti-inflammatory drugs in reducing pain, but have found that electroacupuncture or ultrasound versus analgesics significantly improves pain relief at 4–6 months.
- **Back exercises** Systematic reviews and additional RCTs have found either no significant difference with back exercises versus conservative or inactive treatments in pain or disability, or found that back exercises increase pain or disability.
- **Back schools** One systematic review found limited evidence that back schools versus placebo increased rates of recovery and reduced sick leave in the short term. The review found no significant difference in outcomes with back school versus physiotherapy, and found that back school versus McKenzie exercises increased pain and sick leave.

- **Bed rest** Systematic reviews have found no evidence that bed rest is better, but have found evidence that it could be worse than no treatment, advice to stay active, back exercises, physiotherapy, spinal manipulation, or non-steroidal anti-inflammatory drugs. One systematic review has found that adverse effects of bed rest include joint stiffness, muscle wasting, loss of bone mineral density, pressure sores, and venous thromboembolism.
- **Behavioural therapy** Two RCTs have found that behavioural therapy versus traditional care or electromyographic biofeedback reduces acute low back pain and disability.
- **Epidural steroid injections** One RCT found that epidural steroids versus subcutaneous lidocaine injections increased the proportion of people who were pain free after 3 months. A second RCT found no significant difference in the proportion of people cured or improved with epidural steroids versus epidural saline versus epidural bupivacaine and versus dry needling.
- **Lumbar supports** We found no evidence on the effects of lumbar supports.
- **Massage** Systematic reviews have found no significant difference in pain, functional status, or mobility with massage versus spinal manipulation or electrical stimulation.
- **Multidisciplinary treatment programmes** One systematic review in people with subacute low back pain found limited evidence that multidisciplinary treatment, including a workplace visit, versus usual care reduced sick leave.
- **Muscle relaxants** Systematic reviews have found that muscle relaxants versus placebo reduce pain and muscle tension and increase mobility, but have found no significant difference in outcomes with muscle relaxants versus each other. Adverse effects in people using muscle relaxants were common and included dependency, drowsiness, and dizziness. One RCT found chlormezanone versus methocarbamol significantly increased the proportion of adverse effects (dyspepsia and drowsiness; NNH 6, 95% CI 3 to 90).
- **Non-steroidal anti-inflammatory drugs** Systematic reviews and one additional RCT have found that non-steroidal anti-inflammatory drugs versus placebo significantly increase the proportion of people with overall improvement after 1 week and significantly reduce the proportion of people requiring additional analgesics. Systematic reviews and additional RCTs have found no significant difference in pain relief with non-steroidal anti-inflammatory drugs versus each other or versus other treatments (paracetamol, opioids, muscle relaxants, and non-drug treatments).
- **Spinal manipulation** Systematic reviews found conflicting evidence on the effects of spinal manipulation.
- **Traction** RCTs found conflicting evidence on the effects of traction.
- **Colchicine; electromyographic biofeedback; temperature treatments (short wave diathermy, ultrasound, ice, heat); transcutaneous electrical nerve stimulation (TENS)** We found insufficient evidence on the effects of these interventions.

DEFINITION Low back pain is pain, muscle tension, or stiffness localised below the costal margin and above the inferior gluteal folds, with or without leg pain (sciatica),[1] and is designed as acute when it persists for less than 12 weeks (see definition of chronic low back pain, p 1171).[2] Non-specific low back pain is low back pain not attributed to a recognisable pathology (such as infection, tumour, osteoporosis, rheumatoid arthritis, fracture, or inflammation).[1] This review excludes low back pain or sciatica (see glossary, p 1168) with symptoms or signs at presentation that suggest a specific underlying condition.

INCIDENCE/ PREVALENCE Over 70% of people in developed countries will experience low back pain at some time in their lives.[3] Each year, 15–45% of adults suffer low back pain, and 1/20 people present to hospital with a new episode. Low back pain is most common between the ages of 35–55 years.[3]

AETIOLOGY/ RISK FACTORS Symptoms, pathology, and radiological appearances are poorly correlated. Pain is non-specific in about 85% of people. About 4% of people with low back pain in primary care have compression fractures and about 1% have a tumour. The prevalence of prolapsed intervertebral disc is about 1–3%.[3] Ankylosing spondylitis and spinal infections are less common.[4] Risk factors for the development of back pain include heavy physical work, frequent bending, twisting, lifting, and prolonged static postures. Psychosocial risk factors include anxiety, depression, and mental stress at work.[3,5]

PROGNOSIS Acute low back pain is usually self limiting (90% of people recover within 6 wk), although 2–7% develop chronic pain. One study found recurrent pain accounted for 75–85% of absenteeism from work.[6]

AIMS To relieve pain; to improve function; to develop coping strategies for pain, with minimal adverse effects from treatment; and to prevent the development of chronic back pain (see definition of chronic low back pain, p 1171).[2,7]

OUTCOMES Pain intensity (visual analogue or numerical rating scale); overall improvement (self reported or observed); back pain specific functional status (such as Roland Morris questionnaire, Oswestry questionnaire); impact on employment (days of sick leave, number of people returned to work); medication use; intervention specific outcomes (such as coping and pain behaviour for behavioural treatment, strength and flexibility for exercise, depression for antidepressants, and muscle spasm for muscle relaxants and electromyographic biofeedback [see glossary, p 1168]).

METHODS *Clinical Evidence* search and appraisal October 2001. In addition the authors searched Medline (1966 to December 1998), Embase (1980 to September 1998), and Psychlit (1984 to December 1998), using the search strategy recommended by the Cochrane Back Review Group.[8] Most earlier RCTs of treatments for low back pain were small (< 50 people/intervention group; range 9–169), short term (mostly < 6 months' follow up), and of low overall quality. Problems included lack of power, no description of randomisation procedure, incomplete analysis with failure to account for people who withdrew from trials, and lack of blinding.[9] The quality of the methods used by many recent RCTs is more adequate.

QUESTION What are the effects of oral drug treatments?

OPTION ANALGESICS (PARACETAMOL, OPIOIDS)

Systematic reviews have found no consistent difference with analgesics versus non-steroidal anti-inflammatory drugs in reduction of pain, but have found that electroacupuncture or ultrasound versus analgesics improves pain relief.

Benefits: We found two systematic reviews (search date not stated[2] and 1995;[9] no placebo controlled RCTs; 6 comparative RCTs; no statistical pooling of data). **Versus non-steroidal anti-inflammatory drugs:** The reviews identified two RCTs (110 people), which found no significant difference with meptazinol (an opioid) versus paracetamol or versus diflunisal (a non-steroidal anti-inflammatory drug [NSAID]) in pain relief.[2,9] A third RCT (219 people) identified by the reviews found that paracetamol versus mefenamic acid (an NSAID) increased pain relief.[2,9] **Versus non-drug treatments:** The reviews identified one RCT (40 people) that found that electroacupuncture (see glossary, p 1168) versus paracetamol increased pain relief after 6 weeks, and one RCT (73 people) that found that ultrasound treatment versus analgesics significantly increased the proportion of people who were pain free after 4 weeks.[2,9]

Harms: See paracetamol poisoning, p 1447. RCTs have found adverse effects (constipation and drowsiness) with analgesics in about 50% of people. One systematic review (search date 1995) found that combinations of paracetamol plus weak opioids versus paracetamol alone increased the risk of adverse effects (single dose studies OR 1.1, 95% CI 0.8 to 1.5; multiple dose studies OR 2.5, 95% CI 1.5 to 4.2).[10]

Comment: None.

OPTION COLCHICINE

We found insufficient evidence on the effects of colchicine.

Benefits: We found one systematic review (search date not stated, 1 RCT, 27 people), which found no significant difference with oral colchicine versus placebo in outcomes, although the RCT identified by the review was too small to rule out a clinically important difference.[2]

Harms: The review reported gastrointestinal irritation and skin problems in about 33% of people taking colchicine.[2] Other adverse effects included chemical cellulitis and agranulocytosis.[11]

Comment: The review identified two further RCTs, which did not distinguish between acute and chronic low back pain.[2]

OPTION MUSCLE RELAXANTS

Systematic reviews have found that muscle relaxants versus placebo reduce pain and muscle tension and increase mobility, but found no significant difference with muscle relaxants versus each other in

outcomes. The reviews found that adverse effects in people using muscle relaxants are common and include dependency, drowsiness, and dizziness. One RCT found that chlormezanone versus methocarbamol significantly increased the proportion of adverse effects (dyspepsia and drowsiness).

Benefits: We found two systematic reviews (search date not stated,[2] and search date 1995;[9] 14 RCTs, 1160 people; no statistical pooling of data). **Versus placebo:** The reviews identified nine RCTs (762 people), which compared a muscle relaxant (tizanidine, cyclobenzaprine, dantrolene, carisoprodol, baclofen, orphenadrine, or diazepam) versus placebo.[2,9] Seven of these RCTs found that muscle relaxants versus placebo reduced pain and muscle tension and increased mobility. The remaining two RCTs found no significant difference in outcomes. **Versus each other:** The reviews identified three RCTs (236 people), which found no significant difference with muscle relaxants (cyclobenzaprine, carisoprodol, and diazepam) versus each other in pain intensity, although two of the RCTs found that cyclobenzaprine or carisoprodol versus diazepam increased the proportion of people with overall improvement. One RCT identified by the review found no significant difference with methocarbamol versus chlormezanone in outcomes.

Harms: The reviews found that adverse effects included drowsiness or dizziness in up to 70% of people and a risk of dependency even after 1 week. More people experienced one or more adverse events with muscle relaxants versus placebo (68% of people with baclofen *v* 30% of people with placebo).[2,9] One RCT identified by the reviews found that chlormezanone versus methocarbamol significantly increased the proportion of adverse effects (dyspepsia and drowsiness; 14/52 [27%] with chlormezanone *v* 6/55 [11%] with methocarbamol; RR 2.50, 95% CI 1.02 to 5.93; NNH 6, 95% CI 3 to 90).[2,9]

Comment: None.

OPTION NON-STEROIDAL ANTI-INFLAMMATORY DRUGS (NSAIDS)

Systematic reviews and one additional RCT have found that non-steroidal anti-inflammatory drugs versus placebo significantly increase the proportion of people with overall improvement after 1 week and significantly reduce the proportion of people requiring additional analgesics. Systematic reviews and additional RCTs have found no significant difference with non-steroidal anti-inflammatory drugs versus each other or versus other treatments (paracetamol, opioids, muscle relaxants, and non-drug treatments) in pain relief.

Benefits: We found four systematic reviews (search dates not stated,[2] 1995,[9] 1998,[12] 1994;[13] 45 RCTs, statistical pooling only for non-steroidal anti-inflammatory drugs [NSAIDs] *v* placebo) and three additional RCTs.[14–16] **NSAIDs versus placebo:** The reviews identified nine RCTs, which found that NSAIDs versus placebo increased the proportion of people experiencing global improvement after 1 week (pooled OR 2.0, 95% CI 1.4 to 3.0), and reduced the proportion of people requiring additional analgesics (pooled OR 0.64, 95% CI 0.45 to 0.91).[2,9,12,13] The reviews identified four RCTs (313 people), which found no significant difference with NSAIDs versus placebo in relief of sciatica (see glossary, p 1168). The additional RCT (532 people) found that oral meloxicam (both 7.5 and 15.0 mg) versus placebo increased pain relief after 3 and 7 days.[17] **Versus each other:** The reviews identified 18 RCTs (1982 people), which found no significant difference with NSAIDs versus each other in outcomes.[2,9,12,13] One additional RCT (104 people) found that nimesulide versus ibuprofen improved functional status, but found no significant difference in pain relief after 10 days.[14] A second additional RCT (489 people) found no significant difference with meloxicam versus diclofenac in pain relief.[17] **Versus paracetamol:** The reviews identified two RCTs (93 people), which found no significant difference with mefenamic acid versus paracetamol in recovery rates, and one RCT (60 people), which found that mefenamic acid versus paracetamol increased pain relief.[2,9,12,13] The review identified one RCT (60 people), which found that mefenamic acid versus dextropropoxyphene plus paracetamol improved pain relief. **Versus muscle relaxants plus opioid analgesics:** The reviews identified five RCTs (399 people), which found no significant difference with NSAIDs versus muscle relaxants plus opioids in pain relief or overall improvement.[2,9,12,13] **Versus non-drug treatments:** We found three RCTs (461 people). The first RCT (110 people) found that NSAIDs versus bed rest improved range of movement, although the second RCT (241 people) found no significant difference between treatments in range of movement. Two RCTs (354 people) comparing NSAIDs versus physiotherapy or versus spinal manipulation found no significant difference in pain relief or improvement in mobility. **Versus NSAIDs plus adjuvant treatment:** The reviews identified three RCTs (232 people), which found no significant difference with NSAIDs alone versus NSAIDs plus muscle relaxants in outcomes.[2,9,12,13] One RCT identified by the reviews,[2,9,12,13] and one additional RCT[18] found no significant difference with NSAIDs alone versus NSAIDs plus vitamin B combinations in pain relief, although one of the RCTs found that NSAIDs alone versus NSAIDs plus vitamin B combinations reduced the proportion of people returning to work after 1 week (78% of people with combination treatment *v* 35% with NSAIDs alone).

Harms: NSAIDs may cause gastrointestinal complications (see non-steroidal anti-inflammatory drugs, p 1203). In the reviews, ibuprofen and diclofenac had the lowest gastrointestinal complication rate mainly because of the low doses used in practice (pooled OR for adverse effects versus placebo 1.30, 95% CI 0.91 to 1.80).[2,19] RCTs have found no significant difference with nimesulide versus ibuprofen, and meloxicam versus diclofenac in adverse effects.

Comment: None.

QUESTION What are the effects of local injections?

OPTION EPIDURAL STEROID INJECTIONS

Systematic reviews have identified one RCT that found that epidural steroids versus subcutaneous lidocaine injections increased the proportion of people who were pain free after 3 months. The reviews identified a second RCT that found no significant difference with epidural steroids versus epidural saline, epidural bupivacaine, or dry needling in the proportion of people cured or improved.

Benefits: We found five systematic reviews (search date not stated, 9 RCTs;[2] 1995, 7 RCTs;[9] 1998, 15 RCTs;[20] search date not stated, 11 RCTs;[21] and 1996, 21 RCTs[22]) The first RCT (57 people with acute low back pain and sciatica [see glossary, p 1168]) identified by the reviews found no significant difference with epidural steroids versus subcutaneous lidocaine (lignocaine) injections in pain relief after 1 month, but found that epidural steroids increased the proportion of people who were pain free after 3 months. The second RCT (63 people) identified by the reviews compared four treatments: epidural steroids; epidural saline; epidural bupivacaine; and dry needling. It found no difference between any of the treatments in the proportion of people improved or cured.

Harms: Adverse effects were infrequent and included headache, fever, subdural penetration, and, more rarely, epidural abscess and respiratory depression.[2,20]

Comment: None.

QUESTION What are the effects of non-drug treatments?

OPTION ADVICE TO STAY ACTIVE

Two systematic reviews and one subsequent RCT have found that advice to stay active versus no advice significantly increases the rate of recovery, reduces pain, reduces disability, and reduces time spent off work.

Benefits: We found three systematic reviews (search dates 1999, 9 RCTs;[23] not stated, 8 non-randomised studies;[2] and not stated, 8 RCTs;[24] no statistical pooling of data provided) and one subsequent RCT.[25] Two RCTs (228 people) identified by the third review and the subsequent RCT (457 people) found that advice to stay active versus no advice significantly increased rates of recovery, reduced pain, and reduced disability.[24,25] The reviews identified six RCTs (1957 people), which found that advice to stay active versus traditional medical treatment (analgesics as required, advice to rest, and "let pain be your guide") reduced sick leave and reduced chronic disability (see text, p 1163).[2,23,24]

Harms: The reviews and subsequent RCT did not report harms.[2,23–25]

Comment: Limitations in methods preclude meaningful quantification of effect sizes. Advice to stay active was either provided as a single treatment or in combination with other interventions such as back schools, a graded activity programme, or behavioural counselling.

OPTION BACK SCHOOLS

One systematic review found limited evidence that back schools versus placebo increased rates of recovery and reduced sick leave in the short term. The review found no significant difference with back school versus physiotherapy in outcomes and found that back school versus McKenzie exercises increased pain and sick leave.

Benefits: We found one systematic review (search date 1997, 3 RCTs, no statistical pooling of data provided).[26] The review identified one RCT (145 people), which found that back schools versus placebo (short wave diathermy at lowest intensity) increased rates of recovery and reduced sick leave in the short term. A second RCT (142 people) identified by the review found no difference with back schools versus physiotherapy in short term and long term outcomes. A third RCT (100 people) identified by the review found that ongoing McKenzie exercises (see glossary, p 1168) versus one 45 minute session of back school reduced pain and sick leave for up to 5 years.

Harms: The review did not report harms.[26]

Comment: None.

OPTION BED REST

Systematic reviews have found no evidence that bed rest is better, but have found evidence that it could be worse than no treatment, advice to stay active, back exercises, physiotherapy, spinal manipulation, or non-steroidal anti-inflammatory drugs. One systematic review has found that adverse effects of bed rest include joint stiffness, muscle wasting, loss of bone mineral density, pressure sores, and venous thromboembolism.

Benefits: We found six systematic reviews (search dates not stated, 4 RCTs;[2] 1995, 4 RCTs;[7] 1995, 6 RCTs;[9] 1999, 9 RCTs;[23] not stated, 10 RCTs;[24] not stated, 5 RCTs;[27] no statistical pooling provided). **Versus no treatment:** The reviews identified five RCTs (663 people), which compared bed rest versus no treatment and found either no significant difference between treatments or that no treatment improved outcomes.[2,7,9,23,24,27] **Versus different lengths of bed rest:** The reviews identified two RCTs (254 people), which found no significant difference with 7 days versus 2–4 days of bed rest in outcomes.[2,7,9,23,24,27] **Versus other interventions:** The reviews identified five RCTs (921 people), which compared bed rest versus other interventions (advice to stay active, back exercises, physiotherapy, spinal manipulation, or non-steroidal anti-inflammatory drugs).[2,7,9,23,24,27] They found either no significant difference in outcomes (pain, recovery rate, time to return to daily activities, and sick leave), or an improvement in outcomes with the comparative interventions. The most recent systematic review found no significant difference with bed rest versus advice to stay active in pain intensity after 3 weeks.[23]

Harms: One systematic review found that adverse effects of bed rest included joint stiffness, muscle wasting, loss of bone mineral density, pressure sores, and venous thromboembolism (see thromboembolism, p 209).[24]

Comment: None.

OPTION BEHAVIOURAL THERAPY

Two RCTs have found that behavioural therapy versus traditional care or electromyographic biofeedback reduces acute low back pain and disability.

Benefits: We found five systematic reviews (search dates not stated,[2] 1995,[7] 1995,[9] 1994,[28] and 1999;[29] no statistical pooling of data provided) and one additional RCT.[30] One RCT (107 people) found that behavioural therapy versus traditional care (analgesics plus back exercises until pain had subsided) reduced pain and perceived disability after 9–12 months. A second RCT (50 people with acute low back pain and sciatica) found that risk factor based cognitive behavioural therapy (see glossary, p 1168) versus electromyographic biofeedback (see glossary, p 1168) increased pain relief.

Harms: The reviews and additional RCT did not report on harms.[2,7,9,28,29]

Comment: None.

OPTION ELECTROMYOGRAPHIC BIOFEEDBACK

We found insufficient evidence on electromyographic biofeedback.

Benefits: We found one RCT (50 people with acute low back pain and sciatica [see glossary, p 1168]), which found that risk factor based cognitive behavioural therapy versus electromyographic biofeedback (see glossary, p 1168) improved pain relief.[30]

Harms: The RCT did not report on harms.[30]

Comment: None.

OPTION EXERCISE/BACK EXERCISES

Systematic reviews and additional RCTs have found either no difference with back exercises versus conservative or inactive treatments in pain or disability, or found that back exercises increase pain or disability.

Benefits: We found five systematic reviews (search dates not stated,[2] 1995,[7] 1995,[9] 1995,[31] and 1999;[32] no statistical pooling of data) and two additional RCTs.[16,33] The reviews identified eight RCTs (660 people), which compared specific back exercises (flexion, extension, aerobic, or strengthening programmes such as McKenzie exercises [see glossary, p 1168]) versus other conservative treatments (usual care by the general practitioner, continuation of ordinary activities, bed rest, manipulation, non-steroidal anti-inflammatory drugs, mini back school, or short wave diathermy).[2,7,9,31,32] Seven of these RCTs found either no difference between treatments or that back exercises increased pain intensity and disability. The eighth RCT found that back exercises versus a mini back school improved pain and return to work. The other four RCTs (1234 people) identified by the reviews found no difference between back exercises versus inactive treatments (bed rest, educational booklet, and placebo ultrasound) in pain relief, global improvement, or functional status. The first additional RCT (66 people) found that endurance training back exercises versus no treatment increased improvement in functioning and pain relief after 3 weeks, but found no difference in functioning or pain after 6 weeks.[16] The second additional RCT (41 people) found no significant difference between advice, minimal bed rest, or analgesics versus the same treatment plus specific, localised exercise of the multifidus muscle in pain and disability.[33]

Harms: The reviews and additional RCTs did not report harms.[2,7,9,16,31–33]

Comment: None.

OPTION LUMBAR SUPPORTS

We found no evidence on the effects of lumbar supports.

Benefits: We found no systematic review or RCTs specifically in people with acute low back pain.

Harms: Harms associated with prolonged lumbar support use include decreased strength of the trunk musculature, a false sense of security, heat, skin irritation, and general discomfort.[2]

Comment: None.

OPTION MULTIDISCIPLINARY TREATMENT PROGRAMMES

One systematic review in people with subacute low back pain found limited evidence that multidisciplinary treatment including a workplace visit versus usual care reduced sick leave.

Benefits: We found one systematic review (search date 1998, 2 RCTs, 233 people with subacute low back pain), which found that multidisciplinary treatment (see glossary, p 1168), including a workplace visit, versus usual care reduces sick leave.[34]

Harms: The review did not report harms.[34]

Comment: None.

OPTION TEMPERATURE TREATMENTS (SHORT WAVE DIATHERMY, ULTRASOUND, ICE, AND HEAT)

We found insufficient evidence on the effects of temperature treatments.

Benefits: We found two systematic reviews (search dates not stated[2] and 1992[35]), which found no RCTs.

Harms: The reviews did not report harms.[2,35]

Comment: None.

OPTION MASSAGE

Systematic reviews have found no difference with massage versus spinal manipulation or electrical stimulation in pain, functional status, or mobility.

Benefits: We found two systematic reviews (search dates 1999[36] and 1997;[37] 1 RCT). The reviews identified one RCT (90 people), which compared massage (see glossary, p 1168) versus spinal manipulation or electrical stimulation and found no significant difference in pain relief, functional status, or mobility.[36,37]

Harms: The reviews did not report harms.[36,37]

Comment: None.

OPTION SPINAL MANIPULATION

Systematic reviews found conflicting evidence on the effects of spinal manipulation.

Benefits: We found six systematic reviews (search dates not stated,[2] 1995,[7] 1995,[9] 1995,[38] not stated,[39] and 1997;[40] 18 RCTs; no statistical pooling of data provided). **Versus placebo:** The reviews identified five RCTs (383 people) comparing spinal manipulation versus placebo.[2,7,9,38–40] Two RCTs found that manipulation increased pain relief after 3 weeks, two RCTs found no significant difference in pain relief, and one RCT found that manipulation increased rates of recovery. **Versus other treatments:** The reviews identified 12 RCTs (899 people) comparing spinal manipulation versus other treatments (short wave diathermy, massage (see glossary, p 1168), exercises, back school, or drug treatment). Four of the reviews found that the results of these RCTs were conflicting.[2,7,9,38] The fifth review (7 RCTs, 731 people) found that spinal manipulation significantly increased recovery after 2–3 weeks (NNT 5, 95% CI 4 to 14).[39] The sixth review found limited evidence that spinal manipulation improved outcomes.[40]

Harms: In the RCTs that used a trained therapist to select people and perform spinal manipulation, the risk of serious complications was low (estimated risk: vertebrobasilar strokes 1/20 000–1/1 000 000 people; cauda equina syndrome < 1/1 000 000 people).

Comment: Current guidelines do not advise spinal manipulation in people with severe or progressive neurological deficit.[2,11]

OPTION TRACTION

RCTs found conflicting evidence on the effects of traction.

Benefits: We found three systematic reviews (search dates 1995,[7] 1995,[9] and 1992;[41] 2 RCTs). Two RCTs (225 people) identified by the reviews compared traction versus bed rest plus corset or versus infrared treatment. One RCT found that traction versus both other treatments increased overall improvement after 1 and 3 weeks, but the second RCT found no significant difference in overall improvement after 2 weeks.

Harms: The reviews did not report on harms.[7,9,41] Potential adverse effects include debilitation, loss of muscle tone, bone demineralisation, and thrombophlebitis.[2]

Comment: Of 16 RCTs identified, 12 RCTs (921 people) did not distinguish between acute and chronic low back pain.[7,9,41–43]

OPTION TRANSCUTANEOUS ELECTRICAL NERVE STIMULATION

We found insufficient evidence on the effects of transcutaneous electrical nerve stimulation.

Benefits: We found three systematic reviews (search dates not stated,[2] 1995,[9] and 2000;[44] 2 RCTs, 98 people). One RCT (58 people) compared transcutaneous electrical nerve stimulation alone versus transcutaneous electrical nerve stimulation plus a rehabilitation programme and found no difference in pain and functional status. The second RCT (40 people) found that transcutaneous electrical nerve stimulation versus paracetamol significantly improved pain and mobility after 6 weeks treatment.

Harms: The reviews did not report on harms.[2,9,44]

Comment: The most recent review only included trials on chronic low back pain.[44]

OPTION ACUPUNCTURE

We found no systematic reviews and no RCTs of acupuncture (see glossary, p 1168) specifically in people with acute low back pain.

Benefits: We found two systematic reviews (search dates 1996; see comment below), which found no RCTs in people with acute low back pain.[45,46]

Harms: One systematic review (search date 1996) found that serious, rare, adverse effects included infections (HIV, hepatitis, bacterial endocarditis) and visceral trauma (pneumothorax, cardiac tamponade).[47]

Comment: Three RCTs identified by the systematic reviews combined acute and chronic low back pain and two RCTs did not specify the duration of symptoms. One RCT included people with back and neck pain.[45,46]

Low back pain and sciatica: acute

GLOSSARY

Acupuncture Needle puncture of the skin at traditional "meridian" acupuncture points. Modern acupuncturists also use non-meridian points and trigger points (tender sites occurring in the most painful areas). The needles may be stimulated manually or electrically. Placebo acupuncture is needling of traditionally unimportant sites or non-stimulation of the needles once placed.

Cognitive behavioural therapy This aims to identify and modify peoples understanding of their pain and disability using cognitive restructuring techniques (such as imagery and attention diversion) or by modifying maladaptive thoughts, feelings, and beliefs.

Electroacupuncture Non-penetrative electrical stimulation of classical acupuncture points with low amplitude, pulsed electrical current.

Electromyographic biofeedback A person receives external feedback of their own electromyogram (using visual or auditory scales), and uses this to learn how to control the electromyogram and hence the tension within their own muscles. Electromyogram biofeedback for low back pain aims to relax the paraspinal muscles.

Massage Massage is manipulation of soft tissues (i.e. muscle and fascia) using the hands or a mechanical device, to promote circulation and relaxation of muscle spasm or tension. Different types of soft tissue massage include Shiatsu, Swedish, friction, trigger point, or neuromuscular massage.

McKenzie exercises Extension exercises that use self generated stresses and forces to centralise pain from the legs and buttocks to the lower back. This method emphasises self care.

Multidisciplinary treatment Intensive physical and psychosocial training by a team (e.g. a physician, physiotherapist, psychologist, social worker, and occupational therapist). Training is usually given in groups and does not involve passive physiotherapy.

Sciatica Pain that radiates from the back into the buttock or leg and is most commonly caused by prolapse of an intervertebral disk; the term may also be used to describe pain anywhere along the course of the sciatic nerve.

REFERENCES

1. Van der Heijden GJMG, Bouter LM, Terpstra-Lindeman E. De effectiviteit van tractie bij lage rugklachten. De resultaten van een pilotstudy. *Ned T Fysiotherapie* 1991;101:37–43.
2. Bigos S, Bowyer O, Braen G, et al. Acute low back problems in adults. Clinical Practice Guideline no.14. AHCPR Publication No. 95–0642. Rockville MD: Agency for Health Care Policy and Research, Public Health Service, US, Department of Health and Human Services. December 1994. Search date not stated; primary sources The Quebec Task Force on Spinal Disorders Review to 1984, search carried out by National Library of Medicine from 1984, and references from expert panel.
3. Andersson GBJ. The epidemiology of spinal disorders. In: Frymoyer JW, ed. *The adult spine: principles and practice*. 2nd ed. New York: Raven Press, 1997:93–141.
4. Deyo RA, Rainville J, Kent DL. What can the history and physical examination tell us about low back pain? *JAMA* 1992;268:760–765.
5. Bongers PM, de Winter CR, Kompier MA, et al. Psychosocial factors at work and musculoskeletal disease. *Scand J Work Environ Health* 1993;19:297–312.
6. Frymoyer JW. Back pain and sciatica. *N Engl J Med* 1988;318:291–300.
7. Evans G, Richards S. *Low back pain: an evaluation of therapeutic interventions.* Bristol: Health Care Evaluation Unit, University of Bristol, 1996. Search date 1995; primary sources Medline, Embase, A-Med, Psychlit, and hand searched references.
8. Van Tulder MW, Assendelft WJJ, Koes BW, et al, and the Editorial Board of the Cochrane Collaboration Back Review Group. Method guidelines for systematic reviews in the Cochrane Collaboration back review group for spinal disorders. *Spine* 1997;22:2323–2330.
9. Van Tulder MW, Koes BW, Bouter LM. Conservative treatment of acute and chronic nonspecific low back pain: a systematic review of randomized controlled trials of the most common interventions. *Spine* 1997;22:2128–2156. Search date 1995; primary sources Medline, Embase, Psychlit, and hand searched references.
10. De Craen AJM, Di Giulio G, Lampe-Schoenmaeckers AJEM, et al. Analgesic efficacy and safety of paracetamol–codeine combinations versus paracetamol alone: a systematic review. *BMJ* 1996;313:321–325. Search date 1995; primary sources Medline, Embase, International Pharmaceutical Abstracts, Biosis, contact with pharmaceutical companies, and hand searched references.
11. Waddell G, Feder G, McIntosh A, et al. *Low back pain evidence review.* London: Royal College of General Practitioners, 1996. Search date 1996; primary sources Medline, Embase, Science

Citation Index, Social Sciences Citation Index, correspondence with experts and researchers, and hand searched references.

12. Van Tulder MW, Scholten RJPM, Koes BW, et al. Non-steroidal anti-inflammatory drugs (NSAIDs) for non-specific low back pain. In: The Cochrane Library, Issue 4, 2001. Oxford: Update Software. Search date 1998; primary sources Medline, Embase, Cochrane Controlled Trials Register, and hand searches of reference lists.
13. Koes BW, Scholten RJPM, Mens JMA, et al. Efficacy of non-steroidal anti-inflammatory drugs for low back pain: a systematic review of randomised clinical trials. *Ann Rheum Dis* 1997;56:214–223. Search date 1994; primary sources Medline, Embase, and hand searched references.
14. Pohjolainen T, Jekunen A, Autio L, Vuorela H. Treatment of acute low back pain with the COX-2 selective anti-inflammatory drug Nimesulide: results of a randomised, double-blind comparative trial versus Ibuprofen. *Spine* 2000;25:1579–1585.
15. Laws D. Double blind parallel group investigation in general practice of the efficacy and tolerability of acemetacin, in comparison with diclofenac, in patients suffering with acute low back pain. *Br J Clin Res* 1994;5:55–64.
16. Chok B, Lee R, Latimer J, Tan SB. Endurance training of the trunk extensor muscles in people with subacute low back pain. *Phys Ther* 1999;79:1032–1042.
17. Dreiser RL, LeParc JM, Velicitat P, Lieu PL. Oral meloxicam is effective in acute sciatica: two randomised, double-blind trials versus placebo or diclofenac. *Inflamm Res* 2001;1:S17–S23.
18. Bruggemann G, Koehler CO, Koch EM. Results of a double-blind study of diclofenac + vitamin B1, B6, B12 versus diclofenac in patients with acute pain of the lumbar vertebrae: a multicenter study. *Klinische Wochenschrift* 1990;68:116–120.
19. Henry D, Lim LLY, Rodriguez LAG, et al. Variability in risk of gastrointestinal complications with individual non-steroidal anti-inflammatory drugs: results of a collaborative meta-analysis. *BMJ* 1996;312:1563–1566. Search date 1994; primary sources Medline, contact with study authors, and hand searched references.
20. Koes BW, Scholten RJPM, Mens JMA, Bouter LM. Epidural steroid injections for low back pain and sciatica: an updated systematic review of randomized clinical trials. *Pain Digest* 1999;9:241–247. Search date 1998; primary sources Medline and hand searches from relevant publications.
21. Watts RW, Silagy CA. A meta-analysis on the efficacy of epidural corticosteroids in the treatment of sciatica. *Anaesth Intensive Care* 1995;23:564–569. Search date not stated; primary sources Medline, hand searches from published reviews and clinical trials, and personal contact with published authors in the field and the pharmaceutical manufacturer.
22. Nelemans PJ, de Bie RA, de Vet HCW, Sturmans F. Injection therapy for subacute and chronic benign low back pain. In: The Cochrane Library, Issue 4, 2001. Oxford: Update Software. Search date 1996; primary sources Medline, Embase, and hand searches of reference lists.
23. Hagen KB, Hilde G, Jamtvedt G, Winnem M. Bed rest for acute low back pain and sciatica (Cochrane Review). In: The Cochrane Library, Issue 4, 2001. Oxford: Update Software. Search date 1999; primary sources Cochrane Musculoskeletal Group's trials register, Cochrane Controlled Trials Register (CCTR), Cochrane Library, Medline, Embase, Sport, Scisearch, and hand searches of reference lists and personal contact with the authors of included articles.
24. Waddell G, Feder G, Lewis M. Systematic reviews of bed rest and advice to stay active for acute low back pain. *Br J Gen Pract* 1997;47:647–652. Search date not stated; primary sources Medline, contacted recently published authors and pharmaceutical company, and hand searched references.
25. Hagen EM, Eriksen HR, Ursin H. Does early intervention with a light mobilization program reduce long-term sick leave for low back pain? *Spine* 2000;25:1973–1976.
26. Van Tulder MW, Esmail R, Bombardier C, Koes BW. Back schools for non-specific low back pain. In: The Cochrane Library, Issue 4, 2001. Oxford: Update Software. Search date 1997; primary sources Medline, Embase, and hand searched references.
27. Koes BW, van den Hoogen HMM. Efficacy of bed rest and orthoses of low back pain. A review of randomized clinical trials. *Eur J Phys Med Rehabil* 1994;4:86–93. Search date not stated; primary sources Medline and hand searched references.
28. Turner JA. Educational and behavioral interventions for back pain in primary care. *Spine* 1996;21:2851–2859. Search date 1994; primary sources Medline, Psychlit, hand searches, and inquiries to pharmaceutical companies, and expert researchers in the field.
29. Van Tulder MW, Ostelo R, Vlaeyen JWS, Linton SJ, Morley SJ, Assendelft WJJ. Behavioural treatment for chronic low back pain. In: The Cochrane Library, Issue 4, 2001. Oxford: Update Software. Search date 1999; primary sources Medline, Psychlit, Cochrane Controlled Trials Register, Embase, and hand searches of reference lists.
30. Hasenbring M, Ulrich HW, Hartmann M, et al. The efficacy of a risk factor-based cognitive behavioral intervention and electromyographic biofeedback in patients with acute sciatic pain: an attempt to prevent chronicity. *Spine* 1999;24:2525–2535.
31. Faas A. Exercises: which ones are worth trying, for which patients and when? *Spine* 1996;21:2874–2879. Search date 1995; primary source Medline.
32. van Tulder MW, Malmivaara A, Esmail R, Koes BW. Exercise therapy for non-specific low back pain. In: The Cochrane Library, Issue 4, 2001. Oxford: Update Software. Search date 1999; primary sources Medline, Psychlit, Cochrane Controlled Trials Register, Embase, and hand searches of reference lists.
33. Hides JA, Richardson CA, Jull GA. Multifidus muscle recovery is not automatic after resolution of acute first episode low back pain. *Spine* 1996;21:2763–2769.
34. Karjalainen K, Malmivaara A, van Tulder M, et al. Multidisciplinary biopsychosocial rehabilitation for subacute low back pain among working age adults. In: The Cochrane Library, Issue 4, 2001. Oxford: Update Software. Search date 1998; primary sources Medline, Embase, Psyclit, Cochrane Register of Controlled Clinical Trials, Science Citation Index, and hand searches of reference lists and personal contact with experts.
35. Gam AN, Johannsen F. Ultrasound therapy in musculoskeletal disorders: a meta-analysis. *Pain* 1995;63:85–91. Search date 1992; primary sources Index Medicus, Medline, and hand searched references.
36. Furlan AD, Brosseau L, Welch V, Wong J. Massage for low back pain. In: The Cochrane Library, Issue 4, 2001. Oxford: Update Software. Search date 1999; primary sources Medline, Embase, Cochrane Controlled Trials Register, Healthstar,

Cinahl, Dissertation Abstracts, and hand searches of reference lists and contact with content experts and massage associations.

37. Ernst E. Massage therapy for low back pain: a systematic review. *J Pain Symptom Manage* 1999;17:65–69. Search date 1997; primary sources Medline, Embase, Cochrane Library, and hand searches of personal files, bibliographies, and personal contact with researchers.
38. Koes BW, Assendelft WJJ, van der Heijden GJMG, et al. Spinal manipulation for low back pain. An updated systematic review of randomized clinical trials. *Spine* 1996;21:2860–2871. Search date 1995; primary sources Medline and hand searched references.
39. Shekelle PG, Adams AH, Chassin MR, et al. Spinal manipulation for low back pain. *Ann Intern Med* 1992;117:590–598. Search date not stated; primary sources Medline, Index Medicus, contacted experts, and hand searched references.
40. Mohseni-Bandpei MA, Stephenson R, Richardson B. Spinal manipulation in the treatment of low back pain: a review of the literature with particular emphasis on randomized controlled trials. Phys Ther Rev 1998;3:185–194. Search date 1997; primary sources Medline, Cinhal, and BIDS.
41. Van der Heijden GJMG, Beurskens AJHM, Koes BW, et al. The efficacy of traction for back and neck pain: a systematic, blinded review of randomized clinical trial methods. *Phys Ther* 1995;75:93–104. Search date 1992; primary sources Medline, Embase, Index to Chiropractic Literature, Physiotherapy Index, and hand searched non-indexed journals.
42. Ljunggren E, Weber H, Larssen S. Autotraction versus manual traction in patients with prolapsed lumbar intervertebral discs. *Scand J Rehabil Med* 1984;16:117–124.
43. Werners R, Pynsent PB, Bulstrode CJK. Randomized trial comparing interferential therapy with motorized lumbar traction and massage in the management of low back pain in a primary care setting. *Spine* 1999;24:1579–1584.
44. Milne S, Welch V, Brosseau L, et al. Transcutaneous electrical nerve stimulation (TENS) for chronic low back pain (Cochrane review). In: The Cochrane Library, Issue 4, 2001. Oxford: Update Software. Search date 2000; primary sources Medline, Embase, PEDro, Cochrane Controlled Trials Register, hand searches of bibliographic references, reference lists, Current Contents, abstracts in specialized journals, Conference Proceedings, and personal contact with co-ordinating offices of the trials registries of the Cochrane Field of Physical and Related Therapies and Cochrane Musculoskeletal Group and content experts.
45. Ernst E, White AR. Acupuncture for back pain. A meta-analysis of randomized controlled trials. *Arch Intern Med* 1998;158:2235–2241. Search date 1996; primary sources Medline, Cochrane Controlled Trials Register, CISCOM, contacted authors and experts, and hand searched references.
46. Van Tulder MW, Cherkin DC, Berman B, et al. Acupuncture in low back pain. In: The Cochrane Library, Issue 4, 2001. Oxford: Update Software. Search date 1996; primary sources Medline, Embase, Cochrane Complementary Medicine Field trials register, Cochrane Controlled Trials Register, Science Citation Index, and hand searched references.
47. Ernst E, White A. Life-threatening adverse reactions after acupuncture? A systematic review. *Pain* 1997;71:123–126. Search date 1996; primary sources Medline, CISCOM, other specialised databases, contacted experts, and hand searched references.

Maurits van Tulder
Institute for Research
in Extramural Medicine
Vrije Universiteit Medical Centre
Amsterdam
The Netherlands

Bart Koes
Department of General Practice Erasmus
University
Rotterdam
The Netherlands

Competing interests: None declared.

Low back pain and sciatica: chronic

Search date October 2001

Maurits van Tulder and Bart Koes

QUESTIONS

INTERVENTIONS

See glossary, p 1184.

Key Messages

- **Acupuncture** Two systematic reviews have found no significant difference in outcomes with acupuncture versus placebo or no treatment. One systematic review and one subsequent RCT have found that acupuncture versus transcutaneous electrical nerve stimulation significantly reduces pain intensity and significantly increases overall improvement.
- **Analgesics** One RCT found that tramadol versus placebo decreased pain and increased functional status. A second RCT found that paracetamol versus diflunisal increased the number of people who rated the treatment as good or excellent.
- **Antidepressants** Systematic reviews and additional RCTs have found that antidepressants versus placebo significantly increase pain relief, but have found no significant difference in functioning or depression. Additional RCTs have found conflicting results on pain relief with antidepressants versus each other or versus analgesics.

- **Back schools in occupational settings (*v* no treatment)** One systematic review has found that, in occupational settings, back schools versus no treatment improve pain and reduce disability. Systematic reviews and one subsequent RCT found conflicting evidence on the effects of back schools.
- **Behavioural therapy** Systematic reviews have found that behavioural therapy versus no treatment, placebo, or waiting list control reduces pain and improves functional status and behavioural outcomes. Systematic reviews have found no significant difference with different types of behavioural therapy versus each other in functional status, pain, or behavioural outcomes, and found conflicting results with behavioural therapy versus other treatments in pain, behavioural outcomes, or functional status.
- **Electromyographic biofeedback** One systematic review found no significant difference in pain relief or functional status with electromyographic biofeedback versus placebo or waiting list control, but found conflicting results on the effects of electromyographic biofeedback versus other treatments.
- **Epidural steroid injections** Systematic reviews comparing epidural steroids versus placebo, local anaesthetic, local anaesthetic plus an opioid, or benzodiazepines (midazolam) found insufficient evidence on outcomes. One systematic review has found no difference with epidural steroid injections versus placebo in pain relief after 6 weeks or 6 months. One systematic review has found that epidural steroids versus other treatments significantly increase pain relief in the short term.
- **Exercise (*v* other treatments)** Systematic reviews and additional RCTs have found that exercise versus other treatments (including usual care) improves pain and functional status. RCTs have found conflicting evidence on the effects of exercise versus inactive treatments.
- **Facet joint injections** Two systematic reviews found no significant difference in pain relief with facet joint injections versus placebo or facet joint nerve blocks.
- **Lumbar supports** We found insufficient evidence on the effects of lumbar supports.
- **Massage (*v* other treatments)** Systematic reviews and subsequent RCTs have found that massage versus other treatments reduces pain and improves functioning.
- **Multidisciplinary treatment programmes (*v* non-multidisciplinary treatments)** Systematic reviews have found that intensive multidisciplinary biopsychosocial rehabilitation with functional restoration versus inpatient or outpatient non-multidisciplinary treatments or versus usual care reduces pain and improves function. The reviews found no significant difference in pain or function with less intensive multidisciplinary treatments versus non-multidisciplinary treatments or usual care.
- **Muscle relaxants** We found insufficient evidence on the benefits of muscle relaxants. One RCT found that adverse effects, including dependency, drowsiness, and dizziness, occur in up to 70% of people.
- **Non-steroidal anti-inflammatory drugs** One RCT found that naproxen versus placebo increased pain relief. Systematic reviews and additional RCTs have found no significant difference with non-steroidal anti-inflammatory drugs versus each other in outcomes. Two RCTs found conflicting evidence on the effects of non-steroidal anti-inflammatory drugs versus analgesics.

- **Spinal manipulation** We found four systematic reviews that identified the same 12 RCTs. One of the reviews found that spinal manipulation versus placebo improved outcomes, the other three reviews found that the results of the RCTs were conflicting.
- **Traction** One systematic review and two additional RCTs have found no significant difference in pain relief or functional status with traction versus placebo or with traction plus massage versus interferential treatment (electrotherapy).
- **Transcutaneous electrical nerve stimulation** One systematic review has found no significant difference with transcutaneous electrical nerve stimulation versus control in pain relief. Two systematic reviews found conflicting evidence on the effects of transcutaneous electrical nerve stimulation.versus placebo or conservative treatments.
- **Trigger point and ligamentous injections** One systematic review found limited evidence that steroid plus local anaesthetic injection of trigger points versus local anaesthetic injection alone increased pain relief after 3 months, and that phenol versus saline injection of the lumbar interspinal ligament increased pain relief after 6 months.

DEFINITION Low back pain is pain, muscle tension, or stiffness localised below the costal margin and above the inferior gluteal folds, with or without leg pain (sciatica [see glossary, p 1185]),[1] and is defined as chronic when it persists for 12 weeks or more (see definition of acute low back pain, p 1156).[2] Non-specific low back pain is low back pain not attributed to a recognisable pathology (such as infection, tumour, osteoporosis, rheumatoid arthritis, fracture, or inflammation).[1] This review excludes low back pain or sciatica with symptoms or signs at presentation that suggest a specific underlying condition.

INCIDENCE/ PREVALENCE See incidence of acute low back pain, p 1156

INCIDENCE/ PREVALENCE See aetiology of acute low back pain, p 1156

PROGNOSIS See prognosis of acute low back pain, p 1156

AIMS To relieve pain; to improve function; to develop coping strategies for pain, with minimal adverse effects from treatment.[2,3]

OUTCOMES Pain intensity (visual analogue or numerical rating scale); overall improvement (self reported or observed); back pain specific functional status (such as Roland Morris questionnaire, Oswestry questionnaire); impact on employment (days of sick leave, number of people returned to work); medication use; intervention specific outcomes (such as coping and pain behaviour for behavioural treatment, strength and flexibility for exercise, depression for antidepressants, and muscle spasm for muscle relaxants and electromyographic biofeedback [see glossary, p 1184]).

METHODS *Clinical Evidence* search and appraisal October 2001. In addition the authors searched Medline (1966 to December 1998), Embase (1980 to September 1998), and Psychlit (1984 to December 1998), using the search strategy recommended by the Cochrane Back Review Group.[4] Most earlier RCTs of treatments for low back pain were small (< 50 people/intervention group; range 9–169), short term (mostly < 6 months' follow up), and of low overall quality. Problems included lack of power, no description of randomisation procedure, incomplete analysis with failure to account for people who withdrew from trials, and lack of blinding.[5] The quality of the methods used by many recent RCTs is more adequate.

QUESTION **What are the effects of oral drug treatments?**

OPTION **ANALGESICS (PARACETAMOL, OPIOIDS)**

One RCT found that tramadol versus placebo decreased pain and increased functional status. One RCT found that paracetamol versus diflunisal significantly reduced the proportion of people who rated the treatment as good or excellent at 4 weeks. One RCT found that a lower proportion of people taking paracetamol versus diflusinal rated the treatment as good or excellent at 4 weeks, but the difference was not significant. Another RCT found no significant difference in pain relief with an opioid analgesic versus a parenteral non-steroidal anti-inflammatory.

Benefits: **Analgesics versus placebo:** One RCT (254 people) found that tramadol (an opioid) versus placebo decreased pain and increased functional status.[6] **Analgesics versus non-steroidal anti-inflammatory drugs:** See NSAIDs, p 1203.

Harms: RCTs found adverse effects (constipation and drowsiness) with analgesics in about 50% of people. One systematic review (search date 1995) comparing combinations of paracetamol plus weak opioids versus paracetamol alone found that combination treatment increased the risk of adverse effects (single dose studies OR 1.1, 95% CI 0.8 to 1.5; multiple dose studies OR 2.5, 95% CI 1.5 to 4.2).[7]

Comment: None.

OPTION **ANTIDEPRESSANTS**

Systematic reviews and additional RCTs have found that antidepressants versus placebo significantly increase pain relief, but found no significant difference in functioning or depression. Additional RCTs have found conflicting results with antidepressants versus each other or analgesics on pain relief.

Benefits: We found five systematic reviews (search dates not stated,[2] 1995,[3] 1995,[5] 1992,[8] 2000,[9]) and six additional RCTs.[10–15] **Versus placebo:** The most recent review found that antidepressants versus placebo significantly increased pain relief (standardised mean difference [SMD] 0.41, 95% CI 0.22 to 0.61), but found no significant difference in functioning (SMD +0.24, 95% CI –0.21 to +0.69).[9] We found six RCTs that compared an antidepressant (imipramine, amitriptyline, trazodone, nortriptyline, doxepin, maprotiline, paroxetine, or clomipramine) versus placebo and reported on the outcome of depression. Five of these RCTs found no difference in depression, although the sixth RCT[11,12] found that an antidepressant versus placebo significantly reduced depression. **Versus each**

other: One additional RCT (36 people) compared doxepin versus desipramine and found no differences in pain relief or depression.[12] A second additional RCT (67 people) found that maprotiline versus paroxetine increased pain relief.[14] **Versus analgesics:** A third additional RCT (39 people with mild depression plus chronic low back pain) found that antidepressants versus paracetamol increased pain relief.[13]

Harms: Adverse effects of antidepressants included dry mouth, drowsiness, constipation, urinary retention, orthostatic hypotension, and mania.[2] One RCT found that the prevalence of dry mouth, insomnia, sedation, and orthostatic symptoms was 60–80% with tricyclic antidepressants; however, rates were only slightly lower in the placebo group and none of the differences were significant.[10]

Comment: None.

OPTION MUSCLE RELAXANTS

We found insufficient evidence on the effects of muscle relaxants. One RCT found that adverse effects in people using muscle relaxants are common and include dependency, drowsiness, and dizziness.

Benefits: We found two systematic reviews (search dates not stated[2] and 1995,[5] 1 RCT). The RCT (50 people) identified by the reviews found that tetrazepam versus placebo increased overall improvement (64% *v* 29% of people) and reduced pain after 10 days.[2,5]

Harms: The reviews found that adverse effects of muscle relaxants included drowsiness or dizziness in up to 70% of people and a risk of dependency even after 1 week.[2,5]

Comment: None.

OPTION NON-STEROIDAL ANTI-INFLAMMATORY DRUGS (NSAIDS)

One RCT found that naproxen versus placebo increased pain relief. Systematic reviews and additional RCTs have found no significant differences with non-steroidal anti-inflammatory drugs versus each other in outcomes. One RCT found that a higher proportion of people taking diflusinal versus paracetamol rated the treatment as good or excellent at 4 weeks, but the difference was not significant. Another RCT found no significant difference in pain relief with a parenteral non-steroidal anti-inflammatory versus an opioid analgesic.

Benefits: We found four systematic reviews (search dates not stated,[2] 1995,[5] 1998,[16] and 1994[17]) and two additional RCTs.[18,19] **Versus placebo:** One RCT (37 people) identified by the reviews found that naproxen versus placebo increased pain relief.[2,5,16,17] **Versus each other:** Four RCTs (453 people) identified by the reviews found no difference with different non-steroidal anti-inflammatory drugs (NSAIDs) versus each other in outcomes.[2,5,16,17] One RCT (252 people) identified by the reviews found that diclofenac plus vitamins B_1, B_6, and B_{12} versus diclofenac increased overall improvement.[2,5,16,17] The first additional RCT (196 people) found no significant difference with nimesulide versus diclofenac in pain or functioning.[18] The second additional RCT (155 people) found no significant difference with ketorolac versus meperidine in outcomes.[19] **Versus analgesics:** One RCT (29 people) identified by the reviews found that a higher proportion people taking diflunisal versus paracetamol rated the treatment as good or excellent at 4 weeks, but the difference was not significant (10/16 [62%] *v* 4/12 [33%]; RR 1.87, 95% CI 0.77 to 4.55; calculated by *Clinical Evidence*).[2,5,16,17] A second RCT (155 people) identified by the reviews found no difference with a parenteral NSAID versus a parenteral opioid in pain relief.[2,5,16,17]

Harms: NSAIDs may cause gastrointestinal complications (see non-steroidal anti-inflammatory drugs, p 1203). RCTs have found that ibuprofen and diclofenac have the lowest gastrointestinal complication rate mainly because of the low doses used in practice (pooled OR for adverse effects *v* placebo 1.30, 95% CI 0.91 to 1.80).[2,20,21] The first additional RCT found that nimesulide has a similarly low rate of gastrointestinal adverse effects as diclofenac.[18]

Comment: None.

QUESTION What are the effects of local injections?

OPTION EPIDURAL STEROID INJECTIONS

Three systematic reviews comparing epidural steroids versus either placebo, local anaesthetic, local anaesthetic plus an opioid, or benzodiazepines (midazolam) found insufficient evidence on outcomes. One systematic review has found no significant difference with epidural steroid injections versus placebo in pain relief after 6 weeks or 6 months. One systematic review has found that epidural steroids versus other treatments significantly increase pain relief in the short term.

Benefits: We found five systematic reviews (search dates not stated, 7 RCTs;[2] 1995, 5 RCTs;[5] not stated, 9 RCTs;[21] 1998, 13 RCTs;[22] and 1996, 19 RCTs[23]). The systematic reviews identified 11 RCTs (518 people) comparing epidural steroids versus either placebo (epidural saline), local anaesthetic (epidural bupivacaine or procaine), local anaesthetic plus an opioid (lidocaine [lignocaine] plus morphine), or benzodiazepines (midazolam).[2,5,21–23] Three systematic reviews found insufficient evidence to draw conclusions (no statistical pooling provided).[2,5,22] The most recent systematic review identified four RCTs (302 people) comparing epidural steroid injections versus placebo. It found no significant difference in pain relief after 6 weeks (pooled RR 0.93, 95% CI 0.79 to 1.09) or 6 months (pooled RR 0.92, 95% CI 0.76 to 1.11).[23] One systematic review (of both placebo controlled and comparative RCTs) found that epidural steroids versus other treatments significantly increased pain relief in the short term (pooled OR 2.60, 95% CI 1.90 to 3.80; see comment below).[21]

Harms: The reviews found that adverse effects were infrequent and included headache, fever, subdural penetration, and, more rarely, epidural abscess and respiratory depression.[2,22]

Comment: RCTs identified by the reviews were generally small (range 22 to 73 people) and included people with a variety of conditions (chronic low back pain with and without sciatica alone, lumbar radicular pain syndrome, and post-laminectomy pain syndrome).

OPTION FACET JOINT INJECTIONS

Two systematic reviews found no significant difference in pain relief with facet joint injections versus placebo or facet joint nerve blocks.

Benefits: We found two systematic reviews (search dates not stated[2] and 1996;[23] 3 RCTs; no statistical pooling of data). Two RCTs (206 people) identified by the reviews found no significant difference with intra-articular corticosteroid versus placebo (intra-articular saline) injections in pain relief, disability, and flexibility after 1, 3, or 6 months.[2,23] One RCT (86 people) identified by the reviews found no significant difference with facet joint injections versus facet joint nerve blocks in pain relief after 2 weeks, 1 month, or 3 months.[2,23]

Harms: One of the reviews found that adverse effects included pain at injection site, infection, haemorrhage, neurological damage, and chemical meningitis.[2]

Comment: Two RCTs from one of the reviews,[2] did not distinguish between acute and chronic pain and have not been included in this review.

OPTION TRIGGER POINT AND LIGAMENTOUS INJECTIONS

One systematic review found limited evidence that steroid plus local anaesthetic injection of trigger points versus local anaesthetic injection alone increased pain relief after 3 months and that phenol versus saline injection of the lumbar interspinal ligament increased pain relief after 6 months.

Benefits: We found one systematic review (search date not stated, 2 RCTs, 138 people).[2] One RCT (57 people) identified by the review found that trigger point injection using steroid (methylprednisolone or triamcinolone) plus lidocaine versus lidocaine alone increased the number of people with complete relief of pain after 3 months (60–80% *v* 20%).[2] The other RCT (81 people) identified by the review found that dextrose–glycerine–phenol versus saline injection into the lumbar interspinal ligament increased pain relief after 1, 3, and 6 months.[2]

Harms: The review found that potential harms included nerve or other tissue damage, infection, and haemorrhage.[2]

Comment: None.

QUESTION What are the effects of non-drug treatments?

OPTION BACK SCHOOLS

One systematic review has found that in occupational settings, back schools versus no treatment improve pain and reduce disability. Systematic reviews and one subsequent RCT have found conflicting evidence on the effects of back schools.

Benefits: We found two systematic reviews (search date 1997, 14 RCTs, no statistical pooling of data provided;[24] search date 2000, 18 RCTs and other studies[25]) and one subsequent RCT.[26] Five RCTs (880 people) identified by the first review found that intensive back school programmes in an occupational setting versus no treatment improved pain and reduced disability, but found no difference versus other treatments (physiotherapy, calisthenics group training, or usual care) in outcomes.[24] Six RCTs (529 people) identified by the first review and the subsequent RCT compared back schools versus no treatment, waiting list control, or short wave diathermy. Four of these RCTs found that back schools improved outcomes in the short term,[24] two of these RCTs found no difference in the short term, and the remaining two RCTs found no difference in the long term.[24,26] Five RCTs (861 people) identified by the first review found that back schools versus exercises, manipulation, non-steroidal anti-inflammatory drugs (NSAIDs), or physiotherapy increased pain relief and reduced disability after 6 months, but found no significant difference after 1 year.[24] The second systematic review found that back schools versus no treatment, or versus any other treatment, significantly increased pain relief after 3 months, but found no difference in outcomes in the long term (see comment below).[25]

Harms: The reviews and subsequent RCT did not report on harms.[24–26]

Comment: The second review combined studies (both RCTs, CCTs), which compared back schools versus no treatment and versus other active treatments in the same meta-analysis, and did not take the methodologic quality of the studies into account.[25]

OPTION BEHAVIOURAL THERAPY

Systematic reviews have found that behavioural therapy versus no treatment, placebo, or waiting list control reduces pain and improves functional status and behavioural outcomes. Systematic reviews have found no significant difference in functional status, pain, or behavioural outcomes with different types of behavioural therapy versus each other, and found conflicting results with behavioural therapy versus other treatments.

Benefits: We found five systematic reviews (search dates not stated,[2] 1995,[3] 1995,[5] 1994,[27] and 1999;[28] 20 RCTs, no statistical pooling of data). **Versus placebo, no treatment, or waiting list control:** Eleven RCTs (1223 people) identified by the reviews found that behavioural therapy versus no treatment, placebo, or waiting list control reduced pain intensity and improved functional status and behavioural outcomes.[2,3,5,27,28] **Versus other sorts of behavioural therapy:** The reviews identified nine RCTs (308 people), which found no significant difference with different types of behavioural therapy (cognitive behavioural therapy, operant behavioural treatments, and respondent behavioural treatment (see glossary, p 1185) versus each other in functional status, pain, or behavioural outcomes (including anxiety, depression, pain behaviour, and coping).[2,3,5,27,28] **Versus other treatments:** Two RCTs (202 people) identified by the reviews found that behavioural therapy versus traditional care (rest, analgesics, or physiotherapy) or back exercises increased the number of people who had returned to work after 12 weeks but found no difference in pain or depression after 6 months or 12 months.[2,3,5,27,28] Six RCTs (343 people) identified by the reviews comparing behavioural therapy plus other treatments (physiotherapy and back education, multidisciplinary treatment (see glossary, p 1184) programmes, inpatient pain management programmes, and back exercises) versus other treatments alone found that behavioural therapy plus the other treatments improved functional status in the short term but found no difference in pain or behavioural outcomes.[2,3,5,27,28]

Harms: The reviews did not report on harms.[2,3,5,27,28]

Comment: None.

OPTION ELECTROMYOGRAPHIC BIOFEEDBACK

One systematic review has found no difference in pain relief or functional status with electromyographic biofeedback versus placebo or waiting list control, but found conflicting results on the effects of electromyographic biofeedback versus other treatments.

Benefits: We found one systematic review (search date 1995, 5 RCTs, 168 people, no statistical pooling of data).[5] **Versus placebo or waiting list control:** Three RCTs (102 people) identified by the review found no difference with electromyographic biofeedback (see glossary, p 1184) versus placebo or waiting list control in pain relief or functional status.[5] **Versus other treatments:** Two RCTs (30 people) identified by the review found conflicting results with electromyographic biofeedback versus progressive relaxation training in outcomes.[5] One RCT (30 people) identified by the review found no difference in rehabilitation programmes plus biofeedback versus biofeedback alone in pain or range of movement.[5]

Harms: The review did not report on harms.[5]

Comment: None.

OPTION EXERCISE

Systematic reviews and additional RCTs have found that exercise versus other treatments (including usual care) improves pain and functional status. RCTs have found conflicting evidence on the effects of exercise versus inactive treatments and versus different types of exercise.

Benefits: We found five systematic reviews (search date not stated,[2] 1995,[3] 1995,[5] 1995,[29] and 1999;[30] 23 RCTs, 2240 people; no statistical pooling of data) and 14 additional RCTs.[31–44] **Versus inactive treatment:** Six RCTs (587 people) identified by one review compared exercise versus inactive treatments (hot packs and rest, semi-hot packs plus sham traction, waiting list control, transcutaneous electrical nerve stimulation [TENS], sham TENS, detuned ultrasound, or short wave diathermy).[30] Three of these RCTs found that exercise versus inactive treatments increased overall improvement, whereas the remaining three RCTs found no difference in overall improvement. One additional small RCT (59 people) found that active rehabilitation consisting of 24 exercise sessions during

12 weeks versus inactive treatments improved pain intensity and functional disability.[36] **Versus other treatments:** Nine RCTs (1020 people) identified by the reviews compared exercise versus other treatments.[2,3,5,29,30] Three of these RCTs found no difference with exercise versus conventional physiotherapy in pain, functional status, overall improvement, or return to work. Three RCTs found that exercise versus usual care by the general practitioner improved pain, functional status, and return to work. Three RCTs found that exercise versus back school education plus early morning lumbar flexion control improved both pain and functional status. One additional RCT (132 people) found that a full time, intensive 3 weeks' multidisciplinary programme versus exercise or exercise plus psychological pain management improved ability to work (but not return to work) and disability after 4 and 24 months, and improved pain relief after 4 months.[31,32] A second additional RCT (109 people) found no difference between exercise versus massage (see glossary, p 1184) in pain and disability after 4 weeks (post-treatment).[33] **Versus each other:** One additional RCT (148 people) found no difference with active physiotherapy versus muscle reconditioning on training devices or versus low impact aerobics in pain intensity after 6 months and 1 year, but found that muscle reconditioning and aerobic exercises versus active physiotherapy reduced disability after 6 and 12 months.[38–41] A second additional RCT found that a combined exercise and motivation programme versus exercises alone reduced pain and improved disability after 4 and 12 months.[35] **Extension (including McKenzie exercises [see glossary, p 1184]) exercises:** Three RCTs (153 people) identified by one review compared extension versus flexion back exercises.[30] Two of these RCTs found no difference in pain intensity, and the third RCT found that extension versus flexion exercises reduced global improvement. **Strengthening exercises:** Nine RCTs (899 people) identified by the reviews found no difference with strengthening exercises versus other types of exercise in outcomes and found conflicting evidence on strengthening exercises versus inactive treatment in outcomes.[2,3,5,29,30] **Stabilisation exercises:** One additional RCT (44 people with spondylolysis and spondylolisthesis) found that a 10 week specific stabilising exercise programme versus usual care reduced pain intensity and functional disability after 30 months.[44] **Postural exercises (Mensendieck/ Cesar):** One additional RCT (77 people who had just finished treatment for their last episode of back pain) found that a Mensendieck exercise (see glossary, p 1184) group treatment for 13 weeks versus usual care reduced recurrences of back pain, but found no significant differences in sick leave, pain, or functioning after 1 and 3 years.[42,43] A second additional RCT (222 people) found that Cesar therapy (see glossary, p 1184) versus usual care by the general practitioner increased overall improvement after 3 and 6 months but found no significant difference after 1 year.[34] **Group exercises:** One additional RCT (109 people) found no significant differences with individual versus group exercises in pain and disability after 4 weeks (post-treatment).[33]

Harms: The reviews and RCTs did not report on harms.

Comment: One additional study compared an intensive training programme versus home exercises versus control in people with both acute and chronic low back pain. Randomisation was only successful for the comparison home exercise versus control.[37]

OPTION LUMBAR SUPPORTS

We found insufficient evidence on the effects of lumbar supports.

Benefits: We found four systematic reviews (search dates not stated,[2] 1995,[3] 1995,[5] 1999;[45] 1 RCT). The RCT (19 people) identified by the reviews found that lumbar corset plus a synthetic support versus lumbar corset without synthetic support improved symptom severity and functional disability.

Harms: The reviews did not report on harms.[2,3,5,45] Harms associated with prolonged lumbar support use include decreased strength of the trunk musculature, a false sense of security, heat, skin irritation, and general discomfort.[2]

Comment: Five RCTs (1200 people) identified by the reviews did not differentiate between acute and chronic pain.[2,3,5,45]

OPTION MULTIDISCIPLINARY TREATMENT PROGRAMMES

Systematic reviews have found that intensive multidisciplinary biopsychosocial rehabilitation with functional restoration versus inpatient or outpatient non-multidisciplinary treatments or usual care reduces pain and improves function. The reviews found no difference with less intensive multidisciplinary treatments versus non-multidisciplinary treatment or usual care in pain or function.

Benefits: We found two systematic reviews (search date 1995;[3] 1998;[46] 10 RCTs, 1964 people, which compared multidisciplinary treatment (see glossary, p 1184) versus a control treatment. The reviews found that intensive multidisciplinary biopsychosocial rehabilitation with functional restoration versus inpatient or outpatient non-multidisciplinary treatments or usual care reduced pain and improved function.[3,46] The reviews found no difference with less intensive outpatient multidisciplinary treatments versus non-multidisciplinary outpatient treatment or usual care in pain or function.[3,46]

Harms: The reviews did not report on harms.[3,46]

Comment: None.

OPTION MASSAGE

Systematic reviews and subsequent RCTs have found that massage versus other treatments reduces pain and improves functioning.

Benefits: We found two systematic reviews (search dates 1999[47] and 1997;[48] 2 RCTs; no statistical pooling of data; see comment below) and four subsequent RCTs comparing massage (see glossary, p 1184) versus other treatments.[33,49–51] One RCT (85 people) identified by the reviews found that massage versus spinal manipulation improved functioning.[47,48] The second RCT (41 people) identified by the review found that massage versus transcutaneous electrical nerve stimulation treatment reduced pain relief. The first subsequent RCT (262 people) compared massage versus self care education (see glossary, p 1185) or acupuncture (see glossary, p 1184).[49] It found that massage versus both other treatments significantly improved symptoms and functional status after 10 weeks. The RCT found that massage versus acupuncture also significantly improved symptoms after 1 year. The second subsequent RCT (98 people) compared four treatments: comprehensive massage (soft tissue manipulation, remedial exercise, and posture education); soft tissue manipulation alone; remedial exercise plus posture education; and sham laser treatment.[51] It found that comprehensive massage versus each of the other treatments increased the percentage of people who were pain free after 1 month (63% with comprehensive massage *v* 27% soft tissue manipulation alone, 14% with remedial exercise with posture education, 0% with sham laser treatment).[51] The third subsequent RCT (24 people) found that massage versus progressive muscle relaxation reduced pain, anxiety, and depression after 5 weeks.[50] The last subsequent RCT (109 people in a factorial design) compared acupuncture massage versus Swedish massage and massage versus exercise. It found that acupuncture massage versus Swedish massage reduced pain and improved functional status, but found no difference with massage versus exercise in outcomes.[33]

Harms: The reviews and RCTs did not report on harms.[33,47–51]

Comment: Problems with control group selection in RCTs designed to evaluate the effectiveness of massage in chronic low back pain patients limit the usefulness of their results.[47,48]

OPTION SPINAL MANIPULATION

We found four systematic reviews that identified the same 12 RCTs. One of the reviews found that spinal manipulation versus placebo improved outcomes, but the other three reviews found that the results of the RCTs were conflicting.

Benefits: We found four systematic reviews (search dates 1995,[3] 1995,[5] 1995,[52] and not stated;[53] 12 RCTs; no statistical pooling of data). Four RCTs (514 people) identified by the reviews compared manipulation versus placebo, and eight RCTs (545 people) identified by the reviews compared manipulation versus conservative treatments (usual care, short wave diathermy, massage (see glossary, p 1184), exercises, back schools, and drug treatment).[3,5,52,53] Three of the reviews found that the results of these RCTs were conflicting.[3,52,53] The fourth review (5 RCTs, 543 people) found that spinal manipulation versus placebo improved outcomes.[5]

Harms: In the RCTs identified by the reviews that used a trained therapist to select people and perform spinal manipulation, the risk of serious complications was low (estimated risk: vertebrobasilar strokes 1/20 000 to 1/1 000 000 people; cauda equina syndrome < 1/1 000 000 people).[3,5,52,53]

Comment: Current guidelines do not advise spinal manipulation in people with severe or progressive neurological deficit.[2,54]

OPTION TRACTION

One systematic review and two additional RCTs have found no difference with traction versus placebo or with traction plus massage versus interferential treatment in pain relief or functional status.

Benefits: We found one systematic review (search date 1995,[3] 1 RCT) and two additional RCTs.[55,56] Two RCTs (176 people) found no significant difference with traction versus placebo in global improvement, pain relief, or functional status after 5–9 weeks.[3,56] The second additional RCT (152 people) found no significant difference with lumbar traction plus massage (see glossary, p 1184) versus interferential treatment in pain relief or improvement of disability after 3 weeks (post-treatment) and after 4 months.[55]

Harms: The review and additional RCTs did not report on harms.[3,55,56] Potential adverse effects include debilitation, loss of muscle tone, bone demineralisation, and thrombophlebitis.[2]

Comment: Of the 16 RCTs identified, 12 RCTs (921 people) did not distinguish between acute and chronic low back pain.[3,5,57,58]

OPTION TRANSCUTANEOUS ELECTRICAL NERVE STIMULATION

One systematic review has found no significant difference with transcutaneous electrical nerve stimulation versus control in pain relief. Two systematic reviews found conflicting evidence on the effects of transcutaneous electrical nerve stimulation.

Benefits: We found three systematic reviews (search dates not stated,[2] 1995,[5] and 2000;[59] 5 RCTs; 421 people). Two systematic reviews found conflicting evidence on the effects of transcutaneous electrical nerve stimulation.[2,5] The third systematic review found no difference with transcutaneous electrical nerve stimulation versus control in pain measured using a visual analogue scale (3 RCTs, 171 people; pooled standardised mean difference –0.21; 95% CI –0.51 to +0.1).[59]

Harms: The reviews did not report on harms.[2,5,59]

Comment: None.

OPTION ACUPUNCTURE

Two systematic reviews have found no significant difference with acupuncture versus placebo or no treatment in outcomes. One systematic review and one subsequent RCT have found that acupuncture versus transcutaneous electrical nerve stimulation significantly reduces pain intensity and significantly increasesd overall improvement.

Benefits: We found two systematic reviews (search dates 1996, 12 RCTs; see comment below)[60,61] and one subsequent RCT.[62] The reviews identified seven RCTs (380 people) comparing acupuncture (see glossary, p 1184) versus no treatment, placebo acupuncture, waiting list control, or transcutaneous electrical nerve stimulation.[60,61] One review found no significant difference with acupuncture versus placebo acupuncture or no treatment in outcomes.[61] The second review found that acupuncture versus transcutaneous electrical nerve stimulation increased overall improvement (OR 2.3, 95% CI 1.3 to 4.1), but found no difference with acupuncture versus placebo acupuncture in outcomes (OR 1.4, 95% CI 0.8 to 2.3).[60] The subsequent RCT (60 people) found that acupuncture versus transcutaneous electrical nerve stimulation significantly reduced pain intensity and the number of analgesic tablets consumed a week.[62]

Harms: One systematic review (search date 1996)[61] found that serious, rare, adverse effects included infections (HIV, hepatitis, bacterial endocarditis) and visceral trauma (pneumothorax, cardiac tamponade).

Comment: Three RCTs identified by the systematic reviews combined acute and chronic low back pain and two RCTs did not specify the duration of symptoms.[60,61] One RCT identified by the reviews included people with back and neck pain.[60,61]

GLOSSARY

Acupuncture Acupuncture is needle puncture of the skin at traditional "meridian" acupuncture points. Modern acupuncturists also use non-meridian points and trigger points (tender sites occurring in the most painful areas). The needles may be stimulated manually or electrically. Placebo acupuncture is needling of traditionally unimportant sites or non-stimulation of the needles once placed.

Cesar therapy Cesar therapy is based on the hypothesis that there is an association between postural and movement deficiencies and back pain. The treatment aims to initiate a learning process aimed at correction of postural and movement deficiencies.

Cognitive behavioural therapy Cognitive behavioural therapy aims to identify and modify peoples understanding of their pain and disability using cognitive restructuring techniques (such as imagery and attention diversion) or by modifying maladaptive thoughts, feelings, and beliefs.

Electromyographic biofeedback With electromyographic biofeedback a person receives external feedback of their own electromyogram (using visual or auditory scales), and uses this to learn how to control the electromyogram and hence the tension within their own muscles. Electromyogram biofeedback for low back pain aims to relax the paraspinal muscles.

Massage Massage is manipulation of soft tissues (i.e. muscle and fascia) using the hands or a mechanical device, to promote circulation and relaxation of muscle spasm or tension. Different types of soft tissue massage include Shiatsu, Swedish, friction, trigger point, or neuromuscular massage.

McKenzie exercises McKenzie exercises use self generated stresses and forces to centralise pain from the legs and buttocks to the lower back. This method emphasises self care.

Mensendieck therapy The Mensendieck approach combines postural exercises and education, emphasising "learning by doing". It is based on the assumption that human beings, through insight and guidance, can take responsibility for their own health and thus avoid the consequences of functional disability. Mensendieck therapy has been used for decades in the Netherlands and Scandinavia.

Multidisciplinary treatment Multidisciplinary treatment is intensive physical and psychosocial training by a team (e.g. a physician, physiotherapist, psychologist, social worker, and occupational therapist). Training is usually given in groups and does not involve passive physiotherapy.

Operant behavioural treatments Operant behavioural treatments include positive reinforcement of healthy behaviours and consequent withdrawal of attention from pain behaviours, time contingent instead of pain contingent pain management, and spouse involvement, while undergoing a programme aimed at increasing exercise tolerance towards a preset goal.

Respondent behavioural treatment Respondent behavioural treatment aims to modify physiological responses directly (e.g. reducing muscle tension by explaining the relation between tension and pain, and using relaxation techniques).

Sciatica Sciatica is pain that radiates from the back into the buttock or leg and is most commonly caused by prolapse of an intervertebral disk; the term may also be used to describe pain anywhere along the course of the sciatic nerve.

Self care education Self care education consists of educational materials (book and videotapes) designed for persons with chronic low back pain. Information is provided on, for example, back pain and its treatment, prevention and control of pain, improving quality of life, and coping.

REFERENCES

1. Van der Heijden GJMG, Bouter LM, Terpstra-Lindeman E. De effectiviteit van tractie bij lage rugklachten. De resultaten van een pilotstudy. *Ned T Fysiotherapie* 1991;101:37–43.
2. Bigos S, Bowyer O, Braen G, et al. Acute low back problems in adults. Clinical Practice Guideline no.14. AHCPR Publication No. 95–0642. Rockville MD: Agency for Health Care Policy and Research, Public Health Service, US, Department of Health and Human Services. December 1994. Search date not stated; primary sources The Quebec Task Force on Spinal Disorders Review to 1984, search carried out by National Library of Medicine from 1984, and references from expert panel.
3. Evans G, Richards S. *Low back pain: an evaluation of therapeutic interventions.* Bristol: Health Care Evaluation Unit, University of Bristol, 1996. Search date 1995; primary sources Medline, Embase, A-Med, Psychlit, and hand searched references.
4. Van Tulder MW, Assendelft WJJ, Koes BW, et al, and the Editorial Board of the Cochrane Collaboration Back Review Group. Method guidelines for systematic reviews in the Cochrane Collaboration back review group for spinal disorders. *Spine* 1997;22:2323–2330.
5. Van Tulder MW, Koes BW, Bouter LM. Conservative treatment of acute and chronic nonspecific low back pain: a systematic review of randomized controlled trials of the most common interventions. *Spine* 1997;22:2128–2156. Search date 1995; primary sources Medline, Embase, Psychlit, and hand searched references.
6. Schnitzer TJ, Gray WL, Paster RZ, et al. Efficacy of tramadol in treatment of chronic low back pain. *J Rheumatol* 2000;27:772–778.
7. De Craen AJM, Di Giulio G, Lampe-Schoenmaeckers AJEM, et al. Analgesic efficacy and safety of paracetamol–codeine combinations versus paracetamol alone: a systematic review. *BMJ* 1996;313:321–325. Search date 1995; primary sources Medline, Embase, International Pharmaceutical Abstracts, Biosis, contact with pharmaceutical companies, and hand searched references.
8. Turner JA, Denny MC. Do antidepressant medications relieve chronic low back pain? *J Fam Pract* 1993;37:545–553. Search date 1992; primary sources Medline, Psychlit, hand searches of bibliographies, and enquiries to researchers and drug companies.
9. Salerno SM, Browning R, Jackson JL. The effect of antidepressant treatment in chronic back pain: a meta-analysis. *Arch Intern Med* 2002;162:19–24. Search date 2000; primary sources Medline, Psychlit, Cinahl, Embase, Aidsline, Healthstar, CancerLit, Cochrane Library, Micromedex, Federal Research in Progress databases, and reference lists of articles.
10. Atkinson JH, Slater MA, Williams RA, et al. A placebo-controlled randomized clinical trial of nortriptyline for chronic low back pain. *Pain* 1998;76:287–296.
11. Hameroff SR, Cork RC, Scherer K, et al. Doxepin effects on chronic pain, depression and plasma opioids. *J Clin Psychiatry* 1982;43:22–27.
12. Hameroff SR, Weiss JL, Lerman JC, et al. Doxepin's effects on chronic pain and depression: a controlled study. *J Clin Psychiatry* 1984;45:47–52.
13. Treves R, Montane De La Roque P, Dumond JJ, et al. Prospective study of the analgesic action of clomipramine versus placebo in refractory low back pain and sciatica (68 cases) [French]. *Rev Rhum* 1991;58:549–552.
14. Atkinson JH, Slater MA, Wahlgren DR, et al. Effects of noradrenergic and serotonergic antidepressants on chronic low back pain intensity. *Pain* 1999;83:137–145.
15. Dickens C, Jayson M, Sutton C, Creed F. The relationship between pain and depression in a trial using paroxetine in sufferers of chronic low back pain. *Psychosomatics* 2000;41:490–499.
16. Koes BW, Scholten RJPM, Mens JMA, et al. Efficacy of non-steroidal anti-inflammatory drugs for low back pain: a systematic review of randomised clinical trials. *Ann Rheum Dis* 1997;56:214–223. Search date 1994; primary sources Medline, Embase, and hand searched references.
17. Henry D, Lim LLY, Rodriguez LAG, et al. Variability in risk of gastrointestinal complications with individual non-steroidal anti-inflammatory drugs: results of a collaborative meta-analysis. *BMJ* 1996;312:1563–1566. Search date 1994; primary sources Medline, contact with study authors, and hand searched references.
18. Famaey JP, Bruhwyler J, Vandekerckhove K, Appelboom T. Open controlled randomised multicenter comparison of nimesulide and diclofenac in the treatment of subacute and chronic low back pain. *J Drug Assessment* 1998;1:349–368.

19. Veenema KR, Leahey N, Schneider S. Ketorolac versus meperidine: ED treatment of severe musculoskeletal low back pain. *Am J Emerg Med* 2000;18:404–407.
20. Waddell G, Feder G, McIntosh A, et al. *Low back pain evidence review.* London: Royal College of General Practitioners, 1996. Search date 1996; primary sources Medline, Embase, Science Citation Index, Social Sciences Citation Index, correspondence with experts and researchers, and hand searched references.
21. Watts RW, Silagy CA. A meta-analysis on the efficacy of epidural corticosteroids in the treatment of sciatica. *Anaesth Intensive Care* 1995;23:564–569. Search date not stated; primary sources Medline, hand searches from published reviews and clinical trials, and personal contact with published authors in the field and the pharmaceutical manufacturer.
22. Koes BW, Scholten RJPM, Mens JMA, Bouter LM. Epidural steroid injections for low back pain and sciatica: an updated systematic review of randomized clinical trials. *Pain Digest* 1999;9:241–247. Search date 1998; primary sources Medline and hand searches from relevant publications.
23. Nelemans PJ, de Bie RA, de Vet HCW, Sturmans F. Injection therapy for subacute and chronic benign low back pain. In: The Cochrane Library, Issue 2, 2001. Oxford: Update Software. Search date 1996; primary sources Medline, Embase, and hand searches of reference lists.
24. Van Tulder MW, Esmail R, Bombardier C, Koes BW. Back schools for non-specific low back pain. In: The Cochrane Library, Issue 2, 2001. Oxford: Update Software. Search date 1997; primary sources Medline, Embase, and hand searched references.
25. Maier-Riehle B, Härter M. The effects of back schools: a meta-analysis. *Int J Rehab Res* 2001;24:199–206. Search date April 2000; primary sources Medline, PsychLit, PSYNDEX and hand searches of reference lists from relevant publications.
26. Dalichau S, Scheele K, Perrey RM, et al. Ultraschallgestützte Haltungs-und Bewegungsanalyse der Lendenwirbelsaüle zum Nachweis der Wirksamkeit einer Rückenschule [German]. *Zentralbl Arbeitsmed* 1999;49:148–156.
27. Turner JA. Educational and behavioral interventions for back pain in primary care. *Spine* 1996;21:2851–2859. Search date 1994; primary sources Medline, Psychlit, hand searches, and inquiries to pharmaceutical companies and expert researchers in the field.
28. Van Tulder MW, Ostelo R, Vlaeyen JWS, Linton SJ, Morley SJ, Assendelft WJJ. Behavioural treatment for chronic low back pain. In: The Cochrane Library, Issue 2, 2001. Oxford: Update Software. Search date 1999; primary sources Medline, Psychlit, Cochrane Controlled Trials Register, Embase, and hand searches of reference lists.
29. Faas A. Exercises: which ones are worth trying, for which patients and when? *Spine* 1996;21:2874–2879. Search date 1995; primary source Medline.
30. van Tulder MW, Malmivaara A, Esmail R, Koes BW. Exercise therapy for non-specific low back pain. In: The Cochrane Library, Issue 2, 2001. Oxford: Update Software. Search date 1999; primary sources Medline, Psychlit, Cochrane Controlled Trials Register, Embase, and hand searches of reference lists.
31. Bendix AF, Bendix T, Ostenfeld S, et al. Active treatment programs for patients with chronic low back pain: a prospective, randomized, observer-blinded study. *Eur Spine J* 1995;4:148–152.
32. Bendix AF, Bendix T, Labriola M, et al. Functional restoration for chronic low back pain: two-year follow-up of two randomized clinical trials. *Spine* 1998;23:717–725.
33. Franke A, Gebauer S, Franke K, Brockow T. Acupuncture massage vs Swedish massage and individual exercise vs group exercise in low back pain sufferers–a randomized controlled clinical trial in a 2 x 2 factorial design. [German] *Forsch Komplementarmed Klass Naturheilkd* 2000;7:286–293.
34. Hildebrandt VH, Proper KI, van den Berg R, Douwes M, van den Heuvel SG, van Buuren S. Cesar therapy is temporarily more effective in patients with chronic low back pain than the standard treatment by family practitioner: randomized, controlled and blinded clinical trial with 1 year follow-up. [Dutch]. *Nederlands Tijdschrift voor Geneeskunde* 2000;144:2258–2264.
35. Friedrich M, Gittler G, Halberstadt Y, Cermak T, Heiller I. Combined exercise and motivation program: effect on the compliance and level of disability of patients with chronic low back pain: a randomized controlled trial. *Arch Phys Med Rehabil* 1998;79:475–487.
36. Kankaanpaa M, Taimela S, Airaksinen O, Hanninen O. The efficacy of active rehabilitation in chronic low back pain. Effect on pain intensity, self-experienced disability, and lumbar fatigability. *Spine* 1999;24:1034–1042.
37. Kuukkanen T, Malkia E. Effects of a three-month therapeutic exercise programme on flexibility in subjects with low back pain. *Physiother Res Int* 2000;5:46–61.
38. Mannion AF, Muntener M, Taimela S, Dvorak J. A randomized clinical trial of three active therapies for chronic low back pain. *Spine* 1999;24:2435–2448.
39. Mannion AF, Muntener M, Taimela S, Dvorak J. Comparison of three active therapies for chronic low back pain: results of a randomized clinical trial with one-year follow-up. *Rheumatology* 2001;40:772–778.
40. Mannion AF, Junge A, Taimela S, Muntener M, Lorenzo K, Dvorak J. Active therapy for chronic low back pain: part 3. Factors influencing self-rated disability and its change following therapy. *Spine* 2001;26:920–929.
41. Mannion AF, Taimela S, Muntener M, Dvorak J. Active therapy for chronic low back pain part 1. Effects on back muscle activation, fatigability, and strength. *Spine* 2001;26:897–908.
42. Soukup MG, Glomsrod B, Lonn JH, Bo K, Larsen S. The effect of a Mensendieck exercise program as secondary prophylaxis for recurrent low back pain. A randomized, controlled trial with 12-month follow-up. *Spine* 1999;24:1585–1591.
43. Soukup MG, Lonn J, Glomsrod B, Bo K, Larsen S. Exercises and education as secondary prevention for recurrent low back pain. *Physiother Res Int* 2001;6:27–39.
44. PB, Twomey LT, Allison GT. Evaluation of specific stabilizing exercise in the treatment of chronic low back pain with radiologic diagnosis of spondylolysis or spondylolisthesis. *Spine* 1997;24:2959–2967.
45. Van Tulder MW, Jellema P, van Poppel MNM, et al. Lumbar supports for prevention and treatment of low back pain. In: The Cochrane Library, Issue 2, 2001. Oxford: Update Software. Search date 1999; primary sources Medline, Cinahl, Current

Contents, Cochrane Controlled Trials Register, Embase, Science Citation Index, and hand searches of reference lists.
46. Guzman J, Esmail R, Karjalainen K, Malmivaara A, Irvin E, Bombardier C. Multidisciplinary rehabilitation for chronic low back pain: systematic review. *BMJ* 2001;322:1511–1516. Search date 1998; primary sources Medline, Embase, Psychlit, Cinahl, Health Star, Cochrane Library, citation tracking, and personal contact with content experts.
47. Furlan AD, Brosseau L, Welch V, Wong J. Massage for low back pain. In: The Cochrane Library, Issue 2, 2001. Oxford: Update Software. Search date 1999; primary sources Medline, Embase, Cochrane Controlled Trials Register, Healthstar, Cinahl, Dissertation Abstracts, and hand searches of reference lists and contact with content experts and massage associations.
48. Ernst E. Massage therapy for low back pain: a systematic review. *J Pain Symptom Manage* 1999;17:65–69. Search date 1997; primary sources Medline, Embase, Cochrane Library, and hand searches of personal files, bibliographies, and personal contact with researchers.
49. Cherkin DC, Eisenberg D, Sherman KJ, et al. Randomized trial comparing traditional Chinese medical acupuncture, therapeutic massage, and self-care education for chronic low back pain. *Arch Intern Med* 2001;161:1081–1088.
50. Hernandez-Reif M, Field T, Krasnegor J, Theakston H. Lower back pain is reduced and range of motion increased after massage therapy. *Int J Neurosci* 2001;106:131–145.
51. Preyde M. Effectiveness of massage therapy for subacute low back pain: a randomized controlled trial. *Can Med Ass J* 2000;162:1815–1820.
52. Koes BW, Assendelft WJJ, van der Heijden GJMG, et al. Spinal manipulation for low back pain. An updated systematic review of randomized clinical trials. *Spine* 1996;21:2860–2871. Search date 1995; primary sources Medline and hand searched references.
53. Shekelle PG, Adams AH, Chassin MR, et al. Spinal manipulation for low back pain. *Ann Intern Med* 1992;117:590–598. Search date not stated; primary sources Medline, Index Medicus, contacted experts, and hand searched references.
54. Van Tulder MW, Scholten RJPM, Koes BW, et al. Non-steroidal anti-inflammatory drugs (NSAIDs) for non-specific low back pain. In: The Cochrane Library, Issue 2, 2001. Oxford: Update Software. Search date 1998; primary sources Medline, Embase, Cochrane Controlled Trials Register, and hand searches of reference lists.
55. Werners R, Pynsent PB, Bulstrode CJK. Randomized trial comparing interferential therapy with motorized lumbar traction and massage in the management of low back pain in a primary care setting. *Spine* 1999;24:1579–1584.
56. Beurskens AJ, de Vet HCW, Köke AJ, et al. Efficacy of traction for non-specific low back pain: a randomised clinical trial. *Lancet* 1995;346:1596–1600.
57. Van der Heijden GJMG, Beurskens AJHM, Koes BW, et al. The efficacy of traction for back and neck pain: a systematic, blinded review of randomized clinical trial methods. *Phys Ther* 1995;75:93–104. Search date 1992; primary sources Medline, Embase, Index to Chiropractic Literature, Physiotherapy Index, and hand searched non-indexed journals.
58. Ljunggren E, Weber H, Larssen S. Autotraction versus manual traction in patients with prolapsed lumbar intervertebral discs. *Scand J Rehabil Med* 1984;16:117–124.
59. Milne S, Welch V, Brosseau L, Saginur M, Shea B, Tugwell P, Wells G. Transcutaneous electrical nerve stimulation (TENS) for chronic low back pain (Cochrane review). In: The Cochrane Library, Issue 4, 2001. Oxford: Update Software. Search date 2000; primary sources Medline, Embase, PEDro, Cochrane Controlled Trials Register, hand searches of bibliographic references, reference lists, Current Contents, abstracts in specialised journals, Conference Proceedings, and personal contact with co-ordinating offices of the trials registries of the Cochrane Field of Physical and Related Therapies and Cochrane Musculoskeletal Group and content experts.
60. Ernst E, White AR. Acupuncture for back pain. A meta-analysis of randomized controlled trials. *Arch Intern Med* 1998;158:2235–2241. Search date 1996; primary sources Medline, Cochrane Controlled Trials Register, CISCOM, contacted authors and experts, and hand searched references.
61. Van Tulder MW, Cherkin DC, Berman B, et al. Acupuncture in low back pain. In: The Cochrane Library, Issue 2, 2001. Oxford: Update Software. Search date 1996; primary sources Medline, Embase, Cochrane Complementary Medicine Field trials register, Cochrane Controlled Trials Register, Science Citation Index, and hand searched references.
62. Grant DJ, Bishop-Miller J, Winchester DM, et al. A randomized comparative trial of acupuncture versus transcutaneous electrical nerve stimulation for chronic back pain in the elderly. *Pain* 1999;82:9–13.

Maurits van Tulder
Institute for Research in Extramural Medicine
Vrije Universiteit Medical Centre
Amsterdam
The Netherlands

Bart Koes
Department of General Practice
Erasmus University
Rotterdam
The Netherlands

Competing interests: None declared.

Neck pain

Search date May 2002

Allan Binder

QUESTIONS

INTERVENTIONS

See glossary, p 1200

Key Messages

Uncomplicated neck pain

- **Drug treatments (analgesics, non-steroidal anti-inflammatory drugs, antidepressants, or muscle relaxants)** We found insufficient evidence on the effects of analgesics, non-steroidal anti-inflammatory drugs, antidepressants, or muscle relaxants for neck pain, although they are widely used as a preferred treatment. Some are associated with well documented adverse effects.

Clin Evid 2002;8:1188–1202.

- **Manual treatments (mobilisation and manipulation)** Systematic reviews have found that manipulation or mobilisation versus other treatments improve symptoms. One additional and one subsequent RCT have found no significant difference with mobilisation versus manipulation in pain. Rare but serious adverse effects have been reported after manipulation of the cervical spine.
- **Multidisciplinary (multimodal) treatment** One systematic review and two subsequent RCTs have found no consistent differences in pain or time off work over 18 months with multimodal cognitive behavioural therapy versus other treatments.
- **Patient education** Two systematic reviews and one subsequent RCT found insufficient evidence about the effects of patient education (advice or group instruction).
- **Physical treatments (heat or cold, traction, biofeedback, spray and stretch, acupuncture, laser)** Systematic reviews found insufficient evidence about the effects of these physical treatments.
- **Physical treatments (physiotherapy, pulsed electromagnetic field treatment, exercise)** Systematic reviews and subsequent RCTs have found that pulsed electromagnetic field treatment versus sham treatment, exercise versus stress management, and active physiotherapy versus passive treatment all significantly reduce pain.
- **Soft collars or special pillows** We found no evidence on the effects of soft collars. One RCT found limited evidence that water based pillows versus standard and roll pillows significantly reduced morning pain and improved quality of sleep.

Acute whiplash

- **Early mobilisation** Systematic reviews and subsequent RCTs found limited evidence that early mobilisation versus immobilisation or versus rest plus a collar significantly reduced pain.
- **Early return to normal activity** Systematic reviews and subsequent RCTs found limited evidence that advice to "act as usual" plus anti-inflammatory drugs versus immobilisation plus 14 days sick leave improved mild subjective symptoms.
- **Electrotherapy** One RCT found limited evidence that electromagnetic field treatment versus sham treatment significantly reduced pain after 4 weeks but not after 3 months.
- **Multimodal treatment** One RCT found that multimodal treatment versus physical treatment significantly reduced pain at the end of treatment and after 6 months.

Chronic whiplash

- **Percutaneous radiofrequency neurotomy for zygapophyseal joint pain** One RCT found limited evidence that percutaneous radiofrequency neurotomy versus a sham procedure significantly increased the number of people who were free from pain after 27 weeks.
- **Physiotherapy (v multimodal treatment)** One RCT found no significant difference with physiotherapy alone versus multimodal treatment in disability, pain, or range of movement at the end of treatment or at 3 months.

Neck pain with radiculopathy

- **Drug treatments (epidural steroid injections, analgesics, non-steroidal anti-inflammatory drugs, or muscle relaxants)** We found no RCTs about the effects of epidural steroid injections, analgesics, non-steroidal anti-inflammatory drugs, or muscle relaxants.

- **Surgery versus conservative treatment** One RCT found no significant difference with surgery versus conservative treatment in symptoms after 1 year.

DEFINITION Neck pain can be divided into uncomplicated pain, whiplash, and pain with radiculopathy. Neck pain often occurs in combination with limitation of movement and poorly defined neurological symptoms affecting the upper limbs. The pain can be severe and intractable, and can occur with radiculopathy or myelopathy.

INCIDENCE/ PREVALENCE About two thirds of people will experience neck pain at some time in their lives.[1,2] Prevalence is highest in middle age. In the UK about 15% of hospital based physiotherapy, and in Canada 30% of chiropractic referrals, are for neck pain.[3,4] In the Netherlands, neck pain contributes up to 2% of general practitioner consultations.[5]

AETIOLOGY/ RISK FACTORS Most uncomplicated neck pain is associated with poor posture, anxiety and depression, neck strain, occupational injuries, or sporting injuries. With chronic pain, mechanical and degenerative factors (often referred to as cervical spondylosis) are more likely. Some neck pain results from soft tissue trauma, most typically seen in whiplash injuries. Rarely disc prolapse and inflammatory, infective, or malignant conditions affect the cervical spine and present with neck pain with or without neurological features.

PROGNOSIS Neck pain usually resolves within days or weeks but can recur or become chronic. In some industries, neck related disorders account for as much time off work as low back pain (see low back pain and sciatica: acute, p 1156).[6] The percentage of people in whom neck pain becomes chronic depends on the cause but is thought to be about 10%:[1] similar to low back pain. Neck pain causes severe disability in 5% of affected people.[2] One systematic review (search date 1996) of the clinical course and prognostic factors of non-specific neck pain identified six observational studies and 17 RCTs.[7] In people who had had pain for at least 6 months, a median of 46% (range 22–79%) improved with treatment. Whiplash injuries were more likely to cause disability; up to 40% of sufferers reported symptoms even after 15 years' follow up.[8] Factors associated with a poorer outcome after whiplash are not well defined.[9] The incidence of chronic disability after whiplash varies among countries, although reasons for this variation are unclear.[10]

AIMS To recover from acute episode within 4 weeks; to maintain activities of daily living and reduce absenteeism from work; to prevent development of long term symptoms.

OUTCOMES Pain; range of movement; function; adverse effects of treatment; return to work; level of disability (Neck Disability Index).[11]

METHODS *Clinical Evidence* update search and appraisal May 2002. We also searched the following databases: Chirolars (now called Mantis) for English language articles from 1966 to November 1999; Bioethicsline (1973–1997); Cumulative Index to Nursing and Allied Health (Cinahl) (1982–1997); and Current Contents (1994–1997). Criteria for assessment of RCTs were based on a 100 point scale, including study population, interventions, effects, and data presentation and analysis.[12]

QUESTION What are the effects of treatments for people with uncomplicated neck pain without severe neurological deficit?

OPTION PHYSICAL TREATMENTS

Systematic reviews and RCTs have found that pulsed electromagnetic field treatment versus sham treatment, exercise versus stress management, and active physiotherapy versus passive treatment all significantly reduce pain. Systematic reviews have found insufficient evidence about the effects of most physical treatments (heat or cold, traction, biofeedback, spray and stretch, acupuncture, and laser).

Benefits: We found six systematic reviews[13–18] and four subsequent RCTs.[19–22] Three of the systematic reviews considered all physical treatment modalities,[13,14,18] and the other three considered traction only,[15] or acupuncture only.[16,17] **All physical modalities:** The first systematic review (search date 1993, 13 RCTs, 760 people with neck pain but without neurological deficit) found no significant benefit from any of the following physical treatments: heat or cold, traction, electrotherapy (pulsing electromagnetic field or transcutaneous electrical nerve stimulation), biofeedback, spray and stretch, acupuncture, or laser.[13] The second systematic review (search date 1995, 17 RCTs, 1202 people) found possible benefit for pulsed electromagnetic field treatment and active physiotherapy, but not for traction, acupuncture, or other physical treatments.[14] The third systematic review (search date 2000, 7 CCTs/RCTs, 507 people with chronic neck pain) found some evidence of benefit for proprioceptive and strengthening exercise based on two low quality studies,[23,24] but no evidence that thermotherapy, massage, biofeedback, traction, ultrasound, transcutaneous electrical nerve stimulation, or combined rehabilitation interventions improved symptoms.[18] **Exercise:** One RCT (47 people) included in two reviews[13,14] found that active physiotherapy, including exercise (for 60 min each visit; mean 13 visits) versus passive treatment (heat, massage, and light stretching for 20 min each visit; mean 10 visits) significantly reduced pain immediately after treatment ($P < 0.05$). Pain recurred in both groups by 3 months, but after 1 year the exercise group still had significantly less headache.[25] Three subsequent RCTs examined the effects of exercises.[19,21,22] The first subsequent RCT (103 women with work related neck pain) compared three exercise regimens (strength training, endurance training, and coordination exercises) versus stress management over 10 weeks.[19] It found that exercise versus stress management significantly reduced pain ($P < 0.05$), but found no significant difference between any of the exercise programmes versus each other. The second RCT compared three groups: strengthening exercises plus manipulation; strengthening exercises alone; and manipulation alone, and the third RCT compared intensive training, mobilisation physiotherapy, and manipulation (see benefits of manual treatments: mobilisation and manipulation, p 1193).[21,22] **Traction:** The fourth systematic review (search date 1992, 3 RCTs, 639 people) compared traction versus a range of alternative treatments, including heat, mobilisation, exercise, no treatment, collar, and analgesics.[15] The review found no consistent difference with traction versus any of the other treatments in pain. **Pulsed electromagnetic field treatment:** One RCT included in the second review (81 people with neck pain and radiographic evidence of cervical osteoarthritis and 86 people with osteoarthritis of the knee with symptoms for at least 1 year; see comment below) compared true versus sham pulsed electromagnetic field treatment.[26] It found that in people with chronic neck pain, pulsed electromagnetic field treatment significantly reduced pain ($P < 0.04$) and pain on passive motion ($P = 0.03$), but found no significant difference between treatments in difficulty with activities of daily living, tenderness, self assessment of improvement, or physicians' global assessment after 18 episodes of treatment. The RCT also found that active versus sham pulsed electromagnetic field treatment significantly increased the number of people who had improved in at least three of six variables (57/82 [70%] with active treatment *v* 37/82 [45%] with sham treatment; RR 1.54, 95% CI 1.21 to 1.80; NNT 4, 95% CI 3 to 11). This benefit was sustained up to 1 month (see comment below). **Acupuncture:** Two systematic reviews (search dates 1998; 13 RCTs) compared needle or laser acupuncture versus several different control procedures (sham treatments, diazepam, and physiotherapy) and found no consistent differences between treatments.[16,17] One subsequent RCT (177 people with chronic neck pain mainly because of fibromyalgia or whiplash) compared three groups: acupuncture, massage, and sham laser acupuncture. It found no significant difference between acupuncture versus sham laser acupuncture after 1 week (difference in pain score on a 100 point visual analogue scale: acupuncture *v* sham laser acupuncture +6.9 points, 95% CI –5.0 points to +18.9 points; $P = 0.33$), but found that acupuncture versus massage significantly reduced motion related pain after 1 week (acupuncture reduced pain by 16.3 points more than massage on a 100 point visual analogue scale, 95% CI 4.4 points to 28.3 points; $P = 0.005$). The RCT found no significant difference between treatments after 3 months.[20]

Harms: We found no good data on harms. The incidence of serious adverse events seems to be low for all physical treatments considered.

Comment: The RCT comparing true versus sham pulsed electromagnetic field treatment was double blinded and used random numbers to allocate people to groups.[26] By chance, the baseline characteristics of treated and placebo groups were different: the people allocated to active treatment had higher pain scores, more tenderness, and more difficulty with the activities of daily living than the placebo group. The analysis in the RCT was based on changes from the baseline value, and it is not known how much of the observed effect was caused by bias introduced by the baseline differences.

OPTION MANUAL TREATMENTS: MOBILISATION AND MANIPULATION

Four systematic reviews have found that manipulation or mobilisation versus other treatments improve symptoms. One additional and one subsequent RCT found no significant difference between mobilisation

versus manipulation in pain. One subsequent RCT found limited evidence that manipulation plus strengthening exercises versus either treatment alone significantly reduced pain and increased satisfaction. Rare but serious adverse effects have been reported after manipulation of the cervical spine.

Benefits: We found four systematic reviews (search dates 1990,[12] 1993,[27] 1995,[28] and 1995[14]), one additional RCT,[29] and two subsequent RCTs,[21,22] which assessed mobilisation (any manual treatment to improve joint function that does not involve high velocity movement, anaesthesia, or instrumentation) and manipulation (the use of short or long lever high velocity thrusts directed at 1 or more of the cervical spine joints that does not involve anaesthesia or instrumentation). The four reviews all found that mobilisation or manipulation versus a variety of control procedures improved symptoms.[12,14,27,28] **Mobilisation:** One RCT (included in all 4 systematic reviews; 30 people with acute pain who were all given a collar and allowed to take analgesics) found no significant difference in pain with mobilisation (10 people) versus transcutaneous electrical nerve stimulation (10 people), or versus control (10 people).[30] However, the trial was too small to rule out a beneficial effect. Two other RCTs found modest benefit from mobilisation in the short term.[31,32] The first RCT (63 people) found that mobilisation plus analgesia versus less active physiotherapy plus analgesia significantly reduced pain after 1 month (83% of the mobilisation group improved *v* 60% of the physiotherapy group; $P < 0.05$; CI not provided) but not thereafter.[31] The second RCT (256 people with chronic neck and back pain, 64 having chronic neck pain alone) compared four treatments: manual treatment (mobilisation, manipulation, or both); physical treatment (heat, electrotherapy, ultrasound, shortwave diathermy); usual medical care (analgesics, advice, home exercise, and bed rest); and placebo (detuned shortwave diathermy or ultrasound).[32] It found that manual treatment versus all of the other treatments significantly improved outcomes after 12 months. However, it was not possible to directly compare the effects of the two manual treatments, and more people received manipulation. **Manipulation:** One of the reviews performed a meta-analysis (3 RCTs, 155 people with chronic pain)[32–34] of manipulation versus other treatments (diazepam, anti-inflammatory drugs, usual medical care).[28] It found that manipulation versus the other treatments improved outcomes although the difference was not significant (+12.6 mm on a 100 mm visual analogue scale, 95% CI –0.15 to +25.5).[28] **Mobilisation versus manipulation:** The additional RCT (100 people with mainly chronic neck pain) compared a single mobilisation treatment versus a single manipulation treatment.[29] It found no significant difference between treatments in the number of people reporting immediate improvement in pain (69% with mobilisation *v* 85% with manipulation, RR of improvement in pain with manipulation compared with mobilisation 1.23; $P = 0.16$ after adjusting for pretreatment differences between the groups). The RCT found that people in the manipulation group had improved range of movement, but the result was not significant. The first subsequent RCT (119 people with chronic neck pain) compared three treatments: mobilisation physiotherapy, manipulation, and intensive training.[22] It found no significant difference between groups in pain by the end of treatment ($P = 0.44$) or after 12 months, although median pain on a 30 point scale improved from 12 to 6 with intensive training or mobilisation and from 13 to 6 with manipulation. **Manipulation plus exercise:** The second subsequent RCT (191 people with chronic neck pain who received a home exercise programme and were able to use proprietary medication) compared three treatments: strengthening exercises plus manipulation (combined treatment); strengthening exercises alone; and manipulation alone.[21] The duration of each treatment episode was the same. It found that combined treatment versus both other treatments alone significantly improved participant satisfaction ($P = 0.03$), and that combined treatment versus manipulation significantly improved objective strength and range of movement ($P < 0.05$) after 11 weeks. The RCT also found that both combined treatment and strengthening exercises versus manipulation alone significantly improved pain ($P = 0.02$) and patient satisfaction ($P = 0.002$) after 1 year, although it found no significant differences between treatments in health status, neck disability, or medication use.

Harms: **Mobilisation:** We found occasional reports of increased pain, but no serious adverse effects or deaths. **Manipulation:** Rare but serious adverse effects have been reported, including death and serious disability caused by vertebrobasilar and other strokes, dissection of the vertebral arteries, disc herniation, and other serious neurological complications. The estimated risk from case reports of cerebrovascular accident is 1–3/million manipulations,[35] and of all serious adverse effects is 5–10/10 million manipulations.[28] A non-systematic review of reported cases of injury attributable to manipulation of the cervical spine identified 116 articles published between 1925 and 1997 with 177 cases of injury. The most frequently reported injuries involved arterial dissection or spasm, lesions of the brain stem, and Wallenberg's syndrome (see glossary, p 1200); death occurred in 32 (18%) of the cases. However, the method of data collection and analysis makes it impossible to assess the frequency of complications with this treatment.[36]

Comment: None.

OPTION MULTIDISCIPLINARY (MULTIMODAL) TREATMENT

One systematic review and two subsequent RCTs have found no consistent differences between multimodal cognitive behavioural therapy versus other treatments in pain or time off work.

Benefits: We found one systematic review (search date 1998,[37] 1 RCT[38]) and two subsequent RCTs in people with chronic neck pain.[39,40] The RCT identified by the review (66 people) compared multimodal cognitive behavioural therapy (administered directly by a psychologist) versus exercise plus behavioural modification (with a psychologist acting as an advisor to other therapists).[38] It found no significant difference in time off work or physical function after 18 months. The first subsequent RCT (76 people) compared three treatments: multimodal treatment (which emphasised exercise, relaxation, and behavioural support); supervised home exercises; and a recommendation to exercise.[39] It found that multimodal training or supervised exercise versus a recommendation to exercise significantly reduced pain after 3 months (change in pain score from baseline on 10 cm visual analogue score, –29 mm with multimodal treatment *v* –28 mm with supervised exercise *v* –12 mm with exercise recommendation; multimodal treatment or supervised exercise *v* exercise recommendation; P < 0.001), but found no significant difference between treatments in pain after 12 months. The second subsequent RCT (243 people with chronic spinal pain) compared three treatments: multimodal cognitive behavioural therapy (6 sessions); an educational pamphlet; and a more extensive information programme.[40] It found no significant difference between treatments in pain, but found that multimodal cognitive behavioural therapy versus an educational pamphlet significantly reduced time off work (AR for sick leave of > 30 days in 6 months, 1% with multimodal cognitive behavioural therapy *v* 10% with educational pamphlets; RR 10; P < 0.05).[40]

Harms: None reported.

Comment: None.

OPTION PATIENT EDUCATION

Two systematic reviews and one subsequent RCT have found insufficient evidence about the effect of patient education (advice or group instruction).

Benefits: We found two systematic reviews (search dates 1993[41] and 1998[42]) and one subsequent RCT.[43] One RCT (79 hospital secretaries with chronic neck pain) included in both reviews compared three treatments: group instruction (traditional neck school); neck school plus individual advice; and usual care.[44] It found no significant differences in outcomes. One RCT (93 people) included in only the first review compared individualised education plus analgesic drugs/anti-inflammatory drugs versus placebo.[45] It found no significant difference between treatments in pain. The subsequent RCT (282 nursing aides with neck, shoulder, or back pain) compared three groups: an individualised education and exercise programme; stress management; and no intervention.[43] It found no significant difference between treatments in pain or sick leave at the end of treatment or after 12 or 18 months.

Harms: None reported.

Comment: None.

OPTION SOFT COLLARS AND SPECIAL PILLOWS

We found no evidence on the effects of soft collars. One RCT found limited evidence that water based pillows versus standard and roll pillows significantly reduced morning pain and improved quality of sleep.

Benefits: **Soft collars:** We found no systematic reviews or RCTs. **Special pillows:** We found one crossover RCT (41 people with chronic neck pain), which compared three types of pillow used at night: a water based pillow, a roll type pillow, and a standard pillow.[46] It found that the water based pillow versus both other pillow types significantly reduced morning pain and improved quality of sleep (P < 0.01).[46]

Harms: None reported.

Comment: None.

OPTION DRUG TREATMENTS (ANALGESICS, NON-STEROIDAL ANTI-INFLAMMATORY DRUGS, ANTIDEPRESSANTS, OR MUSCLE RELAXANTS)

We found insufficient evidence on the effects of analgesics, non-steroidal anti-inflammatory drugs, antidepressants, or muscle relaxants for neck pain, although they are widely used as preferred treatment. Several drugs used to treat neck pain are associated with well documented adverse effects.

Benefits: We found three systematic reviews (search dates 1993[9,27] and not stated[47]) and one subsequent RCT.[37] **Simple analgesics (paracetamol, opioids) and oral non-steroidal anti-inflammatory drugs:** The reviews found no RCTs.[9,27,47] **Antidepressants:** The reviews found no RCTs.[9,27,47] RCTs of antidepressants in chronic low back pain syndromes found conflicting results (see antidepressants under low back pain and sciatica: acute, p 1156). **Muscle relaxants and benzodiazepines:** One systematic review identified two RCTs (159 people with chronic neck or back pain with acute spasm), which compared three treatments: cyclobenzaprine, diazepam, and placebo.[27] Both RCTs identified by the review found that cyclobenzaprine versus either of the other treatments significantly improved symptoms after 2 weeks ($P < 0.05$), but measured and follow up pain data could not be extracted.[48,49] One subsequent RCT (157 people with chronic neck pain) found that eperisone versus placebo significantly improved pain control after 6 weeks ($P < 0.05$).[50]

Harms: **Simple analgesics (paracetamol and opioids):** We found no reports of harm from simple analgesics. **Oral non-steroidal anti-inflammatory drugs:** See harms of non-steroidal anti-inflammatory drugs, p 1203. One systematic review found no direct comparisons of harms of manipulation versus non-steroidal anti-inflammatory drugs.[35] Calculations based on indirect comparisons found that the risk of a harm with non-steroidal anti-inflammatory drugs was considerably greater than for manipulation. **Antidepressants:** The reviews found no RCTs (see harms of antidepressants under generalised anxiety disorder, p 980). **Muscle relaxants and benzodiazepines:** The RCTs found minor adverse effects, including weakness, dizziness, drowsiness, and gastrointestinal problems occurring in 4% of people treated with muscle relaxants (see harms of benzodiazepines under generalised anxiety disorder, p 980).

Comment: RCTs of other interventions include the use of analgesics or non-steroidal anti-inflammatory drugs as adjunctive treatments but do not allow for subgroup analysis.[22,26,30,32,34,39] Few RCTs have considered treatment for chronic whiplash, and many people with whiplash are included in general RCTs of chronic mechanical neck pain.

QUESTION What are the effects of treatments for acute whiplash injury?

Systematic reviews and subsequent RCTs have found limited evidence that electromagnetic field treatment versus sham treatment, early mobilisation versus immobilisation or rest plus a collar, and multimodal treatment versus physical treatment significantly reduce pain, and that advice to "act as usual" plus anti-inflammatory drugs versus immobilisation plus 14 days sick leave improves mild subjective symptoms. One RCT found no significant difference between different home exercise programmes versus each other in pain or disability. We found no RCTs of drug treatments in acute whiplash injury.

Benefits: We found four systematic reviews of treatment for acute whiplash injury (search dates 1993,[9,27] 1998,[51] and not stated[47]) and three subsequent RCTs.[52–54] The reviews highlighted the paucity of evidence on all treatment modalities.[9,27,47,51] **Electrotherapy:** One RCT (40 people with acute whiplash who all received analgesia and a neck collar) included in two reviews compared active pulsing electromagnetic field treatment versus sham pulsing electromagnetic field treatment.[55] It found that active pulsing electromagnetic field treatment significantly reduced pain after 4 weeks ($P < 0.05$), but not after 3 months. **Early mobilisation versus immobilisation or less active treatment:** The first review (search date 1993, 2 RCTs, 165 people) plus two subsequent RCTs (104 people)[52,53] compared five treatments: early mobilisation physiotherapy; immobilisation; analgesics; rest; and education. The review found that early mobilisation significantly increased pain relief and improved range of movement after 4 and 8 weeks ($P < 0.01$).[9] The first subsequent RCT, comparing early mobilisation versus immobilisation, found no significant difference in recovery after 12 weeks (see comment below).[52] The second subsequent RCT (97 people) found that active mobilisation versus rest plus a neck collar significantly improved symptoms ($P < 0.001$), but only if started immediately after injury; a 2 week delay resulted in no significant difference between treatments after 6 months.[53] **Early resumption of normal activity versus immobilisation plus rest:** One systematic review found no evidence of benefit from immobilisation, rest, traction, or other physical treatments.[9] One RCT included in the second review (201 people presenting to an emergency department with acute whiplash)[51] compared advice to "act as usual" plus anti-inflammatory drugs versus immobilisation plus 14 days sick leave.[56] It found that advice to "act as usual" plus anti-inflammatory drugs improved subjective symptoms (including pain during daily activities, neck stiffness, memory, concentration, and headache) after 6 months, but found no significant difference between treatments in objective variables such as neck range and length of sick leave. The RCT also found no significant difference in severe symptoms after 6 months (11% with advice to "act as usual" *v* 15% with immobilisation; RR 0.75, 95% CI 0.08 to 1.42). **Home exercise programmes:** The third subsequent RCT (59 people) compared two home mobilisation regimes (a regular exercise treatment regimen or instructions to perform an additional isometric exercise at least 3 times a day) versus each other.[54] It found no significant difference between treatments in disability or pain after 3 or 6 months. **Multimodal treatment:** One RCT (60 people) included in the third review,[51] compared multimodal treatment (postural training, psychological support, eye fixation exercises, and manual treatment) versus physical treatment (electrical, sonic, ultrasound, and transcutaneous electrical nerve stimulation).[57] It found that multimodal treatment significantly reduced pain by the end of treatment ($P < 0.05$) and after 1 and 6 months ($P < 0.001$). The RCT also found that multimodal treatment reduced the time taken to return to work. **Drug treatments:** Two systematic reviews (search date 1993[27] and not stated[47]) found no RCTs. Simple analgesics and non-steroidal anti-inflammatory drugs were adjuvant treatments in many trials of acute whiplash.[51,56,58]

Harms: The reviews and RCTs did not consistently report adverse effects, although one trial has found that early mobilisation physiotherapy is not always well tolerated (see harms of manual treatments, p 1194).[59]

Comment: In the first subsequent RCT comparing early mobilisation versus immobilisation, although early mobilisation led to early benefits in pain relief and movement, at 12 weeks' follow up there was no difference compared with use of a collar.[51] Only the 40% of people most severely affected by whiplash were included in the RCT comparing home exercise programmes, which may have led to a poorer outcome.[54] The management of acute whiplash injury remains controversial and needs further investigation.

QUESTION What are the effects of treatments for chronic whiplash injury?

One RCT found limited evidence that percutaneous radiofrequency neurotomy versus a sham procedure significantly increased the number of people who were free from pain after 27 weeks. A second RCT found no significant difference with physiotherapy alone versus multimodal treatment in disability, pain, or range of movement at the end of treatment or at 3 months.

Benefits: We found one systematic review of treatment of chronic whiplash injury (search date 1993)[9], which highlighted the lack of evidence on all treatment modalities. It identified one RCT (24 people with chronic whiplash; mean age 43 years; in whom the source of pain was confirmed by placebo controlled diagnostic blocks to be the zygapophyseal joints, excluding those between the second and third cervical vertebrae), which compared percutaneous radiofrequency neurotomy versus a sham procedure.[60] The RCT found that neurotomy significantly increased the number of people who were free from pain after 27 weeks (58% with active treatment *v* 8% with placebo; ARR 50%, 95% CI 3% to 85%; NNT 2, 95% CI 1 to 29) and that neurotomy significantly reduced the median time taken for more than half of the pain to return (263 days with radiofrequency neurotomy *v* 8 days with a sham treatment; $P = 0.04$).[60] A subsequent RCT (33 people with chronic whiplash) compared physiotherapy alone versus multimodal treatment (physiotherapy combined with cognitive behavioural therapy; see comment below). It found that although people treated with either physiotherapy or multimodal treatment improved, there were no significant differences between treatments in disability, pain, or range of movement at the end of treatment or at 3 months. However, significantly more people treated with multimodal treatment were satisfied with pain control at the end of treatment and their ability to perform activities at 3 months ($P < 0.05$).[61]

Harms: The RCTs did not report on adverse effects.[60,61]

Comment: Few RCTs have considered treatment for chronic whiplash and many people with whiplash are included in general RCTs of chronic mechanical neck pain. Limitations of the RCT comparing physiotherapy versus multimodal treatment include its small size, and the difference in time spent with the therapist in the two groups.[61]

QUESTION **What are the effects of treatments for neck pain with radiculopathy?**

OPTION **SURGERY VERSUS CONSERVATIVE TREATMENT**

One RCT found no significant difference between surgery versus conservative treatment in symptoms after 1 year.

Benefits: We found one systematic review (search date 2000, 1 RCT).[62] One non-blinded RCT included in the review (81 people with severe radicular symptoms for at least 3 months; see comment below) compared surgery versus conservative treatment (physiotherapy or immobilisation in a neck collar).[63] It found no significant difference between treatments in symptoms after 1 year.

Harms: The RCT did not report adverse effects.[63]

Comment: In the RCT the number of people with prolapsed intervertebral disc was not stated.[63] The RCT reported that people who did not improve between 3 and 12 months were given additional treatments: one person in the physiotherapy group and five in the collar group underwent surgery; eight people in the surgery group underwent a second operation; and 12 people in the surgery group and 11 in the collar group received physiotherapy. The RCT also reported that 41% of people had a high anxiety score and 31% of people had a high depression score, which correlated with pain intensity after but not before treatment. At 1 year, 20% of people were depressed, which suggests that treatment should aim to improve both physical and psychological symptoms.[64] Conservative treatment needs further assessment, particularly in people considered to be poor risk candidates for surgery.

OPTION **DRUG TREATMENTS (EPIDURAL STEROID INJECTIONS, ANALGESICS, NON-STEROIDAL ANTI-INFLAMMATORY DRUGS, OR MUSCLE RELAXANTS)**

We found no evidence about the effects of epidural steroid injections, analgesics, non-steroidal anti-inflammatory drugs, or muscle relaxants.

Benefits: **Periradicular, cervical epidural steroid injections, or both:** We found no systematic review or RCTs. **Simple analgesics (paracetamol and opioids) and oral non-steroidal anti-inflammatory drugs:** We found no systematic review or RCTs. **Antidepressants:** We found no systematic review or RCTs. **Muscle relaxants and benzodiazepines:** We found no systematic review or RCTs.

Harms: **Periradicular, cervical epidural steroid injections, or both:** Case reports have documented occasional complications, such as infection or bleeding after cervical epidural injection. The incidence of adverse events after different cervical injection techniques is unknown.

Comment: None.

GLOSSARY

Wallenberg's syndrome (lateral medullary syndrome) An infarction of the dorsolateral aspect of the medulla oblongata. Manifestations may include loss of pain and temperature sensation in the same side of the face and opposite side of the body.

Substantive changes

Physical treatments One new systematic review;[18] conclusions unchanged.
Treatments for chronic whiplash injury One new RCT;[61] conclusions unchanged.

REFERENCES

1. Mäkelä M, Heliövaara M, Sievers K, et al. Prevalence, determinants, and consequences of chronic neck pain in Finland. *Am J Epidemiol* 1991;134:1356–1367.
2. Cote P, Cassidy D, Carroll L. The Saskatchewan health and back pain survey: the prevalence of neck pain and related disability in Saskatchewan adults. *Spine* 1998;23:1689–1698.
3. Hackett GI, Hudson MF, Wylie JB, et al. Evaluation of the efficacy and acceptability to patients of a physiotherapist working in a health centre. *BMJ* 1987;294:24–26.
4. Waalen D, White P, Waalen J. Demographic and clinical characteristics of chiropractic patients: a 5-year study of patients treated at the Canadian Memorial Chiropractic College. *J Can Chiropract Assoc* 1994;38:75–82.
5. Lamberts H, Brouwer H, Groen AJM, et al. Het transitiemodel in de huisartspraktijk. *Huisart Wet* 1987;30:105–113.
6. Kvarnstrom S. Occurrence of musculoskeletal disorders in a manufacturing industry with special attention to occupational shoulder disorders. *Scand J Rehabil Med Suppl* 1983;8:1–114.
7. Borghouts JA, Koes BW, Bouter LM. The clinical course and prognostic factors of non-specific neck pain: a systematic review. *Pain* 1998;77:1–13. Search date 1996; primary sources Medline and Embase.
8. Squires B, Gargan MF, Bannister GC. Soft-tissue injuries of the cervical spine: 15 year follow-up. *J Bone Joint Surg Br* 1996;78:955–957.
9. Spitzer WO, Skovron ML, Salmi LR, et al. Scientific monograph of the Quebec Task Force on whiplash-associated disorders: redefining "whiplash" and its management. *Spine* 1995;20(suppl 8):1–73. Search date 1993; primary sources Medline, TRIS, NTIS, personal contacts, and Task Force reference lists.
10. Ferrari R, Russell AS. Epidemiology of whiplash: an international dilemma. *Ann Rheum Dis* 1999;58:1–5.
11. Vernon H, Mior S. The neck disability index: a study of reliability and validity. *J Manipulative Physiol Ther* 1991;14:409–415.
12. Koes BW, Assendelft WJ, Van der Heijden GJ, et al. Spinal manipulation and mobilisation for back and neck pain: a blinded review. *BMJ* 1991;303:1298–1303. Search date 1990; primary source Medline.
13. Gross AR, Aker PD, Goldsmith CH, et al. Physical medicine modalities for mechanical neck disorders. In: The Cochrane Library, Issue 2, 2002. Oxford: Update Software. Search date 1993; primary sources Medline, Embase, Chirolars, Index to Chiropractic Literature, Cinahl, and Science Citation Index.
14. Kjellman GV, Skargren EI, Oberg BE. A critical analysis of randomised clinical trials on neck pain and treatment efficacy. A review of the literature.

Scand J Rehabil Med 1999;31:139–152. Search date 1995; primary sources Medline, Cinahl, and hand searches of reference lists.
15. Van der Heijden GJ, Beurskens AJ, Koes BW, et al. The efficacy of traction for back and neck pain: a systematic, blinded review of randomized clinical trial methods. *Phys Ther* 1995;75:93–104. Search date 1992; primary sources Medline, Embase, Index to Chiropractic Literature, and Physiotherapy Index.
16. White AR, Ernst E. A systematic review of randomized controlled trials of acupuncture for neck pain. *Rheumatology* 1999;38:143–147. Search date 1998; primary sources Medline, Embase, Cochrane Library, and CISCOM (a database specialising in complementary medicine).
17. Smith LA, Oldman AD, McQuay HJ, et al. Teasing apart quality and validity in systematic reviews: an example from acupuncture trials in chronic neck and back pain. *Pain* 2000;86:119–132. Search date 1998; primary sources Medline, Embase, Cinahl, Psychlit, Cochrane Library, Oxford Pain Relief Database, and hand searches of reference lists.
18. Philadelphia Panel. Evidence-based clinical practice guidelines on selected rehabilitation interventions for neck pain. *Phys Ther* 2001;81:1701–1717. Search date 2000, primary sources Medline, Embase, Current Contents, Cinahl, Cochrane Controlled Trials Register, Cochrane Field of Rehab and Related Therapies, Cochrane Musculoskeletal Group and PEDro.
19. Waling K, Sundelin G, Ahlgren C, et al. Perceived pain before and after three exercise programs – a controlled clinical trial of women with work-related trapezius myalgia. *Pain* 2000;85:201–207.
20. Irnich D, Behrens N, Molzen H, et al. Randomised trial of acupuncture compared with conventional massage and "sham" laser acupuncture for treatment of chronic neck pain. *BMJ* 2001;322:1574–1578.
21. Bronfort G, Evans R, Nelson B, et al. A randomized clinical trial of exercise and spinal manipulation for patients with chronic neck pain. *Spine* 2001;26:788–797.
22. Jordan A, Bendix T, Nielsen H, et al. Intensive training, physiotherapy, or manipulation for patients with chronic neck pain. A prospective, single-blinded, randomized clinical trial. *Spine* 1998;23:311–319.
23. Goldie I, Landquist A. Evaluation of the effects of different forms of physiotherapy in cervical pain. *Scand J Rehab Med* 1970;2:117–121.
24. Revel M, Minguet M, Gregory P, et al. Changes in cervicocephalic kinesthesia after a proprioceptive rehabilitation program in patients with neck pain: a randomised controlled study. *Arch Phys Med Rehabil* 1994;75:895–899.
25. Levoska S, Keinänen-Kiukaanniemi S. Active or passive physiotherapy for occupational cervicobrachial disorders? A comparison of two treatment methods with a 1-year follow-up. *Arch Phys Med Rehabil* 1993;74:425–430.
26. Trock DH, Bollet AJ, Markoll R. The effect of pulsed electromagnetic fields in the treatment of osteoarthritis of the knee and cervical spine. Report of randomized double-blind placebo controlled trials. *J Rheumatol* 1994;21:1903–1911.
27. Aker PD, Gross AR, Goldsmith CH, et al. Conservative management of mechanical neck pain: systematic overview and meta-analysis. *BMJ* 1996;313:1291–1296. Search date 1993; primary sources Medlars, Embase, Cinahl, and Chirolars.
28. Hurwitz EL, Aker PD, Adams AH, et al. Manipulation and mobilization of the cervical spine: a systematic review of the literature. *Spine* 1996;21:1746–1760. Search date 1995; primary sources Medline, Embase, Chirolars, and Cinahl.
29. Cassidy JD, Lopes AA, Yong-Hing K. The immediate effect of manipulation versus mobilization on pain and range of motion in the cervical spine: a randomised controlled trial. *J Manipulative Physiol Ther* 1992;15:570–575.
30. Nordemar R, Thörner C. Treatment of acute cervical pain: a comparative group study. *Pain* 1981;10:93–101.
31. Brodin H. Cervical pain and mobilization. *Manipulative Med* 1985;2:18–22.
32. Koes BW, Bouter LM, Van Mameren H, et al. Randomised clinical trial of manipulative therapy and physiotherapy for persistent back and neck complaints: results of one year follow up. *BMJ* 1992;304:601–605.
33. Sloop PR, Smith DS, Goldenberg E, et al. Manipulation for chronic neck pain: a double-blind controlled study. *Spine* 1982;7:532–535.
34. Howe DH, Newcombe RG, Wade MT. Manipulation of the cervical spine: a pilot study. *J R Coll Gen Pract* 1983;33:574–579.
35. Dabbs V, Lauretti WJ. A risk assessment of cervical manipulation vs NSAIDS for the treatment of neck pain. *J Manipulative Physiol Ther* 1995;18:530–536.
36. Di Fabio RP. Manipulation of the cervical spine: risks and benefits. *Phys Ther* 1999;79:50–65.
37. Karjalainen K, Malmivaara A, Van Tulder M, et al. Multidisciplinary biopsychosocial rehabilitation for neck and shoulder pain among working age adults: a systematic review within the framework of the Cochrane Collaboration Back Review Group. *Spine* 2001;26:174–181. Search date 1998; primary sources Medline, Psychlit, Embase, and Cochrane.
38. Jensen I, Nygren A, Gamberale F, et al. The role of the psychologist in multidisciplinary treatments for chronic neck and shoulder pain. A controlled cost-effectiveness study. *Scand J Rehabil Med* 1995;27:19–26.
39. Taimela S, Takala EP, Asklof T, et al. Active treatment of chronic neck pain: a prospective randomized intervention. *Spine* 2000;25:1021–1027.
40. Linton SJ, Andersson MA. Can chronic disability be prevented? A randomized trial of a cognitive-behaviour intervention and two forms of information for patients with spinal pain. *Spine* 2000:21:2825–2831.
41. Gross AR, Aker PD, Goldsmith CH, et al. Patient education for mechanical neck disorders. In: The Cochrane Library, Issue 2, 2002. Oxford: Update Software. Search date 1993; primary sources Medline, Embase, Chirolars, Index to Chiropractic Literature, Cinahl, and Science Citation Index.
42. Linton SJ, Van Tulder MW. Preventive intervention for back and neck pain problems. What is the evidence? *Spine* 2001:26:778–787. Search date 1998; primary sources Medline, PsychoInfo, and ArbLine.
43. Horneij E, Hemborg B, Jensen I, et al. No significant differences between intervention programmes on neck, shoulder and low back pain: a prospective randomized study among home-care personnel. *J Rehabil Med* 2001;33:170–176.
44. Kamwendo K, Linton SJ. A controlled study of the effect of neck school in medical secretaries. *Scand J Rehab Med* 1991:23:143–152.
45. Koes BW. *Efficacy of manual therapy for back and neck complaints.* (Thesis) den Haag: Cip-Gegevens Koninklijke Bibliotheek, 1992.

46. Lavin RA, Pappagallo M, Kuhlemeier KV. Cervical pain: a comparison of three pillows. *Arch Phys Med Rehabil* 1997;78:193–198.
47. Bogduk N. Whiplash: why pay for what does not work? *J Musculoskel Pain* 2000;8:29–53. Search date and primary sources not stated.
48. Basmajian JV. Cyclobenzaprine hydrochloride effect on skeletal muscle spasm in the lumbar region and neck: two double-blind controlled clinical and laboratory studies. *Arch Phys Med Rehabil* 1978;59:58–63.
49. Bercel NA. Cyclobenzaprine in the treatment of skeletal muscle spasm in osteoarthritis of the cervical and lumbar spine. *Curr Ther Res* 1977;22:462–468.
50. Bose K. The efficacy and safety of eperisone in patients with cervical spondylosis: results of a randomised double-blind placebo-controlled trial. *Meth Find Exp Clin Pharmacol* 1999:21:209–213.
51. Verhagen AP, Peeters GG, de Bie RA, et al. Conservative treatment for whiplash (Cochrane Review). In: The Cochrane Library, Issue 2, 2002. Oxford: Update Software. Search date 1998; primary sources Medline, Embase, Cinahl, Psychlit, and Cochrane Controlled Trials Register.
52. Bonk AD, Ferrari R, Giebel GD, et al. Prospective, randomized, controlled study of activity versus collar, and the natural history for whiplash injury, in Germany. *J Musculoskel Pain* 2000;8:123–132.
53. Rosenfeld M, Gunnarsson R, Borenstein P. Early intervention in whiplash-associated disorders: a comparison of two treatment protocols. *Spine* 2000;25:1782–1787.
54. Söderlund A, Olerud C, Lindberg P. Acute whiplash-associated disorders (WAD): the effects of early mobilization and prognostic factors in long-term symptomatology. *Clin Rehab* 2000;14:457–467.
55. Foley-Nolan D, Moore K, Codd M, et al. Low energy high frequency pulsed electromagnetic therapy for acute whiplash injuries. A double blind randomised controlled study. *Scand J Rehabil Med* 1992;24:51–59.
56. Borchgrevink GE, Kaasa A, McDonagh D, et al. Acute treatment of whiplash neck sprain injuries: a randomised trial of treatment during the first 14 days after a car accident. *Spine* 1998;23:25–31.
57. Provinciali L, Baroni M, Illuminati L, et al. Multimodal treatment to prevent the late whiplash syndrome. *Scand J Rehabil Med* 1996;28:105–111.
58. McKinney LA, Dornan JO, Ryan M. The role of physiotherapy in the management of acute neck sprains following road-traffic accidents. *Arch Emerg Med* 1989;6:27–33.
59. Pennie BH, Agambar LJ. Whiplash injuries: a trial of early management. *J Bone Joint Surg Br* 1990;72:277–279.
60. Lord SM, Barnsley L, Wallis BJ, et al. Percutaneous radio-frequency neurotomy for chronic cervical zygapophyseal-joint pain. *N Engl J Med*. 1996;335:1721–1726.
61. Söderlund A, Lindberg P. Cognitive behavioural components in physiotherapy management of chronic whiplash associated disorders (WAD) — a randomised group study. *Physiother Theory Pract* 2001;17:229–238.
62. Fouyas IP, Statham PF, Sandercock PA, et al. Surgery for cervical radiculomyelopathy. The Cochrane Library, Issue 2, 2001. Oxford: Update Software. Search date 2000; primary sources Medline, Embase, and Cochrane Controlled Trials Register.
63. Persson LC, Carlsson CA, Carlsson JY. Long-lasting cervical radicular pain managed with surgery, physiotherapy, or a cervical collar: a prospective randomised study. *Spine* 1997;22:751–758.
64. Persson LCG, Lilja A. Pain, coping, emotional state and physical function in patients with chronic radicular neck pain. A comparison between patients treated with surgery, physiotherapy or neck collar — a blinded, prospective randomized study. *Disability Rehabil* 2001;23:325–335.

Allan Binder
Consultant Rheumatologist
Lister Hospital
Stevenage
UK

Competing interests: None declared.

Non-steroidal anti-inflammatory drugs

Search date January 2002

Peter C Gøtzsche

QUESTIONS

INTERVENTIONS

See glossary, p 1210

Key Messages

Differences between non-steroidal anti-inflammatory drugs (NSAIDs)

- **NSAIDs in increased doses** Systematic reviews have found that benefits of NSAIDs increase towards a maximum value at high doses. Recommended doses are close to creating the maximum benefit. In contrast, three systematic reviews found no ceiling for adverse effects, which increased in an approximately linear fashion with dose.
- **Choice between different NSAIDs** Systematic reviews have found no important differences in benefits among different NSAIDs or doses, but found differences in harms related to increased doses and to the nature of the NSAID itself.

Preventing gastrointestinal adverse effects

- **H_2 blockers in people at high risk who cannot avoid NSAIDs** One systematic review in people who had taken NSAIDs for 3 months has found that H_2 blockers versus placebo significantly reduce the development of gastric and duodenal ulcers.

- **Misoprostol in people at high risk who cannot avoid NSAIDs** One systematic review in people who had taken NSAIDs for at least 3 months has found that misoprostol versus placebo significantly reduces the development of gastric or duodenal ulcers. One additional RCT in people with rheumatoid arthritis taking NSAIDs found that misoprostol versus placebo significantly reduced the incidence of serious upper gastrointestinal complications such as perforation, gastric outlet obstruction, or bleeding over 6 months (NNT 265, 95% CI 133 to 6965). However, RCTs have found that misoprostol versus placebo significantly increases minor gastrointestinal adverse effects such as diarrhoea and abdominal pain.
- **Omeprazole in people at high risk who cannot avoid NSAIDs** One systematic review in people who had taken NSAIDs for at least 3 months has found that omeprazole versus placebo significantly reduces the incidence of endoscopically diagnosed gastric and duodenal ulcers.

Topical NSAIDs

- **Topical NSAIDs in acute and chronic pain conditions** One systematic review in people with acute and chronic pain conditions has found that topical NSAIDs versus placebo significantly reduce pain (NNT 5, 95% CI 4 to 6, at 1 wk in acute pain conditions; NNT 4, 95% CI 3 to 4, at 2 wks in chronic pain conditions).
- **Topical versus systemic NSAIDs or versus alternative analgesics** One systematic review found no high quality RCTs of topical NSAIDs versus oral forms of the same NSAID, or versus paracetamol.

DEFINITION Non-steroidal anti-inflammatory drugs (NSAIDs) have anti-inflammatory, analgesic, and antipyretic effects, and inhibit platelet aggregation. The drugs have no documented effect on the course of musculoskeletal diseases, such as rheumatoid arthritis and osteoarthritis.

INCIDENCE/ PREVALENCE NSAIDs are widely used. Almost 10% of people in The Netherlands used a non-aspirin NSAID in 1987, and the overall use was 11 defined daily doses (see glossary, p 1210) per 1000 population per day.[1] In Australia in 1994, overall use was 35 defined daily doses per 1000 population per day, with 36% of the people receiving NSAIDs for osteoarthritis, 42% for sprain and strain or low back pain, and 4% for rheumatoid arthritis; 35% were aged over 60 years.[2]

AIMS To reduce symptoms in rheumatic disorders; to avoid severe gastrointestinal adverse effects.

OUTCOMES **Primary outcomes:** pain intensity; personal preference for one drug over another; global efficacy; clinically significant gastrointestinal complications. **Secondary outcomes:** number of tender joints; perforation; gastrointestinal haemorrhage; dyspepsia; and ulcer detected by routine endoscopy.

METHODS *Clinical Evidence* update search and appraisal January 2002. More than 100 systematic reviews and thousands of RCTs have compared various NSAIDs. Many RCTs are unpublished or published in sources that are not indexed in publicly available databases. The quality of the RCTs is variable and bias is common, both in the design and analysis of the RCTs, to such an extent that a systematic review identified false significant findings favouring new drugs over control drugs in 6% of RCTs.[3] We included only large RCTs that provided clinically important information not already covered in the systematic reviews. We have favoured systematic reviews that have not been sponsored or authored by industry, as bias in such reviews has been repeatedly demonstrated but may be difficult to detect.[4] For example, it is easy to seemingly follow the rules for systematic reviews and yet adopt inclusion and exclusion criteria that omit inconvenient studies. In fact, it is hard to find a systematic review sponsored by, or co-authored by, industry that concludes that the company's product is not better than those of its competitors.

QUESTION Are there any important differences between available non-steroidal anti-inflammatory drugs (NSAIDs)?

Systematic reviews have found no important differences in effect between different NSAIDs or doses, but found differences in toxicity related to increased doses and to the nature of the NSAID itself. We found no large double blind RCTs comparing an NSAID with paracetamol in acute musculoskeletal syndromes. We found no evidence that NSAIDs are more effective than simple analgesics.

Benefits: **Rheumatoid arthritis:** We found two systematic reviews[5,6] and one subsequent RCT.[7] The first systematic review (search date 1985, 37 crossover RCTs, 1416 people) compared indometacin [indomethacin] with 10 newer NSAIDs in people treated for a median of 2 weeks with each drug.[5] Four of the RCTs included a placebo period and one RCT compared four drugs. Only 5% more people (95% CI 0% to 10%) preferred the newer NSAID to indometacin. The second systematic review (search date 1988, 6440 people, 88 RCTs comparing 2 NSAIDs and 27 RCTs comparing an NSAID with placebo) found no significant differences in the number of tender joints among 17 different NSAIDs.[6] The subsequent RCT (1149 people) compared three doses of the cyclo-oxygenase 2 (COX-2) inhibitor celecoxib versus naproxen 1 g.[7] It found a similar beneficial effect, with fewer endoscopically detected ulcers (5% *v* 26%; ARR 21%, 95% CI 13% to 29%). Only one of the ulcers was clinically significant and only 7/692 (1%) people taking celecoxib and 5/225 (2%) people taking naproxen withdrew because of gastrointestinal adverse effects.[7] **Osteoarthritis:** Two systematic reviews (search dates 1994[8] and 1996[9]) found no clear differences between various NSAIDs used to treat osteoarthritis of the hip (39 RCTs)[8] or the knee (16 RCTs).[9] One prespecified meta-analysis (8 RCTs, 5435 people) of rofecoxib versus other NSAIDs found a lower cumulative incidence over 12 months of clinically significant gastrointestinal adverse events with rofecoxlb (1% *v* 2%; RR 0.51, 95% CI 0.26 to 1.00).[10] Fewer people taking rofecoxib withdrew because of gastrointestinal adverse effects (118/3357 [4%] *v* 75/1564 [5%]; ARR 1%; RR 0.73, 95% CI 0.55 to 0.97; NNT with rofecoxib *v* other NSAIDs to avoid 1 additional withdrawal because of gastrointestinal adverse effects 78, 95% CI 46 to 790). **Acute musculoskeletal syndromes:** We found two systematic reviews, which identified generally poor quality RCTs.[11,12] The first systematic review (search date 1998, 17 RCTs for shoulder pain) was inconclusive (see NSAIDs under osteoarthritis, p 1221).[12] The second systematic review (search date 1993, 84 RCTs, 32 025 people with soft tissue injuries of the ankle) was unable to pool data to perform a statistical analysis of the different forms of treatment.[11] **Dose response relation:** One systematic review (search date 1985; 19 RCTs in which participants were randomised to more than 1 dose of 9 different NSAIDs) found a dose response relation that saturated at high doses.[13] This and another systematic review (search date 1992, 1545 people)[14] found that the recommended dosages were close to providing a ceiling effect.[13,14] The review of the 115 RCTs mentioned above found no significant differences between various doses of drugs;[6] 10/21 RCTs of ibuprofen had used a daily dosage of 1200 mg or less.[6]

Harms: **Versus placebo:** One systematic review (search date not stated, 100 RCTs, 12 853 people) found a non-significant tendency towards a higher rate of haemorrhage (ARI for NSAIDs *v* placebo +0.7%, 95% CI –0.1% to +1.5%) and proven ulcer (ARI for NSAIDs *v* placebo +0.05%, 95% CI –0.01% to +0.11%) with NSAIDs compared with placebo.[15] Mean treatment duration was short (2 months).[15] For 40 aspirin RCTs (22 234 people, mean treatment duration 1 year) the review found an increased risk of haemorrhage (ARI 0.6%, 95% CI 0.2% to 1.0%) and for proven ulcer (ARI 0.6%, 95% CI 0% to 1.2%).[15] The number needed to harm was in the range 100–1000. One systematic review (search date 1990, 38 placebo controlled RCTs) found that NSAIDs raised mean blood pressure by 5.0 mm Hg (95% CI 1.2 mm Hg to 8.7 mm Hg).[16] **Versus other NSAIDs:** One meta-analysis of 11 case control studies and one cohort study found that ibuprofen was significantly less toxic than other NSAIDs. The 11 comparator drugs were associated with a 1.6–9.2-fold increase in risk of serious upper gastrointestinal complications.[17] Cyclo-oxygenase 2 (COX-2) inhibitors were associated with less gastrointestinal toxicity than older NSAIDs, but the clinical significance is not clear (see benefits above).[7,10] One systematic review found that COX-2 inhibitors were associated with more serious thrombotic cardiovascular events than older NSAIDs.[18] The difference was significant for rofecoxib versus naproxen (RR 2.38, 95% CI 1.39 to 4.00; ARI 0.6%, 95% CI 0% to 1%), but for celecoxib the difference was not statistically significant (figures presented graphically). However, an indirect comparison in a meta-analysis of thrombosis prevention found a significant increase in the annual rate of myocardial infarction between both rofecoxib and celecoxib versus placebo (0.74% for rofecoxib *v* 0.80% for celecoxib *v* 0.52% for placebo; $P < 0.05$ for both comparisons), which suggests that there may be a class effect. **Dose response relation:** Three systematic reviews (search dates 1992[14,19] and 1994[17]) found no ceiling effect for adverse effects; the incidence of adverse effects increased in an approximately linear fashion with dose.

Comment: Important differences in adverse effects seem to exist between different NSAIDs. In contrast, the beneficial effects of NSAIDs seem similar. People's preferences for particular drugs have not been replicated and could, therefore, be because of chance or natural fluctuations in disease activity.[20,21] The evidence suggests that if the NSAID is unsatisfactory, switching to another NSAID will not solve the problem.[20,21] Likewise, doubling the dose of an NSAID leads to only a small increase in effect, which may not be clinically relevant. In acute musculoskeletal problems it is doubtful whether NSAIDs have any clinically relevant anti-inflammatory effect; we found no large double blind RCT comparing an NSAID with paracetamol. Paracetamol has been studied in osteoarthritis, where it had much the same effect as ibuprofen or naproxen (see simple analgesics *v* NSAIDs under osteoarthritis, p 1221).

QUESTION What are the effects of co-treatments to reduce the risk of gastrointestinal adverse effects of non-steroidal anti-inflammatory drugs (NSAIDs)?

One systematic review has found that misoprostol slightly reduces the incidence of clinically significant gastrointestinal complications of oral NSAIDs. One large RCT has found that omeprazole 20 mg and 40 mg daily and misoprostol 800 µg daily have similar effects in reducing endoscopically diagnosed adverse effects. However, misoprostol causes more adverse effects (mostly diarrhoea and abdominal pain). The review has found that double doses of H_2 blockers reduce the development of endoscopic ulcers compared with placebo. RCTs found H_2 blockers given in standard doses to be inferior to omeprazole and misoprostol, but the effect of H_2 blockers seems to increase with dose. The absolute risk of serious upper gastrointestinal complications is approximately doubled for people over 75 years old, and for those with a history of peptic ulcer, bleeding, or cardiovascular disease.

Benefits: We found one updated systematic review.[22] **Misoprostol versus placebo:** The systematic review (search date 2000, 9 RCTs, 3329 people) included people who had received NSAIDs for at least 3 months and where ulcers were detected by routine endoscopy.[22] Misoprostol reduced the development of endoscopic ulcers compared with placebo (61/1620 [4%] *v* 221/1709 [13%]; ARR 10%, 95% CI 9% to 12% for gastric ulcer; and 46/1301[4%] with misoprostol *v* 85/1394 [6%] with placebo; ARR 4%, 95% CI 2% to 5% for duodenal ulcer). Indirect comparisons of different RCTs suggested a dose response relationship ($P = 0.006$) for gastric ulcers in the dose range 400–800 µg. One additional 6 month RCT (8843 people with rheumatoid arthritis, mean age 68 years, all treated with NSAIDs) with clinically relevant outcomes compared misoprostol 800 µg daily versus placebo.[23] Serious upper gastrointestinal complications (such as perforation, gastric outlet obstruction, or bleeding detected by clinical symptoms or investigation) were reduced by misoprostol compared with placebo (25/4404 [AR 0.6%] with misoprostol *v* 42/4439 [1.0%] with placebo; ARR 0.4%; NNT 265, 95% CI 133 to 6965). The risk of serious upper gastrointestinal complications was approximately doubled for people over 75 years old, and for those with a history of peptic ulcer, bleeding, or cardiovascular disease. People with all four risk factors had an absolute risk of 9% for a major complication in 6 months, corresponding to a number needed to treat with misoprostol rather than placebo of 28 people. **H_2 blockers versus placebo:** The systematic review included five RCTs with 1005 people who had received NSAIDs for at least 3 months.[22] Double doses (see glossary, p 1210) of H_2 blockers significantly reduced the development of endoscopic ulcers compared with placebo (17/151 [11%]

v 38/147 [26%]; ARR 14%, 95% CI 6% to 23% for gastric ulcer; and 5/151 [3%] v 20/147 [14%]; ARR 10%, 95% CI 4% to 17% for duodenal ulcers). **Omeprazole versus placebo:** The systematic review included three RCTs with 774 people who had received NSAIDs for at least 3 months.[22] Omeprazole versus placebo reduced the development of endoscopic ulcers (ARR 13%, 95% CI 8% to 18% for gastric ulcer; ARR 9%, 95% CI 5% to 12% for duodenal ulcer). **Misoprostol versus omeprazole:** We found one RCT in 935 people treated with NSAIDs who had ulcers or more than 10 erosions at endoscopy. Treatment success was defined as fewer than five erosions at each site, no ulcers, and not more than mild dyspepsia.[24] At 8 weeks, treatment was successful in 76% of individuals given omeprazole 20 mg daily, 75% given omeprazole 40 mg daily, and 71% given misoprostol 800 μg daily. A total of 732 people in whom treatment was successful were rerandomised to maintenance treatment for 6 months. A higher percentage of people remained in remission with omeprazole 20 mg than with misoprostol 400 μg (61% v 48% [raw data not available]), and with either drug than with placebo (27% in remission with placebo; ARR for omeprazole v placebo 34%, 95% CI 25% to 43%; NNT 3; ARR for misoprostol v placebo 21%, 95% CI 12% to 30%; NNT 5). **Omeprazole versus H_2 blockers:** In a similarly designed RCT (541 people) treatment was successful in 80% given omeprazole 20 mg, 79% given omeprazole 40 mg, and 63% given ranitidine 300 mg daily.[25] The estimated proportions in remission after 6 months were 72% with omeprazole 20 mg and 59% with ranitidine 300 mg (ARR for omeprazole v ranitidine 13%, 95% CI 4% to 22%; NNT 8). **Misoprostol versus H_2 blockers:** One 8 week RCT (538 people with NSAID related upper gastrointestinal pain without endoscopic evidence of ulcers) compared misoprostol 800 μg versus ranitidine 300 mg daily.[26] A third of the people were excluded from analysis because of problems with adherence and missing endoscopic examinations. Gastric ulcers at least 3 mm in diameter were found in 1% of people taking misoprostol and in 6% of people taking ranitidine (ARR for misoprostol v ranitidine 5%, 95% CI 2% to 9%; NNT 20). Duodenal ulcer rate was 1% with both drugs.

Harms: In one of the large RCTs, significantly more people receiving misoprostol than placebo withdrew from the study because of adverse events, primarily diarrhoea and abdominal pain (1210/4404 [27%] v 896/4439 [20%]; ARI 7%; RR 1.36, 95% CI 1.26 to 1.47; NNH 14, 95% CI 12 to 19).[23] There was no significant difference in the number of deaths (17/4404 [0.4%] deaths in the misoprostol group v 21/4439 [0.5%] in the placebo group; ARR 0.1%; RR 0.82, 95% CI 0.43 to 1.55). One person on placebo died as a direct result of gastrointestinal toxicity. Few adverse events were reported in the RCT comparing omeprazole with ranitidine. Treatment discontinuations (all causes) occurred in 10% of people taking omeprazole 20 mg, 10% taking omeprazole 40 mg, and 14% taking ranitidine.[25] In the RCT comparing misoprostol with ranitidine, adverse events (mostly gastrointestinal) occurred in 77% of people taking misoprostol and 66% taking ranitidine, with withdrawal rates of 13% on misoprostol and 7% on ranitidine (ARR for withdrawal ranitidine v misoprostol 6%, 95% CI 1% to 11%; NNT 17).[26]

Comment: The clinical relevance of these findings is doubtful. The only RCT that used clinically relevant outcomes found little difference between active drug and placebo, except for people at high risk.[23] The rate of ulcers was more than 10 times higher in the studies where the investigators looked for them with regular endoscopy than in earlier RCTs of NSAIDs.[16] These ulcers were sometimes defined as endoscopic lesions with a size of only 3 mm, sometimes as any lesion of an unequivocal depth, and sometimes no definition was provided at all.

QUESTION What are the effects of topical non-steroidal anti-inflammatory drugs (NSAIDs)?

One systematic review has found that topical NSAIDs versus placebo are effective in acute pain conditions (NNT 5 to obtain good pain relief) and chronic pain conditions (NNT 3). We found no high quality RCTs of topical versus oral formulations of the same drug, and found no direct comparisons of topical NSAIDs versus paracetamol. Therefore, it is uncertain whether topical treatment is advantageous over these alternatives.

Benefits: **Versus placebo:** We found one systematic review (search date 1996, 86 RCTs, 10 160 people) that primarily compared a topical NSAID with placebo,[27] and one additional RCT[28] The review was partly sponsored by two manufacturers. Many RCTs of acute pain conditions (soft tissue trauma, strains, and sprains) were small; in 37 RCTs, the average number of actively treated people was 32 and the effect declined significantly with sample size. In seven RCTs with more than 80 people per group, the number of people that would need to be treated for one extra good outcome was five (RR 1.6, 95% CI 1.3 to 1.9; NNT 5, 95% CI 4 to 6). A good outcome included, in the following order: patient global judgement, pain on movement, spontaneous pain, physician global judgement. In 12 RCTs on chronic pain conditions (osteoarthritis, tendinitis) the number of people that would need to be treated for one extra good outcome was three (RR 2.0, 95% CI 1.5 to 2.7; NNT 4, 95% CI 3 to 4). The additional RCT (116 people with osteoarthritis of the hip or knee) compared copper salicylate gel versus placebo applied to the forearm.[28] It found no significant difference in effect (22% *v* 21% of participants reported good effect). **Versus oral NSAIDs:** Five RCTs in the systematic review compared topical versus oral NSAIDs, but they all had inadequate design and power.[27] We found no high quality RCT comparing the same NSAID given orally and topically (see effects of topical agents under osteoarthritis, p 1224). **Versus paracetamol:** We found no RCTs.

Harms: In the systematic review, local adverse effects occurred in 3% of people in both groups and systemic adverse events in 1%.[27] In the additional RCT, more people receiving copper salicylate gel reported adverse reactions, most commonly skin reactions (48/58 [83%] *v* 30/48 [52%]; ARR 31%; RR 1.6, 95% CI 1.2 to 2.1; NNH 3, 95% CI 2 to 7), and more people withdrew from the RCT because of these reactions (10/58 [17%] *v* 1/58 [2%]; ARR 13%; RR 10, 95% CI 1.3 to 75.6; NNH 6, 95% CI 3 to 20).[28]

Comment: Sample size bias hampers the interpretation of the available RCTs. We found no high quality RCTs comparing topical versus systemic administration of the same NSAID, and no RCTs comparing a topical NSAID with paracetamol.

GLOSSARY

Defined daily dose The assumed average daily dose for the main indication of a specified drug. The defined daily dose per 1000 population per day is an estimate of the proportion of that population receiving treatment with that drug.

Double doses Twice the defined daily dose.

Substantive changes

Differences between available non-steroidal anti-inflammatory drugs (NSAIDs) New systematic review found some evidence of increased thrombotic cardiovascular events associated with COX-2 inhibitors.[18]

REFERENCES

1. Leufkens HG, Ameling CB, Hekster YA, et al. Utilization patterns of non-steroidal anti-inflammatory drugs in an open Dutch population. *Pharm Weekbl Sci* 1990;12:97–103.
2. McManus P, Primrose JG, Henry DA, et al. Pattern of non-steroidal anti-inflammatory drug use in Australia 1990–1994. A report from the drug utilization sub-committee of the pharmaceutical benefits advisory committee. *Med J Aust* 1996;164:589–592.
3. Gøtzsche PC. Methodology and overt and hidden bias in reports of 196 double-blind trials of nonsteroidal anti-inflammatory drugs in rheumatoid arthritis (published erratum appears in *Control Clin Trials* 1989;10:356). *Control Clin Trials* 1989;10:31–56. Search date 1985; primary source Medline.
4. Smith GD, Matthias E. Meta-analysis: unresolved issues and future developments. *BMJ* 1998;316:221–225.
5. Gøtzsche PC. Patients' preference in indomethacin trials: an overview. *Lancet* 1989;i:88–91. Search date 1985; primary sources Medline, personal contact with companies that marketed proprietary products, and hand searched reference lists of collected articles.
6. Gøtzsche PC. Meta-analysis of NSAIDs: contribution of drugs, doses, trial designs, and meta-analytic techniques. *Scand J Rheumatol* 1993;22:255–260. Search date 1988; primary source Medline.
7. Simon LS, Weaver AL, Graham DY, et al. Anti-inflammatory and upper gastrointestinal effects of celecoxib in rheumatoid arthritis. *JAMA* 1999;282:1921–1928.
8. Towheed T, Shea B, Wells G, et al. Analgesia and non-aspirin, non-steroidal anti-inflammatory drugs in osteoarthritis of the hip. In: The Cochrane Library, Issue 4, 2001. Oxford: Update Software. Search date 1994; primary sources Cochrane Controlled Trials Register, Medline, and hand searched references.
9. Watson MC, Brookes ST, Kirwan JR, et al. Non-aspirin, non-steroidal anti-inflammatory drugs for treating osteoarthritis of the knee. In: The Cochrane Library, Issue 4, 2001. Oxford: Update Software. Search date 1996; primary sources Medline and Embase.
10. Langman MJ, Jensen DM, Watson DG, et al. Adverse upper gastrointestinal effects of rofecoxib compared with NSAIDs. *JAMA* 1999;282:1929–1933.
11. Ogilvie Harris DJ, Gilbart M. Treatment modalities for soft tissue injuries of the ankle: a critical review. *Clin J Sport Med* 1995;5:175–186. Search date 1993; primary sources Medline and Embase.
12. Green S, Buchbinder R, Glazier R, et al. Interventions for shoulder pain. In: The Cochrane Library, Issue 4, 2001. Oxford: Update Software. Search date 1998; primary sources Cochrane Musculoskeletal Group Trials Register, Cochrane Controlled Trials Register, Medline, Embase, Cinahl, and Science Citation Index.
13. Gøtzsche PC. Review of dose-response studies of NSAIDs in rheumatoid arthritis. *Dan Med Bull* 1989;36:395–399. Search date 1985; primary sources Medline, hand searches of reference lists, and contact with companies marketing proproctary preparations.
14. Eisenberg E, Berkey CS, Carr DB, et al. Efficacy and safety of nonsteroidal antiinflammatory drugs for cancer pain: a meta-analysis. *J Clin Oncol* 1994;12:2756–2765. Search date 1992; primary source Medline.
15. Chalmers TC, Berrier J, Hewitt P, et al. Meta-analysis of randomized controlled trials as a method of estimating rare complications of non-steroidal anti-inflammatory drug therapy. *Aliment Pharmacol Ther* 1988;2(suppl. 1):9–26. Search date not stated; primary source Medline.
16. Johnson AG, Nguyen TV, Day RO. Do nonsteroidal anti-inflammatory drugs affect blood pressure? A meta-analysis. *Ann Intern Med* 1994;121:289–300. Search date 1990; primary sources Medline, Embase, Biosis, Diagenes, Science Citation Abstracts, International Pharmaceutical Abstracts, IOWA Drug Information Service, Combined Health Informatics Database, and hand searched bibliographies, text books, and reference lists.
17. Henry D, Lim LL, Garcia Rodriguez LA, et al. Variability in risk of gastrointestinal complications with individual non-steroidal anti-inflammatory drugs: results of a collaborative meta-analysis. *BMJ* 1996;312:1563–1566. Search date 1994; primary source Medline.
18. Mukherjee D, Nissen SE, Topol EJ. Risk of cardiovascular events associated with selective COX-2 inhibitors. *JAMA* 2001;286:954–959. Search date 2001; primary sources Medline, the internet, and review of relevant submissions to the US Food and Drug Administration by pharmaceutical companies.
19. Cappelleri JC, Lau J, Kupelnick B, et al. Efficacy and safety of different aspirin dosages on vascular diseases in high-risk patients. A metaregression

analysis. *Online J Curr Clin Trials* 1995;Doc No 174. Search date 1992; primary sources Medline and Current Contents.
20. Huskisson EC, Woolf DL, Balme HW, et al. Four new anti-inflammatory drugs: responses and variations. *BMJ* 1976;i:1048–1049.
21. Cooperating Clinics Committee of the American Rheumatism Association. A seven-day variability study of 499 patients with peripheral rheumatoid arthritis. *Arthritis Rheum* 1965;8:302–334.
22. Rostom A, Wells G, Tugwell P, et al. Prevention of chronic NSAID induced upper gastrointestinal toxicity. In: The Cochrane Library, Issue 4, 2001. Oxford: Update Software. Search date 2000; primary sources Medline, Current Contents, Embase, Cochrane Controlled Trials Register, hand searched conference proceedings, and personal contact with experts and companies.
23. Silverstein FE, Graham DY, Senior JR, et al. Misoprostol reduces serious gastrointestinal complications in patients with rheumatoid arthritis receiving nonsteroidal anti-inflammatory drugs. A randomized, double-blind, placebo-controlled trial. *Ann Intern Med* 1995;123:241–249.
24. Hawkey CJ, Karrasch JA, Szczepanski L, et al. Omeprazole compared with misoprostol for ulcers associated with nonsteroidal antiinflammatory drugs. Omeprazole versus misoprostol for NSAID-induced ulcer management (OMNIUM) study group. *N Engl J Med* 1998;338:727–734.
25. Yeomans ND, Tulassay Z, Juhasz L, et al. A comparison of omeprazole with ranitidine for ulcers associated with nonsteroidal antiinflammatory drugs. Acid suppression trial: ranitidine versus omeprazole for NSAID associated ulcer treatment (ASTRONAUT) study group. *N Engl J Med* 1998;338:719–726.
26. Raskin JB, White RH, Jaszewski R, et al. Misoprostol and ranitidine in the prevention of NSAID-induced ulcers: a prospective, double-blind, multicenter study. *Am J Gastroenterol* 1996;91:223–227.
27. Moore RA, Tramer MR, Carroll D, et al. Quantitative systematic review of topically applied non-steroidal anti-inflammatory drugs. *BMJ* 1998;316:333–338. Search date 1996; primary sources Medline, Embase, Oxford Pain Relief Database 1950–1994, contact with pharmaceutical companies, and hand searched references.
28. Shackel NA, Day RO, Kellett B, et al. Copper-salicylate gel for pain relief in osteoarthritis: a randomised controlled trial. *Med J Aust* 1997;167:134–136.

Peter Gøtzsche
Director
The Nordic Cochrane Centre
Copenhagen
Denmark

Competing interests: None declared.

Osteoarthritis

Search date March 2002

David Scott, Claire Smith, Stefan Lohmander, and Jiri Chard

QUESTIONS

INTERVENTIONS

See glossary, p 1232

Key Messages

Non-surgical treatments

- **Analgesic versus non-steroidal anti-inflammatory drugs (NSAIDs)** RCTs found no good evidence that simple analgesics, such as paracetamol (acetaminophen), are significantly different from NSAIDs in pain relief.
- **Chondroitin** One systematic review and two subsequent RCTs found no clear evidence that chondroitin improved symptoms more than placebo.
- **Education** We found insufficient evidence to assess the effects of education and behavioural change in people with hip or knee osteoarthritis.
- **Exercise (pain relief and improved function)** Systematic reviews and subsequent RCTs have found that exercise and physical therapy reduce pain and disability in people with hip or knee osteoarthritis, although many of the trials were limited by poor methods and reporting.
- **Glucosamine** Systematic reviews and subsequent RCTs found limited evidence that glucosamine versus placebo improved symptoms, but publication bias and poor trial quality makes interpretation of results difficult.
- **Glucosamine plus chondroitin** We found no RCTs on glucosamine plus chondroitin alone. We found limited evidence in people with mild or moderate osteoarthritis that glucosamine plus chondroitin plus manganese ascorbate versus placebo significantly improved disease severity scores.
- **Intra-articular glucocorticoid injections of the knee** One systematic review and one subsequent RCT found limited evidence that intra-articular glucocorticoids versus placebo reduced pain for 1–4 weeks.
- **Intra-articular hyaluronan injections of the knee** One systematic review and subsequent non-systematic reviews and RCTs found limited evidence that hyaluronan versus placebo reduced pain for 1–6 months.
- **Other intra-articular injections of the knee** We found limited evidence on other intra-articular treatments such as radioactive isotopes, glycosaminoglycan poly sulphuric acid, orgotein and morphine.
- **Physical aids** RCTs in people with knee osteoarthritis found limited evidence that physical aids (joint braces or taping of the joint) may improve disease specific quality of life.
- **Systemic analgesics in people with existing liver damage** Observational evidence suggests that lower doses of paracetamol (acetaminophen) may cause liver damage in people with liver disease.
- **Systemic analgesics** Systematic reviews in people with osteoarthritis of the hip or knee found limited evidence that simple analgesics, such as paracetamol (acetaminophen), versus placebo reduced pain.
- **Systemic NSAIDs in older people and people at risk of renal disease or peptic ulceration** One RCT found that NSAIDs increased the risk of renal or gastrointestinal damage in older people with osteoarthritis, particularly those with intercurrent disease.
- **Systemic NSAIDs** Systematic reviews in people with osteoarthritis of the hip have found that NSAIDs reduce pain. We found no good evidence that NSAIDs are superior to simple analgesics, such as paracetamol (acetaminophen), or that there are differences between NSAIDs in relieving pain. Serious concerns exist relating to trial quality and commercial bias.

- **Topical agents** One systematic review and one additional RCT have found that topical agents containing NSAIDs versus placebo significantly reduce pain. One systematic review found that systemic adverse events were no more common than with placebo. RCTs found that capsaicin versus placebo significantly improved pain. We found no RCTs comparing different topical agents or comparing topical agents versus other local treatments such as heat or cold packs.

Surgical treatments

- **Hip replacement** One systematic review of observational studies has found that hip replacement is effective for at least 10 years.
- **Hip replacement in obese people** One systematic review of observational studies suggested that people who weigh over 70 kg may have worse outcomes in terms of pain relief and function after hip replacement. One study found lower rates of long term survival of implant in obese people.
- **Hip replacement in older people** One systematic review of observational studies found that people over 75 years may have worse outcomes that people aged 45–75 years in terms of pain relief and function.
- **Hip replacement in younger people** One systematic review of observational studies suggested that people under 45 years old may have worse outcomes in terms of pain relief and function after hip replacement. One cohort study found that younger people were at greater risk of revision.
- **Knee replacement** Systematic reviews have found that knee replacement is effective in relieving pain and improving function. One RCT found limited evidence that unicompartmental knee operations are more effective than tricompartmental replacement. We found limited evidence that unicompartmental knee operations are more effective than bicompartmental operations.
- **Knee replacement in obese people** We found limited and conflicting evidence from observational studies on the effects of obesity on outcomes after knee replacement.
- **Knee replacement in older people** We found limited evidence from observational studies suggesting that knee replacement is effective in older people.
- **Osteotomy** We found no RCTs comparing osteotomy versus conservative treatment. We found limited evidence from two RCTs that osteotomy is as effective as knee replacement.

DEFINITION Osteoarthritis is a heterogeneous condition for which the prevalence, risk factors, clinical manifestations, and prognosis vary according to the joints affected. It most commonly affects hands, knees, hips, and spinal apophyseal joints. It is usually defined by pathological or radiological criteria rather than clinical features, and is characterised by focal areas of damage to the cartilage surfaces of synovial joints, and is associated with remodelling of the underlying bone and mild synovitis. When severe, there is characteristic joint space narrowing and osteophyte formation with visible subchondral bone changes on radiography.

INCIDENCE/ PREVALENCE Osteoarthritis is a common and important cause of pain and disability in older adults.[1,2] Radiographic features are practically universal in at least some joints in people aged over 60 years, but significant clinical disease probably affects 10–20% of people. Knee disease is about twice as prevalent as hip disease in people aged over 60 years (about 10% *v* 5%).[3,4]

AETIOLOGY/ RISK FACTORS The main initiating factors are abnormalities in joint shape or injury. Genetic factors are probably implicated.

PROGNOSIS The natural history of osteoarthritis is poorly understood. Only a minority of people with clinical disease of the hip or knee joint progress to requiring surgery.

AIMS To reduce pain, stiffness, and disability; to limit the risk of progressive joint damage; to improve quality of life, with minimal adverse effects.

OUTCOMES Frequency and severity of joint pain (particularly activity related pain and night pain), stiffness, functional impairment and disability, quality of life, perioperative complications (infection, bleeding, venous thromboembolism, and death), prosthesis survival, and the need for revision surgery. A global knee rating scale that includes measures of pain, function, and range of movement. A modified Knee Society score: this instrument combines three different domains (pain, function, and joint status) into a single score (patient function [i.e. walking ability and stair climbing] accounts for about 50% of the total score, with pain and joint status [i.e. stability and deformity] each accounting for about 25%).[5] The Western Ontario and McMaster osteoarthritis (WOMAC) scale is a validated instrument for assessing lower limb (hip and knee) osteoarthritis and is sensitive to change. It is a self assessment questionnaire and includes questions on pain, stiffness, and physical function (such as walking ability). WOMAC is disease specific but not intervention specific; it can be used to assess any intervention in osteoarthritis.[6–8] The Lequesne Index includes the measurement of pain (5 questions), walking distance (1 question), and activities of daily living (4 questions), with versions available for the hip and knee. Scores for each question are added together to provide a combined disease severity score. Scores of 1–4 are classified as mild osteoarthritis, 5–7 moderate, 8–10 severe, 11–13 very severe, and 14 as extremely severe osteoarthritis.[9] The Arthritis Self-Efficacy (ASE), consists of two subscales, one for Pain (5 items) and one ASE, other symptoms (6 items). Within each, each item is scored from 0 (very uncertain) to 10 (very certain). Scores are summed across the items for each subscale, producing scores of 5–50 for ASE: Pain and 6–60 for ASE: other symptoms. The Multidimensional Health Assessment Questionnaire (MDHAQ). The Brief Pain Inventory (BPI) questionnaire (validated), measures pain intensity and effect (interference) on quality of life. Intensity (worst and least pain in the last week, average pain, pain right now) are recorded on numerical scales from 0 (no pain) to 10 (pain as bad as you can imagine). The effect of the pain are recorded in terms of how much it interferes with general activity, mood, walking ability, normal work, relations with others, sleep, and enjoyment of life, recorded on a numerical scale from 0 (does not interfere) to 10 (completely interferes). The British Orthopedic Association (BOA) score is used as clinical evaluation and has a maximum score of 39 points.

METHODS *Clinical Evidence* update search and appraisal March 2002.

QUESTION What are the effects of exercise and physical therapy?

Systematic reviews and subsequent RCTs have found that exercise and physical therapy reduce pain and disability in people with hip or knee osteoarthritis, although many of the trials were limited by weak methods and poor reporting.

Benefits: We found four systematic reviews,[10–13] one subsequent non-systematic review,[14] and seven subsequent RCTs[15–21] of exercise in people with osteoarthritis of the knee or hip. The first systematic review (search date 1997, 11 RCTs) concluded that exercise regimens were beneficial but that more evidence was needed (see table 1, p 1237).[10] The second systematic review (search date 1993) of non-medicinal and non-invasive treatments for hip and knee osteoarthritis concluded that, of seven modalities reviewed, exercise had the strongest evidence of benefit.[11] The third systematic review (search date 1994) of aerobic exercises for osteoarthritis of the knee found only three admissible RCTs.[12] The review concluded that, despite a favourable impression, the evidence currently available was inadequate. The fourth systematic review (search date 2000) of selected rehabilitation interventions for knee pain concluded that therapeutic exercise and transcutaneous electrical nerve stimulation were beneficial for knee osteoarthritis.[13] The non-systematic review identified 13 RCTs.[14] The review found that there was small to moderate beneficial effects for pain and function from use of strengthening exercise, aerobic exercise interventions, or both. The first subsequent RCT (24 obese people with osteoarthritis, body mass index ≥ 28 kg/m^2) compared an exercise plus weight loss diet versus an exercise programme alone. It found no significant differences in 6 month pain or function scores (no figures available).[15] The second subsequent RCT (179 older people with osteoarthritis, average age 74 years) found that exercise was significantly better than control for pain (Western Ontario and McMaster osteoarthritis [WOMAC] pain subscale; $P = 0.003$), physical activity (WOMAC physical activity subscale; $P = 0.006$), pain at rest (Visual Analogue Scale [VAS]; $P = 0.02$), and pain when walking (VAS; $P = 0.002$).[16] The third subsequent RCT (105 people) compared an education plus exercise package versus no intervention over 6 months.[17] It found that pain and quality of life were significantly better at 6 weeks with the programme but the difference was not significant at 6 months (Impact of Rheumatic Disease on General Health and Lifestyle pain scale, in which a lower score is an improvement: change at 6 wks, –0.4 with treatment *v* +1.2 with control, $P = 0.045$; at 6 months +0.2 with treatment *v* +0.6 with control, P = NS). The fourth subsequent RCT (126 people) compared personal exercise treatment versus small group exercise treatment versus no treatment.[18] Pre-specified analysis combined the results from the two exercise groups and found a significant effect on pain after 8 weeks of treatment versus no treatment (exercise *v* no treatment, $P < 0.01$; change in WOMAC pain scale 10.6, 95% CI 6.3 to 15.0 with exercise *v* –1.5, 95% CI –5.5 to +2.4 with no treatment) and functional improvement (WOMAC function scale 7.7, 95% CI 4.2 to 11.2 with exercise *v* –0.1, 95% CI –3.9 to +3.7 with no treatment). It found no significant difference between individual and group exercise treatment.[18] The fifth subsequent RCT (201 people) compared physiotherapist provided exercise versus standard care (patient education and drug treatment from their general medical practitioner if required). Analysis was by intention to treat.[19] Study inclusion criteria were American College of Rheumatology defined osteoarthritis of the hip or knee. Exclusion criteria were: other conditions that may account for the problem, treatment with exercise within the previous 6 months, problems in fewer than 10 out of 30 days, age under 40 or over 85 years, indication for hip or knee replacement, contraindications for exercise, analgesic or non-steroidal anti-inflammatory drug (NSAID) use, and inability to understand Dutch. It found exercise versus standard care significantly improved pain at 12 and 24 weeks (measured on a VAS 0 mm = no pain, 100 mm = very severe pain: −17.0 difference, 95% CI −23.6 to −10.4 at 12 wks, −11.5, 95% CI −19.7 to −3.3 at 24 wks) but not at 36 weeks, (−6.6, 95% CI −14.7 to +1.6). Observed disability was determined by studying videos of performance of a series of standardised tests. A total score was calculated from five measures: 5 m walking time, stand to sit time, stand to recline time, and levels of caution and rigidity during the performance of the tasks. It found no significant differences between groups (−0.19, 95% CI −0.38 to −0.01 at 12 wks, −0.09, 95% CI −0.30 to +0.12 at 24 wks, and −0.10, 95% CI −0.31 to +0.11 at 36 wks). The RCT suggested decreasing benefit over time may have been because of falling compliance. The sixth subsequent RCT (250 people) compared aerobic exercise versus resistance exercise versus education (including discussions and social gatherings).[20] Inclusion criteria were: age 60 years or more, pain in knees on most days of the month and difficulty with one of the following: walking 400 m, climbing stairs, getting in or out of a car, bath, or bed, rising from a chair, performing shopping, cleaning or self care activities, and radiographic evidence of knee osteoarthritis. Exclusion criteria were: medical conditions that precluded exercise, inflammatory arthritis, already regularly exercising, and inability to walk. Analysis was intention to treat. It found that compared with the education group, the exercise groups had significantly lower risks of loss of activities of daily living for both exercise groups versus education (RR 0.57, 95% CI 0.38 to 0.85), for the resistance exercise group versus education (RR 0.60, 95% CI 0.38 to 0.97), and for the aerobic exercise group versus education (RR 0.53, 95% CI 0.33 to 0.85). The seventh subsequent RCT (69 people) compared physiotherapist led exercise versus no exercise.[21] The results presented were for a subgroup of people who reported osteoarthritis symptoms who were part of a larger RCT (299 people) examining the impact of exercise on sedentary older people. Analysis was intention to treat. If found no significant difference at 12 months using the WOMAC scale.

Harms: We found no evidence about harms. Three subsequent RCTs did not report on harms.[19–21]

Comment: The older reviews reported that many of the trials are limited by methodological and reporting issues.[10–12] The new review reported that most trials were limited by methodological and reporting issues but there was good evidence for transcutaneous electrical nerve stimulation and therapeutic exercise for knee osteoarthritis.

QUESTION What are the effects of education and behavioural change?

We found insufficient evidence to assess the effects of education and behavioural change in people with hip or knee osteoarthritis.

Benefits: We found one systematic review[22] and four subsequent RCTs.[23–26] The systematic review (search date 1993) included 10 controlled trials (see comment below) of education over 2–48 weeks.[22] One trial, which found benefit from a combination of exercise and education, was excluded from the main analysis (see comment below). Effect sizes associated with education were not significant for pain (WMD 0.16, 95% CI –0.69 to +1.02) or disability (WMD 0, 95% CI –0.61 to +0.61). The first subsequent RCT (211 people with osteoarthritis of the knee) compared self care education (see glossary, p 1232) versus attention only education (see glossary, p 1232) over 1 year. The self care education group improved more for both pain and disability.[23] At both 4 and 12 months there was a significant difference for function and pain between self care education versus attention only education. The second subsequent RCT (252 people) assessed methods to improve adherence to treatment plans. The trial compared a targeted education programme versus an information pack, both delivered through a computer over 8 weeks, and found no significant difference in quality of life, pain, or disability between groups. The targeted education programme significantly improved stiffness compared with controls (effect size –0.63, 95% CI –0.81 to –0.45 *v* –0.39, 95% CI –0.53 to –0.25).[24] The third subsequent RCT (113 people) compared an isokinetic exercise regime versus generic information lectures given by health professionals over 12 weeks. It found no significant difference in leg strength, pain, or function between the groups.[25] The fourth subsequent RCT (544 people with all types of arthritis) compared an education programme versus a waiting list control.[26] The intervention comprised of six weekly meetings, each lasting about 2 hours. The meetings involved providing information on arthritis, self management, exercise, cognitive symptom management, dealing with depression, nutrition, communication with family and health professionals, and contracting. Analysis was intention to treat. Inclusion criteria were age greater than 18 years, ability to complete questionnaires, and a diagnosis of arthritis from a general medical practitioner. It found significant differences (99% CI reported, 95% CI not available) in mean values in favour of the intervention group at 4 months follow up on the Arthritis Self-Efficacy (ASE) scale pain (2.65, 99% CI 0.85 to 4.44), ASE other symptoms (3.93, 99% CI 1.66 to 6.19), cognitive symptom management (2.19, 99% CI 1.18 to 3.2), Visual Analogue Scale (VAS) score fatigue (0.48, 99% CI –1 to 0.04, P = 0.020), Hamilton Depression Rating Scale (HAD) anxiety (–0.59, 99% CI –1.2 to +0.03, P = 0.014), HAD depression (–0.86, 99% CI –1.46 to –0.26), Positive and Negative Affect Scale (PANAS) positive effect (1.83, 99% CI 1.65 to 3.50) but not cups of fluid consumed (P = 0.419), Health Assessment Questionnaire (HAQ) (P = 0.351), VAS pain (P = 0.707), or PANAS negative affect (P = 0.429).

Harms: No harms were reported.[22–26] One subsequent RCT did not report on harms.[26]

Comment: We found few well designed RCTs, and the participants in many trials were not representative of those in the general population. Studies of individual education in the systematic review also included biofeedback, exercises, and social support.[22] The systematic review did not state if the controlled trials were RCTs or not.[22] One trial that found a large improvement for pain and disability was excluded from the analysis because its results were so different from the others. It also included exercise in the intervention. The remaining nine trials had no significant heterogeneity of results.

QUESTION What are the effects of physical aids?

RCTs found limited evidence that physical aids versus control treatment improved disease specific quality of life. RCTs found no good evidence of a difference between different physical aids. Physical aids refer to shoe wedges/insoles, walking aids, joint braces, and taping of the joint.

Benefits: We found no systematic reviews. We found four RCTs on physical aids.[27–30] The first RCT (119 people) compared two forms of valgus knee bracing (neoprene sleeve and unloader-brace) against a control group. It found that both the knee brace groups versus the control group significantly improved disease specific quality of life (P = 0.001) and function (P < 0.001). No significant difference was found between Western Ontario and McMaster osteoarthritis (WOMAC) scores for the two braces (P = 0.062).[27] The second small RCT (14 people) found that taping of the knee versus control was associated with a reduction in pain (difference in mean pain score between neutral versus medical taping 15.5, 95% CI 2.4 to 28.6; figures as presented in original paper, units not clear; differences in pain score between neutral and lateral taping –8, 95% CI –22.5 to +6.5; figures as presented in original paper, units not clear).[28] **Versus other physical aids:** The third RCT (90 women, age > 45 years, and with American College of Rheumatology diagnosed osteoarthritis, but not people with a history of congenital foot problems, fused joints, foot deformity, or limitations of range of motion) compared a strapped insole versus an inserted insole.[29] Both groups were also given indometacin (indomethacin) (30 mg) twice daily. The RCT did not test the significance of differences between groups. It found the Lequesne Index significantly improved in both groups from baseline (strapped insole group, from mean 11.1 to 8.2; P = 0.006 *v* inserted insole group, from 10.1 to 8.8, P = 0.009) but pain significantly decreased only for the strapped insole group (VAS mean 43.4 to 21.3, P = 0.041 *v* 42.3 to 46.5, P value not reported). The fourth RCT (156 people) compared laterally elevated insoles versus neutral insoles.[30] Study inclusion criteria were: American College of Rheumatology defined osteoarthritis, aged 18 years or more, pain on daily basis for at least 1 month, pain of greater than 3 on 10 cm VAS after physical activity, evidence of medial femorotibial osteoarthritis on radiograph, functional class of less than IV on Steinbrocker score, greater or similar reduction in lateral than medial joint space. Exclusion criteria were: secondary knee osteoarthritis, hip osteoarthritis, hallux deformity of foot, advanced arthropathy of the hindfoot, any disease treated with insoles in previous 6 months, tibial osteotomy in previous 5 years, joint lavage in previous 3 months, intra-articular corticosteroid injection in previous month, and a change in osteoarthritis drug treatment within previous week. The RCT included people with a range of osteoarthritis severity. No subgroup analysis was specified. At 6 months, the results of the WOMAC subscales showed no significant difference for pain (percentage improved 19.5% with laterally wedged insoles *v* 21.6% with neutrally wedged insoles, P = 0.84), for stiffness (percentage improved 19.5% *v* 25.7%, P = 0.44) and for function (12.2% *v* 13.5%, P = 0.82). Reported compliance with the treatments was 88% for elevated insoles and 74.3% for the neutral insoles at 6 months.

Harms: The third RCT reported that adverse events were more common in the strapped insole group (13%) than in the inserted insole group (2%, significance not reported).[29] In the strapped insole group, three people complained of popliteal pain, two complained of back pain and one reported foot sole pain. One person complained of foot sole pain in the inserted insole group. In no cases was the adverse effect so serious that the participant stopped wearing the insole.

Comment: In addition to the two RCTs identified we found several observational studies, which all found positive effects from using physical aids.

QUESTION What are the effects of oral drug treatments?

OPTION SYSTEMIC ANALGESICS

Systematic reviews in people with osteoarthritis of the hip or knee found limited evidence that simple analgesics, such as paracetamol (acetaminophen), versus placebo reduced pain.

Benefits: We found one systematic review (search date 1994, 3 RCTs) evaluating analgesics in osteoarthritis of the hip[31] and one systematic review (search date 1994)[32] evaluating analgesics in osteoarthritis of the knee. The reviews found limited evidence that simple analgesics versus placebo were effective in controlling pain associated with osteoarthritis. A small RCT included in the review (44 people with osteoarthritis of the knee)[32] found that paracetamol (acetaminophen) was superior to placebo for short term pain relief (improvement in pain at rest in 73% of knees with paracetamol *v* 5% of knees with control) and global responses (improved global response 18/22 [82%] with paracetamol *v* 1/22 [5%] with control; RR 18.0, 95% CI 6.9 to 22.0; NNT 1, 95% CI 1 to 4).[33]

Harms: Liver damage results from overdose of paracetamol (acetaminophen), or at lower doses in people with existing liver damage.[34] See paracetamol (acetaminophen) poisoning, p 1447.

Comment: None.

OPTION NON-STEROIDAL ANTI-INFLAMMATORY DRUGS

Three systematic reviews have found that non-steroidal anti-inflammatory drugs (NSAIDs) versus placebo reduce short term pain in osteoarthritis (see NSAIDs, p 1203). NSAIDs are associated with an increased risk of gastrointestinal haemorrhage.

Benefits: We found three systematic reviews of analgesic and anti-inflammatory treatment in osteoarthritis of the hip (search date 1994, 14 RCTs)[31] and knee (search date 1996, 16 RCTs;[35] search date 1994, 45 RCTs[32]). The reviews found that NSAIDs versus placebo were effective at reducing short term pain. We identified hundreds of RCTs comparing NSAIDs with other NSAIDs or placebo for treatment of osteoarthritis. Most of these trials found benefit from using NSAIDs to treat osteoarthritis. **Oral versus topical NSAIDs:** See topical agents, p 1224.

Harms: One RCT (812 people with osteoarthritis of the knee) found that indometacin may accelerate joint damage in osteoarthritis.[36] A high withdrawal rate made the results difficult to interpret. The RCT also found a risk of gastrointestinal or renal damage in older people with osteoarthritis, particularly those with intercurrent disease.[36] Case control studies of several thousand people suggest that the odds ratio of gastrointestinal haemorrhage when taking any NSAID is about 4–5, the risk increasing with certain drugs and with increased doses.[37,38] A meta-analysis (search date 1994) ranked the risk from different drugs and found it to be dose dependent (see table 2, p 1237).[39] We found insufficient evidence about the gastro-intestinal effects of cyclo-oxygenase-2 (COX-2) inhibitors versus traditional NSAIDs to calculate the comparative risk for more recently introduced NSAIDs (see differences between NSAIDs under NSAIDs, p 1203).

Comment: Despite the many studies of NSAID use in osteoarthritis, the evidence we found on efficacy remains poor and difficult to generalise. Most RCTs suffer from weak methods, including short duration; exclusion of older people, those with intercurrent disease, or those at risk of gastrointestinal and other drug complications; variable outcome measures; comparison of one drug versus another rather than versus placebo; and funding bias.[40,41] In the absence of clear evidence of the superiority of one type of treatment or product, other considerations, such as safety (particularly the risk of gastrointestinal bleeding with NSAIDs) and cost, should determine the choice of drug (see NSAIDs, p 1203).

OPTION ANALGESICS VERSUS NON-STEROIDAL ANTI-INFLAMMATORY DRUGS

Systematic reviews found no good evidence that non-steroidal anti-inflammatory drugs (NSAIDs) are superior to simple analgesics such as paracetamol (acetaminophen) (see NSAIDs, p 1203).

Benefits: We found two systematic reviews (search date 1994,[31] 1 RCT and search date 1994,[32] 5 RCTs[42–46]), one additional study,[47] and one subsequent RCT.[48] The systematic reviews found no evidence for the superiority of NSAIDs over simple analgesics. One RCT (178 people with knee osteoarthritis) in the review compared naproxen versus paracetamol (acetaminophen) over 2 years. The trial found no significant difference in effects.[42] Another RCT (184 people with osteoarthritis) in the review compared two doses of ibuprofen versus paracetamol. It found no significant differences between the three groups.[43] One subsequent study of 20 crossover trials of one person each ("n of 1" trials) compared paracetamol (acetaminophen) versus diclofenac and concluded that although some people's pain was adequately controlled by paracetamol (acetaminophen) alone, others responded better to a NSAID.[47] The subsequent crossover RCT (227 people) compared paracetamol (acetaminophen) versus diclofenac plus misoprostol over a 6 week period.[48] Inclusion criteria were: age over 40 years, Kellgren & Lawrence grade 2–4 osteoarthritis, Visual Analogue Scale (VAS) score pain of greater than or equal to 30 mm. Exclusion criteria were: severe comorbidities and hypersensitivity to test drugs. It found significantly better results with diclofenac plus misoprostol versus paracetamol on the primary outcome of the Western Ontario and McMaster osteoarthritis (WOMAC) score for the target joint, (difference −7.75, $P < 0.001$), and the Multidimensional Health Assessment Questionnaire (MDHAQ) pain score, (difference −14.6, $P < 0.001$). Pre-specified subgroup analysis found the difference on the primary outcome measures increased with disease severity.

Harms: See harms of NSAIDs, p 1221. The subsequent RCT of acetaminophen versus diclofenac plus misoprostol found that acetaminophen was associated with fewer adverse effects, ($P = 0.046$) and gastrointestinal events ($P = 0.006$). The subgroup analysis did not examine the number of adverse effects.[48]

Comment: None.

OPTION GLUCOSAMINE

Systematic reviews and subsequent RCTs found limited evidence that glucosamine improved symptoms more than placebo, but publication bias and poor trial quality makes interpretation of results difficult.

Benefits: We found two systematic reviews[49,50] and three subsequent RCTs.[51–53] The first review (search date 1999, 6 RCTs of glucosamine, 911 people) found a significant effect of glucosamine on symptoms; but it reported that publication bias and trial quality made the results difficult to interpret.[49] The second review (search date 1999, 13 RCTs, 2029 people) of glucosamine versus placebo found that glucosamine was significantly better than placebo (summary random effects SMD of glucosamine *v* placebo 1.40, 95% CI 0.65 to 2.14).[50] It found four RCTs comparing glucosamine versus a non-steroidal anti-inflammatory drug (NSAID).[50] Three of the RCTs reported on pain and these all found greater pain reduction with glucosamine versus a NSAID (see comment below).[50] The first subsequent RCT (998 people) compared glucosamine (500 mg 3 times daily) versus placebo over a 60 day period. It found no significant difference in resting pain ($P = 0.66$) or walking pain ($P = 0.69$).[51] The second RCT (212 people) compared glucosamine (1500 mg sulphate once daily) versus placebo over 3 years.[52] It found glucosamine significantly improved symptoms (Western Ontario and McMaster osteoarthritis [WOMAC] scale mean difference in symptoms at 3 years 21.6%, 95% CI 3.5% to 39.6%). **Versus NSAIDs:** The third subsequent RCT (45 people) compared glucosamine sulphate against ibuprofen for osteoarthritis of the temporomandibular joint.[53] Inclusion criteria were: pain intensity greater than three on Visual Analogue Scale (VAS), for women neither pregnant nor nursing, degenerative joint disease not as a result of trauma, infection or general joint/muscle disease, no history of intra-articular joint injections, no previous use of glucosamine or chondroitin sulfate, no history of congestive heart failure, renal disease or hepatic disease, no history of hypersensitivity to NSAIDs, no history of peptic ulcers or gastrointestinal bleeding, no history of coagulation disorders, no active dental disease, if using an occlusal splint it must have been for at least 3 months, if taking antidepressants it must have been for at least 6 months, willingness to take oral medication, willingness to undergo a 1 week washout period, able to understand English. It found significant differences in favour of glucosamine at 90 days for functional pain, on the Brief Pain Inventory, and paracetamol (acetaminophen) use between 90 and 120 days (for all results $P < 0.05$).

Harms: The second systematic review reported that the safety profile of glucosamine in the 16 RCTs was excellent.[50] Out of the nearly 1000 people randomised to glucosamine treatment in the RCTs, 14 were withdrawn because of toxicity (comparative figures not provided) but it found insufficient evidence on long term tolerance.

Comment: We were unable to replicate the reviews calculation of an effect size for glucosamine versus a NSAID.[50] The first review reported that there was likely to be some benefit from glucosamine but the evidence did not allow us to confidently estimate the size of the effect.[50]

OPTION CHONDROITIN SULPHATE

One systematic review and two subsequent RCTs found no clear evidence that chondroitin improved symptoms more than placebo.

Benefits: We found one systematic review (search date 1999)[49] and two subsequent RCTs.[54,55] The review reported that trial quality and publication bias probably had a major effect on results, making them difficult to interpret.[49] The first subsequent RCT (130 people) found no significant difference between chondroitin sulphate (1 g daily) versus placebo over 6 months on the Lequesne Index ($P = 0.12$).[54] The second RCT (146 men) compared chondroitin sulphate (400 mg 3 times daily) versus diclofenac sodium (50 mg 3 times daily) over 6 months.[55] At the end of the first month, diclofenac was significantly better than chondroitin measured on the Lequesne Index ($P < 0.001$) but by day 60 the chondroitin group was significantly better than the diclofenac group ($P < 0.01$) and people in the diclofenac group were taking placebo by this period, whereas the chondroitin group were still on active treatment (see comment below).[55]

Harms: The review did not report harms.[49]

Comment: During the first month, people in the non-steroidal anti-inflammatory drug group were treated with diclofenac and placebo but from month 2 to 3 they were given placebo only. People in the chondroitin group were given chondroitin and placebo for the first month and then from month 2 to 3 received chondroitin only.[55]

OPTION GLUCOSAMINE PLUS CHONDROITIN

We found limited evidence that glucosamine plus chondroitin plus manganese ascorbate improved disease severity scores more than placebo in mild and moderate cases.

Benefits: We found no RCTs of glucosamine plus chondroitin alone versus placebo. We found two RCTs of glucosamine plus chondroitin plus manganese ascorbate.[56,57] The first RCT (34 people) compared a combination of glucosamine plus chondroitin plus manganese ascorbate versus placebo. It found significant improvement in disease score (–16.3%; $P = 0.05$), self assessment (–0.89; $P < 0.05$), and Visual Analogue Scale pain score (–26.6%; $P < 0.05$).[56] The second RCT (93 people) compared a combination of glucosamine plus chondroitin plus manganese versus placebo over 6 months.[57] It found no overall significant difference in the number of people achieving a 25% improvement on the Western Ontario and McMaster osteoarthritis (WOMAC) or Lequesne Indexes. Pre-specified subgroup analysis of mild and moderate cases found a significant difference in the response rates for WOMAC scores (58% *v* 28%; $P = 0.04$) but not in the Lequesne Index. Subgroup analysis of severe cases found no significant difference in response rates for either the WOMAC or Lequesne Index.

Harms: The second RCT found no significant difference in adverse effects between glucosamine plus chondroitin plus manganese versus placebo (17% with intervention *v* 19% with placebo).[57]

Comment: None.

QUESTION What are the effects of topical agents?

One systematic review and additional RCTs have found that topical non-steroidal anti-inflammatory drugs (NSAIDs) versus placebo provide some pain relief for people with osteoarthritis. One systematic review found that systemic adverse events were no more common with topical NSAIDs than with placebo. We found no RCTs comparing different topical agents or comparing topical agents with other local treatments such as heat or cold packs. We found no RCTs comparing the same NSAID given orally and topically. RCTs have found that capsaicin improves pain more than placebo.

Benefits: **Topical NSAIDs versus placebo:** See NSAIDs, p 1203. We found one systematic review (search date 1996, 86 trials),[58] two subsequent RCTs, and one additional RCT comparing topically applied agents containing NSAIDs versus placebo.[59–61] The systematic review found that these agents reduced pain compared with placebo (RR for relief of chronic musculoskeletal pain because of osteoarthritis and tendinitis 2.0, 95% CI 1.5 to 2.7). The additional RCT (70 people with mild knee osteoarthritis) showed a significant improvement (measured by Western Ontario and McMaster osteoarthritis [WOMAC]) in the treatment group receiving diclofenac gel compared with the control group receiving vehicle gel (P = 0.05).[60] One subsequent RCT (119 people with osteoarthritis) found better pain relief with a topical NSAID (diclofenac–hyaluronan gel) versus placebo gel, but the difference was not significant (P = 0.057).[59] The second subsequent RCT (237 people) compared eltenac gel (3 g 3 times daily) at 0.1%, 0.3%, and 1.0% concentrations or placebo gel over a 6 week period. It found no significant difference between any of the treatment groups versus placebo for pain (differences on a global pain scale eltenac 0.1% *v* placebo –6.1, 90% CI –20.5 to +8.2; eltenac 1.0% *v* placebo –10.8, 90% CI –25.3 to +3.6).[61] **Topical NSAIDs versus oral NSAIDs:** We found no RCT comparing the same NSAID given orally and topically. One good quality RCT (included in the review) in 235 people with mild osteoarthritis of the knee compared topical piroxicam gel versus oral ibuprofen (1200 mg daily) and found no significant difference in pain relief between the two groups (good or excellent relief in 60% *v* 64%; P = 0.56).[62] A second RCT (321 people with osteoarthritis of the fingers) compared diclofenac emulgel plus placebo versus placebo gel plus ibuprofen. It found no significant difference in pain but less people withdrew on the gel (5 on active gel *v* 16 with active tablet).[63] **Capsaicin:** One non-systematic meta-analysis of three RCTs of topically applied capsaicin found that capsaicin cream reduced pain compared with placebo (OR 4.4, 95% CI 2.8 to 6.9; dichotomous outcome not defined).[64] One subsequent RCT (70 people with osteoarthritis) compared 0.025% capsaicin cream versus non-medicated cream. Active treatment resulted in significantly greater pain reduction than placebo (no quantified estimates of benefit available).[65] A second subsequent RCT (200 people) compared topical capsaicin versus glyceryl trinitrate versus topical capsaicin plus glyceryl trinitrate versus placebo gel.[66] It found that pain scores were significantly reduced from baseline with topical capsaicin, glyceryl trinitrate, and topical capsaicin plus glyceryl trinitrate, but not for placebo gel; direct statistical comparisons of the different treatments was not performed. **Versus other local treatments:** We found no systematic review or RCTs comparing agents containing NSAIDs or capsaicin with simple rubefacients (see glossary, p 1232) or local applications such as hot packs.

Harms: The main adverse effect of topical treatment is local skin irritation; systemic adverse effects were no more common than with placebo.[58] We found no reports of gastric or renal problems.

Comment: The evidence is poor, with most studies being short term, including a mixture of patient groups, and comparing different agents with no placebo control. The RCT comparing topical versus oral NSAIDs did not use the same drug so it is difficult to disentangle the effects of this and the different routes of administration.[61]

QUESTION **What are the effects of intra-articular injection of the knee?**

One systematic review and one subsequent RCT found limited evidence of pain reduction over 1–4 weeks but no evidence of long term pain reduction with intra-articular glucocorticoids versus placebo. One systematic review, and subsequent non-systematic reviews and RCTs, found limited evidence of small additional pain reduction with intra-articular hyaluronan versus placebo. We found limited evidence on other intra-articular treatments.

Benefits: **Glucocorticoids:** We found one systematic review (search date not stated, 10 RCTs)[67] and one subsequent RCT.[68] The systematic review found that intra-articular injection of glucocorticoids into the knee (1 trial used 4 injections, the rest used single injections) provided a little additional pain relief compared with placebo. Pain reduction lasted from 1 week to 1 month.[67] The subsequent RCT (89 people randomised to 4 groups) evaluated a single injection with 24 weeks' follow up.[68] It found a short term benefit (1–4 wks) of the steroid injection compared with placebo for both pain and for a functional index.[67] **Hyaluronan:** We found one systematic review (search date not stated),[67] two subsequent non-systematic reviews,[69,70] and three additional RCTs.[71–73] The systematic review identified 10 RCTs of hyaluronan in the knee joint.[67] Treatment consisted of several injections of high molecular weight hyaluronan complexes over several weeks. The review found slightly greater benefit with the injections versus placebo at 1–6 months after treatment. The non-systematic reviews identified four additional RCTs not in the systematic review.[69,70] The first RCT (495 people) compared hyaluronan versus placebo injections (once weekly for 5 wks) or oral naproxen with follow up to 26 weeks.[74] It found a significant difference in walking pain in favour of hyaluronan over placebo (8.8 mm on a 100 mm Visual Analogue Scale [VAS] score; $P = 0.005$). It also found a significant difference in the number of people pain free or with only slight pain with hyaluronate versus placebo (38.9% *v* 33.1%; $P = 0.04$). But approximately a third (162/495 [33%]) of people did not complete the RCT and results were not intention to treat. The second RCT (90 people) found a significant difference between hyaluronan versus 6-methylprednisolone (1 injection weekly for 5 wks) over a 60 day period for pain reduction ($P = 0.003$).[75] The third RCT (52 people) found no significant difference between hyaluronan versus placebo injection (1 injection weekly for 5 wks) over 26 weeks.[76] The fourth RCT (110 people) compared hyaluronate versus placebo injections (4 injections over a 3 wk period) with 52 weeks' follow up.[76] At 3 weeks it found a significant difference in pain after exercise ($P = 0.026$) and function ($P = 0.027$), although no difference in pain at rest ($P = 0.16$). At 1 year there was only a significant difference in functional improvement ($P = 0.046$). The first additional RCT (36 people) compared five administrations of hyaluronic acid versus saline solution.[71] It found no significant difference in pain at day 35, but by day 90 there was significant differences in favour of hyaluronic acid for spontaneous pain ($P < 0.05$), pain on pressure ($P < 0.05$), and pain on movement ($P < 0.05$). But the RCT entered the same four people into the trial twice, making the results difficult to interpret. The second additional RCT (100 people) found significant benefit on the Lequense Index with hyaluronan versus placebo, both at 5 weeks (P = 0.03) and 4 months (P = 0.04).[72] The third additional RCT (120 people) compared four treatments, hyaluronate injection (2 mL at 10 mg/mL) plus placebo tablets, placebo injection (2 mL of saline) plus non-steroidal anti-inflammatory drugs (NSAIDs), hyaluronate injection plus NSAIDs, and placebo injection plus placebo tablets.[73] People were graded 1–3 on Altman radiographic scale (0 mild to 3 severe). Exclusion criteria were: exhibiting non-osteoarthritis arthritis, NSAID intolerance, peptic ulcer disease, avian allergy, consumption of herbal osteoarthritis products (glucosamine), intra-articular injections of hyaluronan or corticosteroid in previous 6 months. The population characteristics were: mean age 65.5 years, mean osteoarthritis grade 2.2, and mean chronic disease score 1. The results showed that on the VAS Western Ontario and McMaster osteoarthritis (WOMAC) pain scale and disability scale, all the active group treatments showed significant reductions (P < 0.05) compared with baseline at week 4. But all groups, including the placebo group, showed significant reductions (P < 0.05) compared with baseline on the VAS WOMAC stiffness scale at week 4. The statistical significance of differences between treatments was not tested.[73] **Other intra-articular treatments:** Several other intra-articular treatments exist, but we found only limited evidence on their effects. Treatments include radioactive isotopes, glycosaminoglycan polysulphuric acid, orgotein, and morphine.[4,77,78]

Harms: We found no reports of serious adverse effects. Localised discomfort after injection is common. A theoretical risk of infection exists, but we found no evidence of this.

Comment: There is little evidence of whether simple aspiration of the knee would be as effective as injection.

QUESTION What are the effects of osteotomy? New

We found no RCTs comparing osteotomy versus conservative treatment. We found limited evidence from two RCTs that osteotomy is as effective as knee replacement.

Benefits: **Versus conservative treatment:** We found no systematic reviews. We found no RCTs. Observational evidence found good results with osteotomy (see comments). **Versus other surgical techniques:** We found two RCTs of osteotomy versus other surgical treatments.[79,80] Subgroup analysis from one RCT (100 people randomised aged 55–70 years with medial osteoarthritis of the knee, grades I–III according to Ahlback's classification, with knee symptoms [mainly pain] regarded as justifying surgical treatment, but not with impairment of hips or ankles; subgroup analysis on 59 people with strictly unilateral knee pain) compared high tibial osteotomy versus unicompartmental prosthetic knee replacement (UKA). Assessment was prior to and 1 year after surgery. It found an overall clinical improvement from baseline on the British Orthopeic Association score, pain during walking, and the ability to ascend and descend steps, but the range of knee flexion and the isokinetic thigh muscle torque remained unchanged after one year with both osteotomy and UKA. On comparing treatments after 1 year, it found no significant difference with osteotomy versus UKA, but walking outcomes were non-significantly better with UKA. The second RCT (60 people) compared high tibial osteotomy versus unicompartmental joint replacement.[79] The inclusion criteria were medial unicompartmental osteoarthritis, age over 60 years, varus malalignment < 10°, flexion contraction < 15°, ligament instability < 2nd degree. It found no significant difference at latest follow up (range 7–10 years) in knee scores (mean scores of 76 [range 29–100] with osteotomy *v* 74 [range 31–94] with unicompartmental joint replacement using the Knee Society Clinical Rating System; higher scores represent a worse outcome; P = 0.77). It found no significant difference in functional score (mean functional score 71 [0 –100] with osteotomy *v* 59 [0–100] with unicompartmental joint replacement; P = 0.22).[80]

Harms: We found no evidence about harms.

Comment: We also identified 18 observational studies. Of the observational studies, only one compared osteotomy with another technique (osteotomy *v* UKA). It found UKA had better results than osteotomy and that these results were sustained over long periods.[81] The other observational studies found that osteotomy was effective in subgroups with appropriate site of osteoarthritis, severity of disease and degree of physical activity.

QUESTION What are the effects of joint replacement surgery?

OPTION TOTAL HIP REPLACEMENT

One systematic review of observational studies has found that hip replacement is effective for at least 10 years. Many uncontrolled, observational studies suggest that even better results can be obtained over longer time periods.

Benefits: We found two systematic reviews.[82,83] In the first systematic review (search date 1995, 17 RCTs, 61 observational studies of hip replacements)[82] mean ages of people in the trials ranged 43–71 years. The review found that at least 70% of people without prosthetic failure were rated "good/excellent" for pain and function at 10 years' follow up (see comment below). A second systematic review (search date 1995) identified 11 RCTs and 180 observational studies comparing different prostheses.[83] It found wide variations in outcome with primary evidence too weak to draw valid conclusions.

Harms: **Death:** We found one systematic review (search date 1995).[84] It pooled data from 130 000 people who had undergone hip replacement and had not received thromboprophylaxis, and found that the rate of fatal pulmonary embolism was 0.1–0.2% and overall mortality was 0.3–0.4%.[84] One retrospective cohort study (11 607 hip replacements) found mortality to be higher in the first 3 months after surgery than in the subsequent 9 months.[85] **Revision and infection:** Two high quality observational studies found that the risk of a revision operation was about 1% per annum, ranging 0.2–2.0%.[82,86] Most studies found that revisions were not required until at least 10 years after implantation. One large study of a patient register in Sweden found that cumulative 10 year proportion of hip replacements that were revised due to infection fell to less that 0.5% between 1978 and 1990. It also found that after the immediate postoperative period, aseptic loosening accounted for about 80% of all requirements for replacement or revision surgery.[87] Observational studies found that the initial results of revision surgery were only slightly worse than primary surgery. But the prostheses deteriorated more quickly.[88–90] One prospective cohort study (39 543 people) on the Norwegian Hip Replacement register found a lower standardised mortality ratio (0.81) for people who had undergone total hip replacement at mean follow up of 5.2 years (range 0–10.4 years).[91]

Comment: One poor quality narrative review of 20 mainly small uncontrolled studies evaluating self assessed quality of life (at least 2 out of the following factors: physical, social, emotional, economic, and overall satisfaction).[92] It found that improvement in non-physical measures occurred most often within 3 months. Benefit was sustained for up to 5 years after surgery. We found no longer term evidence. Most studies did not distinguish between hip replacement for osteoarthritis and hip replacement for other reasons, which may confound data for osteoarthritis. Outcome of hip replacement for osteoarthritis differs significantly from that for other conditions (e.g. hip fracture in the very elderly and frail, or replacement for rheumatoid arthritis). Hundreds of additional uncontrolled observational studies are available. These studies generally find that hip replacement is effective and beneficial. One recent observational study using the Swedish National Total Hip Arthroplasty register (1056 randomly selected people who had not had revision surgery) found that 10 years after surgery people usually had good health (based on SF-36 measures).[93]

OPTION KNEE REPLACEMENT

One systematic review of observational studies has found that tricompartmental knee joint replacement is effective. One systematic review of observational studies has found better outcomes with unicompartmental versus bicompartmental operations. One subsequent RCT has found that unicompartmental knee replacement is more effective than tricompartmental knee replacement at 5 years' follow up. Most studies concentrated on prosthesis survival rather than clinical outcomes.

Benefits: We found one systematic review of tricompartmental prostheses (search date 1992)[94] and one systematic review of bicompartmental and unicompartmental prostheses (search date 1992).[95] **Tricompartmental prostheses:** The review identified 154 studies (4 RCTs, 130 cohort studies, 20 others) of 37 different tricompartmental prostheses in 9879 people (63% with osteoarthritis, mean follow up of 4.1 years).[94] Good or excellent outcomes were reported in 89% of people (improved function 5 years after surgery; pain relief after 5 years; mortality rate at 30 days and at 1 year; thromboembolism by 30 days after surgery; no failure of knee prosthesis).[94] **Bicompartmental prostheses:** The review identified no RCTs but found 18 cohort studies (884 people).[95] The review found that bicompartmental prostheses were effective (based on a global knee rating scale that includes pain, function, and range of movement). **Unicompartmental prostheses:** The review identified no RCTs but 46 cohort studies (2391 people).[95] We found one subsequent RCT.[96] The review found that both unicompartmental and bicompartmental procedures were effective (based on a global knee rating scale that includes measures of pain, function, and range of movement), with better outcomes from unicompartmental operations, particularly since 1987.[95] The subsequent RCT (92 people) found that unicompartmental knee replacement is more effective than tricompartmental knee replacement at 5 years' follow up. Pain relief was good in both groups, but the number of knees able to flex 120° or more was significantly higher in people treated with unicompartmental replacement ($P < 0.001$) and there were more excellent results (90–100 on the Bristol Knee Score) in this group (34/45 [76%] *v* 26/46 [57%], RR 1.3, 95% CI 0.99 to 1.8).[96] **Quality of life:** Two observational studies published since the review found improvement in quality of life after all forms of knee replacement. The first found that knee replacement improved function (measured by Western Ontario and McMaster osteoarthritis, from 58.2 before surgery to 18.4 at time of survey).[97] The second, a cross-sectional community survey, found that more people had moderate to severe pain (assessed using a modified Knee Society score) before surgery (361/487 [74%]) than 1 or more years afterwards (100/487 [21%]).[98]

Harms: **Death:** In one 6 year cohort of 338 736 US Medicare patients, the death rate within 30 days of hospital admission for total knee replacement was 2147 (0.63%).[99] The same cohort study reported a mean mortality of 1.5% per annum (no comparative data available).[99] One observational study (208 people) found no significant increase in the risk of death after knee arthroplasty for women (standardised mortality ratio 1.03, 95% CI 0.76 to 1.37) or men (standardised mortality ratio 1.14, 95% CI 0.68 to 1.80) after a mean follow up of 6 years (range 0–20 years).[100] **Thrombosis:** We found three studies that reported rates of venous thrombosis.[83,101,102] They found that about 24% of people who had a total knee replacement developed a deep vein thrombosis. **Revision and infection:** This is the main long term risk. The first review found a revision rate of 3.8% during 4.1 years' follow up after tricompartmental replacements.[94] The second review found a revision rate of 9.2% over 4.6 years for unicompartmental prostheses and 7.2% over 3.6 years for bicompartmental prostheses.[95] Large patient register based studies in Sweden found that the cumulative 10 year risk for revision surgery because of infection had fallen to less than 1%.[87] Most implant revision surgery was because of aseptic loosening. For unicompartmental osteoarthritis, unicompartmental knee replacement was an effective alternative to total knee replacement.[103,104] **Postoperative pain:** This was rarely recorded, but seemed to be absent or mild in most people. **Wound infection:** We found no good evidence on the frequency of wound infections. One large retrospective cohort study found lower complication rates in centres with a higher volume of procedures.[105]

Comment: We found hundreds of observational studies that reported the time to prosthesis failure or revision surgery, but less evidence on patient related outcomes. The evidence suggests that benefits and harms of knee replacement now seem to be similar to that of hip replacement.

QUESTION Which people are most likely to benefit from hip replacement?

Observational studies have found younger age (< 45 years), old age (> 75 years), and obesity to be associated with worse outcomes from hip replacement in terms of self assessed satisfaction and failure rates.

Benefits: We found no RCTs. One systematic review (search date not stated) identified 40 observational studies (number of people not stated) relating individual characteristics to outcome after hip replacement.[106] It found that the following factors predicted better outcomes in terms of pain relief and function: age 45–75 years; weight less than 70 kg; good social support; higher educational level and less preoperative morbidity. **Obesity:** One prospective cohort study (176 people) found no difference in the quality of life after a primary hip replacement between the non-obese and moderately obese either at 1 or 3 years, but the study reported no results in people with a body mass index greater than 40 kg/m^2.[107] **Age:** We found a few large observational studies. They found conflicting evidence, which suggested that older people had good self reported outcomes in terms of pain and function, but spent longer in hospital, needed more rehabilitation, and experienced more perioperative complications.[92,108–114]

Harms: **Revision and infection:** One Swedish cohort study found that younger people and those doing heavy physical work were at greater risk of revision.[87] Another study found lower rates of long term survival of the implant in obese people.[89]

Comment: Consensus groups have reported from Sweden, the USA, Canada, and New Zealand.[115–118] Constant pain, particularly night or rest pain, with or without substantial functional impairment, were the generally agreed criteria for joint replacement (see table 3, p 1237). In practice, most surgeons prefer to have radiographic evidence of joint damage as well.

QUESTION **Which people are most likely to benefit from knee replacement?**

We found limited and conflicting evidence from observational studies.

Benefits: **Obesity:** We found limited and conflicting evidence from observational studies on the effects of obesity on outcome of knee replacement.[119–122] **Age:** We found limited evidence from observational studies suggesting that knee replacement is effective in elderly people.[114,123,124]

Harms: None found.

Comment: None.

GLOSSARY

Attention only education Information about arthritis but no guidance on self treatment.

Rubefacient An agent that produces mild irritation and redness of the skin.

Self care education Individualised arthritis self care instruction based on patients needs assessment.

Substantive changes

Exercise and physical therapy One new systematic review found that therapeutic exercise and transcutaneous electrical nerve stimulation were beneficial for knee osteoarthritis.[13]

Exercise and physical therapy Three new RCTs.[19–21] One RCT found that exercise versus no treatment significantly improved pain. One RCT found that exercise versus education significantly improved activities of daily living. One RCT found no significant difference between exercise and no exercise on the WOMAC scale.

Education One new RCT found that education versus a waiting list control significantly improved outcomes on the Arthritis Self-Efficacy scale.[26]

Physical aids Two new RCTs found no good evidence of a difference between different physical aids.[29,30]

Analgesics versus NSAIDs One new RCT of paracetamol (acetaminophen) versus diclofenac plus misoprostol found significantly better outcomes on the WOMAC scale with diclofenac plus misoprostol.[48]

Glucosamine One new RCT[53] found that glucosamine versus ibuprofen significantly improved symptoms at 90 days.

Intra-articular injection One new RCT[73] compared four treatments: hyaluronate injection plus placebo tablets, placebo injection plus NSAIDs, hyaluronate injection plus NSAIDs, and placebo injection plus placebo tablets. The statistical significance of differences between treatments was not tested.

REFERENCES

1. Petersson IF. Occurrence of osteoarthritis of the peripheral joints in European populations. *Ann Rheum Dis* 1996;55:659–661.
2. Felson DT. Epidemiology of hip and knee osteoarthritis. *Epidemiol Rev* 1988;10:1–28.
3. Gaffney KL. Intra-articular triamcinolone hexacetonide in knee osteoarthritis: factors influencing the clinical response. *Ann Rheum Dis* 1995;54:379–381.
4. Pavelka JKS. Glycosaminoglycan polysulfuric acid (GAGPS) in osteoarthritis of the knee. *Osteoarthritis Cartilage* 1995;3:15–23.
5. Insall JN, Dorr LD, Scott RD, et al. Rationale of the Knee Society clinical rating system. *Clin Orthopaed Rel Res* 1988;248:13–14.
6. Bellamy N, Buchanan WW, Goldsmith CH, et al. Validation study of WOMAC: a health status instrument for measuring clinically important patient relevant outcomes to antirheumatic drug therapy in patients with osteoarthritis of the hip or knee. *J Rheumatol* 1988;15:1833–1840.
7. Dougados M, Devogelaer JP, Annefeldt M, et al. Recommendations for the registration of drugs used in the treatment of osteoarthritis. *Ann Rheum Dis* 1996;55:552–557.
8. Altman R, Brandt K, Hochberg M, et al. Design and conduct of clinical trials in patients with osteoarthritis: recommendations from a task force of the Osteoarthritis Research Society. *Osteoarthritis Cartilage* 1996;4:217–243.

9. Lequesne M, Mery C, Samson M, et al. Indexes of severity for osteoarthritis of the hip and knee. *Scandinavian J Rheumatol* 1987;65(Suppl):85–89.
10. Van Baar ME, Assendelft WJ, Dekker J, et al. Effectiveness of exercise therapy in patients with osteoarthritis of the hip or knee: a systematic review of randomized clinical trials. *Arthritis Rheum* 1999;42:1361–1369. Search date 1997; primary sources Medline, Embase, Cinahl, and Cochrane Controlled Trials Register.
11. Puett DW, Griffin MR. Published trials of non-medicinal and non-invasive therapies for hip and knee osteoarthritis. *Ann Intern Med* 1994;121:133–140. Search date 1993; primary source Medline.
12. La Mantia K, Marks R. The efficacy of aerobic exercises for treating osteoarthritis of the knee. *NZ J Physiother* 1995;23:23–30. Search date 1994; primary sources Medline, Cinahl, hand searched references, and personal contacts.
13. Tugwell P. Philadelphia panel evidence-based clinical practice guidelines on selected rehabilitation interventions for knee pain. *Phys Ther* 2001;81:1675–1700. Search date: July 2000; primary sources: Medline, Embase, Current Contents, Cinahl, the Cochrane Controlled Trials Register, the Cochrane Field of Rehabilitation and Related Therapies, the Cochrane Musculoskeletal Group Register, the Physiotherapy Evidence Database (PEDro), reference lists of included studies, and contact with experts in the field.
14. Baker K, McAlindon TE. Exercise for knee osteoarthritis. *Curr Opin Rheumatol* 2000;12:456–463.
15. Messier SP, Loeser RF, Mitchell MN, et al. Exercise and weight loss in obese older adults with knee osteoarthritis: a preliminary study. *J Am Geriat Soc* 2000;48:1062–1072.
16. Petrella RJ, Bartha C. Home based exercise therapy for older patients with knee osteoarthritis: a randomized clinical trial. *J Rheumatol* 2000;27:2215–2221.
17. Hopman-Rock M, Westhoff MH. The effects of a health educational and exercise program for older adults with osteoarthritis for the hip or knee. *J Rheumatol* 2000;27:1947–1954.
18. Fransen M, Crosbie J, Edmonds J. Physical therapy is effective for patients with osteoarthritis of the knee: a randomized controlled clinical trial. *J Rheumatol* 2001;28:156–164.
19. Van Baar ME, Dekker J, Oostendorp RA, et al. Effectiveness of exercise in patients with osteoarthritis of hip or knee: nine months' follow up. *Ann Rheum Dis* 2001;60:1123–1130.
20. Penninx BWJH, Messier SP, Rejeski WJ, et al. Physical exercise and the prevention of disability in activities of daily living in older persons with osteoarthritis. *Arch Inter Med* 2001;161:2309–2316.
21. Halbert J, Crotty M, Weller D, et al. Primary care-based physical activity programs: Effectiveness in sedentary older patients with osteoarthritis symptoms. *Arthritis Rheum Arthritis Care Res* 2001;45:228–234.
22. Superio-Cabuslay E, Ward MM, Lorig KR. Patient education interventions in osteoarthritis and rheumatoid arthritis: a meta-analytic comparison with non-steroidal anti-inflammatory drug treatment. *Arthritis Care Res* 1996;9:292–301. Search date 1993; primary sources Medline and hand searched references.
23. Mazzuca SA, Brandt KD, Katz BP, et al. Effects of self-care education on the health status of inner-city patients with osteoarthritis of the knee. *Arthritis Rheum* 1997;40:1466–1474.
24. Edworthy SM, Devins GM. Improving medication adherence through patient education distinguishing between appropriate and inappropriate utilization. Patient Education Study Group. *J Rheumatol* 1999;26:1793–1801.
25. Maurer BT, Stern AG, Kinossian B, et al. Osteoarthritis of the knee: isokinetic quadriceps exercise versus and educational intervention. *Arch Phys Med Rehab* 1999;80:1293–1299.
26. Barlow JH, Turner AP, Wright CC. A randomized controlled study of the Arthritis Self-Management Programme in the UK. *Health Educ Res* 2000;15:665–680.
27. Kirkley A, Websterbogaert S, Litchfield R, et al. The effect of bracing on varus gonarthrosis. *J Bone Joint Surg* 1999;81:539–548.
28. Cushnaghan J, McCarthy C, Dieppe P. Taping the patella medially: a new treatment for osteoarthritis of the knee-joint. *BMJ* 1994;308:753–755.
29. Toda Y, Segal N, Kato A, et al. Effect of a novel insole on the subtalar joint of patients with medial compartment osteoarthritis of the knee. *J Rheumatol* 2001;28:2705–2710.
30. Maillefert JF, Hudry C, Baron G, et al. Laterally elevated wedged insoles in the treatment of medial knee osteoarthritis: a prospective randomized controlled study. *Osteoarthritis Cartilage* 2001;9:738–745.
31. Towheed T, Shea B, Wells G, et al. Analgesia and non-aspirin, non-steroidal anti-inflammatory drugs for osteoarthritis of the hip. In: The Cochrane Library, Issue 1, 2002. Oxford: Update Software. Search date 1994; primary sources Medline, Cochrane Library, and Controlled Clinical Trials Register.
32. Towheed TE, Hochberg MC. A systematic review of randomized controlled trials of pharmacological therapy in osteoarthritis of the knee, with an emphasis on trial methodology. *Semin Arthritis Rheum* 1997;26:755–770. Search date 1994; primary sources Medline and hand searched references.
33. Amadio P, Cummings DM. Evaluation of acetaminophen in the management of osteoarthritis of the knee. *Curr Ther Res Clin Exp* 1983;34:59–66.
34. Hawton K, Ware C, Mistry H, et al. Why patients choose paracetamol for self poisoning and their knowledge of its dangers. *BMJ* 1995;310:164.
35. Watson MC, Brookes ST, Kirwan JR, et al. Osteoarthritis: the comparative efficacy of non-aspirin non-steroidal anti-inflammatory drugs for the management of osteoarthritis of the knee. In: The Cochrane Library, Issue 1, 2002. Oxford: Update Software. Search date 1996, primary sources Medline, BIDS, and Embase.
36. Huskisson EC, Berry H, Gishen P, et al. Effects of anti-inflammatory drugs on the progression of osteoarthritis of the knee. *J Rheumatol* 1995;22;1941–1946.
37. Langman MJ. Non-steroidal anti-inflammatory drugs and peptic ulcer. *Hepatogastroenterology* 1992;39(Suppl 1):37–39.
38. Garcia Rodriguez LA, Williams R, Derby LE, et al. Acute liver injury associated with non-steroidal anti-inflammatory drugs and the role of risk factors. *Arch Intern Med* 1994;154:311–316.
39. Henry D, Lim LL, Garcia Rodriguez LA, et al. Variability in risk of gastrointestinal complications with individual non-steroidal anti-inflammatory drugs: results of a collaborative meta-analysis. *BMJ* 1996;312:1563–1566.
40. Brandt KD. Nonsurgical management of osteoarthritis, with an emphasis on nonpharmacologic measures. *Arch Fam Med* 1995;4:1057–1064.

41. Wollheim FA. Current pharmacological treatment of osteoarthritis. *Drugs* 1996;52(Suppl 3):27–38.
42. Williams HJ, Ward JR, Egger MJ, et al. Comparison of naproxen and acetaminophen in a 2-year study of treatment of osteoarthritis of the knee. *Arthritis Rheum* 1993;36:1196–1206.
43. Bradley JD, Brandt KD, Katz BP, et al. Comparison of an anti-inflammatory dose of ibuprofen, an analgesic dose of ibuprofen, and acetaminophen in the treatment of patients with osteoarthritis of the knee. *N Engl J Med* 1991;325:87–91.
44. Solomon I, Abrams G. Orudis in the management of osteoarthritis of the knee. *S Afr Med J* 1974;48:1526–1529.
45. Muller F, Gosling J, Erdman G. A comparison of tolemetin with aspirin in the treatment of osteoarthritis of the knee. *S Afr Med J* 1977;51:794–796.
46. Valtonen EJ. Clinical comparison of fenbufen and aspirin in osteoarthritis. *Scand J Rheumatol* 1979;27:3–7.
47. March L, Irwig L, Schwarz J, et al. N of 1 trials comparing non-steroidal anti-inflammatory drug with paracetamol in osteoarthritis. *BMJ* 1993;309:1041–1046.
48. Pincus T, Koch GG, Sokka T, et al. A randomized, double-blind, crossover clinical trial of diclofenac plus misoprostol versus acetaminophen in patients with osteoarthritis of the hip or knee. *Arthritis Rheumatism* 2001;44:1587–1598.
49. McAlindon TE, LaValley MP, Gulin JP, et al. Glucosamine and chondroitin for treatment of osteoarthritis: a systematic quality assessment and meta-analysis. *JAMA* 2000;283:1469–1475. Search date 1999; primary sources Medline, Cochrane Controlled Trials Register, and hand searches of review articles, manuscripts, and supplements from rheumatology and osteoarthritis journals, and contact with content experts, study authors, and manufacturers of glucosamine or chondroitin.
50. Towheed TE, Anastassiades TP, Shea B, et al. Glucosamine therapy for treating osteoarthritis. In: The Cochrane Library, Issue 1, 2002. Oxford: Update Software. Search date 1999; primary sources Medline, Embase, Current Contents, Cochrane Controlled Trials Register, and hand searches of reference lists and personal contact with experts.
51. Rindone JP, Hiller D, Collacott E, et al. Randomized, controlled trial of glucosamine for treating osteoarthritis of the knee. *West J Med* 2000;172:91–94.
52. Thie NMR, Prasad NG, Major PW. Evaluation of glucosamine sulfate compared to ibuprofen for the treatment of temporomandibular joint osteoarthritis: A randomized double blind controlled 3 month clinical trial. *J Rheumatol* 2001;28:1347–1355.
53. Reginster JY, Deroisy R, Rovati LC, et al. Long-term effects of glucosamine sulphate on osteoarthritis progression: a randomised, placebo-controlled clinical trial. *Lancet* 2001;357:251–256.
54. Mazieres B, Combe B, Phan Van A, et al. Chondroitin sulfate in osteoarthritis of the knee: a prospective, double blind, placebo controlled multicenter clinical study. *J Rheumatol* 2001;28:173–181.
55. Morreale P, Manopulo R, Galati M, et al. Comparison of the antiinflammatory efficacy of chondroitin sulfate and diclofenac sodium in patients with knee osteoarthritis. *J Rheumatol* 1996;23:1385–1391.
56. Leffler CT, Philippi AF, Leffler SG, et al. Glucosamine, chondroitin, and manganese ascorbate for degenerative joint disease of the knee or low back: a randomized, double-blind, placebo-controlled pilot study. *Mil Med* 1999;164:85–91.
57. Das A Jr, Hammad TA. Efficacy of a combination of FCHG49 glucosamine hydrochloride, TRH122 low molecular weight sodium chondroitin sulfate and manganese ascorbate in the management of knee osteoarthritis. *Osteoarthritis Cartilage* 2000;8:343–350.
58. Moore RA, Tramer MR, Carroll D, et al. Quantitative systematic review of topically applied non-steroidal anti-inflammatory drugs. *BMJ* 1998;316:333–338. Search date 1996; primary sources Embase, Medline, Oxford Pain Relief Database, hand searched references, and librarians and medical directors of 12 pharmaceutical companies asked for reports of their products.
59. Roth SH. A controlled clinical investigation of 3% diclofenac/2.5% sodium hyaluronate topical gel in the treatment of uncontrolled pain in chronic oral NSAID users with osteoarthritis. *Int J Tissue React* 1995;17:129–132.
60. Grace D, Rogers J, Skeith K, et al. Topical diclofenac versus placebo: a double blind, randomized clinical trial in patients with osteoarthritis of the knee. *J Rheumatol* 1999;26:2659–2663.
61. Ottillinger B, Michel BA, Pavelka K, et al. Efficacy and safety of eltenac gel in the treatment of knee osteoarthritis. *Osteoarthritis Cartilage* 2001;9:273–280.
62. Dickson DJ. A double-blind evaluation of topical piroxicam gel with oral ibuprofen in osteoarthritis of the knee. *Curr Ther Res Clin Exp* 1991;49:199–207.
63. Zacher J, Burger K, Färber L, et al. Topical diclofenac versus oral ibuprofen: a double blind, randomized clinical trial to demonstrate efficacy and tolerability in patients with activated osteoarthritis of the finger joints (Heberden and/or Bouchard arthritis). *Aktuelle Rheumatologie* 2001;26:7–14.
64. Zhang WY, Po ALW. The effectiveness of topically applied capsaicin: a meta-analysis. *Eur J Clin Pharmacol* 1994;46:517–522. Search date 1994; primary sources BIDS, Medline, and hand searches of relevant published references.
65. Deal CL, Schnitzer TJ, Lipstein E, et al. Treatment of arthritis with topical capsaicin: a double-blind trial. *Clin Ther* 1991;13:383–395.
66. Weidenhielm L, Olsson E, Brostrom LA, et al. Improvement in gait one year after surgery for knee osteoarthrosis: a comparison between high tibial osteotomy and prosthetic replacement in a prospective randomized study. *Scand J Rehabil Med* 1993;25:25–31.
67. Kirwan JRR. Intra-articular therapy in osteoarthritis. *Baillieres Clin Rheumatol* 1997;11:769–794. Search date not stated; RCTs cited from 1958 to 1996; primary sources Medline and Embase.
68. Ravaud P, Moulinier L, Giraudeau B, et al. Effects of joint lavage and steroid injection in patients with osteoarthritis of the knee: results of a multicenter, randomized, controlled trial. *Arthritis Rheum* 1999;42:475–482.
69. Altman RD. Intra-articular sodium hyaluronate in osteoarthritis of the knee. *Semin Arthrit Rheum* 2000;30:11–18.
70. Hochberg MC. Role of intra-articular hyaluronic acid preparations in medical management of osteoarthritis of the knee. *Semin Arthrit Rheum* 2000;30:2–10.

71. Formiguera SSE. Intra-articular hyaluronic acid in the treatment osteoarthritis of the knee: a short term study. *Eur J Rheumatol Inflamm* 1995;15:33–38.
72. Petrella RJ, DiSilvestro MD, Hildebrand C. Effects of hyaluronate sodium on pain and physical functioning in osteoarthritis of the knee — a randomized, double-blind, placebo-controlled clinical trial. *Arch Inter Med* 2002;162:292–298
73. Huskisson EC, Donnelly S. Hyaluronic acid in the treatment of osteoarthritis of the knee. *Rheumatology* 1999;38:602–607.
74. Altman R, Moskowitz R. Intraarticular sodium hyaluronate in the treatment of patients with osteoarthritis of the knee: a randomized clinical trial. *J Rheum* 1998;25:2203–2212.
75. Pietogrande V, Turchetto L. Hyaluronic-acid versus methylprednisolone intra-articularly injected for treatment of osteoarthritis of the knee. *Curr Ther Res Clin Exp* 1991;50:691–701.
76. Dougados M, Nguyen M, Listrat V, et al. High molecular weight sodium hyaluronate (hyalectin) in osteoarthritis of the knee: a 1 year placebo-controlled trial. *Osteoarthritis Cartilage* 1993;1:97–103.
77. McIlwain HSJ. Intra-articular orgotein in osteoarthritis of the knee: a placebo-controlled efficacy, safety, and dosage comparison. *Am J Med* 1989;87:295–300.
78. Likar RS. Intraarticular morphine analgesia in chronic pain patients with osteoarthritis. *Anesth Analg* 1997;84:1313–1317.
79. Stukenborg-Colsman C, Wirth CJ, Lazovic D, et al. High tibial osteotomy versus unicompartmental joint replacement in unicompartmental knee joint osteoarthritis: 7–10-year follow-up prospective randomised study. *Knee* 2001;8:187–194.
80. Broughton NS, Newman JH, Baily RAJ. Unicompartmental replacement and high tibial osteotomy for osteoarthritis of the knee. A comparative study after 5–10 years follow up. *J Bone Joint Surg* 1986;68-B:447–452.
81. McCleane G. The analgesic efficacy of topical capsaicin is enhanced by glyceryl trinitrate in painful osteoarthritis: a randomized, double blind, placebo controlled study. *Eur J Pain* 2000;4:355–360.
82. Faulkner A, Kennedy LG, Baxter K, et al. Effectiveness of hip prostheses in primary total hip replacement: a critical review of evidence and an economic model. *Health Technol Assess* 1998;2:1–33. Search date 1995; primary sources Embase, Medline, and in-house database on epidemiology and service provision for total hip replacement.
83. Murray DW, Britton AR, Bulstrode CJ. Thromboprophylaxis and death after total hip replacement. *J Bone Joint Surg Br* 1996;78:863–870. Search date 1995; primary source Medline.
84. Seagroatt V, Soon Tan H, Goldacre M, et al. Elective total hip replacement: incidence, emergency readmission rate, and postoperative mortality. *BMJ* 1991;303:1431–1435.
85. Chang RW, Pellissier JM, Hazen GB. A cost-effectiveness analysis of total hip arthroplasty for osteoarthritis of the hip. *JAMA* 1996;275:858–865.
86. Malchau H, Herberts P, Ahnfelt L. Prognosis of total hip replacement in Sweden. Follow up of 92 675 operations performed 1978–1990. *Acta Orthop Scand* 1993;64:497–506.
87. Robinson AH, Palmer CR, Villar RN. Is revision as good as primary hip replacement? A comparison of quality of life. *J Bone Joint Surg Br* 1999;81:42–45.
88. Espehaug B, Havelin LI, Engesaeter LB, et al. Patient-related risk-factors for early revision of total hip replacements. A population register-based case-control study of 674 revised hips. *Acta Orthop Scand* 1997;68:207–215.
89. Johnsson R, Franzen H, Nilsson LT. Combined survivorship and multivariate analyses of revisions in 799 hip prostheses. A 10 to 20-year review of mechanical loosening. *J Bone Joint Surg Br* 1994;76:439–443.
90. Lie SA, Engesaeter LB, Havelin LI, et al. Mortality after total hip replacement: 0–10-year follow-up of 39 543 patients in the Norwegian Arthroplasty Register. *Acta Orthop Scand* 2000;71:19–27.
91. Fitzpatrick R, Shortall E, Sculpher M, et al. Primary total hip replacement surgery: a systematic review of outcomes and modelling of cost-effectiveness associated with different prostheses. *Health Technol Assess* 1998;2:1–64. Search date 1995; primary sources Medline and hand searched references.
92. Towheed TE, Hochberg MC. Health-related quality of life after total hip replacement. *Semin Arthrit Rheum* 1996;26:483–491.
93. Soderman P, Malchau H, Herberts P. Outcome after total hip arthroplasty. Part I. General health evaluation in relation to definition of failure in the Swedish National Total Hip Arthroplasty register. *Acta Orthop Scand* 2000;71:354–359.
94. Callahan CM, Drake BG, Heck DA, et al. Patient outcomes following tricompartmental total knee replacement: a meta-analysis. *JAMA* 1994;271:1349–1357. Search date 1992; primary sources Medlars and hand searched references.
95. Callahan CM, Drake BG, Heck DA, et al. Patient outcomes following unicompartmental or bicompartmental knee arthroplasty: a meta-analysis. *J Arthroplasty* 1995;10:141–150. Search date 1992; primary sources Medlars and hand searched references.
96. Newman JH, Ackroyd CE, Shah NA. Unicompartmental or total knee replacement? Five-year results of a prospective, randomised trial of 102 osteoarthritic knees with unicompartmental arthritis. *J Bone Joint Surg* 1998;80:862–865.
97. Kiebzak GM, Vain PA, Gregory AM, et al. SF-36 general health status survey to determine patient satisfaction at short-term follow up after total hip and knee arthroplasty. *J South Orthop Assoc* 1997;6:169–172.
98. Hawker G, Wright J, Coyte P, et al. Health related quality of life after knee replacement. *J Bone Joint Surg* 1998;80:163–173.
99. Freund DA. *Assessing and improving outcomes: total knee replacement: patient outcomes research team (PORT): final report.* Maryland: Agency for Health Care Policy and Research, 1997.
100. Bohm P, Holy T, Pietsch-Breitfeld B, et al. Mortality after total knee arthroplasty in patients with osteoarthrosis and rheumatoid arthritis. *Arch Orthop Trauma Surg* 2000;120:75–78.
101. Kim YH. The incidence of deep vein thrombosis after cementless and cemented knee replacement. *J Bone Joint Surg Br* 1990;72:779–783.
102. Fauno P, Suomalained O, Rehnberg V, et al. Prophylaxis for the prevention of venous thromboembolism after total knee arthroplasty. *J Bone Joint Surg Am* 1994;76:1814–1818.
103. Knutson K, Lewold S, Robertsson O, et al. The Swedish knee arthroplasty register. A nation-wide study of 30 003 knees. *Acta Orthop Scand* 1994;65:375–386.
104. Robertsson O, Borgquist L, Knutson K, et al. Use of unicompartmental instead of tricompartmental

prostheses for unicompartmental arthrosis of the knee is a cost-effective alternative. 15 437 primary tricompartmental prostheses were compared with 10 624 primary medical or lateral unicompartmental prostheses. *Acta Orthop Scand* 1999;70:170–175.
105. Norton EC, Garfinkel SA, McQuay LJ, et al. The effect of hospital volume on the in-hospital complication rate in knee replacement patients. *Health Serv Res* 1998;33:1191–1210.
106. Young NL, Cheah D, Waddell JP, et al. Patient characteristics that affect the outcome of total hip arthroplasty: a review. *Can J Surg* 1998;41:188–195. Search date not stated; primary sources Medline and hand search of references.
107. Chan CL, Villar RN. Obesity and quality of life after primary hip arthroplasty. *J Bone Joint Surg Br* 1996;78:78–81.
108. Espehaug B, Havelin LI, Engesaeter LB, et al. Patient satisfaction and function after primary and revision total hip replacement. *Clin Orthop* 1998;351:135–148.
109. Garellick G, Malchau H, Herberts P, et al. Life expectancy and cost utility after total hip replacement. *Clin Orthop* 1998;346:141–151.
110. Brander VA, Malhotra S, Jet J, et al. Outcome of hip and knee arthroplasty in persons aged 80 years and older. *Clin Orthop* 1997;345:67–78.
111. Levy RN, Levy CM, Snyder J, et al. Outcome and long-term results following total hip replacement in elderly patients. *Clin Orthop* 1995;316:25–30.
112. Boettcher WG. Total hip arthroplasties in the elderly — morbidity, mortality, and cost-effectiveness. *Clin Orthop* 1992;274:30–34.
113. Jones AC, Voaklander DC, Johnston DWC, et al. The effect of age on pain, function, and quality of life after total hip and knee arthroplasty. *Archi Int Med* 2001;161:454–460.
114. Braeken AM, Lochaas-Gerlach JA, et al. Determinants of 6–12 month postoperative functional status and pain after elective total hip replacement. *Int J Qual Health Care* 1997;9:413–418.
115. Swedish website: http://www.sos.se/sosmenye.htm. (last accessed 27/09/2002).
116. National Institutes of Health. Total hip replacement. NIH consensus development panel on total hip replacement. *JAMA* 1995;273:1950–1956.
117. Naylor CD, Williams JI. Primary hip and knee replacement surgery: Ontario criteria for case selection and surgical priority. *Qual Health Care* 1996;5:20–30.
118. Hardorn DC, Holmes AC. The New Zealand priority criteria project. *BMJ* 1997;31:131–134.
119. Donnell ST, Neyret P, Dejour H, et al. The effect of age on the quality of life after knee replacement. *Knee* 1998;5:125–112.
120. De Leeuw JM, Villar RN. Obesity and quality of life after primary total knee replacement. *Knee* 1998;5:119–23.
121. Lubitz R, Dittus R, Robinson R, et al. Effects of severe obesity on health status 2 years after knee replacement. *J Gen Intern Med* 1996;11:145.
122. Winiarsky R, Barth P, Lotke P. Total knee arthroplasty in morbidly obese patients. *J Bone Joint Surg Am* 1998;80;1770–1774.
123. Ettinger WH Jr, Burns R, Messier SP, et al. A randomized trial comparing aerobic exercise and resistance exercise with a health education program in older adults with knee osteoarthritis. The fitness arthritis and seniors trial (FAST). *JAMA* 1997;277:25–31.
124. Laskin RS. Total knee replacement in patients older than 85 years. *Clin Orthop* 1999;367:43–49.

David Scott
Professor

Claire Smith
Research Fellow

King's College London Medical School
London
UK

Stefan Lohmander
Professor
Department of Orthopaedics
Lund University
Lund
Sweden

Jiri Chard
Research Associate
MRC Health Services Research Collaboration
University of Bristol
Bristol
UK

Competing interests: None declared.

TABLE 1 **Effect sizes (95% CI) of exercise in osteoarthritis of the knee and hip: results of the three best RCTs identified in a systematic review (see text, p 1216).[10] Effectiveness of exercise therapy in patients with osteoarthritis of the hip or knee: a systematice review of randomised controlled trials. Van Baar et al. Arthritis and Rheumatism. Copyright © 1999 John Wiley & Sons. Reprinted by permission of Wiley-Liss, Inc, a subsidiary of John Wiley & Sons, Inc.**

RCT	Pain	Observed disability
1	0.31 (0.28 to 0.34)	0.31 (0.28 to 0.34)
2	0.47 (0.44 to 0.50)	0.89 (0.85 to 0.93)
3	0.58 (0.54 to 0.62)	0.28 (0.24 to 0.32)

TABLE 2 **Estimated relative risk of gastrointestinal adverse effects with the use of individual NSAIDs (pooled data from 12 studies) (see text, p 1221).[39]**

Drug	Pooled RR	95% CI for pooled RR
Ibuprofen (low dose)*	1.0	ND
Fenoprofen	1.6	1.0 to 2.5
Aspirin	1.6	1.3 to 2.0
Diclofenac	1.8	1.4 to 2.3
Sulindac	2.1	1.6 to 2.7
Diflunisal	2.2	1.2 to 4.1
Naproxen	2.2	1.7 to 2.9
Indomethacin	2.4	1.9 to 3.1
Tometin	3.0	1.8 to 4.9
Piroxicam	3.8	2.7 to 5.2
Ketoprofen	4.2	2.7 to 6.4
Azapropazone	9.2	4.0 to 21.0

*Comparative data used low dose ibuprofen as the reference control for calculating the relative risk of other drugs. ND, no data; NSAIDs, non-steroidal anti-inflammatory drugs.

TABLE 3 **Summary of New Zealand priority criteria for joint replacement (see text, p 1231).[118]**

Severity is scored out of a possible 100 on the basis of:

Pain: severity 0–20; duration 0–20
Function: walking difficulty 0–10; other 0–10
Joint damage: pain on passive movement 0–10; other/x ray 0–10
Other: other joints 0–10; work, care giving, independence 0–10

Plantar heel pain (including plantar fasciitis)

Search date May 2002

Fay Crawford

QUESTIONS

INTERVENTIONS

See glossary, p 1248

Key Messages

- **Casted orthoses (custom made insoles)** We found no RCTs on the effects of orthoses versus placebo or no treatment. One systematic review and three RCTs found limited and conflicting evidence about the effects of orthoses versus corticosteroids, corticosteroids plus local anaesthesia, or other physical supports.
- **Corticosteroid injection alone or plus local anaesthetic injection versus placebo (medium to long term)** One small RCT found no significant reduction in pain with hydrocortisone injection versus placebo assessed 6–18 months after the injection. One systematic review identified no RCTs comparing corticosteroid plus local anaesthetic injection versus placebo. Observational studies have found a high rate of plantar fascia rupture and other complications associated with corticosteroid injections, which may lead to chronic disability in some people.
- **Corticosteroid injection alone or plus local anaesthetic injection versus placebo (short term)** We found no RCTs of corticosteroid injections alone versus placebo that assessed short term outcomes. One systematic review identified no RCTs comparing corticosteroid injection plus local anaesthesia versus placebo.

- **Corticosteroid injection plus local anaesthesia versus local anaesthetic injection alone (medium to long term)** One RCT found no significant difference in pain with prednisolone plus lidocaine injection versus lidocaine alone after 3 or 6 months. Observational studies have found a high rate of plantar fascia rupture and other complications associated with corticosteroid injections, which may lead to chronic disability in some people.
- **Corticosteroid injection plus local anaesthesia versus local anaesthetic injection alone (short term)** One RCT found a significant reduction in pain with prednisolone plus lidocaine injection versus lidocaine alone after 1 month.
- **Corticosteroid injection plus local anaesthesia versus pads (medium to long term)** One RCT found no significant difference in pain with triamcinolone plus lidocaine injection versus heel pad after 24 weeks. One RCT found no significant difference in pain with dexamethasone plus local anaesthetic injection plus oral etodolac versus heel pads plus paracetemol at 3 months. Observational studies have found a high rate of plantar fascia rupture and other complications associated with corticosteroid injections, which may lead to chronic disability in some people.
- **Corticosteroid injection plus local anaesthesia versus pads (short term)** One RCT found a significant improvement in pain with triamcinolone plus lidocaine injection versus heel pad after 1 month. One small RCT found no significant difference in pain with triamcinolone plus lidocaine injection versus heel pad at 1, 2, or 12 weeks. One RCT found no significant difference in pain with dexamethasone plus local anaesthetic injection plus oral etodolac versus heel pads plus paracetemol at 3 months.
- **Extracorporeal shock wave therapy** One small RCT found limited evidence that extracorporeal shock wave therapy versus sham treatment improved pain at 6 weeks. Two RCTs found a non-significant reduction in pain with extracorporeal shock wave therapy versus sham treatment after 2 months and 12 weeks, respectively. One RCT found limited evidence of a significant improvement in pain with high dose versus low dose extracorporeal shock wave therapy.
- **Heel pads and heel cups** We found no RCTs on the effects of heel pads and heel cups versus placebo or no treatment. One systematic review and subsequent RCTs found limited and conflicting evidence on the effects of heel pads and heel cups versus other treatment modalities.
- **Lasers** One systematic review of one small RCT found no significant difference with laser treatment versus placebo.
- **Local anaesthetic injection** We found no RCTs on the effects of local anaesthesia versus placebo or no treatment. One RCT found a significant reduction in pain with prednisolone plus lidocaine injection versus lidocaine alone after 1 month; the difference was not significant after 3 or 6 months.
- **Night splints** One RCT found no significant difference with a night splint versus no splint in pain after 3 months.
- **Surgery** One systematic review found no RCTs of surgery for heel pain.
- **Ultrasound** One systematic review of one small RCT found no significant difference in pain with ultrasound versus sham ultrasound.

DEFINITION Plantar heel pain is soreness or tenderness of the heel. It often radiates from the central part of the heel pad or the medial tubercle of the calcaneum, but may extend along the plantar fascia into the medial longitudinal arch of the foot. Severity may range from an irritation at the origin of the plantar fascia, which is noticeable on rising after rest, to an incapacitating pain. This review excludes clinically evident underlying disorders, for example, infection, calcaneal fracture, and calcaneal nerve entrapment, which can be distinguished by their characteristic history and signs. (A calcaneal fracture may present after trauma, whereas calcaneal nerve entrapment gives rise to shooting pains and feelings of "pins and needles" on the medial aspect of the heel.)

INCIDENCE/ PREVALENCE The incidence and prevalence of plantar heel pain is uncertain. Plantar heel pain primarily affects those in mid to late life.[1]

AETIOLOGY/ RISK FACTORS Unknown.

PROGNOSIS One systematic review (search date 1997) found that almost all of the included trials reported an improvement in discomfort regardless of the intervention received (including placebo), suggesting that the condition is at least partially self limiting.[1] A telephone survey of 100 people treated conservatively (average follow up 47 months) found that 82 people had resolution of symptoms, 15 had continued symptoms but no limitations of activity or work, and three had continued symptoms that limited activity or changed work status.[2] Thirty one people said that they would have seriously considered surgical treatment at the time medical attention was sought. The three people still with limitation had bilateral symptoms but no other clear risk factors.

AIMS To reduce pain and immobility, with minimal adverse effects.

OUTCOMES Pain reduction (often measured using visual analogue scales); walking distance.

METHODS *Clinical Evidence* update search and appraisal May 2002.

QUESTION **What are the effects of treatments for plantar heel pain?**

OPTION **CORTICOSTEROID INJECTIONS**

We found no RCTs of corticosteroid injection versus placebo that assessed short term outcomes. One small RCT found no significant reduction in pain with hydrocortisone injection versus placebo assessed 6–18 months after the injection. The RCT may have lacked power to exclude clinically important effects. Observational studies have found a high rate of plantar fascia rupture and other complications associated with corticosteroid injections, which may lead to chronic disability in some people.

Benefits: We found one systematic review (search date 1997).[1] **Versus placebo or no treatment:** The review found one small RCT (19 people with 22 heels with recalcitrant heel pain but not arthritis) of corticosteroid (hydrocortisone acetate 25 mg) injection versus saline injection.[1] Both groups were also given a sponge heel pad (see glossary, p 1248). It found no significant difference with hydrocortisone versus placebo in the number of heels with no relief of pain assessed between 6–18 months after the injection (3/13 [23%] heels *v* 4/9 [44%] heels; RR 0.52, 95% CI 0.15 to 1.79).

Versus orthoses: The review found no RCTs. **Versus pads:** The review found no RCTs. **Versus pain medication alone:** The review found no RCTs. **Corticosteroid injection plus local anaesthesia:** See benefits of corticosteroid injections plus local anaesthesia, p 1242.

Harms: Corticosteroid injections can be painful. In one RCT, participants' heels were injected through the medial aspect of the heel pad. Half of the 106 participants were given a tibial nerve block to reduce discomfort during the injection, but there was no significant difference in pain at time of injection between those who received the nerve block and those who did not.[3] Complications observed from local corticosteroid injection throughout the body include infection, subcutaneous fat atrophy, skin pigmentation changes, fascial rupture, peripheral nerve injury, and muscle damage among others.[4] Observational studies have reported rupture of the plantar fascia in people receiving corticosteroid injections.[5,6] One study reported a 10% incidence of rupture among 122 injected heels.[6] A second study examined 37 people with a presumptive diagnosis of plantar fascia rupture, all of whom had had plantar fasciitis and all of whom had previously been treated with corticosteroid injection.[5] History revealed that in 13/37 (33%) people the rupture had been a sudden event, whereas in the remainder it appeared to be gradual. The study reported the majority had resolution of symptoms, but this often took 6–12 months to occur.[5] The original heel pain may be relieved after rupture, but arch and midfoot strain, lateral plantar nerve dysfunction, stress fracture, deformity, and swelling may result from plantar fascia rupture, and may persist.

Comment: The evidence from observational studies makes it difficult to define the clinical importance of rupture of the plantar fascia, and may be compromised by confounding factors.

OPTION CORTICOSTEROID INJECTIONS PLUS LOCAL ANAESTHESIA

One systematic review identified no RCTs comparing corticosteroid injections plus local anaesthesia versus placebo. One RCT found a significant improvement in pain with triamcinolone plus lidocaine injection versus heel pad after 1 month; the difference was not significant after 24 weeks. One small RCT found no significant difference in pain with triamcinolone plus lidocaine injection versus heel pad at 1, 2, or 12 weeks. One RCT found no significant difference in pain with dexamethasone plus local anaesthetic injection plus oral etodolac versus heel pads plus paracetemol at 3 months, or with dexamethasone plus local anaesthetic injection versus heel pad plus custom made orthoses. One RCT found a significant reduction in pain with prednisolone plus lidocaine injection versus lidocaine alone after 1 month; the difference was not significant after 3 or 6 months. One RCT found a significant reduction in pain with triamcinolone plus lidocaine injection versus triamcinolone plus lidocaine injection and pad after 1 month; the difference was not significant after 24 weeks. Observational studies have found a high rate of plantar fascia rupture and other complications associated with corticosteroid injections, which may lead to chronic disability in some people.

Benefits: We found one systematic review (search date 1997), which included RCTs of injected corticosteroid plus local anaesthetic versus various other treatments.[1] **Versus placebo or no treatment:** The review found no RCTs. **Versus heel pads:** See glossary, p 1248. The review found two RCTs.[1] The first RCT (80 people) in the review included people with pain on the plantar aspect of the heel but excluded people on anti-inflammatory medication, people who had a corticosteroid injection during the past 6 months, people with rheumatoid arthritis, and people with pain that radiated along the plantar fascia more distally. It compared three arms: a heel pad alone versus an injection alone (triamcinolone hexacteonide 20 mg plus 2% lidocaine [lignocaine]) versus injection plus heel pad. Analysis was not by intention to treat, and four people (5%) were lost to follow up. The RCT found that after 1 month the greatest improvement in pain was in people who received the injection alone (22 people), with the least improvement in people who had the pad alone (26 people) (100 mm visual analogue scale: injection alone *v* pad alone, WMD –45 mm, 95% CI –59 to –31). At 24 weeks, there was greater pain reduction with the injection alone versus the pad alone, but the difference was not significant (85% *v* 75%). The second small RCT (17 people) in the review compared triamcinolone (20 mg) plus 2% lidocaine injection versus a prefabricated silicone type heel pad. Although more people improved after treatment with the heel pad (66% *v* 33% at 12 wks), the difference in pain was not significant at 1, 2, or 12 weeks. **Corticosteroid injection plus local anaesthesia plus non-steroidal anti-inflammatory drugs versus heel pad:** The review found no RCTs.[1] We found one subsequent RCT that included 103 people with plantar heel tenderness, a history of pain upon rising in the morning (first step pain), and no history of trauma in the previous 3 months.[7] Analysis was not by intention to treat and 18 people were lost to follow up. It compared three arms: non-steroidal anti-inflammatory drugs plus three corticosteroid plus local anaesthetic injections into the heel (anti-inflammatory, 35 people) versus heel pads plus paracetamol (acetaminophen) as required (accommodative, 33 people) versus a heel pad prior to fitting of custom made orthoses (see glossary, p 1248) (mechanical, 35 people). The anti-inflammatory regimen consisted of etodolac (600 mg) and 0.5 mL dexamethasone sodium phosphate 4 mg/mL plus 1 mL of 0.5% bupivacaine hydrochloride without adrenaline (epinephrine). If there was no response then 0.2 mL of dexamethasone acetate 16 mg/mL injection was added cumulatively to the second (2 wk) and third (4 wk) injections. The RCT found slightly greater pain relief among people treated with the anti-inflammatory regimen versus the accommodative regimen at 3 months, but the difference was not significant (10 cm visual analogue scale: WMD –1.2 cm, 95% CI –2.8 to +0.4). **Corticosteroid injection plus local anaesthesia plus non-steroidal anti-inflammatory drugs versus heel pad plus orthoses:** The review found no RCTs.[1] We found one subsequent RCT comparing an anti-inflammatory regimen versus a mechanical regimen.[7] At 3 months, it found that both the anti-inflammatory regimen and heel pads plus orthoses (mechanical regimen) improved pain, but the difference was not significant (10 cm visual analogue scale: WMD –1 cm, 95% CI –2.5

to +0.5). **Versus orthoses alone:** The review found no RCTs.[1] **Versus local anaesthetic alone:** The review found no RCTs.[1] We found one subsequent RCT (106 heels).[3] It compared a single injection of 1 mL prednisolone acetate 25 mg/mL plus 1 mL lidocaine hydrochloride 2% versus 2 mL lidocaine hydrochloride 2% alone. It found a small benefit in pain with the combined injection at 1 month, the clinical relevance of which is considered small (10 cm visual analogue scale: WMD –0.8 cm, 95% CI –1.5 to –0.2), but no significant difference in pain thereafter (3 months: WMD 0.1 cm, 95% CI –1.2 to +1.3; and 6 months: 0.5 cm, 95% CI –0.8 to +1.7). **Versus corticosteroid alone:** The review found no RCTs. **Versus corticosteroid plus local anaesthetic plus pad:** The review found one RCT (80 people), which found significantly worse results at 1 month after treatment with the heel pad plus injection (triamcinolone hexacetonide 20 mg plus 2% lidocaine) versus injection alone (100 mm visual analogue scale: WMD 1.6 cm, 95% CI 0.07 to 3.12).[1] However, at 24 weeks, people treated with pad plus injection versus injection alone had less pain, but this was not significant (94% *v* 85%). **Corticosteroid plus local anaesthetic plus pad versus pad alone:** The review found one RCT (80 people).[1] It found a significantly better response with injection (triamcinolone hexacetonide 20 mg plus 2% lidocaine) plus pad versus pad alone at 4 weeks (10 cm visual analogue scale: WMD –2.9 cm, 95% CI –4.4 to –1.4) and 12 weeks, but not at 24 weeks (10 cm visual analogue scale: WMD –1.07 cm, 95% CI –2.55 to +0.41; AR for pain reduction 94% *v* 75%).

Harms: No RCTs reported on harms. See harms of corticosteroid injections, p 1241.

Comment: All trials were small. Heterogeneity of interventions prevented data pooling. A survey of UK rheumatologists found that corticosteroid injections are the most common treatment of heel pain and are used by 98% of UK rheumatologists (Crawford F, personal communication, 2000), confirming the results of similar surveys.[4] We found no placebo controlled RCTs of corticosteroid injections plus local anaesthesia, and no evidence of medium to long term efficacy in RCTs comparing this treatment with other options. We found evidence from two observational studies of high rates of moderately severe harms from this treatment (see harms of corticosteroid injections, p 1241). This is also consistent with evidence about harms of corticosteroid injections in other areas.[4] These harms are particularly relevant because the evidence of benefit is poor, and spontaneous resolution of symptoms is common. The RCTs have many flaws (lack of intention to treat analysis, high withdrawal rates, and lack of placebo control). Limitations of the available evidence make the use of corticosteroid injections in heel pain difficult to categorise in terms of benefits and harms.

OPTION CASTED ORTHOSES (CUSTOM MADE INSOLES)

We found no RCTs on the effects of orthoses versus placebo or no treatment. One systematic review and three RCTs found limited and conflicting evidence about the effects of orthoses versus corticosteroids, corticosteroids plus local anaesthesia, or other physical supports.

Benefits: We found one systematic review (search date 1997).[1] **Versus placebo or no treatment:** The review found no RCTs. **Orthoses plus heel pad versus steroid plus pain medication:** The review found no RCTs. We found one subsequent RCT, which found no significant difference in pain improvement (see benefits of corticosteroid injections plus local anaesthesia, p 1242).[7] **Orthoses plus heel pad versus heel pads plus pain medication:** The review found no RCTs. We found one RCT of a heel pad applied for 4 weeks prior to fitting of a custom made orthosis (see glossary, p 1248) heel pad (28 people) versus a viscoelastic heel pad (see glossary, p 1248) plus paracetamol as required (26 people).[7] It found a significantly better pain reduction with pad plus orthoses versus pad plus paracetamol (10 cm visual analogue scale: WMD −2.2 cm, 95% CI −3.8 to −0.5). **Orthoses plus stretching versus heel pad plus stretching:** The review found no RCTs. We found one subsequent RCT (236 people, 5 groups) in people with maximal tenderness over the medial calcaneal tuberosity for which they had received no previous treatment.[8] People with systemic disease, sciatica, or local nerve entrapment were excluded. The RCT compared customised orthoses plus stretching exercises versus prefabricated shoe inserts made from three different materials (silicone, felt, and rubber) plus stretching exercises (achilles and plantar fascial stretching for 10 min twice daily). It found significantly less pain at 8 weeks in people who were assigned to prefabricated inserts (results combined) versus orthoses ($P = 0.007$). **Orthoses plus stretching versus stretching alone:** The review found no RCTs. We found one subsequent RCT of custom made orthoses plus stretching exercises versus stretching exercises alone.[8] It found no significant difference in pain improvement at 8 weeks (100 mm visual analogue scale: WMD −3.2 mm, 95% CI −17.4 to +11.0).

Harms: No RCTs reported on harms.

Comment: Subgroup analysis in the RCT comparing orthoses plus stretching versus heel pads plus stretching found that, among people who stood for more than 8 hours daily, a greater reduction in pain was achieved with stretching alone than with customised insoles.[8] It found no significant difference in people who stood for less than 8 hours a day. This hypothesis requires testing as the primary outcome in an RCT. Only half of the participants in this subgroup analysis responded to the pain questionnaire. We found one RCT comparing heel pads versus custom made orthoses;[9] however, there was a significant difference in weight between the groups at baseline (19 lb) and weight was associated with severity of heel pain. This makes the results difficult to interpret.

OPTION HEEL PADS AND HEEL CUPS

We found no RCTs on the effects of heel pads and heel cups versus placebo or no treatment. One systematic review and subsequent RCTs found limited and conflicting evidence on the effects of heel pads and heel cups versus other treatment modalities.

Benefits: We found one systematic review (search date 1997),[1] which included RCTs of heel pads (see glossary, p 1248) and heel cups (see glossary, p 1248) versus various treatments. **Versus placebo**

or no treatment: The review found no RCTs.[1] **Versus corticosteroid:** The review found no RCTs. **Versus corticosteroid injections plus local anaesthesia:** The review found two RCTs and we found one subsequent RCT, neither of which found evidence of a significant long term benefit (see benefits of corticosteroids plus pain medication versus heel pads, p 1242). **Versus corticosteroid plus pain medication:** We found one RCT, which found no significant difference in pain improvement between corticosteroid injection plus non-steroidal anti-inflammatory drugs versus pads plus paracetamol (see benefits of corticosteroids plus local anaesthesia, p 1242).[7] **Versus custom made orthoses:** The review found one RCT[1] and we found one subsequent RCT.[7] They found conflicting evidence on improvement in pain (see benefits of custom made orthoses, p 1244). **Heel pad plus corticosteroid plus local anaesthetic versus corticosteroid plus local anaesthetic:** The review found one RCT.[1] It found a short term benefit with the corticosteroid plus local anaesthetic injection alone (see benefits of corticosteroids plus local anaesthesia, p 1242).

Harms: None of the RCTs reported harms.

Comment: Heel cups and heel pads can be made from several different materials, but rubber, viscoelastic, and silicone can be bought as prefabricated shoe inserts. Podiatrists or orthotists sometimes use felt and foam to construct heel pads. We found one additional RCT of heel pads versus orthoses but the results were difficult to interpret. See comment on custom made orthoses, p 1244.[9]

OPTION LOCAL ANAESTHETIC INJECTION

We found no RCTs on the effects of local anaesthesia versus placebo or no treatment. One RCT found a significant reduction in pain with prednisolone plus lidocaine injection versus lidocaine alone after 1 month; the difference was not significant after 3 or 6 months.

Benefits: We found one systematic review (search date 1997).[1] **Versus placebo or no treatment:** The review found no RCTs.[1] **Versus corticosteroids plus local anaesthetic:** The review found no RCTs. We found one subsequent RCT (see benefits of corticosteroids plus local anaesthesia, p 1242), which found a short term benefit with lidocaine plus prednisolone injection versus lidocaine injection alone.[3] **Corticosteroid injection plus local anaesthesia:** See benefits of corticosteroid injections plus local anaesthesia, p 1242.

Harms: None of the trials reported on harms.

Comment: Adrenaline is not recommended in local anaesthetics for procedures that involve the appendages because of the risk of ischaemic necrosis.[10]

OPTION EXTRACORPOREAL SHOCK WAVE THERAPY

One small RCT found limited evidence extracorporeal shock wave therapy versus sham treatment improved pain at 6 weeks. Two RCTs found a non-significant reduction in pain with extracorporeal shock wave therapy versus sham treatment at 2 months and 12 weeks, respectively. One RCT found limited evidence of a significant improvement in pain with high dose versus low dose extracorporeal shock wave therapy.

Benefits: **Versus placebo:** We found one systematic review (search date 1997)[1] and two subsequent RCTs of extracorporal shock wave therapy (ESWT) (see glossary, p 1248).[11,12] The review found one single blind RCT (36 people with recalcitrant heel pain), which compared 1000 impulses (0.06 mJ/mm^2) versus placebo (sham ESWT) three times at weekly intervals. It found that pain on manual pressure and pain free walking ability were significantly improved at 6 weeks ($P < 0.005$). Six people withdrew from the trial, and analysis was not intention to treat. The first subsequent RCT (260 people with recalcitrant heel pain) compared ESWT for a total of 1500 pulses at 18 kV power versus sham treatment.[11] It found that more people reported improved pain after 12 weeks (improvement of ≥50% and ≥4 cm on a 10 cm visual analogue scale), but the difference did not reach significance (71/119 [60%] with ESWT *v* 56/116 [48%] with sham treatment; RR 1.24, 95% CI 0.97 to 1.57; results recalculated by *Clinical Evidence*). It also found slightly improved self assessed activity with ESWT, but it was not possible to calculate significance. The second small subsequent RCT (37 people with recalcitrant heel pain) found a non-significant reduction in pain associated with ESWT at 1500 pulses at 3 Hz versus sham treatment at 2 months (100 mm visual analogue scale: WMD –15 mm, 95% CI –45 to +15).[12] **Different doses:** The review identified one non-blinded RCT[1] and we found one additional RCT.[13] The RCT in the review (119 people) compared 1000 impulses versus 10 impulses of 0.08 mJ/mm^2 in people with recalcitrant heel pain. All treatments were given three times at weekly intervals. It found greater improvements in pressure pain between weeks 0–12 with the higher dose (100 mm visual analogue scale: WMD –47 mm, 95% CI –54 to –40). A supplementary report of outcomes from 78/119 (66%) of the original people in the RCT found significantly less pain on manual pressure with high dose versus low dose ESWT after 5 years (100 mm visual analogue scale: WMD –20 mm, 95% CI –28 to –11).[14] The additional RCT (50 people) compared 3 x 500 impulses of ESWT versus 3 x 100 impulses (both at intensity 0.08 mJ/mm^2) in people with recalcitrant heel pain.[13] It found no significant difference in pain on pressure at 6 weeks (10 cm visual analogue scale: WMD –0.4 cm, 95% CI –2.0 to +1.2) or at 12 weeks (WMD –1.4 cm, 95% CI –3.0 to +0.2). It also found no significant difference in walking pain at 6 weeks (WMD –0.8 cm, 95% CI –2.4 to +0.7) or at 12 weeks (WMD –0.9 cm, 95% CI –2.5 to +0.7). Self reported walking pain at 12 months suggested a marginal long term benefit from higher doses of ESWT (10 cm visual analogue scale: WMD –2.0 cm, 95% CI –3.7 to –0.2).

Harms: ESWT without local anaesthetic can be painful.

Comment: All trial participants had recalcitrant heel pain. Availability of ESWT is limited. Pain associated with ESWT and differences in procedures mean the single blinding in the first placebo controlled RCT was probably not maintained.[1] The large RCT reported a large increase in the number of people not using pain medications with ESWT (measured as any use between weeks 10 and 12; 70% with ESWT *v* 35% with sham treatment).[11]

OPTION SURGERY

One systematic review found no RCTs of surgery for heel pain.

Benefits: We found one systematic review (search date 1997),[1] which identified no RCTs of surgery for heel pain.

Harms: We found no RCTs.

Comment: The systematic review identified many observational studies of surgery for chronically painful heels.[1] One of the largest observational studies (76 people) compared postoperative complication rates after endoscopic fasciotomy versus traditional plantar fasciotomy.[15] It found that serious complications (recurrent pain, neuritis, infection) were less common in people treated with endoscopic fasciotomy versus traditional surgery (serious incidents per procedure: 11/66 [17%] with endoscopic fasciotomy *v* 9/26 [35%] with traditional surgery).

OPTION LASERS

One systematic review of one small RCT found no significant difference with laser treatment versus placebo.

Benefits: One systematic review (search date 1997) included one small RCT (32 people) of laser treatment versus placebo (treatment with a disabled laser) in people with pain of at least 1 months' duration, tenderness to pressure at the origin of the plantar fascia, on the mid-anterior inferior border of the calcaneus, and sharp shooting and/or localised inferior foot pain made worse with activity or on rising in the morning.[1] It found no evidence of a significant effect.

Harms: The RCT reported that 96% of people had no adverse effects, and the rest (4%) reported a "mild sensation" during or after treatment.[1]

Comment: None.

OPTION ULTRASOUND

One systematic review of one small RCT found no significant difference in pain with ultrasound versus sham ultrasound.

Benefits: One systematic review (search date 1997) included one small RCT in 19 people (7 with bilateral heel pain) of eight treatments of true ultrasound versus the same number of applications of sham ultrasound.[1] Inclusion criteria were pain radiating from the medial tubercle of the calcaneum in response to both pressure and weight bearing first thing in the morning. It found no significant difference in pain with ultrasound versus sham ultrasound (10 cm visual analogue scale; WMD 0.1 cm, 95% CI −1.8 to +2.1).[1]

Harms: The RCT did not assess harms.[1]

Comment: None.

OPTION **NIGHT SPLINTS**

One RCT found no significant difference in pain with a night splint versus no splint after 3 months.

Benefits: One systematic review (search date 1997) found no good quality trials.[1] We found two subsequent RCTs.[16,17] The first RCT included 116 people with recalcitrant heel pain.[16] All participants received ankle dorsiflexion exercises and piroxicam (20 mg/day for 30 days), with or without a night splint that dorsiflexed the ankle joint by 5°. In people with bilateral complaints, only the most symptomatic foot was studied. The night splint was worn for 3 months. It found no evidence of an effect on pain with night splinting versus no splinting (RR 1.0, 95% CI 0.8 to 1.3). The second RCT (255 people) compared custom made orthoses (see glossary, p 1248) versus night splints. The results were difficult to interpret because there was a large difference in withdrawals between the groups (26% with night splints *v* 7% with orthoses), and we were not able to report intention to treat analysis.[17]

Harms: The RCTs did not assess harms.[16,17]

Comment: The first RCT only studied the most symptomatic foot because of potential inconvenience and poor compliance from wearing two night splints simultaneously.[16]

GLOSSARY

Custom made orthoses Made from polyurethene or similar material to a negative cast of a person's foot.

Extracorporeal shock wave therapy (ESWT) Shock waves are pulsed acoustic waves that dissipate mechanical energy at the interface of two substances with different acoustic impedance.

Heel cups Prefabricated rubber heel cups (firmer than viscoelastic heel pads) that extend up the sides of the heel and enclose the fibro fatty heel pad.

Heel pads Prefabricated viscoelastic heel pads made of malleable material.

Substantive changes

Extracorporeal shock wave therapy Longer term follow up RCT;[14] conclusions unchanged.

REFERENCES

1. Crawford F, Atkins D, Edwards J. Interventions for treating plantar heel pain (Cochrane Review). In: The Cochrane Library, Issue 2, 2002. Oxford: Update Software. Search date 1997; primary sources Medline, Embase, the Cochrane Library, handsearches of *The Foot*, *The Chiropodist* (later *The Journal of British Podiatric Medicine*), and *The British Journal of Podiatric Medicine*. In addition, investigators in the field were contacted to identify unpublished data or research in progress. Non English language reports were excluded from the review.
2. Wolgin M, Cook C, Graham C, et al. Conservative treatment of plantar heel pain: long term follow up. *Foot Ankle Int* 1994;15:97–102.
3. Crawford F, Atkins D, Young P, et al. Steroid injection for heel pain: evidence of short term effectiveness. A randomised controlled trial. *Rheumatology* 1999;38:974–977.

4. Fadale PD, Wiggins MD. Corticosteroid injections: their use and abuse. *J Am Acad Orthop Surg* 1994;2:133–140.
5. Sellman JR. Plantar fascial rupture associated with corticosteroid injection. *Foot Ankle Int* 1994;15:376–381.
6. Acevedo JI, Beskin JL. Complications of plantar fascial rupture associated with steroid injection. *Foot Ankle Int* 1998;19:91–97.
7. Lynch DM, Goforth WP, Martin JE, et al. Conservative treatment of plantar fasciitis. A prospective study. *J Am Podiatr Assoc* 1998;88:375–380.
8. Pfeffer G, Bacchetti P, Deland J, et al. Comparison of custom and prefabricated orthoses in the initial treatment of proximal plantar fasciitis. *Foot Ankle Int* 1999;20:214–221.
9. Turlik M, Donatelli T, Veremis M. A comparison of shoe inserts in relieving mechanical heel pain. *Foot* 1999;9:84–87.
10. McCauley WA, Gerace RV, Scilley C. Treatment of accidental digital injection of epinephrine. *Ann Emerg Med* 1991;6:665–668.
11. Odgen J, Alvarex R, Levitt R, et al. Shock wave therapy for chronic proximal plantar fasciitis. *Clin Orthop Related Res* 2001;1:47–59.
12. Speed CA, Nichols DW, Burnett SP, et al. Extracorporeal shock wave therapy (ESWT) in plantar fasciitis. A pilot double blind randomised placebo controlled study [abstract]. *Rheumatology* 2000;39(suppl 123):230.
13. Krischeck O, Rompe JD, Herbsthrofer B, et al. Symptomatic low-energy shockwave therapy in heel pain and radiologically detected plantar heel spur [in German]. *Z Orthop Ihre Grenzgeb* 1998;136:169–174.
14. Rompe JD, Schoellner C, Nafe B. Evaluation of low-energy extracorporeal shock wave application for treatment of chronic plantar fasciitis. *J Bone Joint Surg Br* 2002; 84-A:335–341.
15. Kinley S, Frascone S, Calderone D, et al. Endoscopic plantar fasciotomy versus traditional heel spur surgery: a prospective study. *J Foot Ankle Surg* 1993;32:595–603.
16. Probe RA, Baca M, Adams R, et al. Night splint treatment for plantar fasciitis. *Clin Orthop* 1999;368:191–195.
17. Martin J, Hosch J, Goforth W, et al. Mechanical treatment of plantar fasciitis. A prospective study. *J Am Pod Med Assoc* 2001;91:55–62.

Fay Crawford
Senior Research Fellow
Dental Health Services Research Unit
Dundee
UK

Competing interests: None declared.

Rheumatoid arthritis

Search date November 2001

Paul Emery, Wednesday Foster, and Maria Suarez-Almazor

QUESTIONS

INTERVENTIONS

Key Messages

- **Antimalarials** One systematic review has found that hydroxychloroquine versus placebo for 6–12 months significantly reduces disease activity and joint inflammation. Two RCTs found no evidence of improved functional status or reduced radiological progression. One systematic review found no consistent differences between antimalarials and other disease modifying antirheumatic drugs. Another systematic review of observational studies and RCTs has found that over 2 years people are less likely to continue treatment with antimalarials than with methotrexate but more likely than with parenteral gold or sulfasalazine. One RCT found significantly fewer people were still taking hydoxychloroquine versus pencillamine at 5 years, but found similar numbers versus parenteral gold and auranofin.
- **Auranofin (less effective than other DMARDs)** One systematic review has found that auranofin (oral gold) versus placebo reduces disease activity and joint inflammation, but found no evidence on radiological progression or long term functional status. Limited evidence from RCTs suggests that auranofin is less effective than DMARDs.

Clin Evid 2002;8:1250–1270.

- **Azathioprine** One systematic review has found that azathioprine versus placebo reduces disease activity in the short term. We found no evidence on radiological progression or long term functional status. A high level of toxicity limits its usefulness.
- **Ciclosporin** One systematic review has found that ciclosporin versus methotrexate for a minimum of 4 months significantly reduces disease activity and joint inflammation, improves functional status, and may decrease the rate of radiological progression. A very high frequency of toxicity limits its usefulness.
- **Cyclophosphamide** One systematic review has found that cyclophosphamide versus placebo significantly reduces disease activity and joint inflammation at 6 months. It may also reduce the rate of radiological progression, but the evidence we found was limited. We found no evidence of its effect on long term functional status. Severe toxicity limits its usefulness.
- **Early intervention with disease modifying antirheumatic drugs (DMARDs)** RCTs found limited evidence that early treatment with DMARDs versus delayed treatment or placebo may reduce pain, joint inflammation, disease activity, and disability. We found insufficient evidence about the effects of early DMARD treatment on radiological progression.
- **Leflunomide (long term safety unclear)** One systematic review has found that leflunomide versus placebo reduces disease activity and joint inflammation, improves functional status and health related quality of life, and decreases radiological progression. We found no good evidence on long term adverse effects.
- **Longer term low dose oral corticosteroids** One systematic review has found that low dose oral corticosteroids versus placebo for at least 3 months significantly reduces pain, joint inflammation, and functional status. One RCT found that prednisolone versus placebo for 2 years may reduce radiological progression. However, long term use is associated with considerable adverse effects.
- **Methotrexate** One systematic review has found that methotrexate versus placebo for 12–18 weeks significantly reduces joint inflammation and radiological progression, and improves functional status. One systematic review has found no consistent differences between methotrexate and other DMARDs, but another systematic review of observational studies and RCTs has found that people are more likely to continue treatment with methotrexate than with other DMARDs.
- **Minocycline** RCTs have found that minocycline versus placebo improves control of disease activity. We found no RCTs comparing minocycline versus other DMARDs.
- **Parenteral gold** One systematic review has found that parenteral gold versus placebo significantly reduces disease activity and joint inflammation, and slows radiological progression over 6 months. We found no evidence on long term functional status. One systematic review and a subsequent RCT found increased withdrawals because of toxicity.
- **Penicillamine** One systematic review has found that penicillamine versus placebo reduces disease activity and joint inflammation. We found no evidence of its effect on radiological progression or long term functional status. Common and potentially serious adverse effects limit its usefulness.
- **Prolonged treatment with DMARDs** One RCT found a significant increase in flare among people in remission who discontinued DMARDs

- **Short term low dose oral corticosteroids** One systematic review has found that low dose oral corticosteroids versus placebo for several weeks significantly reduces disease activity and joint inflammation.
- **Sulfasalazine** Systematic reviews have found that sulfasalazine versus placebo for 6 months significantly reduces disease activity and joint inflammation. We found inadequate evidence on radiological progression and functional status. One systematic review found no consistent differences between sulfasalazine and other DMARDs, but another systematic review of observational studies and RCTs found that over 5 years people were less likely to continue sulfasalazine than methotrexate.
- **Treatment with several DMARDs combined** One systematic review and subsequent RCTs have found that combining certain DMARDs is more effective than using individual drugs alone. However, the balance between benefit and harm varies between combinations.
- **Tumour necrosis factor antagonists (long term safety unclear)** RCTs have found that tumour necrosis factor antibodies (etanercept and infliximab) versus placebo significantly improve symptoms, and reduce long term disease activity and joint inflammation. Short term toxicity is relatively low, but long term safety is less clear. Case reports of reactivation of demyelinating disease and tuberculosis have been published.

DEFINITION Rheumatoid arthritis is a chronic inflammatory disorder. It is characterised by a chronic polyarthritis that primarily affects the peripheral joints and related periarticular tissues. It usually starts as an insidious symmetric polyarthritis, often with non-specific systemic symptoms. Diagnostic criteria include arthritis lasting longer than 6 weeks (although evidence suggests that 12 wks is more specific), positive rheumatoid factor, and radiological damage.[1]

INCIDENCE/ PREVALENCE Prevalence ranges from 0.5–1.5% of the population in industrialised countries.[2,3] Rheumatoid arthritis occurs more frequently in women than men (ratio 2.5 : 1).[2,3] The annual incidence in women was recently estimated at 36/100 000 and in men at 14/100 000.[3]

AETIOLOGY/ RISK FACTORS The evidence suggests that the cause is multifactorial in people with genetic susceptibility.[4]

PROGNOSIS The course of rheumatoid arthritis is variable and unpredictable. Some people experience flares and remissions, and others a progressive course. Over the years, structural damage occurs, leading to articular deformities and functional impairment. About half of people will be unable to work within 10 years.[5] Rheumatoid arthritis shortens life expectancy.[6]

AIMS To relieve symptoms; to improve physical function and slow/arrest progression of structural damage, resulting in improvement in quality of life; to minimise adverse effects of treatment.

OUTCOMES It is now a standard procedure to use composite outcome measures that include subjective and objective measures as well as functional measures. The American College of Rheumatology (ACR) has validated criteria for improvement. ACR20 criteria specify a 20% reduction in swollen and tender joints and 20% improvement in at least three of the following: pain, function, patient and physician global assessments, and acute phase reactants. ACR50 and ACR70 criteria use a 50% and 70% improvement, respectively, in the same parameters. RCTs of many new treatments, such as biological agents, use these aggregate indices as primary end points.[7] However, these are relative improvements and give no indication of the final state of the patient. Consequently, in clinical practice the disease activity score is more commonly used. This uses roughly the same measures of outcome but produces an absolute level of disease activity. A high level of disease activity indicates a need for treatment and low levels indicate a successful outcome approximating to remission. Radiological progression is assessed in many RCTs by reference to standard films. Two scores are commonly used: the Sharp Score, which measures erosion and joint space narrowing separately; and the Larsen score. The former is increasingly used because of its greater sensitivity to change. Most reviews reported results as standardised mean differences, but these have not been included because of difficulties in interpreting clinical relevance. Many small trials found no significant difference between drugs, which may be because no clinically important difference exists or because the trials were too small to detect a real difference. Without power calculations or confidence intervals the two are difficult to distinguish.

METHODS *Clinical Evidence* search and appraisal November 2001.

QUESTION **What are the effects of disease modifying antirheumatic drugs?**

OPTION **METHOTREXATE**

One systematic review has found that methotrexate is more effective than placebo in reducing joint inflammation and radiological progression, and in improving functional status in people with rheumatoid arthritis. One systematic review has found no consistent differences between methotrexate and other disease modifying antirheumatic drugs (DMARDs), but another systematic review of RCTs and observational studies have found that people are more likely to continue treatment with methotrexate than with other DMARDs. One large subsequent RCT found that leflunomide improved outcomes more than methotrexate, but a smaller RCT found no significant difference. One subsequent RCT found no significant difference between parenteral gold and low dose methotrexate.

Benefits: **Versus placebo:** We found one systematic review (search date 1997, 5 RCTs, 161 people) of low dose methotrexate for 12–18 weeks (usually < 20 mg/wk) versus placebo.[8] It found a significant improvement with methotrexate in the number of swollen and tender joints, pain score, physician and patient global assessment, and functional status. There was no significant difference in erythocyte sedimentation rate. We found two subsequent RCTs of methotrexate versus leflunomide versus placebo. **Versus other DMARDs:** We found one systematic review (search dates 1990) of comparative RCTs.[9] It found no consistent difference in effectiveness between methotrexate and other DMARDs. One subsequent RCT (483 people) found that methotrexate was not significantly different from leflunomide over 1 year (see benefits of leflunomide, p 1262).[10,11] Another large subsequent RCT (999 people) found that leflunomide improved outcomes more than did methotrexate (see benefits of leflunomide, p 1262).[12] We found one RCT (141 people from a socially deprived Scottish community) that compared parenteral gold versus low dose methotrexate (median weekly dose 10 mg) over 48 weeks.[13] It found no significant difference in efficacy between the groups.

Harms: One systematic review (search date 1997, 5 RCTs, 161 people) of methotrexate versus placebo found that more people on methotrexate withdrew because of adverse effects (22% *v* 7%).[8] The adverse effects were mainly liver enzyme abnormalities (AR for liver abnormalities: 11% with methotrexate *v* 2.6% with placebo; ARI 9%; RR 4.5, 95% CI 1.6 to 11.0; NNH 11, 95% CI 4 to 65). Other common adverse effects were mucocutaneous, gastrointestinal, or haematological complaints. A systematic review of pancytopenia identified 99 cases, with risk factors being renal failure and coadministration of trimethoprim-sulfamethoxazole (sulphamethoxazole) and salazosulphapyridine. Pulmonary toxicity, hepatic fibrosis, and infections occur occasionally, even at the low dosages usually used in rheumatoid arthritis. Another systematic review (search date 1996) found that concurrent administration of folic acid decreased the risk of gastrointestinal and mucocutaneous adverse effects (AR 51% with folic acid *v* 83% without folic acid; ARR 33%, 95% CI 14% to 51%; NNT 3, 95% CI 2 to 7) with no adverse impact on the efficacy of methotrexate.[14] Although some studies reported an increased risk of tumours with methotrexate, results have not been consistent.[15] One systematic review (search date 1997) of observational studies and RCTs compared withdrawal rates over 60 months.[16] It found that methotrexate was associated with a higher rate of staying on treatment (36%) versus sulfasalazine (sulphasalazine) (22%) and versus parenteral gold (23%). It found the lowest rate of withdrawals because of adverse effects with methotrexate (35%) versus parenteral gold (64%) and versus sulfasalazine (52%). It found no significant difference in withdrawal rates between observational studies and RCTs over 24 months. The subsequent RCT (141 people) of parenteral gold versus low dose methotrexate found that significantly more people withdrew because of adverse effects with gold (31/72 [43%] with parenteral gold *v* 13/69 [19%] with methotrexate; RR 2.3, 95% CI 1.3 to 4.0).[13]

Comment: One systematic review (search date 1991) of observational studies comparing methotrexate versus other DMARDs on radiological progression found a significant benefit from methotrexate only when compared with azathioprine (P = 0.049; CI not provided).[17] It found no significant difference between methotrexate and parenteral gold (results not provided). Systematic reviews included in previous *Clinical Evidence* updates have been removed because they were eclipsed, because they did not directly answer our question, or because they were only available in abstract form.[18–20]

OPTION ANTIMALARIALS

One systematic review has found that hydroxychloroquine versus placebo reduces disease activity and joint inflammation in people with rheumatoid arthritis. Two RCTs found no evidence of a benefit on functional status

and radiological progression. One systematic review found no consistent difference in effectiveness between antimalarials and other disease modifying antirheumatic drugs but another systematic review of observational studies and RCTs has found that over 2 years people were less likely to continue antimalarials than methotrexate but more likely than parenteral gold or sulfasalazine. One RCT found significantly fewer people still taking hydoxychloroquine at 5 years versus pencillamine but similar numbers to parenteral gold and auranofin.

Benefits: **Versus placebo:** We found one systematic review (search date 1997, 4 RCTs of hydroxychloroquine given for 6–12 months, 592 people).[21] It reported a significant improvement in the number of swollen and tender joints, pain score, physician and patient global assessment, and erythrocyte sedimentation rate. One RCT (119 people) assessed functional status and found no significant difference. **Versus other disease modifying antirheumatic drugs (DMARDs):** We found one systematic review (search date 1990).[9] It found no significant difference between antimalarials and other DMARDs. Individual RCTs found no consistent advantage for any one drug, although some found better results with penicillamine and sulfasalazine than with antimalarials. **Hydroxychloroquine versus chloroquine:** We found no RCTs that adequately compared chloroquine versus hydroxychloroquine. One older RCT included both drugs but did not report a direct comparison.[22]

Harms: The systematic review (search date 1997, 4 placebo controlled RCTs) found no significant difference in the number of withdrawals because of adverse effects.[21] **Ocular toxicity:** No participants discontinued treatment because of ocular adverse effects, and mild toxicity was reported in only one person.[21] One long term retrospective observational study (97 people) found that more people receiving chloroquine alone versus hydroxychloroquine developed retinopathy (6/31 [19.4%] *v* 0/66 [0%]).[23] We found no good evidence on the optimal frequency for eye examinations; expert opinion ranges from every 6 months to 2 years. **Non-ocular adverse effects:** One RCT found that the most common non-ocular adverse effects were gastrointestinal disturbances, occurring in about 25% of people.[24] Skin reactions and renal abnormalities occasionally occur. Mild neurological abnormalities include non-specific symptoms such as vertigo and blurred vision. Cardiomyopathy and severe neurological disease are extremely rare. **Withdrawals:** One systematic review (search date 1997) of RCTs and observational studies found that over 2 years people with rheumatoid arthritis were more likely to continue on methotrexate than on antimalarials, but were more likely to continue on antimalarials than on parenteral gold or sulfasalazine.[16] Most people discontinued treatment because of lack of efficacy. One 5 year RCT (541 people) compared hydroxychloroquine versus penicillamine versus parenteral gold versus auranofin.[25] It found that at 5 years significantly more people continued to take pencillamine (53%) than hydroxychloroquine (30%), but similar numbers to parenteral gold (34%) and auranofin (31%).

Comment: Older RCTs of chloroquine versus placebo (not included in the systematic review because of weak methods) found a beneficial effect.

OPTION SULFASALAZINE

Systematic reviews have found that sulfasalazine is more effective than placebo in reducing disease activity and joint inflammation. We found inadequate evidence on radiological progression and functional status. One systematic review found no consistent difference in effectiveness between sulfasalazine and other disease modifying antirheumatic drugs but another systematic review of observational studies and RCTs found that over 5 years people were less likely to continue sulfasalazine than methotrexate.

Benefits: **Versus placebo:** We found two systematic reviews[26,27] and one subsequent RCT.[11] The first review (search date 1997, 6 RCTs, 252 people) of sulfasalazine given for 6 months found improvement in the number of tender and swollen joints, pain score, and erythrocyte sedimentation rate.[26] Only two RCTs (155 people) included global assessments, and they found no significant effect. None evaluated functional status. The second review (search date 1998, 8 RCTs, 903 people) of sulfasalazine versus placebo found better results with sulfasalazine on all outcome measures (decrease in number of swollen joints: 51% in the sulfasalazine group *v* 26% in the placebo group; $P < 0.0001$; CI not provided).[27] The subsequent RCT found that sulfasalazine (133 people) versus placebo (92 people) significantly improved patient and physician global assessment ($P < 0.001$).[11] **Versus other disease modifying antirheumatic drugs (DMARDs):** We found one systematic review (search date 1998, 2 RCTs, 120 people)[27] and three additional RCTs of sulfasalazine versus other DMARDs.[11,28,29] The systematic review found no significant difference between sulfasalazine versus hydroxychloroquine in number of swollen joints (improvement 37% with sulfasalazine *v* 28% with hydroxychloroquine; $P = 0.38$; CI not provided) or erythrocyte sedimentation rate (decreased by 43% with sulfasalazine *v* 26% with hydroxychloroquine; $P = 0.10$). One additional RCT (60 people) comparing sulfasalazine versus hydroxychloroquine found that sulfasalazine was significantly better in controlling radiological damage, although progression occurred with both drugs (median erosion scores at wk 48: 16 with hydroxychloroquine *v* 5 with sulfasalazine; $P < 0.02$; CI not provided).[28] However, hydroxychloroquine was given at a lower dose than is usually recommended. One subsequent RCT (358 people over 24 wks) of sulfasalazine versus leflunomide versus placebo found no significant difference between sulfasalazine and leflunomide in tender joint count, swollen joint count, or pain (on a visual analogue scale).[11] One RCT (200 people) comparing sulfasalazine versus penicillamine found significantly better functional status with sulfasalazine after 12 years.[29] However, differences were small, and many people had changed treatment or died during the 12 years.

Harms: Common adverse effects included gastrointestinal discomfort, rash, and liver enzyme abnormalities.[26] More serious haematological or hepatic toxicity was uncommon. Reversible leucopenia or agranulocytosis was occasionally observed. Treatment was discontinued for adverse effects less often than with other DMARDs, with the exception of antimalarials. One systematic review (search date 1997) found that the proportion of people who remained on the same treatment over 5 years was lower with sulfasalazine than with methotrexate, but was the same as with parenteral gold.[16] More people withdrew because of adverse effects on parenteral gold than with sulfasalazine but less withdrew with methotrexate.

Comment: None.

OPTION PARENTERAL GOLD

One systematic review has found that parenteral gold versus placebo reduces disease activity and joint inflammation, and slows radiological progression in people with rheumatoid arthritis. We found no evidence on long term functional status. One systematic review and an RCT both indicate increased withdrawals because of toxicity.

Benefits: **Versus placebo:** We found one systematic review (search date 1997, 4 RCTs, 309 people) of parenteral gold for 6 months versus placebo.[30] It found significant improvement in the number of swollen joints, patient and physician global assessments, and erythrocyte sedimentation rate. Functional status was not evaluated. One overview (9 RCTs and 1 observational study) that included radiological assessment found that parenteral gold decreased radiological progression versus placebo.[31] **Versus other disease modifying antirheumatic drugs (DMARDs):** We found one systematic review (search date 1990)[9] and one subsequent RCT.[13] They found no consistent differences between parenteral gold and other disease modifying antirheumatic drugs (DMARDs). Some RCTs found that parenteral gold was more effective but also more toxic than its oral counterpart, auranofin. A few RCTs comparing parenteral gold versus methotrexate found no difference in short term efficacy. The subsequent RCT (141 people) found no significant difference between parenteral gold versus methotrexate in terms of efficacy.[13]

Harms: The systematic review (search date 1997, 4 RCTs, 309 people) of parenteral gold versus placebo found that more people receiving gold discontinued treatment because of adverse effects, including dermatitis, stomatitis, proteinuria, and haematological changes (withdrawals because of adverse events with parenteral gold 66/223 [30%] *v* with placebo 29/192 [15%]; RR 1.9; 95% CI 1.3 to 2.8).[30] Life threatening reactions such as aplastic anaemia, although rare, necessitate close monitoring. The subsequent RCT found that more people withdrew with parenteral gold because of toxicity (43% with parenteral gold *v* 19% with methotrexate).[13] One systematic review (search date 1997) found that the proportion of people who remained on the same treatment rates over 5 years were lower with sulfasalazine than with methotrexate but the same as with parenteral gold.[16] More people withdrew because of adverse effects on parenteral gold than with sulfasalazine or methotrexate (see harms of methotrexate, p 1254).

Comment: Use of parenteral gold is limited mainly by toxicity but also by the need for parental administration/frequent toxicity monitoring.

OPTION AURANOFIN (ORAL GOLD)

One systematic review has found that auranofin (oral gold) versus placebo reduces disease activity and joint inflammation, but we found no evidence on radiological progression or long term functional status. Limited evidence from RCTs suggests that auranofin is less effective than other disease modifying antirheumatic drugs.

Benefits: **Versus placebo:** We found one systematic review (search dates 1998, 9 RCTs, 1049 people).[32] It found significantly better results with auranofin for tender joints, swollen joint scores, pain (improved by 4.68, scale 0–100), and erythrocyte sedimentation rate (fell by 9.9 mm). **Versus other disease modifying antirheumatic drugs (DMARDs):** One systematic review (search date 1990) concluded that auranofin was significantly less effective than other DMARDs.[9] A meta-analysis from a non-systematic review found auranofin to be less effective than parenteral gold in controlling disease activity.[33] One subsequent RCT (200 people) of auranofin versus sulfasalazine found that people were more than twice as likely to continue with sulfasalazine than with auranofin (people continuing treatment over 5 years: sulfasalazine 31% *v* auranofin 15%; P < 0.05; CI not provided).[34]

Harms: The review found that the most common adverse effects of auranofin were gastrointestinal (OR 3.0, 95% CI 1.4 to 6.5), particularly diarrhoea (OR 3.0, 95% CI 1.3 to 7.1).[32] It found that withdrawals because of haematological or renal effects were rare (1% each). A review of adverse effects found that serious adverse effects, such as those associated with parenteral gold, were rare with auranofin (participants developing serious organ specific toxicity < 0.5%; blood 0.2%, renal 0.1%, lung 0.1%, and hepatic 0.4%).[35]

Comment: The lack of good comparative efficacy results means that auranofin is now rarely used. Systematic reviews included in previous *Clinical Evidence* updates have been removed because they were eclipsed, because they did not directly answer our question, or because they were only available in abstract form.[18–20]

OPTION MINOCYCLINE

Three RCTs have found that minocycline versus placebo improves control of disease activity in people with rheumatoid arthritis. We found no RCTs versus other disease modifying antirheumatic drugs.

Benefits: **Versus placebo:** We found no systematic review. We found three RCTs of minocycline versus placebo.[36–38] They found that minocycline improved control of disease activity. The largest RCT (219 people) compared minocycline versus placebo over 48 weeks.[36] It found that more people had improvement in swollen joints (54% with minocycline *v* 39% with placebo; P < 0.03; CI not provided) and joint tenderness (56% with minocycline *v* 41% with placebo; P < 0.03; CI not provided). The second RCT (80 people) compared minocycline versus placebo over 24 weeks.[37] It found a significant improvement on a multivariate joint analysis of clinical and laboratory outcomes (P < 0.05; CI not provided). The third RCT found that minocycline versus placebo at least halved the proportion of people who did not improve (13% [3/23] with minocycline *v* 55% [11/20] with placebo; ARR 42%, 95% CI 15% to 52%; RR 0.24, 95% CI 0.06 to 0.73; NNT 2, 95% CI 2 to 7).[38] **Versus other disease modifying antirheumatic drugs:** We found no RCTs.

Harms: The largest RCT reported adverse reactions including nausea (AR at 26 wks 50% with minocycline *v* 13% with placebo), dyspepsia, dizziness (AR 40% with minocycline *v* 15% with placebo), and skin pigmentation.[36] Other important but less frequent reactions include hepatitis and drug induced systemic lupus erythematosus.

Comment: The magnitude of the beneficial effects of minocycline seems moderate, and similar to that observed with antimalarials or sulfasalazine. However, we found no direct comparisons with other disease modifying antirheumatic drugs.

OPTION PENICILLAMINE

One systematic review has found that penicillamine versus placebo reduces disease activity and joint inflammation. We found no evidence of its effect on radiological progression or long term functional status. One systematic review has found no consistent difference with penicillamine versus other disease modifying antirheumatic drugs. Common and potentially serious adverse effects limit its usefulness.

Benefits: **Versus placebo:** We found one systematic review (search date 2000, 6 RCTs of penicillamine *v* placebo, 683 people).[39] It found significant improvement in the number of swollen joints and erythrocyte sedimentation rate. Only some of the RCTs evaluated global assessment and functional status, and results were inconclusive. **Versus other disease modifying antirheumatic drugs (DMARDs):** We found one systematic review (search date 1990, 79 RCTs, 6518 people, 22 treatment arms using penicillamine, 583 people completing the trials).[9] It found no consistent differences in effectiveness between penicillamine and other drugs, although some trials found penicillamine to be superior to antimalarials.

Harms: Adverse effects were common and sometimes serious. Reactions included mucocutaneous reactions, altered taste, gastrointestinal reactions, proteinuria, haematological effects, myositis, and autoimmune induced disease. The most frequent adverse effects responsible for D-penicillamine discontinuation were (all doses combined) haematological 6.6%, mucosal/cutaneous 4.9%, impaired/loss of taste 4.7%, renal 4.1%, and gastrointestinal 2.3%. The review reported withdrawals because of adverse reactions with low dose penicillamine (10/87 [11.5%] with penicillamine 125–500 mg/day *v* 3/52 [5.8%] with placebo; RR 2.0, 95% CI 0.6 to 6.9), with medium dose penicillamine (46/220 [20.1%] penicillamine 500–1000 mg/day *v* 17/195 [8.7%] with placebo; RR 2.4, 95% CI 1.4 to 4.1), and with high dose penicillamine (29/118 [24.6%] with penicillamine ≥ 1000 mg/day or more *v* 6/117 [5.1%] with placebo; RR 4.5, 95% CI 2.0 to 10.0).[39]

Comment: The use of penicillamine is limited by the frequency of serious adverse effects. Observational studies found that most people discontinued the drug within the first 2 years of treatment.[40–43] Use of this drug is declining.

OPTION AZATHIOPRINE

One systematic review has found that azathioprine versus placebo reduces disease activity. We found no evidence on radiological progression or long term functional status. We found no evidence that it is superior to other disease modifying antirheumatic drugs. A high level of toxicity limits its usefulness.

Benefits: **Versus placebo:** We found one systematic review (search date 2000, 3 RCTs of azathioprine versus placebo, 81 people).[44] It found a significant short term benefit in the tender joint score with azathioprine versus placebo. No other outcome was reported by all trials. **Versus other drug modifying antirheumatic drugs (DMARDs):** We found two systematic reviews (search dates 1990[9] and 1998[19]). They found limited evidence that azathioprine had less effect than most other DMARDs, but about the same as that of antimalarials.

Harms: The review found that people on azathioprine were significantly more likely to withdraw than were those on placebo (RR 4.6, 95% CI 1.2 to 17.9).[44] The most common adverse reactions were gastrointestinal (5/34 [15%] with azathioprine *v* 0/30 [0%] with placebo; RR 5.3, 95% CI 0.7 to 42), mucocutaneous (4/15 [26%] with azathioprine *v* 1/13 [7.7%] with placebo; RR 3.5, 95% CI 0.4 to 27), and haematological disturbances (3/34 [9%] with azathioprine *v* 0/30 [0%] with placebo; RR 3.5, 95% CI 0.4 to 30). Serious haematological adverse reactions included leucopenia. The review reported that longer term observational studies found that azathioprine was associated with increased risk of liver function abnormalities, infection, and cancer (quantified results not provided).

Comment: Because of its toxicity profile, azathioprine tends to be reserved for people who have not responded to other DMARDs.

OPTION CYCLOPHOSPHAMIDE

One systematic review has found that cyclophosphamide is more effective than placebo in reducing disease activity and joint inflammation in people with rheumatoid arthritis. We found limited evidence that it reduced the rate of radiological progression. We found no evidence of its effect on long term functional status. Severe toxicity limits its usefulness.

Benefits: **Versus placebo:** We found one systematic review (search date 2000, 2 RCTs of cyclophosphamide given for 6 months, 70 people).[45] Meta-analysis found significant reduction in number of tender and swollen joints versus placebo. One RCT reported radiological progression, which appeared to be delayed in the cyclophosphamide group. We found no evidence of its effect on functional status.

Harms: The review reported adverse effects including nausea or vomiting (58%), alopecia (26%), dysuria (26%), and amenorrhoea (comparative figures not reported).[45] Severe reactions include leucopenia, thrombocytopenia, anaemia, and haemorrhagic cystitis. People on cyclophosphamide were at increased risk of infections such as herpes zoster. One long term (20 years) observational study reported that prolonged use has been associated with increased risk of cancer, in particular bladder cancer.[46]

Comment: Because of its cytotoxic effects, cyclophosphamide is usually reserved for people who have not responded to other disease modifying antirheumatic drugs. Another related drug, chlorambucil, has also been used in people with severe rheumatoid arthritis that is unresponsive to other disease modifying antirheumatic drugs.

OPTION CICLOSPORIN

One systematic review has found that, compared with methotrexate, ciclosporin reduces disease activity and joint inflammation, improves functional status, and may decrease the rate of radiological progression. A very high frequency of toxicity limits its usefulness.

Benefits: **Versus placebo:** We found one systematic review (search date 1997, 3 RCTs of ciclosporin [cyclosproin] given for a minimum of 4 months, 318 people).[47] It found significant improvement in the number of tender and swollen joints, and in pain and functional status. It found limited evidence that radiological progression was also reduced.

Harms: The review reported that ciclosporin was associated with adverse effects including gum hyperplasia (9/98 [9.1%] with ciclosporin v 0/98 [0%] with placebo; RR 10, 95% CI 1.3 to 77), paraesthesia (22/159 [13.8%] with ciclosporin v 10/159 [6.3%] with placebo; RR 2.2, 95% CI 1.1 to 4.5), nausea (41/159 [25.8%] with ciclosporin v 22/159 [13.8%] with placebo; RR 1.9, 95% CI 1.2 to 3.0), headache (10/61 [16.4%] with ciclosporin v 3/61 [4.9%] with placebo; RR 3.3, 95% CI 0.96 to 11.5), and tremor (41/133 [30.8%] with ciclosporin v 8/133 [6.0%] with placebo; RR 5.1, 95% CI 2.5 to 10.5). **Renal toxicity:** People may develop nephropathy, which can be irreversible, and hypertension. **Other adverse reactions:** Dyspepsia, hypertrichosis, gingival hyperplasia, and hepatotoxicity. It has been suggested that ciclosporin may be associated with increased risk of infections and tumours.

Comment: Ciclosporin is usually reserved for people with severe disease or those who do not respond to other less toxic disease modifying antirheumatic drugs.

OPTION LEFLUNOMIDE

One systematic review has found that leflunomide versus placebo reduces disease activity and joint inflammation, improves functional status and health related quality of life, and decreases radiological progression. We found no good evidence on long term adverse effects. One large subsequent RCT found that leflunomide improved outcomes more than methotrexate, but a smaller RCT found no significant difference in outcomes.

Benefits: **Versus placebo:** We found one systematic review (search date 1999, 3 RCTs, 1242 people) of leflunomide versus placebo.[48] It found that leflunomide improved quality of life and radiological progression. The first RCT (402 people with active rheumatoid disease) compared leflunomide (5, 10, or 25 mg daily) versus placebo.[49] Leflunomide (10 and 25 mg daily) was significantly more effective than placebo in reducing the number of swollen joints (–20 with leflunomide 10 mg *v* –20 with leflunomide 25 mg *v* –13 with placebo; $P < 0.05$; CI not provided). The second RCT (358 people) compared leflunomide versus placebo versus sulfasalazine.[11] It found a significant reduction at 6 months in the number of swollen joints with leflunomide (44%) versus placebo (21%; $P < 0.0001$; CI not provided). The third RCT (482 people) compared leflunomide versus methotrexate versus placebo over 24 months.[50,51] Because of the high withdrawal rate with placebo, only 12 month placebo results were reported. It found that 20% improvement (ACR20 criteria) was achieved by 52% with leflunomide versus 26% with placebo; ACR50 response criteria were achieved by 34% with leflunomide, 23% with methotrexate, and 8% with placebo ($P \leq 0.001$; CI not provided). Radiological progression was reduced in people receiving leflunomide compared with placebo. It found significant improvements in the quality of life with leflunomide.[51] **Versus other disease modifying antirheumatic drugs:** We found three RCTs.[10,12,50] One RCT found no evidence of significant differences between leflunomide and sulfasalazine in controlling disease activity or radiological progression.[50] A second RCT (483 people) compared methotrexate versus leflunomide versus placebo.[10] It found no significant difference between methotrexate and leflunomide at 1 year (ACR ≥ 20%: 52% with leflunomide *v* 46% with methotrexate; P value and CI not provided) or at 2 years. The third RCT (999 people) comparing methotrexate versus leflunomide found that, at 1 year, leflunomide reduced the numbers of tender joints (reduction 9.7 *v* 8.3), swollen joints (reduction 9.0 *v* 6.8), and erythrocyte sedimentation rate (reduction 28.2 *v* 14.4), and improved patient and physician global assessments ($P < 0.05$ for all outcomes; CI not provided).[12] At 2 years, radiological disease progression was significantly less with methotrexate, but there was no significant difference in tender joint count and patient global assessment (see benefits of methotrexate, p 1253).

Harms: In one of the RCTs (358 people), adverse effects included diarrhoea (17% with leflunomide v 5% with placebo), nausea (10% with leflunomide v 7% with placebo), rash (10% with leflunomide v 4% with placebo), alopecia (8% with leflunomide v 2% with placebo), and liver enzyme abnormalities (2% with leflunomide v 1% with placebo); significance was not reported.[11] In the second RCT adverse events included diarrhoea (34% with leflunomide v 17% with placebo), nausea (21% with leflunomide v 19% with placebo), alopecia (10% with leflunomide v 1% with placebo), and hypertension (11% with leflunomide v 5% with placebo).[10] Adverse reactions were observed more frequently in the study comparing leflunomide with methotrexate, but the rate of serious adverse events was similar for all three groups (methotrexate, leflunomide, and placebo).[10] We found no evidence on long term adverse effects.

Comment: Leflunomide is a new drug, which seems to be as effective as other disease modifying antirheumatic drugs over 12 months but with different adverse events. Longer term observational studies are being performed.

QUESTION What are the effects of combining disease modifying antirheumatic drugs?

One systematic review and subsequent RCTs have found that combining certain disease modifying antirheumatic drugs is more effective than using individual drugs alone. However, the balance between benefits and harm varies between combinations.

Benefits: We found one systematic review (search date 1997, 20 RCTs, 1956 people)[52] and six subsequent RCTs.[53–58] The review concluded that many combinations of disease modifying antirheumatic drugs (DMARDs) may be useful. Nine of the RCTs (1240 people) compared methotrexate plus another DMARD versus methotrexate or the other DMARD alone. A wide range of other DMARDs was included. The review found that methotrexate combined with most other DMARDs was more beneficial than treatment with a single drug.[52] The six subsequent RCTs found that combinations of different agents (antimalarials, sulfasalazine, methotrexate, ciclosporin, and steroids) have a greater beneficial effect than monotherapy.[53–58] Some RCTs included in the systematic review did not find significant differences between combinations of different agents and monotherapy.[52]

Harms: Toxicity of combination treatments depends on the drugs used with monitoring as for the most toxic part of the combination. The adverse effects of combination treatments may be greater than the sum of individual treatments because of potential interactions.

Comment: An additional meta-analysis (search date 1992) pooled data from RCTs comparing single versus combination drug treatments.[59] However, the analysis did not provide adequate data on specific combinations. We found no evidence that any one or more DMARD combination treatments are more effective than any one of the other combination treatments.

QUESTION When should disease modifying antirheumatic drugs be introduced?

We found limited evidence from RCTs suggesting that people with active rheumatoid arthritis should start treatment with disease modifying antirheumatic drugs early in the course of their disease.

Benefits: We found no systematic review. We found four RCTs.[60–63] One RCT (238 people with recently diagnosed rheumatoid arthritis) compared early treatment with disease modifying antirheumatic drugs (DMARDs) (within 1 year of symptom onset) versus delayed treatment.[60] People who received early treatment had significantly better outcomes at 12 months, including improved measures of disability, pain, joint inflammation, and erythrocyte sedimentation rate. It found no difference in radiological progression between early and delayed treatment. A second RCT (137 people) compared early treatment with auranofin versus placebo for 2 years followed by open treatment with DMARDs for a further 3 years.[61] Five year follow up found better outcomes with auranofin. However, that analysis included only 75 of the original 137 people. A third prospective 3 year follow up of an RCT (119 people with early disease) of hydroxychloroquine versus placebo found that a 9 month delay in instituting DMARD treatment had a significant detrimental effect on pain intensity and patient global wellbeing.[62] A fourth RCT (38 people with disease for < 1 year) compared minocycline versus placebo.[63] All participants were given DMARDs at the end of the 3 month study. After 4 years' follow up, eight people who originally received minocycline were in remission versus one in the placebo group (P = 0.02; CI not provided). The need for DMARDs at 4 years was also reduced in the minocycline group.

Harms: There is concern that people left with active inflammation developed irreversible harm.

Comment: About 10% of people with rheumatoid arthritis experience a short illness that resolves and remains largely quiescent. Early treatment may expose them to adverse effects unnecessarily. The early introduction of DMARDs requires an accurate diagnosis of rheumatoid arthritis. We are aware of one systematic review subsequent to our search date, which will be included in the next *Clinical Evidence* update.[64]

QUESTION For how long should disease modifying antirheumatic drugs be given?

Few RCTs have followed people for more than 1 year, and most people discontinue treatment with an individual drug within a few years because of toxicity or lack of effectiveness. One RCT found a significant increase in flare among people in remission who discontinued disease modifying antirheumatic drugs.

Benefits: We found one non-systematic review of 122 studies of disease modifying antirheumatic drugs (DMARDs) (including 57 single or double blinded RCTs, 35 open label RCTs, and 19 observational studies; 16 071 people).[65] It found that 90% of participants had been followed for 1 year or less. Short term clinical trials in people with rheumatoid arthritis found beneficial effects for most DMARDs, but in the longer term effectiveness of these drugs seemed to decline. Observational studies have found that after a few years most people discontinued the prescribed DMARD, either because of toxicity or lack of effectiveness. We found limited evidence suggesting that discontinuing DMARDs, even for people in remission, may result in disease exacerbation or flare. These effects may vary according to the DMARD being discontinued. One RCT (285 people who had been on second line treatment for a median of 5 years and in remission) compared continuation of second line treatment versus placebo.[66] It found that at 52 weeks significantly more people on placebo had a flare (30/137 [22%] with active treatment *v* 53/139 [38%] with placebo; RR 0.57, 95% CI 0.39 to 0.84). Effects may vary according to DMARDs being discontinued, with some evidence methotrexate has a shorter time to relapse.[67]

Harms: Adverse effects requiring discontinuation are common. The RCT of discontinuation versus active treatment found similar withdrawal rates not due to increased disease activity (5/143 [3.5%] with active treatment *v* 4/142 [2.8%] with placebo) and similar rates of adverse events (52/142 [37%] with active treatment *v* 50/143 [34%] with placebo; significance not tested).[66]

Comment: Clinical practice now means that most people with rheumatoid arthritis are taking a DMARD long term, and this will limit the ability to answer this question.

QUESTION What are the effects of low dose oral corticosteroids?

Two systematic reviews have found benefit from both short and longer term treatment (> 3 months) with low dose oral corticosteroids. Short term treatment reduces disease activity and joint inflammation. Longer term treatment may reduce radiological progression while treatment continues. However, long term use is associated with considerable adverse effects.

Benefits: **Versus placebo or non-steroidal anti-inflammatory drugs:** We found two systematic reviews.[68,69] The first review (search date 1997, 10 RCTs, 402 people) compared short term treatment with low dose prednisolone (15 mg/day for several wks) versus placebo or non-steroidal anti-inflammatory drugs.[68] It found that, in the short term, prednisolone had a greater effect than did placebo or non-steroidal anti-inflammatory drugs in controlling disease activity. Prednisolone versus placebo improved pain, grip strength, and joint tenderness (WMD for the number of tender joints –12, 95% CI –18 to –6). The second review (search date 1998, 7 RCTs, 508 people) evaluated longer term treatment with corticosteroids (for at least 3 months).[69] It found that longer term treatment with prednisolone was superior to placebo (WMD for tender joints –0.37, 95% CI –0.59 to –0.14; swollen joints –0.41, 95% CI –0.67 to –0.16; pain –0.43, 95% CI –0.74 to –0.12; and functional status –0.57, 95% CI –0.92 to –0.22). The review also found that prednisolone was comparable to aspirin or chloroquine. One RCT (128 people) included in the review evaluated radiological damage.[70] It found a significant decrease in the rate of progression in people treated with prednisolone 7.5 mg daily versus placebo over 2 years. One follow up study of people in this RCT found that joint destruction resumed after discontinuing prednisolone.[71] **Versus chloroquine:** One systematic review (search date 1998, 1 RCT, 56 people with rheumatoid arthritis diagnosed at age ≥ 60 years) found no significant difference between oral prednisolone and chloroquine in improving disease activity.[69]

Harms: Serious long term adverse effects of corticosteroids include hypertension, diabetes, osteoporosis, infections, gastrointestinal ulcers, obesity, and hirsutism. Observational studies of people with rheumatoid arthritis have suggested that mortality may be increased by long term treatment with steroids.[72] However, many of those studies included people receiving dosages greater than 7.5 mg daily, which are higher than those currently recommended. One systematic review found that bone loss was limited when lower dosages were prescribed.[73]

Comment: The decision to give oral corticosteroids should balance the potential for increased comorbidity, which is affected by individual risk factors, and the potential improvement in disease activity. One RCT found that dose loading for 6 weeks at a higher dose than that usually recommended when initiating treatment with hydroxychloroquine increased the clinical response.[74]

QUESTION What are the effects of biological agents?

OPTION TUMOUR NECROSIS FACTOR ANTIBODIES

Several RCTs have found that tumour necrosis factor antibodies (etanercept and infliximab) versus placebo improve symptoms, and reduce long term disease activity and joint inflammation. Short term toxicity is relatively low, but long term safety less clear. Problems have been identified with reactivation of demyelinating disease and tuberculosis.

Benefits: **Etanercept:** We found two 6 month placebo controlled RCTs.[75,76] One RCT (234 people who had failed to respond to other disease modifying antirheumatic drugs [DMARDs]) compared two doses of etanercept (25 mg and 10 mg both given 2/wk) versus placebo.[75] More people improved by at least 20% (ACR20 criteria) with etanercept 25 mg than with the lower dose or with placebo (59% with high dose etanercept *v* 51% with low dose etanercept *v* 11% with placebo: 10 mg *v* placebo, $P < 0.001$; 25 mg *v* placebo, $P < 0.001$; 25 mg *v* 10 mg, $P = 0.2$; CI not provided). Improvement by at least 50% (ACR50 criteria) was found in 40% of people with high dose etanercept, in 24% with low dose etanercept, and in 5% with placebo (10 mg *v* placebo; $P < 0.001$; 25 mg *v* placebo; $P < 0.001$; 25 mg *v* 10 mg; $P = 0.032$; CI not provided). The RCT also found that etanercept improved functional status (disability index: 25 mg *v* placebo; $P < 0.05$; CI not provided) and quality of life (general health status: 25 mg *v* placebo; $P < 0.05$; CI not provided). The second RCT (89 people with inadequate response to methotrexate) compared etanercept (25 mg/wk) versus placebo.[76] People were allowed to continue methotrexate. More people achieved ACR20 criteria with etanercept than with placebo (71% *v* 27%; $P < 0.001$; CI not provided). A 12 month RCT (632 people with early rheumatoid arthritis) compared methotrexate versus two doses of etanercept (10 and 25 mg, both given 2/wk).[77] It found significantly more people achieved ACR20, ACR50, and ACR70 responses with etanercept 25 mg versus methotrexate at 6 months. By 12 months there was no significant difference (72% *v* 65%; $P = 0.16$; CI not provided). The higher dose etancercept was significantly better than the lower dose in terms of ACR20, ACR50, and ACR70 response at 12 months ($P < 0.03$ for all comparisons; CI not provided). **Infliximab:** We found three placebo controlled RCTs.[78–80] The first RCT (73 people) compared infliximab 1 mg/kg versus infliximab 10 mg/kg versus placebo over 4 weeks.[78] More people experienced at least 20% improvement in the 10 mg group (79%) than in the 1 mg group (44%) or in the placebo group (8%; placebo *v* 1 mg/kg; $P = 0.008$; placebo *v* 10 mg/kg; $P < 0.0001$; CI not provided). A second RCT (101 people) compared 1, 3, or

10 mg/kg infliximab with or without methotrexate versus placebo. It found a greater improvement with 3 or 10 mg/kg infliximab versus placebo (ACR20 improvement: 60% in people taking 3 or 10 mg/kg infliximab *v* 15% in people taking placebo).[79] A third large multicentre RCT (428 people with active disease not responsive to methotrexate) compared five groups over 7 months: placebo versus infliximab at 3 or 10 mg/kg, administered every 4 or 8 weeks.[80] All continued to receive methotrexate. ACR20 criteria were reached by 50–58% who received infliximab/methotrexate and by 20% of the methotrexate/placebo group. ACR50 was attained by 26–31% of the people receiving infliximab and by 5% in the placebo group ($P < 0.001$; CI not provided). Longer term results at 54 weeks found that all infliximab groups improved versus placebo in terms of ACR20, ACR50, and ACR70 criteria (all results $P < 0.05$; CI no provided).[81]

Harms: **Etanercept:** The most common adverse effect was mild injection site reaction (42–49% in the treated group *v* 7–13% in the placebo group). Other adverse effects included upper respiratory symptoms or infections, headache, and diarrhoea. Autoantibodies to double stranded DNA developed in 5–9% of the treated group. Less than 1% of people developed malignancies or infections in the 6 month trials. Reactivation of demyelinating disease has been described. **Infliximab:** In the RCTs, common adverse reactions were upper respiratory infections, headache, diarrhoea, and abdominal pain. Reactions during or immediately after the injection (headache, nausea, and urticaria) were also observed in the placebo groups, but were more frequent with infliximab. Antibodies to double stranded DNA were found in about 16% of people taking infliximab. The rates of serious adverse effects in treated and placebo groups were not significantly different, but there was insufficient power to detect clinically important differences. Worldwide, over 150 cases of reactivation of tuberculosis have been documented, and people should be screened for previous tuberculosis before treatment (P Emery, personal communication, 2002).

Comment: We found one non-English language review of tumour necrosis factor alpha inhibitors; it will be translated and, if relevant, included in future *Clinical Evidence* updates.[82] These drugs are generally restricted to people who have failed conventional disease modifying antirheumatic drugs and are used in secondary care. The effects on disease activity occurred within weeks, unlike other disease modifying antirheumatic drugs that may take several months to have an effect.

REFERENCES

1. Arnett FC, Edworthy SM, Bloch DA, et al. The American Rheumatism Association 1987 revised criteria for the classification of rheumatoid arthritis. *Arthritis Rheum* 1987;31:315–324.
2. Lawrence RC, Helmick CG, Arnett FC, et al. Estimates of the prevalence of arthritis and selected musculoskeletal disorders in the United States. *Arthritis Rheum* 1998;41:778–781.
3. Symmons DP, Barrett EM, Bankhead CR, Scott DG, Silman AJ. The incidence of rheumatoid arthritis in the United Kingdom: results from the Norfolk Arthritis Register. *Br J Rheumatol* 1994;33:735–739.
4. Winchester R, Dwyer E, Rose S. The genetic basis of rheumatoid arthritis: the shared epitope hypothesis. *Rheum Dis Clin North Am* 1992;18:761–783.
5. Yelin E, Henke C, Epstein W. The work dynamics of the person with rheumatoid arthritis. *Arthritis Rheum* 1987;30:507–512.

6. Mutru O, Laakso M, Isomäki H, Koota K. Ten year mortality and causes of death in patients with rheumatoid arthritis. *BMJ* 1985;290:1797–1799.
7. Felson DT, Anderson JJ, Boers M, et al. American College of Rheumatology preliminary definition of improvement in rheumatoid arthritis. *Arthritis Rheum* 1995;38:727–735.
8. Suarez-Almazor ME, Belseck E, Shea B, Wells G, Tugwell P. Methotrexate for rheumatoid arthritis. In: The Cochrane Library, Issue 3, 2000. Oxford: Update Software. Search date 1997; primary sources Medline, Embase, Cochrane Controlled Trials Register, and hand search of reference lists.
9. Felson DT, Anderson JJ, Meenan RF. Use of short-term efficacy/toxicity trade-offs to select second-line drugs in rheumatoid arthritis: a meta-analysis of published clinical trials. *Arthritis Rheum* 1992;35:1117–1125. Search date 1990; primary sources Medline and hand search of two key journals and reference lists.
10. Strand V, Cohen S, Schiff M, et al. Treatment of active rheumatoid arthritis with leflunomide compared with placebo or methotrexate. *Arch Intern Med* 1999;159:2542–2550.
11. Smolen JS, Kalden JR, Scott, DL, et al. Efficacy and safety of leflunomide compared with placebo and sulfasalazine in active rheumatoid arthritis: A double-blind, randomised, multicentre. Trial. *Lancet* 1999;353:259–266.
12. Emery P, Breedveld FC, Lemmel EM, et al. A comparison of the efficacy and safety of leflunomide and methotrexate for the treatment of rheumatoid arthritis. *Rheumatology* 2000;39:655–665.
13. Hamilton J, McInnes I, Thomson E, et al. Comparative study of intramuscular gold and methotrexate in a rheumatoid arthritis population from a socially deprived area. *Ann Rheum Dis* 2001;60:566–572.
14. Ortiz Z, Shea B, Suarez-Almazor ME, Moher D, Wells GA, Tugwell P. The efficacy of folic acid and folinic acid in reducing methotrexate gastrointestinal toxicity in rheumatoid arthritis: a meta-analysis of randomised controlled clinical trials. *J Rheumatol* 1998;25;36–43. Search date 1996; primary sources Medline, handsearch of bibliographic references, Current Contents, and abstracts selected from rheumatology meetings and journals.
15. Beauparlant P, Papp K, Haroui B. The incidence of cancer associated with the treatment of rheumatoid arthritis. *Semin Arthritis Rheum* 1999;29:145–148.
16. Maetzel A, Wong A, Strand V, Tugwell P, Wells G, Bombardier C. Meta-analysis of treatment termination rates among rheumatoid arthritis patients receiving disease-modifying anti-rheumatic drugs. *Rheumatology* 2000;39:975–981. Search date 1997; primary sources Medline and Embase.
17. Alarcon GS, Lopez-Mendez A, Walter J, et al. Radiographic evidence of disease progression in methotrexate treated and nonmethotrexate disease modifying antirheumatic drug treated rheumatoid arthritis patients: a meta-analysis. *J Rheumatol* 1992;19:1868–1873. Search date 1991; primary sources Medline and hand search of bibliographies and meetings abstract of the American College of Rheumatology 1988–1991.
18. Felson DT, Anderson JJ, Meenan RF. The comparative efficacy and toxicity of second-line drugs in rheumatoid arthritis: results of two meta-analyses. *Arthritis Rheum* 1990;33:1449–1461. Search date 1989; primary sources Medline, and hand search of two key journals and reference lists.
19. Gotzsche PC, Podenphant J, Olesen M, Halberg P. Meta-analysis of second-line antirheumatic drugs: sample size bias and uncertain benefit. *J Clin Epidemiol* 1992;45:587–594. Search date 1988; primary source Medline, hand searching of reference lists, and drug companies contacted for unpublished trials.
20. Suarez-Almazor ME, Belseck E, Wells G, Shea B, Tugwell P. Meta-analyses of placebo controlled trials of disease-modifying antirheumatic drugs (DMARD) for the treatment of rheumatoid arthritis (RA). *Arthritis Rheum* 1998;41:S153. Search date not stated; primary sources Medline and Embase.
21. Suarez-Almazor ME, Belseck E, Shea B, Homik J, Wells G, Tugwell P. Antimalarials for rheumatoid arthritis. In: The Cochrane Library, Issue 3, 2000. Oxford: Update Software. Search date 1997; primary sources Medline, Embase, Cochrane Controlled Trials Register, and hand search of reference lists.
22. Scull E. Chloroquine and hydroxychloroquine therapy in rheumatoid arthritis. *Arthritis Rheum* 1962;5:30–36.
23. Finbloom DS, Silver K, Newsome DA, Gunke R. Comparison of hydroxychloroquine and chloroquine use and the development of retinal toxicity. *J Rheumatol* 1985;12:692–694.
24. The Hera Study Group. A randomized trial of hydroxychloroquine in early rheumatoid arthritis: the Hera study. *Am J Med* 1995;156–158.
25. Jessop JD, O'Sullivan MM, Lewis PA, et al. A long-term five-year randomized controlled trial of hydroxychloroquine, sodium aurothiomalate, auranofin and penicillamine in the treatment of patients with rheumatoid arthritis. *Br J Rheumatol* 1998;37:992–1002.
26. Suarez-Almazor ME, Belseck E, Shea B, Wells G, Tugwell P. Sulfasalazine for rheumatoid arthritis. In: The Cochrane Library, Issue 3, 2000. Oxford: Update Software. Search date 1997; primary sources Medline, Embase, Cochrane Controlled Trials Register, and hand search of reference lists.
27. Weinblatt ME, Reda D, Henderson W, et al. Sulfasalazine treatment for rheumatoid arthritis: a metaanalysis of 15 randomized trials. *J Rheumatol* 1999;26:2123–2130. Search date 1998; primary sources Medline, Excerpta Medica, and Derwent Drug File.
28. Van der Heijde DM, van Riel PL, Nuver-Zwart IH, Gribnau FW, van de Putte LB. Effects of hydroxychloroquine and sulfasalazine on progression of joint damage in rheumatoid arthritis. *Lancet* 1989;1:1036–1038.
29. Capell HA, Maiden N, Madhok R, Hampson R, Thomson EA. Intention-to-treat analysis of 200 patients with rheumatoid arthritis 12 years after random allocation to either sulfasalazine or penicillamine. *J Rheumatol* 1998;25:1880–1886.
30. Clark P, Tugwell P, Bennet K, et al. Injectable gold for rheumatoid arthritis. In: The Cochrane Library, Issue 3, 2000. Oxford: Update Software. Search date 1997; primary sources Medline and hand search of reference lists and bibliographies in selected textbooks.
31. Rau R. Does parenteral gold retard radiological progression in rheumatoid arthritis? *Z Rheumatol* 1996;55:307–318.
32. Suarez-Almazor ME, Spooner CH, Belseck E, Shea B. Auranofin versus placebo in rheumatoid arthritis. In: The Cochrane Library, Issue 4, 2000. Oxford: Update Software. Search date 1998; primary sources Medline, Embase, Cochrane Controlled Trials Register, and hand searches of reference lists of retrieved articles.
33. Berkey CS, Anderson JJ, Hoaglin DC. Multiple outcome meta-analysis of clinical trials. *Stat Med* 1996;15:537–557.

34. McEntegart A, Porter D, Capell HA, Thomson EA. Sulfasalazine has a better efficacy/toxicity profile than auranofin — evidence from a 5 year prospective randomized trial. *J Rheumatol* 1996;23:1887–1890.
35. Singh G, Fieis JF, Williams CA, et al. Toxicity profiles of disease modifying antirheumatic drugs in rheumatoid arthritis. *J Rheumatol* 1991;18:188–194.
36. Kloppenburg M, Breedveld FC, Terwiel JP, Mallee C, Dijkmans BA. Minocycline in active rheumatoid arthritis: a double-blind, placebo-controlled trial. *Arthritis Rheum* 1994;37:629–636.
37. Tilley BC, Alarcon GS, Heyse SP, et al. Minocycline in rheumatoid arthritis: a 48-week, double-blind, placebo-controlled trial. MIRA trial group. *Ann Intern Med* 1995;122:81–89.
38. O'Dell JR, Haire CE, Palmer W, et al. Treatment of early rheumatoid arthritis with minocycline or placebo: results of a randomized, double-blind, placebo-controlled trial. *Arthritis Rheum* 1997;40:842–848.
39. Suarez-Almazor ME, Spooner C, Belseck E. Penicillamine for rheumatoid arthritis. In: The Cochrane Library, Issue 3, 2000. Oxford: Update Software. Search date 2000; primary sources Cochrane Musculoskeletal Group's Trials Register, Cochrane Controlled Trials Register, Medline, Embase, and hand searching of reference lists of trials retrieved.
40. Wolfe F, Hawley DJ, Cathey MA. Termination of slow acting anti-rheumatic therapy in rheumatoid arthritis: a 14 year prospective evaluation of 1017 starts. *J Rheumatol* 1990;17:994–1002.
41. Pincus T, Marcum SB, Callahan LF. Long-term drug therapy for rheumatoid arthritis in seven rheumatology private practices: II. second line drugs and prednisone. *J Rheumatol* 1992;19:1885–1894.
42. Fries JF, Williams CA, Ramey D, Bloch DA. The relative toxicity of disease-modifying antirheumatic drugs. *Arthritis Rheum* 1993;36:297–306.
43. Suarez-Almazor ME, Soskolne CL, Saunders LD, Russell AS. Use of second-line drugs in the treatment of rheumatoid arthritis in Edmonton, Alberta: patterns of prescription and long-term effectiveness. *J Rheumatol* 1995;22:836–843.
44. Suarez-Almazor ME, Spooner C, Bekseck E. Azathioprine for rheumatoid arthritis. In: The Cochrane Library, Issue 3, 2000. Oxford: Update Software. Search date 2000; primary sources Cochrane Musculoskeletal Group's Trials Register, Cochrane Controlled Trials Register, Medline, Embase, and hand searching of reference lists of trials retrieved.
45. Suarez-Almazor ME, Belseck E, Shea B, Wells G, Tugwell P. Cyclophosphamide for rheumatoid arthritis. In: The Cochrane Library, Issue 3, 2000. Oxford: Update Software. Search date 2000; primary sources Cochrane Controlled Trials Register, Medline, Embase, and hand search of reference lists.
46. Radis CD, Kahl LE, Baker GL, et al. Effects of cyclophosphamide on the development of malignancy and on long-term survival of patients with rheumatoid arthritis. A 20-year follow up study. *Arthritis Rheum* 1995;38:1120–1127.
47. Wells G, Haguenauer D, Shea B, Suarez-Almazor ME, Welch VA, Tugwell P. Cyclosporin for rheumatoid arthritis. In: The Cochrane Library, Issue 3, 2000. Oxford: Update Software. Search date 1997; primary sources Medline, hand search of reference lists and consultation with experts.
48. Hewitson PJ, DeBroe S, McBride A, Milne R. Leflunomide and rheumatoid arthritis: a systematic review of effectiveness, safety and cost implications. *J Clin Pharm Ther* 2000;25:295–302. Search date 1999; primary sources Medline, Embase, the Cochrane Library, Econlit, HMIC (Dhdata), HMIC (Helmis), HMIC (King's Fund Database), and Best Evidence3.
49. Mladenovic V, Domljan Z, Rozman B, et al. Safety and effectiveness of leflunomide in the treatment of patients with active rheumatoid arthritis. *Arthritis Rheum* 1995;38:1595–1603.
50. Cohen S, Cannon G, Schiff M, et al. Two-year, blinded, randomized, controlled trial of treatment of active rheumatoid arthritis with leflunomide compared with methotrexate. Utilization of Leflunomide in the Treatment of Rheumatoid Arthritis Trial Investigator Group. *Arthritis Rheum* 2001;44:1984–1992.
51. Strand V, Tugwell P, Bombardier C, et al. Function and health-related quality of life: results from a randomized controlled trial of leflunomide versus methotrexate or placebo in patients with active rheumatoid arthritis. *Arthritis Rheum* 1999;42:1870–1878.
52. Verhoeven AC, Boers M, Tugwell P. Combination therapy in rheumatoid arthritis: updated systematic review. *Br J Rheumatol* 1998;37:612–619. Search date 1997; primary sources Medline and hand searches of article bibliographies.
53. Van den Borne BE, Landewe RB, Goei HS, et al. Combination therapy in recent onset rheumatoid arthritis: a randomized double blind trial of the addition of low dose cyclosporin to patients treated with low dose chloroquine. *J Rheumatol* 1998;25:1493–1498.
54. Boers M, Verhoeven AC, Markusse HM, et al. Randomised comparison of combined step-down prednisolone, methotrexate and sulfasalazine with sulfasalazine alone in early rheumatoid arthritis. *Lancet* 1997;350:309–318.
55. Mottonen T, Hannonen P, Leirisalo-Repo M, et al. Comparison of combination therapy with single-drug therapy in early rheumatoid arthritis: a randomised trial. FIN-RACo trial group. *Lancet* 1999;353:1568–1573.
56. Calguneri M, Pay S, Caliskaner Z, et al. Combination therapy versus monotherapy for the treatment of patients with rheumatoid arthritis. *Clin Exp Rheumatol* 1999;17:699–704.
57. O'Dell JR, Haire CE, Erikson N, et al. Treatment of rheumatoid arthritis with methotrexate alone, sulfasalazine and hydroxychloroquine, or a combination of all three medications. *N Engl J Med* 1996; 334:1287–1291.
58. Proudman S, Conaghan P, Richardson C, et al. Treatment of poor-prognosis early rheumatoid arthritis: a randomized study of treatment with methotrexate, cyclosporin A, and intra-articular corticosteroids compared with sulfasalazine alone. *Arthritis Rheum* 2000;43:1809–1819.
59. Felson DT, Anderson JJ, Meenan RF. The efficacy and toxicity of combination therapy in rheumatoid arthritis: a meta-analysis. *Arthritis Rheum* 1994;37:1487–1491. Search date 1992; primary sources Medline and hand searches of five international rheumatology journals and abstracts of rheumatology society meetings.
60. Van Der Heide A, Jacobs JWG, Bijlsma JWJ, et al. The effectiveness of early treatment with 'second-line' antirheumatic drugs: a randomized, controlled trial. *Ann Intern Med* 1996;124:699–707.
61. Egsmose C, Lund B, Borg G, et al. Patients with rheumatoid arthritis benefit from early second line therapy: 5 year follow up of a prospective double blind placebo controlled study. *J Rheumatol* 1995;22:2208–2213.
62. Tsakonas E, Fitzgerald AA, Fitzcharles MA, et al. Consequences of delayed therapy with second line

agents in rheumatoid arthritis: a 3 year follow up on the hydroxychloroquine in early rheumatoid arthritis (HERA) study. *J Rheumatol* 2000;27:623–629.
63. O'Dell JR, Paulsen G, Haire CE, et al. Treatment of early seropositive rheumatoid arthritis with minocycline: four-year follow up of a double blind, placebo-controlled trial. *Arthritis Rheum* 1999;42:1691–1695.
64. Quinn M, Conaghan P, Emery P. The therapeutic approach of early intervention for rheumatoid arthritis: what is the evidence? *Rheumatology* 2001;40:1211–1220.
65. Hawley DJ, Wolfe F. Are the results of controlled clinical trials and observational studies of second line therapy in rheumatoid arthritis valid and generalizeable as measures of rheumatoid arthritis outcomes? An analysis of 122 studies. *J Rheumatol* 1991;18:1008–1014.
66. ten Wold S, Breedveld F, Hermans J, et al. Randomised placebo-controlled study of stopping second-line drugs in rheumatoid arthritis. *Lancet* 1996;346:347–352.
67. Sander O, Herborn G, Bock E, Rau R. Prospective six year follow up of patients withdrawn from a randomised study comparing parenteral gold salt and methotrexate. *Ann Rheum Dis* 1999;58:281–287.
68. Gotzsche PC, Johansen HK. Meta-analysis of short term low dose prednisolone versus placebo and non-steroidal anti-inflammatory drugs in rheumatoid arthritis. *BMJ* 1998;316:811–818. Search date 1997; primary sources Medline, Cochrane Controlled Trials Register, and hand search of reference lists.
69. Criswell LA, Saag KG, Sems KM, et al. Moderate-term low dose corticosteroids for rheumatoid arthritis. In: The Cochrane Library, Issue 3, 2000. Oxford: Update Software. Search date 1998; primary sources Medline and hand search of selected journals.
70. Kirwan JR. Arthritis and Rheumatism Council low dose glucocorticoid study group: the effect of glucocorticoids on joint destruction in rheumatoid arthritis. *N Engl J Med* 1995;333:142–146.
71. Hickling P, Jacoby RK, Kirwan JR, et al. Joint destruction after glucocorticoids are withdrawn in early rheumatoid arthritis. *Br J Rheumatol* 1998;37:930–936.
72. Wolfe F, Mitchell DM, Sibley JT, et al. The mortality of rheumatoid arthritis. *Arthritis Rheum* 1994;37:481–494.
73. Verhoeven AC, Boers M. Limited bone loss due to corticosteroids: a systematic review of prospective studies in rheumatoid arthritis and other diseases. *J Rheumatol* 1997;24:1495–1503. Search date 1995; primary source Medline.
74. Furst DE, Lindsley H, Baethge B, et al. Dose-loading with hydroxychloroquine improves the rate of response in early, active rheumatoid arthritis: A randomized, double-blind six-week trial with eighteen-week extension. *Arthritis Rheum* 1999;42:357–365.
75. Moreland LW, Schiff MH, Baumgartner SW, et al. Etanercept therapy in rheumatoid arthritis. A randomized, controlled trial. *Ann Intern Med* 1999;130:478–486.
76. Weinblatt ME, Kremer JM, Bankhurst AD, et al. A trial of etanercept, a recombinant tumor necrosis factor receptor: Fc fusion protein, in patients with rheumatoid arthritis receiving methotrexate. *N Engl J Med* 1999;340:253–259.
77. Bathon J, Martin R, Fleischmann R, et al. A comparison of etanercept and methotrexate in patients with early rheumatoid arthritis. *N Engl J Med* 2000;343:1586–1593.
78. Elliott MJ, Maini RN, Feldmann M, et al. Randomised double-blind comparison of chimeric monoclonal antibody to tumour necrosis factor alpha (cA2) versus placebo in rheumatoid arthritis. *Lancet* 1994;344:1105–1110.
79. Maini RN, Breedveld FC, Kalden JR, et al. Therapeutic efficacy of multiple intravenous infusions of anti-tumor necrosis factor α monoclonal antibody combined with low-dose weekly methotrexate in rheumatoid arthritis. *Arthritis Rheum* 1998;41:1552–1563.
80. Maini RN, St Clair EW, Breedweld F, et al. Infliximab (chimeric anti-tumour necrosis factor α monoclonal antibody) versus placebo in rheumatoid arthritis patients receiving concomitant methotrexate: a randomized phase III trial. ATTRACT study group. *Lancet* 1999;354:1932–1939.
81. Lipsky P, van der Heijde D, St Claire W, et al. Infliximab and methotrexate in the treatment of rheumatoid arthritis. *N Engl J Med* 2000;343:1594–1602.
82. Reneses S, Pestana L. Systematic review of clinical trials on the treatment of rheumatoid arthritis with tumour necrosis factor alpha inhibitors [in French]. *Med Clin (Barc)* 2001;116:620–628.

Paul Emery
ARC Professor Head of Academic Unit of Musculoskeletal disease
University of Leeds
Leeds
UK

Wednesday Foster
Research Health Science Specialist
Veterans Affairs Medical Center and Baylor College of Medicine
Houston Texas
USA

Maria Suarez-Almazor
Associate Professor of Medicine
Baylor College of Medicine
Houston Texas
USA

Competing interests: None declared

Shoulder pain

Search date February 2002

Cathy Speed and Brian Hazleman

QUESTIONS

INTERVENTIONS

See glossary, p 1285

Key Messages

- Shoulder pain is not a specific diagnosis. Well designed, double blind RCTs of specific interventions in specific shoulder disorders are needed.
- Systematic reviews have found RCTs mostly with poor methods, and pronounced heterogeneity of study populations and outcome measures.
- We found insufficient evidence on the effects of most interventions in people with non-specific shoulder pain.
- **Arthroscopic laser subacromial decompression** One systematic review found no RCTs on arthroscopic laser treatment.
- **Electrical stimulation** One RCT found no evidence of a significant effect on pain with electrical stimulation versus dummy electrical stimulation. In people with shoulder pain after stroke, one systematic review found no clear evidence of reduced pain with electrical stimulation versus no stimulation, but found limited evidence that electrical stimulation may increase the range of passive external rotation of the shoulder.

- **Extracorporeal shock wave therapy (calcifying tendinitis)** One RCT found limited evidence that extracorporeal shock wave therapy versus placebo significantly improved pain in calcifying tendinitis after two sessions 1 week apart (NNT 2, 95% CI 1 to 21).
- **Hydrodistension and intra-articular corticosteroid injection (frozen shoulder)** One small RCT in people with frozen shoulder found limited evidence that distending the glenohumeral joint in addition to intra-articular steroid injection versus steroid injection alone significantly reduced severity of symptoms (NNT 2, 95% CI 2 to 9) and increased range of movement at 12 weeks.
- **Intra-articular corticosteroid injection** Systematic reviews found no clear evidence of benefit from intra-articular corticosteroid injection versus control treatment.
- **Intra-articular guanethidine** One small RCT found that intra-articular guanethidine versus placebo significantly reduced pain 8 weeks after treatment, but found no evidence of an altered range of abduction.
- **Intra-articular non-steroidal anti-inflammatory drugs** One RCT found insufficient evidence about intra-articular injection of non-steroidal anti-inflammatory drugs versus placebo.
- **Laser treatment** We found conflicting evidence from four small RCTs about laser treatment versus placebo for shoulder pain.
- **Multidisciplinary biopsychosocial rehabilitation** One systematic review of poor quality RCTs found no significant difference in outcomes with multidisciplinary biopsychosocial rehabilitation versus usual care.
- **Oral corticosteroids** Two small RCTs found no evidence of reduced pain or improved abduction with oral corticosteroids versus placebo or versus no treatment at 4–8 months. Adverse effects of corticosteroids are well documented (see rheumatoid arthritis, p 1250 and asthma, p 1506).
- **Oral non-steroidal anti-inflammatory drugs** RCTs found weak evidence that oral non-steroidal anti-inflammatory drugs versus placebo may reduce pain after 2–4 weeks.
- **Phonophoresis** One small RCT found no significant difference in perceived pain or tenderness after 5–10 days from phonophoresis using topical dexamethasone, lidocaine, and aqueous gel versus placebo phonophoresis using only aqueous gel.
- **Physiotherapy (exercises and manual treatments)** Systematic reviews of one small RCT found no significant difference in pain with manual treatment plus exercises versus no treatment at 3 months.
- **Subacromial corticosteroid injection** One systematic review found that subacromial bursa corticosteroid injection versus injection without corticosteroid significantly improved abduction but did not reduce pain at 4 weeks. One additional RCT found no significant pain reduction or improved abduction after 12 weeks with subacromial corticosteroid injection plus local anaesthetic versus local anaesthetic alone.
- **Surgery** We found no RCTs on most surgical interventions. One small RCT in people with frozen shoulder found that forced manipulation versus intra-articular injection of corticosteroid significantly increased the number of people who completely recovered at 3 months.
- **Transdermal glyceryl trinitrate** One small RCT in people with supraspinatus tendinitis found insufficient evidence about pain relief with transdermal glyceryl trinitrate versus placebo.

- **Ultrasound** One systematic review and two subsequent RCTs found no significant difference in pain or abduction with ultrasound versus no treatment.
- **Ice; simple analgesics (paracetamol and opiates); topical non-steroidal anti-inflammatory drugs** We found no RCTs about these interventions.

DEFINITION Shoulder pain arises in or around the shoulder from the glenohumeral, acromioclavicular, sternoclavicular, "subacromial", and scapulothoracic articulations and surrounding soft tissues. Regardless of the disorder, pain is the reason for most consultations. In adhesive capsulitis (frozen shoulder), pain is associated with pronounced restriction of movement. For most shoulder disorders, diagnosis is based on clinical features with imaging studies playing a role in some people.

INCIDENCE/ PREVALENCE Each year in primary care in the UK, about 1% of adults aged over 45 years present with a new episode of shoulder pain.[1] Prevalence is uncertain, with estimates from 4–20%.[2–6] One community survey (392 people) found a 1 month prevalence of shoulder pain of 34%.[7] A second community survey (644 people aged ≥ 70 years) reported a point prevalence of 21%, with a higher frequency in women than men (25% *v* 17%).[8] Seventy per cent of cases involved the rotator cuff. One survey of 134 people in a community based rheumatology clinic found that 65% of cases were rotator cuff lesions; 11% were caused by localised tenderness in the pericapsular musculature; 10% acromioclavicular joint pain; 3% glenohumeral joint arthritis; and 5% were referred pain from the neck.[9] One survey found that in adults the annual incidence of frozen shoulder was about 2%, with those aged 40–70 years most commonly affected.[10] The age distribution of specific shoulder disorders in the community is unknown.

AETIOLOGY/ RISK FACTORS Rotator cuff disorders are associated with excessive overloading, instability of the glenohumeral and acromioclavicular joints, muscle imbalance, adverse anatomical features (narrow coracoacromial arch and a hooked acromion), cuff degeneration with aging, ischaemia, and musculoskeletal diseases that result in wasting of the cuff muscles.[11–14] Risk factors for frozen shoulder include female sex, older age, shoulder trauma, surgery, diabetes, cardiorespiratory disorders, cerebrovascular events, thyroid disease, and hemiplegia.[10,15,16] Arthritis of the glenohumeral joint can occur in numerous forms, including primary and secondary osteoarthritis, rheumatoid arthritis, and crystal arthritides.[11]

PROGNOSIS One survey in an elderly community found that most people with shoulder pain were still affected 3 years after the initial survey.[17] One prospective cohort study of 122 people in primary care found that 25% of people with shoulder pain reported previous episodes, and 49% reported full recovery at 18 months' follow up.[18]

AIMS To reduce pain and to improve range of movement and function, with minimal adverse effects.

OUTCOMES Pain scores (overall score, on activity, at night, at rest, during the day, analgesia count); range of movement measures; assessment of overall severity (self assessed or by blinded assessor); functional score; global improvement scores (self assessed or by blinded assessor); tenderness; strength; stiffness; and adverse effects of treatment. The shoulder pain and disability index is a validated, shoulder related pain and disability questionnaire.[19–24] Other validated participant rated disability scores have been developed.[20]

METHODS *Clinical Evidence* update search and appraisal February 2002. We found some articles that were not published in English; these articles are being translated and, if appropriate, will be included in the next update.

QUESTION What are the effects of treatments on shoulder pain?

OPTION ORAL NON-STEROIDAL ANTI-INFLAMMATORY DRUGS

Two systematic reviews found weak evidence of short term benefits with oral non-steroidal anti-inflammatory drugs in shoulder pain (see acute musculoskeletal syndromes under non-steroidal anti-inflammatory drugs, p 1203).

Benefits: **Non-steroidal anti-inflammatory drugs versus placebo:** We found two systematic reviews of non-steroidal anti-inflammatory drugs (NSAIDs) versus placebo in shoulder pain.[25,26] One of the reviews (search date 1998, 4 RCTs, 151 people with shoulder pain for more than 72 h)[25] pooled results from two small RCTs (90 people with rotator cuff tendinitis) and found no significant reduction of pain after 4 weeks (visual analogue scale, WMD +3%, 95% CI –19% to +25%; positive values represent deterioration) and no significant improvement of abduction (WMD +26°, 95% CI –9° to +61°; positive values represent improvement).[27,28] The third RCT in the review found a small reduction of pain but no change in abduction. The fourth RCT did not assess pain or abduction. The second systematic review (search date 1993) identified three RCTs, including the two pooled in the first review.[26] The other RCT (69 people) compared oral NSAIDs versus placebo for 14 days in acute shoulder pain of less than 96 hours' duration. NSAIDs improved pain relief judged by the investigator (30/35 [86%] *v* 19/32 [59%] with placebo; ARR 26%, CI 5% to 46%; NNT 4, 95% CI 3 to 20).[29]

Harms: One systematic review of NSAIDs in shoulder pain (search date 1993, 5 RCTs, 14 comparative studies) found 10 studies that reported adverse events.[26] The incidence of adverse events ranged widely across the studies (8–76%): most were mild to moderate.[26] Withdrawal because of adverse events occurred in fewer than 10% of people in comparative studies, but in up to 20% of people in RCTs. Adverse events were mostly gastrointestinal symptoms, skin rash, headache, or dizziness. The review found no evidence that the incidence or nature of adverse effects varied among NSAIDs. One RCT (not included in either review, 224 people with musculoskeletal sprains or tendinitis) compared two NSAIDs and found adverse events in 12–18% of people, causing 5–7% to withdraw.[30] We found no systematic review of the adverse effects of cyclo-oxygenase type II selective agents in people with shoulder pain (see differences between NSAIDs under the NSAIDs topic, p 1203).

Comment: Evidence about the effects of NSAIDs in shoulder disorders is limited by the lack of standardised approaches: diverse disorders have been considered under the universal term shoulder pain, different types of NSAIDs were used, and outcome measures and follow up periods vary among RCTs.

OPTION TOPICAL NON-STEROIDAL ANTI-INFLAMMATORY DRUGS

We found no RCTs about the effects of topical non-steroidal anti-inflammatory drugs specifically in shoulder pain (see topical non-steroidal anti-inflammatory drugs under the non-steroidal anti-inflammatory drugs topic, p 1209).

Benefits: We found no systematic review or RCTs of topical non-steroidal anti-inflammatory drugs specifically in shoulder disorders.

Harms: We found no systematic review or RCTs of the harms of topical non-steroidal anti-inflammatory drugs specifically in shoulder disorders.

Comment: See topical non-steroidal anti-inflammatory drugs under osteoarthritis, p 1221.

OPTION INTRA-ARTICULAR NON-STEROIDAL ANTI-INFLAMMATORY DRUGS

One RCT found insufficient evidence about intra-articular injection of non-steroidal anti-inflammatory drugs in people with shoulder pain.

Benefits: We found no systematic review but found one RCT.[31] The RCT (80 people with acute or subacute rotator cuff tendinitis) compared local injection of non-steroidal anti-inflammatory drugs (NSAIDs) versus placebo. People were offered further injections at weekly intervals if the assessor felt this was indicated. There were no differences in the total number of injections per group. After 4 weeks, NSAIDs versus placebo reduced mean pain at rest (visual analogue scale, range not stated: from 4.7 [95% CI 3.8 to 5.6] to 1.7 [95% CI 0.95 to 2.5] with NSAID *v* from 4.8 [95% CI 4.1 to 5.6] to 3.2 [95% CI 2.3 to 4.1] with placebo; no WMD and CI available), mean pain during active movement (from 7.4 [95% CI 6.9 to 7.8] to 2.4 [95% CI 1.5 to 3.2] *v* from 7.0 [95% CI 6.5 to 7.5] to 5.0 [95% CI 4.1 to 5.9]), and mean active abduction (from 111° [95% CI 98° to 124°] to 142° [95% CI 130° to 153°] *v* from 116° [95% CI 105° to 128°] to 129° [95% CI 116° to 142°]). The clinical importance of the benefits found in the trial is uncertain.

Harms: The RCT reported episodes of a vagal reaction (2/38 people [5%] with NSAID injections *v* 0/39 [0%] with placebo), nausea (1/38 [3%] with NSAIDs *v* 1/39 [3%] with placebo), and single separate episodes of hotness, gastric pain, and flu-like symptoms with placebo. There were no withdrawals from the RCT because of adverse events.[31]

Comment: Eight people did not complete the RCT (3 in the treatment group, 5 on placebo) and follow up was limited to 4 weeks after the initial injection.

OPTION PARACETAMOL OR OPIATES

We found no evidence about the effect of paracetamol or opiates specifically for shoulder disorders.

Benefits: We found no systematic review or RCTs of paracetamol or opiates for shoulder pain.

Harms: We found no evidence specifically in people treated for shoulder pain.

Comment: None.

OPTION SUBACROMIAL CORTICOSTEROID INJECTIONS

One systematic review comparing subacromial bursa corticosteroid injection versus injection without corticosteroid found limited evidence of improved abduction but no evidence of pain reduction. One additional RCT found no evidence of pain reduction or improved abduction.

Benefits: **Versus placebo injection:** We found one systematic review (search date 1998, 2 RCTs)[25] and one additional RCT.[32] The first RCT in the review (50 people with rotator cuff tendinitis) involved subacromial bursa injection (triamcinolone 40 mg), and the other RCT (40 people with rotator cuff tendinitis) used subacromial and intra-articular injection (2 mL 0.5% lidocaine [lignocaine] plus 1 mL triamcinolone).[27,28] After 4 weeks, the review found that corticosteroids significantly improved abduction (WMD 35°, 95% CI 14° to 55°) but did not significantly reduce pain (WMD +7%, 95% CI –33% to +47%). The additional RCT (55 people with rotator cuff tendinitis) compared subacromial methylprednisolone plus lidocaine versus lidocaine alone. It found no significant pain reduction or improved abduction after 12 weeks (visual analogue scale 0–30; median pain improved by 8 with active treatment *v* 8 with placebo). The range of abduction did not change from baseline either with active treatment or with placebo.[32]

Harms: One RCT (40 people with rotator cuff tendinitis) found no adverse effects with subacromial corticosteroid injections versus placebo apart from mild discomfort.[27] Another RCT (50 people with rotator cuff tendinitis) found similar adverse events with subacromial corticosteroid injection versus subacromial lidocaine and placebo tablets (3/25 [12%, mild gastrointestinal symptoms; pityriasis rosea 2 days after the injection; increased frequency of urination] with corticosteroid injection *v* 3/25 [12%, mild gastrointestinal symptoms; diarrhoea; vasovagal reaction] with lidocaine injection and placebo tablets).[28]

Comment: Range of movement is not a satisfactory surrogate measure of function. We found no evidence on the accuracy of placement of subacromial injections.

OPTION INTRA-ARTICULAR CORTICOSTEROID INJECTIONS

Two systematic reviews found no clear evidence of benefit from intra-articular corticosteroid injection versus control treatment. We found limited evidence from one small RCT in people with frozen shoulder that distending the glenohumeral joint, in addition to intra-articular steroid injection, could increase range of movement and reduce severity of symptoms.

Benefits: **Versus placebo:** We found two systematic reviews (search dates 1998[25] and 1993;[26] same 2 RCTs[33,34] in each review) and one subsequent RCT (see table 1, p 1288).[35] In the reviews, neither the first RCT (24 people with shoulder pain, 4 wks' follow up) nor the second RCT (30 people with frozen shoulder, 24 wks' follow up) found that intra-articular steroids reduced pain or improved range of movement. The subsequent RCT compared three intra-articular injections of triamcinolone versus three intra-articular injections of saline, and also found no significant difference in pain score, change in mobility, or function.[35] **Different doses:** One RCT compared low dose versus higher dose triamcinolone injections in people with frozen shoulder (10 mg, 32 people; 40 mg, 25 people).[36] After 6 weeks, the RCT found that higher dose versus lower dose significantly reduced pain (change on 100 mm visual analogue scale: 31 mm with low dose *v* 49 mm with high dose; no CI available), movement restriction, and self rated functional impairment (change on 4 point ordinal scale: 0.7 with low dose *v* 1.3 with high dose; no CI available), but did not significantly improve sleep disturbance. The RCT found no significant difference in any outcome after 6 months. **Combined intra-articular and subacromial corticosteroid injections versus placebo:** Two systematic reviews (search dates 1998[25] and 1993;[26] 2 RCTs;[37,38] 42 people with frozen shoulder and 101 people with shoulder pain) compared combined intra-articular and subacromial corticosteroid versus placebo. Results could not be pooled because of diversity in study designs. Both found no significant benefit 6 weeks after injection (figures not available). **Hydrodistension plus corticosteroid versus corticosteroid alone:** We found no systematic review but found one small RCT (22 people with frozen shoulder given weekly intra-articular corticosteroid alone or in combination with hydrodistension for 6 wks or until symptoms resolved).[39] Hydrodistension involved injection of 19 mL of 0.5% lidocaine. Distension of the glenohumeral joint was confirmed by ultrasound. After 12 weeks, hydrodistension significantly improved the number of people with improved external rotation in the affected shoulder (rotation over a range of at least 75% of that in the opposite shoulder: 10/12 [83%] with distension *v* 1/8 [13%] with steroid alone; RR for improvement 7, 95% CI 1 to 42), physicians' impression of symptom severity (number with light or no symptoms 12/12 [100%] with distension *v* 3/8 [38%] with steroid alone; NNT 2, 95% CI 2 to 9), and reduced analgesic use. No significant improvement was found in visual analogue scores of function or pain at rest.

Harms: Intra-articular injections are rarely associated with infection (estimated at 1/14 000–1/50 000 injections).[40,41] An acute self limited synovitis was reported in up to 2% of people. Prevalence of tendon rupture, including rupture of the bicipital tendon and rotator cuff, was reported at fewer than 1% of people after local injection of corticosteroids.[40] Subcutaneous fat necrosis or skin atrophy was found in fewer than 1%. Corticosteroid arthropathy and osteonecrosis were rare (< 0.8%) and seem to affect mostly weight bearing joints.[27] One RCT of corticosteroid injection versus physiotherapy in painful stiff shoulders reported more facial flushing (9/52 [17%] people treated with corticosteroid injections *v* 1/56 [2%] treated with physiotherapy), and more new menstrual irregularities (6/52 [12%] people treated with local corticosteroid injections *v* 0/56 [0%] after physiotherapy).[42] Another RCT found that unacceptable pain was more likely after corticosteroid injection plus hydrodistension versus corticosteroid alone (2/12 [17%] people *v* 0/8 [0%]; P = 0.22).[39] In an RCT of intra-articular triamcinolone acetonide versus saline after stroke, the risk of adverse events was similar in each group (12/18 [67%] with triamcinolone *v* 13/19 [68%] with placebo). The adverse events included increased short term pain (3/18 [17%] with triamcinolone *v* 9/19 [47%] with placebo), local skin lesions (3/18 [17%] *v* 0/19 [0%]), flushing (4/18 [22%] *v* 1/19 [5%]), and postmenopausal haemorrhage (1/18 [6%] *v* 0/19 [0%]).[35]

Comment: Few RCTs of interventions in shoulder pain used high quality methods. One case control study found that clinical outcome correlated with accuracy of injection.[43] Another case control study found that only 10% of intra-articular injections were placed correctly even by experienced operators.[44] Confirmation of injection accuracy can be obtained with fluoroscopy or ultrasound. The RCT of hydrodistension included only 20 people with frozen shoulder, but it used specific inclusion criteria (only 26 people with frozen shoulder were recruited out of 120 referred). They were recruited from a hospital rheumatology clinic and may not be representative of people with frozen shoulder in the community. Twenty two people were randomised, but one dropped out of each group. The reported results were not analysed on an intention to treat basis, but they remain significant even when we reanalysed them in that way. Both groups received intra-articular steroid, so it is not clear whether any effect of hydrodistension versus no hydrodistension depends on the intra-articular steroid injection.[39] We found no other RCTs of hydrodistension. The possibility of publication and other biases cannot be assessed until the results have been replicated in other studies.

OPTION ORAL CORTICOSTEROIDS

Two small RCTs found no evidence of reduced pain or improved abduction with oral corticosteroids versus placebo.

Benefits: **Versus placebo:** We found no systematic review but found two RCTs.[45,46] One RCT (32 people with frozen shoulder) of oral corticosteroids versus placebo found no evidence after 18 weeks of reduced pain (mean improvement of 4 point rating scale [0 = no pain, 3 = severe pain]: from 1.4 at baseline to 0.5 with oral corticosteroids *v* 1.4 at baseline to 0.6 with placebo) or improved abduction (mean range of abduction from 75° at baseline to 154° with oral corticosteroids *v* 82° at baseline to 153° with placebo; no CI available).[45] The other RCT (40 people with frozen shoulder) found no improvement after 8 months with oral corticosteroids for 4 weeks versus no treatment in pain or range of motion (no figures available).[46]

Harms: Adverse effect of corticosteroids are well documented (see rheumatoid arthritis, p 1250, and asthma, p 1506). One RCT (40 people with frozen shoulder) reported mild indigestion in two people that settled after reducing the dose of oral corticosteroids below 10 mg.[46] No other adverse events were reported. The other RCT did not report adverse events.[45]

Comment: None.

OPTION PHYSIOTHERAPY (MANUAL TREATMENT AND EXERCISES)

Systematic reviews of one small RCT found no significant difference in shoulder pain between manual treatment plus exercises versus no treatment.

Benefits: **Versus no treatment:** We found two systematic reviews (search dates 1998[25] and 1993[26]), which identified one small RCT (19 people) of Maitland mobilisation (see glossary, p 1285) versus no treatment for frozen shoulder.[37] It found no significant difference in shoulder pain at 3 months (no figures available).

Harms: One RCT of physiotherapy versus corticosteroid injection in people with painful stiff shoulders found frequent adverse effects in both groups (32/57 [56%] with physiotherapy *v* 30/57 [53%] with corticosteroid injection). After physiotherapy, these effects lasted longer than 2 days in 13% of people.[42] Fever during treatment was found in 1% of people and local skin irritation in 2% of people; 4% of people reported tingling, radiation of pain down the arm, or slight swelling after treatment.

Comment: Studies on the effects of physiotherapy in shoulder disorders are limited by the lack of standardised approaches: diverse disorders are considered under the universal term shoulder pain, diverse forms of physiotherapy have been evaluated, and outcome measures and follow up periods vary.

OPTION ULTRASOUND

One systematic review and two subsequent RCTs found no significant difference in pain or abduction with ultrasound versus no treatment.

Benefits: We found one systematic review[47] and two subsequent RCTs.[48,49] The systematic review (search date 1997, 5 RCTs, 136 people) compared ultrasound versus placebo, sham ultrasound, or versus no treatment for shoulder disorders.[47] Clinical heterogeneity and insufficient description of outcome measures precluded pooling of results, but none of the individual RCTs found evidence of a clinically important effect of ultrasound versus placebo after 4–6 weeks. The first subsequent RCT (180 people with shoulder disorders who had failed to respond to 6 sessions of exercise) compared, in a blinded two by two factorial design, pulsed ultrasound versus dummy ultrasound, and bipolar interferential electrotherapy versus dummy electrotherapy.[48] It also included an additional control group that received no active or dummy treatments (39 people received only pulsed ultrasound and 68 received no active treatment, either no treatment or two dummy treatments). After 6 weeks, ultrasound was not significantly associated with improvement on a 7 point Likert scale (improvement occurred in 7/35 [20%] with no treatment *v* 19/73 [26%] with active ultrasound *v* 14/72 [19%] with dummy ultrasound; ARR for failure to improve with ultrasound *v* control treatments +6%, 95% CI –5% to +22%). Follow up at 12 months found no significant effect of ultrasound versus control treatments on the people reporting substantial improvement in functional status, pain, or range of movement. The second subsequent RCT (63 people, 70 shoulders) found no significant difference between ultrasound versus sham treatment in pain or quality of life scores at 9 months (see table 2, p 1288). Shoulders, not individuals, were randomised to pulsed ultrasound (frequency 890 Hz; intensity 2.5 W/cm^2; pulsed mode 1 : 4) or an indistinguishable sham treatment over the area of calcification. The first 15 treatments were given daily (five times weekly) and the remainder three times weekly for 3 weeks. The treating therapist was blinded. Sixty one shoulders completed the RCT. Nine people (9 shoulders) did not complete the treatment: three in the ultrasound group and six in the sham group, two in the latter because of pain.[49]

Harms: We found no systematic review and no RCTs specifically addressing adverse effects. The RCTs described (see benefits above) gave no information on adverse events.

Comment: In most RCTs, with the exception of the most recent,[49] there was considerable heterogeneity of the groups, interventions, and follow up duration among the RCTs. It is not clear that ultrasound machines were always adequately calibrated before use.

OPTION LASER TREATMENT

We found conflicting evidence from four small RCTs about laser treatment versus placebo in shoulder pain.

Benefits: We found no systematic review but found four placebo controlled RCTs.[50–53] After 8 weeks, one RCT (35 people) found no significant improvement with laser treatment versus no treatment in pain (10 cm visual analogue scale: improved by 3.6 cm with laser *v* 1.2 cm with placebo; $P = 0.34$) or abduction (range of movement improved by 36° with laser *v* 29° with placebo; $P = 0.23$).[50] The second RCT (91 people) found that more people recovered after 1 month with laser than with placebo (42/47 [89%] *v* 18/44 [41%]; ARR 48%, 95% CI 31% to 65%).[51] The third RCT (20 people with rotator cuff tendinitis) found that low level laser versus placebo reduced pain after 2 weeks (mean score difference 2.5%, 95% CI 2.0% to 3.0%).[52] The fourth RCT (24 people with supraspinatus tendinitis) found that low level laser versus placebo had no significant effect on shoulder pain after 12 weeks (no figures available).[53]

Harms: We found no evidence on harms.

Comment: The quality of studies on the effects of laser treatment in shoulder disorders is limited by the lack of standardised approaches.

OPTION ELECTRICAL STIMULATION

One RCT found no evidence of a significant effect of electrical stimulation on shoulder pain. In people with shoulder pain after stroke, one systematic review found no clear evidence of reduced pain with electrical stimulation versus no stimulation, but found limited evidence that electrical stimulation could increase the range of passive external rotation of the shoulder.

Benefits: **Versus control:** We found no systematic review but found two RCTs.[48,54] One RCT (180 people with shoulder disorders not improved by 6 exercise sessions) compared electrical stimulation (bipolar interferential electrical stimulation (see glossary, p 1285)) versus dummy electrical stimulation, and pulsed ultrasound versus dummy ultrasound in a blinded two by two factorial design (see benefits of ultrasound, p 1279).[48] After 6 weeks, it found no significant difference in the proportion of people who reported large improvement (17/73 [23%] with electrical stimulation *v* 16/72 [22%] with control; ARR +1%, 95% CI –13% to +15%). The second RCT (29 people with rotator cuff tendinitis not cured by corticosteroid injection) compared electrical stimulation induced by pulsed electromagnetic fields (5–9 h/day for 4 wks) versus placebo, but it did not report the number of people symptomless after 4 weeks.[54] **Versus control after stroke:** We found one systematic review (search date 1999, 4 RCTs, 170 people with shoulder pain after stroke) of electrical stimulation versus no stimulation.[55] Study designs and electrical stimulation technique varied considerably, precluding the pooling of results. The review found no significant difference in the incidence of pain (OR 0.64, 95% CI 0.19 to 2.14) or in pain intensity after treatment (standardised mean difference treatment *v* control: +0.13, 95% CI –1.00 to +1.24). Electrical stimulation significantly reduced the severity of glenohumeral subluxation (SMD –1.13, 95% CI –1.66 to –0.60), but did not significantly improve upper limb motor function (SMD +0.24, 95% CI –0.14 to +0.62) or upper limb spasticity (WMD +0.05, 95% CI –0.28 to +0.37).

Harms: We found no evidence on harms.

Comment: The quality of studies on the effects of electrical treatments in shoulder disorders is limited by the lack of standardised approaches. We found no good evidence that different forms of electrical stimulation produce different effects.

OPTION ICE

We found no good evidence about the effects of ice.

Benefits: We found no systematic review or RCTs.

Harms: We found no evidence on harms.

Comment: None.

OPTION INTRA-ARTICULAR GUANETHIDINE

One small RCT of intra-articular guanethidine versus placebo found significant pain benefit 8 weeks after treatment, but no evidence of an effect on range of abduction.

Benefits: We found no systematic review but found one RCT (18 people with resistant shoulder pain) of intra-articular sympathetic block with guanethidine versus intra-articular saline.[56] It found greater improvement in pain with guanethidine after 8 weeks (mean reduction in 10 cm visual analogue scale: 36% with guanethidine *v* 16% with placebo; $P < 0.05$), but no significant change in range of movement (mean range of abduction 53° at baseline and 52° at 8 wks with guanethidine *v* 57° at baseline and 56° at 8 wks with placebo; no CI available).

Harms: Adverse effects were not reported.

Comment: This single RCT involved a heterogeneous population, including people with osteoarthritis, frozen shoulder, and rotator cuff tendinitis. The effects of treatment in individual disorders remain uncertain.

OPTION TRANSDERMAL GLYCERYL TRINITRATE

One small RCT found insufficient evidence that transdermal glyceryl trinitrate is superior to placebo for pain relief in people with supraspinatus tendinitis.

Benefits: We found no systematic review but found one small and poor quality RCT (20 people with supraspinatus tendinitis) of local transdermal glyceryl trinitrate versus placebo.[57] The RCT did not report direct comparisons between the treatment and placebo groups (see comment below).

Harms: Headaches were reported in 20% of the treatment group 24 hours after the treatment was started (no comparative figures available).[57]

Comment: The RCT[57] found a significant decrease when comparing pain scores 24 hours after glyceryl trinitrate with pain scores measured at baseline (mean pain intensities with active treatment measured on a 0 to 10 analogue scale: 7.1 at baseline; 4.5 at 24 h, $P < 0.001$; 2.0 at 48 h, $P < 0.001$). Changes in the placebo group were not reported. Relief was maintained after 15 days (figures not available). Mean duration of pain was also significantly reduced with active treatment (figures not available). Mean mobility (assessor rated 4 point scale) significantly improved with active treatment (2.0 at baseline *v* 0.1 at 5 days; $P < 0.0001$), but not with placebo (1.2 at baseline *v* 1.2 at 15 days). The significance figures quoted are not direct comparisons. Significance figures for treatment versus placebo are not stated.

OPTION PHONOPHORESIS

One small RCT found no significant difference between phonophoresis versus placebo in pain or tenderness.

Benefits: We found no systematic review, but found one RCT.[58] The RCT (24 people, 13 with rotator cuff tendinitis, 1 with biceps tendinitis, 1 triceps tendinitis, 9 with knee tendinitis) compared active phonophoresis (see glossary, p 1285) using topical dexamethasone, lidocaine, and aqueous gel versus placebo phonophoresis using aqueous gel only (5 sessions over 5–10 days). It found no significant difference in perceived pain (visual analogue scale [0 cm = no pain, 10 cm = extreme pain]; pain changed from 2.4 cm to 1.3 cm with active treatment *v* from 2.6 cm to 1.5 cm with placebo; not significant, but P value not stated). No significant effect was found in tenderness (localised force in ounces needed to elicit pain: 7.0, 95% CI 5.8 to 8.3 at session 1 to 7.2, 95% CI 6.0 to 8.4 at session 5 with active phonophoresis *v* 6.9, 95% CI 5.4 to 8.3 at session 1 to 8.8, 95% CI 7.8 to 9.7 at session 5 with placebo phonophoresis) (see table 3, p 1289).

Harms: Adverse effects were not reported.

Comment: None.

OPTION EXTRACORPOREAL SHOCK WAVE THERAPY

Limited evidence from one RCT suggests that extracorporeal shock wave therapy versus placebo may improve function in calcifying tendinitis.

Benefits: We found no systematic review but found one RCT with two parts.[59] The first compared three different extracorporeal shock wave therapy regimens (low energy treatment in a single session, a single high energy session, and 2 high energy sessions 1 wk apart) versus placebo in 80 people with calcifying tendinitis. It found that more people experienced subjective improvement of pain after high energy treatment than after low energy treatment or placebo (14/20 [70%] with 2 high energy sessions, 12/20 [60%] with 1 high energy session, 6/21 [29%] with low energy treatment, 0/20 with placebo; NNT 2 for high energy treatment compared with placebo, 95% CI 1 to 21 for single session and 1–14 for 2 session treatment). A combined measure of pain and function in activities of daily living (the Constant score) found significant improvement for both high energy groups versus the placebo group ($P < 0.0001$). The second part compared one versus two high energy sessions in 115 people with calcifying tendinitis (91 followed for 6 months). Fewer people experienced continued pain with two sessions than with a single session, but the result was not significant (23/49 [47%] with 2 sessions *v* 23/42 [55%] with 1 session; RR of continued pain 0.85, 95% CI 0.50 to 1.23). The difference in Constant scores after 6 months was also not significant.

Harms: High intensity extracorporeal shock wave therapy can be painful during treatment. Small haematoma were reported in the RCT, but the incidence was not stated and they could have been related to subcutaneous infiltration of local anaesthetic before treatment.[59]

Comment: The mechanism of action of extracorporeal shock wave therapy remains unclear. There was radiological disappearance or disintegration of calcium deposits in a significantly greater proportion of people who received high energy treatment than placebo; 77% of those receiving two sessions of treatment had radiological disappearance or disintegration of calcium deposits after 6 months compared with 47% who had one session (P = 0.05).

OPTION SURGERY

We found no evidence on most surgical interventions in shoulder pain. One small RCT found that forced manipulation was more effective in the short term management of frozen shoulder (3 months) than intra-articular injection of corticosteroid, although we found no placebo controlled trials.

Benefits: We found one RCT (30 people with frozen shoulder, 15 in each group).[60] It compared forced manipulation and intra-articular hydrocortisone injection versus intra-articular hydrocortisone injection alone. Manipulation and injection versus injection alone increased the number of people who completely recovered (no disability) at 3 months (7/15 [47%] *v* 2/15 [13%]; ARI 33%, 95% CI 1% to 65%).[60]

Harms: Adverse effects were not reported.

Comment: There is a need for RCTs of specific surgical interventions in people with specific shoulder disorders.

OPTION MULTIDISCIPLINARY BIOPSYCHOSOCIAL REHABILITATION

One systematic review found no evidence that multidisciplinary biopsychosocial rehabilitation was effective.

Benefits: We found one systematic review (search date 1998, 1 RCT and 1 controlled trial) of multidisciplinary biopsychosocial rehabilitation (see glossary, p 1285) for neck and shoulder pain among working age adults.[61] Neither trial used adequate methods, and neither found a significant difference with multidisciplinary biopsychosocial rehabilitation versus usual treatment.

Harms: No systematic review and no RCTs were found that specifically addressed this issue.

Comment: The review found that both trials had weak methods. The rehabilitation combined physiotherapy with psychological, behavioural, and educational interventions.

OPTION ARTHROSCOPIC LASER SUBACROMIAL DECOMPRESSION

One systematic review found no RCTs on arthroscopic laser treatment.

Benefits: We found one systematic review (search date 2000) of arthroscopic subacromial decompression with holmium : YAG laser for people with shoulder pain due to impingement syndrome.[62] It identified no RCTs and seven low quality observational studies.

Harms: We found no evidence of harms.

Comment: None.

GLOSSARY

Interferential electrical stimulation Typically a high frequency current (4000 Hz) amplitude modulated at a lower frequency (60–100 Hz) given in bursts of 4 seconds and repeated for up to 15 minutes.[48]
Maitland mobilisation A graded system of manipulations and exercises intended to increase mobility of specific joints.
Multidisciplinary biopsychosocial rehabilitation Combined physical, social, and psychological rehabilitation.
Phonophoresis The application of topical medication followed by ultrasound to the same area; the theory being that the ultrasound energy drives the medication through the skin.

REFERENCES

1. Royal College of General Practitioners; Office of Populations, Censuses and Surveys. Third National Morbidity Survey in General Practice, 1980–1981; Department of Health and Social Security, series MB5 No 1. London: HMSO.
2. Bergunnud H, Lindgarde F, Nilsson B, et al. Shoulder pain in middle age. *Clin Orthop* 1988;231:234–238.
3. McCormack RR, Inman RD, Wells A, et al. Prevalence of tendinitis and related disorders of the upper extremity in a manufacturing workforce. *J Rheumatol* 1990;17:958–964.
4. Allander E. Prevalence, incidence and remission rates of some common rheumatic diseases or syndromes. *Scand J Rheumatol* 1974;3:145–153.
5. Badley EM, Tennant A. Changing profile of joint disorders with age: findings from a postal survey of the population of Calderdale, West Yorkshire, UK. *Ann Rheum Dis* 1992;51:366–371.
6. Andersson HI, Ejlertsson G, Leden I, et al. Chronic pain in a geographically defined general population: studies of differences in age, gender, social class and pain localisation. *Clin J Pain* 1993;9:174–182.
7. Pope DP, Croft PR, Pritchard CM, et al. The frequency of restricted range of movement in individuals with self-reported shoulder pain: results from a population-based survey. *Br J Rheumatol* 1996:35;1137–1141.
8. Chard M, Hazleman R, Hazleman BL, et al. Shoulder disorders in the elderly: a community survey. *Arthritis Rheum* 1991;34:766–769.
9. Vecchio P, Kavanagh R, Hazleman BL, et al. Shoulder pain in a community-based rheumatology clinic. *Br J Rheumatol* 1995;34:440–442.
10. Lundberg B. The frozen shoulder. *Acta Orthop Scand* 1969:suppl 119.
11. Riordan J, Dieppe PA. Arthritis of the glenohumeral joint. *Baillieres Clin Rheumatol* 1989;3:607–626.
12. Bonutti PM, Hawkins RJ. Rotator cuff disorders. *Baillieres Clin Rheumatol* 1989;3:535–550.
13. Jobe FW, Kvitne RS. Shoulder pain in the overhand or throwing athlete: the relationship of anterior instability and rotator cuff impingement. *Orthop Rev* 1989;18:963–975.
14. Soslowsky LJ, An CH, Johnston SP, et al. Geometric and mechanical properties of the coracoacromial ligament and their relationship to rotator cuff disease. *Clin Orthop* 1994;304:10–17.
15. Nash P, Hazleman BL. Frozen shoulder. *Baillieres Clin Rheumatol* 1989;3:551–566.
16. Wohlgethan JR. Frozen shoulder in hyperthyroidism. *Arthritis Rheum* 1987;30:936–939.
17. Vecchio PC, Kavanagh RT, Hazleman BL, et al. Community survey of shoulder disorders in the elderly to assess the natural history and effects of treatment. *Ann Rheumatol Dis* 1995;54:152–154.
18. Croft P, Pope D, Silman A. The clinical course of shoulder pain: prospective cohort study in primary care. *BMJ* 1996;313:601–602.
19. Roach KE, Budiman-Mak E, Songsiridej N, et al. Development of a shoulder pain and disability index. *Arthritis Care Res* 1991;4:143–149.
20. Croft P, Pope D, Zonca M, et al. Measurement of shoulder related disability: results of a validation study. *Ann Rheum Dis* 1994;53:525–528.
21. Beaton DE, Richards RR. Measuring function of the shoulder. A cross-sectional comparison of five questionnaires. *J Bone Joint Surg Am* 1996;78;882–890.
22. Gerber C. Integrated scoring systems for the functional assessment of the shoulder. In: Matsen III FA, Fu EH, Hawkins RJ, eds. *The shoulder: a balance of mobility and stability.* Rosemont, Illinois, US: The American Academy of Orthopaedic Surgeons, 1993:531–550.
23. Richards RR, An KN, Bigliani LU, et al. A standardised method for the assessment of shoulder function. *J Shoulder Elbow Surg* 1994;3:347–352.
24. L'Insalata JC, Warren RF, Cohen SF, et al. A self-administered questionnaire for assessment of symptoms and function of the shoulder. *J Bone Joint Surg* 1997;79:738–748.
25. Green S, Buchbinder R, Glazier R, et al. Interventions for shoulder pain. In: The Cochrane Library, Issue 3, 2001. Oxford: Update Software. Search date 1998; primary sources Cochrane Musculoskeletal Group trials register, Cochrane Controlled Trials Register, Medline, Embase, Cinahl, and Science Citation Index, and hand searches of major textbooks, bibliographies of relevant literature, the fugitive literature, and the subject indices of relevant journals.

26. Van der Windt DAWM, Van der Heijden GJMG, Scholten RJPM, et al. The efficacy of non-steroidal anti-inflammatory drugs (NSAIDs) for shoulder complaints. A systematic review. *J Clin Epidemiol* 1995;48:691–704. Search date 1993; primary sources Medline and hand searched references.
27. Adejabo AO, Nash P, Hazleman BL. A prospective blind dummy placebo controlled study comparing triamcinolone hexacetonide injection with oral diclofenac 50 mg tds in patients with rotator cuff tendinitis. *J Rheumatol* 1990;17:1207–1210.
28. Petri M, Dobrow R, Neiman R, et al. Randomised double blind, placebo controlled study of the treatment of the painful shoulder. *Arthritis Rheum* 1987;30:1040–1045.
29. Mena HR, Lomen PL, Turner LF, et al. Treatment of acute shoulder syndrome with flurbiprofen. *Am J Med* 1986;80:141–144.
30. Auvinet B, Crielaard JM, Manteuffel GE, et al. A double-blind comparison of piroxicam fast-dissolving dosage form and diclofenac enteric-coated tablets in the treatment of patients with acute musculoskeletal disorders. *Curr Ther Res Clin Exp* 1995;56:1142–1153.
31. Itzkowitch D, Ginsberg F, Leon M, et al. Peri-articular injection of tenoxicam for painful shoulders: a double-blind, placebo controlled trial. *Clin Rheumatol* 1996;15:604–609.
32. Vecchio PC, Hazleman BL, King RH. A double-blind trial comparing subacromial methylprednisolone and lignocaine in acute rotator cuff tendinitis. *Br J Rheumatol* 1993;32:743–745.
33. Berry H, Fernandes L, Bloom B, et al. Clinical study comparing acupuncture, physiotherapy, injection and oral anti-inflammatory therapy in the shoulder. *Curr Med Res Opin* 1980;7:121–126.
34. Rizk T, Pinals R, Talaiver A. Corticosteroid injections in adhesive capsulitis: investigation of their value and site. *Arch Phys Med* 1991;72:20–22.
35. Snels IA, Beckerman H, Twisk JW, et al. Effect of triamcinolone acetonide injections on hemiplegic shoulder pain: a randomized clinical trial. *Stroke* 2000;31:2396–2401.
36. De Jong BA, Dahmen R, Hogeweg JA, et al. Intra-articular triamcinolone acetonide injection in patients with capsulitis of the shoulder: a comparative study of two dose regimens. *Clin Rehabil* 1998;12:211–215.
37. Bulgen D, Binder A, Hazleman B, et al. Frozen shoulder: prospective clinical study with an evaluation of three treatment regimes. *Ann Rheum Dis* 1984;43:353–360.
38. Richardson AT. The painful shoulder. *Proc R Soc Med* 1975;68:11–16.
39. Gam AN, Schydlowsky P, Rossel I, et al. Treatment of "frozen shoulder" with distension and glucocorticoid compared with glucocorticoid alone. *Scand J Rheumatol* 1998;27:425–430.
40. Gray RG, Gottlieb NL. Intra-articular corticosteroids. An updated assessment. *Clin Orth* 1983;177:235–263.
41. Hollander JL. The use of intra-articular hydrocortisone, its analogues, and its higher esters in arthritis. *Md Med J* 1970;61:511.
42. Van der Windt DA, Koes BW, Deville W, et al. Effectiveness of corticosteroid injections versus physiotherapy for treatment of painful stiff shoulder in primary care: randomised trial. *BMJ* 1998;317:1292–1296.
43. Eustace JA, Brophy DP, Gibney RP, et al. Comparison of the accuracy of steroid placement with clinical outcome in patients with shoulder symptoms. *Ann Rheum Dis* 1997;56:59–63.
44. Jones A, Regan M, Ledingham J, et al. Importance of placement of intra-articular steroid injections. *BMJ* 1993;307:1329–1330.
45. Blockey N, Wright J. Oral cortisone therapy in periarthritis of the shoulder. *BMJ* 1954;i:1455–1457.
46. Binder A, Hazleman BL, Parr G, et al. A controlled study of oral prednisolone in frozen shoulder. *Br J Rheum* 1986;25:288–292.
47. Van der Windt DAWM, Van der Heijden GJMG, Van der Berg SGM, et al. Ultrasound therapy for musculoskeletal disorders: a systematic review. *Pain* 1999;81:257–271. Search date 1997; primary sources Medline, Embase, and Cochrane Database of Randomised Clinical Trials.
48. Van der Heijden GJMG, Leffers P, Wolters PJMC, et al. No effect of bipolar interferential electrotherapy and pulsed ultrasound for soft tissue shoulder disorders: a randomised controlled trial. *Ann Rheum Dis* 1999;58:530–540.
49. Ebenbichler GR, Erdogmus CB, Resch KL, et al. Ultrasound therapy for calcific tendinitis of the shoulder. *N Engl J Med* 1999;340:1533–1588.
50. Vecchio P, Cave C, King V, et al. A double blind study of the effectiveness of low level laser treatment of rotator cuff tendinitis. *Br J Rheumatol* 1993;32:740–742.
51. Gudmundssen J, Vikne J. Laser treatment for epicondylitis humeri and rotator cuff syndrome. *Nord Tidskr Idrettsmed* 1987;2:6–15.
52. England S, Farrell A, Coppock Jet al. Low laser therapy of shoulder tendonitis. *Scand J Rheumatol* 1989;18:427–443.
53. Saunders L. The efficacy of low level laser therapy in supraspinatus tendinitis. *Clin Rehabil* 1995;9:126–134.
54. Binder A, Parr G, Hazleman B. Pulsed electromagnetic field therapy of persistent rotator cuff tendonitis. *Lancet* 1984;1:695–698.
55. Price CI, Pandyan AD. Electrical stimulation for preventing and treating post-stroke shoulder pain. In: The Cochrane Library, Issue 3, 2001. Oxford: Update Software. Search date 1999; primary sources Medline, Cinahl, Cochrane Controlled Trials Register, and Embase.
56. Gado I, Emery P. Intra-articular guanethidine injection for resistant shoulder pain: a preliminary double blind study of a novel approach. *Ann Rheum Dis* 1996;55:199–201.
57. Berrazueta JR, Losada A, Poveda J, et al. Successful treatment of shoulder pain syndrome due to supraspinatus tendinitis with transdermal nitroglycerin. A double blind study. *Pain* 1996;66:63–67.
58. Penderghest CE, Kimura IF, Gulick DT. Double-blind clinical efficacy study of pulsed phonophoresis on perceived pain associated with symptomatic tendinitis. *J Sport Rehab* 1998;7:9–19.
59. Loew M, Daecke W, Kusnierczak D, et al. Shock-wave therapy is effective for chronic calcifying tendinitis of the shoulder. *J Bone Joint Surg Br* 1999;81:863–867.
60. Thomas D, Williams R, Smith D. The frozen shoulder. A review of manipulative treatment. *Rheumatol Rehab* 1980;19:173–179.
61. Karjalainen K, Malmivaara A, van Tulder M, et al. Multidisciplinary biopsychosocial rehabilitation for neck and shoulder pain among working age adults. In: The Cochrane Library, Issue 3, 2001. Oxford: Update Software. Search date 1998; primary sources Medline, Embase, Cochrane Library, Medic (Finnish medical database), Science Citation Index, and hand searches of reference lists and contact with 24 experts in the field of rehabilitation.

62. Boult M, Wicks M, Watson DI, et al. Arthroscopic Subacromial Decompression with a holmium : YAG laser: review of the literature. *ANZ J Surg* 2001;71:172–177. Search date 2000; primary sources Medline, Embase, Current Contents, and The Cochrane Library.

Cathy Speed
Rheumatologist/Director of Sports and Exercise Medicine Unit

Brian Hazleman
Senior Consultant

Addenbrooke's Hospital
Cambridge
UK

Competing interests: None declared.

TABLE 1 Intra-articular corticosteroid injections (see text, p 1277).

Ref	Pain scale	People	Corticosteroid		Placebo		Duration	P
			Before	After	Before	After		
Pain relief								
33	10 cm VAS	24	3.9	2.7	5.2	2.2	4 wks	> 0.05
34	6 point scale: 0 = no pain, 5 = extreme pain	30	3.9	3.2	4.1	3.0	24 wks	> 0.05
35	Pain score decrease (score range 0–10)	37	2.3		0.2		3 wks	0.06
Abduction								
33	Decrease abduction	24	86	101	92	121	4 wks	> 0.05
34	Decrease of shoulder movement	30	303	351	300	347	24 wks	> 0.05
35	Median improvement passive external rotation	37	2.5°		0°		3 wks	0.71

ref, reference; VAS, visual analogue scale.

TABLE 2 **Ultrasound (see text, p 1279).**

	Score change	Ultrasound (95% CI)	Sham (95% CI)	P
6 weeks				
Improvement in pain	Change in 15 point pain score	6.4 (5.1 to 7.7)	1.6 (0.01 to 3.1)	0.001
Change in quality of life	Change in 10 cm VAS	2.6 (1.7 to 3.6)	0.4 (0.6 to 1.4)	0.002
Change in function	Change in total constant score	17.8 (12.0 to 23.8)	+3.7 (–3.3 to +10.7)	0.002
9 months				
Improvement in pain	Change in 15 point pain score	5.7 (4.0 to 7.3)	4.0 (1.8 to 6.2)	0.23
Change in quality of life	Change in 10 cm VAS	2.4 (1.2 to 3.5)	1.9 (0.8 to 2.9)	0.52
Change in function	Change in total constant score	15.7 (8.5 to 22 .9)	12.4 (4.8 to 19.9)	0.52

VAS, visual analogue scale.

TABLE 3 **Phonophoresis (see text, p 1283).**

	Phonophoresis (95% CI)		Placebo (95% CI)	
Outcome	**Before**	**After**	**Before**	**After**
Pain (10 cm VAS)	2.4 (1.5 to 3.3)	1.3 (0.7 to 1.9)	2.6 (1.4 to 3.8)	1.5 (0.77 to 2.3)
Punctate tenderness (localised force in ounces needed to elicit pain)	7.0 (5.8 to 8.0)	7.2 (6.0 to 8.4)	6.9 (5.4 to 8.3)	8.8 (7.8 to 9.7)

VAS, visual analogue scale.

Tennis elbow (lateral epicondylitis)

Search date August 2002

Willem Assendelft, Sally Green, Rachelle Buchbinder, Peter Struijs, and Nynke Smidt

QUESTIONS

INTERVENTIONS

See glossary, p 1299

Key Messages

- **Acupuncture** One systematic review and one subsequent RCT found insufficient evidence to assess the effects of acupuncture (either needle or laser).
- **Corticosteroid injections** We found one systematic review and two subsequent RCTs of corticosteroid injections, which found limited evidence of a short term improvement in symptoms with steroid injections versus placebo, a local anaesthetic, elbow strapping, or physiotherapy. It found no good evidence on long term effects of corticosteroids versus placebo or local anaesthetic. It found no evidence of a difference with corticosteroid injection versus mobilisation plus massage or versus elbow strapping in overall improvement at 1 year. However, one RCT identified by the review found significantly greater improvement in symptoms with physiotherapy versus an injection at 26 and 52 weeks. The review found limited evidence of greater self perceived improvement at 4 weeks with corticosteroid injection versus an oral non-steroidal anti-inflammatory drug (NSAID), but found greater improvement in pain at 26 weeks with an oral NSAID.
- **Exercise and mobilisation** One systematic review found limited evidence of a better outcome with exercise versus ultrasound plus friction massage at 8 weeks.
- **Extra-corporeal shock wave therapy** One systematic review found conflicting evidence from two RCTs of the effects on symptoms of extra-corporeal shock wave therapy versus sham treatment.
- **Non-steroidal anti-inflammatory drugs for longer term pain relief** We found insufficient evidence to assess the longer term effects of oral or topical NSAID.

Clin Evid 2002;8:1290–1300.

- **Oral NSAIDs** One systematic review found limited evidence of a short term improvement in pain and function with an oral NSAID versus placebo. The review found limited evidence that fewer people receiving an oral NSAID versus a corticosteroid injection had self perceived improvement at 4 weeks, but found that an oral NSAID significantly reduced pain at 26 weeks. We found insufficient evidence to assess the longer term effects of oral or topical NSAIDs.
- **Orthoses** One systematic review found insufficient evidence about the effects of orthoses (braces).
- **Surgery** One systematic review found no RCTs of surgical treatment for tennis elbow.
- **Topical non-steroidal anti-inflammatory drugs for short term pain relief** One systematic review has found that topical non-steroidal anti-inflammatory drugs versus placebo significantly improve pain in the short term. Minor adverse effects have been reported. We found no RCTs comparing oral versus topical non-steroidal anti-inflammatory drugs.

DEFINITION Tennis elbow has many analogous terms, including lateral elbow pain, lateral epicondylitis, rowing elbow, tendonitis of the common extensor origin, and peritendonitis of the elbow. Tennis elbow is characterised by pain and tenderness over the lateral epicondyle of the humerus and pain on resisted dorsi-flexion of the wrist, middle finger, or both. For the purposes of this review, tennis elbow is restricted to lateral elbow pain or lateral epicondylitis.

INCIDENCE/ PREVALENCE Lateral elbow pain is common (population prevalence 1–3%).[1] Peak incidence is 40–50 years, and for women of 42–46 years of age the incidence increases to 10%.[2,3] The incidence of lateral elbow pain in general practice is 4–7/1000 people a year.[3–5]

AETIOLOGY/ RISK FACTORS Tennis elbow is considered to be an overload injury, typically after minor and often unrecognised trauma of the extensor muscles of the forearm. Despite the title tennis elbow, tennis is a direct cause in only 5% of those with epicondylitis.[6]

PROGNOSIS Although lateral elbow pain is generally self limiting, in a minority of people symptoms persist for 18 months to 2 years and in some cases for much longer.[7] The cost is therefore high, both in terms of lost productivity and healthcare use. In a general practice trial of an expectant waiting policy, 80% of the people with elbow pain of already greater than 4 weeks' duration were recovered after 1 year.[8]

AIMS To reduce lateral elbow pain and improve function.

OUTCOMES Pain at rest, with activities and resisted movements (visual analogue scale or Likert scale); function (validated disability questionnaire, includes 30 point Disabilities of the Arm, Shoulder, and Hand questionnaire, or visual analogue scale or Likert scale); quality of life (validated questionnaire); grip strength (dynamometer); return to work, normal activities, or both; overall participant reported improvement; adverse effects (participant or researcher report); Roles-Maudsley subjective pain score where 1 = excellent, no pain, full movement, full activity; 2 = good, occasional discomfort, full movement and full activity; 3 = fair, some discomfort after prolonged activity; and 4 = poor, pain limiting activities.

METHODS *Clinical Evidence* search and appraisal August 2002. Studies were included based on the criteria: all randomised and quasi-RCTs of any of the listed interventions in (1) people older than 16 years of age; (2) lateral elbow pain for greater than 3 weeks' duration; (3) no history of significant trauma or systemic inflammatory conditions such as rheumatoid arthritis; and (4) studies of various soft tissue diseases and pain due to tendinitis at all sites, were included provided that the lateral elbow pain results were presented separately or that greater than 90% of people had lateral elbow pain.

QUESTION What are the effects of treatments for reducing pain and improving function in tennis elbow (lateral epicondylitis)? New

OPTION ACUPUNCTURE

Sally E Green and Rachelle Buchbinder

One systematic review and one subsequent RCT found insufficient evidence to assess the effects of acupuncture (either needle or laser).

Benefits: We found one systematic review (search date 2001, 4 RCTs, 239 people with tennis elbow defined as lateral elbow pain aggravated by wrist and finger dorsiflexion)[9] and one subsequent RCT.[10] The review found that, because of problems with methods of the included trials (particularly small populations, uncertain allocation concealment, and substantial loss to follow up) and clinical differences between trials, results could not be combined in a meta-analysis. The first RCT (48 people) comparing needle acupuncture versus sham acupuncture (with needles not inserted) found significantly longer pain relief with acupuncture (WMD 18.8 h, 95% CI 10.1 to 27.5) and a significantly increased proportion of people with greater than or equal to 50% reduction in pain after one treatment (19/24 [79%] with acupuncture *v* 6/24 [25%] with sham treatment; RR 3.2, 95% 1.5 to 6.5).[11] The second RCT found needle acupuncture versus sham treatment significantly increased the proportion of people with a self reported good or excellent result (22/44 [50%] with needle acupuncture *v* 8/38 [21%] with sham treatment; RR 2.4, 95% CI 1.2 to 4.7) after 10 treatments. However, it found no significant differences in the longer term (after 3 or 12 months).[12] The third RCT compared laser (see glossary, p 1299) acupuncture versus sham treatment. It found no significant difference in participant report of no improvement or worse (after 10 sessions: 13/23 [56.5%] with laser *v* 9/26 [34.6%] with sham treatment, RR 1.36, 95% CI 0.48 to 3.86; at 3 months: 0.38, 95% CI 0.09 to 1.69; after 12 months: 3.47, 95% CI 0.15 to 80.36). The fourth RCT found no significant difference in cure rate (method of defining cure not defined) between vitamin B12 injection plus acupuncture versus vitamin B12 injection alone (risk of cure with B12 injection alone: RR 0.44, 95% CI 0.15 to 1.29). The subsequent RCT (45 people) compared 10 treatments of acupuncture versus sham acupuncture.[10] It found significantly greater reductions in pain intensity and functional impairment with acupuncture versus sham treatment at 2 weeks (on 30 mm visual analogue scale pain improved by 8.43 with acupuncture *v* 4.89 with sham treatment, $P < 0.05$; Disabilities of the Arm, Shoulder, and Hand questionnaire improved by 23.70 with acupuncture *v* 8.54 with sham treatment, $P < 0.05$). At 2 months, only the difference for functional impairment was significant. We found no RCT on the effect of acupuncture on quality of life, strength, or return to work.

Harms: The RCTs identified by the review did not report on adverse events.[9]

Comment: Although statistically significant, an increase of 18 hours in pain relief after needle acupuncture may not be clinically important.[9]

OPTION ORTHOSES (BRACING)

Willem JJ Assendelft and Peter AA Struijs

One systematic review found insufficient evidence about the effects of orthoses (braces).

Benefits: We found one systematic review (search date 1999).[13] Results were not pooled because of large heterogeneity among trials. **Versus placebo or no treatment:** The review identified no RCTs.[13] We found no subsequent RCTs. **Versus corticosteroid injections:** The review found two RCTs comparing orthoses versus corticosteroid injections.[13] The first RCT (16 people) compared an orthotic device versus corticosteroid injections. It found no significant difference in short term improvement in pain (improvement: 27.1 with corticosteroid *v* 13.6 with orthotic device; 100 mm visual analogue score difference +13.5, 95% CI 4.6 to +31.6).[13] The second RCT (70 people, 4 treatment groups) found that corticosteroid injection versus a splint or elbow band significantly increased the proportion of people having a good or excellent self reported outcome at 2 weeks (AR 34/37 [92%] pooled results for splint and elbow band group *v* 6/19 [32%] with injection; RR 2.9; 95% CI 1.8 to 5.7); however, the difference was not significant in the medium or long term (6 months: 19/37 [51%] *v* 14/19 [74%]; RR 0.7, 95% CI 0.46 to 1.05; 12 months: 22/37 [59%] *v* 13/19 [68%]; RR 0.9, 95% CI 0.6 to 1.03).[13] **Versus physiotherapy:** The review found one RCT (84 people) comparing an elbow support versus an unspecified physical therapy.[13] It found no significant difference in short term self reported satisfaction (23/49 [47%] with elbow support *v* 16/35 [46%] with unspecified physical therapy; RR 1.03; 95% CI 0.64 to 1.64). This study had insufficient information to assess pain improvement. It also had a withdrawal rate of 30% and results seem to be completor analysis. **Versus non-steroidal anti-inflammatory cream:** The review found 1 RCT (17 people) comparing a non-steroidal anti-inflammatory cream (AI cream; details of cream not provided in review) versus an elbow strap.[13] It found greater short term pain reduction with AI cream (WMD [scale not specified] 0.38, 95% CI 0.02 to 0.70).

Harms: The systematic review did not report on harms.[13]

Comment: The review reported that validity scores for the RCTs ranged from low to medium.[13] The review identified three RCTs comparing adding an orthotic device to corticosteroid injections or ultrasound. All three RCTs reported only short term results and there was insufficient data or too low power to indicate the effect of orthoses.

OPTION CORTICOSTEROID INJECTIONS

Willem JJ Assendelft and Nynke Smidt

One systematic review and two subsequent RCTs of corticosteroid injections found limited evidence of a short term improvement in symptoms with steroid injections versus placebo, a local anaesthetic, elbow strapping, or physiotherapy. It found no good evidence on long term effects of corticosteroids versus placebo or local anaesthetic. It found no evidence of a difference with corticosteroid injection versus mobilisation plus massage or elbow strapping in overall improvement at 1 year. However, one RCT identified by the review found significantly greater improvement in symptoms with physiotherapy versus an injection at 26 and 52 weeks. The review found limited evidence of greater self perceived improvement at 4 weeks with corticosteroid injections versus an oral non-steroidal anti-inflammatory drug, but found greater improvement in pain at 26 weeks with an oral non-steroidal anti-inflammatory drug.

Benefits: We found one systematic review (search date 1999)[14] and two subsequent RCTs.[15,16] **Versus placebo or no treatment:** The review identified two RCTs comparing steroid injection (1 mL methylprednisolone acetate) versus saline solution. The first RCT (29 people in smallest group) found a significantly lower chance of short term (not specified) global improvement with the placebo (RR 0.11, 95% CI 0.04 to 0.33). The RCT did not measure pain or grip strength. The second RCT (10 people in smallest group) found no significant difference in short term pain, global improvement, or grip strength. We found one subsequent RCT (39 people with symptoms > 4 wks) of corticosteroid injection versus a control injection.[15] All people received rehabilitation. It found that cotricosteroid injection significantly improved pain on a visual analogue scale from 8 weeks to 6 months (100 point visual analogue scale improvement: 24.3 with steroid injection *v* 8.9 with control injection; P = 0.04; CI not available). It found no significant difference in other pain outcomes or grip strength. We found one subsequent RCT (59 people in smallest group) of a corticosteroid injection versus no treatment versus physiotherapy.[16] It found corticosteroid injection versus no treatment significantly improved mean "main complaint" and functional disability at 3 and 6 weeks (at 6 wk mean difference in "main complaint" 24%, 95% CI 14% to 35%). It found no significant difference at 12, 26, and 52 weeks, and the mean was non-significantly worse with steroid injection at 26 and 52 weeks (at 52 wk mean difference in "main complaint" –9%, 95% CI –19% to +2%). **Versus local anaesthetic:** The review identified three RCTs comparing corticosteroid injections versus local anaesthetic alone.[14] Two RCTs (18 and 35 people in smallest groups) found an improvement in short term (4 wks; follow up not stated) global improvement with corticosteroid injections (1 mL hydrocortisone acetate 25 mg and 1 mL methylprednisolone acetate 10 mg), but data could not be pooled because of heterogeneity. The third small RCT (7 people smallest group) only reported medium term results. It found no significant difference in global improvement at 9–17 weeks (chance of not getting a good outcome: RR 0.97, 95% CI 0.41 to 2.32). **Versus elbow support:** See benefits of orthoses, p 1293. **Versus physiotherapies:** The review identified two RCTs

(53 and 12 people in smallest group) comparing corticosteroid injections (1 mL triamcinolone acetate 1% plus 1 mL lidocaine [lignocaine]) versus physiotherapies, and we found one additional RCT.[16] The first RCT (53 people in smallest group) found a significantly lower chance of an overall improvement with friction massage and a manipulation technique versus steroid injection (RR 0.45, 95% CI 0.29 to 0.69), and improvement in pain and grip strength. At 52 weeks, there was no significant difference for any outcome. The review was unable to report measured results for the second RCT. The additional RCT (59 people in smallest group) compared a corticosteroid injection versus no treatment versus physiotherapy (see *v* placebo or no treatment above).[16] It found injection versus physiotherapy (consisting of 9 sessions of ultrasound, deep friction massage, and exercise programme over 6 wk) significantly improved the "main complaint" and functional disability at 3 and 6 weeks (at 6 wks mean difference in "main complaint" 20%, 95% CI 10% to 31%). However, there was no significant difference at 12 weeks, and at 26 and 52 weeks physiotherapy versus injection significantly improved the "main complaint" (at 52 wks mean difference in "main complaint" 15%, 95% CI 5% to 25%). **Versus non-steroidal anti-inflammatory drugs:** See oral non-steroidal anti-inflammatory drugs versus corticosteroids, p 1296. We found no RCTs on the effect of corticosteroid injections on quality of life or return to work.

Harms: The review (8 RCTs) found no significant difference in adverse events between corticosteroid injections and control interventions (including facial flushes, post-injection pain, and local skin atrophy).[14] However, the review did not report measured results.

Comment: The review found that in the longer term there was a high rate of improvement in all groups.[14] It found that in general the quality of the methods of RCTs was poor to modest. The review provided the number of people in the smallest group for each trial rather than the total number of people in the trial. The corticosteroid suspensions used in these trials were methylprednisolone (2 RCTs), triamcinolone (4 RCTs), betamethasone (2 RCTs), hydrocortisone (5 RCTs), and dexamethasone (1 RCT). In one RCT, two different substances were used. The RCTs with longer term results of corticosteroid versus non-steroidal anti-inflammatory drugs and versus physiotherapy suggested that a steroid injection improved outcomes in the short term but increased recurrences in the medium term.

OPTION NON-STEROIDAL ANTI-INFLAMMATORY DRUGS

Sally E Green and Rachelle Buchbinder

One systematic review has found that topical non-steroidal anti-inflammatory drugs (NSAIDs) versus placebo significantly improve pain in the short term. Minor adverse effects have been reported. We found no RCTs comparing oral versus topical NSAIDs. One systematic review found limited evidence of a short term improvement in pain and function with an oral NSAID versus placebo. We found insufficient evidence to assess the longer term effects of NSAIDs. One systematic

review found limited evidence that fewer people receiving an oral NSAID versus a corticosteroid injection had self perceived improvement at 4 weeks, but found that an oral NSAID significantly reduced pain at 26 weeks.

Benefits: **Topical non-steroidal anti-inflammatory drugs versus placebo:** We found one systematic review (search date 2001, 3 RCTs, 130 people).[17] It found that topical non-steroidal anti-inflammatory drugs (NSAIDs) improved pain at up to 4 weeks significantly more than placebo (WMD −1.88, −2.54 to −1.21; scale 0 [no pain] to 10 [maximum pain]) and significantly reduced participant opinion of no benefit (2 RCTs; RR 0.39, 0.23 to 0.66). Inclusion of unblinded trials did not significantly change the results. It found no significant differences between topical NSAIDs and placebo for grip strength (reported as non-significant, further data not provided), or range of motion (RR for limitation of movement 1.01, 95% CI 0.80 to 1.28). It found an improvement in doctor's opinion of effect (RR for poor opinion of effect 0.61, 95% CI 0.37 to 0.99), and in tenderness with NSAIDs versus placebo, which just reached significance (RR for tenderness 0.83, 95% CI 0.70 to 0.99). The topical NSAIDs used were diclofenac (2 RCTs) and benzydamine (1 RCT). **Oral NSAIDs versus placebo:** We found one systematic review (search date 2001, 2 RCTs).[17] The RCTs were not pooled because one reported means and standard deviations and the other medians and ranges. One RCT of diclofenac versus placebo found limited evidence of a short term benefit in pain and function (WMD −13.9, 95% CI −23.2 to −4.6 on 100 point scale), but did not assess long term results. The second RCT found no significant difference in pain over 28 days (median [range] pain score at 4 wks, 4 [2–6] with naproxen *v* 3.5 [2–6] with placebo), or at 6 months or at 1 year (median [range] pain at 6 months: 1 [0–3] with NSAIDs *v* 1 [0–2.2] with placebo; at 12 months: 0 [0–2] with NSAIDs *v* 0 [0–2] with placebo), or for function (at 6 months: 0 [0–2.75] with NSAIDs *v* 0.5 [0–2] with placebo; at 12 months: 1 [0–1] with NSAIDs *v* 0 [0–0] with placebo). **Oral NSAIDs versus corticosteroid injection:** We found one systematic review (search date 2001, 3 RCTs).[17] Only two RCTs were included in the meta-analysis because of incomplete reporting of results. The first of these RCTs compared 20 mg methylprednisolone plus lidocaine versus 500 mg naproxen, and the second compared 6 mg betamethasone plus prilocaine plus placebo tablets versus 500 mg naproxen (initial high dose, then 250 mg). Meta-analysis of self reported perception of benefit found a significant difference in favour of injection at 4 weeks (RR of participant perceived benefit of injection 3.06, 95% CI 1.55 to 6.06). One RCT was not included in the meta-analysis because of skewed data; it found less functional limitation at 4 weeks in the injection group (median [range] 0 [0–2] with injection *v* 3 [1–5] with NSAIDs). The greater benefit of injection versus naproxen was only found in the short term. The largest RCT (53 people in smallest group) found significantly greater chance of improvement in pain at 26 weeks with a NSAID (RR 1.71, 95% CI 1.17 to 2.51). It found no significant difference in grip strength and results were not reported for global improvement. We found no RCTs investigating the effect of NSAIDs (either topical or oral) on return to work or quality of life.

Harms: **Topical NSAIDs:** One RCT found a significantly increased risk of any adverse event with NSAIDs versus placebo (RR 2.26, 95% CI 1.04 to 4.94).[18] Adverse effects were mild and no one was withdrawn from the study. Adverse effects reported in the published trials were foul breath and minor skin irritation. **Oral NSAIDs:** One trial of oral NSAIDs found an increased risk of abdominal pain (RR 3.17, 95% CI 1.35 to 7.41) and diarrhoea (RR 1.92, 95% CI 1.08 to 3.14). One systematic review (search date 1994, 12 RCTs of NSAIDs in a variety of disorders)[19] found the overall relative risk of complications from oral NSAIDs was 3.0–5.0. Adverse effects were predominantly gastrointestinal. See important differences between available NSAIDs under the NSAIDs topic, p 1205.

Comment: Both topical and oral NSAIDs may provide short term relief of pain in tennis elbow, although topical NSAIDs may be associated with less adverse effects. Further placebo controlled and comparative trials of oral versus topical NSAIDs would help clarify the effects of NSAIDs in the treatment of tennis elbow. Few trials used intention to treat analysis, and the sample size of most was small (populations range from 18–128 people for trials included in the meta-analysis).

OPTION EXERCISE AND MOBILISATION

Willem JJ Assendelft and Nynke Smidt

We found limited evidence from one systematic review of a better outcome with exercise versus ultrasound plus friction massage.

Benefits: We found one systematic review (search date 1999, 1 RCT, 19 people).[20] It found one small RCT, which found a significant improvement in symptoms at 8 weeks with exercise versus ultrasound plus friction massage (SMD –0.95, 95% CI –1.64 to –0.26). Four other RCTs were either of poor validity or provided insufficient data on relevant outcome measures.

Harms: In the systematic review no harms were described.[20]

Comment: None.

OPTION EXTRA-CORPOREAL SHOCK WAVE THERAPY

Rachelle Buchbinder and Sally E Green

One systematic review found conflicting evidence from two RCTs about the effects of extra-corporeal shock wave therapy versus sham treatment.

Benefits: We found one systematic review (search date 2001, 2 RCT, 286 people).[21] Both RCTs included similar study populations (mean age 41.9–46.9 years, slightly more women) with chronic symptoms (mean duration 21.9–27.6 months) who had not improved on at least 6 months of conservative treatment, including non-steroidal anti-inflammatory drugs, injections, brace or taping, casting, and physiotherapy. The frequency, doses, and technique of extra-corporeal shock wave therapy (ESWT) application were similar in both trials. In one RCT, the active treatment consisted of 1000 impulses of 0.08 mJ/mm^2 of ESWT at weekly intervals for 3 weeks.[21] The second RCT used "low energy" ESWT with 2000 pulses under local anaesthesia (3 mL mepivacaine 1%) at weekly intervals for 3 weeks using device dependent energy flux density ED+ between 0.07 and 0.09 mJ/mm^2.[21] The review found no significant difference in the risk of treatment failure (defined as Roles-Maudsley subjective pain score of 4) with ESWT versus placebo (6 wks: RR 0.40, 95% CI, 0.08 to 1.91, 1 year: RR 0.44, 95% CI, 0.09 to 2.17 at 1 year). After 6 weeks, it found no significant improvement in pain at rest (WMD pain out of 100, –11.4, 95% CI –26.1 to +3.3), pain with resisted wrist extension (WMD pain out of 100, –16.2, 95% CI –47.8 to +15.4), or pain with resisted middle finger extension (WMD pain out of 100, –20.5, 95% CI –56.6 to +15.6). Combined longer term results (1 measured at 12 wks and 1 at 24 wks) found no significant difference in improvement of pain at rest (WMD pain out of 100, –14.7, 95% CI –35.4 to +6.1), pain with resisted wrist extension (WMD pain out of 100, –14.7, 95% CI –43.4 to +14.0), and pain with resisted middle finger extension (WMD pain out of 100, –21.1, 95% CI –58.3 to +16.1). The effect of ESWT on function, quality of life, and return to work was not reported. The effect of ESWT on grip strength was reported in both trials but the results were difficult to interpret in one RCT. The other RCT found no difference in improvement in grip strength between groups at 6 weeks, 12 weeks, or 1 year.

Harms: One RCT in the review did not report adverse events.[21] The other RCT reported significantly more adverse effects in the EWST group compared with placebo (OR 4.3, 95% CI 2.9 to 6.3). However, there were no treatment discontinuations or dosage adjustments related to adverse effects. The most frequently reported adverse effects in the ESWT treated group were transitory reddening of the skin (21.1% with ESWT *v* 4.7% with placebo); pains (4.8% with ESWT *v* 1.7% with placebo); and petechiae, bleeding, or haematomas (4.5% with ESWT *v* 1.7% with placebo). Migraine occurred in four people and syncope in three people after ESWT compared with no people treated with placebo.

Comment: Two placebo controlled trials of ESWT for chronic lateral elbow pain have yielded conflicting results.[21] When data from both trials are pooled, the benefits observed in the first trial are no longer apparent. This RCT, which found a significant improvement, had uncertain allocation concealment and no analysis of early withdrawals (15/115 [13%]). Further well designed trials are needed to clarify whether ESWT is of value for lateral elbow pain.

OPTION SURGERY

Rachelle Buchbinder and Sally E Green

One systematic review found no RCTs of surgical treatment.

Benefits: We found one systematic review (search date 2001), which identified no RCTs.[22] We found no subsequent RCTs.

Harms: We found no RCTs.

Comment: Various open and percutaneous operations for lateral elbow pain have been described based upon the surgeon's concept of the pathological entity. The most commonly described surgical procedures involve excision of abnormal tissue (comprising microscopic degeneration, rupture, or both, and immature repairative tissue) within the origin of extensor carpi radialis brevis, release of the extensor carpi radialis brevis from the lateral epicondyle region, or both. Additional procedures include release of the anterior capsule, removal of inflamed synovial folds, resection of a third of the orbicular ligament, debridement of articular damage, release of the posterior interosseous nerve, denervation of the lateral epicondyle, denervation of the radiohumeral joint, and excision of a radio-humeral bursa.[23–35]

GLOSSARY

Laser A source of light with a narrow, almost monochromatic, coherent light bundle. It contains a relative high energy intensity.

REFERENCES

1. Allander E. Prevalence, incidence and remission rates of some common rheumatic diseases and syndromes. *Scand J Rheumatol* 1974;3:145–153.
2. Chard MD, Hazleman BL. Tennis elbow – a reappraisal. *Br J Rheumatol* 1989;28:186–190.
3. Verhaar J. Tennis elbow: anatomical, epidemiological and therapeutic aspects. *Int Orthop* 1994;18:263–267.
4. Hamilton P. The prevalence of humeral epicondylitis: a survey in general practice. *J R Coll Gen Pract* 1986;36:464–465.
5. Kivi P. The etiology and conservative treatment of lateral epicondylitis. *Scand J Rehabil Med* 1983;15:37–41.
6. Murtagh J. Tennis elbow. *Aust Fam Physician* 1988;17:90,91,94,95.
7. Hudak P, Cole D, Haines T. Understanding prognosis to improve rehabilitation: the example of lateral elbow pain. *Arch Phys Rehabil* 1996;77:568–593.
8. Smidt N, van der Windt DAWM, Assendelft WJJ, et al. Corticosteroid injections for lateral epicondylitis are superior to physiotherapy and a wait and see policy at short-term follow-up, but inferior at long-term follow-up: results from a randomised controlled trial. *Lancet* 2002;359:657–662.
9. Green S, Buchbinder R, Barnsley L, et al. Acupuncture for lateral elbow pain. In: The Cochrane Library, Issue 3, 2002. Oxford: Update Software. Search date 2001; primary sources Medline, Cinahl, Embase, Scisearch, Cochrane Controlled Trials Register, and Cochrane Musculoskeletal Review Group Specialised Trial Database.
10. Fink M, Wolkenstein E, Karst M, et al. Acupuncture in chronic epicondylitis: a randomized controlled trial. *Rheumatology* 2002;41:205–209.
11. Molsberger A, Hille E. The analgesic effect of acupuncture in chronic tennis elbow pain. *Br J Rheumatol* 1994;33:1162–1165.
12. Haker E, Lundberg T. Acupuncture treatment in epicondylalgia: a comparative study of two acupuncture techniques. *Clin J Pain* 1990;6:221–226.
13. Struijs PAA, Smidt N, Arola H, et al. Orthotic devices for the treatment of tennis elbow. In: The Cochrane Library, Issue 3, 2002. Oxford: Update Software. Search date 1999; primary sources Medline, Embase, Cinahl, Cochrane Controlled Trials Register, Current Contents, hand searches of reference lists from all retrieved articles, and personal contact with subject experts.
14. Smidt N, Assendelft WJJ, van der Windt DAWM, et al. Corticosteroid injections for lateral epicondylitis: a systematic review. *Pain* 2002;96:23–40. Search date 1999; primary sources Medline, Embase, Cinahl, Cochrane Controlled Trials Register, Current Contents, Cochrane Rehabilitation and Related Therapies Field Trials Register, and hand searches of references from retrieved articles.
15. Newcomber K, Laskowski E, Idank D, et al. Corticosteroid injection in early treatment of lateral epicondylitis. *Clin J Sport Med* 2001;11:214–222.
16. Smidt N, van der Windt D, Assendelft W, et al. Corticosteroid injections, physiotherapy, or a wait-and-see policy for lateral epicondylitis: a randomised controlled trial. *Lancet* 2002;359:657–662.
17. Green S, Buchbinder R, Barnsley L, et al. Non-steroidal anti-inflammatory drugs (NSAIDs) for treating lateral elbow pain in adults. In: The Cochrane Library, Issue 3, 2002. Oxford: Update Software. Search date 2001; primary sources Medline, Cinahl, Embase, Scisearch, Cochrane Musculoskeletal Review Group Specialised Trials Register, and Cochrane Controlled Trials Register.
18. Percy E, Carson J. The use of DMSO in tennis elbow and rotator cuff tendonitis: a double blind study. *Med Sci Sports Exerc* 1981;13:215–219.
19. Rodriguez LAG. Nonsteroidal antiinflammatory drugs, ulcers and risk: a collaborative meta-analysis. *Semin Arthritis Rheum* 1997;26:16–20. Search date 1994; primary sources Medline, hand searches of bibliographies of previous meta-analyses, and personal contact with authors of relevant studies.
20. Smidt N. Chapter 2. In: Smidt N. *Conservative treatments for tennis elbow in primary care* [thesis]. Waseningen: Ponsen and Looijen BV, 2001. Search date 1999; primary sources Medline, Embase, Cinahl, Cochrane Controlled Trials Register, Current Contents, Cochrane Rehabilitation and Related Therapies Field Trials Register, and hand searches of references from retrieved articles.
21. Buchbinder R, Green S, White M, et al. Shock wave therapy for lateral elbow pain. In: The Cochrane Library, Issue 3, 2002. Oxford: Update Software. Search date 2001; primary sources of Medline, Cinahl, Embase, Scisearch, Cochrane Controlled Trials Registrar, and Cochrane Musculoskeletal Review Group Specialised Trials Database.
22. Buchbinder R, Green S, Bell S, et al. Surgery for lateral elbow pain. In: The Cochrane Library, Issue 3, 2002. Oxford: Update Software. Search date 2001; primary sources Medline, Cinahl, Embase,

Scisearch, Cochrane Controlled Trials Registrar, and Cochrane Musculoskeletal Review Group Specialised Trials Database.
23. Bosworth DM. Surgical treatment of tennis elbow. A follow-up study. *J Bone Joint Surg Am* 1965;47:1533–1536.
24. Boyd HB, McLeod HC Jr. Tennis elbow. *J Bone Joint Surg Am* 1973;55:1183–1187.
25. Calvert PT, Macpherson IS, Allum RL, et al. Simple lateral release in treatment of tennis elbow. *J R Soc Med* 1985;78:912–915.
26. Coonrad RW, Hooper WR. Tennis elbow: its course, natural history, conservative and surgical management. *J Bone Joint Surg Am* 1973;55:1177–1182.
27. Friden J, Lieber R. Physiological consequences of surgical lengthening of extensor carpi radialis brevis muscle–tendon junction for tennis elbow. *J Hand Surg Am* 1994;19A:269–274.
28. Goldberg EJ, Abraham E, Siegel I. The surgical treatment of chronic lateral humeral epicondylitis by common extensor release. *Clin Orthop* 1988;233:208–212.
29. Kaplan EB. Treatment of tennis elbow (epicondylitis) by denervation. *J Bone Joint Surg Am* 1959;41:147–151.
30. Nirschl RP, Pettrone FA. The surgical treatment of lateral epicondylitis. *J Bone Joint Surg Am* 1979;61:832–839.
31. Posch JN, Goldberg VM, Larrey R. Extensor fasciotomy for tennis elbow: a long term follow-up study. *Clin Orthop* 1978;135:179–182.
32. Verhaar J, Walenkamp G, Kester A, et al. Lateral extensor release for tennis elbow. A prospective long-term follow-up study. *J Bone Joint Surg Am* 1993;75:1034–1043.
33. Wilhelm A. Tennis elbow: treatment of resistant cases by denervation. *J Hand Surg Br* 1996;21:523–533.
34. Wittenberg RH, Schaal S, Muhr G. Surgical treatment of persistent elbow epicondylitis. *Clin Orthop* 1992;278:73–80.
35. Yerger B, Turner T. Percutaneous extensor tenotomy for chronic tennis elbow. *Orthopedics* 1985;8:1261–1263.

Willem Assendelft
Head of Department of Guideline Development and Research Policy
Dutch College of General Practitioners
Utrecht
The Netherlands

Sally Green
Senior Lecturer
Institute of Health Services Research
Monash University
Melbourne
Australia

Rachelle Buchbinder
Director
Department of Clinical Epidemiology
Cabrini Hospital and Monash University
Department of Epidemiology and Preventive Medicine
Melbourne
Australia

Peter Struijs
Academic Medical Center
Amsterdam
The Netherlands

Nynke Smidt
Institute for Research in Extramural Medicine
Amsterdam
The Netherlands

Competing interests: The authors of this piece are the authors of the Cochrane Reviews from which most of the evidence is drawn. WJJ Assendelft has supervised and PAA Struijs has conducted a trial sponsored by Bauerfeind, a manufacturer of orthoses.

Bell's palsy

Search date March 2002

Rodrigo Salinas

QUESTIONS

INTERVENTIONS

See glossary, p 1304

Key Messages

- **Antiviral treatment** Two systematic reviews found no RCTs of aciclovir versus placebo. One RCT found limited evidence that aciclovir plus prednisone versus prednisone alone significantly decreased the number of people with incomplete recovery of facial function after 4 months.
- **Corticosteroids** One systematic review found no clear evidence that corticosteroid versus control improved the recovery of facial motor function or cosmetically disabling sequelae after 6 months.
- **Facial nerve decompression surgery** One systematic review identified no RCTs of facial nerve decompression.

DEFINITION Bell's palsy is an acute, unilateral paresis or paralysis of the face in a pattern consistent with peripheral facial nerve dysfunction, without detectable causes.[1] Additional symptoms may include pain in or behind the ear, numbness in the affected side of the face, impaired tolerance to ordinary levels of noise, and disturbed taste on the anterior part of the tongue.[2–5]

INCIDENCE/ PREVALENCE The incidence is about 23/100 000 people a year, or about 1/60–70 people in a lifetime.[6] Bell's palsy affects men and women more or less equally, with a peak incidence between the ages of 10 and 40 years. It occurs with equal frequency on the right and left sides of the face.[7]

AETIOLOGY/ RISK FACTORS The cause is unclear. Viral infection, ischaemia, autoimmune inflammatory disorders, and heredity factors have been proposed as underlying causes.[2,8,9] A viral cause has gained popularity since the isolation of the herpes simplex virus-1 genome from facial nerve endoneurial fluid in people with Bell's palsy.[10]

PROGNOSIS More than two thirds of people with Bell's palsy achieve full spontaneous recovery. The largest series of people with Bell's palsy who received no specific treatment (1011 people) found the first signs of improvement within 3 weeks of onset in 85% of people.[11] For the other 15%, some improvement occurred 3–6 months later. The same series found that 71% of people recovered normal function of the face, 13% had insignificant sequelae, and the remaining 16% had permanently diminished function, with contracture of facial muscles and synkinesis (see glossary, p 1304). These figures are roughly similar to those of other series of people receiving no specific treatment for Bell's palsy.[7,8,12]

AIMS To maximise recovery of facial function and to reduce the risk of complications, with minimum adverse effects.

OUTCOMES Grade of recovery of motor function of the face; presence of sequelae (motor synkinesis, autonomic dysfunction, hemifacial spasm); time to full recovery.

METHODS *Clinical Evidence* update search and appraisal March 2002. Trials used different scoring systems for reporting outcomes.

QUESTION **What are the effects of treatments in adults and children?**

OPTION **CORTICOSTEROIDS**

One systematic review found no clear evidence that corticosteroid versus control improved the recovery of facial motor function or cosmetically disabling sequelae after 6 months.

Benefits: **Versus placebo or no specific treatment:** We found one systematic review (search date 2000, 3 RCTs, 117 people).[13] In the review, one RCT (26 people aged 12–76 years) compared cortisone acetate versus placebo; one RCT (51 people, ages not specified) compared prednisone plus vitamins versus vitamins alone; and one

RCT (42 children aged 24–74 months) compared methylprednisolone versus no specific treatment. The review found no significant difference with corticosteroid (cortisone acetate, prednisone, methylprednisolone) versus control in the number of people with incomplete recovery of facial motor function after 6 months (3 RCTs: 13/59 [22%] of people with corticosteroid *v* 15/58 [26%] of people with control; RR 0.86, 95% CI 0.47 to 1.59). When data from two quasi-randomised trials found by the review[12,14] were added to the pooled estimate, the result remained non-significant (RR 0.69, 95% CI 0.42 to 1.16; absolute numbers not provided; see comment below). The review also found no significant difference with corticosteroid versus control in the number of people with cosmetically disabling sequelae after 6 months (8/59 [14%] of people with corticosteroid *v* 9/58 [16%] of people with control; RR 0.86, 95% CI 0.38 to 1.98). When data from two quasi-randomised trials found by the review[12,14] were added to the pooled estimate, the result remained non significant (RR 0.82, 95% CI 0.39 to 1.73; absolute numbers not provided). **Versus aciclovir:** See benefits of antiviral treatment, p 1303.

Harms: No adverse effects were reported in the trials.

Comment: Of the two quasi-randomised trials identified by the review, one compared corticosteroids (preparation not stated) versus supportive therapy only, and used alternation in matched participants as the method of allocation.[12] The other compared dexamethasone versus placebo, and used allocation according to the day of admission.[14]

OPTION ANTIVIRAL TREATMENT

Two systematic reviews found no RCTs of aciclovir versus placebo. One RCT found limited evidence that aciclovir plus prednisone versus prednisone alone significantly decreased the number of people with incomplete recovery of facial function after 4 months.

Benefits: We found two systematic reviews (search date 2000, 2 RCTs, 200 people;[15] search date 2000, 3RCTs, 230 people[16]). Neither review included RCTs of aciclovir versus placebo; both included the same RCT (119 people) of aciclovir (400 mg 5 times daily for 10 days) plus prednisone versus prednisone alone (see comment below). The first review found aciclovir plus prednisone versus prednisone alone significantly decreased the number of people with incomplete recovery of facial function (measured using a facial function scoring system) after 4 months (4/53 [8%] of people with aciclovir plus steroid had moderate or moderately severe dysfunction *v* 11/46 [24%] with steroid alone; RR 0.32, 95% CI 0.11 to 0.92; see comment below).[15]

Harms: The RCT reported mild to moderate gastrointestinal complaints, which did not require treatment. No numbers were provided.[15]

Comment: In the RCT, 20/119 (17%) of people enrolled in the trial were lost to follow up. It is not clear to which treatment group these belonged. Results were calculated from the 99/119 (83%) of people who completed the trial. The systematic reviews identified two further RCTs of aciclovir that were not of sufficient quality.

OPTION FACIAL NERVE DECOMPRESSION SURGERY

One systematic review found no RCTs of facial nerve decompression surgery for people with Bell's palsy.

Benefits: We found one systematic review (search date 2000), which found no RCTs of facial nerve decompression surgery for people with Bell's palsy.[16]

Harms: The systematic review found reports of permanent unilateral deafness in four non-randomised prospective studies of facial nerve decompression in people with Bell's palsy.[16] One study of people with complete facial palsy undergoing facial nerve decompression found that 4/41 (10%) people had conductive deafness and 2/41 (5%) people had perceptive deafness after 1 year.[12]

Comment: None.

GLOSSARY

Synkinesis Involuntary movement accompanying a voluntary movement.

Substantive changes

Corticosteroids One new systematic review;[13] conclusions unchanged.

REFERENCES

1. Niparko JK, Mattox DE. Bell's palsy and herpes zoster oticus. In: Johnson RT, Griffin JW, eds. *Current therapy in neurologic disease*. St Louis: Mosby, 1993;355–361.
2. Burgess LPA, Capt MC, Yim DWS, et al. Bell's palsy: the steroid controversy revisited. *Laryngoscope* 1984;94:1472–1476.
3. Knox GW. Treatment controversy in Bell's palsy. *Arch Otolaryngol Head Neck Surg* 1998;124:821–824.
4. May M, Klein SR, Taylor FH. Idiopathic (Bell's) facial palsy: natural history defies steroid or surgical treatment. *Laryngoscope* 1985;95:406–409.
5. Rowland LP. Treatment of Bell's palsy. *N Engl J Med* 1972;287:1298–1299.
6. Victor M, Martin J. Disorders of the cranial nerves. In: Isselbacher KJ, et al, eds. *Harrison's principles of internal medicine* 13th ed. New York: McGraw-Hill, 1994:2347–2352.
7. Prescott CAJ. Idiopathic facial nerve palsy. *J Laryngol Otol* 1988;102:403–407.
8. Adour KK. Diagnosis and management of facial paralysis. *N Engl J Med* 1982;307:348–351.
9. Lorber B. Are all diseases infectious? *Ann Intern Med* 1996;125:844–851.
10. Murakami S, Mizobuchi M, Nakashiro Y, et al. Bell palsy and herpes simplex virus: identification of viral DNA in endoneurial fluid and muscle. *Ann Intern Med* 1996;124:27–30.
11. Peitersen E. The natural history of Bell's palsy. *Am J Otol* 1982;4:107–111.
12. Brown JS. Bell's palsy: a 5 year review of 174 consecutive cases: an attempted double blind study. *Laryngoscope* 1982;92:1369–1373.
13. Salinas RA, Alvarez G, Alvarez MI, et al. Corticosteroids for Bell's palsy (idiopathic facial paralysis) (Cochrane Review). In: The Cochrane Library, Issue 1, 2002. Oxford: Update Software. Search date 2000; primary sources Cochrane Neuromuscular Disease Group register, Medline, Embase, Lilacs, hand searches of reference lists, and personal contact with experts.
14. Akpinar S, Boga M, Yardim M. Akut periferik fasiyel paralizi olgularinda steroid tedavisinin plasebo ile oranlanmasi [Steroid versus placebo treatments in cases of acute peripheral facial paralysis]. *Bulletin of Gulhane Military Medical Academy* 1979;21:45–51.
15. Sipe J, Dunn L. Aciclovir for Bell's palsy (idiopathic facial paralysis) (Cochrane Review). In: The Cochrane Library, Issue 1, 2001. Oxford: Update Software. Search date 2000; primary sources Cochrane neuromuscular disease group register, Medline, Embase, Lilacs hand searches of reference lists, and personal contact with authors and experts.
16. Grogan PM, Gronseth GS. Practice parameter: steroids, acyclovir, and surgery for Bell's palsy (an evidence-based review). *Neurology* 2001;56:830–836. Search date 2000; primary source Medline and hand searches of reference lists.

Rodrigo Salinas
Ministry of Health
Santiago
Chile

Competing interests: None declared.

Chronic tension-type headache

Search date October 2001

Peter Goadsby

QUESTIONS

INTERVENTIONS

See glossary, p 1310

Key Messages

- We found only limited evidence about the treatment of chronic tension-type headache.
- **Amitriptyline (only short term evidence)** Systematic reviews of small, brief RCTs have found that amitriptyline versus placebo improves duration and frequency of chronic tension-type headache (CTTH).
- **Benzodiazepines** RCTs found insufficient evidence about any benefits of benzodiazepines to outweigh the harms associated with their regular use.
- **Regular acute relief medication** One systematic review of observational studies has suggested that regular analgesic medication may lead to a daily headache and reduce the effectiveness of prophylactic medication.
- **Acupuncture; botulinum toxin; cognitive behavioural therapy; relaxation and electromyographic biofeedback therapy; serotonin reuptake inhibitors; tricyclic antidepressants other than amitriptyline** We found insufficient evidence about the effects of these interventions.

DEFINITION The 1988 International Headache Society criteria for chronic tension-type headache (CTTH) are headaches on 15 or more days a month (180 days/year) for at least 6 months; pain that is bilateral, pressing, or tightening in quality, of mild, or moderate intensity, that does not prohibit activities, and that is not aggravated by routine physical activity; presence of no more than one additional clinical feature (nausea, photophobia, or phonophobia); and no vomiting.[1] CTTH is distinguished from chronic daily headache, which is simply a descriptive term for any headache type occurring for 15 days or more a month that may be because of CTTH as well as migraine or analgesic associated headache.[2] In contrast to CTTH, episodic tension-type headache can last for 30 minutes to 7 days and occurs for fewer than 180 days a year. Terms based on assumed mechanisms (muscle contraction headache, tension headache) are not operationally defined, and old studies that used these terms may have included people with many different types of headache. The greatest obstacle to the study of tension-type headache is the lack of any single proven specific or reliable, clinical, or biological defining characteristic of the disorder.

INCIDENCE/ PREVALENCE The prevalence of chronic daily headache from a survey of the general population in the USA was 4.1%. Half of sufferers met the criteria for CTTH.[3] In a survey of 2500 undergraduate students in the USA, the prevalence of CTTH was 2%.[4] The prevalence of CTTH was 2.5% in a Danish population based survey of 975 individuals.[5]

AETIOLOGY/ RISK FACTORS Tension-type headache is more prevalent in women (65% of cases in one survey).[6] Symptoms begin before the age of 10 years in 15% of people with CTTH. Prevalence declines with age.[7] There is a family history of some form of headache in 40% of people with CTTH.[8]

PROGNOSIS The prevalence of chronic tension-type headache declines with age.[7]

AIMS To reduce frequency, severity, and duration of headache, with minimal adverse effects from treatment.

OUTCOMES Headache frequency, intensity, and duration.

METHODS *Clinical Evidence* search and appraisal October 2001 and a hand search of the references in recent books on headache. Unless stated otherwise, we selected studies that used a definition of headache consistent with current International Headache Society criteria[1] and which excluded people with concomitant analgesic or other drug misuse. One systematic review (search date not stated) of chronic daily headache (a term that includes, but is not limited to, chronic tension-type headache) was not included.[9]

QUESTION What are the effects of treatments for chronic tension-type headache?

OPTION PHARMACOLOGICAL TREATMENTS

Small, short duration RCTs have found benefit from amitriptyline compared with placebo for the treatment of chronic tension-type headache. We found insufficient reliable evidence on the effects of other

types of tricyclic antidepressants, serotonin reuptake inhibitors, or benzodiazepines compared with placebo or other treatments. Benzodiazepines are commonly associated with adverse effects if taken regularly.

Benefits: **Tricyclic antidepressants versus placebo:** We found one systematic review (search date 1994, 2 RCTs),[10] a non-systematic review (published in 1997, 4 further RCTs),[11] and two additional RCTs.[12,13] Six of the eight RCTs looked at amitriptyline specifically. All six had important methodological flaws (see web extra table A at www.clinicalevidence.com) (see comment below).[14–18] Treatment duration ranged from 4–32 weeks. Doses of amitriptyline ranged from 10–150 mg daily. Outcomes used in the trials varied considerably. The three RCTs of highest quality[12,13,19] found significant improvement in headache duration and frequency with amitriptyline (see table 1, p 1312). The other four RCTs found variable results. **Serotonin reuptake inhibitors versus tricyclic antidepressants or placebo:** We found one RCT, which found no significant benefit from citalopram versus placebo in headache duration, frequency, or severity.[12] It found that amitriptyline significantly improved headache duration, frequency, and severity more than citalopram (see table 1, p 1312). **Regular analgesics:** We found no RCTs (see comment below). **Benzodiazepines:** We found no systematic review but found two RCTs.[20,21] One small RCT (16 people) found that diazepam versus placebo produced modest improvement over 12 weeks.[20] The dose of diazepam was not stated, and International Headache Society criteria were not used. The other RCT, a crossover study (62 people), compared alprazolam 250 μg three times daily versus placebo over 16 weeks and also found a modest short term improvement ($P < 0.05$).[21] Fourteen people withdrew from the trial at various stages; six of them before the trial started. It was not reported whether analysis was by intention to treat.

Harms: **Tricyclic antidepressants:** One RCT found increased rates of dry mouth (54% with amitriptyline 75 mg daily *v* 17% with placebo; $P < 0.05$), drowsiness (62% *v* 27%; $P < 0.05$), and weight gain (16% *v* 0%; $P > 0.05$).[19] Similar results have been found for amitriptyline[12] and other tricyclic antidepressants.[15,22] **Serotonin reuptake inhibitors:** Four of eight people taking fluvoxamine in a cohort study had transient nausea, two complained of anorexia, and three complained of irritability.[22] **Regular analgesics:** We found no RCTs but found one non-systematic review of 29 observational studies (2612 people),[23] which maintained frequent analgesic use (2–3 times/wk) in people with episodic headache was associated with chronic headache and reduced effectiveness of prophylactic treatment. Many, but not all, people improved over 1–6 months following withdrawal of the acute relief medication (73% of 1101 people, not all of whom had chronic tension-type headache). **Benzodiazepines:** Harms of benzodiazepines found in studies for other indications include increased risk of motor vehicle accidents, falls and fractures, fatal poisonings, depression, dependency, decline in functional status, cognitive decline, confusion, bizarre behaviour, and amnesia.[24]

Comment: Most RCTs were small, short term, and used different outcome measures. Not all studies excluded people taking regular analgesics. The quality of the studies often did not conform to current International Headache Society guidelines. Observational studies are also difficult to interpret. One cohort study found significant benefit from fluvoxamine, but the people recruited were not randomised, and those responding to placebo were excluded before the trial.[22] The available evidence supports the view that prophylactic treatment with amitriptyline is likely to be superior to the habitual use of short term analgesics. It is not clear whether benzodiazepines alone might contribute to the development of a daily headache, but the modest benefit found in the two small RCTs is unlikely to outweigh the risk of dependence with prolonged use.

OPTION RELAXATION AND ELECTROMYOGRAPHIC BIOFEEDBACK

We found no clear evidence that electromyographic biofeedback or relaxation are effective.

Benefits: We found two systematic reviews (search dates 1994[10] and not stated[25]), which did not distinguish between RCTs and observational studies. Appraisal of the papers within the reviews identified 10 relevant RCTs (see web table B at www.clinicalevidence.com).[26–35] We found one subsequent RCT.[4] The RCTs were generally of low quality, and included a variety of different electromyographic biofeedback (see glossary, p 1310) and relaxation (see glossary, p 1310) techniques. Clear conclusions could not be drawn. One larger RCT included people with chronic tension headache and migraine and did not provide intention to treat analysis.[13]

Harms: We found no reported adverse effects of electromyographic biofeedback or relaxation.

Comment: Relaxation and electromyographic biofeedback require additional trained staff and are time consuming.

OPTION COGNITIVE BEHAVIOURAL THERAPY

A systematic review of three small RCTs and one subsequent RCT have found limited evidence that cognitive behavioural therapy versus no treatment reduced the intensity of chronic tension-type headache.

Benefits: **Versus placebo:** We found one systematic review[10] and one subsequent RCT.[13] The systematic review (search date 1994, 3 small RCTs) found greater improvement with cognitive behavioural therapy compared with no treatment, sham treatment, or no usual care.[10] The subsequent RCT (203 adults with chronic tension-type headache [CTTH]) of cognitive behavioural therapy (relaxation (see glossary, p 1310) and cognitive coping) versus antidepressant (amitriptyline up to 100 mg daily or nortriptyline up to 75 mg daily) versus combined cognitive therapy plus antidepressant versus placebo.[13] It found that cognitive behavioural therapy versus placebo significantly reduced the headache index score after 6 months (WMD 0.79 U, 95% CI 0.30 U to 1.28 U; $P < 0.01$), but found a non-significant increase in the frequency of clinically important improvement (at least 50% reduction in headache index score:

17/49 [35%] with cognitive behavioural therapy *v* 14/48 [29%] with placebo; RR 1.19, 95% CI 0.66 to 2.13). **Versus another treatment:** The review found nine additional comparative studies of relaxation or electromyographic biofeedback (see glossary, p 1310) therapy or both compared with either cognitive therapy alone (2 studies) or in combination with relaxation or electromyographic biofeedback therapy (7 studies). Results were inconclusive.[10] **Versus antidepressants:** We found no systematic review but found one RCT (203 adults with CTTH) of cognitive behavioural therapy (relaxation and cognitive coping) versus antidepressant (amitriptyline up to 100 mg daily or nortriptyline up to 75 mg daily) versus combined cognitive therapy plus antidepressant.[13] It found no difference between cognitive behavioural therapy versus antidepressant treatment in either the headache index score after 6 months (WMD −0.13 U, 95% CI −0.61 U to +0.35 U; P = 0.58) or in the frequency of clinically important improvement after 6 months (at least 50% reduction in headache index score: 17/49 [35%] with cognitive behavioural therapy *v* 20/53 [38%] with antidepressant; RR 0.92, 95% CI 0.55 to 1.54).

Harms: We found no reported adverse effects of cognitive behavioural therapy.

Comment: The studies in the systematic review were small and had as few as five people in a group. Although the RCT found the headache index score was reduced, it found no convincing reduction in the number of people who had a clinically important response. The evidence is too limited to define the role of cognitive therapy in CTTH.

OPTION ACUPUNCTURE

One small RCT found no evidence that acupuncture was more effective than placebo in people with episodic or chronic tension-type headache, although the trial was too small to exclude a clinically important effect.

Benefits: We found no systematic review, but found one small RCT (47 people with chronic tension-type headache, 21 people with episodic headache), which compared acupuncture versus sham, non-penetrative acupuncture. Two treatments were given a week over 5 weeks. The RCT found no significant differences with acupuncture versus sham in headache frequency immediately after treatment (mean 13.1 days/month with acupuncture *v* 16.6 days/month with sham) or at 5 months after the end of the treatment (mean 16.7 days/month with acupuncture *v* 17.2 days/month with sham). It also found no significant differences in pain intensity measured by a visual analogue scale.[36]

Harms: Adverse effects were not reported.[36]

Comment: The study was too small to establish or exclude a clinically important difference.

OPTION BOTULINUM TOXIN

Two small RCTs found no evidence that botulinum toxin improved symptoms compared with placebo in people with chronic tension-type headache. Botulinum toxin can cause weakness of the face and can affect swallowing.

Benefits: We found no systematic review but found two double blind RCTs that compared pericranial intramuscular injection of botulinum toxin type A versus placebo in people with chronic tension-type headache.[37,38] The first RCT (59 people) found no significant difference between treatments for pain relief 8 weeks after treatment (> 25% pain relief at 8 wks: 54% with botulinum *v* 38% with placebo; CI not provided; $P > 0.05$).[37] The second, smaller RCT (21 people) also found no significant differences between botulinum versus placebo for headache intensity, duration, and frequency at 4, 8, and 12 weeks.[38]

Harms: The first RCT found no significant difference between treatments.[37] After 4 weeks, the following symptoms were noted: vertigo (1 person with placebo *v* 2 with botulinum); pain at injection site (1 person with placebo *v* 3 with botulinum). By 8 weeks, symptoms had resolved. Botulinum toxin may be associated with facial weakness, difficulty with swallowing, and disturbed local sensation. Adverse effects were not reported in the second RCT.[38]

Comment: The RCTs were too small to exclude a clinically important difference between botulinum and placebo.

GLOSSARY

Electromyographic biofeedback Feedback of the amplified electromyographic signal from forehead and neck muscles through earphones or a loudspeaker to enable people to reduce the amount of muscle contraction.

Relaxation Includes Jacobson's progressive relaxation exercises, meditation, passive relaxation, autogenic training, and functional relaxation.[38]

Headache monitoring People in a study who make daily recordings of headache symptoms without additional therapeutic intervention.

REFERENCES

1. Headache Classification Committee of the International Headache Society. Classification and diagnostic criteria for headache disorders, cranial neuralgias and facial pain. *Cephalalgia* 1988;8:1–96.
2. Silberstein SD, Lipton RB, Sliwinski M. Classification of daily and near-daily headaches: field trial of revised IHS criteria. *Neurology* 1996;47:871–875.
3. Schwartz BS, Stewart WF, Simon D, Lipton RB. Epidemiology of tension-type headache. *JAMA* 1998;279:381–383.
4. Rokicki LA, Semenchuk EM, Bruehl S, Lofland KR, Houle TT. An examination of the validity of the HIS classification system for migraine and tension-type headache in the college student population. *Headache* 1999;39:720–727.
5. Rasmussen BK, Jensen R, Olesen J. A population-based analysis of the diagnostic criteria of the International Headache Society. *Cephalalgia* 1991;11:129–134.
6. Friedman AP, von Storch TJC, Merritt HH. Migraine and tension headaches: a clinical study of two thousand cases. *Neurology* 1954;4:773–788.
7. Lance JW, Curran DA, Anthony M. Investigations into the mechanism and treatment of chronic headache. *Med J Aust* 1965;2:909–914.
8. Russell MB, Ostergaard S, Bendtsen L, Olesen J. Familial occurrence of chronic tension-type headache. *Cephalalgia* 1999;19:207–210.
9. Redillas C, Solomon S. Prophylactic treatment of chronic daily headache. *Headache* 2000;40:83–102. Search date not stated; primary source Medline.
10. Bogaards MC, Moniek M, ter Kuile M. Treatment of recurrent tension-type headache: A meta-analytic review. *Clin J Pain* 1994;10:174–190. Search date March 1994; primary sources Compact Cambridge, Psychlit, and reference lists of relevant articles.
11. Schoenen J, Wang W. Tension-type headache. In: Goadsby PJ, Silberstein SD, eds. *Headache*. 1st ed. Newton: Butterworth-Heinemann, 1997:177–200.

12. Bendtsen L, Jensen R, Olesen J. A non-selective (amitriptyline), but not a selective (citalopram), serotonin reuptake inhibitor is effective in the prophylactic treatment of chronic tension-type headache. *J Neurol Neurosurg Psychiatry* 1996;61:285–290.
13. Holroyd KA, O'Donnell FJ, Lipchik GL, Cordingley GE, Carlson B. Management of chronic tension-type headache with tricyclic antidepressant medication, stress management therapy, and their combination: a randomized controlled trial. *JAMA* 2001;285:2208–2215
14. Diamond S, Baltes BJ. Chronic tension headache treated with amitriptyline: a double-blind study. *Headache* 1971;11:110–116.
15. Fogelholm R, Murros K. Maprotiline in chronic tension headache: a double-blind cross-over study. *Headache* 1985;25:273–275.
16. Langemark M, Loldrup D, Bech P, Oleson J. Clomipramine and mianserin in the treatment of chronic tension headache. A double-blind, controlled study. *Headache* 1990;30:118–121.
17. Pfaffenrath V, Essen D, Islet H, et al. Amitriptyline versus amitriptyline-N-oxide versus placebo in the treatment of chronic tension-type headache: a multi-centre randomised parallel-group double-blind study. *Cephalalgia* 1991;11:329–330.
18. Lance JW. *Mechanism and management of headache*. London: Butterworth, 1973.
19. Gobel H, Hamouz V, Hansen C, et al. Chronic tension type headache: amitriptyline reduces clinical headache-duration and experimental pain sensitivity but does not alter pericranial muscle activity readings. *Pain* 1994;59:241–249.
20. Paiva T, Nunes JS, Moreira A, Santos J, Teixeira J, Barbosa A. Effects of frontalis EMG biofeedback and diazepam in the treatment of tension headache. *Headache* 1982;22:216–220.
21. Shukla R, Nag D, Ahuja RC. Alprazolam in chronic tension-type headache. *J Assoc Physician India* 1996;44:641–644.
22. Manna V, Bolino F, Di Cicco L. Chronic tension-type headache, mood depression and serotonin: therapeutic effects of fluvoxamine and mianserine. *Headache* 1994;34:44–49.
23. Diener H-C, Tfelt-Hansen P. Headache associated with chronic use of substances. In: Oleson J, Tfelt-Hansen P, Welch KMA, eds. *The headaches*. New York: Raven, 1993:721–727.
24. Holbrook AM, Crowther R, Lotter A, Cheng C, King D. The diagnosis and management of insomnia in clinical practice: a practical evidence-based approach. *CMAJ* 2000;162:216–220.
25. Holroyd KA, Penzien DB. Client variables and the behavioural treatment of recurrent tension headache: a meta-analytic review. *J Behav Med* 1986;9:515–536. Search date not stated; primary sources Eric, Medlars, Psycinfo, Psycalert, and hand searches of key journals, book reviews, and conference proceedings.
26. Loew T, Sohn R, Martus P, Tritt K, Rechlin T. Functional relaxation as a somatopsychotherapeutic intervention: a prospective controlled study. *Altern Ther Health Med* 2000;6:70–75.
27. Reich B. Non-invasive treatment of vascular and muscle contraction headache: a comparative longitudinal clinical study. *Headache* 1988;29:34–41.
28. Andrasik F, Holroyd K. A test of specific and nonspecific effects in the biofeedback treatment of tension headache. *J Consult Clin Psychol* 1980;48:575–586.
29. Blanchard E, Appelbaum K, Guarnieri P, et al. Placebo-controlled evaluation of abbreviated progressive muscle relaxation combined with cognitive therapy in the treatment of tension headache. *J Consult Clin Psychol* 1990;58:210–215.
30. Blanchard E, Andrasik F, Appelbaum K, et al. The efficacy and cost-effectiveness of minimal-therapist-contact non-drug treatment of chronic migraine and tension headache. *Headache* 1985;25:214–220.
31. Bruhn P, Olesen J, Melgaard B. Controlled trial of EMG feedback in muscle contraction feedback. *Ann Neurol* 1979;6:34–36.
32. Collett L, Cottrauz J, Juenet C. GSR feedback and Schultz relaxation in tension headaches: a comparative study. *Pain* 1986;25:205–213.
33. Gada M. A comparative study of efficacy of EMG biofeedback and progressive muscular relaxation in tension headache. *Indian J Psychiat* 1984;26:121–127.
34. Holroyd K, Andrasik F, Westbrook T. Cognitive control of tension headache. *Cognitive Ther Res* 1977;1:121–133.
35. Larsson B, Carlsson J. A school-based, nurse-administered relaxation training for children with chronic tension-type headache. *J Pediatr Psychol* 1996;21:603–614.
36. Karst M, Reinhard M, Thum P, Wiese B, Rollnik J, Fink M. Needle acupuncture in tension-type headache: a randomized, placebo-controlled study. *Cephalalgia* 2001;21:637–642.
37. Schmitt WJ, Slowey E, Fravi N, Weber S, Burgunder J-M. Effect of botulinum toxin A injections in the treatment of chronic tension-type headache: a double-blind, placebo-controlled trial. *Headache* 2001;41:658–664.
38. Rollnik JD, Tanneberger O, Schubert M, Schneider U, Dengler R. Treatment of tension-type headache with botulinum toxin type A: a double-blind, placebo-controlled study. *Headache* 2000;40:300–305.

Peter Goadsby
Professor of Clinical Neurology
Institute of Neurology
London
UK

Competing interests: None declared.

TABLE 1 **RCTs evaluating the efficacy of tricyclic antidepressants in the treatment of chronic tension-type headache, including two comparative studies with serotonin reuptake inhibitors (see text, p 1306).**

RCT	Drug	Number in group	CTTH definition	Analgesic overuse excluded	Total duration and type of study	Outcome	Effect of drug compared with placebo
19	Amitriptyline 75 mg *v* placebo	24 29	IHS criteria[1]	Yes	6 week; parallel group	Reduction in mean daily headache duration	At 6 weeks, pain reduced by 3.2 hour/day with amitriptyline *v* 0.28 hour/day with placebo ($P < 0.01$)
12	Amitriptyline 75 mg *v* citalopram 20 mg *v* placebo	34	IHS criteria[1]	Yes	32 week; crossover	Reduction in the product of headache duration and intensity	With amitriptyline: reduced analgesic intake ($P = 0.01$), headache duration, and frequency ($P = 0.002$) but no difference in headache intensity With citalopram: no difference in headache duration, frequency, or severity
13	Amitriptyline or nortriptyline *v* stress management *v* placebo	53 49 48	IHS criteria[1]	Yes	8 months total	Reduction in mean pain scores from daily diary	Antidepressant and stress management both superior to placebo

CTTH, Chronic tension-type headache; IHS, International Headache Society.

Epilepsy

Search date December 2001

Anthony Marson and Sridharan Ramaratnam

QUESTIONS

INTERVENTIONS

* We found no placebo controlled RCTs. However, widespread consensus holds that these drugs are effective.

See glossary, p 1323

Key Messages

- **Antiepileptic monotherapy in generalised epilepsy** We found no placebo controlled trials of the main antiepileptic drugs (carbamazepine, phenobarbital, phenytoin, sodium valproate), but widespread consensus holds that these drugs are effective. Systematic reviews have found no good evidence on which to base a choice among these drugs in terms of seizure control.
- **Antiepileptic monotherapy in partial epilepsy** We found no placebo controlled trials of the main antiepileptic drugs (carbamazepine, phenobarbital, phenytoin, sodium valproate), but widespread consensus holds that these drugs are effective. Systematic reviews have found no good evidence on which to base a choice among these drugs in terms of seizure control. A systematic review has found that phenobarbital versus phenytoin is more likely to be withdrawn, presumably because of side effects.

Clin Evid 2002;8:1313–1328.

- **Addition of second line drugs for drug resistant partial epilepsy** Systematic reviews have found that the addition of second line drugs versus placebo significantly reduces the seizure frequency in people with partial epilepsy who have not responded to usual treatment. Each additional drug increases the frequency of adverse effects, the need for withdrawal of additional treatment, or both. RCTs found no good evidence on which to base a choice among drugs.
- **Antiepileptic drugs after a single seizure** RCTs have found that immediate treatment of single seizures with antiepileptic drugs versus no treatment reduces the risk of further seizures within 2 years by about half, but found no evidence that treatment alters long term prognosis. Long term antiepileptic drug treatment is potentially harmful.
- **Antiepileptic drug withdrawal for people in remission** Long term antiepileptic drug treatment is potentially harmful. One systematic review of observational studies and one RCT have found that antiepileptic drug withdrawal for people in remission is associated with a higher risk of seizure recurrence than continued treatment. Clinical predictors of relapse after drug withdrawal include age, seizure type, number of antiepileptic drugs being taken, whether seizures have occurred since antiepileptic drugs were started, and the period of remission before drug withdrawal.
- **Biofeedback; relaxation therapy; yoga** Systematic reviews have found insufficient evidence on the effects of these interventions.
- **Cognitive behavioural therapy** Two small RCTs found no significant difference with cognitive behavioural therapy versus control in seizure frequency or psychosocial function. Another small RCT found that cognitive behavioural treatment versus control treatment significantly improved a depression score in people with epilepsy plus depressed mood.
- **Educational interventions** RCTs found improvement in knowledge and understanding of epilepsy, adjustment to epilepsy, and improved psychosocial functioning with educational interventions versus control. No information was available regarding reduction in seizure frequency.
- **Family counselling** One small RCT with weak methods found that family counselling versus no treatment significantly improved perceived acceptance by the family, emotional adjustment, interpersonal adjustment, adjustment to seizures, and overall psychosocial function. The RCT gave no information on seizure reduction.
- **Relaxation plus behavioural modification therapy** RCTs found insufficient evidence about the effects of combined relaxation and behavioural modification on seizures. One RCT found that relaxation plus behavioural therapy versus control significantly improved anxiety and adjustment.

DEFINITION Epilepsy is a group of disorders rather than a single disease. Seizures can be classified by type as partial (categorised as simple partial, complex partial, and secondary generalised tonic clonic seizures), or generalised (categorised as generalised tonic clonic, absence, myoclonic, tonic, and atonic seizures).[1] See glossary, p 1324.

INCIDENCE/ PREVALENCE Epilepsy is common, with an estimated prevalence in the developed world of 5–10/1000, and an annual incidence of 50/100 000 people.[2] About 3% of people will be given a diagnosis of epilepsy at some time in their lives.[3]

AETIOLOGY/ RISK FACTORS Epilepsy can also be classified by cause.[1] Idiopathic generalised epilepsies (such as juvenile myoclonic epilepsy or childhood absence epilepsy) are largely genetic. Symptomatic epilepsies result from a known cerebral abnormality — for example, temporal lobe epilepsy may result from a congenital defect, mesial temporal sclerosis, or a tumour. Cryptogenic epilepsies are those that cannot be classified as idiopathic or symptomatic and in which no causative factor has been identified, but is suspected.

PROGNOSIS For most people with epilepsy the prognosis is good. About 70% go into remission, defined as being seizure free for 5 years on or off treatment. This leaves 20–30% who develop chronic epilepsy, often treated with multiple antiepileptic drugs.[4] About 60% of untreated people suffer no further seizures in the 2 years after their first seizure.[5]

AIMS To reduce the risk of subsequent seizures and to improve the prognosis of the seizure disorder; in people in remission, to withdraw antiepileptic drugs without causing seizure recurrence; and to minimise adverse effects of treatment.

OUTCOMES For treatment after a single seizure: time to subsequent seizures, time to achieve remission, proportion achieving remission. For treatment of newly diagnosed epilepsy: retention on allocated treatment or time to withdrawal of allocated treatment, time to remission, time to first seizure after treatment. For treatment of drug resistant epilepsy: percentage reduction in seizure frequency, proportion of responders (response defined as ≥ 50% in reduction in seizure frequency). For drug withdrawal: time to seizure recurrence. Improvement in quality of life, reduction in anxiety, depression, fear of seizures, coping or adjustment to epilepsy (assessed by validated measures).

METHODS *Clinical Evidence* search and appraisal December 2001, *Clinical Evidence* search for systematic reviews November 2001 supplemented by searches of the Cochrane Epilepsy Group to December 2001.

QUESTION Should single seizures be treated?

RCTs have found that treatment with antiepileptic drugs reduces the risk of further seizures by about half. However, we found no evidence that treatment alters long term prognosis. Long term antiepileptic drug treatment is potentially harmful.

Benefits: We found no systematic review. We found three RCTs, the largest of which compared immediate with no treatment in 419 people (42% women, 28% aged ≤ 16 years, 66% aged 16–60 years, 6% aged ≥ 60 years).[6,7] Participants were randomised within 7 days of their first tonic clonic seizure (see glossary, p 1324) and were followed for a minimum of 3 years. At 2 years, there were half as many second seizures in the treatment group compared with the control group (HR 0.36, 95% CI 0.24 to 0.53). However, there was no significant difference in the proportion of people achieving a 2 year remission (AR 60% *v* 68%; RR 0.82, 95% CI 0.64 to 1.03; RR 0.96, 95% CI 0.77 to 1.22).

Harms: The largest RCT gave no information on adverse effects.[6,7] However, these are well known and include idiosyncratic reactions, teratogenesis, and cognitive effects.

Comment: One systematic review of prospective observational studies (search date not stated, about 2500 people, 30% receiving treatment) concluded that, at 2 years from their first seizure, 40% (95% CI 37% to 43%) of people will have had further seizures.[5] The largest RCT was too small to rule out the possibility that treating a first seizure alters the long term prognosis of epilepsy.[6,7]

QUESTION What are the effects of monotherapy in newly diagnosed partial epilepsy?

We found no placebo controlled RCTs of the main antiepileptic drugs (carbamazepine, phenobarbital, phenytoin, sodium valproate) used as monotherapy in people with partial epilepsy but widespread consensus holds that these drugs are effective. Systematic reviews have found no reliable evidence on which to base a choice among drugs in terms of seizure control. A systematic review has found that phenobarbital versus phenytoin is more likely to be withdrawn, presumably because of side effects.

Benefits: **Versus placebo:** We found no systematic reviews or RCTs. **Versus each other:** We found one systematic review (search date 1999, 5 RCTs) of sodium valproate versus carbamazepine (1265 people of which 830 had partial epilepsy and 395 had generalised epilepsy, age 3–83 years, follow up < 5 years).[8] The systematic review included a meta-analysis of the subgroup of people with partial epilepsy (with results expressed as HRs; HR > 1 for an event that is more likely with sodium valproate). It found no significant difference for time to treatment withdrawal (HR 1.00, 95% CI 0.79 to 1.26), an advantage with carbamazepine for time to 12 month remission (HR 0.82, 95% CI 0.67 to 1.00), and a significant advantage with carbamazepine for time to first seizure (HR 1.22, 95% CI 1.04 to 1.44). A test for statistical interaction was performed to test the robustness of these subgroup analyses. This was significant for time to first seizure but not for time to 12 month remission, and so these subgroup analyses must be treated with caution. We found one systematic review (search date 2000, 5 RCTs, 250 people with partial epilepsy, and 419 with generalised epilepsy, age 3–95, follow up < 5 years) of sodium valproate versus phenytoin.[9] This review also included a meta-analysis of the subgroup of people with partial epilepsy with results expressed as HRs (HR > 1 for an event that is more likely with phenytoin). It found no significant difference for time to treatment withdrawal (HR 1.23, 95% CI 0.77 to 1.98), time to 12 month remission (HR 1.02, 95% CI 0.68 to 1.54), or time to first seizure (HR 0.81, 95% CI 0.59 to 1.11). We found one systematic review (search date 1998, 3 RCTs, 599 people with partial or generalised epilepsy, age 3–77 years) of phenobarbital (phenobarbitone) versus phenytoin.[10] Results were expressed as HRs (HR > 1 for an event more likely with phenobarbital), but this review did not undertake subgroup analyses for people with partial or generalised epilepsy. Overall, it found no significant difference for time to 12 month remission (HR 0.93, 95% CI 0.70 to 1.23) or time to first seizure (HR 0.84, 95% CI 0.68 to 1.05). It found that the time to treatment withdrawal was significantly shorter with phenobarbital versus phenytoin, presumably because it was less well tolerated (HR 1.62, 95% CI 1.22 to 2.14).

Harms: Two RCTs found similar prevalence of adverse effects with carbamazepine and sodium valproate.[11,12] Rashes occurred more often in people on carbamazepine than on sodium valproate (11% *v* 1.7%; $P < 0.05$; 6.3% *v* 3.4%; NS).[11,12] More people on valproate reported weight gain (12% *v* 1.1%, $P < 0.05$; 10% *v* 3.9%, NS),[11,12] usually after at least 3 months of treatment. Other adverse events with carbamazepine were dizziness (6.7% *v* 2.9%, NS; 6.3% *v* 0.8%, $P < 0.05$),[11,12] headaches (6.1% *v* 3.4%), ataxia (2.2% *v* 0%), somnolence (20% *v* 9.3%, $P < 0.05$), fatigue (10% *v* 5.1%, NS), diplopia (3.9% *v* 0%, NS), and insomnia (3.9% *v* 0%, NS).[11,12] Other drug related adverse events with sodium valproate were tremor (5.2% *v* 1.7%, NS), alopecia (2.9% *v* 0.6%, NS; 4.2% *v* 1.6%, NS), and appetite increase (2.3% *v* 0%, NS; 9.3% *v* 0%, $P < 0.01$).[11,12] Treatment was withdrawn because of adverse events in 9% of people on sodium valproate compared with 18% on carbamazepine (18 *v* 15 people).[11,12] See also benefits above.

Comment: Placebo controlled trials of these drugs would now be considered unethical. The meta-analysis provides weak evidence in support of the consensus view to use carbamazepine as the drug of choice in people with partial epilepsy.

QUESTION **What are the effects of monotherapy in newly diagnosed generalised epilepsy (generalised tonic clonic seizures with or without other generalised seizure types)?**

We found no placebo controlled trials of the main antiepileptic drugs (carbamazepine, phenobarbital, phenytoin, sodium valproate) used as monotherapy in people with generalised epilepsy but widespread consensus holds that these drugs are effective. Systematic reviews have not found evidence on which to base a choice among drugs in terms of seizure control.

Benefits: **Versus placebo:** We found no systematic reviews or RCTs. **Versus each other:** We found two systematic reviews.[8,9] Trials in both reviews recruited people if they had generalised onset tonic clonic seizures (see glossary, p 1324) with or without other generalised seizures types (e.g. absence or myoclonus). Only generalised onset tonic clonic seizures were documented at follow up and included in analyses. One systematic review compared carbamazepine and sodium valproate (search date 1999, 5 RCTs, 4 of the RCTs included 395 people with generalised epilepsy, age 3–79 years, follow up < 5 years).[8] Results were expressed as HRs (HR > 1 indicates that an event is more likely with valproate). A meta-analysis of the generalised epilepsy subgroup found no significant differences between sodium valproate and carbamazepine for time to treatment withdrawal (HR 0.89, 95% CI 0.62 to 1.29), time to 12 month remission (HR 0.96, 95% CI 0.75 to 1.24), and time to first seizure (HR 0.86, 95% CI 0.68 to 1.67) (see comment below).

The second systematic review compared phenytoin and sodium valproate (search date 2000, 5 RCTs, 419 people aged 3–95 years with generalised epilepsy).[9] Results were expressed as HRs (HR > 1 indicates that an event is more likely with phenytoin). A meta-analysis of the generalised epilepsy subgroup found no significant differences between sodium valproate and phenytoin for time to treatment withdrawal (HR 0.98, 95% CI 0.60 to 1.58), time to 12 month remission (HR 1.06, 95% CI 0.71 to 1.57), and time to first seizure (HR 1.03, 95% CI 0.77 to 1.39) (see comment below).

Harms: See harms under effects of monotherapy in newly diagnosed partial epilepsy, p 1317.

Comment: Although no difference was found in these systematic reviews between sodium valproate and either carbamazepine or phenytoin, the confidence intervals are wide and these results do not establish equivalence of sodium valproate and carbamazepine or phenytoin. Also, the age distribution of people classified as having generalised epilepsy suggests significant errors in the classification of epilepsy type. Failure of the RCTs to document generalised seizures other than tonic clonic seizures is a significant limitation. The meta-analysis does not provide evidence to support or refute the use of sodium valproate for people with generalised tonic clonic seizures as part of generalised epilepsy.

QUESTION Does the addition of second line drugs benefit people with drug resistant partial epilepsy?

Seven systematic reviews have found that the addition of second line drugs significantly reduces the seizure frequency in people with partial epilepsy who have not responded to usual treatment. Each additional drug increases the frequency of adverse effects and the need for withdrawal of additional treatment, or both, compared to placebo. We found no good evidence from RCTs on which to make a choice among drugs.

Benefits: We found seven systematic reviews (search dates 2000[13], 2000[14], 2001[15], 1999[16], 1995[17], 1999[18], 1999[19]) For gabapentin the systematic reviews identified five RCTs (997 people with drug resistant partial epilepsy), for levetiracetam four RCTs (1023 people), for lamotrigine 11 RCTs (1243 people), for oxcarbazepine two RCTs (961 people), for tiagabine three RCTs (769 people), for topiramate six RCTs (743 people), for vigabatrin four RCTs (495 people), and for zonisamide 3 RCTs (499 people). These reviews found that the addition of each drug to usual treatment significantly reduced seizure frequency versus placebo (see table 1, p 1326 and table 2, p 1327).

Harms: Adverse effects were more frequent with additional treatment versus placebo (see table 1, p 1326 and table 2, p 1327).[13,18] Lamotrigine is associated with a rash, which may be avoided by slower titration of the drug. Vigabatrin causes concentric visual field abnormalities in about 40% of people, which are probably irreversible.[20]

Comment: Few RCTs have compared these drugs directly with each other. Because of the irreversible visual field abnormalities associated with vigabatrin, the consensus view among neurologists is not to recommend this drug.

QUESTION Which people are at risk of relapse on withdrawal of drug treatment?

Observational studies have found that nearly a third of people will relapse within 2 years if antiepileptic drugs are withdrawn. Clinical predictors of relapse after drug withdrawal include age, seizure type, number of antiepileptic drugs being taken, whether seizures have occurred since antiepileptic drugs were started, and the period of remission before drug withdrawal.

Benefits: We found no systematic review. The largest single RCT (1013 people who had been seizure free for > 2 years) compared continued antiepileptic treatment with slow antiepileptic drug withdrawal.[21,22] At 2 years, 78% of people who continued treatment remained seizure free compared with 59% in the withdrawal group. Risk reductions with 95% confidence intervals for the main factors predicting recurrence of seizures are tabulated (see table 3, p 1328). One systematic review of observational studies (search date not stated) found that, at 2 years, 29% (95% CI 24% to 34%) of people in remission from all types of epilepsy would relapse if antiepileptic drugs were withdrawn.[23]

Harms: Sixteen people died during the trial, 10 in the continued treatment group and six in the withdrawal group.[21,22] Only two deaths were attributed to epilepsy, and both of these occurred in people randomised to continued treatment.

Comment: There were no significant differences in psychosocial outcomes between groups. People with a seizure recurrence were less likely to be in paid employment at 2 years.[21,22]

QUESTION What are the effects of behavioural and psychological treatments for people with epilepsy?

OPTION RELAXATION THERAPY

We found one systematic review and three small RCTs. The RCTs used weak methods. The effects of relaxation therapy remain unclear.

Benefits: **Seizure frequency:** We found one systematic review (search date 2001,[24] 3 small RCTs,[25–27] 50 people including 32 women). The RCTs used weak methods (see comment below). Two of the studies found a non-significant reduction in seizure frequency with relaxation therapy (see glossary, p 1324) versus no relaxation therapy, and one study found a significantly reduced seizure frequency. The weak methods prevent reliable conclusions being drawn.

Harms: The studies gave no information on adverse effects.

Comment: All three RCTs used weak methods. The randomisation concealment was not optimal. The randomisation methods used in the three studies were strict alternation,[27] alternation in blocks of five,[26] or was not stated.[25] The baseline seizure frequency varied considerably among the randomised groups in all the studies. In one study,[26] two people in the treatment group had new antiepileptic medication added during the study period and one of these had a greater than 50% reduction in seizure frequency; another person discontinued antiepileptic medication. Antiepileptic drug treatment was also adjusted during the trial, making it difficult to conclude whether the observed results were because of changes in drug treatment or because of the intervention. The RCTs were small and were not blinded. The study duration and follow up was short. The possibility of publication bias cannot be excluded. The effects of relaxation therapy remain unclear.

OPTION YOGA

A systematic review identified one study of add on treatment with sahaja yoga. No reliable conclusions could be made.

Benefits: **Seizure frequency:** We found one systematic review (search date 2001, 1 RCT, 32 people[28]).[29] The RCT compared sahaja yoga (10 people) versus control (sham yoga 10 people, no intervention 12 people). The RCT found that yoga versus control treatments reduced seizure frequency but it used weak methods, which prevent reliable conclusions being drawn.

Harms: The study gave no information on adverse effects.

Comment: The number of people included in this quasi-randomised, unblinded study was small. The baseline seizure frequency and duration varied among the groups. These flaws make the results difficult to interpret.

OPTION BIOFEEDBACK

One systematic review identified one RCT of electroencephalographic biofeedback, but inadequate methods and reporting prevent any reliable conclusions being drawn about the effects of electroencephalographic biofeedback.

Benefits: **Seizure frequency:** We found one systematic review (search date 2001,[24] 1 RCT, 24 people with uncontrolled epilepsy[30]) of electroencephalographic (EEG) biofeedback (see glossary, p 1323) versus control treatment. The RCT compared EEG biofeedback versus sham (non-contingent) feedback versus no intervention (8 people in each group). It found a significant reduction in seizure frequency compared with the baseline frequency (median seizure reduction with active treatment 61%; $P < 0.005$ compared with baseline).

Harms: The study did not report any harms.

Comment: The seizure frequency in the control group is not available in the publication. We were unable to compare the EEG biofeedback and control groups. The RCT did not report the number of people who had greater than 50% reduction in seizure frequency. The study was not blinded and the randomisation method is not clear. The duration of follow up was only 6 weeks. The evidence is insufficient to draw reliable conclusions about the effects of EEG biofeedback.

OPTION COGNITIVE BEHAVIOURAL TREATMENT

We found insufficient evidence to define the effects of cognitive behavioural therapy in people with epilepsy. One small RCT of group cognitive behavioural treatment versus control treatment found no significant benefit on seizure frequency. One RCT found no significant improvement in psychosocial function. Another small RCT found that cognitive behavioural treatment versus control treatment significantly improved a depression score in people with epilepsy plus depressed mood.

Benefits: **Seizure frequency:** We found one systematic review (search date2001)[24] that found one RCT (30 people)[31] comparing cognitive behavioural therapy (see glossary, p 1323) versus control treatment. The RCT found no significant difference between cognitive behavioural therapy and control treatment in seizure frequency, but the RCT was too small to exclude a clinically important difference. **Psychosocial functioning:** One RCT[31] found no significant differences between cognitive behavioural therapy and control treatments in various psychological scales, such as the Washington Psycho Social Inventory (WPSI), the Minnesota Multiphasic Inventory (see glossary, p 1324) (MMPI), and the Beck Depression Inventory (see glossary, p 1323). Another RCT (15 people with epilepsy and depression)[32] found that cognitive behavioural therapy versus control treatment significantly reduced depression and self reported anxiety or anger, and significantly increased involvement in social activities. The RCT did not report seizure frequencies, or specify the intervention given to controls or the concomitant antidepressant treatment.

Harms: None reported.

Comment: The method of randomisation concealment is not known for these small RCTs. Publication bias cannot be excluded. The evidence is insufficient to define the effects of cognitive behavioural therapy on people with epilepsy.

OPTION EDUCATIONAL

Two RCTs found improvement in knowledge and understanding of epilepsy, adjustment to epilepsy, and improved psychosocial functioning with educational interventions. No information was available regarding reduction in seizure frequency.

Benefits: We found one systematic review (search date 2001)[24] that found two RCTs.[33,34] **Seizure frequency:** Neither RCT reported the reduction in seizure frequency. **Psychosocial functioning:** One RCT (100 adults with epilepsy)[33] found that a specific 2 day educational programme versus a control intervention significantly improved responses to a 50 item true/false questionnaire (overall understanding of epilepsy, significant decrease in fear of seizures, significant decrease in hazardous medical self management), and significantly improved compliance with current medication (demonstrated by serum antiepileptic drug levels). Another RCT (252 children with epilepsy aged 7–14 years)[34] found that a child centred, family focused, educational program versus control intervention significantly improved questionnaire responses (knowledge about what to do during a seizure, purpose of the electroencephalographic examination and minimal restriction of activities), increased the proportion of children likely to participate in normal activities, improved perceived academic and social competencies of the children, and reduced the anxiety of parents (see comment below).

Harms: None reported.

Comment: In one RCT,[33] randomisation was by random number assignment, but only a proportion of medical records were available to the authors (65% in the experimental group *v* 47% of controls). In the other RCT [34] the method of randomisation was not stated. Only a minority of the people in the first RCT actively participated in the interventions (23/50 in the treatment group *v* 20/50 in the control group), or completed the study (20/50 in the treatment group *v* 18/50 in the control group).[33]

OPTION RELAXATION PLUS BEHAVIOURAL MODIFICATION THERAPY

Two RCTs report insufficient evidence to define the effects of combined relaxation and behavioural modification treatment on seizures. One of the RCTs reported improved anxiety and adjustment.

Benefits: **Seizure frequency:** We found one systematic review[24] that found two RCTs of relaxation plus behaviour therapy.[35–37] One small RCT (18 children with uncontrolled epilepsy)[36,37] found a significant reduction compared to baseline of the median seizure index (the product of the seizure frequency and the seizure duration in seconds) after 1 year and after 8 years with a broad spectrum behaviour modification programme (which included teaching of symptom discrimination, relaxation, and countermeasure techniques to interrupt and abort seizures during early cues of the onset of a seizure). The median seizure index was increased compared to baseline in the control groups after 1 year. The RCT did not report the actual values for these observations, so comparison of groups is not possible. The other RCT (150 adults with uncontrolled epilepsy)[35] compared Jacobson's muscle relaxation plus behavioural therapy versus control treatment. It reported separately the mean seizure frequencies for each seizure type but did not specify the number in each category. It reported separately the mean seizure frequencies for those people with less than 20 seizures and those with more than 20 seizures per month at baseline. We were unable to analyse these results in a meaningful manner. **Psychological outcomes:** One of the RCTs[35] found significant improvements in anxiety and adjustment (home, health, social, and emotional) with combined versus control treatment.

Harms: The studies reported no harms.

Comment: The randomisation method was not stated for one study and was by alternate allocation in the other. The seizure index reported in one study[36,37] is not an ideal outcome measure. One of the RCTs recruited only 18 children and the groups would not be expected to be balanced for baseline characteristics. It is possible that the results of the psychological interventions on psychosocial functioning may depend on the baseline personality of the subjects included in the study, and their education and intelligence.

OPTION FAMILY COUNSELLING

One small RCT with weak methods found that family counselling versus no treatment significantly improved perceived acceptance by the family, emotional adjustment, interpersonal adjustment, adjustment to seizures, and overall psychosocial function. The study gave no information on seizure reduction.

Benefits: We found no systematic review but found one RCT (36 people with epilepsy and job loss),[38] which compared family therapy sessions versus one family session (in which information about the seizure profile was given) versus no intervention. It did not report seizure frequencies, but found a significantly improved psychosocial inventory score with family therapy (Washington Psycho Social Inventory (see glossary, p 1324), 27 completers: improved perceived acceptance by family, emotional adjustment, interpersonal adjustment, adjustment to seizures, and overall psychosocial function).[38] There was a trend towards improvement in job stability.

Harms: The study did not report harms.

Comment: The method of concealment of randomisation is not described in the publication. Nine of the 36 people did not complete the study; withdrawal was uneven across the groups (2 with family therapy, 6 with 1 family session, 1 with no intervention). The available evidence is insufficient to define the effects of family counselling.

GLOSSARY

Absence seizure Previously known as "petit mal", brief episodes of unconsciousness with vacant staring, sometimes with fluttering of the eyelids, as if "daydreaming". No falling to the ground. Rapid recovery. Rare in adults.

Atonic seizure Momentary loss of limb muscle tone causing sudden falling to the ground or drooping of the head.

Beck Depression Inventory Standardised scale to assess depression.

Cognitive behavioural therapy A broad category of interventions designed to promote the identification and control of stress and minimisation of its effects, often by using intellectual experience to correct damaging thoughts and behaviour.

Complex partial seizure Consciousness is impaired, memory of the episode is distorted but the person may not collapse. The subject may exhibit automatic behaviours ("automatisms", such as chewing, scratching the head, undressing). They can spread to the rest of the brain to become a secondary generalised tonic clonic seizure (see below). The electrical abnormality commonly starts in the temporal lobes.

Electroencephalographic (EEG) biofeedback A technique of making EEG activity apparent to a person, who is then taught to produce certain EEG waves, which are believed to increase the threshold for seizures.

Minnesota Multiphasic Personality Inventory A battery of standardised tests to assess personality (psychopathology).
Myoclonic seizure Sudden, symmetrical, shock like limb movements with or without loss of consciousness.
Relaxation therapy Techniques to train people to control muscle tension.
Simple partial seizure Electrical activity confined to one localised part of the brain causing symptoms and signs that depends on the part of the brain affected. The person remains conscious and fully aware.
Tonic clonic seizure Also known as a convulsion or "grand mal" attack. The person will become stiff (tonic) and collapse and have generalised jerking (clonic) movements. Breathing might stop and the bladder might empty. Generalised jerking movements lasting typically for a few minutes are followed by relaxation and deep unconsciousness, before slowly coming round. People are often tired, confused, and may remember nothing. Tonic clonic seizures may follow simple partial or complex partial seizures (see above), where they are classified as secondary generalised tonic clonic seizures. Tonic clonic seizures occurring without warning and in the context of a generalised epilepsy are classified as generalised tonic clonic seizures.
Tonic seizure Stiffening of the whole body with or without loss of consciousness.
Washington Psycho Social Inventory A standardised battery of tests to assess the adjustment in various spheres (measure of psychosocial difficulties) in people with epilepsy.

REFERENCES

1. Commission on classification and terminology of the international league against epilepsy. Proposal for revised classification of epilepsies and epileptic syndromes. *Epilepsia* 1989;30:389–399.
2. Hauser AW, Annegers JF, Kurland LT. Incidence of epilepsy and unprovoked seizures in Rochester, Minnesota 1935–84. *Epilepsia* 1993;34:453–468.
3. Hauser WA, Kurland LT. The epidemiology of epilepsy in Rochester, Minnesota, 1935 through 1967. *Epilepsia* 1975;16:1–66.
4. Cockerell OC, Johnson AL, Sander JW, Hart YM, Shorvon SD. Remission of epilepsy: results from the national general practice study of epilepsy. *Lancet* 1995;346:140–144.
5. Berg AT, Shinnar S. The risk of seizure recurrence following a first unprovoked seizure: a quantitative review. *Neurology* 1991;41:965–972. Search date not stated; primary sources Cumulated Index Medicus, and bibliographies of relevant papers.
6. First Seizure Trial Group (FIRST Group). Randomized clinical trial on the efficacy of antiepileptic drugs in reducing the risk of relapse after a first unprovoked tonic clonic seizure. *Neurology* 1993;43:478–483.
7. Musicco M, Beghi E, Solari A, Viani F, for the FIRST group. Treatment of first tonic clonic seizure does not improve the prognosis of epilepsy. *Neurology* 1997;49:991–998.
8. Marson AG, Williamson PR, Hutton JL, Clough HE, Chadwick DW, on behalf of the epilepsy monotherapy trialists. Carbamazepine versus valproate monotherapy for epilepsy. In: The Cochrane Library, Issue 3, 2000. Oxford: Update Software. Search date 1999; primary sources Medline, Cochrane Library, manufacturers, investigators.
9. Tudur Smith C, Marson AG, Williamson PR. Phenytoin versus valproate monotherapy for partial onset seizures and generalized onset tonic-clonic seizures. In: The Cochrane Library, Issue 4, 2001. Oxford: Update Software. Search date: 2000; primary sources Medline, the Cochrane Library randomized controlled trials register, handsearches of selected articles and the journals *Epilepsia, Epilepsy Research* and *Acta Neurologica Scandinavica*, drug manufacturers of valproate in Europe and USA, and original investigators of relevant trials.
10. Taylor S, Tudur Smith C, Williamson PR, Marson AG. Phenobarbitone versus phenytoin monotherapy for partial onset seizures and generalized onset tonic clonic seizures. The Cochrane Library, Issue 4, 2001. Search date 1998; primary sources Medline, the controlled trials register of the Cochrane Library, hand-searching relevant journals, the pharmaceutical industry, and researchers in the field.
11. Mattson RH, Cramer JA, Collins JF. A comparison of valproate with carbamazepine for the treatment of complex partial seizures and secondarily generalized tonic-clonic seizures in adults. The Department of Veterans Affairs Epilepsy Cooperative Study No. 264 Group. *N Engl J Med* 1992;10:327:765–771.
12. Richens A, Davidson DL, Cartlidge NE, Easter DJ. A multicentre comparative trial of sodium valproate and carbamazepine in adult onset epilepsy: adult EPITEG collaborative group. *J Neurol Neurosurg Psychiatry* 1994;57:682–687.
13. Marson AG, Kadir ZA, Hutton JL, Chadwick DW. Gabapentin for drug resistant partial epilepsy. In: The Cochrane Library, Issue 4, 2001. Oxford: Update Software. Search date 2000; primary Cochrane Epilepsy Group's trial register, the Cochrane Controlled Trials Register, drug manufacturers of gabapentin, and experts in the field.
14. Chaisewikul R, Privitera MD, Hutton JL, Marson AG. Levetiracetam add-on for drug-resistant localization related (partial) epilepsy. In: The Cochrane Library, Issue 3, 2001. Oxford: Update Software. Search date 2000; primary sources the Cochrane Epilepsy Group trials register, the Cochrane Controlled Trials Register, drug manufacturer of levetiracetam, and experts in the field.

15. Ramaratnam S, Baker GA, Marson AG. Lamotrigine for drug resistant partial epilepsy. In: The Cochrane Library, Issue 4, 2001. Oxford: Update Software. Search date April 2001; primary sources the Cochrane Epilepsy Group trials register, the Cochrane Controlled Trials Register, Medline, handsearches of reference lists, and manufacturers of lamotrigine.
16. Castillo S, Schmidt DB, White S. Oxcarbazepine add-on for drug-resistant partial epilepsy. In: The Cochrane Library, Issue 4, 2000. Oxford: Update Software. Search date 1999; primary sources the Cochrane Epilepsy Group's trials register, the Cochrane Controlled Trials Register, Medline, handsearches of reference lists, drug manufacturers, and experts in the field.
17. Marson AG, Kadir ZA, Hutton JL, Chadwick DW. The new antiepileptic drugs: a systematic review of their efficacy and tolerability. *Epilepsia* 1997;38:859–880. Search date 1995, primary sources Medline, hand search of key journals, and contacting pharmaceutical companies.
18. Jette N, Marson AG, Kadir ZA, Hutton JL, Chadwick DW. Topiramate for drug resistant partial epilepsy. In: The Cochrane Library, Issue 4, 2001. Oxford: Update Software. Search date 1999; primary sources The Cochrane Library, the controlled trial register of the Cochrane Epilepsy Group, drug manufacturers, and experts in the field.
19. Chadwick DW, Marson AG. Zonisamide for drug-resistant partial epilepsy. In: The Cochrane Library, Issue 3, 2000. Oxford: Update Software. Search date 1999; primary sources Cochrane Controlled Trials Register, Cochrane Epilepsy Group Trials Register, and personal contact with Dainippon and Elan Pharma, manufacturers of zonisamide, and experts in the field.
20. Kalviainen R, Nousiainen I, Mantyjarvi M, et al. Vigabatrin, a gabaergic antiepileptic drug, causes concentric visual field defects. *Neurology* 1999;53:922–926.
21. Medical Research Council Antiepileptic Drug Withdrawal Study Group. Prognostic index for recurrence of seizures after remission of epilepsy. *BMJ* 1993;306:1374–1378.
22. Medical Research Council Antiepileptic Drug Withdrawal Study Group. Randomised study of antiepileptic drug withdrawal in patients in remission. *Lancet* 1991;337:1175–1180.
23. Berg AT, Shinnar S. Relapse following discontinuation of antiepileptic drugs. *Neurology* 1994;44:601–608. Search date not stated; primary sources Index Medicus and bibliographies of relevant papers.
24. Ramaratnam S, Baker GA, Goldstein LH. Psychological treatments for epilepsy. In: The Cochrane Library, Issue 4, 2001. Oxford: Update Software. Search date 2001; primary sources Cochrane Epilepsy Group Trial Register, Cochrane Library, Issue 2, 2001, Medline, and cross references from identified publications.
25. Dahl J, Melin L, Lund L. Effects of a contingent relaxation treatment program on adults with refractory epileptic seizures. *Epilepsia* 1987;28:125–132.
26. Puskarich CA, Whitman S, Dell J, Hughes JR; Rosen AJ, Hermann BP. Controlled examination of effects of progressive relaxation training on seizure reduction. *Epilepsia* 1992;33:675–680.
27. Rousseau A, Hermann B, Whitman S. Effects of progressive relaxation on epilepsy: Analysis of a series of cases. *Psychol Rep* 1985;57:1203–1212.
28. Panjwani U, Selvamurthy W, Singh SH, Gupta HL, Thakur L, Rai UC. Effect of sahaja yoga practice on seizure control and EEG changes in patients of epilepsy. *Ind J Med Res* 1996;103:165–172.
29. Ramaratnam S, Sridharan K. Yoga for epilepsy. In: The Cochrane Library, Issue 4, 2001. Oxford: Update Software. Search date September 2001; primary sources Cochrane Epilepsy Group Trial Register, Cochrane Library, Issue 3, 2001, Medline, research registries of the research council for complementary medicine, hand searched reference lists, contacts with members of the Neurological Society of India, other neurology institutions, and yoga institutes for unpublished studies.
30. Lantz DL, Sterman MB. Neuropsychological assessment of subjects with uncontrolled epilepsy: effects of EEG feedback training. *Epilepsia* 1988;29:163–171.
31. Tan SY Bruni, J. Cognitive behavior therapy with adult patients with epilepsy: a controlled outcome study. *Epilepsia* 1986,27:225–233.
32. Davis GR, Armstrong HE Jr, Donovan DM, Temkin NR Cognitive-behavioral treatment of depressed affect among epileptics: preliminary findings. *Journal of Clinical Psychology*. 1984;40:930–935
33. Helgeson DC, Mittan R, Tan SY, Chayasirisobhon S. Sepulveda epilepsy education: the efficacy of a psychoeducational treatment program in treating medical and psychosocial aspects of epilepsy. *Epilepsia* 1990;31:75–82.
34. Lewis MA, Salas I, De La Sota A, Chiofalo N, Leake B. Randomized trial of a program to enhance the competencies of children with epilepsy. *Epilepsia* 1990;31:101–109.
35. Sultana SM. A study on the psychological factors and the effect of psychological treatment in intractable epilepsy. PhD Thesis, University of Madras, India 1987.
36. Dahl J, Melin L, Brorson LO, Schollin J. Effects of a broad-spectrum behavior modification treatment program on children with refractory epileptic seizures. *Epilepsia*. 1985; 26: 303–309.
37. Dahl J, Brorson LO, Melin L. Effects of a broad-spectrum behavioral medicine treatment program on children with refractory epileptic seizures: an 8-year follow-up. *Epilepsia* 1992;33:98–102.
38. Earl WL. Job stability and family counseling. *Epilepsia* 1986;27:215–219.

Anthony Marson
Lecturer in Neurology
University of Liverpool
Liverpool
UK

Sridharan Ramaratnam
Senior Consultant Neurologist
Apollo Hospitals
Chennai (Madras)
India

Competing interests: AM has been paid for speaking at meetings by Johnson and Johnson, manufacturers of topiramate, and by Janssen–Cilag, Sanofi, and GlaxoSmithKline for attending conferences. SR, none declared.

TABLE 1 Effects of additional drug treatment in people not responding to usual treatment: results of systematic reviews (see text, p 1318).

Drug	Daily dose (mg)	Percentage responding (95% CI) (> 50% reduction in seizure frequency)	RR treatment withdrawal (95% CI)	RR adverse effects (95% CI)	Comment
Gabapentin	**Adults only**				5 RCTs (1 in children, 4 in adults) Efficacy increased with increasing dose. No plateauing of responce, so doses tested may not have been optimal
	Placebo	9.9 (7.2 to 13.5)	1.4 (0.8 to 2.5)	Dizziness 2.25 (1.3 to 4) Fatigue 2.25 (1.1 to 4.6) Somnolence 2.04 (1.2 to 3.4)	
	600	14.4 (12.0 to 17.3)			
	900	17.3 (14.6 to 20.3)			
	1200	20.6 (17.1 to 24.6)			
	1800	28.5 (21.5 to 36.7)			
	Adults and children		**Adults and children**	**Adults and children**	
	600–1800	1.81 (1.32 to 2.49)	1.04 (0.71 to 1.52)	Dizziness 2.19 (1.24 to 3.89) Fatigue 2.30 (1.11 to 4.75) Somnolence 1.91 (1.20 to 3.05)	
Tiagabine (adults)	Placebo	6.2 (3.9 to 9.7)	1.8 (1.2 to 2.7)	Dizziness 1.69 (1.25 to 2.62)	3 RCTs
	16	9.8 (4.5 to 20.1)			
	30–32	21.6 (17.7 to 26.0)			
	56	29.8 (19.4 to 42.8)			
Topiramate (adults)	Placebo	11.6 (8.0 to 16.6)	2.44 (1.38 to 4.29)	Dizziness 1.79 (1.08 to 2.69) Fatigue 2.02 (1.19 to 3.41) Somnolence 2.57 (1.39 to 4.77) Difficulty thinking 6.42 (1.79 to 23.09)	6 RCTs
	200	26.7 (15.8 to 41.3)			
	400–1000	45.7 (41.3 to 50.1)			
Vigabatrin	Placebo	13.8 (9.7 to 19.2)	2.95 (1.25 to 7.00)	No adverse effects significantly more frequent but 40% develop concentric visual field abnormalities.[18]	3 RCTs
(adults)	1000 or 2000	22.8 (14.5 to 34.9)			
	3000 or 6000	45.9 (39.5 to 52.5)			

Results show percentage responding at particular daily doses, but results for treatment withdrawal and adverse effects are calculated for all doses.

TABLE 2 **Effects of additional drug treatment in people not responding to usual treatment: results of systematic reviews (see text, p 1318).**

Drug	Daily dose (mg)	Percentage responding (95% CI) (> 50% reduction in seizure frequency)	RR treatment withdrawal (95% CI)	RR adverse effects (95% CI)	Comment
Levetiracetam (adults)	1000–3000	3.78 (2.62 to 5.44)	1.21 (0.88 to 1.66)	Dizziness 2.50 (1.16 to 5.41) Infection 1.76 (1.03 to 3.02)	4 RCTs. Results of regression models do not provide reliable estimates for a responce to individual doses.
Lamotrigine (adults)	200–500	2.32 (1.67 to 3.23)	1.10 (0.81 to 1.50)	Ataxia 3.23 (1.93 to 5.42) Diplopia 3.47 (1.91 to 6.31) Dizziness 2.05 (1.52 to 2.78) Nausea 1.76 (1.18 to 2.64)	11 RCTs
Oxcarbazepine (adults and children)	600–2400	2.51 (1.88 to 3.33)	1.72 (1.35 to 2.18)	Ataxia 3.54 (1.75 to 7.13) Dizziness 2.87 (1.82 to 4.52) Fatigue 1.81 (1.00 to 3.29) Nausea 3.09 (1.74 to 5.49) Somnolence 2.36 (1.54 to 3.62) Diplopia 7.25 (3.12 to 16.80)	2 RCTs
Zonisamide	400	RR versus placebo 1.78 (1.26 to 2.51)	2.46 (1.61 to 3.76)	Ataxia 4.50 (1.05 to 19.22) Somnolence 1.91 (1.08 to 3.38) Anorexia 3.00 (1.31 to 6.88)	3 RCTs

All results are calculated for all doses.

TABLE 3 **Relative risks of seizure recurrence within 2 years of treatment withdrawal, according to prognostic variable (see text, p 1319).[21,22]**

Prognostic variable	RR (95% CI) of seizure recurrence within 2 years
Age < 16 years	1.8 (1.3 to 2.4)
Tonic clonic seizures	1.6 (1.1 to 2.2)
Myoclonus	1.8 (1.1 to 3.0)
Treatment with more than one antiepileptic drug	1.9 (1.4 to 2.4)
Seizures since antiepileptic drugs were started	1.6 (1.2 to 2.1)
Any electroencephalographic abnormality	1.3 (1.0 to 1.8)

Risk of recurrence also declined as the seizure free period increased, but in a complex manner.

Essential tremor

Search date January 2002

Joaquim Ferreira and Cristina Sampaio

QUESTIONS

INTERVENTIONS

See glossary, p 1337

Key Messages

- **All treatment options (long term)** We found no RCTs that reported the long term effects of drug treatments for essential tremor.
- **β blockers other than propranolol (atenolol, metoprolol, nadolol, pindolol, sotalol)** Small RCTs found weak evidence that sotalol or atenolol versus placebo significantly improved symptoms and self evaluated measures of tremor at 5 days to 4 weeks.
- **Benzodiazepines** Two brief RCTs found weak evidence that benzodiazepines versus placebo have no significant benefit in people with essential tremor. Adverse effects with benzodiazepines, including sedation and cognitive and behavioural effects, have been well described for other conditions (see panic disorder, p 1003).
- **Botulinum A toxin-haemagglutinin complex (evidence only for short term)** RCTs comparing botulinum A toxin-haemagglutinin complex versus placebo found short term improvement of clinical rating scales, but no consistent improvement of motor task performance or functional disability. Hand weakness, which is dose dependent and transient, is a frequent adverse effect.

Clin Evid 2002;8:1329–1338.

- **Calcium channel blockers (nicardipine, nimodipine)** Poor quality RCTs found insufficient evidence about the effects of dihydropyridine calcium channel blockers versus placebo.
- **Clonidine** One RCT found no significant difference with clonidine versus placebo in the number of people who improved.
- **Flunarizine** One small RCT found weak evidence that flunarizine versus placebo may improve symptoms after 1 month of treatment.
- **Gabapentin** Small crossover RCTs found insufficient evidence about the effects of gabapentin versus placebo.
- **Isoniazid** One RCT found no significant difference with isoniazid versus placebo in clinical score.
- **Methazolamide** One small RCT found no significant difference with methazolamide versus placebo in clinical score, functional tasks, or self evaluation.
- **Phenobarbital (evidence only for short term)** One small RCT found limited evidence that phenobarbital versus placebo significantly improved clinical scores at 5 weeks. Phenobarbital is associated with depression and cognitive and behavioural effects.
- **Primidone (evidence only for short term)** Small RCTs found limited evidence that primidone versus placebo significantly improved clinical scores and self evaluation of tremor at 2–5 weeks. Withdrawal due to adverse effects (including first dose acute toxic reaction, sedation, and depression) was frequent.
- **Propranolol (evidence only for short term)** Small RCTs have found that propranolol versus placebo significantly improves short term clinical scores, tremor amplitude, and self evaluation of severity for up to 6 weeks.

DEFINITION Tremor is a rhythmic, mechanical oscillation of at least one body region. The term essential tremor is used when there is either a persistent bilateral tremor of hands and forearms, or an isolated tremor of the head without abnormal posturing, and when there is no evidence that the tremor arises from another identifiable or separately named cause. The diagnosis is not made if there are abnormal neurological signs, known causes of enhanced physiological tremor, a history or signs of psychogenic tremor, sudden change in severity, primary orthostatic tremor, isolated voice tremor, isolated position specific or task specific tremors, and isolated tongue, chin, or leg tremor.[1]

INCIDENCE/ PREVALENCE Essential tremor is one of the most common movement disorders throughout the world, with a prevalence of 0.4–3.9% in the general population.[2]

AETIOLOGY/ RISK FACTORS Essential tremor is sometimes inherited with an autosomal dominant pattern. About 40% of people with essential tremor have no family history. Alcohol ingestion provides symptomatic benefit in 50–70% of people.[3]

PROGNOSIS Essential tremor is a persistent and progressive condition. It usually begins during young adulthood and the severity of the tremor increases slowly. Only a small proportion of people with essential tremor seek medical advice, but the proportion in different surveys varies from 0.5–11%.[2] Most people with essential tremor are only mildly affected. However, most of the people who seek medical care

are disabled to some extent, and most are socially handicapped by the tremor.[4] A quarter of people receiving medical care for the tremor change jobs or retire because of essential tremor induced disability.[3,5]

AIMS To reduce tremor; to minimise disability and social embarrassment; to improve quality of life, with minimal adverse effects from treatment.

OUTCOMES Severity of symptoms and disability measured by clinical rating scales or patient self evaluation. Clinical rating scales are often composite scores that grade tremor amplitude in each body segment in specific postures or tasks. Few scales have been formally validated. Tremorgraphic recordings are reported in many trials but they are proxy outcomes that have been included in this review only when clinical outcomes were not available.

METHODS *Clinical Evidence* search and appraisal January 2002. We excluded single dose studies and RCTs lasting under 1 week.

QUESTION **What are the effects of drug treatments in people with essential tremor of the hand?**

OPTION **PROPRANOLOL**

Several small RCTs have found that propranolol (60–240 mg) versus placebo for 1 month improves short term clinical scores, tremor amplitude, and self evaluation of severity. We found no RCTs of the long term effects of propranolol in essential tremor.

Benefits: **Propranolol versus placebo:** We found no systematic review but found 10 small (10–24 people), brief (up to 6 wks) RCTs, many of which had a crossover design.[6–15] One RCT[11] compared propranolol versus metoprolol versus placebo, and another RCT[15] compared propranolol versus pindolol versus placebo (see β blockers other than propranolol, p 1332). Seven of the nine RCTs evaluated clinical outcomes, including self evaluations of severity.[6–8,11-14] Propranolol (60–160 mg/day) versus placebo significantly increased the number of people categorised as "responders". The precise definition of responder varied among the RCTs, but the results were similar (22/23 [96%] with propranolol *v* 5/23 [22%] with placebo, ARR 69%, 95% CI 49% to 89%, NNT 2, no CI available;[6] ARR 80%, 95% CI 69% to 91%, NNT 2, no CI available;[7] ARR 64%, 95% CI 33% to 95%, NNT 2, 95% CI 2 to 4;[8] AR 10/16 [63%] with propranolol *v* 5/16 [31%] with placebo, ARR 32%, 95% CI 17% to 47%, NNT 4, 95% CI 2 to 6.[14]). Six RCTs found that propranolol versus placebo significantly improved symptom scores ($P < 0.05$).[7,8,11–14]

Harms: Withdrawals (mainly because of fatigue and bradycardia) were rare (e.g. 1/10 [10%] people in 1 RCT).[8] Depression, diarrhoea, breathlessness, sedation, blurred vision, and sexual problems were each reported in fewer than 5% of people taking propranolol.

Comment: We found no RCTs on the long term effects of propranolol in essential tremor. All trials were analysed as "on treatment" rather than by intention to treat, and this may have biased results.

Accelerometry is a proxy outcome that was reported in six of the RCTs. All six accelerometry results were favourable to propranolol, but there is an inconsistent relationship between accelerometry and clinical measures of effectiveness. People with congestive heart failure, second degree heart block, asthma, severe allergy, and insulin dependent diabetes were generally excluded from the RCTs. All the studies were small. The possibility of publication bias has not been excluded.

OPTION β BLOCKERS OTHER THAN PROPRANOLOL

Four small, brief RCTs found weak evidence that sotalol and atenolol are beneficial for treatment of essential hand tremor. We found no adequate evidence comparing propranolol with other β blockers.

Benefits: **β blockers other than propranolol versus placebo:** We found no systematic review, but found five small (9–24 people), brief (5 days to 4 wks) RCTs of different β blockers (sotalol, atenolol, metoprolol, nadolol, pindolol) versus placebo.[12,15–18] Two RCTs selected participants known to be responders or non-responders to propranolol.[12,17] The RCTs found limited evidence that both sotalol and atenolol versus placebo reduce symptom scores ($P < 0.02$),[12] and that sotalol versus placebo improves self evaluated measures of tremor ($P < 0.05$).[18] A small RCT of nadolol versus placebo found significant results only with a subgroup analysis.[17] The fourth crossover RCT (24 people) compared propranolol versus atenolol versus placebo. It found atenolol versus placebo improved accelerometer readings.[16] A crossover RCT of propranolol (120 mg/day) versus pindolol (30 mg/day) versus placebo found that pindolol versus placebo significantly worsened accelerometer recordings (see glossary, p 1337) ($P < 0.05$).[15] **β blockers other than propranolol versus propranolol:** We found no systematic review but found three small (14–24 participants) crossover, double blind RCTs.[11,15,16] The first RCT compared propranolol (120–240 mg/day) versus metoprolol (150–300 mg/day) versus placebo.[11] The RCT reported three outcomes: a composite clinical score, self evaluation, and accelerometer records. Propranolol (120 mg) versus metoprolol (150 mg) significantly improved clinical scores ($P < 0.05$) and self assessment ($P < 0.01$). Propranolol (240 mg) versus metoprolol (300 mg) significantly improved self assessment ($P < 0.05$). Propranolol was statistically superior to placebo ($P < 0.05$), but metoprolol was not. The second RCT compared propranolol versus atenolol versus placebo. It found no significant difference between propranolol and atenolol in accelerometer readings, but more people preferred propranolol to atenolol (12/24 [50%] *v* 1/24 [4%]).[16] The third crossover RCT (24 people) compared propranolol (120 mg/day) versus pindolol (30 mg/day) versus placebo. It found that pindolol versus propranolol significantly worsened accelerometer recorded tremor amplitude ($P < 0.005$).[15]

Harms: See harms of propranolol, p 1331.

Comment: We found no long term RCTs. People with congestive heart failure, second degree heart block, asthma, severe allergy, and insulin dependent diabetes were generally excluded from the RCTs. All the studies were small. The possibility of publication bias has not been excluded. The weak evidence suggests but does not confirm that β blockers other than propranolol improve essential hand tremor compared with placebo.

OPTION BARBITURATES

Two small, brief RCTs have found that primidone versus placebo improved clinical scores. One small, brief RCT found that phenobarbital versus placebo improved clinical scores. We found no long term RCTs.

Benefits: We found no systematic reviews. **Primidone versus placebo:** We found two crossover RCTs.[19,20] Both were small (8–22 people) and brief (2–5 wks). The first RCT[19] compared primidone (up to 750 mg/day) versus phenobarbital (phenobarbitone) (up to 150 mg/day) versus placebo. Primidone versus placebo significantly improved a clinical score and self evaluation of tremor ($P < 0.05$). In the second RCT (22 people), primidone (up to 750 mg/day) versus placebo significantly improved clinical scores ($P < 0.02$), functional tests ($P < 0.01$), and self evaluation ($P < 0.01$). Only 16/22 (73%) people completed the trial.[20] **Phenobarbital versus placebo:** We found three RCTs.[13,19,21] One crossover RCT (12 people, 5 wks' duration) found that phenobarbital (120 mg/day) versus placebo significantly improved accelerometer recordings (see glossary, p 1337) ($P < 0.01$), symptom rating scale ($P < 0.05$), but found no significant differences for handwriting tests or self evaluation of tremor.[21] More people responded (decrease in tremor score ≥ 15%) to phenobarbital than to placebo (11/11 [100%] with phenobarbital v 6/11 [55%] with placebo; ARR 45%, 95% CI 15% to 75%; NNT 3, 95% CI 2 to 7). The second RCT (double blind, 17 people; only 12 completed the study) compared propranolol (1.7 mg/kg/day) versus phenobarbital (1.25 mg/kg/day) versus placebo.[13] Phenobarbital versus placebo produced no significant differences in a clinical tremor score or functional tests.[13] The third small RCT (8 people) found no significant difference between phenobarbital and placebo.[19]

Harms: **Primidone:** In one RCT[20] 5/12 people taking primidone withdrew because of adverse effects (first dose acute toxic reaction, sedation, daytime sleepiness, tiredness, and depression). **Other barbiturates:** Both primidone (metabolised to phenobarbital) and phenobarbital are associated with depression and cognitive and behavioural effects (particularly in children, elderly people, and people with neuropsychiatric problems). See epilepsy, p 1313.

Comment: The RCTs were short term, small, and many randomised people did not complete the trials. We found no controlled long term RCTs. The possibility of publication bias has not been excluded.

OPTION BENZODIAZEPINES

Two brief RCTs found weak evidence that benzodiazepines versus placebo have no significant clinical benefits in essential hand tremor.

Benefits: We found no systematic reviews. We found two RCTs.[22,23] **Clonazepam versus placebo:** We found one RCT (15 people), which found no significant differences for any outcome.[22] However, nine people withdrew during an open run-in period with clonazepam, so only six entered the double blind phase. Potential selection bias makes it difficult to interpret the results of this RCT. **Alprazolam versus placebo:** We found one double blind RCT (24 people), which found alprazolam (up to 3 mg/day) versus placebo improved investigator global impression, but produced no significant difference in clinical scores, functional tests, or self evaluation of tremor.[23]

Harms: We found no data addressing harms of benzodiazepines specifically in populations with essential tremor. Adverse effects with benzodiazepines, including sedation and cognitive and behavioural effects, have been well described for other conditions (see panic disorder, p 1003).

Comment: None.

OPTION METHAZOLAMIDE

One RCT found no evidence of benefit with methazolamide compared with placebo.

Benefits: We found no systematic review. **Versus placebo:** We found one double blind, crossover RCT (25 people with essential tremor), which found methazolamide (up to 300 mg/day) versus placebo produced no significant differences in clinical score, functional tasks, or self evaluation (7/18 [39%] improved with methazolamide *v* 4/18 [22%] with placebo; ARR +16%, 95% CI −15% to +45%).[24]

Harms: The RCT did not look for adverse effects. Paraesthesias, drowsiness, and headaches are associated with methazolamide.

Comment: Methazolamide is a carbonic anhydrase inhibitor. The RCT was small and limited by being a crossover study. The results were analysed on treatment rather than by intention to treat, but seven people withdrew from the trial.

OPTION DIHYDROPYRIDINE CALCIUM CHANNEL BLOCKERS

Three RCTs with weak methods of calcium channel blockers versus placebo found insufficient evidence.

Benefits: We found no systematic review. **Nicardipine versus placebo:** We found two RCTs.[25,26] One double blind, crossover RCT (11 people) found that nicardipine versus placebo produced no significant differences in accelerometer recordings (see glossary, p 1337) after 1 month.[25] No clinical outcomes were assessed. Another crossover RCT (14 people) compared nicardipine (1 mg/kg/day) for 1 month versus propranolol (160 mg/day) for 1 month versus placebo.[27] Both nicardipine and propranolol versus placebo improved a symptom score. **Nimodipine versus placebo:** We found one double blind, crossover RCT (15 people), which found that nimodipine (90 mg/day) versus placebo produced no difference in clinical scores after 2 weeks of treatment (ARR +20%, 95% CI −15% to +55%).[26]

Harms: Nicardipine and nimodipine can provoke or aggravate heart failure. They are associated with dizziness, flushing, peripheral oedema, lethargy, headache, and fatigue. Adverse gastrointestinal effects (nausea/vomiting, loss of appetite, constipation, weight gain, thirst, indigestion, or altered taste) are reported by 1–3% of people. Abnormalities of laboratory tests (liver function tests) have been observed, usually within 1–8 weeks after starting treatment.

Comment: The RCTs were small, brief, and used crossover design. The possibility of publication bias has not been excluded. The evidence is too weak to assess the role of calcium channel blockers in essential hand tremor.

OPTION FLUNARIZINE

One small RCT found weak evidence that flunarizine compared with placebo may reduce the symptoms of essential hand tremor.

Benefits: We found no systematic review. **Flunarizine versus placebo:** We found one double blind, crossover RCT (17 people), which found that flunarizine (10 mg/day) versus placebo significantly improved clinical scores and tremor amplitude after 1 month of treatment (P = 0.0006).[28] Most of the people who completed the study were considered improved with flunarizine (13/15 [87%]), but the number improving with placebo was not reported.[9]

Harms: Flunarizine is associated with adverse neuropsychiatric effects, and with the development of parkinsonism and other movement disorders.[29–32]

Comment: The RCT was small and brief. The evidence is inconclusive.

OPTION CLONIDINE

One RCT found no improvement of essential hand tremor with clonidine versus placebo.

Benefits: **Versus placebo:** We found no systematic review. One small (10 people), brief crossover RCT of clonidine (up to 0.6 mg/day) versus placebo found no significant difference in the number of people who improved (1/10 [10%] with clonidine *v* 1/10 [10%] with placebo).[33]

Harms: The RCT did not look for adverse effects. Clonidine has been associated in other studies with sedation, lethargy, drowsiness, constipation, dry mouth, headache, dizziness, fatigue, and weakness.

Comment: None.

OPTION ISONIAZID

One RCT found no benefit with isoniazid versus placebo in essential hand tremor.

Benefits: We found no systematic review. **Versus placebo:** We found one small (15 people, 11 with essential tremor), brief, crossover RCT of isoniazid (up to 1200 mg/day) versus placebo.[34] No significant differences were found in clinical scores or in accelerometer recordings (see glossary, p 1337).

Harms: Isoniazid has been associated in other studies with hepatotoxicity and peripheral neuropathy.

Comment: None.

OPTION GABAPENTIN

Three small, brief RCTs found inconsistent evidence about the effects of gabapentin in essential hand tremor

Benefits: We found no systematic review. **Versus placebo:** We found three small, crossover RCTs (16–25 people).[14,35,36] The first RCT of gabapentin (1800 mg/day) versus placebo found no difference in clinical scores, activities of daily living, or self evaluation.[35] The second RCT compared gabapentin (up to 1200 mg/day) versus propranolol (up to 120 mg/day) versus placebo. Compared with placebo, gabapentin improved the number of people who responded (10/16 [63%] with gabapentin *v* 5/16 [31%] with placebo; ARR 32%, 95% CI 17% to 47%; NNT 4, 95% CI 2 to 6), clinical scores ($P < 0.05$), disability ($P < 0.01$), self evaluation ($P < 0.006$), and accelerometer recordings (see glossary, p 1337) ($P < 0.05$).[14] The third RCT (25 people) compared gabapentin (1800 mg/day) versus gabapentin (3600 mg/day) versus placebo. The RCT found no significant differences with high versus low doses of gabapentin in the 20 people who completed the trial. Gabapentin (at either dose) versus placebo significantly improved participants' global assessments ($P < 0.05$), water pouring scores ($P < 0.05$), and scores of activities of daily living ($P < 0.005$). The RCT did not report tremor scores specifically for the hand: it found no significant differences between gabapentin and placebo in accelerometry scores, spirographs, or investigator global impression scores.[36]

Harms: The RCTs reported fatigue, drowsiness, nausea, dizziness, and decreased libido in people taking gabapentin.[14,35,36] See epilepsy, p 1313.

Comment: The results of the three RCTs are contradictory. It is unclear whether the difference arose by chance or whether confounding variables, such as prior use of antitremor medications, baseline severity, or assessment rating scales, explain the difference.

OPTION BOTULINUM A TOXIN-HAEMAGGLUTININ COMPLEX

Two RCTs of botulinum A toxin-haemagglutinin complex versus placebo in essential hand tremor found short term improvement on clinical rating scales but no consistent improvement on motor tasks or functional disability. We found no RCTs addressing long term benefits or harms.

Benefits: We found no systematic review but found two RCTs.[37,38] The first RCT (25 people with essential hand tremor unresponsive to medical treatment)[37] compared botulinum A toxin-haemagglutinin complex versus placebo. Botulinum toxin (50 U) was injected in forearm muscles and repeated if necessary after 1 month (100 U). A successful response to the first injection was more likely with the botulinum toxin than with placebo (12/13 [92%] with botulinum toxin *v* 1/12 [8%] with placebo). After 4 weeks, mild to moderate improvement was more likely with botulinum toxin (75% with botulinum toxin *v* 27% with placebo ARR 48%, 95% CI 30% to 66%; NNT 3, 95% CI 2 to 4). Clinical scores were significantly improved by botulinum toxin versus placebo ($P < 0.05$), but functional tests and accelerometer recordings (see glossary, p 1337) were not significantly different. The second RCT (133 people with essential tremor of the hand by the Tremor Investigation Group criteria, 16 wks follow up) compared single injections of low dose botulinum A toxin-haemagglutinin complex (50 U) versus high dose botulinum A toxin-haemagglutinin complex (100 U) versus placebo into the wrist flexors and extensors. Postural tremor on clinical rating scales was significantly improved after 12 weeks with low dose ($P = 0.004$) and by high dose ($P = 0.0003$) botulinum toxin type A. Both botulinum toxin doses did not significantly improve kinetic tremor, motor task performance, or functional disability.[38]

Harms: The main adverse effect of botulinum A toxin-haemagglutinin complex is dose dependent transient hand weakness.

Comment: None.

GLOSSARY

Accelerometer recording Recording of the movements from a body segment to allow measurement of frequency and amplitude of a tremor.

REFERENCES

1. Deuschl G, Bain P, Brin M, and an Ad Hoc Scientific Committee. Consensus statement of the Movement Disorder Society on Tremor. *Mov Disord* 1998;13(suppl 3):2–23.
2. Louis ED, Ottman R, Hauser WA. How common is the most common adult movement disorder? Estimates the prevalence of essential tremor throughout the world. *Mov Disord* 1988;13:803–808.
3. Koller WC, Busenbark K, Miner K. The relationship of essential tremor to other movement disorders: report on 678 patients. Essential Tremor Study Group. *Ann Neurol* 1994;35:717–723.
4. Auff E, Doppelbauer A, Fertl E. Essential tremor: functional disability vs. subjective impairment. *J Neural Transm Suppl* 1991;33:105–110.
5. Bain PG, Findley LJ, Thompson PD, et al. A study of hereditary essential tremor. *Brain* 1994;117:805–824.
6. Winkler GF, Young RR. Efficacy of chronic propranolol therapy in action tremors of the familial, senile or essential varieties. *N Engl J Med* 1974;290:984–988.
7. Tolosa ES, Loewenson RB. Essential tremor: treatment with propranolol. *Neurology* 1975;25:1041–1044.
8. Morgan MH, Hewer RL, Cooper R. Effect of the beta adrenergic blocking agent propranolol on essential tremor. *J Neurol Neurosurg Psychiatry* 1973;36:618–624.
9. Calzetti S, Findley LJ, Perucca E, Richens A. The response of essential tremor to propranolol evaluation of clinical variables governing its efficacy on prolonged administration. *J Neurol Neurosurg Psychiatry* 1983;46:393–398.
10. Cleeves L, Findley LJ. Propranolol and propranolol-LA in essential tremor: a double blind comparative study. *J Neurol Neurosurg Psychiatry* 1988;51:379–384.
11. Calzetti S, Findley LJ, Perucca E, Richens A. Controlled study of metoprolol and propranolol during prolonged administration in people with essential tremor. *J Neurol Neurosurg Psychiatry* 1982;45:893–897.
12. Jefferson D, Jenner P, Marsden CD. Beta-adrenoreceptor antagonists in essential tremor *J Neurol Neurosurg Psychiatry* 1979;42:904–909.
13. Baruzzi A, Procaccianti G, Martinelli P, et al. Phenobarbitone and propranolol in essential tremor: a double-blind controlled clinical trial. *Neurology* 1983;33:296–300.
14. Gironell A, Kulisevsky J, Barbanoj M, Lopez-Villegas D, Hernandez G, Pascual-Sedano B. A randomized placebo-controlled comparative trial of gabapentin and propranolol in essential tremor. *Arch Neurol* 1999;56:475–480.
15. Teravainen H, Larsen A, Fogelholm R. Comparison between the effects of pindolol and propranolol on essential tremor. *Neurology* 1977;27:439–442.
16. Larsen TA, Teravainen H, Calne DB. Atenolol vs. propranolol in essential tremor. A controlled, quantitative study. *Acta Neurol Scand* 1982;66:547–554.
17. Koller WC. Nadolol in essential tremor. *Neurology* 1983;33:1076–1077.
18. Leigh PN, Jefferson D, Twomey A, Marsden CD. Beta-adrenoreceptor mechanisms in essential tremor; a double-blind placebo controlled trial of metoprolol, sotalol and atenolol. *J Neurol Neurosurg Psychiatry* 1983;46:710–715.
19. Sasso E, Perucca E, Calzetti S. Double-blind comparison of primidone and phenobarbitone in essential tremor. *Neurology* 1988;38:808–810.
20. Findley LJ, Cleeves L, Calzetti S. Primidone in essential tremor of the hands and head: a double-blind controlled clinical study. *J Neurol Neurosurg Psychiatry* 1985;48:911–915.
21. Findley LJ, Cleeves L. Phenobarbitone in essential tremor. *Neurology* 1985;35:1784–1787.

22. Thompson C, Lang A, Parkes JD, Marsden CD. A double-blind trial of clonazepam in benign essential tremor. *Clin Neuropharmacol* 1984;7:83–88.
23. Huber SJ, Paulson GW. Efficacy of alprazolam for essential tremor. *Neurology* 1988;38:241–243.
24. Busenbark K, Pahwa R, Hubble J, Hopfensberg K, Koller W. Double-blind controlled study of methazolamide in treatment of essential tremor. *Neurology* 1993;43:1045–1047.
25. Garcia-Ruiz PJ, Garcia-de-Yebenes-Prous J, Jimenez-Jimenez J. Effect of nicardipine on essential tremor: brief report. *Clin Neuropharmacol* 1993;16:456–459.
26. Biary N, Bahou Y, Sofi MA, Thomas W, al Deeb SM. The effect of nimodipine on essential tremor. *Neurology* 1995;45:1523–1525.
27. Jimenez-Jimenez FJ, Garcia-Ruiz PJ, Cabrera-Valdivia F. Nicardipine versus propranolol in essential tremor. *Acta Neurol (Napoli)* 1994;16:184–188.
28. Biary N, Deeb S, Langenberg P. The effect of flunarizine in essential tremor. *Neurology* 1991;41:311–312.
29. Micheli FE, Pardal MM, Giannaula R, et al. Movement disorders and depression due to flunarizine and cinnarizine. *Mov Disord* 1989;4:139–146.
30. Capella D, Laporte JR, Castel JM, Tristan C, Cos A, Morales-Olivas FJ. Parkinsonism, tremor, and depression induced by cinnarizine and flunarizine. *BMJ* 1988;297:722–723.
31. Chouza C, Scaramelli A, Caamano JL, De Medina O, Aljanati R, Romero S. Parkinsonism, tardive dyskinesia, akathisia and depression induced by flunarizine. *Lancet* 1986;1:1303–1304.
32. Micheli F, Pardal MF, Gatto M. Flunarizine and cinnarizine induced extrapyramidal reactions. *Neurology* 1987;37:881–884.
33. Koller W, Herbster G, Cone S. Clonidine in the treatment of essential tremor. *Mov Disord* 1986;4:235–237.
34. Hallett M, Ravitis J, Dubinsky RM, Gillespie MM, Moinfar A. A double-blind trial of isoniazid for essential tremor and other action tremors. *Mov Disord* 1991;6:253–256.
35. Pahwa R, Lyons K, Hubble JP, et al. Double-blind controlled trial of gabapentin in essential tremor. *Mov Disord* 1998;13:465–467.
36. Ondo W, Hunter C, Vuong KD, Schwartz K, Jankovic J. Gabapentin for essential tremor: a multiple-dose, double-blind, placebo-controlled trial. *Mov Disord* 2000;15:678–682.
37. Jankovic J, Schwartz K, Clemence W, Aswad A, Mordaunt J. A randomised, double-blind, placebo-controlled study to evaluate botulinum toxin type A in essential hand tremor. *Mov Disord* 1996;11:250–256.
38. Brin MF, Lyons KE, Doucette J, et al. A randomized, double masked, controlled trial of botulinum toxin type A in essential hand tremor. *Neurology* 2001;56:1523–1528.

Joaquim Ferreira
Neurologist

Cristina Sampaio
Assistant Professor
Instituto de Farmacologia e Terapêutica
Geral Lisbon School of Medicine
University of Lisbon
Lisbon
Portugal

Competing interests: CS has accepted reimbursement for attending symposia, fees for speaking, fees for organising education, and funds for a member of staff from Allergan (Botox) and IPSEN (Dysport). JF none declared.

Migraine headache

Search date April 2002

Luis Morillo

QUESTIONS

INTERVENTIONS

See glossary, p 1353

Key Messages

- **Diclofenac** Three RCTs using different outcomes found that diclofenac versus placebo significantly improved outcome (measured by treatment success, headache relief, and headache pain). One RCT found that intramuscular diclofenac versus intramuscular paracetamol significantly increased the number of people with partial relief of overall migraine symptoms within 35 minutes.
- **Eletriptan** One systematic review found that eletriptan versus placebo significantly increased headache relief. One subsequent RCT found that eletriptan versus placebo or versus sumatriptan significantly increased headache relief.
- **Ergotamine derivatives** One systematic review found three RCTs in which ergotamine or ergotamine plus caffeine versus placebo significantly improved headache relief, and one RCT that found no significant difference with ergotamine plus caffeine versus placebo. One additional RCT found that ergotamine plus caffeine versus sumatriptan was significantly less effective for headache relief or reducing the need for rescue medication. Another additional RCT found no difference between ergotamine alone versus ergotamine plus metoclopramide in headache intensity. One RCT found a significantly higher migraine intensity with ergotamine plus caffeine plus cyclizine versus naproxen. One RCT found a significantly higher migraine intensity with ergotamine versus naproxen, but another found no significant difference with ergotamine versus naproxen in pain relief after 1 hour. One overview of harms suggested that ergotamine versus placebo increased nausea and vomiting.

- **Ibuprofen** Three RCTs using different outcomes found that ibuprofen versus placebo significantly improved outcome (measured by headache relief, migraine index, and severity of attacks). One RCT found that ibuprofen arginine versus placebo significantly increased the number of people who achieved "considerable" or "complete" relief.
- **Naproxen** One crossover RCT found limited evidence that naproxen versus placebo significantly reduced headache intensity. One crossover RCT found limited evidence that naproxen versus placebo significantly reduced overall pain intensity. One RCT found that naproxen versus ergotamine plus caffeine plus cyclizine significantly reduced migraine intensity. One RCT found that naproxen versus ergotamine significantly reduced migraine intensity, but another RCT found no significant difference with naproxen versus ergotamine in pain relief after 1 hour.
- **Naratriptan** Three RCTs have found that naratriptan versus placebo significantly increases headache relief at 4 hours. One RCT comparing naratriptan versus sumatriptan found no significant difference in headache recurrence.
- **Rizatriptan** One systematic review has found that rizatriptan versus placebo significantly improves headache relief. Two additional RCTs found rizatriptan versus placebo significantly increased headache relief.
- **Salicylates (oral or iv lysine-acetylsalicylate [L-ASA] alone or in combination with metoclopramide; aspirin alone or in combination with metoclopramide; aspirin in combination with paracetamol and caffeine)** Three RCTs have found that oral or intravenous L-ASA (alone or in combination with metoclopramide) versus placebo significantly increases the proportion of people with headache relief. Two RCTs found that effervescent aspirin (alone or in combination with metoclopramide) versus placebo significantly increased headache relief. One large RCT found that aspirin plus paracetamol plus caffeine versus placebo significantly increased headache relief. One RCT found no significant difference between aspirin versus paracetamol plus codeine in headache relief, although both were significantly superior to placebo. One RCT found no significant difference with aspirin plus metoclopramide versus sumatriptan in headache relief. One small crossover RCT found limited evidence that acetylsalicylic acid versus placebo significantly reduced the duration of attack and headache intensity.
- **Sumatriptan** RCTs have found that subcutaneous, oral, or intranasal sumatriptan versus placebo significantly increases headache relief. One RCT found no significant difference with sumatriptan versus aspirin plus metoclopramide in headache relief. One RCT found no significant difference with sumatriptan versus tolfenamic acid in headache relief. One RCT found that sumatriptan versus ergotamine plus caffeine was significantly more effective for headache relief or reducing the need for rescue medication. One RCT comparing sumatriptan versus naratriptan found no significant difference in headache recurrence. One RCT found no significant difference between sumatriptan versus zolmitriptan in headache relief.
- **Tolfenamic acid** One RCT found limited evidence that tolfenamic acid versus placebo significantly increased the proportion of people with headache relief, and found no significant difference between tolfenamic acid versus sumatriptan. One small crossover RCT found limited evidence that tolfenamic acid versus placebo significantly reduced the duration of attack and headache intensity. One RCT found no significant difference between tolfenamic acid versus paracetamol in headache intensity. One crossover RCT found that tolfenamic acid (alone or in combination with either metoclopramide or caffeine) versus placebo significantly reduced headache intensity.

- **Zolmitriptan** Two large RCTs have found that oral zolmitriptan versus placebo significantly increases headache relief. One RCT found no significant difference between zolmitriptan versus sumatriptan in headache relief.

DEFINITION Migraine is a primary headache disorder manifesting as recurring attacks usually lasting for 4–72 hours and involving pain of moderate to severe intensity often with nausea, sometimes vomiting, and/or sensitivity to light, sound, and other sensory stimuli. The 1988 International Headache Society criteria (see glossary, p 1354) include separate criteria for migraine with and without associated aura.[1]

INCIDENCE/ PREVALENCE Migraine is common worldwide. Prevalence has been reported to be between 5% and 25% in women, and 2% and 10% in men. Overall, the highest incidence for migraine without aura has been reported between the ages of 10 and 11 years at 10/1000 person years. The peak incidence of migraine without aura in males is between ages 10 and 11 years (10/1000 person years) and in females between ages 14 and 17 years (19/1000 person years).[2] The incidence of migraine with aura peaks in males around age 5 years (7/1000 person years) and in females around age 12–13 years (14/1000 person years).[2]

AETIOLOGY/ RISK FACTORS Data arising from independent representative samples from Canada,[3,4] the USA,[5,6] several countries in Latin America,[7] several countries in Europe,[8–11] Hong Kong,[12] and Japan[13] demonstrate a female to male predominance and a peak in middle aged women. Migraine has been reported to be 50% more likely in people with a family history of migraine.[14]

PROGNOSIS Acute migraine is self limited and only rarely results in permanent neurological complications. Chronic recurrent migraine may cause disability through pain, and may affect daily functioning and quality of life. Female prevalence of migraine with or without aura has a declining trend after age 45–50 years.

AIMS To reduce frequency of migraine, intensity of accompanying symptoms, and duration of headache, with minimal adverse effects.

OUTCOMES Headache relief (see glossary, p 1354) or being pain free (see glossary, p 1354) at different times after medication. Pain relief at specific post-dose times. Web extra table A at www.clinicalevidence.com specifies those RCTs in which 2 hour or 4 hour headache relief outcome is reported as the preferred clinical outcome measure.[15–36] In this review, headache relief is reported at 2 hours unless expressed otherwise. Some RCTs include the need for rescue medication (see glossary, p 1354) and headache recurrence (see glossary, p 1353) as outcome measures.

METHODS *Clinical Evidence* search and appraisal April 2002.

QUESTION What are the effects of drug treatments of acute migraine?

OPTION SALICYLATES

Three RCTs have found that oral or intravenous lysine acetylsalicylate (alone or in combination with metoclopramide) versus placebo significantly increases the proportion of people with headache relief. Two RCTs found that effervescent aspirin (alone or in combination with metoclopramide) versus placebo significantly increased headache relief. One large RCT found that aspirin plus paracetamol plus caffeine versus placebo significantly increased headache relief. One RCT found no significant difference between aspirin versus paracetamol plus codeine in headache relief, although both were significantly superior to placebo. One RCT found no significant difference with aspirin plus metoclopramide versus sumatriptan in headache relief. One small crossover RCT found limited evidence that acetylsalicylic acid versus placebo significantly reduced the duration of attack and headache intensity.

Benefits: We found no systematic review but found 9 RCTs.[15–20,37–39] **Oral lysine acetylsalicylate (L-ASA):** One RCT (266 people, 475 migraine attacks) found that the proportion with headache relief (see glossary, p 1354) was significantly higher with oral L-ASA (1620 mg) plus metoclopramide (10 mg) than with placebo ($P < 0.001$; AR 56% with L-ASA *v* 28% placebo; RR 2.0, 95% CI 1.6 to 2.5).[15] In one RCT, people were also assigned in a third arm to oral sumatriptan.[16] The groups receiving oral L-ASA (1620 mg) plus metoclopramide (10 mg) or oral sumatriptan (100 mg) attained headache relief more often than the placebo controls ($P < 0.0001$; AR 57% with L-ASA *v* 53% with oral sumatriptan *v* 24% with placebo; RR 2.4, 95% CI 1.7 to 3.3). The difference between active treatment groups was not significant ($P = 0.50$).[16] **Intravenous L-ASA:** One RCT (278 people) compared 1800 mg L-ASA intravenously, to 6 mg of subcutaneous sumatriptan, versus placebo in a third arm.[17] Headache relief with either of the two treatments was better than with placebo ($P < 0.0001$; AR 74% with L-ASA *v* 91% with sumatriptan *v* 24% with placebo; RR L-ASA *v* placebo 3.1, 95% CI 1.8 to 5.4; RR L-ASA *v* sumatriptan 0.8, 95% CI 0.7 to 0.9). Sumatriptan was superior to L-ASA ($P = 0.001$). A smaller RCT (112 attacks in 56 people, crossover design) compared 1000 mg L-ASA given intravenously versus 0.5 mg subcutaneous ergotamine.[37] It found no significant difference between the groups. The primary outcome measure was pain intensity score from a visual analogue scale. **Effervescent aspirin:** One crossover RCT (120 people) compared effervescent aspirin (650 mg) (with and without 10 mg metoclopramide) versus placebo.[38] The 2 hour mean effect on headache was rated lower during the placebo period than during the periods with aspirin alone or in combination. Aspirin alone showed no significant difference from its combination with metoclopramide. Either active treatment was better than placebo ($P < 0.001$). Another RCT (374 people) compared effervescent aspirin (1000 mg) versus placebo. Headache relief was superior with aspirin than with placebo ($P < 0.001$; AR 55% with aspirin *v* 37%; RR 1.5, 95% CI 1.2 to 1.9).[20] **Other combinations:** One large RCT (1357 people with non-disabling migraine) tested a non-prescription combination (oral paracetamol 250 mg, aspirin 250 mg plus caffeine 65 mg) versus placebo.[19] Headache relief was superior with the active treatment ($P < 0.001$; AR 59% with the combination *v* 33% with placebo; RR 1.8, 95% CI 1.6 to 2.1). In a crossover designed RCT (198 people treated for 3 consecutive migraine attacks), aspirin (1000 mg) orally was not significantly different to paracetamol (400 mg) plus codeine (25 mg) in attaining headache relief, although both were superior to placebo ($P = 0.0003$ with aspirin and 0.0002 with paracetamol and codeine).[39] **Versus sumatriptan:** In one RCT (358 people), aspirin (900 mg) plus metoclopramide (10mg) given orally was not significantly different from sumatriptan (100 mg) given orally in attaining headache relief at 2 hours ($P = 0.078$; AR 45% with aspirin plus metoclopramide *v* 56% with sumatriptan).[18] **Versus tolfenamic acid:** See benefits of tolfenamic acid, p 1346.

Harms: One RCT reported adverse effects related to L-ASA in 2%, to sumatriptan in 15%, and to placebo in 2% of people treated.[17] In this trial, severe harms were related to L-ASA in 3%, to sumatriptan 5%, and to the placebo control group in 2% of people treated. Another trial reported premature withdrawal in 2% of placebo, 1% of L-ASA, and 3% of sumatriptan treated people.[16] The most frequently reported harms for L-ASA were somnolence, abdominal pain, nausea or vomiting, fatigue, and headache. The RCT comparing the combination of paracetamol, aspirin, and caffeine versus placebo reported no serious adverse effects.[19]

Comment: None.

OPTION DICLOFENAC

Three RCTs using different outcomes found that diclofenac versus placebo significantly improved outcome (measured by treatment success, headache relief, and headache pain). One RCT found that intramuscular diclofenac versus intramuscular paracetamol significantly increased the number of people with partial relief of overall migraine symptoms within 35 minutes.

Benefits: We found no systematic review. **Versus placebo:** We found two placebo controlled RCTs of oral diclofenac used in three to four consecutive migraine attacks.[21,40] One RCT (170 people) found that diclofenac versus placebo significantly improved treatment success (defined at 2 h as a visual analogue scale score below 10 mm or headache duration of less than 2 h without need of rescue medication [see glossary, p 1354] within this period; AR 27% with diclofenac *v* 19% with placebo; RR 1.5, 95% CI 1.0 to 2.2).[40] The second RCT (72 people) comparing diclofenac 50 mg or 100 mg versus placebo found that either dose significantly increased headache relief (see glossary, p 1354) (AR 39% with 50 mg *v* 44% with 100 mg *v* 22% with placebo; RR diclofenac 50 mg *v* placebo 1.8, 95% CI 1.0 to 3.1; RR diclofenac 100 mg *v* placebo 1.9, 95% CI 1.1 to 3.3). No significant difference was found between 50 mg and 100 mg doses. Diclofenac 100 mg versus placebo significantly reduced the number of people needing rescue medication (AR 37% v 58%; RR 0.64, 95% CI 0.44 to 0.93).[21] The third RCT (156 people meeting International Headache Society criteria (see glossary, p 1354) for migraine with or without aura) compared diclofenac potassium (50–100 mg) versus oral sumatriptan (100 mg) versus placebo.[41] The trial found that diclofenac versus placebo significantly reduced headache pain at 2 hours measured on a visual analogue scale ($P < 0.001$). It found no significant difference between either dose of diclofenac versus sumatriptan.[41] **Versus paracetamol:** One RCT (86 people) compared intramuscular diclofenac 75 mg versus intramuscular paracetamol in people with paroxysmal headaches accompanied by at least two of the following features: (1) unilateral pain; (2) nausea; (3) visual and limb symptoms; and (4) positive family history. The trial found that more people taking diclofenac versus paracetamol had partial relief of overall migraine symptoms (intensity and duration) within 35 minutes (AR 89% with diclofenac v 17% with paracetamol; RR 4.9, 95% CI 2.5 to 9.8).[42]

Harms: In one RCT (72 people), 33% of people reported one or more adverse effects during one or more attacks.[21] Most adverse effects were rated as mild or moderate (gastrointestinal complaints were the most common, followed by tiredness and fatigue), but 12% of people rated adverse experiences as severe. In another RCT (170 people), 14% of people reported at least one side effect, with gastrointestinal effects being the most common (50%). Only three people withdrew because of gastrointestinal symptoms.[40] See non-steroidal anti-inflammatory drugs, p 1203.

Comment: The diversity of outcome measures limits comparisons with the more usual outcome — headache relief. With the exception of one RCT, case definition was not based on International Headache Society criteria.

OPTION IBUPROFEN

Three RCTs using different outcomes found that ibuprofen versus placebo significantly improved outcome (measured by headache relief, migraine index, and severity of attacks). One RCT found that ibuprofen arginine versus placebo significantly increased the number of people who achieved "considerable" or "complete" relief.

Benefits: **Versus placebo:** We found no systematic review but found three RCTs comparing ibuprofen versus placebo,[22,43,44] and one RCT comparing ibuprofen arginine versus placebo.[45] The first RCT (729 people) compared ibuprofen (400 mg and 600 mg) in liquigel formulation versus placebo.[22] The trial found that ibuprofen improved headache relief (see glossary, p 1354) (AR 72% with 400 mg v 72% with 600 mg v 50% with placebo; ibuprofen 400 mg v placebo RR 1.4, 95% CI 1.2 to 1.7; ibuprofen 600 mg v placebo RR 1.4, 95% CI 1.2 to 1.7). There was no significant difference in the need for rescue medication (see glossary, p 1354). The second RCT (25 people, 146 migraines) used outcomes defined using the migraine index (see glossary, p 1354). The trial found that ibuprofen significantly reduced the migraine index (25 ± 28 v 46 ± 27; $P = 0.0014$), and reduced the number of people who required additional medication 4 hours after treatment (26% *v* 56%; P = 0.007).[43] The third RCT (40 people with common and classic migraine, 345 migraines) compared ibuprofen (800–1200 mg orally) versus placebo.[44] The trial found that with ibuprofen versus placebo significantly more attacks were rated as mild (P < 0.001) and significantly fewer attacks were rated as moderate (P < 0.05) or severe (P < 0.05). Ibuprofen versus placebo also reduced the number of migraine attacks requiring rescue medication (AR 22% *v* 81%; RR 0.27, 95% CI 0.20 to 0.36). The fourth RCT (40 people) compared an ibuprofen arginine preparation (400 mg orally) versus placebo.[45] It found that more people taking ibuprofen arginine versus placebo achieved "considerable" or "complete" relief within 2 hours (51% *v* 7%; P < 0.01; insufficient data for RR calculation). Fewer people taking ibuprofen arginine needed rescue medication (31% *v* 48%) but no statistical analysis was performed.

Harms: One RCT did not report adverse effects.[44] Another RCT reported pain and stomach discomfort in 12% of people on treatment, which was not considered serious.[43] See non-steroidal anti-inflammatory drugs, p 1203.

Comment: None.

OPTION NAPROXEN

One crossover RCT found limited evidence that naproxen versus placebo significantly reduced headache intensity. One crossover RCT found limited evidence that naproxen versus placebo significantly reduced overall pain intensity. One RCT found that naproxen versus ergotamine plus caffeine plus cyclizine significantly reduced migraine intensity. One RCT found that naproxen versus ergotamine significantly reduced migraine intensity, but another RCT found no significant difference with naproxen versus ergotamine in pain relief after 1 hour.

Benefits: We found no systematic review. **Versus placebo:** We found one crossover RCT (37 people with classic or common migraine) comparing oral naproxen (750–1250 mg) versus placebo.[46] The RCT found that naproxen reduced headache intensity (see glossary, p 1353) (P = 0.047), but it found no significant difference in the number of people requiring rescue medication (see glossary, p 1354) (absolute numbers not provided; P = 0.13). Headache intensity was defined as (1) none = symptoms absent; (2) mild = symptoms present but not influencing work or recreational activities; (3) moderate = symptoms reducing ability to carry out work or recreational activities; or (4) severe = symptoms hindering work or recreational activities completely. A second crossover RCT (40 people with common or classic migraine) comparing naproxen (750–1000 mg) versus placebo found that naproxen reduced overall pain intensity (rated as mild, moderate, or severe; P = 0.011; time of evaluation not stated).[47] The need for rescue medication after 2 hours was also significantly lower for naproxen (AR 47% *v* 72%; P = 0.002; insufficient data for RR calculation). **Versus ergotamine:** We found three RCTs (256 people), which compared oral naproxen (750–1750 mg) versus ergotamine (2–4 mg) alone or versus ergotamine plus caffeine (91.5 mg) plus cyclizine chlorhydrate (50 mg). The first RCT found that naproxen versus the ergotamine combination significantly reduced migraine intensity (rated as mild, moderate, severe, or incapacitating; P = 0.014), but it found no significant difference in the number of migraine attacks requiring rescue medication.[48] The second RCT compared naproxen versus ergotamine.[49] In this trial, 47% of people were reported to have terminated the study prematurely. The trial found that naproxen versus ergotamine significantly reduced migraine intensity (rated as none, mild, moderate, or severe; P = 0.04), but it found no significant difference in the need for rescue medication (23% *v* 29%). The third RCT compared naproxen versus ergotamine versus placebo.[50] This trial found that people taking naproxen versus placebo had significantly better pain relief 1 hour after the first dose (P = 0.032), but it found no significant difference between ergotamine versus placebo (P = 0.084), or between naproxen versus ergotamine (P = 0.65). The absolute numbers of responders were not provided.

Harms: In the first RCT, adverse effects were reported in 5/32 people taking naproxen; four had stomach pain and dyspepsia, and one withdrew from the trial because of severe stomach pain.[46] One RCT comparing naproxen versus ergotamine found that vomiting was more frequent with ergotamine (34% *v* 10%; P = 0.0083), and more people taking ergotamine withdrew because of severe symptoms (diarrhoea, vomiting, dizziness, nausea, shivering, sweating) compared with those taking naproxen (8% *v* 2%). In another RCT, more people taking naproxen versus ergotamine discontinued medication (6/19 [32%] *v* 2/17 [12%]).[49] A third RCT found that more people taking ergotamine versus naproxen had severe adverse effects (8/48 *v* 1/48), and two people taking ergotamine withdrew from the study.[36] See non-steroidal anti-inflammatory drugs, p 1203.

Comment: The diversity of outcome measures limits comparisons with the more usual outcome — headache relief. Though variable, adverse effects were significant. None of the RCTs used the International Headache Society criteria (see glossary, p 1354) to identify cases.

OPTION TOLFENAMIC ACID

One RCT found limited evidence that tolfenamic acid versus placebo significantly increased the proportion of people with headache relief, and found no significant difference between tolfenamic acid versus sumatriptan. One small crossover RCT found limited evidence that tolfenamic acid versus placebo significantly reduced the duration of attack and headache intensity. One RCT found no significant difference between tolfenamic acid versus paracetamol in headache intensity. One crossover RCT found that tolfenamic acid (alone or in combination with either metoclopramide or caffeine) versus placebo significantly reduced headache intensity.

Benefits: We found no systematic review. **Versus placebo or sumatriptan:** One RCT (141 people, 289 migraine attacks) compared tolfenamic acid (200 mg) versus sumatriptan (100 mg) versus placebo.[23] The trial found that tolfenamic acid versus placebo significantly increased the number of people with headache relief (see glossary, p 1354) (AR 77% *v* 29%; RR 2.6, 95% CI 1.5 to 4.2), but found no significant difference between tolfenamic acid versus sumatriptan. The use of rescue medication (see glossary, p 1354) was not significantly different between any of the three arms. **Versus placebo or acetylsalicylic acid or ergotamine:** One crossover RCT (20 women with common or classic migraine, 160 migraines) compared tolfenamic acid (200 mg), acetylsalicylic acid (500 mg), and ergotamine (1 mg) versus placebo.[51] The RCT found that tolfenamic acid, ergotamine, and acetylsalicylic acid versus placebo significantly reduced the duration of attacks ($P < 0.001$, $P < 0.001$, and $P < 0.005$, respectively) and reduced headache intensity ($P = 0.01$, $P = 0.01$, and $P = 0.05$, respectively; time of evaluation not stated). The mean duration of attack was shortest with tolfenamic acid, but this was not significantly shorter than the mean duration of attack with the other drugs (P value not stated).The need for rescue medication after 2 hours was not significantly different. **Versus paracetamol:** A second RCT (149 people with common or classic migraine) compared tolfenamic acid (400 mg) versus paracetamol (1000 mg).[52] The trial found no significant difference between treatments in headache intensity, side effects, strength, effect duration, or the need for additional medication after 3 hours of test medication. **Combination preparations:** One crossover RCT (49 people with common or classic migraine, 482 migraines) compared tolfenamic acid alone or in combination with either caffeine or metoclopramide versus placebo.[53] The trial found that tolfenamic acid, either alone or in combination, versus placebo significantly reduced headache intensity (measured on a scale of no, slight, moderate, or severe symptoms). All combinations of tolfenamic acid versus placebo significantly reduced the need for rescue medication ($P < 0.01$).

Harms: In one RCT comparing tolfenamic acid versus sumatriptan, the frequency of adverse effects was similar (30% *v* 41%).[50] See non-steroidal anti-inflammatory drugs, p 1203.

Comment: None.

OPTION ERGOTAMINE DERIVATIVES

One systematic review found three RCTs in which ergotamine or ergotamine plus caffeine versus placebo significantly improved headache relief, and one RCT that found no significant difference with ergotamine plus caffeine versus placebo. One additional RCT found that ergotamine plus caffeine versus sumatriptan was significantly less effective for headache relief or reducing the need for rescue medication. Another additional RCT found no significant difference between ergotamine alone versus ergotamine plus metoclopramide in headache intensity. One RCT found a significantly higher migraine intensity with ergotamine plus caffeine plus cyclizine versus naproxen. One RCT found a significantly higher migraine intensity with ergotamine versus naproxen, but another found no significant difference with ergotamine versus naproxen in pain relief after 1 hour. One overview of harms suggested that ergotamine versus placebo increased nausea and vomiting.

Benefits: **Versus placebo:** We found one systematic review (search date 1991, 7 RCTs, 588 people) of ergotamine versus placebo in the acute treatment of headache.[54] Ergotamine was administered orally at doses between 1 mg and 6 mg. Ergotamine was given alone in three RCTs, combined with caffeine in three RCTs, and combined with alkaloids and barbiturates in one RCT. The RCT of ergotamine plus alkaloids plus barbiturates was not evaluable. None of the trials used International Headache Society criteria (see glossary, p 1354) for participant inclusion, and defined responders according to a variety of 3 to 10-point scales. Two RCTs identified by the review found that ergotamine alone versus placebo significantly increased headache relief ($P < 0.01$ in 1 RCT, reported as "significant" in the other RCT; P value not stated) and one RCT found that ergotamine alone versus placebo significantly reduced the duration of attacks ($P < 0.001$). Two RCTs identified by the review found a similar use of escape medication with ergotamine alone versus placebo (P value not stated; no further data provided). Two RCTs identified by the review measuring nausea or vomiting as an efficacy parameter found similar results with ergotamine alone versus placebo (P value not stated). One RCT identified by the review found that ergotamine plus caffeine versus placebo significantly increased headache relief (reported as "significant"; P value not stated), but another RCT found no significant difference (P value not stated). The RCTs comparing ergotamine plus caffeine versus placebo did not assess duration of attack. Two RCTs identified by the review found that ergotamine plus caffeine versus placebo reduced the use of escape medication ($P < 0.05$ in 1 RCT and reported as "significant" in the other; P value not stated). Two RCTs identified by the review measuring nausea or vomiting as an efficacy parameter found placebo superior to ergotamine plus caffeine (no statistical analysis conducted). **Versus sumatriptan:** One RCT (580 people) compared oral ergotamine (2 mg) plus caffeine (100 mg) orally versus oral sumatriptan (100 mg).[55] The trial found that ergotamine plus caffeine versus sumatriptan was significantly less effective in improving headache relief (see glossary, p 1354) (AR 48% *v* 66%; RR 0.73, 95% CI 0.62 to 0.85; $P < 0.001$). Significantly more people required rescue medication (see glossary, p 1354) with ergotamine than with sumatriptan (AR 44% *v* 24%; RR 1.82, 95% CI 1.38 to 2.39). **Plus metoclopramide:** One RCT (24 women with common or classic migraine, 176 migraines) comparing ergotamine alone versus ergotamine plus metoclopramide found no significant difference in headache intensity (see glossary, p 1353) (measured on a 3-point scale as more than usual, usual, or less than usual).[56] There was also no significant difference in the number of people requiring additional medication (timing not stated). **Versus naproxen:** See benefits of naproxen, p 1345.

Harms: In the systematic review comparing ergotamine versus placebo, two RCTs measuring nausea and vomiting as a side effect found placebo superior to ergotamine alone (no statistical analysis conducted), and two RCTs measuring nausea and vomiting as a side effect found placebo superior to ergotamine plus caffeine (no statistical analysis conducted).[54] We found one overview of the safety of dihydroergotamine mesylate (DHE) and ergotamine tartrate.[57] This overview identified two trials (24 and 311 people, respectively), which found that adverse effects with intramuscular DHE occurred in less than 10% of people (with leg cramps and pain at the injection site being most common). Harms resolved within 1 hour. Three RCTs in the overview found that nausea and vomiting were the most common adverse effects, which subsided within 15 minutes. In another open trial (300 people), 32% of people taking DHE complained of nausea. Post-marketing surveillance studies have reported ischaemic complications, nausea, vomiting, seizures, cardiac and non-cardiac vascular disorders such as vasospasm and infarction, liver abnormalities, leg pain, chest pain, hypertensive crisis, injection site reactions, head and shoulder pain, and paraesthesia. Treatment related phenomena were reported in less than 4% of people receiving intranasal DHE. A bitter or unpleasant taste was reported by 2%. Dizziness and muscle pain were reported by less than 1%. Discontinuation of treatment occurred in only 1% of people included in the RCTs. Worsening of baseline nausea or vomiting was suggested in 5 of 7 RCTs comparing acute administration of ergotamine tartrate versus placebo. Single case reports of less common adverse effects include abdominal discomfort, numbness or tingling of fingers or toes, ischaemic complications, swollen fingers, and leg cramps. With chronic use in excessive doses, ischaemic neuropathy, anorectal ulcers following suppository use, habituation, and overuse headaches have been reported.[57]

Comment: With the exception of one RCT, the variety of outcome measures limits comparisons with the more usual outcome, headache relief. Only one of the RCTs used the International Headache Society criteria to identify cases.

OPTION ELETRIPTAN

One systematic review has found that eletriptan versus placebo significantly increases headache relief. One subsequent RCT found that eletriptan versus placebo or versus sumatriptan significantly increased headache relief.

Benefits: We found one systematic review with meta-analysis (search date 2000; 6 unpublished RCTs made available by the manufacturer; 4705 people) comparing eletriptan 20 mg, 40 mg, and 80 mg versus placebo.[24] All doses of eletriptan significantly improved headache relief (see glossary, p 1354). A significant difference was found between 20 mg and 40 mg doses, but not between 40 mg and 80 mg doses for headache relief (pooled data: 20 mg 45% of people had headache relief, RR 2.0, 95% CI 1.6 to 2.6; 40 mg 59%, RR 2.4, 95% CI 2.1 to 2.7; 80 mg 62%, RR 2.5, 95% CI 2.2 to 2.9). One subsequent RCT (857 people) compared eletriptan 20 mg, 40 mg, and 80 mg versus 100 mg sumatriptan versus placebo.[25] Eletriptan versus placebo significantly increased headache relief (20 mg 54%, RR 2.3, 95% CI 1.6 to 3.2; 40 mg 65%, RR 2.7, 95% CI 1.9 to 3.8; 80 mg 77%, RR 3.2, 95% CI 2.3 to 4.5). Eletriptan (80 mg) versus sumatriptan (100 mg) also significantly increased headache relief (AR 77% *v* 55%; RR 1.4, 95% CI 1.2 to 1.7).

Harms: In the first RCT, dizziness and fatigue were the only adverse effects that were significantly more common in people taking eletriptan versus placebo.[24] The first RCT found a dose response relationship between minor and major harms of eletriptan.[24] The risk of major harm with 20 mg eletriptan was 0.7 (95% CI 0.2 to 2.6), with 40 mg 0.6 (95% CI 0.3 to 1.6), and with 80 mg 1.1 (95% CI 0.5 to 2.4). The risk of minor harm with 80 mg eletriptan was 2.0 (95% 1.6 to 2.6) compared with a relative risk of 1.5 (95% CI 1.2 to 1.9) with 40 mg.

Comment: None.

OPTION NARATRIPTAN

Three RCTs have found that naratriptan versus placebo significantly increases headache relief at 4 hours. One RCT comparing naratriptan versus sumatriptan found no significant difference in headache recurrence.

Benefits: We found no systematic review. **Versus placebo:** We found three RCTs.[26,27,58] The first RCT (643 people) found that naratriptan or sumatriptan versus placebo significantly increased the number of people with headache relief (see glossary, p 1354) at 4 hours (63% with naratriptan *v* 80% with sumatriptan *v* 31% with placebo; $P < 0.05$).[26] A second crossover RCT (740 people) compared naratriptan 2.5 mg, 1 mg, and 0.25 mg versus placebo.[27] This trial found that naratriptan (2.5 mg) versus placebo was the most effective dose in producing headache relief at 4 hours (AR 68% *v* 33%; $P < 0.001$; insufficient data for RR calculation). Naratriptan (2.5 mg) significantly reduced the need for rescue medication (see glossary, p 1354) after 4 hours (AR 52% *v* 26%; $P < 0.001$; insufficient data for RR calculation). Headache recurrence (see glossary, p 1353) within 24 hours of initial dosing occurred in fewer people taking naratriptan (2.5 mg) versus placebo (27% *v* 36%; significance not stated). In a third RCT, a subgroup of 206 people with a poor response to sumatriptan (50 mg) in a first attack were randomised 1 week later to either naratriptan (2.5 mg) orally or placebo.[58] Naratriptan versus placebo significantly increased headache relief at 2 hours (AR 25% with naratriptan *v* 10% with placebo; RR 2.5, 95% CI 1.3 to 4.7) and at 4 hours (AR 41% *v* 19%; RR 2.2, 95% CI 1.4 to 3.5). **Versus sumatriptan:** One RCT comparing naratriptan (2.5 mg) orally versus sumatriptan (100 mg) orally found no significant difference in headache recurrence.[59]

Harms: In the crossover RCT (643 people), adverse effects occurred in less than 1% of people with no difference between naratriptan and placebo.[27] The most common adverse effects reported were nausea or vomiting, which could not be differentiated as being caused by naratriptan or being a part of the symptoms accompanying migraine. Blood pressure changes, haemorrhage, bradycardia, tachyarrhythmias, extrasystoles, palpitations, and heart murmurs after the first dose of 2.5 mg naratriptan were reported by 1% of people. Thirteen people withdrew from the study: one (migraine exacerbation) was considered to be related to the administration of naratriptan and five were possibly related. No significant association between dose variation and adverse effects was found. Similar adverse effects were reported in another RCT but were more common (21% with naratriptan 2.5 mg orally v 23% with placebo; significance not stated).[26]

Comment: The benefit of naratriptan in people responding poorly to sumatriptan in a first attack suggests that a different triptan may be useful in the same person to treat a second attack, but the observation needs confirmation in more RCTs.

OPTION RIZATRIPTAN

One systematic review has found that rizatriptan versus placebo significantly improves headache relief. Two additional RCTs found rizatriptan versus placebo significantly increased headache relief.

Benefits: We found one systematic review (search date 2000, 7 RCTs, 3528 people) comparing rizatriptan versus placebo.[28] A meta-analysis in the systematic review found that rizatriptan 5 mg and 10 mg versus placebo significantly increased headache relief (see glossary, p 1354) (AR 59% with 5 mg v 68% with 10 mg v 31% with placebo; RR of rizatriptan 5 mg v placebo 1.8, 95% CI 1.6 to 2.0; RR of rizatriptan 10 mg v placebo 2.2, 95% CI 2.0 to 2.5). One crossover RCT excluded from the meta-analysis above (1538 people) compared oral rizatriptan (5–10 mg) or oral sumatriptan (25–50 mg) versus placebo.[60] It found that rizatriptan (5mg) versus placebo significantly increased headache relief (AR 68% with rizatriptan 5mg v 68% with sumatriptan 50mg v 38% with placebo; $P < 0.05$; insufficient data for RR calculation). Fewer people taking rizatriptan versus placebo needed rescue medication (see glossary, p 1354) (19% v 45%; $P < 0.05$). Another RCT (727 people) comparing rizatriptan (10 mg) versus zolmitriptan (2.5 mg) versus placebo found no significant difference in the number of people who had headache relief with rizatripan versus zolmitriptan ($P = 0.23$). However, both treatments were superior to placebo ($P < 0.05$; AR rizatriptan 10 mg 71%; RR 2.4, 95% CI 1.8 to 3.1).[30]

Harms: The most frequently and consistently reported adverse effects in the RCTs include dizziness, somnolence, nausea, and fatigue.[28–30,60-62] In at least one RCT, these adverse effects were shown to have a dose dependent occurrence.[61]

Comment: None.

OPTION SUMATRIPTAN

RCTs have found that subcutaneous, oral, or intranasal sumatriptan versus placebo significantly increases headache relief. One RCT found no significant difference with sumatriptan versus aspirin plus metoclopramide in headache relief. One RCT found no significant difference with sumatriptan versus tolfenamic acid in headache relief. One RCT found that sumatriptan versus ergotamine plus caffeine was significantly more effective for headache relief or reducing the need for

rescue medication. One RCT comparing sumatriptan versus naratriptan found no significant difference in headache recurrence. One RCT found no significant difference between sumatriptan versus zolmitriptan in headache relief.

Benefits: We found one systematic review (search date 1997, 26 reports on 30 RCTs, 7437 people) comparing different preparations of sumatriptan versus placebo.[31] **Subcutaneous sumatriptan:** Subcutaneous sumatriptan (6 mg) versus placebo significantly increased the number of people with headache relief (see glossary, p 1354) at 1 hour (12 RCTs; 3127 people; 69% *v* 19%; RR 3.7, 95% CI 3.3 to 4.2). **Oral sumatriptan:** Oral sumatriptan (100 mg) versus placebo significantly increased the number of people with headache relief (12 RCTs; 2890 people; 58% *v* 25%; RR 2.3, 95% CI 2.1 to 2.6). One subsequent RCT compared oral sumatriptan (50 mg) versus placebo in the treatment of one migraine attack in 485 people[32] and three consecutive attacks in 1003 people.[63] Sumatriptan significantly increased the number of people with headache relief after 2 hours in people with one attack, and after 4 hours in people with three attacks. **Intranasal sumatriptan:** Intranasal sumatriptan (20 mg) versus placebo significantly increased the number of people with headache relief (6 RCTs; 1420 people; 61% *v* 30%; RR 2.1, 95% CI 1.8 to 2.4). One additional crossover RCT (246 people with up to 12 migraines) comparing subcutaneous sumatriptan (6 mg) versus usual headache treatment (49% combinations, 24% ergotamine, 19% non-steroidal anti-inflammatory drugs, 7% dihydroergotamine)[33] found that sumatriptan significantly improved headache relief (78% *v* 34%; $P < 0.001$). In three additional RCTs (2475 people), intranasal sumatriptan versus placebo significantly increased headache relief (60–64% with sumatriptan *v* 25–35% with placebo).[64–66] **Versus aspirin plus metoclopramide:** See benefits of salicylates, p 1342. **Versus tolfenamic acid:** See benefits of tolfenamic acid, p 1346. **Versus ergotamine:** See benefits of ergotamine, p 1348. **Versus naratriptan:** See benefits of naratriptan, p 1350. **Versus zolmitriptan:** See benefits of zolmitriptan, p 1353.

Harms: One non-systematic review reported that common adverse effects with sumatriptan included sensations of pressure, tightness, heaviness, and tingling affecting any part of the body, and that 3–5% of these symptoms can occur in the chest region.[67] The review found no association between sumatriptan and reported deaths. **Subcutaneous sumatriptan:** In one systematic review (search date 1997), 7/12 RCTs found that more people taking subcutaneous sumatriptan (6 mg) versus placebo reported adverse effects (65% *v* 32%; OR 4, 95% CI 3 to 5; NNH 3).[31] **Oral sumatriptan:** In the same review, 9/12 RCTs found that more people taking oral sumatriptan (100 mg) versus placebo reported adverse effects (36% *v* 24%; OR 1.72, 95% CI 1.48 to 2.08; NNH 8).[31]

Comment: There is a consensus that sumatriptan should not be used in people with ischaemic heart disease nor concomitantly with ergotamine.

OPTION ZOLMITRIPTAN

Two large RCTs have found that oral zolmitriptan versus placebo significantly increases headache relief. One RCT found no significant difference between zolmitriptan versus sumatriptan in headache relief.

Benefits: We found no systematic review. **Versus placebo:** We found two RCTs.[34,35] The first RCT (1144 people) compared oral zolmitriptan 1 mg, 2.5 mg, 5 mg, and 10 mg versus placebo.[34] The trial found that zolmitriptan (2.5 mg) significantly increased the number of people with headache relief (see glossary, p 1354) (AR 65% *v* 34%; RR 1.9, 95% CI 1.5 to 2.5). Zolmitriptan reduced the number of people needing rescue medication (see glossary, p 1354) (AR 38% with zolmitriptan *v* 65% with placebo; RR 0.6, 95% CI 0.5 to 0.7). The second RCT (327 people) compared oral zolmitriptan (2.5 mg) versus placebo.[35] The trial found that zolmitriptan significantly increased headache relief (AR 62% *v* 36%; RR 1.7, 95% CI 1.3 to 2.3) and the number of people needing rescue medication (AR 43% *v* 67%; RR 0.6, 95% CI 0.5 to 0.8). **Versus sumatriptan:** We found one RCT (1445 people) that compared zolmitriptan (2.5–5 mg) versus oral sumatriptan (25–50 mg).[36] The trial found no significant difference in headache relief between treatments at any dose. **Stratified care versus step care:** One RCT (835 people) randomised people into three arms. The first arm, named "stratified care", randomised people with low disability scores to aspirin (800–1000 mg) plus metoclopramide (10 mg) and people with higher disability scores to zolmitriptan (2.5 mg). The second arm, named "step care", involved treating initial attacks with aspirin plus metoclopramide and then switching to zolmitriptan (2.5 mg) for the remaining two to three attacks. The third arm involved "step care within attacks", whereby all attacks were initially treated with aspirin plus metoclopramide, and non-responders were given zolmitriptan after 2 hours. It found that stratified care versus either of the step care groups significantly increased the number of people with headache relief (AR 53% with stratified care *v* 40% with step care *v* 36% with step care within attacks; RR stratified care *v* step care 1.3, 95% CI 1.1 to 1.7; stratified care *v* step care within attacks 1.4, 95% CI 1.2 to 1.7).[68]

Harms: The first RCT found a dose response effect with zolmitriptan, with fewer adverse effects reported with lower doses than with higher doses (39% with 1 mg, 44% with 2.5 mg, 58% with 5 mg and 67% with 10 mg). More than 4% of people reported nausea, dizziness, somnolence, paraesthesia, fatigue, warm sensation, and tightness of throat or chest.[34]

Comment: None.

GLOSSARY

Headache intensity Mild: normal activity allowed. Moderate: disturbing, but not prohibiting normal activity; bed rest not necessary. Severe: normal activity discontinued; bed rest may be necessary.

Headache recurrence In responders, change of headache intensity (see above) from mild/none to moderate/severe within 24 hours of study medication initial dose.

Headache relief Change of headache intensity (see above) score from severe/moderate to mild/none.

International Headache Society criteria (1988) *Migraine without aura (common migraine)* is defined as five or more headache attacks lasting for 4–72 hours with accompanying symptoms of either nausea/vomiting and/or phonophobia and photophobia. Pain should comply with at least two of the following four characteristics: (1) unilateral; (2) throbbing; (3) moderate to severe intensity; and (4) increase with physical activity. For *migraine with aura (classic migraine)*, two or more headache attacks are required that comply with three of the following four characteristics: (1) one or more fully reversible aura symptoms indicating focal cerebral cortical and/or brainstem dysfunction; (2) at least one aura symptom developing gradually over more than 4 minutes or two or more symptoms occurring in succession; (3) no aura symptom should last more than 1 hour; and (4) headache follows aura with a pain free (see below) interval of less than 60 minutes. In both migraine with and without aura, secondary causes of headache should be excluded; if any structural damage is found, it should not explain headache characteristics. Less stringent criteria for migraine without aura can be used. In clinical practice, the so called borderline migraine can be diagnosed when one of the above criteria is not met. International Headache Society criteria were not developed with the intention of identifying potential responders to different medications.

Migraine index Pain scale for migraine resulting from duration times intensity of migraine where intensity is classified as 0 = none, 1 = mild, 2 = moderate, and 3 = severe.

Pain free Change of headache intensity (see above) score from severe/moderate to none.

Rescue medication Additional medications different to study medication permitted in non-responders, usually limited to the habitual medications a person uses to treat their migraine headache.

REFERENCES

1. Headache Classification Committee of the International Headache Society. Classification and diagnostic criteria for headache disorders, cranial neuralgias and face pain. *Cephalalgia* 1988;8:12–96.
2. Stewart W, Linet M, Celentano D, et al. Age and sex specific incidence rates of migraine with and without visual aura. *Am J Epidemiol* 1991;134:1111–1120.
3. O'Brien B, Goerre R, Streiner D. Prevalence of migraine headache in Canada: a population based survey. *Int J Epidemiol* 1994;23:1020–1026.
4. Pryse-Phillips W, Findlay H, Tugwell P, et al. A Canadian population survey on the clinical, epidemiological and societal impact if migraine and tension type headache. *Can J Neurol Sci* 1992;19:333–339.
5. Stewart W, Lipton R, Celentano D, et al. Prevalence of migraine headache in the United States. *JAMA* 1992;267:64–69.
6. Kryst S, Scherl E. A population based survey of social and personal impact of headache. *Headache* 1994;34:344–350.
7. Morillo L, Sanin L, Takeuchi Y, et al. Headache in Latin America: a multination population-based survey. *Neurology* 2001;56(suppl 3):A454.
8. Bank J, Marton S. Hungarian migraine epidemiology. *Headache* 2000;40:164–169.
9. Henry P, Michel P, Brochet B, et al. A nationwide survey of migraine in France: prevalence and clinical features. *Cephalalgia* 1992;12:229–237.
10. Rasmussen B, Jensen R, Schroll, et al. Epidemiology of headache in a general population: a prevalence study. *J Clin Epidemiol* 1991;44:1147–1157.
11. Steiner T, Stewart W, Kolodner K, et al. Epidemiology of migraine in England. *Cephalalgia* 1999;19:305.
12. Cheung RTF. Prevalence of migraine, tension type headache and other headaches in Hong Kong. *Headache* 2000;40:473–479.
13. Sakai F, Igarashi H. Prevalence of migraine in Japan: a nationwide survey. *Cephalalgia* 1997;17:15–22.
14. Stewart W, Staffa J, Lipton R, et al. Familial risk of migraine: a population based study. *Ann Neurol* 1997;41:166–172.
15. Chabriat H, Joire J, Danchot J, et al. Combined oral lysine acetylsalicylate and metoclopramide in the acute treatment of migraine: a multicentre double-blind placebo-controlled study. *Cephalalgia* 2001;14:297–300.
16. Tfelt-Hansen P, Henry P, Mulder L, et al. The effectiveness of combined oral lysine acetylsalicylate and metoclopramide compared with oral sumatriptan for migraine. *Lancet* 1995;346:923–926.
17. Deiner H. Efficacy and safety of intravenous acetylsalicylic acid lysinate compared to subcutaneous sumatriptan and parenteral placebo in the acute treatment of migraine: a double-blind, double-dummy, randomized, multicenter, parallel group study. The ASASUMAMIG Study Group. *Cephalalgia* 1999;19:581–588.

18. The Oral Sumatriptan and Aspirin plus Metoclopramide Comparative Study Group. A study to compare oral sumatriptan with oral aspirin plus metoclopramide in the acute treatment of migraine. *Eur Neurol* 1992;32:177–184.
19. Lipton R, Stewart W, Ryan RJ, et al. Efficacy and safety of paracetamol, aspirin, and caffeine in alleviating migraine headache pain: three double-blind, randomized, placebo-controlled trials. *Arch Neurol* 1998;55:210–217.
20. Lange R, Schwarz JA, Hohn M. Acetylsalicylic acid effervescent 1000 mg (aspirin) in acute migraine attacks; a multicentre, randomized, double-blind, single dose, placebo-controlled parallel group study. *Cephalalgia* 2000;20:663–667.
21. Dahlof C, Bjorkman R. Diclofenac-K (50 and 100 mg) and placebo in the acute treatment of migraine. *Cephalalgia* 1993;13:117–123.
22. Kellstein D, Lipton R, Geetha R, et al. Evaluation of a novel solubilized formulation of ibuprofen in the treatment of migraine headache: a randomized, double-blind, placebo-controlled, dose-ranging study. *Cephalalgia* 2000;20:233–243.
23. Myllyla V, Havanka H, Herrala L, et al. Tolfenamic acid rapid release versus sumatriptan in the acute treatment of migraine: comparable effect in a double-blind, randomized, controlled, parallel-group study. *Headache* 1998;38:201–207.
24. Smith LA, Oldman AD, McQuay HJ, et al. Eletriptan for acute migraine. In: The Cochrane Library, Issue 1, 2002. Oxford: Update Software. Search date 2000; primary sources data from all phase III randomised placebo controlled trials were made available by the manufacturer, Pfizer Inc. To date, these trials comprise the only data on eletriptan relevant to this review in a published or unpublished form; thus searches of electronic databases for further trials of eletriptan were not conducted.
25. Goadsby PJ, Ferrari MD, Olesen J, et al, for the Eletriptan Steering Committee. Eletriptan in acute migraine: a double-blind, placebo-controlled comparison to sumatriptan. *Neurology* 2000;54:156–163.
26. Havanka H, Dahlof C, Pop P, et al. Efficacy of naratriptan tablets in the acute treatment of migraine: a dose-ranging study. *Clin Ther* 2000;22:970–980.
27. Mathew N, Asgharnejad M, Peykamian M, et al. Naratriptan is effective and well tolerated in the acute treatment of migraine. Results of a double-blind, placebo-controlled, crossover study. *Neurology* 1997;49:1485–1490.
28. Oldman Ad, Smith LA, McQuay HJ, et al. Rizatriptan for acute migraine. In: The Cochrane Library, Issue 1, 2002.Oxford: Update Software. Search date 2000; primary sources Medline, Embase, Cochrane Library Issue 3 2000, and Oxford Pain Relief Database.
29. Kramer M, Matzura-Wolfe D, Polis A, et al. A placebo-controlled crossover study of rizatriptan in the treatment of multiple migraine attacks. Rizatriptan Multiple Attack Study Group. *Neurology* 1998;51:773–781.
30. Pascual J, Vega P, Deiner H-C, et al. Comparison of rizatriptan 10 mg vs. zolmitriptan 2.5 mg in the acute treatment of migraine. *Cephalalgia* 2000;20:455–461.
31. Tfelt-Hansen P. Efficacy and harms of subcutaneous, oral, and intranasal sumatriptan used for migraine treatment: a systematic review based on number needed to treat. *Cephalalgia* 2001;18:532–538. Search date 1997; primary sources Medline and hand searches of *Arch Neurol*, *Neurology*, *Headache*, and *Cephalalgia* from 1990.
32. Savani N, Brautaset NJ, Reunanen M, et al. A double-blind placebo-controlled study assessing the efficacy and tolerability of 50 mg sumatriptan tablets in the acute treatment of migraine. Sumatriptan Tablets S2CM07 Study Group. *Int J Clin Pract Suppl* 1999;105:7–15.
33. Boureau F, Chazot G, Emile J, et al. Comparison of subcutaneous sumatriptan with usual acute treatments for migraine. French Sumatriptan Study Group. *Eur Neurol* 1995;35:264–269.
34. Rapoport A, Ramadan N, Adelman J, et al. Optimizing the dose of zolmitriptan (Zomig, 311C90) for the acute treatment of migraine. A multicenter, double-blind, placebo-controlled, dose range-finding study. *Neurology* 1997;49:1210–1218.
35. Solomon G, Cady R, Klappew J, et al. Clinical efficacy and tolerability of 2.5 mg zolmitriptan for the acute treatment of migraine. *Neurology* 1997;49:1219–1225.
36. Gallagher R, Dennidh G, Spierings E, et al. A comparative trial of zolmitriptan and sumatriptan for the acute oral treatment of migraine. *Headache* 2000;40:119–128.
37. Limmroth V, May A, Diener H. Lysine-acetylsalicylic acid in acute migraine attacks. *Eur Neurol* 1999;41:88–93.
38. Tfelt-Hansen P, Olesen J. Effervescent metoclopramide and aspirin (Migravess) versus effervescent aspirin or placebo for migraine attacks: a double-blind study. *Cephalalgia* 1984;4:107–111.
39. Boureau F, Joubert JM, Lasserre V, et al. Double-blind comparison of an paracetamol 400 mg-codeine 25 mg combination versus aspirin 1000 mg and placebo in acute migraine attack. *Cephalalgia* 1994;14:156–161.
40. Massiou H, Serrurier D, Lasserre O, et al. Effectiveness of oral diclofenac in the acute treatment of common migraine attacks: a double-blind study versus placebo. *Cephalalgia* 1991;11:59–63.
41. The Diclofenac-K/Sumatriptan Migraine Study Group. Acute treatment of migraine attacks: efficacy and safety of nonsteroidal anti-inflammatory drug, diclofenac-potassium in comparison to oral sumatriptan and placebo. *Cephalalgia* 1999;19:232–240.
42. Karachalios G, Fotiadou A, Chrisikos N, et al. Treatment of acute migraine attack with diclofenac sodium: a double blind study. *Headache* 1992;32:98–100.
43. Kloster R, Nestvold K, Vilming S. A double-blind study of ibuprofen versus placebo in the treatment of acute migraine attacks. *Cephalalgia* 1992;12:169–171.
44. Havanka-Kanniainen H. Treatment of acute migraine attack: ibuprofen and placebo compared. *Headache* 1989;29:507–509.
45. Sandrini G, Franchini S, Lanfranchi S, et al. Effectiveness of ibuprofen-arginine in the treatment of acute migraine attacks. *Int J Clin Pharmacol Res* 1998;18:145–150.
46. Andersson P, Hinge H, Johansen O, et al. Double-blind study of naproxen v placebo in the treatment of acute migraine attacks. *Cephalalgia* 1989;9:29–32.
47. Nestvold K, Kloster R, Partinen M, et al. Treatment of acute migraine attack: naproxen and placebo compared. *Cephalalgia* 1985;5:115–119.
48. Pradalier A, Rancurel G, Dordain G, et al. Acute migraine attack therapy: comparison of naproxen sodium and an ergotamine tartrate compound. *Cephalalgia* 1985;5:107–112.

49. Treves T, Streiffler M, Korczyn A. Naproxen sodium versus ergotamine tartrate in the treatment of acute migraine attacks. *Headache* 1992;32:280–282.
50. Sargent J, Baumel B, Peters K, et al. Aborting a migraine attack: naproxen v ergotamine plus caffeine. *Headache* 1988;2:263–266.
51. Hakkarainen H, Vapaatalo H, Gothoni G, et al. Tolfenamic acid is as effective as ergotamine during migraine attacks. *Lancet* 1979;2:326–328.
52. Norrelund N, Christiansen L, Plantener S. Tolfenamic acid versus paracetamol in migraine attacks. A double-blind study in general practice. *Ugeskr Laeger* 1989;151:2436–2438.
53. Tokola R, Kangasniemi P, Neuvonen P, et al. Tolfenamic acid, metoclopramide, caffeine and their combinations in the treatment of migraine attacks. *Cephalalgia* 1984;4:253–263.
54. Dahlof C. Placebo-controlled clinical trials with ergotamine in the acute treatment of migraine. *Cephalalgia* 1993;13:166–171. Search date 1991; primary sources Medline, Embase, and hand searched reference lists.
55. Multinational Oral Sumatriptan Cafergot Comparative Study Group. A randomized, double-blind comparison of sumatriptan and Cafergot in the acute treatment of migraine. *Eur Neurol* 1991;31:314–322.
56. Hakkarainen H. Ergotamine vs. metoclopramide vs. their combination in acute migraine attacks. *Headache* 1982;22:10–12.
57. Lipton R. Ergotamine tartrate and dihydroergotamine mesylate: safety profiles. *Headache* 1997;37:S33–41.
58. Stark S, Spierings E, McNeal S, et al. Naratriptan efficacy in migraineurs who respond poorly to oral sumatriptan. *Headache* 2000;40:513–520.
59. Gobel H, Winter P, Boswell D, et al. Comparison of naratriptan and sumatriptan in recurrence-prone migraine patients. *Clin Ther* 2000;22:981–989.
60. Goldstein J, Ryan R, Jaing K, et al. Crossover comparison of rizatriptan 5 mg and 10 mg versus sumatriptan 25 mg and 50 mg in migraine. *Headache* 1998;38:737–747.
61. Teall J, Tuchman M, Cutler N, et al. Rizatriptan (MAXALT) for the acute treatment of migraine and migraine recurrence. A placebo-controlled, outpatient study. *Headache* 1998;38:281–287.
62. Tfelt-Hansen P, Teall J, Rodriguez F, et al. Oral rizatriptan versus oral sumatriptan: a direct comparison study in the acute treatment of migraine. *Headache* 1998;38:748–755.
63. Pfaffenrath V, Cunin G, Sjonell G, et al. Efficacy and safety of sumatriptan tablets (25 mg, 50 mg, and 100 mg) in the acute treatment of migraine: defining the optimum doses of oral sumatriptan. *Headache* 1998;38:184–190.
64. Peikert A, Becker WJ, Ashford EA, et al. Sumatriptan nasal spray: a dose-ranging study in the acute treatment of migraine. *Eur J Neurol* 1999;6:43–49.
65. Diamond S, Elkind A, Jackson RT, et al. Multiple-attack efficacy and tolerability of sumatriptan nasal spray in the treatment of migraine. *Arch Fam Med* 1998;7:234–240.
66. Ryan R, Elkind A, Baker CC, et al. Sumatriptan nasal spray for the acute treatment of migraine. Results of two clinical studies. *Neurology* 1997;49:1225–1230.
67. Ensink F. The efficacy of sumatriptan in the acute treatment of migraine. *Headache Q* 1995;6:280–292.
68. Lipton RB, Stewart WF, Stone AM, et al. Stratified care vs step care strategies for migraine: the Disability in Strategies of Care (DISC) study: a randomized trial. *JAMA* 2000;284:2599–2605.

Luis Morillo
Associate Professor
Javeriana University
Faculty of Medicine Clinical Epidemiology and Biostatistics Unit
Bogota
Colombia

Competing interests: None declared.

Multiple sclerosis

Search date November 2001

Mike Boggild and Helen Ford

QUESTIONS

INTERVENTIONS

Key Messages

Relapse rates and disability

- We found no evidence that any treatment alters long term outcome in multiple sclerosis.
- **Azathioprine** One systematic review in people with relapsing and remitting or progressive multiple sclerosis has found that azathioprine versus placebo has a modest but significant effect on relapse rates over 2 years, but found no significant effect on disability.
- **Glatiramer acetate** One RCT in people with relapsing and remitting multiple sclerosis found that glatiramer acetate versus placebo significantly reduced relapse rates over 2 years, but found no evidence of an effect on disability. We found no good RCTs in people with secondary progressive multiple sclerosis.

- **Interferon beta-1a/b** RCTs in people with a first clinical episode of demyelination have found that interferon beta-1a versus placebo significantly delays a second clinical event. One systematic review in people with active relapsing and remitting multiple sclerosis has found that interferon beta-1a/b versus placebo significantly reduces relapse rates over 2 years, and may delay development of neurological disability. We found conflicting evidence from two RCTs about effects of interferon beta on disease progression in people with secondary progressive multiple sclerosis.
- **Intravenous or oral methylprednisolone or corticotropin (for acute relapses)** One systematic review in people with multiple sclerosis requiring treatment for acute exacerbations has found that corticosteroids (methylprednisolone or corticotropin) versus placebo significantly reduce the risk of deterioration during the first 5 weeks. The optimal dose, route, and duration of treatment are unclear.
- **Intravenous immunoglobulin** One RCT in people with relapsing and remitting multiple sclerosis found limited evidence from baseline comparisons that intravenous immunoglobulin versus placebo may reduce disability over 2 years. We found no good RCTs in people with secondary progressive multiple sclerosis.
- **Methotrexate** One small RCT in people with secondary progressive multiple sclerosis found weak evidence suggesting that low dose, weekly methotrexate versus placebo may significantly delay disease progression.
- **Mitoxantrone** Limited evidence from small RCTs found that pulsed intravenous mitoxantrone improved outcome in people with very active multiple sclerosis, in whom the risk of severe neurological disability may outweigh the risks of cytotoxic treatment.
- **Plasma exchange** We found insufficient evidence about the effects of plasma exchange on neurological disability in people with acute demyelinating episodes who had previously failed to respond to intravenous steroids.

Fatigue

- **Pemoline** One systematic review found no significant difference in self reporting of fatigue with pemoline versus placebo.
- **Treatments for fatigue (amantadine, behaviour modification, exercise)** One systematic review has found that amantadine versus placebo modestly reduces fatigue in multiple sclerosis. We found insufficient evidence on the effects of behavioural modification treatment or exercise.

Spasticity

- **Botulinum toxin (for focal hip adductor spasticity)** One brief RCT found limited evidence that botulinum toxin versus placebo improved adductor spasticity.
- **Treatments for spasticity (oral drug treatments, physiotherapy, intrathecal baclofen)** RCTs found limited evidence that tizanidine versus placebo reduced spasticity, but did not improve mobility. We found insufficient evidence on the effects of other oral drug treatments. One small RCT found that physiotherapy for 8 weeks briefly improved mobility and subjective wellbeing. One small RCT in non-ambulant people with symptomatic spasticity resistant to oral baclofen found that intrathecal baclofen versus intrathecal saline significantly reduced spasticity and spasm frequency.

Multidisciplinary care

- **Multidisciplinary care (rehabilitation)** Two RCTs found limited evidence that 3–4 weeks of inpatient rehabilitation versus remaining on the waiting list or exercises at home improved disability in the short term, despite no reduction in neurological impairment. The duration of this effect is uncertain. One small RCT found that prolonged outpatient rehabilitation versus remaining on the waiting list reduced multiple sclerosis symptom frequency and fatigue.

DEFINITION Multiple sclerosis is a chronic inflammatory disease of the central nervous system. Diagnosis requires evidence of lesions that are separated in both time and space and the exclusion of other inflammatory, structural, or hereditary conditions that might give a similar clinical picture. The disease takes three main forms: relapsing and remitting multiple sclerosis, characterised by episodes of neurological dysfunction interspersed with periods of stability; primary progressive multiple sclerosis, where progressive neurological disability occurs from the outset; and secondary progressive multiple sclerosis, where progressive neurological disability occurs later in the course of the disease.

INCIDENCE/ PREVALENCE Prevalence varies with geography and racial group; it is highest in white populations in temperate regions.[1] In Europe and North America, prevalence is 1/800 people, with an annual incidence of 2 10/100 000, making multiple sclerosis the most common cause of neurological disability in young adults. Age of onset is broad, peaking between 20 and 40 years.[2]

AETIOLOGY/ RISK FACTORS The cause remains unclear, although current evidence suggests that multiple sclerosis is an autoimmune disorder of the central nervous system resulting from an environmental stimulus in genetically susceptible individuals. Multiple sclerosis is currently regarded as a single disorder with clinical variants, but there is some evidence that it may comprise several related disorders with distinct immunological, pathological, and genetic features.[1,3]

PROGNOSIS In 90% of people, early disease is relapsing and remitting. Although some people follow a relatively benign course over many years, most develop secondary progressive disease, usually 6–10 years after onset. In 10% of people, initial disease is primary progressive. Apart from a minority of people with "aggressive" multiple sclerosis, life expectancy is not greatly affected and the disease course is often of more than 30 years' duration.

AIMS To prevent or delay disability; to improve function; to alleviate symptoms of spasticity; to prevent complications (contractures, pressure sores); to optimise quality of life.

OUTCOMES Neurological disability, spasticity, fatigue, general health, relapse rate, quality of life. **Neurological disability:** In clinical trials, disability in multiple sclerosis is usually measured using the disease specific Expanded Disability Status Scale, which ranges from 0 (no disability) to 10 (death from multiple sclerosis) in half point increments.[4] Lower scores (0–4) reflect specific neurological impairments and disability; higher scores reflect reducing levels of mobility (4–7) and upper limb and bulbar function (7–9.5). The scale is non-linear and has been criticised for indicating change poorly, for emphasising neurological examination and mobility, and for failing to reflect other disabilities (e.g. fatigue, sexual disability). Some timed outcomes include ambulation (time taken to walk a specified short distance), the nine-hole peg test (time taken to place some pegs into holes in a block), and the box and block test (time taken to transfer blocks between boxes). **Sustained disease progression:** This is reported when an increase in disability from either disease progression or incomplete recovery from relapse is sustained for 3 or 6 months. A relapse that resolves within this time period constitutes non-sustained progression. **Spasticity:** A variety of clinical measures are used, the most common being the Ashworth scale, which scores muscle tone on a scale of 0–4 with 0 representing normal tone and 4 severe spasticity. For the purposes of this review, the Ashworth scale was considered to represent an appropriate clinical outcome and was selected over other outcome measures for spasticity (e.g. neurophysiological measures, examination ratings) that represent proxy clinical outcomes. **General health:** Attempts have been made to customise generic health status scales, but these scales have not been widely used.[5]

METHODS *Clinical Evidence* search and appraisal November 2001. We included only trials focusing on clinical outcomes (disability, relapses, and symptoms) and commonly used drug treatments.

QUESTION **What are the effects of treatments aimed at reducing relapse rates and disability?**

OPTION **INTERFERON BETA-1A/B**

Two RCTs have found that interferon beta-1a reduces risk of a second clinical event in people experiencing a first demyelinating event. One systematic review has found that interferon beta-1a/b reduces relapse rate and may delay progression of disability at 2 years compared with placebo in people with relapsing and remitting multiple sclerosis. We found conflicting evidence from two RCTs about effects of interferon beta for progression of disability in people with secondary progressive multiple sclerosis. We found insufficient evidence about long term effects of interferon beta on long term outcome and quality of life.

Benefits: **First demyelinating event:** We found two placebo controlled RCTs examining effects of interferon beta-1a in people experiencing a first demyelinating event with evidence of subclinical demyelination on magnetic resonance imaging of the brain.[6,7] Both RCTs found that interferon reduced the risk of a second clinical event and, therefore, conversion to a definite diagnosis of multiple sclerosis (first RCT: 383 people, 30μg/wk intramuscularly, HR interferon *v* placebo 0.56, 95% CI 0.38 to 0.81;[6] second RCT: 308 people, 22μg/wk subcutaneously, OR interferon *v* placebo 0.61, 95% CI 0.37 to 0.99[7]). **Relapsing and remitting multiple sclerosis:** We found one systematic review (search date 2000, 1215 people), which identified seven RCTs comparing interferon beta-1a/b with placebo in people with active (2 relapses in previous 2 or 3 years) relapsing remitting multiple sclerosis.[8] The systematic review found that over 2 years, interferon reduced the risk of exacerbations and disease progression (3 RCTs, 919 people, RR for exacerbation 0.80, 95% CI 0.73 to 0.88; RR for disease progression, defined as

1 point progression on the Expanded Disability Status Scale [EDSS] sustained over 3 or 6 months 0.69, 95% CI 0.55 to 0.87). Results for disease progression were not significant, however, if intention to treat analysis assumed that people lost to follow up experienced disease progression. **Secondary progressive multiple sclerosis:** We found two RCTs.[9,10] The first RCT (718 people) compared interferon beta-1b (8 MIU on alternate days) versus placebo in people with secondary progressive multiple sclerosis and an EDSS score of 3.0–6.5.[9] After a median of 30 months' follow up, the trial found that interferon delayed sustained progression of disability (measured by the EDSS) by 9–12 months, reduced risk of progression, and reduced risk of being wheelchair bound (OR for confirmed progression 0.65, 95% CI 0.52 to 0.83; NNT to prevent 1 additional person becoming wheelchair bound 13, 95% CI 8 to 49). The treatment effect was apparent in people of all levels of baseline disability. There were a large number of withdrawals from both groups (27% placebo and 25% interferon) and no data on quality of life were reported. The second RCT (618 people) compared subcutaneous interferon beta-1a (22 or 44 μg, 3 times/wk) versus placebo. It found no significant difference for confirmed progression of disability, although interferon reduced risk of relapse compared with placebo (HR for progression of disability 0.83, 95% CI 0.65 to 1.07; AR for relapse in 1 year 50% with interferon *v* 71% with placebol; $P < 0.001$).

Harms: The trials did not report any major adverse effects.[9,11–13] Mild to moderate effects included early flu-like symptoms (50% of people) and, rarely, leukopenia and asymptomatic elevation of transaminases. Injection site reactions occurred with subcutaneous administration in 80% of people.

Comment: None.

OPTION GLATIRAMER ACETATE

One RCT found a modest effect on relapse rate over 2 years, but found no evidence of an effect on disability.

Benefits: We found no systematic review. **Relapsing and remitting multiple sclerosis:** We found one placebo controlled RCT in 251 people ([EDSS 0–5).[14] At 2 years, the trial found significantly reduced relapse rates with glatiramer acetate 20 mg daily (ARR 29%; $P = 0.007$). No significant effect on disability was found. **Secondary progressive multiple sclerosis:** We found no good large RCTs.

Harms: Glatiramer acetate seems to be well tolerated. A self limiting allergic type reaction (flushing, chest tightness, and anxiety) lasting up to 30 minutes was reported by 15% of people on active treatment on at least one occasion (maximum 7 reactions).[14]

Comment: None.

OPTION INTRAVENOUS IMMUNOGLOBULIN

We found limited evidence from one RCT in people with relapsing and remitting multiple sclerosis suggesting that monthly intravenous immunoglobulin reduced disability compared with placebo.

Benefits: We found no systematic review. **Relapsing and remitting multiple sclerosis:** We found one RCT (150 people with relapsing and remitting multiple sclerosis) comparing intravenous immunoglobulin 0.2 g/kg monthly versus placebo.[15] Treatment was for a maximum of 2 years, but average duration was 21 months. The level of disability decreased in the experimental group (change in Expanded Disability Status Scale [EDSS] –0.23, 95% CI –0.43 to –0.03) compared with no significant change in the placebo group (change in EDSS +0.12, 95% CI –0.13 to +0.37). The trial did not report the time to development of sustained progression of disability. **Secondary progressive multiple sclerosis:** We found no RCTs meeting our quality criteria.

Harms: No significant adverse effects were reported.[15] However, higher dosages of intravenous immunoglobulin have been associated with aseptic meningitis and several other systemic reactions.[16]

Comment: None.

OPTION AZATHIOPRINE

One systematic review has found a modest reduction in relapse rates but no evidence of a significant effect on disability over 2 years in people with multiple sclerosis.

Benefits: We found one systematic review of azathioprine (search date 1989, 7 RCTs, 793 people with both relapsing and remitting multiple sclerosis and progressive multiple sclerosis).[17] At 2 years, the trial found that azathioprine reduced the relapse rate compared with placebo or no treatment (OR 2.04, 95% CI 1.42 to 2.93), and reduced disability though this did not quite reach significance (Expanded Disability Status Scale mean score difference –0.22, 95% CI –0.43 to +0.003).

Harms: About 10% of people were unable to tolerate therapeutic doses of azathioprine. Well documented adverse effects include hepatotoxicity and bone marrow suppression.[17] There are concerns about long term cancer risk.[18] In one large RCT, 21% of people on azathioprine withdrew after 1 year compared with 12% on placebo.[18]

Comment: The methods used in the multiple sclerosis trials have improved, making it hard to compare older and more recent RCTs. Trials in the review included people with different categories of multiple sclerosis and used different definitions of relapse.[19]

OPTION METHOTREXATE

We found weak evidence from one small RCT suggesting that low dose, weekly methotrexate may delay disease progression in people with secondary progressive multiple sclerosis.

Benefits: We found no systematic review. We found one RCT comparing low dose methotrexate (7.5 mg) versus placebo in 60 people with primary or secondary progressive disease.[20] The trial found that methotrexate reduced the risk of progression (ARR 31%; P = 0.01), defined by a composite outcome measure, including Expanded Disability Status Scale, ambulation, nine-hole peg test, and box and block test.

Harms: No major toxicity was reported in the RCT, but marrow suppression and hepatotoxicity can occur with low dose methotrexate; regular monitoring is advised.[20]

Comment: The findings of the RCT mainly reflected changes in upper limb function.[20] RCTs of other drugs have not used composite outcome measures, which makes comparisons difficult. Relative risks for treatment failure were not reported.

OPTION MITOXANTRONE

Limited evidence from small RCTs suggests that pulsed intravenous mitoxantrone reduces disease activity in people with active multiple sclerosis, in whom the risk of severe neurological disability may outweigh the risks of cytotoxic treatment.

Benefits: We found no systematic review. Several small RCTs have evaluated this cytotoxic antibiotic in people with multiple sclerosis, finding a positive or neutral effect. One non-blinded RCT (42 people with active disease) compared monthly intravenous mitoxantrone (mito zantrone) 20 mg plus methylprednisolone 1 g versus methylprednisolone alone.[21] The trial found mitoxantrone plus methylprednisolone significantly reduced disease activity after 6 months (as assessed by appearance on magnetic resonance imaging), and lowered annual clinical relapse rates compared with methylprednisolone alone (mitoxantrone plus methylprednisolone 0.7 *v* methylprednisolone alone 3.0; P < 0.01).

Harms: The major risk is dose related cardiotoxicity, but this is rare at the doses used in multiple sclerosis. Leukopenia, nausea, and amenorrhoea are commonly reported.[22]

Comment: A larger blinded RCT has recently been completed (Ford H, personal communication, 2002).

QUESTION What are the effects of treatments for acute relapse?

OPTION CORTICOSTEROIDS

One systematic review has found that corticosteroid treatment compared with placebo is associated with improved short term outcome in multiple sclerosis relapses. The optimal dose, route, and duration of treatment are unclear.

Benefits: We found one systematic review (search date 1999, 377 people with multiple sclerosis requiring treatment for acute exacerbations, 4 RCTs of methylprednisolone, 2 RCTs of corticotropin [corticotrophin] versus placebo).[23] The systematic review found that, overall, methylprednisolone or corticotropin reduced the risk of deterioration during the first 5 weeks of treatment (OR 0.37, 95% CI 0.24

to 0.57). No significant differences were found with short (5 days) versus long (15 days) treatment with methylprednisolone. One of the included RCTs (51 people) found no difference with oral methylprednisolone versus placebo in the prevention of new relapses or in disability after 1 year.[23]

Harms: Gastrointestinal symptoms and psychic disorders were significantly more common in people receiving oral, high dose methylprednisolone than in people receiving placebo. Weight gain and oedema were significantly more frequent in people receiving corticotropin than in people receiving placebo.

Comment: None.

OPTION PLASMA EXCHANGE

We found insufficient evidence about plasma exchange in people with acute demyelinating episodes who had previously failed to respond to intravenous steroids.

Benefits: We found no systematic review. We found one, double blind, crossover RCT of plasma exchange versus sham control in people with acute relapses of multiple sclerosis (12 people) or other demyelinating disease (10 people) who had previously failed to respond to intravenous steroids.[24] The trial found moderate or greater improvement in neurological disability in people receiving plasma exchange compared with sham treatment (8/19 [42%] *v* 1/17 [6%]; ARI 36%, 95% CI 1% to 81%; RR 7.2, 95% CI 1.2 to 15; NNT 3, 95% CI 1 to 68).

Harms: The trial reported no major complications.[24]

Comment: At the time of randomisation, all people had failed to respond to standard doses of intravenous corticosteroids and were within 3 months of onset of the acute deficit. The study was small; further studies are needed.

QUESTION What are the effects of treatments for fatigue?

OPTION DRUG TREATMENT: AMANTADINE AND PEMOLINE

One systematic review has found modest evidence that amantadine can alleviate fatigue in multiple sclerosis, although only a proportion of users obtain benefit. It found evidence of benefit from pemoline.

Benefits: We found one systematic review (search date 1999) of amantadine and pemoline.[25] **Amantadine:** The review found one parallel and two crossover RCTs (236 people with multiple sclerosis). All RCTs found a pattern in favour of amantadine compared with placebo.[25] **Pemoline:** The review found one parallel and one crossover RCT (126 people with multiple sclerosis). The review found no significant difference with pemoline versus placebo in the self reporting of fatigue.[25]

Harms: The review found more reports of adverse effects (sleep disturbance, nausea, mood change, palpitations, irritability, insomnia, anorexia) with pemoline than with placebo.

Comment: All RCTs were open to bias (arising from lack of clarity about the randomisation methods, blinding, incompleteness of follow up, and difficulties with interpretation of crossover RCTs).

OPTION BEHAVIOURAL MODIFICATION TREATMENT

We found insufficient evidence about behavioural modification treatment in people with multiple sclerosis related fatigue.

Benefits: We found no systematic review and no RCTs.

Harms: None reported.

Comment: None.

OPTION EXERCISE

We found insufficient evidence about exercise in people with multiple sclerosis related fatigue.

Benefits: We found no systematic review. We found one RCT (46 people, Expanded Disability Status Scale 0–6), which compared 15 weeks of aerobic training versus no exercise.[26] Using a scale that measures mental and physical fatigue, there was a significant reduction in fatigue at 10 weeks but not after completion of the exercise programme. A different scale that measured only physical fatigue remained unchanged in both groups of people. The RCT found significant improvements in other measures of emotional behaviour and quality of life (Profile of Mood States depression and anger score, Sickness Impact profile scores).

Harms: None reported.

Comment: People with moderate disability or severe fatigue may have difficulty adhering to an aerobic exercise programme.

QUESTION What are the effects of treatments for spasticity?

OPTION PHYSIOTHERAPY

One small RCT found that twice weekly physiotherapy, over an 8 week period, briefly improved mobility and subjective wellbeing. Previous RCTs were negative or inconclusive.

Benefits: We found no systematic review. A single blind crossover RCT (40 people) comparing hospital based or home based physiotherapy (45 min, twice weekly for 8 wk) versus no physiotherapy found improved mobility (Rivermead mobility index increased by 1.4–1.5 units, 95% CI 0.6 to 2.1; $P < 0.001$).[27] The treatment effect was short lived, being largely lost 8 weeks post-intervention. A non-blinded RCT compared early versus delayed physiotherapy (9 wk of inpatient treatment) in 45 people with progressive multiple sclerosis.[28] It found no significant difference in measures of mobility (timed walk, Rivermead mobility index) or activities of daily living. Treated people reported reduced mobility related stress ($P < 0.001$).

Harms: None reported.

Comment: None.

OPTION ORAL DRUG TREATMENT

One systematic review found limited evidence in two RCTs that tizanidine reduced spasticity in people with multiple sclerosis, but with no evidence of improved mobility. We found insufficient evidence to assess other oral drug treatments.

Benefits: We found one systematic review (search date 2000, 36 RCTs of duration > 7 days).[29] Of these, only 13 RCTs used an appropriate outcome measure (the Ashworth score). **Oral baclofen versus placebo:** The systematic review identified five RCTs, only one of which utilised an appropriate outcome measure.[30] This crossover study (30 people) used baclofen (20 mg) with or without an exercise programme and found significant beneficial effects comparing exercise plus baclofen versus placebo. It found no significant effect of exercise alone versus placebo. **Dantrolene versus placebo:** Four RCTs were identified, none of which used a validated outcome measure; no conclusions on efficacy could be drawn.[29] **Tizanidine versus placebo:** Three RCTs were identified, two of which used the Ashworth score. One RCT (220 people, tizanidine 2–36 mg/day) found no significant difference in Ashworth score but found that tizanidine reduced self reported clonus and spasm.[31] The other RCT utilising the Ashworth score (187 people, tizanidine 24–36 mg/day) found that tizanidine significantly reduced muscle tone, although the trial found no impact on mobility related activities of daily living.[32] **Baclofen versus tizanidine:** Seven RCTs comparing baclofen and tizanidine were identified, three of which utilised the Ashworth score. No significant differences on this or unvalidated measures of spasticity were found between the two drugs. No other comparative RCTs used validated outcome measures.[29]

Harms: Comparative RCTs of baclofen and tizanidine found similar levels of adverse effects (including muscle weakness, sedation, and dry mouth), but tizanidine may be less likely than baclofen to cause muscle weakness.[33]

Comment: The absolute and comparative efficacy of antispasmodic drugs in multiple sclerosis is poorly documented. The major difficulty in planning and designing future RCTs is the lack of a functionally relevant, well validated measure of spasticity.

OPTION INTRATHECAL BACLOFEN

Limited evidence from one small RCT suggests benefit in non-ambulant people with symptomatic spasticity resistant to oral drug treatment.

Benefits: We found no systematic review. We found one small crossover RCT comparing intrathecal baclofen versus intrathecal saline (19 non-ambulant people, with multiple sclerosis or spinal cord injury, and with spasticity resistant to oral baclofen).[34] Baclofen significantly reduced spasticity and spasm frequency. Average Ashworth scores fell from 4.0 at baseline to 1.2 after 3 days of treatment ($P < 0.0001$), with scores for all people improving from baseline.[34]

Harms: Potential problems include pump failure, infection, and, rarely, baclofen overdose.

Comment: We found no evidence about intrathecal baclofen in ambulant people.

OPTION BOTULINUM TOXIN

Limited evidence from a single brief RCT found that botulinum toxin versus placebo improved focal hip adductor spasticity in multiple sclerosis.

Benefits: We found no systematic review. One double blind, dose ranging RCT (74 people) compared three doses of intramuscular botulinum toxin (500, 1000, and 1500 units) with placebo for the treatment of hip adductor spasticity in multiple sclerosis.[35] Treatment improved passive hip abduction and distance between the knees ($P < 0.02$) over 12 weeks' follow up; hygiene scores were also improved at the 1000 and 1500 units doses.

Harms: No major adverse effects were reported. Botulinum toxin can cause local weakness.

Comment: None.

QUESTION What are the effects of multidisciplinary management?

OPTION INPATIENT REHABILITATION

Two RCTs have found that 3–4 weeks of inpatient rehabilitation improves short term disability, despite no significant evidence of any effect on neurological impairment. The duration of this effect is uncertain.

Benefits: We found no systematic review but found two RCTs.[36,37] The first RCT compared brief inpatient rehabilitation (average 25 days) versus remaining on the waiting list (non-treatment control group) in 66 people with progressive multiple sclerosis who were selected as "good candidates" for rehabilitation.[36] Rehabilitation significantly improved disability, assessed by the functional independence measure and the London handicap scale, despite unchanged levels of neurological impairment (Expanded Disability Status Scale). Benefit persisted for up to 9 months. The second RCT compared 3 weeks of inpatient rehabilitation versus exercises at home in 50 (ambulant) people. The trial found improvements in disability, assessed by the functional independence measure ($P < 0.004$), which persisted at 9 but not at 15 weeks' follow up.[37]

Harms: None reported.

Comment: None.

OPTION OUTPATIENT REHABILITATION

One small RCT has found that prolonged outpatient rehabilitation reduces multiple sclerosis symptom frequency and fatigue.

Benefits: We found no systematic review. We found one RCT comparing outpatient rehabilitation (5 h/wk for 1 year) versus remaining on the waiting list (non-treatment control group) in 46 people with progressive multiple sclerosis. Rehabilitation reduced the frequency of fatigue (effect size –0.27) and multiple sclerosis symptoms (effect size –0.32), despite no significant change in neurological impairment in either group.[38]

Harms: None reported.

Comment: Future trials need to record effects on disability and quality of life as well as impairment.

REFERENCES

1. Compston A. Genetic epidemiology of multiple sclerosis. *J Neurol Neurosurg Psychiatry* 1997;62:553–561.
2. Weinshenker BG, Bass B, Rice GPA, et al. The natural history of multiple sclerosis: a geographically based study. 1. Clinical course and disability. *Brain* 1989;112:133–146.
3. Lucchinetti CF, Bruck W, Rodriguez M, Lassmann H. Distinct patterns of multiple sclerosis pathology indicates heterogeneity in pathogenesis. *Brain Pathol* 1996;6:259–274.
4. Kurtzke JF. Rating neurological impairment in multiple sclerosis: an expanded disability status scale (EDSS). *Neurology* 1983;33:1444–1452.
5. Vickrey BG, Hays RD, Genovese BJ, Myers LW, Ellison GW. Comparison of a generic to disease-targeted health-related quality-of-life measures for multiple sclerosis. *J Clin Epidemiol* 1997;50:557–569.
6. Jacobs LD, Beck RW, Simon JH, et al. Intramuscular interferon beta-1a therapy initiated during a first demyelinating event in multiple sclerosis. *N Engl J Med* 2000;343:898–904.
7. Comi G, Fillipi M, Barkhof F, et al. Effect of early interferon treatment on conversion to definite multiple sclerosis: a randomised study. *Lancet* 2001;357:1576–1582.
8. Rice GA, Incorvaia B, Munari L, et al. Interferon in relapsing-remitting multiple sclerosis. In: The Cochrane Library, Issue 4, 2001. Search date 2000; primary sources Medline, Embase, hand searches of reference lists, and personal contact with researchers and pharmaceutical companies.
9. Kappos L, Polman C, Pozzilli C, et al. Placebo-controlled multicentre randomised trial of interferon beta-1b in treatment of secondary progressive multiple sclerosis. *Lancet* 1998;352:1491–1497.
10. King J, McLeod J, Gonsette RE, et al. Randomised controlled trial of interferon beta-1a in secondary progressive MS: clinical results. *Neurology* 2001;56:1496–1504.
11. Ebers GC, Rice G, Lesaux J, et al. Randomised double-blind placebo-controlled study of interferon beta-1a in relapsing/remitting multiple sclerosis. *Lancet* 1998;352:1498–1504.
12. Duquette P, Girard M, Despault L, et al. Interferon beta-1b is effective in relapsing-remitting multiple sclerosis. Clinical results of a multicenter, randomised, double-blind, placebo-controlled trial. *Neurology* 1993;43:655–661.
13. Jacobs LD, Cookfair DL, Rudick RA, et al. Intramuscular interferon beta-1a for disease progression in relapsing multiple sclerosis. *Ann Neurol* 1996;39:285–294.
14. Johnson KP, Brooks BR, Cohen JA, et al. Copolymer-1 reduces relapse rate and improves disability in relapsing-remitting multiple sclerosis: results of a Phase III multicenter, double-blind, placebo-controlled trial. *Neurology* 1995;45:1268–1276.
15. Fazekas F, Deisenhammer F, Strasser-Fuchs S, et al. Randomised placebo-controlled trial of monthly intravenous immunoglobulin therapy in relapsing–remitting multiple sclerosis. *Lancet* 1997;349:589–593.
16. Stangel M, Hartung HP, Marx P, Gold R. Side-effects of high-dose intravenous immunoglobulins. *Clin Neuropharmacol* 1997;20:385–393.
17. Yudkin PL, Ellison GW, Ghezzi A, et al. Overview of azathioprine treatment in multiple sclerosis. *Lancet* 1991;338:1051–1055. Search date 1989; primary sources Medline and hand searched references.
18. Confavreux C, Saddier P, Grimaud J, Moreau J, Adeleine P, Aimard G. Risk of cancer from azathioprine therapy in multiple sclerosis: a case-control study. *Neurology* 1996;46:1607–1612.
19. Hughes RAC. Double-masked trial of azathioprine in multiple-sclerosis. *Lancet* 1988;2:179–183.
20. Goodkin DE, Rudick RA, VanderBrug Medendorp S, et al. Low-dose (7.5 mg) oral methotrexate reduces the rate of progression in chronic progressive multiple sclerosis. *Ann Neurol* 1995;37:30–40.
21. Edan G, Miller D, Clanet M, et al. Therapeutic effect of mitoxantrone combined with methylprednisolone in multiple sclerosis: a randomised multicentre study of active disease using MRI and clinical criteria. *J Neurol Neurosurg Psychiatry* 1997;62:112–118.
22. MacDonald M, Posner LE, Dukart G, et al. A review of the acute and chronic toxicity of mitoxantrone. *Future Trends Chemother* 1985;6:443–450.
23. Filippini G, Brusaferri F, Sibley WA, et al. Corticosteroids or ACTH for acute exacerbations in multiple sclerosis. In: The Cochrane Library, Issue 3, 2001. Oxford: Update Software. Search date 1999; primary sources Medline, Cochrane

Controlled Trials Register, hand searches of reference lists, main neurology journals, conference abstracts, dissertations, and personal contact with researchers and manufacturers.
24. Weinshenker BG, O'Brien PC, Petterson TM, et al. A randomised trial of plasma exchange in acute central nervous system inflammatory demyelinating disease. *Neurology* 1999;46:878–886.
25. Branas P, Jordan R, Fry-Smith A, Burls A, Hyde C. Treatments for fatigue in multiple sclerosis: a rapid and systematic review. The National Coordinating Centre for Health Technology Assessment (NCCHTA). 13665278. *Health Technol Assess* 2000;4:27:1–73. Search date 1999; primary sources Medline, Embase, hand searches of reference lists, and personal contact with experts.
26. Petajan JH, Gappmaier E, White AT, Spencer MK, Mino L, Hicks RW. Impact of aerobic training on fitness and quality of life in multiple sclerosis. *Ann Neurol* 1996;39:432–441.
27. Wiles CM, Newcombe RG, Fuller KJ, et al. Controlled randomised crossover trial of the effects of physiotherapy on mobility in chronic multiple sclerosis. *J Neurol Neurosurg Psychiatry* 2001;70:174–179.
28. Fuller KJ, Dawson K, Wiles CM. Physiotherapy in chronic multiple sclerosis: a controlled trial. *Clin Rehabil* 1996;10:195–204.
29. Shakespeare DT, Young CA, Boggild M. Anti-spasticity agents for multiple sclerosis (Cochrane Review). In: The Cochrane Library, Issue 1, 2001. Search date 2000; primary sources Medline, Cochrane Controlled Trials Register, Cochrane MS Review Group Specialised Trial Registry, National Health Service National Research Register, Medical Research Council Clinical Trials Directory, hand searches of reference lists, main neurology journals, conference abstracts, dissertations, and personal contact with researchers and manufacturers.
30. Brar S, Smith MB, Nelson LM, Franklin GM, Cobble ND. Evaluation of treatment protocols on minimal to moderate spasticity in multiple sclerosis. *Arch Phys Med Rehabil* 1991;72:186–189.
31. Smith C, Birnbaum G, Carter JL, Greenstein J, Lublin FD. Tizanidine treatment of spasticity caused by multiple sclerosis: results of a double-blind, placebo-controlled trial. *Neurology* 1994;44:34–42.
32. Barnes MP, Bates D, Corston RN, et al. A double-blind, placebo-controlled trial of tizanidine in the treatment of spasticity caused by multiple sclerosis. *Neurology* 1994;44:S70–S78.
33. Groves L, Shellenberger MK, Davis CS. Tizanidine treatment of spasticity: a meta-analysis of controlled, double-blind, comparative studies with baclofen and diazepam. *Adv Ther* 1998;15:241–251. Search date not stated; primary source records of Sandoz (now Novartis).
34. Penn RD, Savoy SM, Corcos D, et al. Intrathecal baclofen for severe spinal spasticity. *N Engl J Med* 1989;320:1517–1521.
35. Hyman N, Barnes M, Bhakta B, et al. Botulinum toxin (Dysport) treatment of hip adductor spasticity in multiple sclerosis: a prospective, randomised, double-blind, placebo controlled, dose ranging study. *J Neurol Neurosurg Psychiatry* 2000;68:707–712.
36. Freeman JA, Langdon DW, Hobart JC, Thompson AJ. The impact of inpatient rehabilitation on progressive multiple sclerosis. *Ann Neurol* 1997;42:236–244.
37. Solari A, Fillipini G, Gasco P, et al. Physical rehabilitation has a positive effect on disability in multiple sclerosis patients. *Neurology* 1999;52:57–62.
38. Di Fabio RP, Soderberg J, Choi T, Hanson CR, Schapiro RT. Extended outpatient rehabilitation: its influence on symptom frequency, fatigue and functional status for persons with progressive multiple sclerosis. *Arch Phys Med Rehabil* 1998;79:141–146.

Mike Boggild
Consultant Neurologist
The Walton Centre for Neurology and Neurosurgery
Liverpool
UK

Helen Ford
Consultant Neurologist
St James's Hospital
Leeds
UK

Competing interests: HF has received financial support for attending scientific meetings by Serono and Biogen, and for speaking at meetings by Scherise and Biogen. MB has received financial support for attending scientific meetings from Biogen, Serono Pharmaceuticals, and Teva Pharmaceuticals, and has organised educational sessions for Serono.

Parkinson's disease

Search date April 2002

Carl Clarke and A Peter Moore

QUESTIONS

INTERVENTIONS

See glossary, p 1382

Key Messages

- **Dopamine agonists versus levodopa* in people with early disease** One systematic review and one subsequent RCT have found that dopamine agonist monotherapy versus levodopa monotherapy reduces the incidence of dyskinesias and fluctuations in motor response. One systematic review and subsequent RCTs have found that dopamine agonist treatment plus levodopa versus levodopa alone reduces dyskinesia. However, some of the RCTs found that levodopa alone versus dopamine agonist plus levodopa improved motor impairments and disability.
- **Dopamine agonists plus levodopa in people with a fluctuating response to levodopa*** Systematic reviews in people with later stage disease taking levodopa have found that adjuvant dopamine agonists reduce "off time", improve motor impairments and activities of daily living, and reduce levodopa dose, but increase dopaminergic adverse effects and dyskinesias.

- **Levodopa* in people with early disease** Experience suggests that levodopa improves motor function, but that dyskinesias and fluctuations in motor response are related to long term levodopa treatment and are irreversible.
- **Modified release levodopa (v immediate release levodopa*) in people with early disease** RCTs found no significant difference with modified versus immediate release levodopa in motor complications or disease control after 5 years.
- **Pallidal surgery in people with later disease** One systematic review found limited evidence that unilateral pallidotomy versus medical treatment improved motor examination and activities of daily living. One RCT found insufficient evidence to assess the effects of pallidotomy versus deep brain stimulation. We found no systematic review or RCTs comparing pallidal deep brain stimulation versus medical treatment. One small RCT found insufficient evidence to assess the effects of pallidal deep brain stimulation versus subthalamic deep brain stimulation. There is a high incidence of adverse effects with pallidotomy.
- **Selegiline in people with early disease** RCTs have found that selegiline versus placebo significantly improves symptoms, but one of the RCTs found increased mortality in people treated with selegiline. One large RCT found that selegiline versus placebo delayed the need for levodopa for 9 months.
- **Subthalamic surgery in people with later disease** One systematic review found no RCTs comparing subthalamic surgery versus medical treatment. One small RCT comparing subthalamic deep brain stimulation versus pallidal deep brain stimulation found no significant difference in motor scores.
- **Thalamic surgery in people with later disease** One systematic review identified no RCTs comparing thalamic surgery versus medical treatment. One RCT found that thalamic deep brain stimulation versus thalamotomy improved functional status and caused fewer adverse effects. Case series found that thalamotomy was associated with permanent complications, including speech disturbance, apraxia, and death in 14–23% of people.
- **Occupational therapy in people with later disease; physiotherapy in people with later disease; speech and language therapy for speech disturbance in people with later disease; swallowing therapy for dysphagia in people with later disease** Systematic reviews of poor quality RCTs found insufficient evidence about the effects of these interventions.

  *We have used the term "levodopa" to refer to a combination of levodopa and a peripheral decarboxylase inhibitor.

DEFINITION Idiopathic Parkinson's disease is an age related neurodegenerative disorder and is the most common cause of the parkinsonian syndrome: a combination of asymmetric bradykinesia, hypokinesia, and rigidity, sometimes combined with rest tremor and postural changes. Clinical diagnostic criteria have a sensitivity of 80% and specificity of 30% compared with the gold standard of diagnosis at autopsy.[1] The primary pathology is progressive loss of cells producing the neurotransmitter dopamine from the substantia nigra in the brainstem. Treatment aims to replace or compensate for the lost dopamine. A good response to treatment supports, but does not confirm, the diagnosis. Several other catecholaminergic neurotransmitter systems are also affected in Parkinson's disease.

INCIDENCE/ PREVALENCE Parkinson's disease occurs worldwide with equal incidence in both sexes. In 5–10% of people who develop Parkinson's disease it appears before the age of 40 years (young onset), with a mean age of onset of about 65 years. Overall age adjusted prevalence is 1% worldwide and 1.6% in Europe, rising from 0.6% at age 60–64 years to 3.5% at age 85–89 years.[2,3]

AETIOLOGY/ RISK FACTORS The cause is unknown. Parkinson's disease may represent different conditions with a final common pathway. People may be affected differently by a combination of genetic and environmental factors (viruses, toxins, 1-methyl-4-phenyl-1,2,3,6-tetrahydropyridine, well water, vitamin E, and smoking).[4–7] First degree relatives of affected people may have twice the risk of developing Parkinson's disease (17% chance of developing the condition in their lifetime) compared with people in the general population.[8–10] However, purely genetic varieties probably affect a small minority of people with Parkinson's disease.[11,12] The parkin gene on chromosome 6 may be associated with Parkinson's disease in families with at least one member with young onset Parkinson's disease, and multiple genetic factors, including the tau gene on chromosome 17q21, may be involved in idiopathic late onset disease.[13,14]

PROGNOSIS Parkinson's disease is currently incurable. Disability is progressive and associated with increased mortality (RR of death compared with matched control populations ranges from 1.6 to 3).[15] Treatment can reduce symptoms and slow progression but rarely achieves complete control. The question of whether treatment reduces mortality remains controversial.[16] Levodopa appeared to reduce mortality in the UK for 5 years after its introduction, before a "catch up" effect was noted and overall mortality rose toward previous levels. This suggested a limited prolongation of life.[17] An Australian cohort study followed 130 people treated for 10 years.[18] The standardised mortality ratio was 1.58 ($P < 0.001$). At 10 years, 25% had been admitted to a nursing home and only four were still employed. The mean duration of disease until death was 9.1 years. In a similar Italian cohort study conducted over 8 years, the relative risk of death for affected people versus healthy controls was 2.3 (95% CI 1.60 to 3.39).[19] Age at initial census date was the main predictor of outcome (for people aged < 75 years: RR of death 1.80, 95% CI 1.04 to 3.11; for people aged > 75 years: RR of death 5.61, 95% CI 2.13 to 14.8).

AIMS To improve symptoms and quality of life; to slow disease progression; to limit short and long term adverse effects of treatment, such as motor fluctuations (see glossary, p 1382).

OUTCOMES Disease severity; severity of drug induced symptoms or signs; rate of progression of symptoms; need for levodopa or other treatment; adverse effects of treatment; withdrawals from treatment; and quality of life measures. There are no universal scales, but commonly used scales are the UPDRS (see glossary, p 1382), the Hoehn and Yahr disability staging scale, Webster scale, the Core Assessment Programme for Intracerebral Transplantation,[20,21] the Parkinson's Disease Quality of Life questionnaire,[22] and the UK Parkinson's Disease Quality of Life questionnaire 39.[23]

METHODS *Clinical Evidence* update search and appraisal April 2002. Unless stated otherwise, we have used the term "levodopa" to refer to a combination of levodopa and a peripheral dopa decarboxylase inhibitor.

QUESTION **What are the effects of drug treatments in people with early Parkinson's disease?**

OPTION **SELEGILINE**

Four large RCTs have found that selegiline versus placebo improves the symptoms of Parkinson's disease, but one of these RCTs found increased mortality in people treated with selegiline. One large RCT found that selegiline versus placebo delayed the need for levodopa for 9 months.

Benefits: We found no systematic review. We found five large RCTs comparing selegiline versus placebo in people with early Parkinson's disease.[24–28] The first RCT (800 people) found that selegiline versus placebo delayed the need for levodopa for 9 months (HR 0.50 for requiring levodopa in each time period, 95% CI 0.41 to 0.62).[24] The second RCT (101 people newly diagnosed with Parkinson's disease) found that selegiline versus placebo significantly improved total Unified Parkinson's Disease Rating Scale (see glossary, p 1382) score after 12 months of treatment and 2 months of washout ($P < 0.001$; CI not stated).[25] The third RCT (782 people) found no significant difference with selegiline versus placebo in disability scores after 4 years ($P = 0.95$; CI not stated).[26] The fourth RCT (116 people) found that selegiline versus placebo significantly reduced the number of people who required a 50% or greater increase in their levodopa dose after 5 years (50% on selegiline *v* 74% on placebo; $P = 0.03$; CI not stated).[27] The fifth RCT (163 people) found that selegiline versus placebo significantly improved motor function after 5 years.[28]

Harms: One non-systematic review (5 RCTs, 589 people) found no significant difference with selegiline versus placebo in mortality at 2.5–4 years (15% with selegiline *v* 6% with placebo; HR 1.02, 95% CI 0.44 to 2.37).[29] One large RCT found no significant difference with selegiline versus placebo in mortality at 35 months (no further data provided).[30] Another RCT found that selegiline versus placebo significantly increased mortality at interim analysis after 5.6 years' follow up (HR 1.57, 95% CI 1.07 to 2.31); the selegiline arm of the trial was terminated early.[26] Updated analysis (including blinded assessment of cause specific mortality) found that the increase in mortality did not quite reach significance (HR 1.30, 95% CI 0.99 to 1.72).[31,32] One retrospective observational study in 12 621 people who had taken an antiparkinsonian drug (excluding those also taking antipsychotic drugs) found increased mortality in people prescribed selegiline, but the increase was of borderline significance (ARI 11%, 95% CI 0% to 23%).[33]

Comment: One RCT (163 people) found that there was no deterioration in symptoms on withdrawal of selegiline after 5 years.[28] This could indicate that it was ineffective. Other studies of early selegiline treatment were either too small or too short to reach a conclusion.[29] A systematic review and a large RCT are under way (Clarke C, personal communication, 2001).

OPTION MODIFIED RELEASE LEVODOPA

Two RCTs in people with early Parkinson's disease found no significant difference with modified versus immediate release levodopa (see methods, p 1372) in motor complications or disease control after 5 years.

Benefits: We found no systematic review but found two RCTs.[34,35] The first RCT (134 people with early Parkinson's disease) compared modified versus immediate release co-beneldopa.[34] It found no significant difference in the incidence of dyskinesia (see glossary, p 1382) at 5 years (41% with modified release *v* 34% with immediate release co-beneldopa; RR 1.21, 95% CI 0.59 to 1.92), motor fluctuations (see glossary, p 1382) (59% *v* 57%; RR 1.03, 95% CI 0.60 to 1.39), motor impairment, or activities of daily living. The second RCT (618 people with early Parkinson's disease) compared modified versus immediate release co-careldopa.[35] It found no significant difference in dyskinesia or motor fluctuations measured by diary data at 5 years (22% of people taking modified release *v* 21% of people taking immediate release) but found that modified versus immediate release co-careldopa significantly improved activities of daily living (scores at 5 years; P = 0.03; CI not stated).

Harms: The RCT of co-careldopa found that immediate versus modified release significantly increased withdrawals because of nausea (P = 0.007; CI not stated).[35]

Comment: The RCT comparing modified versus immediate release co-beneldopa with a 5 year follow up had a withdrawal rate of about 50%.[34]

OPTION DOPAMINE AGONISTS VERSUS LEVODOPA IN EARLY DISEASE

Experience suggests that levodopa improves motor function, but that dyskinesias and fluctuations in motor response are related to long term levodopa treatment and are irreversible. One systematic review and one subsequent RCT have found that dopamine agonist monotherapy versus levodopa monotherapy reduces the incidence of dyskinesias and fluctuations in motor response. One systematic review and subsequent RCTs have found that dopamine agonist treatment plus levodopa versus levodopa alone reduces dyskinesia. However, some of the RCTs found that levodopa alone versus dopamine agonist plus levodopa improved motor impairments and disability. One subsequent RCT found no significant difference with lisuride (lysuride) plus levodopa versus levodopa alone in motor complications at 5 years.

Benefits: Wc found two systematic reviews[36,37] and six subsequent RCTs.[38–43] The first review (search date 1999, 6 RCTs) comparing bromocriptine versus levodopa (see methods, p 1372) found that bromocriptine delayed motor complications and dyskinesias (see glossary, p 1382).[36] The second review (search date 2001, 8 RCTs), which was published as an abstract, compared bromocriptine plus levodopa versus levodopa alone and found a trend toward reduced dyskinesia with combination treatment but no difference in duration of "off time" (see glossary, p 1382) (no further data provided).[37] Neither review reported effects on disability or motor impairment. The first subsequent RCT (268 people) found that ropinirole plus rescue levodopa if needed versus levodopa alone significantly reduced the number of people experiencing dyskinesias after 5 years (20% with ropinirole *v* 45% with levodopa; RR 0.44, 95% CI 0.31 to 0.64).[38] It found no significant difference in disability after 5 years (UPDRS [see glossary, p 1382], activities of daily living scale) and a small increase in motor impairments with ropinirole. The second subsequent RCT (301 people) found that pramipexole plus rescue levodopa versus levodopa alone significantly reduced all motor complications at 2 years (28% *v* 51%; HR 0.45, 95% CI 0.30 to 0.66).[39] Improvements in UPDRS motor and activities of daily living scores were greater in the levodopa group. The third subsequent RCT (419 people), which was published as an abstract, compared cabergoline plus rescue levodopa versus levodopa alone.[40] It found that cabergoline versus levodopa significantly reduced the number of people experiencing motor complications at 5 years (22% *v* 34%; $P < 0.05$; CI not stated). Activities of daily living scores were worse with cabergoline. The fourth subsequent RCT (294 people), which was published as an abstract, compared pergolide alone (without rescue levodopa) versus levodopa.[41] It found that pergolide versus levodopa significantly reduced the number of people experiencing one or more motor complications at 3 years (16% *v* 33%; $P < 0.001$; CI not stated). Motor UPRDS scores were worse in the pergolide group. The fifth subsequent RCT (90 people, unblinded), comparing lisuride plus rescue levodopa versus levodopa alone, found fewer motor complications in the lisuride group after 4 years, although UPDRS motor and activities of daily living scores were worse in those treated with lisuride alone.[42] The sixth subsequent RCT (82 people, partially blinded) found no significant difference with lisuride plus levodopa versus levodopa alone in motor complications after 5 years.[43]

Harms: The RCT comparing ropinirole versus levodopa found that adverse events, including nausea, vomiting, dizziness, confusion, hallucinations, and delusions, were similar in both treatment groups.[38] The RCT comparing pramipexole plus rescue levodopa versus levodopa alone found that pramipexole significantly increased somnolence ($P = 0.003$) and hallucinations ($P = 0.03$; CIs not stated).[39] The RCT comparing pergolide versus levodopa found that significantly more people in the pergolide group withdrew from treatment (18% with pergolide *v* 10% with levodopa; $P < 0.05$; CI not stated).[41]

Comment: Experience suggests that levodopa improves motor function, but that dyskinesias and fluctuations in motor response are related to long term levodopa treatment and are irreversible. The subsequent RCTs with 5 years of follow up had withdrawal rates of about 50%.[38,40,43] In the RCT comparing lisuride plus levedopa versus levodopa alone, the doses used were low.[42] We found no direct comparisons of individual dopamine agonists. A large, UK based RCT is examining quality of life and health economic outcomes of agonist monotherapy in people likely to develop motor complications (Clarke C, personal communication, 2001). A multicentre North American study is investigating the effect of levodopa on dopaminergic cell death.[44]

QUESTION What are the effects of adding a dopamine agonist in people with a fluctuating response to levodopa?

Systematic reviews have found that, in people taking levodopa, certain dopamine agonists significantly reduce "off" time, improve motor impairment and activities of daily living, and reduce requirement for levodopa, but increase dopaminergic adverse effects and dyskinesia.

Benefits: **Versus placebo:** We found six systematic reviews.[45–50] The first review (search date 1998, 7 RCTs, 396 people with later Parkinson's disease taking levodopa; see methods, p 1372) compared adjuvant bromocriptine versus placebo.[45] Heterogeneity in trial design and outcomes made it impossible to draw conclusions. The second review (search date 1998) comparing lisuride versus placebo identified no RCTs.[46] The third review (search date 1999, 1 RCT, 376 people with Parkinson's disease taking levodopa) found that pergolide versus placebo significantly reduced daily off time (see glossary, p 1382) (mean difference 1.6 h; $P < 0.001$), significantly reduced daily levodopa dose (mean 235 mg with pergolide *v* mean 51 mg with placebo; mean difference 184 mg; $P < 0.001$), and improved activities of daily living scores (CIs not stated).[47] The fourth review (search date not stated, 4 RCTs, 669 people with Parkinson's disease taking levodopa) found that pramipexole versus placebo significantly reduced daily "off" time (WMD 1.8 h; 95% CI 1.2 h to 2.3 h), reduced levodopa dose (WMD 115 mg, 95% CI 87 mg to 143 mg), and improved activities of daily living scores.[50] The fifth review (search date not stated, 1 RCT using sufficient dosage of ropinirole [8 mg 3 times daily], 149 people with Parkinson's disease taking levodopa) compared ropinirole versus placebo.[48] It found no significant difference with ropinirole versus placebo in "off" time (WMD 180 mg, 95% CI 106 mg to 253 mg) but found that ropinirole reduced the required dose of levodopa. Complete information on motor impairments and disability was not available. The sixth review (search date not stated, 3 RCTs, 268 people with Parkinson's disease taking levodopa) found no significant difference with cabergoline versus placebo in "off" time (WMD 1.1 h, 95% CI –0.06 h to 2.33 h) but found that cabergoline significantly reduced the required dose of levodopa (WMD 150 mg, 95% CI 94 mg to 205 mg).[49] Small but significant benefits in UPDRS (see glossary, p 1382), activities of daily living, and motor scores were seen with cabergoline in one study only. **Versus each other:** We found five systematic reviews.[51–55] The first systematic review (search date not stated, 1 RCT, 20 people) compared lisuride versus bromocriptine.[51] It found no significant difference with lisuride versus bromocriptine in change in motor fluctuations and the Columbia disability rating scale after 12 weeks (no quantitative data provided). Follow up may have been too short and the study too small to detect significant differences. The second systematic review (search date 1998, 3 RCTs, 293 people) compared pergolide versus bromocriptine.[52] It found that pergolide significantly increased the number of people with "marked or moderate improvement", as measured using a 7 point clinician's global assessment scale, but found no significant difference in reduction in levodopa dose after 8–12 weeks (clinician's global assessment scale: 2 RCTs, "marked or moderate improvement", AR 43% with pergolide v 30% with bromocriptine; RR 1.45, 95% CI 1.08 to 1.95; difference in reduction in levodopa dose: 3 RCTs, WMD 3 mg/day, 95% CI –4 mg/day to +10 mg/day). Two of the RCTs found that pergolide versus bromocriptine significantly improved motor impairment. The third systematic review (search date not stated, 1 RCT, 163 people) compared pramipexole versus bromocriptine.[53] It found that pramipexole reduced "off" time compared with bromocriptine (WMD 1.4 h/day, 95% CI 0 h/day to 2.8 h/day). There were no differences in UPDRS or dyskinesias (see glossary, p 1382) (no quantitative data provided). The fourth systematic review (search date not stated, 3 RCTs, 482 people) compared ropinirole versus bromocriptine.[54] It found that ropinirole versus bromocriptine improved "off" time and levodopa dose reduction after 8–25 weeks, but these differences were not significant (h/day "off" time: WMD 0.8, 95% CI –0.1 to +1.7; difference in levodopa dose reduction: 50 mg/day, 95% CI –49 mg/day to +150 mg/day). The fifth systematic review (search date not stated, 5 RCTs, 1071 people) compared cabergoline versus bromocriptine.[55] Cabergoline improved "off" time compared with bromocriptine after 12–36 weeks, but the difference was not significant (h/day "off" time: WMD 0.3, 95% CI –0.1 to +0.7). Four of the RCTs found no difference in motor scores or activities of daily living scores.

Harms: **Versus placebo:** The systematic reviews found that agonist treatment versus placebo significantly increased dopaminergic adverse effects.[45–50] In particular, dyskinesia was significantly increased with pergolide (OR 4.6, 95% CI 3.1 to 7.0), pramipexole (OR 2.1, 95% CI 1.5 to 2.9), and ropinirole (OR 2.9, 95% CI 1.4 to 6.2).[47,48,50] Withdrawal from treatment was significantly lower with pramipexole versus placebo (OR 0.64, 95% CI 0.44 to 0.93) but not with pergolide, ropinirole, or cabergoline.[47–49] **Versus each other:** Systematic reviews found no significant difference in adverse events with pergolide versus bromocriptine and pramipexole versus bromocriptine,[52,53] but nausea was significantly less frequent with ropinirole (OR 0.5, 95% CI 0.3 to 0.8).[54] Dyskinesias and confusion were reported as adverse events more commonly with cabergoline than bromocriptine, but there was no significant difference in the frequency of other dopaminergic adverse events (dyskinesia: OR 1.6, 95% CI 1.1 to 2.4; confusion: OR 2.0, 95% CI 1.1 to 3.8).[55]

Comment: We found no studies that directly compared the newer dopamine agonists.

QUESTION What are the effects of surgery in people with later Parkinson's disease?

OPTION PALLIDAL SURGERY

One systematic review found limited evidence that unilateral pallidotomy versus medical treatment improved motor examination and activities of daily living. There is a high incidence of adverse effects with pallidotomy. One RCT found insufficient evidence to assess the effects of pallidotomy

versus deep brain stimulation. We found no RCTs comparing pallidal deep brain stimulation versus medical treatment. One small RCT found insufficient evidence to assess the effects of pallidal deep brain stimulation versus subthalamic deep brain stimulation.

Benefits: **Pallidotomy versus medical treatment:** We found one systematic review (search date 1999, 2 RCTs) that evaluated mainly unilateral posteroventral pallidotomy (see glossary, p 1382) in people with advanced Parkinson's disease.[56] The first RCT in the systematic review, published only as an abstract, found that pallidotomy versus medical treatment improved tremor, bradykinesia, rigidity, gait, postural stability, and "off time" (see glossary, p 1382).[57] It found no difference in the need for medical treatment. The second RCT in the systematic review (37 people) compared unilateral pallidotomy versus medical treatment.[58] It found that pallidotomy improved "off" phase motor examination (UPDRS 3 [see glossary, p 1382]), activities of daily living (Barthel Index, UPDRS 2 and Schwab and England scale), but not pain visual analogue score at 6 months (UPDRS 3: decreased from 47 to 33 with pallidotomy *v* increased from 53 to 57 with medical treatment, $P < 0.001$; Barthel Index increased by 2.5 with pallidotomy *v* decreased by 0.5 with medical treatment, $P = 0.004$; UPDRS 2: decreased from 30 to 21 with pallidotomy *v* increased from 32 to 35 with medical treatment, $P = 0.002$; Schwab and England scale: increased from 35 to 70 with pallidotomy *v* decreased from 35 to 30 with medical treatment, $P < 0.001$; pain score: decreased from 27 mm to 14 mm with pallidotomy *v* increased from 15 mm to 22 mm with medical treatment, $P = 0.13$; CIs not stated). **Pallidotomy versus pallidal deep brain stimulation:** We found one systematic review (search date 2000, 1 RCT).[59] The RCT (13 people) in the systematic review found no significant difference with pallidotomy versus deep brain stimulation (see glossary, p 1382) for symptoms, activities of daily living, and adverse effects over 3 months, but was too small to exclude clinically important differences.[60] **Pallidal deep brain stimulation versus medical treatment:** We found one systematic review (search date 2000) that identified no RCTs comparing pallidal deep brain stimulation versus medical treatment.[59] We found no subsequent RCTs. **Pallidal deep brain stimulation versus subthalamic deep brain stimulation:** We found one RCT (10 people) comparing bilateral pallidal deep brain stimulation versus bilateral subthalamic nucleus deep brain stimulation.[61] It found no difference in motor scores after 12 months (UPDRS 3 improvement: 39% with pallidal stimulation *v* 44% with subthalamic stimulation).

Harms: The first RCT in the review comparing pallidotomy versus medical treatment gave no information on adverse effects.[57] In the second RCT in the review, comparing pallidotomy versus medical treatment, 6/19 (31.5%) people who had unilateral pallidotomy had adverse effects persisting for 6 months after surgery, including dysarthria, dysphasia, facial paresis, and urinary incontinence.[58] One controlled study of the cognitive or behavioural effects of pallidotomy versus medical treatment found that left sided, but not right sided, pallidotomy reduced verbal fluency.[62] Another RCT assessing the neuropsychological and psychiatric effects of pallidotomy found subtle changes on measures of frontal lobe function after 6 months in people with unilateral pallidotomy.[63] One systematic review of case series (search date 1998) found that the incidence of permanent adverse effects of unilateral pallidotomy was 4–46%, with a risk of a serious complication (including death) of 3–10%.[64] Another systematic review of case series (search date 1998) estimated a 10–15% incidence of persistent adverse effects with unilateral pallidotomy.[65] One RCT (6 people) compared bilateral pallidotomy versus unilateral pallidotomy plus contralateral pallidal deep brain stimulation.[66] It found that all three bilateral pallidotomy patients experienced severe adverse effects. This led to discontinuation of the study. Complication rates declined as surgeons developed experience in performing pallidotomy.[67] Adverse effects linked with deep brain stimulation include haemorrhage, lead displacement, visual deficit, speech, motor or sensory disturbances, psychosis, confusion, and disorientation. Follow up can be expensive and time consuming. Eventually, equipment or battery replacement may be needed, requiring further surgery.

Comment: One cohort study found that improvement after unilateral pallidotomy was maintained for 12 months.[68] One recent non-systematic review and consensus statement suggested that gait, balance disorders, and hypophonia were less responsive than other features of parkinsonism to surgery (no further data provided).[67] Transplants and implants of dopaminergic tissue remain experimental. Uncontrolled studies and limited RCT information suggest adverse effects may be more frequent after lesioning procedures than deep brain stimulation, and are more likely to be permanent. Bilateral lesioning is likely to carry a high risk of adverse axial effects (see glossary, p 1382). Some surgeons propose that if bilateral procedures are required then deep brain stimulation rather than lesioning should be carried out on one side.

OPTION THALAMIC SURGERY New

One systematic review identified no RCTs comparing thalamic surgery versus medical treatment. One RCT found that thalamic deep brain stimulation versus thalamotomy improved functional status, and caused fewer adverse effects.

Benefits: **Thalamotomy versus medical treatment:** We found two systematic reviews (search date 1999,[56] search date 1998[65]) that identified no RCTs of thalamotomy versus medical treatment for Parkinson's disease (see comment below). **Thalamic deep brain stimulation versus medical treatment:** We found one systematic review (search date 2000).[59] It found no RCTs of thalamic deep brain stimulation (see glossary, p 1382) versus medical treatment. We found no subsequent RCTs. **Thalamotomy versus thalamic deep brain stimulation:** We found one systematic review (search date 2000).[59] It identified one RCT (68 people with tremor, 45 of whom had Parkinson's disease), which compared thalamotomy versus thalamic deep brain stimulation.[69] Subgroup analysis in people with Parkinson's disease found that thalamic deep brain stimulation versus thalamotomy improved functional status after 6 months (change in Frenchay Activities Index: 0.8 with thalamotomy *v* 5.5 with deep brain stimulation, 95% CI for difference 1.2 to 8.0).

Harms: **Thalamotomy versus medical treatment:** Case series included in the second systematic review found that thalamotomy was associated with reversible complications (lasting < 3 months) in 36%–61% of people and permanent complications, including speech disturbance, apraxia, and death, in 14%–23%.[65] Bilateral thalamotomy carries a high risk of speech disturbance.[65] **Thalamotomy versus thalamic deep brain stimulation:** The RCT found that adverse effects were significantly less common with deep brain stimulation versus thalamotomy after 6 months (AR 47% with thalamotomy *v* 18% with deep brain stimulation; P = 0.02; CI not stated).[69]

Comment: The reviews found limited evidence from case series that thalamic surgery may not be as useful as pallidal or subthalamic surgery thalamotomy for parkinsonian features other than tremor.[56,65] The second systematic review did not fully describe the case series it identified, focusing on results from "key studies". See also comment under pallidal surgery, p 1379.

OPTION SUBTHALAMIC SURGERY New

One systematic review found no RCTs comparing subthalamic surgery with medical treatment. One small RCT comparing subthalamic deep brain stimulation with pallidal deep brain stimulation found no significant difference in motor scores.

Benefits: **Subthalamic deep brain stimulation versus medical treatment:** We found one systematic review (search date 2000) that identified no RCTs of subthalamic deep brain stimulation (see glossary, p 1382) versus medical treatment.[59] We found no subsequent RCTs. **Pallidal deep brain stimulation versus subthalamic deep brain stimulation:** See benefits of pallidal surgery, p 1378.

Harms: See comment under pallidal surgery, p 1379.

Comment: Larger and longer term RCTs are needed to compare the effects of pallidal versus subthalamic stimulation. A large RCT comparing quality of life and costs of subthalamic or pallidal lesioning and deep brain stimulation surgery versus best medical treatment is currently under way in the UK (Clarke C, personal communication, 2002).

QUESTION What are the effects of rehabilitation treatments in later Parkinson's disease?

OPTION PHYSIOTHERAPY

Two systematic reviews found insufficient evidence of the effects of physiotherapy in later Parkinson's disease.

Benefits: We found two systematic reviews.[70,71] The first review (search date 2000, 11 RCTs, 280 people with early or later Parkinson's disease) compared physiotherapy versus no treatment or versus inactive physiotherapy.[67] The review was unable to draw conclusions on the effects of physiotherapy in Parkinson's disease because of the small numbers of people, methodological flaws, different types of physiotherapy used, and the wide variety of outcome measures in the

RCTs. The second systematic review (search date 1999, 8 RCTs included in the first review, 4 quasi-randomised studies) compared physiotherapy versus no treatment or versus other treatment (occupational therapy, regular exercises, non-specified psychological treatment).[71] It also found that methodological flaws of trials and trial heterogeneity made it difficult to draw conclusions on the effects of physiotherapy.[71]

Harms: The systematic reviews gave no information on adverse effects.[70,71]

Comment: Further, larger, well designed RCTs are required. A large Anglo–Dutch RCT is in preparation (Clarke C, personal communication, 2001).

OPTION OCCUPATIONAL THERAPY

One systematic review found insufficient evidence of the effects of occupational therapy in later Parkinson's disease.

Benefits: We found one systematic review (search date 2000, 2 RCTs, 84 people with early or later Parkinson's disease).[72] One RCT in the review compared occupational therapy versus no treatment, and the other RCT compared occupational therapy plus physiotherapy versus physiotherapy alone. The review was unable to draw conclusions on the effects of occupational therapy because of the small number of people in the RCTs, methodological flaws, trial heterogenoity, and the variety of outcome measures used.[72]

Harms: The RCTs in the review gave no information on adverse effects.[72]

Comment: Further, larger, well designed RCTs are required. An RCT of occupational therapy in Parkinson's disease is under way (Clarke C, personal communication, 2001).

OPTION SPEECH AND LANGUAGE THERAPY FOR SPEECH DISTURBANCE

One systematic review found insufficient evidence of the effects of speech and language therapy for speech disturbance in later Parkinson's disease.

Benefits: We found one systematic review (search date 2000, 3 RCTs, 63 people) that compared speech and language therapy versus no treatment for speech disturbance.[73] It was unable to draw conclusions on the effects of speech and language therapy because of the small number of people, methodological flaws, and the variety of outcome measures used in the RCTs.

Harms: The RCTs in the review gave no information on adverse effects.[73]

Comment: Further, larger, well designed RCTs are required.

OPTION SWALLOWING THERAPY FOR DYSPHAGIA

One systematic review found no RCTs of swallowing therapy for dysphagia.

Benefits: We found one systematic review (search date 2000) of swallowing therapy for dysphagia that did not identify any RCTs.[74]

Harms: We found no RCTs.

Comment: None.

GLOSSARY

Axial effects Changes affecting axial body sections, such as head and trunk, rather than the limbs.

Deep brain stimulation Prolonged focal electrical brain stimulation through a stereotactically implanted wire.

Dopaminergic adverse effects Include dyskinesia, hallucinations, and psychosis.

Dyskinesia Abnormal or involuntary writhing or jerky movements distinct from tremor.

Motor fluctuations Fluctuations in motor symptoms, such as bradykinesia, rigidity, and tremor, during a day. Response fluctuations are fluctuations in a person's overall response to treatment during a day.

"Off" time Periods when treatment is not working. "On" time is the period when treatment is working.

Pallidotomy Making a permanent surgical lesion, usually thermally or electrically, in the globus pallidum.

Unified Parkinson's Disease Rating Scale (UPDRS) A scale used to measure severity of Parkinson's Disease. It has six parts: mentation, behaviour and mood (UPDRS 1); activities of daily living (UPDRS 2); motor examination (UPDRS 3); complications of treatment (UPDRS 4); a global disability staging score (UPDRS 5); and a global activities of daily living score (UPDRS 6).

Substantive changes

Pallidal surgery New systematic review;[59] conclusions unchanged.

Pallidal surgery New RCT;[61] conclusions unchanged.

Pallidal surgery Two new RCTs[60,63] and one new systematic review of case series;[65] conclusions unchanged.

REFERENCES

1. Hughes AJ, Daniel SE, Blankson S, et al. A clinico-pathologic study of 100 cases of Parkinson's disease. *Arch Neurol* 1993;50:140–148.
2. Zhang Z, Roman G. Worldwide occurrence of Parkinson's disease: an updated review. *Neuroepidemiology* 1993;12:195–208.
3. De Rijk MC, Tzourio C, Breteler MMB, et al. Prevalence of parkinsonism and Parkinson's disease in Europe: the EUROPARKINSON collaborative study. *J Neurol Neurosurg Psychiatry* 1997;62:10–15.
4. Ben-Shlomo Y. How far are we in understanding the cause of Parkinson's disease? *J Neurol Neurosurg Psychiatry* 1996;61:4–16.
5. De Rijk M, Breteler M, den Breeilnen J, et al. Dietary antioxidants and Parkinson's disease: the Rotterdam study. *Arch Neurol* 1997;54:762–765.
6. Hellenbrand W, Seidler A, Robra B, et al. Smoking and Parkinson's disease: a case-control study in Germany. *Int J Epidemiol* 1997;26:328–339.
7. Tzourio C, Rocca W, Breteler M, et al. Smoking and Parkinson's disease: an age-dependent risk effect? *Neurology* 1997;49:1267–1272.
8. Marder K, Tang M, Mejia H, et al. Risk of Parkinson's disease among first degree relatives: a community based study. *Neurology* 1996;47:155–160.
9. Jarman P, Wood N. Parkinson's disease genetics comes of age. *BMJ* 1999;318:1641–1642.
10. Lazzarini A, Myers R, Zimmerman T, et al. A clinical genetic study of Parkinson's disease: evidence for dominant transmission. *Neurology* 1994;44:499–506.
11. Gasser T, Müller-Myhsok B, Wszolek Z, et al. A susceptibility locus for Parkinson's disease maps to chromosome 2p13. *Nat Genet* 1998;18:262–265.
12. Tanner C, Ottman R, Goldman S, et al. Parkinson's disease in twins. An etiologic study. *JAMA* 1999;281:341–346.
13. Scott WK, Nance MA, Watts RL, et al. Complete genomic screen in Parkinson disease: evidence for multiple genes. *JAMA* 2001;286:2239–2244.
14. Martin ER, Scott WK, Nance MA, et al. Association of single-nucleotide polymorphisms of the tau gene with late-onset Parkinson disease. *JAMA* 2001;286:2245–2250.
15. Parkinson Study Group. Mortality in DATATOP: a multicenter trial in early Parkinson's disease. *Ann Neurol* 1998;43:318–325.
16. Rajput A, Uitti J, Offord K. Timely levodopa (LD) administration prolongs survival in Parkinson's disease. *Parkinson Relat Disord* 1997;3:159–165.

17. Clarke CE. Does levodopa therapy delay death in Parkinson's disease? A review of the evidence. *Mov Disord* 1995;10:250–256.
18. Hely MA, Morris JGL, Traficante R, et al. The Sydney multicentre study of Parkinson's disease: progression and mortality at 10 years. *J Neurol Neurosurg Psychiatry* 1999;67:300–307.
19. Morgante L, Salemi G, Meneghini F, et al. Parkinson disease survival. A population-based study. *Arch Neurol* 2000;57:507–512.
20. Fahn S, Elton L, for the UPDRS Development Committee. Unified Parkinson's disease rating scale. In: Fahn S, Marsden C, Calne D, et al, eds. *Recent Developments in Parkinson's Disease*, Vol. 2. Florham Park: Macmillan Healthcare Information, 1987:153–163.
21. Langston JW, Widner H, Goetz CG, et al. Core Assessment Program for Intracerebral Transplantations (CAPIT). *Mov Disord* 1992;7:2–13.
22. De Boer A, Wijker W, Speelman J, et al. Quality of life in people with Parkinson's disease: development of a questionnaire. *J Neurol Neurosurg Psychiatry* 1996;61:70–74.
23. Peto V, Jenkinson C, Fitzpatrick R, et al. The development and validation of a short measure of functioning and well being for individuals with Parkinson's disease. *Qual Life Res* 1995;4:241–248.
24. The Parkinson's Disease Study Group. Effects of tocopherol and deprenyl on the progression of disability in early Parkinson's disease. *N Engl J Med* 1993;328:176–183.
25. Olanow CW, Hauser RA, Gauger L, et al. The effect of deprenyl and levodopa on the progression of Parkinson's disease. *Ann Neurol* 1995;38:771–777.
26. Lees AJ, for the Parkinson's Disease Research Group of the United Kingdom. Comparison of therapeutic effects and mortality data of levodopa and levodopa combined with selegiline in people with early, mild Parkinson's disease. *BMJ* 1995;311:1602–1607.
27. Przuntek H, Conrad B, Dichgans J, et al. SELEDO: a 5-year long-term trial on the effect of selegiline in early Parkinsonian people treated with levodopa. *Eur J Neurol* 1999;6:141–150.
28. Larson JP, Boas J, Erdal JE, et al. Does selegiline modify the progression of early Parkinson's disease? Results from a five-year study. *Eur J Neurol* 1999;6:539–547.
29. Olanow CW, Mylla V, Sotaniemi K, et al. Effect of selegiline on mortality in people with Parkinson's disease. *Neurology* 1998;51:825–830.
30. Parkinson Study Group. Impact of deprenyl and tocopherol treatment for Parkinson's disease in DATATOP people requiring levodopa. *Ann Neurol* 1996;39:37–45.
31. Ben-Shlomo Y, Churchyard A, Head J, et al. Investigation by Parkinson's Disease Research Group of United Kingdom into excess mortality seen with combined levodopa and selegiline treatment in people with early, mild Parkinson's disease: further results of randomised trial and confidential inquiry. *BMJ* 1998;316:1191–1196.
32. Counsell C. Effect of adding selegiline to levodopa in early, mild Parkinson's disease. *BMJ* 1998;17:1586.
33. Thorogood M, Armstrong B, Nichols T, et al. Mortality in people taking selegiline: observational study. *BMJ* 1998;317:252–254.
34. Dupont E, Andersen A, Boas J, et al. Sustained-release Madopar HBS compared with standard Madopar in the long-term treatment of *de novo* Parkinsonian people. *Acta Neurol Scand* 1996;93:14–20.
35. Block G, Liss C, Reines S, et al. Comparison of immediate release and controlled release carbidopa/levodopa in Parkinson's disease. *Eur Neurol* 1997;37:23–27.
36. Ramaker C, van Hilten J. Bromocriptine versus levodopa in early Parkinson's disease. In: The Cochrane Library, Issue 2, 2002. Oxford: Update Software. Search date 1999; primary sources Cochrane Movement Disorders Group Specialised Register, Cochrane Controlled Trials Register, Medline, Embase, pharmaceutical companies, experts for unpublished studies, and hand searched references and selected neurology journals.
37. Ramaker C, Hilten JJ van. Bromocriptine/levodopa combined versus levodopa alone for early Parkinson's disease (Cochrane Review). In: The Cochrane Library, Issue 2, 2002. Oxford: Update Software. Search date 2001; primary sources Cochrane Movement Disorders Group Specialised Register, Cochrane Controlled Trials Register, Medline, Embase, pharmaceutical companies, experts for unpublished studies, and hand searched references and selected neurology journals.
38. Rascol O, Brooks D, Korczyn A, et al. A five-year study of the incidence of dyskinesia in people with early Parkinson's disease who were treated with ropinirole or levodopa. *N Engl J Med* 2000;342:1484–1491.
39. Parkinson Study Group. Pramipexole versus levodopa as initial treatment for Parkinson's disease. *JAMA* 2000;284:1931–1938.
40. Rinne U. A 5-year double-blind study with cabergoline versus levodopa in the treatment of early Parkinson's disease. *Parkinsonism Relat Disord* 1999;5(suppl):84.
41. Oertel WH. Pergolide versus levodopa monotherapy (PELMOPET). *Mov Disord* 2000;15(suppl 3):4.
42. Rinne U. Lisuride, a dopamine agonist in the treatment of early Parkinson's disease. *Neurology* 1989;39:336–339.
43. Allain H, Destee A, Petit H, et al. Five-year follow-up of early lisuride and levodopa combination therapy versus levodopa monotherapy in de novo Parkinson's disease. *Eur Neurol* 2000;44:22–30.
44. Fahn S. Parkinson's disease, the effect of levodopa and the ELLDOPA trial. *Arch Neurol* 1999;56:529–535.
45. Van Hilten J, Beek W, Finken M. Bromocriptine for levodopa-induced motor complications in Parkinson's disease. In: The Cochrane Library, Issue 2, 2002. Oxford: Update Software. Search date 1998; primary sources Cochrane Controlled Trials Register, Medline, Scisearch, pharmaceutical companies, experts for unpublished studies, and hand searched references.
46. Clarke C, Speller J. Lisuride for levodopa-induced complications in Parkinson's disease. In: The Cochrane Library, Issue 2, 2002. Oxford: Update Software. Search date 1998; primary sources Medline, Embase, Cochrane Controlled Trials Register, pharmaceutical companies, and hand searched references.
47. Clarke C, Speller J. Pergolide for levodopa-induced complications in Parkinson's disease. In: The Cochrane Library, Issue 2, 2002. Oxford: Update Software. Search date 1999; primary sources Medline, Embase, Cochrane Controlled Trials Register, pharmaceutical companies, and hand searched references.
48. Clarke C, Deane K. Ropinirole for levodopa-induced complications in Parkinson's disease. In: The Cochrane Library, Issue 2, 2002. Oxford: Update Software. Search date not stated;

primary sources Cochrane Movement Disorders Group Specialised Register, Cochrane Controlled Trials Register, Medline, Embase, pharmaceutical companies, experts for unpublished studies, and hand searched references and selected neurology journals.

49. Clarke C, Deane K. Cabergoline for levodopa-induced complications in Parkinson's disease. In: The Cochrane Library, Issue 2, 2002. Oxford: Update Software. Search date not stated; primary sources Medline, Embase, Cochrane Controlled Trials Register, hand searches of reference lists and selected neurology journals, and contact with Pharmacia Upjohn Ltd.
50. Clarke C, Speller J, Clarke J. Pramipexole for levodopa-induced complications in Parkinson's disease. In: The Cochrane Library, Issue 2, 2002. Oxford: Update Software. Search date not stated; primary sources Cochrane Movement Disorders Group Specialised Register, Cochrane Controlled Trials Register, Medline, Embase, pharmaceutical companies, experts for unpublished studies, and hand searched references and selected neurology journals.
51. Clarke CE, Speller JM. Lisuride versus bromocriptine for levodopa-induced complications in Parkinson's disease. In: The Cochrane Library, Issue 2, 2002. Oxford: Update Software. Search date not stated; primary sources Medline, Embase, Cochrane Controlled Trials Register, hand searches of the neurology literature, reference lists of identified studies, and contact with pharmaceutical companies.
52. Clarke C, Speller J. Pergolide versus bromocriptine for levodopa-induced motor complications in Parkinson's disease. In: The Cochrane Library, Issue 2, 2002. Oxford: Update Software. Search date 1998; primary sources Medline, Embase, Cochrane Controlled Trials Register, pharmaceuticals companies, and hand searched references.
53. Clarke C, Speller J, Clarke J. Pramipexole versus bromocriptine for levodopa-induced complications in Parkinson's disease. In: The Cochrane Library, Issue 2, 2002. Oxford: Update Software. Search date not stated; primary sources Cochrane Movement Disorders Group Specialised Register, Cochrane Controlled Trials Register, Medline, Embase, pharmaceutical companies, experts for unpublished studies, and hand searched references and selected neurology journals.
54. Clarke C, Deane K. Ropinirole versus bromocriptine for levodopa-induced complications in Parkinson's disease. In: The Cochrane Library, Issue 2, 2002. Oxford: Update Software. Search date not stated; primary sources Cochrane Movement Disorders Group Specialised Register, Cochrane Controlled Trials Register, Medline, Embase, pharmaceutical companies, experts for unpublished studies, and hand searched references and selected neurology journals.
55. Clarke C, Deane K. Cabergoline versus bromocriptine for levodopa-induced complications in Parkinson's disease. In: The Cochrane Library, Issue 2, 2002. Oxford: Update Software. Search date not stated; primary sources Cochrane Movement Disorders Group Specialised Register, Cochrane Controlled Trials Register, Medline, Embase, pharmaceutical companies, experts for unpublished studies, and hand searched references and selected neurology journals.
56. Development and Evaluation Committee. Report 105. *Pallidotomy, Thalotomy and Deep Brain Stimulation for Severe Parkinson's Disease*. Southampton: Wessex Institute for Health Research and Development, 1999. Search date 1999; primary sources Cochrane Library, Health Technology Assessment database, Medline, Science Citation Index, BIOSIS, Embase, Index to Scientific and Technical Proceedings, Inspec, and Best Evidence.
57. Vitek J, Bakay R, Freeman A, et al. Randomised clinical trial of pallidotomy for Parkinson's disease. *Neurology* 1998;50(suppl 4):A80.
58. De Bie R, de Haan R, Nijssen P, et al. Unilateral pallidotomy in Parkinson's disease: a randomised, single-blind, multicentre trial. *Lancet* 1999;354:1665–1669.
59. Medical Services Advisory Committee. Deep brain stimulation for Parkinson's disease. Australian Department of Health and Ageing, Canberra, 2001. Search date 2000; primary sources Cochrane library, Medline, Psycinfo, Cinahl, Current Contents, PreMedline, Healthstar, Trip, and Australasian Medical Index.
60. Merello M, Nouzeilles MI, Kuzis G, et al. Unilateral radiofrequency lesion versus electrostimulation of posteroventral pallidum: a prospective randomized comparison. *Mov Disord* 1999;14:50–56.
61. Burchiel K, Anderson V, Favre J, Hammerstad J. Comparison of pallidal and subthalamic nucleus deep brain stimulation for advanced Parkinson's disease: results of a randomized, blinded pilot study. *Neurosurgery* 1999;45:1375–1384.
62. Schmand B, de Bie R, Koning-Haanstra M, et al. Unilateral pallidotomy in PD. A controlled study of cognitive and behavioural effects. *Neurology* 2000;54:1058–1064.
63. Green J, McDonald W, Vitek J, et al. Neuropsychological and psychiatric sequelae of pallidotomy for PD. Clinical trial findings. *Neurology* 2002;58:858–865.
64. Gregory R. Posteroventral pallidotomy for advanced Parkinson's disease: a systematic review. *Neurol Rev Int* 1999;3:8–12. Search date 1998; primary sources not stated.
65. Hallett M, Litvan I. The Task Force on Surgery for Parkinson's Disease. Evaluation of surgery for Parkinson's disease. A report of the Therapeutics and Technology Assessment Subcommittee of the American Academy of Neurology. *Neurology* 1999;53:1910–1921. Search date 1998; primary sources Medline, Embase, Biosis.
66. Merello M, Starkstein S, Nouzeilles M, et al. Bilateral pallidotomy for treatment of Parkinson's disease induced corticobulbar syndrome and psychic akinesia avoidable by globus pallidus lesion combined with contralateral stimulation. *J Neurol Neurosurg Psychiatry* 2001;71:611–614.
67. Bronstein JM, DeSalles A, DeLong MR. Sterotactic pallidotomy in the treatment of Parkinson's disease. *Arch Neurol* 1999;56:1064–1069.
68. De Bie R, Schuurman P, Bosch D, et al. Outcome of unilateral pallidotomy in advanced Parkinson's disease: cohort study of 32 patients. *J Neurol Neurosurg Psychiatry* 2001;71:375–382.
69. Schuurman P, Bosch D, Bossuyt P, et al. A comparison of continuous thalamic stimulation and thalamotomy for suppression of severe tremor. *N Engl J Med* 2000;342:461–468.
70. Deane KHO, Jones D, Clarke CE, et al. Physiotherapy for patients with Parkinson's disease. In: The Cochrane Library. Issue 2, 2002. Oxford: Update Software. Search date 2000; primary sources Medline, Embase, Cinahl, Isi-Sci, Amed, Mantis, Rehabdata, Rehadat, Gerolit, Pascal, Lilacs, MedCarib, Jicst-EPlus, Aim, IMEMR, Sigle, ISI-ISTP, Dissabs, Conference Papers Index, Aslib Index to Theses, Cochrane Library, the CentreWatch Clinical Trials listing service, the metaRegister of Controlled Trials, ClinicalTrials.gov, Crisp, Pedro, Niddr and NRR, and hand searching of reference lists.

71. de Goede CJ, Keus SH, Kwakkel G, et al. The effects of physical therapy in Parkinson's disease: a research synthesis. *Arch Phys Med Rehab* 2001;2:509–515. Search date 1999; primary sources Medline, Cinahl, and hand searches of reference lists.
72. Deane KHO, Ellis-Hill C, Clarke CE, et al. Occupational therapy for patients with Parkinson's disease. In: The Cochrane Library. Issue 2, 2002. Oxford: Update Software. Search date 2000; primary sources Medline, Embase, Cinahl, Isi-Sci, Amed, Mantis, Rehabdata, Rehadat, Gerolit, Pascal, Lilacs, MedCarib, Jicst-EPlus, Aim, IMEMR, Sigle, ISI-ISTP, Dissabs, Conference Papers Index, Aslib Index to Theses, Cochrane Library, the CentreWatch Clinical Trials listing service, the metaRegister of Controlled Trials, ClinicalTrials.gov, Crisp, Pedro, Niddr and NRR, and hand searching of reference lists.
73. Deane KHO, Whurr R, Playford ED, et al. Speech and language therapy for dysarthria in Parkinson's disease. In: The Cochrane Library Issue 2, 2002. Oxford: Update Software. Search date 2000; primary sources Medline, Embase, Cinahl, Isi-Sci, Amed, Mantis, Rehabdata, Rehadat, Gerolit, Pascal, Lilacs, MedCarib, Jicst-EPlus, Aim, IMEMR, Sigle, ISI-ISTP, Dissabs, Conference Papers Index, Aslib Index to Theses, Cochrane Library, the CentreWatch Clinical Trials listing service, the metaRegister of Controlled Trials, ClinicalTrials.gov, Crisp, Pedro, Niddr and NRR, and hand searching of reference lists.
74. Deane KHO, Whurr R, Clarke CE, et al. Non-pharmacological therapies for dysphagia in Parkinson's disease. In: The Cochrane Library Issue 2, 2002. Oxford: Update Software. Search date 2000; Primary sources Medline, Embase, Cinahl, Isi-Sci, Amed, Mantis, Rehabdata, Rehadat, Gerolit, Pascal, Lilacs, MedCarib, Jicst-EPlus, Aim, IMEMR, Sigle, ISI-ISTP, Dissabs, Conference Papers Index, Aslib Index to Theses, Cochrane Library, the CentreWatch Clinical Trials listing service, the metaRegister of Controlled Trials, ClinicalTrials.gov, Crisp, Pedro, Niddr and NRR, and hand searching of reference lists

Carl Clarke
Reader in Clinical Neurology
University of Birmingham
Birmingham
UK

A Moore
Senior Lecturer in Neurology
University of Liverpool
Liverpool
UK

Competing interests: APM has been reimbursed by and/or received fees from various companies producing drugs and surgical equipment for Parkinson's disease, for attending and speaking at conferences, and for advice. CC has been paid by various manufacturers of the drugs dealt with above for speaking at meetings and attending conferences.

Trigeminal neuralgia

Search date November 2001

Joanna Zakrzewska

QUESTIONS

INTERVENTIONS

Key Messages

- **Baclofen** We found insufficient evidence from two small crossover trials on the effects of baclofen versus placebo or versus other active drugs.
- **Carbamazepine** One systematic review of three crossover RCTs has found that carbamazepine versus placebo increases the number of people who have pain relief at 5–14 days (NNT 3, 95% CI 2 to 4), a second systematic review found similar results. The first review found that carbamazepine versus placebo increases drowsiness, dizziness, constipation, and ataxia (NNH 3, 95% CI 2 to 7).
- **Combined streptomycin and lidocaine nerve block** Small poor quality RCTs found insufficient evidence about the effects of nerve block with streptomycin plus lidocaine versus nerve block with lidocaine alone.
- **Lamotrigine** One small crossover trial found limited evidence that lamotrigine versus placebo (added to either carbamazepine or phenytoin) improved pain after 2 weeks.
- **Other drugs (phenytoin, clonazepam, sodium valproate, gabapentin, mexiletine, oxcarbazepine)** We found no RCTs about the effects of other antiepileptic drugs.

Clin Evid 2002;8:1386–1396.

- **Pimozide** One RCT found that pimozide versus carbamazepine significantly reduced pain over 8 weeks, but increased adverse effects including hand tremors, memory impairment, and involuntary movements (NNH 3, 95% CI 2 to 4). The use of pimozide is limited by cardiac toxicity and reports of sudden death.
- **Proparacaine** One RCT found no significant difference in pain at 30 days with single application of proparacaine hydrochloride versus placebo eye drops to the eye on the same side as the pain.
- **Tizanidine** One small RCT found insufficient evidence about the effects of tizanidine.
- **Tocainide** One crossover RCT found no significant difference in the proportion of people improved with tocainide versus carbamazepine. The use of tocainide is limited by considerable harms. The RCT reported a death attributed to haematological effects of tocainide.
- **Cryotherapy of peripheral nerves; peripheral acupuncture; peripheral alcohol injection; peripheral injection of phenol; peripheral neurectomy; peripheral radiofrequency thermocoagulation; peripheral laser treatment** We found no RCTs about the effects of these interventions.

DEFINITION Trigeminal neuralgia is a characteristic pain in the distribution of one or more branches of the fifth cranial nerve. The diagnosis is made on the history alone, based on characteristic features of the pain. It occurs in paroxysms that last a few seconds to 2 minutes. The frequency of paroxysms is highly variable: from hundreds of attacks a day to long periods of remission that can last years. The pain is severe and described as intense, sharp, superficial, stabbing, burning, or like an electric shock. In any individual, the pain has the same character in different attacks. It is often triggered by touch in a specific area or by eating, talking, washing the face, or cleaning the teeth. Between paroxysms the person is asymptomatic. Other causes of facial pain may need to be excluded.[1] In trigeminal neuralgia the neurological examination is usually normal.[2,3]

INCIDENCE/ PREVALENCE Most evidence about the incidence and prevalence of trigeminal neuralgia is from the USA.[4] The annual incidence (when age adjusted to 1980 age distribution of the USA) is 5.9/100 000 women and 3.4/100 000 men. The incidence tends to be slightly higher in women at all ages. The incidence increases with age. In men aged over 80 years the incidence is 45.2/100 000.[5] Other published surveys are small. One questionnaire survey of neurological disease in a single French village found one person with trigeminal neuralgia among 993 people.[6]

AETIOLOGY/ RISK FACTORS The cause of trigeminal neuralgia remains unclear.[7] It is more common in people with multiple sclerosis (RR 20, 95% CI 4.1 to 59).[5] Hypertension is a risk factor in women (RR 2.1, 95% CI 1.2 to 3.4) but the evidence is less clear for men (RR 1.53, 95% CI 0.3 to 4.5).[5] A study in the USA found that people with trigeminal neuralgia smoked less, consumed less alcohol, had fewer tonsillectomies, and were less likely than matched controls to be Jewish or an immigrant.[8]

PROGNOSIS One study found no reduction of 10 year survival with trigeminal neuralgia.[9] We found no evidence about the natural history of trigeminal neuralgia. The illness is characterised by recurrences and remissions. Many people have periods of remission with no pain for months or years.[3] Anecdotal reports suggest that in many people it becomes more severe and less responsive to treatment with time.[10] Most people with trigeminal neuralgia are initially managed medically, and a proportion eventually have a surgical procedure.[5] We found no good evidence about the proportion of people who require surgical treatment for pain control.

AIMS To relieve pain with minimal adverse effects.

OUTCOMES Pain frequency and severity scores; measures of psychological distress; ability to perform normal activities; adverse effects.

METHODS *Clinical Evidence* search and appraisal November 2001. Author performed an additional handsearch of her own bibliography.

QUESTION **What are the effects of medical treatments on trigeminal neuralgia?**

OPTION **CARBAMAZEPINE**

One systematic review of three small crossover RCTs has found that carbamazepine versus placebo increases the number of people who have pain relief (1 in 3 people respond), but one in three people also have adverse effects. A second systematic review found similar results.

Benefits: **Versus placebo:** We found two systematic reviews (see table 1, p 1396).[11,12] The first systematic review (search date 1999, 3 crossover RCTs, 161 people with trigeminal neuralgia) found that treatment with carbamazepine versus placebo (for 5 days to 2 wks) significantly increased the number of people having a good or excellent response (57% with carbamazepine *v* 18% with placebo; OR 4.8, 95% CI 3.4 to 6.9; NNT 3, 95% CI 2 to 4).[11] The second systematic review (search date not stated, 2 RCTs, 107 people with trigeminal neuralgia) found similar results.[12]

Harms: The review found significantly more adverse effects (drowsiness, dizziness, constipation, and ataxia) with carbamazepine than with placebo (NNH 3, 95% CI 2 to 7).[11] In the RCTs, adverse effects were more likely with carbamazepine than with placebo and more people withdrew from the RCTs because of adverse effects (NNH for withdrawal 24, CI 14 to 112).[13] Adverse effects described in observational studies include rashes, leucopenia, and abnormal liver function tests.

Comment: The RCTs used a crossover design, and one RCT[14] used multiple crossovers so that each individual was counted more than once when calculating the estimates of effectiveness in the systematic review.[11,13] The RCTs included in the systematic review were small and short term. All of the RCTs used simple measures for pain outcomes and no quality of life measures. Diagnostic criteria were not clearly stated. Previous treatment and duration of pain varied considerably. Long term effects of carbamazepine have been assessed only in open trials. We found one report (143 people with trigeminal neuralgia followed for up to 16 years) on the long term benefits of carbamazepine.[15] Initially carbamazepine was successful in 69% of participants, but by 5–16 years only 31 participants (22%) were still finding carbamazepine effective and 44% required additional or alternative treatment.

OPTION TIZANIDINE

One small RCT found insufficient evidence about the effects of tizanidine.

Benefits: **Versus placebo:** We found no RCTs. **Versus carbamazepine:** We found one systematic review (search date 1999, 1 double blind RCT, 12 people).[11] It found that tizanidine (up to 18 mg/day) versus carbamazepine (up to 900 mg/day) had no significant effect on the number of people with relief of pain after treatment for 3 weeks (4/6 [67%] with carbamazepine *v* 1/6 [17%] with tizanidine; P = 0.08) (see table 1, p 1396).

Harms: No adverse effects were reported but two people withdrew because of inadequate pain control.

Comment: The RCT was too small to establish or exclude clinically important effects.

OPTION PIMOZIDE

One RCT found pimozide versus carbamazepine reduced pain but caused more adverse effects.

Benefits: **Versus placebo:** We found no RCTs. **Versus carbamazepine:** We found one systematic review (search date 1999) that identified one double blind crossover RCT comparing pimozide versus carbamazepine in 48 people with trigeminal neuralgia who were refractory to other medical treatment.[11] It found that significantly more people achieved a large reduction in pain severity with 8 weeks of pimozide treatment (48/48 [100%] with pimozide *v* 28/48 [56%] with carbamazepine) (see table 1, p 1396).

Harms: The RCT found that more people experienced adverse effects with pimozide than with carbamazepine (40/48 [83%] with pimozide *v* 22/48 [46%] with carbamazepine; OR 7.8, 95% CI 3.7 to 20). Adverse effects included hand tremors, memory impairment, and involuntary movements. The use of pimozide is restricted by its cardiac toxicity and by reports of sudden death.

Comment: This was a well conducted multicentre trial using a variety of outcome measures. The crossover design limits interpretation of the results because untested assumptions are required to perform the statistical analyses.

OPTION TOCAINIDE

One crossover RCT found no significant difference in the proportion of people improved with tocainide versus carbamazepine. The use of tocainide is limited by considerable harms. The RCT reported a death attributed to haematological effects of tocainide.

Benefits: **Versus placebo:** We found no RCTs. **Versus carbamazepine:** We found one systematic review (search date 1999, 1 RCT,[16] 12 people with trigeminal neuralgia).[11] The double blind, crossover RCT had weak methods. It found that tocainide versus carbamazepine had no significant effect on the number of people who improved after 2 weeks of treatment (8/12 [67%] with tocainide *v* 9/12 [75%] with carbamazepine; ARR +8.3%, 95% CI –28% to +45%).

Harms: The RCT found severe adverse effects (1 person withdrew because of a skin rash and 3 others had adverse effects). The postscript to the paper reported a death attributed to haematological effects of tocainide.

Comment: The available evidence is poor, but provides no support for the use of tocainide in trigeminal neuralgia.

OPTION LAMOTRIGINE

One small crossover RCT found limited evidence that lamotrigine versus placebo (added to other anticonvulsants) improved short term pain in trigeminal neuralgia.

Benefits: **Versus placebo:** We found two systematic reviews (search date 1999[11] and search date not stated[12]) that identified one RCT.[17] The RCT (double blind crossover, 14 people with refractory trigeminal neuralgia using either carbamazepine or phenytoin) found that lamotrigine (400 mg) versus placebo in addition to the current medication increased the number of people who improved after 4 weeks of treatment (10/13 [77%] with lamotrigine *v* 8/14 [57%] with placebo; ARI +20%, 95% CI –16% to +55%) (see table 1, p 1396). Although these results show no significant differences, a composite efficacy score based on total pain scores, global evaluations, and use of escape medication was higher with lamotrigine than with placebo (P = 0.01).

Harms: In the RCT, adverse effects with lamotrigine included dizziness, constipation, nausea, and drowsiness. It may also cause serious skin rash and allergic reactions. The total number of people reporting adverse effects was the same as with placebo (7/14 [50%] with lamotrigine *v* 7/14 [50%] with placebo).

Comment: This RCT was a small study and lamotrigine was used in addition to existing treatment. The crossover design and short period of treatment limits interpretation. It is not clear which of the outcomes and analyses were defined *a priori* as the primary outcomes and analyses.

OPTION BACLOFEN

We found insufficient evidence from two small crossover trials on the effects of baclofen versus placebo or versus other active drugs.

Benefits: **Versus placebo:** We found one systematic review (search date not stated)[12] that included one controlled trial.[18] The trial (double blind, crossover, 10 people, 4 using carbamazepine or phenytoin) found that baclofen versus placebo in addition to pre-existing treatment increased the number of people with relief of pain after treatment for 2 weeks (7/10 [70%] with baclofen v 1/10 [10%] with placebo; NNT 2, 95% CI 1 to 6).[18] It is not clear whether treatment allocation was randomised. **Versus other active drugs:** We found one trial (double blind crossover, 15 people, not clearly randomised) that compared racemic baclofen versus L-baclofen over 2 weeks.[19] It found no significant difference in response (9/15 [60%] with L-baclofen v 6/15 [40%] with racemic baclofen; ARI +20%, 95% CI –16% to +56%).

Harms: Baclofen is associated with transient sedation and loss of muscle tone. Abrupt discontinuation may cause seizures and hallucinations. In the second trial more people with racemic baclofen versus L-baclofen reported dizziness, confusion, or lethargy (6/15 [40%] v 1/15 [7%]; ARI 33%, 95% CI 3.1% to 64%).

Comment: Both trials were small and it is not clear whether treatment was randomly allocated. In four people, the baclofen was used as add on treatment to anticonvulsants. In others it was used as monotherapy, making evaluations difficult. Standard baclofen is a racemic mixture. The first RCT,[18] after the initial 2 week period, became an open label trial during which 28/60 people using baclofen were pain free over 1–5 years, although many needed additional phenytoin or carbamazepine. Another small, brief trial of carbamazepine plus baclofen had a low quality score, with 6/30 withdrawals unexplained.

OPTION PROPARACAINE HYDROCHLORIDE DROPS

One RCT found no evidence of benefit from a single application of anaesthetic eye drops to the eye on the same side as the pain.

Benefits: **Versus placebo:** We found no systematic review but found one double blind RCT (47 people with trigeminal neuralgia) of proparacaine hydrochloride versus placebo instilled for 20 minutes on the same side as the trigeminal neuralgia on one occasion only.[20] It found no significant reduction of pain after 3, 10, and 30 days (at 30 days: 6/25 [24%] improved with proparacaine v 5/22 [23%] with placebo; ARI +1.3%, 95% CI –23% to +26%).

Harms: None reported.

Comment: None.

OPTION OTHER DRUGS

We found no evidence about effects of phenytoin, clonazepam, sodium valproate, gabapentin, mexiletine, oxcarbazepine, or topiramate in people with trigeminal neuralgia.

Benefits: We found no systematic reviews and no reliable RCTs examining effects of phenytoin, clonazepam, sodium valproate, gabapentin, mexiletine, oxcarbazepine, or topiramate in people with trigeminal neuralgia.

Harms: See harms of antiepileptic drugs under epilepsy, p 1313. Harms of mexiletine include dizziness, nausea, vomiting, confusion, and tremor.[21]

Comment: We found one double blind crossover RCT (3 people with trigeminal neuralgia) that compared 12 weeks of topiramate (25 mg daily titrated up to 800 mg daily) versus placebo.[22] Titration was by weekly phone assessment of symptoms. Washout period between crossover was 2 weeks. The trial found that topiramate reduced pain (on a 10 point scale) compared with placebo in all three patients (P = 0.04). However, the trial was at high risk of detecting effects by chance.

QUESTION What are the effects of surgical treatments for trigeminal neuralgia?

OPTION CRYOTHERAPY OF PERIPHERAL NERVES

We found insufficient evidence about effects of cryotherapy (see glossary, p 1394) in people with trigeminal neuralgia.

Benefits: We found no RCTs.

Harms: We found insufficient evidence.

Comment: We found many articles that reported studies of limited reliability, duplicated data, or included people with different types of pain.

OPTION NERVE BLOCK

We found insufficient evidence from two small RCTs about effects of combined injection of peripheral nerves with streptomycin and lidocaine compared with lidocaine alone.

Benefits: **Local anaesthetic versus placebo or no treatment:** We found no systematic review and no RCTs. **Local anaesthetic versus streptomycin plus local anaesthetic:** We found two RCTs comparing injections of streptomycin (1 g) and lidocaine (2 mL of 2% solution) versus lidocaine injections alone (one injection weekly for 5 wks).[23,24] The first RCT included 18 people with trigeminal neuralgia who had previously responded poorly to lidocaine injection alone (≤ 24 h pain relief from lidocaine alone). Analysis was biased: one person who did not gain pain relief from allocated treatment was excluded. One week after the final injection, combined streptomycin and lidocaine improved the chance of being pain free compared with lidocaine alone (AR for being pain free: 89% with combined injection *v* 38% with lidocaine alone; ARR 51%; CI not provided; P = 0.04). After 30 months the RCT found no significant difference between treatments (AR for being pain free: 33% with combined injection *v* 25% with lidocaine alone; ARR 8%; CI not reported: P = 0.38).[23] The second RCT compared weekly injections of combined streptomycin (1 g) and lidocaine (3 mL of 2% solution) versus lidocaine alone for 5 weeks in a randomised crossover design involving 20 people with idiopathic or traumatic trigeminal neuralgia. It found no significant short term differences between the groups in severity or frequency of pain as assessed clinically and from pain diaries.[24]

Harms: Patients found the injections painful and some refused to have further injections.[24] No sensory changes or other adverse effects were reported.

Comment: Neither trial reported method of randomisation. One trial had short follow up.[24] Reliability of results may have been limited by selection bias (see Benefits above).[25] Streptomycin was used on the assumption that it causes a long term peripheral nerve block.

OPTION PERIPHERAL ALCOHOL INJECTIONS

We found insufficient evidence about effects of injecting peripheral nerves with alcohol in people with trigeminal neuralgia.

Benefits: We found no RCTs.

Harms: We found insufficient evidence.

Comment: None.

OPTION PERIPHERAL NEURECTOMY

We found insufficient evidence about effects of peripheral neurectomy in people with trigeminal neuralgia.

Benefits: We found no RCTs.

Harms: We found insufficient evidence.

Comment: None.

OPTION PERIPHERAL RADIOFREQUENCY THERMOCOAGULATION

We found insufficient evidence about effects of peripheral radiofrequency thermocoagulation in people with trigeminal neuralgia.

Benefits: We found no RCTs.

Harms: We found insufficient evidence.

Comment: None.

OPTION PERIPHERAL INJECTION OF PHENOL

We found insufficient evidence about effects of peripheral nerve injection with phenol in people with trigeminal neuralgia.

Benefits: We found no RCTs.

Harms: We found insufficient evidence.

Comment: None.

OPTION PERIPHERAL ACUPUNCTURE

We found insufficient evidence about effects of peripheral acupuncture in people with trigeminal neuralgia.

Benefits: We found no RCTs.

Harms: We found insufficient evidence.

Comment: None.

OPTION PERIPHERAL LASER TREATMENT

We found insufficient evidence about effects of peripheral laser treatment (see glossary, p 1394) in people with trigeminal neuralgia.

Benefits: We found no reliable RCTs.

Harms: We found insufficient evidence.

Comment: We found one RCT (35 people with trigeminal neuralgia) comparing helium neon laser (3 treatments weekly for 10 wks, 1 mW, 632.5 nm, 20 Hz applied for 20 s on skin overlying the trigger nerve and 30 s on painful areas of the face) versus sham treatment with apparatus that emitted no light.[25] The trial did not directly compare the two groups. However, it found that mean pain score significantly improved from baseline at weeks 6 and 7 with laser, but did not change significantly from baseline for any week with sham treatment. This *post hoc* analysis has limited reliability.

GLOSSARY

Cryotherapy After surgical exposure of the trigger nerve, three freeze–thaw cycles are applied under local anaesthesia and sedation as necessary.

Peripheral laser treatment Laser irradiation of skin overlying the trigger nerve.

REFERENCES

1. Anonymous. *Classification of chronic pain. Descriptors of chronic pain syndromes and definitions of pain terms.* Seattle: IASP Press, 1994.
2. Katusic S, Williams DB, Beard CM, Bergstralh EJ, Kurland LT. Epidemiology and clinical features of idiopathic trigeminal neuralgia and glossopharyngeal neuralgia: similarities and differences, Rochester, Minnesota, 1945–1984. *Neuroepidemiology* 1991;10:276–281.
3. Zakrzewska JM. *Trigeminal Neuralgia.* London: WB Saunders,1995.
4. Zakrzewska JM, Hamlyn PJ. Facial pain. In: Crombie IKCPR, Linton SJ, LeResche L, Von Korff M, eds. *Epidemiology of Pain.* Seattle: IASP, 1999:171–202.
5. Katusic S, Beard CM, Bergstralh E, Kurland LT. Incidence and clinical features of trigeminal neuralgia, Rochester, Minnesota, 1945–1984. *Ann Neurol* 1990;27:89–95.
6. Munoz M, Dumas M, Boutros-Toni F, et al. A neuro-epidemiologic survey in a Limousin town. *Rev Neurol (Paris)* 1988;144:266–271.
7. Burchiel KJ. Pain in neurology and neurosurgery: tic douloureux (trigeminal neuralgia). In: Campbell JN, ed. *Pain 1996 – an updated review.* Seattle: IASP Press, 1996:41–60.
8. Rothman KJ, Monson RR. Epidemiology of trigeminal neuralgia. *J Chronic Dis* 1973;26:3–12.
9. Rothman KJ, Monson RR. Survival in trigeminal neuralgia. *J Chronic Dis* 1973;26:303–309.
10. Burchiel KJ, Slavin KV. On the natural history of trigeminal neuralgia. *Neurosurgery* 2000;46:152–155.
11. Wiffen P, Collins S, McQuay H, et al. Anticonvulsant drugs for acute and chronic pain. In: The Cochrane Library, Issue 3, 2001. Oxford: Update Software. Search date 1999; primary sources Medline, Embase, Sigle, Cochrane Controlled Trials Register, and handsearches of 40 medical journals and authors of published reports.
12. Sindrup SH, Jensen TS. Efficacy of pharmacological treatments of neuropathic pain: an update and effect related to mechanisms of drug action. *Pain* 1999;83:389–400. Search date not stated but trials included up to 1999; primary sources not stated.
13. McQuay H, Carroll D, Jadad AR, Wiffen P, Moore A. Anticonvulsant drugs for management of pain: a systematic review. *BMJ* 1995;311:1047–1052. Search date 1994; primary sources Medline, and handsearch of 40 medical journals and reference lists, and authors of published reports.
14. Campbell FG, Graham JG, Zilkha KJ. Clinical trial of carbazepine (tegretol) in trigeminal neuralgia. *J Neurol Neurosurg Psychiatry* 1966;29:265–267.
15. Taylor JC, Brauer S, Espir MLE. Long-term treatment of trigeminal neuralgia with carbamazepine. *Postgrad Med J* 1981;57:16–18.
16. Lindstrom P, Lindblom V. The analgesic effect of tocainide in trigeminal neuralgia. *Pain* 1987;28:45–50.
17. Zakrzewska JM, Chaudhry Z, Patton DW, Mullens EL. Lamotrigine in refractory trigeminal neuralgia: results from a double-blind placebo controlled crossover study. *Pain* 1997;73:223–230.
18. Fromm GH, Terrence CF, Chattha AS. Baclofen in the treatment of trigeminal neuralgia: double-blind study and long-term follow-up. *Ann Neurol* 1984;15:240–244.
19. Fromm GH, Terrence CF. Comparison of L-baclofen and racemic baclofen in trigeminal neuralgia. *Neurology* 1987;37:1725–1728.
20. Kondziolka D, Lemley T, Kestle JR, et al. The effect of single-application topical ophthalmic anesthesia in patients with trigeminal neuralgia. A randomized double-blind placebo-controlled trial. *J Neurosurg* 1994;80:993–997.
21. Wooten JM, Earnest J, Reyes J. Review of common adverse effects of selected antiarrhythmic drugs. *Crit Care Nurs Q* 2000;22:23–38.
22. Gilron I, Booher SL, Rowan JS, Max MB. Topiramate in trigeminal neuralgia: a randomized, placebo-controlled multiple crossover pilot study. *Clin Neuropharmacol* 2001;24:109–112

23. Stajcic Z, Juniper RP, Todorovic L. Peripheral streptomycin/lidocaine injections versus lidocaine alone in the treatment of idiopathic trigeminal neuralgia. A double blind controlled trial. *J Craniomaxillofac Surg* 1990;18:243–246.
24. Bittar GT, Graff-Radford SB: The effects of streptomycin/lidocaine block on trigeminal neuralgia: a double blind crossover placebo controlled study. *Headache* 1993;33:155–160.
25. Walker JB, Akhanjee LK, Cooney MM, et al. Laser therapy for pain of trigeminal neuralgia. *Clin J Pain* 1988;3:183–187.
26. Killian JM, Fromm GH. Carbamazepine in the treatment of neuralgia. Use of side effects. *Arch Neurol* 1968;19:129–136.
27. Nicol CF. A four year double blind study of tegretol in facial pain. *Headache* 1969;9:54–57.
28. Vilming ST, Lyberg T, Latase X. Tizanidine in the management of trigeminal neuralgia. *Cephalalgia* 1986;6:181–182.
29. Lechin F, van der Dijs B, Lechin ME, et al. Pimozide therapy for trigeminal neuralgia. *Arch Neurol* 1989;46:960–963.

Joanna M Zakrzewska
Barts and the London Queen Mary's School of Medicine and Dentistry
London
UK

Competing interests: The author has been reimbursed by Glaxo Wellcome (manufacturer of lamotrigine) for attending a conference and for conducting the lamotrigine RCT.

TABLE 1 RCTs of drugs used in the management of trigeminal neuralgia (See text, p 1388).

Ref	Interventions (daily dosage)*		Duration	Design	Diagnostic criteria	Number of people randomised (analysed)	NNT (95% CI)	NNH (95% CI)
	Active arm	Comparison						
14	Carbamazepine (400–800 mg)	Placebo	8 weeks	Crossover	NA	77 (70)	2.8 (2.3 to 3.7)	4.3 (2.6 to 11.7)
26	Carbamazepine (400 mg–1 g)	Placebo	2 weeks to 36 months	Crossover	NA	30 (27)	1.4 (1.14 to 1.88)	1.6 (1.3 to 2.1)
27	Carbamazepine (100 mg–2.4 g)	Placebo	46 months	Partial crossover	NA	54 (44)	NS	3.7 (2.4 to 7.9)
28	Tizanidine (900 mg)	Carbamazepine	3 weeks	Parallel	NA	12 (11)	NS	–
29	Pimozide (4–12 mg)	Carbamazepine (300 mg–1.2 g)	24 weeks	Crossover	NA	48 (48)	2 (2 to 3)	2.9 (2 to 4)
17	Lamotrigine† (400 mg)	Placebo	4 weeks	Crossover	IHS	14 (14)	2.1 (1.3 to 6.1)	NS
18	Baclofen‡ (40–80 mg)	Placebo	2 weeks	Crossover	IHS	10 (10)	1.4 (1 to 2.6)	NS
19	L-Baclofen (6–12 mg)	Racemic baclofen (60 mg)	2 weeks	Crossover	IHS	15 (15)	2 (1 to 4)	2 (1 to 4)
20	Proparacaine (0.5% for 20 min)	Placebo	30 days	Parallel	IHS	47 (47)	NS	–
24	Tocainide	Carbamazepine	2 weeks	Crossover	NA	12 (12)	NS	NS

*All daily doses were given as divided doses; †added to pre-existing treatment; ‡used as add on to other anticonvulsant in 4 of 10 people.
Ref, reference; NA, not available; NS, non-significant; IHS, International Headache Society criteria.

Aphthous ulcers: recurrent

Search date April 2002

Stephen Porter and Crispian Scully

QUESTIONS

INTERVENTIONS

Key Messages

- **Chlorhexidine (but no effect on recurrence rates)** RCTs found that chlorhexidine gluconate mouth rinses versus control preparations increased the number of ulcer free days and reduced the severity of each episode of ulceration, but did not affect the incidence of recurrent ulceration.
- **Hexitidine** One RCT found no significant difference in the incidence or duration of ulceration with hexitidine mouthwash versus a control mouthwash.
- **Topical corticosteroids** Nine small RCTs found no consistent difference in the incidence of new ulcers with topical corticosteroids versus control preparations. They found weak evidence that topical corticosteroids may reduce the duration of ulcers and hasten pain relief.

Aphthous ulcers: recurrent

DEFINITION Recurrent aphthous ulcers are superficial and rounded, with painful mouth ulcers usually occurring in recurrent bouts at intervals of a few days to a few months.[1]

INCIDENCE/ PREVALENCE The point prevalence of recurrent aphthous ulcers in Swedish adults has been reported as 2%.[1] Prevalence may be 5–10% in some groups of children. Up to 66% of young adults give a history consistent with recurrent aphthous ulceration.[1]

AETIOLOGY/ RISK FACTORS The causes of aphthous ulcers remain unknown. Associations with haematinic deficiency, infections, gluten sensitive enteropathy, food sensitivities, and psychological stress have rarely been confirmed. Similar ulcers are seen in Behçet's syndrome.

PROGNOSIS About 80% of people with recurrent aphthous ulcers develop a few ulcers smaller than 1 cm in diameter that heal within 5–14 days without scarring (the pattern known as minor aphthous ulceration). The episodes recur typically after an interval of 1–4 months. One in 10 sufferers has a more severe form (major aphthous ulceration), with lesions larger than 1 cm that may recur after a shorter interval and can cause scarring. Likewise, 1/10 people with such recurrent ulceration may have multiple minute ulcers (herpetiform ulceration).

AIMS To reduce pain, frequency, and duration of ulceration with minimal adverse effects.

OUTCOMES Number of new ulcers appearing within a specified period, usually 4–8 weeks; ulcer day index (the sum of the number of ulcers each day over a period, usually 4–8 wks, which indicates the severity of the episode and reflects the mean prevalence and duration of ulcers); symptom score based on subjective pain severity recorded in categories on a questionnaire (e.g. from 0–3, ranging from no pain to severe pain) or on a 10 cm visual analogue scale; mean duration of individual ulcers (difficult to determine because of uncertainty in detecting the point of complete resolution); number of ulcer free days during a specified period; preference of people for one treatment over another. The diameter of lesions is a proxy measure of these clinical outcomes.

METHODS *Clinical Evidence* update search and appraisal April 2002.

QUESTION What are the effects of treatments for recurrent aphthous ulcers?

OPTION TOPICAL CORTICOSTEROIDS

Nine small RCTs found no consistent effect of topical corticosteroids on the incidence of new ulcers compared with control preparations. They found weak evidence that topical corticosteroids may reduce the duration of ulcers and hasten pain relief without causing notable local or systemic adverse effects.

Benefits: We found no systematic review, but found nine RCTs of corticosteroids versus placebo that reported relevant clinical outcomes in the management of recurrent aphthous ulcers.[2–9] Overall, one RCT found larger effect sizes than the others.[2] **Incidence of new ulcers:** Five randomised crossover RCTs (102 people) found inconsistent effects on the incidence of new ulcers (see table 1, p 1402).[2,4,5] **Ulcer duration:** Six RCTs reported data on ulcer duration, but the data were not in comparable forms.[3,4,6–9] Four RCTs reported the mean duration of ulcers: no consistent effect was seen (see table 1, p 1402).[3,4,7,9] One RCT found topical steroids versus control reduced mean ulcer duration below 6 days (ulcer duration ≤ 6 days, AR 25/33 [76%] people receiving topical steroid *v* 14/30 [47%] with control preparations; ARI 29%, 95% CI 5% to 43%; RR 1.62, 95% CI 1.06 to 2.49; NNT 3, 95% CI 2 to 20).[6] One crossover RCT found that 13/15 people had shorter mean duration with topical steroid versus the control preparation.[8] **Ulcer days index:** Four RCTs found that topical steroids reduced the number of ulcer days compared with control;[2,4,5,7] the reduction was significant in two of the RCTs (see table 1, p 1402). **Symptom scores:** Four RCTs reported symptom scores with topical steroids versus control, but all presented their results in different ways.[6–9] The first RCT found that more people using steroids versus a control preparation had symptom relief (29/33 [88%] *v* 18/30 [60%]; ARI 27%, 95% CI 5% to 43%; RRI 46%, 95% CI 19% to 91%; NNT 4, 95% CI 2 to 20).[6] The second RCT (a crossover trial) found that topical steroids versus a control preparation reduced symptom scores but the results were not significant (2.77 *v* 3.54).[7] Another crossover trial found that 11/15 people using topical steroid versus the control preparation had lower pain scores.[8] A third crossover trial found that the pain score fell with time whether using topical steroids or control applications, but that the rate of fall was significantly faster when using topical steroids.[9] **User preference:** Two crossover trials found that more users preferred topical steroids than control preparations (20/26 [77%] in one study[4] and 10/17 [59%] in the other[6]).

Harms: All nine RCTs reported no serious adverse effects. Long term use of corticosteroid mouth rinses was occasionally associated with oral candidiasis (rate not specified). Limited studies of adrenal function found no evidence that 0.05% fluocinonide in adhesive paste and betamethasone-17-valerate mouth rinse caused adrenal suppression.[8,15] One RCT reported adrenal suppression in one man using betamethasone disodium phosphate.[5]

Comment: The trials differed in many ways: selection of people, type of topical corticosteroid and formulation used, control preparation used (although this was usually a base without topical steroid), duration of treatment, reported outcomes, and design (double or single blind, parallel group or crossover, use of washout period or not). Withdrawal rates were high. Most people in the trials had more severe ulceration than the average person with recurrent aphthous ulceration.

OPTION CHLORHEXIDINE AND SIMILAR AGENTS

RCTs found that chlorhexidine gluconate mouth rinses increased the number of ulcer free days and reduced the severity of each episode of ulceration, but did not effect the incidence of recurrent ulceration. Single RCTs found no significant benefit from hexitidine mouthwash or a proprietary antibacterial mouthwash compared with control mouthwashes.

Benefits: We found no systematic review but found five RCTs (203 people with recurrent aphthous ulceration) of chlorhexidine gluconate or similar preparations versus assumed inactive control preparations.[10–14] Four of the RCTs used a crossover design with a randomised sequence comparing a control preparation versus 1% chlorhexidine gel,[10] 0.2% chlorhexidine gel,[11] 0.2% chlorhexidine mouthwash,[12] or 0.1% hexetidine mouthwash.[13] One trial was a parallel group RCT of a proprietary antibacterial rinse versus a hydroalcoholic control.[14] **Incidence of ulceration:** All RCTs reported the number of ulcers as either the total number of ulcers or the number of new ulcers with each treatment (see table 1, p 1402). Only one of the five RCTs found that active treatment significantly reduced the number of ulcers.[11] Three RCTs found that the number of ulcers fell during the course of the study, irrespective of the treatment received.[12–14] The crossover trial that found a significant difference in numbers of ulcers did not overtly account for this effect.[11] However, data were available from only 12/26 people who were recruited, and it is not clear if there was a balanced sequencing of active and placebo treatments among these people. **Duration of ulceration:** The mean duration of individual ulcers was reported in four of the RCTs (see table 1, p 1402).[10,12–14] The mean duration of individual ulcers was reduced by active treatment in all four RCTs, but the difference was significant in only one RCT and the mean difference was less than 1 day in the others. **Ulcer days index:** Three RCTs reported the ulcer days index. Both studies of chlorhexidine versus control found significant reduction in the ulcer day index.[11,12] One of these RCTs found that chlorhexidine versus an inert preparation significantly increased the number of ulcer free days from a mean of 17.5 to 22.9 over 6 weeks — an extra 5.4 ulcer free days per 6 weeks of treatment.[12] Another RCT found that hexitidine had no significant effect.[13] **Severity of pain:** All five RCTs reported severity scores.[10–14] Two RCTs found that chlorhexidine significantly reduced the mean severity of pain compared with an inert preparation.[10] One RCT of a proprietary antibacterial mouthwash versus the alcohol-containing control preparation found no significant difference between the treatment groups, but found a large improvement in clinical outcomes in both groups compared with baseline levels.[14] The evidence relating to other antibacterial agents such as triclosan will be reviewed in future *Clinical Evidence* updates.

Harms: The RCTs reported few adverse events. One RCT found that chlorhexidine had a bitter taste and was associated with brown staining of teeth and tongue and with nausea.[11]

Comment: Four of the RCTs used a crossover design. A consistent observation was that outcomes improved during the course of the trials irrespective of the treatment received. One of the studies did not make clear if the effect of sequencing had been allowed for.[11] The withdrawal rates in the crossover trials were high. The parallel group trial had fewer withdrawals: 106 people with recurrent aphthous ulceration were recruited and 96 completed the study. Analysis was not by intention to treat and the method of randomisation was not specified.[14] People recruited to the trials might not be typical of the average person with recurrent aphthous ulceration.

REFERENCES

1. Porter SR, Scully C, Pedersen A. Recurrent aphthous stomatitis. *Crit Rev Oral Biol Med* 1998;9:306–321.
2. Cooke BED, Armitage P. Recurrent Mikulicz's aphthae treatment with topical hydrocortisone hemisuccinate sodium. *BMJ* 1960;1:764–766.
3. Walter T, McFall JR. Effect of flurandrenolone on oral aphthae. *J Periodontol* 1968;39:364–365.
4. Browne RM, Fox EC, Anderson RJ. Topical triamcinolone acetonide in recurrent aphthous stomatitis. *Lancet* 1968;1:565–567.
5. MacPhee IT, Sircus W, Farmer ED, et al. Use of steroids in treatment of aphthous ulceration. *BMJ* 1968;2:147–149.
6. Merchant HW, Gangarosa LP, Glassman AB, et al. Betamethasone-17-benzoate in the treatment of recurrent aphthous ulcers. *Oral Surg Oral Med Oral Pathol* 1978;45:870–875.
7. Pimlott SJ, Walker DM. A controlled clinical trial of the efficacy of topically applied fluocinonide in the treatment of recurrent aphthous ulceration. *Br Dent J* 1983;154:174–177.
8. Thompson AC, Nolan A, Lamey P-J. Minor aphthous oral ulceration: a double-blind cross-over study of beclomethasone diproprionate aerosol spray. *Scot Med J* 1989;34:531–532.
9. Miles DA, Bricker SL, Razmus TF, et al. Triamcinolone acetonide versus chlorhexidine for treatment of recurrent stomatitis. *Oral Surg Oral Med Oral Pathol* 1993;75:397–402.
10. Addy M, Carpenter R, Roberts WR. Management of recurrent aphthous ulceration – a trial of chlorhexidine gluconate gel. *Br Dent J* 1976;141:118–120.
11. Addy M. Hibitane in the treatment of recurrent aphthous ulceration. *J Clin Periodontol* 1977;4:108–116.
12. Hunter L, Addy M. Chlorhexidine gluconate mouthwash in the management of minor aphthous stomatitis. *Br Dent J* 1987;162:106–110.
13. Chadwick B, Addy M, Walker DM. Hexetidine mouthrinse in the management of minor aphthous ulceration and as an adjunct to oral hygiene. *Br Dent J* 1991;171:83–87.
14. Meiller TF, Kutcher MJ, Overholser CD, et al. Effect of an antimicrobial mouthrinse on recurrent aphthous ulcerations. *Oral Surg Oral Med Oral Pathol* 1991;72:425–429.
15. Lehner T, Lyne C. Adrenal function during topical oral corticosteroid treatment. *BMJ* 1969;4:138–141.

Stephen Porter
Professor of Oral Medicine

Crispian Scully
Dean and Professor of Special Needs Dentistry

Eastman Dental Institute for Oral Health Care Sciences
UCL
University of London
London
UK

Competing interests: None declared.

TABLE 1 Effects of treatments on different outcomes: results of RCTs (see text, p 1398).

Intervention	Ref	Participants	Treatment duration (wks)	Outcomes: Treatment	Outcomes: Control	Effect (%)* (significance)
Incidence new ulcers (ulcers/wk): topical corticosteroids versus inert preparations	2	17	8	0.51	1.15	–55% (P < 0.05)
	4	26	8	0.84	0.94	–11% (NS)
	5 pilot	8	4	2.07	1.85	+12% (NS)
	5 main	31†	4	0.73	0.82	–11% (NS)
	5	20	6	1.27	1.92	+6% (NS)
Mean ulcer duration (days):	3	50	Until complete healing	6.00	6.00	0% (NS)
topical corticosteroids versus inert preparations	4	26	8	8.07	8.94	–10% (NS)
	7	20	6	4.93	7.83	–37% (P < 0.001)
	9	19	12	5.93	5.92	0% (NS)
Ulcer days index: topical corticosteroids versus inert preparations	2	17	8	26.30	65.90	–60% (P < 0.01)
	4	26	8	58.30	71.30	–18% (NS)
	5 main	25	4	24.00	30.70	–22% (NS)
	7	20	6	48.30	70.60	–32% (P < 0.05)
Number of ulcers (ulcers/person/wk): topical antibacterial versus presumed inert preparations	10	20	5	1.04	1.40	NS
	11	12	5	0.60	1.02	P < 0.05
	12	38	6	1.26	1.38	NS
	13	37	6	1.48	1.39	NS
	14	96	26	0.09	0.13	NS

Mean duration of ulcers (days): topical antibacterial versus inert preparation	10	20	5	4.80	7.80	$P < 0.01$
	12	38	6	5.02	5.78	NS
	13	37	6	6.64	6.80	NS
	14	96	26	Median fall in ulcer duration from start of trial 2.42 days	Median fall in ulcer duration from start of trial 1.58 days	NS
Ulcer days index: topical antibacterial versus inert preparations	11	12	5	9.50	17.00	$P < 0.05$
	12	38	6	42.80	52.30	$P < 0.05$
	13	37	6	79.70	65.70	NS

*Defined as difference between outcome measures for control and treatment, expressed as a fraction of the control.
†Each participant received one treatment for 4 weeks, a blank month, then another treatment with another drug. The trial compared an inert base, two local steroids and two other preparations. The figures given here are those during treatment with local steroids and with the inert base. NS, not significant; ref, reference.

Burning mouth syndrome

Search date February 2002

John Buchanan and Joanna Zakrzewska

QUESTIONS

INTERVENTIONS

Key Messages

- **Cognitive behavioural therapy** One small RCT found that cognitive behavioural therapy in people with resistent burning mouth syndrome versus no cognitive behavioural therapy significantly reduced symptom intensity after 6 months.
- **Antidepressants; benzydamine hydrochloride; dietary supplementation; hormone replacement therapy in postmenopausal women** We found insufficient evidence on the effects of these interventions.

DEFINITION Burning mouth syndrome is a psychogenic or idiopathic burning discomfort or pain affecting people with clinically normal oral mucosa in whom a medical or dental cause has been excluded.[1–3] Terms previously used to describe what is now called burning mouth syndrome include glossodynia, glossopyrosis, stomatodynia, stomatopyrosis, sore tongue, and oral dysaesthesia.[4] A survey of 669 men and 758 women randomly selected from 48 500 people aged between 20 and 69 years found that people with burning mouth also have subjective dryness (66%), take some form of medication (64%), report other systemic illnesses (57%), and have altered taste (11%).[5] Many studies of people with symptoms of burning mouth do not distinguish those with burning mouth syndrome (i.e. idiopathic disease) from those with other conditions (such as vitamin B deficiency), making results unreliable.

INCIDENCE/ PREVALENCE Burning mouth syndrome mainly affects women,[6–8] particularly after the menopause when its prevalence may be 18–33%.[9] One recent study in Sweden found a prevalence of 4% for the symptom of burning mouth without clinical abnormality of the oral mucosa (11/669 [2%] men, mean age 59 years; 42/758 [6%] women, mean age 57 years), with the highest prevalence (12%) in women aged 60–69 years.[5] Reported prevalence in general populations varies from 1%[10] to 15%.[6] Incidence and prevalence vary according to diagnostic criteria,[4] and many studies included people with the symptom of burning mouth rather than with burning mouth syndrome as defined above.

AETIOLOGY/ RISK FACTORS The cause is unknown, and we found no good aetiological studies. Hormonal disturbances associated with the menopause[7–9] and psychogenic factors (including anxiety, depression, stress, life events, personality disorders, and phobia of cancer) are possible causal factors.[11–13] Local and systemic factors (such as infections, allergies, ill fitting dentures,[12] hypersensitivity reactions,[14] and hormone and vitamin deficiencies[15–17]) may cause the symptom of burning mouth and should be excluded before diagnosing burning mouth syndrome.

PROGNOSIS We found no prospective cohort studies or other reliable evidence describing the natural history of burning mouth syndrome.[18] We found anecdotal reports of at least partial spontaneous remission in about half of people with burning mouth syndrome within 6–7 years.[12]

AIMS To alleviate symptoms, with minimal adverse effects.

OUTCOMES Self reported relief of symptoms (burning mouth, altered taste, dry mouth); incidence and severity of anxiety and depression; quality of life using a validated ordinal scale.

METHODS *Clinical Evidence* search and appraisal February 2002 (keywords: burning mouth, burning mouth syndrome, dysaesthesia or dysesthesia, stomatodynia or glossopyrosis, sore tongue, glossodynia or glossalgia).

QUESTION What are the effects of treatments?

OPTION COGNITIVE BEHAVIOURAL THERAPY

One small RCT found that cognitive behavioural therapy relieved symptoms of burning mouth syndrome.

Benefits: We found one systematic review (search date 2000, 5 RCTs, 1 CCT, 384 people).[19] The review identified one small RCT (30 people with resistant burning mouth syndrome), which compared cognitive behavioural therapy (12–15 sessions of 1 h/wk) versus a control group who received similar attention but without the cognitive therapy sessions. It found that cognitive therapy significantly reduced the intensity of symptoms (measured on a visual analogue scale ranging from 1 = endurable to 7 = unendurable), and was still significant at 6 months' follow up (mean pretreatment score 5.0 *v* 4.3 on placebo; mean score 6 months after treatment 1.4 *v* 4.7 on placebo; $P < 0.001$; 4/15 *v* 0/15 people symptom free 6 months after treatment).[19]

Harms: The RCT provided no information on adverse effects.[19]

Comment: The trial was small and individual characteristics of the two groups were not described; therefore, the groups may not have been comparable. The visual analogue scale for assessing oral burning was not validated.[19]

OPTION HORMONE REPLACEMENT THERAPY IN POSTMENOPAUSAL WOMEN

We found insufficient evidence on the effects of hormone replacement therapy in postmenopausal women with burning mouth syndrome.

Benefits: We found one systematic review (search date 2000, 5 RCTs, 1 CCT, 384 people), which identified no RCTs of sufficient quality.[19]

Harms: Adverse effects of hormone replacement therapy are well documented (see oestrogens under menopausal symptoms, p 000).

Comment: We found three non-randomised intervention studies with no clear diagnostic criteria or outcome measures.[20–22]

OPTION DIETARY SUPPLEMENTS

We found no reliable evidence about the effects of dietary supplementation in people with burning mouth syndrome.

Benefits: We found one systematic review (search date 2000, 5 RCTs, 1 CCT, 384 people).[19] The review identified one RCT (42 people with burning mouth syndrome) comparing alphalipoic acid (600 mg daily for 20 days followed by 200 mg daily for 10 days) versus placebo (cellulose starch 100 mg daily for 30 days). It found that alphalipoic acid significantly increased the number of people reported to have "slight" or "decided" improvement in symptoms (AR 16/21 [76%] *v* 3/14 [14%]; RR 0.28, 95% CI 0.13 to 0.61; NNT 2, 95% CI 1 to 3).[19] We found no RCTs in people with vitamin B deficiency and symptoms of burning mouth (see comment below).

Harms: The RCT did not report adverse effects.[19]

Comment: The RCT of alphalipoic acid was unblinded, and the subjective nature of the outcome used means that the results should be interpreted with caution. People with vitamin B group deficiencies and symptoms of burning mouth should no longer be classified as having burning mouth syndrome (see definition, p 1405). One case control study in 70 people found that people with symptoms of burning mouth were more likely to have vitamin B deficiency (28/70 *v* 6/80).[16] One study of 16 people with vitamin deficiencies given vitamins or placebo found no improvement in symptoms.[17]

OPTION ANTIDEPRESSANTS

We found insufficient evidence on the effects of antidepressants in people with burning mouth syndrome.

Benefits: We found one systematic review (search date 2000, 5 RCTs, 1 CCT, 384 people).[19] **Clomipramine and mianserin:** The review identified one short term RCT (253 people with chronic idiopathic pain syndrome, including 77 people with burning mouth syndrome) comparing clomipramine versus mianserin versus placebo for 6 weeks.[19] After 6 weeks there was no significant improvement in any group. **Trazodone:** The review identified one double blind RCT (37 women with burning mouth syndrome) comparing trazodone (200 mg/day) versus placebo.[19] After 8 weeks there was no significant difference in pain or related symptoms between groups measured on a visual analogue scale (0 mm = best score and 100 mm = worst score). The mean pain on a visual analogue scale decreased in both groups at 8 weeks (from 59 to 45 with trazodone and from 47 to 34 with placebo).

Harms: The first RCT did not report adverse effects.[19] In the second RCT, adverse effects caused 7/18 people taking trazodone to withdraw from the trial compared with 2/19 taking placebo. Adverse effects reported with trazodone were dizziness (11 people) and drowsiness (9 people).[19] Adverse effects of clomipramine, mianserin, and other antidepressants are documented elsewhere (see depressive disorders, p 951).

Comment: The trial of clomipramine and mianserin versus placebo was too small to exclude an effect of treatment, did not use adequate diagnostic criteria, was of short duration, and had limited follow up;[19] therefore, it does not provide sufficient evidence to determine the role of antidepressants in treating burning mouth syndrome. Although the trial of trazodone versus placebo was well conducted and used several pertinent outcome measures, including psychological ones, it was too small and brief to detect clinically important effects.[19] The widespread use of antidepressants in burning mouth syndrome may be because of their effects on neuropathic pain,[23] and the association of burning mouth syndrome with generalised anxiety disorder, depression, and adverse life events.[24]

OPTION BENZYDAMINE HYDROCHLORIDE

We found insufficient evidence on the effects of benzydamine hydrochloride in burning mouth syndrome.

Benefits: We found one systematic review (search date 2000, 5 RCTs, 1 CCT, 384 people),[19] which identified one small RCT (30 people with burning mouth syndrome) comparing benzydamine hydrochloride (15 mL of 0.15% for 1 min 3 times daily for 4 wks) versus placebo versus no treatment. It found no significant difference among groups for symptoms (using a visual analogue scale), but the trial was too small to exclude a clinically important difference.[19]

Harms: No adverse effects were reported.

Comment: Inclusion criteria were well defined. The trial was incompletely blinded because the third group received no treatment.

REFERENCES

1. Fox H. Burning tongue glossodynia. *N Y State J Med* 1935;35:881–884.
2. Zakrzewska JM. The burning mouth syndrome remains an enigma. *Pain* 1995;62:253–257.
3. Van der Waal I. *The burning mouth syndrome.* 1st ed. Copenhagen: Munksgaard, 1990.
4. Merksey H, Bogduk N, eds. *Classification of chronic pain.* 2nd ed. Seattle: International Association for the Study of Pain Press, 1994.
5. Bergdahl M, Bergdahl J. Burning mouth syndrome: prevalence and associated factors. *J Oral Pathol Med* 1999;28:350–354.
6. Tammiala-Salonen T, Hiidenkarii T, Parvinen T. Burning mouth in a Finnish adult population. *Community Dent Oral Epidemiol* 1993;21:67–71.
7. Basker RM, Sturdee DW, Davenport JC. Patients with burning mouths. A clinical investigation of causative factors, including the climacteric and diabetes. *Br Dent J* 1978;145:9–16.
8. Grushka M. Clinical features of burning mouth syndrome. *Oral Surg Oral Med Oral Pathol Oral Radiol Endod* 1987;63:30–36.
9. Wardrop RW, Hailes J, Burger H, Reade PC. Oral discomfort at the menopause. *Oral Surg Oral Med Oral Pathol Oral Radiol Endod* 1989;67:535–540.
10. Lipton JA, Ship JA, Larach-Robinson D. Estimated prevalence and distribution of reported orofacial pain in the United States. *J Am Dent Assoc* 1993;124:115–121.
11. Rojo L, Silvestre FJ, Bagan JV, De Vicente T. Psychiatric morbidity in burning mouth syndrome. Psychiatric interview versus depression and anxiety scales. *Oral Surg Oral Med Oral Pathol Oral Radiol Endod* 1993;75:308–311.
12. Grushka M, Sessle BJ. Burning mouth syndrome. *Dent Clin North Am* 1991;35:171–184.
13. Lamey PJ, Lamb AB. The usefulness of the HAD scale in assessing anxiety in patients with burning mouth syndrome. *Oral Surg Oral Med Oral Pathol Oral Radiol Endod* 1989;67:390–392.
14. Bergdahl J, Anneroth G, Anneroth I. Clinical study of patients with burning mouth. *Scand J Dent Res* 1994;102:299–305.
15. Maragou P, Ivanyi L. Serum zinc levels in patients with burning mouth syndrome. *Oral Surg Oral Med Oral Pathol Oral Radiol Endod* 1991;71:447–450.
16. Lamey PJ, Allam BF. Vitamin status of patients with burning mouth syndrome and the response to replacement therapy. *Br Dent J* 1986;168:81–84.
17. Hugoson A, Thorstensson B. Vitamin B status and response to replacement therapy in patients with burning mouth syndrome. *Acta Odontol Scand* 1991;49:367–375.
18. Zakrzewska JM, Hamlyn PJ. Facial pain. In: Crombie IK, Croft PR, Linton SJ, Le Resche L, Von Korff M, eds. *Epidemiology of pain.* Seattle: International Association for the Study of Pain Press, 1999:177–202.
19. Zakrewska JM, Glenny AM, Forsell H. Interventions for the treatment of burning mouth syndrome (Cochrane Review). In: The Cochrane Library, Issue 3, 2001. Oxford: Update Software. Search date 2000; primary sources Medline, Embase, The Cochrane Library, The Cochrane Oral Health Group's Specialised Register, and *Clinical Evidence* Issue 3.
20. Pisanty S, Rafaely B, Polshuk WZ. The effects of steroid hormones on buccal mucosa of menopausal women. *Oral Surg Oral Med Oral Pathol Oral Radiol Endod* 1975;40:346–353.
21. Ferguson MM, Boyle P, Hart D McK, Lindsay R. Oral complaints related to climacteric symptoms in oophorectomized women. *J R Soc Med* 1981;74:492–497.
22. Forabosco A, Crisculo M, Coukos G, et al. Efficacy of hormone replacement therapy in postmenopausal women with oral discomfort. *Oral Surg Oral Med Oral Pathol Oral Radiol Endod* 1992;73:570–574.
23. McQuay HJ, Tramer M, Nye BA, Carroll D, Wiffen PJ, Moore RA. A systematic review of antidepressants in neuropathic pain. *Pain* 1996;68:217–227.
24. Bogetto F, Maina G, Ferro G, Carbone M, Gandolfo S. Psychiatric comorbidity in patients with burning mouth syndrome. *Psychosom Med* 1998;60:378–385.

John Buchanan
Clinical Lecturer in Oral Medicine

Joanna Zakrzewska
Senior Lecturer/Honorary Consultant in Oral Medicine
St Bartholomew's and The Royal London School of Medicine and Dentistry
London, UK

Competing interests: None declared.

Impacted wisdom teeth

Search date June 2002

Stephen Worrall

QUESTIONS

INTERVENTIONS

Likely to be ineffective or harmful

To be covered in future updates

Extraction of symptomatic impacted wisdom teeth

Key Messages

- **Extraction of asymptomatic impacted wisdom teeth** We found limited evidence that the harms of removing asymptomatic impacted wisdom teeth outweigh the benefits.

DEFINITION	Wisdom teeth are third molars that develop in almost all adults by about the age of 20 years. In some people, the teeth become partially or completely impacted below the gumline because of lack of space, obstruction, or abnormal position. Impacted wisdom teeth may be diagnosed because of pain and swelling or incidentally by routine dental radiography.
INCIDENCE/ PREVALENCE	Third molar impaction is common. Over 72% of Swedish people aged 20–30 years have at least one impacted lower third molar.[1] The surgical removal of impacted third molars (symptomatic and asymptomatic) is the most common procedure performed by oral and maxillofacial surgeons. It is performed on about 4/1000 people per year in England and Wales, making it one of the top 10 inpatient and day case procedures.[2–4] Up to 90% of people on oral and maxillofacial surgery hospital waiting lists are awaiting removal of wisdom teeth.[3]
AETIOLOGY/ RISK FACTORS	Impacted wisdom teeth are partly a by-product of improved oral hygiene and changes in diet. Less gum disease and dental caries, and less wear and tear on teeth because of a more refined diet, have increased the likelihood of retaining teeth into adult life, leaving less room for wisdom teeth.
PROGNOSIS	Impacted wisdom teeth can cause pain, swelling, and infection, as well as destroying adjacent teeth and bone. The removal of diseased and symptomatic wisdom teeth alleviates pain and suffering and improves oral health and function. We found no good evidence on what happens without treatment in people with asymptomatic impacted wisdom teeth.
AIMS	To prevent harms and maximise benefits of wisdom teeth removal.
OUTCOMES	Pain; rates of infection; oral health and function.
METHODS	*Clinical Evidence* update search and appraisal June 2002.

QUESTION Should asymptomatic and disease-free impacted wisdom teeth be removed prophylactically?

One systematic review of two RCTs, one of which is still in progress, comparing prophylactic extraction of wisdom teeth versus no extraction found no evidence of benefit with prophylactic extraction. Removal of lower wisdom teeth causes permanent numbness of the lower lip or tongue in about 1/200 people. One systematic review of mainly observational studies found that the use of a lingual nerve retractor significantly increased the incidence of temporary lingual nerve damage, but that permanent damage was rare.

Benefits: We found one systematic review evaluating people with unerupted or impacted third molars (search date 1999, 2 RCTs, 34 reviews).[5] It addressed both clinical preventative and cost effectiveness issues. The first RCT in the review (164 people) investigated the effects of early third molar extraction on late crowding of the lower incisors and randomised people to extraction or to no extraction of third molars.[6] It found no clinically significant difference between the groups. However, the RCT had a low follow up rate (77 people [47%] at an average of 66 months). The second RCT in the review is still in progress, but preliminary results also suggest that no extraction could be the better option in terms of benefits such as functional health status and harms. However, more participants and longer follow up times are needed to establish this preliminary conclusion.

Harms: Pain and swelling are almost universal after removal of impacted wisdom teeth.[7,8] The removal of the lower wisdom teeth carries the risk of damage to the inferior alveolar nerve (injured in 1–8% of people[9,10] with permanent damage in up to 1% of people[11]) and to the lingual nerve (permanently injured in up to 1% of people).[12] The risks appear to be greater with greater depth of impaction. The risks are the same whether the wisdom tooth is symptomatic or asymptomatic. One systematic review (search date 1999, 7 prospective case series, 1 RCT) evaluated the effects of three different surgical techniques on the lingual nerve: buccal approach with lingual nerve retraction (3040 procedures), buccal approach without lingual nerve retraction (1336 procedures), and the lingual split technique with lingual nerve retraction (2077 procedures).[13] It found that, compared to the buccal approach without retraction, temporary lingual nerve injury (lasting < 6 months) was significantly more common with the buccal approach with lingual retraction (RR 8.8, 95% CI 4.3 to 17.8) and the lingual split technique with retraction (RR 13.3, 95% CI 6.6 to 26.9). Permanent lingual nerve injury (lasting > 6 months) occurred in 0.2% of people after the buccal approach without retraction versus 0.6% with the buccal approach with retraction versus 0.1% with lingual split with retraction. The significance of any difference between groups was not calculated because of the low event rates.[13]

Comment: The two RCTs identified by the systematic review were of poor quality. Surgical morbidity is operator and technique sensitive; estimates of the incidence of nerve damage vary widely between reports.[14,15]

REFERENCES

1. Hugoson A, Kugelberg CF. The prevalence of third molars in a Swedish population. An epidemiological study. *Community Dent Health* 1988;5:121–138.
2. Mercier P, Precious D. Risks and benefits of removal of impacted third molars. *Int J Oral Maxillofac Surg* 1992;21:17–27.
3. Shepherd JP, Brickley M. Surgical removal of third molars. *BMJ* 1994;309:620–621.
4. Worrall SF, Riden K, Corrigan AM. UK National Third Molar project: the initial report. *Br J Oral Maxillofac Surg* 1998;36:14–18.
5. Song F, O'Meara S, Wilson P, et al. The effectiveness and cost-effectiveness of prophylactic removal of wisdom teeth. *Health Technol Assess* 2000;4:15. Search date 1999; primary sources Medline, Embase, Science Citation Index, Cochrane Controlled Trials Register, National Research Register, Database of Reviews of Effectiveness, hand searches of paper sources, web-based resources, and contact with relevant organisations and professional bodies.
6. Harradine N, Pearson M, Toth B. The effect of extraction of third molars on late lower incisor crowding: a randomised controlled trial. *Br J Orthodont* 1998;25:117–122.
7. Bramley P. Sense about wisdoms? *J R Soc Med* 1981;74:867–868.
8. Capuzzi P, Montebugnoli L, Vaccaro MA. Extraction of impacted third molars. *Oral Surg Oral Med Oral Pathol Oral Radiol Endod* 1994;77:341–343.
9. Schultze-Mosgau S, Reich RH. Assessment of inferior alveolar and lingual nerve disturbances after dentoalveolar surgery, and recovery of sensitivity. *Int J Oral Maxillofac Surg* 1993;22:214–217.
10. Rood JP. Permanent damage to inferior alveolar nerves during the removal of impacted mandibular third molars: comparison of two methods of bone removal. *Br Dent J* 1992;172:108–110.
11. Blackburn CW, Bramley PA. Lingual nerve damage associated with removal of lower third molars. *Br Dent J* 1989;167:103–107.
12. Robinson PP, Smith KG. Lingual nerve damage during lower third molar removal: a comparison of two surgical methods. *Br Dent J* 1996;180:456–461.
13. Pichler JW, Beirne OR. Lingual flap retraction and prevention of lingual nerve damage associated with third molar surgery: a systematic review of the literature. *Oral Surg Oral Med Oral Pathol Oral Radiol Endod* 2001;91:395–401. Search date 1999; primary sources Medline, Healthstar,

Impacted wisdom teeth

Current Contents, Allied and Alternative Medicine, Life Sciences, Web of Science, Nursing Allied Health, Cochrane Library, and hand searching of references retrieved and the indexes of the journal Oral and Maxillofacial Surgery Clinics of North America 1989–1998.

14. Sisk AL, Hammer WB, Shelton DW, et al. Complications following removal of impacted third molars: the role of the experience of the surgeon. *J Oral Maxillofac Surg* 1986;44:855–859.
15. Moss CE, Wake MJC. Lingual access for third molar surgery: a 20-year retrospective audit. *Br J Oral Maxillofac Surg* 1999;37:255–258.

Stephen Worrall
Consultant Oral and Maxillofacial Surgeon
St Luke's Hospital
Bradford
UK

Competing interests: None declared.

Oropharyngeal candidiasis

Search date October 2001

Caroline Pankhurst

QUESTIONS

INTERVENTIONS

Key Messages

Prevention

- **Antifungal prophylaxis in people with advanced HIV disease** RCTs have found that daily or weekly antifungal prophylaxis with fluconazole, itraconazole, or nystatin significantly reduces the incidence of oropharyngeal candidiasis.

- **Antifungal prophylaxis in people with cancer and neutropenia** One systematic review found that antifungal drugs versus placebo reduced the number of episodes of oropharyngeal candidiasis (NNT 4, 95% CI 4 to 5). Another systematic review comparing oral and topical antifungal prophylaxis versus placebo or no treatment found similar results (NNT 3, 95% CI 3 to 5).
- **Antifungal prophylaxis in immunocompromised infants and children** One RCT has found that fluconazole versus oral polyenes significantly reduces the incidence of oropharyngeal candidiasis.
- **Chlorhexidine oral rinse in neutropenic adults undergoing treatment for cancer** Two RCTs found conflicting evidence about chlorhexidine oral rinse versus placebo or nystatin.
- **Continuous prophylaxis versus intermittent treatment in people with HIV infection and acute episodes of oropharyngeal candidiasis (in preventing antifungal resistance)** One RCT found no significant difference in the emergence of antifungal resistance with continuous antifungal prophylaxis versus intermittent treatment.
- **Preventive interventions in people with diabetes** We found no systematic review or RCTs.

Treatments

- **Antifungal treatment for denture stomatitis** RCTs found conflicting evidence about the effects of antifungal agents versus placebo in clinical improvement or cure of denture stomatitis. Trial methods included professional cleaning of the dentures at the start of the study, combined with advice on denture hygiene and advice not to wear the dentures while asleep at night, which may explain the high clinical cure rate in the placebo groups.
- **Antifungal treatment in immunocompetent and immunocompromised infants and children** In immunocompetent infants, RCTs have found that miconazole gel versus nystatin suspension significantly increases the rate of clinical cure. In immunocompromised infants and children, one RCT has found that fluconazole versus oral nystatin significantly increases clinical cure after 2 weeks (NNT 2, 95% CI 2 to 3).
- **Denture hygiene** Two RCTs found insufficient evidence about the effects of mouth rinses or disinfectants versus placebo in preventing or treating denture stomatitis.
- **Fluconazole versus amphotericin B in adults undergoing treatment for cancer** One small RCT found limited evidence that fluconazole versus amphotericin B lozenges significantly increased clinical cure after 2 weeks (NNT 5, 95% CI 4 to 60).
- **Oral suspension of systemic azoles in people with HIV infection** RCTs have found that topical preparations (suspensions or pastilles) of itraconazole, fluconazole, or clotrimazole effectively treat oropharyngeal candidiasis in people with HIV infection. One RCT found that fluconazole versus topical nystatin significantly reduced symptoms and signs of oropharyngeal candidiasis after 14 days (NNT 3, 95% CI 2 to 5).
- **Treatments in people with diabetes mellitus** We found no RCTs assessing treatments for oral candidiasis in people with diabetes mellitus.

DEFINITION Oropharyngeal candidiasis is an opportunistic mucosal infection caused, in over 85% of cases, by *Candida albicans*. The four main types of oropharyngeal candidiasis are: (1) pseudomembranous (thrush), comprising white discrete plaques on an erythematous background, located on the buccal mucosa, throat, tongue, or gingivae; (2) erythematous, comprising smooth red patches on the hard or soft palate, dorsum of tongue, or buccal mucosa; (3) hyperplastic, comprising white, firmly adherent patches or plaques, usually bilateral on the buccal mucosa; and (4) denture induced stomatitis, presenting as either a smooth or granular erythema confined to the denture-bearing area of the hard palate. Symptoms vary, ranging from none to a sore, painful mouth with a burning tongue and altered taste, which can impair speech, nutritional intake, and quality of life.

INCIDENCE/ PREVALENCE Candida species are commensals in the gastrointestinal tract. Transmission occurs directly between infected people or on fomites (objects that can harbour pathogenic organisims). Candida is found in the mouth of 31–60% of healthy people.[1] Denture stomatitis associated with candida is prevalent in 65% of denture wearers.[1] Oropharyngeal candidiasis affects 15–60% of people with haematological or oncological malignancies during periods of immunosuppression.[2] Oropharyngeal candidiasis occurs in 7–48% of people with HIV infection and in over 90% of those with advanced disease. In severely immunosuppressed people, relapse rates are high (30–50%) and usually occur within 14 days of treatment cessation.[3]

AETIOLOGY/ RISK FACTORS Risk factors associated with symptomatic oropharyngeal candidiasis include local or systemic immunosuppression, haematological disorders, broad spectrum antibiotic use, inhaled or systemic steroids, xerostomia, diabetes, and wearing dentures, obturators, or orthodontic appliances. The same strain may persist for months or years in the absence of infection. In people with HIV infection, there is no direct correlation between the number of organisms and the presence of clinical disease. Symptomatic oropharyngeal candidiasis associated with *in vitro* resistance to fluconazole occurs in 5% of people with advanced HIV disease.[4] Resistance to azole antifungals is associated with severe immunosuppression (≤ 50 CD4 cells/ mm^3), more episodes treated with antifungal drugs, and longer median duration of systemic azole treatment.[5]

PROGNOSIS Untreated candidiasis persists for months or years unless associated risk factors are treated or eliminated. In neonates, spontaneous cure of oropharyngeal candidiasis usually occurs after 3–8 weeks.

AIMS To resolve signs and symptoms of oropharyngeal candidiasis; to prevent or delay relapse in immunocompromised people; and to minimise drug induced resistance, with minimum adverse effects.

OUTCOMES Resolution of signs and symptoms; clinical cure; rate of recurrence on the basis of scoring of signs and symptoms. Many RCTs report the results of mycological culture but, whenever possible, this review has not used these intermediate outcomes because the relation between the clinical and mycological culture findings is uncertain.

METHODS *Clinical Evidence* search and appraisal October 2001, supplemented by a search of the author's library, selecting publications in English, from 1975–2000. We included only systematic reviews and RCTs that specified oropharyngeal candidiasis in the protocol design and outcome measurements; those dealing with oesophagitis and invasive, systemic candidal infections were excluded.

QUESTION **What are the effects of interventions to prevent and treat oropharyngeal candidiasis in people receiving chemotherapy or radiotherapy?**

OPTION **ANTIFUNGAL PROPHYLAXIS**

Two systematic reviews in neutropenic adults and people undergoing treatment for cancer have found that antifungal drugs prevent oropharyngeal candidiasis. Three RCTs found inconsistent results about the effects of azoles versus polyenes, although two RCTs were not sufficiently powered to detect a clinically significant difference. Two RCTs found conflicting evidence about chlorhexidine oral rinse versus placebo or nystatin.

Benefits: **Versus placebo:** We found two systematic reviews[6,7] and one subsequent RCT.[8] The earlier review (search date 1991, 9 RCTs, 710 people with cancer, neutropenia, and immunosuppression) compared systemic or topical antifungal agents versus placebo in the prevention of oropharyngeal candidiasis.[6] Participants were not selected according to their fungal colonisation status before initiation of treatment. Treatments included amphotericin B, clotrimazole, miconazole, ketoconazole, fluconazole, and itraconazole. The duration of the prophylaxis was not stated. No eligible RCTs of nystatin were identified. Continuing colonisation of the throat after starting treatment was found to be a risk factor for development of oropharyngeal candidiasis (OR 3.66, 95% CI 1.74 to 5.18). The review found that antifungal drugs versus placebo reduced the number of episodes of oropharyngeal candidiasis (17/372 [5%] with antifungal *v* 109/338 [32%] with placebo; ARR 26%, 95% CI 23% to 28%; OR 0.15, 95% CI 0.10 to 0.22; NNT 4, 95% CI 4 to 5). The second review (search date 1999, 15 RCTs, 1164 people of all ages with cancer who were receiving chemotherapy, excluding people with head and neck cancer) compared 3–10 weeks of oral and topical antifungal prophylaxis versus placebo or no treatment. The review found a significant reduction of oral candidiasis compared with placebo or no treatment for drugs that were partially absorbed from the gastrointestinal tract (miconazole, clotrimazole: RR 0.13, 95% CI 0.06 to 0.27; NNT 3, 95% CI 3 to 5), and for fully absorbed drugs (fluconazole, itraconazole, metoconazole: RR 0.36, 95% CI 0.19 to 0.69), but not for unabsorbed drugs (nystatin, amphotericin B, natamycin, chlorhexidine: RR 0.81, 95% CI 0.58 to 1.12).[7] One subsequent RCT (210 people with neutropenia) compared itraconazole (100 mg twice daily) versus placebo as antifungal prophylaxis for superficial and systemic infections.[8] The RCT found no significant difference in the incidence of oral candidiasis (1/104 [0.96%] with itraconazole *v* 5/106 [4.7%] with placebo; RR 0.20, 95% 0.02 to 1.72), but fewer cases occurred with itraconazole. **Azoles versus polyenes:** We found no systematic review, but found three RCTs (see table 1, p 1427).[9–11] One multicentre RCT (536 people with cancer and neutropenia associated with chemotherapy, radiotherapy or bone marrow transplant) compared prophylaxis for 30 days with fluconazole 50 mg daily versus the oral polyenes amphotericin B (2 g daily), nystatin (4 times 106 units/day), or both, for the prevention of oropharyngeal candidiasis and invasive fungal infection.[9] Oropharyngeal candidiasis was less likely in people treated with fluconazole. Two smaller RCTs in people with liver transplant compared the prevention of oropharyngeal candidiasis by azoles versus polyenes.[10,11] The first multicentre RCT (143 people given prophylaxis for 28 days after liver transplantation) of fluconazole versus nystatin found a lower incidence of oropharyngeal candidiasis with fluconazole, but the result was not significant.[10] The other RCT found no significant difference between nystatin and clotrimazole for prophylaxis during hospital stay after transplantation.[11] However, the two smaller RCTs had insufficient power individually to show a clinically important difference. **Chlorhexidine oral rinse:** We found two RCTs in people with neutropenia who had received bone marrow transplants.[12,13] One RCT (51 people) compared prophylaxis for 60 days with chlorhexidine oral rinse versus a placebo rinse. All participants received oral nystatin suspension 100 000 units. It found that chlorhexidine versus placebo significantly reduced oropharyngeal candidiasis (2/24 [8%] with chlorhexidine *v* 15/27 [56%] with control; ARR 47%, 95% CI 24% to 54%; RR 15%, 95% CI 3% to 57%; NNT 2, 95% CI 2 to 4) and mucositis.[12] The other RCT (86 adults with leukaemia and bone marrow transplant) comparing rinses containing saline alone, chlorhexidine alone, nystatin alone, or nystatin with chlorhexidine versus each other found no significant difference in the development of oropharyngeal candidiasis (no statistical analysis available).[13]

Harms: In one RCT with no placebo arm, the rates of adverse reactions over 30 days were 5.6% with fluconazole and 5.2% with oral polyenes.[9] The most common adverse events were abdominal pain, nausea and vomiting, and rash. There was no increased hepatotoxicity, ciclosporin (cyclosporin) interaction, or emergence of clinically relevant resistant strains reported in people receiving antifungal prophylaxis after liver transplantation.[10]

Comment: We found no RCTs comparing nystatin versus placebo. The RCTs of chlorhexidine found conflicting results about its effect on oropharyngeal candidiasis and mucositis,[12,13] but the second RCT had four parallel arms and was not powered to detect a clinically important difference.[13]

OPTION ANTIFUNGAL TREATMENT

One small RCT in people undergoing treatment for cancer found limited evidence suggesting that fluconazole versus amphotericin B lozenges increased clinical cure of oropharyngeal candidiasis.

Benefits: We found no systematic review. We found one RCT (73 people with oropharyngeal candidiasis undergoing radiotherapy for head and neck cancer), which compared fluconazole 50 mg tablets daily for 1 week with amphotericin B 10 mg lozenges four times daily for 2 weeks.[14] Fluconazole significantly increased clinical cure (34/37 [92%] *v* 26/36 [72%] with amphotericin; RR of cure 1.27, 95% CI 1.02 to 1.35; NNT 5, 95% CI 4 to 60). For both treatments, cure rate was lower in denture wearers than in people who did not wear dentures.

Harms: The RCT did not give details of adverse effects.

Comment: None.

QUESTION What are the effects of interventions to prevent and treat oropharyngeal candidiasis in infants and children?

OPTION ANTIFUNGAL PREVENTION IN IMMUNOCOMPROMISED INFANTS AND CHILDREN

One RCT in immunocompromised infants and children found that prophylactic fluconazole versus oral polyenes significantly reduced the incidence of oropharyngeal candidiasis.

Benefits: We found no systematic review. We found one large, unblinded, multicentre RCT (502 people) comparing fluconazole 3 mg/kg versus oral polyenes (nystatin 50 000 units/kg 4 times daily, oral amphotericin B 25 mg/kg 4 times daily, or both) for the prevention of fungal infections, including oropharyngeal candidiasis. Participants were immunocompromised infants and children aged 6 months to 17 years, admitted to hospital and scheduled within the next 48 hours to undergo initial or repeat courses of chemotherapy or radiotherapy for haematological or oncological malignancies.[2] The mean duration of prophylaxis was 28 days. The RCT found that fluconazole versus oral polyenes significantly reduced the incidence of oropharyngeal candidiasis (3/236 [1%] for fluconazole *v* 15/249 [6%] for oral polyenes; RR 0.21, 95% CI 0.06 to 0.72; NNT 21, 95% CI 18 to 58).[2] Subsequently 18 of the children from the multicentre RCT[2] were enrolled in a second RCT (25 children in each arm, including the 18 children from the first RCT), which compared fluconazole 3 mg/kg once daily versus oral nystatin 50 000 units/kg four times daily in the prevention of oropharyngeal candidiasis.[15] The RCT found no significant difference in the incidence of oral candidiasis (2/25 [8%] with fluconazole *v* 3/25 [12%] with nystatin; P = 0.63).

Harms: In the first RCT, adverse events caused 8/245 (3%) children on fluconazole to withdraw versus 3/257 (1%) on oral polyenes.[2] In the second RCT, no children were withdrawn from the study, but three treated with fluconazole reported nausea and abdominal discomfort and one reported pruritus.[15]

Comment: None.

OPTION ANTIFUNGAL TREATMENT IN CHILDREN

In immunocompetent infants, two RCTs found that miconazole gel versus nystatin suspension significantly increased the rate of clinical cure of oropharyngeal candidiasis. In immunocompromised infants and children, one RCT found that fluconazole versus nystatin polyenes significantly increased clinical cure of oropharyngeal candidiasis.

Benefits: We found no systematic review. **Immunocompetent infants and children:** We found no placebo controlled RCTs. We found two RCTs in immunocompetent infants, which compared miconazole gel versus nystatin suspension for treatment of oropharyngeal candidiasis.[16,17] Both RCTs found that miconazole increased the rate of

clinical cure. In the larger RCT (183 people), quicker clinical cure was obtained with miconazole (at day 5: cure rate 83/98 [85%] for miconazole gel 25 mg 4 times daily v 18/85 [21%] for nystatin suspension 100 000 units 4 times daily; at day 12: 97/98 [99%] for miconazole v 46/85 [54%] for nystatin).[16]
Immunocompromised infants and children: We found no placebo controlled RCTs. We found one multicentre RCT (32 centres, 182 immunocompromised infants and children aged 6 months to 17 years), which compared fluconazole suspension 3 mg/kg versus nystatin 400 000 units four times daily for 14 days for the treatment of oropharyngeal candidiasis. Participants were immunocompromised for different reasons: 64 were infected with HIV, 92 had a malignancy, and 26 were receiving immunosuppressive treatment.[18] Fluconazole versus nystatin significantly increased the clinical cure rate (78/86 [91%] with fluconazole v 37/73 [51%] with nystatin; RR of cure 1.8, 95% CI 1.6 to 1.9; NNT 2, 95% CI 2 to 3). In subgroup analyses of children with HIV infection, nystatin versus fluconazole significantly increased clinical cure (28/35 [80%] with fluconazole v 6/29 [21%] for nystatin) and for people with malignancy (49/50 [98%] for fluconazole v 30/42 [71%] for nystatin). Clinical relapse rates after 2 weeks were similar (18% for fluconazole v 24% for nystatin).

Harms: **Immunocompetent infants and children:** The most common adverse events with both miconazole and nystatin were vomiting and, more rarely, diarrhoea, affecting less than 4.5% of infants.[16,17]
Immunocompromised infants and children: Adverse events caused 2/94 (2%) children on fluconazole to withdraw versus 0/88 (0%) children on nystatin.[18]

Comment: **Immunocompetent infants and children:** The RCTs were not blinded or placebo controlled.[16,17] There is potential for observer bias, but the clinical results were corroborated by the mycological findings, which were blinded.[16] The larger RCT was carried out in 26 general practices,[16] so it is representative of the context in which most otherwise healthy infants with oropharyngeal candidiasis would be treated, especially regarding compliance and cure rate. **Immunocompromised infants and children:** The RCT showed the benefit of fluconazole for infants and children presenting with a wide range of different haematological malignancies, solid tumours, or HIV infection with no apparent differential effect dependant on age, sex, or race.[18]

QUESTION **What are the effects of interventions to prevent and treat oropharyngeal candidiasis in people with diabetes?**

OPTION **ANTIFUNGAL DRUGS**

We found insufficient evidence in people with diabetes about prevention or treatment of oropharyngeal candidiasis.

Benefits: We found no systematic review or RCTs.

Harms: We found no RCTs.

Comment: None.

QUESTION **What are the effects of interventions for oropharyngeal candidiasis in people with dentures?**

OPTION **ANTIFUNGAL DRUGS**

Five RCTs found conflicting evidence about the effects of antifungal drugs versus placebo in clinical improvement or cure of denture stomatitis. Trial methods included professional cleaning of the dentures at the start of the study, combined with advice on denture hygiene and advice not to wear the dentures while asleep at night, which may explain the high clinical cure rate in the placebo groups. Three RCTs comparing different antifungal drugs found no significant differences in clinical cure rates.

Benefits: We found no systematic review, but found several RCTs. **Versus placebo:** Five RCTs compared topical oral antifungals versus placebo for the treatment of denture stomatitis.[19–23] One RCT (46 people) found that topical oral polyenes (nystatin, amphotericin B) significantly improved the clinical cure of denture stomatitis after 4 weeks' treatment.[20] The second RCT (22 people) found no significant difference between polyenes versus placebo in the clinical appearance of denture stomatitis after 2 weeks of treatment, or 10 days after cessation of treatment.[21] The third RCT (49 people) compared amphotericin B with and without a hydrogen peroxide denture cleanser versus placebo and found no significant difference in clinical cure.[19] The fourth RCT (36 people) compared miconazole dental lacquer applied to the fit surface of an upper denture as a single application versus a placebo lacquer, and found no significant difference in the resolution of palatal symptoms by 14 days (symptom resolution in 54% with lacquer *v* 23% with placebo; RR 2.4, 95% CI 0.89 to 3.8).[22] The fifth RCT (38 people) found that fluconazole versus placebo significantly increased the number of people with clinical improvement or cure at 2 weeks (10/19 [53%] *v* 0/18 [0%]; $P < 0.001$).[23] At 4 weeks, the number of people taking fluconazole who had improvement or cure diminished, but was still significantly more than placebo (5/19 [26%] *v* 0/19 [0%]; $P < 0.02$). **Different antifungal treatments:** We found three RCTs.[24–26] The first RCT (19 elderly, chronically ill, institutionalised people) compared nystatin denture soaking solution (10 000 units/mL) versus tap water as a soaking solution; both groups were given nystatin pastilles (10 000 units/g 3 times daily).[24] The RCT found no additional advantage from the use of nystatin as a soaking agent: all participants in both groups were clinically cured at 7 days.[24] The second RCT (29 people) compared fluconazole 50 mg daily for 14 days versus amphotericin B lozenges plus denture cream for 28 days.[25] There was no significant difference in the clinical cure rate after 28 days (84% for fluconazole *v* 90% for amphotericin B). Clinical relapse was common in both groups at 12 weeks. The third RCT (multicentre, 305 elderly people from 56 investigational sites; 176 wore dentures) compared daily administration of fluconazole (50 mg) suspension versus amphotericin B (0.5 g) oral suspension three times daily for 2 weeks. It found no significant difference between fluconazole and amphotericin in either clinical or mycological cure. Wearing dentures did not affect the response to antifungal treatment (clinical cure rate 151/176 [86%] of denture wearers *v* 102/124 [82%] of non-denture wearers).[26] **Different modes of administration:** Two RCTs (41 people[27] and 33 people[28]) compared a single application of miconazole dental lacquer versus miconazole gel 2% applied to the denture four times daily. Neither RCT found a significant difference in palatal erythema (largest RCT, 14 days after treatment: 13/20 [65%] with lacquer *v* 16/21 [76%] with gel; RR of erythema with lacquer *v* gel 0.85, 95% CI 0.42 to 1.2).[27,28]

Harms: None of the trials exclusively enrolling people with dentures were large enough to report accurately on the incidence of adverse effects. In the large RCT of elderly people, 6/150 (4%) in the fluconazole arm and 0/155 (0%) in the amphotericin arm experienced adverse events, including diarrhoea, buccal bitterness, aggravation of pre-existing renal dysfunction (1, withdrawn from RCT), and increased liver transaminases (1, not withdrawn).[26]

Comment: Trial methods included professional cleaning of the dentures at the start of the study, combined with advice on denture hygiene and advice not to wear the dentures while asleep at night. Because the fit surface of the denture may act as a reservoir of primary and recurrent infection, this cleaning and advice may explain the high clinical cure rate in the placebo groups. There was poor correlation between clinical cure and mycological cure. The RCTs comparing different antifungals were not sufficiently powered to detect clinically important differences.

OPTION DENTURE HYGIENE

Two RCTs found insufficient evidence about the effects of mouth rinses or disinfectants versus placebo in the treatment of denture stomatitis.

Benefits: We found no systematic review, but found two RCTs.[29,30] One small crossover RCT (43 people aged 35–73 years) compared daily soaking of dentures in disinfectant (potassium persulphate 1%) versus placebo (water, peppermint, dye) for 4 weeks.[29] The results provided for the outcome of stomatitis were difficult to interpret and therefore no firm conclusions can be drawn. We found one RCT (78 people with mild to moderate denture stomatitis), which compared mouth rinsing three times daily plus denture soaking once daily with an antimicrobial mouth rinse versus the same procedure with control mouth rinse versus weekly soft relining of the fit surface of the denture (to improve retention and reduce denture trauma) for 4 weeks.[30] It found that antimicrobial versus control mouth rinse significantly reduced symptoms of denture stomatitis ($P < 0.01$; absolute numbers not provided).

Harms: The RCTs did not report on adverse effects.[29,30]

Comment: We found no RCT evaluating the effect of removing dentures at night on preventing denture stomatitis. Two observational studies found a correlation between the prevalence of denture stomatitis and an unhealthy lifestyle (a global measure including dietary habits, physical activity, alcohol consumption and smoking), wearing dentures at night, and poor oral hygiene.[31,32]

QUESTION What are the effects of interventions to prevent and treat oropharyngeal candidiasis in people with HIV infection?

OPTION CONTINUOUS ANTIFUNGAL PROPHYLAXIS

RCTs in people with HIV infection have found that daily or weekly antifungal prophylaxis with fluconazole, itraconazole, or nystatin reduces the incidence of oropharyngeal candidiasis.

Benefits: We found no systematic review. We found eight RCTs using different prophylaxis protocols with follow up from 3–29 months.[33–40] All RCTs enrolled people with AIDS, AIDS related complex, or CD4 cell counts less than or equal to 300 cells/mm^3. **Fluconazole versus placebo:** Five RCTs using daily or weekly regimens found that fluconazole versus placebo significantly reduced oropharyngeal candidiasis.[33,34,36–38] Three of these RCTs compared weekly fluconazole versus placebo. Clinical relapse during 6 months' prophylaxis was reduced by fluconazole 150 mg weekly (relapse: 4/9 with fluconazole *v* 5/5 with placebo;[33] and 13/31 with fluconazole *v* 25/26 with placebo;[36] pooled AR 43% with fluconazole *v* 97% with placebo; RR 0.4, 95% CI 0.1 to 0.9; NNT 2). The third RCT (323 women infected with HIV) compared fluconazole 200 mg weekly versus placebo and found similar results: fluconazole reduced the risk of recurrent oropharyngeal candidiasis over 29 months (RR 0.50, 95% CI 0.33 to 0.74).[34] For people with a history of oropharyngeal candidiasis, the absolute benefit of treatment with weekly fluconazole was higher than in those with no history of infection (ARR 25.6/100 person years for those with previous infection *v* 11.2/100 person years for those with no history of infection).[34] One RCT found that fluconazole versus placebo significantly reduced the median time to relapse (168 days with fluconazole *v* 37 days with placebo; $P \le 0.0001$).[36] We found no RCTs comparing weekly versus daily regimens. No significant difference was found between 50 mg versus 100 mg daily doses (oropharyngeal candidiasis: 2/18 [11%] with 50 mg *v* 4/19 [21%] with 100 mg; RR 0.53, 95% CI 0.09 to 2.09).[37] **Itraconazole versus placebo:** One placebo controlled RCT found that daily prophylaxis with 200 mg of itraconazole for 24 weeks reduced the number of people who relapsed (5/24 [21%] with itraconazole *v* 14/20 [70%] with placebo; ARR 49%, 95% CI 19% to 64%; NNT 2, 95% CI 2 to 5) and increased the time interval before relapse occurred (median time to relapse 10.4 wks with itraconazole *v* 8.0 with placebo; $P = 0.001$).[40] **Nystatin versus placebo:** One RCT found that prophylaxis with nystatin 200 000 unit pastille once daily over 20 weeks versus placebo delayed the onset of oropharyngeal candidiasis (HR 0.56, no 95% CI provided).[35] **Fluconazole versus clotrimazole:** One large RCT (428 people from 29 sites) comparing fluconazole 200 mg daily versus clotrimazole 10 mg five times daily over 35 months found that fluconazole significantly reduced the recurrence of oropharyngeal candidiasis (fluconazole 5.7 episodes/100 person years *v* clotrimazole 38.1 episodes/100 person years; $P \le 0.001$).[39]

Harms: The most commonly reported adverse events were gastrointestinal symptoms, rash, and headache, but data on adverse effects were not presented in all RCTs. No participants withdrew because of adverse changes in liver function or haematological variables. Concomitant medication and severe underlying disease may have confounded attribution of adverse events.

Comment: Many of the RCTs were small and not blinded, and most did not adjust for confounding factors such as anti-retroviral treatment and other established risk factors for oropharyngeal candidiasis. No RCTs used quality of life scores. The optimal dosage schedule and frequency of administration of preventive treatment have not been established.

OPTION TOPICAL ANTIFUNGAL TREATMENT

RCTs have found that topical preparations of itraconazole, fluconazole, and clotrimazole effectively treat oropharyngeal candidiasis in people with HIV infection. One RCT found that fluconazole versus topical nystatin significantly reduced symptoms and signs of oropharyngeal candidiasis.

Benefits: We found no systematic review. We found five RCTs comparing topical (suspensions or pastilles) versus orally absorbed antifungals for treatment of oropharyngeal candidiasis in people with HIV infection.[41–45] Four RCTs found itraconazole oral solution 100 mg or 200 mg used in a swish and swallow mode was as effective as fluconazole 100 mg once daily for 14 days or clotrimazole 10 mg five times a day.[41–43,45] Three of these RCTs achieved clinical response rates over 90%.[41–43] The fifth RCT comparing fluconazole 100 mg daily versus nystatin liquid for 14 days found that fluconazole significantly increased complete resolution of signs and symptoms of oropharyngeal candidiasis (fluconazole 60/69 [87%] *v* 36/69 [52%] for nystatin liquid; ARI 35%, 95% CI 22% to 42%; RR 1.67, 95% CI 1.42 to 1.80; NNT 3, 95% CI 2 to 5).[44]

Harms: The most frequently reported adverse effects were gastrointestinal symptoms (nausea, diarrhoea, vomiting). Altered taste, dry mouth, headache, and rashes were also recorded.[41–44] In the other RCT, there were no withdrawals due to adverse effects.[45] On the basis of data from six RCTs (861 people), in which adverse events were considered to be drug induced and resulted in withdrawal from the study, adverse events were reported with fluconazole (4 people), itraconazole (14 people), clotrimazole (12 people), and nystatin (1 person).[35,39,41–44]

Comment: Once daily dosing is likely to increase adherence to treatment. Non-adherence was reported with clotrimazole because of the inconvenience of taking multiple doses.

QUESTION **Which treatments reduce the risk of acquiring resistance to antifungal drugs?**

OPTION **CONTINUOUS ANTIFUNGAL PROPHYLAXIS VERSUS INTERMITTENT ANTIFUNGAL TREATMENT**

One RCT in people with HIV infection and acute episodes of oropharyngeal candidiasis found no significant difference between continuous antifungal prophylaxis and intermittent antifungal treatment in terms of the emergence of antifungal resistance.

Benefits: We found no systematic review. We found one RCT comparing the effects of different treatment regimens on the development of acquired resistance in people with HIV infection over a mean follow up of 11 months.[46] Antifungal sensitivity testing followed the National Committee for Clinical Laboratory Standards guidelines.[47] The RCT found that continuous prophylaxis with fluconazole versus intermittent treatment with fluconazole 200 mg a day reduced median annual relapse rates (0 episodes/year for continuous prophylaxis *v* 4.1 episodes/year for intermittent treatment; $P \leq 0.001$). It also found that antifungal resistance developed in more people on continuous prophylaxis than on intermittent treatment, but the difference was not significant (9/16 [56%] for continuous *v* 13/28 [46%] for intermittent; $P = 0.75$).

Harms: No adverse reactions were reported.

Comment: Optimal treatment regimens to reduce the risk of acquiring resistance have not been evaluated adequately. In a prospective observational study of protease inhibitor treatment, 93 people with HIV and with a history of recurrent oropharyngeal candidiasis were followed up for 1 year. Oropharyngeal candidiasis was diagnosed in 2/30 people (7%) given protease inhibitors and 23/63 (37%) given other treatment ($P \leq 0.001$; 95% CI not provided).[48] Immunomodulating antiretroviral treatments (e.g. highly active antiretroviral treatment), by reducing the number of recurrences of oropharyngeal candidiasis, are acting indirectly as antifungal sparing agents, thereby reducing exposure to antifungals and the potential risk of resistance.

REFERENCES

1. Webb BC, Thomas CJ, Willcox MD, et al. Candida-associated denture stomatitis. Aetiology and management: a review. Part 3. Treatment of oral candidosis. *Aust Dent J* 1998;43:244–249.
2. Ninane JA. Multicentre study of fluconazole versus oral polyenes in the prevention of fungal infection in children with hematological or oncological malignancies. Multicentre study group. *Eur J Clin Microbiol Infect Dis* 1994;13:330–337.
3. Philips P, Zemcov J, Mahmood W, et al. Itraconazole cyclodextrin solution for fluconazole-refractory oropharyngeal candidiasis in AIDS: correlation of clinical response with in vitro susceptibility. *AIDS* 1996;10:1369–1376.
4. Rex JH, Rinald MG, Pfaler MA. Resistance of candida species to fluconazole. *Antimicrob Agents Chemother* 1995;39:1–8.
5. Maenza JR, Keruly JC, Moore RD, et al. Risk factors for fluconazole-resistant candidiasis in human immuno-deficiency virus-infected patients. *J Infect Dis* 1996;173:219–225.
6. Mcunier F, Paesmans M, Autier P. Value of antifungal prophylaxis with antifungal drugs against oropharyngeal candidiasis in cancer patients. *Eur J Cancer B Oral Oncol* 1994;30:196–199. Search date 1991; primary sources English language papers from Medline and author's library.
7. Clarkson JE, Worthington HV, Eden OB. Prevention of oral mucositis or oral candidiasis for patients with cancer receiving chemotherapy (excluding head and neck cancer). In: The Cochrane Library, Issue 4, 2000. Oxford: Update Software. Search date 1999; primary sources Medline, Embase,

CINAHL, Cancerlit, the Cochrane Controlled Trials Register, and the Cochrane Oral Health Group Specialist Register.
8. Nucci M, Biasoli I, Akiti T, et al. A double-blind, randomized, placebo-controlled trial of itraconazole capsules as antifungal prophylaxis for neutropenic patients. *Clin Infect Dis* 2000;31:300–305.
9. Philpott-Howard JN, Wade JJ, Mufti GJ, et al. Randomized comparison of oral fluconazole versus oral polyenes for the prevention of fungal infection in patients at risk of neutropenia. Multicentre study group. *J Antimicrob Chemother* 1993;31:973–984.
10. Lumbreras C, Cuervas-Mons V, Jara P, et al. Randomized trial of fluconazole versus nystatin for the prophylaxis of candida infection following liver transplantation. *J Infect Dis* 1996;174:583–588.
11. Ruskin JD, Wood RP, Bailey MR, et al. Comparative trial of oral clotrimazole and nystatin for oropharyngeal candidiasis prophylaxis in orthotopic liver transplant patients. *Oral Surg Oral Med Oral Pathol Oral Radiol Endod* 1992;74:567–571.
12. Ferretti GA, Ash RC, Brown AT, Parr MD, Romond EH, Lillich TT. Control of oral mucositis and candidiasis in marrow transplantation: a prospective, double-blind trial of chlorhexidine digluconate oral rinse. *Bone Marrow Transplant* 1988;3:483–493.
13. Epstein JB, Vickars L, Spinelli J, Reece D. Efficacy of chlorhexidine and nystatin rinses in prevention of oral complications in leukemia and bone marrow transplantation. *Oral Surg Oral Med Oral Pathol Oral Radiol Endod* 1992;73:682–689.
14. Finlay PM, Richardson MD, Robertson AG. A comparative study of the efficacy of fluconazole and amphotericin B in the treatment of oropharyngeal candidosis in patients undergoing radiotherapy for head and neck tumours. *Br J Oral Maxillofac Surg* 1996;34:23–25.
15. Groll AH, Just-Nuebling G, Kurz M, et al. Fluconazole versus nystatin in the prevention of candida infections in children and adolescents undergoing remission induction or consolidation chemotherapy for cancer. *J Antimicrob Chemother* 1997;40:855–862.
16. Hoppe J, Burr R, Ebeling H, et al. Treatment of oropharyngeal candidiasis in immunocompetent infants: a randomized multicenter study of miconazole gel vs. nystatin suspension. *Pediatr Infect Dis J* 1997;16:288–293.
17. Hoppe JE, Hahn H. Randomized comparison of two nystatin oral gels with miconazole oral gel for treatment of oral thrush in infants. Antimycotics study group. *Infection* 1996;24:136–139.
18. Flynn PM, Cunningham CK, Kerkering T, et al. Oropharyngeal candidiasis in immunocompromised children: a randomized, multicenter study of orally administered fluconazole suspension versus nystatin. The multicenter fluconazole study group. *J Pediatr* 1995;127:322–328.
19. Walker DM, Stafford GD, Huggett R, et al. The treatment of denture stomatitis: evaluation of two agents. *Br Dent J* 1981;151:416–419.
20. Nairn RI. Nystatin and amphotericin B in the treatment of denture-related candidiasis. *Oral Surg Oral Med Oral Pathol Oral Radiol Endod* 1975;40:68–75.
21. Johnson GH, Taylor TD, Heid DW. Clinical evaluation of a nystatin pastille for treatment of denture-related oral candidiasis. *J Prosthet Dent* 1989;61:699–703.
22. Konsberg R, Axell T. Treatment of candida-infected denture stomatitis with a miconazole lacquer. *Oral Surg Oral Med Oral Pathol Oral Radiol Endod* 1994;78:306–311.
23. Budtz-Jorgensen E, Holmstrup P, and Krogh P. Fluconazole in the treatment of Candida-associated denture stomatitis. *Antimicrob Agents Chemother* 1988;32:1859–1863.
24. Banting DW, Greenhorn PA, McMinn JG. Effectiveness of a topical antifungal regimen for the treatment of oral candidiasis in older, chronically ill, institutionalized adults. *J Can Dent Assoc* 1995;61:199–195.
25. Bissell V, Felix DH, Wray D. Comparative trial of fluconazole and amphotericin B in the treatment of denture stomatitis. *Oral Surg Oral Med Oral Path Oral Radiol Endod* 1993;76:35–39.
26. Taillandier J, Esnault Y, Alemanni M, and the multicentre study group. A comparison of fluconazole oral suspension and amphotericin B oral suspension in older patients with oropharyngeal candidosis. *Age Ageing* 2000;29:117–123.
27. Budtz-Jorgensen E, Carlino P. A miconazole lacquer in the treatment of candida-associated denture stomatitis. *Mycoses* 1994;37:131–135.
28. Parvinen T, Kokko J, Yli-Urpo A. Miconazole lacquer compared with gel in treatment of denture stomatitis. *Scand J Dental Res* 1994;102:361–366.
29. Mahonen K, Virtanen K, Larmas M. The effect of prosthesis disinfection on salivary microbial levels. *J Oral Rehabil* 1998;25:304–310.
30. DePaola LG, Minah GE, Elias SA, Eastwood GW, Walters RA. Clinical and microbial evaluation of treatment regimens to reduce denture stomatitis. *Int J Prosthodont* 1990;3:369–374.
31. Sakki TK, Knuuttila ML, Laara E, Anttila SS. The association of yeasts and denture stomatitis with behavioral and biologic factors. *Oral Surg Oral Med Oral Pathol Oral Radiol Endodont* 1997;84:624–629.
32. Fenlon MR, Sherriff M, Walter JD. Factors associated with the presence of denture related stomatitis in complete denture wearers: a preliminary investigation. *Eur J Prosthodont Restor Dent* 1998;6:145–147.
33. Leen CLS, Dunbar EM, Ellis ME, et al. Once-weekly fluconazole to prevent recurrence of oropharyngeal candidiasis in patients with AIDS and AIDS-related complex: a double-blind placebo controlled study. *J Infect* 1990;21:55–60.
34. Schuman P, Capps L, Peng G, et al. Weekly fluconazole for the prevention of mucosal candidiasis in women with HIV infection. A randomized, double-blind, placebo-controlled trial. Terry Beirn community programs for clinical research on AIDS. *Ann Intern Med* 1997;126:689–696.
35. MacPhail LA, Hilton JF, Dodd CL, et al. Prophylaxis with nystatin pastilles for HIV-associated oral candidiasis. *J Acquir Immune Defic Syndr* 1996;12:470–476.
36. Marriott DJE, Jones PD, Hoy JF, et al. Fluconazole once a week as secondary prophylaxis against oropharyngeal candidiasis in HIV-infected patients. A double-blind placebo-controlled study. *Med J Aust* 1993;158:312–316.
37. Just-Nubling G, Gentschew G, Meissner K, et al. Fluconazole prophylaxis of recurrent oral candidiasis in HIV-positive patients. *Eur J Clin Microbiol Infect Dis* 1991;10:917–921.
38. Stevens DA, Greene SI, Lang OS. Thrush can be prevented in patients with acquired immunodeficiency syndrome and the acquired immunodeficiency syndrome-related complex. Randomized, double-blind, placebo-controlled study of 100 mg oral fluconazole daily. *Arch Intern Med* 1991;151:2458–2464.
39. Powderly WG, Finklestein DM, Feinberg J, et al. A randomised trial comparing fluconazole with

clotrimazole troches for the prevention of fungal infection in patients with advanced human immunodeficiency virus infection. *N Engl J Med* 1995;332:700–705.
40. Smith D, Midgley J, Gazzard B. A randomised, double-blind study of itraconazole versus placebo in the treatment and prevention of oral or oesophageal candidosis in patients with HIV infection. *Int J Clin Pract* 1999;53:349–352.
41. Graybill JR, Vazquez J, Darouiche RO, et al. Randomized trial of itraconazole oral solution for oropharyngeal candidiasis in HIV/AIDS patients. *Am J Med* 1998;104:33–39.
42. Phillips P, De Beule K, Frechette G, et al. A double-blind comparison of itraconazole oral solution and fluconazole capsules for the treatment of oropharyngeal candidiasis in patients with AIDS. *Clin Infect Dis* 1998;26:1368–1373.
43. Murray PA, Koletar SL, Mallegol I, et al. Itraconazole oral solution versus clotrimazole troches for the treatment of oropharyngeal candidiasis in immunocompromised patients. *Clin Ther* 1997;19:471–480.
44. Pons V, Greenspan D, Lozada-Nur F, et al. Oropharyngeal candidiasis in patients with AIDS: randomized comparison of fluconazole versus nystatin oral suspensions. *Clin Infect Dis* 1997;24:1204–1207.
45. Linpiyawan R, Jittreprasert K, Sivayathorn A. Clinical trial: clotrimazole troche vs. itraconazole oral solution in the treatment of oral candidosis in AIDS patients. *Int J Dermatol* 2000;39:859–861.
46. Revankar SG, Kirkpatrick WR, McAtee RK, et al. A randomized trial of continuous or intermittent therapy with fluconazole for oropharyngeal candidiasis in HIV-infected patients: clinical outcomes and development of fluconazole resistance. *Am J Med* 1998;105:7–11.
47. National Committee for Clinical Laboratory Standards. Reference Method for Broth Dilution Antifungal Susceptibility Testing of Yeasts: Approved Standard. Wayne, Penn: NCCLS, 1997 (document M27-A).
48. Cauda R, Tacconelli E, Tumbarello M, et al. Role of protease inhibitors in preventing recurrent oral candidiasis in patients with HIV infections: a prospective case control study. *J Acquir Immune Defic Syndr* 1999;21:20–25.

Caroline Pankhurst
Dr
Guy's, King's College, and St Thomas's Dental Institute
London
UK

Competing interests: None declared.

TABLE 1 RCTs of azoles versus polyenes in prevention of oropharyngeal candidiasis in people with impaired immunity (see text, p 1416).

RCT	AR with azole	AR with nystatin	ARR	RR	NNT
Fluconazole *v* amphotericin and/or nystatin[9]	4/256 (1.6 %)	22/255 (8.6%)	7% (4.2% to 8.1%)	0.18 (0.06 to 0.52)	14 (12 to 24)
Fluconazole *v* nystatin[10]	7/76 (9%)	14/67 (21%)	12%	0.44 (0.18 to 1.01)	ND
Clotrimazole *v* nystatin[11]	1/17 (6%)	1/17 (6%)	0%	1.00 (0.06 to 8.86)	ND
Pooled results	**12/349 (3%)**	**37/339 (11%)**	**7.5% (4.4% to 9.1%)**	**0.32 (0.16 to 0.59)**	**13 (11 to 23)**

ND, no data.

Postoperative pulmonary infections

Search date March 2002

Andrew Smith

QUESTIONS

INTERVENTIONS

See glossary, p 1433

Key Messages

- **Advice to stop smoking preoperatively** We found no RCTs of the effects of preoperative advice to stop cigarette smoking on postoperative pulmonary infection. Two observational studies found that stopping smoking reduced the risk of postoperative pulmonary complications.
- **Chest physiotherapy (incentive spirometry and deep breathing exercises)** One systematic review and one subsequent RCT have found that deep breathing exercises significantly reduce postoperative pulmonary infections. The review also found that incentive spirometry versus control significantly reduces pulmonary complications.
- **Chest physiotherapy (intermittent positive pressure breathing)** One RCT has found that intermittent positive pressure breathing versus control significantly reduces postoperative pulmonary complications (NNT 4, 95% CI 3 to 18).
- **Epidural anaesthesia** Two systematic reviews have found that epidural anaesthesia versus general anaesthesia followed by systemic opioid analgesia significantly reduces postoperative pulmonary infection. Neither review provided information on adverse effects. Three subsequent and one additional RCT found inconsistent results.

Clin Evid 2002;8:1428–1435.

DEFINITION A working diagnosis of postoperative pulmonary infection may be based on three or more new findings from cough, phlegm, shortness of breath, chest pain, temperature above 38°C, and pulse rate above 100/min.[1] In this topic, the diagnosis of pneumonia implies consolidation observed on a chest x ray.[2]

INCIDENCE/ PREVALENCE Reported morbidity for chest complications depends on how carefully they are investigated. One study found blood gas and chest radiograph abnormalities in about 50% of people after open cholecystectomy.[3] However, less than 20% of these had abnormal clinical signs and only 10% had a clinically significant chest infection. Another study estimated the incidence of pneumonia as 20%.[4] Another used a similarly strict definition and found the incidence was 23%.[5]

AETIOLOGY/ RISK FACTORS Risk factors include increasing age (> 50 years), cigarette smoking, obesity, thoracic or upper abdominal operations, and pre-existing lung disease.[6] One multivariate analysis did not confirm the association with cigarette smoking but suggested that longer preoperative hospital stay and higher grading on the American Society of Anesthesiologists' physical status scale (> 2) increased the risk of postoperative pulmonary complications.[5] Depression of the immune system may also contribute.[7]

PROGNOSIS In one large systematic review (search date 1997, 141 RCTs, 9559 people), 10% of people with postoperative pneumonia died.[8] If systemic sepsis ensues, mortality is likely to be substantial.[9] Pneumonia delays recovery from surgery and poor tissue oxygenation may contribute to delayed wound healing.

AIMS To prevent the development of postoperative pulmonary infection; to minimise postoperative pain; to minimise adverse effects of treatment; to reduce mortality.

OUTCOMES Clinically diagnosed pulmonary infection (as in the definition above) and a variety of pain scales. Pulmonary complications are a commonly used outcome, but they combine pulmonary infections with other adverse outcomes.

METHODS *Clinical Evidence* update search and appraisal March 2002.

QUESTION **What are the effects of preoperative advice to stop smoking?**

We found no RCTs of the effects of preoperative advice to stop cigarette smoking on postoperative pulmonary infections. Two observational studies have found that stopping smoking reduces the risk of pneumonia.

Benefits: We found one systematic review (search date 2001), which identified no RCTs.[10] We found no subsequent RCTs.

Harms: We found no evidence.

Comment: One prospective, observational study (200 people undergoing coronary artery bypass surgery) found that smokers were more likely to develop pulmonary complications of all types.[11] People who had stopped smoking 6 months preoperatively reverted to the risk of those who had never smoked. A beneficial effect was seen only in people who had stopped smoking for 2 months or more. A later prospective cohort study (410 people undergoing a variety of elective procedures) found that current smokers were more likely to have postoperative pneumonia than those who had never smoked, but the differences were not tested statistically.[12] For all pulmonary complications, the odds ratio for developing complications for current smokers versus those who have never smoked was 5.5 (95% CI 1.2 to 14.8). One multivariate analysis of postoperative pulmonary infections did not confirm the association with cigarette smoking.[5]

QUESTION What are the effects of different anaesthetic/analgesic techniques?

Two systematic reviews have found that, compared with general anaesthesia followed by systemic opioid analgesia, epidural anaesthesia is associated with a reduced risk of postoperative pulmonary infection. Neither review sought data on adverse effects. Three subsequent RCTs found no significant difference in pulmonary infections or complications between epidural versus general anaesthesia, or versus patient controlled analgesia. One additional RCT has found a significant reduction in pulmonary complications with epidural versus systemic opioid.

Benefits: We found two systematic reviews (search dates 1997[8] and 1996[13]), one additional RCT,[14] and three subsequent RCTs.[15–17] Both systematic reviews found that regional analgesia/anaesthesia versus systemic anaesthesia/analgesia reduced the incidence of pulmonary infections.[8,13] The most recent review (search date 1997) sought to identify all RCTs of intraoperative neuraxial blockade (with epidural or spinal anaesthesia).[8] The other systematic review (search date 1996) made three separate comparisons of epidural versus non-epidural analgesia separately.[13] Sensitivity analysis found there was no clinically significant difference in results after exclusion of low quality trials. **Neuraxial blockade versus general anaesthesia:** The most recent review found that the risk of developing pneumonia was less in people randomised to neuraxial blockade versus general anaesthesia (28 RCTs; 149/4871 [3%] *v* 238/4688 [5%]; ARR 2%; RR 0.60, 95% CI 0.49 to 0.74; NNT 50, 95% CI 36 to 82). The review found some evidence that the relative reduction in pneumonia was greater after thoracic epidural anaesthesia than after lumbar epidural or spinal anaesthesia (P = 0.05). **Epidural local anaesthetic versus systemic opioid:** The older review (search date 1996, 215 people; 3 RCTs in people undergoing cholecystectomy, 1 in upper abdominal and hip surgery, and 1 in upper abdominal surgery) found that the incidence of pulmonary infections was lower in people who had an epidural (RR 0.36, 95% CI 0.21 to 0.65; absolute figures not provided).[13] **Epidural opioids versus systemic opioids:** The older review (search date 1996, 547 people; 2 RCTs of thoracotomies, 2 of abdominal operations, 1 of upper abdominal surgery) found no significant difference in the rate of pulmonary infections (RR of pulmonary infections with epidural opioids 0.53, 95% CI 0.18 to 1.53; absolute figures not provided).[12] **Epidural local anaesthetic plus opioid versus systemic opioid:** The older review (search date 1996) identified only two RCTs (both in abdominal surgery) reporting pulmonary complications.[13] The first RCT (163 people undergoing abdominal surgery for cancer) compared general anaesthesia plus epidural bupivacaine plus morphine for postoperative analgesia versus general anaesthesia plus intravenous fentanyl plus subcutaneous morphine for postoperative analgesia. It found no significant difference in the rate of clinical pulmonary complications (21/78 [31%] with epidural bupivacaine *v* 23/75 [27%] subcutaneous morphine; RR 0.88, 95% CI 0.53 to 1.45; analysis was not intention to treat).[18] The second RCT (53 people undergoing pulmonary resection) compared five different treatment strategies.[19] The RCT found no significant difference in rates of pneumonia (3/12 [25%] with epidural morphine *v* 1/10 [10%] with epidural bupivacaine *v* 2/11 [18%] with epidural morphine plus epidural bupivacaine *v* 2/10 [20%] with epidural saline *v* 1/10 [10%] with morphine; overall P = 0.86). One additional RCT (46 elderly non-smokers undergoing major pancreatic and biliary surgery) comparing epidural local anaesthetic plus opioid versus systemic opioid found a significant reduction in the incidence of pneumonia with epidural versus systemic opioid treatment (2/22 [9%] *v* 8/24 [33%]; P = 0.049).[14] The first subsequent RCT (50 people undergoing thoracotomy) comparing epidural analgesia (local anaesthetic and opioids) versus intravenous patient controlled opioid found no significant difference in postoperative pulmonary complications (1/25 [4%] with epidural analgesia *v* 0/25 [0%] with patient controlled analgesia).[15] Furthermore, pneumonia was not separated out of pulmonary complications as a whole. The second subsequent RCT (24 people with chronic obstructive pulmonary disease undergoing upper abdominal or thoracic surgery) compared general anaesthesia plus epidural anaesthesia versus general anaesthesia alone.[16] It found no significant difference in the incidence of postoperative pulmonary infection. The third subsequent RCT (168 people undergoing elective abdominal aortic surgery) compared thoracic epidural anaesthesia plus light general anaesthesia versus general anaesthesia, both followed by either postoperative patient controlled intravenenous or epidural anaesthesia (4 treatment groups).[17] It found no significant difference between groups in the incidence of postoperative pneumonia.

Harms: These RCTs were not designed to look for information about harms of epidural anaesthesia. However, one found "mild reddening" of the epidural site in 16/25 people after an average of 5.6 days.[15] We found one large prospective French cohort study (30 413 epidural anaesthetics) of the incidence of harms from epidural analgesia.[20] This study estimated the frequency of cardiac arrest (usually owing to inadvertent intravascular injection of local anaesthetic) as 1/10 000; seizures (usually the same cause) as 1.3/10 000; neurological injury as 2/10 000; radiculopathy as 1.6/10 000; and paraplegia as 0.3/10 000.[20] There were no deaths attributable to epidural analgesia in this series. In a large US prospective uncontrolled cohort study (1297 people receiving epidurals), 0.4% of people were judged to need naloxone to reverse the effects of epidural opioids on breathing.[21] One case series reported three cases in which epidural analgesia was thought to contribute to the development of postoperative pressure sores.[22] Inadvertent dural puncture with the epidural needle can cause headache (frequency increases with gauge of needle).[23] Effective pain relief can delay recognition of surgical complications, such as anastomotic breakdown, peritonitis, or compartment compression syndrome of the legs.

Comment: Most of the RCTs were too small to detect a clinically significant difference in postoperative chest infections between treatments, and this may explain why some additional RCTs found no significant difference. Only when these RCTs were combined by meta-analysis was benefit apparent. The two systematic reviews differ in their approach. The more recent review[8] sought aggregated benefit for all types of neuraxial blockade and had more statistical power. However, the other review[13] compared different modalities of epidural anaesthesia; the smaller numbers of RCTs and people in each subgroup probably explain the lack of a significant effect for some of the regimens. Although both reviews examined the effect of epidural anaesthesia on pulmonary infection after all types of surgery, a sensitivity analysis was performed only in the later review.[8] This suggested that the beneficial effects of regional anaesthesia in general, though not necessarily pulmonary infection in particular, held for all types of surgery studied. The overall benefit of regional anaesthesia seemed independent of whether it was combined with general anaesthesia.

QUESTION What are the effects of postoperative chest physiotherapy?

One systematic review has found that physiotherapy reduces postoperative pulmonary infection. We found most evidence for incentive spirometry and deep breathing exercises, but one RCT found evidence of benefit with intermittent positive pressure. One large subsequent RCT has found that deep breathing reduces the risk of pneumonia. We found no evidence about the effects of timing and dosage.

Benefits: We found two systematic reviews (search date 1992, 7 relevant RCTs, 764 people;[24] and search date 2000, 2 relevant RCTs, 212 people[25]) and two subsequent RCTs comparing physiotherapy with no treatment.[26,27] The RCTs compared three methods of physiotherapy (incentive spirometry, deep breathing exercises, and intermittent positive pressure breathing [see glossary, p 1434]) on postoperative pulmonary complications. Only people undergoing any type of upper abdominal surgery were included. Not all of the included RCTs used pneumonia as an outcome. **Incentive spirometry:** Both systematic reviews identified the same two RCTs of incentive spirometry versus no treatment, but only the first review performed meta-analysis. It found that incentive spirometry significantly reduced the risk of postoperative pulmonary complications (212 people; OR 0.44, 95% CI 0.18 to 0.99). **Deep breathing/ coughing exercises:** The first systematic review identified four RCTs (564 people) comparing deep breathing exercises versus control (details of control not stated in review). It found a significant reduction in pulmonary complications with deep breathing exercises (OR 0.43, 95% CI 0.27 to 0.63), but there was significant heterogeneity between trials. However, one of these four RCTs (60 people) used an outcome measure that could not in itself diagnose pulmonary infection. We found two subsequent RCTs.[26,27] The first RCT (368 people undergoing major abdominal surgery) compared instruction to perform deep breathing exercises versus no physiotherapy instruction. Additional resistance training was given to people in the treatment group at high risk (defined as aged > 50 years or with one of the following: smoker or ex-smoker for < 12 months, body mass index > 30, pulmonary disease needing daily medication, or other coexisting medical condition). The trial found that deep breathing significantly reduced the risk of developing pneumonia (1/172 [0.6%] in the physiotherapy group *v* 13/192 [6.8%] in the control group; ARR 6.2%; RR 0.09, 95% CI 0.01 to 0.65; NNT 16, 95% CI 10 to 39). The relative risk of developing pneumonia in people at high risk was not given. The second subsequent RCT (120 people undergoing coronary artery surgery) compared two physiotherapy groups versus no treatment.[27] The RCT found low rates of chest infections in all groups (1/40 [2.5%] with no physiotherapy *v* 4/40 [10%] with instruction to perform deep breathing and coughing exercises *v* 1/40 [2.5%] with instruction to perform deep breathing and coughing exercises and more intensive attention from the physiotherapist). The RCT did not report formal statistical analysis because of the small number of complications. **Intermittent positive pressure breathing:** The first systematic review identified one RCT (89 people) comparing intermittent positive pressure breathing versus control (details of control not stated in the review). It found that intermittent positive pressure breathing significantly reduced pulmonary complications (10/45 [22 %] *v* 21/44 [48%]; ARR 25%; RR 0.5, 95% CI 0.2 to 0.9; NNT 4, 95% CI 3 to 18).[24]

Harms: The RCTs found no evidence of adverse effects.

Comment: Some RCTs in the first systematic review distinguished between people at low and high risk of pulmonary complications. Individual RCTs in low risk people often did not find the beneficial effect of physiotherapy seen when all RCTs were pooled. The two subsequent RCTs were conducted in people at lower risk of pulmonary infection.[26,27] The first systematic review assessed study validity by two independent assessors using the following criteria: reproducibility of patient population and surgical procedure; comparability of groups; clear description of experimental manoeuvre; presence of control group; clear description of outcome measures; random allocation with blinding; withdrawals listed; prior estimate of study power; and some measure of test of compliance with treatment.[24]

GLOSSARY

The following three modalities of physiotherapy all count as methods to increase lung volume. Increasing lung volume is thought to cause a reduction in airways resistance and an improvement in ventilation:[28]

Deep breathing The person is instructed to breathe in deeply, comfortably, and slowly through the nose, and then sigh out through the mouth. Optimum conditions to ensure that deep breaths reach poorly ventilated dependent regions include accurate positioning, ensuring the person is comfortable and relaxed, avoiding distractions, and allowing the person to get their breath back after turning to avoid breathlessness.

Postoperative pulmonary infections

Incentive spirometry The flow and volume achieved by a controlled and sustained deep breath can be encouraged by an incentive spirometer, which gives the person visual feedback on their performance. The same effect can theoretically be obtained without the device, but the incentive of using a tangible object may increase inhaled volume and produce more controlled flow.

Intermittent positive pressure breathing Assisted breathing with a pressure cycled ventilator triggered into inspiration by the user and allowing passive expiration. The user begins to inhale through the machine, which senses the breath and augments it by delivering gas to the user. When a preset pressure is reached, the machine stops delivering gas and allows the user to breathe out. In most devices, the inspiratory sensitivity, flow rate, and pressure can be varied to suit the user's needs, but some devices adjust the sensitivity and flow automatically.

Substantive changes

Advice to stop smoking New systematic review;[10] conclusion unchanged.
Different anaesthetic/analgesic techniques New subsequent RCT;[17] conclusion unchanged.
Postoperative chest physiotherapy New systematic review;[25] conclusion unchanged.

REFERENCES

1. Celli BR, Rodriguez KS, Snider GL. A controlled trial of intermittent positive pressure breathing, incentive spirometry, and deep breathing exercises in preventing pulmonary complications after abdominal surgery. *Am Rev Respir Dis* 1984;130:12–15.
2. Hall JC, Tarala RA, Tapper J, et al. Prevention of respiratory complications after abdominal surgery: a randomised clinical trial. *BMJ* 1996;312:148–152.
3. Wirén FE, Janson L, Hellekant C. Respiratory complications after upper abdominal surgery. *Acta Chir Scand* 1981;147:623–627.
4. Garibaldi RA, Britt MR, Coleman ML, et al. Risk factors for postoperative pneumonia. *Am J Med* 1981;70:677–680.
5. Hall JC, Tarala RA, Hall JL, et al. A multivariate analysis of the risk of pulmonary complications after laparotomy. *Chest* 1991;99:923–927.
6. Christensen EF, Schultz P, Jensen OV, et al. Postoperative pulmonary complications and lung function in high-risk patients: a comparison of three physiotherapy regimens after upper abdominal surgery in general anaesthesia. *Acta Anaesthesiol Scand* 1991;35:97–104.
7. Sabiston DC Jr, ed. *Textbook of surgery: the biological basis of modern surgical practice*. Philadelphia: WB Saunders, 15th ed, 1997:345.
8. Rodgers A, Walker N, Schug S, et al. Reduction of postoperative mortality and morbidity with epidural or spinal anaesthesia: results from overview of randomised trials. *BMJ* 2000;321:1493–1497. Search date 1997; primary sources Medline, Embase, Current Contents, the Cochrane Library, and hand searches of reference lists from all identified papers and of selected conference proceedings and personal contact with authors.
9. Miller G, Ellis ME. Hospital-acquired pneumonia. In: Ellis M, ed. *Infectious diseases of the respiratory tract*. Cambridge: Cambridge University Press, 1998.
10. Møller A, Villebro N, Pedersen T. Interventions for preoperative smoking cessation. In: The Cochrane Library, Issue 1, 2002. Oxford: Update Software. Search date 2001: primary sources: Medline, Embase, and Cinhal.
11. Warner MA, Offord KP, Warner ME, et al. Role of preoperative cessation of smoking and other factors in postoperative pulmonary complications: a blinded prospective study of coronary artery bypass patients. *Mayo Clin Proc* 1989;64:609–616.
12. Bluman LG, Mosca L, Newman N, et al. Preoperative smoking habits and postoperative pulmonary complications. *Chest* 1998;113:148–152.
13. Ballantyne JC, Carr DB, deFerranti S, et al. The comparative effects of postoperative analgesic therapies on pulmonary outcome: cumulative meta-analyses of randomized controlled trials. *Anesth Analg* 1998;86:598–612. Search date 1996; primary sources Medline and hand searches of reference lists from relevant articles.
14. Barzoi G, Bianchi B, Mangiante G, et al. Hepato-biliary-pancreatic surgery in over 70-years-old patients: which is the best anaesthesiologic procedure? *Chir Ital* 1995;47:44–48.
15. Azad SC, Groh J, Beyer A, et al. Continuous epidural analgesia versus patient controlled intravenous analgesia for postthoracotomy pain. *Acute Pain* 2000;3:84–93.
16. Xue Z-G, Bai L, Jiang H. Combined epidural block with general anaesthesia in patients with chronic obstructive pulmonary disease. *J Shanghai Med Univ* 2000;27:302–305, 323.
17. Norris EJ, Beattie C, Perler BA, et al. Double-masked randomized trial comparing alternate combinations of intraoperative anesthesia and postoperative analgesia in abdominal aortic surgery. *Anaesthesiology* 2001;95:1054–1067.
18. Jayr C, Thomas H, Rey A, et al. Postoperative pulmonary complication: epidural analgesia using bupivacaine and opioids versus parenteral opioids. *Anesthesiology* 1993;78:666–676.
19. Logas W, El-Baz N, El-Ganzouri A, et al. Continuous thoracic epidural analgesia for postoperative pain relief following thoracotomy: a randomized prospective study. *Anesthesiology* 1987;67:787–791.
20. Auroy Y, Narchi P, Messiah A, et al. Serious complications related to regional anesthesia. *Anesthesiology* 1997;87:479–486.

21. Scott DA, Beilby DSN, McClymont C. Postoperative analgesia using epidural infusions of fentanyl with bupivacaine. *Anesthesiology* 1995;83:727–737.
22. Shah JL. Postoperative pressure sores after epidural anaesthesia. *BMJ* 2000;321:941–942.
23. Bromage PR. *Epidural analgesia*. Philadelphia: WB Saunders, 1978.
24. Thomas JA, McIntosh JM. Are incentive spirometry, intermittent positive pressure breathing and deep breathing exercises effective in the prevention of postoperative pulmonary complications after upper abdominal surgery? A systematic overview and meta-analysis. *Phys Ther* 1994;74:3–16. Search date 1992; primary sources Medline, Cinahl, and hand searches of reference lists from relevant articles and reference lists, and unpublished abstracts from a Consensus Exercise on Physical Therapy for the Surgical Patient 1989.
25. Overend TJ, Anderson C, Lucy, SD, et al The effect of incentive spirometry on postoperative pulmonary complications: a systematic review. *Chest* 2001;120:971–978. Search date 2000; primary sources Medline, Cinahl, HealthSTAR and Current Contents databases, and handsearches of reference lists from relevant articles.
26. Fagevik-Olsen M, Hahn I, Nordgren S, et al. Randomized controlled trial of prophylactic chest physiotherapy in major abdominal surgery. *Br J Surg* 1997;84:1535–1538.
27. Stiller K, Montarello J, Wallace M, et al. Efficacy of breathing and coughing exercises in the prevention of pulmonary complications after coronary artery surgery. *Chest* 1994;105:741–747.
28. Hough A. *Physiotherapy in respiratory care: a problem-solving approach.* London: Chapman and Hall, 1991.

Andrew Smith
Dept of Anaesthesia
Royal Lancaster Infirmary
Lancaster
UK

Competing interests: None declared.

Acute organophosphorus poisoning

Search date November 2001

Michael Eddleston, Surjit Singh, and Nick Buckley

QUESTIONS

INTERVENTIONS

*Based on consensus, RCTs would be considered unethical.

See glossary, p 1444

Key Messages

- **Atropine** Consensus supports atropine treatment for organophosphorus poisoning. We found no RCTs comparing atropine with placebo, but such an RCT would now be considered unethical.
- **Glycopyrronium bromide** We found one small RCT of glycopyrronium bromide versus atropine, but it was not large enough to find a clinically important difference.
- **Intravenous benzodiazepines** Consensus supports the use of benzodiazepines for organphosporus induced seizures. We found no RCTs comparing a benzodiazepine versus placebo or another anticonvulsant,but RCTs would be considered unethical.
- **Ipecacuanha (ipecac)** The risks of ipecacuanha probably outweigh any possible benefit.
- **Oximes** One systematic review of oximes found insufficient evidence to determine their clinical effectiveness.
- **Washing the poisoned person** with warm water and soap, and removing contaminated clothes after dermal and mucocutaneous exposure appears important and widely recommended, but this intervention has not been assessed in an RCT.

- **Milk or other home remedies soon after ingestion; gastric lavage, activated charcoal (single or multiple dose); sodium bicarbonate; α_2 adrenergic receptor agonists (clonidine); N-methyl-D-aspartate (NMDA) receptor antagonists** We found insufficient evidence about the effects of these interventions.

DEFINITION Acute organophosphorus poisoning occurs following dermal, respiratory, or oral exposure to either low volatility pesticides (e.g. chlorpyrifos, dimethoate) or high volatility nerve gases (e.g. sarin, tabun). Acetylcholinesterase (see glossary, p 1444) inhibition at synapses results in accumulation of acetylcholine and overactivation of acetylcholine receptors at the neuromuscular junction and in the autonomic and central nervous systems.[1] Early clinical features mainly involve the parasympathetic system: bradycardia, bronchorrhoea, miosis, salivation, lachrymation, defecation, urination, and hypotension. Features of neuromuscular junction (muscle weakness and fasciculation) and central nervous system (seizures, coma) involvement are also common at this stage. An intermediate syndrome has been described (cranial nerve palsies and proximal muscle weakness with preserved distal muscle power after resolution of early cholinergic symptoms) but its definition, pathophysiology, and incidence are still unclear. A late motor or motor/sensory peripheral neuropathy may also develop after recovery from acute poisoning with some organophosphorus compounds.[1]

INCIDENCE/ PREVALENCE The vast majority of cases occur in the developing world following occupational or deliberate exposure to organophosphorus pesticides.[2] Although data are sparse, this appears to be the most important cause of death from deliberate self poisoning worldwide.[3] In Sri Lanka, at least 17 000 cases of organophosphorus or carbamate poisoning occurred during 1999, resulting in 1700 deaths; more than 80% were intentional.[4] Case fatality rates across the developing world are commonly greater than 20%.[3] In central America, occupational poisoning is more common than intentional poisoning and deaths are fewer.[5] Extrapolating from very limited data, the World Health Organization has estimated that each year more than 200 000 people worldwide die from pesticide poisoning;[6] however, these figures are old and widely contested.[2] Most deaths occur in Asia, and organophosphorus pesticides probably represent at least 50% of cases.[3] Deaths from organophosphorus nerve gases occurred in Iran during the Iran–Iraq war;[7] military or terrorist action with these chemical weapons remains a possibility. Twelve people died in the Tokyo attack and thousands probably died in Iran after military or terrorist exposure.

AETIOLOGY/ RISK FACTORS The widespread accessibility of pesticides in rural parts of the developing world makes them an easy option for acts of self harm.[3] Occupational exposure follows the use of toxic compounds because insufficient or inappropriate protective equipment is used.[2]

PROGNOSIS There are no validated scoring systems for categorising severity or predicting outcome, although many have been proposed. The highly variable natural history and difficulty in determining the ingested dose make predicting outcome for an individual inaccurate and potentially hazardous, because people admitted in good condition can deteriorate rapidly and require intubation and mechanical ventilation. Prognosis in acute self poisoning is likely to depend on dose and toxicity of the ingested organophosphorus (e.g. neurotoxicity potential, half life, rate of ageing [see glossary, p 1444], whether activation to the toxic compound is required [pro-poison —see glossary, p 1444], and whether dimethylated or diethylated [see comment under oximes, p 1442]).[8,9] Prognosis in occupational exposure is better because the dose is normally smaller and the route is dermal.

AIMS To prevent death, reduced consciousness or respiratory arrest requiring intubation with or without ventilation, pneumonia, the intermediate syndrome (see definition above), and delayed polyneuropathy; and to reduce the period of ventilation and intensive care.

OUTCOMES Rates of death, intubation, pneumonia; the intermediate syndrome; delayed polyneuropathy; and period of time requiring ventilation or intensive care.

METHODS *Clinical Evidence* search and appraisal November 2001. We searched Medline, Embase, and Cochrane databases, handsearched toxicological and Indian journals, and contacted experts in the field to identify unpublished studies.

QUESTION What are the effects of treatments for acute organophosphorus poisoning? New

OPTION WASHING THE POISONED PERSON AND REMOVING CONTAMINATED CLOTHES

We found no studies of washing the poisoned person and removing contaminated clothes. However, this appears to be an obvious way to reduce further dermal and mucocutaneous exposure, and is widely recommended. Care should be taken to protect healthcare workers through the use of gloves, aprons, and eye protection, with careful disposal of contaminated equipment and person's clothes.

Benefits: We found no systematic review and no RCTs.

Harms: We found no study of complications in poisoned people or healthcare workers removing contaminated clothing from poisoned people. However, severe poisoning requiring intubation and mechanical ventilation has been reported in healthcare workers treating poisoned people.[10] No significant complications from the procedure for the initially poisoned person are envisaged.

Comment: Absorption of organophosphorus compounds through the skin varies greatly, according to the volatility of the organophosphorus, its solvent, and the temperature and hydration of the skin.[11] Absorption of pesticides appears to be low, with studies of malathion, chlorpyrifos, and diazinon suggesting that less that 5% is absorbed and excreted in the urine.[12–14]

OPTION DRINKING MILK SOON AFTER ORAL ORGANOPHOSPHORUS EXPOSURE

We found no evidence for the effectiveness of drinking milk soon after oral organophosphorus poisoning.

Benefits: We found no systematic review and no RCTs.

Harms: We found no study of complications. No significant complications are envisaged.

Comment: This practice is widely used in some countries. Although it appears unlikely to cause harm, a mechanism for benefit is not apparent.

OPTION IPECACUANHA (IPECAC)

We found no evidence for the effectiveness of ipecacuanha in acute organophosphorus poisoning. The significant risk of harm, although not quantified, suggests that it should not be used for organophosphorus poisoning.

Benefits: We found no systematic review and no RCTs.

Harms: We found no study of complications in people with acute organophosphorus poisoning receiving ipecacuanha and no large, high quality RCT comparing ipecacuanha with placebo in any form of poisoning that might have allowed calculation of complication rates. Complications of ipecacuanha may include aspiration, diarrhoea, ileus, dysrhythmias during vomiting, dystonia from treatment of vomiting, and haematemesis from vomiting.[15] Use of ipecacuanha in acute organophosphorus poisoning may be particularly hazardous because most organophosphorus compounds are dissolved in aromatic hydrocarbons, which will cause serious harm if aspirated.[15]

Comment: No human simulated overdose studies of ipecacuanha have been reported for organophosphorus poisoning.[15] One non-systematic review of ipecacuanha in all forms of poisoning found no evidence that it improved outcome in poisoned people.[15] Administration of ipecacuanha may delay administration of activated charcoal and specific treatment for organophosphorus poisoning, in addition to increasing the risk of aspiration.

OPTION GASTRIC LAVAGE

We found no evidence for the effectiveness of gastric lavage in acute organophosphorus poisoning.

Benefits: We found no systematic review and no RCTs.

Harms: We found no study of complications in people with acute organophosphorus poisoning receiving gastric lavage and no large, high quality RCTs comparing gastric lavage with placebo in any form of poisoning that might have allowed calculation of complication rates. Complications of gastric lavage may include aspiration, hypoxia, laryngeal spasm, and oesophageal perforation.[16]

Comment: No human simulated overdose studies of gastric lavage have been reported for organophosphorus poisoning.[16] One non-systematic review of gastric lavage in all forms of poisoning found no evidence that it improved outcome in poisoned people.[16] Gastric lavage may delay administration of activated charcoal and specific treatment for organophosphorus poisoning. However, organophosphorus pesticides have been shown to remain in the gut for lengthy periods,[17] suggesting that an RCT to assess the role of gastric lavage, after protection of the airway, may be important.

OPTION ACTIVATED CHARCOAL (SINGLE OR MULTIPLE DOSE)

We found no evidence for the effectiveness of activated charcoal, in either single or multiple dose regimens, in acute organophosphorus poisoning.

Benefits: We found no systematic review and no RCTs.

Harms: We found no study of complications in people with acute organophosphorus poisoning receiving activated charcoal and no large, high quality RCT comparing activated charcoal with placebo in any form of poisoning that might have allowed calculation of complication rates. Complications of activated charcoal may include aspiration pneumonia, vomiting, diarrhoea, constipation, ileus, and reduced absorption of oral medication.[18–20]

Comment: **Single dose regimens:** We found no human simulated overdose studies of single dose activated charcoal in organophosphorus poisoning.[18] Animal studies indicate that activated charcoal can bind to organophosphorus pesticides.[21] One non-systematic review of single dose activated charcoal in all forms of poisoning found no evidence that it improved outcomes in poisoned people.[18] **Multiple dose regimens:** We found no human simulated overdose studies of multiple dose activated charcoal in organophosphorus poisoning.[19] One non-systematic review of multiple dose activated charcoal in all forms of poisoning found no evidence that it improved outcomes in poisoned people.[19] Activated charcoal may reduce the efficacy of treatments given by mouth. A large RCT of single or multiple dose activated charcoal versus placebo in acute organophosphorus pesticide poisoning will start in Sri Lanka during 2002 and the findings are expected to be reported in 2007.

OPTION ATROPINE

Atropine is the mainstay of treatment for organophosphorus poisoning. We found no RCTs comparing atropine versus placebo. It would be considered unethical to perform such an RCT.

Benefits: Many cases series have demonstrated the ability of atropine to reverse the early muscarinic effects of acute organophosphorus poisoning.[22]

Harms: We found no study of complication rates in people with acute organophosphorus poisoning receiving atropine. Excessive treatment with atropine results in toxicity that is characterised by confusion and tachycardia.[22] In hypoxic people, supplemental oxygen may reduce toxicity due to tachycardia with increased myocardial oxygen demand.

Comment: Atropine competes with the excess of acetylcholine at muscarinic acetylcholine receptors. We found no RCTs, but its effectiveness is now considered to be beyond question. The optimum dose of atropine has not been determined but may vary among poisoned people because of the variation in the dose taken and possibly because of coadministration of an oxime (oximes have been proposed to have anticholinergic action at high dose).[8] The first doses are given as boluses to reverse the muscarinic signs; current recommendations are to then set up an atropine infusion.[8] Recent RCTs from India on the use of oximes have used an infusion of atropine sufficient to keep the pupils at mid-point, heart rate greater than 100 beats a minute, normal bowel sounds, clear lungs, and no bronchorrhoea.[23–26] The atropine dose regimen has not been compared with other regimens with different end points of atropinisation (reaching blood levels of atropine sufficiently high to suppress cholinergic signs clinically).

OPTION GLYCOPYRRONIUM BROMIDE (GLYCOPYRROLATE)

Glycopyrronium bromide has been used instead of atropine because of its reduced incidence of central nervous system adverse effects. We found no large RCT comparing glycopyrronium bromide with atropine.

Benefits: We found no systematic review or RCT comparing glycopyrronium bromide with placebo. It is unlikely that such a trial would be considered ethical unless glycopyrronium bromide and placebo were administered in addition to atropine. We found one small RCT (39 people) comparing glycopyrronium bromide versus atropine; it was not powered to detect differences in the rate of death, ventilation, or intermediate syndrome.[27] People receiving atropine had non-significantly fewer deaths (AR 1/22 [5%] with atropine *v* 2/17 [12%] with glycopyrronium; RR 0.39, 95% CI 0.04 to 3.91), similar risk of requiring ventilation (AR 8/22 [36%] with atropine *v* 6/17 [35%] with glycopyrronium; RR 1.03, 95% CI 0.44 to 2.41), and non-significantly increased risk of a respiratory infection (AR 12/22 [55%] with atropine *v* 5/17 [29%] with glycopyrronium; RR 1.86, 95% CI 0.81 to 4.25) compared with those receiving glycopyrronium bromide.

Harms: We found no study of complication rates in people with acute organophosphorus poisoning receiving glycopyrronium bromide. Treatment with glycopyrronium bromide may result in peripheral anticholinergic effects such as tachycardia, dry mouth, and ileus.[28] When these symptoms arise, this is defined as excessive treatment.

Comment: Glycopyrronium bromide is similar to atropine but is more selective for peripheral cholinergic synapses, resulting in less tachycardia and confusion than with atropine.[28] Animal studies have found that it is less effective at controlling bradycardia and central nervous system complications of organophosphorus poisoning. It is not widely used. We find no large RCT that compared atropine with glycopyrronium bromide. In some regions, glycopyrronium bromide is combined with atropine to limit the central stimulation produced by atropine.

OPTION OXIMES

One systematic review of oximes found insufficient evidence about their effects in acute poisoning.

Benefits: One systematic review of oximes (search date 2002, 2 RCTs, 182 people; the inclusion criterion was any RCT of oximes in organophosphorus poisoned people) assessed pralidoxime in pesticide poisoned people.[9] Neither of the two RCTs found any benefit of pralidoxime. The second RCT found an increased risk of death (AR 16/55 [29%] with pralidoxime *v* 3/55 [5%] with placebo; RR 5.3, 95% CI 1.7 to 17.3), intermediate syndrome (36/55 [65%] with pralidoxime *v* 19/55 [35%] with placebo; RR 1.9, 95% CI 1.3 to 2.9), and requirement for ventilation (36/55 [67%] with pralidoxime *v* 22/55 [40%] with placebo; RR 1.7, 95% CI 1.1 to 2.4) in people receiving 12 g pralidoxime as an intravenous infusion over 3 days.[25,26]

Harms: Neither RCT reported the incidence of complications in people with acute organophosphorus poisoning receiving oximes.[23–26] Complications of oximes include hypertension, cardiac dysrhythmias (including cardiac arrest with rapid administration), headache, blurred vision, dizziness, and epigastric discomfort.[29] Such adverse effects with pralidoxime have been reported only with either rapid administration or doses greater than 30 mg/kg bolus. It may be difficult to distinguish these adverse effects from the effects of organophosphorus. In one study of a different oxime (obidoxime), a high dose regimen (8 mg/kg bolus, then 2 mg/kg/h infusion) produced hepatitis in three of 12 people.[7] Two of six deaths were because of liver failure. The use of pralidoxime in eight people in the same study at a dose of 30 mg/kg bolus, then 8 mg/kg an hour infusion, did not produce hepatitis. A more recently developed oxime (HI-6), has also been used in humans with no reported adverse effects.[30] We found no human studies that assessed the harms of giving oximes for carbamate poisoning (which presents with a similar cholinergic crisis but has a better prognosis).[1]

Comment: Oximes (such as pralidoxime, obidoxime, and HI-6) reactivate inhibited acetylcholinesterases (see glossary, p 1444).[8,9] Reactivation is limited by ageing (see glossary, p 1444) of the acetylcholinesterases and high concentrations of pesticides. Ageing takes longer with diethyl organophosphorus compunds than with dimethyl organophosphorus compound (120 h *v* 12 h). Oximes may therefore be effective only for people presenting after about 12 hours if they have taken a diethyl organophosphorus. Treatment may be beneficial if continued for as long as the person is symptomatic because it may take several days for the pesticide concentration to drop below the point at which the rate of reactivation surpasses reinhibition.[8,9] Both RCTs used doses of pralidoxime that are different from the regimen currently recommended by the World Health Organization (at least 30 mg/kg bolus, then 8 mg/kg/h iv infusion).[25,26] The reporting of the methods was poor and baseline differences in the second RCT suggested that more severely poisoned people may have been randomised to the intervention arm.[9] Post hoc analysis of the first RCT suggested that people receiving pralidoxime 1 g in the first 12 hours may be less likely to develop the intermediate syndrome than those receiving less than 1 g in the first 12 hours (29% *v* 51%; RR 0.58, 95% CI 0.27 to 1.26).[23] Studies in poisoned people indicate that oximes can reactivate acetylcholinesterase but have not been able to prove clinical benefit.[31] *In vitro* studies have also revealed mechanisms whereby oximes may be detrimental.[32] A large RCT will start in Sri Lanka during 2002 and the findings are expected to be reported in 2007.

OPTION SODIUM BICARBONATE

We found no evidence for the effectiveness of sodium bicarbonate in acute organophosphorus poisoning.

Benefits: We found no systematic review and no RCTs.

Harms: We found no study of complications in people with acute organophosphorus poisoning receiving sodium bicarbonate. Dose dependent complications of sodium bicarbonate may include sodium and fluid overload, and decreased oxygen delivery.[33]

Comment: Animal studies suggest that increasing the pH, separate from correction of severe acidosis, improves mortality rates.[34,35] Studies in Brazil[35] and Iran[7] have claimed good results in uncontrolled studies. The mechanism of action of sodium bicarbonate in organophosphorus poisoning is unknown. However, it is unclear whether the limited increase in pH that is possible *in vivo* is sufficient to make a significant difference in organophosphorus hydrolysis rates. Further clinical studies are required.

OPTION BENZODIAZEPINES

Diazepam is standard treatment for organophosphorus induced seizures. We found no RCTs comparing diazepam or other benzodiazepines versus placebo or another anticonvulsant; it would now be considered unethical to perform an RCT comparing benzodiazepines with placebo in people with seizures.

Benefits: Many case series have reported that diazepam controls seizures in acute organophosphorus poisoning.[36]

Harms: We found no study of complication rates in people with acute organophosphorus poisoning receiving diazepam. Excessive treatment with diazepam may result in respiratory depression requiring intubation and ventilation. However, this is also a direct complication of organophosphorus poisoning and it is difficult to distinguish between the two.[36]

Comment: Benzodiazepines such as diazepam, lorazepam, and midazolam are widely used for treating organophosphorus induced seizures. However, the seizures are believed to be started by excess acetylcholine in the brain following acetylcholinesterase (see glossary, p 1444) inhibition, with subsequent disruption of other neurotransmitter systems such as glutamate and catecholamine. Sufficient atropinisation may help to manage organophosphorus induced seizures; other anticholinergic drugs may also be useful, and clinical trials are required. The routine use of benzodiazepines before any seizure occurs has support from animal models, but we found no studies in humans.[37]

OPTION CLONIDINE

We found no evidence concerning the use of clonidine in acute organophosphorus poisoning.

Benefits: We found no systematic review and no RCTs.

Harms: We found no study of complications in people with acute organophosphorus poisoning receiving clonidine. Complications of clonidine may include sedation, hypotension, bradycardia, and (with prolonged use) rebound hypertension.[38]

Comment: Clonidine inhibits the release of acetylcholine from cholinergic neurones and has α_2 adrenergic agonist effects. Animal studies have found that clonidine pretreatment improves survival following organophosphorus poisoning; combination with atropine was more than additive.[39] This treatment has not yet been studied in organophosphorus poisoning in humans.

OPTION N-METHYL-D-ASPARTATE RECEPTOR ANTAGONISTS

We found no evidence for the effectiveness of N-methyl-D-aspartate receptor antagonists in acute organophosphorus poisoning.

Benefits: We found no systematic review and no RCTs.

Harms: We found no study of complications in people with acute organophosphorus poisoning receiving N-methyl-D-aspartate (NMDA) receptor antagonists. Complications of NMDA receptor antagonists in humans include dizziness, vomiting, nausea, stupor, agitation, and hallucinations.[40]

Comment: Primate studies have found that treatment with NMDA receptor antagonists, such as gacyclidine, improves clinical recovery, reduces neural death, and improves electroencephalogram activity following organophosphorus poisoning.[41]

GLOSSARY

Acetylcholinesterase An enzyme that cleaves acetylcholine.
Ageing Esterases (such as acetylcholinesterase and neurotoxic target esterase) are inhibited by organophosphorus through phosphorylation. Inhibited acetylcholinesterase reactivates spontaneously at very slow rates; oximes speed up this reaction. However, phosphorylated acetylcholinesterase may lose an alkyl side chain non-enzymatically, leaving a hydroxyl group in its place ("ageing"). Regeneration is then no longer possible.
Pro-poisons Some organophosphorus pesticides require activation *in vivo* to become toxic.
Rates of ageing The rate depends on the identity of the alkyl side chains on each organophosphorus. Those with two methyl groups will age faster than those with two ethyl groups and thus become unresponsive to oximes at an earlier time.

REFERENCES

1. Ballantyne B, Marrs TC. Overview of the biological and clinical aspects of organophosphates and carbamates. In: Ballantyne B, Marrs TC, eds. *Clinical and experimental toxicology of organophosphates and carbamates*. Oxford: Butterworth Heinemann, 1992:3–14.
2. Karalliedde L, Eddleston M, Murray V. The global picture of organophosphate insecticide poisoning. In: Karalliedde L, Feldman F, Henry J, Marrs T, eds. *Organophosphates and health*. London: Imperial Press, 2001:432–471.

3. Eddleston M. Patterns and problems of deliberate self-poisoning in the developing world. *Q J Med* 2000;93:715–731.
4. Sri Lankan Ministry of Health. Annual Health Bulletin, Sri Lanka 1999. Colombo: Ministry of Health, 2001.
5. Wesseling C, McConnell R, Partanen T, Hogstedt C. Agricultural pesticide use in developing countries: health effects and research needs. *Int J Health Serv* 1997;27:273–308.
6. World Health Organization in collaboration with the United Nations Environment Programme. *Public health impact of pesticides used in agriculture.* Geneva: World Health Organization, 1990.
7. Balali-Mood M, Shariat M. Treatment of organophosphate poisoning. Experience of nerve agents and acute pesticide poisoning on the effects of oximes. *J Physiol Paris* 1998;92:375–378.
8. Johnson MK, Jacobsen D, Meredith TJ, et al. Evaluation of antidotes for poisoning by organophosphorus pesticides. *Emerg Med* 2000, 12:22–37.
9. Eddleston M, Szinicz L, Eyer P, Buckley N. Oximes in acute organophosphorus pesticide poisoning: a systematic review of clinical trials. *Q J Med* 2002;95:275–283. Search date 2002; primary sources Medline, Embase, The Cochrane Library, checking of reference lists, contact with experts, and a web search using Google.
10. Anonymous. Nosocomial poisoning associated with emergency department treatment of organophosphate toxicity: Georgia, 2000. *Morb Mortal Wkly Rep MMWR* 2001;49:1156–1158.
11. Riviere JE, Chang SK. Transdermal penetration and metabolism of organophosphate insecticides. In: Chambers JE, Levi PE, eds. *Organophosphates: chemistry, fate and effects*. San Diego: Academic Press, 1992:241–253.
12. Wester RC, Sedik L, Melendres J, et al. Percutaneous absorption of diazinon in humans. *Food Chem Toxicol* 1993;31:569–572.
13. Krieger RI, Dinoff TM. Malathion deposition, metabolite clearance, and cholinesterase status of date dusters and harvesters in California. *Arch Environ Contam Toxicol* 2000;38:546–553.
14. Griffin P, Mason H, Heywood K, Cocker J. Oral and dermal absorption of chlorpyrifos: a human volunteer study. *Occup Environ Med* 1999;56:10–13.
15. American Academy of Clinical Toxicology, European Association of Poison Centres and Clinical Toxicologists. Position statement: ipecac syrup. *J Toxicol Clin Toxicol* 1997;35:699 709.
16. American Academy of Clinical Toxicology, European Association of Poison Centres and Clinical Toxicologists. Position statement: gastric lavage. *J Toxicol Clin Toxicol* 1997;35:711–719.
17. Futagami K, Otsubo K, Nakao Y, et al. Acute organophosphate poisoning after disulfoton ingestion. *J Toxicol Clin Toxicol* 1995;33:151–155.
18. American Academy of Clinical Toxicology, European Association of Poison Centres and Clinical Toxicologists. Position statement: single-dose activated charcoal. *J Toxicol Clin Toxicol* 1997;35:721–741.
19. American Academy of Clinical Toxicology, European Association of Poison Centres and Clinical Toxicologists. Position statement and practice guidelines on the use of multi-dose activated charcoal in the treatment of acute poisoning. *J Toxicol Clin Toxicol* 1999;37:731–751.
20. Mauro LS, Nawarskas JJ, Mauro VF. Misadventures with activated charcoal and recommendations for safe use. *Ann Pharmacother* 1994;28:915–924.
21. Tuncok Y, Gelal A, Apaydin S, Guven H, Fowler J, Gure A. Prevention of oral dichlorvos toxicity by different activated charcoal products in mice. *Ann Emerg Med* 1995;25:353–355.
22. Heath AJW, Meredith T. Atropine in the management of anticholinesterase poisoning. In: Ballantyne B, Marrs TC, eds. *Clinical and experimental toxicology of organophosphates and carbamates*. Oxford: Butterworth Heinemann, 1992:543–554.
23. Samuel J, Thomas K, Jeyaseelan L, Peter JV, Cherian AM. Incidence of intermediate syndrome in organophosphorus poisoning. *J Assoc Physic India* 1995;43:321–323.
24. Samuel J, Peter JV, Thomas K, Jeyaseelan L, Cherian AM. Evaluation of two treatment regimens of pralidoxime (1gm single bolus dose vs 12gm infusion) in the management of organophosphorus poisoning. *J Assoc Physic India* 1996;44:529–531.
25. Cherian AM, Jeyaseelan L, Peter JV, et al. *Effectiveness of pralidoxime in the treatment of organophosphorus poisoning - a randomised, double-blind, placebo-controlled clinical trial.* INCLEN Monograph series on Critical International Health Issues No. 7, 1997.
26. Cherian AM, Peter JV, Samuel J, et al. Effectiveness of P2AM (PAM – pralidoxime) in the treatment of organophosphorus poisoning. A randomised, double-blind, placebo-controlled trial. *J Assoc Physic India* 1997;45:22 24.
27. Bardin PG, van Eeden SF. Organophosphate poisoning: grading the severity and comparing treatment between atropine and glycopyrrolate. *Crit Care Med* 1990;18:956–960.
28. Ali-Melkkila T, Kanto J, Iisalo E. Pharmacokinetics and related pharmacodynamics of anticholinergic drugs. *Acta Anaesthesiol Scand* 1993;37:633–642.
29. Bismuth C, Inns RH, Marrs TC. Efficacy, toxicity and clinical uses of oximes in anticholinesterase poisoning. In: Ballantyne B, Marrs TC, eds. *Clinical and experimental toxicology of organophosphates and carbamates*. Oxford: Butterworth Heinemann, 1992:555–577.
30. Kusic R, Jovanovic D, Randjelovic S, et al. HI-6 in man: efficacy of the oxime in poisoning by organophosphorus insecticides. *Hum Exp Toxicol* 1991;10:113–118.
31. Worek F, Backer M, Thiermann H, et al. Reappraisal of indications and limitations of oxime therapy in organophosphate poisoning. *Hum Exp Toxicol* 1997;16:466–472.
32. Worek F, Eyer P, Kiderlen D, Thiermann H, Szinicz L. Effect of human plasma on the reactivation of sarin-inhibited human erythrocyte acetylcholinesterase. *Arch Toxicol* 2000;74:21–26.
33. Forsythe SM, Schmidt GA. Sodium bicarbonate for the treatment of lactic acidosis. *Chest* 2000;117:260–267.
34. Cordoba D, Cadavid S, Angulo D, Ramos I. Organophosphate poisoning: modifications in acid base equilibrium and use of sodium bicarbonate as an aid in the treatment of toxicity in dogs. *Vet Hum Toxicol* 1983;25:1–3.
35. Wong A, Sandron CA, Magalhaes AS, Rocha LCS. Comparative efficacy of pralidoxime vs sodium bicarbonate in rats and humans severely poisoned with O-P pesticide. *J Toxicol Clin Toxicol* 2000;38:554–555.
36. Sellstrom A. Anticonvulsants in anticholinesterase poisoning. In: Ballantyne B, Marrs TC, eds. *Clinical and experimental toxicology of organophosphates and carbamates*. Oxford: Butterworth Heinemann, 1992:578–586.

37. Murphy MR, Blick DW, Dunn MA, Fanton JW, Hartgraves SL. Diazepam as a treatment for nerve agent poisoning in primates. *Aviat Space Environ Med* 1993;64:110–115.

38. van Zwieten PA. Centrally acting antihypertensive drugs. Present and future. *Clin Exp Hypertens* 1999;21:859–873.

39. Liu WF. A symptomatological assessment of organophosphate-induced lethality in mice: comparison of atropine and clonidine protection. *Toxicol Lett* 1991;56:19–32.

40. Lees KR, Dyker AG, Sharma A, Ford GA, Ardron ME, Grosset DG. Tolerability of the low-affinity, use-dependent NMDA antagonist AR-R15896AR in stroke patients: a dose-ranging study. *Stroke* 2001;32:466–472.

41. Lallement G, Baubichon D, Clarencon D, Galonnier M, Peoc'h M, Carpentier P. Review of the value of gacyclidine (GK-11) as adjuvant medication to conventional treatments of organophosphate poisoning: primate experiments mimicking various scenarios of military or terrorist attack by soman. *Neurotoxicology* 1999;20:675–684.

Michael Eddleston
Centre for Tropical Medicine
University of Oxford
Oxford
UK

Surjit Singh
Department of Internal Medicine
Postgraduate Institute of Medical
Education and Research
Chandigarh
India

Nick Buckley
Department of Clinical Pharmacology
and Toxicology
Canberra Hospital
Canberra
Australia

Competing interests: None declared.

Paracetamol (acetaminophen) poisoning

Search date March 2002

Nick Buckley and Michael Eddleston

QUESTIONS

INTERVENTIONS

Key Messages

- **Acetylcysteine** One small RCT in people with established paracetamol induced liver failure found that acetylcysteine versus placebo significantly reduced mortality at day 21 (NNT 4, 95% CI 2 to 16). One observational study found that people given early treatment with acetylcysteine were less likely to dcvclop liver damage than untreated historical controls.
- **Methionine** One small RCT in people with blood paracetemol concentrations above the UK standard treatment line found that methionine versus supportive care reduced the risk of hepatotoxicity (NNT 2, 95% CI 2 to 6), but was too small to rule out a clinically important effect on mortality.
- **Activated charcoal (single or multiple dose); gastric lavage; ipecacuanha** We found no evidence from systematic review, RCTs, or cohort studies on the effects of these interventions on mortality, liver failure, or hepatotoxicity.

Paracetamol (acetaminophen) poisoning

DEFINITION Paracetamol poisoning occurs as a result of either accidental or intentional overdose with paracetamol (acetaminophen).

INCIDENCE/ PREVALENCE Paracetamol is the most common drug used for self poisoning in the UK.[1] It is also a common means of self poisoning in the rest of Europe, North America, and Australasia. An estimated 41 200 cases of poisoning with products containing paracetamol occurred in 1989–1990 in England and Wales, with a mortality of 0.40% (95% CI 0.38% to 0.46%). Overdoses owing to paracetamol alone result in an estimated 150–200 deaths and 15–20 liver transplants each year in England and Wales.

AETIOLOGY/ RISK FACTORS Most cases in the UK are impulsive acts of self harm in young people.[1,2] In one study of 80 people who had overdosed with paracetamol, 42 had obtained the tablets for the specific purpose of taking an overdose and 33 had obtained them less than 1 hour before the act.[2]

PROGNOSIS People with blood paracetamol concentrations above the standard treatment line (defined in the UK as a line joining 200 mg/L at 4 h and 30 mg/L at 15 h on a semilogarithmic plot) have a poor prognosis without treatment (see figure 1, p 1453).[4,5] In one study of 57 untreated people with blood concentrations above this line, 33 developed severe liver damage and three died.[4] People with a history of chronic alcohol misuse, use of enzyme inducing drugs, eating disorders, or multiple paracetamol overdoses may be at risk of liver damage with blood concentrations below this line.[6] In the USA, a lower line is used as an indication for treatment but we found no data relating this line to prognostic outcomes.[7] **Dose effect:** The dose ingested also indicates the risk of hepatotoxicity. People ingesting less than 125 mg/kg had no significant hepatotoxicity with a sharp dose dependent rise for higher doses.[8] The threshold for toxicity after acute ingestion may be higher in children, where a single dose of less than 200 mg/kg has not been reported to lead to death and rarely causes hepatotoxicity.[9]

AIMS To prevent liver failure, liver transplantation, or death, with minimal adverse effects.

OUTCOMES Mortality, hepatotoxicity (most commonly defined by the objective criterion of blood aspartate aminotransferase > 1000 U/L), liver failure, or liver transplantation.

METHODS *Clinical Evidence* search and appraisal March 2002 (including a cohort study search). We also contacted experts in the field to identify unpublished studies. We evaluated only interventions that are currently in common use (not, for example, mercaptamine, cimetidine, or dimercaprol).

QUESTION **What are the effects of treatments for acute paracetamol poisoning?**

OPTION **ACETYLCYSTEINE**

One small RCT in people with established paracetamol induced liver failure found that acetylcysteine versus placebo significantly reduced mortality when people were followed for 21 days. One observational study found that people given early treatment with acetylcysteine were less likely to develop liver damage than untreated historical controls.

Benefits: We found no systematic review. We found one RCT (50 people with established paracetamol induced liver failure) that compared intravenous acetylcysteine (150 mg/kg over 15 min, 50 mg/kg over 4 h, and then 100 mg/kg diluted in 5% dextrose over 16 h, continued until death or recovery) versus a placebo infusion of 5% dextrose.[10] It found a borderline significant effect in survival favouring acetylcysteine over dextrose after 21 days (12/25 [48%] with acetylcysteine *v* 5/25 [20%] with 5% dextrose; ARI 28%, 95% CI 3% to 53%; RR 2.4, 95% CI 1.0 to 5.8; NNT 4, 95% CI 2 to 16).

Harms: The RCT did not specifically assess adverse outcomes and none were noted.[10] Four case series suggested that the incidence of adverse effects from intravenous acetylcysteine is 5–15%.[11–14] These were predominantly rash, urticaria, and occasionally more serious anaphylactoid reactions occurring with the initial "loading" dose. In most or all cases, adverse effects responded to temporary stopping of infusions and symptomatic treatment, and did not recur when treatment recommenced. Two deaths have been reported due to a 10-fold miscalculation of the dose, although only half of the loading dose was given in one case.[15] Adverse reactions seem to be more common in people with asthma and those who have non-toxic paracetamol concentrations.[13] Vomiting is common after oral acetylcysteine and occurred in 63% of people in one series despite previous administration of metoclopramide.[14] Oral acetylcysteine can also cause hypersensitivity and anaphylactoid reactions.[16]

Comment: In the RCT, allocation was concealed but treatment was not blinded.[10] There were differences between the groups in prognostic variables (prothrombin time, coma grade) and other treatments, but a possible confounding effect could not be adequately assessed because of the small size of the study. One observational study evaluated the effects of intravenous acetylcysteine in people presenting early to hospital.[4] It found that people treated within 10 hours of ingestion were less likely to develop liver damage than untreated historical controls (2% in treated group *v* 58% in controls). As a result, subsequent RCTs were considered unethical. A systematic review of numerous case series found evidence that acetylcysteine is beneficial in paracetamol poisoning.[11] For both oral and intravenous acetylcysteine, overall hepatotoxicity was worse if treatment was delayed beyond 8–10 hours (1% in those treated within 8 h *v* 46% in those treated after 16 h).[4,11] We found no RCTs of different regimens and no evidence of a difference between oral and intravenous routes of administration.[11] The optimal dose, route, and duration of treatment is unknown. Two recent observational studies comparing different protocols for intravenous[17] and oral[18] acetylcysteine did not find marked differences in outcomes.

OPTION METHIONINE

One RCT in people with blood paracetamol concentrations above the UK standard treatment line was too small to detect a clinically important effect of methionine on mortality. The RCT found a lower risk of hepatotoxicity with methionine versus supportive care.

Benefits: We found no systematic review. One RCT (40 people) compared oral methionine (2.5 g 4 hourly for 4 doses), intravenous mercaptamine (cysteamine) (3.6 g over 20 h), and supportive care in people with blood paracetamol concentrations above the UK standard treatment line.[19] It found no significant effect on mortality (0 deaths with methionine *v* 0 deaths with mercaptamine *v* 1 in the supportive care group). Only 27 people had a liver biopsy. Fewer people suffered grade III hepatic necrosis (0/9 [0%] with methionine *v* 6/10 [60%] with supportive care), or had peak aspartate aminotransferase greater than 1000 U (1/13 [8%] with methionine *v* 8/13 [62%] with supportive care; ARR 54%, 95% CI 16% to 61%; RR 0.13, 95% CI 0.02 to 0.86; NNT 2, 95% CI 2 to 6).

Harms: No serious adverse effects associated with treatment were reported in the RCT, but vomiting after administration of methionine occurred in 8/13 people (62%).[19] The incidence of adverse effects in the control group was not reported.

Comment: Interpretation of liver biopsy results from the RCT was difficult as not all people were tested and an intention to treat analysis was not possible. We found one case series in people treated with methionine in early and late paracetamol poisoning, but there was no untreated group for comparison.[20]

OPTION IPECACUANHA

We found no systematic review, RCTs, or cohort studies of the effects of ipecacuanha in paracetamol poisoning.

Benefits: We found no systematic review, RCTs, or cohort study reporting clinical end points.

Harms: We found no large systematic review, RCT, or cohort study of complications in people poisoned with paracetamol receiving ipecacuanha. Specific complications of ipecacuanha may include aspiration, diarrhoea, ileus, arrhythmia during vomiting, dystonia from treatment for vomiting, and haematemesis from vomiting.[21]

Comment: Human simulated overdose studies suggest that ipecacuanha given within 1 hour could reduce paracetamol absorption but no studies have shown a change in clinical outcome.[22] One non-systematic review of ipecacuanha in all forms of poisoning found no evidence that ipecacuanha improved outcome in poisoned people.[22] Administration of ipecacuanha may delay the administration of activated charcoal and oral antidotes.

OPTION ACTIVATED CHARCOAL (SINGLE OR MULTIPLE DOSE)

We found no evidence of the effects of activated charcoal, whether in single or multiple dose regimens, in paracetamol poisoning.

Benefits: We found no studies that reported clinical outcomes.

Harms: We found no large study of complications in paracetamol poisoned people receiving single doses of activated charcoal. We found no large, high quality RCT comparing activated charcoal versus placebo in any form of poisoning that might have allowed calculation of the incidence of complications. Harms may include aspiration pneumonia, vomiting, diarrhoea, constipation, ileus, and interference with regular medications.[22]

Comment: **Single dose regimens:** Studies of simulated overdose studies in human volunteers suggest that activated charcoal given within 2 hours of paracetamol ingestion decreases absorption by a variable amount and that this amount diminishes with time.[23,24] A protocol for a systematic review has been published[25] and the review is under way (N Buckley, personal communication, 2002). One cohort study in 450 consecutive people who had taken 10 g or more of paracetamol found that those who had been given activated charcoal were significantly less likely to have high risk blood paracetamol concentrations (OR 0.36, 95% CI 0.23 to 0.58).[3] The effect was seen only in those treated within 2 hours, and the study was not large enough to assess the effect of numerous potential confounders.[3] One non-systematic review of activated charcoal in all forms of poisoning found no evidence that activated charcoal improved outcome in poisoned people.[23] **Multiple dose regimens:** We found no studies of simulated overdose that evaluated multiple dose regimens in paracetamol poisoning. One non-systematic review of case series and reports of multiple dose regimens in all forms of poisoning found no evidence that multiple dose regimens improve outcomes in poisoned people.[26] The rapid absorption and short half life of paracetamol suggest a beneficial effect is unlikely.

OPTION GASTRIC LAVAGE

We found no evidence of the effects of gastric lavage in paracetamol poisoning.

Benefits: We found no systematic review, RCTs, or cohort studies that reported clinical outcomes.

Harms: We found no large study of complications in paracetamol poisoned people receiving gastric lavage. Harms may include aspiration of stomach contents, hypoxia, and oesophageal perforation.[21]

Comment: A study of simulated overdose in human volunteers suggest that gastric lavage carried out within 1 hour removes a variable number of paracetamol tablets and that the number diminishes with time.[27] A protocol for a systematic review has been published[25] and the review is under way (N Buckley, personal communication, 2002) One cohort study (450 consecutive people who took ≥ 10 g of paracetamol) found that those given activated charcoal were significantly less likely to have high risk blood paracetamol concentrations (OR 0.36, 95% CI 0.23 to 0.58).[3] The addition of gastric lavage did not decrease the risk further (OR 1.12, 95% CI 0.57 to 2.20). One non-systematic review of gastric lavage in all forms of poisoning found no evidence that gastric lavage improved outcome in poisoned people.[27]

REFERENCES

1. Gunnell D, Hawton K, Murray V, et al. Use of paracetamol for suicide and non-fatal poisoning in the UK and France: are restrictions on availability justified? *J Epidemiol Community Health* 1997;51:175–179.
2. Hawton K, Ware C, Mistry H, et al. Paracetamol self-poisoning. Characteristics, prevention and harm reduction. *Br J Psychiatry* 1996;168:43–48.
3. Buckley NA, Whyte IM, O'Connell DL, et al. Activated charcoal reduces the need for N-acetylcysteine treatment after acetaminophen (paracetamol) overdose. *J Toxicol Clin Toxicol* 1999;37:753–757.
4. Prescott LF, Illingworth RN, Critchley JAJH, et al. Intravenous N-acetylcysteine: the treatment of choice for paracetamol poisoning. *BMJ* 1979;2:1097–1100.
5. Rumack BH, Matthew H. Acetaminophen poisoning and toxicity. *Pediatrics* 1975;55:871–876.
6. Vale JA, Proudfoot AT. Paracetamol (acetaminophen) poisoning. *Lancet* 1995;346:547–552.
7. Smilkstein MJ, Knapp GL, Kulig KW, et al. Efficacy of oral N-acetylcysteine in the treatment of acetaminophen overdose. Analysis of the National Multicentre Study (1976–1985). *N Engl J Med* 1988;319:1557–1562.
8. Prescott LF. Paracetamol overdosage. Pharmacological considerations and clinical management. *Drugs* 1983;25:290–314.
9. Caravati EM. Unintentional acetaminophen ingestion in children and the potential for hepatotoxicity. *J Toxicol Clin Toxicol* 2000;38:291–296.
10. Keays R, Harrison PM, Wendon JA, et al. Intravenous acetylcysteine in paracetamol induced fulminant hepatic failure: a prospective controlled trial. *BMJ* 1991;303:1026–1029.
11. Buckley NA, Whyte IM, O'Connell DL, et al. Oral or intravenous N-acetylcysteine: which is the treatment of choice for acetaminophen (paracetamol) poisoning? *J Toxicol Clin Toxicol* 1999;37:759–767.
12. Chan TY, Critchley JA. Adverse reactions to intravenous N-acetylcysteine in Chinese patients with paracetamol (acetaminophen) poisoning. *Hum Exp Toxicol* 1994;13:542–544.
13. Schmidt LE, Dalhoff K. Risk factors in the development of adverse reactions to N-acetylcysteine in patients with paracetamol poisoning. *Br J Clin Pharmacol* 2001;51:87–91.
14. Wright RO, Anderson AC, Lesko SL, et al. Effect of metoclopramide dose on preventing emesis after oral administration of N-acetylcysteine for acetaminophen overdose. *J Toxicol Clin Toxicol* 1999;37:35–42.
15. Mant TG, Tempowski JH, Volans GN, et al. Adverse reactions to acetylcysteine and effects of overdose. *BMJ* 1984;289:217–219.
16. Perry HE, Shannon MW. Efficacy of oral versus intravenous N-acetylcysteine in acetaminophen overdose: results of an open-label, clinical trial. *J Pediatr* 1998;132:149–152.
17. Dougherty T, Greene T, Roberts JR. Acetaminophen overdose: comparison between continuous and intermittent intravenous N-acetylcysteine 48-hour protocols. *Ann Emerg Med* 2000;36:S83.
18. Woo OF, Mueller PD, Olson KR, et al. Shorter duration of oral N-acetylcysteine therapy for acute acetaminophen overdose. *Ann Emerg Med* 2000;35:363–368.
19. Hamlyn AN, Lesna M, Record CO, et al. Methionine and cysteamine in paracetamol (acetaminophen) overdose, prospective controlled trial of early therapy. *J Int Med Res* 1981;9:226–231.
20. Vale JA, Meredith TJ, Goulding R. Treatment of acetaminophen poisoning. The use of oral methionine. *Arch Intern Med* 1981;141:394–396.
21. Pond SM, Lewis-Driver DJ, Williams GM, et al. Gastric emptying in acute overdose: a prospective randomised controlled trial. *Med J Aust* 1995;163:345–349.
22. Krenzelok EP, McGuigan M, Lheur P. Position statement: ipecac syrup. American Academy of Clinical Toxicology and European Association of Poisons Centres and Clinical Toxicologists. *J Toxicol Clin Toxicol* 1997;35:699–709.
23. Chyka PA, Seger D. Position statement: single-dose activated charcoal. American Academy of Clinical Toxicology; European Association of Poisons Centres and Clinical Toxicologists. *J Toxicol Clin Toxicol* 1997;35:721–741.
24. Rose SR, Gorman RL, Oderda GM, et al. Simulated acetaminophen overdose: pharmacokinetics and effectiveness of activated charcoal. *Ann Emerg Med* 1991;20:1064–1068.
25. Brok J, Buckley N, Gluud C. Interventions for paracetamol (acetaminophen) overdose (Protocol for a Cochrane Review). In: The Cochrane Library, Issue 4, 2001. Oxford: Update Software.
26. American Academy of Clinical Toxicology, European Association of Poison Centres, and Clinical Toxicologists. Position statement and practice guidelines on the use of multi-dose activated charcoal in the treatment of acute poisoning. *J Toxicol Clin Toxicol* 1999;37:731–751.(review)
27. Vale JA. Position statement: gastric lavage. American Academy of Clinical Toxicology, European Association of Poisons Centres, and Clinical Toxicologists. *J Toxicol Clin Toxicol* 1997;35:711–719.(review)

Nick Buckley
Consultant Clinical Pharmacologist and Toxicologist
Canberra Hospital
Canberra
Australia

Michael Eddleston
Wellcome Trust Career Development Fellow
Centre for Tropical Medicine
University of Oxford
Oxford
UK

Competing interests: None declared.

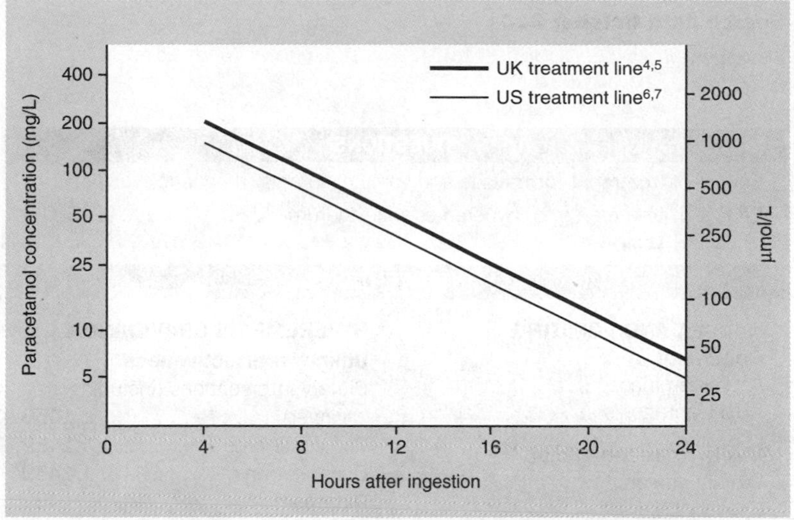

FIGURE 1 **Nomograms used to determine acetylcysteine or methionine treatment, based on the blood concentrations between 4 and 24 hours after ingestion of paracetamol. Published with permission (see text, p 1448).[3]**

Nausea and vomiting in early pregnancy

Search date October 2001

David Jewell

QUESTIONS

INTERVENTIONS

See glossary, p 1460

Key Messages

Nausea and vomiting in pregnancy

- **Antihistamines (H1 antagonists)** One systematic review has found that antihistamines versus placebo significantly reduce the number of women with nausea and vomiting, but increase drowsiness.
- **Cyanocobalamin (vitamin B_{12})** One systematic review has found that cyanocobalamin versus placebo significantly reduces vomiting episodes.
- **Dietary ginger** One RCT found that ginger reduced nausea and vomiting after 4 and 7 days (NNT 2 at 7 days, 95% CI 2 to 3).
- **Dietary interventions (excluding ginger)** We found no RCTs on the effects of other dietary interventions.
- **P6 acupressure** One systematic review including small RCTs found limited evidence that P6 acupressure versus sham acupressure or no intervention significantly reduced self reported morning sickness. One subsequent RCT found that P6 acupressure reduced duration, but not intensity, of nausea and vomiting.
- **Phenothiazines** One systematic review found limited evidence that phenothiazines versus placebo reduced nausea and vomiting.
- **Pyridoxine (vitamin B_6)** One systematic review found limited evidence that pyridoxine versus placebo has no significant effect on vomiting, but may reduce the severity of nausea.

Clin Evid 2002;8:1454–1460.

Hyperemesis gravidarum

- **Corticosteroids** One systematic review found no significant difference in the frequency of hospital admission with corticosteroids versus placebo or antihistamine. The rate of spontaneous resolution of symptoms in control groups was high.
- **Diazepam** One RCT found no significant difference in vomiting with diazepam versus placebo after 2 days, but found that diazepam reduced readmission to hospital.
- **Dietary interventions (including ginger)** One crossover RCT found no significant difference in nausea, vomiting, and weight loss with ginger versus placebo. We found no RCTs on the effects of other dietary interventions.
- **Ondansetron** We found no RCTs of ondansetron versus placebo. One RCT comparing ondansetron versus promethazine found no significant difference in persistence of vomiting.

DEFINITION The severity of nausea and vomiting in early pregnancy varies greatly among women. Hyperemesis gravidarum is persistent vomiting that is severe enough to cause fluid and electrolyte disturbance. It usually requires hospital admission.

INCIDENCE/ PREVALENCE Nausea and vomiting are the most common symptoms experienced in the first trimester of pregnancy, affecting 70–85% of women.[1–3] Only 17% of women report that nausea and vomiting are confined to the morning and 13% are affected beyond 20 weeks' gestation.[2] Hyperemesis is much less common, with an incidence of 3.5/1000 deliveries.[4]

AETIOLOGY/ RISK FACTORS The causes of nausea and vomiting in pregnancy are unknown. One theory, that they are caused by the rise in human chorionic gonadotrophin concentration, is compatible with the natural history of the condition, its severity in pregnancies affected by hydatidiform mole (see glossary, p 1460), and its good prognosis (see below).[4] The aetiology of hyperemesis gravidarum is also uncertain. Again, endocrine and psychological factors are suspected, but evidence is inconclusive.[4]

PROGNOSIS One systematic review (search date 1988, 11 studies) found that nausea and vomiting were associated with a reduced risk of miscarriage (OR 0.36, 95% CI 0.32 to 0.42), but found no relationship with perinatal mortality.[5] Nausea and vomiting and hyperemesis usually improve over the course of pregnancy, but one study found that 13% of women reported nausea and vomiting to persist beyond 20 weeks' gestation.[2]

AIMS To reduce the symptoms of nausea and vomiting in early pregnancy.

OUTCOMES Persistence of nausea and vomiting, or severity of nausea assessed using a nausea score; morbidity and mortality in fetuses and mothers. For hyperemesis, outcomes also included hospital admission.

METHODS *Clinical Evidence* search and appraisal October 2001.

QUESTION **What are the effects of treatment for nausea and vomiting in early pregnancy?**

OPTION **DIETARY**

One RCT found that ginger reduced nausea and vomiting in early pregnancy. We found no evidence about the effects of other dietary interventions.

Benefits: We found no systematic review but found one RCT (70 women) comparing ginger (250 mg in oral capsules taken 4 times daily) versus placebo.[6] The RCT found ginger significantly reduced nausea and vomiting after 4 days (10 point visual analogue scale for nausea: 2.1 reduction with ginger *v* 0.9 reduction with placebo; $P = 0.014$; vomiting episodes: 1.4 reduction with ginger *v* 0.3 reduction with placebo; $P < 0.001$) and after 7 days (AR of reduced nausea on 5 point Lickert scale: 28/32 [88%] with ginger *v* 10/35 [29%] with placebo; ARI 59%, 95% CI 35% to 83%; NNT 2, 95% CI 2 to 3).

Harms: We found no evidence about the harms of ginger. Fewer women had spontaneous abortions with ginger than with placebo, but the difference could have arisen by chance (1/32 [3%] with ginger *v* 3/38 [8%] with placebo; $P = 0.4$).[6]

Comment: None.

OPTION **P6 ACUPRESSURE**

One systematic review has found that P6 acupressure versus sham acupressure (dummy points or placebo wristbands) or no intervention may reduce morning sickness, but that results need to be interpreted with caution.

Benefits: We found one systematic review (search date 2001),[7] which identified the effects of P6 acupressure (see glossary, p 1460) in four RCTs. The review found that acupressure (see glossary, p 1460) reduced the number of women reporting morning sickness (OR 0.35, 95% CI 0.23 to 0.54).[7] However, the authors point out that the odds ratio may be an overestimate as the two trials that could not be included in the summary calculation[8,9] found no evidence of effect and one of these RCTs had the highest completion rate of all four trials (92%). One subsequent RCT of P6 wristband acupressure versus wristband alone (97 women, 8–12 weeks' gestation) found that acupressure reduced duration, but not intensity of nausea and vomiting (WMD 1.89 h/12 h cycle, 95% CI 0.33 to 3.45).[10]

Harms: None reported.

Comment: Conducting high quality trials in this area is difficult, because the condition tends to resolve spontaneously and interventions are difficult to mask and to control with credible placebos. The trial with the largest sample size[11] is subsequently described in a paper[12] that questions the reliability of the randomisation.

OPTION PYRIDOXINE (VITAMIN B_6)

One systematic review of pyridoxine versus placebo in women with nausea and vomiting found a reduction in nausea scores, but not in vomiting.

Benefits: We found one recent systematic review (search date 2001, 2 RCTs, 392 women), which compared pyridoxine versus placebo or no intervention.[7] The review found that pyridoxine did not reduce vomiting (timeframes not specified; OR 0.91, 95% CI 0.60 to 1.38), but that it significantly reduced a nausea score (change in a 10 cm visual analogue scale; WMD 0.9 cm, 95% CI 0.4 cm to 1.4 cm).

Harms: We found a systematic review (search date 1998) that included harms data. It found no increase in major fetal malformations attributable to pyridoxine (RR 1.05, 95% CI 0.60 to 1.84).[13]

Comment: The first review included trials in which the nature of randomisation was unclear.[7]

OPTION CYANOCOBALAMIN (VITAMIN B_{12})

One systematic review has found that cyanocobalamin versus placebo significantly reduces vomiting episodes.

Benefits: We found one systematic review (search date 1998, 2 RCTs, 1018 women), which found that cyanocobalamin (see glossary, p 1460) versus placebo significantly reduced vomiting episodes (timeframes not specified; RR 0.49, 95% CI 0.28 to 0.86).[13]

Harms: The review found no adverse effects.

Comment: The systematic review should be viewed with caution as one RCT accounted for 1000 women and the other RCT only included 18. The review did not provide details on dosing.[13] One of the included RCTs used a dose of cyanocobalamin 25 μg orally, twice daily for 7 days (D Jewell, personal communication, 2001).

OPTION ANTIHISTAMINES (H1 ANTAGONISTS)

One systematic review has found that antihistamines reduce the number of women with nausea and vomiting with no evidence of teratogenicity.

Benefits: We found one systematic review (search date 2001, 7 RCTs, 1 unpublished, 1190 women).[7] It found that antihistamines as a group versus placebo reduced nausea and vomiting (see comment below; timeframes not specified; RR 0.34, 95% CI 0.27 to 0.43).

Harms: We found two systematic reviews (search date 1998[13] and 2001[7]). The first review (24 controlled studies, >200 000 women between 1960 and 1991) found no increase in teratogenicity in women receiving antihistamines (RR 0.76, 95% CI 0.60 to 0.94)[13] The second review (3 RCTs, 179 women) found that antihistamines versus placebo significantly increased drowsiness (23/94 [24%] with antihistamines *v* 9/85 [11%] with placebo; RR 2.3, 95% CI 1.1 to 4.7; NNH 7, 95% CI 3 to 32).[7]

Comment: The trials identified by the second review are old. Detail on randomisation and concealment strategies is not provided.[7] The review combined results from trials in which different antihistamines (e.g. buclizine, dimenhydrinate, doxylamine, hydroxyzine, meclozine) were compared with placebo. Important heterogeneity was found in the meta-analysis, which may be because of the variety of drugs included.[13] One systematic review has found that a combined preparation of doxylamine, dicycloverine (dicyclomine), and pyridoxine reduces nausea and vomiting. This preparation was withdrawn from the market in several countries following publication of papers suggesting teratogenicity, although such claims have subsequently been refuted.

OPTION PHENOTHIAZINES

One systematic review has found that phenothiazines reduce the number of women with nausea and vomiting.

Benefits: One systematic review (search date 1998, 3 RCTs, 398 women) found that phenothiazines versus placebo reduced the number of women with nausea or vomiting (timeframes not specified; RR 0.31, 95% CI 0.24 to 0.42).[13] The results of this review should be interpreted with caution as different phenothiazines were analysed as a group and one of the RCTs recruited women after the first trimester of pregnancy. After excluding this RCT from the review, treatment failure (definition not provided) was found to be reduced with phenothiazines (26/145 [18%] with phenothiazines *v* 89/139 [64%] with placebo; RR 0.28, 95% CI 0.19 to 0.41; NNT 3, 95% CI 2 to 3).

Harms: The review included seven controlled observational trials (78 440 women), which found no evidence of teratogenicity (RR 1.00, 95% CI 0.84 to 1.18).[13] However, harms of different phenothiazines vary, making it difficult to interpret a summary analysis.

Comment: The studies are old and lack sufficient information to appraise the quality of randomisation and allocation concealment. Only two RCTs provide support to the conclusions, and, therefore, conclusions should be drawn with caution.

QUESTION What are the effects of treatments for hyperemesis gravidarum?

OPTION DIETARY

One systematic review found no evidence of benefit from any dietary treatments.

Benefits: We found one systematic review (search date 2001, 1 crossover RCT, 27 women) that compared ginger (250 mg) in oral capsules taken four times daily versus placebo.[7] After 4 days of treatment the RCT found no improvement in a hyperemesis score, which evaluated degree of nausea, vomiting, and weight loss (WMD +3.15, 95% CI –0.92 to +7.22).

Harms: The RCT reported no adverse effects.

Comment: This trial reported results before crossover, but is too small to make reliable conclusions.

OPTION CORTICOSTEROIDS

One systematic review found no evidence of benefit from corticosteroids in hyperemesis.

Benefits: We found one systematic review (search date 1998, 2 RCTs, 71 women) of corticosteroids in hyperemesis.[13] One RCT compared adrenocorticotrophic hormone versus placebo; the second compared oral prednisolone versus promethazine. Meta-analysis of results from the two trials did not find corticosteroids versus either alternative significantly reduced frequency of hospital admissions (RR 1.22, 95% CI 0.35 to 4.17).

Harms: The review, which also included controlled observational studies (8 studies, 109 602 women), did not find evidence of teratogenicity (RR 1.24, 95% CI 0.97 to 1.60).[13]

Comment: Reliable conclusions cannot be drawn from trials included in the review. The rates of spontaneous resolution of symptoms in both control groups were high. Given the difference between treatments in the two RCTs, the appropriateness of pooling results is questionable, although the review did not find significant heterogeneity.

OPTION ONDANSETRON

We found no systematic review or RCT of ondansetron versus placebo. One RCT comparing ondansetron versus promethazine found no difference in persistence of vomiting.

Benefits: We found one systematic review (search date 1998), which identified one RCT (30 women admitted to hospital in the USA) comparing ondansetron (10 mg) versus promethazine (50 mg), both administered by 50 mL solution over 30 minutes.[13] Subsequent doses were given as needed every 8 hours until the person was able to eat a bland diet. The review found no difference in persistence of vomiting between ondansetron and promethazine (OR 0.46, 95% CI 0.06 to 3.35).

Harms: The RCT did not report on adverse effects.

Comment: The small trial[14] was described as a pilot study; it is too small to support reliable conclusions.

OPTION DIAZEPAM

One systematic review found no significant effect on vomiting with diazepam versus placebo.

Benefits: We found one systematic review (search date 2001),[7] which identified one RCT (50 women admitted to hospital in Italy) comparing intravenous fluids containing a multivitamin preparation with or without diazepam 20 mg daily. After symptoms settled, women were randomised to receive oral diazepam 5 mg twice daily for 1 week or placebo. The trial found no difference in persistence of vomiting (assessment not clearly specified) after 2 days of treatment (OR 0.64, 95% CI 0.10 to 4.19), but reported a difference in readmission to hospital (4% with diazepam *v* 27% with placebo; detailed figures not provided).

Harms: The trial did not report on adverse effects or acceptability of treatment.

Comment: The trials were too small to draw reliable conclusions. Rate of resolution in the control group was high.

GLOSSARY

Acupressure Pressure applied to a specific point of the body. It does not require needles and can be administered by women themselves. Commercial products, consisting of an elastic band to fit around the wrist with a plastic disc to apply pressure at the P6 point are available.

Cyanocobalamin Vitamin B_{12} produced for oral administration.

P6 acupressure The P6 (Neiguan) point is an acupuncture point on the volar aspect of the wrist.

Hydatidiform mole A condition in which there is abnormal cystic development of the placenta. The uterus is often large for the duration of pregnancy, and there may be vaginal bleeding, lack of fetal movement and fetal heart sounds, and severe nausea and vomiting. Rarer, but important, complications include haemorrhage, intrauterine infection, raised blood pressure, and persistent gestational trophoblastic disease that may infiltrate local tissues or metastasize to distant sites.

REFERENCES

1. Medalie JH. Relationship between nausea and/or vomiting in early pregnancy and abortion. *Lancet* 1957;2:117–119.
2. Whitehead SA, Andrews PLR, Chamberlain GVP. Characterisation of nausea and vomiting in early pregnancy: a survey of 1000 women. *J Obstet Gynaecol* 1992;12:364–369.
3. Gadsby R, Barnie-Adshead AM, Jagger C. A prospective study of nausea and vomiting during pregnancy. *Br J Gen Pract* 1993;43:245–248.
4. Baron TH, Ramirez B, Richter JE. Gastrointestinal motility disorders during pregnancy. *Ann Int Med* 1993;118:366–375.
5. Weigel MM, Weigel RM. Nausea and vomiting of early pregnancy and pregnancy outcome. A meta-analytical review. *Br J Obst Gynaecol* 1989;96:1312–1318. Search date 1988; primary sources Medline and hand searches of references cited in identified articles.
6. Vutyavanich T, Kraisarin T, Ruangsri R. Ginger for nausea and vomiting in pregnancy: randomized, double-masked, placebo-controlled trial. *Obstet Gynaecol* 97;2001:577–582.
7. Jewell D, Young G. Interventions for nausea and vomiting in early pregnancy. In: The Cochrane Library, Issue 3, 2001. Oxford: Update Software. Search date 2001; primary sources Cochrane Pregnancy and Childbirth Group trials register and the Cochrane Controlled Trials Register.
8. Belluomini J, Litt RC, Lee KA, Katz M. Acupressure for nausea and vomiting of pregnancy: a randomized, blinded study. *Obstet Gynecol* 1994;84:245–248.
9. O'Brien B, Relyea MJ, Taerum T. Efficacy of P6 acupressure in the treatment of nausea and vomiting during pregnancy. *Am J Obstet Gynecol* 1996;174:708–715.
10. Norheim AJ, Pedersen EJ, Fønnebø V, Berge L. Acupressure treatment of morning sickness in pregnancy: a randomised, double-blind, placebo-controlled study. *Scand J Prim Health Care* 2001;19:43–47.
11. Dundee JW, Sourial FBR, Ghaly RG, Bell PF. P6 acupressure reduces morning sickness. *J R Soc Med* 1988;81:456–457.
12. Dundee J, McMillan C. Some problems encountered in the scientific evaluation of acupuncture emesis. *Acupunct Med* 1992;10:2–8.
13. Mazzotta P, Magee LA. A risk-benefit assessment of pharmacological and nonpharmacological treatments for nausea and vomiting of pregnancy. *Drugs* 2000;59:781–800. Search date 1998; primary sources Medline, Pregnancy and Childbirth Module of the Cochrane Database of Systematic Reviews, hand searches of bibliographies of retrieved papers, standard toxicology text (Drugs in Pregnancy and Lactation), and personal contact with pharmaceutical companies, researchers, and clinicians in the fields of pharmacology, toxicology, obstetrics, and paediatrics.
14. Sullivan CA, Johnson CA, Roach H, Martin RW, Stewart DK, Morrison JC. A pilot study of intravenous ondansetron for hyperemesis gravidarum. *Am J Obstet Gynecol* 1996;174:1565–1568.

David Jewell
Honorary Senior Lecturer
University of Bristol
Bristol
UK

Competing interests: None.

Perineal care

Search date April 2002

Chris Kettle and Bazian Ltd (temporary contributors)

QUESTIONS

INTERVENTIONS

See glossary, p 1472

Clin Evid 2002;8:1461–1474.

Perineal care

Key Messages

- **Absorbable synthetic material for perineal repair of first and second degree tears and episiotomies (reduces short term pain)** One systematic review has found that absorbable synthetic suture materials versus catgut sutures significantly reduce analgesia use within 10 days of birth (NNT 18, 95% CI 12 to 35). There was no significant difference between absorbable synthetic suture materials versus catgut sutures in perineal pain or dyspareunia 3 months after birth. One large RCT included in the systematic review found that absorbable synthetic sutures versus catgut sutures significantly reduced dyspareunia at 12 months (NNT 20, 95% CI 11 to 106).
- **Continuous subcutaneous technique of perineal skin closure of first and second degree tears and episiotomies (reduces short term pain)** One systematic review has found that continuous subcutaneous suture versus interrupted, transcutaneous suture of perineal skin significantly reduces pain in the 10 days after birth (NNT 14, 95% CI 10 to 34).
- **Continuous support during labour (reduces instrumental delivery)** One systematic review has found that providing continuous support for women during childbirth versus usual care significantly reduces the rate of instrumental delivery (NNT 41, 95% CI 24 to 239) or episiotomy (NNT 5, 95% CI 3 to 21) but found no significant difference in the risk of perineal trauma.
- **Different methods and materials for repair of third and fourth degree tears** We found no RCTs on the best method or material for repairing third and fourth degree tears and major vaginal lacerations.
- **Epidural anaesthesia (increases instrumental delivery, which is associated with increased rates of perineal trauma)** One systematic review found no direct evidence about the effect of epidural versus other forms of anaesthesia on rates of perineal trauma. However, RCTs found that epidural anaesthesia maintained beyond the first stage of labour versus epidural restricted to the first stage of labour significantly increased risk of instrumental delivery (NNH 10, 95% CI 7 to 20), which in turn is associated with an increased risk of perineal trauma.
- **"Hands poised" versus "hands on" method of delivery (increases pain, no significant difference in rate of perineal trauma and reduces episiotomy rate)** One RCT found that the "hands poised" method (not touching the baby's head or supporting the mother's perineum) versus the conventional "hands on" method (applying pressure to the baby's head during delivery and supporting the mother's perineum) significantly increased perineal pain at day 10 (NNH 33, 95% CI 18 to 212) but reduced episiotomy rates (NNT 38, 95% CI 23 to 106). However, it found no evidence of an effect on the overall risk of perineal trauma or third/fourth degree tears.
- **Midline episiotomy incision (associated with higher risk of third/fourth degree tears compared with mediolateral incision)** We found no evidence that midline episiotomy incision versus mediolateral incision improved perineal pain or wound dehiscence. Limited evidence from one quasi randomised trial suggests that midline incision versus mediolateral incision may increase the risk of third and fourth degree tears (NNH 6, 95% CI 4 to 13).
- **Non-suturing of perineal muscle in second degree tears and episiotomies** One small RCT found no significant difference with non-suturing versus suturing of first and second degree tears in burning sensation or soreness 2–3 days after birth or in healing 2–3 days or 8 weeks after birth.

- **Non-suturing of perineal skin in first and second degree tears and episiotomies (reduces dyspareunia)** One large RCT has found no significant difference between leaving the perineal skin unsutured versus conventional suturing in pain 10 days after birth, but found that non-suturing significantly reduces dyspareunia 3 months after birth.
- **Passive descent in the second stage of labour** One RCT comparing passive fetal descent versus immediate active pushing found no significant difference in perineal trauma.
- **Restrictive use of episiotomy (reduces risk of posterior trauma)** One systematic review has found that restricting episiotomy to specific fetal and maternal indications significantly reduces rates of posterior perineal trauma (NNT 10, 95% CI 8 to 16), need for suturing (NNT 4, 95% CI 4 to 5), and healing complications (NNT 11, 95% CI 7 to 23), but increases the rates of anterior vaginal and labial trauma (NNH 11, 95% CI 9 to 16).
- **Sustained breath holding (Valsalva) method of pushing** One systematic review of two poor quality controlled clinical trials found no significant difference in the extent or rate of perineal trauma when sustained breath holding (Valsalva) versus spontaneous exhalatory methods of pushing are used during the second stage of labour. One additional RCT comparing passive fetal descent with immediate active pushing also found no significant differences in the rates of perineal trauma.
- **Upright versus supine or lateral position during delivery** One systematic review comparing any upright position versus supine or lateral positions for delivery found that an upright position marginally but significantly reduced episiotomies (NNT 17, 95% CI 12 to 35), but this was offset by a significant increase in second degree tears (NNH 40, 95% CI 20 to 574).
- **Vacuum extractor (less perineal trauma than with forceps but newborns have increased risk of cephalhaematoma)** One systematic review has found that the use of the vacuum extractor versus forceps delivery significantly reduces the rate of perineal trauma (NNT 10, 95% CI 8 to 12), but increases the incidence of neonatal cephalhaematoma and retinal haemorrhage (NNH 7, 95% CI 4 to 17).

DEFINITION Perineal trauma is any damage to the genitalia during childbirth that occurs spontaneously or intentionally by surgical incision (episiotomy). Anterior perineal trauma is injury to the labia, anterior vagina, urethra, or clitoris, and is usually associated with little morbidity. Posterior perineal trauma is any injury to the posterior vaginal wall, perineal muscles, or anal sphincter. Depending on severity, posterior perineal trauma is associated with increased morbidity. First degree spontaneous tears involve only skin; second degree involve perineal muscles; third degree partially or completely disrupt the anal sphincter; and fourth degree tears completely disrupt the external and internal anal sphincter and epithelium.[1]

INCIDENCE/ PREVALENCE Over 85% of women having a vaginal birth sustain some form of perineal trauma,[2] and 60–70% receive stitches — equivalent to 400 000 women per year in the UK in 1997.[2,3] There are wide variations in rates of episiotomy: 8% in The Netherlands, 26–67% in the UK, 50% in the USA, and 99% in east European countries.[4–8] Sutured spontaneous tears are reported in about a third of women in the USA[4] and the UK,[6] but this is probably an underestimate because of inconsistency of reporting and classification of perineal trauma. The incidence of anal sphincter tears varies between 0.5% in the UK, 2.5% in Denmark, and 7% in Canada.[9]

AETIOLOGY/ RISK FACTORS Perineal trauma occurs during spontaneous or assisted vaginal delivery and is usually more extensive after the first vaginal delivery.[1] Associated risk factors include parity, size of baby, mode of delivery, malpresentation, and malposition of the fetus. Other maternal factors that may contribute to the extent and degree of trauma are ethnicity, age, tissue type, and nutritional state.[10] Clinicians' practices or preferences in terms of intrapartum interventions may influence the severity and rate of perineal trauma.

PROGNOSIS Perineal trauma affects women's physical, psychological, and social wellbeing in the immediate postnatal period as well as the long term. It can also disrupt breast feeding, family life, and sexual relations. In the UK, about 23–42% of women will continue to have pain and discomfort for 10–12 days post partum, and 7–10% of women will continue to have long term pain (3–18 months after delivery);[2,3,11] 23% of women will experience superficial dyspareunia at 3 months; 3–10% will report faecal incontinence;[12,13] and up to 24% will have urinary problems.[2,3] Complications depend on severity of perineal trauma and on effectiveness of treatment.

AIMS To reduce the rate and severity of trauma; to improve the short and long term maternal morbidity associated with perineal injury and repair.

OUTCOMES Quality of life; incidence and severity of perineal trauma; psychological trauma; short and long term perineal pain; blood loss; infection; wound dehiscence; superficial dyspareunia; stress incontinence; faecal incontinence; adverse effects of treatment.

METHODS *Clinical Evidence* update search and appraisal April 2002, supplemented by a detailed hand search of relevant journals.

QUESTION **What effects do intrapartum surgical interventions have on the risk of perineal trauma?**

OPTION **RESTRICTIVE VERSUS ROUTINE USE OF EPISIOTOMY**

One systematic review has found that restricting the use of episiotomy to specific fetal and maternal indications reduces rates of posterior perineal trauma, need for suturing, and healing complications. Rates of anterior vaginal and labial trauma are slightly increased.

Benefits: We found one systematic review (updated 1999, search date not stated, 6 RCTs, 4850 women) comparing restricted versus routine episiotomy.[14] In the routine episiotomy group 1752/2409 (73%) women had an episiotomy, compared with 673/2441 (28%) women in the restricted group. Restricted use of episiotomy was associated with lower risk of posterior perineal trauma (4 RCTs, 2079 women; 744/1039 [72%] for restricted *v* 849/1040 [82%] for routine; RR 0.88, 95% CI 0.84 to 0.92; NNT 10, 95% CI 8 to 16); less perineal pain at discharge from hospital (1 RCT, 2422 women; 371/1207 [31%] with restricted *v* 516/1215 [42%] with routine; RR 0.72, 95% CI 0.65 to 0.81; NNT 9, 95% CI 7 to 12); less suturing (5 RCTs, 4133 women; 1327/2080 [63.8%] with restricted *v* 1768/2053 [86.1%] with routine; RR 0.74, 95% CI 0.71 to 0.77; NNT 4, 95% CI 4 to 5); and fewer healing complications (1 RCT, 1119 women; 114/555 [21%] with restricted *v* 168/564 [30%] with routine; RR 0.69, 95% CI 0.56 to 0.85; NNT 11, 95% CI 7 to 23). There were no significant differences in the two groups in overall rates of severe vaginal or perineal trauma (3 RCTs, 4284 women; 87/2155 [4%] with restricted *v* 77/2129 [3.6%] with routine; RR 1.11, 95% CI 0.83 to 1.50); dyspareunia within 3 months (1 RCT, 895 women; 96/438 [22%] with restricted *v* 82/457 [18%] with routine; RR 1.22, 95% CI 0.94 to 1.59); suffering dyspareunia in the following 3 years (1 RCT, 674 women; 52/329 [16%] with restricted *v* 45/345 [13%] with routine; RR 1.21, 95% CI 0.84 to 1.75); and urinary incontinence at 3 months (2 RCTs, 1569 women; 140/775 [18%] with restricted *v* 147/794 [19%] with routine; RR 0.98, 95% CI 0.79 to 1.20).

Harms: We found no reports of serious harms associated with restricted use of episiotomy apart from higher rates of anterior perineal trauma, which carries minimal morbidity (4 RCTs, 4342 women; 425/2144 [20%] with restricted *v* 243/2198 [11%] with routine; RR 1.79, 95% CI 1.55 to 2.07; NNH 11, 95% CI 9 to 16).[14]

Comment: The six RCTs included in the review varied in quality. The method of randomisation was not clear in one trial. All trials performed intention to treat analysis. The trials took place in the UK, Canada, and Argentina. The types of episiotomy performed were mediolateral in five of the trials and midline in the sixth.

OPTION TYPE OF EPISIOTOMY INCISION

We found no evidence that midline episiotomy incision improved outcome compared with mediolateral incision. Limited evidence suggests that midline incision may increase the risk of third and fourth degree tears.

Benefits: We found no systematic review comparing mediolateral versus midline episiotomy incisions. However, stratified analysis of data from the systematic review of routine versus restricted episiotomy[14] found no difference in the overall results between midline and mediolateral episiotomies. We found one quasi-randomised trial (407 primigravidas, 24% withdrawals)[15] and one abstract (no detailed data)[16] comparing midline versus mediolateral episiotomies. These were of poor quality and found no evidence of a difference in perineal pain or wound dehiscence.[15,16] Women who had a midline episiotomy experienced significantly less perineal bruising and resumed intercourse earlier.

Harms: The quasi randomised trial found that midline episiotomies increased the risk of third or fourth degree tears (AR 39/163 [24%] with midline episiotomy *v* 22/244 [9%] with mediolateral episiotomy; RR 2.7, 95% CI 1.6 to 4.3; NNH 6, 95% CI 4 to 13).[15] However, these results have to be approached with care because the study limitations compromise their validity. Two retrospective cohort studies, including 5376 primiparous and 341 multiparous women, also found that midline episiotomies were associated with a fourfold increased risk of third and fourth degree tears after allowing for multiple confounders (CI not available).[17,18]

Comment: It is claimed that midline incision is easier to repair and that it is associated with less blood loss, better healing, less pain, and earlier resumption of sexual intercourse. We found no reliable evidence to support these claims. One of the trials had an increased risk of selection bias because of quasi random treatment allocation and because analysis was not by intention to treat.[15] The other trial did not describe the method of treatment allocation.[16]

OPTION EPIDURAL ANAESTHESIA

One systematic review found no direct evidence about the effect of epidural anaesthesia on rates of perineal trauma. However, epidural anaesthesia is associated with an increased risk of instrumental delivery, which in turn is associated with an increased risk of perineal trauma.

Benefits: We found one systematic review (updated 1999, search date not stated, 11 RCTs comparing epidural anaesthesia *v* other forms of analgesia, 3157 women).[19] The RCTs did not report the incidence of perineal trauma. Six trials (1252 women) reported rates of instrumental delivery when the epidural block was maintained beyond the first stage of labour. The women who had epidurals had increased risk of instrumental delivery (8 RCTs, 2 with epidural block in first stage of labour only [131 women] and 6 with block maintained during second stage of labour [1252 women]; 1383 women in total; 186/695 [27%] with restricted *v* 116/688 [17%] with routine; RR 1.56, 95% CI 1.29 to 1.88; NNH 10, 95% CI 7 to 20).

Harms: Analysis of observational evidence found that epidural block was associated with an increased incidence of chronic backache, chronic headache, bladder problems, tingling and numbness, and "sensory confusion".[20]

Comment: The quality of the trials was variable in that the method of randomisation in five of the trials included in the systematic review were not clearly described.

OPTION VACUUM EXTRACTOR VERSUS FORCEPS

One systematic review has found that the use of a vacuum extractor versus forceps delivery reduces the rate of perineal trauma, but increases the incidence of neonatal cephalhaematoma and retinal haemorrhage. One additional case of severe perineal trauma was prevented for every nine occasions that vacuum extraction was used instead of forceps.

Benefits: We found one systematic review (search date 1999, 10 RCTs comparing vacuum extraction *v* forceps, 2885 women).[21] Women allocated to vacuum extraction sustained significantly less perineal injury (7 RCTs, 2582 women; 127/1296 [10%] with vacuum *v*

261/1286 [20%] with forceps; RR 0.46, 95% CI 0.38 to 0.56; NNT 10, 95% CI 8 to 12) and severe perineal pain at 24 hours (1 RCT, 495 women; 21/247 [9%] with vacuum *v* 37/248 [15%] with forceps; RR 0.57, 95% CI 0.34 to 0.94; NNT 16, 95% CI 10 to 119).

Harms: The systematic review found that babies delivered by vacuum extraction were at higher risk of cephalhaematoma (6 RCTs, 1966 women; 98/995 [10%] with vacuum *v* 40/971 [4%] with forceps; RR 2.34, 95% CI 1.64 to 3.35; NNH 17, 95% CI 10 to 35), retinal haemorrhage (5 RCTs, 445 women; 109/224 [49%] with vacuum *v* 74/221 [34%] with forceps; RR 1.46, 95% CI 1.17 to 1.83; NNH 7, 95% CI 4 to 17), and failed delivery with selected instrument (9 RCTs, 2849 women; 166/1436 [12%] with vacuum *v* 102/1413 [7%] with forceps; RR 1.60, 95% CI 1.27 to 2.02; NNH 23, 95% CI 14 to 51).[21]

Comment: The trials in the review varied in quality, some using quasi random treatment allocation.[21] None of the trials attempted to "blind" the allocated intervention during the postnatal assessments. The trials took place in different countries (UK, USA, South Africa, Denmark, Sweden, and Greece), and the procedures in the studies were comparable to everyday practice when an assisted delivery is required. Although some studies were performed in teaching hospitals, they were pragmatic, with wide inclusion criteria. The evidence is likely to be generalisable. We found one new RCT comparing the efficacy and safety of assisted vaginal delivery with forceps and vacuum extractor (awaiting translation and assessment of methodological quality).[22]

QUESTION What effects do intrapartum non-surgical interventions have on the risk of perineal trauma?

OPTION CONTINUOUS SUPPORT DURING LABOUR

One systematic review has found that providing continuous support for women during childbirth versus usual care reduces the rate of instrumental delivery. It found no significant difference in the risk of perineal trauma but could not rule out a clinically important difference.

Benefits: We found one systematic review (search date 2001, 14 RCTs, ≥5000 women) comparing usual care versus continuous support during labour (see glossary, p 1472) from a professional nurse, midwife, or lay person.[23] Women given continuous support versus usual care were less likely to have instrumental delivery (13 RCTs, 4986 women; 351/2424 [15%] with continuous support *v* 433/2562 [17%] with usual care; RR 0.81, 95% CI 0.72 to 0.92; NNT 41, 95% CI 24 to 239) or episiotomy (1 RCT, 145 women; 30/72 [42%] with continuous support *v* 46/73 [63%] with usual care; RR 0.66, 95% CI 0.48 to 0.92; NNT 5, 95% CI 3 to 21), but there was no overall reduction in the risk of perineal trauma (2 RCTs, 588 women; 224/281 [80%] with continuous support *v* 233/277 [84%] with usual care; RR 0.95, 95% CI 0.88 to 1.03).

Harms: We found no evidence of harmful effects. The trials in the review examined a wide range of outcomes, but none revealed harmful effects.[23]

Comment: The trials were of reasonable quality, with 11 using sequentially numbered sealed opaque envelopes for treatment allocation.[23] Only one trial "blinded" the participants to the experimental intervention before randomisation and maintained this throughout the study. Although the experimental intervention was always described as one to one support, the timing and duration varied between trials. The pragmatic trials took place in a wide variety of settings (Europe, Scandinavia, South Africa, and the USA) and found similar results, which suggests that the results are generalisable.

OPTION POSITION DURING DELIVERY

One systematic review comparing any upright position versus supine or lateral positions for delivery found a marginal but significant reduction in episiotomies in the upright group, but this was offset by an increase in second degree tears. Rates of assisted vaginal delivery are slightly reduced in the upright group.

Benefits: We found one systematic review (substantially amended March 1999, search date not stated, 18 RCTs, 5307 women) comparing any upright position for delivery (birthing chairs, stools, cushions, and squatting) versus supine or lateral positions.[24] Fewer episiotomies were performed in the upright group (11 RCTs, 3846 women; 667/1922 [35%] in upright position *v* 782/1924 [41%] in supine or lithotomy position; RR 0.84, 95% CI 0.78 to 0.91; NNT 17, 95% CI 12 to 35), but this was offset by the slight increase in second degree tears in the supine or lithotomy group (10 RCTs, 4257 women; 384/2108 [18%] in upright position *v* 339/2149 [16%] in supine or lithotomy position; RR 1.21, 95% CI 1.07 to 1.37; NNT 40, 95% CI 20 to 574). There was a marginal but significant reduction in assisted vaginal deliveries in the upright group (17 RCTs, 5267 women; 261/2617 [10%] in upright position *v* 308/2650 [12%] in supine or lithotomy position; RR 0.86, 95% CI 0.73 to 1.00) and no significant difference in rates of third and fourth degree tears (4 RCTs, 1478 women; 5/719 [0.7%] in upright position *v* 6/759 [0.8%] in supine or lithotomy position; RR 0.91, 95% CI 0.31 to 2.68).

Harms: Women delivering in the upright position were slightly more at risk of blood loss estimated greater than 500 mL (10 RCTs, 4303 women; 139/2136 [6%] in upright position *v* 82/2167 [4%] in supine or lithotomy position; RR 1.72, 95% CI 1.32 to 2.23; NNH 36, 95% CI 21 to 82) and blood transfusion (2 RCTs, 1747 women; 14/891 [2%] in upright position *v* 8/856 [1%] in supine or lithotomy position; RR 1.66, 95% CI 0.70 to 3.94).[24]

Comment: The findings of this systematic review should be interpreted with caution because of the variable qualities of the trials and diversity of the treatment interventions (squatting, kneeling, Gardosi cushion [see glossary, p 1472], birthing chair).[24] The reviewers state that the main outcome measures may have been affected because of participants being excluded from some of the trials following randomisation, and a number of women allocated to deliver in the upright position had difficulty complying. Further well designed trials are needed with particular attention given to methodological and clinical heterogeneity, observer bias, intention to treat analysis, and standardised objective measurements of blood loss.

OPTION ALTERNATIVE METHODS OF BEARING DOWN (PUSHING)

One systematic review comparing sustained breath holding (Valsalva) versus spontaneous exhalatory methods of pushing during the second stage of labour found no significant difference in the extent or rate of perineal trauma. One additional RCT comparing passive fetal descent versus immediate active pushing also found no significant difference in the rates of perineal trauma.

Benefits: We found one systematic review (search date 1993, 5 trials, 471 women) comparing bearing down by sustained breath holding (Valsalva) versus exhalatory or spontaneous pushing.[25] Only two of the trials provided data on perineal trauma requiring suturing, and they found no significant difference between the two interventions (2 RCTs, 338 women; 57/172 [33%] with sustained Valsalva *v* 66/166 [40%] with exhalatory bearing down; RR 0.83, 95% CI 0.61 to 1.10). One additional RCT (252 women) compared passive fetal descent (see glossary, p 1472) versus active pushing from the start of the second stage of labour.[26] It found no significant difference between bearing down methods for rates of perineal laceration or instrumental delivery (laceration rate in primiparous women 46.9% with passive descent *v* 46.2% with active pushing, P = 0.94; laceration rate in multiparous women 36.4% *v* 33.3%, P = 0.73; rate of instrumental delivery in primiparous women 22.6% *v* 29.7%, P = 0.36; rate of instrumental delivery in multiparous women 3.1% *v* 12.7%, P = 0.078; CIs not reported).

Harms: It is unclear whether the rate of adverse perineal outcomes is affected by different types of bearing down during the second stage of labour.

Comment: The review included published and unpublished trials.[25] Three of the trials were small and of very poor quality. Two of these trials found reduced rates of perineal trauma in the spontaneous bearing down group, but this was not supported by data from the two subsequent more robust controlled trials.

OPTION "HANDS POISED" VERSUS "HANDS ON"

One RCT found that the "hands poised" method (not touching the baby's head or supporting the mother's perineum) versus the conventional "hands on" method (applying pressure to the baby's head during delivery and supporting the mother's perineum) increased short term perineal pain and reduced episiotomy rates. It found no evidence of an effect on the risk of perineal trauma or third/fourth degree tears.

Benefits: We found no systematic review. We found one multicentre RCT (5471 women), which compared the "hands poised" with the "hands on" method of delivery.[2] There was no significant difference between groups in the risk of perineal trauma requiring suturing (1636/2740 [60%] for "hands poised" *v* 1605/2731 [59%] for "hands on"; RR 1.02, 95% CI 0.97 to 1.06) or third/fourth degree tears (40/2740 [1.5%] for "hands poised" *v* 31/2731 [1.2%] for "hands on"; RR 1.3, 95% CI 0.81 to 2.05). In the "hands poised" group, the episiotomy rate was significantly reduced (280/2740 [10%] with "hands poised" *v* 351/2731 [13%] with "hands on"; RR 0.79, 95% CI 0.65 to 0.96; NNT 38, 95% CI 23 to 106), and perineal pain at day 10 was increased (910/2669 [34%] with "hands poised" *v* 823/2647 [31%] with "hands on"; RR 1.10, 95% CI 1.02 to 1.19; NNH 33, 95% CI 18 to 212).

Harms: There was a significant increase in manual removal of placenta in the "hands poised" group (71/2740 [2.6%] with "hands poised" *v* 42/2731 [1.5%] with "hands on"; RR 1.69, 95% CI 1.16 to 2.46; NNH 95, 95% CI 45 to 417).[2]

Comment: This was the only identified trial comparing "hands poised" with "hands on". It was a large robust multicentred pragmatic trial, and the results are likely to be generalisable.

QUESTION What are the effects of different methods and materials for primary repair of perineal trauma, including non-suturing?

OPTION IN FIRST AND SECOND DEGREE TEARS AND EPISIOTOMIES

Two systematic reviews have found that absorbable synthetic suture materials with a continuous subcuticular stitch to appose the skin reduced short term pain compared with catgut sutures. They found no clear difference in the effects on perineal pain or dyspareunia at 3 months post partum. Twelve months' follow up of participants from one large RCT (included in the systematic review) found that absorbable synthetic sutures were associated with reduced dyspareunia. The same RCT found no evidence that leaving the perineal skin unsutured altered short term pain compared with conventional care, which included skin sutures, but dyspareunia was reduced at 3 months post partum.

Benefits: **Non-suturing of perineal skin:** We found no systematic review. We found one RCT carried out in a single centre in the UK in 1780 primiparous and multiparous women who sustained perineal trauma (first and second degree tears or episiotomies) after spontaneous or assisted vaginal delivery.[27] It compared a two stage method of repair (the vagina and perineal muscle was sutured, leaving the perineal skin unsutured but apposed) versus a conventional three stage method (the vagina, perineal muscle, and skin were sutured). It found no significant difference between the two and three stage groups in terms of pain at 10 days post partum (221/886 [25%] with 2 stage suture *v* 244/885 [28%] with 3 stage suture; RR 0.91, 95% CI 0.77 to 1.06), but at 3 months fewer women reported dyspareunia in the two stage group (128/828 [16%] with 2 stage suture *v* 162/836 [19%] with 3 stage suture; RR 0.80, 95% CI 0.64 to 0.99; NNT 26, 95% CI 14 to 345).

Non-suturing of perineal tears: We found no systematic review. We found one small RCT (78 primiparous women in Sweden) comparing non-suturing with suturing of first and second degree tears.[28] Outcomes were assessed after 2–3 days and 8 weeks. The trial found a non-significant difference in "burning sensation" (9/40 [23%] in non-sutured *v* 4/38 [11%] in sutured; RR 0.47, 95% CI 0.16 to 1.39) and in soreness (3/40 [8%] in non-sutured *v* 1/38 [3%] in sutured; RR 0.35, 95% CI 0.04 to 3.23) reported by women at 2–3 days post partum. It reported no significant difference in healing at 2–3 days and 8 weeks post partum (data presented in an unsuitable format for inclusion). **Absorbable synthetic versus catgut sutures:** We found two systematic reviews (search date 1999, 8 RCTs conducted in Europe and the USA, 3681 primiparous and multiparous women;[29] search date 1999, 4 RCTs conducted in Europe, 1864 primiparous and multiparous women[30]). They compared absorbable synthetic versus catgut suture material for repair of episiotomies and second degree tears,[29] and continuous subcuticular versus interrupted sutures to appose the perineal skin.[30] Absorbable synthetic material was associated with less analgesia use within 10 days (5 RCTs, 2820 women; AR 262/1422 [18%] with absorbable synthetic *v* 338/1398 [24%] with catgut; RR 0.74, 95% CI 0.65 to 0.85; NNT 18, 95% CI 13 to 35), and less suture dehiscence, resuturing, and short term pain. There was no clear difference with absorbable synthetic sutures when compared with chromic catgut in perineal pain (2 RCTs; AR 92/1061 [9%] with absorbable synthetic *v* 112/1068 [11%] with chromic catgut; RR 0.86, 95% CI 0.64 to 1.08) or dyspareunia (3 RCTs; AR 171/1086 [16%] with absorbable synthetic *v* 180/1089 [17%] with chromic catgut; RR 0.95, 95% CI 0.79 to 1.15) at 3 months post partum. A follow up for 12 months of one large RCT (793 women),[31] which was included in the systematic review,[29] found that absorbable synthetic sutures (polyglactin 910) was associated with a reduction in dyspareunia when compared with chromic catgut (AR 30/395 [8%] with absorbable synthetic *v* 51/398 [13%] with chromic catgut; RR 0.59, 95% CI 0.39 to 0.91; NNT 20, 95% CI 11 to 106).[32] **Continuous subcutaneous versus interrupted transcutaneous suture:** We found one systematic review (search date 1999).[30] Short term pain was also reduced when a continuous subcutaneous suture was used compared with the interrupted, transcutaneous method of repairing perineal skin (pain up to day 10: 3 RCTs, 1588 women; 160/789 [20%] with continuous sutures *v* 218/799 [27%] with interrupted sutures; RR 0.75, 95% CI 0.63 to 0.89; NNT 14, 95% CI 10 to 34), but there was no clear difference in long term pain (pain at 3 months: 1 RCT, 961 women; 58/465 [13%] with continuous sutures *v* 51/451 [11%] with interrupted sutures; RR 1.1, 95% CI 0.77 to 1.57). Sutures were removed less frequently (suture material removal up to 3 months post partum: 1 RCT, 916 women; 121/465 [26%] with continuous suture *v* 166/451 [37%] with interrupted suture; RR 0.71, 95% CI 0.58 to 0.86; NNT 9, 95% CI 6 to 20), probably as a result of them being less accessible.[30]

Harms: Up to 3 months post partum, suture removal was more common in the absorbable synthetic group than in the catgut group (2 RCTs, 2129 women; 191/1061 [18%] with absorbable synthetic *v* 108/1068 [10%] with catgut; RR 1.78, 95% CI 1.44 to 2.20; NNH 13, 95% CI 8 to 22).[28] We found no reliable evidence that qualifies the harms of leaving perineal muscle unsutured.

Comment: The trials varied in quality and in operator skills and training. It was not possible to "blind" outcome assessment because of the obvious differences in method and materials used. Most of the trials used "intention to treat" as the method of analysis. The RCT comparing "non-suturing of perineal skin to suturing of perineal skin" was a pragmatic study, and the results are likely to be generalisable.[27] An RCT evaluating short term outcomes of non-suturing and suturing in 300 women is in progress (Fleming V, personal communication, 2000). We found no reliable evidence on the effect of leaving minor perineal trauma unsutured (first or second degree tears). Results from the small RCT comparing non-suturing versus suturing must be interpreted with caution because the study limitations compromise the validity of these results.[28] The results of one large RCT (1542 women) comparing an interrupted method of perineal repair with loose continuous technique using two types of absorbable synthetic suture materials should be published next year (Kettle C, personal communication, 2001). Another RCT (pilot study) comparing two different methods for repair of third and fourth degree anal sphincter tears following childbirth is completing a 12 month follow up of participants (Fernando R, personal communication, 2001).

OPTION IN THIRD AND FOURTH DEGREE TEARS

We found no good evidence on the effects of different methods and materials for repair of third and fourth degree tears.

Benefits: We found no systematic review or RCTs.

Harms: We found insufficient data.

Comment: None.

GLOSSARY

Continuous support during labour The presence of a companion (lay person or healthcare worker) who provides continuous social support for the woman during the intrapartum period; social support may include advice, information, assistance, or emotional support.

Gardosi cushion An obstetric aid, used during the second stage of labour, which allows most of the woman's weight to rest on her thighs instead of her feet, while being in a squatting position.

Passive fetal descent An alternative method of bearing down, involving a period of rest to allow passive descent of the fetus before active pushing.

Substantive changes

Alternative methods of bearing down One additional RCT;[26] conclusions unchanged.

REFERENCES

1. Sultan AH, Kamm MA, Bartram CI, et al. Perineal damage at delivery. *Contemp Rev Obstet Gynaecol* 1994;6:18–24.
2. McCandlish R, Bowler U, van Asten H, et al. A randomised controlled trial of care of the perineum during second stage of normal labour. *Br J Obstet Gynaecol* 1998;105:1262–1272.
3. Sleep J, Grant A, Garcia J, et al. West Berkshire perineal management trial. *BMJ* 1984;298:587–690.
4. Graves EJ. 1993 summary: National hospital discharge survey. *Advance Data* 1995;264:1–11.
5. Graham ID, Graham DF. Episiotomy counts: trends and prevalence in Canada, 1981/1982 to 1993/1994. *Birth* 1997;24:141–147.
6. Audit Commission. First class delivery: improving maternity services in England and Wales. London: Audit Commission Publications, 1997.
7. Wagner M. Pursuing the birth machine: the search for appropriate technology. Camperdown: ACE Graphics, 1994;165–174.
8. Williams FL, Florey C du V, Mires GJ, et al. Episiotomy and perineal tears in low-risk UK primigravidae. *J Pub Health Med* 1998;20;422–427.
9. Sultan AH, Monga AK, Kumar D, et al. Primary repair of anal sphincter using the overlap technique. *Br J Obstet Gynaecol* 1999;106:318–323.
10. Renfrew MJ, Hannah W, Albers L, et al. Practices that minimize trauma to the genital tract in childbirth: a systematic review of the literature. *Birth* 1998;25:143–160. Search date 1997; primary sources Cochrane Database of Systematic Reviews, Medline, Cinahl, Miriad, Midirs, Index Medicus, and hand searches of current textbooks of obstetrics, midwifery, and nursing.
11. Glazener CMA, Abdalla M, Stroud P, et al. Postnatal maternal morbidity: extent, causes, prevention and treatment. *Br J Obstet Gynaecol* 1995;102:286–287.
12. Sleep J, Grant A. Pelvic floor exercises in postnatal care. *Br J Midwifery* 1987;3:158–164.
13. Sultan AH, Kamm MA, Hudson CN. Anal sphincter disruption during vaginal delivery. *N Engl J Med* 1993;329:1905–1911.
14. Carroli G, Belizan J. Episiotomy for vaginal birth (Cochrane Review). In: The Cochrane Library, Issue 1, 2002. Oxford: Update Software. Search date not stated; primary sources Cochrane Pregnancy and Childbirth Group Trials Register.
15. Coats PM, Chan KK, Wilkins M, et al. A comparison between midline and mediolateral episiotomies. *Br J Obstet Gynaecol* 1989;87:408–412.
16. Werner CH, Schuler W, Meskendahl I. Midline episiotomy versus mediolateral episiotomy: a randomised prospective study. *Int J Gynaecol Obstet.* Proceedings of 13th World Congress of Gynaecology and Obstetrics (FIGO), Singapore 1991; Book 1:33.
17. Shiono P, Klebanof MD, Carey JC. Midline episiotomies: more harm than good? *Obstet Gynaecol* 1990;75:756–770.
18. Klein MC, Gauthier MD, Robbins JM, et al. Relationship of episiotomy to perineal trauma and morbidity, sexual function, and pelvic floor relaxation. *Am J Obstet Gynecol* 1994;17:591–598.
19. Howell CJ. Epidural versus non-epidural analgesia for pain relief in labour (Review). In: The Cochrane Library, Issue 1, 2002. Oxford: Update Software. Search date not stated; primary source Cochrane pregnancy and Childbirth Group Specialised Register of Controlled Trials.
20. Howell CJ, Chalmers I. A review of prospectively controlled comparisons of epidural with non-epidural forms of pain relief during labour. *Int J Obstet Anaesth* 1992;1:93–110.
21. Johanson RB, Menon BKV. Vacuum extraction versus forceps for assisted vaginal delivery (Cochrane Review). In: The Cochrane Library, Issue 1, 2002. Oxford: Update Software. Search date 1999; primary source Cochrane Pregnancy and Childbirth Group Trials Register.
22. Pliego Perez AR, Moncada Navarro O, Neri Ruz ES, et al. Comparative assessment of efficacy and safety of assisted vaginal delivery with forceps and with vacuum extractor. [Spanish] *Ginecol Obstet Mex* 2000;68:453–459.
23. Hodnett ED. Caregiver support for women during childbirth (Cochrane Review). In: The Cochrane Library, Issue 1, 2002. Oxford: Update Software. Search date 2001; primary sources Cochrane Pregnancy and Childbirth Group Trials Register, CENTRAL, and the Cochrane Controlled Trials Register.
24. Gupta JK, Nikodem VC. Woman's position during second stage of labour (Cochrane Review). In: The Cochrane Library, Issue 1, 2002. Oxford: Update Software. Search date not stated; primary sources Cochrane Pregnancy and Childbirth Group Trials Register, Cochrane Controlled Trials Register, and personal contact with authors of published and unpublished trials.
25. Nikodem VC. Sustained (Valsalva) vs exhalatory bearing down in 2nd stage of labour. In: Enkin MW, Keirse MJNC, Renfrew MJ, et al, eds. Pregnancy and childbirth module. In: The Cochrane Library, Issue 2, 1994. Oxford: Update Software. Search date 1993; primary sources Cochrane Pregnancy and Childbirth Database, Medline, hand search of specialist journals, and conference proceedings.
26. Hansen SL, Clark SL, Foster JC. Active pushing versus passive fetal descent in the second stage of labor: a randomized controlled trial. *Obstet Gynecol* 2002;99:29–34.
27. Gordon B, Mackrodt C, Fern E, et al. The Ipswich Childbirth Study: 1. A randomised evaluation of two stage postpartum perineal repair leaving the skin unsutured. *Br J Obstet Gynaecol* 1998;105:435–440.
28. Lundquist M, Olsson A, Nissen E, et al. Is it necessary to suture all lacerations after a vaginal delivery? *Birth* 2000;27:79–85.
29. Kettle C, Johanson RB. Absorbable synthetic versus catgut suture material for perineal repair (Cochrane Review). In: The Cochrane Library, Issue 1, 2002. Oxford: Update Software. Search date 1999; primary source Cochrane Pregnancy and Childbirth Group Trials Register.
30. Kettle C, Johanson RB. Continuous versus interrupted sutures for perineal repair (Cochrane Review). In: The Cochrane Library, Issue 1, 2002. Oxford: Update Software. Search date 1999; primary source Cochrane Pregnancy and Childbirth Group Specialised Register of Controlled Trials.
31. Mackrodt C, Gordon B, Fern E, et al. The Ipswich childbirth study: 2. A randomised comparison of polyglactin 910 with chromic catgut for postpartum perineal repair. *Br J Obstet Gynaecol* 1998;105:441–445.
32. Grant A, Gordon B, Mackrodt C, et al. The Ipswich childbirth study: one year follow up of alternative methods used in perineal repair. *Br J Obstet Gynaecol* 2001;108:34–40.

Chris Kettle
Midwifery Research Fellow
North Staffordshire Hospital (NHS Trust)
and Keele University
Stoke-on-Trent
UK

Bazian Ltd (temporary contributors)
London
UK

Competing interests: The author was the recipient of a fellowship from the Iolanthe Midwifery Research Trust, which provided funding to enable her to carry out a randomised controlled trial of perineal repair following childbirth — The Methods or Materials Study (MOMS). The Iolanthe Midwifery Research Trust and Ethicon Ltd, UK (manufacturers of suture material) provided funding for employment of a part time data management clerk for the trial. The author has received a Smith & Nephew Fellowship 2001–2002, to provide funding to allow her to complete her research (MOMS) and PhD thesis.

Pre-eclampsia and hypertension

Search date December 2001

Lelia Duley

QUESTIONS

INTERVENTIONS

See glossary, p 1487

Pre-eclampsia and hypertension

Key Messages

Prevention

- **Antiplatelet drugs** One systematic review has found that, in women considered at risk of pre-eclampsia, antiplatelet drugs (mainly aspirin) versus placebo or no treatment significantly reduces the risk of pre-eclampsia (NNT 59, 95% CI 59 to 167), death of the baby (NNT 250, 95% CI 95 to 10 000), and prematurity (NNT 72, 95% CI 44 to 200), with no significant difference in other important outcomes. Two large RCTs of aspirin found no adverse effects in children at 12–18 months old.
- **Calcium supplementation (in high risk women or those with low intake)** One systematic review has found that calcium supplementation (mainly 2g daily) versus placebo reduces the risk of pre-eclampsia and hypertension (NNT 40, 95% CI 28 to 77), and reduces the risk of having a baby with birthweight under 2500 g (NNT 67, 95% CI 36 to 1000). There was no significant effect on the risk of caesarean delivery, preterm delivery, or death of the baby.
- **Other pharmacological interventions** Two small RCTs comparing atenolol or glyceryl trinitrate patches versus placebo were too small to draw reliable conclusions.
- **Magnesium supplementation** One systematic review found insufficient evidence about the effects of magnesium supplements on the risk of pre-eclampsia or its complications.
- **Salt restriction** Limited evidence from one systematic review found no significant difference in the risk of pre-eclampsia with a low salt diet versus a normal diet.
- **Vitamin C and E** One RCT found limited evidence that vitamins C and E versus placebo reduced the risk of pre-eclampsia (NNT 11, 95% CI 8 to 61).
- **Evening primrose oil; fish oil** We found six RCTs of evening primrose and fish oil, which were too small to draw reliable conclusions.

Treatments

- **Aggressive versus expectant management for severe early onset pre-eclampsia** Two RCTs found that a policy of expectant versus agressive management for severe early onset pre-eclampsia reduced the risk of respiratory distress syndrome in the baby. They found insufficient evidence to assess maternal effects.
- **Antihypertensive drugs for mild to moderate hypertension** Two systematic reviews have found that antihypertensive agents versus placebo, no antihypertensive drug or another antihypertensive drug significantly reduce the chance of developing severe hypertension, but found no clear effect on pre-eclampsia and perinatal death. Systematic reviews found that angiotensin converting enzyme inhibitors used in pregnancy were associated with fetal renal failure, and that β blockers increased the risk of the baby being small for its gestational age.
- **Antihypertensive drugs for very high blood pressure (although insufficient evidence on best choice of agent)** One systematic review in women with blood pressures high enough to merit immediate treatment found no evidence of a difference in the control of blood pressure by various antihypertensive drugs, with the possible exceptions of diazoxide and ketanserin, which seem less effective. The studies were too small to draw any further conclusions about the relative effects of different agents.

- **Antioxidants in severe pre-eclampsia** One RCT found insufficient evidence about the effects of a combination of vitamin E, vitamin C, and allopurinol versus placebo.
- **Bed rest/hospital admission** We found insufficient evidence about hospital admission, bed rest, or day care versus outpatient care or normal activities in hospital.
- **Bed rest for proteinuric hypertension** One systematic review found insufficient evidence about the effects of bed rest in hospital versus normal ambulation in hospital.
- **Choice of analgesia during labour with severe pre-eclampsia** One RCT found that epidural analgesia during labour versus intravenous patient controlled analgesia significantly reduced mean pain scores, but the clinical importance of the difference was unclear.
- **Hospital admission for non-proteinuric hypertension** One systematic review found no significant difference in any major outcome with hospital admission versus outpatient clinic assessment.
- **Magnesium sulphate for eclampsia (better than other anticonvulsants)** Systematic reviews have found that magnesium sulphate versus phenytoin, diazepam, or lytic cocktail significantly reduces further fits in women with eclampsia. All reviews found trends towards reduced maternal mortality with magnesium sulphate, although the benefit was not significant.
- **Plasma volume expansion in severe pre-eclampsia** One systematic review found insufficient evidence about the effects of plasma volume expansion versus no expansion.
- **Prophylactic anticonvulsants in severe pre-eclampsia** One systematic review found that prophylactic anticonvulsants may reduce the risk of eclampsia, but found little evidence about the effects on other important outcomes. Limited evidence from case control studies suggests that *in utero* exposure to magnesium sulphate may reduce the risk of cerebral palsy, but it is possible that such exposure may increase infant mortality.

DEFINITION Hypertension during pregnancy may be associated with one of several conditions. **Pregnancy induced hypertension** is a rise in blood pressure, without proteinuria, during the second half of pregnancy. **Pre-eclampsia** is a multisystem disorder, unique to pregnancy, which is usually associated with raised blood pressure and proteinuria. It rarely presents before 20 weeks' gestation. **Eclampsia** is one or more convulsions in association with the syndrome of pre-eclampsia. **Pre-existing hypertension** is known hypertension before pregnancy or raised blood pressure before 20 weeks' gestation. It may be essential hypertension or, less commonly, secondary to underlying disease.[1]

INCIDENCE/ PREVALENCE Pregnancy induced hypertension affects 10% of pregnancies and pre-eclampsia complicates 2–8%.[2] Eclampsia occurs in about 1/2000 deliveries in developed countries.[3] In developing countries, estimates of the incidence of eclampsia vary from 1/100–1/1700.[4,5]

AETIOLOGY/ RISK FACTORS The cause of pre-eclampsia is unknown. It is likely to be multifactorial and may result from deficient placental implantation during the first half of pregnancy.[6] Pre-eclampsia is more common among women likely to have a large placenta, such as those with multiple pregnancy, and among women with medical conditions associated with microvascular disease, such as diabetes, hypertension, and collagen vascular disease.[7,8] Other risk factors include genetic susceptibility, increased parity, and older maternal age.[9] Cigarette smoking seems to be associated with a lower risk of pre-eclampsia, but this potential benefit is outweighed by an increase in adverse outcomes such as low birth weight, placental abruption, and perinatal death.[10]

PROGNOSIS The outcome of pregnancy in women with pregnancy induced hypertension alone is at least as good as that for normotensive pregnancies.[7,11] However, once pre-eclampsia develops, morbidity and mortality rise for both mother and child. For example, perinatal mortality for women with severe pre-eclampsia is double that for normotensive women.[7] Perinatal outcome is worse with early gestational hypertension.[7,9,11] Perinatal mortality also increases in women with severe essential hypertension.[12]

AIMS To delay or prevent the development of pre-eclampsia and eclampsia, and to improve outcomes for women and their children. Once pre-eclampsia has occurred, to minimise morbidity and mortality for the woman and her child, and to ensure that health service resources are used appropriately.

OUTCOMES **For the woman:** Rates of pre-eclampsia (proteinuria and hypertension), eclampsia, death, severe morbidity (such as renal failure, coagulopathy, cardiac failure, liver failure, and stroke), placental abruption, and caesarean section; use of resources (such as dialysis, ventilation, admission to intensive care, or length of stay); adverse effects of treatment. **For the child:** Rates of death, intrauterine growth restriction, prematurity, and severe morbidity (such as intraventricular haemorrhage, respiratory distress syndrome, or asphyxia); measures of infant and child development (such as cerebral palsy or significant learning disability); use of resources (such as admission to special care nursery, ventilation, length of stay in hospital, and special needs in the community); adverse effects of treatment.

METHODS Author search of the register of trials held by the Cochrane Pregnancy and Childbirth Group in November 2000 plus *Clinical Evidence* search and appraisal December 2001. The methods are described in greater detail in the relevant Cochrane reviews.

QUESTION What are the effects of preventive interventions in women at high risk of pre-eclampsia?

OPTION ANTIPLATELET DRUGS

One systematic review has found that, in women considered at risk of pre-eclampsia, antiplatelet drugs (mainly aspirin) versus placebo or no treatment significantly reduces the relative risk of pre-eclampsia (15%), death of the baby (14%), and prematurity (8%), with no significant difference in other important outcomes. Two large aspirin trials that followed children to age 12–18 months have found that aspirin is safe in the short to medium term.

Benefits: We found one systematic review of antiplatelet agents (search date 1999, 39 RCTs, 30 563 women).[13,14] **Versus placebo/no antiplatelet drug:** The systematic review found that, in women considered at risk of pre-eclampsia, antiplatelet agents reduced pre-eclampsia (32 RCTs: 975/14 743 [6.6%] with antiplatelet *v* 1142/14 588 [7.8%] with no antiplatelet; RR 0.85, 95% CI 0.78 to 0.92; NNT 59, 95% CI 59 to 167), premature delivery before 37 completed weeks (23 RCTs: 2447/14 169 [17.3%] with antiplatelet *v* 2621/14 099 [18.6%] with no antiplatelet; RR 0.92, 95% CI 0.88 to 0.97; NNT 72, 95% CI 44 to 200), and baby deaths (30 RCTs: 383/15 091 [2.5%] with antiplatelet v 439/15 002 [2.9%] with no antiplatelet; RR 0.86, 95% CI 0.75 to 0.98; NNT 250, 95% CI 95 to > 10 000). There were no clear effects on other important outcomes. There was no effect of starting treatment before 20 weeks, and no significant difference in the relative risk reduction between women at high and low risk. The benefit was greatest for women given more than 75 mg aspirin daily. **Versus each other:** Trials comparing one antiplatelet agent with another were too small for reliable conclusions.[13]

Harms: The systematic review found no evidence that aspirin increased the risk of bleeding for mother or baby.[13] Two large RCTs that followed up children to age 12–18 months found no differences between the children of mothers given aspirin or placebo.[15,16]

Comment: Almost all studies used low dose aspirin (50–75 mg) and most were placebo controlled. The RCTs included women with a variety of risk factors, including a history of previous early onset disease, diabetes, or chronic hypertension, and were conducted in different countries in the developed and developing world. The number needed to treat values cannot be applied directly to different populations of women; the values stated represent estimates for women with a risk of pre-eclampsia that is an average over all the participants in the RCTs. The absolute benefit was higher (and the NNT lower) in women at higher risk of pre-eclampsia.

OPTION MATERNAL CALCIUM SUPPLEMENTATION

One systematic review has found that calcium supplementation (≥ 1 g daily) versus placebo reduces the risk of pre-eclampsia and hypertension by 30%, and the risk of having a baby with birthweight under 2500 g by 17%. There was no significant effect on the risk of caesarean delivery, preterm delivery, or death of the baby.

Benefits: **Versus placebo:** We found one systematic review of calcium supplementation (search date 2000, 10 RCTs, 7173 women)[17] and one subsequent small RCT.[18] In the review, calcium (mainly 2 g daily) significantly reduced the risk of pre-eclampsia (10 RCTs: 196/3412 [6%] with calcium supplementation *v* 287/3452 [8%] with placebo; RR 0.70, 95% CI 0.58 to 0.83; NNT 40, 95% CI 28 to 77). Subgroup analysis found the strongest effect was for high risk women (8/266 [3%] with calcium supplementation *v* 47/291 [16%] with placebo for high risk women compared with 188/3146 [6%] with calcium supplementation *v* 240/3161 [8%] with placebo for low risk women); and for women with low dietary calcium (27/907

[3%] with calcium supplementation *v* 90/935 [10%] with placebo for low dietary calcium compared with 169/2505 [7%] with calcium supplementation *v* 197/2517 [8%] with placebo for normal dietary calcium). Calcium supplementation significantly reduced the risk of having a baby with birthweight under 2500 g (234/3230 [7.2%] with calcium supplementation *v* 283/3261 [8.7%] with placebo; RR 0.83, 95% CI 0.71 to 0.98; NNT 67, 95% CI 36 to 1000). There was little evidence of effect on the risk of caesarean delivery, preterm delivery, or death of the baby. The small subsequent RCT (placebo controlled, 30 women at high risk of pre-eclampsia) reported results consistent with those of the review.[18] **Calcium and evening primrose oil versus placebo:** One small trial (48 women) did not provide sufficient evidence for reliable conclusions.[19]

Harms: No adverse events were reported in these trials.[17] One large study followed a subgroup of 518 children for 7 years and found no harms associated with long term use of calcium supplementation by their mothers.

Comment: Most trials in the systematic review were of good quality and included a wide range of women. They were conducted largely in the USA and South America. They included mainly women at low risk with adequate dietary calcium, so the number of women in the category who would benefit most from calcium supplementation was small. Several studies reported that adherence to treatment was between 60–90%. The proportion of women taking 90–100% of all allocated treatment was low (20% in 1 study).

OPTION OTHER DIETARY

We found insufficient evidence on the effects of fish oil, or of evening primrose oil plus fish oil plus calcium, on the risk of pre-eclampsia and preterm birth. One RCT found that fish oil was associated with increased risk of post-term delivery and postpartum haemorrhage. One systematic review has found that reduced salt intake (to 20–50 mmol daily) or supplementation with magnesium does not reduce the risk of pre-eclampsia or its complications. One RCT has found that supplementation with vitamins C and E reduces the risk of pre-eclampsia. One small RCT has found that supplementation with protein, fish oil, and calcium, plus rest in the left lateral position, reduces the risk of pre-eclampsia compared with iron supplementation alone.

Benefits: **Fish and evening primrose oil:** We found no systematic review. We found six RCTs of fish and evening primrose oil that were too small to draw reliable conclusions.[20–25] **Protein, fish oil, and calcium, plus rest in left lateral position:** We found one RCT (74 women with a positive roll over test (see glossary, p 1487) at 28–29 weeks).[26] It compared protein (25 mg), fish oil (300 mg), and calcium (300 mg) three times a week plus 15 minutes rest in the left lateral position twice daily versus ferrous sulphate (105 mg) three times a week. It found a reduced risk of pre-eclampsia in the multiple supplements group (2/37 [5%] with multiple supplements *v* 16/37 [46%] with iron alone; RR 0.12, 95% CI 0.03 to 0.51; NNT 3, 95% CI 2 to 6). It was too small for reliable conclusions on other outcomes. **Reduced salt versus normal or high salt:** We found one systematic review (search date 1999, 2 RCTs, 600 women) comparing reduced salt with normal dietary salt.[27] Although these trials were too small for reliable conclusions, together they did not provide any substantive evidence that reducing salt intake during pregnancy affected pre-eclampsia (RR 1.11, 95% CI 0.46 to 2.66). **Magnesium:** We found one systematic review (search date 2001, 2 RCTs, 474 women) reporting pre-eclampsia. The RCTs were too small for reliable conclusions.[28] **Vitamins C and E:** We found one RCT (283 high risk women) that found a reduced risk of pre-eclampsia with vitamin C (1000 mg daily) and vitamin E (400 IU daily) compared with placebo (11/141 [8%] with vitamins *v* 24/142 [17%] with placebo; RR 0.46, 95% CI 0.24 to 0.91; NNT 11, 95% CI 8 to 61).[29] The study was too small to provide reliable evidence about effects on other important outcomes.

Harms: **Fish oil:** One RCT (533 women) found that fish oil compared with either olive oil or no supplement produced an insignificant increase in post-term delivery (RR 1.19, 95% CI 0.73 to 1.93) and postpartum haemorrhage (RR 1.21, 95% CI 0.76 to 1.92).[30] These outcomes were not reported in the other smaller studies. **Fish oil and evening primrose oil:** Vomiting was more commonly reported in the oil treated group, but numbers were not provided.[24] No other adverse events were reported. **Evening primrose oil:** These studies were too small for reliable conclusions. **Reduced salt:** We found no evidence of harmful effects in the trials.[27] **Magnesium:** There was no significant difference between the groups in the number of reported adverse effects (RR 0.84, 95% CI 0.65 to 1.08).[28] **Vitamins C and E:** We found little evidence about the safety of these vitamins at the high doses used in the RCT.[29]

Comment: The fish oil RCTs may have been difficult to blind, because of the distinctive taste of fish oil. One study found that olive oil provided better masking than a no oil placebo.[30] The trials of salt restriction were conducted in the Netherlands, where advice to restrict salt intake during pregnancy has been routine for many years. Such advice is no longer widespread elsewhere. An updated systematic review of fish oil for prevention of pre-eclampsia will be available soon.[31]

OPTION OTHER PHARMACOLOGICAL

We found two small RCTs. One compared atenolol versus placebo and the other compared glyceryl trinitrate patches versus placebo. Both were too small for any reliable conclusions.

Benefits: **Atenolol versus placebo:** We found one small RCT (68 women without hypertension selected because they had a cardiac output > 7.4L/min), which found no significant reduction in the risk of pre-eclampsia with atenolol 100 mg daily (1/28 [4%] with atenolol *v* 5/28 [18%] with placebo; RR 0.20, 95% CI 0.02 to 1.60).[32] **Glyceryl trinitrate versus placebo:** One small RCT (40 women) found no significant difference between glyceryl trinitrate patches versus placebo (RR 1.13, 95% CI 0.35 to 3.60), but the confidence interval was wide.[33]

Harms: The RCT (68 women) of atenolol versus placebo found that mean birthweight was significantly lower with atenolol for a subgroup of primiparous women (mean difference 440 g; P = 0.02).[32]

Comment: Although the possible benefits of atenolol for prevention of pre-eclampsia remain unclear, the reduction in birthweight may be real. Concerns about the possible harmful effects of atenolol on fetal growth and development have been discussed for some time (see harms of antihypertensive agents, p 1484).[34,35]

QUESTION What are the effects of interventions in women who develop hypertension during pregnancy?

OPTION BED REST/HOSPITAL ADMISSION VERSUS DAY CARE

We found inadequate evidence about hospital admission, bed rest, or day care versus outpatient care or normal activities in hospital.

Benefits: **Bed rest/hospital admission versus no hospital admission:** We found two systematic reviews of hospital admission.[36,37] The first systematic review (search date 1993, 3 trials, 408 women) compared hospital admission versus outpatient clinic assessment for non-proteinuric hypertension and found no significant difference for any major outcome.[36] The second systematic review (search date 1993, 2 RCTs, 145 women with proteinuric hypertension) compared bed rest in hospital versus normal ambulation in hospital, but the trials were too small for any reliable conclusions.[37] **Antenatal day care units versus hospital admission:** We found one systematic review (search date 2001, 1 RCT, 54 women).[38] The RCT was too small for reliable conclusions.

Harms: It has been suggested that hospital admission increases the risk of venous stasis, thromboembolic disease, or infection, but we found no evidence in this context. In the trial of day care units, women preferred not to be admitted to hospital. We found no evidence from the other trials about the views of women and their families.

Comment: Trials of hospital admission and bed rest in hospital were conducted before widespread introduction of day care assessment units. Women with hypertension during pregnancy are now often seen in day care units, but only one small trial has compared day care assessment with assessment in an outpatient clinic.

OPTION ANTIHYPERTENSIVE AGENTS

Two systematic reviews have found evidence that antihypertensive agents may reduce by half the chance of developing severe hypertension. The effects of antihypertensive agents on pre-eclampsia and on perinatal death are unclear. We found insufficient evidence for reliable conclusions about any other important outcomes. It remains unclear whether treatment of mild to moderate hypertension during pregnancy is worthwhile with any antihypertensive agent compared with no treatment. Angiotensin converting enzyme inhibitors used in pregnancy are associated with fetal renal failure. β blockers may increase the risk of the baby being small for its gestational age.

Benefits: We found two systematic reviews[39,40] and one subsequent RCT.[41] The first systematic review (search date 2000, 40 RCTs, > 3797 women with mild to moderate hypertension) included studies that compared any antihypertensive versus placebo or versus another antihypertensive.[39] The second systematic review (search date 2000, 27 RCTs, 2400 women) included only studies that compared β blockers versus no antihypertensive drug or versus another antihypertensive drug.[40] **Versus placebo or no antihypertensive:** The only effect was a reduced risk of developing severe hypertension (17 RCTs: RR 0.52, 95% CI 0.41 to 0.64; NNT 12, 95% CI 9 to 17), which was not reflected in other, more substantive, outcomes (pre-eclampsia: RR 0.99, 95% CI 0.84 to 1.18; perinatal death: RR 0.71, 95% CI 0.46 to 1.09).[39] **Versus other antihypertensive agents:** The systematic review[39] found no clear difference between any of these drugs in the risk of developing severe hypertension or pre-eclampsia. The review found that methyldopa versus other antihypertensive agents may increase the risk of the baby dying (14 RCTs: RR 0.49, 95% CI 0.24 to 0.99), but the RCTs were small and used weak methods, so that the difference may have arisen because of random error or bias. The small subsequent RCT (33 women) comparing alternative antihypertensive drugs found no significant differences in the risk of pre-eclampsia.[41]

Harms: The antihypertensive agents included in the systematic reviews[39,40] seem to be well tolerated during pregnancy, but adverse effects have not been reported in many RCTs. All antihypertensive drugs cross the placenta, but few trials reported possible adverse effects for the baby. The baby's risk of being small for its gestational age was increased if a β blocker was used to control the mother's hypertension (13 RCTs: RR 1.34, 95% CI 1.01 to 1.79).[40] Meta regression within a systematic review suggested that lowering blood pressure for women with mild or moderate hypertension may increase the risk of having a baby that is small for its gestational age.[42] One systematic review (search date 1999, 13 small RCTs in women with pre-existing chronic hypertension) found that angiotensin converting enzyme inhibitors used in the second or third trimester are associated with fetal renal failure.[43,44]

Comment: The RCTs were too small to exclude beneficial effects of antihypertensive agents. The trials had problems with their methods. Many were not placebo controlled, and few attempted to blind blood pressure measurement. Many important outcomes were reported by only a few studies. We found little evidence about adherence to treatment. One systematic review found that the effects of antihypertensive agents in women with pre-existing chronic hypertension were similar to those described above for women with pregnancy induced hypertension: the review did not establish or exclude benefit from treatment.[43,44]

QUESTION What are the effects of interventions in women who develop severe pre-eclampsia or very high blood pressure during pregnancy?

OPTION ANTIHYPERTENSIVE DRUGS FOR VERY HIGH BLOOD PRESSURE

One systematic review found no evidence of a difference in the control of blood pressure by various antihypertensive drugs, with the possible exceptions of diazoxide and ketanserin, which seem less effective. Studies were too small for any further conclusions about relative effects of different agents.

Benefits: We found one systematic review (search date 1998, 14 trials, 1200 women), which compared many agents (including hydralazine, labetalol, nifedipine, diazoxide, and ketanserin) mainly with hydralazine.[45] All reduced blood pressure, but there was no significant evidence that any one was better than another.

Harms: The use of ketanserin is associated with more persistent high blood pressure than hydralazine (RR 8.44, 95% CI 2.05 to 34.7), and labetalol is associated with less hypotension requiring treatment than diazoxide (RR 0.06, 95% CI 0.00 to 0.99).[45] Hypotension may compromise fetoplacental blood flow. Only four RCTs reported adverse effects, and frequency varied from 5–50%. Antihypertensives cross the placenta, but we found little evidence about effects on the baby.

Comment: Women in these studies had blood pressures high enough to merit immediate treatment, and many also had proteinuria or "severe pre-eclampsia". The trials were small and reported few outcomes other than control of blood pressure. In most trials there was no blinding after trial entry.

OPTION PLASMA VOLUME EXPANSION

One systematic review of plasma volume expansion versus no expansion found insufficient evidence for reliable conclusions, although the results suggest that benefit is unlikely.

Benefits: We found one systematic review (search date 2000, 3 RCTs, 61 women) evaluating colloid solutions compared with placebo or no infusion. The RCTs were too small for reliable conclusions but suggest that plasma volume expansion is not beneficial.[46]

Harms: RCTs found a non-significant increase in the risk of caesarean section (RR 1.5, 95% CI 0.8 to 2.9), and a non-significant increase in the need for additional treatment (RR 1.5, 95% CI 0.7 to 3.1) with plasma volume expansion versus placebo or no infusion.

Comment: These three RCTs all used a colloid rather than crystalloid solution. Systematic reviews of plasma volume expansion in critically ill men and non-pregnant women have found an increased mortality with albumin (a colloid) when compared with either no expansion or crystalloid.[47,48]

OPTION ANTIOXIDANTS

We found insufficient evidence on the effects of antioxidants.

Benefits: We found no systematic review. We found one RCT (56 women) evaluating combined vitamin E, vitamin C, and allopurinol versus placebo.[49] It was too small for reliable conclusions to be drawn.

Harms: We found insufficient evidence for reliable conclusions.

Comment: Women in this study had severe pre-eclampsia at 24–32 weeks' gestation.

OPTION PROPHYLACTIC ANTICONVULSANTS FOR WOMEN WITH SEVERE PRE-ECLAMPSIA

One systematic review has found that prophylactic anticonvulsants may reduce the risk of eclampsia, but it provides little evidence about effects on other important outcomes. Limited evidence from case control studies suggests that *in utero* exposure to magnesium sulphate may reduce the risk of cerebral palsy, but it is possible that such exposure may increase infant mortality.

Benefits: We found one systematic review (search date 1999, 10 RCTs, 3747 women).[50] **Magnesium sulphate versus placebo or no anticonvulsant:** Four RCTs (1249 women) found reduction in the risk of eclampsia that did not quite reach significance (RR 0.33, 95% CI 0.11 to 1.02). There were no clear effects on other reported outcomes. Limited evidence from case control studies suggests that magnesium sulphate may reduce the risk of cerebral palsy for babies weighing less than 1500 g by as much as 80%.[51,52] One small RCT (59 women) compared diazepam versus no anticonvulsant; it was too small for any reliable conclusions. **Magnesium sulphate versus phenytoin or diazepam:** Five RCTs (2439 women) found that magnesium sulphate was better than phenytoin for preventing eclampsia (RR 0.05, 95% CI 0.00 to 0.84), but there was insufficient evidence for reliable conclusions about magnesium sulphate versus diazepam.[50]

Harms: We found only one RCT (135 women), which reported maternal adverse effects of anticonvulsants. It found a significant increase in flushing (RR 3.81, 95% CI 2.22 to 6.53) and a non-significant increase in slurred speech (RR 3.04, 95% CI 0.13 to 73).[50] Compared with phenytoin, magnesium sulphate was associated with an increased risk of caesarean section (RR 1.21, 95% CI 1.05 to 1.41; NNH 29, 95% CI 12 to 84). One small RCT evaluated magnesium sulphate for preventing and treating preterm labour in women who did not have pre-eclampsia. It found an increase in infant mortality for babies born to these women. Many of the infants had very low birthweight.[53]

Comment: The quality of these RCTs was average to poor. Most trials included women with severe pre-eclampsia. One small study recruited women with mild pre-eclampsia. Results from a large international study (the Magpie Trial) comparing magnesium sulphate with placebo in over 10 000 women with pre-eclampsia will be published in 2002.[54]

OPTION AGGRESSIVE MANAGEMENT FOR SEVERE EARLY ONSET PRE-ECLAMPSIA

Two RCTs found that a policy of expectant or conservative management for severe early onset pre-eclampsia may have substantive benefits for the baby. There was insufficient evidence for reliable conclusions about possible effects for the woman.

Benefits: We found no systematic review. We found two small RCTs (133 women) that, taken together, found expectant management to be associated with reduced risk of respiratory distress syndrome in the baby (RR 2.30, 95% CI 1.39 to 3.81).[55,56] The trials were too small for any reliable conclusions on the effect on perinatal mortality or on maternal morbidity.

Harms: Expectant care aims to gain additional time *in utero* for the baby, but could increase morbidity for the women. We found insufficient evidence for reliable conclusions about possible effects of expectant management on maternal morbidity.

Comment: The women in these trials were at 28–34 weeks' gestation. A systematic review is in preparation.[57]

OPTION CHOICE OF ANALGESIA DURING LABOUR

We found one RCT comparing intravenous patient controlled analgesia during labour with epidural analgesia.

Benefits: We found one RCT (105 women) comparing intravenous patient controlled analgesia versus epidural analgesia.[58] Mean pain scores were significantly lower with an epidural but the clinical importance of the difference is unclear. The trial was too small for a reliable conclusion about other outcomes. We found no RCTs of other forms of intrapartum analgesia for this group of women.

Harms: Neonatal naloxone was more likely to be given following intravenous patient controlled analgesia (28/52 [54%] with intravenous patient controlled analgesia *v* 5/53 [9%] with epidural analgesia; RR 5.71, 95% CI 2.39 to 13.6; NNH 3, 95% CI 2 to 4). No other neonatal outcomes were reported.

Comment: The name of the drug used for patient controlled analgesia was not stated.

QUESTION What is the best choice of anticonvulsant for women with eclampsia?

Systematic reviews have found that magnesium sulphate is better than phenytoin, diazepam, or lytic cocktail for the prevention of further fits in women with eclampsia. Although the effects on maternal mortality are not statistically significant, all reviews have found trends towards reduced risk with magnesium sulphate.

Benefits: **Versus diazepam:** We found one systematic review (search date 1999, 5 RCTs, 1236 women).[59] Magnesium sulphate versus diazepam reduced both maternal mortality (21/617 [3.4%] with magnesium sulphate *v* 36/619 [5.8%] with diazepam; RR 0.59,

95% CI 0.36 to 1.00) and further fits (71/618 [11%] v 160/618 [26%]; RR 0.45, 95% CI 0.35 to 0.58). There was no evidence of any differential effects on any other reported outcome. **Versus phenytoin:** We found one systematic review (search date 1999, 4 RCTs, 823 women)[60] and one subsequent small RCT.[61] Magnesium sulphate versus phenytoin reduced the risks of further fits (23/423 [5.4%] with magnesium sulphate v 73/422 [17%] with phenytoin; RR 0.32, 95% CI 0.21 to 0.50), pneumonia (RR 0.44, 95% CI 0.24 to 0.79), requirement for ventilation (RR 0.66, 95% CI 0.49 to 0.90), and admission to intensive care (RR 0.67, 95% CI 0.50 to 0.89).[60] Fewer babies died or stayed in a special baby care unit for more than 7 days (RR 0.77, 95% CI 0.63 to 0.95). The lower maternal death rate with magnesium sulphate compared with phenytoin was not significant, but the confidence interval was wide and a clinically important effect could not be excluded (RR 0.51, 95% CI 0.25 to 1.06). The small subsequent RCT (50 women) reported results consistent with those of the review.[61] **Versus lytic cocktail:** We found one systematic review (search date 2000, 2 RCTs, 199 women).[62] Magnesium sulphate versus lytic cocktail (see glossary, p 1487) significantly reduced further fits (4/96 [4%] with magnesium sulphate v 49/102 [48%] with lytic cocktail; RR 0.09, 95% CI 0.03 to 0.24), pneumonia (1/51 [2%] v 11/57 [19%]; RR 0.08, 95% CI 0.02 to 0.42), respiratory depression (0/96 [0%] v 8/102 [8%]; RR 0.12, 95% CI 0.02 to 0.91), and fetal or infant death (14/89 [16%] v 30/88 [34%]; RR 0.45, 95% CI 0.26 to 0.79). There was a non-significant reduction in maternal deaths (1/96 [1%] v 6/102 [6%]; RR 0.25, 95% CI 0.04 to 1.43).

Harms: **Versus diazepam:** We found no good evidence from RCTs about harms. **Versus phenytoin:** Clinical experience suggests that magnesium sulphate is safer than phenytoin. **Versus lytic cocktail:** Magnesium sulphate seems to be considerably safer than lytic cocktail.

Comment: Most information about the comparisons with diazepam and phenytoin comes from one large multicentre trial, in which adherence to treatment was 99%. The lytic cocktail trials were conducted in India. Women with both antepartum and postpartum eclampsia were included.

GLOSSARY

Lytic cocktail A mixture of pethidine, chlorpromazine, and promethazine.

Roll over test A test in which a woman lies on her left side for 15 minutes after which blood pressure is recorded. She then rolls into the supine position and, after 5 minutes, blood pressure is measured again. A rise in diastolic blood pressure in the supine position of more than 20 mm Hg is defined as abnormal. The value of this test has been questioned.

REFERENCES

1. Gifford RW, August P, Chesley LC, et al. National high blood pressure education program working group report on high blood pressure in pregnancy. *Am J Obstet Gynecol* 1990;163(5 Pt 1):1691–1712.
2. WHO international collaborative study of hypertensive disorders of pregnancy. Geographic variation in the incidence of hypertension in pregnancy. *Am J Obstet Gynecol* 1988;158:80–83.
3. Douglas K, Redman C. Eclampsia in the United Kingdom. *BMJ* 1994;309:1395–1400.
4. Crowther CA. Eclampsia at Harare maternity hospital. An epidemiological study. *S Afr Med J* 1985;68:927–929.

5. Bergström S, Povey G, Songane F, et al. Seasonal incidence of eclampsia and its relationship to meteorological data in Mozambique. *J Perinat Med* 1992;20:153–158.
6. Roberts JM, Redman CWG. Pre-eclampsia: more than pregnancy-induced hypertension. *Lancet* 1993;341:1447–1451.
7. Taylor DJ. The epidemiology of hypertension during pregnancy. In: Rubin PC, ed. *Hypertension in Pregnancy*. Amsterdam: Elsevier Science, 1988:223–240.
8. Sibai BM, Caritis S, Hauth J. Risks of preeclampsia and adverse neonatal outcomes among women with pregestational diabetes mellitus. National Institute of Child Health and Human Development Network of Maternal-Fetal Medicine Units. *Am J Obstet Gynecol* 2000;182:364–369.
9. MacGillivray I. *Pre-eclampsia. The hypertensive disease of pregnancy*. London: WB Saunders, 1983.
10. Conde-Agudelo A, Althabe F, Belizan JM, Kafury-Goeta AC. Cigarette smoking during pregnancy and risk of preeclampsia: a systematic review. *Am J Obstet Gynecol* 1999;181:1026–1035. Search date 1998; primary sources Medline, Embase, Popline, Cinahl, Lilacs, and hand searches of proceedings of international meetings on pre-eclampsia and reference lists of retrieved articles.
11. Chamberlain GVP, Philip E, Howlett B, Masters K. *British Births*. London: Heinemann, 1970.
12. Sibai B, Lindheimer M, Hauth J, et al. Risk factors for preeclampsia, abruptio placentae, and adverse neonatal outcomes among women with chronic hypertension. *N Engl J Med* 1998;339:667–671.
13. Knight M, Duley L, Henderson-Smart DJ, King JF. Antiplatelet agents for preventing and treating pre-eclampsia. In: The Cochrane Library, Issue 4, 2001. Oxford: Update Software. Search date 1999; primary sources Cochrane Pregnancy and Childbirth Group Trials Register and conference proceedings.
14. Duley L, Henderson-Smart D, Knight M, King J. Antiplatelet drugs for the prevention of pre-eclampsia and its consequences; systematic review. *BMJ* 2001; 322: 329–333. Search date 1999; primary sources Cochrane Pregnancy and Childbirth Group Trials Register and conference proceedings.
15. Grant A, Farrell B, Heineman J, et al. Low dose aspirin in pregnancy and early childhood development: follow up of the collaborative low dose aspirin study in pregnancy. *Br J Obstet Gynaecol* 1995;102:861–868.
16. Parazzini F, Bortolus R, Chatenoud L, Restelli S, Benedetto C. Follow-up of children in the Italian study of aspirin in pregnancy. *Lancet* 1994;343:1235.
17. Atallah AN, Hofmeyr GJ, Duley L. Calcium supplementation during pregnancy for preventing hypertensive disorders and related problems. In: The Cochrane Library, Issue 4, 2001. Oxford: Update Software. Search date 2000; primary source Cochrane Pregnancy and Childbirth Group Trials Register.
18. Niromanesh S, Laghaii S, Mosavi-Jarrahi A. Supplementary calcium in prevention of pre-eclampsia. *Int J Gynaecol Obstet* 2001;74:17–21.
19. Herrera JA, Arevalo-Herrera M, Herrera S. Prevention of pre-eclampsia by linoleic acid and calcium supplementation: a randomized controlled trial. *Obstet Gynecol* 1998;91:585–590.
20. Salvig JD, Olsen SF, Secher NJ. Effects of fish oil supplementation in late pregnancy on blood pressure: a randomised controlled trial. *Br J Obstet Gynaecol* 1996;103:529–533.
21. Onwude JL, Lilford RJ, Hjartardottir H, et al. A randomised double blind placebo controlled trial of fish oil in high risk pregnancy. *Br J Obstet Gynaecol* 1995;102:95–100.
22. Bulstra-Ramakers MTE, Huisjes HJ, Visser GHA. The effects of 3 g eicosapentaenoic acid daily on recurrence of intrauterine growth retardation and pregnancy induced hypertension. *Br J Obstet Gynaecol* 1995;102:123–126.
23. Laivuori H, Hovatta O, Viinikka L, et al. Dietary supplementation with primrose oil or fish oil dose not change urinary excretion of prostacyclin and thromboxane metabolites in pre-eclamptic women. *Prostaglandins Leukot Essent Fatty Acids* 1993;49:691–694.
24. D'Almeida A, Carter JP, Anatol A, Prost C. Effects of a combination of evening primrose oil (gamma linolenic acid) and fish oil (eicosapentaenoic + docahexaenoic acid) versus magnesium, and versus placebo in preventing pre-eclampsia. *Women Health* 1992;19:117–131.
25. Moodley J, Norman RJ. Attempts at dietary alteration of prostaglandin pathways in the management of pre-eclampsia. *Prostaglandins Leukot Essent Fatty Acids* 1989;37:145–147.
26. Herrera JA. Nutritional factors and rest reduce pregnancy-induced hypertension and pre-eclampsia in positive roll-over test primigravidas. *Int J Gynaecol Obstet* 1993;41:31–35.
27. Duley L, Henderson-Smart D. Reduced salt intake compared to normal dietary salt, or high intake, in pregnancy. In: The Cochrane Library, Issue 4, 2001. Oxford: Update Software. Search date 1999; primary source Cochrane Pregnancy and Childbirth Group Trials Register.
28. Makrides M, Crowther CA. Magnesium supplementation in pregnancy. In: The Cochrane Library, Issue 4, 2001. Oxford: Update Software. Search date 2001; primary source Cochrane Pregnancy and Childbirth Group Trials Register.
29. Chappell LC, Seed PT, Briley AL, et al. Effect of antioxidants on the occurrence of pre-eclampsia in women at increased risk: a randomised trial. *Lancet* 1999;354:810–816.
30. Olsen SF, Sorensen JD, Secher NJ, et al. Randomised controlled trial of effect of fish oil supplementation on pregnancy duration. *Lancet* 1992;339:1003–1007.
31. Makrides M, Duley L, Olsen SF. Fish oil and other prostaglandin precursor supplementation during pregnancy for reducing pre-eclampsia, preterm birth, low birth weight and intrauterine growth restriction (Protocol for a Cochrane Review). In: The Cochrane Library, Issue 4, 2001. Oxford: Update Software.
32. Easterling TR, Brateng D, Schucker B, Brown Z, Millard SP. Prevention of preeclampsia: a randomized trial of atenolol in hyperdynamic patients before onset of hypertension. *Obstet Gynecol* 1999;93:725–733.
33. Lees C, Valensise H, Black R, et al. The efficacy and fetal-maternal cardiovascular effects of transdermal glycerol trinitrate in the prophylaxis of pre-eclampsia and its complications: a randomized double blind placebo controlled trial. *Ultrasound Obstet Gynaecol* 1998;12:334–338.
34. Butters L, Kennedy S, Rubin PC. Atenolol in essential hypertension during pregnancy. *BMJ* 1990;301:587–589.
35. Churchill D, Bayliss H, Beevers G. Fetal growth restriction. *Lancet* 1999;355:1366–1367.

36. Duley L. Hospitalisation for non-proteinuric pregnancy hypertension. In: Keirse MJNC, Renfrew MJ, Neilson JP, et al, eds. *Pregnancy and childbirth module*. In: The Cochrane Library, Issue 2, 1995. Oxford: Update Software. Search date 1993; primary source Cochrane Pregnancy and Childbirth Group Trials Register.
37. Duley L. Strict bed rest for proteinuric hypertension in pregnancy. In: Keirse MJNC, Renfrew MJ, Neilson JP, et al, eds. *Pregnancy and childbirth module*. In: The Cochrane Library, Issue 4, 1995. Oxford: Update Software. Search date 1993; primary source Cochrane Pregnancy and Childbirth Group Trials Register.
38. Kröner C, Turnbull D, Wilkinson C. Antenatal day care units versus hospital admission for women with complicated pregnancy. In: The Cochrane Library, Issue 4, 2001. Oxford: Update Software. Search date 2001, primary sources Cochrane Pregnancy and Childbirth Group Trials Register, Cochrane Controlled Trials Register, Cinahl, Current Contents, and conference proceedings.
39. Abalos E, Duley L, Steyn DW, Henderson-Smart DJ. Antihypertensive drug therapy for mild to moderate hypertension during pregnancy. In: The Cochrane Library, Issue 4, 2001. Oxford: Update Software. Search date 2000; primary sources Cochrane Pregnancy and Childbirth Group Trials Register, Cochrane Controlled Trials Register, Medline, and Embase.
40. Magee LA, Duley L. Oral beta-blockers for mild to moderate hypertension during pregnancy. In: The Cochrane Library, Issue 4, 2001. Oxford: Update Software. Search date 2000; primary sources Cochrane Pregnancy and Childbirth Group Trial Register, Medline, and hand searches of reference lists.
41. Rudnicki M, Frolich A, Pilsgaard K, et al. Comparison of magnesium and methyldopa for the control of blood pressure in pregnancies complicated with hypertension. *Gynecol Obstet Invest* 2000;49:231–235.
42. Von Dadelszen P, Ornstein MP, Bull SB, Logan AG, Koren G, Magee LA. Fall in mean arterial pressure and fetal growth restriction in pregnancy hypertension: a meta-analysis. *Lancet* 2000;355:87–92. Search date 1997; primary sources Medline, Embase, hand searches of reference lists, *Hypertension and Pregnancy* 1992–1997, and a standard toxicology text.
43. Ferrer RL, Sibai BM, Mulrow CD, Chiquette E, Stevens KR, Cornell J. Management of mild chronic hypertension during pregnancy: a review. *Obstetrics & Gynecology* 2000; 96: 849–860. Search date 1999; primary sources 16 electronic databases, textbook references, and experts.
44. Mulrow CD, Chiquette E, Ferrer RL, et al. Management of chronic hypertension during pregnancy. Evidence Report/Technology Assessment No 14 (prepared by the San Antonio Evidence-based Practice Center based at the University of Texas Health Science Center at San Antonio under Contract No 290–97-0012). AHRQ Publication No 00-E011. Rockville, MD: Agency for Healthcare Research and Quality. August 2000. http://www.ahrq.gov/clinic/pregsum.htm (accessed 1/3/02) Search date 1999; primary sources 16 electronic databases, textbook references, and experts.
45. Duley L, Henderson-Smart DJ. Drugs for rapid treatment of very high blood pressure during pregnancy. In: The Cochrane Library, Issue 4, 2001. Oxford: Update Software. Search date 1998; primary source Cochrane Pregnancy and Childbirth Group Trials Register.
46. Duley L, Williams J, Henderson-Smart DJ. Plasma volume expansion for treatment of pre-eclampsia. In: The Cochrane Library, Issue 4, 2001. Oxford: Update Software. Search date 2000; primary source Cochrane Pregnancy and Childbirth Group Trials Register.
47. The Albumin Reviewers (Alderson P, Bunn F, Li Wan Po L, Roberts I, Schierhout I). Human albumin solution for resuscitation and volume expansion in critically ill patients. In: The Cochrane Library, Issue 4, 2001. Oxford: Update Software. Search date 1999; primary sources Cochrane Injuries Group Trials Register, Cochrane Controlled Trials Register, Medline, Embase, Bids Scientific and Technical Proceedings, hand searches of reference lists of trials and review articles, and personal contact with authors of identified trials.
48. Alderson P, Schierhout G, Roberts I, Bunn F. Colloids versus crystalloids for fluid resuscitation in critically ill patients. In: The Cochrane Library, Issue 4, 2001. Oxford: Update Software. Search date 1999; primary sources Cochrane Clinical Trials Register, Medline, Embase, Bids Index to Scientific and Technical Proceedings, and reference lists of trials and review articles.
49. Gülmezoglu AM, Hofmeyr GJ, Oosthuizen MMJ. Antioxidants in the treatment of severe preeclampsia: a randomized explanatory study. *Br J Obstet Gynaecol* 1997;104:689–696.
50. Duley L, Gülmezoglu AM, Henderson-Smart D. Anticonvulsants for women with pre-eclampsia. In: The Cochrane Library, Issue 4, 2001. Oxford: Update Software. Search date 1999; primary source Cochrane Pregnancy and Childbirth Group Trials Register.
51. Nelson K, Grether JK. Can magnesium sulfate reduce the risk of cerebral palsy in very low birthweight infants? *Pediatrics* 1995;95:263–269.
52. Schendel DE, Berg CJ, Yeargin-Allsopp M, et al. Prenatal magnesium sulfate exposure and the risk of cerebral palsy or mental retardation among very low-birth-weight children aged 3 to 5 years. *JAMA* 1996;276:1805–1810.
53. Mittendorf R, Covert R, Boman J, et al. Is tocolytic magnesium sulphate associated with increased total paediatric mortality? *Lancet* 1997;350:1517–1518.
54. Anon. The Magpie Trial. http://www.magpietrial.org.uk (accessed 1/3/02)
55. Odendaal HJ, Pattinson RC, Bam R, et al. Aggressive or expectant management for patients with severe preeclampsia between 28–34 weeks gestation: a randomized controlled trial. *Obstet Gynecol* 1990;76:1070–1075.
56. Sibai BM, Mercer BM, Schiff E, et al. Aggressive versus expectant management of severe preeclampsia at 28–32 weeks' gestation: a randomized controlled trial. *Am J Obstet Gynecol* 1994;171:818–822.
57. Churchill D, Duley L. Interventionist versus expectant management of severe pre-eclampsia before term (Protocol for a Cochrane Review). In: The Cochrane Library, Issue 4, 2001. Oxford: Update Software.
58. Hogg B, Owen J, Shih G, Vincent R, Chestnut D, Hauth JC. A randomised trial of intrapartum analgesia in women with severe pre-eclampsia. *Am J Obstet Gynecol* 2000;182:148.
59. Duley L, Henderson-Smart D. Magnesium sulphate versus diazepam for eclampsia. In: The Cochrane Library, Issue 4, 2001. Oxford: Update Software. Search date 1999; primary source Cochrane Pregnancy and Childbirth Group Trials Register.
60. Duley L, Henderson-Smart D. Magnesium sulphate versus phenytoin for eclampsia. In: The Cochrane Library, Issue 4, 2001. Oxford: Update

Software. Search date 1999; primary source Cochrane Pregnancy and Childbirth Group Trials Register.
61. Sawhney H, Sawhney IM, Mandal R, Subramanyam, Vasishta K. Efficacy of magnesium sulphate and phenytoin in the management of eclampsia. *J Obstet Gynaecol Res* 1999;25:333–338.
62. Duley L, Gulmezoglu AM. Magnesium sulphate versus lytic cocktail for eclampsia. In: The Cochrane Library, Issue 4, 2001. Oxford: Update Software. Search date 2000; primary sources Cochrane Pregnancy and Childbirth Group Trials Register and Cochrane Controlled Trials Register.

Lelia Duley
Obstetric Epidemiologist
Institute of Health Sciences
Oxford
UK

Competing interests: None declared.

Preterm birth

Search date May 2002

Bridgette Byrne and John J Morrison

QUESTIONS

INTERVENTIONS

See glossary, p 1503

Key Messages

- **Amnioinfusion for preterm rupture of the membranes** One systematic review found insufficient evidence about the effects of amnioinfusion.

Preterm birth

- **Antenatal corticosteroids** One systematic review in women with anticipated preterm delivery has found that antenatal treatment with corticosteroids versus placebo or no treatment significantly reduces the risk of respiratory distress syndrome, neonatal mortality, and intraventricular haemorrhage in preterm infants.
- **Antibiotic treatment for premature rupture of the membranes (prolongs gestation and may reduce infection, but unknown effect on perinatal mortality)** One systematic review in women with preterm premature rupture of membranes has found that antibiotics versus placebo significantly prolong pregnancy and reduce the risk of neonatal morbidity, such as neonatal infection, requirement for treatment with oxygen, and abnormal cerebral ultrasound. It found that co-amoxiclav (amoxicillin plus clavulanic acid) was associated with a significant increase in the incidence of neonatal necrotising enterocolitis.
- **Antibiotic treatment for preterm labour with intact membranes** One systematic review of women during preterm labour with intact membranes has found that antibiotics versus placebo or no antibiotics significantly prolong pregnancy, and reduce the incidence of maternal infection and necrotising enterocolitis. One large subsequent RCT has found no significant difference in length of pregnancy or neonatal outcomes. The review found that antibiotics versus placebo or no treatment significantly increased perinatal mortality, but the subsequent RCT found no significant difference in perinatal mortality.
- **Elective versus selective caesarean delivery in preterm labour** One systematic review has found limited evidence that elective versus selective caesarean delivery in women with preterm labour increases the risk of maternal morbidity, without clear evidence of benefit in neonatal morbidity or mortality.
- **Enhanced antenatal care programmes for socially deprived population groups/high risk groups** RCTs carried out in a range of countries found no significant difference with enhanced antenatal care versus usual care in reducing the risk of preterm delivery.
- **Prophylactic cervical cerclage for women at risk of cervical incompetence** One large RCT has found that, in women presumed to have cervical incompetence, prophylactic cervical cerclage versus no cerclage significantly reduces preterm birth (< 33 wks' gestation), but significantly increases the risk of puerperal pyrexia (NNH 33, 95% CI 12 to 607). It found that 24 women would need to undergo cerclage to prevent one additional preterm delivery. A second RCT in women with cervix changes detected by ultrasound found that cerclage plus bed rest versus bed rest alone significantly reduced deliveries before 34 weeks (NNT 3, 95% CI 2 to 5). A third RCT found no significant difference in preterm birth with cerclage plus bed rest versus bed rest alone when midtrimester cervical change has been detected by transvaginal ultrasound.
- **Thyrotropin releasing hormone before preterm delivery** One systematic review in women at risk of preterm birth has found no significant difference with thyrotropin releasing hormone plus corticosteroids versus corticosteroids alone in improving neonatal outcomes. Thyrotropin releasing hormone plus corticosteroids versus corticosteroids alone significantly increased maternal and fetal adverse events.
- **Tocolytic treatment in threatened preterm labour** One systematic review has found that atosiban, β mimetics, indometacin, and ethanol versus placebo or no tocolytic significantly prolong pregnancy for women with threatened preterm labour, but do not significantly reduce perinatal mortality or neonatal

morbidity. One subsequent RCT found that atosiban versus placebo significantly prolonged pregnancy for up to 7 days (NNT 6, 95% CI 4 to 14). The systematic review found no significant difference with magnesium sulphate versus placebo or no tocolytic in prolongation of pregnancy or reduction of perinatal mortality or neonatal morbidity. The review has found that tocolytics versus placebo significantly increase maternal adverse effects, such as chest pain, nausea and vomiting, and breathlessness. One systematic review found that calcium channel versus other tocolytics (mainly β mimetics) significantly reduced deliveries within 48 hours, withdrawals owing to maternal adverse effects, and neonatal morbidity.

DEFINITION Preterm or premature birth is defined by the World Health Organization as delivery of an infant before 37 completed weeks of gestation.[1] There is no set lower limit to this definition, but 23–24 weeks' gestation is widely accepted,[1] which approximates to an average fetal weight of 500 g.

INCIDENCE/ PREVALENCE Preterm birth occurs in about 5–10% of all births in developed countries,[2–4] but in recent years the incidence seems to have increased in some countries, particularly the USA.[5] We found little reliable evidence for less developed countries that used the exact definition of premature birth. The rate in northwestern Ethiopia has been reported to vary between 11–22% depending on the age group studied, highest in teenagers.[6]

AETIOLOGY/ RISK FACTORS About 30% of preterm births are unexplained and spontaneous.[4,7,8] The two strongest risk factors for idiopathic preterm labour (see glossary, p 1504) are low socioeconomic status and previous preterm delivery. Multiple pregnancy accounts for about another 30% of cases.[4,7] Other known risk factors include genital tract infection, preterm rupture of the membranes (see glossary, p 1504), antepartum haemorrhage, cervical incompetence, and congenital uterine abnormalities, which collectively account for about 20–25% of cases. The remaining cases (15–20%) are attributed to elective preterm delivery secondary to hypertensive disorders of pregnancy, intrauterine fetal growth restriction, congenital abnormalities, and medical disorders of pregnancy.[4,5,7,8]

PROGNOSIS Preterm labour usually results in preterm birth. One systematic review (search date not stated) of tocolysis versus placebo found that about 27% of preterm labours spontaneously resolved, and about 70% progressed to preterm delivery.[9] Observational studies have found that one preterm birth significantly raises the risk of another in a subsequent pregnancy.[10]

AIMS To prevent preterm birth; to prolong the interval between threatened preterm labour and delivery; to optimise the condition of the fetus in preparation for delivery in order to improve neonatal outcome.

OUTCOMES The main clinical outcome is improved neonatal outcome, as indicated by perinatal (see glossary, p 1504) mortality, neonatal mortality, and morbidity (incidence of respiratory distress syndrome, intraventricular haemorrhage, necrotising enterocolitis, neonatal sepsis, and neonatal convulsions). An additional clinical outcome is incidence of maternal adverse effects. Proxy outcomes include duration of pregnancy, number of hours or days between onset of labour and delivery, and number of deliveries before 37 completed weeks of gestation.

METHODS *Clinical Evidence* update search and appraisal May 2002.

QUESTION What are the effects of preventive interventions in women at high risk of preterm delivery?

OPTION ENHANCED ANTENATAL CARE FOR SOCIALLY DEPRIVED WOMEN AND OTHER HIGH RISK GROUPS

RCTs carried out in a range of countries found no significant difference between enhanced antenatal care versus usual care in reducing the risk of preterm delivery.

Benefits: We found no systematic review. We found eleven RCTs.[11–21] All of the RCTs (carried out in Europe, USA, and Latin America; number of high risk women ranging from 150–2200) found no significant difference between enhanced versus usual antenatal care in reducing preterm birth.

Harms: The RCTs gave no information on adverse effects.[11–21]

Comment: The definition of enhanced antenatal care (see glossary, p 1503) varied.[11–21] Examples of enhanced antenatal care include increased number of antenatal visits, a bed rest programme including rest periods three times daily, home visits by midwives, fortnightly social worker counselling sessions, nutritional education, peer group education, and counselling by a psychologist.

OPTION PROPHYLACTIC CERVICAL CERCLAGE IN WOMEN AT RISK OF CERVICAL INCOMPETENCE

One large RCT has found that, in women presumed to have cervical incompetence, prophylactic cervical cerclage versus no cerclage significantly reduces preterm birth (< 33 wks' gestation), but significantly increases the risk of puerperal pyrexia. It found that 24 women would need to undergo cerclage to prevent one additional preterm delivery. A second RCT in women with cervix changes detected by transvaginal ultrasound found that cerclage plus bed rest versus bed rest alone significantly reduced delivery before 34 weeks. A third RCT found no significant difference in preterm birth with cerclage plus bed rest versus bed rest alone when midtrimester cervical change has been detected by transvaginal ultrasound.

Benefits: We found no systematic review. **When cervical changes have not been identified:** We found one multicentre RCT (1292 women with a history of early delivery or cervical surgery whose obstetricians were uncertain whether to advise cervical cerclage [see glossary, p 1503] or not) comparing cerclage versus no cerclage.[22] It found that cerclage significantly reduced the rate of delivery before 33 weeks' gestation (83/647 [13%] with cerclage *v* 110/645 [17%] with no cerclage; RR 0.75, 95% CI 0.57 to 0.98; NNT 24, 95% CI 14 to 275) but found no significant difference in the rate of deliveries occurring between weeks 33 and 36. **When cervical changes are present:** We found two RCTs of cervical cerclage when cervical change has been detected by transvaginal ultrasound.[23,24] The first RCT (35 women with cervical length < 25 mm and gestational age < 27 wks) found that cerclage plus bed rest versus bed rest alone significantly reduced delivery before 34 weeks (0/19 [0%] with cerclage plus bed rest *v* 7/16 [44%] with bed rest alone; NNT 3, 95% CI 2 to 5; P = 0.002). It found no significant difference in neonatal survival with cerclage plus bed rest versus bed rest alone (19/19 [100%] with cerclage plus bed rest *v* 13/16 [81%] with bed rest alone; ARR 0.19, 95% CI –0.02 to +0.43).[23] The second RCT (113 women between 16 and 24 wks of gestation and distal cervix < 2.5 cm or membrane prolapse into endocervical canal at least 25% of cervical length) found that cerclage plus bed rest versus bed rest alone did not significantly reduce delivery before 34 weeks (35% *v* 36%; P = 0.80), perinatal death (13% *v* 12%; P = 0.90), placental abruption (11% *v* 14%; P = 0.80), or chorioamnionitis (20% *v* 10%; P = 0.20).[24]

Harms: The RCT addressing prophylactic use of cerclage found that insertion of cervical sutures versus no sutures doubled the risk of puerperal pyrexia (24/415 [6%] with cerclage *v* 11/405 [3%] with no cerclage; RR 2.13, 95% CI 1.06 to 4.15; NNH 33, 95% CI 12 to 607).[22] Information about puerperal pyrexia was collected only after 360 women had already been recruited to the trial. The two RCTs looking at the use of cerclage when cervix changes have been detected by ultrasound gave no information on harms.[23,24]

Comment: The most common indication for entry to the trial was a history of preterm delivery or second trimester miscarriage (74% of the cerclage group, 70% of the controls).[18] The two RCTs that examined cervical cerclage in the midtrimester with documented cervical change differed in terms of patient selection and methodology.[23,24] Broad confidence intervals suggest that sample size may have been insufficient to rule out clinically important differences in neonatal mortality.

QUESTION What are the effects of interventions to improve outcome after preterm rupture of the membranes?

OPTION ANTIBIOTICS

One systematic review in women with preterm rupture of membranes has found that antibiotics versus placebo significantly prolong pregnancy and reduce the risk of neonatal morbidity, such as neonatal infection, requirement for treatment with oxygen, and abnormal cerebral ultrasound. It found that co-amoxiclav (amoxicillin [amoxycillin] plus clavulanic acid) was associated with a significant increase in the incidence of neonatal necrotising enterocolitis.

Benefits: One systematic review (search date 2001, 13 RCTs, over 6000 women) found that antibiotics (including erythromycin, co-amoxiclav, benzylpenicillin, ampicillin, piperacillin, or clindamycin) versus placebo significantly reduced the number of babies born within 48 hours (RR 0.7, 95% CI 0.72 to 0.83) and 7 days

(RR 0.88, CI 0.84 to 0.92) following preterm premature rupture of the membranes (see glossary, p 1504).[25] It found that antibiotics versus placebo significantly reduced the incidence of neonatal infection (RR 0.67, 95% CI 0.52 to 0.85), requirement for supplementary oxygen (RR 0.88, 95% CI 0.81 to 0.96), and abnormal cerebral ultrasound (RR 0.82, 95% CI 0.68 to 0.99), but found no significant difference in perinatal mortality with antibiotics versus placebo (RR 0.92, 95% CI 0.75 to 1.12). Antibiotics versus placebo significantly decreased maternal infection after delivery prior to discharge from hospital (RR 0.85, 95% CI 0.76 to 0.96).

Harms: The review found that co-amoxiclav was associated with a significantly increased risk of neonatal necrotising enterocolitis (2 RCTs: RR 4.6, 95% CI 1.98 to 10.72).[25]

Comment: Most of the RCTs in the review did not include antenatal administration of steroids but 77% of the women in one large RCT[26] received steroids. All but one of the RCTs in the review gave data on the percentage of withdrawals, which was always less than 20%.[25]

OPTION AMNIOINFUSION

One systematic review found insufficient evidence from one RCT about the effects of amnioinfusion versus no amnioinfusion in improving neonatal outcomes after preterm rupture of the membranes.

Benefits: We found one systematic review (search date 2001, 1 RCT, 66 women) comparing amnioinfusion (see glossary, p 1503) versus no amnioinfusion.[27] It found no significant difference between amnioinfusion versus no amnioinfusion in rates of caesarean section, low Apgar scores, neonatal mortality, or endometritis.

Harms: No adverse effects were reported in the RCT identified by the review.[27]

Comment: The RCT was too small to detect clinically important changes in some of the outcomes (rates of caesarean section, neonatal mortality, and infectious morbidity) and had shortcomings in methods used (unspecified method of random assignment of women; blinding of treatment not possible).[27]

QUESTION What are the effects of treatments in threatened preterm labour?

OPTION TOCOLYTICS

One systematic review and one subsequent RCT have found that atosiban, β mimetics, indometacin, and ethanol versus placebo or no tocolytic significantly prolong pregnancy, but do not significantly reduce perinatal mortality or neonatal morbidity. The review found no significant difference in prolongation of pregnancy or reduction of perinatal mortality or neonatal morbidity between magnesium sulphate versus placebo or no tocolytic. It has found that tocolytics significantly increase maternal adverse effects, such as chest pain, nausea and vomiting, and dyspnoea.

One systematic review has found that calcium channel versus other tocolytics (mainly β mimetics) significantly reduce deliveries within 48 hours, withdrawals caused by maternal adverse effects, and neonatal morbidity.

Benefits: **Versus placebo or no treatment:** We found one systematic review and one subsequent RCT.[28,29] The systematic review (search date 1998, 18 RCTs, 2785 women in preterm labour) compared different tocolytic drugs (β mimetics, magnesium sulphate, indometacin [indomethacin], atosiban, and ethanol) versus placebo or no tocolytic.[28] Three of the RCTs in the review included women with ruptured membranes. The most frequently evaluated tocolytic agent was the β mimetic, ritodrine (5 RCTs). The review found that β mimetics, indometacin, atosiban, or ethanol versus placebo or no treatment significantly delayed delivery following the onset of preterm labour for greater than 24 hours, 48 hours, and 7 days. **β mimetics versus placebo:** The systematic review (8 RCTs) found no significant difference between β mimetics versus placebo or no treatment in perinatal (see glossary, p 1504) mortality (62/682 [9%] with β mimetics *v* 48/604 [8%] with placebo or no treatment; OR 1.08, 95% CI 0.72 to 1.62), incidence of respiratory distress syndrome (6 RCTs: 117/639 [18%] with β mimetics *v* 140/565 [25%] with placebo or no treatment; OR 0.76, 95% CI 0.57 to 1.01), birth weight less than 2500 g (5 RCTs: 332/601 [55%] with β mimetics *v* 332/525 [63%] with placebo or no treatment; OR 0.79, 95% CI 0.61 to 1.01), patent ductus arteriosus, necrotising enterocolitis, intraventricular haemorrhage, seizures, hypoglycaemia, or neonatal sepsis. **Magnesium sulphate versus placebo:** The review (4 RCTs) found no significant difference between magnesium sulphate versus placebo or no treatment in perinatal mortality (11/169 [6.5%] with magnesium sulphate *v* 7/182 [3.8%] with placebo or no treatment; OR 1.83, 95% CI 0.70 to 4.77) or in the incidence of respiratory distress syndrome (3 RCTs: 22/139 [16%] with magnesium sulphate *v* 22/153 [14%] with placebo or no treatment; OR 1.19, 95% CI 0.61 to 2.31). It also found no significant difference between magnesium sulphate versus placebo or no treatment in birth weight less than 2500 g, patent ductus arteriosus, necrotising enterocolitis, intraventricular haemorrhage, seizures, hypoglycaemia, or neonatal sepsis. The number of newborns assessed for these outcomes was small. **Indometacin versus placebo:** The review (3 RCTs, 100 women) found no significant difference between indometacin versus placebo or no treatment in perinatal mortality, respiratory distress syndrome, bronchopulmonary dysplasia, necrotising enterocolitis, neonatal sepsis, or low birth weight. The number of newborns assessed for these outcomes may be too small to exclude a clinically important difference. **Atosiban:** The systematic review (1 RCT, 114 newborns) found no significant difference with atosiban versus placebo in the incidence of respiratory distress syndrome, patent ductus arteriosus, and hypoglycaemia. The RCT may be too small to exclude a clinically important difference. One subsequent RCT (531 women) compared atosiban versus placebo. It found that in pregnancies of 28 weeks or over, atosiban versus placebo significantly prolonged pregnancy for up to 24 hours (150/203 [74%] with atosiban *v* 128/221 [58%] with placebo; RR 1.28, 95%

CI 1.11 to 1.47; NNT 7, 95% CI 4 to 15), 48 hours (140/203 [69%] with atosiban v 122/221 [55%] with placebo; RR 1.25, 95% CI 1.08 to 1.45; NNT 8, 95% CI 5 to 23), and 7 days (131/203 [65%] with atosiban v 105/220 [48%] with placebo; RR 1.35, 95% CI 1.14 to 1.60; NNT 6, 95% CI 4 to 14).[29] **Calcium channel blockers versus other tocolytics:** We found no RCTs comparing calcium channel blockers versus placebo. We found one systematic review (search date 2002, 11 RCTs, 870 women) comparing calcium channel blockers versus other tocolytics for preterm labour.[30] It found that calcium channel blockers versus other tocolytics (mainly β mimetics) significantly reduced the rate of delivery within 48 hours (7 RCTs: 550 people 58/281 [21%] v 74/269 [27%]; RR 0.73, 95% CI 0.54 to 0.98) and within 7 days (2 RCT: 242 people 55/127 [43%] v 65/115 [56%]; RR 0.76, 95% CI 0.59 to 0.99). It found that calcium channel blockers versus other tocolytics significantly reduced the proportion of babies with respiratory distress syndrome (7 RCTs: 552 people; 41/284 [14%] v 59/268 [22%]; RR 0.64, 95% CI 0.45 to 0.91) and neonatal jaundice (9 RCTs: RR 0.73, 95% CI 0.57 to 0.93). It found that treatment was significantly less likely to be discontinued because of maternal adverse effects with calcium channel blockers versus other tocolytics (9 RCTs: 744 people; 1/374 [0.26%] v 23/370 [6.2%]; RR 0.15, 95% CI 0.06 to 0.43).

Harms: **β mimetics:** In the systematic review,[28] β mimetics versus placebo or no treatment significantly increased maternal adverse effects, such as chest pain (2 RCTs: 39/406 [10%] with β mimetics v 3/408 [1%] with placebo or no treatment; OR 6.2, 95% CI 3.3 to 11.5), palpitations (3 RCTs: 200/420 [48%] with β mimetics v 19/423 [4%] with placebo or no treatment; OR 10.2, 95% CI 7.4 to 13.9), dyspnoea (2 RCTs: 55/406 [14%] with β mimetics v 4/408 [1%] with placebo or no treatment; OR 6.6, 95% CI 3.9 to 11.2), tremor (1 RCT: 138/352 [39%] with β mimetics v 13/356 [4%] with placebo or no treatment; OR 8.3, 95% CI 5.8 to 11.9), nausea (1 RCT: 72/352 [20%] with β mimetics v 42/356 [12%] with placebo or no treatment; OR 1.9, 95% CI 1.3 to 2.8), vomiting (2 RCTs: 48/366 [13%] with β mimetics v 29/371 [8%] with placebo or no treatment; OR 1.8, 95% CI 1.1 to 2.9), headache (2 RCTs: 84/366 [23%] with β mimetics v 22/371 [6%] with placebo or no treatment; OR 4.0, 95% CI 2.6 to 6.0), hyperglycaemia (1 RCT: 106/352 [30%] with β mimetics v 37/356 [10%] with placebo or no treatment; OR 3.4, 95% CI 2.4 to 4.9), and hypokalaemia (1 RCT: 138/352 [39%] with β mimetics v 23/356 [6%] with placebo or no treatment; OR 6.4, 95% CI 4.5 to 9.1), and frequently these adverse effects necessitated discontinuation of treatment (3 RCTs: 25/88 [28%] with β mimetics v 0/86 with placebo or no treatment; OR 11.5, 95% CI 4.8 to 27.5). **Magnesium sulphate:** Significantly increased the need to discontinue treatment (3 RCTs: 10/137 [7%] with magnesium sulphate v 0/144 with placebo or no treatment; OR 8.36, 95% CI 2.36 to 29.61). **Indometacin:** Significantly increased the incidence of postpartum haemorrhage (1 RCT: 7/16 [44%] with indometacin v 2/18 [11%] with placebo or no treatment; OR 5.1, 95% CI 1.1 to 22.9), but there was no significant difference in nausea (1 RCT: 2/18 [11%] with indometacin v 0/18 with placebo or no treatment; OR 7.8, 95% CI 0.5 to 130.5) and chorioamnionitis (1 RCT: 2/15 [13%] with indometacin v 0/15 with placebo or no treatment; OR 7.9, 95% CI 0.5 to 133.3). **Atosiban:** Increased nausea (2 RCTs: 33/306 [11%] with atosiban v 15/307 [5%] with placebo or no treatment; OR 2.3, 95% CI 1.3 to 4.1), but there was no significant difference in vomiting (2 RCTs: 10/306 [3%] with atosiban v 13/307 [4%] with placebo or no treatment; OR 0.8, 95% CI 0.3 to 1.8).[28] Atosiban versus placebo or no treatment significantly reduced chest pain (2 RCTs: 3/306 [1%] with atosiban v 13/307 [4%] with placebo or no treatment; OR 0.3, 95% CI 0.1 to 0.8) and dyspnoea (1 RCT: 1/250 [0.4%] with atosiban v 7/251 [3%] with placebo or no treatment; OR 0.22, 95% CI 0.05 to 0.89). One subsequent RCT found that atosiban versus placebo significantly increased injection site reactions after prolonged use (110/250 [44%] with atosiban v 58/251 [23%] with placebo; RR 1.90, 95% CI 1.46 to 2.48; NNH 4, 95% CI 3 to 7) and significantly increased withdrawal owing to adverse effects (16% with atosiban v 4% with placebo).[29] There was a higher incidence of fetal mortality at less than 26 weeks' gestation with atosiban versus placebo (10/27 [37%] with atosiban v 0/16 [0%] with placebo).[29] **Calcium channel blockers:** Nine of the 11 trials in the systematic review reported discontinuation of treatment related to adverse effects and found a significant reduction of maternal adverse drug reactions with calcium channel blockers (54/313 [17%] with calcium channel blockers v 134/315 [43%] with other tocolytics; OR 0.29, 95% CI 0.20 to 0.40). With the exception of neonatal mortality, neonatal outcomes were less consistently reported, and definitions were often lacking. The systematic review did not report specific adverse effects on calcium channel blockers.[30]

Comment: False preterm labour presents a problem in analysis of effects of tocolytic agents, but in 15/17 RCTs included in the systematic review, the definition of preterm labour used for entry into the study included cervical dilatation, effacement, or change in the cervical condition in addition to uterine contractions.[31] This would minimise the potential confounding effect of spurious preterm labour. Combining results for all tocolytics was reasonable, based on the lack of evidence of the merits of one tocolytic over another.[28] Tocolytic rescue with ritodrine was used in the RCT comparing atosiban with placebo.[29] In this RCT, 24/246 (10%) women randomised to receive atosiban and 13/255 (5%) women randomised to receive placebo were recruited at less than 26 weeks' gestation. This may have contributed to a higher incidence of fetal mortality at less than 26 weeks' gestation in the atosiban group.[29]

QUESTION What are the effects of elective versus selective caesarean delivery for woman in preterm labour? New

One systematic review has found that elective versus selective caesarean delivery increases the risk of maternal morbidity, and does not significantly reduce neonatal morbidity or mortality. The RCTs may have been underpowered to detect a clinically important neonatal benefit.

Benefits: We found one systematic review (search date not stated, 6 RCTs, 122 women).[32] It found no significant difference in neonatal morbidity and mortality with elective caesarean delivery versus selective (see glossary, p 1504) (Low Apgar score at 5 min: OR 0.68, 95% CI 0.29 to 1.60; need for neonatal intubation: OR 0.58, 95% CI 0.26 to 1.31; intracranial haemorrhage 0.86, 95% CI 0.2 to 3.67; perinatal death OR 0.32, 95% CI 0.07 to 1.36).

Harms: The review found that major maternal complications were reported in 7/84 (8%) women, all after caesarean delivery, although one of these women was allocated to expectant management. Maternal complications were therefore significantly higher in women allocated to elective versus selective caesarean delivery (4 RCTs: 84 women; AR 6/44 [14%] with elective caesarean delivery *v* 1/40 [3%] with selective caesarean section; OR 6.18, 95% CI 1.27 to 30.1).[32] Elective caesarean delivery may occasionally result in unnecessary preterm delivery; two women allocated to the selective delivery group did not deliver until some weeks after entry to one trial.

Comment: The neonatal confidence intervals in the systematic review suggest that RCTs were underpowered and no meaningful conclusions can be drawn on the neonatal effects of elective caesarean section.[32] The fetus presented by the breech in three of the studies. Approximately one sixth of each group delivered by an alternative route, but the analysis was by intention to treat. Sample size of trials was small and most of the trials were terminated because of recruitment difficulties.

QUESTION What are the effects of interventions to improve outcome in preterm delivery?

OPTION CORTICOSTEROIDS BEFORE PRETERM DELIVERY

One systematic review in women with anticipated preterm delivery has found that antenatal treatment with corticosteroids versus placebo or no treatment significantly reduces the risk of respiratory distress syndrome, neonatal mortality, and intraventricular haemorrhage in preterm infants.

Benefits: We found one systematic review (search date 1996, 18 RCTs, > 3700 babies) in women experiencing anticipated preterm delivery (elective or after spontaneous onset of preterm labour [see glossary, p 1504]) comparing corticosteroids (β methasone, dexamethasone, or hydrocortisone) versus placebo or no treatment.[33] The review found that antenatal corticosteroids versus placebo or no treatment significantly reduced respiratory distress syndrome (18 RCTs, 3735 neonates, 292/1885 [15%] with corticosteroids *v* 439/1850 [24%] with placebo or no treatment; OR 0.52, 95% CI 0.44 to 0.62). Three RCTs (48 neonates) identified by the review found no significant difference between antenatal corticosteroids versus placebo or no treatment in respiratory distress syndrome in neonates delivered before 28 weeks' gestation (7/17 [41%] with corticosteroids *v* 18/31 [58%] with placebo or no treatment; OR 0.64, 95% CI 0.16 to 2.50). Six RCTs identified by the review (349 neonates) found no significant difference between antenatal corticosteroids versus placebo or no treatment in respiratory distress syndrome in babies delivered within less than 24 hours of initial treatment (45/176 [26%] with corticosteroids *v* 57/173

[33%] with placebo or no treatment; OR 0.70, 95% CI 0.43 to 1.16), and one RCT (42 neonates) identified by the review found no significant difference between antenatal corticosteroids versus placebo or no treatment in respiratory distress syndrome in babies delivered within less than 48 hours of initial treatment (3/23 [13%] with corticosteroids *v* 6/19 [32%] with placebo or no treatment; OR 0.34, 95% CI 0.08 to 1.47). The review found that both β methasone and dexamethasone significantly reduced respiratory distress but not hydrocortisone. The sex of the neonate had no effect on treatment response. The small numbers of evaluable neonates from twin pregnancies did not allow a confident statement about the effects in multiple pregnancy. Antenatal corticosteroids versus placebo or no treatment significantly reduced neonatal mortality (14 RCTs: 129/1770 [7%] with corticosteroids *v* 204/1747 [12%] with placebo or no treatment; OR 0.60, 95% CI 0.48 to 0.75), and risk of intraventricular haemorrhage (diagnosed at autopsy: 7/446 [1.6%] with corticosteroids *v* 23/417 [5.5%] with placebo or no treatment, OR 0.29, 95% CI 0.14 to 0.61; diagnosed by ultrasound: 47/300 [16%] with corticosteroids *v* 77/296 [26%] with placebo or no intervention, OR 0.48, 95% CI 0.32 to 0.72). Antenatal corticosteroids did not significantly reduce the rates of necrotising enterocolitis (17/587 [3%] with corticosteroids *v* 27/567 [5%] with placebo or no treatment; OR 0.59, 95% CI 0.32 to 1.09) or chronic lung disease (38/204 [19%] with corticosteroids *v* 25/207 [12%] with placebo or no treatment; OR 1.57, 95% CI 0.87 to 2.84).[33]

Harms: The RCTs in the review found no strong evidence of any adverse effects of corticosteroids.[33] Subgroup analysis in one RCT in the review suggested that corticosteroids may be associated with death in hypertensive women, but no deaths in hypertensive women were observed in the other three RCTs in the review for which data were available.[33]

Comment: The absence of a significant beneficial effect of corticosteroids on respiratory distress syndrome at less than 28 weeks' gestation may be because of the small numbers available for analysis at this gestation.[33] No RCTs in the review[33] addressed the potentially harmful effects of repeated doses of antenatal corticosteroids, or whether one form of corticosteroid was more harmful than another, as a retrospective cohort study (883 babies delivered between 24 and 31 wks' gestation) suggests.[34]

OPTION **THYROTROPIN RELEASING HORMONE BEFORE PRETERM DELIVERY**

One systematic review in women at risk of preterm birth found no significant difference in neonatal outcomes between thyrotropin releasing hormone plus corticosteroids versus corticosteroids alone, and has found that thyrotropin releasing hormone plus corticosteroids versus corticosteroids alone significantly increase maternal and fetal adverse events.

Benefits: We found one systematic review (search date 1999, 11 RCTs, > 4500 women at risk of preterm birth taking antenatal corticosteroids) comparing thyrotropin releasing hormone (TRH) plus steroids versus steroids alone.[33] It found no significant difference between TRH plus steroids versus steroids alone on gestational age at delivery, admission to the neonatal intensive care unit, respiratory distress syndrome, need for oxygen supplementation at 28 days, intraventricular haemorrhage, necrotising enterocolitis, and perinatal (see glossary, p 1504) mortality.

Harms: The review found that in babies who received TRH plus steroids versus steroids alone, TRH significantly increased the risk of low Apgar score at 5 minutes (OR 1.8, 95% CI 1.14 to 1.92) and increased the requirement for assisted ventilation (OR 1.16, CI 1.02 to 1.29). One RCT included in the review[35] found a significant increase in motor delay (RR 1.31, 95% CI 1.09 to 1.56), motor impairment (RR 1.51, 95% CI 1.02 to 2.24), sensory impairment (RR 1.97, 95% CI 1.10 to 3.53), and social delay after 12 months (RR 1.25, 95% CI 1.03 to 1.51). TRH plus steroids versus steroids alone significantly increased maternal blood pressure (1 RCT: risk of an increase of 25 mm Hg in systolic blood pressure, 36/506 [7%] with TRH plus steroids *v* 20/505 [4%] with steroids alone, RR 1.80, 95% CI 1.05 to 3.06; risk of an increase of 15 mm Hg in diastolic blood pressure, 115/506 [23%] with TRH plus steroids *v* 71/505 [14%] with steroids alone, RR 1.62, 95% CI 1.24 to 2.12). Other maternal adverse effects included nausea (3 RCTs: 303/1175 [26%] with TRH plus steroids *v* 77/1195 [6%] with steroids alone, RR 3.92, 95% CI 3.19 to 4.92), vomiting (1 RCT: 40/506 [8%] with TRH plus steroids *v* 17/505 [3%] with steroids alone, RR 2.35, 95% CI 1.35 to 4.09), light-headedness (1 RCT: 139/506 [27%] with TRH plus steroids *v* 80/505 [16%] with steroids alone, RR 1.73, 95% CI 1.36 to 2.22), urgency of micturition (1 RCT: 115/506 [23%] with TRH plus steroids *v* 48/505 [10%] with steroids alone, RR 2.39, 95% CI 1.75 to 3.27), and facial flushing (3 RCTs: 397/1252 [32%] with TRH plus steroids *v* 149/1271 [12%] with steroids alone, RR 2.67, 95% CI 2.26 to 3.16).[35]

Comment: TRH regimens varied in the RCTs identified by the review.[35] Seven of the RCTs analysed by intention to treat.

OPTION ANTIBIOTICS IN PRETERM LABOUR WITH INTACT MEMBRANES

One systematic review of women during preterm labour with intact membranes has found that antibiotics versus placebo or no antibiotics significantly prolong pregnancy, and reduce maternal infection and necrotising enterocolitis. One large subsequent RCT found no significant difference between antibiotics versus placebo in prolonging pregnancy or improving neonatal outcomes but found that antibiotics versus placebo significantly reduce the rate of maternal antibiotic prescription postnatally. The systematic review has found that antibiotics versus placebo significantly increase perinatal mortality, but the subsequent RCT found no significant difference in perinatal mortality.

Benefits: We found one systematic review[36] and one subsequent RCT.[37] The systematic review (search date not stated, 10 RCTs) in women in preterm labour (see glossary, p 1504) with intact membranes compared single antibiotics (2 RCTs) or combined antibiotics (8 RCTs) versus placebo or no antibiotics.[36] It found that antibiotics versus placebo significantly prolonged pregnancy (4 RCTs: 424 women; mean increase 5.4 days, 95% CI 0.9 to 9.8 days) and significantly reduced the incidence of maternal infection (OR 0.59, 95% CI 0.36 to 0.97) and necrotising enterocolitis (OR 0.33, 95% CI 0.18 to 0.88). It found no significant difference between antibiotics versus placebo in neonatal sepsis (OR 0.67, 95% CI 0.42 to 1.07), mean birth weight, respiratory distress syndrome, or intraventricular haemorrhage.[36] One subsequent RCT (6295 women in preterm labour with intact membranes, found no significant difference between antibiotics versus placebo in delivery within 48 hours (478/4685 [10%] *v* 152/1556 [10%]; RR 1.04, 95% CI 0.88 to 1.24) and within 7 days (724/4685 [15.5%] *v* 237/1556 [15.2%]; RR 1.02, 95% CI 0.89 to 1.16). It found no significant difference between antibiotics versus placebo in perinatal (see glossary, p 1504) mortality (128/4685 [2.7%] with antibiotics *v* 39/1556 [2.5%] with placebo; RR 1.09, 95% CI 0.76 to 1.55), or in a composite outcome of respiratory distress syndrome, abnormal cerebral ultrasound, or perinatal mortality (257/4685 [5.5%] *v* 78/1556 [5.0%]; RR 1.09, 95% CI 0.85 to 1.40).[37] It found that antibiotics versus placebo significantly reduced the need for maternal antibiotic prescription postnatally (433/4685 [9%] *v* 183/1556 [12%]; RR 0.79, 95% CI 0.67 to 0.93).

Harms: The systematic review found that antibiotics versus placebo significantly increased perinatal mortality (8 RCTs: 12/481 [2.5%] with antibiotics *v* 3/486 [0.6%] with no antibiotics; OR 3.36, 95% CI 1.21 to 9.32); a finding that remained significant when only deaths specifically related to prematurity were assessed (OR 2.74, 95% CI 1.02 to 7.35).[36] The subsequent RCT found no significant difference between antibiotics versus placebo in perinatal mortality (128/4685 [2.7%] with antibiotics *v* 39/1556 [2.5%] with placebo; P = 0.63) or necrotising enterocolitis (26/4685 [0.6%] with antibiotics *v* 4/1556 [0.3%] with placebo; P = 0.14).

Comment: The differences in findings between the systematic review and the subsequent RCT may in part be explained by the wide range of antibiotics assessed by the RCTs in the review (ampicillin, erythromycin, metronidazole, sulbactam, mezlocillin, clavulonic acid, clindamycin, and ceftizoxime) compared with the subsequent RCT that assessed erythromycin and co-amoxiclav.[36,37] All of the RCTs in the review used similar definitions of preterm labour, including uterine contractions and cervical dilatation.[36] In the subsequent RCT the diagnosis of preterm labour was made by each clinician.[37]

GLOSSARY

Amnioinfusion Infusion of physiological saline or Ringers lactate through a catheter transabdominally or transcervically into the amniotic cavity.

Cervical cerclage Insertion of a cervical suture, using non-absorbable suture material, circumferentially around the cervix. May be done transvaginally or transabdominally.

Elective caesarean section When the operation is done at a pre-selected time before the onset of labour, usually after 38 weeks of gestation.

Enhanced antenatal care Includes various programmes of increased medical, midwifery, psychological, social, and nutritional support during pregnancy.

Preterm birth

Perinatal Refers to the period after 24 weeks' gestation and includes the first 7 days of postnatal life for the neonate.

Preterm labour Onset of labour (regular uterine contractions with cervical effacement and dilatation) in the preterm period.

Preterm rupture of membranes Leakage of amniotic fluid from the amniotic cavity during the preterm period owing to rupture of the fetal membranes.

Selective caesarean section When the operation is done after the onset of labour.

Substantive changes

Prophylactic cervical cerclage in women at risk of cervical incompetence Two new RCTs included;[23,24] conclusions unchanged.

Antibiotics One systematic review updated;[25] conclusions unchanged.

Amnioinfusion One systematic review updated;[27] conclusions unchanged.

Tocolytics A new comparison addressing calcium channel blockers versus other tocolytics has been added. One systematic review found that calcium channel versus other tocolytics (mainly β mimetics) significantly reduced deliveries within 48 hours, withdrawals due to maternal adverse effects, and neonatal morbidity.[30]

Antibiotics in labour One systematic review updated;[36] conclusions unchanged.

REFERENCES

1. Morrison JJ, Rennie JM. Clinical, scientific and ethical aspects of fetal and neonatal care at extremely preterm periods of gestation. *Br J Obstet Gynaecol* 1997;104:1341–1350.
2. Rush RW, Keirse MJNC, Howat P, et al. Contribution of preterm delivery to perinatal mortality. *BMJ* 1976;2:965–968.
3. Creasy RK. Preterm birth prevention: Where are we? *Am J Obstet Gynecol* 1993;168:1223–1230.
4. Burke C, Morrison JJ. Perinatal factors and preterm delivery in an Irish obstetric population. *J Perinat Med* 2000;28:49–53.
5. Goldenberg RL, Rouse DJ. Prevention of premature birth. *N Engl J Med* 1998;339:313–320.
6. Kumbi S, Isehak A. Obstetric outcome of teenage pregnancy in northwestern Ethiopia. *East Afr Med J* 1999;76:138–140.
7. Iannucci TA, Tomich PG, Gianopoulos JG. Etiology and outcome of extremely low-birth-weight infants. *Am J Obstet Gynecol* 1996;174:1896–1902.
8. Main DM, Gabbe SG, Richardson D, et al. Can preterm deliveries be prevented? *Am J Obstet Gynecol* 1985;151:892–898.
9. King JF, Grant A, Keisre MJNC, et al. β-mimetics in preterm labour: an overview of the randomised controlled trials. *Br J Obstet Gynaecol* 1988;95:211–222. Search date not stated; primary sources Oxford Database of Perinatal Trials, hand searched reference lists, and personal contacts.
10. Keirse MJNC, Rush RW, Anderson AB, et al. Risk of preterm delivery and/or abortion. *Br J Obstet Gynaecol* 1978;85:81–85.
11. Spencer B, Thomas H, Morris J. A randomized controlled trial of the provision of a social support service during pregnancy; the South Manchester Family Worker project. *Br J Obstet Gynaecol* 1989;96:281–288.
12. Mueller-Heubach E, Reddick D, Barrett B, et al. Preterm birth prevention: evaluation of a prospective controlled randomized trial. *Am J Obstet Gynecol* 1989;160:1172–1178.
13. Goldenberg R, Davis R, Copper R, et al. The Alabama birth prevention project. *Obstet Gynecol* 1990;75:933–939.
14. Blondel B, Breart G, Glado J, et al. Evaluation of the home-visiting system for women with threatened preterm labour. Results of a randomized controlled trial. *Eur J Obstet Gynaecol Reprod Biol* 1990;34:47–58.
15. Villar J, Farnot U, Barros F, et al. A randomized trial of psychosocial support during high-risk pregnancies. *N Engl J Med* 1992;327:1266–1271.
16. Collaborative Group on Preterm Birth Prevention. Multicenter randomized controlled trial of a preterm birth prevention program. *Am J Obstet Gynecol* 1993;169:352–366.
17. Moore ML, Meis PJ, Ernest JM, et al. A randomized trial of nurse intervention to reduce preterm and low birth weight births. *Obstet Gynecol* 1998;91:656–661.
18. Olds DL, Henderson CR Jr, Tatelbaum R, et al. Improving the delivery of prenatal care and outcomes of pregnancy: a randomized trial of nurse home visitation. *Pediatrics* 1986;77:16–28.
19. Koniak-Griffin D, Anderson NL, Verzemnieks I, et al. A public health nursing early intervention program for adolescent mothers: outcomes from pregnancy through 6 weeks postpartum. *Nursing Res* 2000;49:130–138.
20. Heins HC, Nance NW, McCarthy BJ, et al. A randomised trial of nurse–midwifery prenatal care to reduce low birth weight. *Obstet Gynecol* 1990;75:341–345.
21. Klerman LV, Ramey SL, Goldenberg RL, et al. A randomised controlled trial of augmented prenatal care for multiple-risk Medicaid eligible African American women. *Am J Public Health* 2001:91:105–111.
22. MRC/RCOG Working party on cervical cerclage. Final report of the Medical Research Council/Royal College of Obstetricians and Gynaecologists multicentre randomised trial of cervical cerclage. *Br J Obstet Gynaecol* 1993;100:516–523.
23. Althuisius SM, Dekker GA, Hummel P, et al. Final results of the Cervical Incompetence Prevention Randomised Cerclage Trial (CIPRACT): therapeutic cerclage with bed rest versus bed rest alone. *Am J Obstet Gynecol* 2001;185:1106 –1112.
24. Rust OA, Atlas RO, Reed J, et al. Revisiting the short cervix detected by transvaginal ultrasound in the second trimester: Why cerclage therapy may not help. *Am J Obstet Gynecol* 2001;185:1098–1105.

25. Kenyon S, Boulvain M. Antibiotics for preterm premature rupture of membranes. In: The Cochrane Library, Issue 2, 2002. Oxford: Update Software. Search date 2001; primary source Cochrane Pregnancy Childbirth Group Trials Register.
26. Kenyon SL, Taylor DJ, Tarnow-Mordi W. Broad-spectrum antibiotics for preterm, prelabour rupture of fetal membranes: the ORACLE I randomised trial. *Lancet* 2001;357:979–988.
27. Hofmeyr GJ. Amnioinfusion for preterm rupture of membranes. In: The Cochrane Library, Issue 2, 2002. Oxford: Update Software. Search date 2001; primary sources Cochrane Pregnancy and Childbirth Group Trials Register and Cochrane Register of Controlled Trials.
28. Gyetvai K, Hannah ME, Hodnett ED, et al. Tocolytics for preterm labor: A systematic review. *Obstet Gynecol* 1999;94:869–877. Search date 1998; primary sources Medline and Cochrane Register of Controlled Trials.
29. Romero R, Sibai BM, Sanchez-Ramos L, et al. An oxytocin receptor antagonist (atosiban) in the treatment of preterm labor: a randomized, double-blind, placebo-controlled trial with tocolytic rescue. *Am J Obstet Gynecol* 2000;182;1173–1183.
30. King JF, Flenady VJ, Papatsonis DNM, et al. Calcium channel blockers for inhibiting preterm labour. In: The Cochrane Library, Issue 2, 2002. Search date 2002; primary sources Cochrane Controlled Trials Register, Medline, Embase, Current Contents, hand searched relevant references, and contact with experts.
31. Hannah M, Amankwah K, Barret J, et al. The Canadian consensus on the use of tocolytics for preterm labour. J SOGC 1995;17:1089–1115.
32. Grant A, Penn ZJ, Steer PJ. Elective or selective caesarean delivery of the small baby? A systematic review of the controlled trials. *Br J Obstet Gynaecol* 1996;103:1197–1200. Search date not stated, primary sources not stated.
33. Crowley P. Prophylactic corticosteroids for preterm birth. In: The Cochrane Library, Issue 2, 2002. Oxford: Update Software. Search date 1996; primary sources Cochrane Pregnancy and Childbirth Group Trials Register.
34. Baud O, Foix-L'Helias L, Kaminski M, et al. Antenatal glucocorticoid treatment and cystic periventricular leukomalacia in very premature infants. *N Engl J Med* 1999;341:1190–1196.
35. Crowther CA, Alfirevic Z, Haslam RR. Prenatal thyrotropin-releasing hormone (TRH) for preterm birth. In: The Cochrane Library, Issue 2, 2002. Oxford: Update Software. Search date 1999; primary source Cochrane Pregnancy and Childbirth Group Trials Register.
36. King J, Flenady V. Antibiotics for preterm labour with intact membranes. In: The Cochrane Library, Issue 2, 2002. Oxford: Update Software. Search date not stated; primary sources Cochrane Pregnancy and Childbirth Group Trials Register, personal contacts, and hand searched reference lists.
37. Kenyon SL, Taylor DJ, Tarnow-Mordi W. Broad-spectrum antibiotics for spontaneous preterm labour: the ORACLE II randomised trial. *Lancet* 2001;357:989–994.

Bridgette Byrne
Senior Lecturer in Obstetrics and Gynaecology
Royal College of Surgeons of Ireland
Coombe Women's Hospital
Dublin
Ireland

John J Morrison
Professor of Obstetrics and Gynaecology
Clinical Science Institute
University College Hospital
Galway
Ireland

Competing interests: None declared.

Asthma

Search date January 2002

Christopher Cates and J Mark FitzGerald

QUESTIONS

INTERVENTIONS

*Highly likely to be effective. RCTs unlikely to be conducted.

See glossary, p 1524

Key Messages

In people with chronic asthma

- **Adding inhaled long acting β_2 agonists to inhaled corticosteroids in poorly controlled asthma (for symptom control)** RCTs have found that, in people with poorly controlled asthma, adding regular doses of long acting, inhaled β_2 agonists to inhaled corticosteroids versus placebo significantly improves symptoms and lung function. Regular use of long acting β_2 agonists has not been linked to deterioration in asthma control.

- **Inhaled short acting β_2 agonists as needed for symptom relief (as effective as regular use) in mild or moderate persistent asthma** One systematic review and one subsequent RCT have found that regular use of inhaled short acting β_2 agonists versus as needed use provides no important clinical benefits.
- **Leukotriene antagonists for people with mild to moderate, persistent asthma** RCTs in people taking short acting β_2 agonists alone have found that the addition of leukotriene antagonists versus placebo significantly reduces asthma symptoms and β_2 agonist use. One systematic review in people taking inhaled corticosteroids found no significant difference in the rate of exacerbations with leukotriene antagonists versus placebo. One systematic review and subsequent RCTs have found no significant difference in the rate of exacerbations with leukotriene antagonists versus inhaled corticosteroids, but have found that inhaled corticosteroids significantly improve quality of life, lung function, and symptom control. One RCT found that an inhaled corticosteroid plus a long acting β_2 agonist versus a leukotriene antagonist significantly improved symptoms, lung function, and exacerbations.
- **Low dose, inhaled corticosteroids in mild, persistent asthma** Systematic reviews and additional RCTs have found that, in people with mild, persistent asthma, low doses of inhaled corticosteroids (250–500 μg of beclometasone dipropionate or equivalent) versus placebo significantly improve symptoms and lung function. One systematic review found that inhaled corticosteroids versus regular β_2 agonists or versus placebo significantly improved lung function.

In people with acute exacerbations of asthma

- **Continuous nebulised delivery of bronchodilators for acute asthma (better than intermittent treatment)** One large RCT found limited evidence that continuous treatment with short acting β_2 agonists versus as needed treatment in people with severe asthma significantly improved forced expiratory volume in 1 second (FEV_1) at 2 hours. Other smaller RCTs found no significant difference in peak expiratory flow rate (PEFR), FEV_1, or hospital admissions. In adults with more severe airflow obstruction, two RCTs have found that continuous nebulised treatment versus intermittent treatment improves lung function.
- **Education about acute asthma** One systematic review has found that education to facilitate self management of asthma in adults versus usual care significantly reduces hospital admission (NNT 38, 95% CI 20 to 382), unscheduled visits to the doctor (NNT 12, 95% CI 8 to 36), and days off work (NNT 7, 95% CI 5 to 13) at the end of the study. One subsequent RCT has found that a structured education asthma management programme versus limited education or versus usual care for 1 year significantly reduces unscheduled visits to the doctor over the final 6 months of treatment.
- **Inhaled corticosteroids for acute asthma** One systematic review in people in the emergency department who were not taking systemic corticosteroids has found that inhaled corticosteroids versus placebo significantly reduce hospital admissions, but has found that in people taking systemic corticosteroids adding inhaled corticosteroids versus placebo does not significantly reduce hospital admissions. A second systematic review found insufficient evidence about the effects of inhaled versus oral corticosteroids. It found no significant difference in relapse rates at 7–10 days with inhaled corticosteroids plus oral corticosteroids versus oral corticosteroids alone.

- **Intravenous versus nebulised delivery of short acting β_2 agonists for acute asthma** One systematic review found that intravenous delivery of short acting β_2 agonists was no more effective than nebulised delivery in improving PEFR in 60 minutes.
- **Ipratropium bromide added to β_2 agonists for acute exacerbations** Three systematic reviews and one subsequent RCT have found that β_2 agonists plus ipratropium bromide versus β_2 agonists alone significantly improve lung function. One of the reviews and the subsequent RCT have found that adding ipratropium bromide to β_2 agonists versus β_2 agonists alone significantly reduces hospital admissions, but the other reviews, which included fewer RCTs in the analysis, found no significant difference.
- **Magnesium sulphate for people with more severe acute asthma** Subgroup analysis from one systematic review suggests that intravenous magnesium sulphate versus placebo may improve PEFR and FEV_1, and reduce rates of hospital admission. Subsequent RCTs found that magnesium sulphate versus saline or versus placebo significantly improved PEFR, but found no significant difference in hospital admissions.
- **Mechanical ventilation for people with severe acute asthma** We found no RCTs of mechanical ventilation, but clinical experience, retrospective cohort studies, and case series suggest that it is likely to reduce death rates.
- **Oxygen supplementation for acute asthma** There is a strong consensus that oxygen should be a key component of acute treatment. We found no RCTs in people with acute exacerbations of asthma of oxygen treatment. Clinical monitoring and case control studies have found that people with near fatal asthma suffer from significant hypoxaemia.
- **Short courses of systemic corticosteroids for acute exacerbations** One systematic review has found that systemic corticosteroids versus placebo taken at the start of an acute exacerbation significantly reduce rates of hospital admission. One systematic review has found that systemic corticosteroids versus placebo taken after discharge from hospital following an acute exacerbation significantly reduce relapses requiring additional care, readmissions to hospital, and the need for additional β_2 agonists. One of the reviews found no significant difference in outcomes with oral corticosteroids versus intramuscular or intravenous corticosteroids. One RCT found no significant difference in morning PEFR with tapering of prednisolone over a week versus abrupt cessation of prednisolone. One small RCT found no difference in PEFR and relapse rates with 1 week versus 2 weeks of oral prednisone, but may have been too small to exclude a clinically important difference.
- **Spacer devices for delivering inhaled medications from pressurised metered dose inhalers in acute asthma (as good as nebulisers)** One systematic review in people with acute, but not life threatening exacerbations of asthma found no significant difference with β_2 agonists delivered by spacer device/holding chamber versus nebulisers in rates of hospital admission, time spent in the emergency department, PEFR, or FEV_1.
- **Specialist versus generalist care for acute exacerbations** One systematic and one non-systematic review of RCTs and observational studies found limited evidence that specialist versus generalist care improved outcomes.

DEFINITION Asthma is characterised by variable airflow obstruction and airway hyperresponsiveness. Symptoms include dyspnoea, cough, chest tightness, and wheezing. The normal diurnal variation of peak expiratory flow rate (see glossary, p 1524) is increased in people with asthma (see table 1, p 1529). **Chronic asthma** is defined here as asthma requiring maintenance treatment. Asthma is classified differently in the USA and UK (see table 1, p 1529): where necessary, the text specifies the system of classification used.[1,2] **Acute asthma** is defined here as an exacerbation of underlying asthma requiring urgent or emergency treatment.

INCIDENCE/ PREVALENCE Reported prevalence of asthma is increasing worldwide. About 10% of people have suffered an attack of asthma.[3–5] Epidemiological studies have also found marked variations in prevalence in different countries.[6,7]

AETIOLOGY/ RISK FACTORS Most people with asthma are atopic. Exposure to certain stimuli initiates inflammation and structural changes in airways causing airway hyperresponsiveness and variable airflow obstruction, which in turn cause most asthma symptoms. There are a large number of such stimuli; the more important include environmental allergens, occupational sensitising agents, and respiratory viral infections.[8,9]

PROGNOSIS **Chronic asthma:** In people with mild asthma, prognosis is good and progression to severe disease is rare. However, as a group, people with asthma lose lung function faster than those without asthma, although less quickly than people without asthma who smoke.[10] People with chronic asthma can improve with treatment. However, for reasons not clearly understood, some people (possibly up to 5%) have severe disease that responds poorly to treatment. These people are most at risk of morbidity and death from asthma. **Acute asthma:** About 10–20% of people presenting to the emergency department with asthma are admitted to hospital. Of these, fewer than 10% receive mechanical ventilation,[11,12] although previous ventilation is associated with a 19-fold increased risk of ventilation for a subsequent episode.[13] It is unusual for people to die unless they have suffered respiratory arrest before reaching hospital.[14] One prospective study of 939 people discharged from emergency care found that 17% (95% CI 14% to 20%) relapsed by 2 weeks.[15]

AIMS To minimise or eliminate symptoms; to maximise lung function; to prevent exacerbations; to minimise the need for medication; to minimise adverse effects of treatment; and to provide enough information and support to facilitate self management of asthma.

OUTCOMES Symptoms (day time and nocturnal); lung function, in terms of peak expiratory flow rate and forced expiratory volume in 1 second (see glossary, p 1524); need for rescue medication such as inhaled β_2 agonists; variability of flow rates; activities of daily living; adverse effects of treatment.

METHODS *Clinical Evidence* update search and appraisal January 2002.

QUESTION What are effects of treatments for chronic asthma?

Christopher Cates

OPTION REGULAR VERSUS AS NEEDED INHALED SHORT ACTING β_2 AGONISTS IN ADULTS WITH MILD OR MODERATE ASTHMA

One systematic review found no significant difference in morning peak expiratory flow rate (PEFR), or rate of exacerbations with "as needed" versus "regular" use of inhaled short acting β_2 agonists. It found that regular versus as needed use significantly increased evening PEFR and reduced the use of rescue medication. As needed versus regular use significantly increased pre-brochodilator forced expiratory volume in 1 second and diurnal variation of PEFR. One subsequent RCT found no significant difference with regular versus as needed salbutamol in the rate of exacerbations or morning PEFR over 1 year, but found that regular salbutamol significantly increased evening PEFR and diurnal variation of PEFR.

Benefits: We found one systematic review (search date not stated, 22 crossover RCTs, 8 parallel group RCTs)[16] and one subsequent RCT[17] comparing regular with as needed β_2 agonists. Results from crossover RCTs and parallel group RCTs were analysed separately; only results from crossover RCTs were suitable for pooling. The majority of the included studies did not allow the use of concurrent inhaled corticosteroids. The review found that morning PEFR (see glossary, p 1524) was not significantly different between regular versus as needed use (5 crossover RCTs, 437 adults: WMD 2.1 L/min, 95% CI –9.5 to +13.6). Regular versus as needed use of β_2 agonists significantly increased evening PEFR (6 crossover RCTs, 874 adults: WMD 13.1 L/min, 95% CI 1.9 to 24.3). As needed versus regular β_2 agonist use significantly increased diurnal variation (see glossary, p 1524) of PEFR (2 crossover RCTs, 170 adults: 4.4%, 95% CI 4.3 to 4.5) and pre-bronchodilator forced expiratory volume in 1 second (FEV_1) (see glossary, p 1524) obtained at clinic visits (303 people: WMD 157 mL, 95% CI 123 to 192). Use of rescue bronchodilator was measured in most of the RCTs that used a short acting β_2 agonist as a rescue agent. Results for an average 24 hour period showed that, when bronchodilators were given regularly, significantly less relief bronchodilator was used (2 crossover RCTs, 45 adults: WMD –0.68 puffs/day, 95% CI –1.30 to –0.07). The two crossover RCTs (174 adults) identified by the review that quantified exacerbation rates found no significant difference between regular versus as needed use of β_2 agonists (SMD 0.10, 95% CI –0.11 to +0.31). One parallel group RCT (117 adults) identified by the review found that as needed versus regular use significantly improved symptom control over a 24 hour period (WMD 0.120 units, 95% CI 0.001 to 0.239). No significant differences were found in quality of life.[16] The subsequent RCT (983 people with asthma in a general practice setting, 90% using regular inhaled corticosteroids) compared as needed versus regular salbutamol (see glossary, p 1525) (400 µg four times daily).[17] It found no significant difference with regular versus as needed salbutamol in the rate of exacerbations over 1 year (RR 0.96, 95% CI 0.8 to 1.15) or in morning PEFR (see comment below). Evening PEFR was significantly higher with regular salbutamol (WMD 10.7 L/min, 95% CI 6.7 to 14.0) and diurnal variation of PEFR was also higher (WMD 3.3%, 95% CI 2.5% to 4.1%).[17]

Harms: The systematic review did not find any significant worsening of airways function after stopping regular treatment with β_2 agonists, and concluded that the small increase in lower airways reactivity with regular treatment was unlikely to be of any clinical significance.[16] Two case control studies found an association between increased asthma mortality and overuse of inhaled short acting β_2 agonists.[18,19] The evidence does not establish causality, as overusing β_2 agonists to treat frequent symptoms may simply indicate severe, uncontrolled asthma in high risk individuals. Other RCTs found that regular use of inhaled β_2 agonists was associated with transient rebound deterioration in airway hyperresponsiveness after stopping the medication,[20] and increased allergen induced bronchoconstriction.[21] Tremor was commonly reported, but tolerance developed with more frequent use.[22]

Comment: In the subsequent RCT, 33% (323/983) of people randomised did not complete the RCT, reducing the power of the RCT to detect a significant difference between regular and as needed salbutamol.[17]

OPTION LOW DOSE INHALED CORTICOSTEROIDS IN PEOPLE WITH MILD, PERSISTENT ASTHMA

Three systematic reviews, five subsequent and five additional RCTs have found that, in people with mild, persistent asthma, low doses of inhaled corticosteroids (250–500 μg of beclometasone dipropionate or equivalent) versus placebo significantly improve symptoms and lung function. One systematic review found that inhaled corticosteroids versus regular β_2 agonists or versus placebo significantly improved lung function. We found no evidence of clinically important adverse effects in adults.

Benefits: **Versus placebo:** We found one systematic review (search date 1999, 6 RCTs, 393 people)[23] and four subsequent RCTs (1026 adults and adolescents)[24–27] of budenoside; one systematic review (search date 1999, 9 RCTs, 1800 people)[28] and one subsequent RCT (304 people aged ≥ 12 years)[29] of fluticasone; and one systematic review (search date 1999, 6 RCTs, 492 people) of beclometasone (beclomethasone).[30] We also found five additional RCTs (2187 adults and adolescents with mild, persistent asthma using the US classification see table 1, p 1529) of low doses of triamcinolone,[31–34] flunisolide,[35] or mometasone.[36] The systematic reviews and RCTs all found that low dose inhaled corticosteroids versus placebo significantly improved lung function and symptoms, and reduced short acting bronchodilator use. The largest systematic review (search date 1999),[28] which compared fluticasone (≥ 100 μg/day) versus placebo found that fluticasone significantly improved forced expiratory volume in 1 second (see glossary, p 1524) from baseline (WMD 0.41 L, 95% CI 0.35 to 0.47), morning peak expiratory flow rate (see glossary, p 1524) (WMD 30 L/min, 95% CI 25 to 35), and significantly reduced the use of inhaled β_2 agonists (WMD 1.36 puffs/day, 95% CI 1.0 to 1.7) and the proportion of people who withdrew because of lack of efficiency over 4–12 weeks (RR 0.32, 95% CI 0.25 to 0.40).[28] **Versus β_2 agonists:** We found one systematic review (search date not stated; 5 RCTs; 3 comparing inhaled corticosteroids *v* placebo; 2 comparing inhaled corticosteroids *v* β_2 agonists; 141 adults with mild persistent asthma).[37] It found that regular inhaled corticosteroids (≤2 drugs) versus regular β_2 agonists or placebo significantly improved lung function (overall weighted effect size for peak expiratory flow rate 0.59, 95% CI 0.32 to 0.84).

Harms: One non-systematic review found no evidence that low doses of inhaled corticosteroids (< 1000 μg/day of beclometasone dipropionate or equivalent) cause important systemic effects in adults.[38] One systematic review (search date 1988) assessing the harms of inhaled corticosteroids found that systemic adverse effects increase with dose and supported tapering the dose of inhaled corticosteroid to the lowest effective dose to minimise adverse effects.[39] It found that, although posterior subcapsular cataracts occur more frequently in people taking oral corticosteroids, most studies in adults provide no evidence that inhaled corticosteroids increase the risk once the confounding effect of oral corticosteroid use is removed.[39] However, one recent population based case control study suggests that, in older people, inhaled high dose beclometasone use is associated with a slightly greater risk of nuclear cataracts (RR 1.5, 95% CI 1.2 to 1.9) and posterior subcapsular cataracts (RR 1.9, 95% CI 1.3 to 2.8).[40] The systematic review assessing harms found no significant effect of low dose inhaled corticosteroids on bruising or skin thickness.[39] Inhaled corticosteroids can cause oral candidiasis or dysphonia, but these are troublesome in fewer than 5% of people.[41] The systematic review of fluticasone found a significant increase in the proportion of people who had oral candidiasis with fluticasone versus placebo (13/653 [2%] *v* 3/645 [0.5%]; RR 3.45, 95% CI 1.29 to 9.26).[28] One non-systematic review (4 RCTs, 1255 people) found no significant difference with budenoside versus placebo in mean intraocular pressure change at 12–20 weeks.[42]

Comment: The case control study on cataract formation[40] did not allow for the confounding effect of allergy, which is also a risk factor for cataract development.[43] Two RCTs have found that inhaled corticosteroids delivered using cholorofluorocarbon-free propellants such as hydrofluoroalkane are effective at low dose for people with mild persistent asthma, but dose equivalence varies with each delivery system.[34,35] It may therefore be necessary to retitrate the dose of inhaled steroids if a cholorofluorocarbon-free propellant is used.

OPTION ADDITION OF LONG ACTING INHALED β_2 AGONISTS IN PEOPLE WITH MILD, PERSISTENT ASTHMA THAT IS POORLY CONTROLLED BY INHALED CORTICOSTEROIDS

Three RCTs have found that, in people with poorly controlled asthma, adding regular doses of long acting, inhaled β_2 agonists to inhaled corticosteroids versus placebo significantly improves symptoms and lung function. One systematic review and two additional RCTs have found that,

in people with poorly controlled asthma, adding regular doses of long acting, inhaled β_2 agonists to inhaled corticosteroids versus increasing the dose of inhaled corticosteroids significantly improves lung function and symptoms, and reduces the use of rescue medication. One RCT found that, in people with poorly controlled asthma, adding a long acting β_2 agonist versus adding a leukotriene antagonist significantly improved symptoms, lung function, the need for rescue medication, and night time awakening. Regular use of long acting β_2 agonists has not been linked to deterioration in asthma control. We found no good evidence about their effect on mortality.

Benefits: **Versus placebo:** We found no systematic review. We found three RCTs (1400 people with moderate persistent asthma, uncontrolled by inhaled corticosteroids 250–2000 μg/day beclometasone dipro-prionate or equivalent) comparing regular long acting inhaled β_2 agonists versus placebo.[44–46] The RCTs found that twice daily salmeterol or formoterol (eformoterol) versus placebo improved quality of life scores, PEFR (see glossary, p 1524), and FEV_1 (see glossary, p 1524) and reduced night awakening. In the largest RCT,[46] salmeterol versus placebo significantly improved the adjusted mean PEFR (398 L/min with salmeterol *v* 386 L/min with placebo; $P < 0.001$), and significantly increased the proportion of people who did not awaken at night (74% with salmeterol *v* 68% with placebo; $P < 0.05$). Exacerbation rates were not significantly different between the two groups in any of the RCTs (proportion of people with severe exacerbations in the largest RCT[46] 20.8% with salmeterol *v* 20.9% with placebo). **Versus increased use of inhaled corticosteroids:** We found one systematic review[47] and two additional RCTs.[48,49] The review (search date 1999, 9 double blind RCTs, 3685 people with symptomatic asthma on their current dose of inhaled steroids, duration 3–6 months) compared adding salmeterol versus increased use of inhaled corticosteroids (at least double the usual dose). It found that morning PEFR was significantly higher with salmeterol (3 months: WMD in PEFR 22 L/min, 95% CI 15 to 30, $P < 0.001$; 6 months: WMD 28 L/min, 95% CI 19 to 36). Salmeterol significantly increased days without symptoms (WMD at 6 months: 15, 95% CI 12 to 18) and nights without symptoms (WMD at 6 months: 5, 95% CI 3 to 7). Salmeterol also significantly reduced the need for rescue medication. No increase in asthma exacerbations of any severity was found in the salmeterol group.[47] The first additional RCT (852 people taking low to moderate dose inhaled corticosteroids) found that additional twice daily formoterol plus as needed terbutaline versus no additional treatment significantly improved symptoms and lung function, and reduced the proportion of people with severe exacerbations from 39% to 30%.[48] The proportion of people with severe exacerbations was reduced further to 28% by a fourfold increase in daily dosage of inhaled corticosteroid, and further still to 19% by a combined, higher dose of budesonide plus formoterol. The second additional RCT (454 people with symptomatic asthma on their current dose of inhaled steroids) compared adding salmeterol 42 μg plus fluticasone 88 μg twice daily versus adding fluticasone 220 μg twice daily.[49] It found that salmeterol plus lower dose fluicasone versus higher dose fluticasone alone improved lung function, reduced the use of rescue β_2 agonists, and increased the proportion of symptom free days. **Versus addition of leukotriene antagonists:** We found one RCT (948 adults with symptomatic asthma on their current dose of inhaled steroids) that compared adding salmeterol (50 μg twice daily) versus adding montelukast (10 mg daily).[50] It found that salmeterol versus montelukast significantly increased the proportion of symptom free days (24% *v* 16%; difference 8%, 95% CI 8 to 12), improved lung function, and reduced the need for rescue medication and night time awakenings, but found no significant difference in the proportion of people with asthma exacerbations (26/476 [6%] *v* 23/472 [5%]; RR 1.12, 95% CI 0.65 to 1.93) over 12 weeks.

Harms: Several studies have found that people taking regular doses of long acting, inhaled β_2 agonists develop tolerance to protection against bronchoconstriction[51–53] and may develop a tremor. Regular use of long acting inhaled β_2 agonists has not been linked to deterioration in asthma control.[46–48]

Comment: We found no RCTs or other studies with sufficient power to assess the effect of regular use of long acting inhaled β_2 agonists on mortality.[54]

OPTION LEUKOTRIENE ANTAGONISTS IN ADULTS WITH MILD TO MODERATE, PERSISTENT ASTHMA

Three RCTs in people taking β_2 agonists alone have found that leukotriene antagonists versus placebo significantly reduce asthma symptoms and β_2 agonist use. One systematic review in people taking inhaled corticosteroids found no significant difference in the rate of exacerbations with leukotriene antagonists versus placebo. One systematic review and three subsequent RCTs have found no significant difference in the rate of exacerbations with leukotriene antagonists versus inhaled corticosteroids, but inhaled corticosteroids significantly improve quality of life, lung function, and symptom control. One RCT found that an inhaled corticosteroid plus a long acting β_2 agonist versus a leukotriene antagonist significantly improved symptoms, lung function, and exacerbations.

Benefits: **Versus placebo in people not taking inhaled corticosteroids:** We found no systematic review. We found three RCTs (1300 adults with asthma taking β_2 agonists alone), which compared the addition of leukotriene antagonists versus placebo for 13 weeks.[55–57] The RCTs all found that the inhaled leukotriene antagonist zafirlukast (20 mg twice daily) versus placebo significantly reduced daytime and night time asthma symptoms and β_2 agonist use. The largest RCT (762 people)[55] found that zafirlukast versus placebo significantly reduced day time symptoms (symptom score 8.05 with zafirlukast *v* 9.45 with placebo; $P < 0.01$), night time awakenings (2.05/wk *v* 2.52/wk; $P < 0.05$), and β_2 agonist use (3.1 puffs/day with zafirlukast *v* 3.9 puffs/day with placebo; $P < 0.01$). Morning FEV (see glossary, p 1524)$_1$ was significantly increased in people taking zafirlukast (morning FEV_1 improved by 7% *v* 3%; $P < 0.01$).[55] **Versus placebo in people taking inhaled corticosteroids:** We found one systematic review (search date 2001, 11 RCTs, 2666 people with symptomatic asthma on their current dose of inhaled steroids).[58] It found no significant different with montelukast (5 mg or 10 mg 4 times daily) versus placebo in the proportion of people with exacerbations requiring systematic steroids at 4–16 weeks (2 RCTs: 20/466 [4%] *v* 33/468 [7%]; RR 0.61, 95% CI 0.36 to 1.05). **Versus inhaled corticosteroids:** We found one systematic review (search date 1999, 8 RCTs, > 2000 adults with asthma)[59] and three subsequent RCTs.[60–62] The review compared various leukotriene antagonists versus inhaled corticosteroids for 6–12 weeks.[59] Doses of corticosteroids were equivalent to beclometasone 250–400 µg daily. It found no significant difference with leukotriene antagonists versus corticosteroids in the proportion of people with exacerbations requiring systemic steroids (4 RCTs; RR 1.3, 95% CI 0.9 to 1.9). However, corticosteroids versus leukotriene antagonists significantly improved lung function (FEV_1: 3 RCTs; SMD 0.3, 95% CI 0.2 to 0.4), morning PEFR (see glossary, p 1524) (3 RCTs; SMD 0.4, 95% CI 0.2 to 0.5), quality of life (3 RCTs; WMD 0.3, 95% CI 0.1 to 0.4), symptoms (3 RCTs; SMD 0.3, 95% CI 0.2 to 0.4), night awakenings (2 RCTs; WMD 0.6 nights/wk, 95% CI 0.3 to 0.9), and reduced the need for rescue β_2 agonists (3 RCTs; SMD 0.3, 95% CI 0.2 to 0.4).[59] The first subsequent RCT (451 adults with asthma, previously treated with β_2 agonists alone) compared fluticasone (88 mg) versus zafirlukast (20 mg), both twice daily for 12 weeks.[60] The second RCT (533 adults with asthma who were symptomatic on β_2 agonists alone) compared fluticasone with montelukast for 24 weeks.[61] The third subsequent RCT (294 adults and children > 11 years of age previously treated with β_2 agonists alone) compared fluticasone (88 µg twice daily) versus zafirlukast (20 µg twice daily).[62] All three RCTs supported the findings of the systematic review with no significant difference in exacerbations between groups, but more effective asthma control with inhaled corticosteroids. **Versus inhaled corticosteroids plus long acting β_2 agonists:** We found no systematic review. We found one RCT (423 adults with symptomatic asthma when taking short acting β_2 agonists) that compared montelukast (20 µg once daily) versus fluticasone (100 µg) plus salmeterol (50 µg twice daily).[63] It found that fluticasone plus salmeterol versus montelukast significantly increased the percentage of symptom free days compared to baseline data (22% with montelukast *v* 49% with fluticasone plus salmeterol; WMD 27%, 95% CI 20% to 35%), reducing the rate of exacerbations (11 with montelukast *v* 0 with fluticasone plus salmeterol; $P < 0.001$), and improving lung function over 12 weeks.

Harms: **Versus placebo in people not taking corticosteroids:** In the RCT comparing zafirlukast versus placebo, the incidence of adverse effects (predominantly pharyngitis and headache) was similar in both groups (350/514 [68%] *v* 160/248 [65%]).[55] **Versus placebo in people taking inhaled corticosteroids:** The systematic review found that higher than licensed dose leukotriene antagonists versus placebo significantly increased the proportion of people with liver enzyme elevation (13/280 [5%] *v* 2/276 [0.7%]; RR 5.36, 95% CI 1.40 to 20.40).[58] **Versus inhaled corticosteroids:** The systematic review found that adverse effects were not significantly different with leukotriene antagonists versus corticosteroids, but leukotriene antagonists significantly increased the risk of "withdrawals for any cause" (RR 1.4, 95% CI 1.1 to 1.9) and "withdrawals due to adverse effects" (RR 1.9, 95% CI 1.1 to 3.3).[49]

Comment: The systematic review comparing leukotriene antagonists versus inhaled corticosteroids advocated caution because of the small number of RCTs so far published in full text.[59]

QUESTION What are the effects of treatments for acute asthma?

Mark FitzGerald

OPTION SPACER DEVICES/HOLDING CHAMBERS VERSUS NEBULISERS FOR DELIVERING β_2 AGONISTS IN ACUTE ASTHMA

One systematic review found no significant difference in forced expiratory volume in 1 second, peak expiratory flow rate, hospital admissions, or time spent in the emergency department with nebulisers versus holding chambers plus metered dose inhalers for delivering β_2 agonists in people with acute but not life threatening asthma.

Benefits: We found one systematic review (search date 1999, 13 RCTs, non-hospitalised adults and children with acute asthma) comparing holding chambers plus metered dose inhalers versus nebulisers for delivering β_2 agonists.[64] Results in adults and children were analysed separately (see asthma in children, p 262). In adults, there was no significant difference in rates of hospital admission (OR 1.12, 95% CI 0.45 to 2.76), length of time spent in the emergency department (WMD +0.02 h, 95% CI –0.40 to +0.44 h), or in PEFR (see glossary, p 1524) and FEV (see glossary, p 1524)$_1$. There was still no significant difference when the three RCTs involving the most severely affected people ($FEV_1 < 30\%$ predicted) were included (WMD for FEV_1 holding chamber *v* nebuliser –1.5% predicted, 95% CI –8.3% to +5.3%). Symptoms were measured on different scales and findings could not be combined.

Harms: The review found no significant difference in heart rates with holding chambers versus nebulisers (WMD with holding chamber *v* nebuliser +1.6% of baseline, 95% CI –2.4% to +5.5% of baseline).[64]

Comment: The review found no evidence of publication bias.[64] To overcome possible dose confounding, the review was confined to studies that used multiple treatment doses titrated against the individuals' responses. As studies excluded people with life threatening asthma (see glossary, p 1524), results may not generalise to such people.

OPTION SYSTEMIC CORTICOSTEROIDS FOR ACUTE ASTHMA

One systematic review has found that systemic corticosteroids versus placebo taken at the start of an acute exacerbation significantly reduce rates of hospital admission. One systematic review has found that systemic corticosteroids versus placebo taken after discharge from hospital following an acute exacerbation significantly reduce relapses requiring additional care, readmissions to hospital, and the need for additional β_2 agonists. One of the reviews found no significant difference in outcomes with oral corticosteroids versus intramuscular or intravenous corticosteroids. One RCT found no significant difference in morning peak expiratory flow rate with tapering of prednisolone over a week versus

abrupt cessation. One small RCT found no difference in peak expiratory flow rate and relapse rates, with 1 week versus 2 weeks of oral prednisone, but may have been too small to exclude a clinically important difference.

Benefits: **Versus placebo:** We found two systematic reviews.[65,66] The first review (search date 1991, 5 RCTs, 422 people) found that early use of systemic corticosteroids (oral, iv, or im) versus placebo in the emergency department significantly reduced hospital admissions (OR 0.47, 95% CI 0.27 to 0.79).[65] The second review (search date 1997, 7 RCTs in about 320 people) compared oral corticosteroids versus placebo (4 RCTs), oral versus intramuscular corticosteroids (2 RCTs), and intramuscular corticosteroids versus placebo (1 RCT) after discharge from the emergency department.[66] It found that systemic corticosteroids (oral or im) versus placebo significantly reduced the proportion of people with relapses requiring additional care (5 RCTs, 345 people, RR of relapse within first wk, systemic corticosteroids *v* placebo 0.39, 95% CI 0.21 to 0.74, NNT 10; 1 RCT, 83 people, RR of relapse with first 21 days 0.47, 95% CI 0.25 to 0.89), and reduced hospital readmissions (4 RCTs, 210 people, RR 0.35, 95% CI 0.13 to 0.95). Corticosteroids significantly reduced the use of β_2 agonists (WMD –3.3 puffs/day, 95% CI –5.5 to –1.0). The review found no clear difference between intramuscular and oral corticosteroids.[66] **Stopping treatment:** We found no systematic review. One RCT (35 people admitted to hospital with acute asthma who received 40 mg prednisolone for 10 days) found no significant difference in morning peak expiratory flow rate (see glossary, p 1524) with tapering of prednisolone over a week versus abrupt cessation (mean increase in peak expiratory flow rate 45 L/min with tapering versus 43 L/min with cessation; P = 0.82).[67] **Optimal dose and duration of treatment:** We found no systematic review. One RCT (20 people) compared 1 week versus 2 weeks of oral prednisone following a 3 day course of intravenous methylprednisolone and found no difference in peak expiratory flow rate and relapse rates.[68] The study is limited by its small sample size. The optimal duration of treatment is likely to depend on the individual, the severity of the exacerbation, and use of concomitant medications.

Harms: Systemic corticosteroids can cause the same adverse effects in asthma as in other diseases, even when administered for a short time (see asthma in children, p 262).

Comment: We found no reliable evidence about the role of oral corticosteroids in acute asthma after admission to hospital, nor is it likely that a placebo controlled RCT would be conducted in acute severe asthma. One RCT (413 adults presenting to general practitioners with acute asthma) found no difference in rates of treatment failure with a short course of oral corticosteroids versus a high dose of inhaled fluticasone.[69]

OPTION INHALED CORTICOSTEROIDS FOR ACUTE ASTHMA

One systematic review in people in the emergency department who were not taking systemic corticosteroids has found that inhaled corticosteroids versus placebo significantly reduce hospital admissions, but has found

that in people taking systemic corticosteroids adding inhaled corticosteroids versus placebo does not significantly reduce hospital admissions. A second systematic review found insufficient evidence of the effects of inhaled versus oral corticosteroids. It found no significant difference in relapse rates at 7–10 days with inhaled corticosteroids plus oral corticosteroids versus oral corticosteroids alone.

Benefits: **Versus placebo:** We found one systematic review (search date 2000, 3 RCTs, 208 people) comparing the early use of inhaled corticosteroids versus placebo in the emergency department.[70] It found that in people not taking systemic corticosteroids, inhaled corticosteroids versus placebo significantly reduced hospital admissions (6/105 *v* 24/103; OR 0.21, 95% CI 0.08 to 0.53). It identified two RCTs in people taking systemic corticosteroids, which compared the addition of inhaled corticosteroids versus placebo.[70] It found that adding inhaled corticosteroids to systemic corticosteroids versus placebo reduced hospital admissions, but the difference was not significant (2 RCTs; 104 adults and children; 10/54 *v* 17/50; OR 0.45, 95% CI 0.18 to 1.12).[70] **Versus oral corticosteroids:** We found one systematic review (search date 1999) that identified seven RCTs (1204 children and adults) comparing inhaled corticosteroids versus oral corticosteroids.[71] In six RCTs, high dose inhaled corticosteroids were compared to tapering oral corticosteroids, whereas in one study the oral corticosteroid dose was fixed. The review found no significant difference in relapse rates at 7–10 days (4 RCTs; 53/343 [15%] *v* 53/341 [15%]; OR 1.0, 95% CI 0.66 to 1.52). **Plus oral corticosteroids versus oral corticosteroids alone:** We found one systematic review (search date 1999) that identified three RCTs (909 adults) comparing inhaled corticosteroids plus oral corticosteroids versus oral corticosteroids alone.[71] It found no significant difference in relapse rates with inhaled plus oral corticosteroid versus oral corticosteroids alone, although the inhaled corticosteroid group did better at day 7–10 (OR 0.72, 95% CI 0.48 to 1.10) and day 20–24 (OR 0.68, 95% CI, 0.46 to 1.02).[71]

Harms: The reviews found no significant differences in adverse effects between the groups, but one review commented that most of the RCTs identified gave little information on adverse effects apart from reporting that they were "rare".[71] See also harms of inhaled corticosteroids under asthma in children, p 271.

Comment: None.

OPTION CONTINUOUS VERSUS AS NEEDED SHORT ACTING β_2 AGONISTS FOR ACUTE ASTHMA

One large RCT found that continuous versus as needed β_2 agonists significantly improved forced expiratory volume in 1 second at 2 hours, but four smaller RCTs found no significant difference in peak expiratory flow rate, forced expiratory volume in 1 second, or rates of admission. In adults with more severe airflow obstruction, two RCTs have found that continuous nebulised treatment versus intermittent treatment improves lung function.

Benefits: We found no systematic review. We found five RCTs.[72–76] One RCT (165 people) compared four regimens of salbutamol (see glossary, p 1524) in a factorial design: high (1.5 mg) versus standard (0.5 mg) doses, and continuous versus as needed delivery. It found significantly greater improvement in forced expiratory volume in 1 second (FEV_1) (see glossary, p 1524) at 2 hours with continuous versus as needed delivery at both high and standard doses ($P < 0.05$).[72] Another RCT (99 people) found no significant difference in PEFR (see glossary, p 1524) or hospital admission over 2 hours with continuous versus as needed β_2 agonists.[73] However, in a subgroup of 69 people with more severe asthma (PEFR ≤ 200 L/min), continuous aerosol delivery versus as needed delivery significantly increased PEFR at 120 minutes (296 L/min, 95% CI 266 to 329 with continuous *v* 244 L/min, 95% CI 216 to 272 with as needed delivery).[73] Hospital admissions in this subgroup were also significantly lower with continuous delivery (11/35 [28%] *v* 19/34 [57%]; P = 0.03). The *post hoc* nature of the analysis weakens these results. A third RCT (38 people) found no significant difference in FEV_1 improvement with continuous versus treatment in people with lower initial FEV_1 as needed salbutamol (see glossary, p 1525), but subgroup analysis in people with lower initial FEV_1 found a greater improvement in FEV_1 with continuous treatment.[74] The other two RCTs found no significant difference in lung function or rate of hospital admission with continuous versus intermittent salbutamol.[75,76]

Harms: Commonly reported mild adverse effects associated with frequent dosing include tachycardia, tremor, and headache. Metabolic abnormalities are less common and include hypokalemia. One RCT found the highest rate of adverse effects with high dose as needed treatment. The most common adverse effect was tremor (24% as needed high dose, 20% continuous high dose, 9% hourly standard dose, and 3% continuous standard dose).[72]

Comment: We found one RCT (46 adults in hospital), which addressed the slightly different, but related, question of regular nebulised salbutamol (5 mg every 4 h) versus on demand salbutamol (2.5 5 mg).[77] It found that on demand dosage significantly reduced hospital stay (3.7 days *v* 4.7 days), the proportion of nebulisations (geometric mean 7.0 *v* 14; P = 0.003), and palpitations (P = 0.05).

OPTION INTRAVENOUS VERSUS NEBULISED DELIVERY OF SHORT ACTING β_2 AGONISTS FOR ACUTE ASTHMA

One systematic review comparing intravenous versus inhaled short acting β_2 agonists in the emergency department found no significant difference in peak expiratory flow rate at 60 minutes.

Benefits: We found one systematic review (search date not stated, 6 RCTs, 337 people) comparing intravenous versus inhaled short acting β_2 agonists.[78] Five of the RCTs used nebulised delivery of inhaled β_2 agonists, and one used intermittent positive pressure breathing. It found that intravenous versus inhaled β_2 agonists lowered peak expiratory flow rate (see glossary, p 1524) at 60 minutes, but the difference was not significant (WMD 24.7 L/min, 95% CI –2.9 to +52). It found no significant difference in heart rate at 60 minutes with intravenous versus inhaled β_2 agonists (WMD 4.5 bpm, 95% CI –4.9 to +14).

Harms: The systematic review found no significant difference in the proportion of people with autonomic adverse effects (including palpitations, tachycardia, hypertension, tremor, headache, nausea and vomiting) with intravenous versus inhaled β_2 agonists (53/153 [35%] *v* 76/144 [53%]; RR 1.46, 95% CI 0.46 to 4.68).[78]

Comment: None.

OPTION ADDITION OF IPRATROPIUM BROMIDE TO β_2 AGONISTS IN ACUTE ASTHMA

Three systematic reviews and one subsequent RCT have found that combining ipratropium bromide with salbutamol versus salbutamol alone significantly improves lung function in people with more severe acute asthma. One of the reviews and the subsequent RCT found that the addition of ipratropium bromide significantly reduced hospital admissions. The other two systematic reviews, which only included three of the five RCTs in first review in their analysis of hospital admissions, found no significant difference with the addition of ipratropium bromide versus salbutamol alone.

Benefits: We found three systematic reviews[79–81] and one subsequent RCT.[82] The first systematic review (search date 1999, 10 RCTs, 1483 people)[79] found that inhaled ipratropium plus salbutamol (see glossary, p 1525) versus salbutamol alone, significantly reduced hospital admissions (5 RCTs, 1186 people; OR 0.62, 95% CI 0.44 to 0.88; NNT 18, 95% CI 11 to 77). Meta-analysis of the four RCTs that evaluated people with severe airflow obstruction (forced expiratory volume in 1 second [FEV_1] < 35%) found that additional treatment with ipratropium significantly improved FEV_1 (see glossary, p 1524) over 90 minutes (effect size 0.38, 95% CI 0.05 to 0.67). The second systematic review (search date not stated) identified the same ten RCTs.[80] It found the same results for improvement in FEV_1 in people with severe airflow obstruction, but included only three of the RCTs in its analysis of hospital admissions (see comment below).[80] It found no significant difference in hospital admissions with ipratropium bromide plus salbutamol versus salbutamol alone (3 RCTs, 1064 people; RR 0.80, 95% CI 0.61 to 1.06). The third systematic review (search date 1997, 10 RCTs including 8 identified by the later reviews, 1377 people) found that adding ipratropium bromide versus salbutamol alone improved lung function, but also found no significant difference in hospital admissions, when assessing the same three RCTs.[81] The subsequent RCT (180 people with acute asthma, mean FEV_1 < 50%) compared salbutamol plus placebo versus salbutamol plus ipratropium.[82] It found that the addition of ipratropium significantly improved peak expiratory flow rate (see glossary, p 1524) (difference in improvement with ipratropium *v* placebo: 21%, 95% CI 2.6% to 38%) and FEV_1 (difference in improvement with ipratropium *v* placebo: 48%, 95% CI 20% to 76%). People taking ipratropium were significantly less likely to require hospital admission at the end of the 3 hour trial period (20% *v* 39%; P = 0.01).

Harms: The reviews and the subsequent RCT found no significant difference in adverse effects with the addition of ipratropium to salbutamol versus salbutamol alone.[79–82]

Comment: The authors of the second and third systematic reviews stated that only three RCTs reported data in sufficient detail to be included in the analysis of hospital admission rates.[80,81]

OPTION OXYGEN SUPPLEMENTATION FOR ACUTE ASTHMA

We found no systematic review or RCTs of oxygen in acute asthma. However, experience and pathophysiology suggest that its role is vital in acute asthma. Small RCTs found mixed evidence that combining oxygen with helium may improve peak expiratory flow rate.

Benefits: **Oxygen alone:** We found no systematic review and no RCTs. **Oxygen with helium:** We found three RCTs of combined helium (70% or 80%) and oxygen (30% or 20%) in adults with acute asthma.[83–85] One RCT included 27 people; peak expiratory flow rate (see glossary, p 1524) less than 250 litres/minutes despite treatment, pulsus paradoxus (see glossary, p 1524) greater than 15 mmHg. Breathing a helium–oxygen mixture (80 : 20) versus breathing room air alone reduced pulsus paradoxus and improved peak flow (results presented only as a graph).[83] The second RCT (23 people) found the helium–oxygen combination versus 30% oxygen increased peak expiratory flow rate (58% with helium–oxygen *v* 10% with oxygen).[84] The third RCT (205 people) found no evidence of benefit from helium plus oxygen, but it was limited by a brief intervention (15 mins), single blinding, and inclusion of people with mild to moderate acute asthma.[85]

Harms: We found no evidence of adverse effects associated with oxygen alone or with helium–oxygen in acute asthma.

Comment: The most severe stages of acute asthma are respiratory failure, cardiopulmonary arrest, and death.[12,13] Studies of near fatal asthma suggest that hypoxia rather than arrhythmias account for asthma deaths. It seems reasonable that supplemental oxygen should continue to form a critical part of management even though we found no RCTs providing direct evidence for this. Peak flow readings vary depending on the viscosity of the gas being delivered (helium is less dense than oxygen so non-standardised measures of peak flow will increase relative to air, even if the mixture has no effect on airway narrowing). It was not clear in all RCTs whether peak flow readings were standardised for air and for helium–oxygen mixtures.

OPTION MAGNESIUM SULPHATE FOR ACUTE ASTHMA

Subgroup analysis from one systematic review suggests that, in people with more severe acute asthma, adding intravenous magnesium sulphate to usual treatment may improve peak expiratory flow rate and forced expiratory volume in 1 second, and reduce rates of hospital admission. Subsequent RCTs found that magnesium sulphate versus saline or versus placebo significantly improved peak expiratory flow rate, but did not reduce hospital admissions.

Benefits: We found one systematic review (search date 1999, 5 RCTs in adults, 3 RCTs in children, 665 people)[86] and three subsequent RCTs.[87–89] The review compared the addition of intravenous magnesium sulphate versus placebo with usual treatment, and found no significant difference in hospital admissions (OR 0.31, 95% CI 0.09 to 1.02). Prespecified subgroup analysis of adults with more severe airflow obstruction (sample size not given; forced expiratory volume in one second (see glossary, p 1524) < 30% at presentation, failure to respond to initial treatment, or failure to improve beyond 60% in forced expiratory volume in one second after 1 h) found that those receiving magnesium sulphate had better PEFR (see glossary, p 1524) and reduced rates of hospital admission. The first subsequent RCT (33 evaluable people) found no significant difference in hospital admissions with magnesium sulphate versus placebo (18% with magnesium sulphate *v* 25% with placebo; RR 0.71, 95% CI 0.19 to 2.67).[88] The second subsequent RCT (35 people) compared salbutamol (see glossary, p 1525) plus saline versus salbutamol plus magnesium sulphate through a nebuliser. It found that magnesium sulphate versus saline significantly increased PEFR (increase in PEFR after 10 mins: 61% *v* 31%; difference 30%, 95% CI 3 to 56%; P = 0.03).[87] The third subsequent RCT (42 people with acute asthma receiving inhaled bronchodilators and intravenous corticosteroids) found that intravenous magnesium sulphate versus placebo significantly improved PEFR at 60 minutes (174 L/min *v* 212 L/min; P = 0.04), but did not reduce the proportion of people admitted to hospital (5/18 [28%] *v* 5/24 [21%]; RR 1.33, 95% CI 0.45 to 3.92).[89]

Harms: RCTs did not specifically address harms.

Comment: Further studies are needed to clarify the role of intravenous magnesium sulphate in acute asthma. Two of the studies involved treatment with aminophylline and one with ipratropium, both of which have been found to affect hospital admission rates without affecting the degree of airflow obstruction.[90] The subgroup analysis involved intergroup and intragroup analyses specified before the trial was conducted, and so provides reasonably strong evidence of an effect.

OPTION MECHANICAL VENTILATION FOR SEVERE ACUTE ASTHMA

We found no RCTs comparing mechanical ventilation versus no ventilation for severe acute asthma. Evidence from cohort studies and case series support its use, despite a high level of morbidity related to the intervention.

Benefits: We found no systematic review or RCTs.

Harms: Mechanical ventilation is associated with hypotension, barotrauma, infection, and myopathy, especially when prolonged paralysis is required with muscle relaxants and systemic corticosteroids.[91] Adverse effects reported in one retrospective study of 88 episodes of mechanical ventilation were hypotension (20%), pulmonary barotrauma (14%), and arrhythmias (10%).[92]

Comment: Experience suggests that mechanical ventilation is a life saving intervention needed by a small minority of people with severe acute asthma. Cohort studies[93,94] and one case series[95] found fewer deaths with controlled hypoventilation versus ventilation in which carbon dioxide levels were normalised (for which historical cohorts and case series have reported mortality rates of 7.5–23%).[92,96–98] Non-invasive ventilation has been used in people with acute exacerbations of chronic obstructive lung disease,[99] but requires prospective validation in people with acute asthma. Future research should also focus on delivery of bronchodilators, optimal use of muscle relaxants, and dose of corticosteroids.

OPTION SPECIALIST VERSUS GENERALIST CARE FOR ACUTE ASTHMA

One systematic and one non-systematic review of RCTs and observational studies suggest that specialist versus generalist care may improve outcomes.

Benefits: We found one systematic review[100] and one non-systematic review.[101] The systematic review (search date 1995, 4 RCTs, 10 observational studies) found limited evidence that specialist care versus generalist care may improve outcomes and that shared care (see glossary, p 1525) may be as effective as usual outpatient care.[100] One non-systematic review of RCTs and observational studies found that "expert based" care versus general care improved outcomes.[101] One quasi-randomised trial (based on day of attendance) identified by the non-systematic review referred people from the emergency department to specialist care versus routine general medical follow up.[102] It found that people receiving specialist care were significantly less likely to wake at night (OR 0.24, 95% CI 0.11 to 0.52), suffer relapse requiring emergency admission by 6 months (for 1 admission RR 0.56, 95% CI 0.34 to 0.95; for 2 admissions RR 0.3, 95% CI 0.16 to 0.6), or suffer multiple relapses. They were more likely to use inhaled corticosteroids (OR 3.6, 95% CI 1.9 to 6.6) and sodium cromoglicate (sodium cromoglycate) (RR 2.2, 95% CI 1.9 to 2.5).

Harms: The reviews gave no information about harms associated with specialist versus generalist care.[100,101]

Comment: Many of the RCTs and observational studies in the systematic review were small.[100]

OPTION EDUCATION ABOUT ACUTE ASTHMA

One systematic review has found that education to facilitate self management of asthma in adults versus usual care significantly reduces hospital admission, unscheduled visits to the doctor, and days off work at the end of the study. One subsequent RCT has found that a structured education asthma management programme versus limited education or versus usual care for 1 year significantly reduces unscheduled visits to the doctor over the final 6 months of treatment.

Benefits: We found one systematic review (search date 1999, 22 RCTs)[103] and one subsequent RCT of adult self management of asthma.[104] The review found that education about asthma to facilitate self management, whether initiated from a specialist or generalist setting, significantly reduced the risk of hospital admission (RR 0.62, 95% CI 0.41 to 0.96; NNT 38, 95% CI 20 to 382), unscheduled visits to the doctor (RR 0.74, 95% CI 0.63 to 0.90; NNT 12, 95% CI 8 to 36), and days off work (RR 0.75, 95% CI 0.63 to 0.90; NNT 7, 95% CI 5 to 13) at the end of the study. Best results were achieved in people who had written care plans.[103] The subsequent RCT (105 people) compared three interventions: limited education (usual care plus teaching inhaler technique plus self care plan); structured education (structured asthma education programme in addition to limited education interventions); and usual care for 1 year.[104] It found no significant difference with limited education versus usual care in the proportion of unscheduled visits to the doctor, but found that structured education versus limited education or versus usual care significantly reduced unscheduled visits over the final 6 months of treatment ($P = 0.03$ with structured versus limited education; $P = 0.01$ with structured education versus usual care; results presented graphically).

Harms: The systematic review and subsequent RCT gave no information on adverse effects.[103,104]

Comment: None.

GLOSSARY

Diurnal variation A characteristic of people with asthma is increased variation in peak flow rates and forced expiratory volume in 1 second during the day. The diurnal variation is sometimes expressed as the difference between maximum and minimum values expressed as a fraction of the maximum value.

Forced expiratory volume in 1 second (FEV_1) The volume breathed out in the first second of forceful blowing into a spirometer, measured in litres.

Life threatening asthma An attack of such severity that the person usually requires management in the emergency department. Some people require endotracheal intubation and, usually in the initial stages of resuscitation, cannot inhale bronchodilator treatment.

Peak expiratory flow rate (PEFR) The maximum rate that gas is expired from the lungs when blowing into a peak flow meter or a spirometer. It is measured at an instant, but the units are expressed as litres per minute.

Pulsus paradoxus A measure of the severity of asthma based on the difference in systolic pressure during inspiration and expiration. The blood pressure normally falls a little during inspiration (< 10 mmHg), but in acute severe asthma (and in some other conditions) the fall of systolic pressure in inspiration is greater.

Salbutamol A short acting β_2 agonist known as albuterol in the USA.
Shared care Involves sharing care between outpatient specialist and general practitioner.

Substantive changes

Low doses of inhaled steroids in people with mild, persistent asthma Two new systematic reviews[23,28] and five new RCTs;[26,27,29,34,35] conclusions unchanged.
Addition of long acting inhaled β_2 agonists in people whose asthma is poorly controlled by inhaled corticosteroids One new RCT comparing adding long acting β_2 agonist versus increased use of corticosteroids;[49] conclusions unchanged.
Addition of long acting inhaled β_2 agonists in people whose asthma is poorly controlled by inhaled corticosteroids One RCT found that, in people with poorly controlled asthma, adding a long acting β_2 agonist versus adding a leukotriene antagonist significantly improved symptoms, lung function, the need for rescue medication, and night time awakening.[50]
Leukotriene antagonists in adults with mild to moderate, persistent asthma One new systematic review in people taking inhaled corticosteroids found no significant difference in the rate of exacerbations with leukotriene antagonists versus placebo.[58]
Leukotriene antagonists in adults with mild to moderate, persistent asthma One new RCT comparing leukotriene antagonists versus corticosteroids;[62] conclusions unchanged.
Leukotriene antagonists in adults with mild to moderate, persistent asthma One new RCT found that an inhaled corticosteroid plus a long acting β_2 agonist improved symptoms, lung function, and exacerbations significantly more than a leukotriene agonist.[63]
Intravenous versus nebulised delivery of short acting β_2 agonists for acute asthma One new systematic review found that intravenous delivery of short acting β_2 agonists was no more effective than nebulised delivery in improving peak expiratory flow rate at 60 minutes.[78]
Addition of ipratropium bromide to β_2 agonists in acute asthma One new systematic review;[80] conclusions unchanged.
Magnesium sulphate One new RCT;[89] conclusions unchanged.
Specialist versus generalist care One new systematic review;[100] conclusions unchanged.
Education about acute asthma One new RCT;[104] conclusions unchanged.

REFERENCES

1. National Heart, Blood and Lung Institute. National Asthma Education and Prevention Program. Expert Panel Report 2. Guidelines for the Diagnosis and Management of Asthma. NIH Publication No. 97 4051;July 1997:20.
2. British Thoracic Society Guidelines. *Thorax* 1997;52:S1–S2.
3. Kaur B, Anderson HR, Austin J, et al. Prevalence of asthma symptoms, diagnosis, and treatment in 12–14 year old children across Great Britain (international study of asthma and allergies in childhood, ISAAC UK). *BMJ* 1998;316:118–124.
4. Woolcock AJ, Peat JK. Evidence for an increase in asthma world-wide. *Ciba Found Symp* 1997;206:122–134.
5. Holgate ST. The epidemic of allergy and asthma. *Nature* 1999;402:B2–4.
6. The International Study of Asthma and Allergies in Childhood (ISAAC) Steering Committee. Worldwide variation in prevalence of symptoms of asthma, allergic rhinoconjunctivitis, and atopic eczema: ISAAC. *Lancet* 1998;351:1225–1232.
7. Burney P, Chinn DJ, Luczynska C, et al. Variations in the prevalence of respiratory symptoms, self-reported asthma attacks, and use of asthma medication in the European Community Respiratory Health Survey. *Eur Respir J* 1996;9:687–695.
8. Duff AL, Platts-Mills TA. Allergens and asthma. *Pediatr Clin North Am* 1992;39:1277–1291.
9. Chan-Yeung M, Malo JL. Occupational asthma. *N Engl J Med* 1995;333:107–112.
10. Lange P, Parner J, Vestbo J, et al. A 15-year follow-up study of ventilatory function in adults with asthma. *N Engl J Med* 1998;339:1194–1200.
11. FitzGerald JM, Grunfeld A. Acute life-threatening asthma. In: FitzGerald JM, Ernst PP, Boulet LP,

O'Byrne PM, eds. *Evidence based asthma management*. Decker: Hamilton, Ontario, 2000:233–244.
12. Nahum A, Tuxen DT. Management of asthma in the intensive care unit. In: FitzGerald JM, Ernst PP, Boulet LP, O'Byrne PM, eds. *Evidence based asthma management*. Decker: Hamilton, Ontario, 2000:245–261.
13. Turner MT, Noertjojo K, Vedal S, et al. Risk factors for near-fatal asthma: a case control study in patients hospitalised with acute asthma. *Am J Respir Crit Care Med* 1998;157:1804–1809.
14. Molfino NA, Nannimi A, Martelli AN, et al. Respiratory arrest in near fatal asthma. *N Engl J Med* 1991;324:285–288.
15. Emmerman CL, Woodruff PG, Cydulka RK, et al. Prospective multi-center study of relapse following treatment for acute asthma among adults presenting to the emergency department. *Chest* 1999;115:919–927.
16. Walters EH, Walters J. Inhaled short acting β_2 agonist use in asthma: regular versus as needed treatment. In: The Cochrane Library, Issue 4, 2001. Oxford: Update Software. Search date not stated; primary sources Cochrane Airways Group Asthma and Wheeze RCT register.
17. Dennis SM, Sharp SJ, Vickers MR, et al. Regular inhaled salbutamol and asthma control: the TRUST randomised trial. *Lancet* 2000;355:1675–1679.
18. Spitzer WO, Suissa S, Ernst P, et al. The use of β-agonists and the risk of death and near death from asthma. *N Engl J Med* 1992;326:501–506.
19. Crane J, Pearce N, Flatt A, et al. Prescribed fenoterol and death from asthma in New Zealand, 1981–1983: case-control study. *Lancet* 1989;1:917–922.
20. Kerrebijn KF, van Essen-Zandvliet EE, Neijens HJ. Effect of long-term treatment with inhaled corticosteroids and β-agonists on the bronchial responsiveness in children with asthma. *J Allergy Clin Immunol* 1987;79:653–659.
21. Cockcroft DW, McParland CP, Britto SA, et al. Regular inhaled salbutamol and airway responsiveness to allergen. *Lancet* 1993;342:833–837.
22. Ahrens RC. Skeletal muscle tremor and the influence of adrenergic drugs. *J Asthma* 1990;27:11–20.
23. Adams N, Bestall J, Jones PW. Budesonide for chronic asthma in children and adults (Cochrane Review). In: The Cochrane Library, Issue 4, 2001. Oxford: Update Software. Search date 1999; primary sources The Cochrane Airways Group Trial Register, reference lists of articles, contact with trialists and handsearch of abstracts of major respiratory society meetings (1997–1999).
24. Kemp J, Wanderer AA, Ramsdell J, et al. Rapid onset of control with budesonide turbuhaler in patients with mild-to-moderate asthma. *Ann Allergy Asthma Immunol* 1999;82:463–471.
25. McFadden ER, Casale TB, Edwards TB, et al. Administration of budesonide once daily by means of turbuhaler to subjects with stable asthma. *J Allergy Clin Immunol* 1999;104:46–52.
26. Miyamoto T, Takahashi T, Nakajima S, et al. A double-blind, placebo-controlled dose-response study with budesonide Turbuhaler in Japanese asthma patients. Japanese Pulmicort Turbuhaler study group. *Respirology* 2000;5:247–256.
27. Banov CH, Howland III WC, Lumry WR. Once-daily budesonide via Turbuhaler improves symptoms in adults with persistent asthma. *Ann Allergy Asthma Immunol* 2001;86:627–632.
28. Adams N, Bestall J, Jones PW. Inhaled fluticasone proprionate for chronic asthma. In: The Cochrane Library, Issue 4, 2001. Oxford: Update Software. Search date 1999; primary sources The Cochrane Airways Group Trial Register, reference lists of articles, contact with trialists, and abstracts of major respiratory society meetings (1997–1999).
29. Wolfe JD, Selner JC, Mendelson LM, et al. Effectiveness of fluticasone propionate in patients with moderate asthma: a dose-ranging study. *Clin Ther* 1996;18:635–646.
30. Adams NP, Bestall JB, Jones PW. Inhaled beclomethasone versus placebo for chronic asthma (Cochrane Review). In: The Cochrane Library, Issue 4, 2001. Oxford: Update Software. Search date 1999; primary sources Cochrane Airways Group Trial Register, handsearching of journals, conference proceedings, and contact with pharmaceutical companies.
31. Bronsky E, Korenblat P, Harris AG, et al. Comparative clinical study of inhaled beclomethasone dipropionate and triamcinolone acetonide in persistent asthma. *Ann Allergy* 1998;80:295–302.
32. Bernstein DI, Cohen R, Ginchansky E, et al. A multicenter, placebo-controlled study of twice daily triamcinolone acetonide (800 μg per day) for the treatment of patients with mild-to-moderate asthma. *J Allergy Clin Immunol* 1998;101:433–438.
33. Ramsdell JW, Fish L, Graft D, et al. A controlled trial of twice daily triamcinolone oral inhaler in patients with mild-to-moderate asthma. *Ann Allergy* 1998;80:385–390.
34. Welch, M Bernstein D. A controlled trial of chlorofluorocarbon-free triamcinolone acetonide inhalation aerosol in the treatment of adult patients with persistent asthma. *Chest* 1999;116:1304–1312.
35. Corren J, Nelson H, Greos LS, et al. Effective control of asthma with hydrofluoroalkane flunisolide delivered as an extrafine aerosol in asthma patients. *Ann Allergy Asthma Immunol* 2001;87:405–411.
36. Nathan RA, Nayak AS, Grant DF, et al. Mometasone furoate; efficacy and safety in moderate asthma compared to beclomethasone dipropionate. *Ann Allergy Asthma Immunol* 2001;86:203–210.
37. Hatoum HT, Schumock GT, Kendzierski DL. Meta-analysis of controlled trials of drug therapy in mild chronic asthma: the role of inhaled corticosteroids. *Ann Pharmacother* 1994;28:1285–1289. Search date not stated; primary source Medline.
38. Barnes PJ, Pedersen S, Busse WW. Efficacy and safety of inhaled corticosteroids: new developments. *Am J Respir Crit Care Med* 1998;157:1–53.
39. Lipworth BJ. Systemic adverse effects of inhaled corticosteroid therapy; a systematic review and meta-analysis. *Arch Intern Med* 1999;159:941–955. Search date 1998; primary sources Medline, Embase, BIDS, and hand searches of bibliographies of retrieved articles and abstracts of respiratory and allergy-based journals.
40. Cumming RG, Mitchell P, Leeder SR. Use of inhaled corticosteroids and the risk of cataracts. *N Engl J Med* 1997;337:8–14.
41. Toogood JH, Jennings B, Greenway RW, et al. Candidiasis and dysphonia complicating beclomethasone treatment of asthma. *J Allergy Clin Immunol* 1980;65:145–153.
42. Duh MS, Walker AM, Lindmark B, et al. Association between intraocular pressure and budesonide inhalation therapy in asthmatic patients. *Ann Allergy Asthma Immunol* 2000;85:356–361.
43. Eckerskorn U, Hockwin O, Müller-Breitenkamp R, et al. Evaluation of cataract-related risk factors

using detailed classification systems and multivariate statistical methods. *Dev Ophthalmol* 1987;15:82–91.
44. Kemp JP, Cook DA, Incaudo GA, et al. Salmeterol improves quality of life in patients with asthma requiring inhaled corticosteroids. *J Allergy Clin Immunol* 1998;101:188–195.
45. FitzGerald JM, Chapman KR, Della Cioppa G, et al. Sustained bronchoprotection, bronchodilatation, and symptom control during regular formoterol use in asthma of moderate or greater severity. *J Allergy Clin Immunol* 1999;103:427–435.
46. D'Urzo AD, Chapman KR, Cartier A, et al. Effectiveness and safety of salmeterol in nonspecialist practice settings. *Chest* 2001;119:714–719.
47. Shrewsbury S, Pyke S, Britton M. Meta-analysis of increased dose of inhaled steroid or addition of salmeterol in symptomatic asthma (MIASMA). *BMJ* 2000;320:1368–1373. Search date 1999; primary sources Medline, Embase, and GlaxoSmithKline databases.
48. Pauwels RA, Lofdahl C-G, Postma DS, et al. Effect of inhaled formoterol and budesonide on exacerbations of asthma. *N Engl J Med* 1997;337:1405–1411.
49. Baraniuk JM-J. Fluticasone alone or in combination with salmeterol vs triamcinolone in asthma. *Chest* 1999;116:625–632
50. Fish JE, Israel E, Murray JJ, et al. Salmeterol powder provides significantly better benefit than montelukast in asthmatic patients receiving concomitant inhaled corticosteroid therapy. *Chest* 2001;120:423–430.
51. Cheung D, Timmers MC, Zwinderman AH, et al. Long-term effects of a long acting β_2-adrenoceptor agonist, salmeterol, on airway hyperresponsiveness in patients with mild asthma. *N Engl J Med* 1992;327:1198–1203.
52. O'Connor BJ, Aikman SL, Barnes PJ. Tolerance to the nonbronchodilating effects of inhaled β_2-agonists in asthma. *N Engl J Med* 1992;327:1204–1208.
53. Nelson JA, Strauss L, Skowronski M, et al. Effect of long-term salmeterol treatment on exercise-induced asthma. *N Engl J Med* 1998;339:141–146.
54. Castle W, Fuller R, Hall J, et al. Serevent nationwide surveillance study: comparison of salmeterol with salbutamol in asthmatic patients who require regular bronchodilator treatment. *BMJ* 1993;306:1034–1037.
55. Fish JE, Kemp JP, Lockey RF, et al. Zafirlukast for symptomatic mild-to-moderate asthma: A 13-week multicenter study. *Clin Ther* 1997;19:675–690.
56. Suissa S, Dennis R, Ernst P, et al. Effectiveness of the leukotriene receptor antagonist zafirlukast for mild-to-moderate asthma. A randomized, double-blind, placebo-controlled trial. *Ann Intern Med* 1997;126:177–183.
57. Nathan RA, Bernstein JA, Bielory L, et al. Zafirlukast improves asthma symptoms and quality of life in patients with moderate reversible airflow obstruction. *Allergy Clin Immunol* 1998;102:935–942.
58. Ducharme F. Addition of anti-leukotriene agents to inhaled corticosteroids for chronic asthma. In: The Cochrane Library. Issue 4, 2001. Oxford: Update Software. Search date 2001; primary sources Medline, Embase, Cinahl, reference lists of review articles and trials, contacted international headquarters of AL manufacturers, and ATS meeting abstracts (1998–2000).
59. Ducharme FM, Hicks GC. Anti-leukotriene agents compared to inhaled corticosteroids in the management of recurrent and/or chronic asthma. In: The Cochrane Library, Issue 4, 2001. Oxford: Update Software. Search date 1999; primary sources Medline, Embase, and Cinahl.
60. Bleecker ER, Welch MJ, Weinstein SE, et al. Low-dose inhaled fluticasone propionate versus oral zafirlukast in the treatment of persistent asthma. *J Allergy Clin Immunol* 2000;105:1123–1229.
61. Busse W, Raphael G, Galant S, et al. Low dose fluticasone propionate compared to montelukast for first-line treatment of persistent asthma: a randomized clinical trial. *J Allergy Clin Immunol* 2001;107:461–468.
62. Nathan RA, Bleecker ER, Kalberg C. A comparison of short-term treatment with inhaled fluticasone propionate and zafirlukast for patients with persistent asthma. *Am J Med* 2001;111:195–202.
63. Calhoun WJ, Nelson HS, Nathan RA, et al. Comparison of fluticasone propionate-salmeterol combination therapy and montelukast in patients who are symptomatic on short-acting β_2 agonists alone. *Am J Respir Crit Care Med* 2001;164:759–763.
64. Cates C. Holding chambers versus nebulisers for β agonist treatment of acute asthma. In: The Cochrane Library, Issue 4, 2001. Oxford: Update Software. Search date 1999; primary sources Cochrane Airways Review Group Register of Trials, Cochrane Controlled Trials Register, bibliographies of all included papers, and authors of included studies.
65. Rowe BH, Keller JL, Oxman AD. Effectiveness of steroid therapy in acute exacerbations of asthma: a meta-analysis. *Am J Emerg Med* 1992;10:301–310. Search date 1991; primary sources Medline, Science Citation Index, review articles, textbooks, experts, and primary authors.
66. Rowe BH, Spooner CH, Duchrame FM, et al. Corticosteroids for preventing relapse following acute exacerbations of asthma. In: The Cochrane Library, Issue 4, 2001. Oxford: Update Software. Search date 1997; primary sources Cochrane Airways Review Group Register of Trials, Asthma, and Wheeze RCT Register.
67. O'Driscoll BR, Kalra S, Wilson M, et al. Double-blind trial of steroid tapering in acute asthma. *Lancet* 1993;341:324–327.
68. Hasegaawa T, Ishihara K, Takakura S, et al. Duration of systemic corticosteroids in the treatment of asthma exacerbation: a randomized study. *Intern Med* 2000;39:794–797.
69. Levy ML, Stevenson C, Maslen T. Comparison of a short course of oral prednisone and fluticasone propionate in the treatment of adults with acute exacerbations of asthma in primary care. *Thorax* 1996;51:1087–1092.
70. Edmonds ML, Camargo CA Jr, Pollack CV, et al. Early use of inhaled corticosteroids in the emergency department treatment of acute asthma. In: The Cochrane Library, Issue 4, 2001. Search date 2000; primary sources The Cochrane Airways Review Group Register of Trials, hand searching of reference lists, conference abstracts, and contact with experts and pharmaceutical companies.
71. Edmonds ML, Camargo CA Jr, Suanders LD, et al. Inhaled steroids in acute asthma following emergency department discharge. The Cochrane Library, Issue 4, 2001. Oxford Software. Search date 1999; primary souces Cochrane Upper Airways Group register of controlled trials, hand searching of bibliographies, 20 respiratory journals, conference proceedings, and contact with authors of articles retrieved and pharmaceutical companies.

72. Shrestha M, Bidadi K, Gourlay S, et al. Continuous vs intermittent albuterol, at high and low doses, in the treatment of severe acute asthma in adults. *Chest* 1996;110:42–47.
73. Rudnitsky GS, Eberlein RS, Schoffstall JM, et al. Comparison of intermittent and continuously nebulized albuterol for treatment of asthma in an urban emergency department. *Ann Emerg Med* 1993;22:1842–1846.
74. Lin RY, Sauter D, Newman T, et al. Continuous versus intermittent nebulization in the treatment of acute asthma. *Ann Emerg Med* 1993;22:1847–1853.
75. Reisner C, Kotch A, Dworkin G. Continuous versus frequent intermittent nebulisations of albuterol in acute asthma: a randomized, prospective study. *Ann Allergy Asthma Immunol* 1995;75:41–47.
76. Khine H, Fuchs SM, Saville AL. Continuous vs intermittent nebulized albuterol for emergency management of asthma. *Acad Emerg Med* 1969;3:1019–1024.
77. Bradding P, Rushby I, Scullion J, et al. As required versus regular nebulized salbutamol for the treatment of acute severe asthma. *Eur Respir J* 1999;13:290–294.
78. Travers A, Jones AP, Kelly K, et al. Intravenous β_2-agonists for acute asthma in the emergency department. The Cochrane Library, Issue 4, 2001. Oxford Software. Search date not stated; primary sources Cochrane Airways Group Register, hand searching of 20 respiratory journals, bibliographies from included studies, and contact with authors and experts to identify eligible studies.
79. Rodrigo G, Rodrigo C, Burschtin O. Ipratropium bromide in acute adult severe asthma: a meta-analysis of randomized controlled trials. *Am J Med* 1999;107:363–370. Search date 1999; primary sources Medline, Current Contents, Science Citation Index, review articles, experts, pharmaceutical companies, Medical Editor's Trial Amnesty Register, and hand searched references.
80. Aaron SD. The use of ipratropium bromide for the management of acute asthma exacerbations in adults and children: a systematic review. *J Asthma* 2001;38:521–530. Search date not stated; primary sources not specified, but electronic and handsearching were performed.
81. Stoodley RG, Aaron SD, Dales RE. The role of ipratropium bromide in the emergency management of acute asthma exacerbation: a metaanalysis of randomized clinical trials. *Ann Emerg Med* 1999;34:8–18. Search date 1997; primary sources Medline, Embase, Cinahl, Biological Abstracts, Cochrane Library, and Current Contents.
82. Rodrigo GJ, Rodrigo C. First-line therapy for adult patients with acute asthma receiving multiple dose protocol of ipratropium bromide plus albuterol in the emergency department. *Am J Respir Crit Care Med* 2000;161:1862–1868.
83. Manthous CA, Hall JB, Caputo MA, et al. Heliox improves pulsus paradoxus and peak expiratory flow in non-intubated patients with severe asthma. *Am J Respir Care Crit Care Med* 1995;151:310 314.
84. Kass JE, Terregino CA. The effect of heliox in acute severe asthma: a randomized controlled trial. *Chest* 1999;116:296–300.
85. Henderson SO, Acharay P, Kilaghbian T, et al. Use of heliox-driven nebulized therapy in the treatment of acute asthma. *Ann Emerg Med* 1999;33:141–146.
86. Rowe BH, Bretzlaff JA, Bourdon C, et al. Magnesium sulfate for treating acute asthmatic exacerbations of acute asthma in the emergency department. In: The Cochrane Library, Issue 4, 2001. Oxford: Update Software. Search date 1999; primary sources Cochrane Airways Review Group Register of Trials, review articles, textbooks, experts, primary authors of included studies, and hand searched references.
87. Nannini LJ, Pendino JC, Corna RA, et al. Magnesium sulfate as a vehicle for nebulized salbutamol in acute asthma. *Am J Med* 2000;108:193–197.
88. Boonyavoroakul C, Thakkinstian A, Charoenpan P. Intravenous magnesium sulfate in acute severe asthma. *Respirology* 2000;5:221–225.
89. Porter RS, Nester S, Braitman LE, et al. Intravenous magnesium is ineffective in adult asthma: a randomised trial. *Eur J Emerg Med* 2001;8:9–15.
90. FitzGerald JM. Commentary: intravenous magnesium in acute asthma. *Evid Based Med* 1999;4:138.
91. Behbehani NA, Al-Mane FD, Yachkova Y, et al. Myopathy following mechanical ventilation for acute severe asthma: the role of muscle relaxants and corticosteroids. *Chest* 1999;115:1627–1631.
92. Williams TJ, Tuxen DV, Sceinkestel CD, et al. Risk factors for morbidity in mechanically ventilated patients with acute severe asthma. *Am Rev Respir Dis* 1992;146:607–615.
93. Darioli R, Perret C. Mechanical controlled hypoventilation in status asthmaticus. *Am Rev Respir Dis* 1984;129:385–387.
94. Menitove SM, Godring RM. Combined ventilator and bicarbonate strategy in the management of status asthmaticus. *Am J Med* 1983;74:898–901.
95. Higgins B, Greening AP, Crompton GK. Assisted ventilation in severe acute asthma. *Thorax* 1986;41:464–467.
96. Lam KN, Mow BM, Chew LS. The profile of ICU admissions for acute severe asthma in a general hospital. *Singapore Med J* 1992;33:460–462.
97. Mansel JK, Stogner SW, Petrini MF, et al. Mechanical ventilation in patients with acute severe asthma. *Am J Med* 1990;89:42–48.
98. Lim TK. Status asthmaticus in a medical intensive care unit. *Singapore Med J* 1989;30:334–338.
99. Keenan SP, Brake D. An evidence based approach to non invasive ventilation in acute respiratory failure. *Crit Care Clin* 1998;14:359–372.
100. Eastwood AJ, Sheldon TA. Organisation of asthma care: what difference does it make? A systematic review of the literature. *Quality Health Care* 1996;5:134–143. Search date 1995; primary sources Medline, CINAHL, HELMIS, Manchester Primary and Secondary Care Interface, Health Planning and Administration, DHSS databases, checking of reference lists, and contact with experts.
101. Bartter T, Pratter MR. Asthma: better outcome at a lower cost? The role of the expert in the care system. *Chest* 1996;110:1589–1596.
102. Zeiger RS, Heller S, Mellon MH, et al. Facilitated referral to asthma specialist reduces relapses in asthma emergency room visits. *J Allergy Clin Immunol* 1991;87:1160–1168.
103. Gibson PG, Coughlan J, Wilson AJ, et al. Self-management education and regular practitioner review for adults with asthma. The Cochrane Library Issue 4, 2001. Search date 1999; primary sources Cochrane Airways Group Register of Trials, and hand searched references.
104. Cote J, Bowie D, Robichaud P, et al Evaluation of two different educational interventions for adult patients consulting with an acute asthma exacerbation. *Am J Respir Crit Care Med* 2001;163:1415–1419.

Christopher Cates
General Practitioner
Manor View Practice
Bushey
UK

J Mark FitzGerald
Respiratory Physician
and Director of Center
for Clinical Epidemiology and
Evaluation
Vancouver General Hospital
Vancouver
Canada

Competing interests: CC, none declared. MF has received honoraria for lectures and research funds from GlaxoSmithKline, Merck, AstraZeneca, Novartis, Boehringer Ingelheim, Byk Canada, Schering Canada, and 3M.

TABLE 1 **Classification of severity for chronic asthma (see text, p 1509).**

In the USA[1]

Asthma is classified by symptoms of severity. Using this system, even people with mild, intermittent asthma can develop severe exacerbations if exposed to appropriate stimuli.

Mild intermittent asthma	Symptoms less than weekly with normal or near normal lung function.
Mild persistent asthma	Symptoms more than weekly but less than daily with normal or near normal lung function.
Moderate persistent asthma	Daily symptoms with mild to moderate variable airflow obstruction.
Severe asthma	Daily symptoms and frequent night symptoms, and moderate to severe variable airflow obstruction.

In the UK[2]

Chronic asthma in ambulatory settings is graded according to the amount of medication required to keep symptoms controlled. People are classified according to whether, for symptom control, they need:

Step 1	Occasional β agonists for symptomatic relief.
Step 2	In addition, regular, inhaled anti-inflammatory agents (such as inhaled corticosteroids, cromoglycate, or nedocromil).
Step 3	In addition, high dose inhaled corticosteroids or low dose inhaled steroids plus long acting inhaled β_2 bronchodilator.
Step 4	In addition, high dose inhaled corticosteroids plus regular bronchodilators.
Step 5	In addition, regular oral corticosteroids.

Chronic obstructive pulmonary disease

Search date February 2002

Huib Kerstjens and Dirkje Postma

QUESTIONS

INTERVENTIONS

To be covered in future updates

Acute exacerbations of chronic obstructive pulmonary disease

Vaccination against influenza and pneumococcus

Programmes to stop smoking

See glossary, p 1543

Key Messages

Short term effects of treatment

- **Inhaled anticholinergic drugs** RCTs have found that inhaled anticholinergic drugs versus placebo for 4–13 weeks significantly improve forced expiratory volume in 1 second (FEV_1) and symptoms.
- **Inhaled β_2 agonists** RCTs have found that short and long acting inhaled β_2 agonists versus placebo for 1–16 weeks significantly improve FEV_1, and symptoms.
- **Inhaled anticholinergics plus β_2 agonists** RCTs have found that combining a β_2 agonist with an anticholinergic drug versus either drug alone for 2–12 weeks significantly improves FEV_1. One RCT found that, when combined with an anticholinergic drug, a long acting β_2 agonist improved FEV_1 and peak expiratory flow rate significantly more than a short acting β_2 agonist.
- **Inhaled corticosteroids** Short term RCTs (10 days to 10 wks) found no significant difference in lung function with inhaled corticosteroids versus placebo.
- **Oral corticosteroids** One systematic review has found that oral corticosteroids versus placebo for 2–4 weeks significantly improve lung function.

- **Theophyllines** Small, short term RCTs (1–8 wks) of theophyllines found limited evidence of a small bronchodilatory effect, but the usefulness of these drugs is limited by adverse effects and the need for frequent monitoring of blood concentrations.
- **Antiobiotics** We found no RCTs for antibiotics or α1 Antitrypsin.

Long term effects of treatment

- **Antibiotics** Two poor quality RCTs found no significant difference with antibiotics versus placebo in frequency of exacerbations or decline in lung function over 5 years.
- **α_1 Antitrypsin augmentation** One RCT in people with α_1 antitrypsin deficiency and moderate emphysema found no significant difference with α_1 antitrypsin versus placebo in the decline in FEV_1 after 1 year.
- **Domiciliary oxygen (in people with hypoxaemia)** RCTs found limited evidence that domiciliary oxygen versus no oxygen improved survival over 2 years in people with COPD and hypoxaemia.
- **Inhaled anticholinergic drugs** One large RCT found that a long term inhaled anticholinergic drug plus a smoking cessation programme versus a smoking cessation programme alone had no significant impact on the decline in FEV_1 over 5 years.
- **Inhaled corticosteroids** Large RCTs lasting at least 6 months have found that inhaled steroids versus placebo increase FEV_1 during the first 3–6 months of use, but found no subsequent effect on decline in lung function.
- **Mucolytics** Systematic reviews have found that mucolytics versus placebo for 3–24 months significantly reduce the frequency and duration of exacerbations.
- **Inhaled β_2 agonists; deoxyribonuclease; oral corticosteroids; theophyllines** We found no RCTs about the long term effects of these interventions.

DEFINITION Chronic obstructive pulmonary disease (COPD) is characterised by chronic bronchitis or emphysema. Emphysema is abnormal permanent enlargement of the air spaces distal to the terminal bronchioles, accompanied by destruction of their walls and without obvious fibrosis. Chronic bronchitis is chronic cough or mucus production for at least 3 months in at least 2 successive years when other causes of chronic cough have been excluded.[1]

INCIDENCE/ PREVALENCE COPD mainly affects middle aged and elderly people. It is one of the leading causes of morbidity and mortality worldwide. In the USA, it affects about 14 million people and is the fourth leading cause of death. Both morbidity and mortality are rising. Estimated prevalence in the USA has risen by 41% since 1982, and age adjusted death rates rose by 71% between 1966 and 1985. All cause age adjusted mortality declined over the same period by 22% and mortality from cardiovascular diseases by 45%.[1] In the UK, physician diagnosed prevalence was 2% in men and 1% in women between 1990 and 1997.[2]

AETIOLOGY/ RISK FACTORS COPD is largely preventable. The main cause is exposure to cigarette smoke. The disease is rare in lifelong non-smokers (estimated incidence 5% in 3 large representative US surveys from 1971–1984), in whom "passive" exposure to environmental tobacco smoke has been proposed as a cause.[3,4] Other proposed causes include airway hyperresponsiveness, air pollution, and allergy.[5–7]

PROGNOSIS Airway obstruction is usually progressive in those who continue to smoke, resulting in early disability and shortened survival. Smoking cessation reverts the rate of decline in lung function to that of non-smokers.[8] Many people will need medication for the rest of their lives, with increased doses and additional drugs during exacerbations.

AIMS To alleviate symptoms; to prevent exacerbations; to preserve optimal lung function; and to improve activities of daily living, quality of life, and survival.[9]

OUTCOMES Short and long term changes in lung function, including changes in forced expiratory volume in 1 second (FEV_1) (see glossary, p 1543); exercise tolerance; peak expiratory flow rate (PEFR) (see glossary, p 1543); frequency, severity, and duration of exacerbations; symptom scores for dyspnoea; quality of life; and survival.

METHODS *Clinical Evidence* update search and appraisal February 2002. This review deals only with treatment of stable COPD and not with treatment of acute exacerbations. We were interested in the maintenance treatment of stable COPD; therefore, we did not include single dose or single day cumulative dose response trials. In this review, short term treatment is defined as less than 6 months and long term as 6 months or over. There is consensus that 6 months is the absolute minimum duration of treatment required to assess effects on decline in lung function. Where RCTs were found, no systematic search for observational studies was performed.

QUESTION What are the effects of maintenance treatment in stable chronic obstructive pulmonary disorder?

OPTION INHALED ANTICHOLINERGIC DRUGS

RCTs have found that inhaled anticholinergic drugs versus placebo for 4–13 weeks significantly improve forced expiratory volume in one second and symptoms. One large RCT found that adding a long term anticholinergic drug to a smoking cessation programme had no significant impact on decline in forced expiratory volume in 1 second over 5 years.

Benefits: We found no systematic review comparing anticholinergic drugs versus placebo. **Short term ipratropium:** We found many small placebo controlled RCTs using different methods and end points. Most included at least some measure of airways obstruction and found a significant effect of ipratropium.[10–13] We found two large RCTs (276 people[14] and 405 people[15]) comparing ipratropium (36 μg four times daily) versus placebo or versus salmeterol for 12 weeks. In both RCTs, ipratropium versus placebo significantly improved baseline FEV_1 but results were only presented graphically. We found one further RCT (780 people) comparing ipratropium (40 μg four times daily) versus placebo and versus formoterol (eformoterol) for 12 weeks.[16] It found that ipratropium versus placebo significantly improved FEV_1 (improvement in average FEV_1 over 12 h after medication 137 mL, 95% CI 88 to 186 mL). There was no difference in morning premedication peak expiratory flow rate (PEFR) (see glossary, p 1543), symptoms or quality of life scores or need for rescue bronchodilators. **Short term tiotropium:** We found three RCTs comparing a long acting (up to 24 h) anticholinergic drug, tiotropium (18 μg/day), versus placebo or versus ipratropium.[17–19] The first RCT (169 people) compared tiotropium versus placebo for 4 weeks. It found that tiotropium versus placebo significantly improved FEV_1 during the first 6 hours after treatment (mean improvement in FEV_1: +0.13 L with tiotropium *v* –0.02 L with placebo; $P < 0.05$), and significantly increased trough FEV_1 24 hours after the last dose (mean FEV_1: +0.07 L *v* –0.03 L with placebo; CI not provided; $P < 0.05$).[17] The second RCT (478 people) compared tiotropium versus placebo for 92 days. It found that tiotropium significantly improved FEV_1 during the first 3 hours after treatment ($P < 0.001$), increased the peak response (CI not provided; $P < 0.001$; results presented graphically) and improved symptoms.[18] The third RCT (288 people, average age 65 years) compared tiotropium (18 μg/day) versus ipratropium (40 μg four times daily) for 13 weeks.[19] It found that tiotropium versus ipratropium significantly increased FEV_1 (mean FEV_1 6 h after treatment on first day: 0.24 L *v* 0.18 L with ipratropium; difference 0.06 L, 95% CI 0.02 to 0.09 L), and significantly increased mean trough FEV_1 (0.15 L *v* 0.01 L with ipratropium; difference 0.13 L, 95% CI 0.09 to 0.18 L). **Long term treatment:** We found one RCT (5887 smokers aged 35–60 years with spirometric signs of early COPD; FEV_1 75% predicted).[8] Three interventions were compared over a 5 year period: usual care, an intensive 12 session smoking cessation programme combining behaviour modification and use of nicotine gum, and the same smoking intervention programme plus ipratropium three times daily. Although decline in FEV_1 was significantly slower in people in the smoking cessation group, the addition of ipratropium had no significant effect (5 year mean cumulative decline in prebronchodilator FEV_1: usual care 249 mL, 95% CI 236 to 262 mL; smoking programme plus ipratropium 188 mL, 95% CI 175 to 200 mL; smoking programme plus placebo 172 mL, 95% CI 159 to 185 mL).

Harms: One RCT (233 people with asthma or chronic obstructive pulmonary disease) found that continuous versus as needed treatment with bronchodilators (both ipratropium and fenoterol) caused a significantly faster decline in lung function (144 people, –0.07 L/year with continuous treatment *v* –0.02 L/year with as needed treatment; $P < 0.05$; CI not provided).[20] In the RCT of long term treatment, there was no significant difference between ipratropium versus placebo in serious adverse events (cardiac symptoms, hypertension, skin rashes, and urinary retention: 1.2% with ipratropium *v* 0.8% with placebo).[8] Dry mouth was the most common mild adverse event. The RCT comparing tiotropium versus ipratropium found no significant difference in the occurrence of dry mouth (14.7% with tiotropium *v* 10.3% with ipratropium).[19]

Comment: The RCT of long term treatment found no evidence that people developed tachyphylaxis in response to the bronchodilating effect of ipratropium over a 5 year period.[8]

OPTION INHALED β_2 AGONISTS

RCTs have found that short and long acting inhaled β_2 agonists versus placebo for at least 1 week significantly improve forced expiratory volume in 1 second and symptoms. We found no RCTs of long term treatment with short or long acting β_2 agonists versus placebo.

Benefits: **Short term treatment with short acting β_2 agonists:** We found one systematic review (search date 2000, 9 crossover RCTs, 264 people with stable chronic obstructive pulmonary disease) comparing short acting β_2 agonists versus placebo for at least 1 week.[21] It found that β_2 agonists delivered by metered dose inhaler versus placebo significantly increased FEV_1 (WMD 0.14 L, 95% CI 0.04 to 0.25 L), and significantly improved the daily dyspnoea score (SMD 1.33, 95% CI 1.01 to 1.65; $P < 0.001$). There was no significant difference between treatments in exercise tolerance. **Short term treatment with long acting β_2 agonists:** We found one systematic review (search date 1998, 3 RCTs of salmeterol)[22] and four subsequent RCTs.[14–16,23] All found significant improvements in symptoms, lung function, and quality of life. The first RCT in the review (674 people) compared salmeterol 50 µg versus 100 µg doses versus placebo twice daily for 16 weeks. It found that both doses of salmeterol versus placebo significantly increased FEV_1 (50 µg: WMD 0.10 L, 95% CI 0.05 to 0.15 L; 100 µg: WMD 0.12 L, 95% CI 0.06 to 0.17 L).[24] The higher but not the lower dose of salmeterol versus placebo significantly improved quality of life.[25] The second RCT in the review (crossover study of 63 smokers) found that salmeterol (50 µg twice daily) versus placebo significantly increased morning FEV_1 after 4 weeks of treatment (mean treatment difference 12 mL, 95% CI 6 to 17 mL). Evening values were not significantly different from placebo.[26] The third RCT in the review (29 people) found that significantly fewer people taking salmeterol (50 µg/day) versus placebo were scored as moderately dyspnoeic or worse (OR 0.60, 95% CI 0.40 to 0.88). There was no significant difference in the mean change from baseline in the 6 minute walking distance (WMD +1.9 m, 95% CI –15.4 m to +19.3 m).[27] The systematic review found no trials of formoterol.[22] The first subsequent RCT (278 people) comparing salmeterol (42 µg twice daily) versus placebo for 12 weeks found that salmeterol significantly improved the average FEV_1 (CI not provided; $P < 0.001$).[14] The second subsequent RCT (97 people) compared salmeterol 50 µg twice daily versus placebo over 12 weeks.[23] Salmeterol significantly increased morning and evening PEFR (see glossary, p 1543), and FEV_1 (mean improvement as a percentage of the predicted FEV_1: 5% *v* 1%; CI not provided; $P < 0.01$), and daytime but not night time symptoms. In the same study, no improvement in quality of life was found with salmeterol compared with placebo.[28] The third subsequent RCT (478 people) found that salmeterol (42 µg twice daily) versus placebo for 12 weeks significantly increased FEV_1 throughout the study period, but results were only presented graphically.[15] The fourth subsequent RCT (780 people) compared formoterol (12 µg *v* 24 µg doses twice daily) versus placebo and versus ipratropium for 12 weeks.[16] It found that both doses of formoterol versus placebo significantly improved FEV_1 (improvement in average FEV_1 over 12 h after medication, 12 µg formoterol *v* placebo 223 mL, 95% CI 174 to 273 mL; 24 µg formoterol *v* placebo 194 mL, 95% CI 145 to 243 mL). It also found that 12 mg or 24 mg formeterol versus placebo significantly improved quality of life scores (improvement in total score on St George's Respiratory Questionnaire, with 12 µg formoterol *v* placebo 5, $P < 0.001$; with 24 µg formoterol *v* placebo about 3–4; difference presented graphically, $P = 0.009$). **Long term treatment with β_2 agonists:** We found no systematic review or RCTs of long term treatment with short or long acting β_2 agonists versus placebo.

Harms: In people with asthma, β_2 agonists have been linked to increased risk of death, worsened control of asthma, and deterioration in lung function.[29] One crossover RCT (53 people with chronic obstructive pulmonary disease, $FEV_1 < 70\%$ predicted) compared regular versus as needed treatment with the short acting inhaled β_2 agonist salbutamol for 3 months.[30] It found that regular versus as needed salbutamol doubled the total daily amount of salbutamol used (13 puffs daily [of which 8 puffs were the allocated regular dose] *v* 6 puffs daily with as needed treatment; significance not stated), with no significant difference in symptoms or lung function. The most common immediate adverse effect is tremor, which is usually worse in the first few days of treatment. High doses of β_2 agonists can reduce plasma potassium, cause dysrhythmias, and reduce arterial oxygen tension.[31] The risk of adverse events may be higher in people with pre-existing cardiac arrhythmias and hypoxaemia.[32] Two of the RCTs comparing salmeterol versus placebo over 12 weeks found no increase in any adverse events, but allowed rescue salbutamol.[14,15]

Comment: Many people report improvement in symptoms with bronchodilators that is not reflected by a change in FEV_1. Long term placebo controlled RCTs of β_2 agonists, looking at adverse effects such as decline in lung function or worsened chronic obstructive pulmonary disorder control, are ethically difficult because of their beneficial effects in the short term.

OPTION INHALED ANTICHOLINERGICS PLUS β_2 AGONISTS

RCTs have found that combining a β_2 agonist with an anticholinergic drug for 2–12 weeks provided small additional bronchodilation compared with either drug alone. One RCT found that, when combined with an anticholinergic drug, a long acting β_2 agonist improved forced expiratory volume in 1 second and peak expiratory flow rate significantly more than a short acting β_2 agonist. We found no RCTs of long term treatment with anticholinergics plus β_2 agonists versus placebo.

Benefits: **Short term treatment with anticholinergics plus short acting inhaled β_2 agonists:** We found six RCTs (705, 195, 652, 863, and 357 people with stable chronic obstructive pulmonary disease; one report combined the results from two RCTs) comparing the addition of ipratropium versus no additional ipratropium in people using standard dose short acting inhaled β_2 for 2 weeks to 3 months.[33–37] All found significant improvements in FEV_1 of about 25% with the combination compared with either drug alone. **Short term**

treatment with anticholinergics plus long acting inhaled β_2 agonists: One RCT (94 people) compared the long acting β_2 agonist salmeterol (50 μg twice daily) plus ipratropium (40 μg four times daily) versus salmeterol (50 μg twice daily) for 12 weeks.[23] It found that the combination versus the β_2 agonist alone significantly improved FEV_1 (mean improvement as a percentage of predicted FEV_1: 8% *v* 5%; CI not provided; $P < 0.01$), and evening but not morning peak expiratory flow rate (PEFR) (see glossary, p 1543). It found no significant difference in daytime or night time symptoms.[28] **Short term treatment with anticholinergics plus long acting β_2 agonists versus anticholinergics plus short acting β_2 agonists:** One crossover RCT (172 people) compared ipratropium (40 μg four times daily) plus formoterol (12 μg twice daily) versus ipratropium (40μg four times daily) plus salbutamol (200 μg four times daily).[38] It found that formoterol plus ipratropium versus salbutamol plus ipratropium significantly improved FEV_1 and PEFR from baseline after 3 weeks treatment (improvement in mean morning PEFR from baseline over the previous 7 days with formoterol 12 L/min, 95% CI 6 to 19; improvement in premedication FEV_1 from baseline 116 mL, 95% CI 83 to 150 mL). **Long term treatment with anticholinergics plus inhaled β_2 agonists:** We found no systematic review or RCTs of long term treatment with anticholinergics plus β_2 agonists versus placebo.

Harms: The RCTs found no significant differences in adverse effects between treatments.[23,28,33–38]

Comment: None.

OPTION INHALED β_2 AGONISTS VERSUS ANTICHOLINERGICS

RCTs have found conflicting evidence on the effects of inhaled β_2 agonists versus anticholinergics over 3 months. We found no RCTs comparing long term treatment with anticholinergic versus β_2 agonists.

Benefits: We found no systematic review. **Short term treatment:** One non-systematic review (7 RCTs, 1445 people) compared ipratropium versus different short acting β_2 agonists for 90 days.[39] Lung function measurements were performed after withholding bronchodilators for at least 12 hours. It found that ipratropium versus β_2 agonists significantly improved mean FEV_1 (28 mL increase *v* 1 mL decrease; CI not provided; $P < 0.05$). We found three subsequent RCTs comparing long acting β_2 agonists versus ipratropium for 12 weeks.[14–16] The first two RCTs compared salmeterol (42 μg twice daily) versus ipratropium (36 μg four times daily).[14,15] The first RCT (411 people) found that salmeterol versus ipratropium significantly improved average FEV_1 at 4 and 8 weeks (CI not provided; $P < 0.005$), but not immediately after treatment or at 12 weeks.[14] The second RCT (405 people) found no significant difference in FEV_1 at any time.[15] The third RCT (780 people) compared formoterol (12 μg v 24 μg doses twice daily) versus placebo and versus ipratropium for 12 weeks.[16] It found that both doses of formoterol versus ipratropium significantly improved FEV_1 (improvement in average FEV_1 over 12 h after medication with formoterol 12 μg *v* ipratropium 86 mL, 95% CI 37 to 136 mL; with formoterol 24 μg *v* ipratropium 57 mL, 95% CI 7 to 106 mL). Lower dose, but not higher dose, formoterol improved quality of life scores compared with ipratropium (improvement in total score on St George's Respiratory Questionnaire with 12 µg formoterol 3.79, $P < 0.001$; with 24 µg formoterol about 2, difference presented graphically; $P = 0.102$). **Long term treatment:** We found no systematic review or RCTs comparing long term treatment with anticholinergics versus β_2 agonists.

Harms: Adverse effects such as tremor and dysrhythmias associated with β_2 agonists seem to be more frequent than the adverse effects associated with anticholinergics, although the review provided no evidence for this.[39] The RCTs comparing salmeterol versus ipratropium found no significant difference in the frequency of adverse effects.[14,15]

Comment: The results of the RCTs comparing anticholinergics versus short acting β_2 agonists may be explained by the design of the RCTs.[39] The measurements were made at least 12 hours after bronchodilation, and the difference between anticholinergics and β_2 agonists may simply reflect the longer duration of action of the anticholinergics. The results may not generalise to measurements at other times. It has been suggested that older people experience greater bronchodilator response with anticholinergic drugs than with β_2 agonists, but we found no evidence for this.

OPTION THEOPHYLLINES

Small RCTs found limited evidence of a small bronchodilatory effect of theophyllines for 1–8 weeks. Adverse effects are frequent. We found no RCTs of long term treatment with theophyllines.

Benefits: We found no systematic review. **Short term treatment:** We found one non-systematic review (11 small RCTs, number of people not specified) of theophyllines. The review provided insufficient detail to specify all comparative or additional interventions used.[40] The RCTs evaluated treatment periods ranging from 1 week to 2 months and found changes in FEV_1 ranging from 0–20%, with equally varied effects on exercise capacity and symptoms (further detail not provided). **Long term treatment:** We found no RCTs.

Harms: The RCTs identified by the review did not report adverse effects.[40] The therapeutic range for theophyllines is small, with blood concentrations of 10–15 mg/litre required for optimal effects. Well documented adverse effects include nausea, diarrhoea, headache, irritability, seizures, and cardiac arrhythmias. These may occur within the therapeutic range.[41]

Comment: Non-bronchodilator effects of theophylline have been found in laboratory settings, including effects on respiratory muscles and improved right ventricular function, but their clinical importance has not been established. Anti-inflammatory effects have been claimed in asthma, especially at lower dosages, but have not been measured in chronic obstructive pulmonary. One RCT found little value from the use of "n of 1" trials to determine objective individualised treatment effects.[42]

OPTION ORAL CORTICOSTEROIDS

One systematic review of short term RCTs (usually 2–4 wks treatment) has found that oral corticosteroids versus placebo significantly improve lung function. We found no RCT of the effects of long term treatment on lung function. Systemic corticosteroids are associated with serious adverse effects including osteoporosis and induction of diabetes.

Benefits: **Short term treatment:** We found one systematic review (search date 1989, 10 RCTs, 445 people), which compared oral corticosteroids versus placebo in people with stable chronic obstructive disease.[43] Treatment usually lasted 2–4 weeks. It found that significantly more people taking oral corticosteroids versus placebo had a 20% or greater improvement in baseline FEV_1 (WMD 10%, 95% CI 2% to 18%). When the other five RCTs were included, the difference in effect size was 11% (95% CI 4% to 18%). **Long term treatment:** We found no long term RCTs examining the effects of oral steroids on decline in lung function.

Harms: Many reviews have described the considerable harms of systemic corticosteroids, including osteoporosis and induction of diabetes.[44]

Comment: None.

OPTION INHALED CORTICOSTEROIDS

RCTs found no significant improvement in lung function (forced expiratory volume in 1 second) with inhaled steroids versus placebo over 10 days to 10 weeks. Large RCTs lasting at least 6 months have found that inhaled steroids increase forced expiratory volume in 1 second during the first 3–6 months of use, but found no subsequent effect on decline in lung function. One RCT also found that inhaled steroids versus placebo reduced the frequency of exacerbations and the rate of deterioration in quality of life.

Benefits: **Short term treatment:** We found no systematic review. We found 10 RCTs of duration less than 6 months, summarised in one non-systematic review.[45] Nine short term trials (10 days to 10 wks, 10–127 people) found no significant improvement in lung function (FEV_1) with inhaled steroids versus placebo. **Long term treatment:** We found one systematic review (search date 1996, 3 long term placebo controlled RCTs of inhaled steroids, 197 people treated for 2–2.5 years)[46] and five large subsequent RCTs.[47–51] The systematic review found that inhaled steroids versus placebo significantly reduced the rate of deterioration in prebronchodilator FEV_1 (WMD 34 mL/year, 95% CI 5 mL to 63 mL/year). It found no significant difference in the rate of deterioration of postbronchodilator FEV_1 (WMD +39 mL/year, 95% CI −6 mL to +84 mL/year) or in the frequency of exacerbations. The first subsequent RCT (281 people with chronic obstructive pulmonary disease [COPD]) found that fluticasone versus placebo significantly reduced moderate and severe exacerbations at 6 months (86% *v* 60%; $P < 0.001$) but not mild exacerbations. Fluticasone versus placebo also significantly improved lung function (adjusted baseline daily peak expiratory flow rate 15 L/min *v* 2 L/min on placebo; $P < 0.001$) and 6 minute walking distance (adjusted mean change in distance walked 27 m *v*

8 m; CI not provided; $P = 0.03$).[47] The second RCT (290 people with mild airways obstruction, FEV_1 86% predicted) found that budesonide (800 μg plus 400 μg daily for 6 months followed by 400 μg twice daily for 30 months) versus placebo had no significant effect on decline in lung function or exacerbation frequency.[48] The third RCT (1277 people, mean FEV_1 77% predicted; 912 people completed the trial) compared 800 μg budesonide daily versus placebo for 3 years.[49] In the first 6 months of the study, FEV_1 improved in the budesonide group but decreased in the placebo group (rate of 17 mL/year with budesonide *v* 81 mL/year with placebo; CI not provided; $P < 0.001$). However, there was no effect on subsequent decline. The fourth RCT (751 people with more severe COPD, FEV_1 50% predicted) compared fluticasone (500 μg twice daily for 3 years) versus placebo.[50] It found no effect on decline in lung function but there was a 25% reduction in exacerbation rate (from 1.32/year on placebo to 0.99 on fluticasone). It also found a significant reduction in the deterioration of quality of life with fluticasone compared with placebo.[50] The fifth RCT (1116 people with COPD, FEV_1 30–90% predicted) compared inhaled triamcinolone 600 μg twice daily versus placebo.[51] It found no significant difference between triamcinolone versus placebo in the rate of decline in FEV_1 after a mean duration of follow up of 40 months (mean 44.2 mL/year *v* 47.0 mL/year; CI not provided; $P = 0.50$). However, people taking triamcinolone had significantly fewer respiratory symptoms (21.1/100 person years *v* 28.2/100 person years; $P = 0.005$), and fewer visits to a physician because of a respiratory illness (1.2/100 person years *v* 2.1/100 person years; $P = 0.03$).

Harms: The fifth subsequent RCT found that people taking triamcinolone versus placebo had significantly lower bone density of the lumbar spine ($P = 0.007$) and femur (CI not provided; $P = 0.001$) after 3 years.[51] Extrapolation from studies in people with asthma is of limited value, as people with COPD are generally at higher risk for osteoporosis because of age, menopausal status, inactivity, and cigarette smoking.[44] One RCT (1277 people) reported skin bruising in 10% of people taking budesonide versus 4% taking placebo.[49] Newly diagnosed hypertension, bone fractures, postcapsular cataracts, myopathy, and diabetes occurred in fewer than 5% of people, with no significant difference between the groups.[49]

Comment: None.

OPTION ORAL VERSUS INHALED STEROIDS

Two RCTs found limited evidence suggesting that 2 weeks of oral prednisolone was more effective than inhaled beclometasone in people with mild to moderate chronic obstructive pulmonary disease; one small RCT found no significant difference in response over 2 weeks with oral prednisolone versus inhaled beclometasone. We found no RCTs of long term treatment with oral versus inhaled corticosteroids.

Benefits: We found no systematic review. **Short term treatment:** We found three RCTs comparing oral prednisolone versus inhaled beclometasone (beclomethasone) (12, 83, and 107 people).[52–54] All were double blind placebo controlled crossover trials, with treatment periods of 2 weeks. One very small RCT found no significant difference between the number of people responding to either or both treatments.[52] The other two RCTs found greater benefit with oral versus inhaled steroids. One found that forced expiratory volume in 1 second (see glossary, p 1543) rose from 0.65 to 1.00 litres with prednisolone versus 0.63 to 0.80 litres with beclometasone (CI not provided; $P < 0.01$). The other found that significantly more people responded to oral treatment (39/107 [36%] *v* 26/107 [24%]; CI not provided; $P < 0.05$).[53,54] **Long term treatment:** We found no RCTs.

Harms: None of the RCTs reported on adverse effects.[52–54]

Comment: The smallest RCT recruited only people known to be responsive to oral steroids, and did not report severity of chronic obstructive pulmonary disease.[53] The other two RCTs included people with chronic obstructive pulmonary disease of duration more than 5 years and forced expiratory volume in 1 second less than 70% predicted.[52,54] All trials excluded people with evidence of reversible airflow obstruction.

OPTION MUCOLYTIC DRUGS

Systematic reviews have found that mucolytics versus placebo for 3–24 months significantly reduce the frequency and duration of exacerbations.

Benefits: **Long term treatment:** We found two systematic reviews.[55,56] The first systematic review (search date 1999, 22 double blind RCTs, > 6000 people) found that mucolytics versus placebo for 3–6 months significantly reduced the average number of exacerbations (WMD −0.067 exacerbations per month, 95% CI −0.079 to −0.055) and days of disability (WMD −0.56 days/month, 95% CI −0.77 to −0.35).[55] The second systematic review (search date 1995, 9 RCTs, 7 of which were included in the first review[55]) compared N-acetylcysteine versus placebo for 3–24 months.[56] It found an overall weighted effect size of 1.37 (95% CI 1.25 to 1.5), corresponding to a 23% reduction in exacerbations compared with placebo.

Harms: The first systematic review found no significant difference between mucolytics and placebo in the total number of adverse events.[55] Adverse effects of N-acetylcysteine were mainly mild gastrointestinal complaints.

Comment: In both reviews there was significant heterogeneity between the RCTs, and symptom scores could not be pooled.[55,56] The effect of N-acetylcysteine in slowing the decline in lung function is being examined in a large European multicentre study (PNR Dekhuijzen, personal communication, 1999).

OPTION ANTIBIOTICS

We found no RCTs of antibiotics in short term treatment of stable chronic obstructive pulmonary disease. Two poor quality RCTs found no significant difference with antibiotics versus placebo in frequency of exacerbations or decline in lung function over 5 years.

Benefits: **Short term treatment:** We found no systematic review or RCTs. **Long term treatment:** We found no systematic review of antibiotics in people with stable chronic obstructive pulmonary disease, but found two RCTs.[57,58] The first RCT (497 people from 13 UK primary care clinics with chronic bronchitis, both with and without obstruction) compared four interventions: oxytetracyline plus chloramphenicol or sulphonamide; chloramphenicol or sulphonamide alone; oxytetracycline alone; or placebo over 5 years with oxytetracycline (0.5 mg/day for 3 years, increased to 0.5 mg twice daily in the fourth year, and 1 mg twice daily in the fifth year) versus chloramphenicol, sulphonamide, or placebo.[57] It found no significant difference in lung function or frequency of exacerbations with oxytetracycline versus chloramphenicol, sulphonamide, or placebo over 5 years (see comment below).[57] The second RCT (79 people) compared four interventions: tetracycline over the winter months for 5 years; placebo over winter for 5 years; tetracycline for two winters plus placebo for three winters; and placebo for two winters plus tetracycline for 3 years.[58] It found no significant difference between any of the treatment groups in mean frequency of exacerbations or decline in lung function, but may have been too small to exclude a clinically important difference.[58]

Harms: We found no good evidence.

Comment: The results of the first RCT should be interpreted with caution as it did not apply specific recruitment criteria and found evidence of heterogeneity in selection of people for the trial by each physician.[57] Doses of oxytetracycline were increased throughout the RCT because of lack of effect, which suggests that the benefits of double blinding may have been lost.[57]

OPTION DOMICILIARY OXYGEN TREATMENT

RCTs found limited evidence that domiciliary oxygen versus no oxygen improved survival over 2 years in people with chronic obstructive pulmonary disease and hypoxaemia. One RCT found that continuous treatment versus nocturnal treatment significantly reduced mortality over 24 months.

Benefits: **Long term treatment:** We found one systematic review (search date 2000, 5 RCTs).[59] The review could not perform a meta-analysis because of differences in trial design and participant selection. The first RCT (87 people), which compared daily oxygen for at least 15 hours versus no oxygen, found that domiciliary oxygen significantly reduced mortality over 5 years.[60] The second RCT (38 people with arterial desaturation at night) comparing nocturnal domiciliary oxygen versus room air found no significant difference in mortality at 3 years (figures not provided).[61] The third RCT (135 people with moderate hypoxaemia) identified by the review comparing oxygen versus no oxygen found no significant difference in survival at 3 years (HR 0.92, 95% CI 0.57 to 1.47; results presented graphically).[62] The fourth RCT (203 people) identified by the review compared continuous versus nocturnal domiciliary oxygen treatment. Continuous oxygen was associated with significant reduction in mortality over 24 months (22% with continuous v 41% with nocturnal oxygen; OR 0.45, 95% CI 0.25 to 0.81).[63] The fifth RCT (76 people with moderate daytime hypoxaemia [7.4–9.2 kPa] and significant nocturnal desaturation) comparing 2 years of nocturnal oxygen treatment versus placebo found no significant difference in survival.[64]

Harms: We found no reports of adverse effects of domiciliary oxygen. Administration is cumbersome.

Comment: Only one of the studies was double blinded. Domiciliary oxygen treatment seems to be more effective in people with severe hypoxaemia (arterial $pO_2 < 8.0$ kPa) than in people with moderate hypoxaemia or those who have arterial desaturation only at night.

OPTION α_1 ANTITRYPSIN INFUSION

We found no RCTs of short term treatment with α_1 antitrypsin. One RCT found no significant difference with α_1 antitrypsin versus placebo in the decline in forced expiratory volume in 1 second after 1 year in people with α_1 antitrypsin deficiency and moderate emphysema.

Benefits: We found no systematic review. **Short term treatment:** We found no RCTs. **Long term treatment:** We found one RCT (56 people with α_1 antitrypsin deficiency and moderate emphysema, FEV_1 30–80% predicted) comparing α_1 antitrypsin infusions (250 mg/kg) versus placebo infusion (albumin) given monthly for at least 3 years. It found no significant difference in the decline in FEV_1 after 1 year (decline in FEV_1 79 mL with α_1 antitrypsin v 59 mL with placebo; CI not provided; P = 0.25).[65]

Harms: The RCT reported no adverse effects in people taking α_1 antitrypsin or placebo.[65]

Comment: We found no clear evidence from observational studies on the effect of α_1 antitrypsin; for example, one cohort study (1048 people either homozygous for α_1 antitrypsin deficiency or with an α_1 antitrypsin concentration $\leq 11\,\mu M$, with mean FEV_1 49% ± 30% predicted) comparing weekly infusions of α_1 antitrypsin 60 mg/kg versus placebo for 3.5–7 years.[66] It found that α_1 antitrypsin significantly reduced mortality after an average of 5 years (RR of death 0.64, 95% CI 0.43 to 0.94). It found no significant difference between treatments in the decline in FEV_1, but in a subgroup of people with a mean FEV_1 35–49% predicted, α_1 antitrypsin significantly reduced the decline in FEV_1 (mean difference in FEV_1 0.08 L/year, 95% CI 0.003 to 0.500 L/year; CI not provided; P = 0.03). A second cohort study (295 people homozygous for α_1 antitrypsin deficiency with $FEV_1 < 65\%$ predicted) compared 198 people who received weekly infusions of α_1 antitrypsin 60 mg/kg (duration not stated) versus 97 people who had never received α_1 antitrypsin. It found that α_1 antitrypsin significantly reduced the decline in FEV_1 (0.05 L/year v 0.08 L/year; CI not provided; P = 0.02).[67]

OPTION DEOXYRIBONUCLEASE

We found no RCTs of deoxyribonuclease in people with chronic obstructive pulmonary disease.

Benefits: We found no systematic review or RCTs of deoxyribonuclease (dnase) specifically in people with chronic obstructive pulmonary disease (see comment below).

Harms: We found no evidence.

Comment: We found one RCT (349 people with bronchiectasis but not necessarily chronic airway obstruction) comparing DNase versus placebo given twice daily for 24 weeks.[68] It found that DNase significantly reduced FEV_1 decline (CI not provided; $P \leq 0.05$), but found no significant difference in the frequency of exacerbations over 168 days (0.66/person with DNase *v* 0.56/person with placebo; RR 1.7, 95% CI 0.85 to 1.65). In people with cystic fibrosis, DNase treatment is used to degrade DNA that increases the viscosity of pulmonary secretions. However, we found no evidence that this mechanism is useful to people with chronic obstructive pulmonary disease and chronic sputum production.

GLOSSARY

Forced expiratory volume in 1 second (FEV_1) The volume breathed out in the first second of forceful blowing into a spirometer, measured in litres.

Peak expiratory flow rate (PEFR) The maximum rate that gas is expired from the lungs when blowing into a peak flow meter or a spirometer; the units are expressed as litres per minute.

Substantive changes

Short term treatment with long acting β_2 agonists One new RCT;[16] conclusions unchanged.

Anticholinergics plus inhaled β_2 agonists One new RCT found that, when combined with an anticholinergic drug, a long acting β_2 agonist improved forced expiratory volume in 1 second and peak expiratory flow rate significantly more than a short acting β_2 agonist.[38]

Antibiotics Two new RCTs found no significant difference with maintenance antibiotics versus placebo in frequency of exacerbations or decline in lung function, but were of poor quality.[57,58]

REFERENCES

1. American Thoracic Society. Standards for the diagnosis and care of patients with chronic obstructive pulmonary disease: ATS statement. *Am J Respir Crit Care Med* 1995;152(5 pt 2)(suppl):77–120.
2. Soriano JB, Maier WC, Egger P, et al. Recent trends in physician diagnosed COPD in women and men in the UK. *Thorax* 2000;55:789–794.
3. Whittemore AS, Perlin SA, DiCiccio Y. Chronic obstructive pulmonary disease in lifelong nonsmokers: results from NHANES. *Am J Public Health* 1995;85:702–706.
4. Brunekreef B, Fischer P, Remijn B, et al. Indoor air pollution and its effects on pulmonary function of adult non-smoking women: III passive smoking and pulmonary function. *Int J Epidemiol* 1985;14:227–230.
5. Rijcken B, Weiss ST. Longitudinal analyses of airway responsiveness and pulmonary function decline. *Am J Respir Crit Care Med* 1996;154(suppl):246–249.
6. Dockery DW, Brunekreef B. Longitudinal studies of air pollution effects on lung function. *Am J Respir Crit Care Med* 1996;154(suppl):250–256.
7. O'Connor GT, Sparrow D, Weiss ST. The role of allergy and non-specific airway hyperresponsiveness in the pathogenesis of chronic obstructive pulmonary disease: state of the art. *Am Rev Respir Dis* 1989;140:225–252.
8. Anthonisen NR, Connett JE, Kiley JP, et al. Effects of smoking intervention and the use of an inhaled anticholinergic bronchodilator on the rate of decline of FEV_1: the lung health study. *JAMA* 1994;272:1497–1505.
9. Siafakas NM, Vermeire P, Pride NB, et al. Optimal assessment and management of chronic obstructive

pulmonary disease (COPD): a consensus statement of the European Respiratory Society. *Eur Respir J* 1995;8:1398–1420.

10. Braun SR, McKenzie WN, Copeland W, et al. A comparison of the effect of ipratropium bromide and albuterol in the treatment of chronic obstructive airway disease. *Arch Intern Med* 1989;149:544–547.
11. Higgins BG, Powell RM, Cooper S, et al. Effect of salbutamol and ipratropium bromide on airway calibre and bronchial reactivity in asthma and chronic bronchitis. *Eur Respir J* 1991;4:415–420.
12. Ikeda A, Nishimura K, Koyama H, et al. Bronchodilating effects of combined therapy with clinical dosages of ipratropium bromide and salbutamol for stable COPD: comparison with ipratropium bromide alone. *Chest* 1995;107:401–405.
13. Ikeda A, Nishimura K, Koyama H, et al. Comparative dose-response study of three anticholinergic agents and fenoterol using a metered dose inhaler in patients with chronic obstructive pulmonary disease. *Thorax* 1995;50:62–66.
14. Mahler DA, Donohue JF, Barbee RA, et al. Efficacy of salmeterol xinafoate in the treatment of COPD. *Chest* 1999;115:957–965.
15. Rennard SI, Anderson W, ZuWallack R, et al. Use of a long-acting inhaled beta2-adrenergic agonist, salmeterol xinafoate, in patients with chronic obstructive pulmonary disease. *Am J Respir Crit Care Med* 2001;163:1087–1092.
16. Dahl R, Greefhorst LA, Nowak D, et al. Inhaled formoterol dry powder versus ipratropium bromide in chronic obstructive pulmonary disease. *Am J Respir Crit Care Med* 2001;164:778–784.
17. Littner MR, Ilowite JS, Tashkin DP, et al. Long-acting bronchodilation with once-daily dosing of tiotropium (Spiriva) in stable chronic obstructive pulmonary disease. *Am J Respir Crit Care Med* 2000;161:1136–1142.
18. Casaburi R, Briggs DD Jr, Donohue JF, et al. The spirometric efficacy of once-daily dosing with tiotropium in stable COPD: a 13-week multicenter trial. *Chest* 2000;118:1294–1302.
19. Van Noord JA, Bantje TA, Eland ME, et al. A randomised controlled comparison of tiotropium and ipratropium in the treatment of chronic obstructive pulmonary disease. The Dutch Tiotropium Study Group. *Thorax* 2000;55:289–294.
20. Van Schayck CP, Dompeling E, van Herwaarden CLA, et al. Bronchodilator treatment in moderate asthma or chronic bronchitis: continuous or on demand? A randomised controlled study. *BMJ* 1991;303:1426–1431.
21. Sestini P, Renzoni E, Robinson S, et al. Short-acting beta 2 agonists for stable chronic obstructive pulmonary disease. In: The Cochrane Library, Issue 1, 2002. Oxford: Update Software. Search date 2000; primary sources Cochrane Airways Group database, and reference lists of review articles and retrieved studies.
22. Appleton S, Smith B, Veale A, et al. Long-acting beta-2 adrenoceptor agonists in stable chronic obstructive airways disease. In: The Cochrane Library, Issue 1, 2002. Oxford: Update Software. Search date 1999; primary sources Cochrane Airways Group Register to October 1998, hand searched references, and pharmaceutical companies contacted for unpublished studies.
23. Van Noord JM, de Munck DR, Bantje TA, et al. Long-term treatment of chronic obstructive pulmonary disease with salmeterol and the additive effect of ipratropium. *Eur Respir J* 2000;15:878–885.
24. Boyd G, Morice AH, Pounsford JC, et al. An evaluation of salmeterol in the treatment of chronic obstructive pulmonary disease (COPD). *Eur Respir J* 1997;10:815–821.
25. Jones PW, Bosh TK. Quality of life changes in COPD patients treated with salmeterol. *Am J Respir Crit Care Med* 1997;155:1283–1289.
26. Ulrik CS. Efficacy of inhaled salmeterol in the management of smokers with chronic obstructive pulmonary disease: a single centre randomised, double blind, placebo controlled, crossover study. *Thorax* 1995;50:750–754.
27. Grove A, Lipworth BJ, Reid P, et al. Effects of regular salmeterol on lung function and exercise capacity in patients with chronic obstructive airways disease. *Thorax* 1996;51:689–693.
28. Rutten van Molken M, Roos B, van Noord JA. An empirical comparison of the St George's Respiratory Questionnaire (SGRQ) and the Chronic Respiratory Disease Questionnaire (CRQ) in a clinical trial setting. *Thorax* 1999;54:995–1003.
29. O'Byrne PM, Kerstjens HAM. Inhaled β_2-agonists in the treatment of asthma. *N Engl J Med* 1996;335:886–888.
30. Cook D, Guyatt G, Wong E, et al. Regular versus as-needed short-acting inhaled beta-agonist therapy for chronic obstructive pulmonary disease. *Am J Respir Crit Care Med* 2001;163:85–90.
31. Hall IP, Tattersfield AE. Beta-agonists. In: Clark TJH, Godfrey S, Lee TH, eds. *Asthma*. 3rd ed. London: Chapman and Hall Medical, 1992:341–365.
32. Cazzola M, Imperatore F, Salzillo A, et al. Cardiac effects of formoterol and salmeterol in patients suffering from COPD with preexisting cardiac arrhythmias and hypoxemia. *Chest* 1998;114:411–415.
33. Friedman M, Serby C, Menjoge S, et al. Pharmoeconomic evaluation of a combination of ipratropium plus albuterol compared with ipratropium alone and albuterol alone in COPD. *Chest* 1999;115:635–641.
34. Levin DC, Little KS, Laughlin KR, et al. Addition of anticholinergic solution prolongs bronchodilator effect of beta 2 agonists in patients with chronic obstructive pulmonary disease. *Am J Med* 1996;100(1A;suppl):40–48.
35. Combivent Inhalation Solution Study Group. Routine nebulized ipratropium and albuterol together are better than either alone in COPD. *Chest* 1997;112:1514–1521.
36. Gross N, Tashkin D, Miller R, et al. Inhalation by nebulization of albuterol-ipratropium combination (Dey combination) is superior to either agent alone in the treatment of chronic obstructive pulmonary disease. Dey combination solution study group. *Respiration* 1998;65:354–362.
37. Campbell S. For COPD a combination of ipratropium bromide and albuterol sulfate is more effective than albuterol base. *Arch Intern Med* 1999;159:156–160.
38. D'Urzo AD, De Salvo MC, Ramirez-Rivera A, et al. In patients with COPD, treatment with a combination of formoterol and ipratropium is more effective than a combination of salbutamol and ipratropium: a 3-week, randomized, double-blind, within-patient, multicenter study. *Chest* 2001;119:1347–1356.
39. Rennard SI, Serby CW, Ghafouri M, et al. Extended therapy with ipratropium is associated with improved lung function in patients with COPD: a retrospective analysis of data from seven clinical trials. *Chest* 1996;110:62–70.
40. Calverley PMA. Symptomatic bronchodilator treatment. In: Calverley PMA, Pride N, eds. *Chronic obstructive pulmonary disease*. London: Chapman and Hall, 1995:419–446.
41. Ramsdell J. Use of theophylline in the treatment of COPD. *Chest* 1995;107(suppl):206–209.

42. Mahon JL, Laupacis A, Hodder RV, et al. Theophylline for irreversible chronic airflow limitation: a randomized study comparing n of 1 trials to standard practice. *Chest* 1999;115:38–48.
43. Callahan CM, Dittus RS, Katz BP. Oral corticosteroid therapy for patients with stable chronic obstructive pulmonary disease: a meta-analysis. *Ann Intern Med* 1991;114:216–223. Search date 1989; primary source Medline.
44. McEvoy CE, Niewoehner DE. Adverse effects of corticosteroid therapy for COPD: a critical review. *Chest* 1997;111:732–743.
45. Postma DS, Kerstjens HAM. Are inhaled glucocorticosteroids effective in chronic obstructive pulmonary disease? *Am J Respir Crit Care Med* 1999;160:66–71.
46. Van Grunsven PM, van Schayck CP, Derenne JP, et al. Long term effects of inhaled corticosteroids in chronic obstructive pulmonary disease: a meta-analysis. *Thorax* 1999;54:714–729. Search date 1996; primary sources Medline, Biosis, Online Contents, Glin, Cochrane Library, and Embase.
47. Paggiaro PL, Dahle R, Bakran I, et al. Multicentre randomised placebo-controlled trial of inhaled fluticasone propionate in patients with chronic obstructive pulmonary disease. *Lancet* 1998;351:773–780.
48. Vestbo J, Sorensen T, Lange P, et al. Long-term effect of inhaled budesonide in mild and moderate chronic obstructive pulmonary disease: a randomised controlled trial. *Lancet* 1999;353:1819–1823.
49. Pauwels RA, Lofdahl CG, Laitinen LA, et al. Long term treatment with inhaled budesonide in persons with mild chronic obstructive pulmonary disease who continue smoking. European Respiratory Society study on chronic obstructive pulmonary disease. *N Engl J Med* 1999;340:1948–1953.
50. Burge PS, Calverley PM, Jones PW, et al. Randomised, double blind, placebo controlled study of fluticasone propionate in patients with moderate to severe chronic obstructive pulmonary disease: the ISOLDE trial. *BMJ* 2000;320:1297–1303.
51. Anonymous. Effect of inhaled triamcinolone on the decline in pulmonary function in chronic obstructive pulmonary disease. *N Engl J Med* 2000;343:1902–1909.
52. Robertson AS, Gove RI, Wieland GA, et al. A double-blind comparison of oral prednisolone 40 mg/day with inhaled beclomethasone dipropionate 1500 g/day in patients with adult onset chronic obstructive airways disease. *Eur J Respir Dis* 1986;69(suppl 146):565–569.
53. Shim CS, Williams MH. Aerosol beclomethasone in patients with steroid-responsive chronic obstructive pulmonary disease. *Am J Med* 1985;78:655–658.
54. Weir DC, Gove RI, Robertson AS, et al. Corticosteroid trials in non-asthmatic chronic airflow obstruction: a comparison of oral prednisolone and inhaled beclomethasone dipropionate. *Thorax* 1990;45:112–117.
55. Poole PJ, Black PN. Mucolytic agents for chronic bronchitis or chronic obstructive pulmonary disease. In: The Cochrane Library, Issue 1, 2002. Oxford: Update Software. Search date 1999; primary sources Cochrane Airways Group Register and hand searched references. www.update-software.com/abstracts/ab001287.htm
56. Grandjean EM, Berthet P, Ruffmann R, et al. Efficacy of oral long-term N-acetylcysteine in chronic bronchopulmonary disease: a meta-analysis of published double-blind, placebo-controlled clinical trials. *Clin Ther* 2000;22:209–221. Search date 1995; primary sources Medline, hand searches of reference list, and personal contact with two experts.
57. Anonymous. Value of chemoprophylaxis and chemotherapy in early chronic bronchitis. A report to the Medical Research Council by their working party on trials of chemotherapy in early chronic bronchitis. *BMJ* 1966;5499:1317–1322.
58. Johnston RN, McNeill RS, Smith DH, et al. Five-year winter chemoprophylaxis for chronic bronchitis. *BMJ* 1969;4:265–269.
59. Crockett AJ, Moss JR, Cranston JM, et al. Domiciliary oxygen in chronic obstructive pulmonary disease. In: The Cochrane Library, Issue 1, 2002. Oxford: Update Software. Search date 2000; primary source Cochrane Airways Group Register.
60. Medical Research Council Working Party. Long term domiciliary oxygen therapy in chronic hypoxic cor pulmonale complicating chronic bronchitis and emphysema. *Lancet* 1981;1:681–686.
61. Fletcher EC, Luckett RA, Goodnight-White S, et al. A double-blind trial of nocturnal supplemental oxygen for sleep desaturation in patients with chronic obstructive pulmonary disease and a daytime PaO_2 above 60 mm Hg. *Am Rev Respir Dis* 1992;145:1070–1076.
62. Gorecka D, Gorzelak K, Sliwinski P, et al. Effect of long-term oxygen therapy on survival in patients with chronic obstructive pulmonary disease with moderate hypoxaemia. *Thorax* 1997;52:674–679.
63. Nocturnal Oxygen Therapy Trial Group. Continuous or nocturnal oxygen therapy in hypoxemic chronic obstructive lung disease: a clinical trial. *Ann Intern Med* 1980;93:391–398.
64. Chaouat A, Weitzenblum E, Kessler R, et al. A randomized trial of nocturnal oxygen therapy in chronic obstructive pulmonary disease patients. *Eur Respir J* 1999;14:1002–1008.
65. Dirksen A, Dijkman JH, Madsen F, et al. A randomized clinical trial of alpha$_1$-antitrypsin augmentation therapy. *Am J Respir Crit Care Med* 1999;160:1468–1472.
66. Anonymous. Survival and FEV_1 decline in individuals with severe deficiency of alpha1-antitrypsin. The Alpha-1-Antitrypsin Deficiency Registry Study Group. *Am J Respir Crit Care Med* 1998;158:49–59.
67. Seersholm N, Wencker M, Banik N, et al. Does alpha1-antitrypsin augmentation therapy slow the annual decline in FEV_1 in patients with severe hereditary alpha1-antitrypsin deficiency? Wissenschaftliche Arbeitsgemeinschaft zur Therapie von Lungenerkrankungen (WATL) alpha1-AT study group. *Eur Respir J* 1997;10:2260–2263.
68. O'Donnell AE, Barker AF, Ilowite JS, et al. Treatment of idiopathic bronchiectasis with aerosolized recombinant human DNase I. rhDNase Study Group. *Chest* 1998;113:1329–1334.

Huib Kerstjens
Pulmonary Physician

Dirkje Postma
Professor of Pulmonary Medicine
University Hospital Groningen
Groningen
The Netherlands

Competing interests: Both authors have received funding from the following manufacturers: AstraZeneca, the manufacturer of budesonide, terbutaline, formoterol; GlaxoSmithKline, the manufacturer of beclometasone, salbutamol, salmeterol, and fluticasone; Boehringer Ingelheim, the manufacturer of fenoterol, ipratropium, and tiotropium; and Novartis, the manufacturer of formoterol. DP has also received funding from Zambon, the manufacturer of N-acetylcysteine.

Community acquired pneumonia

Search date April 2002

Mark Loeb

QUESTIONS

INTERVENTIONS

Key Messages

Treatment

- **Antibiotics (amoxicillin, cephalosporins, macrolides, penicillin, quinolones) in hospital** RCTs evaluating different oral antibiotics in people admitted to hospital found cure or improvement in 73–96% of people, regardless of the antibiotic taken. RCTs found no significant difference in cure with cephalosporins versus penicillin or quinolones versus amoxicillin or versus cephalosporins. However, most trials were small and were designed to show equivalence between treatments rather than superiority of one over another.

- **Antibiotics (amoxicillin, cephalosporins, macrolides, penicillin, quinolones) in outpatient settings** One systematic review evaluating different oral antibiotics in outpatient settings has found clinical cure or improvement in over 90% of people, regardless of antibiotic taken. Another systematic review found that azithromycin versus other macrolides, cephalosporins, or penicillin significantly reduced clinical failures over 6–21 days. A third systematic review found no significant difference in clinical cure or improvement with quinolones versus amoxicillin, cephalosporins, or macrolides. Most trials were designed to show equivalence between treatments rather than superiority of one over another.
- **Bottle blowing** One unblinded RCT in people receiving antibiotics and usual medical care found that bottle blowing physiotherapy plus early mobilisation plus encouragement to regularly sit up and take deep breaths versus early mobilisation alone significantly reduced mean hospital stay.
- **Guidelines for treating pneumonia (for clinical outcomes)** One systematic review found no significant difference with the use of guidelines (incorporating early switch from intravenous to oral antibiotics and early discharge strategies, or both) versus usual care in improving clinical outcomes in community acquired pneumonia.
- **Intravenous versus oral antibiotics in immunocompetent people in hospital without life threatening illness** Two RCTs found that in immunocompetent people admitted to hospital who were not suffering life threatening illness, intravenous versus oral co-amoxiclav (amoxicillin plus clavulanic acid) or cefuroxime did not increase cure rates or reduce mortality. Intravenous antibiotics increased the length of hospital stay.
- **Prompt versus delayed administration of antibiotics in people severely ill with community acquired pneumonia** Retrospective studies found that prompt administration of antibiotics significantly improved survival. It would probably be unethical to perform an RCT of delayed antibiotic treatment.
- **Specific combinations of antibiotics in intensive care settings** We found no RCTs comparing one combination of antibiotics versus another in intensive care units.

Prevention

- **Influenza vaccine in elderly people** One RCT in people aged 60 years or over found that influenza vaccine versus placebo significantly reduced the incidence of influenza at 5 months.
- **Pneumococcal vaccine in chronically ill, immunosuppressed, or elderly people** One systematic review found no significant difference with pneumococcal vaccination versus no vaccination in the incidence of pneumonia in elderly people or people likely to have an impaired immune system.
- **Pneumococcal vaccine in immunocompetent adults** One systematic review in immunocompetent people has found that over one winter season, pneumococcal vaccination versus no vaccination significantly reduces pneumococcal pneumonia.

DEFINITION Community acquired pneumonia is pneumonia contracted in the community rather than in hospital. It is defined by clinical symptoms and signs with radiological confirmation.

INCIDENCE/ PREVALENCE In the northern hemisphere, community acquired pneumonia affects about 12/1000 people a year, particularly during winter and at the extremes of age (incidence: < 1 year old 30–50/1000 a year; 15–45 years 1–5/1000 a year; 60–70 years 10–20/1000 a year; 71–85 years 50/1000 a year).[1–6]

AETIOLOGY/ RISK FACTORS Over 100 microorganisms have been implicated in community acquired pneumonia, but most cases are caused by *Streptococcus pneumoniae* (see table 1, p 1557).[4–7] Smoking is probably an important risk factor.[8]

PROGNOSIS Severity varies from mild to life threatening illness within days of the onset of symptoms. One systematic review (search date 1995, 33 148 people) of prognosis studies for community acquired pneumonia found overall mortality to be 13.7%, ranging from 5.1% for ambulant people to 36.5% for people requiring intensive care.[9] The following prognostic factors were significantly associated with mortality: male sex (OR 1.3, 95% CI 1.2 to 1.4); pleuritic chest pain (OR 0.5, 95% CI 0.3 to 0.8, i.e. lower mortality); hypothermia (OR 5.0, 95% CI 2.4 to 10.4); systolic hypotension (OR 4.8, 95% CI 2.8 to 8.3); tachypnoea (OR 2.9, 95% CI 1.7 to 4.9); diabetes mellitus (OR 1.3, 95% CI 1.1 to 1.5); neoplastic disease (OR 2.8, 95% CI 2.4 to 3.1); neurological disease (OR 4.6, 95% CI 2.3 to 8.9); bacteraemia (OR 2.8, 95% CI 2.3 to 3.6); leucopenia (OR 2.5, 95% CI 1.6 to 3.7); and multilobar radiographic pulmonary infiltrates (OR 3.1, 95% CI 1.9 to 5.1).

AIMS **Treatment:** to clinically cure infection; to prevent death; to alleviate symptoms; to enable return to normal activities; and to prevent recurrence, whilst minimising adverse effects of treatments. **Prevention:** to prevent onset of pneumonia.

OUTCOMES Clinical cure (defined as return to premorbid health status); relief of symptoms; admission to hospital; complications (empyema, endocarditis, lung abscess); death; adverse effects of antibiotics.

METHODS *Clinical Evidence* update search and appraisal April 2002.

QUESTION What are the effects of antibiotics in outpatient settings?

OPTION ANTIBIOTICS

One systematic review evaluating different oral antibiotics in outpatient settings has found clinical cure or improvement in over 90% of people regardless of antibiotic taken. Another systematic review found that azithromycin versus other macrolides, cephalosporins, or penicillin significantly reduced clinical failures over 6–21 days. A third systematic review found no significant difference in clinical cure or improvement with quinolones versus amoxicillin, cephalosporins, or macrolides. Most trials were designed to show equivalence between treatments rather than superiority of one over another.

Benefits: We found three systematic reviews.[10–12] The first systematic review (search date not stated, 9 RCTs, 1164 people) compared different oral antibiotics in outpatient settings.[10] Antibiotics evaluated were amoxicillin (amoxycillin) with and without clavulanate, macrolides, cephalosporins, and quinolones. The review did not perform a meta-analysis directly comparing antibiotics. Clinical cure or improvement was reported in over 90% of people regardless of antibiotic taken (no further data provided). **Azithromycin versus other macrolides, cephalosporins, or penicillin:** The second systematic review (search date 2000, 18 RCTs, 2 of which were included in the first review, 1664 people) found that azithromycin versus other macrolides (clarithromycin, erythromycin, or roxithromycin, 13 RCTs) versus cefaclor (2 RCTs) or versus penicillin (co-amoxiclav [amoxicillin plus clavulanic acid] or penicillin, 3 RCTs) significantly reduced clinical failures over 6–21 days (56/928 [6%] with azithromycin *v* 72/736 [10%] with other oral antibiotics; OR 0.63, 95% CI 0.42 to 0.95).[11] These results should be interpreted with caution as most of the RCTs were not blinded. **Quinolones versus amoxicillin, macrolides, or cephalosporins:** The third systematic review (search date 1999, 8 RCTs, none of which were included in the first or second review, 3131 people) found no significant difference in cure or improvement with quinolones (gatifloxacin, levofloxacin, moxifloxacin, sparfloxacin, and trovafloxacin) versus high dose amoxicillin, cefaclor, cefpodoxime, ceftriaxone, ceftriaxone plus clarithromycin, cefuroxime axetil, clarithromycin, co-amoxiclav, erythromycin, or roxithromycin (ARR 1.7%, 95% CI –1.4% to +4.8%; no further data provided).[12]

Harms: Antibiotics can cause allergic reactions (including anaphylaxis), rash, gastrointestinal intolerance (nausea, vomiting, and diarrhoea), vaginal or oral candidiasis, and *Clostridium difficile* diarrhoea (including pseudomembranous colitis). Frequency of adverse effects varies with the antibiotic used. Most trials are designed to show equivalence between treatments rather than superiority of one over another.

Comment: Most trials were designed to show equivalence between treatments rather than superiority of one over another.

QUESTION What are the effects of treatments in people admitted to hospital?

OPTION ANTIBIOTICS

RCTs comparing different oral antibiotics in people admitted to hospital found clinical cure or improvement in 73–96% of people, regardless of antibiotic taken. The RCTs found no significant difference in clinical cure or improvement with cephalosporins versus penicillin or quinolones versus amoxicillin or versus cephalosporins. However, most trials were small and were designed to show equivalence between treatments rather than superiority of one over another.

Benefits: We found no systematic review. **Cephalosporins versus penicillin:** We found several RCTs that were too small, too old, or both, to be reliable given the changing sensitivity of organisms to antibiotics. One RCT (378 people) compared intravenous co-amoxiclav (amoxicillin plus clavulanic acid) followed by oral co-amoxiclav versus intravenous ceftriaxone followed by intramuscular ceftriaxone.[13] People in both groups also received intravenous erythromycin as decided by their physician (17/184 [9.2%] people taking co-amoxiclav *v* 25/194 [12.9%] people taking ceftriaxone). It found no significant difference in clinical cure at long term follow up, which was not specified (136/184 [73.9%] with co-amoxiclav *v* 144/194 [74.2%] with ceftriaxone; RR 0.99, 95% CI 0.88 to 1.12).

Quinolones versus high dose amoxicillin: We found two multicentre double blind RCTs.[14,15] The first RCT (329 people in hospital in France, South Africa, and Switzerland) comparing sparfloxacin 400 mg on day 1 followed by 200 mg once daily versus amoxicillin 1000 mg three times daily found no significant difference in clinical cure at 14–21 days (133/159 [83.6%] with sparfloxacin *v* 144/170 [84.7%] with amoxicillin; ARR +1.1%, 95% CI –5.5% to +10.8%; RR 0.99, 95% CI 0.87 to 1.07).[14] It found that fewer people treated with sparfloxacin versus amoxicillin discontinued the drug at days 3, 4, or 5 because of a lack of response, but the difference did not reach significance (3/126 [2.4%] *v* 11/140 [7.9%]; ARR +5.5%, 95% CI –0.4% to +7.2%; RR 0.30, 95% CI 0.08 to 1.05). The second RCT (411 people with suspected pneumococcal pneumonia, 285 of whom were admitted to hospital) compared oral moxifloxacin 400 mg once daily versus oral amoxicillin 1000 mg three times daily.[15] It found no significant difference in clinical cure at 3–4 weeks after the end of 5–7 days' treatment (154/200 [77.0%] with moxifloxacin *v* 164/208 [78.8%] with amoxicillin; RR 0.97, 95% CI 0.86 to 1.07). **Quinolones versus cephalosporins:** We found one unblinded RCT (590 people, 280 of whom had been admitted to hospital) comparing oral or intravenous levofloxacin or both versus intravenous ceftriaxone or oral cefuroxime axetil or both.[16] It found that levofloxacin versus cephalosporins significantly increased the proportion of people clinically cured or improved at 5–7 days (96.5% with levofloxacin *v* 90.4% with cephalosporins; ARR 6.1%, 95% CI 1.3% to 10.7%).

Harms: See harms of antibiotics, p 1549.

Comment: Most trials were small and were designed to show equivalence between treatments rather than superiority of one over another. Although detection of penicillin resistant and multidrug resistant *S pneumoniae* is commonly reported, it is hard to enrol people with this infection in randomised studies. One study was carried out in areas with high prevalence of penicillin resistant *S pneumoniae*.[14] However, only 8/135 (6.9%) isolates tested were resistant to penicillin, and none showed high level resistance. The trials in uncomplicated pneumonia may not apply to people with comorbidities such as meningitis.[17] There are also concerns about macrolide resistant *S pneumoniae* but, so far, treatment failure in ambulatory people with community acquired pneumonia is uncommon.[18] In the RCT comparing levofloxacin versus cephalosporins, the route of administration was decided by the physician and it is unclear whether all participants receiving intravenous antibiotics were admitted to hospital.[16] We found one retrospective review (12 945 people ≥ 65 years old in hospital with community acquired pneumonia).[19] It found that initial treatment with a second generation cephalosporin plus a macrolide, a non-pseudomonal third generation cephalosporin plus a macrolide, or a fluoroquinolone alone versus a β-lactam/β-lactamase inhibitor plus a macrolide, and an aminoglycoside plus another agent reduced mortality at 30 days.[19] One retrospective cohort study found that people infected with penicillin resistant versus non-penicillin resistant *S pneumoniae* were at greater risk of death in hospital (RR 2.1, 95% CI 1.0 to 4.3) and suppurative complications (RR 4.5, 95% CI 1.0 to 19.3).[20]

From national surveillance data, penicillin resistant versus non-penicillin resistant pneumonia was associated with significantly higher mortality after the first 4 days in hospital.[21] However, these results should be interpreted with caution as they may not account for confounding factors.

OPTION INTRAVENOUS VERSUS ORAL ANTIBIOTICS

Two RCTs found that, in immunocompetent people admitted to hospital who were not suffering life threatening illness, intravenous versus oral co-amoxiclav (amoxicillin plus clavulanic acid) or cefuroxime did not increase cure rates or reduce mortality, and increased the length of hospital stay.

Benefits: We found no systematic review. We found two RCTs comparing oral versus intravenous antibiotics in people admitted to hospital with community acquired pneumonia.[22,23] The first RCT (541 people with lower respiratory tract infections, 40% of whom had chest radiographs that were compatible with pneumonia) compared 7 days of treatment with oral co-amoxiclav versus intravenous co-amoxiclav for 3 days followed by oral co-amoxiclav versus intravenous cefotaxime for 3 days followed by oral cefuroxime.[22] People were excluded if they had life threatening infection or were immunocompromised. The RCT found no significant difference in cure rates or mortality among the three groups at discharge, but hospital stay was significantly shorter in those on oral treatment than in those on intravenous treatment ($P < 0.001$). The second RCT (73 people, no intention to treat analysis) compared intravenous versus oral cefuroxime.[23] People were randomised to 2 days of intravenous followed by 8 days of oral treatment (group 1) versus 5 days of each treatment (group 2) versus 10 days of intravenous treatment (group 3). The only significant difference was in the length of hospital stay (6 days with group 1 *v* 8 days with group 2 *v* 11 days with group 3; no P value stated).

Harms: The RCTs gave no information on adverse effects.[22,23]

Comment: Intravenous antibiotics are used in people who cannot take oral medication because of severe nausea or vomiting. A follow up study (96 people admitted to hospital with community acquired pneumonia) found clinical cure of pneumonia at 30 days in people who were switched from intravenous to oral antibiotics when they had been afebrile for 8 hours, symptoms of cough and shortness of breath were improving, white blood cell counts were returning to normal, and they could tolerate oral medication.[24]

OPTION BOTTLE BLOWING

One unblinded RCT in people receiving antibiotics and usual medical care found that bottle blowing physiotherapy plus early mobilisation plus encouragement to sit up regularly and take deep breaths versus early mobilisation alone significantly reduced mean hospital stay.

Benefits: We found no systematic review. We found one RCT (145 people in hospital with community acquired pneumonia) comparing three groups: early mobilisation; early mobilisation and encouragement to sit up 10 times a day and take 20 deep breaths; and early mobilisation and encouragement to sit up 10 times a day and blow bubbles through a plastic tube for 20 breaths into a bottle containing 10 cm of water (bottle blowing).[25] Participants concurrently received benzylpenicillin or phenoxymethylpenicillin and usual medical care independently of the study interventions. It found that bottle blowing plus early mobilisation plus encouragement versus early mobilisation alone significantly reduced mean hospital stay (5.3 *v* 3.9 days; P = 0.01).

Harms: The RCT gave no information on adverse effects.[25]

Comment: Neither study participants nor clinicians were blinded to the intervention.

QUESTION What are the effects of treatments in people with community acquired pneumonia receiving intensive care?

OPTION SPECIFIC COMBINATIONS OF ANTIBIOTICS

We found no RCTs comparing one combination of antibiotics versus another in intensive care units.

Benefits: We found no systematic review and no RCTs.

Harms: We found no RCTs.

Comment: Using a combination of antibiotics is regarded as current best practice.

OPTION PROMPT VERSUS DELAYED ANTIBIOTIC TREATMENT

Two retrospective studies found that prompt administration of antibiotics significantly improved survival. It would probably be regarded as unethical to perform an RCT of delayed antibiotic treatment.

Benefits: We found no systematic review and no RCTs. One multicentre retrospective review (medical records of ≥ 14 000 people aged ≥65 years who were severely ill with community acquired pneumonia) found that giving antibiotics within 8 hours of admission to hospital was associated with lower 30 day mortality (OR 0.85, 95% CI 0.75 to 0.96).[26] The review did not specify whether oral or intravenous antibiotics were given. Another retrospective study (39 people with serologically confirmed Legionnaires' disease) examined outcome and time to start of treatment.[27] For the 10 people who died, the median delay between diagnosis of pneumonia and start of intravenous erythromycin was 5 days (range 1–10 days), and for those who survived it was 1 day (range 1–5 days; P < 0.001).

Harms: None reported.

Comment: It would probably be regarded as unethical to perform an RCT of delayed antibiotic treatment.

QUESTION **What are the effects of guidelines on the treatment of community acquired pneumonia?**

One systematic review comparing a guideline incorporating early switch from intravenous to oral antibiotics and early discharge strategies (or both) versus usual care has found no significant difference in clinical outcomes.

Benefits: We found one systematic review (search date 2000, 3 RCTs, 7 cohort studies) comparing a guideline incorporating early switch from intravenous to oral antibiotics and early discharge or both versus usual care.[28] It found no significant difference in therapeutic success (not defined), readmission to hospital, intensive care unit admission, complications, mortality, or any adverse outcome (no further data provided). It also found no significant difference between a guideline versus usual care in mean length of hospital stay (mean 6.0 days for guideline *v* 7.6 days for usual care; P = 0.05).

Harms: The review found no significant difference in "any adverse outcome" (not specified) with a guideline versus usual care (no further data provided).[28]

Comment: None.

QUESTION **What are the effects of preventive interventions?**

OPTION **INFLUENZA VACCINE**

One RCT found that influenza vaccine versus placebo significantly reduced the incidence of influenza in people aged 60 years or over. Another RCT found that intranasal live vaccine plus parenteral vaccine versus parenteral vaccine alone significantly reduced the incidence of influenza A in elderly people. Two RCTs found that the offer of vaccination of healthcare workers versus no offer of vaccination significantly reduced mortality in elderly people in long term care hospitals.

Benefits: **Effects in vaccinated people:** We found one systematic review (search date 2000,[29] 1 RCT[30]) and one additional RCT.[31] The RCT (> 1800 people aged ≥ 60 years) identified by the review[29] compared split virion vaccine versus saline solution.[30] It found that vaccine versus placebo significantly reduced the incidence of clinical influenza at 5 months (AR 17/927 [1.8%] *v* AR 31/911 [3.4%]; RR 0.53, 95% CI 0.39 to 0.73).[30] The additional RCT (324 elderly residents of nursing homes) compared parenteral trivalent inactivated vaccine plus intranasal live attenuated cold adapted vaccine versus parenteral trivalent inactivated vaccine alone. It found that inactivated vaccine plus live attenuated vaccine versus inactivated vaccine alone significantly reduced the incidence of influenza A (9/162 [5.5%] for inactivated vaccine plus live attenuated vaccine *v* 24/169 [14.2%] for inactivated vaccine alone; ARR 8.6%, 95% CI 2.6% to 11.6%; RR 0.39, 95% CI 0.18 to 0.81; NNT 12, 95% CI 9 to 38).[31] **Effects of vaccinating healthcare workers:** We found no systematic review but found two RCTs, which are difficult to interpret (see comment below).[32,33] The first RCT (12 long term elderly care hospitals) compared the offer of vaccination of healthcare workers versus no offer of vaccination.[32] Of the healthcare workers offered vaccination, 653/1078 (60.6%) were vaccinated. In the hospitals where vaccination was offered to healthcare workers, more than 85% of residents had already been vaccinated compared to only one resident in the hospitals where vaccination was not offered to healthcare workers. The RCT found that vaccination of healthcare workers versus no vaccination significantly reduced all cause mortality of elderly residents during one winter (50/490 [10.0%] residents in vaccine hospitals *v* 98/569 [17.2%] in non-vaccine hospitals; ARR 7.0%, 95% CI 3.2% to 9.9%; RR 0.59, 95% CI 0.42 to 0.82).[32] Another RCT (20 elderly care hospitals) compared influenza vaccination of healthcare workers versus no vaccination in a similar design to the previous RCT.[33] Of the healthcare workers offered vaccination, 620/1217 (50.9%) were vaccinated. In vaccine hospitals, 48% of residents versus 33% of residents in non-vaccine hospitals were already vaccinated. The RCT found that influenza vaccination of healthcare workers versus no vaccination significantly reduced all cause mortality of elderly people over 6 months (102/749 [13.6%] in vaccine hospitals *v* 154/688 [22.4%] in non-vaccine hospitals; RR 0.60, 95% CI 0.48 to 0.77; NNT 11; 95% CI 9 to 19).[33]

Harms: Two of the RCTs found that adverse effects included pain and tenderness at the site of injection.[32,33] Guillain-Barré syndrome was associated with 1/100 000 influenza vaccinations during the national vaccination programme against swine influenza in the USA in 1976, during which 45 million people were vaccinated.[34]

Comment: One systematic review of cohort studies (search date not stated, 20 studies) comparing influenza vaccine versus no vaccine found that influenza vaccine significantly reduced the incidence of pneumonia (24 774 people; ARR 53%, 95% CI 35% to 66%) and significantly reduced mortality (29 928 people; ARR 68%, 95% CI 56% to 76%).[35] Time scales were not provided for any outcomes. Analysis of an administrative database (≥ 25 000 people aged ≥ 64 years) suggested that influenza vaccination reduced the rate of admission to hospital in people with pneumonia or influenza by 48–57% ($P < 0.01$).[36] A reduction in rates of influenza does not necessarily imply a reduction in rates of pneumonia. The RCTs of the effects of vaccination in healthcare workers seemed to find a reduction in mortality in elderly people in long term care hospitals.[32,33] However, the groups were not comparable.

OPTION PNEUMOCOCCAL VACCINE

One systematic review has found that pneumococcal vaccination versus no vaccination significantly reduces pneumococcal pneumonia in immunocompetent people, but found no significant difference between pneumococcal vaccination versus no vaccination in the incidence of pneumonia in elderly people or people likely to have an impaired immune system.

Benefits: We found one systematic review (search date 2000, 13 RCTs, > 45 000 people) comparing pneumococcal vaccination versus no vaccination.[37] It found that in immunocompetent people (3 RCTs,

21 152 African gold workers and Papua New Guinea highlanders), pneumococcal vaccination versus no vaccination significantly reduced all cause pneumonia (3.1% *v* 6.5%; RR 0.56, 95% CI 0.47 to 0.66), pneumococcal pneumonia (0.5% *v* 3.1%; RR 0.16, 95% CI 0.11 to 0.23), pneumococcal bacteraemia (0.7% *v* 3.8%; RR 0.18, 95% CI 0.09 to 0.34), and pneumonia related mortality during one winter (1.1 *v* 1.6; RR 0.70, 95% CI 0.50 to 0.96). In elderly people or people likely to have an impaired immune system (10 RCTs, 24 074 people), the review found no significant difference between pneumococcal vaccination versus no vaccination in all cause pneumonia (7.0% *v* 6.5%; RR 1.08, 95% CI 0.92 to 1.27), pneumococcal pneumonia (1.7% *v* 1.9%; RR 0.88, 95% CI 0.72 to 1.07), pneumococcal bacteraemia (0.8% *v* 1.4%; RR 0.53, 95% CI 0.14 to 1.94), and pneumonia related mortality (1% *v* 1.1%; RR 0.93, 95% CI 0.72 to 1.20).

Harms: The systematic review found few RCTs that gave information on adverse effects.[37] One RCT in the review found that pneumococcal vaccination versus no vaccination was associated with erythema and induration. Another RCT in the review found that pneumococcal vaccination versus no vaccination increased sore arm, swollen arm, and fever.

Comment: A fifth of healthy elderly adults (mean age 71 years) do not have an antibody response to vaccination.[38] New conjugate pneumococcal vaccines are being evaluated. These have been shown to stimulate an antibody response in infants and have decreased the rate of carriage of resistant strains of *S pneumoniae*.[39,40] One retrospective cohort study (1898 elderly members of a staff healthcare organisation) found that pneumococcal vaccination was associated with lower risks of admission to hospital for pneumonia (adjusted RR 0.57, 95% CI 0.38 to 0.84) and for death (adjusted RR 0.71, 95% CI 0.56 to 0.91).[41] The study found evidence of an additive effect for people who received both pneumococcal and influenza vaccinations during the influenza season (RR 0.28, 95% CI 0.14 to 0.58 for admission to hospital for pneumonia and influenza; RR 0.18, 95% CI 0.11 to 0.31 for death).

Substantive changes

Antibiotics (outpatients) Two new systematic reviews comparing azithromycin versus other macrolides, penicillin, and cephalosporins;[11] and quinolones versus amoxicillin, macrolides, or cephalosporins,[12] found insufficient evidence on the effects of different classes of antibiotics.

Influenza vaccine One new systematic review;[29] conclusions unchanged

REFERENCES

1. Foy HM, Cooney MK, Allan I, et al. Rates of pneumonia during influenza epidemics in Seattle, 1964–1975. *JAMA* 1979;241: 253–258.
2. Murphy TF, Henderson FW, Clyde WA, et al. Pneumonia: an 11 year study in a pediatric practice. *Am J Epidemiol* 1981;113:12–21.
3. McConnochie KM, Hall CB, Barker WH. Lower respiratory tract illness in the first two years of life: epidemiologic patterns and costs in a suburban pediatric practice. *Am J Public Health* 1988;78:34–39.
4. Porath A, Schlaeffer F, Lieberman D. The epidemiology of community-acquired pneumonia among hospitalized adults. *J Infect* 1997;34:41–48.
5. Jokinen C, Heiskanen L, Juvonen H, et al. Incidence of community-acquired pneumonia in the population of four municipalities in eastern Finland. *Am J Epidemiol* 1993;137:977–988.
6. Houston MS, Silverstein MD, Suman VJ. Risk factors for 30-day mortality in elderly patients with lower respiratory tract infection. *Arch Intern Med* 1997;157:2190–2195.

7. Bartlett JG, Mundy LM. Community-acquired pneumonia. *N Engl J Med* 1995;333:1618–1624.
8. Almirall J, Gonzalez CA, Balanco X, et al. Proportion of community-acquired pneumonia attributable to tobacco smoking. *Chest* 1999;116:375–379.
9. Fine MJ, Smith MA, Carson CA, et al. Prognosis and outcomes of patients with community-acquired pneumonia: a meta-analysis. *JAMA* 1995;274:134–141. Search date 1995; primary sources Medline and handsearching of reference lists.
10. Pomilla PV, Brown RB. Outpatient treatment of community-acquired pneumonia in adults. *Arch Intern Med* 1994;154:1793–1802. Search date not stated; primary source Medline.
11. Contopoulos-Ioannidis DG, Ioannidis JPA, Chew P, et al. Meta-analysis of randomized controlled trials on the comparative efficacy and safety of azithromycin against other antibiotics for lower respiratory tract infections. *J Antimicrob Chemother* 2001;48:691–703. Search date 2000; primary sources Embase, Medline, Cochrane Controlled Trials Registry.
12. Metge CJ, Vercaigne L, Carrie A, et al. The new fluoroquinolones in community-acquired pneumonia: clinical and economic perspectives. Ottawa: Canadian Coordinating Office for Health Technology Assessment; 2001. Technology Overview No 5. Search date 1999; primary sources Medline and Embase.
13. Roson B, Carratala J, Tubau F, et al. Usefulness of betalactam therapy for community-acquired pneumonia in the era of drug-resistant *Streptococcus pneumoniae*: a randomized study of amoxicillin-clavulanate and ceftriaxone. *Microb Drug Resist* 2001;7:85–96.
14. Aubier M, Verster R, Regamey C, et al and the Sparfloxacin European Study Group. Once-daily sparfloxacin versus high-dosage amoxicillin in the treatment of community-acquired, suspected pneumococcal pneumonia in adults. *Clin Infect Dis* 1998;26:1312–1320.
15. Petitpretz P, Arvis P, Marel M, et al. Oral moxifloxacin vs high-dosage amoxicillin in the treatment of mild-to-moderate, community-acquired, suspected pneumococcal pneumonia in adults. *Chest* 2001;119:185–195.
16. File TM Jr, Segreti J, Dunbar L, et al. A multicenter, randomized study comparing the efficacy and safety of intravenous and/or oral levofloxacin versus ceftriaxone and/or cefuroxime axetil in treatment of adults with community-acquired pneumonia. *Antimicrob Agents Chemother* 1997;41:1965–1972.
17. Friedland IR, McCracken GH Jr. Management of infections caused by antibiotic-resistant *Streptococcus pneumoniae*. *N Engl J Med* 1994;331:377–382.
18. Siegel RE. The significance of serum vs. tissue levels of antibiotics in the treatment of penicillin-resistant *Streptococcus pneumoniae* and community-acquired pneumonia. Are we looking in the wrong place? *Chest* 1999;116:535–538.
19. Gleason PP, Meehan TP, Fine JM, et al. Associations between initial antimicrobial therapy and medical outcomes for hospitalized elderly patients with pneumonia. *Arch Intern Med* 1999;159:2562–2572.
20. Metlay JP, Hofmann J, Cetron MS, et al. Impact of penicillin susceptibility on medical outcomes for adult patients with bacteremic pneumococcal pneumonia. *Clin Infect Dis* 2000;30:520–528.
21. Faikin DR, Schuchat A, Kolczak M, et al. Mortality from invasive pneumococcal pneumonia in the era of antibiotic resistance, 1995–1997. *Am J Public Health* 2000;90:223–229.
22. Chan R, Hemeryck L, O'Regan M, et al. Oral versus intravenous antibiotics for community-acquired lower respiratory tract infection in a general hospital: open randomised controlled trial. *BMJ* 1995;310:1360–1362.
23. Siegel RE, Halperin NA, Almenoff PL, et al. A prospective randomized study of inpatient IV antibiotics for community-acquired pneumonia: the optimal duration of therapy. *Chest* 1996;110:965–971.
24. Ramirez JA, Ahkee S. Early switch from intravenous antimicrobials to oral clarithromycin in patients with community acquired pneumonia. *Infect Med* 1997;14:319–323.
25. Bjorkqvist M, Wiberg B, Bodin L, et al. Bottle-blowing in hospital-treated patients with community-acquired pneumonia. *Scand J Infect Dis* 1997;29:77–82.
26. Meehan TP, Fine MJ, Krumholz HM, et al. Quality of care, process, and outcomes in elderly patients with pneumonia. *JAMA* 1997;278:2080–2084.
27. Heath CH, Grove DI, Looke DFM. Delay in appropriate therapy of *Legionella pneumonia* associated with increased mortality. *Eur J Clin Microbiol Infect Dis* 1966;15:286–290.
28. Rhew DC, Tu GS, Ofman J, et al. Early switch and early discharge strategies in patients with community-acquired pneumonia: a meta-analysis. *Arch Intern Med* 2001;161:722–727. Search date 2000; primary sources Medline, Healthstar, Embase, Cochrane Library, and Best Evidence.
29. Vu T, Farish S, Jenkins M, et al. A meta-analysis of influenza vaccine in persons aged 65 years and over living in the community. *Vaccine* 2002;20:1831–1836. Search date 2000; primary sources Medline, Biosis, Firstsearch, Bandolier, Cochrane Library, Current Contents, Effectiveness Matters, Derwent Drug File, American College of Physicians Journal Club, Database of Abstracts of Effectiveness, FluNet, CDC Influenza Home Page, Influenza Bibiography, several government Internet sites, and hand searches of reference lists and contact with prominent researchers in the field.
30. Govaert TM, Thijs CT, Masurel N, et al. The efficacy of influenza vaccination in elderly individuals: a randomized double-blind placebo-controlled trial. *JAMA* 1994;272:1661–1665.
31. Treanor JJ, Mattison HR, Dumyati G, et al. Protective efficacy of combined live intranasal and inactivated influenza A virus vaccines in the elderly. *Ann Intern Med* 1992;117:625–633.
32. Potter J, Stott DJ, Roberts MA, et al. Influenza vaccination of health care workers in long-term-care hospitals reduces the mortality of elderly patients. *J Infect Dis* 1997;175:1–6.
33. Carmen WF, Elder AG, Wallace LA, et al. Effects of influenza vaccination of health-care workers on mortality of elderly people in long-term care: a randomized controlled trial. *Lancet* 2000;355:93–97.
34. Betts RF. Influenza virus. In: Mandell GL, Bennett JE, Dolin R, eds. *Principles and practice of infectious diseases*. 4th edn. New York: Churchill Livingstone, 1995.
35. Gross PA, Hermogenes AW, Sacks HS, et al. The efficacy of influenza vaccine in elderly persons: a meta-analysis and review of the literature. *Ann Intern Med* 1995;123:518–527. Search date not stated; primary source Medline.
36. Nichol KL, Margolis KL, Wuorenma J, et al. The efficacy and cost effectiveness of vaccination

against influenza among elderly persons living in the community. *N Engl J Med* 1994;331:778–784.

37. Moore RA, Wiffen PJ, Lipsky BA. Are the pneumococcal polysaccharide vaccines effective ? Meta-analysis of the prospective trials. *BMC Family Practice* 2000;1. http://www.biomedcentral.com/1471–2296/1/1 (last accessed 5 Sept 2002). Search date 2000; primary sources Cochrane Library, Medline, Embase, and handsearches of reference lists.
38. Rubins JB, Puri AKG, Loch J, et al. Magnitude, duration, quality and function of pneumococcal vaccine responses in elderly adults. *J Infect Dis* 1998;178:431–440.
39. Mbelle N, Wasas A, Huebner R, et al. Immunogenicity and impact on carriage of 9-valent pneumococcal conjugate vaccine given to infants in Soweto, South Africa. *Proceedings of the 37th Interscience Conference on Antimicrobial Agents and Chemotherapy; 1997 September*. Toronto, Herndon VA: ASM Press, 1997.
40. Gesner M, Desidero D, Kim M, et al. *Streptococcus pneumoniae* in human immunodeficiency virus type 1 infected children. *Pediatr Infect Dis J* 1994;13:697–703.
41. Nichol KL, Baken L, Wuorenma J, Nelson A. The health and economic benefits associated with pneumococcal vaccination in elderly people with chronic lung disease. *Arch Intern Med* 1999;159:2437–2442.

Mark Loeb
Associate Professor
Departments of Pathology & Molecular Medicine and Clinical Epidemiology & Biostatistics
McMaster University
Hamilton
Canada

Competing interests: The author has received a research grant from Bayer and has attended conferences sponsored by Janssen Ortho and Aventis.

TABLE 1 **Causes of community acquired pneumonia (see text, p 1548).**

	USA (% of participants)*	UK (% of participants)†	Susceptibility (laboratory results)‡
Streptococcus pneumoniae	20–60	60–75	25% penicillin resistant, sensitive to quinolones
Haemophilus influenzae	3–10	4–5	30% ampicillin resistant, sensitive to cephalosporins or co-amoxiclav
Staphylococcus aureus	3–5	1–5	Methicillin resistant *S aureus* rare as cause of community acquired pneumonia
Chlamydia pneumoniae	4–6	ND	Sensitive to macrolides, tetracyclines, quinolones
Mycoplasma pneumoniae	1–6	5–18	Sensitive to macrolides, tetracyclines, quinolones
Legionella pneumophila	2–8	2–5	Sensitive to macrolides, tetracyclines, quinolones
Gram-negative bacilli	3–10	Rare	
Aspiration	6–10	ND	
Viruses	2–15	8–16	

*Pooled data from 15 published reports from North America;[7] †Data from British Thoracic Society;[7] ‡Susceptibility data from recent studies. ND, no data.

Lung cancer

Search date May 2002

Alan Neville

QUESTIONS

INTERVENTIONS

See glossary, p 1571

Key Messages

Non-small cell lung cancer

- **Hyperfractionated radiation treatment versus conventional radiotherapy in unresectable stage 3 non-small cell lung cancer** One systematic review in people with stage 3 non-small cell lung cancer has found no significant difference with standard hyperfractionation versus conventional radiotherapy in survival at 2 years. One RCT in people with stage 3 non-small cell lung cancer found that continuous, hyperfractionated, accelerated radiotherapy versus conventional radiotherapy significantly increased survival at 2 years.

Clin Evid 2002;8:1558–1574.

- **Newer single drug or combined drug regimens in stage 4 non-small cell lung cancer (not clearly better than cisplatin or docetaxel based regimens)** One systematic review and subsequent RCTs in people with stage 3 and 4 non-small cell lung cancer found conflicting evidence on the effects of single versus combined chemotherapy. One RCT in people with stage 3 and 4 non-small cell lung cancer found no significant difference in survival at 1 year with first line platinum based versus non-platinum based chemotherapy.
- **Palliative chemotherapy with cisplatin or docetaxel containing regimens in stage 4 non-small cell lung cancer** Systematic reviews in people with stage 4 non-small cell lung cancer have found that the addition of chemotherapy regimens containing cisplatin to best supportive care significantly increase survival at 1 year. Limited evidence from RCTs suggests that the addition of chemotherapy to best supportive care versus best supportive care alone may improve quality of life.
- **Postoperative chemotherapy in people with resected stage 1–3 non-small cell lung cancer** Systematic reviews and one subsequent RCT in people with completely resected stage 2 and 3 non-small cell lung cancer have found no significant difference in survival at 5 years with postoperative cisplatin based chemotherapy versus surgery with or without concomitant radiotherapy. One systematic review has found that postoperative alkylating agents increase mortality compared with no chemotherapy.
- **Preoperative chemotherapy in people with resectable stage 3 non-small cell lung cancer** One systematic review of two small RCTs in people with technically resectable stage 3A non-small cell lung cancer found that preoperative chemotherapy versus no preoperative chemotherapy significantly improved survival at 2 years (NNT 4, 95% CI 2 to 11). One additional RCT found that preoperative chemotherapy versus no preoperative chemotherapy non-significantly improved survival at 4 years in people with resectable stages 1–3 non-small cell lung cancer.
- **Thoracic irradiation plus chemotherapy versus irradiation alone in unresected stage 3 non-small cell lung cancer** Systematic reviews and one subsequent RCT in people with unresectable stage 3 non-small cell lung cancer have found that adding chemotherapy to thoracic irradiation significantly improves survival at 2–5 years. Another subsequent RCT has found no significant difference in median survival with radical radiotherapy plus chemotherapy versus radiotherapy alone.

Small cell lung cancer

- **Chemotherapy plus thoracic irradiation versus chemotherapy alone in limited stage small cell lung cancer** Two systematic reviews in people with limited stage small cell lung cancer have found that adding thoracic irradiation to chemotherapy significantly improves survival at 3 years. However, one of these reviews has found that chemotherapy plus thoracic irradiation significantly increases deaths related to treatment.
- **Dose intensive chemotherapy versus standard chemotherapy** Two RCTs found that dose intensification versus standard chemotherapy significantly increased deaths related to toxicity, and did not improve progression free survival. One RCT in people with limited disease found that early dose intensification of chemotherapy alternating with radiotherapy versus no early intensification of chemotherapy significantly increased survival at 2 years. One RCT found that cisplatin plus irinotecan versus cisplatin plus etoposide may improve survival over 2 years. Two RCTs found conflicting evidence about the effects of dose intensification plus growth factor support.

- **Oral etoposide in extensive stage small cell lung cancer** RCTs in people with extensive stage small cell lung cancer have found that oral etoposide improves survival at 1 year significantly less than combination chemotherapy. One RCT found that etoposide versus combination chemotherapy caused less nausea and vomiting in the short term but found no evidence that etoposide offers significantly better quality of life overall.
- **Prophylactic cranial irradiation for people in complete remission with limited or extensive stage small cell lung cancer** One systematic review in people in with small cell lung cancer in complete remission has found that prophylactic cranial irradiation versus no irradiation significantly improves survival at 3 years and reduces the risk of developing brain metastases. Long term cognitive dysfunction following cranial irradiation has been described, but longer follow up studies are needed to assess its significance and importance.

DEFINITION Lung cancer (bronchogenic carcinoma) is an epithelial cancer arising from the bronchial surface epithelium or bronchial mucous glands (see table 1, p 1574).

INCIDENCE/ PREVALENCE Lung cancer is the leading cause of cancer death in both men and women, affecting about 100 000 men and 80 000 women annually in the USA, and about 40 000 men and women in the UK. Small cell lung cancer constitutes about 20–25% of all lung cancers, the remainder being non-small cell lung cancers of which adenocarcinoma is now the most prevalent form.[1]

AETIOLOGY/ RISK FACTORS Smoking remains the major preventable risk factor, accounting for about 80–90% of all cases.[2]

PROGNOSIS Lung cancer has an overall 5 year survival rate of 10–12%.[3] At the time of diagnosis, 10–15% of people with lung cancer have localised disease. Of these, half will have died at 5 years despite potentially curative surgery. Over half of people have metastatic disease at the time of diagnosis. People with non-small cell cancer who undergo surgery have a 5 year survival of 60–80% for stage 1 disease and 25–50% for stage 2 disease.[3] In people with small cell cancer, those with limited stage disease who undergo combined chemotherapy and mediastinal irradiation have a median survival of 18–24 months, whereas those with extensive stage disease who are given palliative chemotherapy have a median survival of 10–12 months.[3] About 5–10% of people with small cell lung cancer present with central nervous system involvement, and half develop symptomatic brain metastases by 2 years. Of these, only half respond to palliative radiation, and their median survival is less than 3 months.[3]

AIMS To prolong life; to improve quality of life; and to provide palliation of symptoms, with minimum adverse effects of treatment.

OUTCOMES Survival; clinical response rates; disease related symptoms; adverse effects of treatment; quality of life. Despite recent progress in the development of valid instruments, measuring quality of life in people with lung cancer remains a serious challenge.[4,5]

METHODS *Clinical Evidence* update search and appraisal May 2002. Unless stated otherwise, we have used the term stage 3 non-small cell lung cancer to refer to both stage 3A and stage 3B.

QUESTION What are the effects of treatments for non-small cell lung cancer?

OPTION PRE- AND POSTOPERATIVE CHEMOTHERAPY IN RESECTABLE NON-SMALL CELL LUNG CANCER

One systematic review of two small RCTs in people with technically resectable stage 3A non-small cell lung cancer found that preoperative chemotherapy versus no chemotherapy significantly improved survival at 2 years. One additional RCT found that preoperative chemotherapy versus no preoperative chemotherapy non-significantly improved survival in people with resectable stages 1–3 non-small cell lung cancer at 4 years. Systematic reviews and one subsequent RCT in people with completely resected stage 2 and 3 non-small cell lung cancer have found no significant difference in survival at 5 years with postoperative cisplatin based chemotherapy versus surgery with or without concomitant radiotherapy. One systematic review found that postoperative alkylating agents increased mortality compared with no chemotherapy.

Benefits: **Preoperative chemotherapy:** We found one systematic review,[6] one non-systematic review,[7] and one subsequent RCT.[8] The systematic review (search date 1997, 4 RCTs, 204 people with technically resectable stage 3A non-small cell lung cancer) compared preoperative cisplatin based chemotherapy versus no chemotherapy.[6] It found that preoperative chemotherapy versus no chemotherapy significantly reduced mortality at 2 years (2 fully reported RCTs; AR 34/58 [59%] with preoperative chemotherapy *v* 54/62 [87%] with no chemotherapy; RR 0.67, 95% CI 0.42 to 0.89; NNT 4, 95% CI 2 to 11). One non-systematic review which identified the same RCTs suggested that this evidence is limited because the trials were small, staging was clinical rather than pathological, and treatment groups were not balanced for prognostic factors such as K-Ras mutations.[7] We found one subsequent RCT (355 people with resectable stages 1 [except T1N0] to 3A non-small cell lung cancer), which compared preoperative chemotherapy (two cycles of ifosfamide plus mitomycin plus cisplatin) versus primary surgery alone.[8] It found no significant difference in survival between groups in people with any disease stage and in people with stage 3 disease after 4 years follow up (median survival for any disease stage 37 months, 95% CI 26.7 to 48.3 months with preoperative chemotherapy *v* 26.0 months, 95% CI 19.8 to 33.6 months, P = 0.15; RR for survival in people with stage 3 disease 1.04, 95% CI 0.68 to 1.60; P = 0.85). **Postoperative chemotherapy:** We found two systematic reviews[9,10] and one subsequent RCT.[11] The most recent review (search date 1998, 1 earlier systematic review)[9] did not fully describe the earlier review it identified comparing postoperative cisplatin based chemotherapy versus no chemotherapy.[10] The earlier review (search date 1991, 14 RCTs, 1394 people with resected stage 1–3 non-small cell lung cancer) found no significant difference with postoperative cisplatin based chemotherapy versus surgery alone in mortality at 5 years (8 RCTs; ARR +5%, 95% CI –1% to +10%; HR 0.87, 95% CI 0.74 to 1.02; P = 0.08).[10] However, it found that postoperative alkylating agents increased risk of death compared with surgery alone

(5 RCTs; HR 1.15; CI not stated; P = 0.005; ARR of death at 5 years +5%). **Postoperative chemotherapy plus radiotherapy versus postoperative radiotherapy:** We found one systematic review (search date 1991, 7 RCTs, 807 people)[10] and one subsequent RCT.[11] The review found that adding postoperative chemotherapy to postoperative radiotherapy did not significantly improve survival (overall HR 0.98, CI not stated, P = 0.76; HR for 6 RCTs that added cisplatin based chemotherapy HR 0.94, CI not stated, P = 0.46; ARR for death at 5 years +2%, 95% CI –3% to +8%).[7] The subsequent RCT (488 people with completely resected stage 2 or 3A non-small cell lung cancer) compared postoperative radiotherapy with or without cisplatin plus etoposide.[11] It found no significant difference with postoperative chemotherapy plus radiotherapy versus radiotherapy alone in median survival (37.9 months *v* 38.8 months; P = 0.56).

Harms: One RCT identified by the review comparing preoperative chemotherapy versus no chemotherapy found that chemotherapy was associated with grade III or IV neutropenia in 80% of people, nausea and vomiting, diarrhoea, hypomagnesaemia, and alopecia (no further data provided).[6] The systematic review of postoperative cisplatin based chemotherapy gave no information on adverse effects.[10] One RCT (269 people) identified by the review, which compared four postoperative courses of cyclophosphamide plus adriamycin plus cisplatin versus no postoperative chemotherapy, found that only 53% of people allocated to postoperative chemotherapy completed all four courses.[12] Mild to severe gastrointestinal toxicity was reported in 88% of people taking postoperative chemotherapy. A second RCT identified by the review reported similar toxicity.[13] Many adjuvant chemotherapy studies were published before serotonin receptor antagonist antiemetics were available.

Comment: The systematic review[6] examining effects of pre-operative chemotherapy identified one interim report[14] of an RCT in 27 people, which was unsuitable for inclusion in the meta-analysis. The RCT found that pre-operative chemotherapy versus no pre-operative chemotherapy significantly improved median survival after about 30 months follow up (median survival 28.7 months with pre-operative chemotherapy *v* 15.6 months without, P = 0.095).[14] Larger trials of preoperative chemotherapy in people with stage 3A non-small cell lung cancer are needed. Most of the chemotherapy regimens in the postoperative studies are no longer used, and trials examining newer agents are needed.

OPTION ADDING CHEMOTHERAPY TO THORACIC RADIATION FOR UNRESECTABLE STAGE 3 NON-SMALL CELL LUNG CANCER

Systematic reviews and one subsequent RCT in people with unresectable stage 3 non-small cell lung cancer have found that adding chemotherapy to irradiation versus irradiation alone significantly improves survival at 2–5 years. Another subsequent RCT has found no significant difference in median survival with radical radiotherapy plus chemotherapy versus radiotherapy alone. Observational evidence suggests that in people aged

over 70 years with unresectable stage 3 non-small cell lung cancer, chemotherapy plus radiotherapy versus radiotherapy alone may significantly reduce quality adjusted survival. We found insufficient evidence about effects on quality of life.

Benefits: We found three systematic reviews[10,15,16] and two subsequent RCTs.[17,18] The first review (search date 1991, 22 RCTs, 3033 people with unresected stage 3 non-small cell lung cancer) found that chemotherapy plus thoracic irradiation versus radiotherapy alone significantly reduced mortality (HR 0.90, 95% CI 0.83 to 0.97) with an absolute survival benefit of 3% with combined treatment versus radiotherapy alone at 2 years.[10] The second review (search date 1995, 14 RCTs, 1887 people) found that a cisplatin based regimen plus radiotherapy versus radiotherapy alone significantly reduced mortality at 2 years (OR 0.7, 95% CI 0.5 to 0.9).[15] The third review (search date 1995, 14 RCTs, 2589 people) found that chemotherapy (primarily cisplatin based) plus radiotherapy versus radiotherapy alone significantly reduced mortality at 3 years (RR 0.83, 95% CI 0.77 to 0.90).[16] The first subsequent RCT (458 people) compared 2 months of cisplatin plus vinblastine followed by standard radiotherapy versus either standard or hyperfractionated radiotherapy alone. It found that combined treatment versus radiotherapy significantly improved 5 year survival (AR 8% with combined treatment *v* 5% with standard radiotherapy *v* 6% with hyperfractionated radiotherapy; P = 0.04 for combined *v* either comparison).[17] The second subsequent RCT (446 people) compared radical radiotherapy plus four cycles of mitomycin, ifosfamide, and cisplatin versus radical radiotherapy alone.[18] It found no significant difference in median survival (11.7 months with combined treatment *v* 9.7 months with radiotherapy alone; P = 0.14). We found insufficient evidence about the effects of combining thoracic irradiation with chemotherapy on quality of life.

Harms: The reviews and RCTs gave no information on long term adverse effects of treatment.[10,15–18]

Comment: Radioprotector drugs and three-dimensional conformal radiotherapy are being investigated to reduce the toxicities of combined modality treatment.[19] One meta-analysis (6 prospective phase II or phase III studies) found that in people aged over 70 years with unresectable stage 3 non-small cell lung cancer, chemotherapy plus radiotherapy versus radiotherapy alone significantly reduced quality adjusted survival (10.8 months with chemotherapy plus radiotherapy *v* 13.1 months with standard radiotherapy; P < 0.01).[20]

OPTION HYPERFRACTIONATED RADIATION TREATMENT FOR UNRESECTABLE STAGE 3 NON-SMALL CELL LUNG CANCER

One systematic review in people with stage 3 non-small cell lung cancer has found no significant difference with standard hyperfractionation versus conventional radiotherapy in 2 year survival. One RCT in people with stage 1–3B non-small cell lung cancer found that continuous, hyperfractionated, accelerated radiotherapy versus conventional radiotherapy significantly increased 2 year survival.

Benefits: **Hyperfractionation:** We found one systematic review (search date 1999, 3 RCTs, 442 people with unresectable stage 3 non-small cell lung cancer) comparing standard hyperfractionation (not continuous, hyperfractionated, accelerated radiotherapy [CHART] — see glossary, p 1571) versus conventional radiotherapy.[21] It found no significant difference in 2 year survival (OR 0.67, 95% CI 0.42 to 1.07; P = 0.09).[21] **CHART:** We found no systematic review or RCTs exclusively in people with stage 3 non-small cell lung cancer. One RCT (563 people with non-small cell lung cancer; 61% with stage 3A or 3B; 39% with stage 1 or stage 2) compared CHART versus conventional radiotherapy.[19] It found that CHART versus conventional radiotherapy significantly reduced the risk of death at 2 years (AR 71% with CHART *v* 80% with conventional radiotherapy, HR 0.78, 95% CI 0.65 to 0.94; P = 0.008) and significantly improved local tumour control at 2 years (HR 0.79, 95% CI 0.63 to 0.98; P = 0.03).

Harms: Additional evidence on adverse effects was published subsequent to the RCT on CHART.[22] Significantly more people receiving CHART versus conventional radiotherapy experienced pain on swallowing, heartburn (both of which were of brief duration), cough (P = 0.01), shortness of breath (P = 0.03), and dizziness (P = 0.03). There was no significant difference in long term morbidity.[19,22]

Comment: RCTs comparing CHART versus conventional radiotherapy versus chemotherapy plus radiotherapy in people with stage 3 non-small cell lung cancer are under way.[21]

OPTION CHEMOTHERAPY IN STAGE 4 NON-SMALL CELL LUNG CANCER

Systematic reviews in people with stage 4 non-small cell lung cancer have found that chemotherapy regimens containing cisplatin plus supportive care versus supportive care alone significantly increase survival at 1 year. Limited evidence from RCTs suggests that chemotherapy plus best supportive care versus best supportive care alone may improve quality of life. One systematic review and five subsequent RCTs in people with advanced non-small cell lung cancer have found conflicting evidence on the effects of single versus combined chemotherapy. One RCT in people with stage 3 or 4 non-small cell lung cancer found no significant difference with first line platinum based versus non-platinum based chemotherapy in survival at 1 year. We found insufficient evidence to assess the effects of second line chemotherapy, although one systematic review found limited evidence that single agent docetaxel versus best supportive care or other chemotherapy may improve survival at 1 year in people who are resistant to platinum chemotherapy.

Benefits: **First line chemotherapy versus supportive care:** We found three systematic reviews.[9,10,23] The most recent systematic review (search date 1998, 4 earlier systematic reviews)[9] did not fully describe the four earlier systematic reviews it identified, three of which included the same RCTs. The review did not perform a meta-analysis. The first review that performed a meta-analysis (search date 1991, 11 RCTs, 1190 people with advanced non-small cell lung cancer) compared supportive care plus chemotherapy versus supportive care alone.[10] It found that, in trials from the 1970s, long term alkylating agents plus supportive care versus supportive care alone did not significantly improve survival (HR 1.26, 95% CI 0.96 to 1.66; P = 0.095). However, cisplatin containing regimens plus supportive care versus supportive care alone significantly increased survival at 1 year (HR 0.73; P < 0.0001) and increased median survival (5.5 months with cisplatin containing regimens plus supportive care *v* 4 months with supportive care alone). It is not possible to deduce from these studies to what extent the observed effects are due to the cisplatin or to all the other drugs in the combinations studied. The second review[23] that performed a meta-analysis (search date not stated, 8 RCTs, 7 of which were included in the first review,[10] 712 people with advanced non-small cell lung cancer) comparing chemotherapy plus best supportive care versus best supportive care alone found that chemotherapy significantly reduced mortality at 6 months (OR 0.44, 95% CI 0.32 to 0.59).[23] The third review[9] identified four RCTs that compared single agent chemotherapy plus best supportive care versus best supportive care alone, and assessed effects on quality of life.[24–27] Chemotherapeutic agents used were vinorelbine (191 people aged > 70),[24] gemcitabine (300 people),[25] docetaxel (207 people),[26] and paclitaxel (157 people).[27] Overall, the trials consistently found that chemotherapy plus best supportive care improved quality of life compared with best supportive care alone.

First line single agent versus combined chemotherapy: We found one systematic review (search date 1995–1996, 25 RCTs, 5156 people with stage 4 non-small cell lung cancer)[28] and five subsequent RCTs.[29–33] The review found no significant difference with platinum analogue or vinorelbine containing combination chemotherapy versus platinum analogue or vinorelbine alone in 1 year survival (RR 1.10, 95% CI 0.94 to 1.43).[28] The first subsequent RCT (120 people with advanced non-small cell lung cancer aged > 70 years) found that gemcitabine plus vinorelbine versus vinorelbine alone significantly improved survival at median 14 months (median survival 29 wks with combined treatment *v* 18 wks with single treatment; P < 0.01).[29] The second subsequent RCT (522 chemotherapy naive people with stage 3 or 4 non-small cell lung cancer) found that gemcitabine plus cisplatin versus cisplatin alone significantly improved survival (median survival 9.1 months with combination treatment *v* 7.6 months; P = 0.004).[30] The third subsequent RCT (415 people) found that cisplatin plus vinorelbine versus cisplatin alone significantly improved survival (median survival 8 months with combination *v* 6 months; P = 0.002).[31] The fourth subsequent RCT (147 people with stage 3 or 4 non-small cell lung cancer) found no difference in median survival with cisplatin plus etoposide versus gemcitabine (6.6 months with gemcitabine *v* 7.6 months with cisplatin plus etoposide).[32] The fifth RCT (169 people) compared single agent gemcitabine versus cisplatin plus vindesine.[33] It found that clinical benefit (based on visual analogue symptom scores, Karnofsky performance status and weight) was significantly greater with gemcitabine versus cisplatin plus vindesine (AR for clinical benefit 48.1% with gemcitabine *v* 28.9% with cisplatin plus vindesine, P = 0.003).[33] **First line platinum based versus non-platinum based chemotherapy:** One RCT (441 people with stage 3 or 4 non-small cell lung cancer) comparing docetaxel plus cisplatin versus docetaxel plus gemcitabine found no significant difference in 1 year survival (86/205 [42%] with docetaxel plus cisplatin *v* 78/201 [39%] with docetaxel plus gemcitabine; RR 1.08, 95% CI 0.84 to 1.33).[34] **Any second line chemotherapy:** We found one systematic review (search date not stated, 34 single agent studies and 24 combination regimen studies).[35] The review found that results from RCTs were conflicting and was unable to draw conclusions because of the heterogeneity of participant selection in the RCTs, and the different definitions of people considered sensitive or refractory to treatment. **Second line single agent docetaxel:** We found one systematic review (search date 2000, 2 RCTs, 477 people resistant to platinum based combination chemotherapy).[36] Results of the trials were not combined because of trial heterogeneity. The first RCT identified by the review found that docetaxel 75 mg/m^2 versus best supportive care significantly improved survival at 1 year (37% with docetaxel *v* 11% with supportive care; P = 0.003).[37] The second RCT identified by the review found that docetaxel versus vinorelbine or ifosfamide significantly improved survival at 1 year (32% with docetaxel *v* 19% with vinorelbine or ifosfamide; P = 0.025).[38]

Harms: Some studies have reported improvement in lung cancer symptoms with chemotherapy, but over 50% of people with advanced lung cancer patients treated with chemotherapy reported alopecia, and gastrointestinal and haematological toxicity.[39] One non-systematic review found greater toxicity in people with Eastern Cooperative Oncology Group (ECOG) scale performance status 3 or 4 (see glossary, p 1571).[40] The RCT comparing docetaxel plus cisplatin versus docetaxel plus gemcitabine found that docetaxel plus cisplatin significantly increased neutropenia (P = 0.01), nausea and vomiting (P = 0.001), and diarrhoea (P = 0.001).[34] Subgroup analysis (64 people with ECOG scale performance status 2) from an RCT comparing four cisplatin based chemotherapy regimens found high rates of haematologic and gastrointestinal toxicity and low response rates after 1 year; as a result the enrollment of people with ECOG performance status 2 was discontinued (proportion of people who had any grade 3–4 toxicity: 30–60% of people taking paclitaxel plus cisplatin; 8–67% of people taking gemcitabine plus cisplatin; 12–59% of people taking docetaxel plus cisplatin; 27–33% of people taking paclitaxel plus carboplatin; response rate with any type of chemotherapy 14%, 95 CI 5.6% to 22.6%; median survival 4.1 months, 95% CI 0.2 to 31.0 months).[41]

Comment: For people with stage 4 non-small cell lung cancer, treatment options consist of either chemotherapy or symptomatic care, including palliative radiation. People with ECOG scale performance status 3 or 4 have usually been excluded from RCTs of lung cancer chemotherapy. One non-systematic review has found that carboplatin has comparable response rate to, but a better toxicity profile than, cisplatin in people with stage 4 non-small cell lung cancer.[42] Newer agents such as vinorelbine, gemcitabine, irinotecan, paclitaxel, and docetaxel produce objective responses in more than 20%

of people with advanced lung cancer.[42] One RCT (408 people) comparing carboplatin plus paclitaxel versus vinorelbine plus cisplatin found no significant difference in survival at 1 year (36% *v* 38%; reported as non-significant), but found that vinorelbine plus cisplatin significantly increased withdrawal owing to toxicity (28% with vinorelbine plus cisplatin *v* 15% with carboplatin plus paclitaxel; P = 0.001).[43] Measuring quality of life in people with lung cancer remains a serious challenge. The systematic review comparing second line chemotherapy versus supportive care recommended that RCTs of second line chemotherapy report and analyse details of patient characteristics, response to first line treatment, and interval between last chemotherapy and recurrence.[35]

QUESTION What are the effects of treatments for small cell lung cancer?

OPTION DOSE INTENSIVE CHEMOTHERAPY VERSUS STANDARD CHEMOTHERAPY

Two RCTs found that dose intensification versus standard chemotherapy significantly increased deaths related to toxicity, and did not improve progression free survival. One RCT in people with limited disease found that early dose intensification of chemotherapy alternating with radiotherapy versus no early intensification of chemotherapy significantly increased survival at 2 years. One RCT found that cisplatin plus irinotecan versus cisplatin plus etoposide may improve survival over 2 years. Two RCTs found conflicting evidence about the effects of dose intensification plus growth factor support.

Benefits: We found no systematic review but found six RCTs.[44–49] The first RCT (229 people with extensive stage small cell lung cancer) comparing dose intensive (cisplatin plus vincristine plus doxorubicin plus etoposide) versus standard chemotherapy (alternating cyclophosphamide, doxorubicin, vincristine plus cisplatin) found no significant difference in progression free survival (median 0.66 years in each group) or overall survival (0.98 *v* 0.91 years).[44] The second RCT (59 people with limited stage and 74 people with extensive stage small cell lung cancer) found no significant difference with paclitaxel plus cisplatin plus etoposide versus cisplatin plus etoposide in survival at 1 year (AR 38.2% *v* 37%; P = 0.09).[45] The third RCT (105 people with limited stage disease receiving alternating cycles of radiotherapy) compared one cycle of high versus low dose cisplatin plus cyclophosphamide (along with standard dose doxorubicin and etoposide).[46] It found that high versus standard dose chemotherapy significantly improved overall survival and disease free survival at 2 years (overall survival 43% with high dose chemotherapy *v* 26% with low dose chemotherapy, CI not stated, P = 0.02; disease free survival 28% *v* 8%, P = 0.02). The fourth RCT (154 people with extensive stage small cell lung cancer) compared cisplatin plus irinotecan versus cisplatin plus etoposide.[47] It found that cisplatin plus irinotecan versus cisplatin plus etoposide improved survival over 2 years (2 year survival; 19.5%, 95% CI 10.6 to 28.3%, with cisplatin plus irinotecan *v* 5.2%, 95%

CI 0.2 to 10.2% with cisplatin plus etoposide; significance not stated).[47] The fifth RCT (403 people) compared low intensity (3 weekly) cycles of doxorubicin, cyclophosphamide and etoposide versus higher intensity (2 weekly) cycles of the same chemotherapy supported with granulocyte colony stimulating factor.[48] It found that high intensity treatment improved overall survival compared with lower dose treatment at 2 years (HR 0.8, 95% CI 0.65 to 0.99, P = 0.04; overall survival at 2 years 13% with high intensity *v* 8% with low intensity treatment). The sixth RCT (233 people with extensive disease) found no significant difference in survival over 2 years with three different schedules of epirubicin, vindesine and ifosfamide (six 3 weekly cycles; six accelerated 2 weekly cycles with granulocyte macrophage colony stimulating factor [GM–CSF] support, and six accelerated 2 weekly cycles with oral co-trimoxazole) (2 year survival 5%–6%, P = 0.86).[49]

Harms: Except in people with widespread extensive stage small cell lung cancer, adverse effects of chemotherapy were of short duration. However, the first RCT found that dose intense chemotherapy versus standard chemotherapy significantly increased deaths related to toxicity (9/110 [8%] with dose intense treatment *v* 1/109 [1%] with standard chemotherapy; RR 8.9, 95% CI 1.1 to 69; NNH 14, 95% CI 7 to 60).[44] The second RCT also found that paclitaxel plus cisplatin plus etoposide versus cisplatin plus etoposide significantly increased deaths related to toxicity (8/62 [13%] *v* 0/71 [0%]; P = 0.001).[45] The third RCT found no deaths related to toxicity with one cycle of high versus low chemotherapy.[46] The fourth RCT found no difference in deaths related to toxicity with cisplatin plus irinotecan versus cisplatin plus etoposide (3/77 [4%] *v* 1/77 [1%]; RR 1.30, 95% CI 0.14 to 12.35).[47] The fifth RCT found no significant difference in deaths related to toxicity with higher intensity versus lower intensity chemotherapy with doxorubicin, cyclophosphamide and etoposide (6/197 [3%] *v* 9/197 [5%]; RR 0.67, 95% CI 0.24 to 1.83).[48]

Comment: None.

OPTION ADDING THORACIC IRRADIATION TO CHEMOTHERAPY IN LIMITED STAGE SMALL CELL LUNG CANCER

Two systematic reviews in people with limited stage small cell lung cancer have found that adding thoracic irradiation to chemotherapy versus chemotherapy alone significantly improves survival at 3 years. However, one of these reviews has found that thoracic radiation plus chemotherapy versus chemotherapy alone significantly increases death related to treatment. One systematic review and five additional RCTs have found insufficient evidence on the best timing, dose, and fractionation of radiation.

Benefits: We found two systematic reviews.[50,51] The first review (search date not stated, 13 RCTs, 2573 people with limited stage small cell lung cancer, range 52–426 people) found that radiation plus chemotherapy versus chemotherapy alone significantly increased 3 year survival (AR 15% *v* 10%; P = 0.001).[50] The second review (search date not stated, 11 RCTs, 10 of which were included in the first review, 1911 people with limited stage small cell lung cancer) pooled data from nine of the RCTs (1521 people) and found that thoracic radiation plus chemotherapy versus chemotherapy alone significantly improved local control (50% *v* 25%; ARR 25%, 95% CI 17% to 34%).[51] **Timing of radiation:** We found one systematic review (search date 2000, 4 RCTs, 927 people)[52] and two additional RCTs that compared early versus late addition of thoracic radiotherapy to chemotherapy.[53,54] The review found no significant difference with early versus late addition of radiotherapy in 5 year survival (AR 66/455 [14.5 %] *v* 63/472 [13.2 %]; RR 1.09, 95% CI 0.78 to 1.48).[52] One additional RCT, included in the review but not in the meta-analysis, found that early versus late addition of radiotherapy significantly increased 5 year survival (30% *v* 15%; P = 0.03).[53] The second additional RCT (81 people with limited stage small cell lung cancer) compared early radiotherapy (given with the first cycle of chemotherapy) versus late radiotherapy (given with the fourth cycle of chemotherapy).[54] It found no significant difference with early versus late chemotherapy in median survival after median follow up of 35 months (17.5 months with early radiotherapy v 17 months with late radiotherapy). **Dose:** One RCT (333 people) found no significant difference with standard dose radiotherapy (25 Gy over 2 wks) versus high dose radiotherapy (37.5 Gy over 3 wks) in overall survival over 3 years (P = 0.18; results presented graphically).[55] **Fractionation:** We found two RCTs.[56,57] One RCT found that hyperfractionation (twice daily treatment) versus conventional fractionation (once daily treatment) significantly improved 5 year survival (26% with hyperfractionation *v* 16% with conventional fractionation; P = 0.04).[56] Another RCT comparing once daily irradiation versus twice daily irradiation found no significant difference in 3 year survival (34% with 50.4 Gy in 28 fractions daily *v* 29% with 48 Gy in 32 fractions twice daily; P = 0.46).[57]

Harms: The second systematic review found that thoracic radiation plus chemotherapy versus chemotherapy alone significantly increased death related to treatment (29/884 [3.3%] *v* 12/841 [1.4%]; OR 2.54, 95% CI 1.90 to 3.18).[51] One RCT found that hyperfractionation versus conventional fractionation increased the incidence of oesophagitis.[56]

Comment: Interest in adding thoracic irradiation to chemotherapy derives from the observation that local recurrence in the chest is a major cause of first treatment failure and carries an extremely poor prognosis. A non-systematic review found that median survival in limited stage disease has improved over the past 10 years from 14–16 months to 20–24 months.[58] The reasons for this improvement have not been established but may include the early use of radiation plus chemotherapy rather than improvements in either modality alone.[59] The RCTs of early versus late addition of radiotherapy used different methods and do not provide strong evidence.[52,53] The different results may be explained by different rates of early toxicity from treatment and different rates of relapse in the central nervous system.

OPTION PROPHYLACTIC CRANIAL IRRADIATION IN LIMITED STAGE SMALL CELL LUNG CANCER

One systematic review in people with small cell lung cancer in complete remission has found that prophylactic cranial irradiation versus no irradiation improves survival and reduces the risk of developing brain metastases. Long term cognitive dysfunction following cranial irradiation has been described, but longer follow up studies are needed to assess its significance and importance.

Benefits: We found one systematic review (search date 2000, 7 RCTs, 987 people with small cell lung cancer in complete remission) comparing cranial radiation versus no cranial radiation.[60] Of the people in the RCTs, 12% in the irradiation group and 17% in the no irradiation group had extensive stage small cell lung cancer at presentation. It found that cranial irradiation versus no cranial irradiation significantly improved survival (RR of death at 3 years 0.84, 95% CI 0.73 to 0.97, corresponding to a 5.4% increase in survival) and increased disease free survival (RR of recurrence or death at 3 years 0.75, 95% CI 0.65 to 0.86). Subgroup analysis identified survival benefit only for men and not for women, but the difference in survival was not significant ($P = 0.07$). The review found that cranial irradiation versus no cranial irradiation significantly reduced the cumulative incidence of brain metastases (RR 0.46, 95% CI 0.38 to 0.57). Larger doses of radiation significantly reduced brain metastases ($P = 0.02$), but did not significantly improve survival ($P = 0.89$).

Harms: The review could not assess whether prophylactic cranial irradiation leads to neuropsychological sequelae because adequate assessments were carried out in only two of the seven RCTs.[60] These RCTs and other non-randomised studies found that 24–60% of participants may have neuropsychological problems before treatment, and other studies have not accounted for potential confounding factors such as age, tobacco use, paraneoplastic syndromes, and neurotoxic chemotherapy effects.

Comment: The clinical significance of cognitive impairment after prophylactic cranial irradiation remains unclear.

OPTION ORAL ETOPOSIDE IN EXTENSIVE STAGE SMALL CELL LUNG CANCER

Two RCTs in people with extensive stage small cell lung cancer found that oral etoposide improves survival significantly less than combination chemotherapy at 1 year. One RCT found that etoposide reduced nausea and vomiting in the short term, but found no evidence that it offers significantly better quality of life overall.

Benefits: **Versus combination chemotherapy:** We found no systematic review but found two RCTs.[61,62] The first RCT (155 people with extensive stage small cell lung cancer) compared oral etoposide 100 mg daily for 5 days versus combination chemotherapy.[61] It found that etoposide improved survival significantly less than combined chemotherapy at 1 year (9.8% with etoposide *v* 19.3 % with combined chemotherapy; $P < 0.05$). It found no significant difference with etoposide versus combination chemotherapy in median survival (4.8 months *v* 5.9 months) and found conflicting results on quality of life. Acute nausea was significantly worse with combination chemotherapy ($P < 0.01$), but pain, appetite, general well-being, and mood were worse with oral etoposide ($P < 0.001$). Palliation of lung cancer symptoms was of shorter duration with etoposide ($P < 0.01$).[61] The second RCT (339 people with extensive stage small cell lung cancer) comparing oral etoposide versus combination chemotherapy found that etoposide significantly reduced survival at mean 21 months (HR 1.35, 95% CI 1.03 to 1.70; $P = 0.03$; absolute numbers not provided).[62]

Harms: The first RCT found that treatment related symptoms were significantly worse with combination chemotherapy versus etoposide ($P < 0.01$).[61] The second RCT found that etoposide versus combination chemotherapy reduced alopecia and numbness but increased haematological adverse effects, particularly anaemia.[62]

Comment: Because treatment of extensive stage disease is palliative, and because age has been identified as a prognostic factor in small cell lung cancer, studies have looked at outcomes in elderly people with limited and extensive stage disease and in people of all ages with a poor prognosis. Although small cell lung cancer is relatively sensitive to chemotherapy, extensive stage disease remains incurable. Median survival with treatment is 10–12 months, and as yet has been unaffected by high dose combination chemotherapy. Because of its lower acute toxicity, etoposide may be considered for elderly people with extensive stage disease or people with a poor prognosis.

GLOSSARY

Continuous, hyperfractionated, accelerated radiotherapy Radiotherapy given at a rate of two or more radiation fractions a day (each of smaller dose than conventionally fractionated doses). The number of fractions a week is gradually increased to shorten overall duration of treatment.

Performance status Expression used to describe functional status or wellness of participants in studies of cancer. There are two widely accepted scales: the Eastern Cooperative Oncology Group scale (0 = no symptoms; 1 = symptomatic but no extra time in bed; 2 = in bed less than 50% of the day, no work, can care for self; 3 = in bed more than 50% of day, not bedridden, minimal self care; 4 = completely bedridden), and the Karnofsky Scale of symptoms and disability (from 100% = no symptoms to 0% = dead).

Substantive changes

Preoperative chemotherapy for non-small cell lung cancer One new RCT;[8] conclusions unchanged.

Chemotherapy in stage 4 non-small cell lung cancer One new RCT;[33] conclusions unchanged.

Chemotherapy in stage 4 non-small cell lung cancer One new systematic review found limited evidence that single agent docetaxel may improve survival compared with best supportive care or other chemotherapy in people who are resistant to platinum chemotherapy.[36]

Dose intensive chemotherapy versus standard chemotherapy for small cell lung cancer Four new RCTs;[46–49] conclusions unchanged.

Adding thoracic irradiation to chemotherapy in limited stage small cell lung cancer One new RCT;[54] conclusions unchanged.

REFERENCES

1. Travis WD, Travis LB, Devesa SS. Lung cancer. *Cancer* 1995;75(suppl 1):191–202.
2. American Thoracic Society/European Respiratory Society Pre-treatment evaluation of non-small cell lung cancer *Am J Respir Crit Care* 1997;156:320–332.
3. Ihde DC, Pass HI, Glatstein E. Lung cancer. In: DeVita VT Jr, Hellman S, Rosenberg SA, eds. *Cancer, principles and practice of oncology*, 5th ed. Philadelphia: Lippincott-Raven, 1997;849–959.
4. Montazeri A, Gillis CR, McEwen J. Quality of life in people with lung cancer: a review of literature from 1970 to 1995. *Chest* 1998;113:467–481.
5. Grilli R, Oxman AD, Julian JA. Chemotherapy for advanced non-small-cell lung cancer: how much benefit is enough? *J Clin Oncol* 1993;11:1866–1872. Search date 1991; primary source Medline.
6. Goss G, Paszat L, Newman T, et al. Use of preoperative chemotherapy with or without postoperative radiotherapy in technically resectable stage IIIA non-small cell lung cancer. *Cancer Prev Control* 1998;2:32–39. Search date 1997; primary sources Medline, hand searches of reference lists, and contact with experts.
7. Ramnath N, Hernandez FJ, Bepler G. Neoadjuvant chemotherapy for non-small-call lung cancer: Will the answer be in targeted chemotherapy. *Oncol Spect* 2002:1;27–34.
8. Depierre A, Milleron B, Moro-Sibilot D, et al. Pre-operative chemotherapy followed by surgery compared with primary surgery in resectable Stage I (except T1N0), II and IIIA non-small cell lung cancer. *J Clin Oncol* 2002;20:247–253.
9. Sorenson S, Glimelius B, Nygren P, et al. A systematic overview of chemotherapy effects in non-small cell lung cancer. *Acta Oncol* 2001;40:327–339. Search date 1998; primary sources Medline, Cancerlit, PDQ database, and handsearching of reference lists and the grey literature.
10. Non-Small Cell Lung Cancer Collaborative Group. Chemotherapy for non-small cell lung cancer. In: The Cochrane Library, Issue 1, 2002. Oxford: Update Software. Search date 1991; primary sources Medline, Cancerlit, hand search of meetings abstracts, bibliographies of books and specialist journals, consultation of trials registers of National Cancer Institute, UK Coordinating Committee for Cancer Research, the Union Internationale Contre le Cancer, and discussion with trialists.
11. Keller SM, Adak S, Wagner H, et al. A randomized trial of postoperative adjuvant therapy in patients with completely resected stage II or IIIA non-small-cell lung cancer. *N Engl J Med* 2000:343:1217–1222.
12. Feld R, Rubinstein L, Thomas PA, et al. Adjuvant chemotherapy with cyclophosphamide, doxorubicin, and cisplatin in patients with completely resected stage I non-small-cell lung cancer. *J Natl Cancer Inst* 1993;85:299–306.
13. Niiranen A, Niitamo-Korhonen S, Kouri M, et al. Adjuvant chemotherapy after radical surgery for non-small cell lung cancer: a randomized study. *J Clin Oncol* 1992;10:1927–1932.
14. Pass HI, Pogrebniak HW, Steinberg SM, et al. Randomized trial of neoadjuvant therapy for lung cancer: Interim analysis. *Ann Thoracic Surg* 1992;53:992–998.
15. Marino P, Preatoni A. Randomized trials of radiotherapy alone versus combined chemotherapy and radiotherapy in stages IIIa and IIIb non small cell lung cancer. *Cancer* 1995;76:593–601. Search date 1995; primary sources Medline and manual search of references of review articles and abstracts.
16. Pritchard RS, Anthony SP. Chemotherapy plus radiotherapy compared with radiotherapy alone in the treatment of locally advance, unresectable, non-small-cell lung cancer. *Ann Intern Med* 1996;125:723–729. Search date 1995; primary sources Medline and hand search of references of review articles and abstracts.
17. Sause W, Kolesar P, Taylor S, et al. Final results of phase III trial in regionally advanced unresectable non-small cell lung cancer: Radiation Therapy Oncology Group, Eastern Cooperative Oncology Group, and Southwest Oncology Group. *Chest* 2000;117:358–364.
18. Cullen MH, Billingham CM, Woodroffe AD, et al. Mitomycin, ifosfamide, and cisplatin in unresectable non-small cell lung cancer: effects on survival and quality of life. *J Clin Oncol* 1999;17:3188–3194.
19. Saunders M, Dische S, Barrett A, et al. Continuous, hyperfractionated, accelerated radiotherapy (CHART) versus conventional radiotherapy in non-small cell lung cancer: mature data from the randomised multicentre trial. *Radiother Oncol* 1999;52:137–148.
20. Mousas B, Scott C, Sause W, et al. The benefit of treatment intensification is age and histology-dependent in patients with locally advanced non-small cell lung cancer (NSCLC): a quality-adjusted survival analysis of Radiation Therapy Oncology Group (RTOG) chemoradiation studies. *Int J Radiat Oncol Biol Phys* 1999;45:1143–1149.
21. Yu E, Lochrin C, Dixon P, et al. Altered fractionation of radical radiation therapy in the management of unresectable non-small-cell lung cancer. *Curr Oncol* 2000;7:98–109. Search date 1999; primary sources Medline, Cancerlit, PDQ database, and The Cochrane Library.
22. Bailey AJ, Parmar MKB, Stephens RJ. Patient-reported short-term and long-term physical and psychological symptoms: results of the continuous hyperfractionated accelerated radiotherapy (CHART) randomized trial in non-small cell lung cancer. *J Clin Oncol* 1998;16:3082–3093.
23. Marino P, Pampallona S, Preatoni A, et al. Chemotherapy versus supportive care in advanced non-small cell lung cancer: results of a meta-analysis of the literature. *Chest* 1994;106:861–865. Search date not stated; primary sources Medline and hand search of references from review articles and abstracts.
24. Elderly Lung Cancer Vinorelbine Study Group. Effects of vinorelbine on quality of life and survival of elderly patients with non-small cell lung cancer. *J Natl Cancer Inst* 1999;91:66–72.
25. Anderson H, Hopwood P, Stephens RJ, et al. Gemcitabine plus best supportive care (BSC) versus BSC in inoperable non-small cell lung cancer in a randomised trail with quality of life as the primary outcome. *Br J Cancer* 2000;83:447–453.
26. Roszkowski K, Pluzanska A, Krzakowski M, et al. A multicenter, randomised phase III study of docetaxel plus best supportive care versus best supportive care in chemo-naive patients with metastatic or non-resectable localised non-small cell lung cancer (NSCLC). *Lung Cancer* 2000;27:145–157.
27. Ranson M, Davidson N, Nicolson M, et al. Randomised trial of paclitaxel plus supportive care

versus supportive care for patients with advanced non-small cell lung cancer. *J Natl Cancer Inst* 2000;92:1074–1080.

28. Lilenbaum RC, Langenberg P, Dickersin K. Single agent versus combination chemotherapy in patients with advanced non-small cell lung cancer: a meta-analysis of response, toxicity and survival. *Cancer* 1998;82:116–126. Search dates 1995–1996; primary sources Medline, Embase, handsearching of references, Physician Data Query from the National Cancer Institute, and expert consultation.
29. Frasci G, Lorusso V, Panza N, et al. Gemcitabine plus vinorelbine versus vinorelbine alone in elderly patients with advanced non-small cell lung cancer. *J Clin Oncol* 2000;18:2529–2536.
30. Sandler AB, Nemunaitis J, Denham C, et al. Phase III trial of gemcitabine plus cisplatin versus cisplatin alone in patients with locally advanced or metastatic non-small cell lung cancer. *J Clin Oncol* 2000;18:122–130.
31. Wozniak AG, Crowley JJ, Balcerzak SP, et al. Randomised trial comparing cisplatin with cisplatin plus vinorelbine in the treatment of advanced non-small cell lung cancer: a Southwest Oncology Group study. *J Clin Oncol* 1998;16:2459–2465.
32. Bokkel-Huinink WW, Bergman B, Chemaissani A, et al. Single-agent gemcitabine: an active and better tolerated alternative to standard cisplatin-based chemotherapy in locally advanced or metastatic non-small cell lung cancer. *Lung Cancer* 1999;26:85–94.
33. Vansteenkiste JF, Vanderbroek JE, Nackaerts KL, et al. Clinical-benefit response in advanced non-small cell lung cancer: A multicentre prospective randomized phase III study of single agent gemcitabine versus cisplatin-vindesine. *Ann Oncol* 2001;12:1221–1230.
34. Georgoulias V, Papadakis E, Alexopoulos A, et al. Platinum-based and non-platinum-based chemotherapy in advanced non-small cell lung cancer: a randomised multicentre trial. *Lancet* 2001;357:1478–1484.
35. Huisman C, Smit EF, Postmus PE. Second-line chemotherapy in relapsing or refractory non-small cell lung cancer: a review. *J Clin Oncol* 2000;18:3722–3730. Search date not stated; primary sources Medline and hand searches of the past five conference abstracts of the American Society of Clinical Oncology, European Cancer Conference, and the European Society of Medical Oncology.
36. Logan D, Laurie S, Markman BR, et al. The role of single-agent docetaxel as second-line treatment for advanced non-small cell lung cancer. *Curr Oncol* 2001;8:50–58. Search date 2000; primary sources Medline, Cancerlit, Cochrane Library, and hand search of reference lists of relevant articles.
37. Shepherd FA, Dancey J, Ramlau, et al. Prospective randomized trial of docetaxel versus best supportive care in patients with non-small-cell lung cancer previously treated with platinum-based chemotherapy. *J Clin Oncol* 2000;18:2095–2103.
38 Fossella FV, DeVore R, Kerr RN. Randomized phase III trial of docetaxel versus vinorelbine or ifosphamide in patients with advanced non-small cell lung cancer previously treated with platinum-containing regimens. *J Clin Oncol* 2000;18:2354–2362.
39. Le Chevalier T, Brisgand D, Douillard J-Y, et al. Randomized study of vinorelbine and cisplatin versus vindesine and cisplatin versus vinorelbine alone in advanced non-small cell lung cancer: results of a European multicenter trial including 612 people. *J Clin Oncol* 1994;12:360–367.
40. Bunn PA Jr, Kelly K. New chemotherapeutic agents prolong survival and improve quality of life in non-small cell lung cancer: a review of literature and future directions. *Clin Cancer Res* 1998;4:1087–1100.
41. Sweeney CJ, Zhu J, Sandler AB, et al. Outcome of patients with a performance status of 2 in Eastern Cooperative Oncology Group Study E1594. A Phase III trial in patients with metastatic non-small cell lung carcinoma. *Cancer* 2001;982:2639–2647.
42. Bunn PA Jr. Review of therapeutic trials of carboplatin in lung cancer. *Semin Oncol* 1989;16(suppl 5):27–33.
43. Kelly K, Crowley J, Bunn PA, et al. Randomised phase III trial of paclitaxel plus carboplatin versus vinorelbine plus cisplatin in the treatment of patients with advanced non-small-cell lung cancer: a Southwest Oncology Group trial. *J Clin Oncol* 2001;19:3210–3218.
44. Murray N, Livingston RB, Shepherd FA, et al. Randomised study of CODE versus alternating CAV/EP for extensive-stage small-cell lung cancer: an intergroup study of the National Cancer Institute of Canada clinical trials group and the Southwest Oncology Group. *J Clin Oncol* 1999;17:2300–2308.
45. Mavroudis D, Papadakis E, Veslemes M, et al. A multicenter randomized clinical trial comparing paclitaxel-cisplatin-etoposide versus cisplatin-etoposide as first-line treatment in patients with small-cell lung cancer. *Ann Oncol* 2001;12.463–470.
46. Arriagada R, LeChevalier T, Pignon JP. Initial chemotherapeutic doses and survival in patients with limited small-cell lung cancer. *NEJM* 1993;329:1848–1852.
47. Noda K, Nishikaa Y, Kawahara M, et al. Irinotecan plus cisplatin compared with etoposide plus cisplatin for extensive small cell lung cancer. *NEJM* 2002;346:85–91.
48. Thatcher N, Girling DJ, Hopwood P, et al. Improving survival without reducing quality of life in small cell lung cancer patients by increasing the dose-intensity of chemotherapy with granulocyte colony-stimulating factor support: Results of a British Medical Research Council multicentre randomized trial. *J Clin Oncol* 2000;18:395–404.
49. Sculier JP, Paessmans M, Reconte J, et al. A three-arm Phase III randomized trial assessing in patients with extensive disease small cell lung cancer, accelerated chemotherapy with support of hematological growth factor or oral antibiotics. *Br J Cancer* 2001;85:1444–1451.
50. Pignon JP, Arriagada R, Ihde DC, et al. A meta-analysis of thoracic radiotherapy for small-cell lung cancer. *N Engl J Med* 1992;327:1618–1624. Search date not stated; primary sources Medline and hand search of proceedings of key oncology meetings.
51. Warde P, Payne D. Does thoracic irradiation improve survival and local control in limited-stage small cell carcinoma of the lung? A meta-analysis. *J Clin Oncol* 1992;10:890–895. Search date not stated; primary sources Medline and Cancerline.
52. Okawara G, Gagliardi A, Evans WK, et al. The role of thoracic radiotherapy as an adjunct to standard chemotherapy in limited-stage small-cell lung cancer. *Curr Oncol* 2000;7:162–172. Search date 2000; primary sources Medline, Cochrane Library, Physician Data Query File, Cancerlit, and hand searches of conference proceedings.
53. Jeremic B, Shibamoto Y, Acimovic L, et al. Initial versus delayed accelerated hyperfracationated radiation therapy and concurrent chemotherapy in limited small-cell lung cancer. A randomised study. *J Clin Oncol* 1997;15:893–900.

54. Skarlos DV, Samantas E, Briassoulis E, et al. Randomized comparison of early versus late hyperfractionated thoracic irradiation concurrently with chemotherapy in limited disease small-cell lung cancer: A randomized phase II study of the Hellenic Cooperative Oncology Group (HeCOG). *Ann Oncol* 2001;12:1231–1238.
55. Coy P, Hodson I, Payne DG, et al. The effect of dose of thoracic irradiation on recurrence in patients with limited stage small cell lung cancer. Initial results of a Canadian Multicentre Randomized Trial. *Int J Radiat Oncol Biol Phys* 1988;14:219–226.
56. Turrisi AT, Kim K, Blum R, et al. Twice-daily compared with once-daily thoracic radiotherapy in limited small-cell lung cancer treated concurrently with cisplatin and etoposide. *N Engl J Med* 1999;340:265–271.
57. Bonner JA, Sloan JA, Shanahan TG, et al. Phase III comparison of twice-daily split-course irradiation versus once-daily irradiation for patients with limited stage small-cell lung carcinoma. *J Clin Oncol* 1999;17:2681–2691.
58. Kumar P. The role of radiotherapy in the management of limited-stage small cell lung cancer: past, present, and future. *Chest* 1997;112(suppl):259–265.
59. Murray N, Coy P, Pater JL, et al. Importance of timing for thoracic irradiation in the combined modality treatment of limited-stage small-cell lung cancer. *J Clin Oncol* 1993;11:336–344.
60. Prophylactic Cranial Irradiation Overview Collaborative Group. Cranial irradiation for preventing brain metastasis of small cell lung cancer in patients in complete remission. In: The Cochrane Library, Issue 1, 2002. Oxford: Update Software. Search date 2000; primary sources Medline, Cancerlit, Excerpta Medica, Biosis, hand searches of meeting proceedings, the Physician Data Query clinical trial registry, and personal contact with investigators and experts.
61. Souhami RL, Spiro SG, Rudd RM, et al. Five day oral etoposide treatment for advanced small cell lung cancer: randomized comparison with intravenous chemotherapy. *J Natl Cancer Inst* 1997;89:577–580.
62. Medical Research Council Lung Cancer Working Party. Comparison of oral etoposide and standard intravenouis multidrug chemotherapy for small-cell lung cancer: a stopped multicentre randomised trial. *Lancet* 1996;348:563–566.

Alan Neville
Professor
McMaster University
Hamilton
Canada

Competing interests: None declared.

TABLE 1 **Staging lung cancer (see text, p 1560).**

Non-small cell lung cancer

Stage	Definition*	5 year survival (%)
1	T1–T2, N0, M0	55–75
2	T1–T2, N1, M0	25–50
3A	T3, N0–N1, M0 or T1–T3, N2, M0	20–40
3B	T4, any N, M0 or any T, N3, M0	≤5
4	Any M1	≤5

Small cell lung cancer

Stage	Definition	Median survival
Limited stage disease	Tumour confined to one side of the chest, supraclavicular lymph nodes, or both	18–24 months†
Extensive stage disease	Defined as anything beyond limited stage	10–12 months‡

*M, metastases; N, nodes; T, tumour. †With combined chemotherapy and mediastinal irradiation. ‡With palliative chemotherapy.

Spontaneous pneumothorax

Search date April 2002

John Cunnington

QUESTIONS

INTERVENTIONS

See glossary, p 1581

Key Messages

Treatment

- We found insufficient evidence to determine whether any intervention is more effective than no intervention for spontaneous pneumothorax.
- **Chest tube drainage** We found no sufficiently large RCTs comparing chest tube drainage versus observation. Two small RCTs found that resolution is faster with chest tube drainage than with needle aspiration, but found no difference in recurrence rate. One of the RCTs found that chest tube drainage versus needle aspiration significantly increased pain and increased the time spent in hospital by an average of 2 days.
- **Chest tube drainage plus suction** One small RCT found no significant difference in the rate of resolution whether chest tube drainage bottles were connected to suction or not, but the trial was too small to exclude a clinically important difference.
- **Needle aspiration** One small RCT found no good evidence of an improved rate of resolution with needle aspiration versus observation alone. Two small RCTs found that resolution is slower with needle aspiration than with chest tube drainage, but found no difference in recurrence rate. One of the RCTs found that people treated with needle aspiration versus chest tube drainage experienced significantly less pain and spent an average of two fewer days in hospital.
- **One way valves on chest tubes versus bottles with underwater seal** One small RCT found no significant difference in the rate of resolution with one way valves versus drainage bottles with an underwater seal, 48 hours after treatment, but the trial was too small to exclude a clinically important different but people treated with one way valves required less analgesia and spent less time in hospital.

Spontaneous pneumothorax

- **Small versus standard sized chest tubes** We found no RCTs comparing small versus standard sized chest tubes.

Preventing recurrence

- **Chemical pleurodesis** Two RCTs have found that chest tube drainage plus chemical pleurodesis versus chest tube drainage alone significantly reduces the rate of recurrence of spontaneous pneumothorax, but one of the RCTs found that treatment can be painful. The RCTs found no significant difference in length of hospital stay with pleurodesis versus chest tube drainage alone. One non-randomised prospective study found no significant difference in recurrence rate with chemical versus surgical pleurodesis. We found no RCTs or high quality cohort studies about the optimal timing of chemical pleurodesis.
- **Surgical pleurodesis** We found no RCTs comparing surgical pleurodesis versus chest tube drainage alone or versus chemical pleurodesis. One small RCT found that video-assisted thoracoscopic surgery versus thoracotomy significantly reduced hospital stay. It found no significant difference in the rate of recurrence, but the limited evidence cannot exclude a clinically important difference.
- **Optimal timing of pleurodesis (after first, second, or third spontaneous pneumothorax)** We found no RCTs or high quality cohort studies assessing whether pleurodesis should take place after the first, second, or subsequent episodes of spontaneous pneumothorax.

DEFINITION A pneumothorax is air in the pleural space. A spontaneous pneumothorax occurs when there is no provoking factor, such as trauma, surgery, or diagnostic intervention. It implies a leak of air from the lung parenchyma through the visceral pleura into the pleural space.

INCIDENCE/ PREVALENCE In a survey in Minnesota, USA, the incidence of spontaneous pneumothorax was 7/100 000 for men and 1/100 000 for women.[1] Smoking increases the likelihood of spontaneous pneumothorax by 22 times for men and eight times for women. A dose–response relationship has been observed.[2]

AETIOLOGY/ RISK FACTORS Spontaneous pneumothorax can be primary (typically in young fit people and thought to be because of a congenital abnormality of the pleura) or secondary (caused by underlying lung disease, typically occurring in older people with emphysema or pulmonary fibrosis).

PROGNOSIS Death from spontaneous pneumothorax is rare and in some cases a consequence of tension pneumothorax. Morbidity with pain and shortness of breath is common. Published recurrence rates vary; one cohort study in Denmark found that, after a first episode of primary spontaneous pneumothorax, 23% of people suffered a recurrence within 5 years, most within a year.[3] Recurrence rates had been thought to increase substantially after the first recurrence, but one case control study of military personnel found that 28% of men with a first spontaneous pneumothorax had a recurrence; 23% of the 28% had a second recurrence; and only 14% of that 23% had a third recurrence, giving a total recurrence rate of 35%.[4]

AIMS To reduce morbidity; to restore normal function as quickly as possible; to prevent recurrence and mortality, with minimum adverse effects.

OUTCOMES Proportion of people with successful resolution of spontaneous pneumothorax after a stated period; time to full expansion of the lung; duration of hospital stay; time off work; harmful effects of treatments (pain, surgical emphysema, wound and pleural space infection); and rate of recurrence.

METHODS *Clinical Evidence* update search and appraisal April 2002. Most of the literature comprised uncontrolled case series.

QUESTION **What are the effects of treatments?**

OPTION **NEEDLE ASPIRATION**

One small RCT found no evidence of an improved rate of resolution with needle aspiration versus observation alone. Two small RCTs found significantly faster resolution of pneumothorax with chest tube drainage versus needle aspiration, but found no significant difference in recurrence rate. One of the RCTs found that people treated with needle aspiration had less pain and spent less time in hospital than those treated with a chest tube.

Benefits: We found no systematic review. **Versus observation alone:** We found one small RCT (21 people) comparing needle aspiration versus no treatment.[5] It found no good evidence of faster resolution with needle aspiration (time to full expansion was 3.2 wks in 10 people with conservative treatment *v* 1.6 wks in 8 people successfully treated with needle aspiration, but 2 people randomised to needle aspiration required a chest tube). **Versus chest tube drainage:** We found two small RCTs.[6,7] The first RCT found that needle aspiration versus a chest tube reduced resolution of the pneumothorax in the short term (28/35 resolved with needle aspiration *v* 38/38 with a chest tube; time not provided; 7 people initially treated with needle aspiration required subsequent chest tube drainage) and found no significant difference in recurrence at 1 year (5/30 [17%] with needle aspiration *v* 10/35 [29%] with a chest tube; ARR 12%, 95% CI −9% to +32%; RR 0.58, 95% CI 0.22 to 1.52).[6] The second RCT found that needle aspiration versus a chest tube significantly reduced resolution of the pneumothorax by 24 hours (22/33 [67%] with needle aspiration *v* 26/28 [93%] with a chest tube; ARR 26%, 95% CI 6% to 47%) and did not significantly change recurrence (9/41 [22%] with needle aspiration *v* 7/24 [29%] with needle aspiration; ARR 7%, 95% CI −14% to +28%; RR 0.75, 95% CI 0.32 to 1.76).[7] The RCT was not designed to find a difference in duration of hospital stay because chest tube drainage was done on admission, whereas in most people needle aspiration was performed after 3 days of observation in hospital.

Harms: The RCT of needle aspiration versus observation did not report details of the harmful effects of needle aspiration. **Versus chest tube drainage:** In one RCT, people treated with needle aspiration versus chest tube drainage experienced significantly less pain on daily total pain scores during their hospital stay and on average spent two fewer days in hospital (3.2 days *v* 5.3 days; P = 0.005).[6]

Comment: The RCT of needle aspiration versus observation[5] is consistent with a large case series in which 88/119 (74%) people presenting to an outpatient chest clinic with spontaneous pneumothorax were managed successfully without intervention or hospital admission.[8]

OPTION CHEST TUBE DRAINAGE

We found insufficient evidence on the effects of chest tube drainage compared with observation. Two small RCTs found faster resolution with chest tube drainage than needle aspiration, but found no evidence of a difference in recurrence rate. One of the RCTs found that chest tube drainage versus needle aspiration caused more pain and longer hospital stay. We found no RCTs assessing small versus standard size tubes for chest drainage.

Benefits: We found no systematic review. **Versus observation:** We found no sufficiently large RCTs. **Versus needle aspiration:** See text, p 1577. **Small versus standard sized chest tubes:** We found no RCTs. One non-randomised trial (44 people) compared small gauge (8 French gauge — see glossary, p 1581) catheters versus standard chest tubes.[9] It found no significant difference in duration of drainage between groups. In people with large pneumothoraces (> 50% lung volume), successful resolution was more likely with standard chest tubes than small gauge catheters (100% *v* 57%; $P < 0.05$). No such difference was found in people with small (< 50%) pneumothoraces.

Harms: **Versus needle aspiration:** See text, p 1577. **Small versus standard sized chest tubes:** The RCT found that conventional chest tubes versus small gauge catheters significantly increased the risk of subcutaneous emphysema (9/23 *v* 0/21; $P < 0.05$) and pain.[9]

Comment: Small gauge chest tubes are usually easier to insert.

OPTION ONE WAY VALVES ON CHEST TUBES

One small RCT found no significant difference in rates of resolution with one way valves versus drainage bottles with underwater seals, but the trial was too small to exclude a clinically important difference. People treated with one way valves used less analgesia and spent less time in hospital.

Benefits: We found no systematic review. We found one RCT (30 people with spontaneous pneumothorax and respiratory distress) comparing a chest tube (13 French gauge — see glossary, p 1581) connected to a one way valve versus a chest tube (14 French gauge) connected to a drainage bottle with an underwater seal.[10] It found no significant difference in pneumothorax resolution between groups (complete or nearly complete expansion 48 h after treatment: 15/17 [88%] with one way valve *v* 11/13 [85%] with drainage bottle; ARI 4%, 95% CI –21% to +28%), but fewer people treated with a one way valve required analgesia (5/17 [29%] *v* 10/13 [77%]; RR 0.38, 95% CI 0.17 to 0.85).[10]

Harms: The RCT found that, compared with drainage using an underwater seal, there was no significant difference in the rate of complications (need for a second drain: 3/17 with one way valve *v* 1/13; skin emphysema 3/17 *v* 3/13).[10]

Comment: One way valves often allow people to be treated at home. Admission to hospital was less likely with one way valves than with drainage bottle treatment (5/17 [29%] *v* 13/13 [100%]; RR 0.29, 95% CI 0.14 to 0.61).[10]

OPTION CHEST TUBE DRAINAGE PLUS SUCTION

One RCT found no significant difference in rate of resolution regardless of whether chest tube drainage bottles were connected to suction or not. However, the trial was too small to rule out a clinically important difference.

Benefits: We found no systematic review, but found one RCT (53 people) comparing chest tube drainage using an underwater seal only versus drainage plus suction. Suction pressures ranged from 8–20 cm H_2O.[11] It found no significant difference in the proportion of people with full lung expansion by 10 days (13/23 [57%] with suction *v* 15/30 [50%] without; ARI 7%, 95% CI –21% to +34%).

Harms: We found no reports of adverse effects due to suction.

Comment: We found one RCT comparing suction versus no suction in 80 people with traumatic pneumothorax, but because the mechanism of injury is different the results could not be extrapolated to spontaneous pneumothorax.[12]

QUESTION What are the effects of interventions to prevent recurrence?

OPTION CHEMICAL PLEURODESIS

Two RCTs have found that chest tube drainage plus chemical pleurodesis versus chest tube drainage alone significantly reduces the rate of recurrence of spontaneous pneumothorax, but one of the RCTs found that treatment can be painful. The RCTs found no significant difference in length of hospital stay with pleurodesis versus chest tube drainage alone. We found no RCTs or high quality cohort studies about the optimal timing of pleurodesis.

Benefits: **Versus chest tube drainage alone:** We found no systematic review but found two RCTs[13,14] and one non-randomised trial (see comment below).[15] The first RCT (unblinded, 229 men with pneumothorax successfully treated by chest tube; mean age 54 years; 55% with chronic obstructive pulmonary disease) found that a chest tube plus intrapleural instillation of tetracycline versus a chest tube alone significantly reduced the recurrence rate over 30 months (26/104 [25%] with tetracycline *v* 44/108 [41%] with the chest tube alone; ARR 16%, 95% CI 3% to 28%; RR 0.61, 95% CI 0.41 to 0.92) but had no significant effect on length of hospital stay (5 days with tetracycline *v* 7 days with chest tube alone) or 5 year mortality (40/113 [35%] deaths with tetracycline *v* 42/116 [36%] with chest tube alone; RR 0.98, 95% CI 0.62 to 1.38). It found no effect on pulmonary function at 2 years' follow up.[13] The second RCT (96 people treated with a chest tube) compared three groups: no further treatment; tetracycline pleurodesis; and talc pleurodesis.[14] Mean follow up was 4.6 years. It found that the pneumothorax recurrence rate of the treated lung was significantly higher in people receiving no treatment (9/25 [36%] with no treatment *v* 2/24 [8%] with talc *v* 3/23 [13%] with tetracycline; ARR with either form of pleurodesis 25%, 95% CI 6% to 45%), but found no significant difference in mean length of hospital stay (mean 7 days with tetracycline *v* mean 6 days with talc or with chest tube alone). **Versus surgical pleurodesis:** We found no RCTs but found one non-randomised prospective study (see comment below). **Optimal timing of pleurodesis:** We found no systematic review, RCTs, or high quality cohort studies comparing pleurodesis undertaken at different times (after the first, second, or subsequent episodes of spontaneous pneumothorax).

Harms: In the first unblinded RCT, 61/105 (58%) people reported intense chest pain on injection of tetracycline.[13] The second RCT found no significant difference in the proportion of people reporting pain with chemical pleurodesis versus chest tube alone (17/33 [74%] with tetracycline *v* 14/29 [58%] with talc *v* 18/34 [69%] with chest tube; no further data provided). The non-randomised study (see comment below) gave no information on adverse effects.[15]

Comment: We found one non-randomised prospective study (204 people) comparing four interventions: chest tube drainage plus tetracycline pleurodesis (78 people); chest tube drainage alone (66 people); thoracotomy (28 people); and observation (32 people).[15] The mean follow up was 45 months. It found that chest tube drainage plus tetracycline pleurodesis versus chest tube drainage alone or versus observation significantly reduced recurrence (6/66 [9%], 8 treatment failures, 4 lost to follow up with tetracycline pleurodesis *v* 18/51 [36%], 15 lost to follow up with chest tube alone v 10/28 [36%], 3 lost to follow up with observation; $P < 0.05$ for both comparisons), but found no significant difference in recurrence rate with tetracycline pleurodesis versus thoracotomy (6/66 [9%] *v* 0/26 [0%], 2 deaths, 10 lost to follow up; $P = 0.13$). It found that chemical pleurodesis versus chest tube drainage or versus observation alone significantly increased the duration of hospital stay (mean 10 days *v* 4 days; $P < 0.01$). The study provided no data on length of hospital stay with thoracotomy.[15] The 5 year recurrence rate after a first pneumothorax is about 28%, so there could be little reason to perform pleurodesis after the first episode of pneumothorax.[4] There has been a consensus that pleurodesis is warranted after the second or third episode of pneumothorax, but this convention may be questioned if only 23% of this 28% will have a second recurrence and only 14% of that 23% will have a third recurrence.[4] Even though the probability of success with pleurodesis is high, clinicians will have to weigh the likelihood of recurrence against the morbidity associated with the procedure.

OPTION SURGICAL PLEURODESIS

We found no RCTs comparing surgical pleurodesis versus chest tube drainage alone or versus chemical pleurodesis. One small RCT has found that video-assisted thoracoscopic surgery versus thoracotomy significantly reduces hospital stay. It found no significant difference in the rate of recurrence after 3 years, but the limited evidence cannot exclude a clinically important difference.

Benefits: We found no systematic review. **Versus chemical pleurodesis:** See text, p 1579. **Video-assisted thoracoscopic surgery:** We found one RCT (60 people with primary spontaneous pneumothorax, either first recurrence or non-resolving first episode) that compared video-assisted thoracoscopic surgery versus thoracotomy.[16] It found that video-assisted surgery versus thoracotomy significantly reduced the use of analgesia and hospital stay (hospital stay 6.5 *v* 10.7 days; $P < 0.0001$). It found no significant difference in the rate of recurrence after 3 years (3/30 [10%] people after thoracoscopic surgery *v* 0/30 [0%] after thoracotomy; ARR 10%, 95% CI –1% to +21%).

Harms: The RCT and non-randomised study gave no information on adverse effects.[16,15]

Comment: The RCT comparing thoracoscopic surgery versus thoracotomy was too small to exclude a clinically important difference in recurrence rate.[16]

GLOSSARY

French gauge A measure of the size of a catheter or drainage tube defined (in France by JFB Charrière in 1842) to be the outside diameter of the tube in units of 1/3 mm. A 12 French gauge tube has an outer diameter of 4 mm. Sometimes the French gauge is called the Charrière (Ch) gauge.

REFERENCES

1. Melton LJ, Hepper NG, Offord KP. Incidence of spontaneous pneumothorax in Olmsted County, Minnesota: 1950–1974. *Am Rev Respir Dis* 1979;120:1379–1382.
2. Bense L, Eklung G, Wiman LG. Smoking and the increased risk of contracting spontaneous pneumothorax. *Chest* 1987;92:1009–1012.
3. Lippert HL, Lund O, Blegvad S, et al. Independent risk factors for cumulative recurrence rate after first spontaneous pneumothorax. *Eur Respir J* 1991;4:324–331.
4. Voge VM, Anthracite R. Spontaneous pneumothorax in the USAF aircrew population: a retrospective study. *Aviat Space Environ Med* 1986;57:939–949.
5. Flint K, Al-Hillawi AH, Johnson NM. Conservative management of spontaneous pneumothorax. *Lancet* 1984;1:687–688.
6. Harvey J, Prescott RJ. Simple aspiration versus intercostal tube drainage for spontaneous pneumothorax in patients with normal lungs. British Thoracic Society Research Committee. *BMJ* 1994;309:1338–1339.
7. Andrivet P, Djedaini K, Teboul JL, et al. Spontaneous pneumothorax. Comparison of thoracic drainage vs immediate or delayed needle aspiration. *Chest* 1995;108:335–339.
8. Stradling P, Poole G. Conservative management of spontaneous pneumothorax. *Thorax* 1966;21:145–149.
9. Kang YJ, Koh HG, Shin JW, et al. The effect of 8 French catheter and chest tube on the treatment of spontaneous pneumothorax. *Tuber Respir Dis* 1996;43:410–419.
10. Roggla M, Wagner A, Brunner C, et al. The management of pneumothorax with the thoracic vent versus conventional intercostal tube drainage. *Wien Klin Wochenschr* 1996;108:330–333.
11. So SY, Yu DYC. Catheter drainage of spontaneous pneumothorax: suction or no suction, early or late removal? *Thorax* 1982;37:46–48.
12. Davis JW, Mackersie RC, Hoyt DB, et al. Randomized study of algorithms for discontinuing tube thoracostomy drainage. *J Am Coll Surg* 1994;179:553–557.
13. Light RW, O'Hara VS, Moritz TE, et al. Intrapleural tetracycline for the prevention of recurrent spontaneous pneumothorax. Results of a Department of Veterans Affairs cooperative study. *JAMA* 1990;264:2224–2230.
14. Almind M, Lange P, Viskum K. Spontaneous pneumothorax: comparison of simple drainage, talc pleurodesis, and tetracycline pleurodesis. *Thorax* 1989;44:627–630.

15. Alfageme I, Moreno L, Huertas C, Vargas A, Hernandez J, Beiztegui A. Spontaneous pneumothorax. Long-term results with tetracycline pleurodesis. *Chest* 1994;106:347–350.

16. Ayed AK, Al-Din HJ. Video-assisted thoracoscopy versus thoracotomy for primary spontaneous pneumothorax: A randomized controlled trial. *Med Principles Pract* 2000;9:113–118.

John Cunnington
Associate Professor Medicine
McMaster University
Hamilton, Ontario
Canada

Competing interests: None declared.

Upper respiratory tract infection

Search date October 2001

Chris Del Mar and Paul Glasziou

QUESTIONS

INTERVENTIONS

Key Messages

- **Analgesia/anti-inflammatories for symptom relief** One systematic review has found that analgesics and anti-inflammatory drugs versus placebo significantly reduce sore throat at 1–5 days. One RCT in people with acute sinusitis taking antibiotics found that steroid spray versus placebo significantly improved symptoms over 21 days.
- **Antibiotics for decreasing time to recovery in people with proven infection with Haemophilus influenzae, Moraxella catarrhalis, or Streptococcus pneumoniae** In a minority of people, the upper respiratory tract infection is found to be caused by *H influenzae*, *M catarrhalis*, or *S pneumoniae*. One RCT found that in these people antibiotics versus placebo significantly increased recovery at 5 days (NNT 4, CI not provided, for people with a positive nasopharyngeal culture at first consultation). However, we have no methods currently of easily identifying this subgroup within the majority of people with negative nasopharyngeal cultures.
- **Antibiotics for reducing time to recovery in people with acute bronchitis, pharyngitis, and sinusitis** Systematic reviews have found that antibiotics versus placebo slightly but significantly improve symptoms. Adverse effects (nausea, vomiting, headache, rash, vaginitis) were more common with antibiotics.

Upper respiratory tract infection

- **Antibiotics for preventing (rare) complications of β haemolytic streptococcal pharyngitis** One systematic review has found that antibiotics versus no antibiotics can prevent non-suppurative complications of β haemolytic streptococcal pharyngitis, but in industrialised countries such complications are rare.
- **Antihistamines for runny nose and sneezing** One systematic review has found that antihistamines versus placebo reduce runny nose and sneezing after 2 days, but the clinical benefit is small.
- **Antibiotics in people with colds, coughs, and sore throat** Systematic reviews found no significant difference between antibiotics versus placebo in cure or general improvement.
- **β Agonists for reducing duration of cough** Two RCTs in people with acute bronchitis have found that salbutamol versus erythromycin significantly increases the number of people who are cough free at 7 days, although a third RCT, comparing fenoterol versus placebo, found that this benefit may be limited to people with bronchial hyperresponsiveness, wheeze, or airflow limitation.
- **Decongestants for long term relief of congestive symptoms** One systematic review found no good evidence on the effects of repeated use over several days.
- **Decongestants for short term relief of congestive symptoms** One systematic review has found limited evidence that a single dose of decongestant versus placebo may reduce congestion in the short term.
- **Echinacea for prevention** One systematic review found limited evidence that echinachea versus no treatment significantly reduced the number of people who had one infection episode, but found insufficient evidence of the effects of echinachea versus placebo.
- **Echinacea for treatment** Systematic reviews found limited evidence that some preparations of echinacea versus placebo may improve symptoms, but we found insufficient evidence about the effects of any specific product.
- **Steam inhalation** One systematic review found conflicting evidence about the effects of steam inhalation.
- **Vitamin C** One systematic review has found that vitamin C versus placebo slightly but significantly reduces the duration of cold symptoms, but the benefit was small and may be explained by publication bias.
- **Zinc intranasal gel for reducing the duration of cold symptoms** Two RCTs have found conflicting evidence about the effects of intranasal zinc versus placebo on the duration of cold symptoms.
- **Zinc lozenges** Two systematic reviews found inconsistent evidence on the effects of zinc gluconate or acetate lozenges versus placebo on duration of symptoms.

DEFINITION Upper respiratory tract infection involves inflammation of the respiratory mucosa from the nose to the lower respiratory tree, but not including the alveoli. In addition to malaise, it causes localised symptoms that constitute several overlapping syndromes: sore throat (pharyngitis), rhinorrhoea (common cold), facial fullness and pain (sinusitis), and cough (bronchitis).

INCIDENCE/ PREVALENCE Upper respiratory tract infections, nasal congestion, throat complaints, and cough are responsible for 11% of general practice consultations in Australia.[1] Each year, children suffer about five such infections and adults two to three infections.[1]

AETIOLOGY/ RISK FACTORS Infective agents include over 200 viruses (with 100 rhinoviruses) and several bacteria. Transmission is mostly through hand to hand contact with subsequent passage to the nostrils or eyes rather than, as commonly perceived, through droplets in the air.[2]

PROGNOSIS Upper respiratory tract infections are usually self limiting. Although they cause little mortality or serious morbidity, upper respiratory tract infections are responsible for considerable discomfort, lost work, and medical costs. Clinical patterns vary and overlap between infective agents. In addition to nasal symptoms, half of sufferers experience sore throat and 40% experience cough. Symptoms peak within 1–3 days and generally clear by 1 week, although cough often persists.[2]

AIMS To relieve symptoms and to prevent suppurative and non-suppurative complications of bacterial infection, with minimal adverse effects from treatments.

OUTCOMES Cure rate; duration of symptoms; incidence of complications; incidence of adverse effects of treatment.

METHODS *Clinical Evidence* search and appraisal October 2001.

QUESTION **What are the effects of treatments?**

OPTION **ANTIBIOTICS**

We found no evidence that antibiotics have a clinically important effect on colds. Systematic reviews have found a minimal to modest effect of antibiotics in people with acute bronchitis, sore throat, and sinusitis. Antibiotics can prevent non-suppurative complications of β haemolytic streptococcal pharyngitis, but in industrialised countries such complications are rare.

Benefits: **Colds:** We found two systematic reviews. The first review (search date 1998, 7 RCTs in people with acute upper respiratory infections without complications) found no effect of antibiotics on general improvement or cure (RR 0.95, 95% CI 0.70 to 1.25).[3] The second review (search date not stated, 12 RCTs of antibiotics in children) found no change in clinical outcomes in the six trials with adequate data (RR 1.01, 95% CI 0.90 to 1.13), or in complications or progression (RR 0.71, 95% CI 0.45 to 1.12).[4] Similarly, one additional RCT (314 adults) comparing amoxicillin (amoxycillin)/clavulanic acid (co-amoxiclav) (375 mg 3 times daily) versus placebo found no overall difference in "cure" rates.[5] However, in the 61 people (20%) who were found to have positive sputum cultures for *Haemophilus influenzae*, *Moraxella catarrhalis*, or *Streptococcus pneumoniae*, there was a significant difference in recovery of 27% with co-amoxiclav versus 4% with placebo at 5 days. If such people could be identified at first consultation, then treating four of these people with antibiotic rather than placebo would result in an average of one more recovery at 5 days (NNT 4; CI not provided). **Acute bronchitis:** We found two systematic reviews (search date 2000[6] and 1996,[7] including 8 RCTs, 750 people aged 8 to > 65 years with acute bronchitis) comparing doxycycline (4 RCTs), erythromycin (3 RCTs), and trimethoprim/sulfamethoxazole (sulphamethoxazole) (co-trimoxazole) (1 RCT) versus placebo. The most recent review found that people receiving antibiotics were less likely to report cough at a follow up visit (RR for reporting cough at follow up antibiotics *v* placebo 0.64, 95% CI 0.49 to 0.85; see comment below). There was a small but significant difference with antibiotics in time to return to work or usual activities (WMD 0.74 days earlier with antibiotics *v* placebo, 95% CI 0.16 to 1.32).[6] **Sore throat:** We found one systematic review (search date 1999, 25 controlled trials, 10 863 people with sore throat).[8] The combined effects from seven trials found that antibiotics reduced the risk of rheumatic fever compared with no antibiotic (RR 0.30, 95% CI 0.20 to 0.45). There were too few events to detect any possible protective effect of antibiotics against acute glomerulonephritis (2/1834 cases among controls *v* 0/2558 treated with antibiotics). Suppurative complications were also significantly reduced (otitis media: RR 0.22, 95% CI 0.11 to 0.43; quinsy: RR 0.16, 95% CI 0.07 to 0.35). Acute sinusitis was not significantly reduced (RR 0.46, 95% CI 0.10 to 2.05). To prevent one case of otitis media, 30 children or 145 adults suffering from sore throat would need to be treated. Antibiotics shortened symptom duration but only by a mean of about 8 hours overall. **Sinusitis:** We found one systematic review (search date 1998, 6 RCTs, 761 people with sinusitis) comparing antibiotics versus placebo.[9] It found that antimicrobial agents (amoxicillin in 3 RCTs, other agents in 3 RCTs) were effective in treating uncomplicated acute sinusitis. Symptoms improved or disappeared in significantly fewer people taking placebo versus antibiotics (69% *v* 84%; RR 1.33, 95% CI 1.02 to 1.74). The same review analysed head to head trials of different antibiotics and found no advantage for other antibiotics over amoxicillin.

Harms: Adverse effects such as nausea, vomiting, headache, rash, or vaginitis were more common in people taking antibiotics than placebo. For example, in the review in people with bronchitis, the absolute risk increase for adverse effects was 6% (95% CI 0.1% to 11%), or a rate of one extra adverse effect per 16 people treated.[6] We found no evidence of the size of the risk of antibiotic resistance or pseudomembranous colitis.

Comment: Because most upper respiratory tract infections are viral, the potential benefit from antibiotics is limited. Until rapid identification of those people likely to benefit is possible, the modest effects seen in trials must be weighed against the adverse effects of antibiotics, costs, and potential for inducing antibiotic resistance. One of the reviews reported that some of the RCTs only reported detailed information on outcomes that were statistically significant.[6]

OPTION β AGONISTS

Two RCTs have found that β agonists reduce the duration of cough in acute bronchitis compared with placebo or erythromycin, although limited evidence from a third RCT suggests that this beneficial effect may be only in people with bronchial hyperresponsiveness, wheeze, or airflow limitation.

Benefits: We found no systematic review. We found three RCTs of β agonists.[10–12] In the first RCT comparing liquid salbutamol versus erythromycin, significantly more people taking salbutamol were cough free at 7 days (59% *v* 12%; NNT 3).[10] In the second RCT comparing inhaled salbutamol versus erythromycin, more people using salbutamol were cough free at 7 days (39% *v* 9%; NNT 4).[11] In the third RCT comparing fenoterol versus placebo, subgroup analysis found that benefits may be confined to people with bronchial hyperresponsiveness, wheezes, or baseline forced expiratory volume in 1 second less than 80% of predicted.[12]

Harms: Short term use of a β agonist may cause tachycardia and anxiety.

Comment: The cough associated with acute bronchitis is self limiting, so treatment is for symptomatic relief; therefore, it is important to consider the degree of disturbance caused and peoples' preferences and interpretation of cough. A new systematic review on β agonists is expected to be published soon.

OPTION VITAMIN C

One systematic review has found evidence that vitamin C reduces the duration of symptoms in people with upper respiratory tract infections. However, the beneficial effect is small and may be explained by publication bias.

Benefits: We found one systematic review.[13] The review (search date not stated, 30 RCTs) compared vitamin C versus placebo for prophylaxis and treatment of colds. Three RCTs used 1 g daily or more of vitamin C taken at symptom onset. It found that in people taking vitamin C, the duration of symptoms was around half a day less (WMD 0.44 days/cold episode, 95% CI 0.23 to 0.64) representing about 15% fewer symptomatic days per episode.

Harms: The RCTs found no evidence of adverse effects potentially caused by vitamin C.

Comment: The beneficial effect reported in the review was small and might be explained by publication bias.

OPTION ZINC

Two systematic reviews found no clear evidence that zinc gluconate or acetate lozenges are beneficial in people with upper respiratory tract infections. Two RCTs have found conflicting evidence about effects of zinc nasal gel on duration of symptoms.

Benefits: **Zinc lozenges:** We found two systematic reviews (search date 1997,[14] 7 RCTs and search date 1998,[15] 8 controlled trials) comparing zinc lozenges (gluconate or acetate) versus placebo for the treatment of naturally acquired colds. Symptoms were unchanged at 3 and 5 days. However, at 7 days, the reviews found conflicting effects. The first review found that zinc reduced risk of continuing symptoms at 7 days (RR zinc *v* control 0.69 at 7 days; NNT 7, 95% CI 5 to 15), but the second review found that the reduction in risk was not significant (OR for continuing symptoms, zinc *v* placebo 0.5, 95% CI 0.25 to 1.2). The results at 7 days were statistically heterogeneous, which may be because of the zinc formulation, the type of virus, or to other unknown factors. **Intranasal zinc:** Two RCTs (213 and 160 people) of intranasal zinc versus placebo found conflicting results.[16,17] The first found that intranasal zinc significantly reduced symptom duration compared with placebo (mean duration 9.0 days with placebo *v* 2.3 days with intranasal zinc; $P < 0.05$).[16] The second trial found no significant difference for symptom duration (mean duration of nasal symptoms 6 days for each group).[17]

Harms: Adverse outcomes were not reviewed systematically, but individual trials found that nausea, altered taste, dry mouth, abdominal pain, and headache were increased in the zinc group.

Comment: None.

OPTION ECHINACEA

Systematic reviews found limited evidence that some preparations of echinacea may be better than placebo for cold treatment and prevention, but we found insufficient evidence about effects of a specific echinacea product compared with other or no interventions for treating or preventing common colds.

Benefits: **Treatment:** We found two systematic reviews (search date 1998,[18] 8 RCTs; search date 2000,[19] additional 5 RCTs included). All RCTs included in the first review were double blind except one that was single blind. The first review found most RCTs to be of poor quality.[18] Quantitative results could be extracted for only two RCTs on duration of illness, three RCTs for runny nose, and five RCTs for a summary symptom score. Data pooling was not possible because of trial heterogeneity. There were nine comparisons (8 *v* placebo and, in 1 RCT, an additional comparison of high *v* low dose treatment) from the eight RCTs. Six comparisons found significantly better results associated with echinacea. One RCT found significant results for a subgroup only, and two RCTs found no difference after treatment.[18] The second review identified five further trials published after 1997. It also found that trials were heterogeneous and of poor quality and it reached the same conclusions as the first review.[19] **Prevention:** The first systematic review identified eight RCTs, with a total of almost 4000 people.[18] The placebo-controlled RCTs varied considerably in quality of methods and preparation used, so results were not combined. Of the five placebo controlled RCTs, two found a significantly lower incidence of infection in people taking echinacea. One of these had large loss to follow up. The other placebo-controlled RCTs found a non-significant reduction in the rate of infection. Meta-analysis of the three RCTs comparing echinacea versus no treatment found that significantly fewer people had one infection episode after taking echinacea (167/571 [29%] *v* 292/566 [52%]; OR 0.36, 95% CI 0.28 to 0.46). The three uncontrolled studies all found a significant benefit, but were not randomised or blinded.

Harms: Three of the eight treatment RCTs and four of the eight prevention RCTs reported adverse events. These were generally infrequent and not significantly different between echinacea and placebo. However, outside the trials, anaphylaxis has been reported with echinacea.[20]

Comment: Echinacea is not a single product. There are more than 200 different preparations based on different plants, different parts of the plant (roots, herbs, whole plant), and different methods of extraction. None of the trials were published in a Medline listed journal. The weakness of trial methods and differences in interventions make drawing conclusive evidence of effectiveness impossible. Large studies may be difficult because echinacea is not patentable, and each producer controls a small share of the market. The authors of the systematic review received personal information about several unpublished studies that they were not able to include.

OPTION STEAM INHALATION

One systematic review found conflicting evidence for the efficacy of steam inhalation.

Benefits: We found one systematic review (search date 1999, 6 RCTs, 319 people) of steam inhalation at 40–47°C.[21] Some RCTs found benefit and none found any harm. Benefits included increased patency of the nose following exposure to hot, humid steam.

Harms: The RCTs found no evidence of harms. There may be a danger from spilling very hot water and from nosocomial infections related to humidifier units.

Comment: None.

OPTION DECONGESTANTS

One systematic review found evidence for limited short term benefit following a single dose, but no evidence of benefit with longer use of decongestants for symptomatic relief.

Benefits: We found one systematic review (search dates 1999, 4 RCTs, 246 adults).[22] The review found that in the common cold, a single dose of nasal decongestant versus placebo was only moderately effective for the short term relief of congestion in adults (reducing subjective symptom scores by 13%). We found no good evidence on the effects of repeated use over several days.

Harms: Information about harms was not sought actively or reported in RCTs. One case control study compared the use of cold preparations containing phenylpropanolamine among 702 people with a history of haemorrhagic stroke versus 1376 control participants with no history of stroke. The study found a non-significant trend towards increased risk of haemorrhage stroke with phenylpropanolamine (RR 1.5, 95% CI 0.85 to 2.65).[23] However, the study was too small to make definitive conclusions.

Comment: The review found no RCTs in children.

OPTION ANTIHISTAMINES

One systematic review has found evidence that antihistamines produce small clinical benefits for the symptoms of runny nose and sneezing.

Benefits: One well conducted systematic review of previously unpublished individual patient data (search date not stated, 9 RCTs, 1757 adults) of antihistamines versus placebo found antihistamines reduced the symptoms of runny nose and sneezing for the first

2 days of both natural and experimentally induced colds.[24] The effects were small. On a severity scale ranging from 0 (no symptoms) to 3 or 4 (severe symptoms), antihistamines reduced the score by 0.25 (95% CI 0.12 to 0.73) for runny nose on days 1 and 2, 0.14 (95% CI 0.0 to 0.3) for sneezing on day 1, and 0.3 (95% CI 1.5 to 4.5) for sneezing on day 2.

Harms: Harms were not actively looked for in RCTs, but known harms of antihistamines include drowsiness and dry mouth.

Comment: None.

OPTION ANALGESICS AND ANTI-INFLAMMATORY AGENTS

One systematic review has found that analgesics and anti-inflammatory agents significantly relieve the symptoms of sore throat. One RCT has found that steroid spray provides additional benefit to antibiotics for acute sinusitis.

Benefits: **Sore throat:** We found one systematic review (search date 1999, 12 RCTs of non-steroidal anti-inflammatory drugs [NSAIDs], 3 of paracetamol, 1 of steroids).[25] The RCTs found that all interventions were superior to placebo. Six RCTs (493 people) assessed the effects of NSAIDs only over 24 hours or less. The RCTs found consistently that NSAIDs reduced throat pain. Five RCTs (646 people) assessed the effects of NSAIDs over more than 24 hours. All the RCTs found a significant reduction in symptoms over the length of the trials (2–5 days). Two RCTs (158 people) assessed the effects of paracetamol over 24 hours or less. One of these RCTs found a significant reduction in throat pain at 6 hours; the other found no significant difference. One RCT (154 people) assessed the effects of paracetamol over 2 days. It found a significant reduction in sore throat symptoms after 2 days ($P < 0.01$). One RCT comparing corticosteroid injection (dexamethasone 10 mg) versus placebo over 24 hours found a significant reduction in mean pain at 24 hours ($P < 0.05$). **Acute sinusitis:** We found one RCT (407 people all receiving antibiotics) of intranasal steroid versus placebo.[26] The RCT found that intranasal corticosteroid significantly improved symptoms of acute sinusitis over 21 days. Over days 1–15, mean total symptom scores decreased by 5.9 with steroids versus 5.1 with placebo ($P < 0.01$).

Harms: NSAIDs increase the risk of gastrointestinal haemorrhage (see NSAIDs, p 1203). One review of aspirin trials (40 RCTs; 22 234 people; mean treatment duration 1 year) found an increased risk of gross haemorrhage (over 1 year ARI 0.6%, 95% CI 0.2% to 1.2%).

Comment: None.

REFERENCES

1. Fry J, Sandler G. *Common diseases. Their nature prevalence and care.* Dordrecht, The Netherlands: Kluwer Academic, 1993.
2. Lauber B. The common cold. *J Gen Intern Med* 1996;11:229–236.
3. Arroll B, Kenealy T. The use of antibiotics versus placebo in the common cold. In: The Cochrane Library, Issue 3, 2001. Oxford: Update Software. Search date 1998; primary sources Cochrane Controlled Trials Register, Medline, Embase, Family Medicine Database, reference lists in articles, and principal investigators.
4. Fahey T, Stocks N, Thomas T. Systematic review of the treatment of upper respiratory tract infection. *Arch Dis Child* 1998;79:225–230. Search date not stated; primary sources Medline, Embase, Science Citation Index, Cochrane Controlled Trials

Register, authors of published RCTs, drug manufacturers, and hand searched references.

5. Kaiser L, Lew D, Hirschel B, et al. Effects of antibiotic treatment in the subset of common-cold patients who have bacteria in nasopharyngeal secretions. *Lancet* 1996;347:1507–1510.
6. Smucny J, Fahey T, Becker L, Glazier R. Antibiotics for acute bronchitis. In: The Cochrane Library, Issue 3, 2001. Oxford: Update Software. Search date 2000; primary sources Medline, Embase, Science Citation Index, hand search of reference lists of relevant trials, textbooks, and review articles.
7. Chandran R. Should we prescribe antibiotics for acute bronchitis? *Am Fam Physician* 2001:64;135–138. Search date 1996; primary sources Medline, Embase, personal collections, and Sci-search.
8. Del Mar CB, Glasziou PP, Spinks AB. Antibiotics for sore throat. In: The Cochrane Library, Issue 3, 2001. Oxford: Update Software. Search date 1999; primary sources Medline, Cochrane Library, and hand search of reference lists of relevant articles.
9. De Ferranti SD, Ionnidis JPA, Lau J, et al. Are amoxycillin and folate inhibitors as effective as other antibiotics for acute sinusitis? A meta-analysis. *BMJ* 1998;317:632–637. Search date 1998; primary sources Medline, hand search of Excerpta Medica, recent abstracts for Interscience Conference on Antimicrobial Agents and Chemotherapy, and references of all trials, review articles, and special issues for additional studies.
10. Hueston WJ. A comparison of albuterol and erythromycin for the treatment of acute bronchitis. *J Fam Pract* 1991;33:476–480.
11. Hueston WJ. Albuterol delivered by metered-dose inhaler to treat acute bronchitis. *J Fam Pract* 1994;39:437–440.
12. Melbye H, Aasebo U, Straume B. Symptomatic effect of inhaled fenoterol in acute bronchitis: a placebo-controlled double-blind study. *Fam Pract* 1991;8:216–222.
13. Douglas RM, Chalker EB, Treacy B. Vitamin C for preventing and treating the common cold. In: The Cochrane Library, Issue 3, 2001. Oxford: Update Software. Search date not stated; primary sources reviews by Kleinjon[27] and Hemila.[28]
14. Marshall I. Zinc in the treatment of the common cold. In: The Cochrane Library, Issue 3, 2001. Oxford: Update Software. Search date 1997; primary sources Medline, Embase, The Cochrane Library, and hand searched journals.
15. Jackson JL, Lesho E, Peterson C. Zinc and the common cold: a meta-analysis revisited. *J Nutrition* 2000;130(Suppl):1512S–1515S. Search date: 1998; primary sources Medline, National Institute of Health database of funded studies, the Cochrane randomised clinical trial database, and relevant papers.
16. Hirt M, Nobel S, Barron E. Zinc nasal gel for the treatment of common cold symptoms: a double-blind, placebo-controlled trial. *Ear Nose Throat J* 2000;79:778–782.
17. Belongia EA, Berg R, Liu K. A randomized trial of zinc nasal spray for the treatment of upper respiratory illness in adults. *Am J Med* 2001;111:103–108.
18. Melchart D, Linde K, Fischer P, Kaesmayr J. Echinacea for the prevention and treatment of the common cold. In: The Cochrane Library, Issue 3, 2001. Oxford: Update Software. Search date 1998; primary sources Medline, Embase, database of the Cochrane Acute Respiratory Infections Group, database of the Cochrane Field Complementary Medicine, Phytodok, bibliographies of existing reviews, and personal communications.
19. Giles JT, Palat CT III, Chien SH, Chang ZG, Kennedy DT. Evaluation of echinacea for treatment of the common cold. *Pharmacotherapy* 2000;20:690–697. Search date 2000; primary sources Medline, International Pharmaceutical Abstracts, Cambridge Scientific Abstracts Biological Sciences, Alt-Health Watch, Embase, and references from published articles.
20. Mullins RJ. Echinacea associated anaphylaxis. *Med J Aust* 1998;168:170–171.
21. Singh M. Heated, humidified air for the common cold. In: The Cochrane Library, Issue 3, 2001. Oxford: Update Software. Search date 1999; primary sources Medline, Embase, Current Contents, hand search of review articles and reference lists, and contact with manufacturers.
22. Taverner D, Bickford L, Draper M. Nasal decongestants for the common cold. In: The Cochrane Library, Issue 3, 2001. Oxford: Update Software. Search date 1999; primary sources Medline, Embase, Current Contents, Cochrane Acute Respiratory Infectious Group's trials register, hand search of reference lists, and personal contacts with known investigators and pharmaceutical companies.
23. Kernan WN, Viscoli CM, Brass LM, et al. Phenylpropanolamine and the risk of hemorrhagic stroke. *N Engl J Med* 2000;343:1826–1832.
24. D'Agostino RB Sr, Weintraub M, Russell HK, et al. The effectiveness of antihistamines in reducing the severity of runny nose and sneezing: a meta-analysis. *Clin Pharmacol Ther* 1998;64:579–596. Search date not stated; primary sources Medline and FDA unpublished clinical trials.
25. Thomas M, Del Mar C, Glaziou P. How effective are treatments other than antibiotics for acute sore throat? *Br J Gen Pract* 2000;50:817–820. Search date 1999; primary sources Medline and Cochrane Controlled Trials Registry.
26. Meltzer EO, Charous BL, Busse WW, Zinreich SJ, Lorber RR, Danzig MR. Added relief in the treatment of acute recurrent sinusitis with adjunctive mometasone furoate nasal spray. *J Allergy Clin Immunol* 2000;106:630–637.
27. Kleijnen J, Ter Riet G, Knipschild PG. Vitamin C and the common cold; review of a megadoses literature [in Dutch]. *Ned Tijdschr Geneeskd* 1989;133:1532–1535. Search date 1998; primary sources Medline and hand searched references.
28. Hemila H. Vitamin C and the common cold. *Br J Nutr* 1992;67:3–16. Search date not stated; primary sources not stated.

Chris Del Mar
Professor of General Practice
University of Queensland
Brisbane
Australia

Paul Glasziou
Professor of Evidence-Based Practice
University of Queensland
Brisbane
Australia

Competing interests: None declared.

Bacterial vaginosis

Search date March 2002

M Joesoef and George Schmid

QUESTIONS

INTERVENTIONS

Key Messages

- Bacterial vaginosis may resolve spontaneously.

In non-pregnant women

- **Antianaerobic treatment in symptomatic non-pregnant women** One systematic review has found no significant difference between oral and intravaginal antianaerobic drugs in cure rates after 5–10 days or at 4 weeks. Another systematic review has found that a 7 day course of twice daily oral metronidazole versus a single 2 g dose significantly increases cure rates at 3–4 weeks. Limited evidence from RCTs found no significant difference in cure rates with oral clindamycin versus oral metronidazole twice daily for 7 days, and no difference between once and twice daily dosing with intravaginal metronidazole gel. One RCT found no difference in cure rates at 35 days with intravaginal clindamycin ovules for 3 days versus intravaginal clindamycin cream for 7 days.

In pregnant women

- **Antianaerobic treatment (except clindamycin) in low risk pregnancy** Two systematic reviews of antianaerobic treatment versus placebo have found no significant difference in the risk of preterm delivery.

Clin Evid 2002;8:1592–1600.

- **Antianaerobic treatment (except clindamycin) in pregnant women who have had a previous preterm birth** Limited evidence from a subgroup analysis in pregnant women with bacterial vaginosis who had a previous preterm birth found that oral antianaerobic treatment versus placebo significantly reduced the risk of premature delivery (NNT 4, 95% CI 3 to 7).
- **Treating pregnant women with intravaginal clindamycin** Four RCTs found that intravaginal clindamycin cream versus placebo was associated with an increased risk of preterm delivery and low birth weight, but the increase was not significant.
- **Treating pregnant women without bacterial vaginosis** Subgroup analysis in two RCTs of pregnant women without bacterial vaginosis found that both intravaginal clindamycin cream and oral metronidazole plus erythromycin versus placebo were associated with an increased risk of preterm delivery before 34 weeks' gestation, although the difference was significant in only one of the RCTs.

Preventing recurrence

- **Treating a woman's one steady male sexual partner** One systematic review has found that, in women with one steady male sexual partner, treating the partner with an oral antianaerobic agent does not reduce the woman's risk of recurrence.

Treatment before procedures

- **Antianaerobic treatment before gynaecological procedures (other than abortion)** We found no RCTs on the effects of antianaerobic treatment in women with bacterial vaginosis about to undergo gynaecological procedures other than abortion.
- **Oral antianaerobic treatment before surgical abortion** RCTs consistently found that oral antianaerobic treatment versus placebo in women with bacterial vaginosis about to undergo surgical abortion was associated with a lower risk of pelvic inflammatory disease, but the difference was only significant in the largest RCT.

DEFINITION Bacterial vaginosis is a microbial disease characterised by an alteration in the bacterial flora of the vagina from a predominance of *Lactobacillus* species to high concentrations of anaerobic bacteria. Diagnosis requires three out of four features: the presence of clue cells; a homogenous discharge adherent to the vaginal walls; pH of vaginal fluid > 4.5; and a "fishy" amine odour of the vaginal discharge before or after addition of 10% potassium hydroxide. The condition is asymptomatic in 50% of infected women. Women with symptoms have an excessive white to grey, or malodorous vaginal discharge, or both; the odour may be particularly noticeable during sexual intercourse.

INCIDENCE/ PREVALENCE Bacterial vaginosis is the most common infectious cause of vaginitis, being about twice as common as candidiasis.[1] Prevalences of 10–61% have been reported among unselected women from a range of settings.[2] Data on incidence are limited but one study found that, over a 2 year period, 50% of women using an intrauterine contraceptive device had at least one episode, as did 20% of women using oral contraceptives.[3] Bacterial vaginosis is particularly prevalent in lesbians.[4]

AETIOLOGY/ RISK FACTORS The cause of bacterial vaginosis is not understood fully. Risk factors include new or multiple sexual partners[1,3,5] and early age of sexual intercourse,[6] but no causative microorganism has been shown to be transmitted between partners. Use of an intrauterine contraceptive device[3] and douching[5] has also been reported as risk factors. Infection seems to be most common around the time of menstruation.[7]

PROGNOSIS The course of bacterial vaginosis varies and is poorly understood. Without treatment, symptoms may persist or resolve in both pregnant and non-pregnant women. Recurrence after treatment occurs in about a third of women. The condition is associated with complications of pregnancy: low birth weight; preterm birth (pooled OR from 10 cohort studies: 1.8, 95% CI 1.5 to 2.6);[8] preterm labour; premature rupture of membranes; late miscarriage; chorioamnionitis (48% *v* 22%, OR 2.6, 95% CI 1.0 to 6.6);[9] endometritis after normal delivery (8.2% *v* 1.5%, OR 5.6, 95% CI 1.8 to 17.2);[10] endometritis after caesarean section (55% *v* 17%, OR 5.8, 95% CI 3.0 to 10.9);[11] and surgery to the genital tract. Women who have had a previous premature delivery are especially at risk of complications in pregnancy, with a sevenfold increased risk of preterm birth (24/428 [5.6%] in all women *v* 10/24 [41.7%] in women with a previous preterm birth).[12] Bacterial vaginosis can also enhance HIV acquisition and transmission.[13]

AIMS To alleviate symptoms and to prevent complications relating to childbirth, termination of pregnancy, and gynaecological surgery, with minimal adverse effects; to reduce adverse neonatal outcomes.

OUTCOMES Preterm delivery; puerperal and neonatal morbidity and mortality; clinical or microbiological cure rates, usually at 1–2 weeks or 4 weeks after completing treatment.

METHODS *Clinical Evidence* update search and appraisal March 2002. In addition, the authors used information from drug manufacturers.

QUESTION **What are the effects of different antianaerobic regimens in non-pregnant women with symptomatic bacterial vaginosis?**

One systematic review found no significant difference in cure rates at 5–10 days or 4 weeks between oral and intravaginal antianaerobic drugs. Another systematic review has found that a 7 day course of twice daily oral metronidazole versus a single 2 g dose significantly increases cure rates. Limited evidence from RCTs found no significant difference in cure rates between oral clindamycin and oral metronidazole, and no difference between once and twice daily dosing with intravaginal metronidazole gel. One RCT found no difference in cure rates at 35 days between 3 day treatment with intravaginal ovules versus 7 day treatment with intravaginal clindamycin cream.

Benefits: **Oral versus intravaginal antianaerobic treatment:** We found one systematic review (search date 1996, 5 RCTs) comparing oral and intravaginal formulations of metronidazole and clindamycin,[14] and one subsequent RCT.[15] Three RCTs were in symptomatic non-pregnant women and two were in symptomatic and asymptomatic non-pregnant women. There was no significant difference in cumulative cure rates 5–10 days after completing treatment (86% for oral metronidazole 500 mg twice daily for 7 days *v* 85% for clindamycin vaginal cream 5 g at bedtime for 7 days *v* 81% for metronidazole vaginal gel 5 g twice daily for 5 days; P values and CI not provided). Four weeks after completing treatment, the cumulative cure rates were 78% for oral metronidazole versus 82% for clindamycin vaginal cream versus 71% for metronidazole vaginal gel. The subsequent RCT (399 women) of clindamycin vaginal cream versus oral metronidazole also found no significant difference in cure rates (68% for clindamycin cream *v* 67% for oral metronidazole; P = 0.81).[15] However, a large number of women were not included in the efficacy analysis, making interpretation of the results difficult (results reported on 233 women, many exclusions for different reasons). **Different oral antianaerobic regimens:** We found one systematic review (search date 1996, 4 RCTs) comparing metronidazole 500 mg twice daily for 7 days versus a single 2 g dose of metronidazole, and two additional RCTs comparing metronidazole 500 mg twice daily for 7 days versus clindamycin 300 mg twice daily for 7 days.[14,16,17] It found significantly higher cumulative cure rates at 3–4 weeks after completing treatment with 7 day metronidazole (82% with 7 days of metronidazole *v* 62% with single dose metronidazole; P < 0.05). The first additional RCT (143 symptomatic non-pregnant women) found no significant difference in cure rates within 7–10 days of starting treatment (women cured: 46/49 [94%] with clindamycin *v* 48/50 [96%] with metronidazole; RR 0.98, 95% CI 0.89 to 1.07).[16] A quarter of women were lost to follow up. The second RCT (96 non-pregnant women) found no significant difference in cure rates (39/41 [95%] with clindamycin *v* 41/44 [93%] with metronidazole; ARI 2%; RR 1.0, 95% CI 0.92 to 1.14).[17] **Different intravaginal antianaerobic regimens:** We found two RCTs.[18,19] The first RCT (514 women) found no significant difference in effectiveness between once daily versus twice daily dosing of intravaginal metronidazole gel (118/207 [57%] with once daily gel *v* 129/209 [62%] with twice daily gel; RR 0.92, 95% CI 0.79 to 1.08).[18] The second RCT (662 women) compared 3 day treatment with intravaginal clindamycin ovules versus 7 day treatment with intravaginal clindamycin cream.[19] It found no significant difference in cure rates at 35 day assessment (134/238 [56%] with 3 day regimen *v* 113/224 [50%] with 7 day regimen; ARI 6%; RR 1.10, 95% CI 0.94 to 1.30). **Recurrence:** One RCT (139 women treated with 12 weeks' clindamycin vaginal cream) found no significant difference between treating the women's partners with clindamycin capsules versus placebo (30% with clindamycin capsules *v* 32% with placebo, P > 0.05).[20] A second RCT (61 women, 19 withdrew) of clindamycin vaginal cream versus oral metronidazole found that more than 50% of women in both groups had recurrent bacterial vaginosis 2 months after treatment (exact figures or statistical analysis not provided).[21] We found no good studies of maintenance regimens for recurrent bacterial vaginosis.

Harms: The review of different oral antianaerobic regimens found that adverse effects occurred in between a quarter and two thirds of women taking oral metronidazole, including mild to moderate nausea/dyspepsia, unpleasant metallic taste, headache, and dizziness.[14] Infrequent adverse effects from oral clindamycin included heartburn, nausea, vomiting, diarrhoea, constipation, headache, dizziness, and vertigo; the trials gave no data on frequency. Intravaginal clindamycin has been associated, rarely, with mild to severe colitis[22] and vaginal candidiasis. The RCT of once versus twice daily intravaginal metronidazole gel found no significant difference in frequency of adverse effects.[18] Comparison of results across RCTs found that yeast vulvovaginitis might be less common with intravaginal metronidazole than with oral metronidazole (4% for intravaginal[23] *v* 8–22% for oral[24]).

Comment: Intravaginal administration reduces systemic absorption and systemic adverse effects. Some women may prefer oral medication because it is more convenient.

QUESTION What are the effects of treatments in pregnant women with bacterial vaginosis?

Two systematic reviews of antianaerobic treatment of bacterial vaginosis during pregnancy have found no significant difference in the risk of preterm delivery. Subgroup analysis in women with bacterial vaginosis who had a previous preterm delivery found heterogeneous results, but most RCTs found that oral antianaerobic treatment significantly reduced the risk of preterm delivery. Four RCTs found an increase in preterm birth and low birth weight in women with bacterial vaginosis treated with clindamycin cream versus placebo.

Benefits: **In low risk pregnancy:** We found two systematic reviews (search date 1999, 7 RCTs, 3613 women;[25] and search date not stated, 5 RCTs, 1508 women[26]). The first review included one RCT not in the second review and the second review contained three RCTs not in the first review, two of these were published subsequent to the first review's search date. Both reviews found no significant difference in the general population of women with bacterial vaginosis of antianaerobic treatment versus placebo on the rate of preterm delivery (< 37 weeks) (ARR +0.1%, 95% CI –1.7% to +1.9%),[25] and (RR 0.83, 95% CI 0.67 to 1.03).[26] **In women with previous preterm birth:** The first systematic review (5 RCTs, 440 women) included subgroup analysis in women with a previous preterm birth from RCTs in general populations.[25] Four RCTs reported results for preterm delivery at less than 37 weeks. It found clustered results. Three RCTs found a reduction in the risk of preterm delivery (ARR 22%, 90% CI 13% to 31%; 95% CI not available), but one RCT found no reduction (ARI +8%, 90% CI –4% to +19%; 95% CI not available).

Harms: The second review found adverse effects occurred in 4% of women receiving antibiotics for bacterial vaginosis.[26] **In women without bacterial vaginosis:** Two RCTs of antibiotic administration[27,28] found an increase in preterm birth (before 34 weeks' gestation) in a subgroup of women without bacterial vaginosis who received intravaginal clindamycin cream versus placebo[27] or oral metronidazole and erythromycin versus placebo.[28] In the first RCT, differences between groups did not reach statistical significance (9/72 [12.5%] with clindamycin *v* 3/74 [4.1%] with placebo; recalculation by *Clinical Evidence*: ARI 8.4%; RR 3.1, 95% CI 0.9 to 10.9).[27] However, this RCT found a significantly increased risk of neonatal sepsis with clindamycin cream (5/83 [6%] with clindamycin *v* 0/85 [0%] with placebo; ARI 6.0%, 95% CI 0.5% to 13.3%). Subgroup analysis in the second RCT found no significant difference for preterm birth before 37 weeks' gestation (56/254 [22%] with metronidazole and erythromycin *v* 26/104 [25%] with placebo; RR 0.98, 95% CI 0.57 to 1.30), but found a significant difference for preterm birth before 34 weeks' gestation (34/254 [13%] with metronidazole and erythromycin *v* 5/104 [5%] with placebo; RR 2.8, 95% CI 1.2 to 6.0; NNH 12, 95% CI 4 to 136).[28] **In women with bacterial vaginosis:** Four RCTs[29–32] found an increase in preterm birth and low birth weight of women with bacterial vaginosis who received intravaginal clindamycin cream versus placebo. In all RCTs, the increase was not significant. In the second trial, the rate of preterm birth (< 32 weeks' gestation) was higher with clindamycin cream than with placebo (16/340 [5%] with clindamycin *v* 9/341 [3%] with placebo; ARI +2.1%, 95% CI –0.8% to +5.1%; RR 1.78, 95% CI 0.80 to 3.98). The rate of low birth weight was higher with clindamycin but the difference was not significant (30/334 [9%] with clindamycin cream *v* 23/338 [7%] with placebo; RR 1.32, 95% CI 0.78 to 2.22).[30] In the third RCT the rate of preterm birth (< 37 weeks' gestation) was higher with clindamycin cream than placebo (7/51 [14%] with clindamycin cream *v* 3/50 [6%] with placebo; RR 2.3, 95% CI 0.6 to 8.4).[31] In the fourth RCT the rate of preterm birth (< 37 weeks' gestation) was slightly higher with clindamycin cream than placebo (9/187 [5%] with clindamycin cream *v* 7/188 [4%] with placebo; RR 1.29, 95% CI 0.49 to 3.40).[32] One large RCT (1953 women) found significantly more adverse effects with oral metronidazole versus placebo, particularly gastrointestinal symptoms (20.0% with metronidazole *v* 7.5% with placebo; CI not provided).[33]

Comment: The average quality of the trials in the systematic reviews was good. All trials reported loss to follow up between 1–17% for the various treatment groups.[26] In addition to an increased risk of preterm birth and neonatal sepsis with intravaginal clindamycin treatment,[27] one RCT reported an alteration of normal vaginal flora to bacterial vaginosis among women at high risk of preterm birth who were treated with clindamycin cream. The finding of two different clusters of results for oral treatment of bacterial vaginosis among high risk women may be due to differences in treatment regimens. Of the three RCTs that found a reduction of preterm birth, two used the US Centers for Disease Control and Prevention recommended treatment of bacterial vaginosis in pregnancy (metronidazole 250 mg three times daily for 7 days). The other RCT used a lower dose of metronidazole (400 mg twice daily for 2 days), but found a reduction of preterm birth in a small subgroup analysis (17 women in each group). The only RCT that found no reduction of preterm birth also used a lower dose of metronidazole (2 g single dose, repeated 48 h later). Thus, the difference in dose of treatment regimen may be responsible for differing results. To a lesser degree differences in study population (symptomatic *v* asymptomatic), timing of treatment (early *v* late gestational age), and diagnosis of bacterial vaginosis (clinical *v* Gram stain diagnosis) may also have contributed to the differing results. Because bacterial vaginosis is a condition of altered vaginal flora there is no clear cut category of diagnosis, but a continuum of flora condition. Given this uncertainty, screening of bacterial vaginosis may result in the treatment of some women who do not have bacterial vaginosis. Thus, it is important to evaluate the harm of the bacterial vaginosis treatment among women who do not have bacterial vaginosis.

QUESTION Does treating male partners prevent recurrence?

One systematic review has found that, in women with one steady male sexual partner, treating the partner with an oral antianaerobic agent does not reduce the woman's risk of recurrence.

Benefits: We found one systematic review (search date not stated, 5 RCTs) with a variety of treatment regimens and populations.[34] It found that treatment of a sexual partner with metronidazole or clindamycin had no significant effect on recurrence rates.

Harms: No harmful effects were reported.

Comment: The lack of evidence of effectiveness of both metronidazole and clindamycin suggests that anaerobes are unlikely to be the sole pathogenic agents linking bacterial vaginosis with sexual intercourse.

QUESTION What are the effects of treatment before gynaecological procedures?

In women with bacterial vaginosis who are about to undergo surgical abortion, three RCTs found a lower rate of pelvic inflammatory disease with oral or intravaginal antianaerobic treatment versus placebo but the difference was only significant in the largest RCT. We found no RCTs on the effects of treatment before other gynaecological procedures, including abdominal hysterectomy, caesarean section, or insertion of an intrauterine contraceptive device.

Benefits: We found no systematic review. **Before surgical abortion:** We found three RCTs.[35–37] The first RCT (174 women with bacterial vaginosis) compared oral metronidazole 500 mg three times daily for 10 days versus placebo in women about to undergo surgical abortion.[35] Fewer women taking metronidazole developed pelvic inflammatory disease than those taking placebo, although the result did not reach significance (3/84 [4%] with metronidazole *v* 11/90 [12%] with placebo; RR 0.29, 95% CI 0.08 to 1.01). The second RCT (1655 women) compared intravaginal clindamycin cream versus placebo in women about to undergo surgical abortion. It found that significantly less women treated with clindamycin had an infection after abortion (recalculation by *Clinical Evidence*: infection after abortion 3/181 [2%] with clindamycin cream *v* 12/181 [7%] with placebo; RR 0.25, 95% CI 0.07 to 0.87; NNT 20, 95% CI 11 to 409).[36] The third RCT compared a single dose metronidazole suppository 2 mg versus placebo.[37] It found that metronidazole suppository was associated with a non-significantly lower rate of postoperative upper genital tract infection (12/142 [8%] with metronidazole *v* 21/131 [16%] with placebo; RR 0.52, 95% CI 0.27 to 1.02). **Before gynaecological surgery:** Bacterial vaginosis is associated with an increased risk of endometritis after caesarean section and vaginal cuff cellulitis after abdominal hysterectomy,[11,38] but we found no RCTs of antianaerobic treatment in women before such surgery. **Before insertion of an intrauterine contraceptive device:** Bacterial vaginosis has been associated with pelvic inflammatory disease (see pelvic inflammatory disease, p 1649) in women using intrauterine contraceptive devices,[3] but we found no RCTs of antianaerobic treatment in women with bacterial vaginosis before insertion of these devices.

Harms: The RCTs provided no information on adverse effects.[35]

Comment: None.

Substantive changes

Effects of treating pregnant women New systematic review;[25] found no significant difference in the risk of preterm delivery.

REFERENCES

1. Barbone F, Austin H, Louv WC, et al. A follow-up study of methods of contraception, sexual activity, and rates of trichomoniasis, candidiasis, and bacterial vaginosis. *Am J Obstet Gynecol* 1990;163:510–514.
2. Mead PB. Epidemiology of bacterial vaginosis. *Am J Obstet Gynecol* 1993;169:446–449.
3. Avonts D, Sercu M, Heyerick P, et al. Incidence of uncomplicated genital infections in women using oral contraception or an intrauterine device: a prospective study. *Sex Transm Dis* 1990;17:23–29.
4. Berger BJ, Kolton S, Zenilman JM, et al. Bacterial vaginosis in lesbians: a sexually transmitted disease. *Clin Infect Dis* 1995;21:1402–1405.
5. Hawes SE, Hillier SL, Benedetti J, et al. Hydrogen peroxide-producing lactobacilli and acquisition of vaginal infections. *J Infect Dis* 1996;174:1058–1063.
6. Hillier SL, Nugent RP, Eschenbach DA, et al. Association between bacterial vaginosis and preterm delivery of a low-birth-weight infant. *N Engl J Med* 1995;333:1737–1742.
7. Schwebke JR, Morgan SC, Weiss HL. The use of sequential self obtained vaginal smears for detecting changes in the vaginal flora. *Sex Transm Dis* 1997;24:236–239.
8. Flynn CA, Helwig AL, Meurer LN. Bacterial vaginosis in pregnancy and the risk of prematurity: a meta-analysis. *J Fam Pract* 1999;48:885–892.
9. Hillier SL, Martius J, Krohn MA, et al. Case-control study of chorioamnionic infection and chorioamnionitis in prematurity. *N Engl J Med* 1988;319:972–975.
10. Newton ER, Prihoda TJ, Gibbs RS. A clinical and microbiologic analysis of risk factors for puerperal endometritis. *Obstet Gynecol* 1990;75:403–406.
11. Watts D, Krohn M, Hillier S, et al. Bacterial vaginosis as a risk factor for postcesarean endometritis. *Obstet Gynecol* 1990;75:52–58.
12. McDonald HM, O'Loughlin JA, Vigneswaran R, et al. Impact of metronidazole therapy on preterm birth in women with bacterial vaginosis flora (*Gardnerella vaginalis*): a randomised, placebo controlled trial. *Br J Obstet Gynaecol* 1997;104:1391–1397.
13. Schmid G, Markowitz L, Joesoef R, et al. Bacterial vaginosis and HIV infection [editorial]. *Sex Transm Infect* 2000;76:3–4.
14. Joesoef MR, Schmid GP. Bacterial vaginosis: review of treatment options and potential clinical indications for therapy. *Clin Infect Dis* 1999;28(suppl 1):72–79. Search date 1996; primary sources Medline, hand searches of text books about sexually transmitted diseases, meeting abstracts, and contact with drug manufacturers.
15. Paavonen J, Mangioni C, Martin MA, et al. Vaginal clindamycin and oral metronidazole for bacterial vaginosis: a randomized trial. *Obstet Gynecol* 2000;96:256–260.
16. Greaves WL, Chungafung J, Morris B, et al. Clindamycin versus metronidazole in the treatment of bacterial vaginosis. *Obstet Gynecol* 1988;72:799–802.
17. Aubert JM, Oliete S, Leira J. Treatment of bacterial vaginosis: clindamycin versus metronidazol. *Prog Obst Gin* 1994;37:287–292.
18. Livengood CH, Soper DE, Sheehan KL, et al. Comparison of once daily and twice daily dosing of 0.75% metronidazole gel in the treatment of bacterial vaginosis. *Sex Transm Dis* 1999;26:137–142.
19. Sobel J, Peipert JF, McGregor JA, et al. Efficacy of clindamycin vaginal ovule (3-day treatment) versus clindamycin vaginal cream (7-day treatment) in bacterial vaginosis. *Infect Dis Obstet Gynecol* 2001;9:9–15.
20. Colli E, Landoni M, Parazzini F. Treatment of male partners and recurrence of bacterial vaginosis: a randomised trial. *Genitourin Med* 1997;73:267–270.
21. Sobel JD, Schmitt C, Meriwether C. Long-term follow-up of patients with bacterial vaginosis treated with oral metronidazole and topical clindamycin. *J Infect Dis* 1993;167:783–784.
22. Trexler MF, Fraser TG, Jones MP. Fulminant pseudomembranous colitis caused by clindamycin phosphate vaginal cream. *Am J Gastroenterol* 1997;92:2112–2113.

23. Hillier SL, Lipinski C, Briselden AM, et al. Efficacy of intravaginal 0.75% metronidazole gel for the treatment of bacterial vaginosis. *Obstet Gynecol* 1993;81:963–967.
24. Schmitt C, Sobel JD, Meriwether C. Bacterial vaginosis: treatment with clindamycin cream versus oral metronidazole. *Obstet Gynecol* 1992;79:1020–1023.
25. Guise J-M, Mahon SM, Aickin M, et al. Screening for bacterial vaginosis in pregnancy. *Am J Prevent Med* 2001;20:62–72. Search date 1999; primary sources Medline, Cochrane Controlled Trials Register, the Cochrane Library, hand searches of reference lists of selected publications, and personal contact with national experts.
26. Brocklehurst P, Hannah M, McDonald H. Interventions for treating bacterial vaginosis in pregnancy. In: The Cochrane Library, Issue 1, 2002. Oxford: Update Software. Search date not stated; primary sources Cochrane Pregnancy and Childbirth Group Specialised Register of Controlled Trials and Cochrane Controlled Trials Register.
27. Vermeulen GM, Bruinse HW. Prophylactic administration of clindamycin 2% vaginal cream to reduce the incidence of spontaneous preterm birth in women with an increased recurrence risk: a randomized placebo-controlled double-blind trial. *Br J Obstet Gynaecol* 1999;106:652–657.
28. Hauth JC, Goldenberg RL, Andrews WW, et al. Reduced incidence of preterm delivery with metronidazole and erythromycin in women with bacterial vaginosis. *N Engl J Med* 1995;333:1732–1736.
29. McGregor JA, French JI, Jones W, et al. Bacterial vaginosis is associated with prematurity and vaginal fluid mucinase and sialidase: results of a controlled trial of topical clindamycin cream. *Am J Obstet Gynecol* 1994;170:1048–1059.
30. Joesoef MR, Hillier SL, Wiknjosastro G, et al. Intravaginal clindamycin treatment for bacterial vaginosis: effect on preterm delivery and low birth weight. *Am J Obstet Gynecol* 1995;173:1527–1531.
31. Kurkinen-Raty M, Vuopala S, Koskela M, et al. A randomised controlled trial of vaginal clindamycin for early pregnancy bacterial vaginosis. *BJOG* 2000;107:1427–1432.
32. Kekki M, Kurki T, Pelkonen J, et al. Vaginal clindamycin in preventing preterm birth and peripartal infections in asymptomatic women with bacterial vaginosis: a randomized, controlled trial. *Obstet Gynecol* 2001;97:643–648.
33. Carey JC, Klebanoff MA, Hauth JC, et al. Metronidazole to prevent preterm delivery in pregnant women with asymptomatic bacterial vaginosis. *N Engl J Med* 2000;342:534–540.
34. Hamrick M, Chambliss ML. Bacterial vaginosis and treatment of sexual partners. *Arch Fam Med* 2000;9:647–648. Search date not stated; primary sources Medline and the Cochrane Library.
35. Larsson PG, Platz-Christensen JJ, Thejls H, et al. Incidence of pelvic inflammatory disease after first-trimester legal abortion in women with bacterial vaginosis after treatment with metronidazole: a double-blind, randomized study. *Am J Obstet Gynecol* 1992;166:100–103.
36. Larsson PG, Platz-Christensen JJ, Dalaker K, et al. Treatment with 2% clindamycin vaginal cream prior to first trimester surgical abortion to reduce signs of postoperative infection: a prospective, double-blinded, placebo-controlled, multicenter study. *Acta Obstet Gynecol Scand* 2000;79:390–396.
37. Crowley T, Low N, Turner A, et al. Antibiotic prophylaxis to prevent post-abortal upper genital tract infection in women with bacterial vaginosis: randomised controlled trial. *BJOG* 2001;108:396–402.
38. Soper DE, Bump RC, Hurt WG. Bacterial vaginosis and trichomoniasis vaginitis are risk factors for cuff cellulitis after abdominal hysterectomy. *Am J Obstet Gynecol* 1990;163:1016–1021.

M Joesoef
Medical Epidemiologist
National Center for HIV STD
and TB Prevention
Atlanta
USA

George Schmid
Medical Epidemiologist
World Health Organization
Geneva
Switzerland

Competing interests: None declared.

Genital chlamydial infection

Search date January 2002

Nicola Low and Frances Cowan

QUESTIONS

INTERVENTIONS

Key Messages

- Short term microbiological cure is the outcome used in most RCTs, but this may not mean eradication of *Chlamydia trachomatis*. Long term cure rates have not been studied extensively because of high default rates and difficulty in distinguishing persistent infection from reinfection due to re-exposure.

In men and non-pregnant women

- **Azithromycin (single dose)** One systematic review and meta-analysis of short term RCTs found no significant difference in cure rate between a single dose of azithromycin versus a 7 day course of doxycycline.
- **Ciprofloxacin (multiple dose)** Two RCTs found that ciprofloxacin cured 63–92% of people. Meta-analysis found that ciprofloxacin versus doxycycline significantly increased microbiological failure.
- **Doxycycline, tetracycline, rosaramicin (multiple dose)** Small RCTs with short term follow up and high withdrawal rates comparing different antibiotic regimens have found that multiple dose regimens of tetracyclines (doxycycline, tetracycline) and macrolides (rosaramicin) achieve micrological cure in at least 95% of people with genital chlamydia.

- **Erythromycin (multiple dose regimens)** Three small RCTs found that erythromycin achieved microbiological cure in 77–100% of people, with the highest cure rate with a 2 g versus a 1 g daily dose.
- **Ofloxacin, trovafloxacin, minocycline, lymecycline, clarithromycin, ampicillin, rifampicin (multiple dose regimens)** We found limited evidence on the effects of these regimens.

In pregnant women

- **Erythromycin, amoxicillin (multiple dose regimens)** Two systematic reviews have found that both amoxicillin and erythromycin versus placebo significantly increase microbiological cure.
- **Azithromycin (single *v* multiple dose antibiotics)** One systematic review has found that a single dose of azithromycin versus a 7 day course of erythromycin significantly increases microbiological cure.
- **Clindamycin (multiple dose)** One small RCT has found no significant difference in cure between clindamycin versus erythromycin.

DEFINITION Uncomplicated genital chlamydia is a sexually transmitted infection of the urethra in men, and of the endocervix, urethra, or both, in women, that has not ascended to the upper genital tract. Infection is asymptomatic in up to 80% of women, but may cause non-specific symptoms, including vaginal discharge and intermenstrual bleeding. Infection in men causes urethral discharge and urethral irritation or dysuria, but may also be asymptomatic in up to half of cases.[1]

INCIDENCE/ PREVALENCE Genital chlamydia is the commonest bacterial sexually transmitted infection in developed countries. In the USA, over 642 000 cases of chlamydia were reported in the year 2000.[2] The prevalence of uncomplicated genital chlamydia in women attending general practice surgeries in the UK is reported to be 3–5%.[3] Prevalence is highest in young adults. Reported rates in 16–19 year old women are about 940/100 000 in the UK,[4] 1000/100 000 in Sweden,[1] and 2500/100 000 in the USA.[5]

AETIOLOGY/ RISK FACTORS Infection is caused by the bacterium *C trachomatis* serotypes D–K. It is transmitted primarily through sexual intercourse.

PROGNOSIS In women, untreated chlamydial infection that ascends to the upper genital tract causes pelvic inflammatory disease in an estimated 30–40% of women (see pelvic inflammatory disease, p 1649).[6] Tubal infertility has been found to occur in about 11% of women after a single episode of pelvic inflammatory disease, and the risk of ectopic pregnancy is increased six- to sevenfold.[7] Ascending infection in men causes epididymitis, but evidence that this causes male infertility is limited.[8] Maternal to infant transmission can lead to neonatal conjunctivitis and pneumonitis in 30–40% of cases.[1] Chlamydia may coexist with other genital infections and may facilitate transmission and acquisition of HIV infection.[1] Untreated chlamydial infection persists symptomatically in most women for at least 60 days and for a shorter period in men.[9] Spontaneous remission also occurs but data are insufficient to determine the rate of clearance.[9]

AIMS To eradicate *C trachomatis*; to prevent the development of upper genital tract infection; and to prevent further sexual transmission, with minimal adverse effects of treatment.

OUTCOMES Microbiological cure rate (calculated as the percentage of people attending a follow up visit at least 1 week after the end of antibiotic treatment who had a negative test for *C trachomatis*); adverse effects of treatment, including effects on the fetus; pelvic inflammatory disease; infertility. Short term microbiological cure may not mean eradication of *C trachomatis* because of the organism's prolonged life cycle. Some studies using DNA amplification techniques found that persistence of infection after successful antibiotic treatment does not appear to occur in people followed for up to 20 weeks[9] but long term cure rates have not been studied extensively because of high default rates and difficulty in distinguishing persistent infection from reinfection owing to re-exposure.

METHODS *Clinical Evidence* update search and appraisal January 2002. All relevant systematic reviews and masked clinical RCTs were included. We present the range of cure rates (with exact binomial CIs) or, if there was no evidence of statistical heterogeneity between RCTs, the summary cure rate (95% CIs) weighted by the standard error. Summary rates do not include cure rates of 100% because the standard error cannot be computed if there are no treatment failures. Where two or more RCTs compared the same regimens with no evidence of statistical heterogeneity, we used a fixed effects meta-analysis to calculate the summary odds ratio with 95% confidence intervals. Trial quality was assessed in terms of randomisation, blinding, and numbers of withdrawals from analysis.[10] RCTs with methodological limitations have been included but relevant problems are mentioned in the text. **Categorising interventions:** We considered a regimen beneficial if the summary cure rate from two or more RCTs was 95% or greater, as previously suggested,[11] and if the lower confidence limit was also above 90%. We found insufficient data to differentiate reinfections from persistent infections. We considered regimens to be likely (or unlikely) to be beneficial on the basis of positive (or negative) results from two or more RCTs, and of unknown effectiveness if there was only one RCT or if results were conflicting.

QUESTION **What are the effects of antibiotic treatment for men and non-pregnant women with uncomplicated genital chlamydial infection?**

OPTION **MULTIPLE DOSE ANTIBIOTICS VERSUS OTHER MULTIPLE DOSE ANTIBIOTICS**

Small RCTs, with short term follow up and high withdrawal rates, have found that tetracyclines (doxycycline and tetracycline) and macrolides (rosaramicin) achieve microbiological cure in 95% or more cases of genital chlamydia. We found no differences in microbiological cure rates between men and women or between those with proven or presumed infection. We found limited evidence on the effectiveness of other macrolides, quinolones, and penicillins.

Benefits: We found no systematic review. We found 22 RCTs reported to be double blind or with blinded outcome assessment comparing 19 different antibiotic regimens (see web extra table A at www.clinicalevidence.com).[12–33] Results were similar in men and women and in populations with proven and presumed infection, so data were combined. **Doxycycline:** We found 11 RCTs (1434 men and women) comparing doxycycline with another antibiotic.[12–14,16–23] The cure rate was 100% in six RCTs and the weighted average 98% (95% CI 96% to 99%) in the other five. We found no RCTs comparing different regimens for doxycycline, but the most frequent schedule (in 6 RCTs) was 100 mg twice daily for 7 days. **Tetracycline:** The summary cure rate in four RCTs (201 men and women) comparing tetracycline hydrochloride (500 mg 4 times daily for 7 days) versus another antibiotic was 97% (95% CI 94% to 99%).[24–27] A *Clinical Evidence* meta-analysis of three RCTs[25–27] found that rates of treatment failure with rosaramicin compared with tetracycline were similar (OR 1.57, 95% CI 0.51 to 4.7; see web extra figure A at www.clinicalevidence.com). **Erythromycin:** Cure rates with erythromycin stearate 1 g daily for 7 days (3 RCTs, 191 people) ranged from 77–95%,[30–32] and with erythromycin 2 g daily for 7 days (2 RCTs, 40 people) from 94–100%.[29,32] **Ciprofloxacin:** In two RCTs (190 men and women) the cure rate for ciprofloxacin ranged from 63–92%.[20,21] A meta-analysis by *Clinical Evidence* found that failure of microbiological cure was more frequent with ciprofloxacin than doxycycline (OR 5.0, 95% CI 1.2 to 10.0). A variety of other antibiotics were studied in single RCTs (see web extra table A at www.clinicalevidence.com). No trial measured the effect of antibiotics on pelvic inflammatory disease or infertility.

Harms: Reported adverse effects varied widely between RCTs but were mostly gastrointestinal (see web extra table A at www.clinicalevidence.com).

Comment: Most RCTs were conducted in sexually transmitted diseases clinics, where follow up is difficult; in 7 of 14 RCTs with available data, more than 15% of randomised participants were not included in the analysis.[15,22,29–33] Most RCTs were small (3 had fewer than 40 people with chlamydia)[16,24,29] and many antibiotic regimens were compared so it is difficult to draw conclusions about relative efficacy. Only five RCTs reported that sexual partners of participants were offered treatment. Amoxicillin (amoxycillin) and ampicillin have not been adequately assessed in the treatment of genital chlamydia infection (see web extra table A at www.clinicalevidence.com) because *in vitro* studies suggest that amoxicillin does not eradicate *C trachomatis*,[34] raising the concern that infection may persist and recrudesce *in vivo*.

OPTION SINGLE DOSE VERSUS DIFFERENT MULTIPLE DOSE ANTIBIOTICS

One systematic review and meta-analysis of short term RCTs has found that a single dose of azithromycin may be as effective in achieving microbiological cure of *C trachomatis* as a 7 day course of doxycycline. Rates of adverse effects were similar.

Benefits: We found one systematic review (search date 1996, 9 blinded and unblinded RCTs, 1800 people) comparing azithromycin (1 g as a single dose) versus doxycycline (100 mg twice daily for 7 days) in people with proven or presumed genital chlamydia.[35] Data about laboratory diagnosed infection were available for five RCTs (554 men and women). Cure rates for azithromycin ranged from 90–100% and for doxycycline from 93–100%. Microbiological failure tended to be more frequent with azithromycin than with doxycycline, but this did not reach statistical significance (AR 22/301 *v* 10/253; OR recalculated from data in the paper 1.8, 95% CI 0.9 to 3.9; P = 0.11).

Harms: Short term adverse effects of both azithromycin and doxycycline were reported to be mild.

Comment: Azithromycin can be given in a single dose as directly observed therapy. More comparisons of azithromycin and doxycycline are needed to rule out a clinically important difference between them.

QUESTION What are the effects of treatment for pregnant women with uncomplicated genital chlamydial infection?

OPTION MULTIPLE DOSE ANTIBIOTICS VERSUS OTHER MULTIPLE DOSE ANTIBIOTICS

Two systematic reviews have found that both amoxicillin and erythromycin are likely to be effective in achieving microbiological cure of genital chlamydia in pregnant women. One small RCT has found that clindamycin and erythromycin have a similar effect on cure rates.

Benefits: We found one systematic review (search date 1998, 11 blinded and unblinded RCTs, 1449 people).[36] **Erythromycin and amoxicillin:** It found high rates of microbiological cure with both drugs but there was a non-significant higher rate of cure with amoxicillin (cure rates 182/199 [91%] with amoxicillin 500 mg 3 times daily for 7 days *v* 163/191 [85%] with erythromycin 500 mg 4 times daily for 7 days; OR for failure of cure with amoxicillin compared with erythromycin 0.54, 95% CI 0.28 to 1.02), and treatment with any antibiotic was better than placebo (OR for failure of cure 0.06, 95% CI 0.03 to 0.12). **Clindamycin:** One small RCT found no significant difference in cure rates between clindamycin and erythromycin (38/41 [93%] *v* 31/37 [84%]; RR for failure of cure 0.45, 95% CI 0.12 to 1.7).

Harms: Rates of adverse effects were similar for clindamycin and erythromycin, but adverse effects sufficient to stop treatment were less frequent with amoxicillin than erythromycin (OR 0.16, 95% CI 0.09 to 0.30). None of the RCTs gave information on adverse clinical outcomes in the offspring.

Comment: We found no long term follow up data.

OPTION SINGLE DOSE VERSUS DIFFERENT MULTIPLE DOSE ANTIBIOTICS

One systematic review has found that, in pregnant women, a single dose of azithromycin is as effective in achieving microbiological cure of *C trachomatis* as a 7 day course of erythromycin.

Benefits: We found one systematic review (search date 1998, 4 non-blinded RCTs, 290 pregnant women) comparing a single dose of azithromycin (1 g) versus erythromycin (500 mg 4 times daily) for 7 days.[36] At first follow up visit, failure of microbiological cure was less frequent with azithromycin than erythromycin (11/145 [8%] *v* 27/145 [19%]; OR 0.38, 95% CI 0.19 to 0.74).[36] There was no significant difference in the rate of premature delivery (OR 0.73, 95% CI 0.24 to 2.20).

Harms: The RCTs found that azithromycin was associated with fewer adverse effects. Fetal anomaly was reported in one infant in each group.[36] Effects of azithromycin in pregnancy have not been extensively studied.

Comment: None.

REFERENCES

1. Holmes KK, Sparling PF, M rdh PA, et al, eds. *Sexually transmitted diseases*. 3rd ed. New York: McGraw Hill Inc, 1999.
2. Anonymous. Notifiable diseases/deaths in selected cities weekly information. *MMR Morb Mortal Wkly Rep* 2001;49:1168.
3. Stokes T. Screening for chlamydia in general practice: a literature review and summary of the evidence [review]. *J Public Health Med* 1997;19:222–232.
4. http://www.phls.co.uk/topics_az/hiv_and_sti/sti-chlamydia/epidemiology/epidemiology.htm (last accessed 16 September 2002).
5. US Department of Health and Human Services, Public Health Service. *Sexually Transmitted Disease Surveillance, 1999*. Atlanta: Centers for Disease Control and Prevention (CDC), September 2000.
6. Cates W Jr, Rolfs RT Jr, Aral SO. Sexually transmitted diseases, pelvic inflammatory disease, and infertility: an epidemiologic update. *Epidemiol Rev* 1990;12:199–220.
7. Weström L, Bengtsson LP, M rdh PA. Incidence, trends, and risks of ectopic pregnancy in a population of women. *BMJ* 1981;282:15–18.
8. Ness RB, Markovic N, Carlson CL, et al. Do men become infertile after having sexually transmitted urethritis? An epidemiologic examination [review]. *Fertil Steril* 1997;68:205–213.
9. Golden MR, Schillinger JA, Markowitz L, et al. Duration of untreated genital infections with *Chlamydia trachomatis*. A review of the literature. *Sex Transm Dis 2000;27:329–337.*
10. Chalmers I, Adams M, Dickersin K, et al. A cohort study of summary reports of controlled trials. *JAMA* 1990;263:1401–1405.
11. Clinical Effectiveness Group. National guideline for the management of *Chlamydia trachomatis* genital tract infection. *Sex Transm Infect* 1999;75(Suppl 1):4–8.
12. Nilsen A, Halsos A, Johansen A, et al. A double blind study of single dose azithromycin and doxycycline in the treatment of chlamydial urethritis in males. *Genitourin Med* 1992;68:325–327.
13. Steingr msson , lafsson JH, Thórarinsson H, et al. Single dose azithromycin treatment of gonorrhea and infections caused by *C trachomatis* and *U urealyticum* in men. *Sex Transm Dis* 1994;21:43–46.
14. Stamm WE, Hicks CB, Martin DH, et al. Azithromycin for empirical treatment of the nongonococcal urethritis syndrome in men. A randomized double-blind study. *JAMA* 1995;274:545–549.
15. Brihmer C, M rdh PA, Kallings I, et al. Efficacy and safety of azithromycin versus lymecycline in the treatment of genital chlamydial infections in women. *Scand J Infect Dis* 1996;28:451–454.
16. Stein GE, Mummaw NL, Havlichek DH. A preliminary study of clarithromycin versus doxycycline in the treatment of nongonococcal urethritis and mucopurulent cervicitis. *Pharmacotherapy* 1995;15:727–731.
17. Romanowski B, Talbot H, Stadnyk M, et al. Minocycline compared with doxycycline in the treatment of nongonococcal urethritis and mucopurulent cervicitis. *Ann Intern Med* 1993;119:16–22.
18. Boslego JW, Hicks CB, Greenup R, et al. A prospective randomized trial of ofloxacin vs. doxycycline in the treatment of uncomplicated male urethritis. *Sex Transm Dis* 1988;15:186–191.
19. Phillips I, Dimian C, Barlow D, et al. A comparative study of two different regimens of sparfloxacin versus doxycycline in the treatment of non-gonococcal urethritis in men. *J Antimicrob Chemother* 1996;37(suppl A):123–134.
20. Hooton TM, Rogers ME, Medina TG, et al. Ciprofloxacin compared with doxycycline for nongonococcal urethritis. Ineffectiveness against *Chlamydia trachomatis* due to relapsing infection. *JAMA* 1990;264:1418–1421.
21. Jeskanen L, Karppinen L, Ingervo L, et al. Ciprofloxacin versus doxycycline in the treatment of uncomplicated urogenital *Chlamydia trachomatis* infections. A double-blind comparative study. *Scand J Infect Dis Suppl* 1989;60:62–65.
22. McCormack WM, Dalu ZA, Martin DH, et al. Double-blind comparison of trovafloxacin and doxycycline in the treatment of uncomplicated Chlamydial urethritis and cervicitis. Trovafloxacin Chlamydial Urethritis/Cervicitis Study Group. *Sex Transm Dis* 1999;26:531–536.
23. Lassus AB, Virrankoski T, Reitamo SJ, et al. Pivampicillin versus doxycycline in the treatment of chlamydial urethritis in men. *Sex Transm Dis* 1990;17:20–22.
24. Lassus A, Juvakoski T, Kanerva L. Comparison between rifampicin and tetracycline in the treatment of nongonococcal urethritis in males with special reference to *Chlamydia trachomatis*. *Eur J Sex Transm Dis* 1984;2:15–17.

25. Lassus A, Allgulander C, Juvakoski T. Efficacy of rosaramicin and tetracycline in chlamydia-positive and -negative nongonococcal urethritis. *Eur J Sex Transm Dis* 1982;1:29–31.
26. Juvakoski T, Allgulander C, Lassus A. Rosaramicin and tetracycline treatment in *Chlamydia trachomatis*-positive and -negative nongonococcal urethritis. *Sex Transm Dis* 1981;8:12–15.
27. Brunham RC, Kuo CC, Stevens CE, et al. Therapy of cervical chlamydial infection. *Ann Intern Med* 1982;97:216–219.
28. Batteiger BE, Zwickl BE, French ML, et al. Women at risk for gonorrhea: comparison of rosaramicin and ampicillin plus probenecid in the eradication of *Neisseria gonorrhoeae*, *Chlamydia trachomatis* and genital mycoplasmas. *Sex Transm Dis* 1985;12:1–4.
29. Robson HG, Shah PP, Lalonde RG, et al. Comparison of rosaramicin and erythromycin stearate for treatment of cervical infection with *Chlamydia trachomatis*. *Sex Transm Dis* 1983;10:130–134.
30. Worm AM, Hoff G, Kroon S, et al. Roxithromycin compared with erythromycin against genitourinary chlamydial infections. *Genitourin Med* 1989;65:35–38.
31. Worm AM, Avnstorp C, Petersen CS. Erythromycin against *Chlamydia trachomatis* infections. A double blind study comparing 4- and 7-day treatment in men and women. *Dan Med Bull* 1985;32:269–271.
32. Linnemann CCJ, Heaton CL, Ritchey M. Treatment of *Chlamydia trachomatis* infections: comparison of 1- and 2-g doses of erythromycin daily for seven days. *Sex Transm Dis* 1987;14:102–106.
33. Paavonen J, Kousa M, Saikku P, et al. Treatment of nongonococcal urethritis with trimethoprim-sulphadiazine and with placebo. A double-blind partner-controlled study. *Br J Venereal Dis* 1980;56:101–104.
34. Kuo CC, Wang SP, Grayston JT. Antimicrobial activity of several antibiotics and a sulfonamide against *Chlamydia trachomatis* organisms in cell culture. *Antimicrob Agents Chemother* 1977;12:80–83.
35. Chlamydial STD treatment. *Bandolier* 1996;28:4–6. Search date 1996; primary source Medline. http://www.jr2.ox.ac.uk/bandolier/band28/b28-4.html (last accessed 16 September 2002).
36. Brocklehurst P, Rooney G. Interventions for treating genital *Chlamydia trachomatis* infection in pregnancy. In: The Cochrane Library, Issue 4, 1999. Oxford: Update Software. Search date 1998; primary sources Cochrane Pregnancy and Childbirth Review Group Specialised Register of Controlled Trials, and Cochrane Controlled Trials Register.

Nicola Low
Department of Social Medicine
University of Bristol
Bristol
UK

Frances Cowan
Department of Sexually
Transmitted Diseases
Royal Free and
University College Medical School
London
UK

Competing interests: FC has received research and symposium funding from Glaxo Wellcome in relation to HSV research. NL, none declared.

Genital herpes

Search date March 2002

Anna Wald

QUESTIONS

INTERVENTIONS

*Categorisation based on observational evidence

Key Messages

Treating first and recurrent episodes of genital herpes

- **Daily oral antiviral treatment in people with high rates of recurrence** RCTs have found that daily maintenance treatment with oral antiviral agents versus placebo reduces the frequency of recurrences and improves psychosocial morbidity.
- **Oral antiviral treatment in first episodes** RCTs in people with first episode genital herpes have found that oral antiviral treatment versus placebo reduces the duration of symptoms, lesions, and viral shedding but found no significant difference in the time to recurrence or frequency of subsequent recurrences.
- **Oral antiviral treatment in people with HIV infection** RCTs found insufficient evidence on the effects of antiviral treatment in people with HIV infection.

- **Oral antiviral treatment taken at the start of a recurrence** RCTs have found that oral antiviral treatment versus placebo taken at the start of a recurrence reduces the duration of lesions, symptoms, and viral shedding in people with recurrent genital herpes. RCTs found no evidence of significant differences in effectiveness or adverse events between aciclovir, valaciclovir, and famciclovir.
- **Psychotherapy to reduce recurrence** One systematic review found insufficient evidence on the effects of psychotherapy on genital herpes recurrence.

Preventing transmission of herpes simplex virus

- **Abdominal delivery in women with genital lesions at term** We found insufficient evidence of the effects of abdominal delivery on mother to baby transmission of genital herpes. The procedure carries the risk of increased maternal morbidity and mortality.
- **Antiviral treatment to prevent transmission** We found no good evidence on the effects of antiviral treatments to prevent tranmission.
- **Condom use to prevent transmission to men** One prospective cohort study found no significant difference between male condom use versus no condom use in preventing acquisition of herpes simplex virus type 2 in men who had sexual partners with genital herpes. We found no good evidence on the effects of female condom use.
- **Daily oral antiviral treatment in late pregnancy (36 or more wks of gestation) in women with a history of genital herpes** Limited evidence from RCTs in pregnant women near term with genital herpes suggests that antiviral treatment may reduce the risk of genital herpes at term. Because women with genital lesions at term are usually offered abdominal deliveries, antiviral treatment may reduce the rate of abdominal delivery.
- **Male condom use to prevent sexual transmission to women** Limited evidence from a prospective cohort study suggested that male condom use reduced the risk of acquisition of herpes simplex virus type 2 in women who had sexual partners with herpes simplex virus 2.
- **Recombinant glycoprotein vaccine (gB2 and gD2)** One RCT found no significant difference between a glycoprotein vaccine versus placebo in acquisition rates of herpes simplex virus 2. We found no good evidence on other forms of immunisation.
- **Serological screening and counselling in late pregnancy** The highest risk of mother to baby transmission is in women newly infected with genital herpes in late pregnancy. We found insufficient evidence of the effects of interventions to prevent infection in late pregnancy (such as serological screening and counselling).

DEFINITION Genital herpes is an infection with herpes simplex virus type 1 or type 2, causing ulceration in the genital area. Herpes simplex virus infections can be defined on the basis of virological and serological findings. Types of infection include **first episode primary infection,** which is herpes simplex virus in a person without prior herpes simplex virus type 1 or type 2 antibodies; **first episode non-primary infection,** which is herpes simplex virus type 2 in a person with prior herpes simplex virus type 1 antibodies or vice versa; **first recognised recurrence,** which is herpes simplex virus type 2 (or type 1) in a person with prior herpes simplex virus type 2 (or type 1) antibodies; and **recurrent genital herpes,** which is caused by reactivation of latent herpes simplex virus.

INCIDENCE/ PREVALENCE Genital herpes infections are among the most common sexually transmitted diseases. Seroprevalence studies show that 22% of adults in the USA have herpes simplex virus type 2 antibodies.[1] A UK study found that 23% of adults attending sexual medicine clinics and 7.6% of blood donors in London had antibodies to herpes simplex virus type 2.[2] However, herpes simplex type 2 can cause other herpes infections such as ocular herpes.

AETIOLOGY/ RISK FACTORS Both herpes simplex virus type 1 and 2 can cause a first episode of genital infection, but herpes simplex virus type 2 is more likely to cause recurrent disease.[3] Most people with herpes simplex virus type 2 infection are not aware that they have genital herpes, as their symptoms are mild. However, these people can pass on the infection to sexual partners and newborns.[4,5]

PROGNOSIS Sequelae of herpes simplex virus infection include neonatal herpes simplex virus infection, opportunistic infections in immunocompromised people, recurrent genital ulceration, and psychosocial morbidity. Herpes simplex virus type 2 infection is associated with an increased risk of HIV transmission and acquisition.[6] The most common neurological complications are aseptic meningitis (reported in about a quarter of women during primary infection) and urinary retention. The absolute risk of neonatal infection is high (41%, 95% CI 26% to 56%) in babies born to women who acquire infection near the time of labour[7,8] and low (< 3%) in women with established infection, even in those who have a recurrence at term. About 15% of neonatal infections result from postnatal transmission from oral lesions.

AIMS To reduce the morbidity of the first episode; to reduce the risk of recurrent disease after a first episode; to prevent further transmission, with minimal adverse effects of treatment.

OUTCOMES Severity and duration of symptoms; healing time; duration of viral shedding; recurrence rates; psychosocial morbidity; rates of transmission; adverse effects of treatment.

METHODS *Clinical Evidence* update search and appraisal March 2002, using the terms herpes simplex virus, aciclovir, valaciclovir, famciclovir, cidofovir, trifluridine, and neonatal herpes. We also included preliminary results of clinical trials published in the abstracts of the Interscience Conference on Antimicrobial Agents and Chemotherapy and International Society for STD Research.

QUESTION **What are the effects of antiviral treatment in people with a first episode of genital herpes?**

RCTs have found that oral antiviral treatment versus placebo decreases the duration of lesions, symptoms, and viral shedding, and reduces neurological complications in people with first episode genital herpes. Limited data provide no evidence that oral antiviral treatment reduced the rate of recurrence compared with placebo. RCTs have found no evidence of a significant difference in terms of clinical outcomes of a first episode of genital herpes between aciclovir, valaciclovir, and famciclovir treatments.

Benefits: We found no systematic review. **Immediate effects:** We found five RCTs (350 men and women) of oral aciclovir for the treatment of first episode genital herpes.[9–13] The largest RCT (180 people) compared aciclovir (200 mg 5 times daily) versus placebo. It excluded 30 people from analysis (see comments below). Subgroup analysis (131 people with primary first episode genital herpes) found that aciclovir decreased the duration of viral shedding (median 2 days with aciclovir *v* 9 days with placebo), pain (5 days with aciclovir *v* 7 days with placebo), time to healing of lesions (12 days with aciclovir *v* 14 days with placebo), and reduced formation of new lesions (18% with aciclovir *v* 62% with placebo).[11] The other RCTs found similar results.[9,10,12,13] Neurological complications (aseptic meningitis and urinary retention) were also reduced. Numbers were small so no firm estimates of effectiveness were available. **Different regimens:** We found two RCTs.[14,15] The first RCT (643 otherwise healthy adults with first episode genital herpes) compared oral valaciclovir (1000 mg twice daily) versus oral aciclovir (200 mg 5 times daily) for 10 days.[14] It found no significant differences between the two medications in any clinical or virological variables. The second RCT (951 adults with first episode genital herpes) compared three different doses of oral famciclovir (125, 250, or 500 mg 3 times daily) versus oral aciclovir (200 mg 5 times daily).[15] It found no significant differences. **Recurrence rates:** A meta-analysis of two small placebo controlled RCTs (61 people with first episode genital herpes) found no significant difference in time to recurrence or frequency of recurrence between people given oral aciclovir and those given placebo.[16] **Systemic versus topical treatment:** We found no direct randomised comparisons of oral, intravenous, or topical antiviral treatment.

Harms: Adverse effects (mostly headache and nausea) were rare and frequency was similar for aciclovir, valaciclovir, famciclovir, and placebo.

Comment: Oral aciclovir has the advantage of convenience over intravenous aciclovir.[17] A non-randomised comparison of results from different trials performed at one institution suggests that systemic treatment is more effective than topical.[17] The largest RCT of immediate treatment excluded 10 people for not completing the study protocol, 12 because of suspected past infection, and 8 because HSV was not isolated.[11]

QUESTION What interventions reduce the impact of recurrence?

OPTION ANTIVIRAL TREATMENT AT THE START OF RECURRENCE

One systematic review has found that oral antiviral treatment taken at the start of a recurrence reduces the duration of lesions, symptoms, and viral shedding in people with recurrent genital herpes. RCTs found no significant differences between different antivirals.

Benefits: **Famciclovir versus placebo:** We found one systematic review (search date 1997, 1 RCT, 467 people with recurrent genital herpes) of famciclovir versus placebo.[18] The RCT found that oral famciclovir (125–500 mg twice daily) significantly reduced the duration of lesions (5 days with famciclovir *v* 4 days with placebo) and viral shedding (3 days with famciclovir *v* 2 days with placebo). **Valaciclovir versus placebo:** We found one systematic review (search date 1997, 1 RCT, 986 people) of valaciclovir versus placebo.[18] The RCT (987 people with recurrent genital herpes) found that self initiated oral valaciclovir (500 or 1000 mg twice daily) for 5 days versus placebo decreased the episode duration (4 days with valaciclovir *v* 6 days with placebo) and viral shedding (2 days with valaciclovir *v* 4 days with placebo), and increased the rate of aborted recurrences (31% with valaciclovir *v* 21% with placebo). **Aciclovir versus placebo:** We found one non-systematic review of several RCTs (more than 650 healthy adults with recurrent genital herpes).[19] These evaluated 5 days of oral aciclovir (200 mg 5 times daily or 800 mg twice daily), started at the first sign of recurrence. Aciclovir versus placebo reduced the period of viral shedding (1 with aciclovir *v* 2 days with placebo) and duration of lesions (5 with aciclovir *v* 6 days with placebo). **Valaciclovir versus aciclovir:** We found one systematic review (search date 1997, 2 RCTs, 1939 people) of oral valaciclovir versus aciclovir.[18] It found no significant difference between oral valaciclovir and aciclovir. **Famciclovir versus aciclovir:** We found one RCT (204 people with recurrent genital herpes), which found no significant difference in time to healing between oral famciclovir versus aciclovir (mean lesion healing time 5.1 days with famciclovir *v* 5.4 days with aciclovir, mean difference 0.3 days, 95% CI –0.3 to +0.8 days).[20]

Harms: Adverse effects (mostly headache and nausea) were rare, and frequency was similar for aciclovir, valaciclovir, famciclovir, and placebo.[18]

Comment: The benefit was found to be greater if the person with recurrent herpes initiated treatment at the first symptom or sign of a recurrence.[21] People can learn to recognise recurrences early on and should have an adequate supply of medication at home.

OPTION DAILY MAINTENANCE ANTIVIRAL TREATMENT

One systematic review of famciclovir and valaciclovir and one non-systematic review and one large subsequent RCT of aciclovir have found that daily maintenance treatment with oral antiviral agents versus placebo reduces the frequency of recurrences with genital herpes. One large RCT found that daily maintenance treatment with aciclovir improves psychosocial morbidity; one small RCT found that daily maintenance treatment with aciclovir reduces viral shedding.

Benefits: **Recurrence rates:** We found one systematic review of famciclovir and valaciclovir (search date 1997, 4 placebo controlled RCTs).[18] Two RCTs in the review evaluated treatment for one year. The first RCT (1479 people with frequently recurring genital herpes) compared valaciclovir 250 mg (4 times a day), valaciclovir 250 mg (2 times a day), valaciclovir 500 mg (4 times a day), valaciclovir 1000 mg (4 times a day), aciclovir 400 mg (2 times a day), versus placebo. It found freedom from recurrence in 48–50% of people who received valaciclovir (250 mg 2 times a day, or 1000 mg 4 times a day), and aciclovir (400 mg 2 times a day), 40% of people who received valaciclovir (500 mg 4 times daily), 22% who received valaciclovir (250 mg 4 times daily) versus 5% who received placebo.[22] The second RCT (455 people with frequently recurring genital herpes) compared famciclovir (250 mg 2 times a day), famciclovir (125 mg 3 times a day), famciclovir (250 mg 3 times a day) versus placebo. It found median time to first recurrence of 11 months with famciclovir (250 mg twice daily), 10 months with famciclovir (250 mg 3 times a day), 8 months with famciclovir (125 mg 3 times a day), versus 1.5 months with placebo.[23] One non-systematic review identified small two RCTs of aciclovir versus placebo for one year or more (107 people with a history of frequent recurrence ≥6/year).[19] The first RCT (32 people) of aciclovir (800 mg daily) versus placebo found a significantly greater proportion recurrence free with aciclovir over 2 years (5/18 [28%] with aciclovir *v* 0/14 [0%] with placebo; ARR 28%, 95% CI 1% to 51%). The second RCT compared aciclovir (400 mg, 2 times a day) versus placebo found a significantly greater proportion recurrence free with aciclovir over one year (21/48 [44%] with aciclovir *v* 0/28 [0%] with placebo; ARR 44%, 95% CI 26% to 56%). We found one subsequent double blind, placebo controlled RCT (1146 adults), which found significantly fewer recurrences during the first year with aciclovir (1.7 with aciclovir *v* 12.5 with placebo; $P < 0.0001$).[24] Of 210 adults in the trial who completed 5 years of continuous treatment with aciclovir (400 mg twice daily), 53–70% were free of recurrence each year. **Viral shedding:** We found one RCT (34 women with recently acquired genital herpes simplex virus type 2 infection) of daily maintenance with aciclovir treatment versus placebo that assessed viral shedding in women.[25] Women obtained swabs for viral cultures daily for 70 days while receiving aciclovir (400 mg twice daily) or placebo. It found that aciclovir reduced viral shedding by 95% on days with reported lesions and by 94% on days without lesions. **Psychosocial morbidity:** We found one RCT (1479 people) that evaluated the effect of daily oral antiviral treatment on a genital herpes quality of life scale.[26] People receiving daily aciclovir or valaciclovir had significantly greater mean improvements from baseline than those receiving placebo.[27]

Harms: Daily treatment with aciclovir, famciclovir, and valaciclovir was well tolerated.[28] People taking aciclovir were followed for up to 7 years, and those taking famciclovir and valaciclovir for up to 1 year. Nausea and headache were infrequent, and participants rarely discontinued treatment because of adverse effects. We found no studies evaluating whether daily maintenance treatment increases high risk sexual behaviour. We found no evidence that daily treatment with aciclovir results in emergence of aciclovir resistant herpes simplex virus during or after stopping treatment in healthy adults.[28]

Comment: Viral shedding is an intermediate outcome, but may be important to people with herpes as it reflects the risk of transmitting infection.

OPTION PSYCHOTHERAPY

One systematic review found that the effects of psychotherapy on the rate of genital herpes recurrence have not yet been adequately studied.

Benefits: We found one systematic review (search date 1991), which identified six poor quality studies of psychotherapeutic interventions in 69 people (4 studies had < 10 participants).[29] Interventions varied from hypnotherapy and progressive muscle relaxation to cognitive therapy and multifaceted intervention. The largest RCT (31 people with > 4 recurrences a year) compared psychosocial intervention, versus social support, versus waiting list. Participants receiving psychosocial intervention had significantly lower recurrence rates (6 recurrences/year) as compared with the pretreatment frequency (11/year) and with the other groups (11/year).

Harms: No adverse effects were noted.[29]

Comment: Small numbers of people, inadequate controls, and subjective and retrospective assessment of recurrence frequency at baseline limit the usefulness of these studies.[29] Controlled studies that include prospective clinical evaluation of disease activity are needed.

QUESTION What are the effects of interventions to prevent transmission of herpes simplex virus?

OPTION CONDOMS

Limited evidence from one prospective cohort study suggested that male condom use may decrease the risk of sexual transmission of herpes simplex virus 2 among women who have a sexual partner disconcordant for herpes simplex virus 2. However, no benefit was found among men.

Benefits: We found no RCTs. In a prospective cohort study (528 couples discordant for herpes simplex virus [HSV] type 2 infection and followed for 18 months), the male use of condoms in more than 25% of sexual acts was associated with a lower risk of HSV-2 acquisition among women (adjusted HR 0.09, 95% CI 0.01 to 0.67) but not among men (adjusted HR 2.02, 95% CI 0.32 to 12.5).[30] Only 61% of couples ever used condoms during the study and only 8% used them consistently. One person acquired HSV-2 despite consistent condom use.

Harms: None reported.

Comment: Controlled trials of condoms for prevention of HSV-2 transmission are impractical. Even with routine counselling, many couples do not regularly use condoms. Trials of different methods of advising people to use condoms or providing condoms could be performed.

OPTION ANTIVIRAL TREATMENT

We found no good evidence on the effects of antiviral treatments.

Benefits: We found no RCTs with transmission rates as outcomes. However, RCTs have shown that daily antiviral treatment decreases the frequency of clinical and subclinical viral shedding (see text, p 1611).

Harms: As for individual interventions (see harms of daily maintenance antiviral treatment, p 1613).

Comment: None.

OPTION IMMUNISATION

One RCT found no significant difference between a glycoprotein vaccine versus placebo in acquisition of genital herpes.

Benefits: We found one double blind RCT (2393 HSV-2 and HIV seronegative people) of recombinant glycoprotein vaccine (gB2 and gD2) versus placebo.[31] It found no significant difference in vaccine efficacy (4.6 cases per 100 person years with placebo v 4.2 cases per 100 person years with glycoprotein vaccine; $P = 0.58$). It found no significant difference in the duration of initial genital herpes, or the frequency of subsequent recurrences in people who acquired genital HSV infection.

Harms: We found no good evidence on harms.

Comment: None.

OPTION ABDOMINAL DELIVERY TO PREVENT NEONATAL HERPES

We found insufficient evidence for the effect of abdominal delivery on the risk of neonatal herpes. The procedure carries a risk of increased maternal morbidity and mortality.

Benefits: We found no systematic review and no RCTs that assessed the effects of abdominal delivery on the risk of mother to child transmission of herpes simplex virus. In the Netherlands, women with recurrent genital herpes at delivery have been allowed vaginal birth since 1987. This policy has not resulted in an increase in neonatal herpes: 26 cases from 1981–1986 and 19 cases from 1987–1991.[8]

Harms: Abdominal delivery is associated with significant maternal morbidity and mortality. A study pooling data from different studies estimated that, for every two neonatal deaths from herpes simplex virus infection prevented by abdominal delivery, one maternal death may be caused.[32]

Comment: Countries vary in their approach to obstetric management of women with recurrent genital herpes at term. In the USA and the UK, these women are advised to undergo abdominal delivery, with its attendant risks to the mother. The absolute risk of neonatal infection is high (AR 41%, 95% CI 26% to 56%) in babies born to women who acquired infection near the time of labour[7,8] and low (AR < 3%) in women with established infection, even in those who have recurrence at term. Most women who acquired infection toward the end of pregnancy are undiagnosed, and most cases of neonatal herpes simplex virus infection are acquired from women without a history of genital herpes. The available evidence suggests that efforts to prevent neonatal herpes simplex virus infection should focus on preventing the acquisition of infection in late pregnancy.

OPTION ANTIVIRAL TREATMENT DURING PREGNANCY

We found limited evidence from one systematic review suggesting that aciclovir reduces the rate of genital lesions at term in women with first or recurrent episodes of genital herpes simplex virus during pregnancy. We found that adverse effects have not been adequately studied.

Benefits: We found one systematic review (search date 1996, 2 RCTs and 1 controlled study, 210 pregnant women near term with genital herpes),[8,33–35] of daily aciclovir versus placebo. The trials differed in terms of the dose and duration of aciclovir and the populations enrolled. Abdominal delivery was performed in women with genital lesions at term. All three studies found lower rates of abdominal delivery in women treated with aciclovir, although in two studies the effect was not significant (AR of abdominal delivery 4/21 [19%] in women receiving aciclovir *v* 10/25 [40%] in women receiving placebo, RR 0.48, 95% CI 0.17 to 1.30;[33] AR of abdominal delivery 6/46 [13%] in women receiving aciclovir *v* 15/46 [33%] in women receiving no treatment, RR 0.4, 95% CI 0.17 to 0.94, NNT 6, 95% CI 3 to 43;[35] and AR of abdominal delivery 7/31 [23%] in women receiving aciclovir *v* 10/32 [31%] in women receiving placebo, RR 0.72, 95% CI 0.32 to 1.66).[34]

Harms: No adverse effects for women or newborns were reported, but the number of women was small. Rare adverse events, such as an increase in asymptomatic viral shedding or aciclovir related obstructive uropathy in the newborns, would be difficult to detect.

Comment: None.

OPTION SEROLOGICAL SCREENING AND COUNSELLING TO PREVENT ACQUISITION OF HERPES SIMPLEX VIRUS DURING PREGNANCY

We found insufficient evidence on the effects of serological screening and counselling during pregnancy on infection rates.

Benefits: We found no systematic review or RCTs that assessed either serological screening with type specific assays to identify women at risk for acquisition of herpes simplex virus infection in late pregnancy, or counselling to avoid genital–genital and oral–genital contact in late pregnancy.

Harms: We found insufficient evidence.

Comment: None.

QUESTION What are the effects of treatments in people with genital herpes and HIV infection?

OPTION ANTIVIRAL TREATMENTS

We found limited evidence of the effect of antiviral treatment for genital herpes in people immunocompromised with HIV infection. However, evidence from other settings suggests that antivirals may be effective treatment of genital herpes in immunocompromised people.

Benefits: We found no systematic review and no RCTs on the treatment of first episode genital herpes in people with HIV infection. **Treatment of recurrence:** We found two RCTs.[36,37] One RCT (193 people on stable antiretroviral treatment) compared famciclovir (500 mg twice daily) versus aciclovir (400 mg 5 times daily) for 1 week.[36] It found no difference between the two drugs in mucocutaneous recurrence of herpes simplex virus. The other RCT (467 people) compared valaciclovir (1 g twice daily) versus aciclovir (200 mg 5 times daily) for 5 days.[37] It found no significant differences between the two drugs. **Prevention of recurrence:** We found two RCTs.[37,38] One crossover RCT (48 people with antibodies to HIV and herpes simplex virus; 38 with a history of genital herpes) compared famciclovir versus placebo over 8 weeks.[38] The conclusions of that study are difficult to interpret (see comment below). The other RCT (1062 people with a median CD4 count of 320/mm^3) compared valaciclovir (500 mg twice daily) versus valaciclovir (1000 mg once daily) versus aciclovir (400 mg twice daily) over 1 year.[37] It found no significant difference between either dose of valaciclovir versus aciclovir, although recurrence was less likely with valaciclovir (500 mg twice daily) than with the valaciclovir (1000 mg once daily; 82% *v* 71% recurrence free at 48 weeks; $P < 0.05$).

Harms: Adverse effects (mostly headache and nausea) occurred with similar frequencies with aciclovir, valaciclovir, and famciclovir. Thrombotic microangiopathy, which has been reported in people receiving valaciclovir (8 g daily), has not been reported among 713 HIV infected persons who received oral valaciclovir in daily doses ranging from 250–1000 mg for up to 1 year (Wald A, personal communication, 2000).

Comment: Three of the four RCTs did not have a placebo control. Most studies compared new treatments with aciclovir rather than placebo. The crossover trial of famciclovir versus placebo was difficult to interpret because the withdrawal rate was high.[38] Although we found only limited evidence of an effect of antivirals for treatment of genital herpes in people with HIV infection, there was a consensus that antiviral treatment may be helpful, based on evidence from immunocompromised people who do not have HIV. Aciclovir has been found effective in immunocompromised populations. With the availability of effective treatments for HIV, trials of antiviral (anti-herpes simplex virus) versus placebo may now be conducted. A trial of valaciclovir versus placebo has now been completed and results will be included in the future updates of this chapter (Wald A, personal communication, 2002). In HIV infected people, there is a markedly increased rate of herpes simplex virus shedding.[39] HIV has been recovered from genital herpes lesions.[40] We found no evidence on the effect of daily antiviral treatment on transmission of HIV to sexual partners.

REFERENCES

1. Fleming DT, McQuillan GM, Johnson RE, et al. Herpes simplex virus type 2 in the United States, 1976 to 1994. *N Engl J Med* 1997;337:1105–1111.
2. Cowan FM, Johnson AM, Ashley R, et al. Antibody to herpes simplex virus type 2 as serological marker of sexual lifestyle in populations. *BMJ* 1994;309:1325–1329.
3. Benedetti J, Corey L, Ashley R. Recurrence rates in genital herpes after symptomatic first-episode infection. *Ann Intern Med* 1994;121:847–854.
4. Mertz GJ, Schmidt O, Jourden JL, et al. Frequency of acquisition of first-episode genital infection with herpes simplex virus from symptomatic and asymptomatic source contacts. *Sex Transm Dis* 1985;12:33–39.
5. Whitley RJ, Kimberlin DW, Roizman B. Herpes simplex viruses. *Clin Infect Dis* 1998;26:541–553.
6. Wald A, Link K. Risk of HIV infection in HSV-2 seropositive persons: A meta-analysis. *J Infect Dis* 2002;185:45–52.
7. Brown ZA, Selke SA, Zeh J, et al. Acquisition of herpes simplex virus during pregnancy. *N Engl J Med* 1997;337:509–515.
8. Smith J, Cowan FM, Munday P. The management of herpes simplex virus infection in pregnancy. *Br J Obstet Gynaecol* 1998;105:255–268. Search date 1996; primary source Medline.
9. Nilsen AE, Aasen T, Halsos AM, et al. Efficacy of oral acyclovir in treatment of initial and recurrent genital herpes. *Lancet* 1982;2:571–573.
10. Corey L, Fife K, Benedetti JK, et al. Intravenous acyclovir for the treatment of primary genital herpes. *Ann Intern Med* 1983;98:914–921.
11. Mertz G, Critchlow C, Benedetti J, et al. Double-blind placebo-controlled trial of oral acyclovir in the first episode genital herpes simplex virus infection. *JAMA* 1984;252:1147–1151.
12. Mindel A, Adler MW, Sutherland S, et al. Intravenous acyclovir treatment for primary genital herpes. *Lancet* 1982;2:697–700.
13. Bryson YJ, Dillon M, Lovett M, et al. Treatment of first episodes of genital herpes simplex virus infections with oral acyclovir: a randomized double-blind controlled trial in normal subjects. *N Engl J Med* 1983;308:916–1920.
14. Fife KH, Barbarash RA, Rudolph T, et al. Valaciclovir versus acyclovir in the treatment of first-episode genital herpes infection: results of an international, multicenter, double-blind randomized clinical trial. *Sex Transm Dis* 1997;24:481–486.
15. Loveless M, Harris W, Sacks S. *Treatment of first episode genital herpes with famciclovir. Programs and abstracts of the 35th Interscience Conference on Antimicrobial Agents and Chemotherapy*. San Francisco, California, 1995.
16. Corey L, Mindel A, Fife KH, et al. Risk of recurrence after treatment of first episode genital herpes with intravenous acyclovir. *Sex Transm Dis* 1985;12:215–218.
17. Corey L, Benedetti J, Critchlow C, et al. Treatment of primary first-episode genital herpes simplex virus infections with acyclovir: results of topical, intravenous and oral therapy. *J Antimicrob Chemother* 1983;12(suppl B):79–88.
18. Wald A. New therapies and prevention strategies for genital herpes. *Clin Infect Dis* 1999;28:S4–13. Search date 1997; primary source Medline.
19. Stone K, Whittington W. Treatment of genital herpes. *Rev Infect Dis* 1990;12(suppl 6):610–619.
20. Chosidow O, Drouault Y, Leconte-Veyriac F, et al. Famciclovir versus aciclovir in immunocompetent patients with recurrent genital herpes infections: a parallel-groups, randomised, double-blind clinical trial. *Br J Dermatol* 2001;144:818–824.
21. Reichman RC, Badger GJ, Mertz GJ, et al. Treatment of recurrent genital herpes simplex infections with oral acyclovir: a controlled trial. *JAMA* 1984;251:2103–2107.
22. Reitano M, Tyring S, Lang W, et al. Valaciclovir for the suppression of recurrent genital herpes simplex virus infection: a large-scale dose range finding study. *J Infect Dis* 1998;178:603–610.
23. Diaz-Mitoma F, Sibbald RG, Shafran SD. Oral famciclovir for the suppression of recurrent genital herpes: a randomized controlled trial. *JAMA* 1998;280:887–892.
24. Goldberg L, Kaufman R, Kurtz T, et al. Continuous five-year treatment of patients with frequently recurring genital herpes simplex virus infection with acyclovir. *J Med Virol* 1993(suppl 1);45–50.
25. Wald A, Zeh J, Barnum G, et al. Suppression of subclinical shedding of herpes simplex virus type 2 with acyclovir. *Ann Intern Med* 1996;124:8–15.
26. Doward LC, McKenna SP, Kohlmann T, et al. The international development of the RGHQoL: a quality of life measure for recurrent genital herpes. *Qual Life Res* 1998;7:143–153.
27. Patel R, Tyring S, Strand A, et al. Impact of suppressive antiviral therapy on the health related quality of life of patients with recurrent genital herpes infection. *Sex Transm Infect* 1999;75:398–402.
28. Fife KH, Crumpacker CS, Mertz GJ. Recurrence and resistance patterns of herpes simplex virus following stop of ≥ 6 years of chronic suppression with acyclovir. *J Infect Dis* 1994;169:1338–1341.
29. Longo D, Koehn K. Psychosocial factors and recurrent genital herpes: a review of prediction and psychiatric treatment studies. *Int J Psychiatry Med* 1993;23:99–117. Search date 1991; primary sources Psychological Abstracts, Medline, and hand searches of reference lists.
30. Wald A, Langenberg A, Link K, et al. Effect of condoms on reducing the transmission of herpes simples virus type 2 from men to women. *JAMA* 2001;285:3100–6.
31. Corey L, Langenberg AG, Ashley R, et al. Recombinant glycoprotein vaccine for the prevention of genital HSV-2 infection: two randomised controlled trials. *JAMA* 1999;282:331–340.
32. Randolph A, Washington A, Prober C. Cesarean delivery for women presenting with genital herpes lesions. *JAMA* 1993;270:77–82.
33. Scott LL, Sanchez PJ, Jackson GL, et al. Acyclovir suppression to prevent cesarean delivery after first-episode genital herpes. *Obstet Gynecol* 1996;87:69–73.
34. Brocklehurst P, Kinghorn G, Carney O, et al. A randomised placebo controlled trial of suppressive

acyclovir in late pregnancy in women with recurrent genital herpes infection. *Br J Obstet Gynaecol* 1998;105:275–280.
35. Stray-Pedersen B. Acyclovir in late pregnancy to prevent neonatal herpes simplex [Letter] [see comments]. *Lancet* 1990;336:756.
36. Romanowski B, Aoki FY, Martel AY, et al. Efficacy and safety of famciclovir for treating mucocutaneous herpes simplex infection in HIV-infected individuals. Collaborative Famciclovir HIV Study Group. *AIDS* 2000;14:1211–1217.
37. Conant MA, Schacker TW, Murphy RL, et al. International Valaciclovir HSV Study Group. Valaciclovir versus aciclovir for herpes simplex virus infection in HIV-infected individuals: two randomized trials. *Int J of STD AIDS* 2002;13:12–21.
38. Schacker T, Hu HL, Koelle DM, et al. Famciclovir for the suppression of symptomatic and asymptomatic herpes simplex virus reactivation in HIV-infected persons. A double-blind, placebo-controlled trial. *Ann Intern Med* 1998;128:21–28.
39. Schacker T, Zeh J, Hu HL, et al. Frequency of symptomatic and asymptomatic HSV-2 reactivations among HIV-infected men. *J Infect Dis* 1998;178:1616–1622.
40. Schacker T, Ryncarz A, Goddard J, et al. Frequent recovery of HIV from genital herpes simplex virus lesions in HIV infected persons. *JAMA* 1998;280:61–66.

Anna Wald
Associate Professor of Medicine and Epidemiology
University of Washington
Seattle
USA

Competing interests: The author has received research support from GlaxoSmithKline, Wyeth Lederly Vaccines and Pediatrics, and 3M. The author is a consultant to GlaxoSmithKline.

Genital warts

Search date January 2002

DJ Wiley

QUESTIONS

INTERVENTIONS

Key Messages

- **Bi- and trichloroacetic acid** We found insufficient evidence to evaluate the efficacy of bi- and trichloroacetic acid versus placebo.
- **Cryotherapy (as effective as podophyllin, trichloroacetic acid, or electrosurgery)** We found no RCTs comparing cryotherapy versus placebo or no treatment. One RCT found limited evidence that cryotherapy versus podophyllin significantly increased clearance after 6 weeks' treatment, but follow up of the people with successful wart clearance found no significant difference in the proportion of people who had warts at 3–5 months. Two RCTs found no significant difference with cryotherapy versus trichloroacetic acid in clearance of warts after 6–10 weeks' treatment, and one of the RCTs found no significant difference in recurrence of warts at 2 months after the end of treatment. One RCT found limited evidence that cryotherapy was significantly less effective for clearance than electrosurgery after 6 weeks' treatment, but follow up of the people with successful wart clearance found no significant difference in the proportion of people who had warts at 3–5 months. Another RCT found no significant difference in wart clearance at 3 months with cryotherapy versus electrosurgery.

Clin Evid 2002;8:1620–1632.

- **Electrosurgery (more effective than intramuscular or subcutaneous interferon; as effective as cryotherapy)** We found no RCTs comparing electrosurgery versus no treatment. One RCT found limited evidence suggesting that electrosurgery may be more effective than intramuscular or subcutaneous interferon. One RCT found limited evidence that electrosurgery versus cryotherapy or podophyllin significantly improved clearance after 6 weeks' treatment, but follow up of the people with successful wart clearance found no significant difference in the proportion of people who had warts at 3–5 months. Another RCT found no significant difference in wart clearance at 3 months with electrosurgery versus cryotherapy.
- **Imiquimod** One systematic review has found that imiquimod cream versus placebo significantly increases wart clearance (NNT 3, 95% CI 2 to 3) and reduces recurrence over 16 weeks (NNT 10, 95% CI 3 to 91) in people without human immunodeficiency virus (HIV). One RCT in people with HIV identified by the review found no signifcant difference in wart clearance over 16 weeks with imiquimod cream versus placebo.
- **Interferon, intralesional injection** RCTs have found that intralesional injection of interferon versus placebo significantly increases partial or total wart clearance
- **Interferon, topical** RCTs have found that topical interferon versus placebo significantly increases wart clearance at 4 weeks.
- **Interferon, topical as adjuvant treatment to laser surgery** RCTs found insufficient evidence on the effects of this intervention.
- **Laser surgery (as effective as surgical excision)** We found no RCTs comparing laser surgery versus placebo or no treatment. One RCT found no significant difference with laser versus surgical excision in wart clearance at 36 months.
- **Podophyllin (as effective as podophyllotoxin, cryotherapy, or electrosurgery)** We found no RCTs comparing podophyllin versus placebo. RCTs have found that podophyllin resin is as effective in clearing warts as podophyllotoxin, cryotherapy, and electrosurgery, but is significantly less effective than surgical excision.
- **Podophyllotoxin** RCTs have found that podophyllotoxin versus placebo significantly increases wart clearance within 16 weeks.
- **Surgical excision (as effective as laser surgery)** We found no RCTs comparing surgical excision versus placebo or no treatment. One RCT found no significant difference with surgical excision versus laser surgery in wart clearance.
- **Systemic interferon** RCTs found no significant difference with systemic interferon versus placebo in wart clearance after 3 months and found that it is associated with a range of adverse effects.
- **5-Fluorouracil cream; condoms in preventing human papillomavirus transmission; treatments to prevent human papillomavirus transmission** We found no RCTs on the effects of these interventions.

DEFINITION External genital warts are benign epidermal growths on the external perianal and perigenital region. There are four morphological types: condylomatous, keratotic, papular, and flat warts.

INCIDENCE/ PREVALENCE In 1996, external and internal genital warts accounted for over 180 000 initial visits to private physicians' offices in the USA: about 60 000 fewer than were reported for 1995.[1] In the USA, 1% of sexually active men and women aged 18–49 years are estimated to have external genital warts.[2]

AETIOLOGY/ RISK FACTORS External genital warts are caused by the human papillomavirus (HPV). Although more than 70 types of HPV have been identified, most external genital warts in immunocompetent people are caused by HPV types 6 and 11.[3,4] HPV infections and, more specifically, external genital warts are sexually transmissible.

PROGNOSIS Clinical trials have found that recurrences are frequent and may necessitate repeated treatment. Without treatment, external genital warts may remain unchanged, may increase in size or number, or may completely resolve. They rarely, if ever, progress to cancer.[5] Juvenile laryngeal papillomatosis, a rare and sometimes life threatening condition, occurs in children of women with a history of genital warts. Its rarity makes it hard to design studies that can evaluate whether treatment in pregnant women alters the risk.[6,7]

AIMS To eliminate symptomatic warts from the external genitalia; to prevent recurrence; and to avoid sequelae, with minimal adverse effects.

OUTCOMES Wart clearance (generally accepted as complete eradication of warts from the treated area); recurrence; sequelae; adverse effects of treatment; quality of life; transmission.

METHODS *Clinical Evidence* search and appraisal 1985 to January 2002. We also performed selected Medline searches for papers published before 1985. Other data came from abstract booklets, conference proceedings, references identified from bibliographies of pertinent articles and books, and manufacturers of therapeutic agents. This review is limited to systematic reviews and subsequent RCTs, unless no RCTs were found for a particular treatment. This limitation may have biased the review in favour of newer and heavily marketed treatments.

QUESTION **What are the effects of non-surgical treatments?**

OPTION **PODOPHYLLOTOXIN**

RCTs have found that podophyllotoxin versus placebo significantly increases wart clearance within 16 weeks, and have found no significant difference in wart clearance with podophyllotoxin versus podophyllin.

Benefits: We found no systematic review. **Versus placebo:** Eight RCTs (1035 people) compared podophyllotoxin versus placebo.[8–15] All found that, within 16 weeks of treatment, podophyllotoxin was more effective for clearance than placebo (RR of clearance *v* placebo ranged between 2.0, 95% CI 0.9 to 4.3 and 48.0, 95% CI 3.0 to 773.0). RCTs of 0.5% cream or solution found recurrence rates ranging from 4%[15] to 33%.[9] One RCT (57 people) of 0.5% podophyllotoxin solution as prophylaxis against recurrence of external genital warts (initially treated in an open label study) found fewer recurrences among people taking placebo.[16] **Versus podophyllin:** Five RCTs compared podophyllotoxin versus podophyllin.[17–21] They found no significant difference in wart clearance (RR values for podophyllin v podophyllotoxin ranging between 0.7, 95% CI 0.4 to 1.1[18] and 1.7, 95% CI 0.9 to 3.2).[20] One RCT used a 2% solution in a limited study of self treatment for penile warts and found no significant difference with podophyllotoxin versus podophyllin (RR for podophyllin v podophyllotoxin 0.6, 95% CI 0.3 to 1.3).[21]

Harms: Safety during pregnancy is unknown. Podophyllotoxin does not contain the mutagenic flavonoid compounds, quercetin and kaempherol, which are contained in podophyllin resin preparations.[22] Local inflammation or irritation, erosion, burning, pain, and itching are reported in most trials. Balanoposthitis,[23,24] dyspareunia, bleeding, scarring, and insomnia are reported rarely.[8] One large RCT reported burning and inflammation in 75% and bleeding in 25% of treated people.[12] Although rare, preputial tightening has been reported.[17]

Comment: RCTs examined the efficacy of podophyllotoxin solutions more often than cream preparations, but cream or gel preparations may be easier to apply than solutions. This and other differences may cause variable efficacy.

OPTION IMIQUIMOD

One systematic review in people without human immunodeficiency virus (HIV) has found that imiquimod cream versus placebo significantly increases wart clearance and reduces recurrence. One RCT in people with HIV identified by the review found no significant difference in wart clearance over 16 weeks with imiquimod cream versus placebo.

Benefits: We found one systematic review (search date 2000, 5 RCTs in 588 people with genital warts without HIV infection, 1 RCT in 100 people with HIV).[25] **Clearance:** The review found that in people without HIV, imiquimod cream (1–5%) versus placebo significantly increased clearance rates over 16 weeks (5 RCTs, AR for clearance 51% with imiquimod v 6% with placebo; RR 8.3, 95% CI 5.2 to 13.0; NNT 3, 95% CI 2 to 3).[25] One included RCT (100 people with HIV) found no significant difference in clearance at 16 weeks with imiquimod cream 5% versus placebo (11% with imiquimod v 6% with placebo; P = 0.48).[25] **Recurrence:** The review found that in people without HIV, imiquimod (1% or 5%) versus placebo significantly increased the proportion of people with no recurrence at 10–16 weeks after treatment (AR of no recurrence after clearance 37% with imiquimod [5% dose] v 28% with imiquimod [1% dose] v 4%–5% with placebo; RR for imiquimod 5% v placebo 9.0, 95% CI 4.9 to 17.0; NNT 3, 95% CI 3 to 4; RR for imiquimod 1% v placebo 2.9, 95% CI 1.5 to 5.9; NNT 10, 95% CI 3 to 91).[25]

Harms: The systematic review found no significant difference with imiquimod versus placebo in withdrawal from treatment because of adverse effects (4 RCTs; AR 1.8% with imiquimod v 0% with placebo; RR 1.7, 95% CI 0.4 to 9.9).[25] The largest included RCT found that moderate to severe erythema, erosion, excoriation, oedema, and scabbing were more common with imiquimod 5% than with imiquimod 1% or placebo (erythema: 40% *v* 4% *v* 3%; erosion: 10% *v* 1% *v* 2%; excoriation: 7% *v* 0% *v* 0%; oedema: 2% *v* 0% *v* 0%; scabbing: 5% *v* 2% *v* 0%: no further data provided).[25]

Comment: We found one subsequent RCT (60 men) of imiquimod 2% versus placebo, but excluded it pending review of its methods.[26]

OPTION CRYOTHERAPY

We found no RCTs comparing cryotherapy versus placebo or no treatment. One RCT found limited evidence that cryotherapy versus podophyllin significantly increased clearance after 6 weeks' treatment, but follow up of the people with successful wart clearance found no significant difference in the proportion of people who had warts at 3–5 months. Two RCTs found no significant difference with cryotherapy versus trichloroacetic acid in clearance of warts after 6–10 weeks' treatment, and one of the RCTs found no significant difference in recurrence of warts at 2 months after the end of treatment. One RCT found limited evidence that cryotherapy was significantly less effective for clearance than electrosurgery after 6 weeks' treatment, but follow up of the people with successful wart clearance found no significant difference in the proportion of people who had warts at 3–5 months. Another RCT found no significant difference in wart clearance at 3 months with cryotherapy versus electrosurgery.

Benefits: We found no systematic review. We found no RCTs comparing cryotherapy with placebo or no treatment. **Clearance:** One RCT found that cryotherapy versus podophyllin significantly increased wart clearance after 6 weeks' treatment (68/86 [79%] *v* 26/63 [41%]; RR 1.9, 95% CI 1.4 to 2.6; see comment below).[27] Two RCTs found no significant difference in wart clearance with cryotherapy versus trichloroacetic acid at the end of treatment at 6 weeks (1 RCT; 86 people; 37/53 [70%] *v* 21/33 [64%]; RR 1.1, 95% CI 0.8 to 1.5),[28] and 10 weeks (1 RCT; 130 men; 46/57 [81%] *v* 43/49 [89%]; RR 0.9, 95% CI 0.8 to 1.1).[29] One RCT found that cryotherapy was slightly less effective than electrosurgery after 6 weeks' treatment but follow up of the people with successful wart clearance found no significant difference in the proportion of people who had warts at 3–5 months.[27] Another RCT found no significant difference in wart clearance at 3 months with cryotherapy versus electrosurgery (see benefits of electrosurgery, p 1629).[30] **Recurrence:** The RCT comparing cryotherapy versus podophyllin or versus electrosurgery followed up people who had successful wart clearance after 6 weeks' treatment (177 people), and found no significant difference in the proportion of people who had warts at 3–5 months after treatment (10/46 [22%] with cryotherapy *v* 9/42 [21%] with electrosurgery *v* 7/16 [44%] with podophyllin resin; RR with cryotherapy *v* podophyllin 0.49, 95% CI 0.22 to 1.09; RR with cryotherapy *v* electrosurgery 0.99, 95% CI 0.44 to 2.19).[27] One of the RCTs comparing cryotherapy versus trichloreacetic acid found no significant difference in recurrence at 2 months after the end of 10 weeks' treatment (15/38 [40%] with cryotherapy *v* 14/39 [36%] with trichloreacetic acid; RR 1.1, 95% CI 0.61 to 1.95).[29]

Harms: Discomfort, ulceration, and scabbing were reported in nearly a fifth of people after cryotherapy.[27,30] One RCT reported local infection in 1/86 (1%) people taking cryotherapy versus 0/149 (0%) people taking podophyllin resin or electrosurgery.[27]

Comment: The results of the RCT comparing cryotherapy versus podophyllin should be interpreted with caution as they are not intention to treat and 213/450 (47%) of people withdrew from the trial.[27] One case series of 34 pregnant women who received three or fewer treatments of cryotherapy found no subsequent infection or premature rupture of membranes.[31]

OPTION PODOPHYLLIN

We found no RCTs comparing podophyllin versus placebo. RCTs have found that podophyllin resin is as effective in clearing warts as podophyllotoxin, cryotherapy, and electrosurgery, but is significantly less effective than surgical excision.

Benefits: We found no systematic review. **Versus placebo:** We found no RCTs. **Versus podophyllotoxin:** We found five RCTs that found no significant difference in wart clearance with podophyllin versus podophyllotoxin (see benefits of podophyllotoxin, p 1622).[17–21] **Versus cryotherapy or electrosurgery:** We found one RCT.[27] It found no significant difference in wart clearance with podophyllin versus cryotherapy (see benefits of cryotherapy, p 1624) or podophyllin versus electrosurgery at 3 months (see benefits of electrosurgery, p 1629). **Versus systemic interferon:** One RCT found that podophyllin versus interferon significantly improved clearance at 3 months (see benefits of systemic interferon, p 1628).[32] **Podophyllin plus intralesional interferon versus podophyllin alone:** One RCT found that combined treatment versus podophyllin alone improved clearance at 3 weeks (see benefits of intralesional interferon, p 1627).[33] **Podophyllin plus systemic interferon versus podophyllin alone:** One RCT (124 people with anogenital warts) compared 6 weeks of combined treatment with podophyllin plus systemic interferon versus podophyllin alone.[33] It found no significant difference between treatments for clearance at 10 weeks, although the withdrawal rate was high (85/124 [69%] participants included in analysis; AR for clearance 15/42 [36%] with combined treatment *v* 11/43 [26%] with podophyllin alone; RR 1.40, 95% CI 0.73 to 2.69).[34] **Podophyllin plus trichloroacetic acid versus podophyllin alone:** One RCT comparing podophyllin with and without trichloroacetic acid found no significant difference in clearance rates at 3 months (see benefits of bi- and trichloroacetic acid, p 1626).[35] **Versus surgical excision:** Two RCTs have found that podophyllin is less effective than surgical excision for clearance and for preventing recurrence (see benefits of surgical excision, p 1629).[36,37] **Different doses of podophyllin:** One RCT compared podophyllin 10% versus podophyllin 25% in 140 men with anogenital warts.[38] It found no significant difference between treatments for clearance rates at 3 months (AR 22% in both groups).

Harms: Eight RCTs reported pain, erythema, irritation, and tenderness in 3–17% of people treated with podophyllin.[17,18,20,27,32,33,36,37] Skin burns (1–3%),[36] bleeding (4%),[37] and erosion or ulcerations (1[18]–11%[31]) were also reported. Faecal incontinence (4%)[37] and preputial tightening (1%)[17] were reported rarely.

Comment: Safety during pregnancy is unknown. Podophyllin may contain the mutagenic flavonoid compounds, quercetin and kaempherol.[22]

OPTION BI- AND TRICHLOROACETIC ACID

We found no RCTs comparing bi- and trichloroacetic acid versus placebo. Two RCTs found no significant difference with trichloroacetic acid versus cryotherapy in clearance of warts after 6–10 weeks' treatment, and one of the RCTs found no significant difference in recurrence of warts at 2 months after the end of treatment. One RCT found no significant difference in wart clearance at 3 months with trichloroacetic acid plus podophyllin versus podophyllin alone.

Benefits: We found no systematic review. **Versus placebo:** We found no RCTs. **Versus cryotherapy:** We found two RCTs (192 people) comparing trichloroacetic acid versus cryotherapy.[28,29] See benefits of cyrotherapy, p 1624. **Trichloroacetic acid plus podophyllin versus podophyllin alone:** One RCT (73 people) found no significant difference in wart clearance at 3 months with trichloroacetic acid plus podophyllin versus podophyllin alone.[35]

Harms: The RCTs gave no information on harms.[28,29,35]

Comment: Small numbers of participants and inadequate study designs make it difficult to evaluate effectiveness. In pregnant women, only case series are available: 31/32 (97%) pregnant women treated with trichloroacetic acid had wart clearance, and 2/31 (6%) had recurrence.[39] The evidence is inadequate to evaluate adverse effects of trichloroacetic acid in pregnancy.

OPTION TOPICAL INTERFERON

Three RCTs have found increased wart clearance with topical interferon versus placebo. One of the RCTs also found that interferon versus podophyllotoxin significantly increased wart clearance at about 4 weeks after treatment.

Benefits: We found no systematic review. **Versus placebo:** We found three RCTs (223 men and women). Complete wart clearance 4 weeks after treatment occurred in more people using interferon versus placebo (6% *v* 3%, P value not provided;[40] 73% *v* 10%, $P < 0.0001$;[41] 90% *v* 20%, P value not provided[11]). About a third of people in each group in the first study had cleared their warts by 16 weeks.[40] Recurrence rates were not evaluated. **Versus podophyllotoxin:** One of the RCTs also compared topical interferon versus podophyllotoxin and found that interferon significantly increased wart clearance at about 4 weeks after treatment (RR compared with podophyllotoxin 1.5, 95% CI 1.0 to 1.6).[11] **As adjuvant to other treatment:** One RCT compared recombinant β interferon at two doses plus CO_2 laser versus CO_2 laser alone, electrotherapy, and liquid nitrogen. Recurrences occurred in 21/36 (58%) of people treated with 1.0 MU/g interferon, in 19/35 (54%) treated with 0.15 MU/g interferon, and 27/36 (75%) treated with laser alone.[42]

Harms: One placebo controlled study reported local burning and itching in 39% of treated people.[40] Another RCT reported fever, headache, and itching in 18% of people treated with interferon.[11]

Comment: Differences in the RCTs' findings may be attributable to the preparations used; one preparation was incorporated into a methyl cellulose aqueous base[40] and the other was instilled into a cream base.[11]

OPTION INTRALESIONAL INJECTION OF INTERFERON

RCTs have found that intralesional injection of interferon versus placebo increases wart clearance. One RCT found that podophyllin and intralesional interferon together were more effective for wart clearance than podophyllin alone 3 weeks after treatment.

Benefits: We found no systematic review. We found eight placebo controlled trials[43–51] and one RCT (1000 people) comparing interferon plus podophyllin versus podophyllin alone.[33] Doses and follow up intervals varied. Two of the placebo controlled RCTs randomised treatment to lesions rather than to people.[46,48] **Versus placebo:** In studies using 1 MU/mL, intralesional interferon was between twofold (95% CI 0.8 to 4.6)[47] and 3.5-fold (95% CI 1.4 to 8.8)[44] more likely to achieve complete wart clearance than placebo. One RCT found no significant difference for complete wart clearance between 1 MU/ml intralesional interferon and placebo. However, it found a twofold improvement if complete and partial responders were grouped together for analysis (RR of clearance 2.3, 95% CI 1.2 to 4.3).[51] **Added to podophyllin:** One RCT found that podophyllin plus intralesional interferon versus podophyllin alone increased wart clearance 3 weeks after treatment (RR 2.0, 95% CI 1.1 to 3.6); however, no significant difference was observed at 11 weeks (RR 2.3, 95% CI 0.9 to 5.8).[33]

Harms: Flu like symptoms (dizziness, fever, malaise, myalgia, nausea and vomiting, headache, and pain) were reported in 0–100% of people. Eight of nine studies reported local irritation and one reported hypopigmentation among treated individuals.[51] Several studies reported a fall in white cell counts,[33,43-45,47-50] thrombocytopenia (1%),[43] and raised serum aspartate transaminase concentrations (6%)[33] in people on interferon.

Comment: None.

OPTION SYSTEMIC INTERFERON

RCTs have found no clear evidence that systemic interferon is more effective than placebo at wart clearance, and it is associated with a range of adverse effects.

Benefits: We found no systematic review. **Versus placebo:** We found six RCTs.[52–57] Five of these found a significant difference in rates of wart clearance at 3 months. One of the RCTs found that people taking systemic interferon showed greater wart clearance than people treated with placebo, which was significant at 8 weeks' follow up (51% *v* 29%; $P < 0.05$), but no difference was detected 12 months after treatment.[55] **Versus podophyllin:** One RCT (154 people with condylomata acuminata of < 6 months' duration) found that podophyllin improved clearance compared with interferon at 3 months (AR for clearance 23% with interferon *v* 45% with podophyllin; $P = 0.003$).[32] **Systemic interferon plus podophyllin versus podophyllin alone:** We found one RCT.[34] See benefits of podophyllin, p 1625.

Harms: Flu-like symptoms were reported at variable frequencies. Headache, fatigue and malaise, myalgia, nausea and vomiting, fever, chills, and dizziness were reported in 0.5–100% of people on interferon.[32,52–59] Anaphylactic reaction occurred in 2% of people in one RCT;[60] leukopenia in 6–28% and thrombocytopenia in 3–4% of people in another RCT;[54] and raised liver enzymes in 3% of people in two RCTs.[54,58]

Comment: None.

OPTION TOPICAL 5-FLUOROURACIL

We found no RCTs of topical 5-fluorouracil in people with external genital warts.

Benefits: We found no systematic review or RCTs.

Harms: One case series found that 5-fluorouracil 1% was associated with minor local erosions (48% of people), urinary meatus erosions (5%), vulvar irritation (10%), burning (10%), and dysuria (4%).[61]

Comment: We found three case series in 224 men and women treated with 1% and 5% cream and solution preparations in various doses.[61–63] Wart clearance was reported in 10–50% of people within 3 months of treatment. One case series found that recurrence at 6–9 months occurred in 2/20 (10%) people who had wart clearance after 10 weeks' treatment with 5-fluorouracil.[62] 5-Fluorouracil has teratogenic and mutagenic properties in animals, and its safety in pregnancy has not yet been established. One case report[64] in a pregnant woman with breast cancer taking 5-fluorouracil up to 3 weeks prior to delivery found no adverse effects in the infant at 24 months, and one case series (5 people)[65] of accidental exposure to 5-fluorouracil during early pregnancy (up to 16 weeks' gestation) reported no fetal adverse effects.

QUESTION What are the effects of surgical treatments?

OPTION ELECTROSURGERY

We found no RCTs comparing electrosurgery versus no treatment. One RCT found limited evidence suggesting that electrosurgery is more effective than intramuscular or subcutaneous interferon. One RCT found

limited evidence that electrosurgery versus cryotherapy or podophyllin significantly improved clearance after 6 weeks' treatment, but follow up of the people with successful wart clearance after 6 weeks' treatment found no significant difference in the proportion of people who had warts at 3–5 months after treatment. Another RCT found no significant difference in wart clearance at 3 months with electrosurgery versus cryotherapy.

Benefits: We found no systematic review. **Clearance:** We found no RCTs versus no treatment or sham treatment, but found three RCTs (482 men and women) comparing electrosurgery versus interferon, cryotherapy, or podophyllin resin.[27,30,60] The first RCT (450 people) compared three treatments: electrosurgery, cryotherapy, and podophyllin resin (see comment below).[27] It found that electrosurgery versus cryotherapy or versus podophyllin resin significantly increased wart clearance after 6 weeks' treatment (83/88 [94%] with electrosurgery *v* 68/86 [79%] with cryotherapy *v* 26/63 [41%]; RR of wart clearance with electrosurgery *v* cryotherapy 1.2, 95% CI 1.1 to 1.3; RR of wart clearance with electrosurgery *v* podophyllin 2.3, 95% CI 1.7 to 3.0). The second RCT (42 people) compared electrosurgery versus cryotherapy given at 2 weekly intervals as necessary until warts were completely cleared.[30] It found no significant difference in wart clearance at 3 months' follow up with electrosurgery versus cryotherapy (10/24 [42%] with electrosurgery *v* 10/18 [56%] with cryotherapy; RR 0.75, 95% CI 0.40 to 1.40). The third RCT found that electrosurgery was more effective than intramuscular interferon (RR *v* intramuscular 3.3, 95% CI 1.8 to 5.9) or subcutaneous interferon (RR *v* subcutaneous 6.9, 95% CI 2.8 to 17.1).[60] **Recurrence:** The first RCT followed up people who had successful wart clearance after 6 weeks' treatment (177 people), and found no significant difference in the proportion of people who had warts at 3–5 months after treatment (10/46 [22%] with electrosurgery *v* 9/42 [21%] with cryotherapy *v* 7/16 [44%] with podophyllin resin; RR with electrosurgery *v* cryotherapy 1.0, 95% CI 0.8 to 1.2; RR electrosurgery *v* podophyllin 0.49, 95% CI 0.23 to 1.09).[27]

Harms: The first RCT found that pain and local irritation were reported in 17% of treated people given electrosurgery.[27]

Comment: The results of the first RCT should be interpreted with caution as they are not intention to treat and 213/450 (47%) of people withdrew from the trial.[27]

OPTION SURGICAL EXCISION

We found no RCTs comparing surgical excision versus no treatment. RCTs have found that surgical (scissor) excision is as effective as laser surgery for clearance and more effective than podophyllin.

Benefits: We found no systematic review. **Clearance:** We found no RCTs versus no treatment or sham treatment, but found three RCTs comparing surgical excision versus CO_2 laser[66] or podophyllin.[36,37] Two studies found that podophyllin was less effective than surgery for clearance (RR values of clearance 0.3, 95% CI 0.2 to 0.7).[36,37] One trial found no significant difference in clearance between laser versus surgical excision (RR 1.2, 95% CI 0.6 to 2.4).[66] **Recurrence:** Recurrence occurred in 19–29% of people after excision versus 60–65% after podophyllin.[36,37] The trial comparing conventional and laser surgery found no significant difference in recurrence rates between the two treatments.[66]

Harms: All surgically treated participants experienced pain. Scar formation (9%)[66] and bleeding (37%)[37] were less frequent.

Comment: None.

OPTION LASER SURGERY

We found no RCTs comparing laser surgery versus no treatment. One RCT found no evidence of a significant difference in wart clearance or recurrence rates between laser versus surgical excision.

Benefits: We found no systematic review. We found no RCTs comparing laser surgery versus no treatment or sham treatment. One RCT (50 people) compared laser surgery versus conventional surgical excision.[66] It found no significant difference between treatments for clearance or recurrence rates (see benefits of surgical excision, p 1629).[66]

Harms: The RCT comparing laser with surgical excision found no significant difference in the rate of local scar formation (28% after laser surgery v 9% after surgical excision; $P > 0.2$).[66] Postoperative pain was reported equally in both groups.

Comment: We found two case series of laser surgery, which included 47 pregnant women.[39,67] These reported premature rupture of membranes (2/32 [6%] women), prolonged rupture of membranes (1/32 [3%]), the need for postoperative suprapubic catheterisation (7/32 [22%]), pyelonephritis (1/32 [3%]), prolonged healing time (1/52 [2%]), and rectal perforation with secondary abscess (1/52 [2%]).

QUESTION Does treatment of external genital warts or the use of barrier contraceptives prevent transmission of human papillomavirus?

We found no RCTs about barrier contraceptives or treatment of external genital warts to prevent transmission of human papillomavirus.

Benefits: We found no RCTs about the effects of barrier contraceptives or treatment of external genital warts on the rate of transmitting human papillomavirus.

Harms: We found no RCTs.

Comment: Penetrative intercourse may not be required for transmission of human papillomavirus infection, and it is unclear whether sexual contact with any infected and uninfected perigenital tissues is sufficient to cause external genital warts.

Substantive changes

Imiquimod One new systematic review;[25] conclusions unchanged.

REFERENCES

1. US Department of Health and Human Services, Public Health Service. Division of STD Prevention. *Sexually transmitted disease surveillance*. Atlanta: Centers for Disease Control and Prevention, 1996.
2. Koutsky LA, Galloway DA, Holmes KK. Epidemiology of genital human papillomavirus infection. *Epidemiol Rev* 1988;10:122–163.
3. Gissmann L, zur Hausen H. Partial characterization of viral DNA from human genital warts (condylomata acuminata). *Int J Cancer* 1980;25:605–609.
4. Gissmann L, Boshart M, Durst M, et al. Presence of human papillomavirus in genital tumors. *J Invest Dermatol* 1984;83(suppl 1):26–28.
5. IARC Working Group on Evaluation of Carcinogenic Risks to Humans. *IARC monographs on the evaluation of carcinogenic risks to humans: human papillomaviruses.* Lyon, France: World Health Organization, International Agency for Research on Cancer, 1995.
6. Bonnez W, Kashima HK, Leventhal B, et al. Antibody response to human papillomavirus (HPV) type 11 in children with juvenile-onset recurrent respiratory papillomatosis (RRP). *Virology* 1992;188:384–387.
7. Hallden C, Majmudar B. The relationship between juvenile laryngeal papillomatosis and maternal condylomata acuminata. *J Reprod Med* 1986;31:804–807.
8. Greenberg MD, Rutledge LH, Reid R, et al. A double blind, randomized trial of 0.5% podofilox and placebo for the treatment of genital warts in women. *Obstet Gynecol* 1991;77:735–739.
9. Beutner KR, Conant MA, Friedman-Kien AE, et al. Patient-applied podofilox for treatment of genital warts. *Lancet* 1989;i:831–834.
10. Kirby P, Dunne King D, Corey L. Double-blind randomized clinical trial of self-administered podofilox solution versus vehicle in the treatment of genital warts. *Am J Med* 1990;88:465–469.
11. Syed TA, Khayyami M, Kriz D, et al. Management of genital warts in women with human leukocyte interferon-α vs podophyllotoxin in cream: a placebo-controlled, double-blind, comparative study. *J Mol Med* 1995;73:255–258.
12. Tyring S, Edwards L, Cherry LK, et al. Safety and efficacy of 0.5% podofilox gel in the treatment of anogenital warts. *Arch Dermatol* 1998;134:33–38.
13. Von Krogh G, Hellberg D. Self-treatment using a 0.5% podophyllotoxin cream of external genital condylomata acuminata in women. A placebo-controlled, double-blind study. *Sex Transm Dis* 1992;19:170–174.
14. Von Krogh G, Szpak E, Andersson M, et al. Self-treatment using 0.25%–0.50% podophyllotoxin-ethanol solutions against penile condylomata acuminata: a placebo-controlled comparative study. *Genitourin Med* 1994;70:105–109.
15. Syed TA, Lundin S, Ahmad SA. Topical 0.3% and 0.5% podophyllotoxin cream for self-treatment of condylomata acuminata in women: a placebo-controlled, double-blind study. *Dermatology* 1994;189:142–145.
16. Bonnez W, Elswick RK Jr, Bailey-Farchione A, et al. Efficacy and safety of 0.5% podofilox solution in the treatment and suppression of anogenital warts. *Am J Med* 1994;96:420–425.
17. Edwards A, Atma-Ram A, Thin RN. Podophyllotoxin 0.5% v podophyllin 20% to treat penile warts. *Genitourin Med* 1988;64:263–265.
18. Hellberg D, Svarrer T, Nilsson S, et al. Self-treatment of female external genital warts with 0.5% podophyllotoxin cream (Condyline) vs weekly applications of 20% podophyllin solution. *Int J STD AIDS* 1995;6:257–261.
19. Kinghorn GR, McMillan A, Mulcahy F, et al. An open, comparative, study of the efficacy of 0.5% podophyllotoxin lotion and 25% podophyllotoxin solution in the treatment of condylomata acuminata in males and females. *Int J STD AIDS* 1993;4:194–199.
20. Lassus A, Haukka K, Forsstrom S. Podophyllotoxin for treatment of genital warts in males: a comparison with conventional podophyllin therapy. *Eur J Sex Transm Dis* 1984;2:31–33.
21. White, DJ, Billingham C, Chapman S, et al. Podophyllin 0.5% or 2.0% v podophyllotoxin 0.5% for self treatment of penile warts: a double blind randomised study. *Genitourin Med* 1997;73:184–187.
22. Petersen CS, Weismann K. Quercetin and kaempherol: an argument against the use of podophyllin? *Genitourin Med* 1995;71:92–93.
23. Von Krogh G. Topical self-treatment of penile warts with 0.5% podophyllotoxin in ethanol for four or five days. *Sex Transm Dis* 1987;14:135–140.
24. Von Krogh G. Penile condylomata acuminata: an experimental model for evaluation of topical self-treatment with 0.5–1.0% ethanolic preparations of podophyllotoxin for three days. *Sex Transm Dis* 1981;8:179–186.
25. Moore RA, Edwards JE, Hopwood J, et al. Imiquimod for the treatment of genital warts: a quantitative systematic review. *BMC Infect Dis* 2001;1:3. Search date 2000; primary sources Medline, Cochrane Library, and hand searches of review articles and reference lists.
26. Syed TA, Hadi SM, Qureshi ZA, et al. Treatment of external genital warts in men with imiquimod 2% in cream. A placebo-controlled, double-blind study. *J Infect* 2000;41:148–51
27. Stone KM, Becker TM, Hadgu A, et al. Treatment of external genital warts: a randomised clinical trial comparing podophyllin, cryotherapy, and electrodesiccation. *Genitourin Med* 1990;66:16–19.
28. Abdullah AN, Walzman M, Wade A. Treatment of external genital warts comparing cryotherapy (liquid nitrogen) and trichloroacetic acid. *Sex Transm Dis* 1993;20:344–345.
29. Godley MJ, Bradbeer CS, Gellan M, et al. Cryotherapy compared with trichloroacetic acid in treating genital warts. *Genitourin Med* 1987;63:390–392.
30. Simmons PD, Langlet F, Thin RN. Cryotherapy versus electrocautery in the treatment of genital warts. *Br J Venereal Dis* 1981;57:273–274.
31. Bergman A, Bhatia NN, Broen EM. Cryotherapy for treatment of genital condylomata during pregnancy. *J Reprod Med* 1984;29:432–435.
32. Condylomata International Collaborative Study Group. A comparison of interferon alfa-2a and podophyllin in the treatment of primary condylomata acuminata. *Genitourin Med* 1991;67:394–399.
33. Douglas JM Jr, Eron LJ, Judson FN, et al. A randomized trial of combination therapy with intralesional interferon α 2b and podophyllin versus podophyllin alone for the therapy of anogenital warts. *J Infect Dis* 1990;162:52–59.
34. Armstrong DK, Maw RD, Dinsmore WW, et al. A randomised, double-blind, parallel group study to compare subcutaneous interferon α-2a plus podophyllin with placebo plus podophyllin in the treatment of primary condylomata acuminata. *Genitourin Med* 1994;70:389–393.

Genital warts

35. Gabriel G, Thin RN. Treatment of anogenital warts. Comparison of trichloroacetic acid and podophyllin versus podophyllin alone. *Br J Venereal Dis* 1983;59:124–126.
36. Khawaja HT. Podophyllin versus scissor excision in the treatment of perianal condylomata acuminata: a prospective study. *Br J Surg* 1989;76:1067–1068.
37. Jensen SL. Comparison of podophyllin application with simple surgical excision in clearance and recurrence of perianal condylomata acuminata. *Lancet* 1985;2:1146–1148.
38. Simmons PD. Podophyllin 10% and 25% in the treatment of ano-genital warts: a comparative double-blind study. *Br J Venereal Dis* 1981;57:208–209.
39. Schwartz DB, Greenberg MD, Daoud Y, et al. Genital condylomas in pregnancy: use of trichloroacetic acid and laser therapy. *Am J Obstet Gynecol* 1988;158(6 pt 1):1407–1416.
40. Keay S, Teng N, Eisenberg M, et al. Topical interferon for treating condyloma acuminata in women. *J Infect Dis* 1988;158:934–939.
41. Syed TA, Ahmadpour OA. Human leukocyte derived interferon-α in a hydrophilic gel for the treatment of intravaginal warts in women: a placebo-controlled, double-blind study. *Int J STD AIDS* 1998;9:769–772.
42. Gross G, Rogozinski T, Schofer H, et al. Recombinant interferon β gel as an adjuvant in the treatment of recurrent genital warts: results of a placebo-controlled double blind study of 120 patients. *Dermatology* 1998;196:330–334.
43. Eron LJ, Judson F, Tucker S, et al. Interferon therapy for condylomata acuminata. *N Engl J Med* 1986;315:1059–1064.
44. Friedman-Kien AE, Eron LJ, Conant M, et al. Natural interferon alfa for treatment of condylomata acuminata. *JAMA* 1988;259:533–538.
45. Friedman-Kien A. Management of condylomata acuminata with Alferon N injection, interferon alfa-n3 (human leukocyte derived). *Am J Obstet Gynecol* 1995;172(4 pt 2):1359–1368.
46. Monsonego J, Cessot G, Ince SE, et al. Randomised double-blind trial of recombinant interferon-β for condyloma acuminatum. *Genitourin Med* 1996;72:111–114.
47. Reichman RC, Oakes D, Bonnez W, et al. Treatment of condyloma acuminatum with three different interferons administered intralesionally: a double-blind, placebo-controlled trial. *Ann Intern Med* 1988;108:675–679.
48. Scott GM, Csonka GW. Effect of injections of small doses of human fibroblast interferon into genital warts: a pilot study. *Br J Venereal Dis* 1979;55:442–445.
49. Vance JC, Bart BJ, Hansen RC, et al. Intralesional recombinant α-2 interferon for the treatment of patients with condyloma acuminatum or verruca plantaris. *Arch Dermatol* 1986;122:272–277.
50. Welander CE, Homesley HD, Smiles KA, et al. Intralesional interferon alfa-2b for the treatment of genital warts. *Am J Obstet Gynecol* 1990;162:348–354.
51. Bornstein J, Pascal B, Zarfati D, et al. Recombinant human interferon-β for condylomata acuminata: a randomized, double-blind, placebo controlled study of intralesional therapy. *Int J STD AIDS* 1997;8:614–621.
52. Armstrong DK, Maw RD, Dinsmore WW, et al. Combined therapy trial with interferon α-2a and ablative therapy in the treatment of anogenital warts. *Genitourin Med* 1996;72:103–107.
53. Condylomata International Collaborative Study Group. Recurrent condylomata acuminata treated with recombinant interferon alfa-2a: a multicenter double-blind placebo-controlled clinical trial. *JAMA* 1991;265:2684–2687.
54. Condylomata International Collaborative Study Group. Recurrent condylomata acuminata treated with recombinant interferon α-2a: a multicenter double-blind placebo-controlled clinical trial. *Acta Derm Venereol* 1993;73:223–226.
55. Gall SA, Constantine L, Koukol D. Therapy of persistent human papillomavirus disease with two different interferon species. *Am J Obstet Gynecol* 1991;164(1 pt 1):130–134.
56. Olmos L, Vilata J, Rodriguez Pichardo A, et al. Double-blind, randomized clinical trial on the effect of interferon-β in the treatment of condylomata acuminata. *Int J STD AIDS* 1994;5:182–185.
57. Reichman RC, Oakes D, Bonnez W, et al. Treatment of condyloma acuminatum with three different interferon-α preparations administered parenterally: a double-blind, placebo-controlled trial. *J Infect Dis* 1990;162:1270–1276.
58. Kirby PK, Kiviat N, Beckman A, et al. Tolerance and efficacy of recombinant human interferon γ in the treatment of refractory genital warts. *Am J Med* 1988;85:183–188.
59. Reichman RC, Micha JP, Weck PK, et al. Interferon α-n1 (Wellferon) for refractory genital warts: efficacy and tolerance of low dose systemic therapy. *Antiviral Res* 1988;10(1–3):41–57.
60. Benedetti Panici P, Scambia G, Baiocchi G, et al. Randomized clinical trial comparing systemic interferon with diathermocoagulation in primary multiple and widespread anogenital condyloma. *Obstet Gynecol* 1989;74(3 pt 1):393–397.
61. Von Krogh G. The beneficial effect of 1% 5-fluorouracil in 70% ethanol on therapeutically refractory condylomas in the preputial cavity. *Sex Transm Dis* 1978;5:137–140.
62. Krebs H. Treatment of extensive vulvar condylomata acuminata with topical 5-fluorouracil. *South Med J* 1990;83:761–764.
63. Haye KR. Treatment of condyloma acuminata with 5 per cent 5-fluorouracil (5-FU) cream [letter]. *Br J Vener Dis* 1974;50:466.
64. Dreicer R, Love RR. High total dose 5-fluorouracil treatment during pregnancy. *Wis Med J* 1991;90:582–583.
65. Van Le L, Pizzuti DJ, Greenberg M, et al. Accidental use of low-dose 5-fluorouracil in pregnancy. *J Reprod Med* 1991;36:872–874.
66. Duus BR, Philipsen T, Christensen JD, et al. Refractory condylomata acuminata: a controlled clinical trial of carbon dioxide laser versus conventional surgical treatment. *Genitourin Med* 1985;61:59–61.
67. Kryger-Baggesen N, Falck Larsen J, Hjortkjaer Pedersen P. CO_2 laser treatment of condylomata acuminata. *Acta Obstet Gynecol Scand* 1984;63:341–343.

DJ Wiley

Assistant Professor in Residence

School of Nursing Primary Care, University of California, Los Angeles, USA

Competing interests: DJW has been a consultant to 3M Pharmaceuticals and has received research funding from Merck and Co.

Gonorrhoea

Search date May 2002

John Moran

QUESTIONS

INTERVENTIONS

Beneficial

Single dose regimens using selected fluoroquinolones, selected cephalosporins, or spectinomycin in uncomplicated infection* 1635

Single dose regimens using selected cephalosporins or spectinomycin in uncomplicated infection in pregnant women 1636

Likely to be beneficial

Selected injectable fluoroquinolones or selected injectable cephalosporins in disseminated infection** . .1637

Unknown effectiveness

Dual treatment for gonorrhoea and chlamydia infections in all people diagnosed with gonorrhoea .1637

*Based on comparisons of results across arms of different trials.

**Based only on non-RCT evidence and consensus.

Key Messages

- **Dual treatment for gonorrhoea and chlamydia infections in all people diagnosed with gonorrhoea** Dual treatment for gonorrhoea and chlamydia infections is based on theory and expert opinion rather than on evidence from RCTs. The balance between benefits and harms will vary with the prevalence of co-infection in each population.
- **Selected injectable fluoroquinolones or selected injectable cephalosporins in disseminated infection** We found no RCTs assessing treatments for disseminated gonococcal infection published in the last 20 years, but there is strong consensus that multidose regimens using injectable cephalosporins or quinolones are the most effective treatment. We found no reports of treatment failures with these regimens.
- **Single dose regimens using selected cephalosporins or spectinomycin in uncomplicated infection in pregnant women** RCTs comparing different antimicrobial agents have found that ceftriaxone and spectinomycin cure 89–97% of rectal, cervical, and pharyngeal infections.

- **Single dose regimens using selected fluoroquinolones, selected cephalosporins, or spectinomycin in uncomplicated infection in men and non-pregnant women** One systematic review found limited evidence by combining cure rates across different arms of RCTs. It found that single dose regimens based on an antimicrobial agent other than a penicillin or a tetracycline achieve cure rates of 95% or higher in urogenital or rectal infection. Cure rates were lower (≤80%) for pharyngeal infection. Resistance is now widespread to penicillins, tetracyclines, and sulphonamides.

DEFINITION Gonorrhoea is caused by infection with *Neisseria gonorrhoeae*. In men, uncomplicated urethritis is the most common manifestation, with dysuria and urethral discharge. Less typically, signs and symptoms are mild and indistinguishable from chlamydial urethritis. In women, the most common manifestation is cervicitis, which produces symptoms (e.g. vaginal discharge, lower abdominal discomfort, and dyspareunia) in only half of the women. Co-infection with chlamydia is reported in 20–40% of people.[1]

INCIDENCE/ PREVALENCE Between 1975 and 1997, the incidence of reported gonorrhoea in the USA fell by 74%, reaching a level in 1996 of 122/100 000 people. Since 1997, between 122 and 132 cases have been reported per 100 000 people each year.[2] In the UK, diagnoses of gonorrhoea have increased since 1994, reaching 218/100 000 for 20–24 year old males and 184/100 000 for 16–19 year old females in 2001.[3] In poor communities, rates may be higher: the estimated incidence in people aged 15–59 years living in three inner London boroughs in 1994–1995 was 138/100 000 women and 292/100 000 men.[4] Rates are highest in younger people. In the USA in 2000, incidence was highest in women aged 15–19 years (716/100 000) and men aged 20–24 years (590/100 000).[2]

AETIOLOGY/ RISK FACTORS Most infections result from penile-vaginal, penile-rectal, or penile-pharyngeal contact. An important minority of infections are transmitted from mother to child during birth, which can cause ophthalmia neonatorum. Less common are ocular infections in older children and adults as a result of sexual exposure, poor hygiene, or the medicinal use of urine.

PROGNOSIS The natural history of untreated gonococcal infection is spontaneous resolution after weeks or months of unpleasant symptoms. During this time, there is a substantial likelihood of transmission to others and of complications developing in the infected individual.[5] Symptoms in most men are severe enough to cause them to seek treatment, but an estimated 1–3% of infected men remain asymptomatic. These men, and men who are infectious but not yet symptomatic, are largely responsible for the spread of the disease. In many women, the lack of readily discernible signs or symptoms of cervicitis means that infections go unrecognised and untreated. An unknown proportion of untreated infections causes local complications, including lymphangitis, periurethral abscess, bartholinitis, and urethral stricture; epididymitis in men; and in women involvement of the uterus, fallopian tubes, or ovaries causing pelvic inflammatory disease (see pelvic inflammatory disease, p 1649). It is the association of gonorrhoea with pelvic inflammatory disease — a major cause of secondary infertility, ectopic pregnancy, and chronic pelvic pain — that makes gonorrhoea an important public health issue. Manifestations of disseminated infection are petechial or pustular skin lesions; asymmetrical arthropathies, tenosynovitis or septic arthritis; and, rarely, meningitis or endocarditis.

AIMS To relieve symptoms; avoid complications; and prevent further transmission, with minimal adverse effects of treatment.

OUTCOMES Microbiological cure rates (number of infected people or infected sites culture-negative 1–14 days after treatment, divided by number of infected people or infected sites cultured 1–14 days after treatment).

METHODS *Clinical Evidence* update search and appraisal May 2002. Additional author PubMed search October 2001. Key words: gonorrhoea and *N gonorrhoeae* infections, plus a search of references of key articles and books. Studies were excluded if they defined possible treatment failures as "reinfections", if they did not use end points based on microbiological cure, or if they were based on drug regimens unlikely to be of general use (e.g. those using antibiotic regimens that are toxic or to which resistance is now widespread).[6]

QUESTION What are the effects of treatments for uncomplicated infections in men and non-pregnant women?

One systematic review has found that many antimicrobial agents other than penicillin and tetracycline achieve cure rates of 97% or higher in urogenital or rectal infection (see table 1, p 1640). Cure rates are lower (≤ 80%) for pharyngeal infection. Most regimens cause few adverse effects. Resistance to penicillins, tetracyclines, and sulphonamides is now widespread.

Benefits: **Uncomplicated urogenital, rectal, and pharyngeal infections:** We found one systematic review (search date 1993).[6] The results were updated to 2002 by the author of the review using the original methods and are tabulated (see table 1, p 1640) (Moran JS, personal communication, 2002). The original review identified studies (both RCTs and other clinical trials) published from 1981–1993 that used a single dose regimen based on an antimicrobial other than a β lactamase sensitive penicillin or a tetracycline.[6] The search retrieved studies with a total of 24 383 evaluable people or infections. Combining results across arms of trials, 96% were cured on the basis of culture results. Sites of infection, when specified, included the cervix, urethra, rectum, and pharynx. Comparison of cure rates by site of infection found that cure rates were over 95% for all sites except the pharynx, for which they were about 80% (see table 1, p 1640).[9] **Eye infections:** We found no systematic review or RCTs. We found only one study of the treatment of gonococcal conjunctivitis, in which all 12 participants responded well to a single 1 g dose of ceftriaxone.[10]

Harms: Single dose regimens using fluoroquinolones, third generation and extended spectrum cephalosporins, or spectinomycin are generally safe and well tolerated. The most important adverse effects are rare hypersensitivity reactions. Minor adverse effects are most troublesome for the 800 mg cefixime regimen,[11,12] and the 2 g azithromycin regimen;[13] both cause frequent gastrointestinal upset. All the other doses found effective are associated with a low incidence of adverse outcomes. One large observational cohort study of azithromycin, cefixime, ciprofloxacin, and ofloxacin "in everyday use" found few serious adverse effects.[14] Quinolones may cause arthropathy in animals. No evidence of joint toxicity has been observed in clinical use, even with prolonged, multiple dose regimens used for the management of children with cystic fibrosis.[15–19]

Comment: There is good agreement between antigonococcal activity of antimicrobials *in vitro* and their efficacy in clinical trials. A large number of people were evaluated in a range of settings, suggesting that the results can be generalised. However, comparative results from different settings were not provided. Single dose regimens may make adherence more likely. The ceftriaxone and spectinomycin regimens require intramuscular injection. Resistance is now widespread for all penicillins, sulphonamides, and tetracyclines, and is becoming common for fluroquinolones in parts of Asia and the Pacific including Hawaii and California. Resistance to third generation and extended spectrum cephalosporins or spectinomycin is rarely reported (see table 2, p 1641).

QUESTION What are the effects of treatments for uncomplicated infections in pregnant women?

One systematic review has found that antibiotic treatment in pregnancy is effective. We found no reports of serious adverse effects.

Benefits: We found one systematic review (search date 2001; 2 RCTs) of treatments of gonococcal infection during pregnancy.[25] One of the RCTs (267 pregnant women with positive cultures for gonorrhoea) compared amoxicillin (amoxycillin) plus probenecid versus spectinomycin, versus ceftriaxone. Overall, it found no significant difference between regimens (failure to achieve cure 9/84 [10.7%] with amoxicillin *v* 4/84 [4.8%] with spectinomycin, RR 2.25, 95% CI 0.72 to 7.02; 9/84 [10.7%] with amoxicillin *v* 4/84 [4.8%] with ceftriaxone, RR 2.25, 95% CI 0.72 to 7.02). By site of infection amoxicillin 3 g cured 91% of cervical infections, 85% of rectal infections, and 80% of pharyngeal infections; single dose ceftriaxone 250 mg cured 95% of rectal and cervical infections and 100% of pharyngeal infections; spectinomycin 2 g cured 97% of rectal and cervical infections and 83% of pharyngeal infections.[26] The second RCT (95 women with positive cultures for gonorrhoea) compared a single dose of ceftriaxone intramuscularly versus a single dose of cefixime orally.[25] It found that eradication rates were similar in the two groups: ceftriaxone 125 mg eradicated 96.8% (95% CI 89.0% to 99.6%) of cervical and rectal infections and 100% (95% CI 47.8% to 100%) of pharyngeal infections; cefixime 400 mg eradicated 96% (95% CI 88.8% to 99.6%) of cervical and rectal infections and 100% (95% CI 54.1% to 100%) of pharyngeal infections.

Harms: The systematic review reported vomiting after treatment in 1/267 (0.4%) women included in one trial.[25] The second RCT reported soreness at the injection site among women receiving ceftriaxone and some "minor" malformations among their children, generally cosmetic (e.g. nevus, café au lait spots, skin tag; 10/60 [16.7%]

with ceftriaxone *v* 7/62 [11.3%] with cefixime).[27] Because quinolones cause arthropathy in animals, their use is not recommended in pregnancy, although we found no reports of adverse effects of quinolones on pregnancy outcome in humans. One multicentre, prospective, controlled study (200 exposed women) found no evidence of adverse effects.[28] We found no evidence that the non-quinolone regimens listed above are less safe or less well tolerated by pregnant women than by men or non-pregnant women.

Comment: None.

QUESTION What are the effects of treatments for disseminated gonococcal infection?

We found no recent RCTs evaluating treatment for disseminated gonococcal infection. We found no reports of treatment failures with multidose regimens using injectable cephalosporins or quinolones.

Benefits: We found no systematic review and no RCTs of the treatment of disseminated gonococcal infection published in the last 20 years.

Harms: We found no reports of adverse effects of multidose regimens using injectable cephalosporins or quinolones in this context.

Comment: More than a hundred clinical trials involving over 20 000 people have found that many single dose antimicrobial regimens cure uncomplicated infections more than 90% of the time.[6] Given the protracted natural history without treatment, this evidence suggests that treatment with these antimicrobial regimens is beneficial. Which regimens are most beneficial cannot be determined precisely because direct randomised comparisons of the best different regimens have not been performed. However, analysis of available trials supports the consensus that the most effective regimens are those using selected third generation or expanded spectrum cephalosporins and, except where resistance is common, those using selected fluoroquinolones or spectinomycin. We found no RCTs of antibiotic treatment in complicated gonorrhoea, but there is a strong consensus supporting the view that the most effective treatments for these conditions are multidose regimens using injectable cephalosporins or quinolones. Although we found no published data establishing the efficacy of this treatment, we found no reports of treatment failures.

QUESTION What are the effects of dual treatment for gonorrhoea and chlamydia infection?

Dual treatment with an antimicrobial effective against *Chlamydia trachomatis* is based on theory and expert opinion rather than evidence. The balance between benefits and harms from controlled trials will vary with the prevalence of coinfection in each population.

Benefits: We found no systematic review or RCTs.

Harms: We found no good evidence on the harms of dual treatment. Treatment for chlamydia can cause mild gastrointestinal distress, and there is the possibility that using a second drug could stimulate the emergence or spread of resistance in *N gonorrhoeae* or other bacteria.

Comment: Routine dual treatment has been advocated and implemented for the last 19 years, and is believed to have two potential benefits. Firstly, it is believed by some to have contributed to the decline in the prevalence of chlamydia infection observed in some populations. We found no evidence for any direct effect of dual treatment on chlamydia prevalence. Other factors may have contributed to reduced chlamydia prevalence (including widespread screening for asymptomatic chlamydia infection and changes in sexual behaviour), making it difficult to attribute decreases in the prevalence of chlamydia infection to any specific cause. Secondly, routine dual treatment may retard the spread of resistant gonococcal strains. Limited data from case reports support this belief. In the past, chlamydia testing was often unavailable, expensive, time consuming, and not highly sensitive, whereas dual treatment with a tetracycline, such as doxycycline, was safe and inexpensive. Chlamydia testing has now become more widely available, more affordable, quicker, and more sensitive, and the prevalence of chlamydia has fallen in some populations. Nevertheless, chlamydia is still found in 20–40% of people with gonorrhoea in many clinics.[1]

Substantive changes

Treatments for uncomplicated infections Updated systematic review;[25] conclusions unchanged.

REFERENCES

1. Centers for Disease Control and Prevention. Sexually transmitted diseases treatment guidelines 2002. *Morb Mortal Wkly Rep* 2002;51(RR-6):36–42.
2. Division of STD Prevention, Centers for Disease Control and Prevention, Sexually transmitted diseases surveillance, 2000. Atlanta, GA: US Department of Health and Human Services, Centers for Disease Control and Prevention, September 2001. http://www.cdc.gov/std/stats (last accessed 26/09/2002).
3. PHLS, DHSS and PS, Scottish ISD(D)5 Collaborative Group. Trends in sexually transmitted infections in the United Kingdom, 1996 to 2001. London: Public Health Laboratory Service, 2002. http://www.phls.co.uk/topics_az/hiv_and_sti/sti-gonorrhoea/epidemiology/epidemiology.htm (last accessed 26/09/2002).
4. Low N, Daker-White G, Barlow D, et al. Gonorrhoea in inner London: results of a cross-sectional study. *BMJ* 1997;314:1719–1723.
5. Hook EW, Handsfield HH. Gonococcal infections in the adult. In: Holmes KK, Mardh P-A, Sparling PF, et al, eds. *Sexually Transmitted Diseases* 3rd ed. New York: McGraw-Hill, 1999.
6. Moran JS, Levine WC. Drugs of choice for the treatment of uncomplicated gonococcal infections. *Clin Infect Dis* 1995;20(suppl 1):47–65. Search date 1993; primary sources Medline, reference lists from retrieved articles, abstracts from the annual Interscience Conference on Antimicrobial Agents and Chemotherapy, and meetings of the International Society for Sexually Transmitted Disease Research 1990–1993.
7. Aplasca de los Reyes MR, Pato-Mesola V, et al. A randomized trial of ciprofloxacin versus cefixime for treatment of gonorrhea after rapid emergence of gonococcal ciprofloxacin resistance in the Philippines. *Clin Infect Dis* 2001;32:1313–1318.
8. Rahman M, Alam A, Nessa K, et al. Treatment failure with the use of ciprofloxacin for gonorrhea correlates with the prevalence of fluoroquinolone-resistant *Neisseria gonorrhoeae* strains in Bangladesh. *Clin Infect Dis* 2001;32:884–889.
9. Moran JS. Treating uncomplicated *Neisseria gonorrhoeae* infections: is the anatomic site of infection important? *Sex Transm Dis* 1995;22:39–47.
10. Haimovici R, Roussel TJ. Treatment of gonococcal conjunctivitis with single-dose intramuscular ceftriaxone. *Am J Ophthalmol* 1989;107:511–514.
11. Handsfield HH, McCormack WM, Hook EW III, et al. The Gonorrhea Treatment Study Group. A comparison of single-dose cefixime with ceftriaxone as treatment for uncomplicated gonorrhea. *N Engl J Med* 1991;325:1337–1341.
12. Megran DW, LeFebvre K, Willets V, et al. Single-dose oral cefixime versus amoxicillin plus probenecid for the treatment of uncomplicated gonorrhea in men. *Antimicrob Agents Chemother* 1990;34:355–357.
13. Handsfield HH, Dalu ZA, Martin DH, et al. Azithromycin Gonorrhea Study Group. Multicenter

trial of single-dose azithromycin vs. ceftriaxone in the treatment of uncomplicated gonorrhea. *Sex Transm Dis* 1994;21:107–111.
14. Wilton LV, Pearce GL, Mann RD. A comparison of ciprofloxacin, norfloxacin, ofloxacin, azithromycin and cefixime examined by observational cohort studies. *Br J Clin Pharmacol* 1996;41:277–284.
15. Green SD. Indications and restrictions of fluoroquinolone use in children. *Br J Hosp Med* 1996;56:420–423.
16. Grenier B. Use of fluoroquinolones in children. An overview. *Adv Antimicrob Antineoplastic Chemother* 1992;11–12:135–140.
17. Schaad UB. Use of quinolones in children and articular risk. *Arch Pediatr* 1996;3:183–184.
18. Hampel B, Hullmann R, Schmidt H. Ciprofloxacin in pediatrics: worldwide clinical experience based on compassionate use. Safety report. *Pediatr Infect Dis J* 1997;16:127–129.
19. Warren RW. Rheumatologic aspects of pediatric cystic fibrosis patients treated with fluoroquinolones. *Pediatr Infect Dis J* 1997;16:118–122.
20. Ye SZ. Survey on antibiotic sensitivity of Neisseria gonorrhoeae strains isolated in China, 1987–1992. *Sex Transm Dis* 1994;21:237–240.
21. Guoming L, Qun C, Shengchun W. Resistance of Neisseria gonorrhoeae epidemic strains to antibiotics: report of resistant isolates and surveillance in Zhanjiang, China: 1998–1999. *Sex Transm Dis* 2000;27:115–118.
22. The WHO Western Pacific Region Gonococcal Antimicrobial Surveillance Programme. Surveillance of antibiotic resistance in *Neisseria gonorrhoeae* in the WHO Western Pacific Region, 2000. *Commun Dis Intell* 2001;25:274–276.
23. Public Health Laboratory Service. The Gonococcal Resistance to Antimicrobials Surveillance Programme Annual Report, Year 2000 Collection. http://www.phls.co.uk/topics_az/hiv_and_sti/sti_gonorrhoea/epidemiology/grasp_report.pdf (last accessed 26/09/2002).
24. Fiorito S, Galarza P, Pagano I, et al. Emergence of high level ciprofloxacin resistant *Neisseria gonorrhoeae* strain in Buenos Aires, Argentina. Sex *Transm Infect* 2001;77:77.
25. Brocklehurst P. Antibiotics for gonorrhoea in pregnancy (Cochrane Review). In: The Cochrane Library, Issue 2, 2002. Oxford: Update Software. Search date 2001; primary sources Cochrane Pregnancy and Childbirth Group Register and The Cochrane Controlled Trials Register.
26. Cavenee M, Farris J, Spalding T. Treatment of gonorrhea in pregnancy. *Obs Gyn* 1993;81:33–38.
27. Ramus RM, Sheffield JS, Mayfield JA, et al. A randomized trial that compared oral cefixime and intramuscular ceftriaxone for the treatment of gonorrhea in pregnancy. *Am J Obstet Gynecol* 2001;185:629–632.
28. Loebstein R, Addis A, Ho E, et al. Pregnancy outcome following gestational exposure to fluoroquinolones: a multicenter prospective controlled study. *Antimicrob Agents Chemother* 1998;42:1336–1339.

John Moran
Medical Epidemiologist
Centers for Disease Control and Prevention
Atlanta
USA

Competing interests: None declared.

TABLE 1 Effectiveness of selected single dose regimens in published clinical trials[6] and updated to 2002 (see text, p 1635).

	Pharyngeal infections		Urogenital and rectal infections	
Drug and dose	**% cured**	**95% CI**	**% cured**	**95% CI**
Ceftriaxone 250 mg	98.9	94.0 to 100	99.2	98.8 to 99.5
Ciprofloxacin 500 mg*	97.2	85.5 to 99.9	99.8	98.7 to 100
Ciprofloxacin 250 mg	88.5	88.8 to 95.2	98.7	98.0 to 99.4
Ceftriaxone 125 mg	94.1	85.6 to 98.4	98.8	97.9 to 99.8
Gatifloxacin 600 mg	100	82.3 to 100	99.6	97.7 to 100
Spectinomycin 2 g*	51.8	38.7 to 64.9	98.2	97.6 to 99.9
Azithromycin 2 g	100	82.3 to 100	99.2	97.2 to 99.9
Ofloxacin 400 mg	88.7	68.8 to 97.8	98.6	97.8 to 99.4
Gatifloxacin 400 mg	100	63.1 to 100	99.2	97.1 to 99.9
Cefixime 800 mg	80.0	51.9 to 95.7	98.4	95.9 to 99.6
Cefixime 400 mg	92.3	74.9 to 99.1	97.4	95.9 to 98.6

Data have been updated to include those from eligible studies published between 1993 and 2001. Only those regimens that are available in the USA, and have been shown in published studies to cure more than 95% of uncomplicated urogenital and rectal infections (with a lower 95% confidence limit > 95%), have been selected.

* Excludes two published clinical trials among people known to be at high risk of harbouring fluoroquinolone resistant strains; ciprofloxacin 500 mg cured only 48/72 (67%) of cervical infections in one trial[7] and 41/66 (62%) in the other.[8]

TABLE 2 Reported resistance of *N gonorrhoeae* to antimicrobials (see text, p 1635).

Drug	Resistance
Sulphonamides	Widespread
Penicillins	Widespread
Tetracyclines	Widespread
Third generation cephalosporins (e.g. ceftriaxone, cefixime)	Two reports from China[20,21]
Spectinomycin	Rare
Quinolones	Parts of Asia: common[22]
	USA: in 2000, resistance to ciprofloxacin was reported in 0.2% of isolates from the mainland and in 14% of isolates from Hawaii[2]
	UK: among 3166 gonorrhoeae isolates tested in 2000, 1.8% were flouroquinolone resistant and a further 2.4% showed decreased susceptibility[23]
	Australia, New Zealand, and Pacific Islands: 0–14%[22]
	South America: one fluoroquinolone resistant isolate reported[24]

Partner notification

Search date March 2002

Catherine Mathews, Nicol Coetzee, Merrick Zwarenstein, and Sally Guttmacher

QUESTIONS

INTERVENTIONS

See glossary, p 1648

Key Messages

- We found no good evidence on the effects of partner notification on relationships between patients and partners and, in particular, on the rate of violence, abuse, and abandonment of patient or partner.
- We found no studies comparing the effects of an intervention across different groups, such as people with different diseases or combinations of diseases, or people from different settings.
- **Contract referral (as effective as provider referral in people with syphilis)** One systematic review of one RCT comparing different partner notification strategies in people with syphilis found no significant difference in the proportion of partners notified between provider referral and contract referral, when people receiving the contract referral option were given only 2 days to notify their partners.
- **Provider referral, contract referral, or offering a choice between provider and patient referral (v patient referral alone) in people with HIV, gonorrhoea, or chlamydia** One systematic review comparing different partner notification strategies found that in people with HIV, offering a choice between provider referral (where the identity of the index patient was not revealed) and patient referral was more effective than offering patient referral alone. It found that in people with gonorrhoea infections, contract referral versus patient referral significantly increases the number of partners presenting for treatment. In chlamydia infections, provider referral versus patient referral significantly increased the proportion of partners assessed per patient (NNT 2, 95% CI 1 to 3) and the rate of positive partners detected per patient (NNT 17, 95% CI 10 to 50). The systematic review found no good evidence on the effects of these strategies on relationships between patients and partners and, in particular, on the rate of violence, abuse, and abandonment of patient or partner.

Clin Evid 2002;8:1642–1648.

■ **Adding telephone reminders and contact cards to patient referral; patient referral with educational videos; patient referral by different types of healthcare professionals** We found insufficient evidence about the effects of these interventions in improving partner notification.

DEFINITION Partner notification is a process whereby the sexual partners of people with a diagnosis of sexually transmitted infection are informed of their exposure to infection. The main methods are patient referral, provider referral, contract referral, and outreach assistance (see glossary, p 1648).

INCIDENCE/ PREVALENCE A large proportion of people with sexually transmitted infections will have neither symptoms nor signs of infection. For example, 22–68% of men with gonorrhoea who were identified through partner notification were asymptomatic.[1] Partner notification is one of the two strategies to reach such individuals, the other strategy being screening. Managing infection in people with more than one current sexual partner is likely to have the greatest impact on the spread of sexually transmitted infections.[2]

PROGNOSIS Studies showing that partner notification results in a health benefit, either to the partner or to future partners of infected partners, are not available. Obtaining such evidence would be technically and ethically difficult. One RCT in asymptomatic women compared identifying, testing, and treating women at increased risk for cervical chlamydial infection versus usual care. It found these reduced incidence of pelvic inflammatory disease (RR 0.44, 95% CI 0.20 to 0.90).[3] This evidence suggests that partner notification, which also aims to identify and treat people who are largely unaware of infection, would provide a direct health benefit to partners who are infected.

AIMS To prevent complications of infection in the partner; to prevent transmission to others; to prevent reinfection; and to identify social networks of people practising risky sexual behaviours.

OUTCOMES Partners identified; partners notified; partners presenting for care; partners testing positive; partners treated; rates of reinfection in the patient; incidence of sexually transmitted diseases in the population; harms to patient or partner, such as domestic violence and abuse; ethical outcomes (patient autonomy versus beneficence). The main outcome presented in each option is the ratio of the number of partners notified to the number of index patients.

METHODS *Clinical Evidence* update search and appraisal March 2002. We included RCTs comparing at least two alternative partner notification strategies. The outcome used in this summary was the absolute difference between the ratio of partners identified, notified, presenting for care, testing positive, or treated per index case. Assuming a Poisson distribution for the outcomes, the 95% confidence intervals were calculated using the normal approximation to the Poisson distribution. We excluded studies that did not allow us to extract data on people with specific sexually transmitted diseases, rather than on one of a range of sexually transmitted diseases.

QUESTION **What are the effects of different partner notification strategies in different groups of people?**

OPTION **IN PEOPLE WITH HIV INFECTION**

One systematic review of one RCT found that, for people with HIV infection, offering index patients a choice between provider referral (where the identity of the index patient is not revealed to the partner) and patient referral resulted in more partners being notified than offering patient referral alone.

Benefits: We found one systematic review (search date 2001, 1 RCT, 162 people who tested positive for HIV).[4] **Offering a choice between provider and patient referral versus patient referral:** The RCT (162 people who tested positive for HIV) compared provider referral (see glossary, p 1648) with patient referral (see glossary, p 1648). It was conducted at three public health departments in North Carolina, USA. Of those approached, the 46% who agreed to participate in the study were mostly men (69%), of whom most were homosexual or bisexual (76%). The choice between provider referral and patient referral significantly increased the likelihood that partners would be notified (rate of number of partners notified to number of index patients 78/39 [2.00] for the group with choice *v* 10/35 [0.29] for the patient referral group; rate reduction 1.71, 95% CI 1.35 to 2.07). Thus, for every person offered provider referral compared with using patient referral there will be more than one additional partner notified (see web extra figure A at www.clinicalevidence.com). **Contract referral:** We found no RCTs assessing contract referral (see glossary, p 1648) in people with HIV infection. **Outreach assistance:** The systematic review found one RCT, comparing patient referral versus outreach assistance (see glossary, p 1648) in people with HIV who were injecting drug users, the findings of which have yet to be fully reported.[4]

Harms: People's reluctance to disclose their HIV status to partners (see comment below) suggests expectation of harms from doing so. These and other potential harms are poorly understood. The results of the RCT comparing patient referral with outreach assistance[5] are expected to be published soon, and these will include comparisons of the risk of domestic violence and suicide.

Comment: The number of partners notified is an intermediate outcome. The number of infections in partners that are prevented or treated has not been assessed. Thus, the true benefits and harms of HIV partner notification are unknown. **Rates of disclosure:** One descriptive study (276 people attending for initial primary care for HIV infection in the USA) found that 40% of the respondents had not disclosed their HIV status to all partners over the preceding 6 months.[6] Individuals with more than one partner were significantly less likely to disclose to all partners. Only 42% of the non-disclosers reported that they used condoms all the time, which indicates that many partners were at risk of HIV infection. Another descriptive study conducted in the USA found that, even after repeated individual counselling of people with HIV infection and a 6 month opportunity to disclose HIV status, 30% had not informed any of their past partners and 29% had not informed any of their present partners.[7] **Patient preferences:** The RCT (162 people) comparing offering people a choice between provider and patient referral with patient referral alone found that, in the group with the choice, most partners (90%) were notified by the provider and only eight people by the index patient.[4] The RCT comparing patient referral versus outreach assistance[5] found, among people allocated to a choice, 82% chose to have the outreach team notify at least one partner, and the team was asked to notify 71% of all partners named by this group. One group in the USA attempted to compare contract referral with provider referral, but contamination between comparison groups made this impossible.[8] The results were therefore analysed as a cohort study without comparison groups, where all patients were assigned to provider referral. The study included 1070 people, who reported having had 8633 partners in the past year. Of these partners, 1035 were successfully located, of whom 248 had previously tested positive for HIV, 560 were tested by the disease intervention specialist, 69 refused testing, and 158 were located by record search only. Of the 560 partners tested, 122 tested positive.

OPTION IN PEOPLE WITH GONORRHOEA OR CHLAMYDIA

One systematic review has found that, for people with gonorrhoea, contract versus patient referral increases the rate of partners presenting for treatment. One RCT also found that contract versus patient referral increased the rate of positive partners detected. For people with non-gonococcal urethritis, one RCT found that provider versus patient referral increased the proportion of partners notified and of positive partners detected per patient.

Benefits: We found one systematic review (search date 2001, 2 RCTs of partner notification in people with gonorrhoea and 1 in people with non-gonococcal urethritis).[4] **Gonorrhoea:** The two RCTs (2085 people with gonorrhoea) compared patient referral with contract referral (see glossary, p 1648). The first RCT (1898 people) found that contract referral significantly increased the number of partners assessed per index patient (392/632 [0.62 partners per index patient] with contract referral *v* 469/1266 [0.37] with patient referral; rate difference 0.25 partners per index patient, 95% CI 0.18 to 0.32). Positive gonorrhoea culture was significantly more likely in the contract referral group than in the patient referral group (233/632 [0.37 positive partners per index patient] with contract referral v 315/1266 [0.25] with patient referral; rate difference 0.12, 95% CI 0.06 to 0.18). The second RCT (187 index patients) found contract referral was associated with a non-significantly higher proportion of partners assessed per index patient (119/94 [1.27] with contract referral *v* 107/93 [1.15] in the patient referral group; rate difference +0.12, 95% CI –0.2 to +0.44), and found no significant difference in the number of partners with positive gonorrhoea cultures per index patient.[4] (See web extra figure B at www.clinicalevidence.com.) **Chlamydia:** One RCT (678 people with non-gonococcal urethritis) compared patient referral with provider referral (see glossary, p 1648). It found that provider referral significantly increased the proportion of partners assessed per patient (159/221 [0.72] with provider referral *v* 91/457 [0.20] with patient referral; rate difference 0.52, 95% CI 0.40 to 0.64). In this study, provider referral also significantly increased the proportion of partners with positive culture per index patient (20/221 [0.09] with provider referral *v* 14/457 [0.03] with patient referral; rate difference 0.06, 95% CI 0.02 to 0.10). Provider referral would have to be offered to two index patients with non-gonococcal urethritis for one additional partner to be assessed (NNT 2, 95% CI 1 to 3), and to 17 index patients to identify one additional partner with a positive culture (NNT 17, 95% CI 10 to 50). These findings are likely to over estimate the difference, as partners referred by index patients may have been assessed elsewhere.[4] See web extra figure C at www.clinicalevidence.com.

Harms: These are poorly understood.

Comment: One cohort study (265 urban, adolescent girls attending a clinic in Alabama, USA) found that, given the choice, people with gonorrhoea or chlamydia are about as likely to choose provider referral as patient referral.[9]

OPTION IN PEOPLE WITH SYPHILIS

One systematic review of one large RCT found no significant difference between provider referral versus contract referral, when people receiving the contract referral option were given only 2 days in which to notify their partners. We found no RCTs assessing patient referral.

Benefits: We found one systematic review (search date 2001, 1 RCT, 1966 people diagnosed with syphilis in 3 US states).[4] It compared the proportion of partners per patient who were located, tested, tested positive, and treated, using three types of referral process: contract referral (see glossary, p 1648) (patients were given 2 days to notify partners themselves, before disease intervention specialists would notify them); provider referral (see glossary, p 1648) (immediate notification by an intervention specialist); and provider referral with the option of a blood test (immediate notification by an intervention specialist who had the option of performing a blood test if he or she thought that the partner would not seek medical attention despite being notified of exposure). There were no significant differences between the three groups: 1.2, 1.1, and 1.1 partners per patient were located; 0.92, 0.87, and 0.86 were tested; and 0.67, 0.61, and 0.62 were treated (CI not provided).[4]

Harms: These are poorly understood.

Comment: In the RCT, the investigators had no way of determining whether disease intervention specialists began actively seeking partners in the contract referral group before waiting 2 days, and they found some evidence of such contamination.[4] Furthermore, the investigators speculated that people may have been allocated to groups not according to the randomisation schedule. These problems may compromise the validity of the study. The use of disease intervention specialists is an approach that may not be generalisable to other settings.

QUESTION **What can be done to improve the effectiveness of patient referral?**

One systematic review found one small RCT, which found no significant difference between counselling plus contract referral cards and telephone follow up versus counselling alone. One RCT found no difference in the effects of patient referral by different healthcare professionals. One RCT found no difference in the effects of providing an information pamphlet versus routine counselling alone, but the RCT was potentially subject to confounding. One RCT found no significant difference between educational versus standard care, but the outcome reported was potentially inappropriate.

Benefits: We found one systematic review (search date 2001, 4 published RCTs and 1 unpublished RCT).[4] **Counselling plus contract referral cards and telephone follow up:** One RCT (38 students from a university clinic in the USA) compared the use of counselling plus contact referral cards and telephone follow up of the index case with counselling alone. It found no difference between the strategies in the rate of partners presenting for care. The trial also assessed adding a \$3 incentive to the referral card. Charges for clinic visits for patients and partners would be waived after successful recruitment of partners for treatment. This had no effect on the number of partners presenting for care.[4] **Different health professionals:** One RCT (678 index patients) found that there was no difference between patient referral (see glossary, p 1648) using nurses who did not ask for partners' names and gave referral letters, and disease intervention specialists who took partners' names but no contact details, in terms of the number of partners with positive cultures who were identified (rate difference 0, 95% CI –0.03 to +0.03).[4] **Information pamphlets:** One unpublished RCT (1898 index patients), conducted in the USA, investigated the use of information pamphlets compared with a routine counselling interview alone. Providing patients with information pamphlets was as effective as the interview alone (rate difference 0, 95% CI –0.07 to +0.07). The two strategies were also equally effective in terms of the number of partners identified with a positive culture per index patient. However, the RCT combined two interventions: different health professionals and asking for partners' names, either of which may have affected the results.[4] **Educational videos:** The review identified one RCT (902 people in the USA) comparing a video taped story promoting partner notification versus standard care. No differences in the number of partners assessed were reported (figures not provided).[4] The RCT counted returned contact cards as the main outcome, which has not been shown to be a sensitive enough surrogate indicator for partners presenting for assessment.[10]

Harms: None reported.

Comment: None.

Partner notification

GLOSSARY

Contract referral (also known as conditional referral). Index patients are encouraged to inform their partners, with the understanding that health service personnel will notify those partners who do not visit the health service within a contracted time period.

Outreach assistance At the request of patients, partners are notified by members of an outreach team indigenous to the community, who do not disclose the name of the patient to the partners.

Patient referral Health service personnel encourage index patients to inform partners directly of their possible exposure to sexually transmitted infections.

Provider referral Third parties (usually health service personnel) notify partners identified by index patients, without disclosing the name of the patient to the partners.

REFERENCES

1. Holmes KK, Mardh PA, Sparling PF, et al, eds. *Sexually Transmitted Diseases*, 2nd edn. New York: McGraw-Hill, 1990:1083.
2. Fenton KA, Peterman TA. HIV partner notification: taking a new look. *AIDS* 1997;11:1535–1546.
3. Scholes D, Stergachis A, Heidrich FE, et al. Prevention of pelvic inflammatory disease by screening for cervical chlamydial infection. *N Engl J Med* 1996;21:1399–1401.
4. Mathews C, Coetzee N, Zwarenstein M, et al. Strategies for partner notification for sexually transmitted diseases. Cochrane Library, Issue 1, 2002. Search date 2001; primary sources Medline, Embase, Psychological Abstracts, Sociological Abstracts, Cochrane Controlled Trials Register, hand searching of the proceedings of International AIDS Conferences and the International Society for STD Research meetings, and personal contact with key experts.
5. Levy JA, Fox SE. The outreach-assisted model of partner notification with IDUs. *Public Health Rep* 1998;113(suppl 1):160–169.
6. Stein MD, Freedberg KA, Sullivan LM, et al. Sexual ethics: disclosure of HIV-positive status to partners. *Arch Intern Med* 1998;158:253–257.
7. Perry SW, Card CAL, Moffatt M, et al. Self-disclosure of HIV infection to sexual partners after repeated counseling. *AIDS Educ Prev* 1994;6:403–411.
8. Toomey KE, Peterman TA, Dicker LW, et al. Human immunodeficiency virus partner notification. *Sex Transm Dis* 1998;25:310–316.
9. Oh MK, Boker JR, Genuardi FJ, et al. Sexual contact tracing in adolescent chlamydial and gonococcal cervicitis cases. *J Adolesc Health* 1996;18:4–9.
10. Potterat JJ, Rothenberg R. The case-finding effectiveness of self-referral system for gonorrhea: a preliminary report. *Am J Public Health* 1977;67:174–176.

Nicol Coetzee
Senior Lecturer and Consultant
Department of Public Health University of Cape Town
Cape Town
South Africa

Sally Guttmacher
Department of Health Studies
New York University
New York
USA

Catherine Mathews
Senior Scientist
Health Systems Unit
South African Medical Research Council
University of Cape Town
Cape Town
South Africa

Merrick Zwarenstein
Director, Health Systems Research Unit
Medical Research Council
Tygerberg
South Africa

Competing interests: None declared.

Pelvic inflammatory disease

Search date April 2002

Jonathan Ross

QUESTIONS

INTERVENTIONS

Key Messages

- **Antibiotics (symptoms improved and microbiological clearance in women with confirmed pelvic inflammatory disease)** One systematic review of observational studies and RCTs has found that several different regimens of antibiotic treatment are effective in relieving the symptoms of pelvic inflammatory disease and achieve high rates of microbiological cure.
- **Different durations of antibiotic treatment** Systematic reviews found no good evidence on the optimal duration of treatment.
- **Empirical antibiotic treatment** We found no RCTs comparing empirical treatment with antibiotics (before receiving results of microbiological tests) versus delaying treatment until test results are available.
- **Oral versus parenteral antibiotics** Two RCTs found no significant difference between oral ofloxacin versus parenteral cefoxitin and doxycycline.
- **Routine antibiotic prophylaxis prior to intrauterine device insertion** One systematic review found no significant difference between routine prophylaxis with doxycycline versus placebo prior to intrauterine contraceptive device insertion in pelvic inflammatory disease. The absolute risk of pelvic inflammatory disease following intrauterine contraceptive device insertion was low. However, the systematic review may have lacked power to rule out a clinically important difference. We found no good evidence on the effects in people likely to be at high risk for pelvic inflammatory disease.

Pelvic inflammatory disease

DEFINITION Pelvic inflammatory disease (PID) is inflammation and infection of the upper genital tract in women, typically involving the fallopian tubes, ovaries, and surrounding structures.

INCIDENCE/ PREVALENCE The exact incidence of PID is unknown because the disease cannot be diagnosed reliably from clinical symptoms and signs.[1–3] Direct visualisation of the fallopian tubes by laparoscopy is the best single diagnostic test, but it is invasive and not used routinely in clinical practice. PID is the most common gynaecological reason for admission to hospital in the USA, accounting for 49/10 000 recorded hospital discharges and a diagnosis of PID is made in 1/62 (1.6%) women aged 16–45 years attending their primary care physician in England and Wales.[4] However, because most PID diseases are asymptomatic, this figure underestimates the true prevalence.[1,5] A crude marker of PID in developing countries can be obtained from reported hospital admission rates, where it accounts for 17–40% of gynaecological admissions in sub-Saharan Africa, 15–37% in Southeast Asia, and 3–10% in India.[6]

AETIOLOGY/ RISK FACTORS Factors associated with PID mirror those for sexually transmitted infections: young age, reduced socioeconomic circumstances, African/Afro-Caribbean ethnicity, lower educational attainment, and recent new sexual partner.[2,7,8] Infection ascends from the cervix and initial epithelial damage caused by bacteria (especially *Chlamydia trachomatis* and *Neisseria gonorrhoeae*) allows the opportunistic entry of other organisms. Isolates from the upper genital tract are polymicrobial, including *Mycoplasma hominis* and anaerobes.[9] The spread of infection to the upper genital tract may be increased by vaginal douching and instrumentation of the cervix, but reduced by the barrier method and oral contraceptives compared with other forms of contraception.[10–13]

PROGNOSIS PID has high morbidity; about 20% of affected women become infertile, 20% develop chronic pelvic pain, and 10% of those who conceive have an ectopic pregnancy.[2] We found no placebo controlled trials of antibiotic treatment. Uncontrolled observations suggest that clinical symptoms and signs resolve in a significant number of untreated women.[14] Repeated episodes of pelvic inflammatory disease are associated with a four to six times increase in the risk of permanent tubal damage.[15] One case control study (76 cases and 367 controls) found that delaying treatment by even a few days is associated with impaired fertility (OR 2.6, 95% CI 1.2 to 5.9).[16]

AIMS To alleviate the pain and systemic malaise associated with infection; to achieve microbiological cure; to prevent development of permanent tubal damage with associated sequelae, such as chronic pelvic pain, ectopic pregnancy, and infertility; and to prevent the spread of infection to others.

OUTCOMES Incidence and severity of acute symptoms and signs; microbiological cure of the upper genital tract; incidence of chronic pelvic pain, ectopic pregnancy, and infertility; rate of transmission to others.

METHODS *Clinical Evidence* update search and appraisal April 2002.

QUESTION **What are the effects of empirical treatment versus treatment delayed until the results of microbiological investigations are known?**

OPTION **EMPIRICAL ANTIBIOTIC TREATMENT**

We found no good evidence on the effects of empirical treatment versus delayed antibiotic treatment for suspected pelvic inflammatory disease.

Benefits: We found no systematic review or RCTs comparing empirical versus delayed treatment.

Harms: We found no reliable evidence on harms.

Comment: Because there are no reliable clinical diagnostic criteria for pelvic inflammatory disease, early empirical treatment is common.[3] The positive predictive value of a clinical diagnosis is 65–90% compared with laparoscopy.[1–3] The absence of infection from the lower genital tract, where samples are usually taken, does not exclude pelvic inflammatory disease[2] and so may not influence the decision to treat. One case control study (76 cases and 367 controls) found that delaying treatment is associated with impaired fertility (OR 2.6, 95% CI 1.2 to 5.9).[16]

QUESTION **How do different antimicrobial regimens compare?**

One systematic review of observational trials and RCTs has found that several different regimens of parenteral followed by oral antibiotic treatment are effective in resolving the acute symptoms and signs associated with pelvic inflammatory disease. We found no good evidence on the optimal duration of treatment. Two RCTs found no significant difference between oral ofloxacin versus parenteral cefoxitin and doxycycline.

Benefits: We found one systematic review (search date 1992, 21 studies),[17] aspects of which were subsequently updated (search date 1997, 26 studies, 1925 women).[18] These reviews answer different questions and cover different aspects. They evaluated 16 different antimicrobial regimens. The identified studies included case series, and it is not possible from the aggregated data published in the reviews to ascertain how many studies were RCTs. Inclusion criteria were a diagnosis of pelvic inflammatory disease (clinical, microbiological, laparoscopic, or by endometrial biopsy) and microbiological testing for *C trachomatis* and *N gonorrhoeae*. The reviews found antibiotics were effective in relieving the symptoms associated with pelvic inflammatory disease, with clinical and microbiological cure rates of 88–100% (see table 1, p 1654). The only regimen that appeared to perform less well was oral metronidazole with doxycycline (see table 1, p 1654). **Duration of treatment:** The duration of treatment was not addressed, although the most common treatment period was 14 days. **Oral versus parenteral treatment:** The reviews did not analyse outcomes by oral or parenteral route of administration. Most regimens started with parenteral treatment and continued with oral treatment at different points. Two RCTs (249 and 72 women) compared oral ofloxacin versus parenteral cefoxitin and doxycycline. The RCTs found no significant difference in cure rates between groups (clinical cure rates about 95% for all treatments).[19,20]

Harms: The harms associated with treatment were not specifically addressed by the systematic reviews.[17,18] In two RCTs reporting adverse effects, withdrawal from treatment was uncommon (2/20 for doxycycline/metronidazole; 0/20 for pefloxacin/metronidazole; 0/16 for ciprofloxacin).[21,22]

Comment: We found little evidence about long term sequelae of pelvic inflammatory disease, adverse effects of treatment, treatment of pelvic inflammatory disease of differing severity, the effect of ethnicity, or the effects of tracing sexual contacts (see partner notification, p 1642). The risks of tubal occlusion and subsequent infertility relate to the severity of pelvic inflammatory disease prior to starting treatment,[23] and clinical improvement may not translate into preserved fertility.[24,25] The inclusion of observational studies in the systematic review without a sensitivity analysis may compromise the validity of the conclusions.

QUESTION **What are the effects of routine antibiotic prophylaxis to prevent pelvic inflammatory disease prior to intrauterine contraceptive device insertion?**

One systematic review found that routine prophylaxis with doxycycline versus placebo prior to intrauterine contraceptive device insertion did not reduce the risk of pelvic inflammatory disease. The absolute risk of pelvic inflammatory disease following intrauterine contraceptive device insertion was low. We found no good evidence on the effects in groups likely to be at high risk.

Benefits: We found one systematic review (search date 2000, 4 RCTs, 3598 women requesting intrauterine contraceptive device insertion).[26] The RCTs compared a single dose of doxycycline (200 mg), 1 hour prior to intrauterine device insertion, versus placebo. Meta-analysis in the review found no significant difference in the incidence of pelvic inflammatory disease (doxycycline *v* placebo OR 0.89, 95% CI 0.53 to 1.51). The rate of pelvic inflammatory disease in all women was low (0.5–1.6%). We found no RCTs on the effects in people likely to be at high risk.

Harms: The harms associated with treatment were not specifically addressed by the systematic review.[26] Nausea and vomiting has been reported with 17–28% of healthy volunteers on doxycycline, depending on the formulation administered.[27] See harms of antimicrobial regimens, p 1652.

Comment: In the populations included in the systematic review, the risk of pelvic inflammatory disease following intrauterine device insertion was low.[26] The occurrence of pelvic inflammatory disease in this group usually reflects the introduction of infection into the uterus during intrauterine device insertion and therefore will vary with the prevalence of sexually transmitted infections in the population. The confidence intervals are wide, suggesting that the study may have insufficient power to rule out a clinical important difference.

REFERENCES

1. Morcos R, Frost N, Hnat M, et al. Laparoscopic versus clinical diagnosis of acute pelvic inflammatory disease. *J Reprod Med* 1993;38:53–56.
2. Metters JS, Catchpole M, Smith C, et al. *Chlamydia trachomatis: summary and conclusions of CMO's expert advisory group*. London: Department of Health, 1998.
3. Centers for Disease Control. *1998 guidelines for treatment of sexually transmitted diseases*. Bethesda, Maryland: CDC, 1998. http://www.cdc.gov/epo/mmwr/preview/mmwrhtml/00050909.htm (last accessed 23 Sept 2002).
4. Simms I, Rogers P, Charlett A. The rate of diagnosis and demography of pelvic inflammatory disease in general practice: England and Wales. *International Journal of STD and AIDs* 1999;10:448–455.
5. Velebil P, Wingo PA, Xia Z, et al. Rate of hospitalization for gynecologic disorders among reproductive-age women in the United States. *Obstet Gynecol* 1995;86:764–769.
6. Kani J, Adler MW. Epidemiology of pelvic inflammatory disease. In: Berger GS, Weström L, eds. *Inflammatory disease*. New York: Raven Press, 1992.
7. Simms I, Catchpole M, Brugha R, et al. Epidemiology of genital *Chlamydia trachomatis* in England and Wales. *Genitourin Med* 1997;73:122–126.
8. Grodstein F, Rothman KJ. Epidemiology of pelvic inflammatory disease. *Epidemiology* 1994;5:234–242.
9. Bevan CD, Johal BJ, Mumtaz G, et al. Clinical, laparoscopic and microbiological findings in acute salpingitis: report on a United Kingdom cohort. *Br J Obstet Gynaecol* 1995;102:407–414.
10. Wolner-Hanssen P, Eschenbach DA, Paavonen J, et al. Association between vaginal douching and acute pelvic inflammatory disease. *JAMA* 1990;263:1936–1941.
11. Jacobson L, Westrom L. Objectivized diagnosis of acute pelvic inflammatory disease. Diagnostic and prognostic value of routine laparoscopy. *Am J Obstet Gynecol* 1969;105:1088–1098.
12. Kelaghan J, Rubin GL, Ory HW, et al. Barrier-method contraceptives and pelvic inflammatory disease. *JAMA* 1982;248:184–187.
13. Wolner-Hanssen P, Eschenbach DA, Paavonen J, et al. Decreased risk of symptomatic chlamydial pelvic inflammatory disease associated with oral contraceptive use. *JAMA* 1990;263:54–59.
14. Curtis AH. Bacteriology and pathology of fallopian tubes removed at operation. *Surg Gynecol Obstet* 1921;33:621.
15. Hillis SD, Owens LM, Marchbanks PA, et al. Recurrent chlamydial infections increase the risks of hospitalization for ectopic pregnancy and pelvic inflammatory disease. *Am J Obstet Gynecol* 1997;176:103–107.
16. Hillis SD, Joesoef R, Marchbanks PA, et al. Delayed care of pelvic inflammatory disease as a risk factor for impaired fertility. *Am J Obstet Gynecol* 1993;168:1503–1509.
17. Walker CK, Kahn JG, Washington AE, et al. Pelvic inflammatory disease: metaanalysis of antimicrobial regimen efficacy. *J Infect Dis* 1993;168:969–978. Search date 1992; primary sources Medline, and bibliographies from reviews, textbooks, and references.
18. Walker CK, Workowski KA, Washington AE, et al. Anaerobes in pelvic inflammatory disease: implications for the Centers for Disease Control and Prevention's guidelines for treatment of sexually transmitted diseases. *Clin Infect Dis* 1999;28(suppl):29–36. Search date 1997; primary sources Medline, and bibliographies from reviews, textbooks, and references.
19. Martens MG, Gordon S, Yarborough DR, et al. Multicenter randomized trial of ofloxacin versus cefoxitin and doxycycline in outpatient treatment of pelvic inflammatory disease. Ambulatory PID Research Group. *South Med J* 1993;86:604–610.
20. Wendel GD, Cox SM, Bawdon RE, et al. A randomized trial of ofloxacin versus cefoxitin and doxycycline in the outpatient treatment of acute salpingitis. *Am J Obstet Gynecol* 1991;164:1390–1396.
21. Witte EH, Peters AA, Smit IB, et al. A comparison of pefloxacin/metronidazole and doxycycline/metronidazole in the treatment of laparoscopically confirmed acute pelvic inflammatory disease. *Eur J Obstet Gynecol Reprod Biol* 1993;50:153–158.
22. Heinonen PK, Teisala K, Miettinen A, et al. A comparison of ciprofloxacin with doxycycline plus metronidazole in the treatment of acute pelvic inflammatory disease. *Scand J Infect Dis* 1989;60(suppl):66–73.
23. Soper DE, Brockwell NJ, Dalton HP. Microbial etiology of urban emergency department acute salpingitis: treatment with ofloxacin. *Am J Obstet Gynecol* 1992;167:653–660.
24. Buchan H, Vessey M, Goldacre M, et al. Morbidity following pelvic inflammatory disease. *Br J Obstet Gynaecol* 1993;100:558–562.
25. Brunham RC, Binns B, Guijon F, et al. Etiology and outcome of acute pelvic inflammatory disease. *J Infect Dis* 1988;158:510–517.
26. Grimes DA, Schulz KF. Antibiotic prophylaxis for intrauterine contraceptive device insertion. In: The Cochrane Library, Issue 2, 2001. Oxford: Update Software. Search date 2000; primary sources Medline, Embase, hand search of journals through CENTRAL, lists of references, and contact with experts in the field.
27. Story MJ, McCloud PI, Boehm G. Doxycycline tolerance study. Incidence of nausea after doxycycline administration to healthy volunteers: a comparison of 2 formulations (Doryx' vs Vibramycin'). *Eur J Clin Pharmacol* 1991;40:419–421.

Jonathan Ross
Honorary Senior Lecturer
University of Birmingham
Birmingham, UK

Competing interests: None declared.

TABLE 1 **Cure rates for the antibiotic treatment of acute pelvic inflammatory disease: aggregated data from systematic reviews of RCTs and case series (see text, p 1651).[17,18]**

Drug regimen	Number of studies	Number of women	Cure rate (%) clinical/ microbiological*
Inpatient treatment (initially parenteral switching to oral)			
Clindamycin + aminoglycoside	11	470	91/97
Cefoxitin + doxycycline	8	427	91/98
Cefotetan + doxycycline	3	174	95/100
Ceftizoxime + tetracycline	1	18	88/100
Cefotaxime + tetracycline	1	19	94/100
Ciprofloxacin	4	90	94/96
Ofloxacin	1	36	100/97
Sulbactam/ ampicillin + doxycycline	1	37	95/100
Co-amoxiclav	1	32	93/–
Metronidazole + doxycycline	2	36	75/71
Outpatient treatment (oral unless indicated otherwise)			
Cefoxitin (im) + probenecid + doxycycline	3	219	89/93
Ofloxacin	2	165	95/100
Co-amoxiclav	1	35	100/100
Sulbactam/ampicillin	1	36	70/70
Ceftriaxone (im) + doxycycline	1	64	95/100
Ciprofloxacin + clindamycin	1	67	97/94

**N gonorrhoeae*, *C trachomatis*, or both, when detected in lower genital tract; im, intramuscular.

Athlete's foot and fungally infected toe nails

Search date October 2001

Fay Crawford

QUESTIONS

INTERVENTIONS

Key Messages

- **Oral allylamines for athlete's foot** One RCT identified by a systematic review found limited evidence that oral terbinafine versus placebo for 6 weeks significantly improved cure rates at 8 weeks. One RCT found that oral terbinafine versus oral itraconazole for 2 weeks significantly increased cure rates, but found no significant difference in cure rates with 2 weeks of oral terbinafine versus 4 weeks of oral itraconazole.
- **Oral azoles for athlete's foot** One RCT identified by a systematic review found that oral itraconazole versus placebo for 1 week significantly increased cure rates at 8 weeks. The review found no significant difference in cure rates between individual azoles and oral allylamines, or between oral azoles and oral griseofulvin.
- **Topical acidified nitrite cream for athlete's foot** One systematic review of one RCT found limited evidence that topical nitrate plus salicylic acid versus salicylic acid alone for 4 weeks significantly improved cure rate.
- **Topical allylamines for athlete's foot** One systematic review and two subsequent RCTs have found that allylamines versus placebo significantly increase the proportion of people cured at 6–16 weeks. One systematic review and two additional RCTs have found that allylamines produce a faster response than azoles, but the cure rates are similar.
- **Topical azoles for athlete's foot** One systematic review has found that azole creams versus placebo administered for 4–6 weeks significantly increase cure rates at 6–10 weeks (NNT 2, 95% CI 1 to 4). One systematic review and two additional RCTs have found that azoles produce a slower response than allylamines, but the cure rates are similar.

Athlete's foot and fungally infected toe nails

- **Topical butenafine for fungal nail infections** RCTs found limited evidence that butenafine cream in combination with either urea or tea tree oil versus placebo significantly improved cure rates at 16–36 weeks.
- **Topical ciclopiroxolamine for athlete's foot** One systematic review of one RCT found that topical ciclopiroxolamine versus placebo for 4 weeks significantly reduced treatment failure at 6 weeks (NNT 2, 95% CI 1 to 4).
- **Topical ciclopiroxolamine for fungal nail infections** RCTs found that ciclopiroxolamine lacquer versus placebo significantly improved cure rates at 48 weeks.
- **Topical griseofulvin for athlete's foot** One systematic review of one RCT found that topical griseofulvin versus placebo significantly reduced treatment failure after 4 weeks (NNT 2, 95% CI 2 to 4).
- **Topical tolnaftate for athlete's foot** One systematic review has found that tolnaftate versus placebo for 4 weeks significantly reduces treatment failure after 5–8 weeks (NNT 2, 95% CI 2 to 4).
- **Topical undecenoic acid for athlete's foot** One systematic review has found that undecenoic acid versus placebo significantly reduces treatment failure at 4–6 weeks (NNT 2, 95% CI 2 to 3).

DEFINITION Athlete's foot is a cutaneous fungal infection that causes the skin to itch, flake, and fissure. Nail involvement is characterised by ungual thickening and discolouration.

INCIDENCE/ PREVALENCE In the UK, athlete's foot is present in about 15% of the general population,[1] and 1.2 million people have fungally infected toe nails.[2]

AETIOLOGY/ RISK FACTORS Swimming pool users and industrial workers may have increased risk of fungal foot infection. However, one survey found fungal foot infection in only 9% of swimmers, with the highest incidence (20%) in men aged 16 years and over.[1]

PROGNOSIS Fungal infections of the foot are not life threatening in people with normal immunity, but in some people they cause persistent symptoms. Others are apparently oblivious of persistent infection. The infection can spread to other parts of the body and to other individuals.

AIMS To control symptoms and prevent recurrence, with minimal adverse effects.

OUTCOMES Rates of fungal eradication, shown by negative microscopy and culture, and resolution of clinical signs and symptoms at follow up.

METHODS *Clinical Evidence* search and appraisal October 2001. We initially searched Medline, Embase, and the Cochrane Controlled Trials Register to May 2000 for systematic reviews and subsequent RCTs (all languages). Studies were excluded if foot specific data could not be extracted. We excluded studies that did not use microscopy and culture (skin infections) or culture (nail infections) for diagnosis and as an outcome measure. The evidence is presented for classes of treatment (allylamines, azoles, etc); individual members of each class are described in the text and listed in table 1 (see table 1, p 1663).

QUESTION What are the effects of topical antifungals for athlete's foot?

OPTION TOPICAL ALLYLAMINES (NAFTIFINE, TERBINAFINE)

One systematic review and two subsequent RCTs have found that allylamines versus placebo significantly increase the proportion of people cured at 6–16 weeks. One systematic review and two additional RCTs have found that allylamines produce a faster response than azoles, but the cure rates are similar.

Benefits: **Versus placebo:** We found one systematic review,[3,4] and three subsequent RCTs.[5–7] The systematic review (search date 1997, 12 RCTs, 1433 people with fungal infections of the foot) found that topical allylamines versus placebo for 1–4 weeks significantly reduced the risk of treatment failure assessed by culture or microscopy after 6–8 weeks (192/724 [27%] *v* 570/709 [80%] for placebo; ARR 55%, 95% CI 41% to 70%; RR 0.30, 95% CI 0.24 to 0.38; NNT 2 at 6 wks). The first subsequent RCT (70 people with interdigital tinea pedis and positive fungal culture) found a significant increase in the cure rate after 7 weeks with 7 days of 1% terbinafine cream versus placebo (mycological cure: 91% with terbinafine *v* 37% with placebo; CI not provided; $P < 0.001$).[5] The second subsequent RCT (60 people with moccasin type tinea pedis) compared 1% terbinafine cream versus 1% butenafine (a benzylamine derivative) cream versus placebo.[6] People receiving butenafine applied the cream for 1 week. Placebo and terbinafine were applied for 2 weeks. The RCT found significantly more people cured after 16 weeks with both terbinafine versus placebo and with butenafine versus placebo. The third subsequent RCT (153 people with interdigital tinea pedis) found significantly increased clinical cure after 8 weeks with terbinafine (1% solution) versus placebo (35/56 [65%] terbinafine *v* 1/23 [4%] with placebo; ARR 60%, 95% CI 45% to 75%). **Different allylamines:** The systematic review identified one small RCT (60 people), which found no significant difference in treatment failure with naftifine versus terbinafine (75% with naftifine *v* 81% with terbinafine; ARR 5%, 95% CI –17% to +21%). **Versus topical azoles:** See topical azoles, p 1658. **Versus butenafine**: We found one RCT (60 people with moccasin type tinea pedis), which compared 1% terbinafine cream versus 1% butenafine cream versus placebo.[6] The RCT found no significant difference in cure rate with terbinafine versus butenafine after 16 weeks (ARR 10%, 95% CI –12% to +32%).

Harms: The systematic review[3,4] did not report frequency of adverse effects. We found few reports of local irritation in any of the trials.

Comment: The systematic review assessed the quality of reporting in the trials. Out of a possible 12 points, the mean quality score for all 72 included studies was 6.3. Few demographic details of participants were reported.[3]

OPTION TOPICAL AZOLES

One systematic review has found that azole creams versus placebo administered for 4–6 weeks significantly increase cure rates at 6–10 weeks. One systematic review and two additional RCTs have found that azoles produce a slower response than allylamines, but the cure rates are similar.

Benefits: **Versus placebo:** We found one systematic review (search date 1997, 17 RCTs, 1259 people with fungal skin infections of the foot).[3,4] Interventions lasted for 4–6 weeks. The review found a significant reduction of the risk of treatment failure (determined by culture or microscopy after 6–10 wks) with azoles versus placebo (126/664 [19%] with azoles *v* 362/595 [61%] with placebo; ARR 42%, 95% CI 38% to 48%; RR 0.31, 95% CI 0.25 to 0.38; NNT 2, 95% CI 2 to 3). **Different azoles:** The systematic review (12 RCTs, 584 people) found no consistent difference over 3–10 weeks with one azole for 3–4 weeks versus another.[3,4] **Versus topical allylamines:** We found one systematic review (search date 1997, 12 RCTs, 1487 people with fungal infections of the foot)[3,4] and two additional RCTs.[8,9] The systematic review found a significant reduction after 3–12 weeks in the risk of treatment failure with 1–6 weeks of topical allylamine versus at least 4 weeks of topical azole (146/773 [19%] with topical allylamine *v* 224/714 [31%] for topical azole; ARR 13%, 95% CI 9% to 16%; RR 0.60, 95% CI 0.49 to 0.73; NNT 8, 95% CI 6 to 12). Four included RCTs found that a 1 week course of allylamine had similar failure rates as a 4 week course of azoles (53/464 [11%] with 1 wk of allylamine *v* 71/448 [16%] with 4 weeks of azole; ARR 4.4%, 95% CI 0% to 8%).[3,4] The first additional RCT (429 people with interdigital athlete's foot) found no significant difference in mycological cure after 8 weeks with 1% terbinafine solution (twice daily for 1 wk followed by 3 wks of placebo) versus 4 weeks of 1% clotrimazole solution (83% with terbinafine *v* 82% with clotrimazole; ARR +1%, 95% CI –5% to +8%).[8] The second RCT (48 people) also found no significant difference for mycological cure with 1% terbinafine cream (for 1 wk) versus 4 weeks of 2% clotrimazole cream after 10 weeks (ARR –2%, 95% CI –33% to +28%).[9]

Harms: One subsequent RCT found similar adverse events with 1% terbinafine solution and 1% clotrimazole solution.[8] About 5% of the people experienced mild to moderate local skin reactions, such as itching, erythema, or scaling.

Comment: See table 1 for a list of compounds categorised as topical azoles, p 1663.

OPTION OTHER TOPICAL AGENTS

One systematic review of one RCT found that topical ciclopiroxolamine versus placebo for 4 weeks significantly reduced treatment failure at 6 weeks. RCTs found that topical griseofulvin, undenoic acid, tolnaftate, or acidified nitrate cream versus placebo significantly reduced treatment failure after 4–8 weeks. One systematic review of one RCT found limited evidence that topical nitrate plus salicylic acid versus salicylic acid alone for 4 weeks significantly improved cure rate.

Benefits: We found one systematic review (search date 1997).[3] **Topical ciclopiroxolamine versus placebo:** The review identified one RCT (144 people with fungal skin infection of the foot).[4] It found a significant reduction of treatment failure after 6 weeks with topical ciclopiroxolamine versus placebo for 4 weeks (31/71 [44%] with ciclopiroxolamine *v* 67/73 [92%] with placebo; ARR 48%, 95% CI 25% to 69%; RRR 0.48, 95% CI 0.25 to 0.73; NNT 2, 95% CI 1 to 4). **Topical griseofulvin versus placebo:** The review identified one RCT (94 people), which found a significant reduction of treatment failure at 4 weeks with griseofulvin versus placebo (9/47 [19%] with griseofulvin *v* 31/47 [66%] with placebo; ARR 47%, 95% CI 28% to 58%; RR 0.29, 95% CI 0.13 to 0.57; NNT 2, 95% CI 2 to 4). **Topical undecenoic acid versus placebo:** The review identified four RCTs (223 people), which found a significant reduction of treatment failure at 4–6 weeks with undecenoic acid versus placebo (40/123 [33%] with undecenoic acid *v* 81/103 [79%] with placebo; ARR 46%, 95% CI 32% to 58%; RRR 0.41, 95% CI 0.27 to 0.60; NNT 2, 95% CI 2 to 3). **Topical tolnaftate versus placebo:** The review identified three RCTs (148 people), which found a significant reduction after 5–8 weeks in treatment failure with tolnaftate for 4 weeks versus placebo (20/78 [26%] with tolnaftate *v* 49/70 [70%] with placebo; ARR 44%, 95% CI 29% to 56%; RR 0.37, 95% CI 0.21 to 0.59; NNT 2, 95% CI 2 to 4). **Topical acidified nitrite cream and salicylate versus salicylate:** The review identified one RCT (60 people with interdigital athlete's foot), which found a significant improvement in cure rate with 3% nitrite plus 3% salicylic acid cream for 4 weeks versus 3% salicylic acid alone (completer analysis: 18/19 [95%] with nitrite plus salicylate *v* 11/16 [69%] with salicylate; ARR 26%, 95% CI 1% to 51%).[10]

Harms: The systematic review did not report frequency of adverse effects. The RCT comparing nitrite plus salicylate found no drug associated adverse events in active or salicylate only groups.[10]

Comment: In the RCT of nitrite plus salicylate versus salicylate alone, only 58% [36/60] of those randomised completed the RCT.

QUESTION What are the effects of oral antifungal treatments for athlete's foot?

OPTION ORAL AZOLES

One RCT identified by a systematic review found that oral itraconazole versus placebo for 1 week significantly increased cure rates at 8 weeks. The review found no significant difference in cure rates between individual azoles and oral allylamines, or between oral azoles and oral griseofulvin.

Benefits: **Versus placebo**: We found one systematic review (search date 2000, 1 RCT, 72 people with tinea pedis).[11] The RCT found a significantly improved cure rate with 1 week of oral itraconazole (200 mg) versus placebo (mycological cure after 8 wks: 20/36 [56%] *v* 3/36 [8%]; ARR 47%, 95% CI 28% to 65%).[12] **Versus oral allylamines:** See benefits of oral allylamines, p 1660. **Versus other azoles:** We found one systematic review (search date 2000,

2 RCTs) of oral fluconazole (50 mg daily for 4 wks) versus another azole.[11] Results were not pooled. The first RCT (35 people with tinea pedis) found no significant difference in cure rate with fluconazole versus itraconazole (100 mg daily) (ARR –5%, 95% CI –24% to +13%).[13] The second RCT (42 people) also found no significant differences in cure rate with fluconazole versus ketoconazole (200 mg daily) (ARR 4%, 95% CI –4% to +12%).[14] **Versus griseofulvin:** We found one systematic review (search date 2000, 1 RCT, 29 people with tinea pedis).[11] The RCT found no significant difference in cure rate with ketoconazole (200 mg daily for 4 wks) versus griseofulvin (1000 mg daily) (ARR –4%, 95% CI –40% to +32%).[15]

Harms: The systematic review[11] found that all RCTs of oral antifungal drugs reported adverse events, mainly gastrointestinal effects. Fluconazole had a lower frequency of adverse events (11%), but the rate was not significantly lower than the rates for griseofulvin or oral allylamines (18%).

Comment: None.

OPTION ORAL ALLYLAMINES

One RCT identified by a systematic review found limited evidence that oral terbinafine versus placebo for 6 weeks significantly improved cure rates at 8 weeks. One RCT found that oral terbinafine versus oral itraconazole for 2 weeks significantly increased cure rates, but found no significant difference in cure rates with 2 weeks of oral terbinafine versus 4 weeks of oral itraconazole.

Benefits: **Versus placebo:** We found one systematic review (search date 2000, 1 RCT, 41 people with athlete's foot).[11] It found significantly improved cure rates after 8 weeks with terbinafine (250 mg daily for 6 wks) versus placebo (15/23 [65%] with terbinafine *v* 0/18 [0%] with placebo; ARR 65%, 95% CI 46% to 85%; RR 23.5, 95% CI 2.8 to 226; NNT 2).[16] **Versus azoles:** We found one systematic review (search date 2000, 4 RCTs, 339 people with cutaneous fungal infections of the foot).[11] One of the included RCTs found a significant difference between 2 wks of terbinafine (250 mg daily) and 2 weeks of itraconazole (100mg daily) (ARR 32%, 95% CI 16% to 47%), but the other 3 RCTs (comparing 2 wks of terbinafine versus 4 wks of itraconazole) found no significant difference. Overall, the review found no significant difference in cure rate with oral allylamines (terbinafine 250 mg for 2 wks) versus oral azoles (itraconazole 100 mg for 2 or 4 wks) after 4–16 weeks (128/161 [80%] with terbinafine *v* 116/178 [65%] with itraconazole; ARR 5%, 95% CI –6% to +17%). **Versus griseofulvin:** We found one systematic review (search date 2000, 2 RCTs, 81 people with tinea pedis).[11] One RCT included only people with interdigital infection; the other included only those with plantar tinea pedis. Pooled analysis found a significantly improved cure rate with terbinafine (250 mg daily) versus griseofulvin (500 mg daily) after 4–6 weeks (35/38 [92%] with terbinafine *v* 13/33 [39%] with griseofulvin; ARR 52%, 95% CI 33% to 70%).

Harms: The systematic review found all oral antifungal drugs were associated with adverse events (mainly gastrointestinal).[11] Terbinafine was associated with a greater risk of adverse events (18%), but the rate was not significantly different from that for griseofulvin or oral azoles.

Comment: None.

QUESTION What are the effects of topical antifungals for nail infections?

OPTION FUNGAL NAILS: TOPICAL AGENTS

RCTs found limited evidence that butenafine cream in combination with either urea or tea tree oil versus placebo significantly improved cure rates at 16–36 weeks in people with fungally infected toenails. RCTs found that ciclopiroxolamine lacquer versus placebo significantly improved cure rates at 48 weeks.

Benefits: We found one systematic review (search date 1997, 2 RCTs, 153 people),[3,4] and four subsequent RCTs.[17–19] The systematic review found insufficient evidence to draw conclusions. **Butenafine plus urea:** One subsequent RCT[17] (60 people with fungally infected toenails) found significantly improved cure rate (based on microscopy and culture after 36 wks) with 2% butenafine plus 20% urea cream (twice daily for 1 wk) versus placebo (44/50 [88%] with butenafine plus urea cream *v* 0/10 [0%] with placebo; ARR 88%, 95% CI 79% to 97%; NNT 2).[17] **Butenafine plus tea tree oil:** One subsequent RCT (60 people, mean age 30 years, mean duration of disease 15 months) found significantly improved cure rates at 16 weeks with 2% butenafine plus 5% tea tree oil versus 5% tea tree oil alone (placebo) (32/40 [80%] with active cream *v* 0/20 [0%] with placebo; ARR 80%, 95% CI 54% to 90%).[18] **Ciclopiroxolamine versus placebo:** Two subsequent RCTs were reported together.[19] Both found significantly improved mycological cure rates at 48 weeks with 8% ciclopiroxolamine nail lacquer versus placebo (intention to treat analysis, first trial: 211 people, 29% with ciclopiroxolamine *v* 11% with placebo; ARR 17%, 95% CI 7% to 27%; second trial: 229 people, 36% with ciclopiroxolamine *v* 9% with placebo; ARR 26% 95% CI 16% to 37%).

Harms: In the RCT of butenafine plus tea tree oil versus tea tree oils alone (placebo), four people reported mild inflammation in the active arm, although adherence to treatment was not affected.[18] The RCTs of ciclopiroxolamine versus placebo found no significant difference in the frequency of adverse events between intervention and control groups except for rash (10% with ciclopiroxolamine *v* 2% with placebo).[19] Butenafine plus urea cream was associated with mild inflammation in 10% of people.[17]

Comment: Ciclopiroxolamine nail lacquer (8%) is not currently available in the UK. The article describing the RCTs of ciclopiroxolamine referred to 13 other trials of ciclopiroxolamine nail lacquer in people with fungally infected toenails or fingernails, but details were not stated. Reported mycological cure rates with ciclopiroxolamine ranged from about 30% to about 80%.

Athlete's foot and fungally infected toe nails

REFERENCES

1. Gentles JC, Evans EGV. Foot infections in swimming baths. *BMJ* 1973;3:260–262.
2. Roberts DT. Prevalence of dermatophyte onychomycosis in the UK: results of an omnibus survey. *Br J Dermatol* 1992;126(suppl 39):23–27.
3. Crawford F, Hart R, Bell-Syer S, Torgerson D, Young P, Russell I. Topical treatments for fungal infections of the skin and nails of the foot. In: The Cochrane Library, Issue 3, 2001. Oxford: Update Software. Search date 1997; primary sources Medline, Embase, Cinahl, Cochrane Controlled Trials Register, Science Citation Index, Biosis, CAB-Health, Healthstar, DARE, the NHS Economic Evaluation Database, Econlit, hand searched references and key journals, and pharmaceutical companies contacted.
4. Hart R, Bell-Syer EM, Crawford F, Torgerson DJ, Young P, Russell I. Systematic review of topical treatments for fungal infections of the skin and nails of the feet. *BMJ* 1999;319:79–82. Search date 1997; primary sources Medline, Embase, Cinahl, Cochrane Controlled Trials Register, Science Citation Index, Biosis, CAB-Health, Healthstar, DARE, the NHS Economic Evaluation Database, Econlit, hand searched references and key journals, and pharmaceutical companies contacted.
5. Korting HC, Tietz HJ, Brautigam M, Mayser P, Rapatz G, Pauls C, for the LAS-INT-06 study group. *Med Mycology* 2000;39:335–340.
6. Syed TA, Hadi SM, Quereshi ZA, Ali SA, Ahamed SA. Butenafine 1% versus terbinafine 1% in cream for the treatment of Tinea Pedis. A placebo controlled double-blind comparative study. *Clin Drug Invest* 2000;19:393–397.
7. Lebwohl M, Elewski B, Eisen D, Savin RC. Efficacy and safety of terbinafine 1% solution in the treatment of interdigital tinea pedis and tinea corporis or tinea cruris. *Cutis* 2001;67:261–266.
8. Schopf R, Hettler O, Brautigam M, et al. Efficacy and tolerability of terbinafine 1% topical solution used for 1 week compared with 4 weeks clotrimazole 1% topical solution in the treatment of interdigital tinea pedis: a randomised controlled clinical trial. *Mycoses* 1999;42:415–420.
9. Leenutaphong V, Tangwiwat S, Muanprasat C, Niumpradit N, Spitaveesuawan R. Double-blind study of the efficacy of 1 week topical terbinafine cream compared to 4 weeks miconazole cream in patients with tinea pedis. *J Med Assoc Thailand* 1999;82:1006–1009.
10. Weller R, Omerod AD, Hobson RP, Benjamin NJ. A randomised trial of acidified nitrite cream in the treatment of tinea pedis. *J Am Acad Dermatol* 1998;38:559–563.
11. Bell-Syer SEM, Hart R, Crawford F, et al. A systematic review of oral treatments for fungal infections of the skin of the feet. *J Dermatol* 2001;12:69–74. Search date 2000; primary sources DARE, Ecolit, Embase, Healthstar, NHS Economic Evaluation Database, BIDS, Cinahl, Cochrane Controlled Trials Register, Embase, Medline, hand searching of *Brit Podiatr Med*, *The Foot*, *Foot Ankle Int*, and *J Am Podiatr Med Assoc*. Pharmaceutical companies and UK podiatry schools were contacted for unpublished material.
12. Svejgaard E, Avnstorp C, Wanscher B, et al. Efficacy and safety of short-term itraconazole in tinea pedis: a double blind, randomised, placebo controlled trial. *Dermatology* 1998;197:368–372.
13. Difonzo EM, Papini M, Cilli P, et al. A double-blind study comparison of itraconazole and fluconazole in tinea pedis and tinea manuum. *J Eur Acad Dermatol Venereol* 1995;4:148–152.
14. Fischbein A, Haneke E, Lacner K. Comparative evaluation of oral fluconazole and oral ketoconazole in the treatment of fungal infections of the skin. *Int J Dermatol* 1992;31(suppl 2):12–16.
15. Roberts DT, Cox NH, Gentles JC, et al. Comparison of ketoconazole and griseofulvin in the treatment of tinea pedis. *J Med Vet Mycology* 1987;25:347–350.
16. Savin RC, Zaias N. Treatment of chronic moccasin-type tinea pedis with terbinafine: a double-blind placebo-controlled trial. *J Am Acad Dermatol* 1990;23:804–807.
17. Syed TA, Ahamadpour OA, Ahamad SA, et al. Management of toenail onychomycosis with 2% butenafine and 20% urea cream: a placebo controlled trial. *J Dermatol* 1998;25:648–652.
18. Syed TA, Qureshi ZA, Ali SM, Ahmad SA. Treatment of toenail onychomycosis with 2% butenafine and 5% melaleuca (tea tree) oil in cream. *Trop Med Internat Health* 1999;4:284–287.
19. Gupta AK, Fleckman P, Baran R. Ciclopirox nail lacquer topical solution 8% in the treatment of toenail onychomycosis. *J Am Acad Dermatol* 2000;43;S70–S80.

Fay Crawford
Senior Research Fellow
Dental Health Services Research Unit
Dundee
UK

Competing interests: None declared.

TABLE 1 **Antifungal drugs and antifungal drug classes cited in this topic (see text, p 1656).**

Antifungal drug classes	Topical compounds	Oral drugs
Azoles	Bifonazole Clotrimazole Econazole Fenticonazole Ketoconazole Miconazole Oxiconazole Sulconazole Tioconazole	Fluconazole Itraconazole Ketoconazole
Allylamines	Naftifine Terbinafine	Terbinafine
Polyenes	Nystatin	Amphotericin B Nystatin
Benzylamine derivative	Butenafine	
Morpholines	Amorolfine	
Miscellaneous	Ciclopiroxolamine Tea Tree Oil Tolnaftate Undecanoates	Griseofulvin

Atopic eczema

Search date May 2002

Dominic Smethurst and Sarah Macfarlane

QUESTIONS

INTERVENTIONS

See glossary, p 1678

Key Messages

Treatments

- **Control of house dust mite** RCTs found limited evidence suggesting that controlling house dust mite significantly reduced severity of symptoms at 6–12 months, but only if very low levels of mites were achieved. We found conflicting evidence about the effects on eczema severity of reducing dust mites in people with atopic eczema and positive mite radioallergosorbent test scores.
- **Dietary manipulation** One systematic review in children and adults with atopic eczema found inconclusive evidence about the effects of dietary manipulation, such as exclusion of egg and cows' milk.
- **Emollients** One systematic review has found that moisturising cream plus topical corticosteroid versus topical corticosteroid alone significantly improves clinical signs and symptoms of atopic eczema after 3 weeks.

Clin Evid 2002;8:1664–1682.

Skin disorders

- **Topical antimicrobial plus steroid combinations** One systematic review has found no significant difference with topical antimicrobial agents plus steroids versus topical steroids alone in improving the clinical signs and symptoms of atopic eczema.
- **Topical steroids** One systematic review has found that topical corticosteroids versus placebo improve atopic eczema after 1–4 weeks. Another systematic review comparing a variety of topical steroids versus each other found significant improvement in 22–100% of people after 1–6 weeks. One subsequent RCT in people with mild to moderate eczema found no significant difference in mean scratch free days over 18 weeks with 3 day treatment with betamethasone (a potent topical steroid) versus 7 day treatment with hydrocortisone (a mild topical steroid). Short term RCTs and one longer term cohort study found no serious systemic adverse effects or skin atrophy associated with topical steroids. Small studies in volunteers who did not have eczema have found that potent topical steroid preparations cause skin thinning after twice daily application for up to 6 weeks, although skin thickness returns to normal within 4 weeks of stopping treatment. One RCT found insufficient evidence of the effects of topical steroids in preventing relapse.
- **Wet wrap dressing and bandaging** One systematic review identified no RCTs on the effects of wet wrap or other forms of bandaging.

Prevention in predisposed infants

- **Dietary manipulation during lactation in mothers of predisposed infants** Limited evidence from one systematic review suggests that maternal dietary restriction during lactation may protect against the development of eczema at 12–18 months in infants with a family history of atopy.
- **Dietary manipulation during pregnancy in mothers of predisposed infants** One systematic review found no significant difference with maternal diet restriction during pregnancy versus no restriction in development of atopic eczema in the infant at 12–18 months.
- **Prolonged breast feeding in predisposed infants** One systematic review of prospective cohort studies suggests that exclusive breast feeding for at least 3 months may reduce the risk of eczema in infants with a family history of atopy.

Avoidance of provoking factors

- **Avoidance of biological washing detergents** One systematic review found no significant difference with washing detergents that contain enzymes versus washing detergents without enzymes in eczema severity at 1 month.
- **Avoidance of certain clothing textiles** RCTs found limited evidence that, in people with atopic eczema, the roughness of clothing textiles is a more important factor for skin irritation than the type of textile fibre (synthetic or natural). One RCT in infants with atopic eczema comparing cotton nappy/diaper versus cellulose core nappy/diaper versus cellulose core nappy/diaper containing absorbent gelling found no significant difference in eczema scores after 26 weeks.
- **Avoidance of animal contact; avoidance of vaccination/immunisation; avoidance of all washing detergents** We found no RCTs about the effects of these preventive interventions.

DEFINITION Atopic eczema (atopic dermatitis) is an inflammatory skin disease characterised by an itchy erythematous poorly demarcated skin eruption with a predilection for skin creases.[1]

INCIDENCE/ PREVALENCE	Atopic eczema affects 15–20% of school children in the UK and 2–3% of adults.[2] Prevalence has increased substantially over the past 30 years,[3] possibly because of environmental and lifestyle changes.
AETIOLOGY/ RISK FACTORS	Aetiology is believed to be multifactorial. Recent interest has focused on airborne allergens (house dust mites, pollen, and animal dander), outdoor pollution, climate, diet, and prenatal/early life factors such as infections.
PROGNOSIS	Although there is currently no cure, several interventions can help to control symptoms. Atopic eczema clears in 60–70% of children by their early teens, although relapses may occur.
AIMS	To prevent atopic eczema in predisposed infants and children; to minimise the impact of atopic eczema on quality of life in children and adults.
OUTCOMES	Severity of symptoms (itching, sleep disturbance) and signs (erythema, oozing/crusting, lichenification, cracking, oedema/papulation, excoriation, and dryness); quality of life; area of skin involvement. Trials used a range of atopic eczema scoring systems, including scoring of atopic dermatitis (SCORAD), six area six sign atopic dermatitis severity score (SASSAD), Rajka and Langeland scoring system, and the dermatology life quality index.
METHODS	*Clinical Evidence* update search and appraisal May 2002. The authors also performed hand searches of conference proceedings and personal contact with experts. Because of the limited studies available for many questions, we included some with shortcomings in methods, which we mention in the text.

QUESTION **What are the effects of treatments in adults and children with atopic eczema?**

OPTION **TOPICAL STEROIDS**

One systematic review has found that topical corticosteroids versus placebo improve atopic eczema after 1–4 weeks. Another systematic review comparing a variety of topical steroids versus each other found significant improvement in 22–100% of people after 1–6 weeks. One subsequent RCT in people with mild to moderate eczema found no significant difference in mean scratch free days over 18 weeks with 3 day treatment with betamethasone (a potent topical steroid) versus 7 day treatment with hydrocortisone (a mild topical steroid). Short term RCTs and one longer term cohort study found no serious systemic adverse effects or skin atrophy associated with topical steroids. Small studies in volunteers who did not have eczema have found that potent topical steroid preparations cause skin thinning after twice daily application for up to 6 weeks, although skin thickness returns to normal within 4 weeks of stopping treatment. One RCT found insufficient evidence of the effects of topical steroids in preventing relapse.

Benefits: **Versus placebo:** We found one systematic review (search date 1999, 11 RCTs[4–14] in children and adults with atopic eczema) comparing topical steroids versus placebo cream.[15] All of the RCTs found that topical steroid versus placebo significantly improved clinical signs and symptoms of eczema (see table 1, p 1681). **Versus each other:** One systematic review (search date 1999, 40 RCTs in children and adults with atopic eczema) comparing a wide variety of topical steroids versus each other found significant improvements in 22–100% of people after 1–6 weeks of treatment.[15] Many of the RCTs identified by the review were of poor quality and the review was unable to draw conclusions about differences in effectiveness between different corticosteroids. One subsequent RCT (207 children with mild to moderate atopic eczema, 174 in primary care and 33 in a hospital outpatient clinic) compared betamethasone valerate 0.1% (a potent steroid) for 3 days plus base ointment for 4 days versus hydrocortisone 1% (a mild steroid) for 7 days.[16] It found that both bethamethasone and hydrocortisone significantly improved disease severity and quality of life from baseline, and found no significant difference in the mean number of scratch free days over 18 weeks with bethamethasone versus hydrocortisone (118.0 *v* 117.5 days; mean difference 0.5, 95% CI –3.0 to +2.0; P = 0.53).[16] **Prevention of relapse:** We found one systematic review (search date 1999),[15] which identified one RCT.[17] The RCT (56 adults with atopic eczema that had "completely healed" with a 4 wk course of fluticasone propionate) compared fluticasone propionate (2 consecutive days a wk for 16 wks) versus placebo.[17] It found that fluticasone propionate versus placebo significantly maintained improvement of atopic dermatitis scores at 16 weeks (P = 0.018; no further data provided).[17]

Harms: **Versus placebo:** The short term RCTs identified by the review[4–14] and one longer term cohort study[18] (14 prepubertal children, median treatment 6.5 years taking mild to moderate dose topical steroids) found no serious systemic effects or cases of skin atrophy. Minor adverse effects, such as burning, stinging, irritation, folliculitis, hypertrichosis, contact dermatitis, and pigmentary disturbances, occurred in less than 10% of people. **Versus each other:** The subsequent RCT found no difference with betamethasone versus hydrocorticosone in the proportion of people with worse symptoms (9/104 [9%] with betamethasone *v* 5/103 [5%] with hydrocortisone), spots or rashes (2/104 [2%] with betamethasone *v* 0/103 [0%] with hydrocortisone), or hair growth (1/104 [0.10%] with betamethasone *v* 0/103 [0%] with hydrocortisone).[16] One person taking betamethasone was admitted to hospital with viral encephalitis. **Skin thinning:** The subsequent RCT (207 children) comparing betamethasone for 3 days versus hydrocortisone for 7 days obtained ultrasound measurements from 106 (51%) children and assessed skin thinning over 18 weeks.[16] It found that 11 children (3 taking betamethasone and 4 taking hydrocortisone) had a greater than 25% reduction in skin thickness at 12 body sites. However, most of these children had active eczema with baseline skin thickness 20–50% higher than the mean for the site (see comment below). Skin thickness was within the normal range at baseline for all children after 18 weeks. The RCT examining prevention of relapse in people with atopic eczema found no significant difference between corticosteroids twice weekly to healed lesions versus placebo in histological evidence of skin atrophy after 16 weeks.[17] We found no further RCTs looking at skin thinning in people with atopic eczema. Four very small RCTs in healthy volunteers (12 people) used ultrasound to evaluate skin thickness.[19–22] The RCTs found that clobetasol 17-propionate 0.05% twice daily versus placebo significantly increased skin thinning after 1 week, and that triamcinolone acetate 0.1% or betamethasone 17-valerate 0.1% twice daily versus placebo significantly increased skin thinning after 3 weeks. They found no significant difference between hydrocortisone prednicarbate twice daily or mometasone furoate once daily versus placebo in skin thinning after 6 weeks. All preparations were used for up to 6 weeks, and skin thinning reversed within 4 weeks of stopping treatment.

Comment: Studies that did not specify the type of eczema, or those that included other dermatoses in the overall analysis, were excluded. The RCTs identified by the review used different clinical scoring systems, making it difficult to compare results.[15] In the RCT (56 adults) comparing fluticasone propionate versus placebo to prevent relapse, participants using fluticasone propionate were advised to apply cream to both known "healed" sites and any newly occurring sites of eczema and improvement in scoring of atopic dermatitis scores was measured overall;[17] therefore, it is uncertain whether improvements in scoring of atopic dermatitis scores were because of prevention of relapse or improvement in newly occurring sites of eczema. Interpretation of ultrasound data to assess skin thinning is difficult as many variables affect skin thickness (e.g. body site, temperature, humidity). Skin affected by eczema is often abnormally thick (lichenified) and reduction in thickness may reflect resolution of active eczema and a return to a normal level of thickness. There is inadequate long term data about the effects of topic steroids on skin thinning.

OPTION TOPICAL ANTIMICROBIAL PLUS STEROID COMBINATIONS

One systematic review has found no significant difference between topical antimicrobial agents plus steroids versus topical steroids alone in improving the clinical signs and symptoms of atopic eczema. One systematic review and three additional RCTs have found no significant difference between different antimicrobial agents plus steroids in improving the clinical signs and symptoms of atopic eczema.

Benefits: **Versus topical steroid alone:** We found one systematic review (search date 1999, 3 RCTs, 329 people with atopic dermatitis) comparing topical antimicrobial plus steroid combinations versus topical steroid alone.[15] It found no significant difference between betamethasone valerate plus fusidic acid, hydrocortisone acetate plus fusidic acid, or betamethasone valerate plus gentamicin versus topical steroid alone in clinical signs and symptoms of eczema (no further data provided). **Versus each other:** We found one systematic review (search date 1999, 4 RCTs, 322 people)[15] and three additional RCTs[23–25] in people with clinically infected eczema (atopic eczema not specified) comparing different topical antimicrobial plus steroid combinations with each other. The systematic review and subsequent RCTs found clinical improvement in 54–95%

of participants, with no significant difference between the various preparations with respect to improvement in clinical signs and symptoms. People treated with fusidic acid plus hydrocortisone showed a more rapid clinical response than those treated with miconazole plus hydrocortisone.[15,23–25]

Harms: Overall, the RCTs identified by the review reported minor adverse effects comprising itching, stinging, burning, and irritation in fewer than 2% of people.[15]

Comment: Only two of the RCTs identified by the review specified a degree of infection in most participants at recruitment.[15] One of these also included people with contact dermatitis in the overall analysis, and the use of left/right comparisons within individual participants may have reduced the difference between groups because of systemic absorption of the antimicrobial agent. One additional RCT (44 adults), published only as an abstract, compared tetracycline 3% plus triamcinolone acetonide 0.1% ointment versus triamcinolone 0.1% ointment alone daily over 2 weeks, followed by a maintenance period using triamcinolone 0.1% ointment alone.[26] It found no significant difference in disease severity as assessed by SCORAD and SASSAD at 2, 4, or 8 weeks with tetracycline plus triamcinolone versus triamcinolone alone (reported as non-significant; no further data provided).[26]

OPTION EMOLLIENTS

One systematic review has found that emollient plus topical corticosteroid versus topical corticosteroid alone significantly improves clinical signs and symptoms of atopic eczema. One additional controlled clinical trial found no significant difference in signs and symptoms after 3 weeks with emollient cream once daily plus hydrocortisone 2.5% cream once daily versus hydrocortisone 2.5% cream twice daily.

Benefits: **Emollient plus topical steroid versus topical steroid alone:** We found one systematic review (search date 1999, 2 RCTs,[27,28] 130 people)[15] and one additional controlled clinical trial[29] comparing topical corticosteroid plus moisturising cream versus topical corticosteroid alone. The first RCT identified by the review (80 people with mild to moderate atopic eczema) compared moisturising cream three times daily plus a topical corticosteroid (desonide 0.05%) twice daily versus topical corticosteroid alone.[27] It found that the combined regimen significantly improved clinical signs and symptoms of eczema at 3 weeks (70% *v* 55%; $P < 0.01$). The second RCT identified by the review (50 people with atopic eczema) compared emollient cream once daily plus hydrocortisone 2.5% cream once daily versus emollient lotion once daily plus hydrocortisone 2.5% cream once daily.[28] It found significant improvement in signs and symptoms with both treatment regimens after 3 weeks. One additional controlled clinical trial (25 children, randomisation not mentioned) found no significant difference between emollient cream once daily plus hydrocortisone 2.5% cream once daily versus hydrocortisone 2.5% cream twice daily in signs and symptoms after 3 weeks ($P > 0.545$).[29]

Harms: Minor adverse effects, such as a burning sensation, were reported in fewer than 2% of people in the RCTs identified by the review.[15]

Comment: We excluded many of the studies located in our search as they did not specify the type of eczema, or they included people with other forms of eczema. We have not included studies looking at bath additives.

OPTION WET WRAP DRESSINGS AND BANDAGING

One systematic review found no RCTs on the effects of wet wrap or other forms of bandaging in people with atopic eczema.

Benefits: We found one systematic review (search date 1999), which identified no RCTs on the effects of wet wraps or other forms of bandaging in people with atopic eczema.[15]

Harms: Uncontrolled studies have found enhanced topical steroid absorption and adverse effects have been found with earlier forms of wet wrap dressings (see glossary, p 1678).[30]

Comment: We found two small RCTs[31,32] and three uncontrolled studies.[30,33,34] The first pilot RCT (19 infants), published only as an abstract, compared hydrocortisone ointment plus Tubifast® bandages twice daily for 1 week, followed by hydrocortisone ointment once daily plus Tubifast® bandages once daily for 1 week versus hydrocortisone ointment twice daily for 2 weeks.[31] It found no difference in disease severity (as measured by SASSAD) or quality of life with wet wrap dressings plus hydrocortisone plus versus hydrocortisone alone at 2–3 weeks.[31] The second RCT (20 children aged 2–17 years with exacerbated atopic eczema) compared wet wraps plus mometasone furoate 0.1% versus wet wrap dressings plus placebo cream in a left/right design. It found that wet wrap dressings plus mometasone furoate versus wet wrap dressings plus placebo significantly improved SCORAD scores at 3 and 5 days ($P < 0.01$).[32] The RCT gave no information about adverse effects.[32] The first uncontrolled study used wet wrap dressings in 30 children with acute erythrodermic eczema.[30] All children responded well to treatment after 2–5 days, with no relapses 2 weeks later (no quantitative results provided). The second uncontrolled study (21 children with chronic severe atopic eczema treated with wet wrap dressings ≤ 2/wk for 3 months) found that in all children the eczema improved after starting treatment and sleep disturbance was reduced. Most parents reported a reduction in topical steroid requirements (no quantitative results provided).[33] The third uncontrolled study (40 children) compared topical mometasone furoate for 2 weeks followed by an additional 2 weeks of mometasone furoate applied with or without wet wraps versus fluticasone proprionate for 2 weeks followed by an additional 2 weeks of fluticasone proprionate applied with or without wet wraps.[34] It found that wet wraps versus no wet wraps improved eczema severity but as most of the improvement occurred in the first 2 weeks, prior to application of wet wraps, it is impossible to isolate the effects of wet wraps. As these studies were uncontrolled, the improvement may have been attributable to the additional medical or nursing input during the study rather than to the effect of the wet wraps.

OPTION CONTROL OF HOUSE DUST MITE

Three RCTs in people with atopic eczema found that extreme reduction in dust levels (achieved by measures such as synthetic mattress covers, acaricidal spraying, and high filtration vacuuming) versus placebo significantly reduced eczema severity score. However, one RCT and one controlled clinical trial found no significant difference between polyurethane coated cotton covers versus placebo in eczema severity scores. The clinical relevance of the reduction in severity score in the RCTs is uncertain. One small RCT comparing natamycin spray plus vacuuming versus placebo found no correlation between improvement in eczema severity score and reduction in mite levels, but the reduction in mite numbers was only 68%. Two RCTs and one controlled clinical trial in people with atopic eczema or dermatitis and positive mite radioallergosorbent test scores found conflicting evidence of the effects of reducing the number of dust mites in improving eczema severity.

Benefits: We found one systematic review (search date 1999,[15] 5 RCTs[35–39]), two additional controlled clinical trials that were excluded from the review because of lack of explicit randomisation,[40,41] and one subsequent RCT.[42] The review could not perform a meta-analysis because of differences between the trials in methods used to control house dust mite.[15] The first RCT identified by the review (24 atopic adults and 24 atopic children > 7 years old, skin prick, and radioallergosorbent [RAST] status not specified) compared extreme reduction in dust levels (achieved by a trained nurse visiting to apply bed covers made of a breathable synthetic material plus benzyltannate spray and high filtration vacuuming) versus placebo (nurse visit to apply cotton bedcovers plus placebo spray and standard vacuum cleaners).[35] It found that extreme reduction in dust levels versus placebo significantly reduced eczema severity scores at 6 months ([maximum score 108 units], mean difference in severity score 4.3 units, 95% CI 1.3 to 7.3). This was associated with a 98% reduction in mean mattress dust load versus 16% in the placebo group (P = 0.002) and a 91% reduction in the concentration of mite allergen Der p1 on bedroom carpet and 76% reduction on living room carpet versus 89% reduction (P = 0.94) and 38% reduction (P = 0.27) in the placebo group.[35] The second RCT identified by the review (28 people with atopic dermatitis) compared extreme reduction in dust levels (achieved by nurse visits to apply bed covers made of a breathable synthetic material plus mitocidal spray plus high filtration vacuuming) versus placebo (nurse visits to apply cotton bed covers plus water spraying plus low filtration vacuuming).[39] It found that extreme reduction in dust levels versus placebo significantly reduced eczema surface area (mean difference in area 10%, 95% CI 3 to 17; P = 0.0006) and significantly improved eczema severity score after 6 months (mean improvement in score 4.2 *v* 12.6; P = 0.006; results presented graphically).[39] The third RCT identified by the review (20 atopic dermatitis patients, aged 12–47 years with positive skin prick and RAST tests to house dust mite) compared four groups: natamycin spray alone; natamycin spray plus vacuuming; placebo spray alone; and placebo spray plus vacuuming.[36] It found no correlation between improvement in clinical score and lowered mite numbers. However, the maximum reduction in mite numbers in mattresses was only 68%. The fourth RCT identified by the review (57 infants with atopic dermatitis, unblinded) compared reduction in house mite levels (achieved by special pillows, washing of bedding, removal of pets and soft toys, and intensive vacuuming) plus mite blocking bedding versus reduction in house mite levels plus regular bedding.[37] The RCT did not assess the effects on atopic eczema severity. It found that mite reduction bedding versus regular bedding significantly reduced serum and skin prick responses to dust mite allergens after 1 year (17/27 [63%] *v* 8/26 [31%]; $P < 0.02$).[37] The fifth RCT identified by the review (30 children aged 3–12 years with stable eczema, unblinded) compared intensive versus gentle cleaning of mattresses, quilts, and floors every 3 weeks by a team of dust mite specialists. Both groups also received advice to clean either intensively or gently. It found that intensive versus gentle cleaning significantly improved clinically scored eczema after 1 year ($P < 0.01$; results presented graphically).[38] The first controlled clinical trial (51 people with atopic eczema; randomisation not mentioned) compared three groups: 3 weeks in a "clean room" with reduced dust levels in people with positive mite RAST scores; 3 weeks in an ordinary hospital room in people with positive mite RAST scores; and 3 weeks in a "clean room" in people with negative RAST scores. It found that "clean room" treatment in people with high RAST scores resulted in induction of an itch free period and prolonged remission but found no itch free period in people with positive RAST scores treated in an ordinary hospital room or in people with negative RAST scores treated in a "clean room".[40] The second controlled clinical trial (40 people with atopic dermatitis; randomisation not mentioned) compared polyurethane coated cotton bed covers plus monthly vacuuming of mattresses and bedroom carpets versus placebo (cotton covers without monthly vacuuming).[41] It found no significant difference between polyurethane coated cotton covers versus placebo in eczema severity at 12 months as measured by SCORAD (reduction in SCORAD from baseline 45% with polyurethane covers *v* 39% with placebo). The subsequent RCT (20 adults with moderate to severe atopic dermatitis and positive mite RAST scores) compared allergen impermeable polyurethane mattress covers plus an acaricide spray containing tannic acid and benzylbenzoate versus placebo (allergen permeable cotton bed covers plus a water/ethanol spray).[42] It found no significant difference with an allergen impermeable polyurethane cover plus acaricide spray versus placebo in eczema severity SCORAD scores after 1 year (results presented graphically; $P = 0.90$), although an allergen impermeable mattress plus spray significantly reduced the level of Der p1 allergen exposure ($P = 0.0008$).

Harms: The RCTs gave no information on adverse effects.[35–42]

Comment: In the first RCT of extreme reduction of dust levels, the clinical importance of the reduction in eczema severity score is uncertain.[35] The extreme dust control measures in the RCTs, such as home visits for intensive cleaning and removal of all pets and toys, may not be applicable to the general population.[35,37–39] In the first controlled clinical trial, where people spent 3 weeks in a "clean room" with reduced dust levels, participants were only allowed out of the room for toilet and shower breaks.[40] The use of bedding covers seems to be the simplest and most effective measure to reduce house dust mite levels in the home (see table 2, p 1682).

OPTION DIETARY MANIPULATION

One systematic review in children or adults with atopic eczema found inconclusive evidence of the effects of dietary manipulation, such as exclusion of egg and cows' milk.

Benefits: **In children:** We found one systematic review (search date 1999,[15] 4 RCTs[43–46]) of the effects of an egg and milk exclusion diet in unselected children with eczema. The review could not perform a meta-analysis because of trial heterogeneity.[15] The first RCT identified by the review (20 children aged 2–8 years; crossover trial) compared an egg and cows' milk exclusion diet with soya milk substitution versus a control diet with egg and cows' milk.[43] It found that an egg and cows' milk exclusion diet versus control diet significantly improved eczema severity (14/20 [70%] treated children improved *v* 1/20 [5%] controls; RR 7.5, 95% CI 4.85 to 9.73).[43] The second RCT identified by the review (40 children and young adults) found no significant difference between an egg and cows' milk exclusion diet with soya milk substitution versus a control diet with egg and cows' milk in mean eczema area score, itch score, or use of topical corticosteroids (reported as non-significant; no further data provided).[44] The third RCT identified by the review (55 children with proven sensitivity to eggs; positive mite radioallergosorbent) comparing an egg exclusion diet versus general dietary advice found that an egg free diet significantly reduced the surface area affected by eczema (mean reduction 8.7 *v* 3.0; P = 0.02). It also found that an egg exclusion diet versus general dietary advice significantly improved mean eczema severity score (9.9 with egg exclusion *v* 3.2 with general advice; P = 0.04).[45] The fourth RCT identified by the review (85 children, 46 evaluable) comparing a "few foods diet" (in which all but a handful of foods were excluded) versus usual diet found no significant difference in eczema severity.[46] **In adults:** We found one systematic review (search date 1999)[15] that identified two RCTs.[44,47] The first RCT identified by the review (18 adults aged 16–23 years) found no significant difference between an egg and cows' milk exclusion diet with soya milk substitution versus a control diet with egg and cows' milk in mean eczema area score, itch score, or use of topical corticosteroids (no raw data provided).[44] The second RCT identified by the review (33 adults in hospital) found no significant difference between a liquid elemental diet (containing amino acids, essential fatty acids, glucose, trace elements, sorbic acid, and vitamins) versus placebo diet in the number of people with an improvement eczema severity score over 3 weeks (5/16 [31%] with elemental diet *v* 4/9 [44%] with placebo; RR 1.02, 95% CI 0.34 to 3.03).[48]

Harms: The RCTs gave no information on adverse effects.[43–46]

Comment: Calcium, protein, and calorie deficiency are risks of dairy free diets in children. The clinical importance of changes in severity scores obtained in many studies is unknown. We have not included studies looking at the role of food additives, fatty acid supplementation, or trace elements in eczema. Two of the RCTs identified by the review used potentially allergenic soya based milk substitute during the trial period.[43,44] One of the RCTs identified by the review included both children and adults but assessed them separately.[44] Double blind placebo controlled food challenges have been used to identify people with food allergy, but the clinical relevance of positive reactions (which may include gastrointestinal, respiratory, or cutaneous symptoms) to subsequent eczema control is unclear. One retrospective diagnostic study examined hypersensitivity reactions up to 48 hours after double blind, placebo controlled food challenges in 107 children aged 5 months to 12 years with moderate to severe atopic dermatitis and a history suggestive of food allergy.[49] This study found positive reactions in 81% of children, with 70% of reactions occurring within 2 hours. Egg and cows' milk accounted for 83% of the positive reactions.[49] In three further studies, double blind, placebo controlled food challenges caused hypersensitivity reactions (all within 2 h of the challenge) in 63% of children with moderate to severe atopic eczema (320 children) and in 33–39% of children with mild to severe atopic eczema (211 children). Egg, milk, and peanut accounted for 67–78% of the reactions. The effect of subsequent dietary elimination was studied in only 27 of these children. A greater improvement was found in children on exclusion diets than in non-randomly selected controls, using a crude scoring system.[47]

QUESTION What are the effects of preventive interventions in predisposed infants?

OPTION PROLONGED BREAST FEEDING IN PREDISPOSED INFANTS

We found no RCTs and it is unlikely that an RCT would be conducted in this area. One systematic review of prospective cohort studies suggests that exclusive breast feeding for at least 3 months may reduce the risk of eczema in infants with a family history of atopy.

Benefits: We found no RCTs (see comment below). We found one systematic review (search date 2000, 18 prospective cohort studies, 4158 infants) that assessed the effects of exclusive breast feeding during the first 3 months after birth.[50] It found that exclusive breast feeding during the first 3 months after birth or longer significantly reduced the risk of eczema after a mean 4.5 years (OR 0.68, 95% CI 0.52 to 0.88; no raw data provided). Subgroup analysis found that the preventive effect was greater in children with a family history of atopy (OR 0.58, 95% CI 0.41 to 0.92 for children who had first degree relative with an atopic condition), and found no significant difference in the risk of eczema in children without a family history of atopy (OR 1.43; 95% CI 0.72 to 2.86).

Harms: The systematic review gave no information on harms.[50]

Comment: It is unlikely that an RCT would be conducted in this area. Much of the available evidence was limited by weak methods, for example selection and information bias, short duration of breast feeding, and inadequate control for confounding factors, such as introducing supplemental milk or solid foods. Prolonged self selected breast feeding may be associated with unknown protective factors, leading to bias. One large cohort/nested case control study not included in the systematic review identified 370 children with visible eczema (as recognised by a medical officer) out of 14 862 children taking part in the 1958 National Child Development Survey. Odds ratio analysis found no evidence to support a protective effect of breast feeding.[51] Another large prospective study (14 000 families), published only as an abstract and not included in the systematic review, found that breast feeding (duration not specified) was associated with a significantly increased risk of atopic dermatitis at 30 months (OR 1.3, 95% CI 1.1 to 1.5).[52] Cases of very early eczema were excluded from the analysis. Although the evidence to date suggests a protective effect for breast feeding against developing atopic eczema in individuals with a family history of atopy, the evidence is not strong, and the degree of protection may be small. Breast feeding may be actively encouraged for other health reasons.

OPTION MATERNAL DIETARY RESTRICTION

We found limited evidence from one systematic review that maternal dietary restriction during lactation may protect against the development of eczema in infants with a family history of atopy. One systematic review found no significant difference between maternal diet restriction during pregnancy versus no restriction in development of atopic eczema in the infant at 12–18 months.

Benefits: We found one systematic review (search date 1999;[15] 2 earlier systematic reviews[53,54]). **During lactation:** The review[15] did not fully describe the earlier review it identified.[53] The earlier review (search date not stated, 3 RCTs, 194 women) found that maternal antigen avoidance diet versus normal diet during lactation (range 36 weeks' gestation to 6 months' lactation) significantly reduced the number of breast-fed infants who developed atopic eczema at 12–18 months.[53] **During pregnancy:** The review[15] did not fully describe the earlier systematic review it identified.[54] The earlier review (search date not stated, 3 RCTs, 504 women at high risk of giving birth to an atopic child) compared a maternal antigen avoidance diet during pregnancy versus no restricted diet.[54] It found no significant difference between maternal diet restriction versus no restriction in development of atopic eczema in the infant at 12–18 months (47/77 [26%] v 52/195 [27%]; RR 0.97, 95% CI 0.71 to 1.34).

Harms: **During lactation:** The systematic review gave no information on adverse effects.[53] **During pregnancy:** One RCT (212 women) identified by the review found that mean birth weight was lower with a resticted diet versus no restricted diet (mean 3% lower; no further data provided), but the difference may not be clinically important.[54]

Comment: All of the RCTs identified by thc review of antigen diets during lactation were limited by weak methods; therefore, the results should be interpreted with caution.[53]

QUESTION What are the effects of avoidance of provoking factors in adults and children with atopic eczema?

OPTION CLOTHING TEXTILES

RCTs found limited evidence that, in people with atopic eczema, the roughness of clothing textiles is a more important factor for skin irritation than the type of textile fibre (synthetic or natural). It found that polyester and cotton of similar textile fineness seemed to be equally well tolerated. One RCT in infants with atopic eczema comparing cotton nappy/diaper versus cellulose core nappy/diaper versus cellulose core nappy/diaper containing absorbent gelling found no significant difference in eczema scores. We found no RCTs on the long term effects of different textiles on the severity of atopic eczema.

Benefits: We found one systematic review (search date 1999)[15] that identified three RCTs[55–57]) and one additional RCT.[58] The first RCT identified by the review (20 people with atopic eczema and 20 healthy controls; mean age 25 years, double blind) compared cotton and polyester shirts of different fabric structure and coarseness at rest and after exercise to induce sweating.[55] It found no significant difference between fabrics in comfort ratings. Knitted fabrics (polyester or cotton) were better tolerated than woven fabrics (all polyester). Of the knitted fabrics, polyester was as well tolerated by people with eczema as the comparable cotton shirt of similar textile fineness. At rest, people with eczema tolerated the less coarse knitted polyester better than the other polyester knitted fabrics, although there was no significant difference during exercise. Of the woven fabrics, the finer polyester was better tolerated by people with eczema than the coarser fabrics, both at rest and during exercise, although controls showed no significant difference. The second RCT identified by the review (55 people with atopic dermatitis) compared four different shirts: one cotton and three synthetic with differing fibre structure.[56] It found that cotton shirts versus synthetic shirts that were rougher or heavier in fibre composition significantly improved comfort as measured by a comfort score ($P < 0.0001$).[56] The third RCT identified by the review (85 infants) comparing cotton nappy/diaper versus cellulose core nappy/diaper (conventional disposable nappy/diaper) versus cellulose core nappy/diaper containing absorbent gelling found no significant difference in eczema scores after 26 weeks (no further data provided).[56] One additional RCT (25 women with atopic eczema, aged 15–20 years, with a history of wool irritation) compared the effects of two different wool fibres on itching.[58] It found that coarser 36 μm wool fibre versus thin 20 μm wool fibre increased the frequency of wool induced itching after 12 hours. Visible skin changes, disappearing within 24 hours in all cases, were seen in more women wearing thick versus thin fibre wool but the difference was not significant (6/9 [67%] *v* 11/16 [69%]; RR 0.97, 95% CI 0.55 to 1.71).[58]

Harms: With the exception of short term skin irritation, no harmful effects were reported in the RCTs.[55–58]

Comment: The RCT comparing cotton nappy/diaper versus cellulose core nappy/diaper (conventional disposable nappy/diaper) versus cellulose core nappy diaper containing absorbent gelling stratified randomisation by severity of nappy rash and atopic eczema (assessed by a grading scale) and by age, weight, and maturity.[57]

OPTION WASHING DETERGENTS

One systematic review found no significant difference between washing detergents that contain enzymes versus washing detergents without enzymes in eczema severity at 1 month. We found no RCTs of the effect of avoidance of all contact with washing detergents.

Benefits: **Biological versus non-biological detergents:** One systematic review (search date 1999, 1 RCT, 25 people with atopic eczema, aged 17–59 years) comparing washing detergents with enzymes versus detergents without enzymes found no significant difference in clinical disease severity (score on scoring of atopic dermatitis [SCORAD] scale 29 with detergents with enzymes *v* 29 with detergents without enzymes), subjective symptoms, or corticosteroid use after detergent use for 1 month.[15] **Avoidance of all washing detergents:** We found no RCTs.

Harms: No harmful effects were reported in the RCT identified by the review.[15]

Comment: None.

OPTION VACCINATION/IMMUNISATION

We found no evidence about the effects of vaccination on atopic eczema severity.

Benefits: We found no systematic review, RCTs, or cohort studies.

Harms: One observational study in 134 allergic children (with atopic eczema, asthma, or cows' milk allergy) reported transient mild generalised urticaria and fever in two children with atopic eczema within 24 hours of vaccination against measles, mumps, and rubella.[59]

Comment: The study found that the lowest rate of positive skin prick tests to measles, mumps, and rubella vaccine was in the 68 children with atopic eczema (4% positive), compared with the 47 children with asthma (9% positive), and the 11 children with cows' milk allergy (18% positive).[58] The 64 children with atopic eczema who were subsequently vaccinated had no serious reactions, although the long term effect on eczema severity was not studied.

OPTION ANIMAL CONTACT

We found no evidence on the effects of avoiding animal contact on the severity of atopic eczema.

Benefits: We found no systematic review, RCTs, or cohort studies of the effects of avoiding animal contact on the severity of atopic eczema.

Harms: We found no evidence.

Comment: Observational studies have suggested that keeping pets is associated with an increased prevalence of atopic eczema. Following removal of animals from the home it may take many months for the allergen load to decrease because of widespread distribution in carpets and soft furnishings.

GLOSSARY

Wet wrap dressings Wet occlusive tubifast dressings that are applied over topical steroid or emollient.

Substantive changes

Topical steroids One new RCT;[16] conclusions unchanged.

Prolonged breast feeding in predisposed infants One new systematic review of prospective cohort studies;[50] conclusions unchanged.

REFERENCES

1. Williams HC, Burney PGJ, Pembroke AC, et al. The UK working party's diagnostic criteria for atopic dermatitis. III Independent hospital validation. *Br J Dermatol* 1994;131:406–417.
2. Kay J, Gawkrodger DJ, Mortimer MJ, et al. The prevalence of childhood atopic eczema in a general population. *J Am Acad Dermatol* 1994;30:35–39.
3. Williams HC. Is the prevalence of atopic dermatitis increasing? *Clin Exp Dermatol* 1992;17:385–391.
4. Lawlor F, Black AK, Greaves M. Prednicarbate 0.25% ointment in the treatment of atopic dermatitis: A vehicle-controlled double-blind study. *J Dermatol Treat* 1995;6:233–235.
5. Roth HL, Brown EP. Hydrocortisone valerate. Double-blind comparison with two other topical steroids. *Cutis* 1978;21:695–698.
6. Maloney JM, Morman MR, Stewart DM, et al. Clobetasol propionate emollient 0.05% in the treatment of atopic dermatitis. *Int J Dermatol* 1998;37:128–144.
7. Sears HW, Bailer JW, Yeadon A. Efficacy and safety of hydrocortisone buteprate 0.1% cream in patients with atopic dermatitis. *Clin Ther* 1997;19:710–719.
8. Vanderploeg DE. Betamethasone dipropionate ointment in the treatment of psoriasis and atopic dermatitis: a double-blind study. *South Med J* 1976;69:862–863.
9. Lupton ES, Abbrecht MM, Brandon ML. Short-term topical corticosteroid therapy (halcinonide ointment) in the management of atopic dermatitis. *Cutis* 1982;30:671–675.
10. Stalder JF, Fleury M, Sourisse M, et al. Local steroid therapy and bacterial skin flora in atopic dermatitis. *Br J Dermatol* 1994;131:536–540.
11. Sefton J, Loder JS, Kyriakopoulos AA. Clinical evaluation of hydrocortisone valerate 0.2% ointment. *Clin Ther* 1984;6:282–293.
12. Wahlgren CF, Hägermark O, Bergström R, et al. Evaluation of a new method of assessing pruritus and antipruritic drugs. *Skin Pharmacol* 1988;1:3–13.
13. Sudilovsky A, Muir JG, Bocobo FC. A comparison of single and multiple applications of Halcinonide cream. *Int J Dermatol* 1981;20:609–613.
14. Lebwohl M. Efficacy and safety of fluticasone propionate ointment, 0.005%, in the treatment of eczema. *Cutis* 1996;57(2 suppl):62–68.
15. Hoare C, Li Wan PA, Williams HC. A systematic review of treatments for atopic eczema. *Health Technol Assess* 2000;4:1–203. Search date 1999; primary sources Medline, Embase, Cochrane Library, and Cochrane Skin Group Specialised Trials Register.
16. Thomas KS, Armstrong S, Avery T, et al. Randomised controlled trial of short bursts of a potent topical corticosteroid versus prolonged use of a mild preparation for children with mild or moderate atopic eczema. *BMJ* 2002;324:768–771.
17. Van der Meer JB, Glazenburg EJ, Mulder PGH, et al. The management of moderate to severe atopic dermatitis in adults with topical fluticasone propionate. *Br J Dermatol* 1999;140:1114–1121.
18. Patel L, Clayton PE, Addison GM, et al. Adrenal function following topical steroid treatment in children with atopic dermatitis. *Br J Dermatol* 1995;132:950–955.
19. Kerscher MJ, Hart H, Korting HC, et al. In vivo assessment of the atrophogenic potency of mometasone furoate, a newly developed chlorinated potent topical glucocorticoid as compared to other topical glucocorticoids old and new. *Int J Clin Pharmacol Ther* 1995;33:187–189.
20. Kerscher MJ, Korting HC. Comparative atrophogenicity potential of medium and highly

potent topical glucocorticoids in cream and ointment according to ultrasound analysis. *Skin Pharmacol* 1992;5:77–80.
21. Kerscher MJ, Korting HC. Topical glucocorticoids of the non-fluorinated double-ester type. *Acta Derm Venereol* 1992;72:214–216.
22. Korting HC, Vieluf D, Kerscher M. 0.25% prednicarbate cream and the corresponding vehicle induce less skin atrophy than 0.1% betamethasone-17-valerate cream and 0.05% clobetasol-17-propionate cream. *Eur J Clin Pharmacol* 1992;42:159–161.
23. Hill VA, Wong E, Corbett MF, et al. Comparative efficacy of betamethasone/clioquinol (Betnovate-C) cream and betamethasone/fusidic acid (Fucibet) cream in the treatment of infected hand eczema. *J Dermatol Treat* 1998;9:15–19.
24. Poyner TF, Dass BK. Comparative efficacy and tolerability of fusidic acid/hydrocortisone cream (Fucidin H cream) and miconazole/hydrocortisone cream (Daktacort cream) in infected eczema. *J Eur Acad Dermatol Venereol* 1996;7(suppl 1):23–30.
25. Jaffe GV, Grimshaw JJ. A clinical trial of hydrocortisone/potassium hydroxyquinolone sulphate (Quinocort) in the treatment of infected eczema and impetigo in general practice. *Pharmatherapeutica* 1986;4:628–636.
26. Schuttelar M-L, Coenraads P. Randomised, double-blind study to assess the efficacy of addition of tetracycline to triamcinolone acetonide (class II corticosteroid) in the treatment of moderate to severe atopic dermatitis. Abstract presented at national meeting: *"Treatments for Atopic Dermatitis: An Evidence-Based Update"*. Nottingham 2002.
27. Hanifin JM, Hebert AA, Mays SR, et al. Effects of a low-potency corticosteroid lotion plus a moisturizing regimen in the treatment of atopic dermatitis. *Curr Ther Res* 1998;59:227–233.
28. Kantor I, Milbauer J, Posner M, et al. Efficacy and safety of emollients as adjunctive agents in topical corticosteroid therapy for atopic dermatitis. *Today Ther Trend* 1993;11:157–166.
29. Lucky AW, Leach AD, Laskarzewski P, et al. Use of an emollient as a steroid-sparing agent in the treatment of mild to moderate atopic dermatitis in children. *Pediatr Dermatol* 1997;14:321–324.
30. Goodyear HM, Spowart K, Harper JI. "Wet wrap" dressings for the treatment of atopic eczema in children. *Br J Dermatol* 1991;125:604.
31. Lewis-Jones S. Keeping wet wraps under wraps. Abstract presented at national meeting: *"Treatments for Atopic Dermatitis: An Evidence-Based Update"*. Nottingham 2002.
32. Schnopp C, Holtman C, Stock S, et al. Topical steroids under wet wrap dressings in atopic dermatitis: a vehicle controlled trial. *Dermatology* 2002;204:56–59.
33. Mallon E, Powell S, Bridgman A. "Wet-wrap" dressings for the treatment of atopic eczema in the community. *J Dermatol Treat* 1994;5:97–98.
34. Pei AYS, Chan HL, Ho KM. The effectiveness of wet wrap dressings using 0.1% mometasone furoate and 0.005% fluticasone proprionate ointments in the treatment of moderate to severe atopic dermatitis in children. *Pedriatr Dermatol* 2001;18:343–348.
35. Tan B, Weald D, Strickland I, et al. Double-blind controlled trial of effect of house dust-mite allergen avoidance on atopic dermatitis. *Lancet* 1996;347:15–18.
36. Colloff MJ, Lever RS, McSharry C. A controlled trial of house dust mite eradication using natamycin in homes of patients with atopic dermatitis: effect on clinical status and mite populations. *Br J Dermatol* 1989;121:199–208.
37. Nishioka K, Yasueda H, Saito H. Preventative effect of bedding encasement with microfine fibres on mite sensitisation. *J Allergy Clin Immunol* 1998; 101; 28–32.
38. Endo K, Fukuzumi T, Adachi J, et al. Effect of vacuum cleaning of floors and bed clothes of patients on house dust mite counts and clinical scores of atopic dermatitis. A double blind control trial. [Japanese]. *Aerrerugi* 1997;46:1013–1024.
39. Friedmann PS, Tan BB. Mite elimination — clinical effect on eczema. *Allergy* 1998; 53 Suppl 48:97–100.
40. Sanda T, Yasue T, Oohashi M, et al. Effectiveness of house dust-mite allergen avoidance through clean room therapy in patients with atopic dermatitis. *J Allergy Clin Immunol* 1992;89:653–657.
41. Holm L, Ohman S, Bengtsson A, et al. Effectiveness of occlusive bedding in the treatment of atopic dermatitis — a placebo-controlled trial of 12 months' duration *Allergy* 2001;56:152–158.
42. Gutgesell C, Heise S, Seubert S, et al. Double-blind placebo-controlled house dust mite control measures in adult patients with atopic dermatitis. *Br J Dermatolol* 2001;145:70–74.
43. Atherton DJ, Sewell M, Soothill JF, et al. A double-blind controlled crossover trial of an antigen avoidance diet in atopic eczema. *Lancet* 1978;1:401–403.
44. Neild VS, Marsden RA, Bailes JA, et al. Egg and milk exclusion diets in atopic eczema. *Br J Dermatol* 1986;114:117–123.
45. Lever R, MacDonald C, Waugh P, et al. Randomised controlled trial of advice on an egg exclusion diet in young children with atopic eczema and sensitivity to eggs. *Pediatr Allergy* 1998;9:13–19.
46. Mabin DC, Sykes AE, David TJ. Controlled trial of a few foods diet in severe atopic dermatitis. *Arch Dis Child* 1995;73:202–207.
47. Sampson HA, McCaskill CM. Food hypersensitivity and atopic dermatitis: evaluation of 113 patients. *J Pediatr* 1985;107:669–675.
48. Munkvad M, Danielsen L, Høj L, et al. Antigen-free diet in adult patients with atopic dermatitis. *Acta Derm Venereol* 1984;64:524–528.
49. Niggemann B, Sielaff B, Beyer K, et al. Outcome of double-blind, placebo-controlled food challenge tests in 107 children with atopic dermatitis. *Clin Exp Allergy* 1999;29:91–96.
50. Gdalevich M, Mimouni D, David M, et al. Breast-feeding and the onset of atopic dermatitis in childhood: A systematic review and meta-analysis of prospective studies. *J Am Acad Dermatol* 2001;45 (4):520–527. Search date 2000; prmary sources Medline and hand searches of reference lists.
51. Williams HC. *Predictors of childhood eczema.* MSc Thesis. University of London 1991:48–50.
52. Wadanda N, Golding J, Kennedy CTC, et al. Breast-feeding, high social class and maternal smoking influence the risk of atopic dermatitis. (Abstract) *Br J Dermatol* 2001;145(Suppl 59):21.
53. Kramer MS. Maternal antigen avoidance during lactation for preventing atopic disease in infants of women at high risk. In: The Cochrane Library, Issue 4, 2000. Oxford: Update Software. Search date not stated; primary sources The Cochrane Pregnancy and Childbirth Group Trials Register and contact with authors of studies.
54. Kramer MS. Maternal antigen avoidance during pregnancy for preventing atopic disease in infants of women at high risk. In: The Cochrane Library, Issue 3, 2001. Oxford: Update Software. Search date not stated; primary sources The Cochrane Pregnancy and Childbirth Group Trials Register.

55. Diepgen TL, Salzer B, Tepe A, et al. A study of skin irritations caused by textiles under standardized sweating conditions in patients with atopic eczema [German]. *Melliand Deutsch/English* 1995;12:E268–E269.
56. Diepgen TL, Stabler A, Tepe A, et al. A study of skin irritation by textiles under standardised sweating conditions in patients with atopic eczema [German]. *Z Hautkrankheiten* 1990;65:907–910.
57. Seymour JL, Keswick BH, Hanifin JM, et al. Clinical effects of diaper types on the skin of normal infants and infants with atopic dermatitis. *J Am Acad Dermatol* 1987;17:988–997.
58. Bendsöe N, Björnberg A, Åsnes H. Itching from wool fibres in atopic dermatitis. *Contact Dermatitis* 1987;17:21–22.
59. Juntunen-Backman K, Peltola H, Backman A, Salo OP. Safe immunisation of allergic children against measles, mumps and rubella. *Am J Dis Child* 1987;141:1103–1105.

Dominic Smethurst
Clinical Research Fellow
Department of Evidence-based Dermatology
Nottingham
UK

Sarah Macfarlane
Specialist registrar in dermatology
Department of Dermatology
Queen's Medical Centre
Nottingham
UK

Competing interests: None declared.

TABLE 1 Topical steroids versus placebo in atopic eczema: results of RCTs* (see text, p 1666).[4–13]

	Number of participants (age in years)	Outcome
Prednicarbate ointment, 0.25% twice daily for 4 weeks.[4]	51 (18–60)	Reduced dermatitis: 87% active treatment, 8% controls. Significantly reduced patient-assessed pruritis on active treatment.
Hydrocortisone valerate cream, 0.2% three times daily for 2 weeks.[5]	20 (2–75)	Excellent or better: 75% active treatment, 20% controls.
Clobetasol propionate cream, 0.05% twice daily for 4 weeks.[6]	81 (≥ 12)	Good, excellent, or clear: 82% active treatment, 29% controls.
Hydrocortisone buteprate cream, 0.1% once daily for 2 weeks.[9]	194 (17–76)	Excellent or good: 69% active treatment, 26% controls.
Betamethasone dipropionate ointment, 0.05% twice daily for 3 weeks.[8]	36 (2–63)	Good or excellent: 94% active treatment, 13% controls.
Halcinonide ointment, 0.1% three times daily for 2 weeks.[7]	233 (2–67)	Good or excellent: 85% active treatment, 44% controls.
Desonide cream once daily for 1 week.[10]	40 (0.4–15)	Improvement or resolution: 67% active treatment, 16% controls.
Hydrocortisone valerate 0.2% ointment twice daily for 2 weeks.[11]	64 (> 12)	Disease severity score: 70% reduction with active treatment, 15% controls.
Betamethasone dipropionate twice daily for 4 days.[12]	30 (19–57)	Itch free on days 3–4: 36% active treatment, 22% controls.
Halcinonide cream, 0.1% twice daily for 3 weeks.[13]	58 (0.8–86)	57% of people achieved a better response with active treatment than control treatment ("better response" was not defined).
Fluticasone propionate, 0.005% twice daily for 4 weeks[14]	203 (12–82)	Good, excellent or clear at 28 days: 80% active treatment, 38% controls
Fluticasone propionate, 0.005% twice daily for 4 weeks[14]	194 (12–84)	Good, excellent or clear at 28 days: 80% active treatment 34% controls

*Confidence intervals not reported.

TABLE 2 Methods for reducing house dust mite levels: results of controlled trials (see text, p 1672).

Methods	Results*
Mattress, pillow and duvet covers (micro-porous or polyurethane coated)	Very effective (4 RCTs). Dust mite allergen levels 1–25% of control levels after 3–12 months; 44–98% reduction in dust load after 3 months.
Washing bedding at 55°C	Effective (2 RCTs). Reduces levels of dust mite allergen by > 95% and kills 100% of mites.
Removal of carpets and curtains	Unknown.
Acaricides (e.g. benzyl benzoate)	Conflicting results from RCTs — better when used on carpets than on mattresses. Effect may be short lived.
Intensive vacuuming	Small effect on mite levels in mattresses (1 RCT, 1 crossover trial) but not correlated with improvement in symptoms, possibly because conventional rather than high filtration cleaners may increase levels of airborne mite allergens, which may aggravate atopic disease (1 RCT in 16 rooms).
Air filters and dehumidifiers	Conflicting results from RCTs.

*Trials have tended to use a combination of control measures, making it difficult to see which measures were responsible for beneficial effects.

Cellulitis and erysipelas

Search date October 2001

Andrew Morris

QUESTIONS

INTERVENTIONS

Key Messages

- **Antibiotics** We found no RCTs comparing antibiotics versus placebo. RCTs comparing different single antibiotic regimens found clinical cure in 50–100% of people at 4–30 days. The RCTs were not designed to detect a clinically important difference between antibiotics.
- **Treatment of predisposing factors to prevent recurrence** We found no RCTs or observational studies on the effects of treatment of predisposing factors on recurrence of cellulitis or erysipelas.
- **Different antibiotic regimens; oral versus intravenous antibiotics; short versus long courses of antibiotics** We found no RCTs comparing oral versus intravenous antibiotics, or different durations of treatment. RCTs comparing different antibiotics regimens were not designed to detect clinically significant differences.

Cellulitis and erysipelas

DEFINITION Cellulitis is a spreading bacterial infection of the dermis and subcutaneous tissues. It causes local signs of inflammation such as warmth, erythema, pain, and lymphangitis, and frequently systemic upset with fever and raised white blood cell count. Erysipelas differs from cellulitis in that it tends to be more superficial, with a clearly demarcated edge. The lower limbs are by far the commonest sites, but any area can be affected.

INCIDENCE/ PREVALENCE We found no specific data on the incidence of cellulitis. However, in the UK in 1991, cellulitis and abscess infections were responsible for 158 consultations per 10 000 person years at risk. In 1985, skin and subcutaneous tissue infections resulted in 29 820 hospital admissions and a mean occupancy of 664 hospital beds each day.[1,2]

AETIOLOGY/ RISK FACTORS The commonest infective organisms in adults are *Streptococci* (particularly *S pyogenes*) and *Staphylococcus aureus.*[3] In children, *Haemophilus influenzae* is a frequent cause. Several risk factors for cellulitis/erysipelas have been identified in a case control study (167 cases and 294 controls): lymphoedema (OR 71.2, 95% CI 5.6 to 908.0), leg ulcer (OR 62.5, 95% CI 7.0 to 556.0), toe web intertrigo (OR 13.9, 95% CI 7.2 to 27.0), and traumatic wounds (OR 10.7, 95% CI 4.8 to 23.8).[4]

PROGNOSIS Cellulitis can spread through the bloodstream and lymphatic system. A retrospective case note study of people admitted to hospital with cellulitis found that systemic symptoms such as fever and raised white blood cell count were present in up to 42% of cases at presentation.[5] Lymphatic involvement can lead to obstruction and damage that predisposes to recurrent cellulitis. Recurrence can occur rapidly or after months or years. One study found that 29% of people with erysipelas had a recurrent episode within 3 years.[6] Local necrosis and abscess formation can also occur. It is not known whether the prognosis of erysipelas differs from that of cellulitis. We found no evidence about factors that predict recurrence, or a better or worse outcome. We found no good evidence on the prognosis of untreated cellulitis.

AIMS To reduce the severity and duration of infection; to relieve pain and systemic symptoms; to restore the skin to its premorbid state; to prevent recurrence; to minimise adverse effects of treatment.

OUTCOMES Duration and severity of symptoms (pain, swelling, erythema, and fever); clinical cure (defined as the absence of pain, swelling, and erythema); recurrence; adverse effects of treatment. We found no standard scales of severity in cellulitis or erysipelas.

METHODS *Clinical Evidence* search and appraisal October 2001. Where we found no RCTs, we included observational studies retrieved by the contributor's own search June 1999.

QUESTION What are the effects of antibiotics?

We found no RCTs comparing antibiotics versus placebo, oral versus intravenous antibiotics, different combinations of antibiotics, or different durations of treatment. RCTs comparing different antibiotic regimens found clinical cure in 50–100% of people at 4–30 days, but only one of

the RCTs found a significant difference between different antibiotics in clinical cure. However, most of the RCTs included only a small number of people with cellulitis or erysipelas and were not designed to detect a clinically significant difference between antibiotics.

Benefits: We found no systematic review. **Versus placebo:** We found no RCTs. **Oral versus intravenous antibiotics:** One small quasi-randomised trial (73 people with erysipelas in hospital with a body temperature >38.5 °C and no suspected septicaemia) comparing oral versus intravenous penicillin found no significant difference in clinical efficacy, which was assessed by indirect measures such as temperature fall, length of hospital stay, and absence from work.[7] No results were provided on relapse. **Combinations of antibiotics:** We found no RCTs. **Different antibiotic regimens:** We found eight RCTs comparing different antibiotic regimens in people with a variety of skin infections (see table 1, p 1687).[8–15] Only one of the RCTs found a significant difference between different antibiotics in clinical cure at 4–30 days.[14] However, most of the RCTs only included small numbers of people with cellulitis or erysipelas and were not designed to detect a clinically significant difference between antibiotics.[8–13,15] **Short versus long courses of antibiotics:** We found no RCTs comparing different durations of treatment.

Harms: In the quasi-randomised trial (73 people) comparing oral versus intravenous penicillin, adverse events occurred in 15 people taking oral penicillin (exanthem 4, diarrhoea 7, abscess 4) and in 10 people taking intravenous penicillin (exanthem 2, diarrhoea 4, cannula phlebitis 4).[7] The RCT (58 people with moderate to severe cellulitis) comparing flucloxacillin versus ceftriaxone found no significant difference in the number of people experiencing diarrhoea, nausea and vomiting, abdominal pain, or vaginal candidiasis (6/22 [27%] with flucloxacillin *v* 3/22 [14%] with ceftriaxone; RR 2.00, 95% CI 0.57 to 7.00).[14] The RCT (69 people with erysipelas) comparing penicillin versus roxithromycin found no significant difference in the number of people experiencing drug related rashes (2/38 [5%] with penicillin *v* 0/31 [0%] people with roxithromycin).[11] The RCTs that compared different antibiotics in a variety of skin infections gave no discrete information on adverse effects in people with cellulitis.[8–10,12,13,15]

Comment: None.

QUESTION Does the treatment of predisposing factors reduce recurrence?

We found no RCTs or observational studies on the effects of treatment of predisposing factors on recurrence of cellulitis or erysipelas.

Benefits: We found no systematic review, RCTs, or observational studies.

Harms: We found no good evidence.

Comment: Although there is a consensus that successful treatment of the predisposing factors reduces the risk of developing cellulitis/erysipelas (see aetiology, p 1684), we found no evidence to support this.

Cellulitis and erysipelas

REFERENCES

1. Office of Population Censuses and Surveys. *Morbidity statistics from general practice*. Fourth National Study. London: HMSO (series MB5), 1992, 272.
2. Department of Health, Department of Health and Social Security. *Hospital in-patient enquiry*. London: HMSO (series MB4), 1985, 16, 28.
3. Bernard P, Bedane C, Mounier M, Denis F, Catanzano G, Bonnetblanc JM. Streptococcal cause of erysipelas and cellulitis in adults. *Arch Dermatol* 1989;125:779–782.
4. Dupuy A, Benchikhi H, Roujeau J-C, et al. Risk factors for erysipelas of the leg (cellulitis): case-control study. *BMJ* 1999;318:1591–1594.
5. Aly AA, Roberts NM, Seipol K, MacLellan DG. Case survey of management of cellulitis in a tertiary teaching hospital. *Med J Aust* 1996;165:553–556.
6. Jorup-Ronstrom C, Britton S. Recurrent erysipelas: predisposing factors and costs, of prophylaxis. *Infection* 1987;15:105–106.
7. Jorup-Ronstrom C, Britton A, Gavlevik K, Gunnarsson K, Redman AC. The course, costs and complications of oral versus intravenous penicillin therapy of erysipelas. *Infection* 1984;12:390–394.
8. Daniel R, Austad J, Debersaques J, et al. Azithromycin, erythromycin and cloxacillin in the treatment of infections of skin and associated soft tissues. *J Int Med Res* 1991;19:433–445.
9. Kiani R. Double-blind, double-dummy comparison of azithromycin and cephalexin in the treatment of skin and skin structure infections. *Eur J Clin Microbiol Infect Dis* 1991;10:880–884.
10. Tack KJ, Littlejohn TW, Mailloux G, Wolf MM, Keyserling CH. Cefdinir versus cephalexin for the treatment of skin and skin-structure infections. *Clin Ther* 1998;20:244–255.
11. Bernard P, Plantin P, Roger H, et al. Roxithromycin versus penicillin in the treatment of erysipelas in adults: a comparative study. *Br J Dermatol* 1992;127:155–159.
12. Parish LC, Jungkind DL. Systemic anti-microbial therapy for skin and skin structure infections: comparison of fleroxacin and ceftazidime. *Am J Med* 1993;94:166S–173S.
13. Tassler H. Comparative efficacy and safety of oral fleroxacin and amoxicillin/clavulanate potassium in skin and soft tissue infections. *Am J Med* 1993;94:159S–165S.
14. Vinen J, Hudson B, Chan B, Fernandes C. A randomized comparative study of once-daily ceftriaxone and 6-hourly flucloxacillin in the treatment of moderate to severe cellulitis. Clinical efficacy, safety and pharmacoeconomic implications. *Clin Drug Invest* 1996;12:221–225.
15. Chan JC. Ampicillin-sulbactam versus cefazolin or cefoxitin in the treatment of skin and skin-structure infections of bacterial etiology. *Adv Ther* 1995;12:139–146.

Andrew Morris
Specialist Registrar in Dermatology
University Hospital
Nottingham
UK

Competing interests: None declared.

TABLE 1 **Different antibiotic regimens: results of comparative RCTs** **(see text, p 1685).**

Ref	Regimen	Participants	Clinical cure (significance)
8	Oral azithromycin total dose 1.5 g over 5 days *v* oral erythromycin 500 mg qds for 7 days	128 people with cellulitis	52/72 (72%) *v* 37/50 (74%) after 4–11 days (RR 0.97, 95% CI 0.78 to 1.21)
8	Oral azithromycin total dose 1.5 g over 5 days *v* oral cloxacillin 500 mg qds for 7 days	62 people with cellulitis	27/41 (66%) *v* 11/21 (52%) after 4–9 days (RR 1.26, 95% CI 0.79 to 2.00)
9	Oral azithromycin total dose 750 mg over 5 days *v* cefalexin 500 mg bd for 10 days	95 people with suspected cellulitis, 47 of whom had microbiologically proven cellulitis	12/24 (50%) *v* 14/23 (61%) after 11 days (RR 0.82, 95% CI 0.49 to 1.38)
10	Cefdinir 300 mg bd for 10 days *v* cefalexin 500 mg qds for 10 days	78 people with suspected cellulitis, 34 of whom had microbiologically proven cellulitis	In the 34 people with microbiologically proven cellulitis: 13/17 (76%) *v* 14/17 (82%) after 7–16 days (RR 0.93, 95% CI 0.66 to 1.31)
11	iv penicillin 2.5 MU 8 times daily followed by 6 MU orally od for mean 13 days *v* oral roxithromycin 150 mg bd for mean 13 days	69 people with erysipelas	29/38 (76%) *v* 26/31 (84%) after 30 days (RR 0.91, 95% CI 0.72 to 1.15)
12	iv fleroxacin 400 mg od *v* iv ceftazidime 0.52 g bd/tds	39 people with cellulitis	26/27 (96%) *v* 9/12 (75%) after 21 days (RR 1.28, 95% CI 0.92 to 1.78)
13	Oral amoxicillin/clavulanate potassium 125–500 mg tds *v* oral fleroxacin 400 mg od	11 people with cellulitis or erysipelas	7/7 (100%) *v* 4/4 (100%) after 3–9 days
14	iv ceftriaxone 1g od for 7 days *v* iv flucloxacillin 1 g qds for a mean of 9 days	58 people with cellulitis	21/23 (92%) *v* 14/22 (64%) after 4–6 days (RR 1.43, 95% CI 1.02 to 2.02; NNT 4, 95% CI 2 to 17)
15	iv ampicillin/sulbactam 0.5–1g qds *v* iv cefazolin 500 mg qds for 6–7 days	20 people with cellulitis	8/8 (100%) *v* 9/12 (75%) after 10 days

bd, twice daily; iv, intravenous; od, once daily; qds, four times daily; ref, reference tds, three times daily; ref, reference.

Chronic plaque psoriasis

Search date May 2002

Luigi Naldi and Berthold Rzany

QUESTIONS

INTERVENTIONS

See glossary, p 1706

Key Messages

- **Alefacept** One RCT found limited evidence that alefacept versus placebo may improve psoriasis. Adverse effects included dizziness, accidents, chills, and cough.
- **Ciclosporin** One systematic review has found optimal clearance rates with a ciclosporin dose of 5.0 mg/kg daily. Any advantage of doses greater than 5.0 mg/kg daily may be offset by an increase in dose related side effects, particularly increased renal toxicity.
- **Dithranol** Small RCTs have found that dithranol versus placebo improves chronic plaque psoriasis.
- **Emollients and keratolytics** We found no clear evidence on the effects of emollients and keratolytics.
- **Etanercept** One small RCT found limited evidence that etanercept versus placebo may improve psoriasis. Reported adverse effects include skin reactions, urticarial manifestations, and upper respiratory tract infections.

Clin Evid 2002;8:1688–1708.

- **Fumaric acid derivatives** One systematic review found limited evidence that oral fumaric acid esters provided short term improvement or complete clearing of psoriasis. Monoethylfumarate on its own has not been found to have a beneficial effect. The incidence of acute adverse effects (flushing and gastrointestinal symptoms) is high; 30–40% of people discontinue treatment because of adverse effects, non-compliance, or both. We found no evidence on the effects of fumaric acid derivatives as maintenance treatment.
- **Goeckerman treatment** We found no good evidence on the effects of the Goeckerman treatment.
- **Infliximab** One RCT found limited evidence that infliximab versus placebo may improve psoriasis. Reported adverse effects include lupus-like syndrome and severe infections.
- **Ingram regimen** One large RCT has found that the Ingram regimen is of similar effectiveness to psoralen plus ultraviolet A in clearing moderate to severe psoriasis.
- **Methotrexate** Limited evidence from one small RCT in people with psoriatic arthritis suggests that methotrexate may improve skin lesions in psoriasis. Non-randomised evidence suggests that clearance can be maintained as long as treatment is continued. About half of people relapse within 6 months of stopping treatment. Methotrexate can induce acute myelosuppression. Long term methotrexate carries the risk of hepatic fibrosis and cirrhosis, which is related to the dose regimen employed.
- **Oral retinoids (etretinate, acitretin, liarazole)** RCTs found limited evidence that oral retinoids alone may achieve complete clearance in people with plaque psoriasis. The number of people with complete clearance is increased by combination with psoralen ultraviolet A or ultraviolet B. We found insufficient evidence on the effects of liarozole. We found little reliable evidence on the effects of oral retinoids as maintenance treatment. Adverse effects lead to discontinuation of treatment in 10–20% of people. Teratogenicity renders oral retinoids less acceptable.
- **Psoralen plus ultraviolet A** One systematic review has found that clearing of psoriasis is more likely with higher versus lower doses of psoralen, and that the mean cumulative dose of ultraviolet A required for clearance is significantly reduced. Long term treatment risks include photoageing and skin cancer (mainly squamous cell carcinoma).
- **Tacrolimus** One RCT found limited evidence that tacrolimus versus placebo may improve psoriasis. Adverse effects are reported to be similar to those of ciclosporin.
- **Tars** Small RCTs have found conflicting results on the effects of tars in combination with ultraviolet B exposure.
- **Topical retinoids (tazarotene)** RCTs have found that tazarotene versus placebo improves chronic plaque psoriasis in the short term. One RCT has found that tazarotene plus topical steroids versus calcipotriol improves short term outcomes.
- **Topical steroids** RCTs have found that topical steroids improve psoriasis in the short term. Topical steroids may cause striae and atrophy, which increase with clinical potency and use of occlusive dressings. Continuous use may lead to adrenocortical suppression, and case reports suggest that severe flares of the disease may occur on withdrawal.

- **Ultraviolet B** There is a consensus that ultraviolet B is effective, but one systematic review has found insufficient evidence on the effects of ultraviolet B versus other treatments, or on the effects of narrow band versus broad band ultraviolet B for either clearance or maintenance treatment.
- **Vitamin D derivatives** Systematic reviews and additional long term uncontrolled studies have found that calcipotriol versus placebo improves plaque psoriasis and is at least as effective as topical steroids, coal tars, and dithranol. One review found that calcipotriol monotherapy caused more irritation than potent topical steroids.
- **Acupuncture; antistreptococcal treatments; balneotherapy; fish oil; heliotherapy; lifestyle changes; oral vitamin D; stress reduction; sunbeds** We found insufficient evidence on the effects of these interventions.

DEFINITION Chronic plaque psoriasis is a chronic inflammatory skin disease that is characterised by well demarcated erythematous scaly patches on the extensor surfaces of the body and scalp. The lesions may itch, sting, and occasionally bleed. Dystrophic nail changes are found in more than a third of people with chronic plaque psoriasis, and psoriatic arthropathy occurs in 1–3%. The condition waxes and wanes, with wide variations in course and severity among individuals. Other varieties of psoriasis include guttate, inverse, pustular, and erythrodermic psoriasis. This review deals with treatments for chronic plaque psoriasis.

INCIDENCE/ PREVALENCE Psoriasis affects 1–2% of the general population. It is believed to be less frequent in people from Africa and Asia, but we found no reliable epidemiological data.[1]

AETIOLOGY/ RISK FACTORS About a third of people with psoriasis have a family history of psoriasis, but physical trauma, acute infection, and some medications (e.g. lithium salts and β blockers) are believed to trigger the condition. A few observational studies have linked the onset or relapse of psoriasis with stressful life events and personal habits, including cigarette smoking and, less consistently, alcohol consumption. Others have found an association of psoriasis with body mass index (see glossary, p 1706) and an inverse association with intake of fruit and vegetables.

PROGNOSIS We found no long term prognostic studies. With the exceptions of erythrodermic and acute generalised pustular psoriasis (severe conditions that affect less than 1% of people with psoriasis and that require intensive hospital care), psoriasis is not known to affect mortality. Psoriasis may substantially affect quality of life.[2] At present there is no cure for psoriasis.

AIMS To achieve short term suppression of symptoms and long term modulation of disease severity; to improve quality of life, with minimal adverse effects of treatment.

OUTCOMES State of lesions over time; use of routine treatments; duration of remission; patient satisfaction and autonomy; disease related quality of life; adverse effects of treatment. We found no documented evidence that clinical activity scores, such as the Psoriasis Area Severity Index (PASI) score (see glossary, p 1706), are reliable proxies for these outcomes. Many clinical studies provide no explicit criteria for severity.[3]

METHODS *Clinical Evidence* update search and appraisal May 2002. The authors additionally hand searched a number of dermatological and medical journals for the years 1976–1996 as a project of the European Dermatoepidemiology Network. These were the *Journal of Investigative Dermatology, British Journal of Dermatology, Dermatology, Acta Dermo-Venereologica, Archives of Dermatology, Journal of the American Academy of Dermatology, Annales de Dermatologie et de Vénéréologie, Giornale Italiano di Dermatologia e Venereologia, Hautarzt, British Medical Journal, Lancet, Journal of the American Medical Association,* and *New England Journal of Medicine.*

QUESTION What are the effects of non-drug treatments?

We found insufficient evidence on the effects of non-drug treatments.

Benefits: **Heliotherapy:** We found one RCT (2 year, crossover design, 95 people), which compared 4 weeks of supervised heliotherapy versus no intervention.[4] Compared with no intervention, heliotherapy significantly improved psoriasis and reduced use of routine treatment by 30% in the year after treatment. **Sunbeds:** We found one small RCT (38 people with chronic stable plaque psoriasis) comparing ultraviolet A (UVA) light versus placebo (visible light).[5] In each person, one side of the body was exposed to UVA light and the other to placebo. The trial found a small improvement in the modified Psoriasis Area and Severity Index (PASI) score (see glossary, p 1706) (mean PASI score 3.9 UVA treated side *v* 4.2 placebo treated side; CI not provided; P = 0.04). **Fish oil supplementation:** We found six RCTs, which reported conflicting results. The largest RCT (145 people) found no significant benefit from fish oil versus corn oil.[6] **Oral vitamin D:** One RCT (50 people) found no significant difference between oral colecalciferol (cholecalciferol) and placebo.[7] **Stress reduction:** We found two small RCTs, which found that psychological interventions for stress improved psoriasis. The largest RCT (51 people) found a slight but significant improvement in psoriasis activity scores.[8] **Lifestyle change:** We found no RCTs of smoking cessation or dietary change in people with psoriasis. **Antistreptococcal treatments:** We found one systematic review (search date 1999, 1 RCT, 20 people) of antistreptococcal interventions for guttate and chronic plaque psoriasis.[9] The review found no evidence that tonsillectomy (or antibiotics) is beneficial as compared with placebo or no treatment. **Balneotherapy:** We found one systematic review (search date 1999)[10] and two additional RCTs of salt water baths.[11,12] The systematic review identified five small RCTs comparing phototherapy combined with salt water versus tap water baths. The included RCTs found conflicting results and the review did not report any summary effect estimate. The first additional RCT (71 people) found no significant difference between saline spa water combined with phototherapy compared with phototherapy alone.[11] The second, and weaker, additional RCT (50 people) found clinical improvement in more people with a thermal bath (bicarbonate, calcium, and magnesium rich water) than with a tap water bath (64% *v* 11%).[12] **Acupuncture:** We found one RCT (56 people), which found no significant difference between classic acupuncture and sham (placebo) acupuncture.[13]

Harms: We found no good evidence on harms.

Comment: Because several trigger and perpetuating factors for psoriasis have been recognised, including physical trauma, acute infections, smoking, diet, and stress, disease severity might be modulated by non-drug treatments. However, we found no good evidence on the effects of non-drug treatments.

QUESTION What are the effects of topical drug treatments?

OPTION EMOLLIENTS AND KERATOLYTICS

We found no clear evidence on the effects of emollients and keratolytics.

Benefits: We found two systematic reviews of emollients and keratolytics[14,15] and five additional RCTs. The first systematic review (search date 1994, 4 RCTs, 245 people) found that capsaicin versus other treatments had a beneficial effect on itching, scaling, and erythema.[14] However, there was significant unexplained heterogeneity in the results from individual trials. The second systematic review (search date 1998, 10 RCTs) evaluated aloe vera for a large variety of conditions, including psoriasis. It found no clear evidence of effectiveness, but did not exclude the possibility of a clinically important effect.[15] The largest of the additional RCTs (43 people) found that emollients temporarily improved psoriasis when they were combined with ultraviolet B radiation.[16]

Harms: Local irritation and contact dermatitis have been reported with emollients and keratolytics.

Comment: Emollients and keratolytics are usually used as adjuncts to other treatments.

OPTION TARS

Small RCTs found conflicting results on the effects of tars in combination with ultraviolet B exposure.

Benefits: We found no systematic review. We found one small RCT (18 people), which found that coal tar was more effective than the emollient base in improving disease activity scores.[17] One additional small RCT (20 people; one treatment applied to the right side of the body and the other treatment to the left, the sides determined randomly) found no significant difference between coal tar plus esterified essential fatty acids versus coal tar alone.[18] Four small RCTs found conflicting results about the effects of coal tar when combined with ultraviolet B exposure and dithranol (see benefits of Ingram regimen, p 1699).

Harms: Smell, staining, and burning are the main adverse effects of coal tar.

Comment: These RCTs were probably underpowered.

OPTION DITHRANOL

Small RCTs have found that dithranol versus placebo improves chronic plaque psoriasis. The best evidence relates to its use in the Ingram regimen (see benefits of Ingram regimen, p 1699).

Benefits: **Versus placebo:** We found no systematic review. We found two small RCTs, which found that dithranol was more effective than placebo in improving psoriasis. **Conventional versus short contact treatment:** One survey of published studies (search date 1989, 22 small RCTs) compared conventional dithranol treatment versus dithranol short contact treatment (shorter contact time at higher concentrations).[19] It found no significant differences, but the trials were too small to rule out clinically important differences.

Harms: Smell, staining, and burning are the main adverse effects of dithranol.

Comment: Few trials examined participant satisfaction, so it remains unclear whether short contact treatment is easier and more convenient for people at home compared with conventional dithranol treatment.

OPTION TOPICAL STEROIDS

RCTs have found that topical steroids improve psoriasis in the short term. Topical steroids may cause striae and atrophy, which increase with clinical potency and use of occlusive dressings. Continuous use may lead to adrenocortical suppression, and case reports suggest that severe flares of the disease may occur on withdrawal.

Benefits: We found no systematic review. **Clearance:** More than 30 short term, mainly small, vehicle controlled RCTs, often involving within-person comparisons, found that topical mid to high potency steroids temporarily improved psoriatic lesions. The study duration was usually no longer than 8 weeks and improvement was judged mainly in terms of reduced erythema and scaling. The largest parallel group RCTs have evaluated the more recently developed molecules (such as mometasone). **Maintenance:** One RCT (90 people with 1 target area cleared or nearly cleared of psoriasis by betamethasone dipropionate) found better control at 6 months with topical steroids applied once a week than with placebo (AR for maintenance of clearance in the target area 60% *v* 20%).[20] **Occlusive dressings:** Twelve small RCTs, mostly using people as their own controls, found that occlusive polyethylene or hydrocolloid dressings enhanced clinical activity.

Harms: Topical steroids can cause striae and atrophy, which increase with clinical potency and use of occlusive dressings. Continuous use may lead to adrenocortical suppression,[21] and case reports suggest that severe flares of the disease may occur on withdrawal. Diminishing clinical response with repeated use (tachyphylaxis) has been described, but we found no estimates of its frequency.

Comment: The RCT assessed effects of treatment on lesions rather than on people.[20]

OPTION **VITAMIN D DERIVATIVES**

Systematic reviews and additional long term uncontrolled studies have found that calcipotriol improves plaque psoriasis compared with placebo and is at least as effective as topical steroids, coal tars, and dithranol. One review has found that calcipotriol monotherapy causes more irritation than potent topical steroids.

Benefits: We found one systematic review comparing calcipotriol versus placebo (search date 1999, 37 RCTs, 6038 people),[22] one systematic review of combination regimens (search date 1999, 11 RCTs, 756 people),[23] and nine additional RCTs of calcipotriol. **Versus placebo:** The systematic review identified eight RCTs, which found benefit in people with mild to moderately severe plaque psoriasis (mean difference in the percentage change in severity index was 44%, 95% CI 28% to 60%).[22] Long term uncontrolled studies found that treatment gains were maintained in about 70% of people for as long as the treatment was continued.[24] **Versus each other:** We found six RCTs comparing calcipotriol versus another vitamin D derivative. Five were of tacalcitol, the largest of which (287 people) found that tacalcitol once daily was slightly less effective than calcipotriol twice daily in clearing psoriasis.[25] Another RCT (144 people) found that maxacalcitol once daily compared favourably with calcipotriol once daily (55% *v* 46% of people reporting large improvement or clearance). However, the established dosage of calcipotriol is twice daily.[26] **Versus topical steroids:** In four short term comparative RCTs (largest one involving 345 people) calcipotriol was either as effective or slightly more effective than topical steroids.[27] **Versus dithranol short contact treatment:** Four RCTs (largest one involving 478 people) found that calcipotriol was either as effective or slightly more effective than dithranol short contact treatment.[28] However, one recent RCT (171 people) found that, of people who initially improved on treatment, more stayed in remission with dithranol than with calcipotriol.[29] One RCT (114 people) found no significant difference between twice daily calcitriol ointment and short contact treatment.[30] The treatment acceptability was rated as good by 47% with calcitriol and only 22% with dithranol. Twenty eight people (24%) terminated the study prematurely. **Versus coal tar:** Two RCTs (largest one involving 122 people)[31] found that calcipotriol was more effective than coal tar. **With other treatments:** Six RCTs (largest involving 169 people) found that a combination of calcipotriol with topical steroids provided better clearance and maintenance.[32] One systematic review (search date 1999, 11 RCTs, 756 people) found significant improvement in Psoriasis Area and Severity Index score (see glossary, p 1706) with calcipotriol plus acitretin, ciclosporin (cyclosporin) or psoralen plus ultraviolet A versus acitretin, ciclosporin, or psoralen plus ultraviolet A alone.[23] It found no significant difference in the rate of marked improvement (at 12 wks for acitretin plus calcipotriol v acitretin RR 1.4, 95% CI 1.0 to 1.9; at 6 wks for ciclosporin plus calcipotriol *v* ciclosporin RR 1.2, 95% CI 0.9 to 1.6; at 12 wks for PUVA plus calcipotriol *v* PUVA RR 1.2, 95% CI 0.9 to 1.6; at 8 wks for ultraviolet B plus calcipotriol v ultraviolet B RR 1.0, 95% CI 0.8 to 1.1), in cumulative exposure to phototherapy, or in use of systemic treatment.

Harms: The review found that calcipotriol monotherapy caused more irritation than potent topical steroids (NNH 10, 95% CI 6 to 34).[22] Perilesional irritation from calcipotriol has been reported in as many as 25% of people, the face and skin folds being more susceptible. In the short term, the combination of a topical steroid may reduce the incidence of skin irritation.[33] Hypercalcaemia and hypercalciuria are dose-related adverse effects.

Comment: There is a consensus that the dosage of calcipotriol should be limited to 100 g a week.

OPTION TOPICAL RETINOIDS (TAZAROTENE)

RCTs have found that tazarotene versus placebo improves chronic plaque psoriasis in the short term. One RCT has found that tazarotene plus topical steriods versus calcipotriol improves short term outcomes.

Benefits: We found no systematic review. **Versus placebo:** Three RCTs have found that tazarotene was more effective than placebo in people with chronic plaque psoriasis. In the largest RCT (318 evaluable people), clinical response was judged after 12 weeks of treatment to be good, excellent, or completely cleared in 60% of those on tazarotene 0.1% strength, in 50% of those on tazarotene 0.05% strength, and in 30% of those on vehicle control (RRR for tazarotene 0.1% strength *v* placebo 43%, 95% CI 30% to 60%).[34] **Versus steroids:** One RCT (275 evaluable people) found that tazarotene was nearly as effective in clearing psoriasis as the high potency topical steroid flucinonide.[35] **Plus steroids:** Three RCTs, the largest one involving 398 people, found that topical mid or high potency steroids added to tazarotene, or alternated on a daily basis with tazarotene, increased the response rate as compared with tazarotene alone.[36,37] **Versus calcipotriol:** One RCT (120 people) compared tazarotene 0.1% in conjunction with topical mometasone furoate 0.1% once daily versus calcipotriol 0.005% twice daily for 8 weeks.[38] The trial found significant improvements with the tazarotene and mometasone combination versus calcipotriol in terms of the number of people showing marked improvement (≥ 75% global improvement) after 2 weeks, and for scaling, erythema, and percentage of body surface coverage after 4 weeks. It found no significant difference in the number of people attaining complete or almost complete clearance (≥ 90% clearance) at any time during follow up.

Harms: The RCTs found that some perilesional irritation was reported in most people. Addition of steroids reduced the withdrawal rate and treatment related adverse effects.[36,37]

Comment: Tazarotene is contraindicated in women who are, or intend to become, pregnant because it is potentially teratogenic.

QUESTION **What are the effects of treatments with ultraviolet light?**

OPTION **ULTRAVIOLET B**

One systematic review found insufficient evidence on the effects of ultraviolet B versus other treatments, or on the effects of narrow band versus broad band ultraviolet B for either clearance or maintenance treatment.

Benefits: **Ultraviolet B (UVB) versus no UVB on clearance:** We found no systematic review and no RCTs. **UVB plus retinoids versus acitretin alone on clearance:** We found one systematic review (search date 1999, 2 small RCTs, 78 people).[39] One of the small RCTs found that significantly more people achieved 80% clearance of lesions with UVB plus acitretin versus acitretin alone (89% with combined treatment *v* 22% with acitretin alone; ARR 67%, 95% CI 33% to 100%). The other small RCT compared narrow band UVB alone versus narrow band UVB plus etretinate versus psoralen plus ultraviolet A (PUVA) plus etretinate, but was too small to draw conclusions. It found no significant difference in the number of people achieving a satisfactory response with PUVA plus etretinate versus narrow band UVB plus etretinate (100% with PUVA and etretinate *v* 93% with narrow band UVB and etretinate; ARR +7%, 95% CI –6% to +20%). It found that significantly fewer people achieved a satisfactory response with narrow band UVB alone versus PUVA plus etretinate (100% with PUVA and etretinate *v* 80% with narrow band UVB and etretinate; ARR 20%, 95% CI 0% to 40%). **Narrow band UVB versus broad band UVB on clearance:** We found one systematic review (search date 1999, 3 small crossover RCTs, 146 people) of narrow band UVB versus broad band UVB.[39] It was not possible to calculate response rates from the results reported by the RCTs. **UVB versus PUVA on clearance:** We found no systematic review but found two RCTs.[40,41] The first RCT (183 people with moderate to severe psoriasis) found no significant difference in clearance rates with PUVA versus UVB (88% cleared with PUVA *v* 80% with UVB; RR of non-clearance with PUVA *v* broad band UVB 0.62, 95% CI 0.29 to 1.22).[40] Subgroup analysis found that UVB radiation was significantly less effective in people with more than 50% body involvement. The second RCT (100 people) found that more people achieved clearance with PUVA versus narrow band UVB (84% cleared with PUVA *v* 63% with UVB).[41] **Maintenance:** We found no systematic review but found one RCT.[42] The RCT (104 people with initial clearance of symptoms) found significantly more people were still clear of symptoms after 181 days with weekly UVB versus no maintenance treatment (> 50% with UVB *v* 28% with no UVB; RR relapse 0.67, 95% CI 0.41 to 0.92).[42]

Harms: UVB radiation may increase photoageing and risk of skin cancer. One systematic review (search date 1996) estimated that the excess annual risk of non-melanoma skin cancer associated with UVB radiation was likely to be less than 2%.[43]

Comment: We found only weak evidence from RCTs on the effects of UVB.

OPTION PSORALEN PLUS ULTRAVIOLET A

One systematic review has found that clearing of psoriasis is more likely with 40 mg versus 10 mg of 8-methoxypsoralen. The mean cumulative dose of ultraviolet A required for clearance is significantly reduced by 40 mg versus 10 mg of 8-methoxypsoralen; 1.2 mg/kg versus 0.6 mg/kg of 5-methoxypsoralen; 0.6 mg/kg of 8-methoxypsoralen versus 1.2 mg/kg 5-methoxypsoralen; topical (bath) 8-methoxypsoralen versus oral 8-methoxypsoralen; and by basing the ultraviolet A dose used in each treatment on skin type rather than using the minimal phototoxic dose. No significant difference was found with liquid versus crystalline oral 8-methoxypsoralen or with topical 8-methoxypsoralen versus topical 5-methoxypsoralen. One RCT found that psoralen plus ultraviolet A was slightly more effective in clearing psoriasis than dithranol. Long term treatment risks include photoageing and skin cancer (mainly squamous cell carcinoma).

Benefits: We found one systematic review of phototherapy and photochemotherapy (search date 1999, 51 RCTs).[39] Results could not be pooled because of trial heterogeneity. **Psoralen plus ultraviolet A (PUVA) versus no PUVA:** The systematic review found no RCTs.[39] **Comparison of different doses of psoralen:** The systematic review (2 RCTs, 167 people) found significantly greater success (major improvement in or full remission of psoriasis) with higher versus lower dose psoralen (ARR 72%, 95% CI 54% to 90%; NNT 2).[39] The first RCT compared 40 mg versus 10 mg of 8-methoxypsoralen. The second RCT compared 1.2 mg/kg versus 0.6 mg/kg 5-methoxypsoralen. Both RCTs also found a lower mean cumulative ultraviolet A (UVA) dose to achieve success (54 J/cm^2 with 40 mg of 8-methoxypsoralen *v* 77 J/cm^2 with the lower dose; 53 J/cm^2 with 1.2 mg/kg 5-methoxypsoralen *v* 132 J/cm^2 with the lower dose). **Comparison of different oral psoralens:** The systematic review included two RCTs that compared different oral psoralens.[39] One RCT (169 people) found no significant difference with 5-methoxypsoralen (1.2 mg/kg) versus 8-methoxypsoralen (0.6 mg/kg) in the mean cumulative UVA dose needed for clearance (53 J/cm^2 with 5-methoxypsoralen *v* 45 J/cm^2 with 8-methoxypsoralen). The other RCT (38 people) found that people treated with 8-methoxypsoralen (0.6 mg/kg) required a lower mean cumulative UVA dose to achieve success (155 J/cm^2 with 8-methoxypsoralen *v* 187 J/cm^2 with 1.2 mg/kg 5-methoxypsoralen; CI not provided; $P < 0.05$). **Comparison of different topical psoralens:** The systematic review included one RCT (38 people), which found no significant difference with 5-methoxypsoralen versus 8-methoxypsoralen in the mean total dose of UVA required for clearance (56.8 J/cm^2 with 5-methoxypsoralen *v* 59.1 J/cm^2 with 8-methoxypsoralen). **Comparison of different oral psoralen formulations:** The systematic review included one RCT (47 people), which found no significant difference between liquid versus crystalline forms of oral 8-methoxypsoralen in the number of people with marked improvement or clearance of psoriasis (liquid *v* crystalline: ARI 25%, 95% CI −1% to +51%; mean UVA dose to achieve clearance 68.7 J/cm^2 with liquid psoralen *v* 80.8 J/cm^2 with crystalline psoralen).[39] **Comparison of oral versus bath psoralen formulations:** The systematic review found two RCTs (137 people), which found no significant difference in the success rate (major improvement or clearance), but found significantly greater mean cumulative UVA dose for clearance with oral versus topical psoralens (in the first RCT: 14.5 J/cm^2 with bath 8-methoxypsoralen *v* 60.1 J/cm^2 with oral 8-methoxypsoralen; in the other RCT: 23.5 J/cm^2 with bath 8-methoxypsoralen *v* 131.1 J/cm^2 with oral 8-methoxypsoralen).[39] **Comparison of dose setting strategies:** The systematic review included two RCTs (157 people) that compared the routine use of the minimal phototoxic dose of UVA at each treatment versus a strategy of setting the UVA dose according to skin type (see glossary, p 1706).[39] Neither study found any significant difference for success rate (clearance). One RCT found that the minimal phototoxic dose strategy (see glossary, p 1706) had a significantly higher median cumulative UVA dose for clearance (62.9 J/cm^2 with the minimal phototoxic dose *v* 39.5 J/cm^2 with the dose set on the basis of skin type). The second RCT found similar differences, but they were not significant. **Comparison of PUVA with other phototherapies:** The systematic review included five RCTs (285 people).[39] The largest RCT (100 people) found no significant difference with PUVA twice weekly versus psoralen plus narrow band UVB twice weekly (ARR for clearance 12%, 95% CI –4% to +28%). **Comparison of PUVA and other treatments:** The systematic review included 25 RCTs (1268 people) that compared different combinations of ultraviolet radiation versus systemic or topical treatments, including dithranol, tar, vitamin D_3 analogues, steroids, and fish oil.[39] The RCTs were mostly small and underpowered to detect clinically important differences. The largest of the RCTs (224 people) found that PUVA cleared psoriasis slightly more often than did dithranol (ARR 9%, 95% CI 0% to 18%). **Maintenance:** One large RCT (1005 people whose psoriasis had been cleared by PUVA) found that maintenance treatment with PUVA versus no maintenance treatment reduced relapse at 18 months (AR of flares 27% with treatment once a week *v* 34% with treatment once every 3 weeks *v* 62% with no treatment; RR for relapse with once weekly treatment *v* no treatment 0.44, 95% CI 0.32 to 0.56).[44]

Harms: The best evidence on chronic toxicity comes from an ongoing study of more than 1300 people who first received PUVA treatment in 1975.[45] The study found a dose dependent increased risk of squamous cell carcinoma, basal cell carcinoma, and possibly malignant melanoma compared with the risk in the general population. A systematic review (search date 1998) of eight additional studies has confirmed the findings concerning non-melanoma skin cancer.[46] Premature photoageing is another expected adverse effect. After less than 15 years, about a quarter of people exposed to 300 or more treatments of PUVA had at least one squamous cell carcinoma of the skin, with particularly high risk in people with skin types I and II. In people who wear UVA opaque glasses for 24 hours after psoralen ingestion, the risk of cataract development seems negligible. A combined analysis of two cohort studies (944 people treated with bath PUVA) excluded a threefold excess risk of squamous cell carcinoma after a mean follow up of 14.7 years, suggesting that bath PUVA is possibly safer than conventional PUVA.[47]

Comment: People receiving PUVA need close monitoring for acute toxicity and long term cutaneous carcinogenic effects.

OPTION COMBINATION REGIMENS

One RCT has found that the Ingram regimen was of similar effectiveness to psoralen plus ultraviolet A in clearing moderate to severe psoriasis. We found no good evidence on effectiveness of the Goeckerman treatment.

Benefits: We found one systematic review (search date 1999) of calcipotriol plus phototherapy (see benefits of vitamin D derivatives, p 1694),[23] and one systematic review (search date 1999) examining treatment for severe psoriasis,[39] which compared different combinations of ultraviolet radiation versus systemic or topical treatments, including dithranol, tar, vitamin D derivatives, steroids, and fish oil (see benefits of psoralen plus ultraviolet A, p 1697). **Ingram regimen:** One RCT (224 people) compared an inpatient Ingram regimen (see glossary, p 1706) (dithranol concentration 0.01–1.0%) versus psoralen plus ultraviolet A (PUVA) in people with at least 10% of body surface involvement.[48] It found that clearance rates were 82% (95% CI 77% to 89%) with the Ingram regimen versus 91% (95% CI 86% to 96%) with PUVA. Five small RCTs (largest one involving 53 people)[39] found conflicting results on the added efficacy of dithranol when combined with ultraviolet B (UVB) exposure. However, the trials were too small to rule out a clinically important difference. **Goeckerman treatment:** See glossary, p 1706. We found no good evidence on the effects of combining coal tar and UVB radiation. **Other combinations:** We found one systematic review (search date 1999; see benefits of vitamin D derivatives, p 1694)[23] and an additional RCT[49] of calcipotriol plus UVB or PUVA. The RCT (164 people) found that fewer UVB treatments were required to achieve clearance with calcipotriol plus UVB versus UVB alone (median number of UVB treatments: 22 with calcipotriol plus UVB *v* 25 with UVB alone; no statistical analysis for a continuous variable was reported).[49]

Harms: Adverse effects vary with the treatments being combined. Local irritation often occurs.

Comment: None.

QUESTION What are the effects of systemic drug treatments?

OPTION ORAL RETINOIDS (ETRETINATE, ACITRETIN, LIAROZOLE)

We found limited evidence that oral retinoids alone may achieve complete clearance in people with plaque psoriasis. The number of people with complete clearance is increased by combination with psoralen plus ultraviolet A or ultraviolet B. We found insufficient evidence on the effects of liarozole. We found little reliable evidence on the effects of oral retinoids as maintenance treatment. Adverse effects lead to discontinuation of treatment in 10–20% of people. Teratogenicity renders oral retinoids less acceptable.

Benefits: We found one systematic review of people with severe psoriasis (search date 1999, 32 RCTs: 13 of etretinate, 11 of acitretin, 8 of acitretin *v* etretinate),[39] one systematic review (search date 2000) of people with psoriatic arthropathy,[50] and one (search date 1999) on the combination of acitretin with calcipotriol.[23] The main outcome was treatment success, as indicated by a specific decrease in Psoriasis Area and Severity Index (PASI) score (see glossary, p 1706) or the extent of body surface area involved, or by a global improvement. Hetereogeneity among trials often prevented pooling of data. **Retinoids versus placebo:** The review[39] found 11 RCTs (455 people) and we found one additional RCT.[51] Three RCTs allowed concomitant topical steroids. Heterogeneity prevented pooling. Overall, the review found limited evidence that symptoms improved (marked improvement or complete remission) with retinoids versus placebo. The three RCTs of etretinate (1 mg/kg) versus placebo all found a greater response rate with etretinate (the largest of these RCTs found almost or complete clearance in 35% with etretinate *v* 5% with placebo; ARR 30%; 95% CI 7% to 53%). However, an RCT of etretinate (50 mg) versus placebo found no significant difference in clearance rate (complete remission: 17% with etretinate *v* 6% with placebo; ARR +11%; 95% CI –2% to +24%). Results were extractable for only two of the RCTs of acitretin versus placebo. One (38 people) was underpowered and detected no differences between acitretin and placebo. The other RCT (80 people) found no significant difference in achieving 75% or greater decrease in PASI or a PASI score of less than 8 with acitretin (10 mg) versus placebo (40% of people with acitretin *v* 25% with placebo; ARR +15%; 95% CI –14% to +44%). Higher doses of acitretin versus placebo increased the number of people who achieved 75% or greater decrease in PASI or a PASI score of less than 8 (60% with acitretin [25 mg] *v* 25% with placebo, ARR 35%, 95% CI 6% to 64%; 70% with acitretin [50 mg] *v* 25% with placebo, ARR 45%, 95% CI 17% to 73%). The additional RCT (139 people) compared liarozole 50 mg daily versus 75 mg versus 150 mg versus placebo.[51] A total of 116 people completed the 12 week study period. Only 150 mg increased the proportion of people in the "marked improvement or better" categories versus placebo (38% with liarozole 150 mg daily *v* 6% with placebo; ARR 32%; CI not stated; $P < 0.001$). **Acitretin versus etretinate:** The review identified six RCTs (598 people), which found no significant difference in the proportion of people achieving a marked improvement (≥ 75% decrease in PASI or Psoriasis Severity Index [a modified PASI], or a marked or total clearance) with acetretin versus etretinate (for the largest study, 74% of people achieved clearance with 40 mg acitretin *v* 76% with 40 mg etretinate; ARR +2%, 95% CI –17% to +13%).[39] **Etretinate versus ciclosporin:** The review found two RCTs (286 people).[39] Results could not be pooled. The RCT using the higher dose of etretinate (0.7 mg/kg) found that significantly fewer people treated with etretinate than with ciclosporin (5 mg/kg) achieved a marked response (≥ 75% decrease in PASI, 97% of people with ciclosporin *v* 73% people with etretinate; ARR 24%, 95% CI 39% to 9%). **Retinoid plus psoralen plus ultraviolet A (PUVA) versus PUVA alone:** The review identified six RCTs (305 people).[39] Results could not be pooled. Only one RCT (30 people) found a significant increase in clearance rates with retinoid plus PUVA versus PUVA alone (93% with etretinate 0.75 mg/kg plus PUVA *v* 60% with PUVA plus placebo; ARR 33%, 95% CI 5% to 61%). **Retinoid plus PUVA versus retinoid alone:** We found no

RCTs. **Retinoid plus ultraviolet B (UVB) (broad band or narrow band) versus UVB alone or retinoid alone:** The review included four RCTs (245 people).[39] Results could not be pooled. In each RCT the combined treatment was superior to UVB alone. The largest RCT (82 people) found that significantly more people with acitretin (3 mg daily) plus UVB versus UVB alone achieved 75% or greater decrease in PASI (57% with the combination *v* 23% with UVB alone; ARR 34%, 95% CI 14% to 54%). One small RCT (18 people) found that significantly more people with acitretin plus UVB versus acitretin alone achieved 80% or greater clearance (89% with the combination *v* 22% with acitretin alone; ARR 67%, 95% CI 33% to 100%). **Retinoid combination with other treatments:** The systematic review included four RCTs (511 people), which found that a retinoid plus topical steroid was superior to the single treatments in improving subjective end points.[39] Another systematic review (search date 1999) found insufficient evidence on the combination of acitretin with calcipotriol (see benefits of vitamin D derivatives, p 1694).[23] **Maintenance:** One systematic review included two RCTs.[39] One of the RCTs (36 people achieving clearance with PUVA plus etretinate) found significant reduction with low dose etretinate (half of the maximum dose tolerated) versus placebo in the relapse rate over 1 year (44% with etretinate *v* 85% with placebo; ARR 41%, 95% CI 12% to 70%). The second RCT found no significant difference with three dosages of acitretin (10 *v* 25 *v* 50 mg daily) versus placebo for 6 months.

Harms: Most people experience mucocutaneous adverse effects, such as dry skin, cheilitis, and conjunctivitis. Mucocutaneous effects were generally mild. Increased serum cholesterol and triglyceride concentrations occurred in about half of the people. Low grade hepatotoxicity was observed in about 1% of people treated with etretinate.[52] Two people treated with liarozole were withdrawn because of liver enzyme abnormalities. Occasionally, acute hepatitis occurred as a purported idiosyncratic hypersensitivity reaction. Radiographic evidence of extraspinal tendon and ligament calcifications has been documented. In one cohort study, a quarter of 956 people treated with etretinate attributed a joint problem or its worsening to the drug.[52] Etretinate is a known teratogen and may be detected in the plasma for 2–3 years after treatment stops. Acitretin can undergo esterification to etretinate.

Comment: Women of childbearing age are given effective contraception for 1 month before starting etretinate and acitretin, throughout treatment, and after stopping treatment for at least 3 years because it is potentially teratogenic. Etretinate is no longer available in many countries.

OPTION METHOTREXATE

Limited evidence from one small RCT in people with psoriatic arthritis suggests that methotrexate improves skin lesions in psoriasis. Non-randomised evidence suggests that clearance can be maintained as long as treatment is continued. About half of people relapse within 6 months of stopping treatment. Methotrexate can induce acute myelosuppression. Long term methotrexate carries the risk of hepatic fibrosis and cirrhosis, which is related to the dose regimen employed.

Benefits: We found two systematic reviews (search dates 1999[39] and 2000[50]). **Oral methotrexate; clearance:** The first systematic review identified no RCTs. The second systematic review identified one small RCT (37 people with psoriatic arthritis), which found that methotrexate versus placebo significantly reduced the surface area of psoriasis after 12 weeks (CI not provided; $P = 0.04$).[53] **Oral methotrexate; maintenance:** We found no RCTs. In one uncontrolled case series (113 people with severe psoriasis), maintenance treatment with low dose methotrexate (weekly dose not exceeding 15 mg) provided satisfactory control of skin lesions in 81% of people (mean treatment duration 8 years).[54] When treatment was stopped, 45% of people experienced a full relapse within 6 months.

Harms: In the uncontrolled case series, treatment was stopped in 33/113 (29%) people because of adverse effects.[54] The most serious acute reaction, particularly in elderly people, is dose related myelosuppression. In the long term, major adverse events included liver fibrosis and pulmonary toxicity. One systematic review (search date not stated) found that about 28% (95% CI 24% to 32%) of people taking long term methotrexate for psoriasis and rheumatoid arthritis developed liver fibrosis of histological grade 1 or higher on liver biopsy, whereas 5% developed advanced liver disease (histological grade IIIB or IV).[55] The risk was dose related and was higher with increased alcohol consumption. A limitation of the systematic review was the lack of untreated control groups. Pulmonary disease associated with methotrexate has been described as an acute or chronic interstitial pneumonitis.[56] Adverse pulmonary effects of treatment are considered much rarer in psoriasis than in rheumatoid arthritis, but we found no published evidence to support this claim. Several drug interactions that increase methotrexate toxicity have been described (e.g. with sulphonamides). Methotrexate appears to double the risk of developing squamous cell carcinoma in people exposed to psoralen plus ultraviolet A and may be an independent risk factor for this cancer in people with psoriatic arthritis.[45] A higher risk of lymphoproliferative diseases in long term users has been suggested by a few case reports. On the basis of data from a large case series (248 people), the cumulative incidence of lymphoma is not expected to be much higher than 1%.[57]

Comment: People using methotrexate are closely monitored for liver toxicity[39] and advised to limit their consumption of alcohol. The most reliable test of liver damage remains needle biopsy of the liver. It is rare for life threatening liver disease to develop with the first 1.0–1.5 g of methotrexate.

OPTION CICLOSPORIN

One systematic review has found optimal clearance rates with a ciclosporin dose of 5.0 mg/kg daily. Any advantage of doses greater than 5.0 mg/kg daily may be offset by an increase in dose related side effects, particularly increased renal toxicity. Maintenance treatment required a dose of 3.0–3.5 mg/kg daily.

Benefits: We found one systematic review (search date 1999, 18 RCTs: 13 on induction of remission, 5 on maintenance of remission).[39] Success was defined mostly as reduction in Psoriasis Area and

Severity Index (PASI) score (see glossary, p 1706) or clinical criteria such as "clearance". Dosages of ciclosporin ranged from 1.25–14 mg/kg daily. Duration of treatment ranged from 4–12 weeks. Data could not be pooled. **Ciclosporin versus placebo for clearance:** The review included six RCTs (289 people).[39] Results for the proportions of people responding to each treatment were not extractable from each RCT (the largest study reported an ARR of 22%, 95% CI 7% to 37%). **Ciclosporin versus etretinate for clearance:** The review included two RCTs (286 people).[39] The review found a significant increase in the number of people who achieved greater than 70% decrease in PASI with ciclosporin 2.5 mg/kg daily versus etretinate 0.5 mg/kg daily (62% with ciclosporin *v* 16% with etretinate; ARR 46%, CI 34% to 58%). Ciclosporin 5 mg/kg daily was more effective than 0.75 mg/kg daily etretinate (97% with ciclosporin *v* 73% with etretinate; ARR 24%, CI 9% to 39%). **Comparison of different ciclosporin doses:** Two non-blinded RCTs compared different dosages of ciclosporin (468 people), both finding that ciclosporin (5 mg/kg daily) versus ciclosporin (2.5 mg/kg daily) increased the proportion of people achieving a 75% decrease in PASI (89% with 5 mg/kg daily *v* 48% with 2.5 mg/kg daily; ARR 41%, 95% CI 31% to 51%). **Ciclosporin plus calcipotriol versus ciclosporin:** We found one RCT (69 people), but the proportion of people responding to each treatment were not extractable. **Comparison of ciclosporin formulations:** Two RCTs (345 people, 12 wks, one with a crossover design) found no significant differences in the proportion of people achieving a marked response (≥ 75% decrease in PASI) with conventional oil-based ciclosporin formulation versus the microemulsion preconcentrate formulation (the larger, parallel group RCT results: 78% of the people treated with the oil-based formulation *v* 80% with the microemulsion; ARI +2%; 95% CI −7% to +11%). **Maintenance:** The review included five RCTs.[39] One RCT found that significantly more people achieved a good response (< 50% of baseline body surface area affected) with ciclosporin (3 mg/kg daily) versus ciclosporin (1.5 mg/kg daily) versus placebo (58% with 3 mg/kg daily *v* 16% with placebo; ARR 42%; CI not provided). Another RCT of 24 week maintenance treatment found no significant differences in response with the conventional oil-based ciclosporin formulation versus the microemulsion preconcentrate formulation.

Harms: Ciclosporin is associated with dose-related hypertension (diastolic blood pressure > 90 mm Hg over 12 wks: 4/36 [11%] with 1.25 mg/kg daily *v* 25/121 [21%] with 2.5 mg/kg daily *v* 16/60 [26%] with 5 mg/kg daily) and renal impairment (creatinine ≥ 130% of baseline value: 1% *v* 5% *v* 13%, respectively).[39] The incidence of these adverse events increases over time. In a case series follow up study of 122 consecutive people treated continuously with ciclosporin for 3–76 months at a dose not exceeding 5 mg/kg daily, 104 people discontinued treatment.[58] The mean percentage of people who discontinued treatment because of adverse effects (mostly renal dysfunction and hypertension) rose from 14% at 12 months to 41% at 48 months. One RCT (400 people) found that intermittent treatment with a microemulsion formulation for 1 year (with maximum treatment periods of 12 wks as 1–4 courses) was well tolerated and produced no clinically significant change in blood pressure or creatinine concentration.[39] With this regimen only 10 (2.5%) people withdrew because of adverse events. Long term follow up studies are needed to confirm this finding.

Comment: None.

OPTION IMMUNOSUPPRESSIVE DRUGS OTHER THAN CICLOSPORIN

We found limited evidence on the effects of immunosuppressive drugs other than ciclosporin, including tacrolimus, anti-CD4 monoclonal antibodies, and alefacept.

Benefits: We found no systematic review. **Tacrolimus:** We found one RCT (50 people), which found a significant increase with tacrolimus versus placebo in the proportion of people with 70% or greater reduction in Psoriasis Area and Severity Index (PASI) score (see glossary, p 1706) after treatment for 9 weeks (63% with tacrolimus *v* 25% with placebo; RR 0.62; 95% CI not provided).[59] One RCT (70 people) of topical tacrolimus versus placebo in the treatment of a single plaque found that tacrolimus was no better than placebo in improving psoriasis (local Psoriasis Severity Index score reduced by 33% with tacrolimus *v* 43% with placebo; P = 0.77; CI not provided).[60] **Humanised anti-CD4 monoclonal antibody:** We found one RCT (28 people with moderate to severe psoriasis), which compared an anti-CD4 monoclonal antibody (OKTcdr4a) at low dose (250 mg) versus high dose (750 mg) versus placebo.[61] No significant differences were found (mean decrease in the PASI score at 15 days: 4% with low-dose OKTcdr4a *v* 17% with high-dose *v* 11% with placebo). **Alefacept:** One RCT (229 people) compared intravenous alefacept (0.025, 0.075, or 0.150 mg/kg of body weight) versus placebo weekly for 12 weeks with follow up for 12 additional weeks.[62] Twelve weeks after treatment, alefacept versus placebo significantly increased the proportion of people with 75% or greater decrease in baseline PASI score (33% with alefacept 0.025 mg/kg *v* 11% with placebo; ARR 22%; P = 0.02; CI not provided).[62]

Harms: Most of the evidence concerning the safety of tacrolimus comes from studies in people with transplant. Despite major differences in their chemical structure, tacrolimus and ciclosporin appear to have a notably similar profile of side effects.[63] We found no evidence on the long term safety of other immunosuppressive drugs. The RCT of alefacept versus placebo[62] found an increased frequency of adverse effects with alefacept (dizziness, accidents, nausea, chills, and cough).

Comment: The benefit and risk profile of these drugs in psoriasis is still poorly defined. Alefacept is a recombinant protein that binds to CD2 receptor on memory effector T lymphocytes.

OPTION CYTOKINE BLOCKING AGENTS

We found limited evidence on the effects of cytokine blocking agents in people with plaque psoriasis.

Benefits: We found no systematic review. **Etanercept:** We found one RCT (60 people mainly with psoriatic arthropathy; 19 with skin lesions).[64] A subgroup analysis for the 19 people with skin lesions found a significant increase with etanercept versus placebo in the proportion of people with 75% or greater improvement in Psoriasis Area and Severity Index (PASI) score (see glossary, p 1706) (26% with etanercept *v* 0% with placebo; P = 0.015; CI not provided). The results of that subgroup analysis are too weak to allow any generalisable conclusion. **Infliximab:** We found one RCT (33 people with severe psoriasis), which compared weekly intravenous infliximab 5 mg/kg versus infliximab 10 mg/kg versus placebo.[65] At 10 weeks, significantly more people achieved a good, excellent, or clear rating on physician's global assessment with both doses of infliximab than with placebo (91% with infliximab 10 mg/kg *v* 82% with infliximab 5 mg/kg *v* 18% with placebo; ARR for 10 mg/kg 73%, 95% CI 30% to 94%; ARR for 5 mg/kg 64%, 95% CI 20% to 89%).

Harms: Most of the evidence on the safety of etanercept and infliximab is from studies in people with rheumatoid arthritis or Crohn's disease. Cutaneous reactions to etanercept have been reported with a frequency of up to 5%, including reactions at the injection site and urticarial manifestations.[66] Upper respiratory tract infections have been reported. A few cases of lupus-like syndrome and severe infections have been reported with infliximab treatment.[67]

Comment: We found insufficient evidence to draw conclusions on the effects of cytokine blocking agents in people with plaque psoriasis.

OPTION FUMARIC ACID DERIVATIVES

One systematic review found short term good improvement or complete clearing with oral fumaric acid esters. Monoethylfumarate on its own has not been found to have a beneficial effect. The incidence of acute adverse effects (flushing and gastrointestinal symptoms) is high; 30–40% of patients discontinue treatment because of adverse effects, non-compliance, or both. We found no evidence on the effects of fumaric acid derivatives as maintenance treatment.

Benefits: **Versus placebo:** We found one systematic review (search date 1999, 4 RCTs, 203 people).[39] Fumaric acid esters versus placebo significantly increased the proportion of people who achieved improvement or complete clearing at 16 weeks (in the largest study: 57% with fumaric acid *v* 10% with placebo; ARR 47%, 95% CI 33% to 61%). One RCT found no significant difference with monoethylfumarate versus placebo in the proportion of people with greater than 50% improvement in Psoriasis Area and Severity Index (PASI) score (see glossary, p 1706) (5% with monoethylfumarate *v* 10% with placebo; ARR +5%, 95% CI –22% to +21%).

Harms: All large RCTs on fumaric acid esters have found large withdrawal rates; 39% in the drug group of one RCT terminated the treatment prematurely, mostly because of gastrointestinal side effects.[68]

Acute adverse effects, including flushing and gastrointestinal symptoms, were reported in up to 75% of people. In one RCT (50 people) of fumaric acid esters versus placebo for 16 weeks, diarrhoea was reported 27 times, stomach ache or stomach cramps 35 times, flush 21 times, and skin burning twice.[68] Another open study (101 people) reported adverse effects in 69% of people (mainly gastrointestinal [56%] and flushing [31%]).[39] Eosinophilia was often reported.[39] There have been case reports of renal failure, but one recent systematic review found no evidence of significant renal impairment.[39]

Comment: We found limited evidence on the effects of fumaric acid derivatives in people with plaque psoriasis. Gastrointestinal adverse effects are frequent.

GLOSSARY

Body mass index A measure of obesity, defined as the weight (in kilograms) divided by the square of the height (in metres).

Goeckerman treatment A daily application of coal tar followed by ultraviolet B irradiation.

Ingram regimen A daily coal tar bath, ultraviolet B irradiation, and dithranol.

Psoriasis Area and Severity Index (PASI score) Composite score grading severity of psoriasis in six body regions according to erythema, scaling, thickness, and the total area of skin affected.

Skin types A clinical classification of an individual's burning and tanning tendencies. Usually ranges from skin phototype I (which always burns and never tans) to skin phototype VI (marked constitutive pigmentation).

Skin type regimen and minimal phototoxic dose regimen The four parameters of psoralen plus ultraviolet A are the dose of psoralen, the frequency of treatment, the initial dose of ultraviolet A (UVA), and the incremental UVA dose. The initial and incremental UVA doses are described by at least two regimens. In the minimal phototoxic dose regimen, the initial UVA dose is a fraction of the minimal phototoxic dose. Weekly increments in dose occur until the maximum dose is reached. In the skin type regimen, the initial dose is based on skin phototype. Weekly dose increments are decreased if erythema develops.

REFERENCES

1. Naldi L. Psoriasis. In: Williams HC, Strachan DP, eds. *The Challenge of Dermato-Epidemiology*. Boca Raton: CRC Press, 1997;175–190.
2. O'Neill P, Kelly P. Postal questionnaire of disability in the community associated with psoriasis. *BMJ* 1996;313:919–921.
3. Petersen LI, Kristensen JK. Selection of patients for psoriasis clinical trials: a survey of the recent dermatological literature. *J Dermatol Treat* 1992;3:171–176.
4. Snellman E, Aromaa A, Jansen CT, et al. Supervised four-week heliotherapy alleviates the long-term course of psoriasis. *Acta Derm Venereol* 1993;73:388–392.
5. Turner RJ, Walshaw D, Diffey BL, et al. A controlled study of ultraviolet A sunbed treatment of psoriasis. *Br J Dermatol* 2000;143:957–963.
6. Soyland E, Funk J, Rajka G, et al. Effect of dietary supplementation with very-long-chain n-3 fatty acids in patients with psoriasis. *N Engl J Med* 1993;328:1812–1816.
7. Siddiqui MA, Al Khawajah MM. Vitamin D and psoriasis: a randomised double-blind placebo-controlled study. *J Dermatol Treat* 1990;1:243–245.
8. Zachariae R, Oster H, Bjerring P, et al. Effects of psychologic intervention on psoriasis: a preliminary report. *J Am Acad Dermatol* 1996;34:1008–1015.
9. Owen CM, Chalmers RJG, O'Sullivan T, et al. Antistreptococcal interventions for guttate and chronic plaque psoriasis. In: The Cochrane Library, Issue 3, 2001. Oxford: Update Software. Search date 1999; primary sources Cochrane Clinical Trials Register, Medline, Embase, Salford Database of Psoriasis Trials and European Dermato-Epidemiology Network Psoriasis Trials Database.
10. Gambichler T, Kreuter JA, Altmeyer P, et al. Meta-analysis of the efficacy of balneotherapy. *Aktuelle Dermatologie* 2000;26:402–406. Search date 1999; primary sources Medline and Embase/Excerpta Medica.
11. Leaute-Labreze C, Saillour F, Chene G, et al. Saline spa water or combined water and UVB for psoriasis vs conventional UVB: lessons from the Salies de Bearn randomized study. *Arch Dermatol* 2001;137:1035–1039.
12. Zumiani G, Zanoni M, Agostini G. Evaluation of the efficacy of Comano thermal baths water versus

tap water in the treatment of psoriasis. *G Ital Dermatol Venereol* 2000;135:259–263.
13. Jerner B, Skogh M, Vahlquist A. A controlled trial of acupuncture in psoriasis: no convincing effect. *Acta Derm Venereol* 1997;77:154–156.
14. Zhang WY, Li Wan Po A. The effectiveness of topically applied capsaicin: a meta-analysis. *Eur J Clin Pharmacol* 1994;46:517–522. Search date 1994; primary sources BIDS and Medline.
15. Vogler BK, Ernst E. Aloe vera: a systematic review of its clinical effectiveness. *Br J Gen Pract* 1999;49:823–828. Search date 1998; primary sources Medline, Embase, Biosis, and Cochrane Library, Issue 2, 1998.
16. Berne B, Blom I, Spangberg S. Enhanced response of psoriasis to UVB therapy after pretreatment with a lubrificating base. *Acta Derm Venereol* 1990;70:474–477.
17. Kanzler MH, Gorsulowsky DC. Efficacy of topical 5% liquor carbonis detergens vs. its emollient base in the treatment of psoriasis. *Br J Dermatol* 1993;129:310–314.
18. Smith CH, Jackson K, Chinn S, et al. A double-blind randomized controlled clinical trial to assess the efficacy of a new coal tar preparation (Exorex) in the treatment of chronic, plaque type psoriasis. *Clin Exp Dermatol* 2000;25:580–583.
19. Naldi L, Carrel CF, Parazzini F, et al. Development of anthralin short-contact therapy in psoriasis: survey of published clinical trials. *Int J Dermatol* 1992;31:126–130. Search date 1989; primary sources Medline, Index Medicus, and Excerpta Medica.
20. Katz HI, Prawer SE, Medansky RS, et al. Intermittent corticosteroid treatment of psoriasis: a double-blind multicenter trial of augmented betamethasone dipropionate ointment in a pulse dose treatment regimen. *Dermatologica* 1991;183:269–274.
21. Wilson L, Williams DI, Marsh SD. Plasma corticosteroid levels in outpatients treated with topical steroids. *Br J Dermatol* 1973;88:373–380.
22. Ashcroft DM, Li Wan Po A, Williams HC, et al. Systematic review of comparative efficacy and tolerability of calcipotriol in treating chronic plaque psoriasis. *BMJ* 2000;320:963–967. Search date 1999; primary sources Medline, Embase, Cochrane Controlled Trials Register, BIDs, hand searches of reference lists, and manufacturer of calcipotriol contacted.
23. Aschcroft DM, Li Wan Po A, Williams HC, et al . Combination regimens of topical calcipotriene in chronic plaque psoriasis: systematic review of efficacy and tolerability. *Arch Dermatol* 2000;136:1536–1543. Search date 1999; primary sources Medline and Embase.
24. Ramsay CA, Berth-Johnes J, Brundin J, et al. Long-term use of topical calcipotriol in chronic plaque psoriasis. *Dermatology* 1994;189:260–264.
25. Veien NK, Bjerke JR, Rossmann Ringdahl I, et al. Once daily treatment of psoriasis with tacalcitol compared with twice daily treatment with calcipotriol: a double-blind trial. *Br J Dermatol* 1997;137:581–586.
26. Barker JN, Ashton RE, Marks R, et al. Topical maxacalcitol for the treatment of psoriasis vulgaris: a placebo controlled, double-blind, dose-finding study with active comparator. *Br J Dermatol* 1999;141:274–278.
27. Kragballe K, Gjertsen BT, De Hoop D, et al. Double-blind, right/left comparison of calcipotriol and betamethasone valerate in treatment of psoriasis vulgaris. *Lancet* 1991;337:193–196.
28. Berth-Jones J, Chu AC, Dodd WAH, et al. A multicentre, parallel-group comparison of calcipotriol ointment and short-contact therapy in chronic plaque psoriasis. *Br J Dermatol* 1992;127:266–271.
29. Christensen OB, Mork NJ, Ashton R, et al. Comparison of a treatment phase and a follow-up phase of short contact dithranol and calcipotriol in outpatients with chronic plaque psoriasis. *J Dermatol Treat* 1999;10:261–265.
30. Hutchinson PE, Marks R, White J. The efficacy, safety, and tolerance of calcitriol 3 mcgr/g ointment in the treatment of plaque psoriasis. A comparison with short-contact therapy. *Dermatology* 2000;201:139–245.
31. Pinheiro N. Comparative effects of calcipotriol ointment (50 micrograms/g) and 5% coal tar/2% allantoin/0.5% hydrocortisone cream in treating plaque psoriasis. *Br J Clin Pract* 1997;51:16–19.
32. Ruzicka T, Lorenz B. Comparison of calcipotriol monotherapy and a combination of calcipotriol and betamethasone valerate after 2 weeks' treatment with calcipotriol in the topical therapy of psoriasis vulgaris: a multicentre, double-blind, randomized study. *Br J Dermatol* 1998;138:254–258.
33. Kragballe K, Barnes L, Hamberg K, et al. Calcipotriol cream with or without concurrent topical corticosteroid in psoriasis. Tolerability and efficacy. *Br J Dermatol* 1998;139:649–654.
34. Weinstein GD, Krueger GG, Lowe NJ, et al. Tazarotene gel, a new retinoid, for topical therapy of psoriasis: vehicle-controlled study of safety, efficacy, and duration of therapeutic effect. *J Am Acad Dermatol* 1997;37:85–92.
35. Lebwohl M, Ast E, Callen JP, et al. Once-daily tazarotene gel versus twice-daily fluocinonide cream in the treatment of plaque psoriasis. *J Am Acad Dermatol* 1998;38:705–711.
36. Lebwohl MG, Breneman DL, Goffe BS, et al. Tazarotene 0.1% gel plus corticosteroid cream in the treatment of plaque psoriasis. *J Am Acad Dermatol* 1998;39:590–596.
37. Gollnick H, Menter A. Combination therapy with tazarotene plus a topical corticosteroid for the treatment of plaque psoriasis. *Br J Dermatol* 1999;140(suppl):18–23.
38. Guenther LC, Poulin YP, Pariser DM. A comparison of tazarotene 0.1% gel once daily plus mometasone furoate 0.1% cream once daily versus calcipotriene 0.005% ointment twice daily in the treatment of plaque psoriasis. *Clin Ther* 2000;22:1225–1238.
39. Griffiths GEM, Clark CM, Chalmers RJG, et al. A systematic review of treatments for severe psoriasis. *Health Technol Assess* 2000;4:1–125. Search date 1999; primary sources Medline, Embase, and Cochrane Register of RCTs.
40. Boer J, Hermans J, Schothorst AA, et al. Comparison of phototherapy (UVB) and photochemotherapy (PUVA) for clearing and maintenance therapy of psoriasis. *Arch Dermatol* 1984;120:52–57.
41. Gorden PM, Diffey BL, Mathews JN, et al. A randomised comparison of narrow-band TL-01 phototherapy for psoriasis. *J Am Acad Dermatol* 1999;41:728–732.
42. Stern RS, Armstrong RB, Anderson TF, et al. Effect of continued ultraviolet B phototherapy on the duration of remission of psoriasis. A randomized study. *J Am Acad Dermatol* 1986;15:546–552.
43. Pieternel CM, Pasker-de-Jong M, Wielink G, et al. Treatment with UV-B for psoriasis and nonmelanoma skin cancer. A systematic review of the literature. *Arch Dermatol* 1999;135:834–840. Search date 1996; primary sources Medline, Biosis, and Online Contents.

44. Melski JW, Tanenbaum L, Parrish JA, et al. Oral methoxsalen photochemotherapy for the treatment of psoriasis. A cooperative clinical trial. *J Invest Dermatol* 1977;68:328–324.
45. Stern RS, Laird N. The carcinogenic risk of treatments for severe psoriasis. Photochemotherapy follow-up study. *Cancer* 1994;73:2759–2764.
46. Stern RS, Lunder EJ. Risk of squamous cell carcinoma and methoxsalen (psoralen) and UV-A radiation (PUVA). A meta-analysis. *Arch Dermatol* 1998;134:1582–1585. Search date 1998; primary sources Medline, Healthstar, Aidsline, and Cancerlit.
47. Hannuksela-Svahn A, Sigurgeirsson B, Pukkala E, et al. Trioxsalen bath PUVA did not increase the risk of squamous cell skin carcinoma and cutaneous malignant melanoma in a joint analysis of 944 Swedish and Finnish patients with psoriasis. *Br J Dermatol* 1999;141:497–501.
48. Rogers S, Marks J, Shuster S, et al. Comparison of photochemotherapy and dithranol in the treatment of chronic plaque psoriasis. *Lancet* 1979;i:455–458.
49. Ramsay CA, Schwartz BE, Lowson D, et al. Calcipotriol cream combined with twice weekly broad-band UVB phototherapy: a safe, effective and UVB-sparing antipsoriatic combination treatment. The Canadian Calcipotriol and UVB Study Group. *Dermatology* 2000;200:17–24.
50. Jones G, Crotty M, Brooks P. Interventions for treating psoriatic arthritis. An overview of therapy and toxicity. In: The Cochrane Library, Issue 3, 2001. Oxford: Update Software. Search date 2000; primary sources Medline, Excerpta Medica, and Cochrane Clinical Trials Register.
51. Berth-Jones J, Todd G, Hutchinson PE, et al. Treatment of psoriasis with oral liarozole: a dose ranging study. *Br J Dermatol* 2000;143:1170–1176.
52. Stern RS, Fitzgerald E, Ellis CN, et al. The safety of etretinate as long-term therapy for psoriasis. Results of the etretinate follow-up study. *J Am Acad Dermatol* 1995;33:44–52.
53. Wilkens RF, Williams HJ, Ward JR, et al. Randomized, double-blind, placebo controlled trial of low-dose pulse methotrexate in psoriatic arthritis. *Arthritis Rheum* 1984;27:376–381.
54. Van Dooren-Greebe RJ, Kuijpers AL, Mulder J, et al. Methotrexate revisited: effects of long-term treatment of psoriasis. *Br J Dermatol* 1994;130:204–210.
55. Whiting-O'Keefe QE, Fye KH, Sack KD. Methotrexate and histologic hepatic abnormalities. *Am J Med* 1991;90:711–716. Search date and primary sources not stated.
56. Cottin V, Tebib J, Souquet PJ, Bernard JP. Pulmonary function in patients receiving long-term low-dose methotrexate. *Chest* 1996;109:933–938.
57. Nyfors A, Jensen H. Frequency of malignant neoplasms in 248 long-term methotrexate-treated psoriatics. A preliminary study. *Dermatologica* 1983;167:260–261.
58. Grossman RM, Chevret S, Abi-Rached J, et al. Long-term safety of ciclosporin in the treatment of psoriasis. *Arch Dermatol* 1996;132:623–629.
59. The European FK 506 Multicentre Psoriasis Study Group. Systemic tacrolimus (FK 506) is effective for the treatment of psoriasis in a double-blind, placebo-controlled study. *Arch Dermatol* 1996;132:419–423.
60. Zonneveld IM, Rubins A, Jablonska S, et al. Topical tacrolimus is not effective in chronic plaque psoriasis: A pilot study. *Arch Dermatol* 1998;134:1101–1102.
61. Gottlieb AB, Lebwohl M, Shirin S, et al. Anti-CD4 monoclonal antibody treatment of moderate to severe psoriasis vulgaris: results of a pilot, multicenter, multiple-dose, placebo-controlled study. *J Am Acad Dermatol* 2000;43:595–604.
62. Ellis CN, Krueger GG, and Alefacept Clinical Study Group. Treatment of chronic plaque psoriasis by selective targeting of memory effector T lymphocytes. *N Engl J Med* 2001;345:248–255.
63. Mihatsch MJ, Kyo M, Morozumi K, et al. The side-effects of ciclosporin A and tacrolimus. *Clin Nephrol* 1998;49:356–363.
64. Mease PJ, Goffe BS, Metz J, et al. Etanercept in the treatment of psoriatic arthritis and psoriasis: a randomised trial. *Lancet* 2000;356:385–390.
65. Chaudhari U, Romano P, Mulcahy LD, et al. Efficacy and safety of infliximab monotherapy for plaque-type psoriasis: a randomised trial. *Lancet* 2001;357:1842–1847.
66. Skytta E, Pohjankoski H, Savolainen A. Etanercept and urticaria in patients with juvenile idiopathic arthritis. *Clin Exp Rheumatol* 2000;18:533–534.
67. Kalden JR. How do the biologics fit into the current DMARD armamentarium? *J Rheumatol* 2001;28(suppl 62):27–35.
68. Altmeyer PJ, Matthes U, Pawlak F, et al. Antipsoriatic effect of fumaric acid derivatives: results of a multicenter double-blind study in 100 patients. *J Am Acad Dermatol* 1994;30:977–981.

Luigi Naldi
Dermatologist Ospedali Riuniti Bergamo
Bergamo, Italy

Berthold Rzany
Dermatologist
Klinik für Dermatologie Universitätsklinikum Mannheim
Mannheim, Germany

Competing interests: The research activities of the Italian Group for Epidemiologic Research in Dermatology, which is coordinated by one of the authors (LN), have been supported by grants from GlaxoWellcome, Roche, Novartis, Schering and Schering-Plough. BR, none declared.

Head lice

Search date June 2002

Ian Burgess

QUESTIONS

INTERVENTIONS

Key Messages

- **Insecticide based pharmaceutical products** One systematic review found that permethrin or malathion versus placebo significantly reduced the number of people with head lice at 1 week (malathion: NNT 2, 95% CI 1 to 3) and at 2 weeks (permethrin: NNT 2, 95% CI 1 to 2). Limited evidence from another systematic review suggests that permethrin versus lindane significantly reduces the number of people with head lice.
- **Mechanical removal of lice or viable eggs by combing** We found two RCTs comparing combing with an insecticide treatment. The larger RCT found that wet combing with conditioner was significantly less effective than malathion in eradicating head lice 7 days after treatment. A smaller RCT found limited evidence that wet combing with conditioner was marginally more effective than phenothrin lotion plus combing in eradicating head lice after 14 days.
- **Essential oils and other chemicals used as repellents; herbal treatments** We found insufficient evidence on the effects of these interventions.

Head lice

DEFINITION Head lice are obligate ectoparasites of socially active humans. They infest the scalp and attach their eggs to the hair shafts. Itching, resulting from multiple bites, is not diagnostic but may increase the index of suspicion. Infestation can be diagnosed only by finding living lice. Eggs glued to hairs, whether hatched (nits) or unhatched, are not proof of active infection, because eggs may retain a viable appearance for weeks after death.

INCIDENCE/ PREVALENCE We found no studies on incidence and no recent published prevalence results from any developed country. Anecdotal reports suggest that prevalence has increased in the past few years in most communities in the UK and USA.

AETIOLOGY/ RISK FACTORS Observational studies indicate that infections occur most frequently in school children, although there is no proof of a link with school attendance.[1,2] We found no evidence that lice prefer clean hair to dirty hair.

PROGNOSIS The infection is almost harmless. Sensitisation reactions to louse saliva and faeces may result in localised irritation and erythema. Secondary infection of scratches may occur. Lice have been identified as primary mechanical vectors of scalp pyoderma caused by streptococci and staphylococci usually found on the skin.[3]

AIMS To eliminate infestation by killing or removing all head lice and their eggs.

OUTCOMES Treatment success is given as the percentage of people completely cleared of head lice. There are no standard criteria for judging treatment success. Trials used different methods and, in many cases, the method was not stated. Few studies are pragmatic.

METHODS *Clinical Evidence* update search and appraisal June 2002. The initial search was performed by the Cochrane Infectious Diseases Group at the Liverpool School of Tropical Medicine for a systematic review compiled in July 1998.[4]

QUESTION **What are the effects of treatment for head lice?**

OPTION **INSECTICIDE BASED PHARMACEUTICAL PRODUCTS**

We found two systematic reviews of insecticide based pharmaceutical products. One systematic review has found that permethrin and malathion were significantly more effective than placebo, and synergised pyrethrins and permethrin were of similar effectiveness. An earlier systematic review found that permethrin was more effective than lindane, but the RCTs had flawed methods. One RCT found that malathion versus wet combing significantly increased eradication of head lice (see mechanical removal of lice or viable eggs by combing, p 1712).

Benefits: We found two systematic reviews.[4,5] The first systematic review (search date 1995, 7 RCTs, 1808 people) assessed 11 insecticide products, including lindane, carbaryl, malathion, permethrin, and other pyrethroids in various vehicles.[4] The subsequent systematic review (search date 2001, 4 RCTs, 345 children and adults) set stricter criteria for RCTs and rejected all but four RCTs,[5] and excluded studies on which the earlier review was based. **Versus**

placebo: The second systematic review identified one RCT (63 people) comparing permethrin versus placebo.[5] It found that permethrin (1% cream rinse) versus placebo was significantly increased the number of people with no head lice after 7 days (29/29 [100%] with permethrin *v* 3/34 [9%] with placebo; RR 11.3, 95% CI 3.9 to 33.4). Two weeks after permethrin treatment, more people had no head lice compared with placebo (28/29 [97%] with permethrin *v* 2/24 [8%] with placebo; RR 11.6, 95% CI 3.1 to 43.8; NNT 2, 95% CI 1 to 2). The second systematic review also identified one RCT (115 people) comparing malathion (0.5% alcoholic lotion) versus placebo.[5] At 1 week, significantly more people treated with malathion versus placebo were free of head lice (62/65 [95%] with malathion *v* 21/47 [45%] with placebo; RR 2.1, 95% CI 1.5 to 2.9; NNT 2, 95% CI 1 to 3). **Versus each other:** The first systematic review (7 RCTs, 726 people, search date 1995) found that permethrin (1% cream) versus lindane (1% shampoo) produced clinically significant differences in the rate of treatment success (lindane *v* permethrin; 2 RCTs; OR for not clearing head lice 15.2, 95% CI 8.0 to 28.8).[4]

Harms: Only minor adverse effects have been reported for most insecticides. The exception is lindane, where there are extensive reports of effects related to overdosing (treatment of scabies) and absorption (treatment of head lice). Transdermal passage of lindane occurs during treatment of head lice,[6] but we found no reports of adverse effects in this setting. We found no confirmed reports of adverse effects from the organophosphate malathion when used therapeutically. One observational study (32 people) found that 0.2–3.2% of the applied dose of 0.1–0.2 g of malathion, given in the form of head louse products, was excreted in urine as metabolites, suggesting limited transdermal absorption. No effect was observed on plasma or erythrocyte cholinesterase activity.[7]

Comment: Follow up for 6 days is inadequate, as the eggs take 7 days to hatch. Most investigators agree that a final examination after 14 days is appropriate for primary end point determination of cure. The three trials included in the most recent systematic review were conducted in developing countries where insecticide treatments were not regularly available.[5] This may have resulted in greater efficacy, because the insects may have had no previous exposure to the therapeutic agent. Studies *in vitro* suggest that other components of products (e.g. terpenoids and solvents) may be more effective pediculicides than the insecticide itself.[8] Resistance to one or more insecticides is now common.[9–11] One RCT (193 people) investigating resistance compared malathion (0.5% lotion with terpenoids) versus phenothrin (0.3% lotion) in a community where lice were identified *in vitro* as being tolerant of phenothrin.[12] One day after treatment significantly more people treated with malathion versus phenothrin were louse free (87/95 [92%] with malathion *v* 39/98 [40%] with phenothrin; RR 2.3, 95% CI 1.7 to 2.9) and this difference had increased by day 7 (90/95 [95%] with malathion *v* 38/98 [39%] with phenothrin; RR 2.4, 95% CI 1.8 to 3.2). However, some children not free from lice on day 1 had become louse free by day 7 in both groups, suggesting some parental intervention had influenced the results. This study suggests that resistance to pyrethroid insecticide may have influenced about 60% of the treatments.

OPTION MECHANICAL REMOVAL OF LICE OR VIABLE EGGS BY COMBING

We found two RCTs comparing combing versus an insecticide treatment. The larger RCT found that wet combing with conditioner was significantly less effective than malathion in eradicating head lice. A smaller RCT found a marginally significant reduction in head lice with "bug busting" versus a single application of phenothrin. Removal of viable eggs was not specifically addressed.

Benefits: We found two RCTs.[13,14] The first RCT (72 people) compared "bug busting" (wet combing with conditioner) versus two applications of 0.5% malathion 7 days apart.[13] Significantly more people treated with malathion had no lice compared with "bug busting" 7 days after treatment (12/32 [38%] with "bug busting" *v* 31/40 [78%] with malathion; RR 0.48, 95% CI 0.30 to 0.78; NNH 3, 95% CI 2 to 5).[13] The second RCT (30 people) compared "bug busting" versus two weekly applications of phenothrin lotion (concentration not specified) plus combing. A marginally significant reduction in head lice was found after 14 days (eradication of head lice: 8/15 [53%] with "bug busting" *v* 2/15 [13%] with phenothrin group; RR 4.0, CI 1.01 to 15.8; NNT 3, 95% CI 2 to 17).[14] We found three RCTs comparing different pediculicides in combination with nit combing, but none included a non-combing control group.[15–17]

Harms: Apart from discomfort, we found no evidence of harms due to combing. Wet combing with conditioner may risk adverse reactions, which have been observed during normal cosmetic use, to hair conditioning agents.[18–22]

Comment: The first RCT was designed to be a pragmatic RCT with results that are applicable to normal practice.[13] In the second RCT interventions were applied by trained nurses. "Bug busting" involved the use of different graded combs and specific hair conditioner, while people in the phenothrin group used a single head lice comb and unspecified hair conditioners. The follow up strategy for the combing group differed from that offered to the lotion group.[14] This difference may introduce bias and confounding.

OPTION HERBAL TREATMENTS

We found no systematic review, RCTs, or cohort studies on the effects of herbal treatments.

Benefits: We found no systematic review, RCTs, or cohort studies evaluating herbal treatments.

Harms: We found no evidence of harms.

Comment: None.

OPTION **ESSENTIAL OILS AND OTHER CHEMICALS USED AS REPELLENTS**

We found no systematic review, RCTs, or cohort studies on the effects of essential oils or other chemicals used as repellents (such as piperonal).

Benefits: We found no systematic review, RCTs, or cohort studies evaluating repellents.

Harms: We found no evidence of harms, although a potential for toxic effects has been recognised for several essential oils.[23]

Comment: None.

Substantive changes

Mechanical removal of lice or viable eggs by combing One new RCT;[14] conclusions unchanged.

REFERENCES

1. Burgess IF. Human lice and their management. *Adv Parasitol* 1995;36:271–342.
2. Gratz NG. *Human lice. Their prevalence, control and resistance to insecticides.* Geneva: World Health Organization, 1997.
3. Taplin D, Meinking TL. Infestations. In: Schachner LA, Hansen RC, eds. *Pediatric dermatology*, vol 2. New York: Churchill Livingstone, 1988:1465–1493.
4. Vander Stichele RH, Dezeure EM, Bogaert MG. Systematic review of clinical efficacy of topical treatments for head lice. *BMJ* 1995;311:604–608. Search date 1995; primary sources Medline, International Pharmaceutical Abstracts, and Science Citation Index.
5. Dodd CS. Interventions for treating head lice (Cochrane Review). In: The Cochrane Library, Issue 3, 2001. Oxford: Update Software. Search date 2001; primary sources Cochrane Infectious Diseases Group Trials Register, Cochrane Controlled Trials Register, Medline, Embase, Science Citation Index, Biosis, Toxline and hand searches of reference lists from relevant articles and personal contact with pharmaceutical companies and UK and US Regulatory Authorities.
6. Ginsburg CM, Lowry W. Absorption of gamma benzene hexachloride following application of Kwell shampoo. *Pediatr Dermatol* 1983;1:74–76.
7. Dennis GA, Lee PN. A phase I volunteer study to establish the degree of absorption and effect on cholinesterase activity of four head lice preparations containing malathion. *Clin Drug Invest* 1999;18:105–115.
8. Burgess I. Malathion lotions for head lice: a less reliable treatment than commonly believed. *Pharm J* 1991;247:630–632.
9. Burgess IF, Brown CM, Peock S, et al. Head lice resistant to pyrethroid insecticides in Britain [letter]. *BMJ* 1995;311:752.
10. Pollack RJ, Kiszewski A, Armstrong P, et al. Differential permethrin susceptibility of head lice sampled in the United States and Borneo. *Arch Pediatr Adolesc Med* 1999;153:969–973.
11. Lee SH, Yoon KS, Williamson M, et al. Molecular analyses of *kdr*-like resistance in permethrin-resistant strains of head lice, *Pediculus capitis*. *Pestic Biochem Physiol* 2000;66:130–143.
12. Chosidow O, Chastang C, Brue C, et al. Controlled study of malathion and *d*-phenothrin lotions for *Pediculus humanus* var *capitis*-infested schoolchildren. *Lancet* 1994;334:1724–1727.
13. Roberts RJ, Casey D, Morgan DA, et al. Comparison of wet combing with malathion for treatment of head lice in the UK: a pragmatic randomised controlled trial. *Lancet* 2000;356:540–544.
14. Plastow L, Luthra M, Powell R, et al. Head lice infestation: bug busting vs. traditional treatment. *J Clin Nurs* 2001;10:775–783.
15. Bainbridge CV, Klein GI, Neibart SI, et al. Comparative study of the clinical effectiveness of a pyrethrin-based pediculicide with combing versus a permethrin-based pediculicide with combing. *Clin Pediatr (Phila)* 1998;37:17–22.
16. Clore ER, Longyear LA. A comparative study of seven pediculicides and their packaged nit combs. *J Pediatr Health Care* 1993;7:55–60.
17. Hipolito RB, Mallorca FG, Zuniga-Macaraig ZO, et al. Head lice infestation: single drug versus combination therapy with one percent permethrin and trimethoprim/sulfamethoxazole. *Pediatrics* 2001;107:E30.
18. Korting JC, Pursch FM, Enders F, et al. Allergic contact dermatitis to cocamidopropyl betaine in shampoo. *J Am Acad Dermatol* 1992;27:1013–1015.
19. Niinimaki A, Niinimaki M, Makinen-Kiljunen S, et al. Contact urticaria from protein hydrolysates in hair conditioners. *Allergy* 1998;53:1070–1082.
20. Schalock PC, Storrs FJ, Morrison L. Contact urticaria from panthenol in hair conditioner. *Contact Dermatitis* 2000;43:223.
21. Pasche-Koo F, Claeys M, Hauser C. Contact urticaria with systemic symptoms caused by bovine collagen in hair conditioner. *Am J Contact Dermatol* 1996;7:56–57.
22. Stadtmauer G, Chandler M. Hair conditioner causes angioedema. *Ann Allergy Asthma Immunol* 1997;78:602.
23. Veal L. The potential effectiveness of essential oils as a treatment for headlice, *Pediculus humanus capitis*. *Complement Ther Nurs Midwifery* 1996;2:97–101.

Head lice

Ian Burgess
Director
Insect Research
& Development Limited
Cambridge
UK

Competing interests: The author has been a consultant to several companies involved in development and marketing of pediculicides and has received payment for professional services, including development of educational materials.

Herpes labialis

Search date April 2002

Graham Worrall and Bazian Ltd (temporary contributors)

QUESTIONS

INTERVENTIONS

Key Messages

Prevention

- **Oral aciclovir** Limited evidence from RCTs suggests that prophylactic oral aciclovir versus placebo may reduce the frequency and severity of attacks, but the optimal timing and duration of treatment is uncertain.
- **Sunscreen** Two small crossover RCTs found that ultraviolet sunscreen versus placebo significantly reduced herpes recurrence.
- **Topical antiviral agents** We found no RCTs on the effects of topical antiviral agents used as prophylaxis.

Treatment

- **Oral aciclovir for first attack** One small RCT in children found that oral aciclovir versus placebo marginally but significantly reduced the mean duration of pain. One small RCT in children found that oral aciclovir versus placebo significantly reduced the median time to healing.
- **Oral aciclovir for recurrent attack** Two RCTs have found that oral aciclovir versus placebo (if taken early in the attack) marginally but significantly reduces the duration of symptoms and pain.
- **Topical anaesthetic agents** One small RCT found limited evidence that topical tetracaine versus placebo significantly reduced the mean time to scab loss.
- **Topical antiviral agents for first attack** We found no RCTs on the effects of topical antiviral agents in the first attack.
- **Topical antiviral agents for recurrent attacks** RCTs found conflicting evidence on the effects of topical antiviral agents.
- **Zinc oxide cream** One small RCT found limited evidence that zinc oxide cream versus placebo significantly reduced time to resolution of skin lesions.

Herpes labialis

DEFINITION Herpes labialis is a mild self limiting infection with herpes simplex virus type 1. It causes pain and blistering on the lips and perioral area (cold sores); fever and constitutional symptoms are rare. Most people have no warning of an attack, but some experience a recognisable prodrome.

INCIDENCE/ PREVALENCE Herpes labialis accounts for about 1% of primary care consultations in the UK each year; 20–40% of people have experienced cold sores at some time.[1]

AETIOLOGY/ RISK FACTORS Herpes labialis is caused by herpes simplex virus type 1. After the primary infection, which usually occurs in childhood, the virus is thought to remain latent in the trigeminal ganglion.[2] A variety of factors, including exposure to bright sunlight, fatigue, or psychological stress, can precipitate a recurrence.

PROGNOSIS In most people, herpes labialis is a mild, self limiting illness. Recurrences are usually shorter and less severe than the initial attack. Healing is usually complete in 7–10 days without scarring.[3] Rates of reactivation are unknown. Herpes labialis can cause serious illness in immunocompromised people.

AIMS To reduce the frequency and severity of recurrent attacks; to speed healing of lesions; and to reduce pain, with minimal adverse effects.

OUTCOMES Severity of symptoms; duration of symptoms; time to crusting of lesions; time to healing; rate of recurrence; adverse effects of treatment.

METHODS *Clinical Evidence* update search and appraisal April 2002. Keywords: herpes labialis, treatment, prevention, prophylaxis, controlled trial, and effectiveness.

QUESTION **What are the effects of interventions aimed at preventing attacks?**

OPTION **ORAL/TOPICAL ANTIVIRAL AGENTS**

Limited evidence from RCTs suggests that prophylactic oral aciclovir versus placebo may reduce the frequency and severity of attacks, but the optimal timing and duration of treatment is uncertain. We found no RCTs on the effects of topical antiviral agents used as prophylaxis.

Benefits: We found no systematic review. **Topical antiviral agents:** We found no good quality RCTs. **Oral antiviral agents:** We found four double blind, placebo controlled RCTs.[4–7] The first RCT (147 American skiers with a history of herpes labialis precipitated by ultraviolet light) found that people given prophylactic oral aciclovir (400 mg twice daily, beginning 12 h before ultraviolet exposure) had significantly fewer attacks and shorter duration of symptoms ($P < 0.05$).[4] The second RCT (239 Canadian skiers) found no significant difference between aciclovir (800 mg twice daily, starting on the day before exposure to ultraviolet light for a minimum of 3 days to a maximum of 7 days) versus placebo.[5] The third RCT (20 people with recurrent herpes labialis) found that aciclovir (400 mg twice daily for 4 months) led to 53% fewer clinical recurrences and 71% fewer virus culture positive recurrences ($P = 0.05$).[6] The fourth RCT (248 adults with a history of sun induced recurrent herpes labialis) compared three different dosages of famciclovir (125 mg, 250 mg, and 500 mg) versus placebo.[7] Treatment was given three times daily for 5 days, beginning 48 hours after exposure to artificial ultraviolet light. There was no significant difference in the number of lesions in the four groups, but increasing the dose of famciclovir significantly reduced the mean size ($P = 0.04$) and duration of lesions, in a dose–response relation. Compared with placebo, the 500 mg dose reduced the mean time to healing by 2 days ($P < 0.01$).

Harms: See harms under the effects of antiviral treatment for the first attack, p 1718.

Comment: None.

OPTION SUNSCREEN

Two small RCTs found that ultraviolet sunscreen versus placebo significantly reduced herpes recurrence.

Benefits: We found no systematic review. We found two small, crossover RCTs.[8,9] The first RCT (38 people with a history of recurrent herpes) found that sunscreen use versus placebo significantly reduced recurrence at 6 days (recurrence 0/35 [0%] with sunscreen *v* 27/38 [71%] with placebo; ARR 0.71, 95% CI 0.52 to 0.83; NNT 2, 95% CI 1 to 2).[8] The second RCT (19 people exposed to a pre-established dose of ultraviolet light in a laboratory) comparing sunscreen versus placebo found that significantly more people taking placebo suffered recurrence at 6 days (11/19 [58%] with placebo *v* 1/19 [5%] with sunscreen; $P < 0.01$; see comment below).[9]

Harms: None reported.

Comment: The conclusions from the RCTs should be considered with care.[8,9] Crossover studies have important limitations, and the second RCT was conducted under artificial conditions.[9]

QUESTION What are the effects of antiviral treatment for the first attack of herpes labialis?

We found no RCTs on the effects of topical antiviral agents. One small RCT in children found that oral aciclovir versus placebo marginally but significantly reduced the mean duration of pain. Another small RCT in children found that oral aciclovir versus placebo significantly reduced the median time to healing.

Benefits: We found no systematic review. **Topical antiviral agents:** We found no RCTs. **Oral antiviral agents:** We found two small RCTs in children.[10,11] One double blind RCT (20 children having their first attack) compared oral aciclovir (200 mg 5 times daily) versus placebo.[10] It found that aciclovir versus placebo significantly reduced mean duration of pain from 5.0 to 4.3 days, and mean duration of excess salivation from 5.0 to 3.3 days ($P < 0.05$). The second RCT (72 children aged 1–6 years with herpes simplex gingivostomatitis of less than 3 days' duration) compared oral aciclovir (15 mg/kg five times daily for 7 days) versus placebo. It found that aciclovir versus placebo significantly reduced the median time to healing from 10 to 4 days (median difference 6 days, 95% CI 4 to 8 days).[11] We found no RCTs in adults.

Harms: Topical aciclovir causes rash, pruritus, and irritation in some people, but no more frequently in trials than placebo.[12–14] It has also caused head and tail abnormalities in fetal rats, but we found no recorded cases of teratogenicity in humans. Oral aciclovir is excreted in breast milk. Aciclovir has been used to treat pregnant women with genital herpes, and one systematic review (search date 1996, 3 studies) found no evidence of adverse effects in women or newborn children (see antiviral treatment during pregnancy under genital herpes, p 1608).[14] However, the evidence is limited, and clinically significant adverse effects cannot be ruled out.

Comment: Research in this area is difficult because people do not usually consult clinicians until after they have had several attacks of herpes labialis.

QUESTION **Do treatments taken at the beginning or during a recurrent attack reduce the duration or severity of symptoms?**

OPTION **ORAL/TOPICAL ANTIVIRAL AGENTS**

RCTs found conflicting evidence on the effects of topical antiviral agents. Two RCTs have found that oral aciclovir versus placebo (if taken early in the attack) marginally but significantly reduces the duration of symptoms and pain.

Benefits: We found no systematic review. **Topical antiviral agents:** We found several RCTs of antiviral creams or ointments.[12,13,15–21] The largest RCT (double blind, 2209 people) compared penciclovir cream (twice hourly for 4 days) versus placebo.[18] It found that penciclovir cream versus placebo reduced healing times by 0.7 days and duration of pain by 0.6 days (CIs could not be calculated from the published report). One small RCT (31 people aged > 17 years with recurrent herpes labialis) compared 5% aciclovir cream (10 people) versus 5% aciclovir in a liposomal vehicle (12 people) versus the drug free vehicle (9 people).[20] It found that aciclovir in liposomal vehicle versus drug free vehicle significantly reduced the mean time to crusting of the lesions (1.6 days for aciclovir in liposomes *v* 4.8 days for control; $P < 0.05$) but found no significant difference with aciclovir cream versus the drug free vehicle (4.3 days for aciclovir cream *v* 4.8 days for control). Fifteen people then took part in a crossover study in which they received the two forms of aciclovir (in random order) separated by a washout period of at least 1 month. It found aciclovir in liposomes versus aciclovir cream significantly reduced the time to crusting of lesions (1.8 *v* 3.5 days; $P < 0.05$). Too few people in the study experienced pain to analyse the impact of the preparations on discomfort statistically. A further double blind RCT (534 people) compared 1% penciclovir cream versus placebo.[21] It found that penciclovir versus placebo significantly reduced the mean healing time of lesions from 8.8 to 7.6 days ($P < 0.01$). Four of the remaining RCTs, including one trial in 208 people, found no evidence that aciclovir cream or ointment versus placebo improved clinical endpoints.[12,16,17,19] The other two remaining small RCTs found that aciclovir versus placebo significantly reduced the duration of lesions.[13,15] **Oral antiviral agents:** We found two RCTs.[22,23] One double blind RCT (174 adults with recurrent herpes labialis) compared oral aciclovir (400 mg 5 times daily for 5 days) versus placebo.[22] Oral aciclovir taken early in the attack (when the person first experienced tingling) reducing the duration of symptoms from 12.5 to 8.1 days (CIs could not be calculated from the published report). If treatment was initiated later (when the vesicular rash appeared), there was no benefit compared with placebo. A second double blind RCT (149 people) compared oral aciclovir within 12 hours of onset of symptoms versus placebo.[23] It found a significant but clinically small effect; oral aciclovir reduced healing time by 0.98 days and duration of pain by 0.04 days ($P < 0.05$).

Harms: See harms under the effects of antiviral treatment for the first attack, p 1718.

Comment: We found no RCTs comparing early versus delayed intervention, so no firm conclusions regarding timing of treatment can be drawn.

OPTION TOPICAL ANAESTHETIC AGENTS

One small RCT found limited evidence that topical tetracaine versus placebo significantly reduced the mean time to scab loss.

Benefits: We found no systematic review. One double blind RCT (72 people) found that 1.8% tetracaine (amethocaine) cream versus placebo, applied six times daily until scab loss occurred, significantly reduced mean time to scab loss from 7.2 to 5.1 days ($P = 0.002$), and increased a composite symptom benefit index from 5.9 to 7.3 ($P = 0.036$).[24]

Harms: None reported.

Comment: See comment under antiviral agents for recurrent attacks, p 1719.

OPTION ZINC OXIDE CREAM

One small RCT found limited evidence that zinc oxide cream versus placebo significantly reduced time to resolution of skin lesions.

Benefits: One double blind RCT (46 people) compared zinc oxide/glycine applied twice hourly during waking hours as soon as possible after the onset of an attack versus placebo.[25] It found that zinc oxide cream versus placebo significantly reduced time to resolution of skin lesions (5.0 days, SD 1.7 days with cream *v* 6.5 days, SD 2.5 days with placebo; $P = 0.018$).

Harms: The RCT reported adverse effects consisted of transient mild to moderate sensations of burning (7 [22%] people with zinc *v* 2 [7%] with placebo), itching (3 [9%] people with zinc *v* 1 [4%] with placebo), stinging (1 [3%] person with zinc *v* 1 [4%] with placebo), and tingling (1 [3%] person with zinc *v* 0 [0%] with placebo).[25] The RCT reported that all adverse effects resolved spontaneously. One person discontinued the active medication because of burning. One person discontinued the placebo because of lack of improvement.

Comment: See comment under antiviral agents for recurrent attacks, p 1719.

REFERENCES

1. Hodgkin K. *Towards earlier diagnosis: a guide to general practice*. Edinburgh: Churchill Livingstone, 1973.
2. Baringer SR, Swoveland P. Recovery of herpes simplex virus from human trigeminal ganglions. *N Engl J Med* 1973;288:648–650.
3. Bader C, Crumpacker CS, Schnipner LE, et al. The natural history of recurrent facial-oral infections with the herpes simplex virus. *J Infect Dis* 1978;138:897–905.
4. Spruance SL, Hammil ML, Hoge WS, et al. Acylovir prevents reactivation of herpes labialis in skiers. *JAMA* 1988;260:1597–1599.
5. Raborn GW, Martel AY, Grace MG, et al. Oral acyclovir in prevention of herpes labialis: a randomized, double-blind, placebo controlled trial. *Oral Surg Oral Med Oral Pathol Oral Radiol Endod* 1998;85:55–59.
6. Rooney JF, Strauss SE, Mannix ML, et al. Oral acyclovir to suppress frequently recurrent herpes labialis: a double-blind, placebo controlled trial. *Ann Intern Med* 1993;118:268–272.
7. Spruance SL, Rowe NH, Raborn GW, et al. Peroral famciclovir in the treatment of experimental ultraviolet radiation-induced herpes simplex labialis: a double-blind, dose-ranging, placebo-controlled, multicenter trial. *J Infect Dis* 1999;179:303–310.
8. Rooney JF, Bryson Y, Mannix ML, et al. Prevention of ultraviolet-light-induced herpes labialis by sunscreen. *Lancet* 1991;338:1419–1421.
9. Duteil L, Queille-Roussel C, Loesche C, et al. Assessment of the effect of a sunblock stick in the prevention of solar-simulating ultraviolet light-induced herpes labialis. *J Dermatol Treat* 1998;9:11–14.
10. Ducoulombier H, Cousin J, DeWilde A, et al. La stomato-gingivite herpetique de l'enfant: essai a contolle aciclovir versus placebo [in French]. *Ann Pediatr* 1988;35:212–216.
11. Amir J, Harel L, Smetana Z, et al. Treatment of herpes simplex gingivostomatitis with aciclovir in children: a randomised double blind placebo controlled trial. *BMJ* 1997;314:1800–1803.
12. Raborn GW, Martel WT, Grace M, et al. Herpes labialis treatment with acyclovir modified aqueous cream: a double-blind randomized trial. *Oral Surg Oral Med Oral Pathol* 1989;67:676–679.
13. Fiddian AP, Ivanyi L. Topical acyclovir in the management of recurrent herpes labialis. *Br J Dermatol* 1983;109:321–326.
14. Smith J, Cowan FM, Munday P. The management of herpes simplex virus infection in pregnancy. *Br J Obstet Gynaecol* 1998;105:255–268. Search date 1996; primary sources Medline and hand searched references.
15. Van Vloten WA, Swart RNJ, Pot F. Topical acyclovir therapy in patients with recurrent orofacial herpes simplex infections. *J Antimicrob Chemother* 1983;12(suppl B):89–93.
16. Shaw M, King M, Best JM, et al. Failure of acyclovir ointment in treatment of recurrent herpes labialis. *BMJ* 1985;291:7–9.
17. Spruance SL, Schnipper LE, Overall JC, et al. Treatment of herpes simplex labialis with topical acyclovir in polyethylene glycol. *J Infect Dis* 1982;146:85–90.
18. Spruance SL, Rea TL, Thoming C, et al. Penciclovir cream for the treatment of herpes simplex labialis. *JAMA* 1997;277:1374–1379.
19. Raborn GW, McGraw WT, Grace MG, et al. Herpes labialis treatment with acyclovir 5 per cent ointment. *Sci J* 1989;55:135–137.
20. Horwitz E, Pisanty S, Czerninski R, et al. A clinical evaluation of a novel liposomal carrier for acyclovir in the topical treatment of recurrent herpes labialis. *Oral Surg Oral Med Oral Pathol Oral Radiol Endod* 1999;87:700–705.
21. Boon R, Goodman JJ, Martinez J, et al. Penciclovir cream for the treatment of sunlight-induced herpes simplex labialis: a randomized, double-blind, placebo-controlled trial. Penciclovir Cream Herpes Labialis Study Group. *Clin Ther* 2000;22:76–90.
22. Spruance SL, Stewart JC, Rowe NH, et al. Treatment of recurrent herpes simplex labialis with oral acyclovir. *J Infect Dis* 1990;161:185–190.
23. Raborn WG, McGraw WT, Grace M, et al. Oral acyclovir and herpes labialis: a randomized, double-blind, placebo-controlled study. *J Am Dental Assoc* 1987;115:38–42.
24. Kaminester LH, Pariser RJ, Pariser, et al. A double-blind, placebo-controlled study of topical tetracaine in the treatment of herpes labialis. *J Am Acad Dermatol* 1999;41:996–1001.
25. Godfrey H, Godfrey N, Godfrey J, et al. A randomized clinical trial on the treatment of oral herpes with topical zinc oxide/glycine. *Altern Ther Health Med* 2001;7:49–56.

Graham Worrall
Professor of Family Medicine
Memorial University of Newfoundland
Whitbourne
Canada

Bazian Ltd (temporary contributors)
London
UK

Competing interests: None declared.

Malignant melanoma: non-metastatic

Search date October 2001

David Crosby, Thomas Crosby, and Malcolm Mason

QUESTIONS

INTERVENTIONS

See glossary, p 1727

Key Messages

- **High dose adjuvant alfa-2b interferon** RCTs have found that high dose alfa-2_b interferon versus no adjuvant treatment significantly extends the time to relapse and may improve overall survival, but have found that toxicity (myelosuppression, hepatotoxicity, and neurotoxicity) and withdrawal rates are high.
- **Low dose adjuvant alfa-2b interferon** RCTs found inconsistent evidence on the effects on survival of low dose alfa-2_b interferon versus no adjuvant treatment. Toxicity occurred in 10% of people.
- **Other adjuvant treatments (non-specific immunotherapy and chemotherapy)** RCTs found no evidence of improved survival with non-specific immunotherapy (e.g bacille Calmette-Guérin or *Corynebacterium parvum).* RCTs found no difference in survival with single agent cytotoxic agents (especially dacarbazine), chemoimmunotherapy, and multi-agent cytotoxic treatments versus placebo.
- **Prophylactic lymph node dissection** Four RCTs found no significant difference in overall survival with elective lymph node dissection versus surgery deferred until clinical recurrence, but an effect within subgroups cannot be ruled out.
- **Sunscreens in prevention** We found no RCTs about the preventive effects of sunscreens. However, the correct use of sunscreen seems a sensible measure to avoid excessive exposure to sunlight.
- **Wide primary excision (no better than less radical surgery)** RCTs have found no difference in survival or local recurrence with wide primary excision (4–5 cm margins) versus narrow incision (1–2 cm margins). Wide excision increases the need for skin grafting.

Malignant melanoma: non-metastatic

DEFINITION Cutaneous malignant melanoma is a tumour derived from melanocytes in the basal layer of the epidermis. After undergoing malignant transformation, it becomes invasive by penetrating into and beyond the dermis.

INCIDENCE/ PREVALENCE Incidence in developed countries has increased by 50% in the past 20 years. Incidence varies in different populations (see table 1, p 1728) and is about 10-fold higher in white than in non-white populations. Despite the rise in incidence, mortality has plateaued and even fallen in some populations (e.g. in women and young men in Australia).[1,2] During the same period there has been a sixfold increase in the incidence of melanoma *in situ*, suggesting earlier detection.

AETIOLOGY/ RISK FACTORS The number of common, atypical, and dysplastic naevi on a person's body correlates closely with the risk of developing malignant melanoma. A genetic predisposition probably accounts for 5–10% of all cases. Although the risk of developing malignant melanoma is higher in fair skinned white populations living close to the equator, the relation between sun exposure, sunscreen use, and skin type is not clear cut. Exposure to excessive sunlight and severe sunburn in childhood are associated with an increased risk of developing malignant melanoma in adult life. However, people do not necessarily develop tumours at sites of maximum exposure to the sun.

PROGNOSIS The prognosis of early malignant melanoma (stages I–III) (see table 2, p 1729) relates to the depth of invasion of the primary lesion, the presence of ulceration, and involvement of the regional lymph nodes, with the prognosis worsening with the number of nodes involved.[3] A person with a thin lesion (Breslow depth [see glossary, p 1727] < 0.75 mm) and without lymph node involvement has a 3% risk of developing metastases and a 95% chance of surviving 5 years.[4] If regional lymph nodes are macroscopically involved there is a 20–50% chance of surviving 5 years. Most studies have shown a better prognosis in women and in people with lesions on the extremities compared with those with lesions on the trunk.

AIMS To prevent melanoma; to detect melanoma earlier; to minimise mutilating surgical treatment while still achieving cure of local disease; to optimise quality of life; and to eradicate occult micrometastatic disease, with minimum adverse effects.

OUTCOMES **Prevention:** Rates and severity of sunburn (proxy measure); incidence of malignant melanoma; mortality from malignant melanoma. **Primary excision:** Local recurrence; overall survival; requirement for skin grafting. **Lymph node dissection and adjuvant treatment:** Overall survival; disease free survival; quality of life; morbidity of disease treatment.

METHODS *Clinical Evidence* search and appraisal October 2001, and searches of reference lists of all review articles found and the main oncological and dermatological textbooks.

QUESTION **Does the use of sunscreens help to prevent malignant melanoma?**

OPTION **SUNSCREENS**

We found no RCTs assessing the effect of sunscreens on the incidence of, or mortality from, malignant melanoma. However, the correct use of sunscreen seems a sensible measure to avoid excessive exposure to sunlight.

Benefits: We found no systematic review. Although one RCT found that sunscreens reduced the incidence or progression of solar keratosis,[5] we found no similar evidence for malignant melanoma. Retrospective case control studies and questionnaire based surveys, all of which have potential biases and confounding factors, have found conflicting results.[6–8] One case control study found that adults with melanoma were less likely to have been protected from sunlight as children,[7] whereas some questionnaire based surveys found no such effect.[6,8]

Harms: Sunscreens can irritate the skin and cause allergic contact dermatitis. Some questionnaire based surveys have suggested that sunscreen may have contributed to the development of malignant melanoma.[6,8] A possible mechanism for this suggestion may be that because some sunscreens protect predominantly against ultraviolet B (UVB, which induces sunburn) people may spend more time exposed to higher doses of ultraviolet A (UVA). One placebo controlled RCT found that a sunscreen with a high sun protection factor (SPF 30) was associated with significantly longer recreational sun exposure.[9]

Comment: Although we found no prospective evidence, it would seem reasonable to take sensible precautions to avoid excessive exposure to sunlight, particularly in children and fair skinned individuals. Sunscreens may have a role if used appropriately (SPF of at least 15 and a star rating for UVA protection of 3–4), rather than being used to prolong the time spent in direct sunlight.

QUESTION **Is there an optimal margin for primary excision of melanoma of different Breslow thicknesses?**

Three RCTs found that more radical local surgery (4–5 cm excision margins) provided no greater benefit than less radical surgery (1–2 cm excision margins).

Benefits: **Radical local surgery versus less radical surgery:** We found no systematic review. We found three RCTs in people with thin (< 1 mm) and intermediate thickness (1–4 mm) malignant melanoma.[10–12] The first RCT randomised 612 people with lesions less than 2 mm thick to surgical excision with either 1 or 3 cm margins.[10] The second RCT randomised 486 people with intermediate thickness lesions (1–4 mm) to either 2 or 4 cm margins. The third RCT randomised 989 people with lesions 0.8–2.0 mm to either 2 or 5 cm margins.[12] None of the trials found that wide margins reduced local recurrence rates or increased overall survival compared with narrow excision margins (see table 3, p 1730).

Harms: Narrower excision margins reduced skin grafting (in 1 RCT by 75%), anaesthetic requirements, and inpatient stay.[10] Narrow margin surgery can usually be performed on outpatient day surgery lists. Of concern is the possibility of higher local recurrence rates using 1 cm margins for tumours 1–2 mm. One RCT (612 people) comparing narrow margin with wide margin surgery reported three local recurrences, all in people with tumours 1–2 mm treated with narrow (1 cm) margin excision; local cure was achieved in two people with further surgery.[10] Although not measured, there is potential for psychological and physical morbidity associated with further surgery after local recurrence.

Comment: The evidence relating to survival is good, but we found no good evidence relating to quality of life or physical and psychological morbidity caused by extent of surgery or local recurrence.

QUESTION Does elective lymph node dissection improve outcomes in people with clinically uninvolved lymph nodes?

Four RCTs found no benefit from elective lymph node dissection in people with clinically uninvolved lymph nodes, although an effect within particular subgroups cannot be ruled out.

Benefits: We found no systematic review. We found four RCTs (a total of 1718 people with no clinical evidence of lymph node metastases) comparing elective lymph node dissection with surgery deferred until the time of clinical recurrence.[13–16] None of the studies found a significant overall survival benefit for people receiving elective lymph node dissection. Retrospective subgroup analyses found non-significant trends in favour of elective lymph node dissection in certain groups of people (those with intermediate thickness tumours, especially those < 60 years of age), but such analyses are subject to bias.

Harms: Lymph node dissection has several complications. In one retrospective case series these included temporary seroma (17%), wound infection (9%), wound necrosis (3%), and lymphoedema (20%).[17]

Comment: In about 20% of people who do not have clinically apparent lymph node involvement, the lymph nodes will contain occult micrometastases. None of the RCTs gave data on morbidity and quality of life in people undergoing lymph node dissection. An alternative to elective lymph node dissection, sentinel lymph node excision, which can accurately determine the specific nodes draining the primary lesion and their involvement with metastatic disease,[18] is currently being evaluated in clinical trials (T Crosby, personal communication, 2001).

QUESTION **Does adjuvant treatment improve prognosis after curative surgery of cutaneous malignant melanoma, and at what stage?**

OPTION **ALFA-2_B INTERFERON**

RCTs have found that high dose alfa-2_b interferon significantly extends the time to relapse compared with no adjuvant treatment and may improve overall survival. We found conflicting results for low dose alfa-2_b interferon. Toxicity and withdrawal rates are high. Less toxic regimens for interferon treatment are being evaluated.

Benefits: We found no systematic review. **High dose:** We found four RCTs.[19–22] All found that high dose alfa-2_b interferon improved relapse free survival, although effects on overall survival were not consistent. One RCT (287 people with primary lesions > 4 mm or resectable stage III disease) compared high dose alfa-2_b interferon (20 MU/m^2 iv/day for 1 month, followed by 10 MU/m^2 sc 3 times/wk for 11 months) versus observation.[19] At a median follow up of 6.9 years, an intention to treat analysis found a significant improvement in disease free survival (median 1.7 *v* 1.0 years) and overall survival (median 3.8 *v* 2.8 years; no CI available). Retrospective analysis by the authors found prolonged quality of life adjusted survival in people receiving alfa interferon. The significance of this gain varied with the values assigned by people for the impact of treatment toxicity and time with relapsed disease.[23] The second RCT (642 people) found no survival benefit with high or low dose adjuvant alfa interferon at a median follow up of 4.3 years.[20] The third RCT (262 people with completely resected melanomas, primary tumours > 0.7 mm, lymph node negative) compared short course, high dose interferon (20 MU/m^2 3 times/wk for 12 wks) versus no interferon and found no significant difference in disease free survival ($P = 0.19$) or overall survival ($P = 0.40$).[21] The fourth RCT compared high dose interferon versus ganglioside GM2 vaccine in 880 people with resected stage IIB and III melanoma.[22] It found that interferon improved both relapse free survival and overall survival compared with control (HR for relapse free survival with interferon *v* control 1.47, 95% CI 1.14 to 1.90; HR for overall survival 1.52, 95%CI 1.07 to 2.15). The vaccine control intervention may not have been an inactive comparator. However, response to vaccine was associated with a trend towards improvement, which supports the conclusion that interferon would improve outcomes compared with inactive control. **Low dose:** We found five RCTs,[24–28] three of them studying people with stage II melanoma (primary tumours > 1.5 mm and lymph node negative).[25–27] The largest and most recent RCT (830 people with primary tumours > 3 mm or lymph node involvement) compared low dose gamma or alfa interferon versus no adjuvant and found no significant difference in disease free or overall survival.[24] The second RCT (499 people) compared low dose interferon (3 MU 3 times/wk for 18 months) versus surgery alone. It showed a significant extension of the relapse free interval (HR 0.75, 95% CI 0.57 to 0.98; $P = 0.038$) and a trend towards extension of overall survival (HR 0.72, 95%

CI 0.51 to 1.0; P = 0.059).[25] The third RCT (311 people) compared alfa-2_b interferon (3 MU/day for 3 wks and 3 times/wk for 12 months) versus no interferon after excision of the primary tumour. At 41 months' follow up there was prolonged relapse free survival (P = 0.02; no CI available) but no effect on overall survival.[26] The fourth RCT (abstract only) found no significant difference for relapse free survival between interferon (3 MU 3 times/wk) versus observation in people with stage II melanoma.[27] The fifth RCT (95 people with primary melanomas of at least 3 mm Breslow thickness (see glossary, p 1727), or with evidence of regional node involvement) similarly found no significant effect of interferon (3 MU twice/wk) on relapse free survival, although the study may have lacked power to exclude clinically important effects.[28]

Harms: Interferons commonly cause malaise, fevers, and flu-like symptoms. In the first RCT, high dose alfa interferon also caused significant (> grade 3) myelosuppression in 24% of people, hepatotoxicity in 15% (including 2 deaths), and neurotoxicity in 28%. At 11 months, only 25% of participants were receiving more than 80% of the planned dose.[19] In one of the RCTs of low dose interferon, 10% of people suffered significant toxicity.[25]

Comment: RCTs investigating the effects of more tolerable alfa interferon regimens are under way (T Crosby, personal communication, 2001).

OPTION OTHER ADJUVANT TREATMENTS

We found no evidence of improved survival with other adjuvant treatments (non-specific immunotherapy and chemotherapy). Surveillance, specific immunotherapy, hormones, coumarin, and retinoids have not been evaluated adequately.

Benefits: We found no systematic review but found 60 RCTs of adjuvant systemic treatment. Most were too small or too brief to detect a clinically significant benefit, and involved heterogeneous groups of participants (see table 4, p 1729). **Non-specific immunostimulation:** A total of 24 RCTs (mainly small, ranging from 26–400 people) evaluated non-specific immunostimulation with agents such as bacille Calmette-Guerin or *Corynebacterium parvum*. These RCTs found no beneficial effect on survival, although most were too small to exclude a beneficial effect. **Active specific immunostimulation:** Results from RCTs are awaited. **Chemotherapy:** About 15 RCTs (mostly small, ranging from 15–258 people) compared single agent cytotoxic agents, especially dacarbazine, chemoimmunotherapy, and multi-agent cytotoxic treatments versus placebo. No beneficial effect on survival was found. The regimen believed to be most powerful in advanced disease — cisplatin, bischloroethylnitrosourea, dacarbazine, and tamoxifen (the Dartmouth regimen) — has not yet been tested in RCTs. **Hormones, coumarins, and retinoids:** Several small RCTs of hormones (megesterol acetate) and coumarins found mixed results. Several small RCTs all found no benefit from retinoids. **Surveillance:** We found no RCTs (see comment below).

Harms: Certain types of immunostimulation may be associated with flu-like symptoms such as fever, arthralgia, and rigor. Chemotherapy toxicities are well known and include nausea and vomiting, myelosuppression, and alopecia, depending on the cytotoxic agents used. Hormonal treatment can cause weight gain and lead to an increased risk of thromboembolism. Long term adverse effects of retinoids are less well known, but they may possibly be carcinogenic in certain circumstances. Although surveillance can do little physical harm, the possibility of inducing anxiety has not been excluded.

Comment: **Surveillance:** Retrospective studies found that people presented with symptomatic recurrent disease regardless of whether they were taking part in an intensive follow up programme.[29] Thinner lesions (< 0.75 mm) may require longer surveillance as recurrences peak at 5–10 years.[30] **Active specific immunostimulation:** Small pilot studies in single institutions found encouraging results compared with historical controls, especially from allogeneic tumour cell vaccines, viral oncolysates, gangliosides, or melanoma associated peptide vaccines.

GLOSSARY

Breslow thickness The vertical depth (in mm) to which the tumour has penetrated.

REFERENCES

1. Armstrong BK, Kricker A. Cutaneous melanoma. *Cancer Surv* 1994;19:219–240.
2. Giles GG, Armstrong BK, Burton RC, et al. Has mortality from melanoma stopped rising in Australia? Analysis of trends between 1931 and 1994. *BMJ* 1996;312:1121–1125.
3. Balch CM, Soong SJ, Shaw HM, et al. An analysis of prognostic factors in 8500 patients with cutaneous melanoma. In: Balch CM, Houghton Anilton GW, Sober AJ, Soong SJ, eds. *Cutaneous melanoma.* 2nd ed. New York: Ellis Horwood, 1992.
4. Balch CM, Smalley RV, Bartolucci AA, et al. A randomised prospective clinical trial of adjuvant *C. parvum* immunotherapy in 260 patients with clinically localized melanoma (stage I): prognostic factor analysis and preliminary results of immunotherapy. *Cancer* 1982;49:1079–1084.
5. Thompson SC, Jolley D, Marks R. Reduction of solar keratoses by regular sunscreen use. *N Engl J Med* 1993;329:1147–1151.
6. Autier P, Dore J-F, Lejeune FJ, et al. Sun protection in childhood or early adolescence and reduction of melanoma risk in adults: an EORTC case-control study in Germany, Belgium and France. *J Epidemiol Biostat* 1996;1:51–57.
7. Holly EA, Aston DA, Cress RD, et al. Cutaneous melanoma in women. *Am J Epidemiol* 1995;141:923–933.
8. Wolf P, Quehenberger F, Mullegger R, et al. Phenotypic markers, sunlight-related factors and sunscreen use in patients with cutaneous melanoma: an Austrian case-control study. *Melanoma Res* 1998;8:370–378.
9. Autier P, Dore JF, Negrier S, et al. Sunscreen use and duration of sun exposure: a double-blind, randomized trial. *J Natl Cancer Inst* 1999;91:1304–1309.
10. Veronesi U, Cascinelli N, Adamus J, et al. Thin stage I primary cutaneous malignant melanoma: comparison of excision with margins of 1 or 3 cm. *N Engl J Med* 1988;318:1159–1162.
11. Balch CM, Urist MM, Karakousis CP, et al. Efficacy of 2 cm surgical margins for intermediate-thickness melanomas (1 to 4 mm): results of a multi-institutional randomized surgical trial. *Ann Surg* 1993;218:262–267.
12. Cohn-Cedermark G, Rutqvist LE, Andersson R, et al. Long term results of a randomized study by the Swedish melanoma study group on 2- versus 5 cm resection margins for patients with cutaneous melanoma with a tumour thickness of 0.8–2.0 mm. *Cancer* 2000,89:1495–1501.
13. Balch CM, Soong SJ, Bartolucci AA, et al. Efficacy of an elective regional lymph node dissection of 1–4 mm thick melanomas for patients 60 years of age and younger. *Ann Surg* 1996;224:255–263.
14. Cascinelli N, Morabito A, Santinami M, et al. Immediate or delayed dissection of regional nodes in patients with melanoma of the trunk: a randomised trial. WHO Melanoma Programme. *Lancet* 1998;351:793–796.
15. Sim FH, Taylor WF, Ivins JC, et al. A prospective randomized study of the efficacy of routine elective lymphadenectomy in management of malignant melanoma: preliminary results. *Cancer* 1978;41:948–956.
16. Veronesi U, Adamus J, Bandiera DC, et al. Inefficacy of immediate node dissection in stage I melanoma of the limbs. *N Engl J Med* 1977;297:627–630.
17. Baas PC, Schraffordt KH, Koops H, et al. Groin dissection in the treatment of lower-extremity melanoma: short-term and long-term morbidity. *Arch Surg* 1992;127:281–286.
18. Ross MI. Surgical management of stage I and II melanoma patients: approach to the regional lymph node basin. *Semin Surg Oncol* 1996;12:394–401.
19. Kirkwood JM, Strawderman MH, Erstoff MS, et al. Interferon alfa-2_b adjuvant therapy of high-risk resected cutaneous melanoma: The eastern cooperative oncology group trial EST 1684. *J Clin Oncol* 1996;14:7–17.

20. Kirkwood JM, Ibrahim JG, Sondak VK. High- and low-dose interferon Alfa-2_b in high risk melanoma: First analysis of intergroup trial E1690/S9111/C9190. *J Clin Oncol* 2000;18:2444–2458.
21. Creagan ET, Dalton RJ, Ahmann DL. Randomized, surgical adjuvant clinical trial of recombinant interferon alfa-2_b in selected patients with malignant melanoma. *J Clin Oncol* 1995;13:2776–2783.
22. Kirkwood JM, Ibrahim JG, Sosman JA, et al. High-dose interferon alfa2_b significantly prolongs relapse-free and overall survival compared with GM2-KLH/QS-21 vaccine in patients with resected stage IIB–III melanoma: results of the intergroup trial E1694/S9512/C509801. *J Clin Oncol* 2001;19:2370–2380.
23. Cole BF, Gelber RD, Kirkwood JM, et al. Quality-of-life-adjusted survival analysis of high-risk resected cutaneous melanoma: the eastern cooperative oncology group study. *J Clin Oncol* 1996;14:2666–2673.
24. Kleeberg UR, Brocker EB, Lejeune F. Adjuvant trial in melanoma patients comparing rIFN-alfa to rIFN-gamma to Iscador to a control group after curative resection high risk primary (> 3 mm) or regional lymph node metastasis (EORTC 18871). *Eur J Cancer* 1999;35:S82.
25. Grob JJ, Dreno B, de la Salmoniere P, et al. Randomised trial of interferon alpha-2_a as adjuvant therapy in resected primary melanoma thicker than 1.5 mm without clinically detectable node metastases. French cooperative group on melanoma. *Lancet* 1998;351:1905–1910.
26. Pehamberger H, Peter Soyer H, Steiner A, et al. Adjuvant interferon alfa-2_a treatment in resected primary stage II cutaneous melanoma. *J Clin Oncol* 1998;16:1425–1429.
27. Hancock BW, Wheatley K, Harrison G, Gore M. Aim high adjuvant interferon in melanoma (high risk), a United Kingdom Co-ordinating Committee on Cancer Research (UKCCCR) randomised study of observation versus adjuvant low dose extended duration interferon alfa 2_a in high risk resected malignant melanoma. *Proc Am Soc Clin Oncol* 2001;20:1393.
28. Cameron DA, Cornbleet MC, Mackie RM, et al. Adjuvant interferon alpha 2b in high risk melanoma — the Scottish study. Br J Cancer 2001;84:1146–1149.
29. Shumate CR, Urist MM, Maddox WA. Melanoma recurrence surveillance: patient or physician based? *Ann Surg* 1995;221:566–559.
30. Rogers GS, Kopf AW, Rigel DS, et al. Hazard-rate analysis in stage I malignant melanoma. *Arch Dermatol* 1986;122:999–1002.

David Crosby
Consultant Surgeon
Cardiff Community Healthcare Trust
Cardiff
UK

Thomas Crosby
Consultant Clinical Oncologist

Malcolm Mason
Professor of Clinical Oncology

Velindre Hospital
Cardiff
UK

Competing interests: None declared.

TABLE 1 Melanoma incidence and mortality in different populations (see text, p 1722).[1]

Population	Incidence/ 100 000 people	New cases/year	Deaths/year
Asian/Oriental	0.2	NA	NA
UK	8	4000	1500
USA	12	32 000	6700
Caucasians in Queensland, Australia	40	NA	NA

NA, not available.

TABLE 2 **Stage of malignant melanoma and 5 year survival (see text, p 1722).[3]**

Stage	Description	Approximate 5 year survival (%)
I	Primary tumour < 0.75 mm (T1) or 0.75–1.5 mm (T2), no lymphadenopathy (N0)	95
II	Primary tumour > 1.5–4 mm (T3), no lymphadenopathy (N0)	50–70
III	Primary tumour > 4 mm or satellite(s) within 2 cm; lymphadenopathy < 3 cm (N1); lymphadenopathy > 3 cm or in transit metastasis (N2).* No metastases (M0)	20–50
IV	Presence of metastases (M1)	0–5

*In transit metastasis, a metastasis located between the primary tumour and the closest lymph node region.

TABLE 4 **Effects of non-cytokine adjuvant treatment (see text, p 1726)**

Intervention	Examples	Evidence
Non-specific immunotherapy	BCG *Corynebacterium parvum*	Many RCTs found no evidence of improved overall or disease free survival
Active specific immunotherapy	Melanoma cell vaccines Viral oncolysates Defined antigen vaccines Dendritic cells	No evidence from RCTs (although some are under way)
Chemotherapy	Single agents Combination treatments	RCTs found no evidence of benefit. The most powerful regimen (DTIC, cisplatin, BCNU, and tamoxifen) has not been evaluated in RCTs
Others	Hormones (megesterol acetate) Coumarin Retinoids	Small RCTs found survival benefit from hormones and coumarin, but not from retinoids. Findings have not yet been replicated in larger studies
Surveillance	Follow up programme (e.g. every 3 months for first 2 years)	Standard management for stage I (thin lesions < 0.75 mm). Thinner lesions may require longer follow up to detect later relapses. Has not been evaluated in RCTs

BCG, Bacille Calmette-Guérin; BCNU, bischloroethylnitrosourea; DTIC, dimethyltriazeno-imidazole carboxamide (dacarbazine).

TABLE 3 **RCTs addressing radical versus less radical local surgery for malignant melanoma (see text, p 1723).**[10–12]

Ref	Randomisation	Excision margin	Population	Relapse rates	Overall survival
10	Sealed envelopes, stratified blocks according to centre and previous treatment	(a) 1 cm margin (b) 3 cm margin	International multicentre study, 612 people with lesions < 2 mm thick	Local recurrence: 3/321 (1%) with 1 mm margin *v* 0/272 (0%) with 3 mm margin Regional node metastases as first relapse: 14/305 (5%) with 1 mm margin *v* 20/307 (7%) with 3 mm margin Distant metastases: 7/321 (2%) with 1 mm margin *v* 8/272 (3%) with 3 mm margin	4 year actuarial survival rate: 96.8% (305 people) with 1 cm margin *v* 96.0 (307 people) with 3 cm margin; P = 0.66
11	Strategy not described	(a) 2 cm margin (b) 2 cm margin plus elective node dissection (c) 4 cm margin (d) 4 cm margin plus elective node dissection	Multicentre study, 486 people in USA with 1–4 mm thickness lesion and no evidence of metastatic melanoma	Recurrence at median follow up of 72 months: 2/242 (0.8%) with 2 cm margin *v* 4/244 (1.7%) with 4 cm margins; P = NS A subgroup of all these people had elective node dissection as a co-intervention	Overall 5 year survival: 79.5% with 2 cm margin *v* 83.7% with 4 cm margin; P = NS
12	Telephone allocation using randomisation lists	(a) 2 cm margin (b) 5 cm margin	Multicentre study with 989 people in Sweden, with lesions 0.8–2.0 mm, followed for a median time of 11 years for survival, and 8 years for recurrence	First event local recurrence: 1/476 (0.2%) with 2 cm excision *v* 4/513 (1%) with 5 cm excision Distant metastases: 24/479 (5%) with 2 cm excision *v* 34/513 (7%) with 5 cm excision; HR 0.76, 95% CI 0.45 to 1.28; P = 0.29	Overall survival at a median of 8 year follow up: 117/476 (25%) with 2 cm margin: 134/513 (26%) with 5 cm margin; HR 0.96, 95% CI 0.75 to 1.24; P = 0.77

NS, not significant; ref, reference.

Non-genital warts

Search date May 2002

Mike Bigby, Sam Gibbs, Ian Harvey, and Jane Sterling

QUESTIONS

INTERVENTIONS

To be covered in future updates
5-Fluorouracil
Formaldehyde
Imiquimod
Intralesional interferon α
Podophyllin
Systemic retinoids

Covered elsewhere in *Clinical Evidence*
See genital warts, p 1620

See glossary, p 1743

Key Messages

Treatments

- **Carbon dioxide laser** One systematic review identified no RCTs about the effects of carbon dioxide laser.
- **Cimetidine** Three small RCTs found insufficient evidence about the effects of cimetidine versus placebo in the number of people with wart clearance after 12 weeks, and one RCT found insufficient evidence about the effects of cimetidine versus local treatments.
- **Contact immunotherapy (dinitrochlorobenzene)** One systematic review has found that contact immunotherapy with dinitrochlorobenzene versus placebo significantly increases the number of people with wart clearance.
- **Cryotherapy** One systematic review found limited evidence from two small RCTs that cryotherapy is no more effective than placebo in increasing the proportion of people with wart clearance after 2–4 months. But the review also identified two larger RCTs that found cryotherapy was as effective as salicylic acid in wart clearance at 3–6 months.
- **Distant healing** One RCT found insufficient evidence about the effects of distant healing on wart clearance.
- **Homeopathy** Two RCTs found no significant difference with homeopathy versus placebo in the number of people with wart clearance after 18 weeks.

Clin Evid 2002;8:1731–1744.

- **Hypnotic suggestion** We found no RCTs on the effects of hypnotic suggestion in clearance of warts.
- **Inosine pranobex** One RCT found insufficient evidence about the effects of inosine pranobex on wart clearance.
- **Intralesional bleomycin** RCTs found conflicting evidence about the effects of intralesional bleomycin. Two RCTs found that intralesional bleomycin versus placebo significantly increased the number of warts cured after 6 weeks. One RCT found no significant difference with bleomycin versus placebo in the number of people with wart clearance after 30 days, and another RCT found that bleomycin cured fewer warts than placebo after 3 months. One RCT found no significant difference between different concentrations of bleomycin in the number of warts cured after 3 months.
- **Levamisole** Two RCTs and one controlled clinical trial found insufficient evidence about the effects of levamisole versus placebo on the clearance of warts. One RCT found that levamisole plus cimetidine versus cimetidine alone significantly increased the number of people with wart clearance.
- **Photodynamic treatment** RCTs found insufficient evidence about the effects of photodynamic treatment on wart clearance.
- **Pulsed dye laser** One RCT found insufficient evidence about the effects of pulsed dye laser in number of warts cured.
- **Surgical procedures** One systematic review identified no RCTs about the effects of surgical procedures on wart clearance.
- **Systemic interferon α** We found no RCTs of sufficient quality about systemic interferon α.
- **Topical treatments containing salicylic acid** One systematic review has found that simple topical treatments containing salicylic acid versus placebo significantly increase the number of people with complete wart clearance, successful treatment, or loss of one or more warts after 6–12 weeks (NNT 4, 95% CI 3 to 6).

DEFINITION Non-genital warts are an extremely common, benign, and usually self limiting skin disease. Infection of epidermal cells with the human papillomavirus results in cell proliferation and a thickened, warty papule on the skin. Any area of skin can be infected, but the most common sites involved are the hands and feet. Genital warts are not covered in this review (see topic, p 1620).

INCIDENCE/ PREVALENCE There are few reliable, population based data on the incidence and prevalence of common warts. Prevalence probably varies widely between different age groups, populations, and periods of time. Two large population based studies found prevalence rates of 0.84% in the USA[1] and 12.9% in Russia.[2] Prevalence rates are highest in children and young adults, and two studies in school populations have shown prevalence rates of 12% in 4–6 year olds in the UK[3] and 24% in 16–18 year olds in Australia.[4]

AETIOLOGY/ RISK FACTORS Warts are caused by human papillomavirus, of which there are over 70 different types. They are most common at sites of trauma, such as the hands and feet, and probably result from inoculation of virus into minimally damaged areas of epithelium. Warts on the feet can be acquired from common bare foot areas. One observational study (146 adolescents) found that the prevalence of warts on the feet was 27% in those that used a communal shower room versus 1.3% in those that used the locker room.[5] Hand warts are also an occupational risk for butchers and meat handlers. One cross-sectional survey (1086 people) found that the prevalence of hand warts was 33% in abattoir workers, 34% in retail butchers, 20% in engineering fitters, and 15% in office workers.[6] Immunosuppression is another important risk factor. One observational study in immunosuppressed renal transplant recipients found that at 5 years or longer after transplantation 90% had warts.[7]

PROGNOSIS Non-genital warts in immunocompetent people are harmless and usually resolve spontaneously as a result of natural immunity within months or years. The rate of resolution is highly variable and probably depends on a number of factors, including host immunity, age, human papillomavirus type, and site of infection. One cohort study (1000 institutionalised children) found that two thirds of warts resolved without treatment within a 2 year period.[8] One systematic review (search date 2000, 17 RCTs) comparing local treatments versus placebo found that about 30% of people using placebo (range 0–73%) had no warts after about 10 weeks (range 4–24 wks).[9]

AIMS To eliminate warts, with minimal adverse effects.

OUTCOMES Wart clearance (generally accepted as complete eradication of warts from the treated area); adverse effects of treatment; recurrence.

METHODS *Clinical Evidence* update search and appraisal May 2002, and hand searches by the contributors.

QUESTION What are the effects of treatments?

OPTION INTRALESIONAL BLEOMYCIN

Sam Gibbs, Ian Harvey, and Jane Sterling

Five RCTs found conflicting evidence on the effects of intralesional bleomycin. Two RCTs found that intralesional bleomycin versus placebo significantly increased the number of warts cured after 6 weeks. One RCT found no significant difference between bleomycin versus placebo in the number of people with wart clearance after 30 days, and another RCT found that bleomycin cured fewer warts than placebo after 3 months. One RCT found no significant difference between different concentrations of bleomycin in the number of warts cured after 3 months.

Benefits: We found one systematic review (search date 2000, 5 RCTs, 159 people).[9] The review did not perform a meta-analysis because of trial heterogeneity. **Versus placebo:** Four RCTs (133 people) identified by the review compared intralesional bleomycin versus placebo.[10–13] The first RCT (24 adults with warts unsuccessfully treated for > 3 months) compared bleomycin 0.1% versus saline placebo.[10] Matched pairs of warts on the left and right hand side of the body were injected with bleomycin or saline. It found that bleomycin versus placebo significantly increased the number of people with a more favourable response (not defined) after 6 weeks (21/24 [87.5%] *v* 3/24 [13%]; $P < 0.001$) and increased the number of warts cured after 6 weeks (34/59 [58%] of warts *v* 6/59 [10%] of warts; $P < 0.001$).[10] The second RCT (16 people) found that bleomycin 0.1% versus placebo significantly increased the number of warts cured at 6 weeks (31/38 [82%] of warts *v* 16/46 [34%] of warts; $P < 0.001$).[11] The third RCT (62 adults) compared four groups: bleomycin 0.1% in saline; bleomycin 0.1% in oil; saline placebo; and sesame oil placebo. It found that bleomycin cured fewer warts than placebo after 3 months (4/22 [18%] with bleomycin in saline *v* 5/22 [23%] with bleomycin in oil *v* 8/19 [42%] with saline placebo *v* 5/11 [46%] with sesame oil placebo).[12] The fourth RCT (31 people), which compared 0.1% bleomycin versus placebo, found no significant difference in the number of people with wart clearance after 30 days (15/16 [94%] *v* 11/15 [73%]; RR 1.28, 95% CI 0.92 to 1.78).[13] **Different concentrations of bleomycin:** One RCT (26 adults) found no significant difference between bleomycin 0.25% versus bleomycin 0.5% versus bleomycin 1.0% in the proportion of warts cured after 3 months (11/15 [73%] *v* 26/30 [86%] *v* 25/34 [74%]; $P > 0.05$).[14]

Harms: **Versus placebo:** In the first RCT, one person withdrew because of pain during injection and one withdrew because of pain after injection.[10] The third RCT reported dullness, pain, swelling, or bleeding in 19/62 (31%) of all participants but did not specify which treatment they received.[12] The other RCTs found that pain was experienced by most participants (no further data provided).[10,11,14] In two of the RCTs, local anaesthetic was used routinely before the injection of bleomycin.[11,13] **Different concentrations of bleomycin:** The RCT comparing different concentrations of bleomycin reported pain at the injection site in most participants, irrespective of dose (no further data provided).[14]

Comment: The results of two of the RCTs should be interpreted with caution as they randomised people but analysed number of warts cured rather than number of people cured.[11,12] In the RCT comparing different concentrations of bleomycin, the disparity in the number of warts assessed in each group could be explained by the exclusion of warts that spontaneously regressed from the analysis, and by a high withdrawl rate in participants receiving bleomycin 0.25%.[14]

OPTION CARBON DIOXIDE LASER

Sam Gibbs, Ian Harvey, and Jane Sterling

One systematic review identified no RCTs on the effects of carbon dioxide laser.

Benefits: One systematic review (search date 2000) identified no RCTs.[9]

Harms: We found no evidence of harms.

Comment: None.

OPTION CIMETIDINE

Michael Bigby

Three small RCTs found insufficient evidence on the effects of cimetidine versus placebo in the number of people with wart clearance after 12 weeks, and one RCT found insufficient evidence on the effects of cimetidine versus local treatments.

Benefits: We found no systematic review. **Versus placebo:** We found three small RCTs.[15–17] The first RCT (39 people aged > 15 years), which compared cimetidine (2400 mg/day) versus placebo, found no significant difference in the number of people with wart clearance after 12 weeks (5/19 [26%] with cimetidine *v* 1/20 [5%] with placebo; RR 3.14, 95% CI 0.75 to 5.66).[15] The second RCT (54 people), which compared cimetidine (400 mg three times daily) versus placebo, found no significant difference in the proportion of people with wart clearance after 12 weeks (10/36 [27%] with cimetidine *v* 4/18 [22%] with placebo; RR 1.3, 95% CI 0.5 to 3.4).[16] The third RCT (70 women and children), which compared cimetidine (25–40 mg/kg) versus placebo, found no significant difference in the proportion of people with wart clearance after 3 months (9/35 [26%] with cimetidine *v* 8/35 [23%] with placebo; RR 1.1, 95% CI 0.5 to 2.6).[17] **Versus local treatments:** One RCT (13 people) compared cimetidine (30–40 mg/kg) versus topical treatment (cryotherapy, salicylic acid and other [not specified]).[18] It found no significant difference between cimetidine versus topical treatments in the number of people with wart clearance after 8 weeks (2/6 [33%] with cimetidine *v* 3/7 [42%] with topical treatments; RR 0.78, 95% CI 0.19 to 3.21). **Cimetidine plus levamisole**: See levamisole, p 1740.

Harms: Two of the RCTs, which compared cimetidine versus placebo, found no adverse effects associated with cimetidine.[16,17] The third RCT found no significant difference between cimetidine versus placebo in the number of people with gastrointestinal symptoms, fatigue, dyspnoea, or hair thinning (5/19 with cimetidine *v* 5/21 with placebo).[15] In the RCT comparing cimetidine with local treatments, 1/6 people taking cimetidine developed watery, green diarrhoea, and 1/6 had a rash and abdominal pain.[18]

Comment: The RCTs may have been too small to exclude a clinically important difference between treatments.[15–18]

OPTION CRYOTHERAPY

Sam Gibbs, Ian Harvey, and Jane Sterling

One systematic review found limited evidence from two small RCTs that cryotherapy is no more effective than placebo in increasing the number of people with wart clearance after 2–4 months. However, the review also identified two larger RCTs that found no significant difference between cryotherapy versus salicylic acid in wart clearance at 3–6 months.

Benefits: We found one systematic review (search date 2000, 13 RCTs, 1389 people).[9] **Versus placebo or versus no treatment:** The review found no significant difference between cryotherapy (see glossary, p 1743) versus topical placebo cream or no treatment in the number of people with wart clearance at 2–4 months (2 RCTs, 69 people: 11/31 [35%] *v* 13/38 [34%]; RR 0.95, 95% CI 0.49 to 1.84).[9] **Versus photodynamic treatment:** One RCT (28 adults receiving topical salicylic acid) identified by the review compared cryotherapy versus four different types of photodynamic treatment (see glossary, p 1743) (white light photodynamic treatment 3 times; white light photodynamic treatment once; red light photodynamic treatment 3 times; and blue light photodynamic treatment 3 times).[19] It found that cryotherapy reduced the number of warts significantly less than white light or red light photodynamic treatment after 4–6 weeks (20% with cryotherapy *v* 73% with white photodynamic treatment 3 times, P < 0.01; 20% *v* 71% with white photodynamic treatment once, P value not provided; 20% *v* 42% with red light photodynamic treatment 3 times, P = 0.03). **Versus salicylic acid:** The review found no significant difference with cryotherapy versus salicylic acid in the number of people with wart clearance at 3–6 months (2 RCTs, 320 people: 107/165 [65%] *v* 96/155 [62%]; RR 1.05, 95% CI 0.89 to 1.24).[9] **Aggressive versus gentle cryotherapy (defined by length of freeze):** Four RCTs (592 adults) identified by the review found that aggressive versus gentle cryotherapy significantly increased the number of people with wart clearance after 1–3 months (159/304 [52%] *v* 89/288 [31%]; RR 1.68, 95% CI 1.37 to 2.06; NNT 5, 95% CI 4 to 7).[9] Definitions of aggressive and gentle differed and some RCTs included warts that were resistant to treatment and others did not. **Interval between freezes:** Three RCTs (313 people) identified by the review found no significant difference between cryotherapy at 2, 3, or 4 weekly intervals in wart clearance at the end of the trial (not specified).[9] **Number of freezes:** One RCT (115 people not cured after 3 months of 3 weekly cryotherapy) identified by the review found no significant difference between no further treatment versus prolonging cryotherapy for a further 3 months in the number of people with wart clearance (after a total of 6 months: 43% *v* 38%; no further data available to calculate RR).[9]

Harms: **Versus photodynamic treatment:** In the RCT comparing cryotherapy versus photodynamic treatment, one person receiving cryotherapy withdrew because of pain.[19] Photodynamic treatment was associated with burning and itching during the first few minutes of treatment and mild discomfort throughout treatment in all participants. **Interval between freezes:** One RCT identified by the review found that cryotherapy at 1, 2, and 3 weekly intervals was associated with pain and/or blistering in 29%, 7%, and 0% of people, respectively (no further data provided).[20] **Aggressive versus gentle cryotherapy:** One RCT identified by the review found that aggressive versus gentle cryotherapy significantly increased pain or blistering (64/100 [64%] *v* 44/100 [44%]; RR 1.44, 95% CI 1.14 to 1.75; NNH 5, 95% CI 3 to 16).[21] Five participants withdrew from the aggressive group and one from the gentle group because of pain and blistering.

Comment: The evidence from available RCTs about the effectiveness of cryotherapy for warts is both limited and contradictory. Heterogeneity of study design, methodology, and the populations included make it extremely difficult to draw firm conclusions.[9] For instance, some RCTs identified by the review included all types of warts on the hands and feet in all age groups, whereas others were more selective and simply looked at hand warts, or excluded certain groups such as mosaic plantar warts or warts that were resistant to treatment. Of particular note is the likelihood that wart clinic populations used for these studies might have had very different characteristics in different periods of time. For instance, hospital based studies carried out in the 1970s in the UK would have included a higher proportion of participants with warts that had never been treated before, which have a greater chance of cure and/or spontaneous resolution. In the 1980s and 1990s more people with warts were being treated in primary care; consequently the people included in hospital based RCTs were more likely to have warts that were resistant to treatment, with correspondingly lower cure rates.

OPTION DISTANT HEALING

Michael Bigby

One RCT found insufficient evidence on the effects of distant healing on wart clearance.

Benefits: We found no systematic review. One RCT (84 people) compared distant healing versus no treatment (see comment below).[22] Wart clearance was not reported. It found no significant difference between distant healing versus placebo in number of warts at 6 weeks (increase of 0.2 warts with healing *v* decrease of 1.1 warts with no treatment; $P = 0.25$) or in mean change in size of three representative warts.

Harms: The RCT gave no information on adverse effects.[22]

Comment: Ten experienced healers located within 150 miles of the area in which participants lived performed distant healing for 6 weeks, which was defined as a flow/channelling/projection of energy between healer and participant at a distance.[22]

OPTION HOMEOPATHY

Michael Bigby

Two RCTs found no significant difference between homeopathy versus placebo in the number of people with wart clearance after 18 weeks.

Benefits: We found no systematic review but found two RCTs comparing homeopathy versus placebo.[23,24] The first RCT (172 people), which compared homeopathy (Thuya 30CH, amtimony crudum 7CH, nitricium acidum 7CH for 6 wks) versus placebo found no significant difference in the number of people with wart clearance after 18 weeks (16/86 [19%] *v* 20/88 [23%]; RR 0.82, 95% CI 0.46 to 1.47).[23] The second RCT (67 people) found no significant difference between homeopathy (10 different regimens) versus placebo in the number of people with wart clearance after 8 weeks (5/34 [15%] with homeopathy *v* 1/33 [3%] with placebo; RR 4.85, 95% CI 0.60 to 39.35).[24]

Harms: The first RCT found no significant difference between homeopathy versus placebo in the number of people with stomach ache, loose stools, fatigue, and acne (2/86 [2%] with homeopathy *v* 4/88 [5%] with placebo; RR 0.61, 95% CI –0.51 to 1.7).[23] The second RCT gave no information on adverse effects.[24]

Comment: Performing RCTs of homeopathic treatment is difficult because a major principle of homeopathy is to individualise treatment to the overall condition of the patient. One RCT overcame this difficulty by allowing practitioners to evaluate all participants prior to randomisation and select homeopathic regimens appropriate to each of their overall conditions.[24] Participants were then randomised to their individually selected regimen (10 different regimens were used) or to placebo.

OPTION HYPNOTIC SUGGESTION

Michael Bigby

We found no RCTs on the effects of hypnotic suggestion in the clearance of warts.

Benefits: **Wart clearance:** We found no systematic review or RCTs that assessed the effects of hypnotic suggestion on complete wart clearance. **Loss of one wart:** Three RCTs, two of which are reported in the same article, assessed the effects of hypnotic suggestion on the loss of one wart.[25,26] The first RCT (40 people) compared four treatments: hypnotic suggestion; topical salicylic acid; topical placebo; or no treatment (see comment below).[25] It found that hypnotic suggestion versus salicyclic acid, topical placebo, or no treatment, significantly increased the number of people with loss of one wart at 6 weeks (6/10 [60%] with hypnosis *v* 0/10 [0%] with salicylic acid *v* 1/10 [10%] with topical placebo *v* 3/10 [30%] with no treatment; $P < 0.05$). The second RCT (64 people) compared hypnotic suggestion versus cold laser placebo versus no treatment (see comment below).[26] It found that hypnosis versus laser or no treatment significantly increased the number of people with loss of one wart after 6 weeks (11/22 [50%] with hypnosis *v* 6/24 [25%] with placebo; $P = 0.06$; 6/12 [25%] with placebo *v* 2/17 [12%] with no treatment; $P < 0.01$). Participants who lost warts had significantly more warts at baseline than those who did not lose warts ($P < 0.01$). The third RCT (76 people) compared four groups: hypnotic suggestion; hypnotic suggestion plus relaxation; suggestion alone; and no treatment (see comment below).[26] It found that hypnotic suggestion versus no treatment significantly increased the number of people who lost warts after 6 weeks (4/19 [21%] *v* 0/19 [0%]; $P < 0.05$), but found no significant difference between hypnotic suggestion plus relaxation versus no treatment (2/19 [11%] *v* 0/19 [0%]; no further data provided).

Harms: The RCTs gave no information on adverse effects.[25,26]

Comment: In the first RCT, participants were given a 10 minute hypnotic induction procedure involving inter related suggestions for sleep, drowsiness, and entering hypnosis, followed by a 2 minute suggestion of wart regression imagery repeated again after 30 seconds. Participants were then awakened and instructed to practice their wart regression imagery twice daily for 6 weeks.[25] The second RCT used the same procedure for hypnotic suggestion, except people were given a 5 minute hypnotic induction.[26] The cold laser placebo group in the RCT received two 4 minute treatments with a simulated laser and were told to count their warts daily and assess whether they experienced any sensations in their warts. The third RCT used the same hypnotic suggestion as the second RCT. The hypnotic suggestion plus relaxation group received a 5 minute relaxation procedure involving interrelated suggestions for relaxation and comfort instead of the induction procedure, and the suggestion alone group received suggestions for wart regression without the hypnotic induction procedure.[26]

OPTION CONTACT IMMUNOTHERAPY

Sam Gibbs, Ian Harvey, and Jane Sterling

One systematic review has found that contact immunotherapy (see glossary, p 1743) with dinitrochlorobenzene versus placebo significantly increases the number of people with wart clearance.

Benefits: We found one systematic review (search date 2000, 2 RCTs, 80 people), which found that dinitrochlorobenzene 2% solution followed by 1% solution versus placebo significantly increased the number of people with wart clearance at the end of the trial, which was 4 months in one trial and unspecified in the other (32/40 [80%] *v* 15/40 [38%]; RR 1.88, 95% CI 1.27 to 2.79).[9]

Harms: The systematic review gave no information on adverse effects.[9] One of the RCTs identified by the review found that 6/20 (30%) of participants developed an inflammatory reaction to dinitrochlorobenzene 2% solution only after the second application, but that all of these people subsequently experienced significant local irritation with or without blistering when they were treated with dinitrochlorobenzene 1% solution.[27] None withdrew from the study.

Comment: None.

OPTION INOSINE PRANOBEX

Michael Bigby

One RCT found insufficient evidence about the effects of inosine pranobex on wart clearance.

Benefits: We found no systematic review. One RCT (50 people aged > 12 years receiving topical salicylic acid and cryotherapy [see glossary, p 1743]), which compared inosine pranobex (1 g three times daily for 1 month) versus placebo, found no significant difference in the number of people with wart clearance at 6 months (9/24 [38%] with inosine pranobex *v* 9/26 [35 %] with placebo; RR 1.08, 95% 0.5 to 2.27).[28]

Harms: One person taking inosine pranobex developed a sore throat.[28]

Comment: The RCT could have been too small to exclude a clinically important difference between treatments.

OPTION SYSTEMIC INTERFERON α

Michael Bigby

We found no RCTs of sufficient quality on systemic interferon α.

Benefits: We found no systematic review and no RCTs of sufficient quality.

Harms: We found no RCTs.

Comment: None.

OPTION LEVAMISOLE

Michael Bigby

Two RCTs and one controlled clinical trial found insufficient evidence on the effects of levamisole versus placebo on clearance of warts. One RCT found that levamisole plus cimetidine versus cimetidine alone significantly increased the number of people with wart clearance.

Benefits: We found no systematic review. **Versus placebo:** We found two RCTs and one controlled clinical trial.[29–31] The first RCT (60 people), which compared levamisole (150 mg three times weekly for 10 wks) versus placebo, found no significant difference in the number of people with wart clearance after 3 months (5 /29 [17%] with levamisole *v* 6/31 [19%] with placebo; RR 0.89, 95% CI 0.30 to 2.61).[29] The second RCT (32 people), which compared levamisole (2.5 mg/kg 2 days/wk) versus placebo, found no significant difference in wart clearance after 8 weeks (7/14 [50%] with levimasole *v* 10/18 [55%] with placebo; RR 0.90, 95% CI 0.46 to 1.75).[30] One controlled clinical trial (40 people), which compared levamisole (5 mg/kg for 3 days every 2 wks) versus placebo, found that levamisole significantly increased the number of people with wart clearance after 5 months (12/20 [60%] with levamisole *v* 1/20 [5%] with placebo; RR 12.0; 95% CI 1.7 to 83.8).[31] **Levamisole plus cimetidine:** One RCT (48 people) found that levamisole (150 mg twice weekly) plus cimetidine (30 mg/kg) versus cimetidine alone (50 mg/kg/day) significantly increased the number of people with wart clearance at 12 weeks (15/24 [62%] with cimetidine plus levamisole *v* 8/24 [33%] with cimetidine alone; RR 1.78, 95% CI 1.01 to 2.49).[32]

Harms: The RCTs and controlled clinical trial of levamisole versus placebo gave no information on adverse effects.[29–31] In the RCT that compared cimetidine plus levamisole versus cimetidine alone, two people taking cimetidine plus levamisole withdrew because of severe nausea.[32] One person taking cimetidine plus levamisole and one person taking cimetidine alone experienced change in taste and constitutional symptoms (fatigue, weakness, and myalgia).[32]

Comment: The RCTs may have been too small to detect a clinically important difference between treatments.[29,30] The lack of randomisation in the controlled clinical trial means that the results should be interpreted with caution.[31]

OPTION PHOTODYNAMIC TREATMENT

Sam Gibbs, Ian Harvey, and Jane Sterling

RCTs found insufficient evidence on the effects of photodynamic treatment on wart clearance.

Benefits: We found one systematic review (search date 2000, 4 RCTs, 240 people)[9] and one subsequent RCT.[33] **Versus placebo:** The review could not perform a meta-analysis because of trial heterogeneity; one of the RCTs identified assessed complete wart clearance, the others assessed number of warts cured.[9] The first RCT (52 people) in the review compared proflavine photodynamic treatment (see glossary, p 1743) or neutral red photodynamic treatment versus placebo in a left/right hand design.[34] Matched pairs of warts on the left and right hands were treated with photodynamic treatment or placebo. It found no significant difference between proflavine photodynamic treatment versus neutral red photodynamic treatment in the number of people with wart clearance after 8 weeks (10/27 [43%] v 10/23 [37%]; RR 0.85, 95% CI 0.43 to 1.68). In all those who responded to treatment, the warts on the placebo treated side also resolved.[34] The second RCT in the review (45 adults with warts unsuccessfully treated for > 3 months), which compared aminolaevulinic acid photodynamic treatment versus placebo photodynamic treatment, found that aminolaevulinic acid photodynamic treatment significantly increased the number of warts cured after 18 weeks (64/114 [56%] of warts v 47/113 [42%] of warts; $P < 0.05$).[35] One subsequent RCT (67 people with warts unsuccessfully treated for > 12 months who had received keratolytic ointment under an occlusive dressing for 7 days) compared aminolaevulinic acid photodynamic treatment three times versus placebo photodynamic treatment.[33] It found that aminolaevulinic acid photodynamic treatment versus placebo significantly increased the number of warts cured after 4 months (48/64 [75%] of warts v 13/57 [23%] of warts; $P < 0.01$). **Versus cryotherapy:** See glossary, p 1743 The review identified one RCT (see cryotherapy v photodynamic treatment, p 1735). Versus salicylic acid: One RCT (120 people) identified by the review found no significant difference between methylthioninium chloride (methylene blue)/dimethyl sulfoxide (dimethyl sulphoxide) photodynamic treatment versus salicylic acid plus creosote in the number of people with wart clearance after 8 weeks (5/65 [8%] v 8/55 [15%]; RR 0.54, 95% CI 0.19 to 1.55).[36]

Harms: **Versus placebo:** One of the RCTs identified by the review found that aminolaevulinic acid photodynamic treatment versus placebo significantly increased the number of painful warts (light–unbearable pain) immediately after treatment.[35] Burning and itching continued for up to 48 hours in some participants and 3/30 (10%) withdrew because of pain during treatment. The subsequent RCT found that participants receiving aminolaevulinic acid photodynamic treatment experienced a burning sensation or slight pain during treatment, and moderate swelling and mild erythema of the treated area 24 hours after treatment.[33] **Versus cryotherapy:** See cryotherapy versus photodynamic treatment, p 1736.

Comment: Differences in trial methodology makes it difficult to draw conclusions from these RCTs.[9]

OPTION PULSED DYE LASER

Sam Gibbs, Ian Harvey, and Jane Sterling

One RCT found insufficient evidence on the effects of pulsed dye laser in number of warts cured.

Benefits: We found one systematic review (search date 2000, 1 RCT).[9] The RCT (40 people using daily topical salicylic acid, 194 warts) in the review compared pulsed dye laser versus cryotherapy (see glossary, p 1743) or cantharidin.[37] All treatments were used at monthly intervals up to a maximum of four times. The RCT did not assess complete wart clearance. It found no difference between pulsed dye laser versus cryotherapy or cantharidin in the number of warts cured at the end of the study, which was not specified (66% of warts with pulsed dye laser *v* 70% of warts with either cryotherapy or cantharidin). Fifteen of the 35 participants were contacted by telephone at an average of 11 months after treatment. There was no significant difference between pulsed dye laser versus cryotherapy or cantharidin in the proportion of people who had recurrence of at least one wart (3/10 [30%] *v* 2/5 [40%]; RR 1.05, 95% CI 0.23 to 4.73).[37]

Harms: The RCT found that participants experienced mild discomfort and blistering but did not specify whether the adverse effects were associated with pulsed dye laser, cryotherapy, or cantharidin.[37]

Comment: None.

OPTION TOPICAL TREATMENTS CONTAINING SALICYLIC ACID

Sam Gibbs, Ian Harvey, and Jane Sterling

One systematic review has found that simple topical treatments containing salicylic acid versus placebo significantly increase the number of people with either complete wart clearance, successful treatment, or loss of one or more warts after 6–12 weeks.

Benefits: We found one systematic review (search date 2000, 9 RCTs, 816 people) of topical salicylic acid.[9] **Versus placebo or versus no treatment:** The review (6 RCTs, 376 people) found that salicylic acid versus placebo significantly increased the number of people with either complete wart clearance, successful treatment (not defined), or loss of one or more warts after 6–12 weeks (144/191 [75%] *v* 89/185 [48%]; RR 1.55, 95% CI 1.32 to 1.82; NNT 4, 95% CI 3 to 6). **Versus cryotherapy:** See glossary, p 1743. We found two RCTs (see cryotherapy v salicylic acid, p 1735). **Versus photodynamic treatment:** See glossary, p 1743. We found one RCT (see photodynamic treatment v salicylic acid, p 1740).

Harms: Some of the RCTs identified by the review found that salicylic acid was associated with minor skin irritation.[9]

Comment: Trial heterogeneity and poor quality of the RCTs included in the review mean that the pooled results should be treated with caution.[9]

OPTION SURGICAL PROCEDURES

Sam Gibbs, Ian Harvey, and Jane Sterling

One systematic review identified no RCTs on the effects of surgical procedures on wart clearance.

Benefits: One systematic review (search date 2000) identified no RCTs.[9]

Harms: We found no evidence.

Comment: None.

GLOSSARY

Contact immunotherapy Contact sensitisers such as dinitrochlorobenzene, diphencyprone, and squaric acid dibutyl ester result in allergic dermatitis, which stimulates an immune reaction in close proximity to the wart and results in its eradication.

Cryotherapy A destructive treatment based on the targeted freezing of tissue using liquid nitrogen, dimethyl ether propane, or carbon dioxide snow. Liquid nitrogen achieves the lowest temperatures and is now the most commonly used agent.

Photodynamic treatment Combines the application of a photosensitising substance (usually aminolaevulinic acid) to the wart and subsequent irradiation with wavelengths of light that are absorbed by the photosensitising substance and lead to destruction of the target tissue.

REFERENCES

1. Johnson ML, Roberts J. Skin conditions and related need for medical care among persons 1–74 years. *US Department of Health Education and Welfare Publication* 1978;1660:1–26.
2. Beliaeva TL. The population incidence of warts. *Vestn Dermatol Venerol* 1990;2:55–58.
3. Williams HC, Pottier A, Strachan D. The descriptive epidemiology of warts in British schoolchildren. *Br J Dermatol* 1993;128:504–511.
4. Kilkenny M, Merlin K, Young R, et al. The prevalence of common skin conditions in Australian school students: 1. Common, plane and plantar viral warts. *Br J Dermatol* 1998;138:840–845.
5. Johnson LW. Communal showers and the risk of plantar warts. *J Fam Pract* 1995;40:136–138.
6. Keefe M, al-Ghamdi A, Coggon D, et al. Cutaneous warts in butchers. *Br J Dermatol* 1995;132:166–167.
7. Leigh IM, Glover MT. Skin cancer and warts in immunosuppressed renal transplant recipients. *Recent Results Cancer Res* 1995;139:69–86.
8. Massing AM, Epstein WL. Natural history of warts. *Arch Dermatol* 1963;87:303–310.
9. Gibbs S, Harvey I, Sterling J, et al. Local treatments for cutaneous warts. In: The Cochrane Library, Issue 3, 2001. Oxford: Update Software. Search date 2000; primary sources Medline, Embase, Cinahl, Cochrane Controlled Trials Register, Science Citation Index, CAB-Health, Heathstar, DARE, NHS Economic Evaluation Database, EconLit, Amed, hand search of selected journals, reference lists, and pharmaceutical companies, and authors contacted.
10. Bunney MH, Nolan MW, Buxton PK, et al. The treatment of resistant warts with intralesional bleomycin: a controlled clinical trial. *Br J Dermatol* 1984;111:197–207.
11. Rossi E, Soto JH, Battan J, et al. Intralesional bleomycin in verruca vulgaris. Double-blind study. *Dermatol Rev Mex* 1981;25:158–165.
12. Munkvad M, Genner J, Staberg B, et al. Locally injected bleomycin in the treatment of warts. *Dermatologica* 1983;167:86–89.
13. Perez Alfonzo R, Weiss E, Piquero Martin J. Hypertonic saline solution vs intralesional bleomycin in the treatment of common warts. *Dermatol Venez* 1992;30:176–178.
14. Hayes ME, O'Keefe EJ. Reduced dose of bleomycin in the treatment of recalcitrant warts. *J Am Acad Dermatol* 1986;15:1002–1006.
15. Rogers CJ, Gibney MD, Siegfried EC, et al. Cimetidine therapy for recalcitrant warts in adults: is it any better than placebo? *J Am Acad Dermatol* 1999;41:123–127.
16. Karabulut AA, Sahin S, Eksioglu M. Is cimetidine effective for nongenital warts: a double-blind, placebo-controlled study [letter]. *Arch Dermatol* 1997;133:533–534.
17. Yilmaz E, Alpsoy E, Basaran E. Cimetidine therapy for warts: a placebo-controlled, double-blind study. *J Am Acad Dermatol* 1996;34:1005–1007.
18. Bauman C, Francis JS, Vanderhooft S, et al. Cimetidine therapy for multiple viral warts in children [see comments]. *J Am Acad Dermatol* 1996;35:271–272.
19. Stender IM, Lock-Anderson J, Wulf HC. Recalcitrant hand and foot warts successfully treated with photodynamic therapy with topical 5-aminolaevulinic acid: a pilot study. *Clin Exp Dermatol* 1999;24:154–159.
20. Bourke JF, Berth-Jones J, Hutchinson PE. Cryotherapy of common viral warts at intervals of 1, 2 and 3 weeks. *Br J Dermatol* 1995;132:433–436.
21. Connolly M, Basmi K, O'Connell M, et al. Cryotherapy of viral warts: a sustained 10-s freeze is more effective than the traditional method. *Br J Dermatol* 2001;145:554–557.
22. Harkness EF, Abbot NC, Ernst E. A randomized trial of distant healing for skin warts [see comments]. *Am J Med* 2000;108:448–452.
23. Labrecque M, Audet D, Latulippe LG, et al. Homeopathic treatment of plantar warts [see comments]. *CMAJ* 1992;146:1749–1753.
24. Kainz JT, Kozel G, Haidvogl M, et al. Homoeopathic versus placebo therapy of children with warts on the hands: a randomized, double-blind clinical trial [see comments]. *Dermatology* 1996;193:318–320.
25. Spanos NP, Williams V, Gwynn MI. Effects of hypnotic, placebo, and salicylic acid treatments on wart regression. *Psychosom Med* 1990;52:109–114.
26. Spanos NP, Stenstrom RJ, Johnston JC. Hypnosis, placebo, and suggestion in the treatment of warts. *Psychosom Med* 1988;50:245–260.
27. Rosado-Cancino MA, Ruiz-Maldonado R, Tamayo L, et al. Treatment of multiple and stubborn warts in children with 1-chloro-2,4-dinitrobenzene (DNCB) and placebo. *Dermatol Rev Mex* 1989;33:245–252.
28. Benton EC, Nolan MW, Kemmett D, et al. Trial of inosine pranobex in the management of cutaneous viral warts. *J Dermatol Treat* 1991;1:295–297.
29. Morales-Caballero HG, Ruiz MR, Tamayo L. Levamisole in the treatment of warts (double blind study). *Dermatologia* 1978;22:20–25.
30. Saul A, Sanz R, Gomez M. Treatment of multiple viral warts with levamisole. *Int J Dermatol* 1980;19:342–343.

31. Amer M, Tosson Z, Soliman A, et al. Verrucae treated by levamisole. *Int J Dermatol* 1991;30:738–740.
32. Parsad D, Saini R, Negi KS. Comparison of combination of cimetidine and levamisole with cimetidine alone in the treatment of recalcitrant warts. *Australas J Dermatol* 1999;40:93–95.
33. Fabbrocini G, Di Constanzo MP, Riccardo AM, et al. Photodynamic therapy with topical delta-aminolaevulinic acid for the treatment of plantar warts. *J Photochem Photobiol* 2001;61:30–34.
34. Veien NK, Genner J, Brodthagen H, et al. Photodynamic inactivation of verrucae vulgares. II. *Acta Derm Venereol* 1977;57:445–447.
35. Stender IM, Na R, Fogh H, et al. Photodynamic therapy with 5-aminolaevulinic acid or placebo for recalcitrant foot and hand warts: randomised double-blind trial. *Lancet* 2000;355:963–966.
36. Stahl D, Veien NK, Wulf HC. Photodynamic inactivation of virus warts: a controlled clinical trial. *Clin Exp Dermatol* 1979;4:81–85.
37. Robson KJ, Cunningham NM, Kruzan KL. Pulsed dye laser versus conventional therapy for the treatment of warts: a prospective randomized trial. *J Am Acad Dermatol* 2000;43:275–280.

Michael Bigby
Assistant Professor of Dermatology
Harvard Medical School
Boston, Massachusetts
USA

Sam Gibbs
Consultant Dermatologist
Ipswich Hospital NHS Trust
Ipswich
UK

Ian Harvey
Professor of Epidemiology
and Public Health
University of East Anglia
Norwich
UK

Jane Sterling
Honorary Consultant Dermatologist
Addenbrooke's NHS Trust
Cambridge
UK

Competing interests: None declared.

Scabies

Search date May 2002

Godfrey Walker and Paul Johnstone

QUESTIONS

INTERVENTIONS

Key Messages

- **Benzyl benzoate** One systematic review identified one small RCT that found no significant difference with benzyl benzoate versus ivermectin in clinical cure rates at 30 days. One subsequent RCT found a significantly lower proportion of people with clinical cure with benzyl benzoate versus ivermectin at 30 days. One systematic review identified one RCT that found no significant difference with benzyl benzoate versus sulphur ointment in clinical cure at 8 or 14 days.
- **Crotamiton** One systematic review has found a significantly lower proportion of people with clinical and parasitic cure with crotamiton versus permethrin after 28 days. One systematic review identified one RCT that found no significant difference with crotamiton versus lindane in clinical cure rates at 28 days.
- **Lindane** One systematic review identified one RCT that found no significant difference with lindane versus crotamiton in clinical cure rates at 28 days. The systematic review found conflicting results with lindane versus permethrin after 28 days. Another small RCT identified by the review found no significant difference with lindane versus ivermectin in cure rates at 15 days. One subsequent RCT found no significant difference with lindane versus ivermectin in failed clinical cure rates at 2 weeks, but found a significantly higher proportion of people with failed clinical cure with lindane versus ivermectin at 4 weeks. We found reports of rare side effects such as convulsions and other severe adverse effects.
- **Malathion** One systematic review found no RCTs on the effects of malathion. Case series have reported cure rates in scabies of over 80% of people.
- **Oral ivermectin** One systematic review identified one RCT that found that ivermectin versus placebo significantly increased clinical cure rates after 7 days. Another small RCT identified by the review found no significant difference with ivermectin versus benzyl benzoate in clinical cure rates at 30 days. One subsequent RCT found that ivermectin versus benzyl benzoate significantly increased clinical cure rates at 30 days. One systematic review identified one small RCT that found no significant difference with ivermectin versus lindane in

cure rates at 15 days. One subsequent RCT found no significant difference with ivermectin versus lindane in failed clinical cure rates at 2 weeks, but found that ivermectin significantly decreased failed clinical cure rates at 4 weeks. One RCT found limited evidence that ivermectin versus permethrin reduced clinical cure rates at 14 days. Experience of the use of oral ivermectin in onchocerciasis suggests that it is safe in younger adults, but no such experience exists for children, and there have been reports of increased risk of death in elderly people.

- **Permethrin** One systematic review has found that permethrin versus crotamiton significantly increases clinical and parasitic cure after 28 days. The systematic review found conflicting results with permethrin versus lindane. One subsequent RCT found limited evidence that permethrin versus ivermectin significantly increased clinical cure at 14 days.
- **Sulphur compounds** One systematic review identified one RCT that found no significant difference with sulphur ointment versus benzyl benzoate in clinical cure at 8 or 14 days.

DEFINITION Scabies is an infestation of the skin by the mite *Sarcoptes scabiei*.[1] Typical sites of infestation are skin folds and flexor surfaces. In adults, the most common sites are between the fingers and on the wrists, although infection may manifest in elderly people as a diffuse truncal eruption. In infants and children, the face, scalp, palms, and soles are also often affected.

INCIDENCE/ PREVALENCE Scabies is a common public health problem with an estimated prevalence of 300 million cases worldwide, mostly affecting people in developing countries where prevalence can exceed 50%.[2] In industrialised countries it is most common in institutionalised communities. Case studies suggest that epidemic cycles occur every 7–15 years and that these partly reflect the population's immune status.

AETIOLOGY/ RISK FACTORS Scabies is particularly common where there is social disruption, overcrowding with close body contact, and limited access to water.[3] Young children, immobilised elderly people, people with HIV/AIDS, and other medically and immunologically compromised people are predisposed to infestation and have particularly high mite counts.[4]

PROGNOSIS Scabies is not life threatening, but the severe, persistent itch and secondary infections may be debilitating. Occasionally, crusted scabies develops. This form of the disease is resistant to routine treatment and can be a source of continued reinfestation and spread to others.

AIMS To eliminate the scabies mites and ova from the skin; to cure pruritus (itching); to prevent reinfestation; to prevent spread to other people.

OUTCOMES **Clinical cure:** number of visible burrows and papular and vesicular eruptions; pruritus. **Parasitic cure:** presence of mites, ova, or faecal pellets in skin scrapings under a magnifying lens or microscope. Outcomes should be assessed 28–30 days after start of treatment, which is the time it takes for lesions to heal and for any eggs and mites to reach maturity if treatment fails.

METHODS *Clinical Evidence* update search and appraisal May 2002.

QUESTION What are the effects of topical treatments?

OPTION PERMETHRIN

One systematic review has found that permethrin versus crotamiton significantly increases clinical and parasitic cure after 28 days. The systematic review found conflicting results with permethrin versus lindane after 28 days. One subsequent RCT found limited evidence that permethrin versus ivermectin significantly increased clinical cure at 14 days.

Benefits: We found no RCTs comparing permethrin versus placebo. We found one systematic review (search date 1999, 6 RCTs)[5] and one subsequent RCT[6] comparing permethrin versus other topical and oral agents. **Versus crotamiton:** The review (2 RCTs, 194 people) found that permethrin versus crotamiton significantly increased clinical cure rates after 28 days (2 RCTs; OR for failed clinical cure with permethrin *v* crotamiton 0.21, 95% CI 0.10 to 0.47) and significantly increased parasitic cure after 28 days (1 RCT; 94 people; OR for failed parasitic cure with permethrin *v* crotamiton 0.21, 95% CI 0.08 to 0.53). It found no significant difference between permethrin and crotamiton in self reported pruritus (1 RCT: OR for itch persistence with permethrin *v* with crotamiton 0.38, 95% CI 0.12 to 1.19).[5] **Versus lindane:** The systematic review identified four RCTs comparing permethrin versus lindane.[5] Overall, the review found that permethrin versus lindane appeared to be more effective in clinical cure after 28 days. However, it found significant trial heterogeneity ($P < 0.005$). Two RCTs (100 people; 52 people) included in the review found permethrin versus lindane significantly reduced clinical failure (OR for failed clinical cure of permethrin *v* lindane 0.14, 95% CI 0.05 to 0.43, and 0.19, 95% CI 0.05 to 0.70, respectively) whereas two RCTs (99 people; 467 people), including the largest RCT, found no significant difference with permethrin versus lindane (OR for failed clinical cure of permethrin *v* lindane 0.8, 95% CI 0.21 to 3.14, and 0.93, 95% CI 0.60 to 1.42, respectively).[5] **Versus oral ivermectin:** We found one subsequent RCT that compared topical permethrin versus oral ivermectin.[6] The RCT (85 people attending an outpatient clinic in India) assessed clinical cure at 14 days, and if not assessed as completely cured at that time the same treatment was repeated. It found that permethrin versus ivermectin significantly increased clinical cure rate at 14 days (OR for failed clinical cure of permethrin *v* ivermectin 0.12, 95% CI 0.04 to 0.39).[6]

Harms: One RCT identified by the review reported five people with adverse effects: two in the permethrin group (rash and possible diarrhoea) and three in the lindane group (pruritic rash, papules, and diarrhoea).[7] During 1990–1995, six adverse events were reported per 100 000 units distributed in the USA (1 central nervous system adverse effect reported per 500 000 units of permethrin distributed).[8] Resistance to permethrin seems to be rare[8] (see harms of lindane, p 1748).

Comment: None.

OPTION LINDANE

One systematic review identified one RCT that found no significant difference with lindane versus crotamiton in clinical cure rates at 28 days. The systematic review found conflicting results with lindane versus permethrin after 28 days. Another small RCT identified by the review found no significant difference with lindane versus ivermectin in cure rates at 15 days. One subsequent RCT found no significant difference with lindane versus ivermectin in failed clinical cure rates at 2 weeks, but found a significantly higher proportion of people with failed clinical cure with lindane at 4 weeks. We found reports of rare side effects such as convulsions and other severe adverse effects with lindane.

Benefits: We found no RCTs comparing lindane versus placebo. We found one systematic review (search date 1999, 6 RCTs)[5] comparing lindane versus other topical and oral agents, and one subsequent RCT comparing lindane versus ivermectin.[9] **Versus crotamiton:** One RCT (100 adults and children) identified by the review found no significant difference in clinical cure rates at 28 days (OR for failed clinical cure with crotamiton *v* lindane 0.41, 95% CI 0.15 to 1.10).[5] However, confidence intervals are broad and a clinically important difference cannot be ruled out. **Versus permethrin:** See benefits of permethrin, p 1747. **Versus oral ivermectin:** One RCT[10] (53 adults referred to hospital with scabies) identified by the review found no significant difference between lindane versus ivermectin in clinical cure rates at 15 days (failed clinical cure 14/27 [52%] with lindane *v* 12/26 [46%] with oral ivermectin; RR 0.89, 95% CI 0.51 to 1.55).[5] One subsequent RCT compared topical lindane versus ivermectin.[9] It found no significant difference in failed clinical cure rates with lindane versus ivermectin at 2 weeks (failed clinical cure rate 70/100 [70%] with ivermectin *v* 81/100 [81%] with lindane; RR 0.86, 95% CI 0.74 to 1.01) but found ivermectin versus lindane significantly increased clinical cure rates at 4 weeks (failed clinical cure rate 43/100 [43%] with ivermectin *v* 64/100 [64%] with lindane; RR 0.67, 95% CI 0.51 to 0.88).

Harms: One RCT identified by the review reported five people with adverse effects: two in the permethrin group (rash and possible diarrhoea) and three in the lindane group (pruritic rash, papules, and diarrhoea).[7] One RCT identified by the review reported that six people taking lindane had headaches, and 1 person each had headache, hypotension, abdominal pain, and vomiting in the ivermectin group.[10] Case reports have reported rare severe adverse effects (e.g. convulsions, other long term neurological complications, and aplastic anaemia) particularly when lindane was applied to people with extensive skin diseases and to children.[11–13] Figures from the World Health Organization Collaborating Centre for International Drug Monitoring covering summary reports from 47 countries suggest that lindane is more toxic than other preparations (see comment below).[14] Five convulsions were reported in people on benzyl benzoate, two in people on crotamiton, 48 in people on lindane, two in people on malathion, and 19 in people on permethrin. Deaths reported on benzyl benzoate were none, crotamiton one, lindane four, malathion none, and permethrin five.[14] Resistance to lindane has been reported in many countries.[15]

Comment: Lindane was withdrawn from the market in the UK in 1995 because of concern about possible adverse effects. The evidence linking lindane with convulsions is suggestive but not conclusive.[11–14] It is difficult to draw firm conclusions on the relative occurrence of severe side effects of different preparations reported to the World Health Organization Collaborating Centre for International Drug Monitoring because of incomplete information on incidence in relation to use; however lindane and permethrin appear possibly to be more likely to be related to rare severe side effects. Safety results from trials and observational studies need to be summarised, particularly regarding additional risks in infants and pregnant women.

OPTION CROTAMITON

One systematic review has found that crotamiton versus permethrin significantly reduced clinical and parasitic cure after 28 days. One systematic review identified one RCT that found no significant difference with crotamiton versus lindane in clinical cure rates at 28 days.

Benefits: We found no RCTs comparing crotamiton versus placebo. We found one systematic review (search date 1999, 3 RCTs) comparing crotamiton versus other topical agents.[5] **Crotamiton versus permethrin:** See benefits of permethrin, p 1747. **Crotamiton versus lindane:** See benefits of lindane, p 1748.

Harms: The RCTs reported no serious adverse effects[5] (see harms of lindane, p 1748).

Comment: None.

OPTION MALATHION

One systematic review found no RCTs on the effects of malathion. Case series have reported cure rates in scabies of over 80% of people.

Benefits: We found one systematic review (search date 1999) that identified no RCTs.[5] Case series suggest that malathion is effective in curing infestation with scabies, with a cure rate of over 80% of people at 4 weeks.[16–18]

Harms: We found no RCTs (see harms of lindane, p 1748).

Comment: The safety results from trials and observational studies need to be summarised, particularly with regard to additional risks in infants and pregnant women.

OPTION BENZYL BENZOATE

One systematic review identified one small RCT that found no significant difference with benzyl benzoate versus ivermectin in clinical cure rates at 30 days. One subsequent RCT found that benzyl benzoate versus ivermectin significantly reduced clinical cure at 30 days. One systematic review identified one RCT that found no significant difference with benzyl benzoate versus sulphur ointment in clinical cure at 8 or 14 days.

Benefits: We found no RCTs comparing benzyl benzoate versus placebo. We found one systematic review (search date 1999, 2 RCTs, 202 people) comparing benzyl benzoate versus other agents[5] and one subsequent RCT comparing ivermectin and benzyl benzoate.[19] **Versus oral ivermectin:** The systematic review identified one RCT[20] and we found one subsequent RCT[19] (see benefits of oral ivermectin, p 1751). **Versus sulphur ointment:** One RCT identified by the review compared benzyl benzoate versus sulphur ointment (158 adults and children identified in a house-to-house survey of a semi-urban area of India).[21] It found no significant difference in the number of people with apparently cured lesions by 8 days (AR 68/89 [76%] with benzyl benzoate *v* 45/69 [65%] with sulphur ointment; RR 1.17, 95% CI 0.95 to 1.33) or by 14 days (AR 81/89 [91%] with benzyl benzoate *v* 67/69 [97%] with sulphur ointment; RR 0.94, 95% CI 0.86 to 1.01).

Harms: Both RCTs comparing benzyl benzoate versus oral ivermectin found that about a quarter of people treated with benzyl benzoate reported a transient increase in pruritus and dermatitis.[19,20] See harms of lindane, p 1748.

Comment: Non-randomised trials suggest benzyl benzoate has variable effectiveness (as low as 50%).[22,23] The low cure rate may be related to the concentration of the preparation and resistance of the mite to benzyl benzoate.

OPTION SULPHUR COMPOUNDS

One systematic review identified one RCT that found no significant difference with sulphur ointment versus benzyl benzoate in clinical cure at 8 or 14 days.

Benefits: We found no RCTs comparing sulphur compounds versus placebo. **Versus benzyl benzoate:** We found one RCT (see benefits of benzyl benzoate, p 1750).[21]

Harms: Use of sulphur has been associated with increased local irritation in about a quarter of cases.[13]

Comment: None.

QUESTION What are the effects of systemic treatments?

OPTION ORAL IVERMECTIN

One systematic review identified one RCT that found that ivermectin versus placebo significantly increased clinical cure rates after 7 days. Another small RCT identified by the review found no significant difference with ivermectin versus benzyl benzoate in clinical cure rates at 30 days. One subsequent RCT found that ivermectin versus benzyl benzoate significantly increased clinical cure rates at 30 days. One systematic review identified one small RCT that found no significant difference with ivermectin versus lindane in cure rates at 15 days. One subsequent RCT found no significant difference with ivermectin versus lindane in failed clinical cure rates at 2 weeks, but found that ivermectin significantly increased clinical cure rates at 4 weeks. One RCT found limited evidence that ivermectin versus permethrin

significantly reduced clinical cure at 14 days. Experience of the use of oral ivermectin in onchocerciasis suggests that it is safe in younger adults, but no such experience exists for children and there have been reports of increased risk of death in elderly people.

Benefits: We found one systematic review (search date 1999, 3 RCTs)[5] and three subsequent RCTs[6,9,19] comparing oral ivermectin versus placebo or other agents. **Versus placebo:** One RCT (55 young adults and children aged > 5 years) identified by the review found that oral ivermectin versus placebo significantly increased clinical cure rates after 7 days (23/29 [79%] with oral ivermectin *v* 4/26 [15%] with placebo; RR 5.2, 95% CI 2.1 to 12.9; NNT 2, 95% CI 1 to 3).[5] **Versus benzyl benzoate:** One small RCT (44 adults and children) identified by the review found no significant difference in clinical cure rates at 30 days (16/23 [70%] with oral ivermectin *v* 10/21 [48%] with benzyl benzoate; RR 1.5, 95% CI 0.9 to 2.5).[20] One subsequent small RCT (58 adults and children) found significantly increased clinical cure rates at 30 days with oral ivermectin versus benzyl benzoate (27/29 [93%] with oral ivermectin *v* 14/29 [48%] with benzyl benzoate; RR 1.9, 95% CI 1.3 to 2.8).[19] **Versus lindane:** See benefits of lindane, p 1748. **Versus permethrin:** See benefits of permethrin, p 1747.

Harms: One RCT identified by the review reported that six people had headaches in the lindane group, and one person each had headache, hypotension, abdominal pain, and vomiting in the ivermectin group.[10] One RCT reported no side effects for oral ivermectin, whilst 7/29 (24%) people taking benzyl benzoate had a mild to moderate increase of skin irritation by day 2 of treatment.[19] One RCT comparing ivermectin versus lindane reported one headache in the ivermectin group.[9] Oral ivermectin has been used widely in adults with onchocerciasis and even with repeated doses serious adverse effects have been rare.[24,25] Summary reports to the World Health Organization Collaborating Centre for International Drug Monitoring from five countries indicate that it is associated with rare severe side effects, including three convulsions and eight deaths.[26] We found no good evidence about its safety in children. An increased risk of death has been reported among elderly people taking oral ivermectin for scabies in a long term care facility.[27] It is not clear whether this was caused by oral ivermectin, interactions with other scabicides (including lindane and permethrin), or other treatments such as psychoactive drugs. Other studies reported no such complications from its use in elderly people.[28]

Comment: Case series suggest that oral ivermectin may be effective when included in the treatment of hyperkeratotic crusted scabies (also known as Norwegian scabies)[29–31] and in people with concomitant HIV disease.[4] The RCT comparing oral ivermectin versus placebo assessed outcomes 7 days after the intervention was administered, which may be insufficient time to achieve cure.[5]

Substantive changes

Permethrin New RCT permethrin versus ivermectin;[6] conclusions unchanged.

Lindane New RCT lindane versus ivermectin;[9] conclusions unchanged.

Ivermectin New RCT ivermectin versus benzyl benzoate;[19] conclusions unchanged.

REFERENCES

1. Meinking TL, Taplin D. Infestations. In: Schachner LA, Hansen RC, eds. *Pediatric dermatology*. New York: Churchill Livingston, 1995.
2. Stein DH. Scabies and pediculosis. *Curr Opin Pediatr* 1991;3:660–666.
3. Green M. Epidemiology of scabies. *Epidemiol Rev* 1989;11:126–150.
4. Meinking TL, Taplin D, Hermida JL, et al. The treatment of scabies with ivermectin. *N Engl J Med* 1995;333:26–30.
5. Walker GJA, Johnstone PW. Interventions for treating scabies. In: The Cochrane Library, Issue 2, 2002. Oxford: Update Software. Search date 1999; primary sources Medline, Embase, records of military trials from UK, USA, and Russia, and specialist register of the Cochrane Diseases Group.
6. Usha V, Gopalakrishnan Nair TV. A comparative study of oral ivermectin and topical permethrin cream in the treatment of scabies. *J Am Acad Dermatol* 2000;42:236–240.
7. Schultz MW, Gomez M, Hansen RC, et al. Comparative study of 5% permethrin cream and 1% lindane lotion for the treatment of scabies. *Arch Dermatol* 1990;126:167–170.
8. Meinking TL, Taplin D. Safety of permethrin vs lindane for the treatment of scabies. *Arch Dermatol* 1996;132:959–962.
9. Madan V, Jaskiran K, Gupta U, et al. Oral ivermectin in scabies patients: a comparison with 1% topical lindane lotion. *J Dermatol* 2001;28:481–484.
10. Chouela EN, Abeldano AM, Pellerano O, et al. Equivalent therapeutic efficacy and safety of ivermectin and lindane in the treatment of human scabies. *Arch Dermatol* 1999;135:651–655.
11. Hall RC, Hall RC. Long-term psychological and neurological complications of lindane poisoning. *Psychosomatics* 1999;40(6):513–517.
12. Nordt SP, Chew G. Acute lindane poisoning in three children. *J Emerg Med* 2000;18(1):51–53.
13. Elgart ML. A risk benefit assessment of agents used in the treatment of scabies. *Drug Saf* 1996;14386–393.
14. WHO Collaborating Centre for International Drug Monitoring. Reported adverse reactions to ectoparasiticodes, including scabicides, insecticides and repellents. Uppsala, Sweden, 2002. The WHO Collaborating Centre receives summary clinical reports from National Centres in countries participating in a collaborative programme. The information is not homogenous at least with respect to origin or likelihood that the pharmaceutical product caused the adverse reaction. The information does not represent the opinion of the World Health Organization.
15. Brown S, Belcher J, Brady W. Treatment of ectoparasitic infections: review of the English-language literature. *Clin Infect Dis* 1995;20(suppl 1):104–109.
16. Hanna NF, Clay JC, Harris JRW. *Sarcoptes scabiei* infestation treated with malathion liquid. *Br J Vener Dis* 1978;54:354.
17. Thianprasit M, Schuetzenberger R. Prioderm lotion in the treatment of scabies. *Southeast Asian J Trop Med Public Health* 1984;15:119–120.
18. Burgess I, Robinson RJF, Robinson J, et al. Aqueous malathion 0.5% as a scabicide: clinical trial. *BMJ* 1986;292:1172.
19. Nnoruka EN, Agu CE. Successful treatment of scabies with oral ivermectin in Nigeria. *Trop Doct* 2001;31(1):15–18.
20. Glaziou P, Cartel JL, Alzieu P, et al. Comparison of ivermectin and benzyl benzoate for treatment of scabies. *Trop Med Parasitol* 1993;44:331–332.
21. Gulati PV, Singh KP. A family based study on the treatment of scabies with benzyl benzoate and sulphur ointment. *Indian J Dermatol Venereol Lepr* 1978;44:269–273.
22. Kaur GA, Nadeswary K. Field trials on the management of scabies in Jengka Triangle, Pahang. *Med J Malaysia* 1980;35:14–21.
23. Haustein UF, Hlawa B. Treatment of scabies with permethrin versus lindane and benzyl benzoate. *Acta Derm Venereol* 1989;69:348–351.
24. Pacque M, Munoz B, Greene BM, et al. Safety of and compliance with community-based ivermectin therapy. *Lancet* 1990;335:1377–1380.
25. De Sole G, Remme J, Awadzi K, et al. Adverse reactions after large-scale treatment of onchocerciasis with ivermectin: combined results from eight community trials. *Bull World Health Organ* 1989;67:707–719.
26. WHO Collaborating Centre for International Drug Monitoring. Reported adverse reactions to ivermectin. Uppsala, Sweden, 2002. The WHO Collaborating Centre receives summary clinical reports from National Centres in countries participating in a collaborative programme. The information is not homogenous at least with respect to origin or likelihood that the pharmaceutical product caused the adverse reaction. The information does not represent the opinion of the World Health Organization
27. Barkwell R, Shields S. Deaths associated with ivermectin treatment of scabies. *Lancet* 1997;349:1144–1145.
28. Diazgranados JA, Costa JL. Deaths after ivermectin treatment. *Lancet* 1997;349:1698.
29. Sullivan JR, Watt G, Barker B. Successful use of ivermectin in the treatment of endemic scabies in a nursing home. *Australas J Dermatol* 1997;38:137–140.
30. Aubin F, Humbert P. Ivermectin for crusted (Norwegian) scabies. *N Engl J Med* 1995;332:612.
31. Haas N, Henz BM, Ohlendorf D. Is single oral dose of ivermectin sufficient in crusted scabies? *International Journal of Dermatology* 2001;40:599.

Godfrey Walker
Specialist in Reproductive Health
UNFPA Country Technical Services
Team for Eastern Europe and Central Asia
Bratislava
Slovak Republic

Paul Johnstone
Director of Public Health Visiting
Professor in Public Health
University of Teesside
Middlesbrough
UK

Competing interests: None declared.

Squamous cell carcinoma of the skin: non-metastatic

Search date January 2002

Adèle Green and Robin Marks

QUESTIONS

INTERVENTIONS

See glossary, p 1757

Key Messages

Prevention

- **Sunscreen (daily versus discretionary use)** One RCT in adults in a subtropical Australian community found that daily versus discretionary use of sunscreen to the head, neck, arms, and hands significantly reduced the incidence of squamous cell carcinoma after 4.5 years.
- **Sunscreens to prevent development of new solar keratoses (better than placebo)** One RCT in people with previous solar keratoses aged > 40 years and living in Victoria, Australia found that daily sunscreen versus placebo sunscreen significantly reduced the incidence of new solar keratoses after 7 months use.

Treatment

- **Micrographically controlled surgery (unknown benefit compared with standard surgical excision)** We found no RCTs comparing micrographically controlled surgery versus standard excision in primary treatment.
- **Primary excision (unknown optimal margin of excision)** We found insufficient evidence relating size of primary excision margin to local recurrence rate.
- **Radiotherapy after surgery (unknown benefit compared with surgery alone)** We found no RCTs comparing the addition of radiotherapy to surgery versus surgery alone.

Clin Evid 2002;8:1753–1758.

DEFINITION Cutaneous squamous cell carcinoma is a malignant tumour of keratinocytes arising in the epidermis, showing histological evidence of dermal invasion.

INCIDENCE/ PREVALENCE Incidence rates are often derived from special surveys because few cancer registries routinely collect notifications of squamous cell carcinoma of the skin. Incidence rates on exposed skin vary markedly around the world according to skin colour and latitude, and range from negligible rates in black populations and white populations living at very high latitudes to rates of about 1000/100 000 in white residents of tropical Australia.[1]

AETIOLOGY/ RISK FACTORS People with fair skin colour who sunburn easily without tanning, people with xeroderma pigmentosum (see glossary, p 1757),[2–4] and those who are immunosuppressed[5] are susceptible to squamous cell carcinoma. The strongest environmental risk factor for squamous cell carcinoma is chronic sun exposure. Cohort and case control studies have found that clinical signs of chronic skin damage, especially solar keratoses, are also determinants of cutaneous squamous cell carcinoma.[3,4] For example, the risk of squamous cell carcinoma in people with the propensity to severe sunburn or with a history of multiple sunburns is three times greater than in people with no such propensity. In people with multiple solar keratoses (> 15), the risk of squamous cell carcinoma is 10–15 times greater than in people with no solar keratoses.[3,4]

PROGNOSIS Prognosis is related to the location and size of tumour, histological pattern, depth of invasion, perineural involvement, and whether the person is immunosuppressed.[6,7] A worldwide review of 95 case series, each comprising at least 20 people, found the overall metastasis rate for squamous cell carcinoma on the ear is 11% and on the lip 14%, compared with an average over all sites of 5%.[7] A review of 71 case series found that lesions less than 2 cm in diameter compared with lesions greater than 2 cm have less than half the local recurrence rate (7% *v* 15%), and less than one third of the rate of metastasis (9% *v* 30%).[7]

AIMS To prevent the occurrence of squamous cell carcinoma; to achieve cure by eradicating local disease including microinvasive disease; and to reduce mortality.

OUTCOMES **Prevention:** Incidence of cutaneous squamous cell carcinoma; mortality from squamous cell carcinoma. **Primary excision:** Local recurrence; survival; cosmetic outcome. **Radiotherapy after surgery:** Local recurrence; regional recurrence; survival.

METHODS *Clinical Evidence* search and appraisal January 2002, and supplementary search of reference lists of all identified review articles and relevant sections of dermatology textbooks.

QUESTION Does the use of sunscreen help to prevent cutaneous squamous cell carcinoma?

Adèle Green

One RCT in people with previous solar keratoses aged > 40 years and living in Victoria, Australia found that daily sunscreen versus placebo sunscreen significantly reduced the incidence of new solar keratoses

after 7 months use. One RCT in adults in a subtropical Australian community found that daily versus discretionary use of sunscreen to the head, neck, arms, and hands significantly reduced the incidence of squamous cell carcinoma after 4.5 years.

Benefits: We found no systematic review. **Versus placebo:** One RCT (588 people with previous solar keratoses, aged > 40 years, and living in Victoria, Australia) found a significant decrease in new solar keratoses after 7 months' use of daily sunscreen versus placebo (mean number of new lesions per person: 1.6 with sunscreen *v* 2.3 with placebo; RR for developing new lesions 0.62, 95% CI 0.54 to 0.71), and a significantly greater chance of lesion remission (OR 1.5, 95% CI 1.3 to 1.8).[8] **Daily versus discretionary use:** One community based RCT (1621 adults in a subtropical Australian community) compared daily use of a sunscreen (sun protection factor 15+) versus sunscreen use at their usual discretionary rate.[9] People allocated to daily use of sunscreen were told to apply it to the head, neck, arms, and hands every morning and reapplication was advised after heavy sweating, bathing, or long sun exposure. They were reminded every 3 months by research staff when sunscreen supplies were replenished. There was a significantly lower incidence of squamous cell carcinoma tumours after 4.5 years (22 people with 28 new squamous cell carcinomas with daily sunscreen use *v* 25 people with 46 new squamous cell carcinomas with discretionary sunscreen use; RR of developing new tumours 0.61, 95% CI 0.46 to 0.81). Subgroup analysis found no significant difference between those with a history of skin cancer and those without.[9] However, confidence intervals were wide, suggesting that the study may have had insufficient power to rule out such a difference.

Harms: Daily sunscreen use in two RCTs caused contact allergy in a small proportion of users (< 10%)[10] and skin irritation in a variable proportion of users (2–15%).[9,10] No people tested were allergic to the active ingredients of sunscreen, whereas irritant reactions both to active sunscreen and the control base cream were observed in the placebo controlled RCT.[8] The RCT of regular versus discretionary use found that daily sunscreen use was not associated with greater sun exposure, including recreational exposure.[9] However, another RCT among young adults who used sunscreen while intentionally exposing themselves to the sun ("sunbathing") found that use of a sun protection factor 30 sunscreen compared with a sun protection factor 10 sunscreen was associated with significantly longer exposure times.[11]

Comment: In a long term prevention trial using skin cancer as the outcome, placebo sunscreen may be regarded as unethical. It would also be difficult to mask treatment allocation. The subgroup analysis comparing people with and without a history of skin cancer had insufficient power to rule out important differences between groups.

Squamous cell carcinoma of the skin: non-metastatic

QUESTION What is the optimal margin for primary excision of cutaneous squamous cell carcinoma?

Robin Marks

We found no RCTs relating size of primary excision margin to local recurrence rate.

Benefits: We found no systematic review or RCTs assessing different excision margins at any sites measuring local recurrence.

Harms: We found no quantified evidence. As with all kinds of surgery, there is a potential for tissue destruction and scarring — particularly of vital structures such as eyelids, lip margins, and motor and sensory nerves.

Comment: One prospective case series using micrographically controlled surgery (see glossary, p 1757) related excision margins to histological extension of the tumour and found a 95% clearance rate of squamous cell carcinomas less than 2 cm in diameter with a margin of 4 mm of normal skin, and a 96% clearance rate of tumours greater than 2 cm with a margin of 6 mm.[12] The sites of scalp, ears, eyelid, nose, and lip were found to have more deeply invasive tumours. Numerous case series suggest that primary excision of cutaneous squamous cell carcinoma has a likelihood of local recurrence varying from 5–20% depending on tumour size, site, histopathological differentiation, perineural involvement, and depth of invasion.[7,13–18]

QUESTION Does micrographically controlled surgery result in lower rates of local recurrence than standard primary excision?

We found no RCTs comparing micrographically controlled (Mohs') surgery (see glossary, p 1757) with standard surgical excision.

Benefits: We found no systematic review or RCTs.

Harms: Although we found no quantified evidence, it is thought that with all kinds of surgery there is potential for tissue destruction and scarring particularly of vital structures such as eyelids, lip margins, and motor and sensory nerves. However, Mohs' microscopic surgery is considered more tissue sparing because of its specificity in determining the amount of normal surrounding tissue removed.

Comment: A review of case series since 1940 suggested a local recurrence rate of 3% for Mohs' surgery compared with 8% for primary excision of cutaneous squamous cell carcinoma. However, the evidence must be treated with caution because of differing study quality, the long time period covered, and potential differences between people referred for Mohs' surgery and those treated with non-Mohs' surgery.[7] A site specific comparison found lower 5 year local recurrence rates after Mohs' surgery for primary squamous cell carcinoma of the lip (2% with Mohs' *v* 16% with primary excision) and of the ear (5% with Mohs' *v* 19% with primary excision).[7]

QUESTION **Does radiotherapy after surgery effect local recurrence of cutaneous squamous cell carcinoma?**

Adèle Green

We found RCTs about the effects of radiotherapy after surgery versus surgery alone on recurrence rates.

Benefits: We found no systematic review or RCTs.

Harms: Although not measured, there is the potential for long term scar deterioration with post-radiation depigmentation and gradual development of chronic radiodermatitis, including telangiectasiae, thinning of the skin, and hyperkeratosis (see glossary, p 1757).

Comment: In rare instances, squamous cell carcinomas cannot be excised completely and these have recurrence rates of over 50%.[19,20] Case series of inadequately excised squamous cell carcinomas, especially those with microscopic perineural invasion (see glossary, p 1757) found at the time of curative surgery, have reported recurrence rates of 20–25% after 5 years when surgery was followed by radiotherapy.[21,22] Ability to detect advanced perineural invasion can be enhanced by the use of computerised tomography or magnetic resonance imaging.[23]

GLOSSARY

Hyperkeratosis Increased scaling on the surface of the skin.

Micrographically controlled surgery does not use standard excision margins as the basis for achieving tumour clearance. The visible tumour and a thin margin of apparently normal skin are removed, mapped, and examined microscopically using a specialised sectioning technique at the time of surgery, and the surgery continues until there is microscopic confirmation of complete tumour clearance, at which stage the wound is closed.[24]

Perineural invasion Tumour invasion along (not in) a nerve.

Radiodermatitis Chronic non-malignant changes in the skin due to excessive radiation.

Telangiectasiae Permanently dilated small blood vessels in the skin.

Xeroderma pigmentosum An inherited disorder with defective repair of DNA damage caused by ultraviolet radiation, resulting in sun related skin cancers of all types at a very early age.

REFERENCES

1. Buettner PG, Raasch BA. Incidence rates of skin cancer in Townsville, Australia. *Int J Cancer* 1998;78:587–593.
2. Bouwes Bavinck JN, Claas FH, Hardie DR, Green A, Vermeer BJ, Hardie IR. The risk of skin cancer in renal transplant recipients in Queensland, Australia: a follow-up study. *Transplantation* 1996;15:715–721.
3. English DR, Armstrong BK, Kricker A, Winter MG, Heenan PJ, Randell PL. Demographic characteristics, pigmentary and cutaneous risk factors for squamous cell carcinoma: a case-control study. *Int J Cancer* 1998;76:628–634.
4. Green A, Battistutta D, Hart V, Leslie D, Weedon D, the Nambour Study Group. Skin cancer in a subtropical Australian population: incidence and lack of association with occupation. *Am J Epidemiol* 1996;144:1034–1040.
5. Kraemer KH, Lee MM, Andrews AD, Lambert WC. The role of sunlight and DNA repair in melanoma and nonmelanoma skin cancer. The xeroderma pigmentosum paradigm. *Arch Dermatol* 1994;130:1018–1021.
6. Johnson TM, Rowe DE, Nelson BR, Swanson NA. Squamous cell carcinoma of the skin (excluding lip and oral mucosa). *J Am Acad Dermatol* 1992;26:467–484.
7. Rowe DE, Carroll RJ, Day CL. Prognostic factors for local recurrence, metastasis, and survival rates in squamous cell carcinoma of the skin, ear, and lip. *J Am Acad Dermatol* 1992;26:976–990.
8. Thompson SC, Jolley D, Marks R. Reduction of solar keratoses by regular sunscreen use. *N Engl J Med* 1993;329:1147–1151.
9. Green A, Williams G, Neale R, et al. Daily sunscreen application and betacarotene supplementation in prevention of basal cell and

squamous-cell carcinomas of the skin: a randomised controlled trial. *Lancet* 1999;354:723–729.

10. Foley P, Nixon R, Marks R, Frowen K, Thompson S. The frequency of reactions to sunscreens: results of a longitudinal population-based study on the regular use of sunscreens in Australia. *Br J Dermatol* 1993;128:512–518.
11. Autier P, Dore JF, Negrier S, et al. Sunscreen use and duration of sun exposure: a double blind randomised trial. *J Natl Cancer Inst* 1999;15:1304–1309.
12. Brodland DG, Zitelli JA. Surgical margins for excision of primary cutaneous squamous cell carcinoma. *J Am Acad Dermatol* 1992;27:241–248.
13. de Visscher JGAM, Botke G, Schakenradd JACM, van der Waal I. A comparison of results after radiotherapy and surgery for stage 1 squamous cell carcinoma of the lower lip. *Head Neck* 1999:526–530.
14. Ashby MA, Smith J, Ainslie J, McEwan L. Treatment of nonmelanoma skin cancer at a large Australian Center. *Cancer* 1989;6:1863–1871.
15. Eroglu A, Berberoglu U, Berreroglu S. Risk factors related to locoregional recurrence in squamous cell carcinoma of the skin. *J Surg Oncol* 1996;61:124–130.
16. McCombe D, MacGill, Ainslie J, Beresford J, Matthews J. Squamous cell carcinoma of the lip: A retrospective review of the Peter MacCallum Cancer Institute experience 1979–88. *Aust NZ J Surg* 2000;70:358–361.
17. Yoon M, Chougule P, Dufresne R, Wanebo HJ. Localised carcinoma of the external ear is an unrecognised aggressive disease with a high propensity for local regional recurrence. *Am J Surg* 1992;164:574–577.
18. Zitsch RP, Park CW, Renner GJ, Rea JL. Outcome analysis for lip carcinoma. *Otolaryngol Head Neck Surg* 1995;113:589–596.
19. Glass RL, Perez-Mesa C. Management of inadequately excised epidermoid carcinoma. *Arch Surg* 1974;108:50–51.
20. Glass RL, Spratt JS, Perez-Mesa C. The fate of inadequately excised epidermoid carcinoma of the skin. *Surg Gynaecol Obstet* 1966;122:245–248.
21. Shimm DS, Wilder RB. Radiation therapy for squamous cell carcinoma of the skin. *Am J Clin Oncol* 1991;14:381–386.
22. McCord MW, Mendenhall WM, Parsons JT, et al. Skin cancer of the head and neck with clinical perineural invasion. *Int J Radiat Oncol Biol Phys* 2000;47:89–93.
23. Williams LS, Mancuso AA, Mendenhall WM. Perineural spread of cutaneous squamous and basal cell carcinoma: CT and MR detection and its impact on patient management and prognosis. *Int J Radiat Oncol Biol Phys* 2001;49:1061–1069.
24. Holmkvist KA, Roenigk RK. Squamous cell carcinoma of the lip treated with Mohs' micrographic surgery: outcome at 5 years. *J Am Acad Dermatol* 1998;38:960–966.

Adèle Green
Professor
Queensland Institute of Medical Research
Brisbane
Australia

Robin Marks
Professor
University of Melbourne
Melbourne
Australia

Competing interests: AG, none declared. RM has undertaken studies in association with 3M Pharmaceuticals on the value of topically applied imiquimod in the management of actinic (solar) keratoses and basal cell carcinoma.

Search date August 2002

Miny Samuel, Rebecca Brooke, and Christopher Griffiths

QUESTIONS

INTERVENTIONS

See glossary, p 1769

Key Messages

Prevention

- **Sunscreens; vitamins (vitamin C and vitamin E)** We found no RCTs on the effects of these interventions in preventing wrinkles.

Treatment

- **Carbon dioxide (CO_2) laser** We found no RCTs comparing CO_2 laser versus placebo or no treatment. Three small RCTs in women with perioral wrinkles found no significant difference with CO_2 laser versus dermabrasion in improvement in wrinkles at 4–6 months. One small RCT found limited evidence that CO_2 laser reduced the wrinkle score significantly less than chemical peel at 6 months. Two small RCTs found that CO_2 laser improved wrinkles more than erbium YAG laser at 2 months and 6 months. Another RCT found no significant difference in wrinkle improvement with CO_2 laser versus erbium YAG laser, but may have been too small to exclude a clinically important difference. One small RCT found no significant difference with CO_2 laser plus YAG laser versus CO_2 laser alone in improvement in upper lip wrinkles at 4 months. Erythema was common but there were no clear difference between treatments.

- **Dermabrasion** We found no RCTs of dermabrasion versus placebo or no treatment. Three small RCTs in women with perioral wrinkles found no significant difference with dermabrasion versus CO_2 laser in improvement in wrinkles at 4–6 months. Adverse effects were commonly reported. Erythema was reported in all three RCTs, two of which found that erythema was significantly more common with laser versus dermabrasion.
- **Facelift** We found no RCTs on the effects of facelifts.
- **Isotretinoin** Two RCTs found that isotretinoin versus vehicle cream significantly improved fine and coarse wrinkles after 36 weeks in people with mild to severe photodamage. Severe facial irritation occurred in 5–10% of people using isotretinoin.
- **Oral natural cartilage polysaccharides** One RCT found limited evidence that an oral commercial preparation of cartilage polysaccharide was no more effective than placebo at reducing wrinkles at 3 months. Another RCT found that a different oral commercial preparation of cartilage polysaccharide versus placebo significantly reduced the number of women with moderate or severe wrinkles at 90 days. We found limited evidence that some commercial preparations may be more effective than others.
- **Retinyl esters** We found no systematic review or RCTs of retinyl esters that evaluated clinical outcomes.
- **Topical antioxidants (ascorbic acid)** One poor quality RCT found limited evidence that an ascorbic acid formulation versus a vehicle cream applied daily to the face for 3 months significantly improved fine and coarse wrinkles. Stinging and erythema were common but were not analysed by treatment.
- **Topical natural cartilage polysaccharides** One small RCT found that a topical commercial preparation of natural cartilage polysaccharide versus placebo significantly reduced the number of fine and coarse wrinkles at 120 days.
- **Tretinoin (for fine wrinkles after 6 months)** RCTs in people with mild to moderate photodamage have found that topical tretinoin versus vehicle cream applied for an average of 6 months significantly improves fine wrinkles. The effect of tretinoin on coarse wrinkles was inconsistent. Common short term adverse effects with tretinoin include itching, burning, and erythema. Skin peeling is the most common persistent adverse effect, which peaks at 12–16 weeks.

DEFINITION Wrinkles, also known as rhytides, are visible creases or folds in the skin. Wrinkles less than 1 mm in width and depth are defined as fine wrinkles and those greater than 1 mm are coarse wrinkles. Most RCTs have studied wrinkles on the face, forearms, and hands.

INCIDENCE/ PREVALENCE We found no information on the incidence of wrinkles alone, only on the incidence of skin photodamage (see glossary, p 1769), which includes a spectrum of features such as wrinkles, hyperpigmentation, tactile roughness, and telangiectasia. The incidence of ultraviolet light associated skin disorders increases with age and develops over several decades. One Australian study (1539 people aged 20–55 years living in Queensland) found moderate to severe photoaging in 72% of men and 47% of women under 30 years of age.[1] The severity of photoaging was significantly greater with increasing age, and was independently associated with solar keratoses ($P < 0.01$) and skin cancer ($P < 0.05$). Wrinkling was more common in people with white skin, especially skin phototypes I and II. One study reported that the incidence of photodamage in European and North American populations with Fitzpatrick skin types I, II, and III (see glossary, p 1769) is about 80–90%.[2] We found few reports of photodamage in black skin (phototypes V and VI).

AETIOLOGY/ RISK FACTORS Wrinkles may be caused by intrinsic factors (e.g. aging, hormonal status, and intercurrent diseases) and by extrinsic factors (e.g. exposure to ultraviolet radiation and cigarette smoke). These factors contribute to epidermal thinning, loss of elasticity, skin fragility, and creases and lines in the skin. The severity of photodamage varies with skin type, which includes skin colour and the capacity to tan.[3] One review of five observational studies found that facial wrinkles in men and women were more common in smokers than in non-smokers.[4] It also found that the risk of moderate to severe wrinkles in lifelong smokers was more than twice that in current smokers (RR 2.57, 95% CI 1.83 to 3.06). Oestrogen deficiency may contribute to wrinkles in postmenopausal women.[5]

PROGNOSIS Although wrinkles cannot be considered a medical illness requiring intervention, concerns about aging that affect quality of life are becoming increasingly common. Such concerns are likely to be influenced by geographical differences, culture, and personal values. In some cases, concerns about physical appearance can lead to difficulties with interpersonal interactions, occupational functioning, and self esteem.[6] In societies in which the aging population is growing and a high value is placed on the maintenance of a youthful appearance, there is a growing preference for interventions that ameliorate the visible signs of aging.

AIMS To prevent skin wrinkling; to improve fine and coarse wrinkling in adults; to minimise adverse effects of treatment; to improve quality of life.

OUTCOMES Physician and patient evaluation of wrinkles, and adverse effects of treatment. We excluded RCTs based solely on non-clinical outcomes such as histological assessment, photography, or optical profilometry. Quality of life was not reported in any trials.

METHODS *Clinical Evidence* update search and appraisal August 2002. Most RCTs recruited people with moderate to severe photodamage and wrinkles, rather than people with wrinkles alone.

QUESTION **What are the effects of interventions to prevent skin wrinkles?**

OPTION **SUNSCREENS**

We found no RCTs on the effects of sunscreens in preventing wrinkles.

Benefits: We found no systematic review or RCTs.

Harms: We found no RCTs.

Comment: We found two non-systematic reviews that reported the effects of sunscreens on the incidence of photodamage and skin cancer, but did not assess the effect of sunscreens in preventing wrinkles.[7,8]

OPTION VITAMINS

We found no RCTs on the effects of vitamins C or E on wrinkles.

Benefits: We found no systematic review or RCTs.

Harms: We found no RCTs.

Comment: None.

QUESTION What are the effects of treatments for skin wrinkles?

OPTION TOPICAL ANTIOXIDANTS

One poor quality RCT found limited evidence that an ascorbic acid formulation versus a vehicle cream applied daily to the face for 3 months significantly improved fine and coarse wrinkling. Stinging and erythema were common but were not quantified according to treatment.

Benefits: We found no systematic review. We found one small and brief RCT (28 people, age 36–72 years, with mild to moderate photodamage [see glossary, p 1769]) comparing topical L-ascorbic acid (0.5 mL) in a vehicle cream versus the vehicle cream alone applied once daily for 12 weeks.[9] Only 19 people completed the trial. Participants were randomly assigned to treatments to the left and right sides of the face. Improvement was assessed by investigators with reference to pretreatment photographs, and graded as "much improved", "improved", "no change", or "worse". Non-intention to treat analysis found that significantly more people had improvement in fine and course wrinkles with ascorbic acid at 12 weeks (16/19 [84%] *v* 3/19 [15.8%]; P = 0.02; coarse wrinkles 13/19 [68%] *v* 6/19 [32%]; P = 0.01). The RCT also found that significantly more participants reported improvement in wrinkles with ascorbic acid versus vehicle cream (number of people reporting wrinkles as being "slightly improved", "improved", or "much improved": 16/19 [84%] *v* 3/19 [16%]; RR 5.33, 95% CI 1.85 to 15.34).

Harms: Adverse effects in the RCT, which were not quantified by treatment given, included stinging in 11 people (55%), erythema in five people (24%), and dry skin in one person (0.05%).[9] Symptoms responded to moisturisation and usually resolved within the first 2 months of treatment.

Comment: The RCT is limited by its small sample size and short duration, and by the high withdrawal rate (9/28 [32%]), which compromises the validity of the results.[9]

OPTION TRETINOIN

RCTs in people with mild to moderate photodamage have found that topical tretinoin versus vehicle cream applied for up to 48 weeks significantly improves fine wrinkles. The effect of tretinoin on coarse wrinkles is inconsistent. Common short term adverse effects with tretinoin included itching, burning, and erythema. Skin peeling was the most common persistent adverse effect, which peaks at 12–16 weeks.

Benefits: We found no systematic review. **Versus vehicle cream:** We found 10 double blind, vehicle controlled RCTs (see web extra table A at www.clinicalevidence.com).[10–19] Seven of these included people with mild to moderate photodamage with Fitzpatrick skin types I–III (see glossary, p 1769). Of the remaining three RCTs, one included people with moderate to severe photodamage (see glossary, p 1769),[19] and the other two did not clearly define the extent of photodamage. The RCTs compared tretinoin (0.1%, 0.05%, 0.01%, 0.025%, and 0.001%) once daily, three times weekly, or once weekly versus a vehicle cream for 12–48 weeks. All of the RCTs found that higher concentrations of tretinoin (0.1% and 0.05%) versus vehicle cream significantly improved fine wrinkles. Of three RCTs comparing lower doses of tretinoin (0.01% and 0.001%),[15,17,18] two found a significant reduction in fine wrinkles[15,18] and one found no significant difference.[17] Assessment of improvement by the participants and investigators was consistent, although the degree of improvement varied. The effect of tretinoin on coarse wrinkles was inconsistent.

Harms: Overall, the most common adverse effects reported after the application of tretinoin were dry skin/peeling, which peaked after 12–16 weeks and tended to be persistent; and itching, burning/stinging, and erythema, which peaked during the first 2 weeks and decreased with time. One RCT found that erythema and scaling occurred in significantly more people taking tretinoin 0.1% versus 0.025% (16/36 [44%] *v* 5/39 [13%]; RR 3.47, 95% CI 1.41 to 8.49).[19] We found individual case reports of congenital defects associated with topical tretinoin used during the first trimester of pregnancy.[20,21] We found one observational study that identified 215 case histories of women who used tretinoin cream for acne during the first trimester of pregnancy and compared them with 430 age matched, non-exposed women who delivered infants at the same hospital.[22] It found no significant difference in the incidence of major congenital disorders (1.9% *v* 2.6%; RR 0.7, 95% CI 0.2 to 2.3).

Comment: The RCTs were limited by small sample sizes, short duration, and inconsistencies among investigator and participant assessments.[10–19]

OPTION RETINYL ESTERS

We found no RCTs of retinyl esters that evaluated clinical outcomes.

Benefits: We found no systematic review or RCTs that evaluated clinical outcomes.

Harms: We found no RCTs.

Comment: None.

OPTION ISOTRETINOIN

In people with mild to severe photodamage, two RCTs found that isotretinoin versus vehicle cream significantly improved fine and coarse wrinkles after 36 weeks. Severe facial irritation occurred in 5–10% of people using isotretinoin.

Benefits: We found no systematic review. We found two RCTs (see web extra table B at www.clinicalevidence.com).[23,24] The first RCT (776 people in 17 US centres, aged 20–76 years, with mild to moderate facial photodamage [see glossary, p 1769]) compared isotretinoin 0.05% applied once daily for 12 weeks followed by 0.1% for another 24 weeks versus vehicle cream for 36 weeks.[23] Baseline assessment of photodamage performed by a physician was graded on a 100 mm visual analogue scale (0 = no change from baseline; +50 mm = improvement; and –50 mm = worse). In addition, photographs taken at baseline were compared after 12, 24, and 36 weeks. Only 613 (79%) people remained in the study at 36 weeks and analysis was not by intention to treat. Physician assessment at 36 weeks found that isotretinoin versus vehicle cream significantly improved overall skin appearance and fine wrinkles (see web extra table B at www.clinicalevidence.com). Participant assessment found no significant difference between treatments in overall skin appearance, but isotretinoin significantly improved fine wrinkles. Pretreatment and post-treatment photographs were also assessed by five dermatologists; all found that isotretinoin significantly improved fine wrinkles (see web extra table B at www.clinicalevidence.com). The second RCT (800 people in 20 European centres, mean age 53.5 years, Fitzpatrick skin types I–IV [see glossary, p 1769] with moderate/severe facial photodamage, mild to severe photodamage of the forearms and hands) compared isotretinoin 0.1% versus vehicle cream for 36 weeks.[24] The methods of the trial were the same as those in the first RCT. Physician assessment at 36 weeks found that isotretinoin versus vehicle cream significantly improved overall appearance, fine and coarse wrinkles of the face, and fine wrinkles of the forearms and hands (see web extra table B at www.clinicalevidence.com). Participant and panel assessment found consistent results.

Harms: The first RCT reported that severe tolerability reactions, which were unspecified, occurred in "less than 5% of people" taking isotretinoin.[23] More people using isotretinoin withdrew from the study because of local irritation (5 *v* 1). The second RCT found that facial symptoms were more common in people using isotretinoin versus vehicle cream: erythema (65% *v* 26%), peeling (54% *v* 8%), burning (64% *v* 16%), and pruritus (45% *v* 13%).[24] Severe facial irritation occurred in 5–10% of people, causing 3.6% of people to discontinue treatment. Irritation usually occurred during the first few weeks of treatment, and was alleviated by emollients or brief interruption of treatment.

Comment: None.

OPTION TOPICAL NATURAL CARTILAGE POLYSACCHARIDES

One small RCT found that a topical commercial preparation of natural cartilage polysaccharide versus placebo significantly reduced the number of fine and coarse wrinkles at 120 days.

Benefits: We found no systematic review. **Versus placebo:** We found one double blind RCT (30 women, aged 40–60 years, with moderate to severe facial wrinkles) comparing application of a commercial preparation of natural cartilage polysaccharide 1% twice daily for 120 days on one side of the face versus placebo on the other.[25] It found that active treatment significantly increased the number of women with no shallow (< 1 mm), moderate (1 mm), or deep (> 1 mm) wrinkles after 120 days (treatment *v* placebo: no shallow wrinkles, 30/30 *v* 0/30; no moderate wrinkles, 27/30 *v* 0/30; no deep wrinkles, 5/30 *v* 2/30; overall P < 0.001).

Harms: No adverse effects were reported by any of the participants in the RCT.[25]

Comment: The RCT is limited by its small sample size and by potential difficulties with concealment of allocation.[25] Application of creams to each side of the face may result in contamination (one side receiving treatment intended for the other side).

OPTION ORAL NATURAL CARTILAGE POLYSACCHARIDES

One RCT found limited evidence that an oral commercial preparation of cartilage polysaccharide was no more effective than placebo at reducing wrinkles at 3 months. Another RCT found that a different oral commercial preparation of cartilage polysaccharide versus placebo significantly reduced the number of women with moderate or severe wrinkles at 90 days. We found limited evidence that some commercial preparations may be more effective than others.

Benefits: We found no systematic review. **Versus placebo:** We found two RCTs.[26,27] The first double blind RCT (144 people, aged 35–50 years, with Fitzpatrick skin type of II or III and mild to moderate photoaging [see glossary, p 1769]) compared a commercial preparation of a cartilage polysaccharide (Imedeen® 400 or 200 mg daily) versus placebo for 3 months.[26] It found no significant difference between either dose of active treatment versus placebo in face or eye wrinkles, as assessed by investigator or subject analyses on a 10 cm visual analogue and by assessment of photographs by a dermatologist. The second RCT (30 women, aged 40–60 years, with moderate to severe wrinkles) compared a different commercial oral cartilage polysaccharide preparation (Vivida® 500 mg daily) versus placebo for 90 days.[27] Assessment of wrinkles by the investigator was measured on a three-point scale (0 = absent; 1 = moderate; 2 = severe). It found that treatment versus placebo significantly reduced the number of women with moderate or severe wrinkles at 45 days (overall P < 0.01) and at 90 days (P < 0.001). **Versus each other:** One double blind RCT (30 women, aged 40–60 years, with moderate to severe wrinkles) compared two commercial preparations.[28] Participants were given Vivida® 500 mg daily or Imedeen® 380 mg daily for 90 days. At 90 days, the RCT found that Vivida® versus Imedeen® significantly increased the number of women with no wrinkles (10/15 [66%] *v* 3/15 [20%]) and reduced the number of women with severe wrinkles (0/15 [0%] *v* 7/15 [47%]; overall P < 0.01). It found no significant difference in the number of women with moderate wrinkles (5/15 [33%] *v* 5/15 [33%]; RR 1.0, 95% CI 0.4 to 2.7).

Harms: The first RCT found no significant difference between Imedeen® and placebo in adverse effects (23/96 [24%] *v* 10/48 [21%]; P > 0.05).[26] Acne and seborrhoea were the most common skin related events (24/38 [63%]), and oedema and weight increase were the most frequently reported non-skin related events (18/47 [38%]), but the proportions attributable to active treatment or placebo were not specified. The second RCT reported that "some" people taking Vivida® developed mild pimples during the first 3–4 weeks.[27] In the third RCT, 5/30 (33%) of people using Vivida® had mild facial pimples during the first 3–4 weeks versus no adverse effects in the Imedeen group.[28]

Comment: In the RCT of Vivida® versus placebo, the grading of wrinkling is unusual in that wrinkles were only graded as severe, moderate, or absent.[27] One might have expected that wrinkles would have reduced from moderate/severe to mild rather than to absent. The RCTs are small, and the possibility of publication bias cannot be excluded. The available evidence is inadequate to assess accurately the effects of oral cartilage preparations.

OPTION DERMABRASION

We found no RCTs of dermabrasion versus placebo or no treatment. Three small RCTs in women with perioral wrinkles found no significant difference between dermabrasion versus carbon dioxide (CO_2) laser in improvement of wrinkles at 4–6 months. Adverse effects were commonly reported. Erythema was reported in all three RCTs, two of which found that erythema was significantly more common with laser versus dermabrasion.

Benefits: **Versus placebo/control:** We found no RCTs. **Versus CO_2 laser:** We found three RCTs comparing dermabrasion versus a CO_2 laser.[29–31] The first RCT (20 women, 48–76 years old with moderate/severe wrinkles of the upper lip, Fitzpatrick skin types I–III [see glossary, p 1769]) compared dermabrasion with a coarse diamond fraize versus CO_2 laser to the left or right upper lip.[29] Upper lip wrinkles were graded as 0 (none) to 5 (severe) by an independent investigator before treatment and 6 months later. The average pretreatment wrinkle score was 4.3 for the laser side and 4.4 for the dermabrasion side. The RCT found no significant difference in wrinkle score between treatments at 6 months (areas retaining wrinkle score of 4/5: 1/19 [5%] with dermabrasion *v* 2/19 [11%] laser; P = 0.22). The second RCT (15 women, 46–73 years old with perioral wrinkles, Fitzpatrick skin types I–III) compared dermabrasion versus a CO_2 laser to the left and right sides of the perioral area.[30] The mean pretreatment wrinkle score on both sides of the perioral area was 3.73 (1 = mild; 5 = severe). The RCT found no significant difference in mean post-treatment wrinkle score at 4 months, as assessed by the investigator (2.64 with laser *v* 2.79 with dermabrasion; P = 0.35). The third RCT (20 women, 44–74 years old with perioral wrinkles, moderate to severe photodamage [see glossary, p 1769], Fitzpatrick skin type not specified) compared dermabrasion versus a CO_2 laser to the left or right sides of the perioral area.[31] Photographs of participants assessed by plastic surgeons were graded in terms of improvement in wrinkles (0 = no improvement to 5 = best improvement) at 1 and 6 months after treatment. The RCT found that laser versus dermabrasion significantly improved the wrinkle score at 1 month (2.33 *v* 2.01;

P = 0.002) but not at 6 months (2.55 *v* 2.22; P = 0.02). The RCT also found that significantly more people rated a greater improvement in wrinkles with laser versus dermabrasion at 6 months (13/20 [65%] *v* 3/20 [15%]; P = 0.001; 4 people reported no difference).

Harms: In the first RCT, 85% of women had erythema on the upper lip, which was similar on CO_2 laser and dermabrasion sides 1 month after treatment.[29] In 10% of people the erythema was worse on the laser treated side, and in 5% it was worse on the dermabraded side. The average duration of erythema was 2.5 months for both treatments. One woman developed a hypertrophic scar on the dermabraded side. Three people developed herpetic lesions several days after treatment, despite being given prophylaxis with valaciclovir. Other complications such as pain, oedema, eczema, and whiteheads resolved either spontaneously or with minimal treatment. The second RCT found that erythema was significantly increased on the laser versus dermabrasion side at 1 month (P = 0.003) but not at 4 months (P = 0.15).[30] The third RCT found that laser versus dermabrasion significantly increased erythema at 1 month (P < 0.001).[31] Also, significantly more people reported that "post-treatment drainage" was worse with laser versus dermabrasion (10/20 [50%] *v* 2/20 [10%]; P = 0.002).

Comment: The RCTs found inconsistent results, were small, and may not have been powered to detect a significant difference between treatments.[29–31] The RCTs varied in their grading of wrinkles, and in participant and investigator assessments. The available evidence is insufficient to define the effects of dermabrasion for wrinkles.

OPTION CARBON DIOXIDE LASER

We found no RCTs of carbon dioxide (CO_2) laser versus placebo or no treatment. Three small RCTs in women with perioral wrinkles found no significant difference with CO_2 laser versus dermabrasion in improvement in wrinkles at 4–6 months.One small RCT found limited evidence that CO_2 laser reduced the wrinkle score significantly less than chemical peel at 6 months. Two small RCTs found that CO_2 laser improved wrinkles more than erbium YAG laser at 2 months and 6 months. Another RCT found no significant difference in wrinkle improvement with CO_2 laser versus erbium YAG laser, but it may have been too small to exclude a clinically important difference. One small RCT found no difference between CO_2 laser plus YAG laser in improvement of upper lip wrinkles at 4 months. Erythema was common, but there was no clear difference between treatments.

Benefits: We found no systematic review. **Versus placebo/no treatment:** We found no RCTs. **Versus dermabrasion:** See benefits of dermabrasion, p 1766. **Versus chemical peel:** We found one double blind RCT (20 women, aged 51–71 years, with upper lip wrinkles, Fitzpatrick skin types I–III [see glossary, p 1769]) comparing a CO_2 laser versus a phenol chemical peel.[32] At the start of the RCT, photographs of each participant were graded by an independent investigator in terms of the severity of upper lip wrinkles (0 = none; 5 = severe). Participants were then randomised to receive laser treatment on one side of the upper lip versus chemical peel on the other. The RCT found that CO_2 laser reduced the wrinkle score significantly less than chemical peel at 6 months (wrinkle score reduced from 4.30 to 1.11 with laser *v* 4.20 to 0.47 with chemical peel; mean difference in post treatment score 0.54, $P < 0.03$; see comment). **Versus erbium:YAG laser:** We found three RCTs.[33–35] The first RCT (21 women, aged 39–74 years, with upper lip wrinkles, Fitzpatrick skin types I–IV, double blind) comparing variable pulse erbium:YAG laser (see glossary, p 1769) versus CO_2 laser to the left or right sides of the upper lip.[33] Photographs and digital images of participants were recorded preoperatively and at intervals up to 2 months after treatment. The RCT found that there was a greater overall improvement (which was not defined) in wrinkles with CO_2 laser versus YAG laser (improvement: 63% *v* 54%; P value not stated). The second RCT (13 people [12 were women] aged 30–80 years, with perioral or periorbital wrinkles, Fitzpatrick skin types I–III) compared treatment with one pass pulsed CO_2 laser versus four passes erbium:YAG laser to periorbital or perioral sites or both.[34] Each participant received CO_2 on one side of the face and erbium:YAG laser on the other by random allocation. Wrinkles were graded from zero (absent) to eight (severe) based on photographs. The RCT found no significant difference between treatments for wrinkle improvement (time to outcome not stated; average improvement in wrinkle scores from baseline about 1–2 points in both groups; P value not provided for difference). However, it may have been too small to exclude a clinically important difference. The third RCT (21 people [19 were women] aged 18–90 years, with perioral or periorbital wrinkles, Fitzpatrick skin types I–III) compared variable pulse erbium:YAG laser versus CO_2 laser to the left or right sides of the face by alternate allocation.[35] Photographs of participants were taken preoperatively and at 1 week, 2 weeks, 2 months, and 6 months. Investigators and participants were not blinded to treatment allocation, but a blinded panel of dermatologists also assessed outcomes. The RCT found that CO_2 laser improved wrinkles significantly more than erbium:YAG laser at 6 months (measured by aggregate of investigators', participants' and panel's combined assessment; $P < 0.03$; further data not provided; see comment). **Plus variable pulse erbium:YAG laser:** We found one double blind RCT (20 people, aged 42–72 years with upper lip wrinkles, Fitzpatrick skin types I–III) comparing CO_2 laser versus CO_2 laser plus variable pulse erbium:YAG laser to right or left sides of the upper lip.[36] Photographs recorded before treatment and at intervals after treatment for up to 4 months were graded by investigators, but no details of grading were provided. The RCT found no significant difference in improvement in perioral wrinkles at 4 months (67.5% with laser alone *v* 68.5% with combination; P value not stated).

Harms: **Versus chemical peel:** The RCT found that 55% of people had erythema and/or coagulum on the upper lip; in 35% of people this was more severe on the chemical peel side, and in 10% it was more severe on the laser treated side.[32] One person developed an 8 mm hypertrophic scar on the phenol treated side. Herpes simplex infection was reported in three people, which responded to valaciclovir (treatment side not reported). **Versus erbium:YAG laser:** In the first RCT, postoperative erythema occurred with both treatments, but there was no significant difference (P values not provided).[33] Only one person was reported to have mild hyperpigmentation at around 4 weeks after treatment with erbium:YAG laser, which had cleared by 3 months. The second RCT found that postoperative erythema was significantly less frequent with CO_2 laser versus erbium:YAG laser at 2 weeks ($P < 0.04$), but rates were similar at 2 and 6 months.[34] The RCT found no significant difference between treatments for rates of hyperpigmentation. The third RCT found that both treatments were associated with erythema (at 2 weeks: AR 67% with erbium:YAG laser *v* 95% with CO_2 laser; at 2 months: AR 24% with erbium:YAG laser *v* 62% with CO_2 laser; at 6 months: AR for mild erythema 0% with erbium:YAG laser *v* 10% with CO_2 laser).[35] Hypopigmentation (5% with erbium:YAG laser *v* 43% with CO_2 laser; $P < 0.05$) and hyperpigmentation (24% with erbium:YAG laser *v* 29% with CO_2 laser) were seen. Hyperpigmentation resolved spontaneously in all cases within 6 months. **Plus variable pulse erbium:YAG laser:** The RCT reported no significant difference between treatments in erythema or pain.[36]

Comment: The effects of chemical peels and CO_2 lasers are likely to be dependent on the expertise of the dermatological surgeon, and therefore results may not generalise to different populations.[32] The difference in outcomes was not expressed dichotomously, and the clinical importance of the mean "0.54 units" difference in wrinkle score with CO_2 laser versus chemical peel is difficult to interpret. The available evidence is too weak to define the effects of CO_2 laser on wrinkles.[32] The results of the third RCT comparing CO_2 versus erbium:YAG laser should be interpreted with caution as the participants and investigators were not blinded to treatment allocation.

OPTION FACELIFT

We found no systematic review or RCTs on the effects of facelifts.

Benefits: We found no systematic review and no RCTs.

Harms: We found no RCTs.

Comment: The effectiveness and safety of facelift surgery is likely to depend on the expertise of the surgeon.

GLOSSARY

Erbium:YAG laser An yttrium aluminium garnet laser.

Fitzpatrick skin phototype classification I = always burns easily, never tans; II = always burns easily, tans minimally; III = burns moderately, tans gradually (light brown); IV = burns minimally, always tans well (brown); V = rarely burns, tans profusely (dark brown); VI = never burns, deeply pigmented (black).

Mild/moderate/severe photodamage A spectrum of features including wrinkles, hyperpigmentation, tactile roughness, and telangiectasia. Usually measured on a scale from 0 to 9 (0 = none; 1–3 = mild; 4–6 = moderate; and 7–9 = severe).

Substantive changes

Carbon dioxide laser Two new RCTs;[35,36] conclusions unchanged.

REFERENCES

1. Green AC. Premature aging of the skin in a Queensland population. *Clin Exp Dermatol* 1991;155:473–478.
2. Maddin S, Lauharanta J, Agache P, et al. Isotretinoin improves the appearance of photodamaged skin: results of a 36-week, multicenter, double-blind, placebo-controlled trial. *J Am Acad Dermatol* 2000;42:56–63.
3. Nagashima H, Hanada K, Hashimoto I. Correlation of skin phototype with facial wrinkle formation. *Photodermatol Photoimmunol Photomed* 1999;15:2–6.
4. Grady D, Ernster V. Does cigarette smoking make you ugly and old? *Am J Epidemiol* 1992;135:839–842.
5. Affinito P, Palomba S, Sorrentino C, et al. Effects of postmenopausal hypoestrogenism on skin collagen. *Maturitas* 1999;15:239–247.
6. Gupta MA, Gupta AK. Photodamaged skin and quality of life: reasons for therapy. *J Dermatol Treat* 1996;7:261–264.
7. Alsarraaf R. Outcomes research in facial plastic surgery: a review and new directions. *Aesthetic Plast Surg* 2000;24:192–197.
8. Boyd AS, Naylor M, Cameron GS, et al. The effects of chronic sunscreen use on the histologic changes of dermatoheliosis. *J Am Acad Dermatol* 1995;33:941–946.
9. Traikovich SS. Use of topical ascorbic acid and its effects on photodamaged skin topography. *Arch Otolaryngol Head Neck Surg* 1999;125:1091–1098.
10. Weiss JS, Ellis CN, Headington JT, et al. Topical tretinoin improves photoaged skin. *JAMA* 1988;259:527–532.
11. Leyden JJ, Grove GL, Grove MJ, et al. Treatment of photodamaged facial skin with topical tretinoin. *J Am Acad Dermatol* 1989;21:638–644.
12. Lever L, Kumar P, Marks R. Topical retinoic acid for treatment of solar damage. *Br J Dermatol* 1990; 122:91–98.
13. Barel AO, Delune M, Clarys P, et al. Treatment of photodamaged facial skin with topical tretinoin: a blinded, vehicle-controlled half-side study. *Nouv Dermatol* 1995;14:585–591.
14. Lowe PM, Woods J, Lewis A, et al. Topical tretinoin improves the appearance of photo damaged skin. *Australas J Dermatol* 1994;35:1–9.
15. Weinstein GD, Nigra TP, Pochi PE, et al. Topical tretinoin for treatment of photodamaged skin. *Arch Dermatol* 1991;127:659–665.
16. Salagnac V, Leonard F, Lacharriere Y, et al. Topical treatment of actinic aging with vitamin A acid at various concentrations. *Rev Fr Gynecol Obstet* 1991;86:458–460.
17. Olsen EA, Katz HI, Levine N, et al. Tretinoin emollient cream: a new therapy for photodamaged skin. *J Am Acad Dermatol* 1992;26:215–224.
18. Andreano J, Bergfeld WF, Medendorp SV. Tretinoin emollient cream 0.01% for the treatment of photoaged skin. *Cleve Clin J Med* 1993;60:49–55.
19. Griffiths CEM, Kang S, Ellis CN, et al. Two concentrations of topical tretinoin (retinoic acid) cause similar improvement of photoaging but different degrees of irritation. *Arch Dermatol* 1995;131:1037–1044.
20. Lipson AH, Collins F, Webster WS. Multiple congenital defects associated with maternal use of topical tretinoin. *Lancet* 1993;341:1352–1353.
21. Camera G, Pregliasco P. Ear malformation in baby born to mother using tretinoin cream. *Lancet* 1992;339:687.
22. Jick SS, Terris BZ, Jick H. First trimester topical tretinoin and congenital disorders. *Lancet* 1993;341:1181–1182.
23. Sendagorta E, Lesiewicz J, Armstrong RB. Topical isotretinoin for photodamaged skin. *J Am Acad Dermatol* 1992;27:S15–S18.
24. Maddin S, Lauharanta J, Agache P, et al. Isotretinoin improves the appearance of photodamaged skin: results of a 36-week, multicenter, double blind, placebo-controlled trial. *J Am Acad Dermatol* 2000;42:56–63.
25. Lassus A, Eskelinen A, Santalahti J. The effect of Vivida® cream as compared with placebo cream in the treatment of sun-damaged or age-damaged facial skin. *J Int Med Res* 1992;20:381–391.
26. Kieffer ME, Efsen J. Imedeen® in the treatment of photoaged skin: an efficacy and safety trial over 12 months. *J Eur Acad Dermatol Venereol* 1998;11:129–136.
27. Eskelinen A, Santalahti J. Special natural cartilage polysaccharides for the treatment of sun-damaged skin in females. *J Int Med Res* 1992;20:99–105.
28. Eskelinen A, Santalahti J. Natural cartilage polysaccharides for the treatment of sun-damaged skin in females: a double-blind comparison of Vivida® and Imedeen®. *J Int Med Res* 1992; 20:227–233.
29. Gin I, Chew J, Rau KA, et al. Treatment of upper lip wrinkles: a comparison of the 950 μsec dwell time carbon dioxide laser to manual tumescent dermabrasion. *Dermatol Surg* 1999;25:468–474.
30. Holmkvist KA, Rogers GS. Treatment of perioral rhytides. *Arch Dermatol* 2000;136:725–731.
31. Kitzmiller WJ, Visscher M, Page DA, et al. A controlled evaluation of dermabrasion versus CO_2 laser resurfacing for the treatment of perioral wrinkles. *Plast Reconstr Surg* 2000;106:1366–1372.
32. Chew J, Gin I, Rau KA, et al. Treatment of upper lip wrinkles: a comparison of 950 μsec dwell time carbon dioxide laser with unoccluded baker's phenol chemical peel. *Dermatol Surg* 1999; 25:262–266.
33. Newman JB, Lord JL, Ash K, et al. Variable pulse erbium:YAG laser skin resurfacing of perioral rhytides and side-by-side comparison with carbon dioxide laser. *Lasers Surg Med* 2000;26:208–214.
34. Ross EV, Miller C, Meehan K, et al. One-pass CO_2 versus multiple-pass Er:YAG laser resurfacing in the treatment of rhytides: a comparison side-by-side study of pulsed CO_2 and Er:YAG lasers. *Dermatol Surg 2001;27:709–715.*
35. Khatri KA, Ross V, Grevelink LM, et al. Comparison of Erbium:YAG and carbon dioxide lasers in resurfacing of facial rhytides. *Arch Dermatol* 1999;135:391–397.
36. McDaniel DH, Lord J, Ash K, et al. Combined CO_2/Erbium:YAG laser resurfacing of peri-oral rhytides and side-by-side comparison with carbon dioxide laser alone. *Dermatol Surg* 1999;25:285–293.

Miny Samuel
EBM Analyst
NMRC Clinical Trials & Epidemiology
Research Unit
Singapore

Rebecca Brooke
Research Fellow
Dermatology Centre
University of Manchester
School of Medicine
Manchester
UK

Christopher Griffiths
Professor of Dermatology
University of Manchester
Manchester
UK

Competing interests: MS none declared. CG has been a paid consultant to Johnson & Johnson, the manufacturers of Tretinoin; he has also received fees for speaking from Johnson & Johnson.

Sleep apnoea (obstructive sleep apnoea-hypopnoea syndrome)

Search date August 2001

Michael Hensley

QUESTIONS

INTERVENTIONS

See glossary, p 1781

Key Messages

- **Nasal continuous positive airway pressure in moderate to severe obstructive sleep apnoea-hypopnoea syndrome (OSAHS)** Systematic reviews and subsequent RCTs have found that nasal continuous positive airway pressure (CPAP) versus control or no treatment reduces daytime sleepiness, improves vigilance and cognitive functioning, and reduces depression after 1–3 months.
- **Nasal continuous positive airway pressure in mild OSAHS** One systematic review has found no significant difference with nasal continuous positive airway pressure versus conservative treatment or placebo tablets in daytime sleepiness, but found significant improvement in some measures of cognitive performance at about 4 weeks.
- **Oral appliance in mild OSAHS** One RCT found a significant reduction in apnoea/hypopnoea index with oral appliances, but found no significant difference in daytime sleepiness or quality of life at 12 months with oral appliances that produce anterior advancement of the mandible versus uvulopalatopharyngoplasty.
- **Oral appliance in moderate to severe OSAHS** RCTs have found that oral appliances that produce anterior advancement of the mandible versus no treatment or versus control oral appliances significantly reduce daytime sleepiness and sleep disordered breathing at 1–2 weeks.
- **Weight loss in mild OSAHS** One systematic review found no RCTs on the effects of weight loss in people with mild obstructive sleep apnoea-hypopnoea syndrome.
- **Weight loss in moderate to severe OSAHS** One systematic review found no RCTs on the effects of weight loss in people with moderate to severe OSAHS.

Clin Evid 2002;8:1772–1784.

DEFINITION Obstructive sleep apnoea-hypopnoea syndrome (OSAHS) is abnormal breathing during sleep that causes recurrent arousals, sleep fragmentation, and nocturnal hypoxaemia. It is associated with daytime sleepiness, impaired vigilance and cognitive functioning, and reduced quality of life.[1,2] The diagnosis is made when a person with daytime symptoms has significant sleep disordered breathing (see glossary, p 1782) revealed by polysomnography (study of sleep state, breathing, and oxygenation) or by more limited studies. Criteria for the diagnosis of significant sleep disordered breathing have not been rigorously assessed, but have been set by consensus and convention.[3,4] The criteria are based on the finding of sleep disordered breathing, reported as the number of abnormal breathing events in 1 hour of sleep (for full polysomnography) or in 1 hour in bed for home based monitoring systems that do not include electroencephalography recordings. There are differences in the measurement techniques and the criteria used: the criteria for hypopnoea (see glossary, p 1782) may or may not include associated hypoxaemia or arousal and the criteria vary for a significant obstructive event that is not apnoea (see glossary, p 1781) or hypopnoea. In OSAHS, apnoeas and hypopnoeas are associated with absent or reduced airflow despite normal or increased inspiratory effort, but may also involve reduced inspiratory effort. However, many healthy people, especially the elderly, can have frequent apnoeas and hypopnoeas. Diagnostic tests are not completely sensitive or specific. For example, an apnoea/hypopnoea index (see glossary, p 1781) of 5–20 episodes an hour is often used to define borderline to mild OSAHS, 20–35 to define moderate OSAHS, and more than 35 to define severe OSAHS,[5] but people with upper airway resistance syndrome (see glossary, p 1782) have an index below 5 episodes an hour[6] and many healthy elderly people have an index greater than 5 episodes an hour.[7] In an effort to obtain an international consensus, some new criteria were proposed but these have not been widely adopted.[8] The ultimate test for clinically significant OSAHS is to demonstrate clinical improvement in daytime symptoms after correction of sleep disordered breathing by a treatment. Clinically important sleep disordered breathing can also occur without apnoeas or hypopnoeas (upper airway resistance syndrome).[6] In this topic, the criteria for OSAHS include apnoeas and hypopnoeas caused by upper airway obstruction. Central sleep apnoea and sleep associated hypoventilation syndromes are not covered here.

INCIDENCE/ PREVALENCE The Wisconsin Sleep Cohort Study of over 1000 people (mean age 47 years) in North America found a prevalence of apnoea/hypopnoea index greater than five episodes an hour in 24% of men and 9% of women, and of OSAHS with an index greater than 5 plus excessive sleepiness in 4% of men and 2% of women.[9] There are international differences in the occurrence of OSAHS for which obesity is considered to be an important determinant.[10] Ethnic differences in prevalence have also been found after adjustment for other risk factors.[7,10] Little is known about the burden of illness in developing countries.

AETIOLOGY/ RISK FACTORS The site of the upper airway obstruction in the OSAHS is around the level of the tongue, soft palate, or epiglottis. Disorders that predispose to either narrowing of the upper airway or reduction in its stability (e.g. obesity, certain craniofacial abnormalities, vocal cord abnormalities, and enlarged tonsils) have been associated with an increased risk of OSAHS. It has been estimated that a 1 kg/m^2 increase in body mass index (3.2 kg for a person 1.8 m tall) leads to a 30% increase (95% CI 13% to 50%) in the relative risk of developing abnormal sleep disordered breathing (apnoea/hypopnoea index ≥5/h) over a period of 4 years.[10] Other strong associations include increasing age and sex (the male to female ratio is 2 : 1); weaker associations include menopause, family history, smoking, and night time nasal congestion.[10]

PROGNOSIS The long term prognosis of people with untreated severe OSAHS is poor with respect to quality of life, likelihood of motor vehicle accidents, hypertension, and possibly cardiovascular disease and premature mortality.[11] Unfortunately the prognosis of both treated and untreated OSAHS is unclear.[7] The limitations in the evidence include bias in the selection of subjects, short duration of follow up, and variation in the measurement of confounders (e.g. smoking, alcohol use, and other cardiovascular risk factors). The widespread use of treatments complicates the evidence on prognosis for untreated OSAHS. Observational studies support a causal association between OSAHS and systemic hypertension, which increases with the severity of OSAHS (OR 1.21 for mild OSAHS to 3.07 for severe OSAHS).[11] OSAHS increases the risk of motor vehicle accidents three- to sevenfold.[11,12] It is associated with increased risk of premature mortality, cardiovascular disease, and impaired neurocognitive functioning.[11]

AIMS To minimise or eliminate symptoms of daytime sleepiness; to improve vigilance and quality of life; to reduce or abolish the increased risk of motor vehicle accidents and cardiovascular events; to enhance compliance with treatment; to minimise adverse effects of treatment.

OUTCOMES **Daytime sleepiness:** subjective and objective measures such as Epworth Sleepiness Scale, Multiple Sleep Latency Test, and Maintenance of Wakefulness Test. **Quality of life:** general measures such as the Medical Outcomes Study 36-item Short Form Health Survey and the General Health Questionnaire; measures of mood such as the Hospital Anxiety and Depression Scale, the Beck Depression Inventory, and the Profile of Mood States; measures of energy and vitality such as the 36-item Short Form SF-36 energy scale, the UWIST Mood Adjective Checklist, and the energy and vitality scale of the Nottingham Health Profile. Disease specific quality of life measures include the Functional Outcomes of Sleep Questionnaire. **Cognitive performance measures:** Steer Clear, Trailmaking Test B, Digit Symbol Substitution, and Paced Auditory Serial Addition-2 Second Timing. **Mortality and morbidity:** for example, road traffic accidents, hypertension, stroke, cardiac failure, and ischaemic heart disease. **Intermediate outcomes:** measures of the degree of disturbed breathing during sleep, such as the number of apnoeas and hypopnoeas an hour (apnoea/hypopnoea index), the frequency of arousals, and the degree of sleep fragmentation. Details of individual scales will be expanded in future *Clinical Evidence* updates.

METHODS *Clinical Evidence* search and appraisal August 2001 plus an additional hand search. Different RCTs have used slightly different definitions of OSAHS. An attempt has been made to provide some details of the definitions used. Further clarification will be attempted in future *Clinical Evidence* updates.

QUESTION **What are the effects of treatment of moderate to severe obstructive sleep apnoea-hypopnoea syndrome?**

OPTION **NASAL CONTINUOUS POSITIVE AIRWAY PRESSURE IN MODERATE TO SEVERE OBSTRUCTIVE SLEEP APNOEA-HYPOPNOEA SYNDROME**

Systematic reviews and subsequent RCTs have found that nasal continuous positive airway pressure versus control or no treatment reduces daytime sleepiness, improves vigilance and cognitive functioning, and reduces depression in people with moderate to severe obstructive sleep apnoea-hypopnoea syndrome.

Benefits: **Versus no treatment:** We found one systematic review (search date 1999, 1 RCT) comparing nasal continuous positive airway pressure (CPAP) (see glossary, p 1781) versus control for 3 months.[5] The RCT (105 people with severe obstructive sleep apnoea-hypopnoea syndrome [OSAHS], mean [apnoea/hypopnoea index — see glossary, p 1781] 56/h and mean Epworth Sleepiness Scale 12) found that nasal CPAP versus control significantly reduced daytime sleepiness (mean Epworth Sleepiness Scale was reduced from 12.1 to 5.6 with nasal CPAP, $P < 0.01$, CI not provided; and was reduced from 11.4 to 10.6 with control, NS).[13] The RCT also found significant improvement in the sleepiness and social isolation subsets of an energy and vitality scale (Nottingham Health Profile) (see table 1, p 1784). **Versus sham/subtherapeutic nasal CPAP:** We found one systematic review (search date 1999, 1 RCT)[5] and two subsequent RCTs[15,16] that compared nasal CPAP versus sham/subtherapeutic nasal CPAP (see glossary, p 1782). The RCT identified by the systematic review (101 people with moderate to severe OSAHS) found that nasal CPAP versus sham/subtherapeutic nasal CPAP significantly improved daytime sleepiness (Epworth Sleepiness Scale 7.0, $P < 0.0001$, CI not provided; Maintenance of Wakefulness Test 6.75 min, $P = 0.005$, CI not provided).[18] The first subsequent RCT (55 people with moderate to severe [sleep disordered breathing — see glossary, p 1782], all with an apnoea/hypopnoea index > 30/h [average > 50/h], but with no or very little complaint of excessive daytime sleepiness [average Epworth Sleepiness Scale was 7/24, normal is < 10/24]) found no significant difference with nasal CPAP versus sham nasal CPAP in daytime sleepiness after 6 weeks (change in Epworth Sleepiness Scale: 1, 95% CI 0 to 2 with nasal CPAP *v* 1, 95% CI 0 to 2 with sham nasal CPAP).[15] It also found no significant difference in a range of measures of cognitive functioning or in 24 hour blood pressure readings. The second subsequent RCT (59 men with an Epworth Sleepiness Scale > 10 and moderate to severe OSAHS; 48 people included in this RCT were also included in the RCT described above)[18] compared the effects of nasal CPAP versus sham nasal CPAP on simulated driving performance for 1 month.[16] It found that nasal CPAP versus sham nasal CPAP significantly improved daytime sleepiness (subjective measures, $P = 0.0006$; objective measures, $P = 0.003$; CI not provided) (see table 1, p 1784). **Versus oral placebo tablets:** We found two systematic reviews[5,14] and one subsequent RCT[17] comparing nasal CPAP versus oral placebo tablets. One systematic review (search date 1996,[14] 1 crossover RCT,[19] 32 people) compared nasal CPAP versus oral placebo tablet in people with moderate OSAHS. All RCTs in that systematic review were found to have some methodological shortcomings and a meta-analysis was not done. The RCT found significant improvement with nasal CPAP versus oral placebo tablets for sleep latency (Multiple Sleep Latency Test 7.2 min *v* 6.1 min, $P = 0.03$; CI not provided), cognitive functioning (Trailmaking Test B, $P = 0.02$; Steer Clear, $P = 0.01$; Digit Symbol Substitution, $P = 0.05$; intelligence quotient decrement, $P = 0.04$; CI not provided), anxiety (Hospital Anxiety and Depression Scale, $P = 0.02$; CI not provided), depression (Hospital Anxiety and Depression Scale, $P = 0.002$; CI not provided), and general health (General Health Questionnaire, $P = 0.003$; Nottingham Health Profile, $P = 0.002$; CI not provided). The other systematic review (search date 1999,[5] 1 RCT[20]) found that nasal CPAP versus oral placebo tablet significantly improved cognitive performance on two measures (Paced Auditory Serial Addition-2 Second Timing, $P = 0.001$; and Steer Clear, $P = 0.03$; CI not provided) but not on two others (Trailmaking Test B and Digit Symbol Substitution). It also found a significant improvement in depression (Hospital Anxiety Depression Scale, $P = 0.02$; CI not provided). The subsequent RCT (68 people with moderate to severe OSAHS, apnoea/hypopnoea index range 15–129/h, Epworth Sleepiness Scale range 6–24) compared the effect of nasal CPAP versus oral placebo tablet on 24 hour blood pressure over 4 weeks.[17] It found that nasal CPAP versus oral placebo tablet significantly decreased the mean 24 hour diastolic blood pressure (77.8 mmHg with nasal CPAP *v* 79.2 mmHg with placebo tablet; mean difference –1.5 mmHg, 95% CI –3.0 to –0.1 mmHg; $P = 0.04$), improved daytime sleepiness (Epworth Sleepiness Scale 10.1 with nasal CPAP *v* 12.5 with placebo tablet; $P = 0.001$), and quality of life (Functional Outcomes of Sleep Questionnaire total score 12.4 with nasal CPAP *v* 11.6 with placebo tablet; $P = 0.01$) (see table 1, p 1784).[17] **Versus oral appliances:** We found one systematic review (search date 1996,[14] 60 people, 3 RCTs[21–23]) comparing nasal CPAP versus oral appliances (see glossary, p 1782) (removable mandibular advancement devices). It found that nasal CPAP versus oral appliance significantly improved apnoea/hypopnoea index (WMD –7.3/h, –10.0 to –4.7/h). One RCT included in the review found no significant difference in sleepiness with nasal CPAP versus oral appliances.[23] Overall, the review found that people preferred an oral appliance over nasal CPAP (OR 9.5, 95% CI 4.3 to 21.1; heterogeneity between trials observed) (see table 1, p 1784).[14]

Harms: Neither of the systematic reviews summarised any harmful effects found in the RCTs that were reviewed.[5,14] One systematic review (search date 1999) reported a high prevalence of minor side effects from nasal CPAP treatment, the most common being dry mouth, nose, and throat (40%).[5] We found a case series (52 consecutive people with severe OSAHS, mean oxygen desaturation index 43/h) in which the occurrence of nasopharyngeal symptoms was studied systematically before and after nasal CPAP.[24] It found that nasopharyngeal symptoms were common before nasal CPAP in OSAHS (nasal dryness 74%, sneezing 51%, blocked nose 43%, and rhinorrhoea 37%) and increased during nasal CPAP (sneezing 75% and rhinorrhoea 57%), with greater discomfort in winter. Other adverse effects of nasal CPAP include local effects of the mask on the nasal bridge, mask discomfort, nasal congestion, rhinitis, sore eyes, headache, chest discomfort, and noise disturbance.

Comment: The OSAHS RCTs have problems with their methods. The evaluation of severity of sleep disordered breathing (using apnoea/hypopnoea index, etc) is not a good guide to severity of daytime sleepiness.[15] Some RCTs have compared nasal CPAP against a variety of "placebo" interventions, most recently sham or subtherapeutic nasal CPAP. RCT evidence reports short term outcomes not mortality, motor vehicle accident rate, hypertension, stroke, and ischaemic heart disease.

OPTION WEIGHT LOSS IN MODERATE TO SEVERE OBSTRUCTIVE SLEEP APNOEA-HYPOPNOEA SYNDROME

We found no RCTs on the effect of weight loss in people with moderate to severe obstructive sleep apnoea-hypopnoea syndrome.

Benefits: We found one systematic review (search date 2000), which found no RCTs on the effect of weight loss in people with obstructive sleep apnoea-hypopnoea syndrome (OSAHS).[25]

Harms: We found no RCTs on the effects of weight loss in people with OSAHS.

Comment: One review of the effect of body weight in OSAHS found no RCT but included a number of case series in which weight loss, especially that achieved by surgery, was associated with improvement in people with mostly severe OSAHS.[26] Large relative improvements in apnoea/hypopnoea index (–72% to –98%) were found after a weight loss of 30–70% of initial weight.[26] It seems that weight loss has the potential to benefit obese persons with OSAHS. There is consensus that advice about weight reduction is an important component of management. However, weight loss is difficult with conservative techniques and may need to be combined with nasal continuous positive airway pressure in people with moderate and severe OSAHS.

OPTION ORAL APPLIANCES IN MODERATE TO SEVERE OBSTRUCTIVE SLEEP APNOEA-HYPOPNOEA SYNDROME

RCTs have found that oral appliances that produce anterior advancement of the mandible versus no treatment or versus control oral appliances significantly reduce daytime sleepiness and sleep disordered breathing at 1–2 weeks in people with moderate to severe obstructive sleep apnoea-hypopnoea syndrome.

Benefits: **Versus no treatment:** We found no systematic review but found one RCT.[27] The RCT (crossover; 24 people with moderate obstructive sleep apnoea-hypopnoea syndrome [OSAHS]; mean apnoea/hypopnoea index [see glossary, p 1781] 26.7, 95% CI 20.6 to 33.2] and significant daytime sleepiness [Epworth Sleepiness Scale 11.9, 95% CI 10.3 to 13.5]) compared use of two different oral appliances (see glossary, p 1782) (A and B, which produced mandibular advancement) versus no treatment for 1 week each. It found that after 1 week, the two oral appliances significantly reduced subjective daytime sleepiness (Epworth Sleepiness Scale 9, 95% CI 6.5 to 11 with oral appliance A; 9, 95% CI 6.5 to 10.0 with oral appliance B; and 13.5, 95% CI 9.5 to 16 with no oral appliance; $P < 0.01$ for each oral appliance *v* no oral appliance) and sleep disordered breathing (see glossary, p 1782) (apnoea/hypopnoea index 8.7, 95% CI 5.8 to 11.6 with oral appliance A; 7.9, 95% CI 4.8 to 11.0 with oral appliance B; 22.6, 95% CI 16.5 to 28.7 with no oral appliance; $P < 0.05$ for each oral appliance *v* no oral appliance). It also found that oral appliance versus no treatment significantly reduced interference with daily tasks, snoring frequency and loudness, and improved performance ability and energy level. **Versus control oral appliances:** We found two RCTs comparing an oral appliance that produced anterior advancement of the mandible (removable mandibular advancement device) versus an oral appliance that did not (control).[28,29] The first RCT (24 adults with loud snoring and severe OSAHS) found that, after 2 weeks, mandibular advancement device versus control oral appliance significantly reduced daytime sleepiness (Epworth Sleepiness Scale –3.8 with mandibular advancement device *v* –0.5 with control oral appliance; $P < 0.005$).[28] There was a significant withdrawal rate, with only 10 mandibular advancement device and 8 control subjects providing outcome data after 2 weeks of treatment. The second RCT (crossover study, 28 people with moderate to severe OSAHS [average apnoea/hypopnoea index 27/h]) compared a mandibular advancement splint versus control (oral appliance that did not advance the mandible) for 1 week each.[29] It found that mandibular advancement splint versus control oral appliance significantly improved daytime sleepiness (Epworth Sleepiness Scale 3.9 with mandibular advancement splint *v* 10.1 with control oral appliance; $P < 0.01$; CI not provided) and apnoea/hypopnoea index (14/h with mandibular advancement splint *v* 30/h with control oral appliance; $P < 0.0001$; CI not provided). It also found that with the mandibular advancement splint there was a complete response (resolution of symptoms plus an apnoea/hypopnoea index < 5/h) in nine (37.5%), a partial response (improved symptoms plus ≥ 50%

reduction in apnoea/hypopnoea index) in six (25%), and failure in nine (37.5%). The treatment outcome was not related to the baseline severity of OSAHS. **Versus nasal continuous positive airway pressure:** See benefits of nasal continuous positive airway pressure in moderate to severe OSAHS, p 1775.

Harms: **Versus no treatment:** The RCT did not report on adverse effects.[27] A cohort study (22 people involved in the RCT) investigated adverse effects over 12–30 months.[30] It found that adverse effects were common (mucosal dryness [86%], tooth discomfort [59%], and hypersalivation [55%]) but did not require discontinuation of treatment. **Versus control oral appliances:** The first RCT did not report on adverse effects.[28] The second RCT reported the following adverse effects: excessive salivation (50%), gum irritation (20%), mouth dryness (46%), jaw discomfort (12.5%), and tooth grinding (12.5%).[29] Those adverse effects were described as mild to moderate, lasting less than 3 weeks, and not preventing the use of the mandibular advancement splint.

Comment: Oral appliances are commonly used for snoring. We found one systematic review (search date 1994, 304 people with mean apnoea/hypopnoea index in the severe range, 21 publications, 19 case series studies), which found that about 70% of people had a 50% or greater reduction in apnoea/hypopnoea index.[31] There is insufficient evidence about long term effectiveness and adverse effects.

QUESTION **What are the effects of treatment for mild obstructive sleep apnoea-hypopnoea syndrome?**

OPTION **NASAL CONTINUOUS POSITIVE AIRWAY PRESSURE IN MILD OBSTRUCTIVE SLEEP APNOEA-HYPOPNOEA SYNDROME**

One systematic review found no significant difference with nasal continuous positive airway pressure versus conservative treatment or placebo tablets in daytime sleepiness, but found significant improvement in some measures of cognitive performance in people with mild obstructive sleep apnoea-hypopnoea syndrome.

Benefits: **Versus no treatment:** We found no RCTs. **Versus conservative treatment or oral placebo tablets:** We found one systematic review (search date 1999, 4 RCTs, 208 people with mild obstructive sleep apnoea-hypopnoea syndrome [OSAHS]) reporting on effects of nasal continuous positive airway pressure (CPAP) versus conservative treatment (sleep hygiene and advice about weight reduction) or oral placebo tablet for at least 4 weeks.[5] The review found no significant difference with nasal CPAP versus conservative treatment or oral placebo tablet for daytime sleepiness (1 RCT:[32] mean reduction in Epworth Sleepiness Scale –0.57, 95% CI –1.39 to +0.25; 3 RCTs:[33–35] Multiple Sleep Latency Test, graphical representation; mean effect around 0 with 95% CI of about ±0.7). It found no significant difference with nasal CPAP versus conservative treatment or oral placebo tablets for two measures of cognitive performance (Steer Clear, 2 RCTs;[32,33] or Digit Symbol Substitution,

2 RCTs[32,34]) but found significant improvement in two other measures of cognitive performance (3 RCTs, Trailmaking Test B:[32–34] P = 0.003; 2 RCTs, Paced Auditory Serial Addition-2 Second Timing:[32,33] P < 0.0001; CI not provided). The review found no significant difference with nasal CPAP versus oral placebo tablet for quality of life (2 RCTs, 36-item Short Form general perception)[32,34] and anxiety measures (2 RCTs, Hospital Anxiety and Depression Scale),[32,33] but found significant improvement for depression (2 RCTS, Hospital Anxiety and Depression Scale;[32,33] 1 RCT, Beck Depression Inventory;[34] combined P = 0.0004) and for energy and vitality (2 RCTs, 36-item Short Form vitality;[32,34] 1 RCT, UWIST Mood Adaptive Checklist Energetic Arousal Score;[33] combined P = 0.013; 1 RCT, energy/fatigue subscore of MOD;[35] P < 0.05). The three RCTs that reported a symptom score (in-house questionnaires using an analogue scale) showed a significant benefit (combined P = 0.006).[32–34]

Harms: The systematic review grouped mild and moderate to severe OSAHS for reporting of side effects (See harms of nasal CPAP in moderate to severe OSAHS, p 1777).

Comment: People with mild OSAHS find nasal CPAP less acceptable. People with an apnoea/hypopnoea index (see glossary, p 1781) below 15/hour have been found to have half the long term use of nasal CPAP compared with people with an apnoea/hypopnoea index greater than 15/hour.[36]

OPTION WEIGHT LOSS IN MILD OBSTRUCTIVE SLEEP APNOEA-HYPOPNOEA SYNDROME

One systematic review found no RCTs on the effect of weight loss in people with mild obstructive sleep apnoea-hypopnoea syndrome.

Benefits: We found one systematic review (search date 2000) that found no RCTs on the effect of weight loss on in people with obstructive sleep apnoea-hypopnoea syndrome (OSAHS).[25]

Harms: We found no RCTs on the effect of weight loss in people with mild OSAHS.

Comment: We found one large population based cohort study (690 people with sleep disordered breathing, including those who did not qualify for diagnosis of obstructive sleep apnoea-hypopnoea syndrome) that evaluated sleep disordered breathing at 4 year intervals over 10 years.[37] It found an association between changes in weight and apnoea/hypopnoea index (see glossary, p 1781): a weight gain of 10% was associated with an increase in apnoea/hypopnoea index of 32% (95% CI 20% to 45%) and a weight loss of 10% was associated with a decrease in apnoea/hypopnoea index of 26% (95 % CI 18% to 34%).

OPTION ORAL APPLIANCES IN MILD OBSTRUCTIVE SLEEP APNOEA-HYPOPNOEA SYNDROME

One RCT found no significant difference in daytime sleepiness or quality of life with oral appliances that produce anterior advancement of the mandible versus uvulopalatopharyngoplasty, but found a significant reduction in apnoea/hypopnoea index with oral appliances in people with mild obstructive sleep apnoea-hypopnoea syndrome.

Benefits: **Versus surgical treatment (uvulopalatopharyngoplasty):** We found three RCTs comparing an oral appliance (see glossary, p 1782) (producing anterior advancement of the mandible) versus uvulopalatopharyngoplasty;[38–40] however, they were all related to the same RCT of 95 people with mild obstructive sleep apnoea-hypopnoea syndrome (mean [apnoea/hypopnoea index — see glossary, p 1781] 18.2/h, 95% CI 15.7/h to 20.8/h in oral appliance group; 20.4/h, 95% CI 17.4/h to 23.3/h in the uvulopalatopharyngoplasty group). Successful treatment was defined as a reduction in apnoea/hypopnoea index to less than 10/hour. The RCT found significant improvement in apnoea/hypopnoea index with oral appliance versus uvulopalatopharyngoplasty at 12 months (78% with oral appliance *v* 51% with uvulopalatopharyngoplasty; $P < 0.05$; CI not provided). The RCT found no significant difference between oral appliance versus uvulopalatopharyngoplasty in daytime sleepiness (as measured using 5 questions, with a 5 point scale for each),[38] quality of life (Minor Symptoms Evaluation Profile), or vitality, contentment, and sleep.[40] The uvulopalatopharyngoplasty group had a better contentment score.

Harms: The RCTs on oral appliances have generally been too brief to evaluate significant side effects. See harms of oral appliances in moderate to severe obstructive sleep apnoea-hypopnoea syndrome, p 1779.

Comment: Oral appliances are used commonly for people with snoring with or without mild sleep apnoea. Although the number and duration of trials are not ideal, there is consensus oral appliances are effective.[41]

GLOSSARY

Apnoea Cessation of airflow at the nose and mouth for at least 10 seconds. Sometimes defined indirectly in terms of oxygen desaturation index (impact on pulse oximetry saturation is measured as the number of occasions an hour when oxygen saturation falls by ≥ 4%). Apnoeas may be "central", in which there is cessation of inspiratory effort, or "obstructive", in which inspiratory efforts continue but are ineffective because of upper airway obstruction.

Apnoea/hypopnoea index The sum of apnoeas and hypopnoeas per hour of sleep. Although the generally accepted cutpoint for "normal" is an index of 5/hour, there are a number of definitions of normal of which at least four are applicable to the situation of sleep disordered breathing: levels that are inside the range found in a "normal" (i.e. healthy) population; levels that are well removed from those found in a target disorder such as obstructive sleep apnoea-hypopnoea syndrome; levels that are not associated with a significant risk of disease and disability; and levels for which there is evidence of a significant benefit of treatment.[4]

Continuous positive airway pressure (CPAP) Involves the application of positive pressure from a blower motor to the upper airway through tubing and a soft nasal mask or a face mask. It provides a "pneumatic splint" to the upper airway. Because nasal delivery is the most common in the published literature, we refer to "nasal CPAP". There appears to be little or no difference in effectiveness between nasal or facial delivery of CPAP.

Hypopnoea A major reduction (> 50%) in airflow at the nose and mouth for at least 10 seconds. A smaller reduction in airflow may be accepted as hypopnoea if it is associated with either an arousal or a reduction in oxygen saturation of 4% or more.

Oral appliance The term "oral appliance" is generic for devices that are placed in the mouth in order to change the position of the mandible, tongue, and other structures in the upper airway to reduce snoring or the upper airway obstruction of obstructive sleep apnoea-hypopnoea syndrome. Specific types are referred to as mandibular advancement devices or splints.

Sham/subtherapeutic nasal continuous positive airway pressure This involves the use of the nasal mask and continuous positive airway pressure machine, but with inadequate pressure generated to overcome upper airway obstruction during sleep.

Sleep disordered breathing Can be described as apnoeas (no airflow for 10 s or more) or hypopnoeas (markedly reduced airflow for 10 s or more). The choice of 10 seconds is by convention. The usual measure of the degree of sleep disordered breathing is the apnoea/hypopnoea index. Features of sleep disordered breathing include snoring, witnessed episodes of absent breathing (apnoeas), abnormal breathing during sleep, nocturnal hypoxaemia, and abnormal sleep architecture.

Upper airway resistance syndrome Measurement of inspiratory effort by oesophageal pressure shows recurrent episodes of increased inspiratory effort that maintain stable ventilation but are associated with arousals and sleep fragmentation. These episodes are also referred to as respiratory effort related arousal events.[8] More recent techniques of measuring nasal air flow can show changes consistent with upper airway resistance syndrome without the need for an oesophageal pressure catheter.[42]

REFERENCES

1. Gastaut H, Tassarini CA, Duron B. Polygraphic study of the episodic diurnal and nocturnal (hypnic and respiratory) manifestations of the Pickwick syndrome. *Brain Res* 1965;2:167–186.
2. Bassari AG, Guilleminault C. Clinical features and evaluation of obstructive sleep apnea hypopnea syndrome. In: Kryger MH, Roth T, Dement WC, eds. *Principles and practice of sleep medicine*. Philadelphia, PA: WB Saunders, 2000: 869–878.
3. Ross SD, Sheinhait IA, Harrison KJ, et al. Systematic review and meta-analysis of the literature regarding the diagnosis of sleep apnea. *Sleep* 2000;23:519–532.
4. Sackett DL, Straus SE, Richardson WS, Rosenberg W, Haynes RB. *Evidence-based medicine. How to practice and teach EBM*. Edinburgh: Churchill Livingstone, 2000:69–70.
5. National Health and Medical Research Council of Australia. *Effectiveness of nasal continuous airway pressure (nCPAP) in obstructive sleep apnoea in adults*. National Health and Medical Research Council of Australia, 2000. http://www.health.gov.au/nhmrc/publications/pdf/hpr21.pdf Search date 1999; primary sources Medline, Cochrane Library, some HTA websites, CRD website, Veteran Affairs Research website, hand searches of reference lists of review articles, and personal contact with experts.
6. Guilleminault C, Stoohs R, Clerk A, Cetel M, Maistros P. A cause of excessive daytime sleepiness. The upper airway resistance syndrome. *Chest* 1993;104:781–787
7. Lindberg E, Gislason T. Epidemiology of sleep-related obstructive breathing. *Sleep Med Reviews* 2000;4:411–433.
8. American Academy of Sleep Medicine Task Force (Flemons W, Chair). Sleep-related breathing disorders in adults: recommendations for syndrome definition and measurement techniques in clinical research. *Sleep* 1999;22:667–689.
9. Young T, Palta M, Dempsey J, Skatrud J, Weber S, Badr S. The occurrence of sleep-disordered breathing among middle-aged adults. *N Engl J Med* 1993;328:1230–1235.
10. Young TB, Peppard P. Epidemiology of obstructive sleep apnea. In: McNicholas WT, Phillipson EA, eds. *Breathing disorders in sleep*. London, UK: WB Saunders, 2002:31–43.
11. Redline S. Morbidity, mortality and public health burden of sleep apnea. In: McNicholas WT, Phillipson EA, eds. *Breathing disorders in sleep*. London, UK: WB Saunders, 2002:222–235.
12. George CFP. Reduction in motor vehicle collisions following treatment of sleep apnoea with nasal CPAP. *Thorax* 2001;56:508–512.
13. Ballester E, Badia JR, Hernandez L, et al. Evidence of the effectiveness of continuous positive airway pressure in the treatment of sleep apnea/hypopnea syndrome. *Am J Respir Crit Care Med* 1999;159:495–501.
14. Wright J, White J. Continuous positive airways pressure for obstructive sleep apnoea (Cochrane Review). In: The Cochrane Library, Issue 3, 2000. Oxford: Update Software. Search date 1996; primary sources Medline, Embase, Cinahl, hand searches of reference lists of identified papers, and personal contact with researchers and clinical experts.

15. Barbe F, Mayoralas LR, Duran J, et al. Treatment with continuous airway pressure is not effective in patients with sleep apnea but no daytime sleepiness. A randomised, controlled trial. *Ann Int Med* 2001;134:1015–1023.
16. Hack M, Davies RJ, Mullins R, et al. Randomised prospective parallel trial of therapeutic versus subtherapeutic nasal continuous positive airway pressure on simulated steering performance in patients with obstructive sleep apnoea. *Thorax* 2000;55:224–231.
17. Faccenda JF, Mackay TW, Boon NA, Douglas NJ. Randomised placebo-controlled trial of continuous positive airway pressure on blood pressure in the sleep apnea-hypopnea syndrome. *Am J Respir Crit Care Med* 2001;163:344–348.
18. Jenkinson C, Davies RJO, Mullins R, Stradling JR. Comparison of therapeutic and subtherapeutic nasal continuous positive airway pressure for obstructive sleep apnoea: a randomised prospective parallel trial. *Lancet* 1999;353:2100–2105.
19. Engleman HM, Martin SE, Deary IJ, Douglas NJ. Effect of continuous positive airway pressure treatment on daytime function in sleep apnoea/hypopnoea syndrome. *Lancet* 1994;343:572–575.
20. Douglas NJ. Systematic review of the efficacy of nasal CPAP. *Thorax* 1998;53:414–415.
21. Clark GT, Blumenfeld I, Yoffe N, Peled E, Lavie P. A crossover study comparing the efficacy of continuous airway pressure with anterior mandibular positioning devices on patients with obstructive sleep apnea. *Chest* 1996;109:1477–1483.
22. Ferguson KA, Ono T, Lowe AA, Keenan SP, Fleetham JA. A randomized crossover study of an oral appliance vs nasal-continuous positive airway pressure in the treatment of mild-moderate obstructive sleep apnea. *Chest* 1996;109:1269–1275.
23. Ferguson KA, Ono T, Lowe AA, al-Majed S, Love LL, Fleetham JA. A short term controlled trial of an adjustable oral appliance for the treatment of mild to moderate obstructive sleep apnoea. *Thorax* 1997;52:362–368.
24. Brander PE, Soirinsuo M, Lohela P. Nasopharyngeal symptoms in patients with obstructive sleep apnea syndrome. *Respiration* 1999;66:128–135.
25. Shneerson J, Wright J. Lifestyle modification ofr obstructive sleep apnoea (Cochrane Review). In: The Cochrane Library, Issue 1, 2001. Oxford: Update Software. Search date 2000; primary sources Cochrane Airways Group Trials Register, Medline, Embase, Cinahl and hand searches of reference lists of review articles.
26. Barvaux VA, Aubert G, Rodenstein DO. Weight loss as a treatment for obstructive sleep apnoea. *Sleep Med Rev* 2000;4:435–452.
27. Bloch KE, Iseli A, Zhang JN, et al. A randomized, controlled crossover trial of two oral appliances for sleep apnea treatment. *Am J Respir Crit Care Med* 2000;162:246–251.
28. Hans MG, Nelson S, Luks VG, Lorkovich P, Baek S-J. Comparison of two dental devices for treatment of obstructive sleep apnea syndrome (OSAS). *Am J Orthod Dentofac Orthop* 1997;111:562–570.
29. Mehta A, Qian J, Petocz P, Darendeliler MA, Cistulli PA. A randomized controlled study of a mandibular advancement splint for obstructive sleep apnea. *Am J Respir Crit Care Med* 2001;163:1457–1461.
30. Fritsch KM, Iselli A, Russi EW, Bloch KE. Side effects of mandibular advancement devices for sleep apnea treatment. *Am J Respir Crit Care Med* 2001;164:813–818.
31. Schmidt-Nowra W, Lowe A, Wiegand L, Cartwright R, Perez-Guerra F, Menn S. Oral appliance for the treatment of snoring and obstructive sleep apnea: a review. *Sleep* 1995;18:501–510. Search date 1994; primary sources Medline, and consultation with experts.
32. Engleman HM, Kingshott RN, Wraith PK, Mackay TW, Deary IJ, Douglas NJ. Randomised placebo-controlled crossover trial of continuous positive airway pressure for mild sleep apnea/hypopnea syndrome. *Am J Respir Crit Care Med* 1999;159:461–467.
33. Engleman HM, Martin SE, Deary IJ, Douglas NJ. Effect of CPAP therapy on daytime function in patients with mild sleep apnoea/hypopnoea syndrome. *Thorax* 1997;52:114–119.
34. Barnes M, Houston D, Worsnop CJ, et al. A randomised controlled trial of CPAP in mild obstructive sleep apnea. *Am J Resp Crit Care Med* 2002;165:773–780.
35. Redline S, Adams N, Strauss ME, Roebuck T, Winters M, Rosenberg C. Improvement of mild sleep-disordered breathing with CPAP compared with conservative therapy. *Am J Respir Crit Care Med* 1998;157:858–865.
36. McArdle N, Dvereux G, Heidarnejad H, Engleman HM, Mackay TW, Douglas NJ. Long-term use of CPAP therapy for sleep apnea/hypopnea syndrome. *Am J Respir Crit Care Med* 1999;159:1108–1114.
37. Peppard PE, Young T, Dempsey J, Skatrud. Longitudinal study of moderate weight change and sleep-disordered breathing. *JAMA* 2000;284:3015–3021.
38. Wilhelmsson B, Tegelberg A, Walker-Engstrom ML, et al. A prospective randomized study of a dental appliance compared with uvulopalatopharyngoplasty in the treatment of obstructive sleep apnoea. *Acta Otolaryngol* 1999;119:503–509.
39. Tegelberg A, Wilhelmsson B, Walker-Engstrom ML, et al. Effects and adverse events of a dental appliance for treatment of obstructive sleep apnoea. *Swed Dent J* 1999;23:117–126.
40. Walker Engstrom ML, Wilhelmsson B, Tegelberg A, Dimenas E. Ringqvist I. Quality of life assessment of treatment with dental appliance or UPPP in patients with mild to moderate obstructive sleep apnoea. A prospective randomized 1-year follow-up study. *J Sleep Res* 2000;9:303–308.
41. Ferguson K. Oral appliance therapy for obstructive sleep apnea. Finally evidence you can sink your teeth into (editorial). *Am J Resp Crit Care Med* 2001;163:1294–1295.
42. Ayappa I, Norman RG, Krieger AC, Rosen A, O'Malley RL, Rapoport DM. Non-invasive detection of respiratory effort-related arousals (RERAs) by a nasal cannula/pressure transducer system. *Sleep* 2000;23:763–761.

Michael Hensley
Professor of Medicine
University of Newcastle
Newcastle
Australia

Competing interests: None declared

TABLE 1 Effects of nasal continuous positive airway pressure in moderate to severe obstructive sleep apnoea-hypopnoea syndrome(see text, p 1775).

Ref	Evidence type	Intervention/control	Outcome measure	Treatment effect and accuracy
14	SR	CPAP/placebo	Patient preference placebo/CPAP (OR)	0.4 (95% CI 0.2 to 0.8)
	SR	CPAP/oral appliance	Patient preference oral appliance/CPAP (OR)	9.5 (95% CI 4.3 to 21.1)
5	SR	CPAP/no or minimal other treatment	ESS	–5.84 (95% CI –8.3 to –3.38)
			MSLT	1.7 ($P < 0.001$; CI not provided)
15	RCT (no or minimal daytime sleepiness)	CPAP/sham CPAP	Change in ESS in CPAP group	1 (95% CI 0 to 2)
			Change in ESS in sham CPAP group	1 (95% CI 0 to 2)
			Change in MSLT (min) in CPAP group	1 (95% CI –1 to +3)
			Change in MSLT (min) in sham CPAP group	1 (95% CI –1 to +3)
			Change in FOSQ in CPAP group	7 (95% CI 2 to 12)
			Change in FOSQ in sham CPAP group	3 (95% CI –3 to +9)
16	RCT	CPAP/sham CPAP	ESS change in sham CPAP group	–3.0 (95% CI –11.8 to + 1.8)
			ESS change in CPAP group	–9.0 (95% CI –16.8 to –2.0)
			MWT change in sham CPAP group	0.0 (95% CI –9.9 to +15.6)
			MWT change in CPAP group	7.1 (%% CI – to +28.5)
17	RCT	CPAP/oral placebo	24 hour diastolic blood pressure mean difference (mmHg; CPAP minus placebo)	–1.5 (95% CI –3.0 to –0.1; $P = 0.04$)
			ESS difference (CPAP minus placebo)	–2.4 ($P = 0.001$; CI not provided)
			FOSQ score difference (CPAP minus placebo)	0.8 ($P = 0.01$)

CPAP, continuous positive airway pressure; ESS, Epworth Sleepiness Scale; FOSQ, Functional Outcomes in Sleep Questionnaire; MSLT, Multiple Sleep Latency Test; MWT, Maintenance of Wakefulness Test; SR, systematic review.

Breast cancer: metastatic

Search date April 2002

Stephen Johnston and Justin Stebbing

QUESTIONS

INTERVENTIONS

* Not based on RCT evidence

See glossary, p 1804

Breast cancer: metastatic

Key Messages

- **Anthracycline based regimens (CAF) containing doxorubicin as first line treatment** RCTs have found that combination chemotherapy regimens containing an anthracycline, such as doxorubicin (CAF), versus other regimens as first line treatment significantly increase response rates, time to progression, and survival.
- **Bisphosphonates for bone metastases** RCTs in women receiving standard chemotherapy for bone metastases secondary to metastatic breast cancer have found that bisphosphonates versus placebo significantly reduce and delay skeletal complications. None of the RCTs found an impact on overall survival.
- **Classical combination chemotherapy (CMF)** One systematic review has found that classical combination chemotherapy versus modified regimens as first line treatment significantly increases response rate and survival.
- **Combined gonadorelin analogues and tamoxifen in premenopausal women** RCTs (in premenopausal women with oestrogen receptor positive metastatic breast cancer) have found that first line treatment with gonadorelin analogues plus tamoxifen versus gonadorelin analogues alone significantly improves response rates, overall survival, and progression free survival.
- **First line chemotherapy plus monoclonal antibody (in women with overexpressed HER2 neu oncogene)** One RCT found that, in women whose tumours overexpress HER2, standard chemotherapy plus the monoclonal antibody trastuzumab versus standard chemotherapy alone as first line treatment significantly increased the time to disease progression, objective response, and overall survival.
- **High dose chemotherapy (*v* conventional chemotherapy) as first line treatment** One RCT (in women who had complete or partial response to standard induction chemotherapy) found no significant difference in overall survival at 3 years with additional high dose versus standard dose chemotherapy as first line treatment.
- **New cytotoxic drugs in anthracycline resistant disease (such as taxanes and semisynthetic vinca alkaloids) as second line treatment** RCTs suggest that second line treatment with the docetaxel or vinorelbine versus standard relapse regimens may improve response rates, especially in women with anthracycline resistant disease.
- **Ovarian ablation as first line treatment in premenopausal women (*v* tamoxifen)** One systematic review and one subsequent RCT in premenopausal women found no significant difference in response rate, duration of response, or survival with ovarian ablation (surgery or irradiation) versus tamoxifen as first line treatment. Ovarian ablation is associated with substantial adverse effects such as hot flushes and "tumour flare".
- **Progestins as first line treatment (*v* tamoxifen, beneficial in women with bone pain or anorexia)** RCTs found no significant difference in response rates, remission rates, or survival between progestins versus tamoxifen as first line treatment, but found that progestins increased adverse effects, including nausea, weight gain, and exacerbations of hypertension. One RCT found that medroxyprogesterone versus tamoxifen significantly improved bone pain. Observational evidence suggests that progestins may increase appetite, weight gain, and well being.

- **Progestins (v aromatase inhibitors) as second line treatment** RCTs have found that in postmenopausal women with metastatic breast cancer who have relapsed on adjuvant tamoxifen or progressed during first line treatment with tamoxifen, the selective aromatase inhibitors anastrozole, letrozole, and exemestane prolong survival compared with progestins or aminoglutethimide, with minimal adverse effects.
- **Radiotherapy for spinal cord compression** We found no RCTs. Retrospective analyses found that early radiotherapy improved outcomes, but fewer than 10% of people walked again if severe deterioration of motor function occurred before radiotherapy.
- **Radiotherapy plus appropriate analgesia** We found no RCTs comparing radiotherapy versus no treatment or versus bisphosphonates. We found limited evidence from non-randomised studies that persistent and localised bone pain can be treated successfully in over 80% of women with radiotherapy plus concomitant appropriate analgesia (from non-steroidal anti-inflammatory drugs to morphine and its derivatives). RCTs found no evidence that short courses are less effective for pain relief than long courses of radiotherapy. One RCT found that different fractionation schedules can be used to treat neuropathic bone pain effectively.
- **Radiotherapy plus high dose steroids in spinal cord compression** One small RCT found that adding high dose steroids to radiotherapy improved the chance of walking after 6 months.
- **Radiotherapy to control cerebral and choroidal metastases** We found no RCTs. Retrospective studies suggest that whole brain radiation produces general improvement in neurological function in 40–70% of women with brain metastases secondary to breast cancer, and that radiotherapy benefits 70% of women with choroidal metastases.
- **Selective aromatase inhibitors as first line hormonal treatment in postmenopausal women** RCTs have found that the aromatase inhibitor anastrozole as first line treatment in metastatic postmenopausal breast cancer is at least as effective as tamoxifen in reducing time to disease progression, and found that the aromatase inhibitor letrozole was superior to tamoxifen in reducing time to disease progression.
- **Selective aromatase inhibitors as second line hormonal treatment in postmenopausal women** RCTs in postmenopausal women who have relapsed during or after treatment with tamoxifen have found that the selective aromatase inhibitors anastrozole, letrozole, and exemestane versus progestins or aminoglutethimide significantly increase overall survival at 2–3 years, and are associated with fewer adverse effects.
- **Tamoxifen as first line treatment in oestrogen receptor positive disease** RCTs have found prolonged remission with tamoxifen in the first line treatment of women with oestrogen receptor positive metastatic breast cancer.

DEFINITION Metastatic or advanced breast cancer is the presence of disease at distant sites such as the bone, liver, or lung. It is not treatable by primary surgery and is currently considered incurable. However, young people with good performance status may survive for 15 to 20 years.[1] Symptoms may include pain from bone metastases, breathlessness from spread to the lung, and nausea or abdominal discomfort from liver involvement.

INCIDENCE/ PREVALENCE Breast cancer is the second most frequent cancer in the world (1.05 million people) and is by far the most common malignant disease in women (22% of all new cancer cases). Worldwide, the ratio of mortality to incidence is about 36%. It ranks fifth as a cause of death from cancer overall (although it is the leading cause of mortality in women — the 370 000 annual deaths represent 13.9% of cancer deaths in women). In the USA, metastatic breast cancer causes 46 000 deaths, and in the UK causes 15 000 deaths.[2] It is the most prevalent cancer in the world today and there are an estimated 3.9 million women alive who have had breast cancer diagnosed in the past 5 years (compared, for example, with lung cancer, where there are 1.4 million alive). The true prevalence of metastatic disease is high because some women live with the disease for many years. Since 1990, there has been an overall increase in incidence rates of about 1.5% annually.[3]

AETIOLOGY/ RISK FACTORS The risk of metastatic disease relates to known prognostic factors in the original primary tumour. These factors include oestrogen receptor negative disease, primary tumours 3 cm or more in diameter, and axillary node involvement — recurrence occurred within 10 years of adjuvant chemotherapy for early breast cancer (see glossary, p 1805) in 60–70% of node positive women and 25–30% of node negative women in one large systematic review.[4]

PROGNOSIS Prognosis depends on age, extent of disease, and oestrogen receptor status. There is also evidence that overexpression of the product of the HER2/neu oncogene, which occurs in about a third of women with metastatic breast cancer, is associated with a worse prognosis.[5] A short disease free interval (see glossary, p 1805) (e.g. < 1 year) between surgery for early breast cancer and developing metastases suggests that the recurrent disease is likely to be resistant to the drug used for adjuvant treatment (see glossary, p 1804).[6] In women who receive no treatment for metastatic disease, the median survival from diagnosis of metastases is 12 months.[7] The choice of first line treatment (see glossary, p 1805) (hormonal or chemotherapy) is based on a variety of clinical factors (see table 1, p 1810).[8–11] In many countries there is evidence of a decrease in death rates in recent years, evident in the USA, Canada, and some European countries. This probably reflects improvements in treatment (and therefore improved survival) as well as earlier diagnosis.[2,12]

AIMS To relieve symptoms, prolong life, and improve quality of life, with minimal adverse effects.

OUTCOMES Symptoms; progression free survival; overall objective response rate; complete response; partial response (see glossary, p 1805); duration of response; disease stabilisation; time to progression of disease (progression defined > 25% increase in lesion size or the appearance of new lesions); quality of life;[13] improvement in performance status (according to validated scales of daily functioning/activity);[14] adverse effects and toxicity of treatment;[15] and overall survival. Response to treatment is a surrogate outcome measure for assessing the effects of treatment on survival or quality of life. The link between clinical and proxy outcomes has not been clearly validated. Women who respond to treatment are more likely to experience improved symptomatic relief, performance status, and survival.[16–18] One recent prospective study (300 women with metastatic breast cancer) found a significant relationship between improvement and objective response for three symptoms, in particular cancer pain, shortness of breath, and abnormal mood. Symptom improvement was greatest in those women who had a complete or partial response.[19]

METHODS *Clinical Evidence* update search and appraisal April 2002. We looked for good quality systematic reviews that used the outcome measures listed above. Where we found no good systematic reviews, we selected relevant randomised phase III trials using these outcomes. Studies presented only in abstract form were discarded. Response to treatment is often assessed in an unblinded fashion, introducing the possibility of bias. We found few trials of good quality that reported on symptoms or quality of life.

QUESTION **What are the effects of first line treatments?**

OPTION **ANTIOESTROGENS (TAMOXIFEN)**

RCTs have found that antioestrogens such as tamoxifen prolong remission in women with oestrogen rcceptor positive metastatic breast cancer.

Benefits: We found no systematic review. Non systematic reviews published in 1986 and 1991 identified 86 RCTs in 5353 women with metastatic breast cancer unselected for oestrogen receptor status. The overall objective response rate to tamoxifen (see glossary, p 1805) was 34%. Disease stabilisation was achieved in a further 20%, and overall the median duration of response was 12–18 months.[8,9] The likelihood of responding to tamoxifen was highest (60–70%) in postmenopausal women with oestrogen receptor positive disease (see comment below).[10,11] **Versus ovarian ablation in premenopausal women:** See ovarian ablation in premenopausal women, p 1790.

Harms: **Minor adverse effects:** Tamoxifen is well tolerated in women with metastatic breast cancer; fewer than 3% of women discontinued tamoxifen as a result of toxicity.[20] Reported adverse effects included minor gastrointestinal upset (8%), hot flushes (27%), and menstrual disturbance in premenopausal women (13%).[21] **Tumour flare:** During the first few weeks of treatment tumour flare occurred in fewer than 5% of women. For those with bone metastases, this may have resulted in increased pain or symptomatic hypercalcaemia. **Relapse:** Most women who initially respond to tamoxifen eventually progress and develop acquired resistance to tamoxifen, although they may still respond to further hormonal interventions.[22]

Comment: The choice of first line treatment (hormonal or chemotherapy — see glossary, p 1805) is based on a variety of clinical factors (see table 1, p 1810).[8–11] **Antioestrogens:** An emerging problem is that many women have already received adjuvant tamoxifen for early breast cancer or have developed metastatic disease while still on tamoxifen, and are thus considered resistant to it. Effective second line treatment (see glossary, p 1805) hormonal drugs, such as selective aromatase inhibitors (see glossary, p 1804), are now used after tamoxifen failure (see selective aromatase inhibitors in postmenopausal women, p 1793), and RCTs have compared these drugs with tamoxifen as first line treatment (see selective aromatase inhibitors as first line treatment in postmenopausal women, p 1792). New non-steroidal antioestrogens (toremifene, idoxifene, raloxifene) and steroidal antioestrogens (fulvestrant) are more selective than tamoxifen and may have fewer long term adverse effects. RCTs comparing some of these drugs with tamoxifen as first line hormonal treatment in metastatic breast cancer are in progress. So far, one RCT in 658 women has found no evidence of clear clinical superiority of toremifene over tamoxifen.[23]

OPTION PROGESTINS (MEDROXYPROGESTERONE; MEGESTROL)

RCTs have found that progestins are as effective as tamoxifen in first line treatment of metastatic breast cancer, but they are not as well tolerated. Specific beneficial effects can make progestins useful in women with bone pain or anorexia.

Benefits: We found one systematic review (search date 1991, 7 RCTs, 801 women with metastatic breast cancer) comparing medroxyprogesterone versus tamoxifen (see glossary, p 1805),[24] and one subsequent RCT.[25] The review found no significant difference in response rates (35–54%), remission rates, or survival between the two groups. Benefits of progestins (see glossary, p 1805) included an analgesic effect (assessed using questionnaires), especially on painful bone metastases,[26] increased appetite, weight gain, and a feeling of wellbeing. The subsequent RCT (166 women) found that the rate of response of bone metastases was significantly higher with medroxyprogesterone than with tamoxifen (33% *v* 13%; $P = 0.01$), although there was no significant difference in survival.[25]

Harms: Women taking medroxyprogesterone experienced more adverse effects than women taking tamoxifen.[27] These were common at higher doses and included nausea (14%), weight gain (56%), vaginal bleeding (10%), and exacerbation of hypertension. In women with lymphangitis carcinomatosis, progestins may exacerbate symptoms of breathlessness.[28]

Comment: In view of the lack of evidence of greater benefit, and the evidence of greater harm, progestins are reserved for second or third line hormonal treatment (see glossary, p 1805) in women with advanced breast cancer who have not responded to tamoxifen.

OPTION OVARIAN ABLATION IN PREMENOPAUSAL WOMEN

One systematic review and one subsequent RCT in premenopausal women found no significant difference in response rate, duration of response, or survival with ovarian ablation (surgery or irradiation) versus tamoxifen as first line treatment. Ovarian ablation is associated with substantial adverse effects such as hot flushes and "tumour flare".

Benefits: **Versus tamoxifen:** We found one systematic review (search date not stated, 4 RCTs, 220 premenopausal women) comparing tamoxifen (see glossary, p 1805) versus ovarian ablation (carried out by either surgery or irradiation),[29] and one subsequent RCT.[30] There was no significant difference between treatments in terms of response rate, response duration, or survival. The subsequent RCT (39 premenopausal women) comparing initial treatment with tamoxifen or ovarian ablation confirmed these findings (OR for progressive disease [see glossary, p 1805] 0.71, 95% CI 0.37 to 1.38; median survival 2.35 years with tamoxifen, 2.46 years with ovarian ablation; P = 0.98; OR for death 1.07, 95% CI 0.55 to 2.06).[30] **Different methods of ovarian ablation:** We found two RCTs comparing gonadorelin analogues (see glossary, p 1805) versus surgical ovariectomy or irradiation. They found no significant difference in survival between treatments.[31,32]

Harms: Adverse effects include hot flushes (75% with gonadorelin analogues, 46% with surgical ovariectomy) and "tumour flare" (16% with gonadorelin analogues).[31] In addition, surgical ovariectomy requires an operation and anaesthetic in someone with an incurable disease.

Comment: None.

OPTION COMBINED GONADORELIN ANALOGUES PLUS TAMOXIFEN IN PREMENOPAUSAL WOMEN

Stephen Johnston

One non-systematic review has found that in premenopausal women combined treatment with a gonadorelin analogue and tamoxifen versus a gonadorelin analogue alone significantly improves response rates, overall survival, and progression free survival.

Benefits: We found one non-systematic review (4 RCTs, 506 women) that found combined endocrine treatment with gonadorelin analogues plus tamoxifen (see glossary, p 1805) versus a gonadorelin analogue alone significantly improved both progression free survival (see glossary, p 1805) (HR 0.70, 95% CI 0.58 to 0.85; P = 0.0003) and overall survival (HR 0.78, 95% CI 0.63 to 0.96; P = 0.02).[33] The overall response rate was also significantly higher for combined treatment (OR 0.67; P = 0.03).

Harms: Although the meta-analysis did not analyse differences in tolerability, the largest of the individual trials found there was no significant difference in the incidence of expected hormonal effects (hot flushes, vaginal discharge) for the combined treatment versus gonadorelin analogues alone.

Comment: We found that combined endocrine treatment in metastatic breast cancer has been shown to be beneficial over single agent treatment. Attention is now turning to see if there is any additional benefit for complete oestrogen deprivation in premenopausal women using ovarian ablation with gonadorelin analogues combined with aromatase inhibitors (see glossary, p 1804).

OPTION **SELECTIVE AROMATASE INHIBITORS AS FIRST LINE HORMONAL TREATMENT IN POSTMENOPAUSAL WOMEN**

Stephen Johnston and Justin Stebbing

Two RCTs have found that the aromatase inhibitor anastrozole is at least as effective as tamoxifen as first line treatment in metastatic postmenopausal breast cancer, and one RCT found that the aromatase inhibitor letrozole was superior to tamoxifen.

Benefits: **Anastrozole:** We found two RCTs comparing anastrozole versus tamoxifen (see glossary, p 1805).[34,35] The larger RCT (668 women) showed no significant difference in time to disease progression (HR 0.99, 95% CI 0.86 to 1.12) or response rate (32.9% anastrozole *v* 32.6% tamoxifen).[34] The smaller RCT (353 women) found that anastrozole significantly prolonged the time to progression (HR 1.44, 95% CI 1.16 to 1.82).[35] Neither trial reported on the effect on survival. **Letrozole:** One RCT (907 women) found that letrozole versus tamoxifen significantly improved the time to disease progression (HR 0.70, 95% CI 0.60 to 0.82; P = 0.0001) and tumour response rate (OR 1.71, 95% CI 1.26 to 2.31; P = 0.0006).[36] For women who had received prior adjuvant tamoxifen but stopped at least 12 months prior to study entry, there was a significantly greater chance of response to letrozole compared with tamoxifen rechallenge (HR 0.64, 95% CI 0.41 to 0.98). Women with visceral disease as the dominant site of metastases had a significantly greater chance of response to letrozole than tamoxifen (HR 0.37, 95% CI 0.26 to 0.53).[36]

Harms: In both anastrozole trials the incidence of thromboembolic events was less in women receiving anastrozole than in those receiving tamoxifen (4.8 *v* 7.3%;[34] 4.1% *v* 8.2%[35]). There were fewer reported events of vaginal bleeding (1.2 % with anastrazole *v* 3.8% with tamoxifen,[34] and 1.2% with anastrazole *v* 2.4% with tamoxifen[35]). In the letrozole trial the frequency of adverse events was similar between letrozole and tamoxifen.[36]

Comment: These RCTs with anastrozole and letrozole[34–36] have confirmed that the selective third generation aromatase inhibitors (see glossary, p 1804) are superior in efficacy to tamoxifen, with an equal if not better safety profile. As a consequence, these treatments may replace tamoxifen as the first line endocrine treatment of choice for postmenopausal women with oestrogen receptor positive metastatic breast cancer. Results from the letrozole trials suggest an early survival advantage for women treated with letrozole rather than tamoxifen, which was not seen on further follow up owing to the prospective crossover of a large number of patients at progression (Mouridsen H et al, San Antonio Breast Cancer Symposium, 2001).[37]

QUESTION What are the effects of second line hormonal treatment in women who have not responded to tamoxifen?

OPTION PROGESTINS

RCTs have found that progestins are less effective in second line treatment than selective aromatase inhibitors and have more adverse effects.

Benefits: **Versus selective aromatase inhibitors:** See selective aromatase inhibitors in postmenopausal women, p 1793.

Harms: **Versus selective aromatase inhibitors:** See selective aromatase inhibitors in postmenopausal women, p 1794.

Comment: In women who are not responding to tamoxifen, progestins (see glossary, p 1805) may have a role in increasing feelings of wellbeing and relieving anorexia.

OPTION SELECTIVE AROMATASE INHIBITORS IN POSTMENOPAUSAL WOMEN

RCTs have found that in postmenopausal women with metastatic breast cancer who have relapsed on adjuvant tamoxifen or progressed during first line treatment with tamoxifen, the selective aromatase inhibitors anastrozole, letrozole, and exemestane prolong survival compared with progestins or aminoglutethimide, with minimal adverse effects. The evidence suggests that selective aromatase inhibitors are significantly more effective and better tolerated than previous standard second line treatment with a progestin or the non-selective aromatase inhibitor aminoglutethimide, and are most effective in oestrogen receptor positive women.

Benefits: **Anastrozole versus progestins:** A meta-analysis of the two randomised phase III trials comparing anastrozole versus megestrol (764 postmenopausal women with metastatic breast cancer unresponsive to tamoxifen [see glossary, p 1805], median age 65 years, 70% oestrogen receptor positive, 30% oestrogen receptor status unknown) found no significant difference in objective response rates (10.3% *v* 7.9%), or in the proportion of women whose disease was stabilised for 6 months (25.1% *v* 26.1%).[38] A subsequent analysis after a median of 31 months' follow up found a significant improvement in overall survival with anastrozole (HR 0.78; P = 0.02), with an absolute improvement in 2 year survival from 46–56% (P = 0.02) and an improvement in median survival of 4 months (from 22.5–26.7 months).[39] **Exemestane versus progestins:** Exemestane is currently being evaluated in phase III trials.[40] One RCT (769 women) found that median survival time was significantly longer with exemestane (median not reached) than with megestrol (123 wks; P = 0.039), as were the median duration of overall success (complete response/partial response or stable disease ≥ 24 wks; 60.1 *v* 49.1 wks; P = 0.025) and time to tumour progression (20.3 *v* 16.6 wks; P = 0.037).[41] Compared with megestrol, there were similar or greater improvements in pain control, tumour related signs and symptoms, and quality of life with exemestane.[41] **Letrozole versus progestins or aminoglutethimide:** Two large RCTs compared letrozole (0.5 mg or 2.5 mg) versus megestrol (551 women)[42] and aminoglutethimide (555 women).[43] Both trials were in postmenopausal women with metastatic breast cancer unresponsive to tamoxifen (median age 64–65 years, 55% oestrogen receptor positive, 45% oestrogen receptor status unknown). Letrozole 2.5 mg versus megestrol significantly increased the response rate (HR 1.82, 95% CI 1.02 to 3.25), the duration of response (HR 0.42, 95% CI 0.2 to 0.86), and the time to treatment failure (HR 0.77, 95% CI 0.61 to 0.99).[42] Compared with aminoglutethimide, letrozole achieved better overall survival (HR 0.64, 95% CI 0.49 to 0.85) and time to progression (HR 0.72, 95% CI 0.57 to 0.92).[43]

Harms: The selective aromatase inhibitors (see glossary, p 1804) were generally well tolerated and associated with fewer adverse events than aminoglutethimide or progestins. **Anastrozole:** In the RCTs, anastrozole 1 mg was associated with a higher incidence of minor gastrointestinal disturbance (nausea or change in bowel habit) than megestrol (29% *v* 21%; $P = 0.005$), but a significantly lower incidence of greater than 5% gain in weight (13% *v* 34%; $P < 0.0001$).[38] **Exemestane:** In the RCTs more women treated with progestin had adverse events (45.8% *v* 39.1%). The most frequently reported adverse events with exemestane were low grade hot flushes (12.6%), nausea (9.2%), and fatigue (7.5%). In the RCT against megestrol, both drugs were well tolerated, although grade 3 or 4 weight changes (> 10% weight gain) were more common with megestrol (17.1% *v* 7.6%; $P = 0.001$).[41] **Letrozole:** Compared with megestrol, letrozole (2.5 mg) was associated with a significantly lower incidence of serious cardiovascular adverse events (2% *v* 11%) and greater than 5% weight gain (19% *v* 30%).[42] Compared with aminoglutethimide, letrozole (2.5 mg) had a significantly lower incidence of skin rash (3% *v* 11%) and serious drug related adverse events (0% *v* 3%).[43]

Comment: The evidence indicates greater efficacy and tolerability of anastrozole and letrozole over megestrol acetate or aminoglutethimide. There is a consensus that they are agents of choice as second line hormonal treatment in postmenopausal women no longer responding to tamoxifen. An ongoing RCT is comparing anastrozole versus letrozole in this context (Rose C, et al, personal communication, 1999). A trial conducted in 2000 has evaluated the activity of exemestane in metastatic breast cancer after failure of non-steroidal aromatase inhibitors.[44] A total of 241 people were enrolled; 56% had received aminoglutethimide, 19% anastrozole, and 17% letrozole. Exemestane produced objective responses in 7% of treated women, including 8% of women after failure of treatment with aminoglutethimide and 5% after failure of other non-steroidal aromatase inhibitors (anastrozole, letrozole, and vorozole), and an overall success rate (complete response plus partial response plus no change for 24 wks or longer) of 24%. Women who do not respond to anastrozole or letrozole may respond to exemestane.

QUESTION What are the effects of first line chemotherapy?

OPTION COMBINATION CHEMOTHERAPY

We found no RCTs comparing combination chemotherapy versus no chemotherapy in women with metastatic breast cancer. Trials comparing one type of chemotherapy versus another found that first line chemotherapy was associated with an objective tumour response in 40–60% of women, with a median response duration of 6–12 months irrespective of menopausal or oestrogen receptor status. A small proportion of women achieve complete remission, which may persist for an extended length of time (see high dose chemotherapy, p 1797). We found limited evidence from one systematic review and subsequent RCTs that CAF regimens increased time to progression and survival time compared with CMF regimens.

Benefits: **Versus best supportive care:** We found no systematic review and no RCTs comparing first line chemotherapy versus palliative (best supportive) care in women with metastatic breast cancer. **Different chemotherapy regimens:** We found one systematic review (search date 1997, 189 RCTs, 31 510 women) evaluating different chemotherapy (see glossary, p 1805) and endocrine regimens.[20] **"Classical" versus modified CMF:** In the largest RCT (254 postmenopausal women with metastatic breast cancer who had received no prior chemotherapy) the classical CMF (see glossary, p 1805) regimen versus a modified version in which all three drugs were given intravenously every 3 weeks significantly improved survival and response rate (response rate 48% *v* 29%; P = 0.03: median survival 17 *v* 12 months; P = 0.016).[45] One RCT (133 women who had received no prior chemotherapy) found that standard dose CMF versus low dose CMF significantly improved both response rate (30% *v* 11%; P = 0.03) and symptom control.[46] **CAF versus CMF:** One systematic review (search date not stated) found that regimens containing doxorubicin versus other regimens increased response rate, time to progression, and survival.[47] However, two RCTs comparing CAF (see glossary, p 1805) versus non-anthracycline based regimens (CMF) found no evidence of improved survival.[48,49] **Standard versus modified CAF regimens:** Two large multicentre trials of CAF (containing doxorubicin) versus FEC (see glossary, p 1805), a modified anthracycline based regimen containing epirubicin, found no significant difference in response rates (263 women, response rate 52% *v* 50%;[50] 497 women, response rate 56% *v* 54%[51]). One RCT (249 women) comparing standard CAF (containing doxorubicin) versus a modified better tolerated anthracycline based regimen containing mitoxantrone (mitozantrone) found that the regimen containing doxorubicin significantly prolonged the time to progression (3.2 *v* 5.3 months; P = 0.03) and increased median survival (10.9 *v* 15.2 months; P = 0.003).[52] **CAF or modified CAF versus mitoxantrone and vinorelbine (MV):** One RCT (281 women) compared MV versus either CAF or FEC. No significant differences in response rates were seen (35% for MV *v* 33% for CAF or FEC), but MV appeared more effective in people who had received prior adjuvant treatment (33% *v* 13%; P = 0.025) with an improved progression free survival (9 months *v* 6 months; P = 0.014).[53]

Harms: The toxicity profiles of different combination chemotherapy regimens vary. In RCTs, anthracycline based regimens (CAF) and non-anthracycline based regimens (CMF) are equally associated with haematological toxicity,[49] but CAF is more likely to be associated with alopecia (34% *v* 22%) and severe nausea and vomiting (17% *v* 7%; P = 0.05). Other studies reported the incidence of greater than grade 3 alopecia (complete hair loss) to be 55–61% with CAF, which was significantly higher than with either mitoxantrone or epirubicin (FEC).[51,52] In one of the trials comparing CAF versus FEC, FEC was associated with fewer episodes of greater than or equal to grade 2 neutropenia (10% *v* 13.1%), and significantly lower rates of nausea and vomiting (7.8% *v* 13.3%; P < 0.01), and no cardiotoxicity (8 women taking CAF discontinued treatment because of cardiac dysfunction compared with none taking FEC).[50] MV was associated with less nausea and vomiting and alopecia than CAF or FEC although myelosuppression was greater (P = 0.001).

Comment: The optimal duration of chemotherapy for metastatic breast cancer is unknown, although a more recent systematic review (search date not stated; 65 publications reporting 97 treatment comparisons) has found that more, rather than fewer, cycles of chemotherapy given at appropriate doses improved survival (ratio of median survivals 1.23, 95% CI 1.01 to 1.49; P = 0.01).[54] The choice of first line treatment (see glossary, p 1805) (hormonal or chemotherapy) is based on a variety of clinical factors (see table 1, p 1810).[8–11] In one RCT (231 women undergoing first line treatment, 60% oestrogen receptor positive, remainder unknown) women were randomised to receive either chemotherapy (CAF) or chemotherapy plus hormonal treatment (see glossary, p 1805) (CAF plus tamoxifen and fluoxymesterone). Response rates and time to treatment failure were similar for women who received chemo–hormonal therapy compared with chemotherapy alone (time to treatment failure 13.4 months *v* 10.3 months; P = 0.087).[55] The effect on time to treatment failure was just significant for women who were oestrogen receptor positive compared with those who were negative (17.4 *v* 10.3 months; P = 0.048). Oestrogen receptor status had no effect on overall survival. The choice of a specific drug or regimen is based on what drugs have already been given as adjuvant treatment (see glossary, p 1804), together with the likelihood of benefit balanced against a given drug's adverse effects and tolerability profile. Retrospective series in sequential decades (from 1950–1980) have compared the survival of women from the time of diagnosis with metastatic breast cancer. They suggest that the introduction of chemotherapy has improved median survival by about 9 months (from 12 months without treatment to 21 months with treatment).[7,56] This median survival conceals a bimodal distribution of benefit, with the 40–60% of women who respond to treatment achieving survival of 1 year or greater, and the non-responders experiencing little or no survival benefit. With the increasing use of adjuvant chemotherapy,[57] more women who develop metastatic disease will have received combination chemotherapy. In the treatment of metastatic breast cancer, better quality of life scores predict better outcome (this is not the case in adjuvant treatment).[58] In one RCT (283 women with metastatic breast cancer) evaluating quality of life as a primary end point, no significant differences were found between women randomised to receive either docetaxel or sequential methotrexate and fluorouracil. This suggests that choice of treatment should be based on expected clinical effect.[59] This may influence the likelihood of response to further treatment.[6,60] The prevention of nausea and vomiting caused by chemotherapy has been studied in one RCT (619 women). It compared placebo versus dexamethasone versus dexamethasone plus ondansetron following chemotherapy. In people who did not have acute nausea and vomiting with chemotherapy, dexamethasone alone was found to provide adequate protection against delayed nausea and vomiting.[61]

OPTION HIGH DOSE VERSUS STANDARD DOSE CHEMOTHERAPY

One RCT found no evidence that high dose chemotherapy improved time to progression or overall survival.

Benefits: We found no systematic review. We found one RCT (533 women aged 18–60 who had complete response or partial response to induction chemotherapy — see glossary, p 1805). It compared high dose chemotherapy (single course of high doses of carboplatin, thiotepa, and cyclophosphamide) plus haematopoietic stem cell rescue versus prolonged course of monthly conventional dose chemotherapy (cyclophosphamide, methotrexate, and fluorouracil). It found no significant difference in overall survival at 3 years (32%, 95% CI 21% to 42% *v* 38%, 95% CI 26% to 50%) or in median progression free survival (see glossary, p 1805) (9.6 months *v* 9.0 months; CI not provided).[62]

Harms: Although haematological support with colony stimulating growth factors (see glossary, p 1805) has lessened complications from high dose chemotherapy, non-haematological toxicity to the gastrointestinal tract, and nervous system remain dose limiting. There is a recognised mortality with high dose chemotherapy (3%), although this is lower than in the early days of this approach.

Comment: Fifteen years' follow up of women with metastatic breast cancer treated with standard dose FAC (see glossary, p 1805) chemotherapy found that 263/1581 (16.6%) women achieved a complete response and had a median time to progression of 2 years, and that 19% of these women remained free of disease at 5 years.[18] Any long term remissions associated with high dose chemotherapy in metastatic disease must be interpreted in the context of these figures. It remains to be seen if certain women, for example those with a complete response after standard dose chemotherapy, may benefit from high dose treatment as a "coup de grace" for any remaining cancer cells.[63,64]

QUESTION **What are the effects of first line chemotherapy in combination with a monoclonal antibody?**

OPTION **TRASTUZUMAB**

One RCT found that trastuzumab increased the clinical benefit of first line chemotherapy in metastatic breast cancer in those women whose tumours overexpress HER2. The main adverse effect observed was cardiac dysfunction in women who received an anthracycline plus trastuzumab.

Benefits: We found no systematic review and no RCTs comparing treatment with no treatment. **Versus chemotherapy alone:** One RCT (469 women) compared standard chemotherapy alone versus standard chemotherapy (see glossary, p 1805) plus trastuzumab. Women who had not previously received adjuvant (postoperative) chemotherapy with an anthracycline were treated with doxorubicin (or epirubicin) and cyclophosphamide with or without trastuzumab. Women who had previously received adjuvant anthracycline were treated with paclitaxel with or without trastuzumab. The addition of trastuzumab to chemotherapy significantly prolonged the time to disease progression (7.4 months *v* 4.6 months; $P < 0.001$), increased objective response (50% *v* 32%; $P < 0.001$), and improved overall survival (25.1 months *v* 20.3 months; $P = 0.046$).[65]

Harms: Cardiac dysfunction occurred in 27% of the group given an anthracycline, cyclophosphamide, and trastuzumab versus 8% of the group given an anthracycline and cyclophosphamide alone versus 13% of the group given paclitaxel and trastuzumab versus 1% of those given paclitaxel alone. Symptoms here usually improved with standard medical management, although two women died from cardiac dysfunction. About 25% of women had chills, fever, or both during the initial infusion; no episodes of anaphylaxis occurred.

Comment: Trastuzumab based combination treatment was effective at reducing the relative risk of death by 20% at a median follow up of 30 months. Few studies have demonstrated a survival advantage of this magnitude in association with addition of a single agent. Cardiac toxicity, the most noteworthy side effect, appears only significant in those concurrently receiving an anthracycline. The most appropriate treatment duration in responders is unclear. We found one RCT, which compared two different dosing regimens of trastuzumab as first line treatment in 114 women with HER2 overexpressing metastatic breast cancer. It found no significant difference between the high dose regimen (8 mg/kg loading dose followed by 4 mg/kg weekly) and low dose regimen (4 mg/kg loading dose followed by 2 mg/kg weekly) for time to progression or time to death (median time to progression 3.5 months with high dose, 95% CI 3.3 to 5.5 months *v* 3.8 months, 95% CI 2.4 to 5.5 months; median survival 22.9 months, 95% CI 16.0 months to 37.1 months *v* 25.8 months, 95% CI 13.3 to 34.7 months).[66] Adverse effects included asthenia (23%), fever (22%), nausea (14%), and cardiac dysfunction (2%).

QUESTION What are the effects of second line chemotherapy?

The response rates to further chemotherapy when women relapse after standard dose chemotherapy are generally poor, with objective response rates of only 20–30%, and median durations of response ranging from 3–6 months. We found limited evidence that the taxanes and semisynthetic vinca alkaloids may improve response rates compared with CMF or continued doxorubicin, especially in anthracycline resistant disease. One RCT found no evidence of a difference between paclitaxel and capecitabine for time to progression and survival.

Benefits: We found no systematic review and no RCTs comparing treatment with no treatment. **Taxanes:** See glossary, p 1806. One non-systematic review of RCTs and other studies concluded that, in women with anthracycline resistant (see glossary, p 1804) disease, second line treatment (see glossary, p 1805) with paclitaxel was associated with response rates ranging from 6–48%.[67] The taxane paclitaxel has been compared in two RCTs with both doxorubicin (331 women)[68] and CMF based chemotherapy (see glossary, p 1805) (209 women).[69] The response rates were higher with doxorubicin than paclitaxel (41% v 25%; $P = 0.003$), yet compared with CMF based chemotherapy there was a modest survival advantage for the use of paclitaxel in a multivariate analysis (median survival 17.3 v 13.9 months; $P = 0.025$). One RCT (392 women with anthracycline resistant metastatic disease) compared the taxane docetaxel (100 mg/m^2 iv every 3 wks) versus a standard relapse treatment of mitomycin (12 mg/m^2) plus vinblastine (6 mg/m^2).[70] Docetaxel was associated with a significantly higher response rate (30% v 11.6%; $P < 0.001$), longer time to progression (median 19 wks v 11 wks; $P = 0.001$), and longer overall survival (11.4 v 8.7 months; $P = 0.0097$). Another RCT (283 women with anthracycline resistant metastatic disease) comparing docetaxel versus methotrexate and fluorouracil found a similar improvement for docetaxel both in response rate (42% v 19%; $P < 0.001$) and time to progression (median 6 months v 3 months; $P = 0.006$).[71] In a separate RCT (326 women who had not responded to an alkylating regimen [CMF] either in the adjuvant setting or as first line treatment) docetaxel was associated with a significantly higher response rate than single drug doxorubicin (43% v 21%; $P = 0.003$).[72] **Semisynthetic vinca alkaloids:** We found no RCTs comparing vinorelbine versus a taxane for second line treatment. One RCT (303 women, first or second line treatment, no previous vinca alkaloid or anthracycline) compared doxorubicin combined with vinorelbine versus doxorubicin alone. The response rates, quality of life scores, and overall survival were not significantly improved with combined chemotherapy in this setting.[73] Vinorelbine has single agent activity with response rates of 20–33%, including in women with anthacycline resistant metastatic disease.[67] One RCT (183 women with anthracycline resistant disease) found increased time to progression and survival with vinorelbine 30 mg/m^2 weekly compared with intravenous melphalan (median survival 35 v 31 wks; $P < 0.001$).[74] **Capecitabine:** We found one systematic review (search date 2000) assessing the oral fluoropyrimidine capecitabine in metastatic breast cancer,[75] which identified one RCT (42 women) comparing capecitabine versus paclitaxel as second or third line treatment following anthracycline failure. It found no significant difference between treatments in response rate or time to disease progression.

Harms: **Taxanes:** Paclitaxel was better tolerated than doxorubicin with a lower incidence of febrile neutropenia (7% *v* 20%; $P < 0.001$) and grade 3/4 vomiting (2% *v* 13%; $P < 0.001$), although there was a higher incidence of sensory neurotoxicity (5% *v* 0%; $P < 0.001$).[68] Likewise, compared with CMF based chemotherapy, paclitaxel was associated with significantly less febrile neutropenia and infection (10% *v* 27%; $P = 0.001$), and nausea and vomiting, but significantly more alopecia, sensory neuropathy, and myalgia and arthralgia ($P < 0.0001$).[69] Docetaxel is associated with moderate to severe haematological toxicity; 89% of women experienced grade 3/4 neutropenia in the phase III study compared with 69% given mitomycin plus vinblastine,[70] although the incidence of febrile neutropenia with docetaxel was only 9%. Other specific toxicities associated with docetaxel include alopecia, neurotoxicity, arthralgia, and occasionally fluid retention. Hypersensitivity reactions can be avoided by premedication with corticosteroids and histamine H_2 receptor antagonists. **Semisynthetic vinca alkaloids:** Vinorelbine is associated with minimal toxicity compared with anthracycline based chemotherapy (FAC/FEC — see glossary, p 1805), with considerably lower rates of nausea (8% *v* 16%; $P = 0.03$) and grade 3 alopecia (7% *v* 30%; $P = 0.0001$), although haematological toxicity that delayed treatment was more frequent (27% *v* 17%).[76] **Capecitabine:** The most commonly reported grade 3/4 toxicities were hand-foot syndrome (13%), diarrhoea (12%), and stomatitis (4%).[75]

Comment: The taxanes, paclitaxel and docetaxel, have an established role as second line treatment in advanced breast cancer, especially in people with disease progression despite a previous anthracycline based regimen, with evidence in some RCTs for a survival advantage over other available options. Trials are in progress to determine the efficacy and tolerability of taxanes in combination with anthracyclines as first line treatment (see glossary, p 1805), although there are concerns about cardiac toxicity. At present the indication for docetaxel remains as a single drug for second line treatment, especially in anthracycline resistant disease, although definitive results on improvement in quality of life are awaited. Vinorelbine seems to have a favourable toxicity profile, but results from phase III trials are awaited. Promising activity has been seen with capecitabine in paclitaxel–refractory heavily pretreated women,[77] and the low toxicity profile, together with evidence of efficacy, all warrant further investigation of this drug as an alternative to more toxic second or third line chemotherapy schedules. It has been suggested that the effectiveness of docetaxel may be increased by the addition of capecitabine,[78] and RCTs are under way. Vinorelbine associated with protracted infusional fluorouracil is an active and well tolerated regimen (overall response rate 61.4%, 95% CI 50.9 to 70.9), and further trials are under way.[79] One uncontrolled study of vinorelbine plus gemcitabine twice weekly found an objective response rate of 54%.[80]

QUESTION **What are the effects of treatments for bone metastases?**

OPTION **BISPHOSPHONATES**

Three placebo controlled RCTs in women with metastatic breast cancer and bone involvement have found that bisphosphonates given in conjunction with standard treatment significantly reduces and delays skeletal complications, but have no effect on survival.

Benefits: We found no systematic review. **Versus placebo:** Three double blind RCTs in women with metastatic breast cancer who had bone involvement compared bisphosphonates (see glossary, p 1805) with placebo given in conjunction with standard treatment (either chemotherapy or hormonal treatment — see glossary, p 1805).[81–83] The first RCT (380 women with at least 1 lytic bone lesion who also received chemotherapy) found that intravenous pamidronate (90 mg as a 2 h infusion every month for 12 cycles) significantly prolonged the median time to the first skeletal complication (13.1 months *v* 7.0 months; P = 0.005).[81] Significantly fewer women taking pamidronate developed skeletal complications (43% *v* 56%; P = 0.008), and there was a significantly reduced requirement for radiotherapy to treat painful sites of bone disease (19% *v* 33%; P = 0.01). In an updated analysis in women who completed 2 years of treatment, those taking placebo were more than twice as likely to suffer a fracture than those taking pamidronate (OR 2.3, 95% CI 1.5 to 3.5).[84] The second RCT (173 women with bone metastases who may also have received either chemotherapy or hormonal treatment) found that the addition of oral clodronate (1600 mg daily) significantly reduced the number of hypercalcaemic episodes (23% *v* 35%; P < 0.01) and the incidence of vertebral fractures (84 *v* 124 per 100 women years; P < 0.025).[82] The third RCT (372 women with at least 1 lytic bone lesion who also received hormonal treatment) found that pamidronate significantly prolonged the median time to the first skeletal complication (10.4 months *v* 6.9 months; P = 0.049).[83] Significantly fewer women taking pamidronate developed skeletal complications (2.4 *v* 3.8 events a year; P = 0.008), and there was a significantly reduced requirement for radiotherapy to treat painful sites of bone disease (25% *v* 34%; P = 0.042). None of the three trials found an impact on overall survival. **Versus radiotherapy:** We found no RCTs.

Harms: In the first RCT, intravenous pamidronate was well tolerated with no serious adverse events in women treated for up to 2 years.[81] One of the 185 women taking pamidronate developed symptomatic hypocalcaemia. Myalgia and arthralgia were more common in women taking pamidronate. Oral clodronate can be associated with minor gastrointestinal disturbance, but the RCT reported this in fewer than 5% of women.[81]

Comment: Large RCTs are in progress in the adjuvant setting to see whether these agents may delay or prevent the development of bone metastases. The American Society of Clinical Oncology released recent guidelines on the use of bisphosphonates, stating that this treatment reduces the rate of bone complications (although not mortality) in women with lytic bone disease who may or may not also be receiving systemic treatment (chemotherapy or endocrine treatment).[85] It remains unclear exactly when to start or stop treatment, which may impact on the costs involved.[86] Although these effects are likely to improve quality of life, this outcome has not been formally evaluated. We found no evidence that bisphosphonates improve survival.

OPTION RADIOTHERAPY

We found limited evidence from non-randomised studies that persistent and localised bone pain can be successfully treated with radiotherapy and concomitant analgesics in over 80% of cases. Longer courses and wide fields are rarely required, and adverse effects are minimal. The RCTs found no evidence that single fraction regimens (usually 8 Gy) were less effective than fractionated regimens.

Benefits: We found no systematic review and no RCTs comparing radiotherapy versus no treatment or versus bisphosphonates (see glossary, p 1805) (see comment below). **Pain control:** Questionnaire studies found that control of pain was successful in over 80% of women who received radiotherapy for bone metastases, with concomitant use of appropriate analgesia according to the World Health Organization ladder, which moves upwards from non-steroidal anti-inflammatory drugs and paracetamol to opiate containing analgesia (codeine based products) through to morphine and its derivatives (diamorphine, hydromorphone).[87] **Cranial nerve compression:** In people with skull base metastases causing cranial nerve involvement, retrospective studies suggest that radiotherapy leads to improvement in 50–80% of women, which is usually maintained.[88] **Different radiotherapy regimens:** We found two RCTs comparing different radiotherapy regimens. These found no significant differences between short courses (8 Gy as a single fraction) and longer courses (e.g. 20 Gy/5 fractions or 30 Gy/10 fractions).[89,90] Studies of accelerated fractionation schedules (e.g. twice daily treatments for 5 days) have failed to show any benefit over conventional regimens in the control of disease secondary to metastatic breast cancer.[91] Published interim results from one RCT (270 women) have found that different fractionation regimens can be used to effectively treat neuropathic bone pain.[92]

Harms: Adverse effects of radiotherapy for bone metastases include nausea and vomiting.[91] Higher dose fractions a day produce more toxic effects.

Comment: Randomised comparisons against no treatment or placebo would be considered unethical in palliative care, and even RCTs comparing one treatment versus another are difficult to undertake because it is reasonable to try many different options in order to make a woman comfortable. Rating of success of end of life care is difficult. Usual outcomes, such as response rates and survival duration, do not apply.[93]

QUESTION **What are the effects of treatments for spinal cord, cerebral, and choroidal metastases?**

OPTION **SPINAL CORD COMPRESSION**

Spinal cord compression is an emergency. Retrospective studies suggest that early radiotherapy preserves function. One small RCT suggested that adding high dose steroids improved the chance of walking 6 months after radiotherapy for spinal cord compression.

Benefits: We found no systematic review. **Radiotherapy:** Retrospective analyses found an improvement with early radiotherapy, but fewer than 10% of people walked again if severe deterioration of motor function occurred before radiotherapy.[94] **Addition of high dose steroids:** One blinded RCT (57 women) evaluated addition of high dose steroids to radiotherapy. It found that more women were walking 6 months after receiving intravenous dexamethasone 96 mg bolus followed by 96 mg orally for 3 days compared with those who received no steroids (59% *v* 33%).[95]

Harms: In the RCT of high dose steroids, significant adverse effects caused withdrawal from treatment in 11% of people.[95] Use of lower doses of glucocorticoids in the control of symptoms from cerebral metastases may result in short term agitation and the longer term development of Cushingoid facies.

Comment: See comment under radiotherapy, p 1803.

OPTION **CEREBRAL METASTASES**

Evidence from retrospective studies suggests that symptoms from cerebral metastases can be successfully controlled with radiotherapy.

Benefits: We found no systematic review and no RCTs comparing one form of treatment with another. **Radiotherapy:** Retrospective studies suggest that whole brain radiation produces general improvement in neurological function in 40–70% of women with brain metastases secondary to breast cancer.[96] **Different radiotherapy regimens:** One RCT (544 symptomatic people) that compared two whole brain radiotherapy schedules (30 Gy/10 fractions *v* 12 Gy/2 fractions) found no evidence that the response rate or duration of response in people with multiple brain metastases were improved with higher doses of radiation compared with the shorter regimen.[91] **Surgical resection:** A retrospective cohort study nested in one RCT (859 women) found that there may be some beneficial effect in a small subgroup of people.[97] **Intrathecal chemotherapy:** We found no evidence that meningeal infiltration responds to intrathecal chemotherapy.

Harms: Adverse effects of radiotherapy in the treatment of cerebral metastases include hair loss and somnolence.[91] Higher dose fractions a day produce more toxic effects.

Comment: See comment under radiotherapy, p 1803. There is a consensus that raised intracranial pressure associated with cerebral metastases is best managed by dexamethasone given immediately with anticonvulsants to control seizures if necessary.

OPTION CHOROIDAL METASTASES

Evidence from retrospective studies suggests that symptoms from choroidal metastases can be successfully controlled with radiotherapy.

Benefits: We found no systematic review and no RCTs. External beam radiotherapy prevents functional loss and doses of about 40 Gy in total are used.[98] Retrospective studies suggest that radiotherapy benefits 70% of people.[99]

Harms: People with choroidal metastases who are treated with radiotherapy may lose the sight in that eye. Optic atrophy and proliferative radiation retinopathy are possible late complications.

Comment: See comment under radiotherapy, p 1803. Generally, choroidal metastases occur later than metastases to other organs. Choroidal metastasis is considered a poor prognostic sign; most people die within 6 months of diagnosis. Systemic chemotherapy can induce partial or complete remission of metastatic choroidal breast carcinoma.[100] Recent retrospective studies have shown that krypton red or argon green laser photocoagulation is feasible, easy, rapid, and effective for small choroidal breast carcinoma.[101] Women with deteriorating vision are likely to benefit from emergency assessment and treatment for choroidal metastases.

GLOSSARY

Adjuvant treatment This usually refers to systemic chemotherapy or hormonal treatment, or both, taken after removal of a primary tumour (in this case, surgery for early breast cancer), with the aim of killing any remaining micrometastatic tumour cells and thus preventing recurrence.

Anthracycline resistance This applies to people who have received at least one chemotherapeutic regimen with anthracyclines (doxorubicin or epirubicin) in either an adjuvant setting or for metastatic disease. Primary resistance to an anthracycline is defined as progressive disease during or within 6 months after completion of adjuvant anthracycline. People without any documented tumour response to first line chemotherapy that included anthracyclines for metastatic disease are also classified as having primary resistance. Secondary resistance is defined as disease progression after a documented clinical response to first line chemotherapy with anthracyclines for metastatic disease. Secondary resistance can be further divided into three categories, as follows: (1) absolute resistance, or disease progression during treatment with regimens that contained anthracyclines after a period of response; (2) relative resistance, or disease progression within 6 months after completion of the chemotherapy; and (3) sensitive regrowth, or disease progression more than 6 months after completion of the chemotherapy.[102]

Aromatase inhibitors Block the conversion of androgens into oestrogens. Aminoglutethimide, anastrozole, and letrozole are non-steroidal aromatase inhibitors. Formestane and exemestane are steroidal aromatase inhibitors. Anastrozole, formestane, exemestane, and letrozole are selective inhibitors of oestrogen synthetase, which is a part of the aromatase enzyme system. Aminoglutethimide also inhibits adrenal steroid production. These drugs cause oestrogen suppression in postmenopausal women.

Bisphosphonates (pamidronate, clodronate) Bone specific palliative drugs that inhibit osteoclast induced bone resorption associated with breast cancer metastases.

Chemotherapy Treatment with cytotoxic drugs.

Colony stimulating growth factors Naturally occurring cytokines that stimulate development of different cell lines.

Combination chemotherapy regimens Use of different combinations of cytotoxic drugs:

CAF Cyclophosphamide (500 mg/m^2 iv), doxorubicin (50 mg/m^2 iv), and fluorouracil (500 mg/m^2 iv) every 3 weeks for up to six cycles of treatment are given, depending on response.

Classical CMF Cyclophosphamide (100 mg/m^2 orally days 1–14), methotrexate (40 mg/m^2 iv days 1 and 8), and fluorouracil (600 mg/m^2 iv days 1 and 8) every 4 weeks for up to six cycles of treatment are given, depending on response.

FAC Fluorouracil, doxorubicin, and cyclophosphamide every 3 weeks for up to six cycles of treatment are given, depending on response.

FEC Fluorouracil, epirubicin, and cyclophosphamide every 3 weeks for up to six cycles of treatment are given, depending on response.

Complete response Disappearance of all known lesions on two separate measurements at least 4 weeks apart.

Disease free interval Time between surgery for early breast cancer (see below) and metastatic breast cancer developing.

Early breast cancer Operable disease, restricted to the breast and sometimes to local lymph nodes.

First line treatment Initial treatment for a particular condition that has previously not been treated. For example, first line treatment for metastatic breast cancer may include chemotherapy or hormonal treatment, or both.

Gonadorelin analogues (also called LHRH agonists) These are synthetic peptides that occupy the receptors for gonadorelin in the pituitary gland. Continuous administration of gonadorelin agonists may initially increase the release of luteinising hormone, but continuous administration blocks the physiological pulsatile luteinising hormone release and this causes a fall in oestrogen levels.

Hormonal treatment Includes treatment with antioestrogens such as tamoxifen, aromatase inhibitors, and progestins.

Overall objective response rate The proportion of treated people in whom a complete (see above) or partial response (see below) is observed.

Partial response More than a 50% reduction in the size of lesions.

Progestins (medroxyprogesterone, megestrol) The antitumour effects of progestins may be mediated by a direct action on tumour cells, or an indirect effect on the pituitary–ovarian/adrenal axes.

Progression free survival (or time to progression) Interval between diagnosis of metastatic disease and diagnosis of progression (see below).

Progressive disease More than a 25% increase in the size of lesions, or the appearance of new lesions.

Second line treatment Treatment given after relapse following first line treatment (see above).

Tamoxifen An oral, non-steroidal, competitive oestrogen receptor antagonist.

Taxanes Drugs derived from the Pacific yew tree *Taxus brevifolia*, such as paclitaxel and docetaxel.

REFERENCES

1. Hortobagyi GN. Can we cure limited metastatic breast cancer? *J Clin Oncol* 2002;20:620–623.
2. Pisani P, Parkin DM, Ferlay J. Estimates of the worldwide mortality from eighteen major cancers in 1985. Implications for prevention and projections of future burden. *Int J Cancer* 1993;55:891–903.
3. Parkin MD. Global Cancer Statistics in the Year 2000. *Lancet Oncol* 2001;2:533–543.
4. Early Breast Cancer Trialists' Collaborative Group. Polychemotherapy for early breast cancer: an overview of the randomised trials. *Lancet* 1998;352:930–942. Search date 1995; studies were identified using lists prepared by three international cancer research groups, by searching the international Cancer Research Data Bank, meeting abstracts and references of published trials, and by consulting experts.
5. Slamon DJ, Clark GM, Wong SG, et al. Human breast cancer: correlation of relapse and survival with amplification of the HER-2/neu oncogene. *Science* 1987;235:177–182.
6. Rubens RD, Bajetta E, Bonneterre J, et al. Treatment of relapse of breast cancer after adjuvant systemic therapy. *Eur J Cancer* 1994;30A:106–111.
7. Cold S, Jensen NV, Brincker H, et al. The influence of chemotherapy on survival after recurrence in breast cancer: a population based study of patients treated in the 1950s, 1960s, and 1970s. *Eur J Cancer* 1993;29A:1146–1152.
8. Jackson IM, Litherland S, Wakeling AE. Tamoxifen and other antioestrogens. In: Powels TJ, Smith IE, eds. *Medical management of breast cancer*. London: Martin Dunitz, 1997:51–59.
9. Arafah BM, Pearson OH. Endocrine treatment of advanced breast cancer. In: Jordan VC, ed. *Estrogen/antiestrogen action and breast cancer therapy*. Madison: University of Wisconsin Press, 1986:417–429.
10. McGuire WL. Hormone receptors: their role in predicting prognosis and response to endocrine therapy. *Semin Oncol* 1978;5:428–443.
11. Kuss JT, Muss HB, Hoen H, Case LD. Tamoxifen as initial endocrine therapy for metastatic breast cancer: long term follow-up of two Piedmont Oncology Association (POA) trials. *Breast Cancer Res Treat* 1997;42:265–274.
12. Olsen O, Gotzsche PC. Cochrane review on screening for breast cancer with mammography. *Lancet* 2001;358:1340–1342.
13. Coates A, Gebski V, Signori D. Prognostic value of quality-of-life scores during chemotherapy for advanced breast cancer. *J Clin Oncol* 1992;10:1833–1838.
14. European Organisation for Research and Treatment of Cancer (EORTC). *A practical guide to EORTC studies*. Brussels: EORTC Data Center, 1996:126.
15. Miller AB, Hoogstraten B, Staquet M, et al. Reporting results of cancer treatment. *Cancer* 1981;47:207–214.
16. Baum M, Priestman T, West RR, et al. A comparison of subjective responses in a trial comparing endocrine with cytotoxic treatment in advanced carcinoma of the breast. In: Mouridsen HT, Palshof T, eds. *Breast cancer – experimental and clinical methods*. London: Pergamon Press, 1980:223–228.
17. Bernhard J, Thurlimann B, Schmitz SF, et al. Defining clinical benefit in postmenopausal patients with breast cancer under second-line endocrine treatment: Does quality of life matter? *J Clin Oncol* 1999;17:1672–1679.
18. Greenberg PA, Hortobagyi GN, Smith TL, et al. Long-term follow-up of patients with complete remission following combination chemotherapy for metastatic breast cancer. *J Clin Oncol* 1996;14:2197–2205.
19. Geels P, Eisenhauer E, Bezjak A, et al. Palliative effect of chemotherapy: objective tumor response is associated with symptom improvement in patients with metastatic breast cancer. *J Clin Oncol* 2000;18:2395–2405.
20. Fossati R, Confalonieri C, Torri V, et al. Cytotoxic and hormonal treatment for metastatic breast cancer: a systematic review of published randomised trials involving 31 510 women. *J Clin Oncol* 1998;16:3439–3460. Search date 1997; primary sources Medline, Embase, and hand search of reference lists from retrieved articles and lists from relevant meetings.
21. Litherland S, Jackson IM. Antioestrogens in the management of hormone-dependent cancer. *Cancer Treat Rev* 1988;15:183–194.
22. Johnston SRD. Acquired tamoxifen resistance in human breast cancer – potential mechanisms and clinical implications. *Anti Cancer Drugs* 1997;8:911–930.
23. Hayes DF, Van Zyl JA, Goedhals L, et al. Randomised comparison of tamoxifen and two separate doses of toremifene in postmenopausal patients with metastatic breast cancer. *J Clin Oncol* 1995;13:2556–2566.
24. Parazzini F, Colli E, Scatigna M, Tozzi L. Treatment with tamoxifen and progestins for metastatic breast cancer in postmenopausal women: a quantitative review of published randomised clinical trials. *Oncology* 1993;50:483–489. Search date 1991; primary sources Medline and hand searching reference lists of articles identified.
25. Muss HB, Case DL, Atkins JN, et al. Tamoxifen versus high-dose oral medroxyprogesterone acetate as initial endocrine therapy for patients with metastatic breast cancer: a Piedmont Oncology Association study. *J Clin Oncol* 1994;12:1630–1638.
26. Pannuti F, Martoni A, Murari G, et al. Analgesic activity of medroxyprogesterone acetate in cancer patients: an anti-inflammatory mediated activity? *Int J Tissue React* 1985;7:505–508.
27. Ingle JN, Ahmann DL, Green SJ. Randomised clinical trial of megesterol acetate versus tamoxifen in paramenopausal or castrated women with advanced breast cancer. *Am J Clin Oncol* 1982;5:155–160.
28. Panutti F, Martoni A, Zamagni C, et al. Progestins. In: Powles TJ, Smith IE, eds. *Medical management of breast cancer*. London: Martin Dunitz, 1997:95–107.
29. Crump M, Sawka CA, DeBoer G, et al. An individual patient-based meta-analysis of tamoxifen versus ovarian ablation as first-line endocrine therapy for premenopausal women with metastatic breast cancer. *Breast Cancer Res Treat* 1997;44:201–210. Search date not stated; primary sources Medline, CancerLit, hand searches of bibliographies of related publications, and personal contact with principal investigators of unpublished trials.
30. Sawka CA, Pritchard KI, Shelley W, et al. A randomised crossover trial of tamoxifen versus

ovarian ablation for metastatic breast cancer in premenopausal women: a report of the National Cancer Institute of Canada clinical trials group trial MA1. *Breast Cancer Res Treat* 1997;44:211–215.
31. Taylor CW, Green S, Dalton WS, et al. Multicenter randomised clinical trial of goserelin versus surgical ovariectomy in premenopausal patients with receptor-positive metastatic breast cancer: an intergroup study. *J Clin Oncol* 1998;16:994–999.
32. Boccardo F, Rubagotti A, Perotta A, et al. Ovarian ablation versus goserelin with or without tamoxifen in pre-perimenopausal patients with advanced breast cancer: results of a multicentric Italian study. *Ann Oncol* 1994;5:337–342.
33. Klijn JGN, Blamey RW, Boccardo F, et al. Combined tamoxifen and luteinising hormone-releasing hormone (LHRH) agonist versus LHRH agonist alone in premenopausal advanced breast cancer; a meta-analysis of four randomised trials. *J Clin Oncol* 2001;19:343–353.
34. Bonneterre J, Thurlimann B, Robertson JFR, et al. Anastrozole versus tamoxifen as first-line therapy for advanced breast cancer in 668 postmenopausal women: results of the tamoxifen or Arimidex randomised group efficacy and tolerability study. *J Clin Oncol* 2000;18:3748–3757.
35. Nabholtz JM, Buzdar A, Pollak M, et al. Anastrozole is superior to tamoxifen as first-line therapy for advanced breast cancer in postmenopausal women: results of a North American multicentre randomised trial. *J Clin Oncol* 2000;18:3758–3767.
36. Mouridsen H, Gershanovich M, Sun Y, et al. Superior efficacy of letrozole (Femara) versus tamoxifen as first-line therapy for post-menopausal women with advanced breast cancer; results of a phase III study of the International Letrozole Breast Cancer Group. *J Clin Oncol* 2001:19;2596–2606.
37. Mouridsen H, Sun Y, Gershanovich M, et al. Final survival analysis of the double-blind, randomized, multinational phase III trial of letrozole (Femara®) compared to tamoxifen as first-line hormonal therapy for advanced breast cancer. Program of the 24th Annual San Antonio Breast Cancer Symposium, San Antonio, December 10–13, 2001. http://www.sabcs.org/Program.html.
38. Buzdar A, Jonat W, Howell A, et al. Anastrozole, a potent and selective aromatase inhibitor, versus megesterol acetate in post-menopausal women with advanced breast cancer; results of overview analysis of two phase III trials. *J Clin Oncol* 1996;14:2000–2011.
39. Buzdar A, Jonat W, Howell A, et al. Significant improved survival with Arimidex (anastrozole) versus megesterol acetate in postmenopausal advanced breast cancer; updated results of two randomised trials. *Proc Am Soc Clin Oncol* 1997;16:A545.
40. Jones S, Vogel C, Arkhipov A, et al. Multicenter phase II trial of exemestane as third-line hormonal therapy of postmenopausal women with metastatic breast cancer. *J Clin Oncol* 1999;17:3418–3425.
41. Kaufman M, Bajetta E, Dirix LY, et al. Exemestane is superior to megestrol acetate after tamoxifen failure in postmenopausal women with advanced breast cancer: results of a phase III randomised double-blind trial. *J Clin Oncol* 2000;18:1399–1411.
42. Dombernowsky P, Smith IE, Falkson G, et al. Letrozole, a new oral aromatase inhibitor for advanced breast cancer: double-blind randomised trial showing a dose effect and improved efficacy and tolerability compared with megesterol acetate. *J Clin Oncol* 1998;16:453–461.
43. Gershanovich M, Chaudri HA, Campos D, et al. Letrozole, a new oral aromatase inhibitor: randomised trial comparing 2.5 mg daily, 0.5 mg daily and aminoglutethimide in postmenopausal women with advanced breast cancer. *Ann Oncol* 1998;9:639–645.
44. Lønning PE, Bajetta E, Murray R, et al. Activity of exemestane in metastatic breast cancer after failure of nonsteroidal aromatase inhibitors: a phase II trial. *J Clin Oncol* 2000;18:2234–2244.
45. Engelsman E, Klijn JCM, Rubens RD, et al. "Classical" CMF versus a 3-weekly intravenous CMF schedule in postmenopausal patients with advanced breast cancer. *Eur J Cancer* 1991;27:966–970.
46. Tannock IF, Boyd NF, DeBoer G, et al. A randomised trial of two dose levels of cyclophosphamide, methotrexate and fluorouracil chemotherapy for patients with metastatic breast cancer. *J Clin Oncol* 1988;6:1377–1387.
47. A'Hern RP, Smith IE, Ebbs SR. Chemotherapy and survival in advanced breast cancer: the inclusion of doxorubicin in Cooper type regimens. *Br J Cancer* 1993;67:801–805. Search date not stated; primary sources CancerLit and communication with colleagues.
48. Cummings FJ, Gelman R, Horton J. Comparison of CAF versus CMFP in metastatic breast cancer: analysis of prognostic factors. *J Clin Oncol* 1985;3:932–940.
49. Smalley RV, Lefante J, Bartolucci A, et al. A comparison of cyclophosphamide, adriamycin, and 5-fluorouracil (CAF) and cyclophosphamide, methotrexate, 5-fluorouracil, vincristine, and prednisolone (CMFVP) in patients with advanced breast cancer. *Breast Cancer Res Treat* 1983;3:209–220.
50. French Epirubicin Study Group. A prospective randomised phase III trial comparing combination chemotherapy with cyclophosphamide, fluorouracil, and either doxorubicin or epirubicin. *J Clin Oncol* 1988;6:679–688.
51. Italian Multicentre Breast Study with Epirubicin. Randomised phase III study of fluorouracil, doxorubicin, and cyclophosphamide in advanced breast cancer: an Italian multicentre trial. *J Clin Oncol* 1988;6:976–982.
52. Stewart DJ, Evans WK, Shepherd FA, et al. Cyclophosphamide and fluorouracil combined with mitozantrone versus doxorubicin for breast cancer: superiority of doxorubicin. *J Clin Oncol* 1997;15:1897–1905.
53. Namer M, Soler-Michel P, Turpin F. Results of a phase III prospective randomised trial comparing mitoxantrone and vinorelbine in combination with standard FAC/FEC in front-line therapy of metastatic breast cancer. *Eur J Cancer* 2001;37:1132–1140.
54. Stockler M, Wilcken NR, Ghersi D, et al. Systematic reviews of chemotherapy and chemotherapy and endocrine therapy in metastatic breast cancer. *Cancer Treat Rev* 2000;26:151–168. Search date not stated; primary source Medline.
55. Sledge GW, Hu P, Torney D, et al. Comparison of chemotherapy with chemohormonal therapy as first-line therapy for metastatic, hormone sensitive breast cancer. An Eastern Cooperative Oncology Group Study. *J Clin Oncol* 2000;18:262–266.
56. Ross MB, Buzdar AU, Smith TL, et al. Improved survival of patients with metastatic breast cancer receiving combination chemotherapy. *Cancer* 1985;55:341–346.

57. Goldhirsch A, Glick JH, Gelber RD, et al. International consensus panel on the treatment of primary breast cancer. *J Natl Cancer Inst* 1998;90:1601–1608.
58. Coates AS, Hurny C, Peterson HF, et al. Quality of life scores predict outcome in metastatic but not early breast cancer. *J Clin Oncol* 2000;18:3768–3774.
59. Hakamies-Blomquist L, Luoma M, Sjostrom J, et al. Quality of life in patients with metastatic breast cancer receiving either docetaxel or sequential methotrexate and 5-fluorouracil. A multicenter randomised phase III trial by the Scandinavian breast group. *J Clin Oncol* 2000;36:1411–1417.
60. Houston SJ, Richards MA, Bentley AE, et al. The influence of adjuvant chemotherapy on outcome after relapse for patients with breast cancer. *Eur J Cancer* 1993;29A:1513–1518.
61. The Italian Group for Antiemetic Research. Dexamethasone alone or in combination with ondansetron for the prevention of delayed nausea and vomiting induced by chemotherapy. *N Engl J Med* 2000;342:1554–1559.
62. Stadtmauer E, O'Neill A, Goldstein L. Conventional-dose chemotherapy compared with high-dose chemotherapy plus autologous hematopoietic stem-cell transplantation for metastatic breast cancer. *N Engl J Med* 2000; 342: 1069–76 http://www/nejm.org/content/stadmauer/1.asp.
63. Hortobagyi GN, Bodey GP, Buzdar AU, et al. Evaluation of high-dose versus standard FAC chemotherapy for advanced breast cancer in protected environment units; a prospective randomised trial. *J Clin Oncol* 1987;5:354–364.
64. Bastholt L, Dalmark M, Gjedde S, et al. Dose-response relationship of epirubicin in the treatment of post-menopausal patients with metastatic breast cancer: a randomised study of epirubicin at four different dose-levels performed by the Danish Breast Cancer Co-operative Group. *J Clin Oncol* 1996;14:1146–1155.
65. Slamon DJ, Leyland-Jones B, Shak S, et al. Use of chemotherapy plus a monoclonal antibody against HER2 for metastatic breast cancer that overexpresses HER2. *New Engl J Med* 2001;344:783–792.
66. Vogel CL, Cobleigh MA, Tripathy D, et al. Efficacy and safety of trastuzumab as a single agent in first-line treatment of HER2-overexpressing metastatic breast cancer. *J Clin Oncol* 2002;20:719–726.
67. Vermoken JB, Ten Bokkel Huinick WW. Chemotherapy for advanced breast cancer: the place of active new drugs. *Breast* 1996;5:304–311.
68. Paridaens R, Bignazoli L, Bruning P, et al. Paclitaxel versus doxorubicin as first-line single agent chemotherapy for metastatic breast cancer; an EORTC randomised study with cross-over. *J Clin Oncol* 2000;18:724–733.
69. Bishop JF, Dewar J, Toner GC, et al. Initial paclitaxel improves outcome compared with CMFP combination chemotherapy as front-line therapy in untreated metastatic breast cancer. *J Clin Oncol* 1999;17:2355–2364.
70. Nabholtz JM, Senn HJ, Bezwoda WR, et al. Prospective randomised trial of docetaxel vs mitomycin plus vinblastine in patients with metastatic breast cancer progressing despite previous anthracycline-containing chemotherapy. *J Clin Oncol* 1999;17:1413–1424.
71. Sjosrom J, Blomqvist C, Mouridsen H, et al. Docetaxel compared with sequential methotrexate and 5-fluorouracil in patients with advanced breast cancer after anthracycline failure; a randomised phase III study with cross-over on progression by the Scandinavian Breast Group. *Eur J Cancer* 1999;35:1194–1201.
72. Chan S, Friedrichs K, Noel D, et al. Prospective randomised trial of docetaxel versus doxorubicin in patients with metastatic breast cancer. *J Clin Oncol* 1999;35:2341–2354.
73. Norris B, Pritchard KI, James K, et al. Phase III comparative study of vinorelbine combined with doxorubicin versus doxorubicin alone in disseminated metastatic/recurrent breast cancer: National Cancer Institute of Canada Clinical Trials Group Study MA8. *J Clin Oncol* 2000;18:2385–2394.
74. Jones S, Winer E, Vogel C, et al. Randomised comparison of vinorelbine and melphalan in anthracycline-refractory advanced breast cancer. *J Clin Oncol* 1995;13:2567–2574.
75. Tomiak E, Verma S, Levine M, et al. Use of capecitabine in stage IV breast cancer: an evidence summary. *Curr Oncol* 2000;7:84–90. Search date 2000; primary sources Medline, Cancerlit, Cochrane, PubMed, United States Food and Drug Administration website, Physician Query Database, Clinical Trials Listing service, hand searches of proceedings of the American Society of Clinical Oncology, and contact with Hoffmann-La Roche.
76. Namer M, Soler-Michel P, Mefti F, et al. Is the combination FAC/FEC always the best regimen in advanced breast cancer? Utility of mitoxantrone and vinorelbine association as an alternative: results from a randomised trial [abstract]. *Breast Cancer Res Treat* 1997;46:94(A406).
77. Blum JL, Jones SE, Buzdar AU, et al. Multicenter phase II study of capecitabine in paclitaxel-refractory metastatic breast cancer. *J Clin Oncol* 1999;17:485–493.
78. Diasio RB. An evolving role for oral fluoropyrimidine drugs. *J Clin Oncol* 2002;20:894–896.
79. Berruti A, Sperone P, Bottini A. Phase II study of vinorelbine with protracted fluorouracil infusion as a second or third line approach for advanced breast cancer patients previously treated with anthracyclines. *J Clin Oncol* 2000;18 (19):3370–3377.
80. Stathopoulus GP, Rigatos SK, Pergantas N, et al. Phase II trial of biweekly administration of vinorelbine and gemcitabine in pretreated advanced breast cancer. *J Clin Oncol* 2002;20:37–41.
81. Hortobagyi GN, Theriault RL, Porter L, et al. Efficacy of pamidronate in reducing skeletal complications in patients with breast cancer and lytic bone metastases. *N Engl J Med* 1996;335:1785–1791.
82. Paterson AHG, Powles TJ, Kanis JA, et al. Double-blind controlled trial of oral clodronate in patients with bone metastases from breast cancer. *J Clin Oncol* 1993;11:59–65.
83. Theriault RL, Lipton A, Hortobagyi GN. Pamidronate reduces skeletal morbidity in women with advanced breast cancer and lytic bone lesions; a randomised placebo controlled trial. *J Clin Oncol* 1999;17:846–854.
84. Hortobagyi GN, Theriault RL, Lipton A, et al. Long-term prevention of skeletal complications of metastatic breast cancer with pamidronate. *J Clin Oncol* 1998;16:2038–2044.
85. Hillner BE, Ingle JN, Berenson JR, et al. American Society of Clinical Oncology guideline on the role of bisphosphonates in breast cancer: American Society of Oncology Bisphosphonates Expert Panel. *J Clin Oncol* 2000;18:1378–1391.

86. Hillner BE, Weeks JC, Desch CE, et al. Pamidronate in prevention of bone complications in metastatic breast cancer; a cost-effectiveness analysis. *J Clin Oncol* 2000;18:72–79.
87. World Health Organization. *Cancer pain relief*. Geneva: WHO, 1996.
88. Hall SM, Budzar AV, Blumenschein GR. Cranial nerve palsies in metastatic breast cancer due to osseous metastasis without intracranial involvement. *Cancer* 1983;52:180–184.
89. Bone Trial Working Party. 8 Gy single fraction radiotherapy for the treatment of metastatic skeletal pain: randomised comparison with a multifraction schedule over 12 months of patient follow-up. *Radiother Oncol* 1999;52:111–121.
90. Price P, Hoskin PJ, Easton D, et al. Prospective randomised trial of single and multifraction radiotherapy schedules in treatment of painful bony metastases. *Radiother Oncol* 1986;6:247–255.
91. Priestman TJ, Dunn J, Brada M, et al. Final results of the Royal College of Radiologists' trial comparing two different radiotherapy schedules in the treatment of brain metastases. *Clin Oncol* 1996;8:308–315.
92. Roos DE, O'Brien PC, Smith JG, et al. A role for radiotherapy in neuropathic bone pain: preliminary response rates from a prospective trial. *Int J Radiat Oncol Biol Phys* 2000;46:975–981.
93. Bretscher N. Care for dying patients: what is right? *J Clin Oncol* 2000;18:233–234.
94. Rades D, Blach M, Nerreter V, et al. Metastatic spinal cord compression. Influence of time between onset of motor deficits and start of irradiation on therapeutic effect. *Strahlenther Onkol* 1999;175:378–381.
95. Sorensen S, Helweg-Larsen S, Mouridsen H, et al. Effect of high-dose dexamethasone in carcinomatous metastatic spinal cord compression treated with radiotherapy: a randomised trial. *Eur J Cancer* 1994;30A:22–27.
96. Cancer Guidance Subgroup of the Clinical Outcomes Group. *Improving outcomes in breast cancer. The research evidence*. London: NHS Executive, 1996.
97. Diener-West M, Dobbins TW, Phillips TL, et al. Identification of an optimal subgroup for treatment evaluation of patients with brain metastases using RTOG study 7916. *Int J Radiat Oncol Biol Phys* 1989;16:669–673.
98. Ratanatharathorn V, Powers WE, Grimm J, et al. Eye metastasis from carcinoma of the breast: radiation treatment and results. *Cancer Treat Rev* 1991;18:261–276.
99. Piccone MR, Maguire AM, Fox KC, et al. Choroidal metastases. Case 1: breast cancer. *J Clin Oncol* 1999;17:3356–3358.
100. Hortobagyi GN. Treatment of breast cancer. *N Engl J Med* 1998;339:974–984.
101. Levinger S, Merin S, Seigal R, et al. Laser therapy in the management of choroidal breast tumor metastases. *Ophthalmic Surg Lasers* 2001;32:294–299.
102. Ando M, Watanabe T, Nagata K, et al. Efficacy of docetaxel 60 mg/m^2 in patients with metastatic breast cancer according to the status of anthracycline resistance. *J Clin Oncol* 2001;19:336–342.

Stephen Johnston
Senior Lecturer in Medical Oncology

Justin Stebbing
MRC Clinical Training Fellow

The Royal Marsden NHS Trust
London
UK

Competing interests: None declared.

TABLE 1 Clinical factors that predict response to hormonal treatment in metastatic breast cancer, based on results of RCTs (see text, p 1788).[8–11]

Factors predictive of good response to hormonal treatment

Postmenopausal status

Disease limited to soft tissue sites (skin, nodes)

Oestrogen receptor positive tumour

Long disease free interval since primary treatment for early breast cancer (> 18–24 months).

Factors making initial hormonal treatment less appropriate

Symptomatic visceral metastases (e.g. lymphangitis carcinomatosis or progressive liver metastases)

Oestrogen receptor negative tumour

Short disease free interval (12–18 months)

Relapse on adjuvant tamoxifen (unless oestrogen receptor positive tumour and other features predictive of good response).

Breast cancer: non-metastatic

Search date February 2002

J Michael Dixon, Kate Gregory, Stephen Johnston, and Alan Rodger

QUESTIONS

INTERVENTIONS

Breast cancer: non-metastatic

Key Messages

Ductal carcinoma *in situ*

- **Radiotherapy after breast conserving surgery (reduces recurrence)** RCTs found that radiotherapy reduced the risk of local recurrence and invasive carcinoma, with no evidence of an effect on survival.
- **Tamoxifen plus radiotherapy after breast conserving surgery (reduces recurrence)** One RCT has found that adjuvant tamoxifen significantly reduces breast cancer events in women who have undergone wide excision and radiotherapy, but found no significant difference in overall survival at 6 years.

Primary operable breast cancer

- **Adjuvant chemotherapy** One systematic review has found that adjuvant chemotherapy versus no chemotherapy significantly reduces rates of recurrence and improves survival at 10 years. The benefit seems to be independent of nodal or menopausal status, although the absolute improvements are greater in those women with node positive disease, and probably greater in younger women.
- **Adjuvant tamoxifen** One systematic review has found that adjuvant tamoxifen taken for up to 5 years reduces the risk of recurrence and death in women with oestrogen receptor positive tumours irrespective of age, menopausal status, nodal involvement, or the addition of chemotherapy. Tamoxifen slightly increases the risk of endometrial cancer, but we found no evidence of an overall adverse effect on non-breast cancer mortality.
- **Anthracycline regimens as adjuvant chemotherapy** One systematic review has found that adjuvant regimens containing an anthracycline versus a standard multidrug chemotherapy (CMF) regimen significantly reduce recurrence, and significantly improve survival at 5 years.

- **Axillary clearance (no evidence of survival benefit and increased morbidity compared with axillary sampling)** RCTs found no significant difference in survival at 5–10 years between axillary clearance versus axillary sampling, axillary radiotherapy, or sampling plus radiotherapy combined. One systematic review of mainly poor quality evidence found that the risk of arm lymphoedema was highest with axillary clearance plus radiotherapy, lower with axillary sampling plus radiotherapy, and lowest with sampling alone.
- **Axillary radiotherapy** One systematic review has found that axilliary radiotherapy versus axilliary clearance significantly reduces isolated local recurrence, and has found no significant difference in mortality or overall recurrence at 10 years.
- **Breast conserving surgery (similar survival to more extensive surgery)** Systematic reviews have found that, providing all local disease is excised, more extensive surgery does not increase survival at 10 years. More extensive local resection in breast conserving surgery gives worse cosmetic results.
- **Chemotherapy plus tamoxifen** One RCT found that adding chemotherapy (CMF) to tamoxifen significantly improves survival at 5 years.
- **Enhanced dose regimens of adjuvant chemotherapy** RCTs found no significant improvement from enhanced dose regimens.
- **Neoadjuvant chemotherapy (reduces mastectomy rates *v* adjuvant chemotherapy; no evidence of effect on survival)** RCTs have found that neoadjuvant versus adjuvant chemotherapy reduces mastectomy rates, but found no significant difference in survival at 4–10 years.
- **Ovarian ablation in premenopausal women** One systematic review has found that in women less than 50 years of age, ovarian ablation versus no ablation significantly improves survival for at least 15 years.
- **Prolonged chemotherapy (8–12 months *v* 4–6 months)** One systematic review found no additional benefit from prolonging adjuvant chemotherapy from 4–6 to 8–12 months.
- **Radical mastectomy (no greater survival than less extensive surgery)** Systematic reviews have found no significant difference between radical, total, supraradical, or simple mastectectomy in survival at 10 years. More extensive surgery results in greater mutilation.
- **Radiotherapy after breast conserving surgery (reduces local recurrence; no evidence of effect on survival)** One systematic review has found that the addition of radiotherapy to breast conserving surgery significantly reduces the risk of isolated local recurrence and loss of a breast, but does not increase survival at 10 years. Similar rates of survival and local recurrence are achieved with radiotherapy plus either breast conserving surgery or mastectomy.
- **Radiotherapy after mastectomy in women at high risk of local recurrence** RCTs in high risk women receiving adjuvant chemotherapy after mastectomy have found that radiotherapy versus no radiotherapy significantly reduces local recurrence and increases survival at 10–15 years.
- **Radiotherapy after mastectomy in node positive disease, large tumours, or where lymphovascular invasion is present** One systematic review has found that radiotherapy to the chest wall after mastectomy reduces the risk of local recurrence by about two thirds and the risk of death from breast cancer at 10 years, but found no evidence of effect on overall 10 year survival. One review of retrospective data found that greater axillary node involvement, larger tumour size, higher histological grade, presence of lymphovascular invasion, and involvement of tumour margins reduced the chance of successful treatment.

- **Radiotherapy after mastectomy in women not at high risk of local recurrence** One systematic review has found that radiotherapy to the chest wall after mastectomy reduces the risk of local recurrence by about two thirds and the risk of death from breast cancer at 10 years, but found no evidence of effect on overall 10 year survival. Radiotherapy may be associated with late adverse effects, which are rare, including pneumonitis, pericarditis, arm oedema, brachial plexopathy, and radionecrotic rib fracture.
- **Radiotherapy to the internal mammary chain** One RCT found no significant difference in overall survival or breast cancer specific survival at 2–3 years between radiotherapy versus no radiotherapy to the internal mammary chain. Treatment may increase radiation induced cardiac morbidity.
- **Radiotherapy to the ipsilateral supraclavicular fossa** We found insufficient evidence about the effects of irradiation of the ipsilateral supraclavicular fossa on survival. RCTs have found that radiotherapy reduces the risk of supraclavicular fossa nodal recurrence.
- **Total mastectomy** Systematic reviews have found no significant difference between total, supraradical, radical, or simple mastectectomy in survival at 10 years. More extensive surgery results in greater mutilation.
- **Total nodal radiotherapy in high risk disease** RCTs have found that in women with high risk disease total nodal irradiation versus no irradiation improves survival. An earlier systematic review found reduced locoregional recurrence, but no evidence of improved survival.

Locally advanced breast cancer

- **Chemotherapy (cyclophosphamide/methotrexate/fluorouracil [5-FU] or anthracycline based regimens)** We found no evidence that the cytotoxic, multidrug chemotherapy regimen (CMF) improves survival, disease free survival, or long term locoregional control.
- **Radiotherapy** For locally advanced breast cancer that is rendered operable, small RCTs found that radiotherapy or surgery as sole local treatments have similar effects on response rates, duration of response, and overall survival.
- **Radiotherapy after attempted curative surgery** One RCT found weak evidence that radiotherapy after attempted curative surgery versus no further local treatment may reduce local and/or regional recurrence.
- **Surgery** For locally advanced breast cancer that is rendered operable, small RCTs found that surgery or radiotherapy as sole local treatments have similar effects on response rates, duration of response, and overall survival.
- **Tamoxifen plus radiotherapy (*v* radiotherapy)** One RCT found that hormone treatment plus radiotherapy versus radiotherapy alone significantly improved locoregional recurrence at 6 years and improved median survival at 8 years.

DEFINITION **Ductal carcinoma *in situ*** is a non-invasive tumour characterised by the presence of malignant cells in the breast ducts but with no evidence that they breach the basement membrane and invade into periductal connective tissues. **Invasive breast cancer** can be separated into three main groups: early or operable breast cancer, locally advanced disease, and metastatic breast cancer (see metastatic breast cancer, p 1785). **Operable breast cancer** is apparently restricted to the breast and sometimes to local lymph nodes and can be surgically removed. Although these women do not have overt metastases at the time of staging, they remain at risk of local recurrence and of metastatic spread. They can be divided into those with tumours greater than 4 cm or multifocal cancers that can be treated by mastectomy, and those with tumours less than 4 cm with unifocal cancers that can be treated by breast conserving surgery (see glossary, p 1834). **Locally advanced breast cancer** is defined according to the TNM staging system (see glossary, p 1835) of the UICC TNM system (see glossary, p 1835)[1] as stage III B (includes T4 a–d; N2 disease, but absence of metastases). It is a disease presentation with evidence (clinical or histopathological) of skin and/or chest wall involvement and/or axillary nodes matted together by tumour extension. **Metastatic breast cancer** is presented in a separate topic (see metastatic breast cancer, p 1785).

INCIDENCE/ PREVALENCE Breast cancer affects 1/10–1/11 women in the UK and causes about 21 000 deaths per year. Prevalence is about five times higher, with over 100 000 women living with breast cancer at any one time. Of the 15 000 new cases of breast cancer per annum in the UK, the majority will present with primary operable disease.[2]

AETIOLOGY/ RISK FACTORS The risk of breast cancer increases with age, doubling every 10 years up to the menopause. Risk factors include an early age at menarche, older age at menopause, older age at birth of first child, family history, atypical hyperplasia, excess alcohol intake, radiation exposure to developing breast tissue, oral contraceptive use, postmenopausal hormone replacement therapy, and obesity. Risk in different countries varies fivefold. The cause of breast cancer in most women is unknown. About 5% of breast cancers can be attributed to mutations in the genes BRCA1 and BRCA2.[3]

PROGNOSIS **Primary carcinoma** of the breast is potentially curable. The risk of relapse depends on various clinicopathological features, including axillary node involvement, oestrogen receptor status, and tumour size. Tumour size, axillary node status, histological grade, and oestrogen receptor status provide the most significant prognostic information. Seventy per cent of women with operable disease are alive 5 years after diagnosis and treatment (adjuvant drug treatment is given to most women after surgery). Risk of recurrence is highest during the first 5 years, but the risk remains even 15–20 years after surgery. Those with node positive disease have a 50–60% chance of recurrence within 5 years, compared with 30–35% for node negative disease. Recurrence at 10 years, according to one large systematic review,[4] is 60–70% compared with 25–30% of node negative women. The prognosis for a disease free survival (see glossary, p 1834) at 5 years is worse for stage III B (33%) than that for stage III A (71%). Five year overall survival is 44% and 84%, respectively.[5] Poor survival and high rates of local recurrence characterise locally advanced breast cancer (see glossary, p 1834).

AIMS To improve survival; to prevent local or regional node recurrence; to obtain prognostic information on the type and extent of tumour and the status of the axillary lymph nodes; to optimise cosmetic results and minimise psychosocial impact; to minimise adverse effects of treatment; and to maximise quality of life.

OUTCOMES Survival; rates of local and regional recurrence; rates of mastectomy after breast conserving treatment; rates of development of metastases; cosmetic outcomes; quality of life; incidence of adverse effects of treatment, including upper limb lymphoedema.

METHODS *Clinical Evidence* update search and appraisal February 2002.

QUESTION What are the effects of interventions after breast conserving surgery for ductal carcinoma *in situ*?

OPTION RADIOTHERAPY

Alan Rodger and Mike Dixon

Two RCTs found that radiotherapy is associated with a reduced risk of local recurrence and invasive carcinoma, but with no evidence of an effect on survival.

Benefits: We found no systematic review but found two RCTs comparing with no radiotherapy after surgery for ductal carcinoma *in situ* (DCIS). The first RCT (814 women) found no significant difference in survival at 8 years with radiotherapy, but a significant reduction in risk of local recurrence (survival 95% *v* 94%; local recurrence 12.1% *v* 26.8%; P = < 0.000005; risk of recurrent DCIS 8.2% *v* 13.4%; P = 0.007; risk of invasive carcinoma 3.9% *v* 13.4%; P < 0.0001).[6] The second RCT (1002 women) found, at median follow up of 4.25 years, significantly lower recurrence of DCIS in women given radiotherapy.[7] At 4 years, local relapse free survival was more likely with surgery plus radiotherapy than with surgery alone (91% *v* 84%; P = 0.005; HR 0.62, 95% CI 0.44 to 0.87). More women were free of DCIS recurrence after 4 years with radiotherapy but the difference was not significant (95% *v* 92%; HR 0.65, 95% CI 0.43 to 1.03). There was a significant reduction in invasive recurrence (96% *v* 92%; HR 0.60, 95% CI 0.37 to 0.97).

Harms: One RCT found an increase in contralateral breast cancer associated with radiotherapy at 4 years (3% *v* 1%; HR 2.57, 95% CI 1.24 to 5.33).[7]

Comment: Ongoing RCTs are evaluating radiotherapy in all grades of DCIS. Subset analyses may be required to identify subgroups of women who benefit most from radiotherapy after breast conserving surgery.

OPTION TAMOXIFEN PLUS RADIOTHERAPY

Mike Dixon and Alan Rodger

One RCT found that adjuvant tamoxifen reduced breast cancer events in women who have undergone wide excision and radiotherapy, but found no evidence of an effect on survival.

Benefits: We found no systematic review. We found one RCT in women with ductal carcinoma *in situ* treated with wide excision and radiotherapy (see glossary, p 1835), which compared adjuvant tamoxifen (see glossary, p 1835) 20 mg daily with placebo for 5 years in 1804 women.[8] At median follow up of 74 months, there were fewer breast cancer events with tamoxifen than placebo (OR 0.63, 95% CI 0.47 to 0.83), and fewer invasive ipsilateral or contralateral breast cancers (OR 0.57, 95% CI 0.38 to 0.85). However, there was no significant difference in overall survival (RR 0.88, 95% CI 0.33 to 2.28).

Harms: One RCT found a higher, but non-significant rate of endometrial cancers associated with tamoxifen (RR 3.4, 95% CI 0.6 to 33.4).[8]

Comment: RCTs of tamoxifen in ductal carcinoma *in situ* are under way. Results of one of these RCTs are expected to be published shortly (Dixon M, personal communication, 2002).

QUESTION What are the effects of neoadjuvant chemotherapy in the management of primary breast cancer?

Kate Gregory and Stephen Johnston

Five RCTs found no difference in survival with neoadjuvant chemotherapy versus adjuvant chemotherapy.

Benefits: We found no systematic review. We found five RCTs of neoadjuvant chemotherapy (see glossary, p 1835) versus adjuvant chemotherapy.[9–13] The first RCT (272 women with tumours > 3 cm in whom mastectomy was indicated) compared preoperative (neoadjuvant) EVMTV (epirubicin, vincristine, mitomycin-C, thiotepa, vindesine) chemotherapy versus mastectomy followed by EVMTV regimen. At an initial median follow up of 34 months, a significant survival difference was reported in favour of neoadjuvant chemotherapy (85% *v* 95%; P = 0.04).[9] However, the final analysis at 124 months showed that the survival improvement was no longer significant, with survival of about 55% in both groups.[14] The second RCT (414 women) compared four cycles of FAC chemotherapy (see glossary, p 1835) given either pre- or postoperatively. At 54 months' follow up, the primary (neoadjuvant) chemotherapy group had a better overall survival (86% *v* 68%; P = 0.039);[10] however, a subsequent analysis at 105 months did not demonstrate a long term survival benefit.[15] The third RCT (309 women) compared four cycles of MM (mitoxantrone [mitozantrone], methotrexate) chemotherapy, then surgery, then four cycles of MM versus surgery, then eight cycles of MM. At 48 months' follow up, there was no difference in survival between the neoadjuvant and adjuvant groups (84% *v* 82%, not significant).[11] The third, and largest RCT (NSABP-18), in which 1523 women were randomised to four cycles of AC (adriamycin, cyclophosphamide) either pre- or postoperatively, found identical survival rates (67%) in the two groups at 60 months.[12] The fifth RCT (698 women) compared four cycles of flurouracil, epirubicin, and cyclophosphamide given either pre- or postoperatively. It found no significant difference between preoperative versus postoperative chemotherapy in overall survival (82% *v* 84%, HR 1.16, 95% CI 0.83 to 1.63), progression free survival (65% *v* 70%; HR 1.15, 95% CI 0.89 to 1.48), or locoregional recurrence at 4 years (21.5% *v* 17.8%; HR 1.13, 95% CI 0.70 to 1.81).[13]

Harms: We found no evidence that neoadjuvant chemotherapy has a negative impact on survival.

Comment: We found no evidence to support the use of neoadjuvant chemotherapy to improve the chances of survival for operable breast cancers outside the context of an RCT.

QUESTION What is the effect of neoadjuvant chemotherapy on mastectomy rates?

Several RCTs have found that neoadjuvant chemotherapy leads to a marked reduction in the mastectomy rate.

Benefits: **Neoadjuvant versus adjuvant chemotherapy:** We found no systematic review but found three RCTs, which found a lower rate of mastectomy in women who had received neoadjuvant chemotherapy (see glossary, p 1835) compared with women receiving adjuvant chemotherapy. **MM regimen:** One RCT in the UK (309 women receiving MM [mitoxantrone methorexate] chemotherapy) found that neoadjuvant versus adjuvant chemotherapy significantly reduced the mastectomy rate (13% *v* 28%; $P < 0.005$).[16] **AC (adriamycin, cyclophosphamide) regimen:** In the NSABP-18 study (1523 women), breast conservation rates were lower in the adjuvant arm (60% *v* 67%), although this was not significant.[12] **FAC regimen:** See glossary, p 1835. One RCT assessed 272 women at diagnosis in terms of the recommended surgical procedure, and two of three women who were initially advised to have mastectomy were able to have breast conserving surgery after neoadjuvant chemotherapy.[17]

Harms: None of the RCTs reported a significantly higher local recurrence rate with neoadjuvant chemotherapy compared with adjuvant chemotherapy.[9,11,12]

Comment: With an increased number of conservative operations being performed after downstaging by neoadjuvant chemotherapy for large primary tumours, there are theoretical concerns that this may result in an increased rate of local recurrence. Neoadjuvant chemotherapy can lead to a reduction in the requirement for mastectomy and as such an increase in breast conservation surgery. In the three RCTs of women with operable breast cancer receiving breast conserving surgery, this has not been associated with a significant increase in the rate of local recurrence.[12,16,17]

QUESTION What are the effects of different regimens used in the neoadjuvant setting?

We found no evidence that any one of the commonly used chemotherapy regimens is superior in the neoadjuvant setting.

Benefits: We found no systematic review. We found one non-systematic review and five additional RCTs comparing adjuvant to neoadjuvant chemotherapy (see glossary, p 1835) using a variety of regimens.[11,12,18–21] Most studies used anthracycline based regimens, which are of proven benefit in the adjuvant setting.[18] **AC regimen:** The NSABP-18 RCT treated women with AC (adriamycin, cyclophosphamide) and found an objective response rate (complete or partial clinical response) of 79%.[12] **MM regimen:** MM (mitoxantrone, methotrexate) in the UK RCT gave an overall objective response rate (see glossary, p 1835) of 85%.[11] Three RCTs compared different neoadjuvant regimens. **FAC regimen versus paclitaxel:** An RCT (174 women in the US) compared conventional FAC versus single agent paclitaxel, and found similar response rates in both groups: FAC 79%, paclitaxel 80%, with no significant difference in survival rates.[19] **Comparison between MPEMi, MPEpiE and MPEpiV regimens:** A European RCT (101 women treated with three different combinations: MPEMi [methotrexate, cisplatin, etoposide, mitomycin-C], MPEpiE [methotrexate, cisplatin, epirubicin, etoposide], and MPEpiV [methotrexate, cisplatin, epirubicin, vincristine]) found the response to be 89%, with no significant differences between the groups.[20] **Comparison between routes of administration:** We found one Japanese study comparing routes of administration.[21] It compared no neoadjuvant treatment, neoadjuvant intravenous epirubicin, or intra-arterial epirubicin. Response rates were higher in women receiving intra-arterial epirubicin versus intravenous epirubicin (68% compared with 36%; $P < 0.05$); however, this was not associated with a survival benefit.

Harms: **FAC versus paclitaxel:** In the RCT in the US comparing FAC with paclitaxel, rates of septic neutropenia (53% *v* 21%) and granulocyte colony stimulating factor usage (56% *v* 25%) were higher in women taking paclitaxel.[19]

Comment: More work is needed to determine the optimal regimen for neoadjuvant treatment. We found little evidence in the literature comparing different combinations, but anthracycline-based combinations probably remain the treatment of choice. Ongoing RCTs are investigating the role of taxane sequencing after anthracycline based therapy (NSABP-27), and anthracycline in combination with infusional fluorouracil (5-FU).

QUESTION Is the extent of surgery related to outcome in early invasive breast cancer?

Mike Dixon and Alan Rodger

Two systematic reviews have found that more extensive surgery is not associated with better outcomes, providing that all local disease is excised. The more extensive the local resection in breast conserving surgery, the worse the cosmetic result.

Benefits: **Comparisons between supraradical, radical, and total mastectomy (see glossary, p 1835):** We found one systematic review (search date not stated, 5 RCTs, 2090 women with operable breast cancer) comparing supraradical mastectomy with radical mastectomy, radical with total mastectomy, and supraradical with total mastectomy.[22] It found no significant difference in risk of death over 10 years (ARR of more extensive *v* less extensive surgery 0.02, 95% CI –0.04 to +0.08). **Comparisons between radical, total, and simple mastectomy:** The same review included four RCTs comparing either radical with simple mastectomy (3 RCTs) or total with simple mastectomy (1 RCT) in 1296 women with operable breast cancer.[22] Meta-analysis found no significant difference in risk of death over 10 years (ARR for more extensive *v* less extensive surgery 2%, 95% CI –5% to +9%). **Mastectomy versus breast conservation:** We found two systematic reviews.[22,23] One review (search date 1995)[23] analysed data on 10 year survival from six RCTs comparing breast conservation with mastectomy. Meta-analysis of data from five of the RCTs (3006 women) found no significant difference in the risk of death at 10 years (OR *v* mastectomy 0.91, 95% CI 0.78 to 1.05). The sixth RCT used different protocols. Where more than half of node positive women in both mastectomy and breast conservation groups received adjuvant nodal radiotherapy, both groups had similar survival rates. Where fewer than half of node positive women in both groups received adjuvant nodal radiotherapy, survival was better with breast conservation (OR *v* with mastectomy 0.69, 95% CI 0.49 to 0.97). In the second review (search date not stated), 9 RCTs, 4981 women potentially suitable for breast conserving surgery (see glossary, p 1834) all participants received postoperative radiotherapy (see glossary, p 1835).[22] Meta-analysis found no significant difference in risk of death over 10 years (RRR for breast conservation compared with mastectomy 0.02, 95% CI –0.05 to +0.09). It also found no significant difference in rates of local recurrence (6 RCTs in 3107 women; RRR mastectomy *v* breast conservation 0.04, 95% CI –0.04 to +0.12). **Different extents of local excision in breast conservation:** We found no systematic review. We found one RCT (705 women) comparing lumpectomy (see glossary, p 1835) with quadrantectomy (see glossary, p 1835).[24] There were significantly more local recurrences with lumpectomy than with quadrantectomy (7% *v* 2%), but a major factor associated with local recurrence in the lumpectomy group was incomplete excision (see comment below).[25] We found no RCTs comparing wide local excision (complete excision microscopically) with quadrantectomy.

Harms: More extensive surgery results in greater mutilation. Between 60–90% of women having breast conservation have an excellent or good cosmetic result (median 83%, 95% CI 67% to 87%).[24,26–34] The single most important factor influencing cosmetic outcome is the volume of tissue excised; the larger the amount of tissue excised the worse the cosmetic result.[24] The RCT of different extents of local excision in breast conservation found that, in a subset of 148 women, there was a significantly higher rate of poor cosmetic outcome with quadrantectomy (RR *v* lumpectomy 3.11, 95% CI 1.2 to 8.1).[24] Only isolated small studies have shown no correlation between extent of surgical excision and cosmesis.[32]

Comment: The link between completeness of excision and local recurrence after breast conservation has been evaluated in 16 centres. In 13 of these, incomplete excision was associated with an increased relative risk of local recurrence compared with complete excision (estimated median RRI 3.4, 95% CI 2.6% to 4.6%).[25] The three centres not reporting increased rates of local recurrence after incomplete excision gave much higher doses of local radiotherapy (65–72 Gy) to people with involved margins. Two centres also used re-excision, and women with involved margins had only focal margin involvement.

QUESTION What are the effects of different radiotherapy regimens in operable breast cancer?

Alan Rodger and Mike Dixon

OPTION RADIOTHERAPY AFTER BREAST CONSERVING SURGERY

One systematic review has found that radiotherapy reduces the risk of isolated local recurrence and loss of a breast, but does not increase 10 year survival compared with breast conserving surgery alone. Similar rates of survival and local recurrence are achieved with breast conserving surgery plus radiotherapy as with mastectomy.

Benefits: **Versus breast conserving surgery alone:** See glossary, p 1834. We found one systematic review (search date not stated, 4 RCTs, 382–1450 women),[22] comparing surgery plus radiotherapy (see glossary, p 1835) with surgery alone. All four RCTs began before 1985 and used megavoltage x rays. Pooled data from RCTs reporting sites of local recurrence (781 women) found that women with isolated local recurrence were less likely to have received radiotherapy (OR 0.25, 95% CI 0.16 to 0.34). Even an RCT limited to "good prognosis disease" (tumour ≤2 cm, node negative, 381 people) found a significantly lower local relapse rate with radiotherapy at 5 and 10 years (5 years: relapse rate with radiotherapy 2.3%, 95% CI 1% to 4.3% *v* no radiotherapy 18.4%, 95% CI 12.5% to 24.2%).[35] Ten year data found that radiotherapy was associated with significantly lower local recurrence rates (8.5%, 95% CI 3.9% to 13.1% *v* 24%, 95% CI 17.6% to 30.4%; P = 0.0001), but no significant difference in overall survival (77.5% *v* 78%).[36] One subsequent RCT (585 people) also found that after 6 years the proportion of women free of locoregional disease and with breast conservation was higher with radiotherapy (93.8% *v* 81.3%).[37] Pooled data from all four RCTs found no significant difference in 10 year survival (80.1% *v* 78.9%). **Versus mastectomy:** The systematic review identified nine RCTs (4891 women) comparing breast radiotherapy after breast conserving surgery with simple or modified radical mastectomy (see glossary, p 1835) in women with invasive breast cancer.[22] It found no difference in survival rates at 10 years (22.9% *v* 22.9%; no CIs provided) or in local recurrence (6.2% *v* 5.9% from pooled data from 6 RCTs, 3107 women).[22]

Harms: The RCTs and systematic review included in a consensus document published in 1998 (mainly of women undergoing breast conserving surgery or mastectomy with variation in radiotherapy techniques, doses, and fractionation) reported two severe adverse effects of radiotherapy: acute pneumonitis (0.7%–7.0%) and pericarditis (0%–0.3%); and the following long term adverse effects: significant arm oedema (1% without axillary dissection), radionecrotic rib fracture (1.1%–1.5%), and brachial plexopathy (0%–1.8%).[38] The risk and severity of adverse effects increased with volume irradiated, total dose received, dose per fraction, previous surgery (e.g. axillary dissection), and radiotherapy techniques that caused overlap in irradiated tissues. The review found an increased risk of non-breast cancer death (OR 1.24, 95% CI 1.09 to 1.43).[22] One systematic review (search date not stated)[39] of 10 RCTs found that the excess of non-breast cancer deaths after chest wall radiotherapy was caused by cardiac deaths resulting from the radiotherapy, but recent RCTs with data beyond 10 years did not find an excess of cardiac deaths.[40–42] A more recent systematic review (search date not stated, 40 RCTs in early breast cancer with meta-analysis of 10 and 20 year results) confirms a reduction in local recurrence of two thirds, a reduction in breast cancer mortality, but an increase in other, particularly vascular, mortality.[43] Overall, 20 year survival was 37.1% with radiotherapy versus 35.9% for controls (two sided P value = 0.06). Studies assessing cosmetic results have mainly been retrospective using poorly validated outcomes. The effects of social, psychological, and financial disruptions from attending 5–6 weeks of radiotherapy have not been clearly addressed. There is an extremely low reported incidence of radiation induced malignancy, usually soft tissue sarcomas, in the irradiated breast.

Comment: The four RCTs comparing breast conserving surgery with and without radiotherapy, as well as retrospective case series, found that prognostic factors for local recurrence after breast conserving surgery include positive tumour margins, an extensive intraduct component, younger age, lymphovascular invasion, histological grade, and systemic treatment. The only consistent independent risk factor is avoiding radiotherapy. Although there is no published evidence of a difference in survival at 10 years, recent results from the Fifth Early Breast Cancer Trialists' Group meeting suggest a reduction in breast cancer death in women having breast surgery with radiotherapy versus no radiotherapy (6100 women; 3.9% [SE 1.2%] increase in survival) (Dixon M, personal communication 2001).

OPTION RADIOTHERAPY AFTER MASTECTOMY

RCTs have found that radiotherapy to the chest wall after mastectomy reduces the risk of local recurrence by about two thirds, and reduces the risk of death from breast cancer at 10 years compared with mastectomy alone.

Benefits: We found one systematic review (search date not stated, 32 RCTs) comparing mastectomy with mastectomy followed by radiotherapy (see glossary, p 1835) to the chest wall.[22] Five RCTs were of mastectomy alone (4541 women), four of mastectomy and axillary clearance (see glossary, p 1834) (3286 women), and 23 of mastectomy and axillary clearance (6699 women). The review found that radiotherapy reduced local recurrence by two thirds and slightly reduced breast cancer mortality (OR 0.94, 95% CI 0.88 to 1.00), but found no significant difference in overall survival (OR 0.98, 95% CI 0.93 to 1.03).[22] **Versus mastectomy plus adjuvant chemotherapy or tamoxifen alone:** Two subsequent RCTs in high risk women receiving adjuvant chemotherapy (CMF) (see glossary, p 1835) after mastectomy compared irradiation to the chest wall and peripheral lymphatics with no radiotherapy.[40,41] One found radiotherapy reduced relative locoregional relapse rates by 56% (RR 0.44, 95% CI 0.26 to 0.77), and the other by 76% (AR 58% *v* 14%).[40,41] One RCT found that survival at 10 years was higher with radiotherapy (54%, 95% CI 51% to 58% *v* 45%, 95% CI 42% to 48%).[41] The other, smaller RCT found a 29% relative reduction in mortality at 15 years with radiotherapy (RR 0.71, CI 0.51 to 0.99), although when these results were pooled with the results of the review no significant difference in overall mortality was detected (OR 0.96, 95% CI 0.91 to 1.01).[22,40,44,45] Another RCT in high risk postmenopausal women who underwent mastectomy and received tamoxifen (see glossary, p 1835) 30 mg daily for 1 year, compared irradiation of the chest wall and peripheral lymphatics versus no radiotherapy. It found that radiotherapy reduced local or regional recurrence (as first site of recurrence) from 35%–8%. Overall survival at 10 years was higher with radiotherapy (45%, 95% CI 41% to 49% *v* 36%, 95% CI 33% to 40%).[44] We found no evidence that reduction in relative risk of local recurrence was affected by age, nodal status, receptor status, tumour grade, or tumour size, nor that the effect of radiotherapy on mortality varied significantly with extent of surgery, type of radiotherapy (megavoltage or orthovoltage), years the RCTs commenced or completed recruitment, or whether systemic treatment was given.[45]

Harms: See harms of radiotherapy after breast conserving surgery, p 1821. Three RCTs of postmastectomy total nodal irradiation (see glossary, p 1835) in high risk disease found no significant increase in cardiac mortality.[40–42,44]

Comment: The RCTs in the large systematic review were heterogeneous, in part because they began when RCT methods were less developed.[22] They varied in randomisation processes, areas irradiated, use of systemic treatment, radiotherapy doses, fractionation, and treatment schedules. We found little good evidence to identify which women should have postmastectomy radiotherapy to prevent local recurrence. One review of retrospective data found that extent of axillary node involvement, larger tumour size, higher histological grade, presence of lymphovascular invasion, and involvement of tumour margins reduced the chance of successful treatment.[45–48]

OPTION RADIOTHERAPY TO THE INTERNAL MAMMARY CHAIN

We found no direct evidence that radiotherapy to the internal mammary chain improved overall survival or breast cancer specific survival. Treatment may increase radiation induced cardiac morbidity.

Benefits: We found no systematic review. We found one RCT (270 women treated with breast conserving surgery and radiotherapy — see glossary, p 1835), which compared internal mammary chain irradiation with no internal mammary chain irradiation.[49] At median follow up of 2.7 years there was no significant difference in relapse or survival (figures not provided).

Harms: See harms of radiotherapy after breast conserving surgery, p 1821. Radiotherapy to the internal mammary chain is more likely to affect the heart compared with other types of radiotherapy.

Comment: The risk of internal mammary chain node involvement is related to the location and size of the primary tumour and, most importantly, histopathological axillary nodal status. Up to 30% of women with axillary involvement will also exhibit internal mammary chain nodal metastases. Central or medial breast cancers are more likely to metastasise to the internal mammary chain, as are larger tumours.[50,51] The risk of internal mammary chain recurrence is low, and after modified radical mastectomy (see glossary, p 1835) alone is 2%.[52] Modern radiotherapy planning and delivery should involve an assessment of the position and depth of the internal mammary chain nodes to be treated (using computerised tomography or ultrasound), and computer assisted placement, arrangement, and determination of dose distribution, technologies unavailable at the time of most RCTs included in the reviews.[22,39] Recent indirect evidence from RCTs suggests improved survival from nodal irradiation (including radiation to the internal mammary chain) after modified radical mastectomy combined with systemic treatment.[40,41,44] Another RCT of internal mammary chain irradiation has recently started (sponsored by the European Organisation for Research and Treatment of Cancer [EORTC]).

OPTION RADIOTHERAPY TO THE IPSILATERAL SUPRACLAVICULAR FOSSA

We found insufficient evidence to assess the impact on survival of irradiation of the ipsilateral supraclavicular fossa. RCTs have found that radiotherapy is associated with reduced risk of supraclavicular fossa nodal recurrence. Morbidity associated with irradiation of the supraclavicular fossa is rare and, where it occurs, is mild and temporary.

Benefits: We found no systematic review or RCTs on radiotherapy (see glossary, p 1835) to the ipsilateral supraclavicular fossa. One systematic review (search date not stated) found that postoperative radiotherapy was associated with reduced locoregional recurrence: see radiotherapy after breast conserving surgery, p 1821; radiotherapy after mastectomy, p 1822; and radiotherapy to internal mammary chain irradiation, p 1823.[22] RCTs indicate reduced recurrence in the supraclavicular fossa. One RCT in postmenopausal women at high risk of local recurrence who received tamoxifen (see glossary, p 1835) after mastectomy found that radiotherapy was associated with lower recurrence in the supraclavicular fossa (37/686 [5.4%] *v* 9/689 [1.3%]) at median follow up of 123 months.[44]

Harms: The acute morbidity of irradiation to the supraclavicular fossa is mild and includes temporary upper oesophagitis in nearly all women. The risk of radiation pneumonitis increases with the volume of lung irradiated. Treatment irradiates the lung apex in addition to any lung included in the breast or chest wall fields. Possible late morbidity includes brachial plexopathy but this should not exceed 1.8% if attention is paid to limiting total dose to 50 Gy, the limiting of the dose per fraction to 2 Gy or less, and avoiding field junction overlaps.[38,53] Late apical lung fibrosis is common and usually of no clinical importance. Demyelination of the cervical cord is an extremely rare complication of supraclavicular fossa radiotherapy.

Comment: None.

OPTION TOTAL NODAL RADIOTHERAPY

Three RCTs found that total nodal irradiation improved survival in high risk disease. An earlier systematic review found reduced locoregional recurrence, but no evidence of improved survival.

Benefits: One systematic review (search date not stated) included RCTs of total nodal irradiation to the internal mammary chain, supraclavicular fossa, and axilla.[22] It found that postoperative radiotherapy (see glossary, p 1835) was associated with reduced locoregional recurrence, but no evidence of improved 10 year survival.[22] However, three recent RCTs found improved overall survival in women with high risk disease who underwent mastectomy, axillary dissection, and systemic adjuvant therapy, if total nodal postoperative radiotherapy was given.[40,41,44]

Harms: See radiotherapy to the internal mammary chain, p 1823, supraclavicular fossa, p 1824, and axilla, p 1829. The three RCTs found no increase in cardiac mortality due to radiotherapy.[40–42,44]

Comment: None.

QUESTION What are the effects of adjuvant systemic treatment?

Stephen Johnston

OPTION ADJUVANT COMBINATION CHEMOTHERAPY

One systematic review has found that adjuvant chemotherapy reduces rates of recurrence and improves survival for women with early breast cancer. The benefit seems to be independent of nodal or menopausal status, although the absolute improvements are greater in those with node positive disease, and probably greater in younger women. The review found no evidence of a survival advantage from additional months of combination chemotherapy using two or more drugs, nor did RCTs find survival advantage from increased or reduced dosages of combination chemotherapy. Regimens containing anthracycline may modestly improve outcomes compared with the standard CMF regimen.

Benefits: **Versus no chemotherapy:** We found one systematic review (search date not stated, 47 RCTs, 18 000 women) comparing prolonged combination chemotherapy (see glossary, p 1834) with no chemotherapy.[54] Chemotherapy was associated with significantly lower rates of any kind of recurrence (women aged under 50 years, OR 0.65, 95% CI 0.61 to 0.69; women aged 50–69 years, OR 0.80, 95% 0.72 to 0.88), and death from all causes (women aged under 50 years, OR 0.73, 95% CI 0.68 to 0.78; women aged 50–69 years, OR 0.89, 95% CI 0.86 to 0.92). Proportional benefits were similar for women with node negative and node positive disease. Ten year survival according to nodal and age group is summarised (see table 1, p 1839). **Duration of treatment:** The same review identified 11 RCTs (6104 women), which compared longer regimens (doubling duration of chemotherapy from between 4 and 6 months to 8 and 12 months) with shorter regimens.[54] It found no additional benefit from longer treatment duration.

Different doses: Several RCTs found no significant improvement from enhanced dose regimens, whereas others found little difference from untreated controls when suboptimal doses were used.[55,56] **Anthracycline regimens versus standard CMF regimen:** The systematic review identified 11 RCTs (5942 women) comparing regimens containing anthracycline (see glossary, p 1834) (including the drugs doxorubicin or 4-epidoxorubicin) with standard CMF regimens (see glossary, p 1835).[54] It found a significant reduction in recurrence rates in those on anthracycline regimens (P = 0.006), and a modest but significant improvement in 5 year survival (69% *v* 72%; P = 0.02).

Harms: **Acute adverse effects:** Adverse effects include nausea and vomiting, hair loss, bone marrow suppression, fatigue, and gastrointestinal disturbance. Prolonged chemotherapy is more likely to be associated with lethargy and haematological toxicity (anaemia and neutropenia), and anthracycline regimens cause complete hair loss. **Long term adverse effects:** Fertility and ovarian function may be permanently affected by chemotherapy, especially in women aged over 40 years, although for some women with hormone dependent cancer, reduced ovarian function may contribute to the benefit of adjuvant treatment (see glossary, p 1834). Other potential long term risks include induction of second cancers (especially haematological malignancies, although the risk is very low), and cardiac impairment with cumulative anthracycline dosages. Provided the cumulative dose of doxorubicin does not exceed 300–350 mg/m^2, the risk of congestive heart failure is less than 1%.

Comment: The absolute benefits of these regimens need to be balanced against their toxicity for different women. RCTs of high dose chemotherapy with haematological support (bone marrow transplantation or peripheral stem cell support) are under way in women with high risk disease (at least 10 positive lymph nodes), although a recent RCT did not find survival advantage for high dose treatment.[57,58] New and highly active cytotoxic agents such as the taxanes are being examined with anthracyclines either in combination or sequence. Alternating sequences of cytotoxic agents may prove an effective way of circumventing acquired drug resistance and thus enhancing the efficacy of a regimen, such as the Milan regimen (see glossary, p 1835) of single agent anthracycline followed by standard CMF chemotherapy.[59]

OPTION ADJUVANT TAMOXIFEN

One systematic review has found that adjuvant tamoxifen taken for up to 5 years reduces the chance of recurrence and death in postmenopausal women, and in women with oestrogen receptor positive tumours irrespective of age, menopausal status, nodal involvement, or the addition of chemotherapy. Five years of treatment seems better than shorter durations, but available evidence does not find benefit associated with prolongation beyond 5 years. Tamoxifen carries a slightly increased risk of endometrial cancer, but we found no evidence of an overall adverse effect on non-breast cancer mortality.

Benefits: **Versus placebo:** We found one systematic review (search date not stated, 55 RCTs, 37 000 women), which compared adjuvant tamoxifen (see glossary, p 1835) with placebo.[60] It found that 5 years of adjuvant tamoxifen had a similar effect on recurrence and long term survival in all age groups, irrespective of menopausal status or age. Overall tamoxifen for 5 years reduced the annual risk of recurrence by 47%, and of death by 26%. **Oestrogen receptor status:** Five years of tamoxifen treatment was associated with a greater reduction in the recurrence rate for women with oestrogen receptor positive rather than negative tumours (RRR 50% *v* 6%), and with a slightly greater reduction in the risk of 10 year recurrence in women with node positive compared with node negative disease (ARR 14.9% *v* 15.2%). **Duration of treatment:** The review found significantly greater reductions in recurrence with increasing duration of adjuvant tamoxifen (RRR 26% for 5 years of tamoxifen use *v* 12% for 1 year; $P < 0.00001$).[60] The absolute improvement in 10 year survival from 5 years of tamoxifen is tabulated (see table 2, p 1839). One RCT (3887 women) comparing 2 and 5 years of treatment found similar results.[61] The effects of prolonged treatment beyond 5 years are unclear. In the largest RCT in the systematic review, 1153 women who had completed 5 years of tamoxifen were randomised to either placebo or 5 more years of tamoxifen.[60,62] Disease free survival (see glossary, p 1834) after 4 years of further follow up was greater for those who switched to placebo rather than continued tamoxifen (92% *v* 86%, $P = 0.003$), although there was no significant difference in overall survival. Other studies found no detrimental effect or improvement in continuing tamoxifen beyond 5 years.[63]

Harms: One systematic review found an increased hazard ratio for endometrial cancer with tamoxifen (average HR 2.58, 95% CI 2.23 to 2.93).[60] For 5 years of tamoxifen treatment, this resulted in a cumulative risk over 10 years of two deaths (95% CI 0 to 4) per 1000 women. There was no evidence of an increased incidence of other cancers, nor of non-breast cancer related deaths (i.e. cardiac or vascular), although one extra death per 5000 women years of tamoxifen was attributed to pulmonary embolus. Bone loss was found in premenopausal women (1.4% bone loss per annum) but not in postmenopausal women, because of tamoxifen's partial agonist effects.[64] There were mixed effects on cardiovascular risk, with significant reductions in low density lipoprotein cholesterol associated with a reduced incidence of myocardial infarction in some studies, but an increased risk of thrombosis. Overall, no effect has been found on non-breast cancer mortality (HR 0.99 95% CI 0.88 to 1.16).[60]

Comment: The risk to benefit ratio may vary between women, with oestrogen receptor negative women deriving little benefit. Even in oestrogen receptor positive women, any benefit on breast cancer could be offset with prolonged treatment (beyond 5 years), by drug resistance, and by adverse effects on the endometrium. Two multicentre RCTs of tamoxifen duration are in progress (Cancer Research Campaign, personal communication, 2000); however, because of concerns about long term toxicity with tamoxifen (see above) and in the absence of further definitive data, current clinical practice has been to recommend tamoxifen for 5 years.[65] For women with completely oestrogen receptor negative disease, the overall benefit of adjuvant tamoxifen needs further research.

OPTION COMBINED CHEMOTHERAPY PLUS TAMOXIFEN

One RCT has found that adding chemotherapy to tamoxifen improved survival.

Benefits: We found no systematic review. We found one RCT (2306 women with lymph node negative, oestrogen receptor positive early breast cancer), which compared tamoxifen (see glossary, p 1835) alone versus tamoxifen plus CMF (see glossary, p 1835) chemotherapy.[66] It found that adding chemotherapy to tamoxifen caused a further absolute improvement in disease free survival (at 5 years' follow up 90% *v* 85%; P = 0.006), and in overall survival (97% *v* 94%; P = 0.03).

Harms: Adding CMF chemotherapy to tamoxifen was associated with a greater incidence of grade 3/4 neutropenia (9% *v* 0%), greater than or equal to grade 2 nausea (35% *v* 4%), moderate/severe alopecia (35.6% *v* 0.4%), and thromboembolism/phlebitis (7.5% *v* 2.1%).[66]

Comment: None.

OPTION OVARIAN ABLATION

One systematic review has found that ovarian ablation significantly improves long term survival in women aged under 50 years with early breast cancer.

Benefits: We found one systematic review (search date not stated, 12 RCTs with at least 15 years' follow up, 2102 premenopausal women) comparing ovarian ablation (see glossary, p 1835) by irradiation or surgery with no ablation.[67] Significantly more women with ovarian ablation survived (52% *v* 46%; P = 0.001), and survived recurrence free (45% *v* 39%; P = 0.0007). Benefit was independent of nodal status.

Harms: We found no good evidence on long term adverse effects. Concerns exist about late sequelae of ovarian ablation, especially effects on bone mineral density and cardiovascular risk. Acute adverse effects are likely to be menopausal symptoms.

Comment: Five of the RCTs compared ovarian ablation plus chemotherapy with chemotherapy alone.[67] In these, the absolute benefit of ablation was smaller than in RCTs of ovarian ablation alone. It may be that cytotoxic chemotherapy itself suppresses ovarian function, making the effect of ablation difficult to detect in combined RCTs. When only premenopausal women were considered in the absence of chemotherapy, there was a 27% improvement in the odds of recurrence free survival. RCTs are under way of reversible oophorectomy using gonadotrophin releasing hormone analogues, which would allow preservation of fertility in younger women with oestrogen receptor positive tumours.

QUESTION What are the effects of axillary clearance, sampling, or radiotherapy in women with operable primary breast cancer?

Mike Dixon and Alan Rodger

RCTs found no evidence that axillary clearance is associated with improved survival compared with axillary node sampling, axillary radiotherapy, or sampling plus radiotherapy combined. One systematic review of mainly poor quality evidence found that the risk of arm lymphoedema was highest with axillary clearance plus radiotherapy, lower with axillary sampling plus radiotherapy, and lowest with sampling alone.

Benefits: **Versus axillary sampling:** We found no systematic review but found one RCT (466 women) in women undergoing breast conserving surgery (see glossary, p 1834). It found that axillary sampling (see glossary, p 1834) was associated with improved survival compared with axillary clearance, but the difference was not significant (estimated 5 year survival 88.6% v 82.1%).[68] Rates of node positivity were similar in both groups. **Versus axillary radiotherapy:** We found one systematic review (search date not stated, 8 RCTs, 4370 women) comparing axillary clearance (level I, II, and III dissection) versus axillary radiotherapy (see glossary, p 1834). It found no significant difference in mortality at 10 years (54.7% v 54.9%), or in rates of recurrence (OR 1.01). Radiotherapy was associated with fewer isolated local recurrences (OR 15%, 95% CI 7% to 22%).[22] **Versus sampling plus radiotherapy:** We found no systematic review. Two RCTs compared axillary clearance (level I, II, and III dissection) with sampling followed by radiotherapy (see glossary, p 1835) in women with involved axillary nodes. They found no significant difference in local, axillary, or distant recurrence.[68,69] **Axillary clearance plus radiotherapy:** We found no studies assessing the effect of radiotherapy in addition to axillary clearance (level I and II, or level I, II, and III dissection) in regional control of disease.

Harms: **Axillary clearance:** Adverse effects of axillary surgery include seroma formation, arm swelling, damage to the intercostobrachial nerve, and shoulder stiffness. We found one RCT comparing the morbidity of different axillary procedures.[68] It compared complete axillary clearance (level I, II, and III dissection) with four node axillary sampling followed by radiotherapy if the nodes were involved. The rate of arm swelling was higher after clearance than after sampling whether or not women received postoperative radiotherapy (at 3 years, forearm girth was significantly greater; $P = 0.005$). After removal of axillary drains, between a quarter and half of women who had undergone a level I and II, or level I, II, and III axillary dissection developed seromas requiring aspiration. **Axillary radiotherapy:** One RCT comparing clearance with sampling plus radiotherapy for node positive disease found significantly reduced shoulder movement with radiotherapy, even though the shoulder joint was not irradiated.[68] At 6 months, both groups had significantly reduced shoulder movement compared with women receiving axillary sampling alone ($P < 0.004$). However, by 3 years, the axillary clearance group had improved and was not significantly different from the sampling group. **Arm lymphoedema:** One Australian systematic review (search date 1996) of lymphoedema prevalence, risks, and management found that, although current information is of poor quality, the combination of axillary dissection (to or beyond level II) and axillary radiotherapy was associated with a risk of lymphoedema of between 12% and 60%, with most studies suggesting that at least a third of women are affected.[70] Studies of axillary sampling followed by irradiation found lower rates (between 6% and 32%), and for axillary sampling alone, lower still (between 0% and 21%). Studies of dissection beyond level I found rates between 0% and 42%, with most studies reporting a rate of 20–30% 1 year after operation.[70] In women who receive axillary radiotherapy without axillary surgery, the overall lymphoedema rate is about 8%.

Comment: **Axillary staging:** Both clearance and sampling provide important prognostic information on which decisions on local and systemic treatment can be based. Further RCTs of less invasive and potentially less morbid staging procedures such as sentinel node biopsy are under way. A decision on axillary management should be based on the risk of involvement of axillary nodes (which varies according to tumour size, grade, and the presence of vascular/lymphatic invasion), and potential treatment related morbidity. Two retrospective cohort studies found that level I dissection accurately assessed axillary lymph node status, providing that at least 10 nodes were removed.[71,72] One RCT found that a sample of four nodes provided sufficient information to categorise an axilla as histologically positive or negative.[73] Removal of nodes at level I and level II, or removal of all nodes below the axillary vein (level I, II, and III), accurately stages the axilla.[71,72] RCTs comparing sentinel node biopsy with axillary node clearance and sampling are currently under way, and results of these will be incorporated in *Clinical Evidence* updates (Dixon M, personal communication, 2000).

QUESTION What are the effects of interventions in locally advanced breast cancer (stage III B)?

Alan Rodger

OPTION LOCAL TREATMENT FOR LOCALLY ADVANCED BREAST CANCER

Two small RCTs including women with locally advanced disease (stage III B) found that, for locally advanced breast cancer that is rendered operable, radiotherapy or surgery as sole local treatments have similar effects on response rates, duration of response, and overall survival. One RCT found weak evidence that, if surgery is possible and is carried out, postoperative radiotherapy will reduce locoregional recurrence. Local skin toxicity (acute and late) after radiotherapy is greater in locally advanced breast cancer than after treatment for less advanced disease, because of the need for a higher radiation dose to skin.

Benefits: We found no systematic review of the role of radiotherapy (see glossary, p 1835) in locally advanced (stage III B) breast cancer. We found seven RCTs, including women with stage III B, which compared radiotherapy versus no radiotherapy.[41,44,74–78] Other management options varied across these RCTs. Most RCTs were small, but included more than stage III B women. **Postoperative radiotherapy versus no further local treatment after surgery:** We found two RCTs.[74,77] In one of these RCTs[74] pre- and postoperative chemo-endocrine treatment was administered to all women who also underwent mastectomy while half the women were randomised to postmastectomy radiotherapy to the chest wall and regional lymphatics (45–50 Gy in 5 wks). However, 43% of the 184 women were excluded with more exclusions in the radiotherapy group, and it is impossible to ascertain what percentage of women were stage III B. There were numerous chemotherapy complications, including one death. The RCT found no significant difference in local or distant failures, but found that overall crude survival was significantly higher with no radiotherapy versus radiotherapy (28.7 months *v* 21.7 months; $P < 0.05$). Conclusions cannot be drawn from this RCT. The second RCT of operable locally advanced breast cancer (332 women who were recurrence free after modified radical mastectomy [see glossary, p 1835]) and 6 cycles of chemohormone treatment; 38% stage T4 and 14% N2)[76] compared postoperative radiotherapy versus no further treatment. It found no significant difference in time to relapse (4.7 years for radiotherapy *v* 5.2 years for no further treatment), and median overall survival (8.3 years *v* 8.1 years). Radiotherapy reduced locoregional sites as first recurrence by 9%. **Postmastectomy radiotherapy in women having systemic treatment after surgery:** Two RCTs of "high risk breast cancer" (including women with stage III B disease) studied postmastectomy radiotherapy in women having systemic treatment after surgery.[41,44] The postmenopausal RCT separated some T4 tumours by skin invasion (14%).[44] For those receiving postmastectomy radiotherapy with tamoxifen (see glossary, p 1835), 8% developed local recurrence versus 34% receiving tamoxifen alone (5 year disease free survival: 41% *v* 37%; 10 year disease free survival: 23% *v* 22%; 5 year survivals: 51% *v* 61%; 10 year survivals: 31% *v* 27%). However, the studies used small and retrospective subgroups, making conclusions uncertain. **Surgery alone versus radiotherapy alone:** Two RCTs compared surgery alone versus radiotherapy alone as local treatment.[75,76] In one RCT (113 women with stage III breast cancer, 67% stage III B) women were given chemotherapy and 81% became operable; then 87 women were randomised to surgery or to radiotherapy.[75] After local treatment, a further 2 years of chemotherapy was given. Both groups had similar duration of disease control (29.2 months with surgery *v* 24.4 months with radiation; $P = 0.5$), similar overall median survival (39.3 *v* 39 months), and similar sites of first relapse. In the other RCT (132 women, 91% stage III B, 9% stage III A) all women received chemotherapy before randomisation to either surgery or radiotherapy.[75] Total response rate was 75% in each group. Duration of remission was not significantly different (15 months with surgery *v* 22 months with radiotherapy; $P = 0.58$). Survival was similar at 4 years (52 months with radiotherapy *v* 49.1 months with surgery). **Low dose radiotherapy versus tamoxifen:** A small RCT (143 women)[78] compared low dose radiotherapy (40 Gy in 15 fractions) versus tamoxifen (20 mg twice daily). Women were given the alternative treatment on relapse. The RCT found no significant difference in response rates (P = 0.34), duration of response (P = 0.76), or survival (P = 0.38).

Harms: The type of harms from radiotherapy for locally advanced breast cancer were similar to those from radiotherapy after mastectomy or breast conserving surgery (see glossary, p 1834). However, in stage III B disease with skin involvement (T4 b, c, d), the skin is usually given a higher dose of radiotherapy. In addition, a higher dose (60 Gy) is often given to more of the breast volume. Acute skin toxicity (including moist desquamation) and late skin toxicity (pigmentation and telangiectasia) are also more likely than in women without skin involvement.

Comment: The lack of good quality, large RCTs addressing directly stage III B breast cancer and the role of radiotherapy render it difficult to draw firm conclusions on its value. Such RCTs are small and have varying approaches to management. From the results of two RCTs,[75,76] it can be concluded that in terms of overall response (which includes the response from local treatments such as surgery, radiotherapy, or both, and the effects of any initial systemic treatment), duration of that response, and overall survival, there is no advantage of either surgery alone or radiotherapy alone as sole local treatment over the other. It is more difficult to detail the possible benefits of postoperative radiotherapy in women whose locally advanced breast cancers have been rendered operable by systemic treatment and who have undergone surgery, usually modified radical mastectomy. It is likely that such postoperative radiotherapy will reduce the risk of local (and regional if nodal areas are irradiated) recurrence. It is not possible to conclude that it will affect survival.

OPTION — SYSTEMIC TREATMENT FOR LOCALLY ADVANCED BREAST CANCER

We found no evidence that cytotoxic chemotherapy of cyclophosphamide, methotrexate, and fluorouracil (5-FU), or an anthracycline based multidrug regimen improved survival, disease free survival, or long term locoregional control in locally advanced breast cancer. One RCT found evidence that hormone treatment plus radiotherapy versus radiotherapy alone improves survival in locally advanced breast cancer. One RCT found that chemotherapy, hormone therapy, or both, delayed locoregional recurrence.

Benefits: We found no systematic review. **Radiotherapy versus radiotherapy plus systemic chemotherapy:** We found three RCTs,[79–81] which compared radiotherapy versus radiotherapy (see glossary, p 1835) plus systemic treatment (hormone therapy, chemotherapy, or both). One RCT (410 women, most stage III B)[79] compared radiotherapy versus radiotherapy plus chemotherapy (CMF — see glossary, p 1835) (for 12 cycles) versus radiotherapy plus hormone therapy (ovarian irradiation for premenopausal women, tamoxifen for postmenopausal women) versus radiotherapy plus both chemotherapy and hormone therapy. Both chemotherapy (P = 0.0002) and hormone therapy (P = 0.0007) significantly delayed locoregional recurrence. Combined chemotherapy and hormone therapy had the largest effect (P = 0.0001). Locoregional recurrence at 6 years was reduced (59%–48% with chemotherapy *v* 61%–47% with hormone therapy). The effect on distant metastases was similar but less marked. Significantly increased median survival was found only with hormone therapy (4.3 years with hormone therapy *v* 3.3 years without hormone therapy, after 8 years HR death 0.75, 95% CI 0.59 to 0.96; median survival 3.8 years with chemotherapy *v* 3.6 years without, HR 0.84, 95% CI 0.66 to 1.08). Another RCT (118 women with stage III B breast cancer)[80] compared radiotherapy versus radiotherapy plus chemotherapy (cyclophosphamide, methrotrexate, and fluorouracil [5-FU]–CMF for 12 cycles) plus tamoxifen versus chemotherapy (CMF alternating with adriamycin and vincristine [AV]) followed by radiotherapy and then further similar chemotherapy and tamoxifen. The radiotherapy in the third arm delivered a lower dose to the skin and a lower total dose. After a minimum follow up of 14 years, the RCT found no significant difference in survival, disease free survival (see glossary, p 1834), or locoregional control. The 10 year survival rates were 13% with radiotherapy alone, 21% with radiotherapy, CMF, and tamoxifen, and 28% for radiotherapy plus CMF/AV/tamoxifen. Differences in 10 year survival were 8% (95% CI –9% to +25%) for radiotherapy versus radiotherapy, CMF, and tamoxifen; and 15% (95% CI 3% to 33%) for radiotherapy versus radiotherapy plus CMF/AV/tamoxifen. There was no significant difference between the two arms with chemotherapy. The disease free survival at 10 years for radiotherapy alone was 4%; 15% for radiotherapy plus CMF/tamoxifen; and 15% for radiotherapy plus CMF/AV/tamoxifen. The difference in this at 10 years was 12% (95% CI 1% to 25%) between radiotherapy and radiotherapy plus CMF; and 12% (95% CI 1.4% to 25.4%) for radiotherapy versus the third arm. Local recurrence was similar in the three arms (42% *v* 45% *v* 49%). The third RCT (52 women with T4 breast cancer)[81] compared an anthracycline (see glossary, p 1834) chemotherapy regimen before radiotherapy versus similar radiotherapy alone. The combined therapy arm achieved a higher initial locoregional control rate (complete response 78.6% *v* 45.8%; P = 0.03). However, the number of women free of locoregional spread at death or last follow up was similar (57% combined *v* 50% radiotherapy alone). Overall survival and time to distant recurrence were not significantly different. **Multimodal treatment versus hormone treatment:** One RCT (108 women)[82,83] compared multimodal treatment (preoperative chemotherapy, surgery, radiotherapy, and tamoxifen) versus initial hormone treatment plus subsequent salvage treatments upon tumour progression. The objective remission after 6 months was higher with multimodal treatment than with tamoxifen alone (31/54 [57%] *v* 19/53 [36%]; OR 2.4, 95% CI 1.1 to 5.0; P = 0.03).[82] However, at a median follow up of 52 months, there was no significant difference in survival, the development of metastases, the time to metastases, or uncontrolled local disease. Women with oestrogen receptor positive tumours had a higher objective response rate (49% with oestrogen receptor positive *v* 7% with oestrogen receptor negative tumours; P value not provided), and increased survival (numbers not provided).[83]

Harms: In many RCTs harms of treatment were not reported.

Comment: The lack of large RCTs and the frequent inclusion of less locally advanced disease (T3) with locally advanced breast cancer defined here as stage III B make it difficult to draw conclusions. There is, however, no evidence from the studies using CMF chemotherapy or various regimens incorporating anthracyclines that cytotoxic chemotherapy improves survival, disease free survival, or long term locoregional control in stage III B breast cancer.

GLOSSARY

Adjuvant treatment This usually refers to systemic chemotherapy or hormonal treatment, or both, taken by people after removal of a primary tumour (in this case, surgery for early breast cancer), with the aim of killing any remaining micrometastatic tumour cells and thus preventing recurrence.

Advanced breast cancer Operable locally advanced breast cancer (stage III A) is T3 (tumours > 5 cm) and N1 (non-matted involved axillary nodes). Locally advanced breast cancer (stage III B) is M0 with T4 (skin or chest wall infiltration by tumour) and/or N2 (matted axillary nodes)/N3 (internal mammary node involvement) disease, not classified as non-invasive or early invasive breast cancer. Metastatic breast cancer (stage IV) is M1 (any supraclavicular fossa node involvement or distant metastases to bone, lung, liver, etc.) with any combination of tumour and node parameters.

Anthracyclines Are also known as cytotoxic antibiotics, and are used as adjuvant treatment with radiotherapy. Examples of anthracyclines are aclarubicin, daunorubicin, doxorubicin, epirubicin, and idarubicin.

Axillary clearance Clearance of level I, II, and usually level III axillary lymph nodes. Level I nodes are lateral to the pectoralis minor muscle, level II nodes are under it, and level III nodes are medial to it at the apex of the axilla.

Axillary radiotherapy This usually includes irradiation of the supraclavicular fossa. Irradiation of this area incorporates some underlying lung that increases the risk of radiation pneumonitis. By increasing the volume of the lung irradiated, compared with chest wall or breast radiotherapy alone, the risk of acute pneumonitis is increased.

Axillary sampling Aims to remove the four largest, most easily palpable axillary lymph nodes, for histological examination.

Breast conserving surgery Surgery that consists of lumpectomy (minimal free margins), wide local excision (wider free margins), or segmental or quadrant resection (usually with very wide free margins).

CMF (classical) Chemotherapy regimen containing cyclophosphamide, methotrexate, and fluorouracil (5-FU).

Combination chemotherapy Two or more cytotoxic drugs given intravenously every 3–4 weeks for 4–6 months.

Disease free survival Means being alive with no local or distant recurrence or contralateral disease.

Early invasive breast cancer (stage I or II) is M0 with T1 or T2 (tumour diameter ≤ 5 cm, no involvement of skin or chest wall) and N0 or N1 (mobile axillary nodes); or M0 with T3 (tumour diameter > 5 cm, no skin or chest wall involvement), but only N0.

FAC Chemotherapy regimen containing fluorouracil (5-FU), doxorubicin, and cyclophosphamide.

Lumpectomy Gross tumour excision.

Milan regimen A sequential regimen of single agent anthracycline followed by CMF.

Neoadjuvant chemotherapy (Also known as primary medical therapy) involves the use of chemotherapy to treat breast cancer before locoregional therapy (surgery and or radiotherapy) to the breast to downstage large primary cancers that would require mastectomy to improve chances of survival.

Non-invasive breast cancer (stage 0) is Tis (carcinoma *in situ*, intraductal carcinoma, lobular carcinoma *in situ*, or Paget's disease of the nipple with no associated tumour); N0 (no axillary nodal involvement); and M0 (no metastases).

Ovarian ablation Surgical, medical, or radiation induced suppression of ovarian function in premenopausal women.

Overall objective response rate The proportion of treated people in whom a complete response (disappearance of all known lesions on 2 separate measurements at least 4 wks apart), or partial response (> 50% reduction in the size of lesions) is observed.

Quadrantectomy Tumour excised with at least 2 cm of normal surrounding breast tissue and with a segment of breast tissue from the periphery of the breast to the nipple.

Radical mastectomy Removal of breast and pectoralis major and minor muscles and axillary contents.

Radiotherapy Part of initial local and regional treatment. In early stage disease it may be an adjunct to surgery; in locally advanced disease (T4, N2) it may be the sole locoregional treatment. Radiotherapy may be delivered to the breast or postmastectomy chest wall, as well as to the lymphatic areas of the axilla, supraclavicular fossa, or internal mammary node chain.

Staging of breast cancer A detailed description by tumour, nodal, and metastatic parameters at a particular time (TNM).[1] These are amalgamated into broader categories called stages (0 to IV). Stages can be aggregated into even broader categories (non-invasive, early invasive, and advanced breast cancer) (see table 3, p 1839).

Supraradical mastectomy Removal of breast, pectoralis major and minor muscles, axillary contents, and internal mammary chain of nodes.

Tamoxifen A non-steroidal anti-oestrogen taken as daily oral tablets, usually for between 2–5 years.

TNM staging system See "staging of breast cancer" above.

Total mastectomy Removal of breast.

Total nodal irradiation Radiotherapy to the regional lymph nodes, including supraclavicular, infraclavicular, axillary nodes, and internal mammary nodes in the upper intercostal spaces.

UICC system International Union against Cancer.

Substantive changes

Systemic treatment for locally advanced breast cancer Longer term results of existing RCT[82] published;[83] conclusion unchanged.

Neoadjuvant chemotherapy One new RCT;[15] conclusions unchanged.

REFERENCES

1. UICC International Union Against Cancer. *TNM classification of malignant tumours* 5th ed. Sobin LH, Wittekind CH, eds. New York:Wiley–Liss Inc, 1997.
2. CRC. Breast Cancer Factsheet. 1996.
3. Easton D, Ford D. Breast and ovarian cancer incidence in BRCA-1 mutation carriers. *Am J Hum Genet* 1995;56:265–271.
4. Carter CL, Allen C, Henson DE. Relation of tumour size, lymph node status and survival in 24 740 breast cancer cases. *Cancer* 1989;63: 181–187.
5. Hortobagyi GN, Ames FC, Buzdar AU, et al. Management of stage III primary breast cancer with primary chemotherapy, surgery and radiation therapy. *Cancer* 1988;62:2507–2516.

6. Fisher B, Dignam J, Wolmark N, et al. Lumpectomy and radiation therapy for the treatment of intraductal breast cancer: findings of the National Surgical Adjuvant Breast and Bowel Project B-17. *J Clin Oncol* 1998;16:441–452.
7. Julien JP, Bijker N, Fentiman IS, et al. Radiotherapy in breast-conserving treatment for ductal carcinoma *in situ*; first results of EORTC randomised phase III trial 10853. *Lancet* 2000;355:528–533.
8. Fisher B, Dignam J, Wolmark N, et al. Tamoxifen in treatment of intraductal breast cancer: National Surgical Adjuvant Breast and Bowel Project B-24 randomised controlled trial. *Lancet* 1999;353:1993–2000.
9. Mauriac L, Durand M, Avril A, et al. Effects of primary chemotherapy in conservative treatment of breast cancer patients with operable tumours larger than 3 cm: results of a randomised trial in a single centre. *Ann Oncol* 1991;2:347–354.
10. Scholl SM, Fourquet A, Asselain B, et al. Neoadjuvant versus adjuvant chemotherapy in premenopausal patients with tumours considered too large for breast conserving surgery: preliminary results of a randomised trial. *Eur J Cancer* 1994; 30A:645–652.
11. Powles TJ, Hickish TF, Makris A, et al. Randomized trial of chemoendocrine therapy started before or after surgery for treatment of primary breast cancer. *J Clin Oncol* 1995;13:547–552.
12. Fisher B, Bryant J, Wolmark N, et al. Effect of preoperative chemotherapy on the outcome of women with operable breast cancer. *J Clin Oncol* 1998;16:2672–2685.
13. Van der Hage JA, van de Velde CJ, Julien JP, et al. Pre-operative chemotherapy in primary operable breast cancer: Results from the European Organisation for Research and Treatment of Cancer Trial 10902. *J Clin Oncol 2001;19:4224–4237.*
14. Mauriac L, MacGrogan G, Avril A, et al. Neoadjuvant chemotherapy for operable breast carcinoma larger than 3 cm: a unicentre randomized trial with a 124-month median follow-up. Institut Bergonie Bordeaux Groupe Sein (IBBGS). *Ann Oncol* 1999;10:47–52.
15. Broet P, Scholl S, De la Rochrfordiere A, et al. Short and long term effects on survival in breast cancer patients treated by primary chemotherapy: an updated analysis of a randomised trial. *Breast Cancer Res Treat* 1999;58:151–156.
16. Makris A, Powles TJ, Ashley SE, et al. A reduction in the requirements for mastectomy in a randomized trial of neoadjuvant chemoendocrine therapy in primary breast cancer. *Ann Oncol* 1998;9:1179–1184.
17. Avril A, Faucher A, Bussieres E, et al. Resultats a 10 ans d'un essai randomise de chimiotherapie neo-adjuvante dans les cancers du sein de plus de 3 cm. *Chirurgie* 1998;123:247–256.
18. Early Breast Cancer Trialists Collaborative Group. Polychemotherapy for early breast cancer: an overview of the randomised trials. *Lancet* 1998;352:930–942.
19. Buzdar AU, Singletary SE, Theriault RL, et al. Prospective evaluation of paclitaxel versus combination chemotherapy with fluorouracil, doxorubicin, and cyclophosphamide as neoadjuvant therapy in patients with operable breast cancer. *J Clin Oncol* 1999;17:3412–3417.
20. Cocconi G, Bisagni G, Ceci G, et al. Three new active cisplatin-containing combinations in the neoadjuvant treatment of locally advanced and locally recurrent breast carcinoma: a randomized phase II trial. *Breast Canc Res Treat* 1999;56:125–132.
21. Takatsuka Y, Yayoi E, Kobayashi T, et al. Neoadjuvant intra-arterial chemotherapy in locally advanced breast cancer: a prospective randomised study. *Jpn J Clin Oncol* 1994;24:20–25.
22. Early Breast Cancer Trialists' Collaborative Group. Effects of radiotherapy and surgery in early breast cancer: an overview of the randomised trials. *N Engl J Med* 1995;333:1444–1455. Search date not stated; primary sources individual patient data from trials that began before 1985, trials identified from lists from national cancer bodies, the International Cancer Research Data Bank, handsearches of conference proceedings and reference lists, and personal contact with investigators.
23. Morris AD, Morris RD, Wilson JF, et al. Breast conserving therapy versus mastectomy in early stage breast cancer: a meta-analysis of 10 year survival. *Cancer J Sci Am* 1997;3:6–12. Search date 1995, primary source Medline.
24. Sacchini V, Luini A, Tana S, et al. Quantitative and qualitative cosmetic evaluation after conservative treatment for breast cancer. *Eur J Cancer* 1991;27:1395–1400.
25. Smitt NC, Nowels KW, Zdeblick MJ, et al. The importance of the lumpectomy surgical margin status in long-term results of breast conservation. *Cancer* 1995;76:259–267.
26. Wazer DE, DiPetrillo T, Schmidt-Ullrich R, et al. Factors influencing cosmetic outcome and complication risk after conservative surgery and radiotherapy for early-stage breast carcinoma. *J Clin Oncol* 1992;10:356–363.
27. Abner AL, Recht A, Vicini FA, et al. Cosmetic results after surgery, chemotherapy and radiation therapy for early breast cancer. *Int J Radiat Oncol Biol Phys* 1991;21:331–338.
28. Dewar JA, Benhamou S, Benhamou E, et al. Cosmetic results following lumpectomy axillary dissection and radiotherapy for small breast cancers. *Radiother Oncol* 1988;12:273–280.
29. Rochefordiere A, Abner A, Silver B, et al. Are cosmetic results following conservative surgery and radiation therapy for early breast cancer dependent on technique? *Int J Radiat Oncol Biol Phys* 1992;23:925–931.
30. Sneeuw KA, Aaronson N, Yarnold J, et al. Cosmetic and functional outcomes of breast conserving treatment for early stage breast cancer 1: comparison of patients' ratings, observers' ratings and objective assessments. *Radiother Oncol* 1992;25:153–159.
31. Ash DV, Benson EA, Sainsbury JR, et al. Seven year follow-up on 334 patients treated by breast conserving surgery and short course radical postoperative radiotherapy: a report of the Yorkshire breast cancer group. *Clin Oncol* 1995;7:93–96.
32. Lindsey I, Serpell JW, Johnson WR, et al. Cosmesis following complete local excision of breast cancer. *Aust N Z J Surg* 1997;67:428–432.
33. Touboul E, Belkacemi Y, Lefranc JP, et al. Early breast cancer: influence of type of boost (electrons vs iridium-192 implant) on local control and cosmesis after conservative surgery and radiation therapy. *Radiother Oncol* 1995;34:105–113.
34. Halyard MY, Grado GL, Schomber PJ, et al. Conservative therapy of breast cancer: the Mayo Clinic experience. *Am J Clin Oncol* 1996;19:445–450.
35. Liljegren G, Holmberg L, Adami HO, et al, for the Uppsala– rebro Breast Cancer Study Group. Sector resection with or without postoperative radiotherapy for stage I breast cancer: five year results of a randomised trial. *J Natl Cancer Inst* 1994;86:717–722.
36. Liljegren G, Holmberg J, Bergh, J, et al, and the Uppsala– rebro Breast Cancer Study Group. 10-year results after sector resection with or without postoperative radiotherapy for stage I breast cancer: a randomized trial. *J Clin Oncol* 1999;17:2326–2333.

37. Forrest AP, Stewart HJ, Everington D, et al, on behalf of the Scottish Cancer Trials Breast Group. Randomised controlled trial of conservation therapy in breast cancer: 6 year analysis of the Scottish trial. *Lancet* 1996;348:708–713.
38. Steering Committee on Clinical Practice Guidelines for the Care and Treatment of Breast Cancer. A Canadian consensus document. *Can Med Assoc J* 1998;158(suppl 3):1–84.
39. Cuzick J, Stewart H, Rutqvist L, et al. Cause-specific mortality in long term survivors of breast cancer who participated in trials of radiotherapy. *J Clin Oncol* 1994;12:447–453. Search date not stated; primary source cause-specific mortality data from unconfounded randomised trials began before 1975 (trial identification methods not stated.).
40. Ragaz J, Jackson SM, Le N, et al. Adjuvant radiotherapy and chemotherapy in node-positive premenopausal women with breast cancer. *N Engl J Med* 1997;337:956–962.
41. Overgaard M, Hansen PS, Overgaard J, et al. Postoperative radiotherapy in high-risk premenopausal women with breast cancer who receive adjuvant chemotherapy. *N Engl J Med* 1997;337:949–955.
42. Hojris I, Overgaard M, Christensen JJ, et al. Morbidity and mortality of ischaemic heart disease in high-risk breast-cancer patients after adjuvant postmastectomy systemic treatment with or without radiotherapy: analysis of DBCG 82b and 82c randomised trials. Radiotherapy Committee of the Danish Breast Cancer Cooperative Group. *Lancet* 1999;354:1425–1430.
43. Early Breast Cancer Trialists Collaborative Group. Favourable and unfavourable effects on long-term survival of radiotherapy for early breast cancer: an overview of the randomised trials. Early Breast Cancer Trialists' Collaborative Group. *Lancet* 2000;355:1757–1770. Search date not stated; primary sources individual patient data from trials that began before 1990, trials identified from lists from national cancer bodies, the International Cancer Research Data Bank, handsearches of conference proceedings and reference lists, and personal contact with investigators.
44. Overgaard M, Jensen MB, Overgaard J, et al. Postoperative radiotherapy in high risk postmenopausal breast cancer patients given adjuvant tamoxifen: Danish Breast Cancer Cooperative Group DBCG 82c randomised trial. *Lancet* 1999;353:1641–1648.
45. Ghersi D, Simes J. Draft report of effectiveness of postmastectomy radiotherapy and risk factors for local recurrence in early breast cancer. Report to NHMRC National Breast Cancer Centre, Sydney, 1998.
46. O'Rourke S, Gaba MH, Morgan D, et al. Local recurrence after simple mastectomy. *Br J Surg* 1994;81:386–389.
47. Fowble B, Gray R, Gilchrist K, et al. Identification of a subset of patients with breast cancer and histologically positive nodes who may benefit from postoperative radiotherapy. *J Clin Oncol* 1988;6:1107–1117.
48. Houghton J, Baum M, Haybittle JL. Role of radiotherapy following total mastectomy in patients with early breast cancer: the closed trials working party of the CRC breast cancer trials group. *World J Surg* 1994;18:117–122.
49. Kaija H, Maunu P. Tangential breast irradiation with or without internal mammary chain irradiation: results of a randomised trial. *Radiother Oncol* 1995;36:172–176.
50. Handley R. Carcinoma of the breast. *Ann R Coll Surg Engl* 1975;57:59–66.
51. Veronesi U, Cascinelli NM, Bufalino R, et al. Risk of internal mammary lymph node metastases and its relevance on prognosis in breast cancer patients. *Ann Surg* 1983;198:681–684.
52. Veronesi U, Valagussa P. Inefficacy of internal mammary node dissection in breast cancer surgery. *Cancer* 1981;47:170–175.
53. Bates T, Evans RGB. Report of the Independent Review commissioned by The Royal College of Radiologists into brachial plexus neuropathy following radiotherapy for breast cancer. London: Royal College of Radiologists, 1995.
54. Early Breast Cancer Trialists' Collaborative Group. Polychemotherapy for early breast cancer: an overview of the randomised trials. *Lancet* 1998;352:930–942. Search date not stated; primary sources individual patient data from trials that began before 1990, trials identified from lists from national cancer bodies, the International Cancer Research Data Bank, handsearches of conference proceedings and reference lists, and personal contact with investigators.
55. Fisher B, Anderson S, Wickerham DL, et al. Increased intensification and total dose of cyclophosphamide in a doxorubicin-cyclophosphamide regimen for the treatment of primary breast cancer: findings from national surgical adjuvant breast and bowel project B-22. *J Clin Oncol* 1997;15:1858–1869.
56. Wood WC, Budman DR, Korzun AH. Dose and dose intensity of adjuvant chemotherapy for stage II, node-positive breast carcinoma. *N Engl J Med* 1994;330:1253–1259.
57. Peters WP, Ross M, Vredenburgh JJ, et al. High-dose chemotherapy and autologous bone marrow support as consolidation after standard-dose adjuvant chemotherapy for high-risk primary breast cancer. *J Clin Oncol* 1993;11:1132–1143.
58. Rodenhuis S, Richel DJ, Van der Wall E, et al. Randomised trial of high-dose chemotherapy and haemopoietic progenitor-cell support in operable breast cancer with extensive axillary lymph-node involvement. *Lancet* 1998;352:515–521.
59. Bonadonna G, Zambeti M, Valagussa P. Sequential or alternating doxorubicin and CMF regimens in breast cancer with more than three positive nodes. *JAMA* 1995;273:542–547.
60. Early Breast Cancer Trialists' Collaborative Group. Tamoxifen for early breast cancer: an overview of the randomised trials. *Lancet* 1998;351:1451–1467. Search date not stated; primary sources individual patient data from trials that began before 1990, trials identified from lists from national cancer bodies, the International Cancer Research Data Bank, handsearches of conference proceedings and reference lists, and personal contact with investigators.
61. Swedish Breast Cancer Cooperative Group. Randomised trial of two versus five years of adjuvant tamoxifen for post-menopausal early stage breast cancer. *J Natl Cancer Inst* 1996;88:1543–1549.
62. Fisher B, Dignam J, Bryant J, et al. Five versus more than five years of tamoxifen therapy for breast cancer patients with negative lymph nodes and estrogen receptor-positive tumours. *J Natl Cancer Inst* 1996;88:1529–1542.
63. Stewart HJ, Forrest AP, Everington D, et al. Randomised comparison of 5 years of adjuvant tamoxifen with continuous therapy for operable breast cancer. *Br J Cancer* 1996;74:297–299.
64. Powles TJ, Hickish T, Kanis JA, et al. Effect of tamoxifen on bone mineral density measured by dual-energy x-ray absorptiometry in healthy premenopausal and postmenopausal women. *J Clin Oncol* 1996;14:78–84.
65. Swain SM. Tamoxifen: the long and short of it. *J Natl Cancer Inst* 1996;88:1510–1512.

66. Fisher B, Dignam J, Wolmark N, et al. Tamoxifen and chemotherapy for lymph node-negative, estrogen receptor-positive breast cancer. *J Natl Cancer Inst* 1997;89:1673–1682.
67. Early Breast Cancer Trialists' Group. Ovarian ablation in early breast cancer: overview of the randomised trials. *Lancet* 1996;348:1189–1196. Search date not stated; primary sources individual patient data from trials that began before 1990, trials identified from lists from national cancer bodies, the International Cancer Research Data Bank, handsearches of conference proceedings and reference lists, and personal contact with investigators.
68. Chetty U, Jack W, Prescott RJ, et al. A. Management of the axilla in operable breast cancer treated by breast conservation: a randomised controlled trial. *Br J Surg* 2000;87:163–169.
69. Stelle RJC, Forrest APM, Gibson R, Stuart HJ, Chetty U. The efficacy of lower axillary sampling in obtaining lymph node status in breast cancer: a controlled randomised trial. *Br J Surg* 1985;72:368–369.
70. Browning C, Redman S, Pillar C, Turner J, Boyle F. NHMRC National Breast Cancer Centre, Sydney 1998. Lymphoedema: prevalence risk factors and management: a review of research. Search date 1996; primary sources Medline, hand searches of article references, personal contact with key resources of article references, and personal contact with key resources.
71. Axelsson CK, Mouridzsen HT, Zedeler K. Axillary dissection at level I and II lymph nodes is important in breast cancer classification. *Eur J Cancer* 1992;28A:1415–1418.
72. Kiricuta CI, Tausch J. A mathematical model of axillary lymph node involvement based on 1446 complete axillary dissections in patients with breast carcinoma. *Cancer* 1992;69:2496–2501.
73. Steele RJC, Forrest APM, Givson T, et al. The efficacy of lower axillary sampling in obtaining lymph node status in breast cancer: a controlled randomised trial. *Br J Surg* 1985;72:368–369.
74. Papaioannou A, Lissaios B, Vasilaros S, et al. Pre- and post-operative chemoendocrine treatment with or without post-operative radiotherapy for locally advanced breast cancer. *Cancer* 1983;51:1284–1290.
75. Perloff M, Lesnick G J, Korzun A, et al. Combination chemotherapy with mastectomy or radiotherapy for stage III breast carcinoma: a Cancer and Leukaemia Group B Study. *J Clin Oncol* 1988;6:261–269.
76. De Lena M, Varini M, Zucali R, et al. Multimodal treatment for locally advanced breast cancer. Results of chemotherapy–radiotherapy versus chemotherapy–surgery. *Cancer Clin Trials* 1981;4:229–236.
77. Olson JE, Neuberg D, Pandya KJ, et al. The role of radiotherapy in the management of operable locally advanced breast carcinoma: results of a randomised trial by the Eastern Co-operative Oncology Group. *Cancer* 1997;79:1138–1149.
78. Willsher PC, Robertson JF, Armitage NC, et al. Locally advanced breast cancer: long term results of a randomised trial comparing primary treatment with tamoxifen or radiotherapy in post-menopausal women. *Eur J Surg Oncol* 1996;22:34–37.
79. Bartelink H, Rubens RD, Van der Schueren E, et al. Hormonal therapy prolongs survival in irradiated locally advanced breast cancer: a European Organisation for Research and Treatment of Cancer randomised phase III trial. *J Clin Oncol* 1997;15:207–215.
80. Koning C, Hart G. Long term follow up of a randomised trial on adjuvant chemotherapy and hormonal therapy in locally advanced breast cancer. *Int J Rad Oncol Biol Phys* 1998;41:397–400.
81. Rodger A, Jack WJL, Hardman PDJ, et al. Locally advanced breast cancer: report of a phase II study and subsequent phase III trial. *Br J Cancer* 1992;65:761–765.
82. Willsher PC, Robertson JF, Chan SY, et al. Locally advanced breast cancer: early results of a randomised trial of multimodal therapy versus initial hormone therapy. *Eur J Cancer* 1997;33:45–49.
83. Tan SM, Cheung KL, Willsher PC, et al. Locally advanced primary breast cancer: medium term results of a randomised trial of multimodal therapy versus initial hormone therapy. *Eur J Cancer* 2001;37:2331–2338.

J Michael Dixon
Senior Lecturer in Surgery
Western General Hospital
Edinburgh
UK

Stephen Johnston
Senior Lecturer in Medical Oncology
The Royal Marsden NHS Trust
London
UK

Kate Gregory
Consultant Medical Oncologist
Royal Southampton Hospital
Southampton
UK

Alan Rodger
Professor of Radiation Oncology
William Buckland Radiotherapy Centre
The Alfred Hospital Monash University
Melbourne
Australia

Competing interests: MD see last issue, SJ none declaredm AR none declared. KG has been reimbursed by Pierre Fabre the manufacturer of vinorelbrne, for attending a conference. She has also received a fee for speaking from Bristol-Myers-Squibb, the manufacturer of Packtaxer.

TABLE 1 **Ten year survival with combination chemotherapy versus placebo, according to nodal and age/menopausal status: results of a systematic review of RCTs (see text, p 1825).[54]**

	Control (%)	Chemotherapy (%)	Absolute benefit (%)	SD (%)	Significance (two sided)
Age < 50 years					
Node +ve	41.4	53.8	+12.4	2.4	P < 0.00001
Node –ve	71.9	77.6	+5.7	2.1	P = 0.01
Age 50–69 years					
Node +ve	46.3	48.6	+2.3	1.3	P = 0.001
Node –ve	64.8	71.2	+6.4	2.3	P = 0.0025

SD, standard deviation.

TABLE 2 **Ten year survival in women treated with tamoxifen for 5 years compared with control treatment (no tamoxifen): results of a systematic review (see text, p 1826).[60]**

	Control (%)	Tamoxifen (%)	Absolute benefit (%)	SD (%)	Significance (two sided)
Node +ve	50.5	61.4	+10.9	2.5	P < 0.00001
Node –ve	73.3	78.9	+5.6	1.3	P < 0.00001

SD, standard deviation.

TABLE 3 **Staging of breast cancer (the individual terms are explained in the glossary).[1]**

	TNM			Stage
Non-invasive	Tis	N0	M0	0
Early invasive	T1–2	N0–1	M0	I, II A or B
	T3	N0	M0	II B
Advanced				
Locally advanced	Tany	N2	M0	III A
	T3	N1–2	M0	III A
	T4	N0–3	M0	III B
	Tany	N3	M0	III B
Metastatic	Tany	Nany	M1	IV

Breast pain

Search date March 2002

Nigel Bundred

QUESTIONS

INTERVENTIONS

Key Messages

- **Bromocriptine** Two RCTs found that bromocriptine versus placebo significantly reduced breast pain but one of these RCTs found that bromocriptine significantly increased adverse effects (including nausea, dizziness, postural hypotension, and constipation; NNH 7, 95% CI 4 to 29).
- **Danazol** One RCT found that danazol versus placebo significantly reduced cyclical breast pain after 12 months (NNT 3, 95% CI 2 to 5), but significantly increased adverse effects (weight gain, deepening of the voice, menorrhagia, and muscle cramps). It found no significant difference in pain relief with danazol versus tamoxifen.
- **Gestrinone** One RCT found that gestrinone versus placebo significantly reduced breast pain after 3 months, but significantly increased adverse effects (greasy skin, hirsutism, acne, reduction in breast size, headache, and depression).
- **Hormone replacement therapy** One small RCT found limited evidence that women taking hormone replacement therapy had significantly more breast pain after 1 year than women taking tibolone.
- **Lisuride maleate** One RCT found limited evidence that lisuride maleate versus placebo significantly reduced breast pain over 2 months (NNT 2, 95% CI 2 to 3).
- **Low fat, high carbohydrate diet** One RCT found limited evidence that advice to follow a low fat, high carbohydrate diet versus general dietary advice significantly reduced breast swelling (NNT 2, 95% CI 2 to 5) and breast tenderness (NNT 3, 95% CI 2 to 9) at 6 months.
- **Progesterones** Limited evidence from two crossover RCTs found no significant difference between progesterones versus placebo in breast pain.

- **Tamoxifen** One RCT found that tamoxifen versus placebo significantly reduced breast pain after 3 months (NNT 3, 95% CI 2 to 13); another found that tamoxifen versus placebo significantly increased the number of women with greater than 50% reduction in mean pain score after 12 months (NNT 3, 95% CI 1 to 10). Tamoxifen increased adverse effects such as hot flushes, vaginal discharge, and gastrointestinal disturbances. Fewer adverse effects were found with the lower dose of 10 mg given between days 15 and 25 of the menstrual period.
- **Tibolone** One small RCT found limited evidence that tibolone versus hormone replacement therapy significantly reduced breast pain after 1 year.
- **Antibiotics; diuretics; evening primrose oil; gonadorelin analogues (luteinising hormone releasing hormone analogues); progestogens; pyridoxine; vitamin E** We found no RCTs on the effects of these interventions.

DEFINITION Breast pain can be differentiated into cyclical mastalgia (worse before a menstrual period) or non-cyclical mastalgia (unrelated to the menstrual cycle).[1,2] Cyclical pain is often bilateral, usually most severe in the upper outer quadrants of the breast, and may refer to the medial aspect of the upper arm.[1-3] Non-cyclical pain may be caused by true breast pain or chest wall pain located over the costal cartilages.[1,2,4] Specific breast pathology and referred pain unrelated to the breasts are not included in this definition.

INCIDENCE/ PREVALENCE Up to 70% of women develop breast pain in their lifetime.[1,2] Of 1171 US women attending a gynaecology clinic, 69% suffered regular discomfort, which was judged as severe in 11% of women, and 36% had consulted a doctor about breast pain.[2]

AETIOLOGY/ RISK FACTORS Breast pain is more common in women aged 30–50 years.[1,2]

PROGNOSIS Cyclical breast pain resolves spontaneously within 3 months of onset in 20–30% of women.[5] The pain tends to relapse and remit, and up to 60% of women develop recurrent symptoms 2 years after treatment.[1] Non-cyclical pain responds poorly to treatment but may resolve spontaneously in about 50% of women.[1]

AIMS To reduce breast pain and improve quality of life.

OUTCOMES Breast pain score based on the number of days of severe (score 2) or moderate (score 1) pain experienced in each menstrual cycle; visual analogue score of breast pain, heaviness, or breast tenderness; questionnaires.

METHODS *Clinical Evidence* update search and appraisal March 2002 using the following keywords: breast tenderness; discomfort; pain; mastalgia; and mastodynia. Overall the evidence was poor and some studies with weaker methods were included when higher quality evidence was not found, as indicated in the text. Studies were included whatever the definition of breast pain, as indicated in the text.

QUESTION **What are the effects of treatments for breast pain?**

OPTION **LOW FAT, HIGH CARBOHYDRATE DIET**

One small RCT found that advice to follow a low fat, high carbohydrate diet reduced self reported breast swelling and tenderness significantly more than general dietary advice.

Benefits: We found no systematic review. We found one RCT (21 women attending a clinic in Canada with severe cyclical mastalgia for at least 5 years), which compared instruction to reduce fat content of the diet (to 15% of total calorie intake, while increasing complex carbohydrates to maintain caloric intake) versus general dietary advice (the principles for a healthy diet based on Canada's Food Guide, but not counselled to modify the fat content of their diet) for 6 months.[6] One woman in each group withdrew and was excluded from the analysis. Over 6 months, self reported breast swelling was significantly reduced in women with low fat, high carbohydrate diet versus general dietary advice (breast swelling at 6 months: 5/10 [50%] with low fat diet *v* 9/9 [100%] with general diet; NNT 2, 95% CI 2 to 5). Tenderness was significantly reduced in women receiving low fat dietary advice compared with those receiving general dietary advice (tenderness reported: 6/10 [60%] with low fat diet *v* 9/9 [100%] with general diet; NNT 3, 95% CI 2 to 9). However, no significant difference in breast swelling, tenderness, and nodularity was found on physical examination 6 months after allocation (breast swelling, tenderness, and nodularity on physical examination: 6/10 [60%] with low fat diet *v* 2/9 [22%] with general diet; RR 2.7, 95% CI 0.8 to 4.1).[6]

Harms: The small RCT reported no adverse effects.[6]

Comment: Diets can be difficult to sustain in the long term.

OPTION **EVENING PRIMROSE OIL**

We found insufficient evidence on the effects of evening primrose oil.

Benefits: We found no systematic review and no good quality RCTs.

Harms: Poor quality RCTs found that adverse effects causing treatment discontinuation were similar with evening primrose oil and placebo (3%), and largely caused by abdominal bloating.[5,7]

Comment: In one RCT, 72 women received evening primrose oil or placebo for 3 months followed by 3 months of evening primrose oil.[7] It reported that pain, tenderness, and lumpiness improved in cyclical but not non-cyclical breast pain. However, the methodology of the trial was poor and included post hoc revision of the inclusion criteria, subgroup analysis, exclusion of withdrawals, and the use of baseline comparisons (with the best response seen in women who were symptomatically worse at baseline). We found one survey of randomised and open studies; however, data were reported as overall summary figures, which makes specific data extraction impossible.[5]

OPTION DANAZOL

One RCT found that danazol versus placebo significantly reduced cyclical breast pain after 12 months, but with increased adverse effects. It found no significant difference in pain relief with danazol versus tamoxifen.

Benefits: We found no systematic review. We found one good quality three arm outpatient based RCT in 93 women with severe cyclical mastalgia.[8] **Versus placebo:** The RCT compared danazol (200 mg daily) versus tamoxifen (10 mg daily) versus placebo over 6 months. It found that significantly more women achieved greater than 50% pain relief at the end of treatment with danazol versus placebo (pain relief: 21/32 [66%] with danazol *v* 11/29 [38%] with placebo; RR 1.7, 95% CI 1.0 to 2.9; NNT 4, 95% CI 2 to 29). After 12 months of treatment the difference remained significant (pain relief after 1 year: 12/32 [38%] with danazol *v* 0/29 [0%] with placebo; NNT 3, 95% CI 2 to 5). **Versus tamoxifen:** See tamoxifen, p 1845. The same RCT found no significant difference in pain relief after treatment with danazol versus tamoxifen (21/32 [66%] with danazol *v* 23/32 [72%] with tamoxifen; RR 0.9, 95% CI 0.7 to 1.3).[8]

Harms: Adverse effects were reported in more women taking danazol than placebo.[8] These included a significant increase in weight gain (10/32 [31%] with danazol *v* 1/29 [3%] with placebo; Fisher extract test; P = 0.006), and non-significant increases for deepening of the voice (4/32 [13%] with danazol *v* 0/29 [0%] with placebo; P = 0.11), menorrhagia (4/32 [13%] with danazol *v* 0/29 [0%] with placebo; P = 0.11), and muscle cramps (3/32 [9%] with danazol *v* 0/29 [0%] with placebo; P = 0.24).[8]

Comment: Although we found no direct evidence, there is consensus that once a response is achieved adverse effects can be avoided by reducing the dose of danazol to 100 mg daily and confining treatment to the 2 weeks preceding menstruation.[8,9] Non-hormonal contraception is essential with danazol when given in 200 mg doses, as danazol has deleterious androgenic effects in the fetus.[10] An additional RCT comparing tamoxifen with placebo was identified and is being translated.[11]

OPTION BROMOCRIPTINE

Two RCTs found limited evidence that bromocriptine (a dopamine agonist) versus placebo significantly reduced breast pain. One RCT found a high incidence of adverse effects.

Benefits: We found no systematic review but found two RCTs.[12,13] The first outpatient based, European RCT (272 premenopausal women with diffuse fibrocystic disease of the breast) compared bromocriptine (2.5 mg twice daily) with placebo.[12] After 3 and 6 months it found that bromocriptine versus placebo significantly improved symptoms on self assessed visual analogue scoring of breast pain, tenderness, and heaviness (results presented graphically).[12] Results have to be approached with care as overall withdrawal rates were high (see comment below). The second RCT (10 women) used a crossover design, and also found that bromocriptine reduced pain compared with placebo ($P < 0.02$).[13]

Harms: The larger RCT found that adverse effects were significantly more frequent with bromocriptine than with placebo (61/135 [45%] with bromocriptine *v* 41/137 [30%] with placebo; RR 1.5, 95% CI 1.1 to 1.9; NNH 7, 95% CI 4 to 29). Withdrawals related to adverse effects were more frequent in women taking bromocriptine (15/135 [11%] with bromocriptine *v* 8/137 [6%] with placebo; RR 1.9, 95% CI 0.8 to 4.3). Adverse reactions included nausea (32% with bromocriptine *v* 13% with placebo), dizziness (12% with bromocriptine *v* 7% with placebo), postural hypertension, and constipation.[12] Overall withdrawal rates were high (see comment below). The second RCT found that nausea and dizziness occurred in 8/10 (80%) women on bromocriptine compared with 0/10 (0%) on placebo.[13] Strokes and death have been reported after use of bromocriptine to inhibit lactation, and the US Food and Drug Administration has withdrawn its license for this indication.[14]

Comment: Bromocriptine is now used rarely because frequent and intolerable adverse effects at the therapeutic dose outweigh the benefits for this indication. In the larger RCT, analysis was not intention to treat and overall withdrawal rates were high (withdrawals: 49/135 [36%] with bromocriptine *v* 36/137 [26%] with placebo; RR 1.4, 95% CI 1.0 to 2.0).[12]

OPTION LISURIDE MALEATE

One small RCT found that lisuride maleate (a dopamine agonist) versus placebo significantly relieved breast pain over 2 months.

Benefits: One double blind RCT (60 women with premenstrual breast pain) comparing lisuride maleate (200 μg daily) versus placebo over 2 months found significant improvement in visual analogue scores for pain (improved scores in 27/30 [90%] with lisuride maleate *v* 10/30 [33%] with placebo; RR 2.7, 95% CI 1.6 to 4.5; NNT 2, 95% CI 2 to 3).[15]

Harms: During the first month of treatment, nausea was more frequently reported by women taking lisuride maleate; however the difference was not significant (women reporting nausea: 5/30 [17%] with lisuride maleate *v* 3/30 [10%] with placebo; RR 1.7, 95% CI 0.4 to 6.4).[15]

Comment: Allocation was carried out in blocks of ten consecutive women. Tablet coding for active treatments and placebo differed. Response to treatment was considered when the scale was marked with a reduction greater than 25% with respect to the baseline score during the first month, or greater than 50% during the second month.[15]

OPTION HORMONE REPLACEMENT THERAPY IN BREAST PAIN

One small RCT found that hormone replacement therapy versus tibolone significantly increased breast pain.

Benefits: We found no systematic review. **Versus placebo:** We found no RCTs. **Versus tibolone:** One RCT (44 postmenopausal women) compared hormone replacement therapy (transdermal oestrogen patches 50 μg twice weekly for 3 wks/month, plus progestogen 5 mg daily for 12 days/month/cycle) versus tibolone (2.5 mg daily) versus no treatment.[16] The RCT found that breast pain was significantly increased in women on hormone replacement therapy versus tibolone after 1 year (increase of breast pain as assessed by questionnaire: 53% with hormone replacement therapy *v* 5% with tibolone; $P < 0.02$).[16]

Harms: The RCT did not report on adverse effects.[16] See harms of hormone replacement therapy under secondary prevention of ischaemic cardiac events, p 129.

Comment: Tibolone is a synthetic steroid reported to have oestrogenic, progestogenic, and weak androgenic properties, which can be used as a form of hormone replacement therapy.[17]

OPTION TAMOXIFEN

Two RCTs found limited evidence that tamoxifen is more effective than placebo at reducing breast pain. One RCT found no significant difference between tamoxifen and danazol. Tamoxifen increased hot flushes, vaginal discharge, and the risk of venous thromboembolism. Fewer adverse effects were found with the lower dose of 10 mg given between days 15–25 of the menstrual period.

Benefits: We found no systematic review. **Versus placebo:** We found two RCTs.[8,17] One double blind crossover RCT (60 premenopausal women with cyclical breast pain) compared tamoxifen (20 mg) with placebo.[18] It found that more women experienced pain relief (measured by visual analogue scale over 3 months) with tamoxifen versus placebo (71% with tamoxifen *v* 38% with placebo; RR 1.9, 95% CI 1.2 to 1.9; NNT 3, 95% CI 2 to 13). The second RCT (93 women) compared tamoxifen versus danazol versus placebo.[8] It found that significantly more women with tamoxifen versus placebo achieved a good outcome (> 50% reduction in mean pain score) at the end of treatment, 6 months later, and 12 months later (pain relief after 6 months of treatment: 23/32 [72%] with tamoxifen *v* 11/29 [38%] with placebo; RR 1.9, 95 CI 1.1 to 3.2; NNT 3, 95% CI 1 to 10). **Dose response:** One RCT (301 women with cyclical breast pain for > 6 months) compared 10 mg versus 20 mg of tamoxifen from days 15–25 in the menstrual cycle for 3 months. It found no significant difference in pain relief (127/155 [82%] with 10 mg dose *v* 107/142 [75%] with 20 mg dose; RR 1.09, 95% CI 0.96 to 1.18).[19] Another RCT (60 women) compared 10 mg versus 20 mg daily doses of tamoxifen for 3 and 6 months in cyclical and non-cyclical mastalgia.[20] Three month response rates were similar (pain relief: 12/14 [86%] with 10 mg *v* 14/15 [93%] with 20 mg; RR 0.9, 95% CI 0.4 to 1.1). **Versus other treatments:** One RCT found no significant difference in pain relief between tamoxifen and danazol (see versus other drugs under benefits of danazol, p 1843).[8]

Harms: One RCT found more women taking 20 mg of tamoxifen versus placebo experienced hot flushes (26% with tamoxifen *v* 10% with placebo; ARI 16%; RRI +1.49, 95% CI –0.34 to +3.33) and vaginal discharge (16% with tamoxifen *v* 7% with placebo; ARI 9.2%; RRI +1.34, 95% CI –0.97 to +3.64), but these differences were not significant.[18] See adverse effects of tamoxifen under treatment of breast cancer, p 1811. **Dose response:** Adverse effects occurred more frequently with the 20 mg dose than with the 10 mg dose between days 15–25 of the menstrual cycle.[19,20] The largest RCT found that adverse effects were reported more frequently with the 20 mg versus 10 mg dose (adverse effects: 94/142 [66%] with 20 mg daily *v* 80/155 [52%] with 10 mg daily; RR 1.28, 95% CI 1.06 to 1.56; NNT 6, 95% CI 3 to 28).[18] Adverse effects were primarily hot flushes (AR 54/142 [38%] with 20 mg dose of tamoxifen *v* 33/155 [21%] with the 10 mg dose; RR 1.79, 95% CI 1.24 to 2.58; NNH 6, 95% CI 3 to 16) and gastrointestinal disturbances (AR 54/142 [38%] with 20 mg *v* 30/155 [19%] with 10 mg tamoxifen; RR 1.97, 95% CI 1.34 to 2.88; NNH 6, 95% CI 4 to 12).

Comment: Tamoxifen is not licensed for mastalgia in the UK or the USA. There is consensus because of the high incidence of adverse effects to limit its use to no more than 6 months at a time under expert supervision and with appropriate non-hormonal contraception. Tamoxifen is contraindicated in pregnancy because of potential teratogenicity.[21]

OPTION GONADORELIN ANALOGUES (LUTEINISING HORMONE RELEASING HORMONE ANALOGUES)

We found no systematic review or RCTs on the effects of gonadorelin analogues (e.g. goserelin) in women with breast pain.

Benefits: We found no systematic review or RCTs.

Harms: Adverse effects of goserelin can include hot flushes (90%), headaches (57%), nausea and vomiting (29%), depression and irritability (24%), loss of libido (37%), and amenorrhoea (100%).[22]

Comment: None.

OPTION SYNTHETIC STEROIDS (GESTRINONE, TIBOLONE)

One RCT found that gestrinone relieved breast pain significantly more than placebo, but significantly increased adverse effects (greasy skin, hirsutism, acne, reduction in breast size, headache, and depression). One small RCT found that tibolone reduced breast pain significantly more than hormone replacement therapy after 1 year.

Benefits: We found no systematic review. **Versus placebo:** We found one double blind, outpatient based RCT (145 premenopausal women with cyclical breast pain) comparing gestrinone (2.4 mg twice weekly) with placebo.[23] It found that gestrinone reduced breast pain more than placebo after 3 months (using visual analogue score where 0 = no pain, 100 = worst pain; pain score reduced from 59.5 to 11.0 with gestrinone *v* 58.2 to 36.7 with placebo; $P < 0.0001$). **Versus hormone replacement therapy:** See hormone replacement therapy versus tibolone, p 1844.[16]

Harms: **Versus placebo:** The RCT found that significantly more women taking gestrinone versus placebo had adverse effects (at least 1 adverse effect, 41% with gestrinone *v* 14% with placebo; ARI 0.27; RR 2.96, 95% CI 1.70 to 4.40). Adverse effects included greasy skin (13 with gestrinone *v* 2 with placebo); hirsutism (10 with gestrinone *v* 3 with placebo); acne (9 with gestrinone *v* 2 with placebo); intermenstrual bleeding (7 with gestrinone *v* 0 with placebo); voice change (5 with gestrinone v 1 with placebo); reduced libido (5 with gestrinone v 3 with placebo); reduction in breast size (3 with gestrinone v 0 with placebo); headache (4 with gestrinone v 0 with placebo); depression (2 with gestrinone v 0 with placebo); and tiredness (2 with gestrinone v 0 with placebo).[23] **Versus hormone replacement therapy:** The RCT comparing tibolone versus hormone replacement therapy did not report adverse effects.[16]

Comment: Gestrinone is a synthetic steroid, reported to have androgenic, antioestrogenic, and antiprogestogenic properties.[17]

OPTION PROGESTERONES New

Two small crossover RCTs found significant difference in breast pain with progesterones versus placebo.

Benefits: We found two RCTs.[24,25] The first RCT (crossover, 26 women with cyclical breast pain of at least 6 months' duration) treated all included women with daily 20 mg tablets of medroxyprogesterone acetate for 6 months, followed by a 2 month observation period. Women with persistent symptoms were then randomly allocated to oral medroxyprogesterone acetate (20 mg tablets) versus placebo given from day 10–26 of the menstrual cycle, for 3 months and then switched group (crossover) for the remaining 3 months.[24] The RCT found no significant differences in the visual analogue scale for pain at the end of each phase before and after the crossover (data presented graphically). The overall withdrawal rate was 15%.[24] The second RCT (crossover, 80 women with breast pain of at least 2 months' duration) identified women who were able to keep an updated diary with visual analogue scales of pain for 2 months and then randomised them to daily applications of cream with progesterone 1% versus placebo, from the 10th day of the cycle to the beginning of the next cycle, for 3 months. The pre-crossover analysis found no significant difference in pain scores with progesterone versus placebo cream (figures not available).[25]

Harms: The first RCT found that five women reported adverse effects while on medroxyprogesterone acetate, five while on placebo, and one with both. Symptoms were mostly vague premenstrual symptoms.[24] No further details were provided. The second RCT did not report harms.[25]

Comment: The second RCT provided insufficient details about the analysis. Withdrawals involved 7/32 (22%) women.[25] Both RCTs have small sample size, significant withdrawals, and a selection phase, which may restrict the generalisibility of the evidence.[24,25]

OPTION PROGESTOGENS

We found no RCTs on the effects of progestogens in women with breast pain.

Benefits: We found no systematic review or good quality RCTs.

Harms: We found no RCTs.

Comment: None.

OPTION OTHER AGENTS

We found no RCTs of the effects of pyridoxine, diuretics, antibiotics, or vitamin E compared with placebo for the treatment of breast pain.

Benefits: We found no systematic review or good quality RCTs.

Harms: We found no RCTs.

Comment: None.

REFERENCES

1. Gateley CA, Mansel RE. Management of the painful and nodular breast. *Br Med Bull* 1991;47:284–294.
2. Ader DN, Shriver CD. Cyclical mastalgia: prevalence and impact in an outpatient breast clinic sample. *J Am Coll Surg* 1997;185:466–470.
3. Harding C, Osundeko O, Tetlow L, et al. Hormonally-regulated proteins in breast secretions are markers of target organ sensitivity. *Br J Cancer* 2000;2:354–360.
4. Maddox PR, Harrison BJ, Mansel RE, et al. Non-cyclical mastalgia: improved classification and treatment. *Br J Surg* 1989;76:901–904.
5. Pye JK, Mansel RE, Hughes LE. Clinical experience of drug treatments for mastalgia. *Lancet* 1985;1:373–377.
6. Boyd NF, McGuire V, Shannon P, et al. Effect of a low-fat high-carbohydrate diet on symptoms of cyclical mastopathy. *Lancet* 1988;2:128–132.
7. Preece PE, Hanslip JI, Gilbert L, et al. Evening primrose oil (Efamol) for mastalgia. In: Horrobin D, ed. *Clinical uses of essential fatty acids*. Montreal: Eden Press Inc, 1982:147–154.
8. Kontostolis E, Stefanidis K, Navrozoglou I, et al. Comparison of tamoxifen with danazol for treatment of cyclical mastalgia. *Gynecol Endocrinol* 1997;11:393–397.
9. Maddox PR, Harrison BJ, Mansel RE. Low-dose danazol for mastalgia. *Br J Clin Pract* 1989;68:43–47.
10. Anonymous. Danazol. In: *The ABPI compendium of data sheets and summaries of product characteristics*. London: Datapharm Publications Ltd, 1999–2000:1395.
11. Grio R, Cellura A, Geranio R, et al. Clinical efficacy of tamoxifen in the treatment of premenstrual mastodynia. *Minerva Ginecol* 1998;50:101–103.
12. Mansel RE, Dogliotti L. European multicentre trial of bromocriptine in cyclical mastalgia. *Lancet* 1990;335:190–193.
13. Blichert-Toft M, Anderson AN, Henrikson OB, et al. Treatment of mastalgia with bromocriptine: a double blind crossover study. *BMJ* 1979;1:237.
14. Arrowsmith-Lowe T. Bromocriptine indications withdrawn. *FDA Med Bull* 1994;24:2.
15. Kaleli S, Aydin Y, Erel CT, et al. Symptomatic treatment of premenstrual mastalgia in premenopausal women with lisuride maleate: a double-blind placebo-controlled randomized study. *Fertil Steril* 2001;75:718–723.
16. Colacurci N, Mele D, De Franciscis P, et al. Effects of tibolone on the breast. *Eur J Obs Gynae Rep Bio* 1998;80:235–238.
17. Parfitt K, ed. *Martindale. The complete drug reference*, 32nd ed. London: Pharmaceutical Press, 1999:1447–1448.
18. Fentiman IS, Caleffi M, Brame K, et al. Double blind controlled trial of tamoxifen therapy for mastalgia. *Lancet* 1986;1:287–288.
19. GEMB Group. Tamoxifen therapy for cyclical mastalgia: dose randomised trial. *Breast* 1997;5:212–213.
20. Fentiman IS, Hamed H, Caleffi M, et al. Dosage and duration of tamoxifen treatment for mastalgia: a controlled trial. *Br J Surg* 1988;75:845–846.
21. Anonymous. Nolvadex. In: *The ABPI compendium of data sheets and summaries of product characteristics*. London: Datapharm Publications Ltd, 1999–2000:1799.
22. Hamed H, Caleffi M, Chaudary MA, et al. LHRH analogue for treatment of recurrent and refractory mastalgia. *Ann R Coll Surg Engl* 1990;72:221–224.
23. Peters F. Multicentre study of gestinone in cyclical breast pain. *Lancet* 1992;339:205–208.
24. Maddox PR, Harrison BJ, Horobin JM, et al. A randomised controlled trial of medroxyprogesterone acetate in mastalgia. *Ann R Coll Surg Engl* 1990;72:71–76.
25. McFadyen IJ, Raab GM, Macintyre CC, et al. Progesterone cream for cyclic breast pain. *BMJ* 1989;298:931.

Nigel Bundred
Professor in Surgical Oncology
University of Manchester Department of Surgery/
South Manchester University Hospital
Manchester, UK

Competing interests: The author has received reimbursement by AstraZeneca, the maker of tamoxifen, for attending several conferences and running education programmes. The author has also received support by Searle Pharmacia for attending and speaking at symposia.

Dysmenorrhoea

Search date October 2001

Cynthia Farquhar and Michelle Proctor

QUESTIONS

INTERVENTIONS

See glossary, p 1860

Key Messages

- **Acupuncture** One small RCT found limited evidence that acupuncture versus placebo acupuncture or versus no treatment significantly reduced pain after 3 months.
- **Aspirin, paracetamol, and compound analgesics** One systematic review has found that aspirin is significantly more effective for pain relief than placebo (NNT 10, 95% CI 5 to 50 over at least 1 menstrual cycle), but less effective than naproxen or ibuprofen. The review found no significant difference with paracetamol versus either placebo, aspirin, or ibuprofen in pain relief. It found limited evidence that co-proxamol versus placebo significantly reduced pain, but compared to naproxen reduced pain significantly less and was associated with significantly more adverse effects. It also found that co-proxamol reduced dysmenorrhoea related symptoms significantly less than mefenamic acid.
- **Behavioural interventions** Two RCTs found insufficient evidence about the effects of behavioural interventions.
- **Combined oral contraceptives** One systematic review found insufficient evidence about the effects of combined oral contraceptives versus placebo for pain relief.
- **Dietary supplements (other than magnesium or thiamine)** RCTs found insufficient evidence about the effects of fish oil, dietary change, or vitamin E.
- **Herbal remedies** One systematic review found insufficient evidence of the effects of herbal remedies.

Clin Evid 2002;8:1849–1863.

- **Magnesium** Two RCTs found limited evidence that magnesium versus placebo significantly reduced pain, and another RCT found no significant difference with magnesium versus placebo in pain relief.
- **Non-steroidal anti-inflammatory drugs (other than aspirin)** One systematic review has found that naproxen, ibuprofen, and mefenamic acid are significantly more effective than placebo for pain relief over at least one menstrual cycle .The review found some evidence of increased adverse effects with naproxen versus placebo.
- **Spinal manipulation** Two RCTs found no significant difference in pain after one menstrual cycle with spinal manipulation versus placebo manipulation or no treatment, and two RCTs found that spinal manipulation versus placebo manipulation reduced pain after one menstrual cycle. One RCT comparing spinal manipulation versus placebo manipulation for 3 months found no significant difference in pain intensity at 3 months, but found that spinal manipulation significantly reduced pain intensity at 6 months.
- **Surgical interruption of pelvic nerve pathways** One small RCT found limited evidence suggesting that laparoscopic uterine nerve ablation versus diagnostic laparoscopy significantly increased pain relief at 3 and 12 months. Another RCT comparing laparoscopic uterine nerve ablation versus laparoscopic presacral neurectomy found no significant difference in pain relief at 3 months, but found that laparoscopic presacral neurectomy significantly reduced pain at 12 months.
- **Thiamine** One large RCT has found that thiamine versus placebo significantly reduces pain after 60 days.
- **Transcutaneous electrical nerve stimulation** Two small RCTs have found that high frequency transcutaneous electrical nerve stimulation versus placebo significantly increased pain relief. One RCT found no significant difference with low frequency transcutaneous electrical nerve stimulation versus placebo in pain relief. Two RCTs found insufficient evidence about the effects of transcutaneous electrical nerve stimulation versus non-steroidal anti-inflammatory drugs in pain relief.

DEFINITION Dysmenorrhoea comprises painful menstrual cramps of uterine origin. It is commonly divided into primary dysmenorrhoea (pain without organic pathology) and secondary dysmenorrhoea (pelvic pain associated with an identifiable pathological condition, such as endometriosis or ovarian cysts). The initial onset of primary dysmenorrhoea is usually shortly after menarche (6–12 months) when ovulatory cycles are established. The pain duration is commonly 8–72 hours and is usually associated with the onset of the menstrual flow. Secondary dysmenorrhoea may arise as a new symptom during a woman's fourth and fifth decade.[1]

INCIDENCE/ PREVALENCE Variations in the definition of dysmenorrhoea make it difficult to determine the precise prevalence. However, various types of study have found a consistently high prevalence in women of different ages and nationalities. A systematic review (search date 1996) of the prevalence of chronic pelvic pain, summarising both community and hospital surveys, estimated the prevalence at 45–95%.[2] Reports focus on adolescent girls and generally include only primary dysmenorrhoea, although this is not always specified. Studies of prevalence are summarised in table 1, p 1862.

AETIOLOGY/ RISK FACTORS A longitudinal study of a representative sample of women born in 1962 found that severity of dysmenorrhoea was significantly associated with duration of menstrual flow (average duration of menstrual flow was 5 days for women with no dysmenorrhoea and 5.8 days for women with severe dysmenorrhoea; $P < 0.001$; WMD −0.8, 95% CI −1.36 to −0.24); younger average menarcheal age (13.1 years in women without dysmenorrhoea *v* 12.6 years in women with severe dysmenorrhoea; $P < 0.01$; WMD 0.5, 95% CI 0.09 to 0.91); and cigarette smoking (41% of smokers and 26% of non-smokers experienced moderate or severe dysmenorrhoea).[9] There is also some evidence of a dose-response relationship between exposure to environmental tobacco smoke and increased incidence of dysmenorrhoea.[10]

PROGNOSIS Primary dysmenorrhoea is a chronic recurring condition that affects most young women. Studies of the natural history of this condition are sparse. One longitudinal study in Scandinavia found that primary dysmenorrhoea often improves in the third decade of a woman's reproductive life, and is also reduced following childbirth.[9]

AIMS To relieve pain from dysmenorrhoea, with minimal adverse effects.

OUTCOMES Pain relief, measured either by a visual analogue scale (see glossary, p 1861), other pain scales, or as a dichotomous outcome (pain relief achieved yes/no); overall improvement in dysmenorrhoea measured by change in dysmenorrhoeic symptoms either self reported or observed, quality of life scales, or other similar measures such as the Menstrual Distress or Menstrual Symptom Questionnaires; adverse effects of treatment (incidence and type of adverse effects); proportion of women requiring analgesics in addition to their assigned treatment; proportion of women reporting activity restriction or absences from work or school and hours or days of absence as a more selective measure.

METHODS *Clinical Evidence* search and appraisal October 2001.

QUESTION What are the effects of drug treatments?

OPTION ASPIRIN, PARACETAMOL, AND COMPOUND ANALGESICS

One systematic review has found that aspirin is significantly more effective for pain relief than placebo, but less effective than naproxen or ibuprofen. The review found no significant difference between paracetamol versus placebo, aspirin, or ibuprofen in pain relief. It found limited evidence that co-proxamol versus placebo significantly reduced pain, but reduced pain significantly less and was associated with significantly more adverse effects than naproxen. It also found that co-proxamol reduced dysmenorrhoea-related symptoms significantly less than mefenamic acid.

Benefits: We found one systematic review (search date 1997, 13 RCTs) of the effects of analgesics in primary dysmenorrhoea (see table 2, p 1863), which compared analgesics versus placebo, versus each other, or versus non-steroidal anti-inflammatory drugs.[11] **Aspirin versus placebo:** The review identified eight RCTs comparing aspirin versus placebo (486 women, 650 mg 4 times daily). Aspirin was significantly more effective than placebo for pain relief (5 RCTs; RR 1.60, 95% CI 1.12 to 2.29; NNT 10, 95% CI 5 to 50). There was no significant difference between aspirin versus placebo in the need for additional medication (3 RCTs; RR 0.79, 95% CI 0.58 to 1.08), or restriction of daily activity and absence from work (3 RCTs: RR 0.82, 95% CI 0.64 to 1.04; 1 RCT: RR 1.28, 95% CI 0.24 to 6.76). **Paracetamol versus placebo:** One RCT identified by the review found no significant difference between paracetamol 500 mg four times daily versus placebo in pain relief (35 women; RR 1.0, 95% CI 0.3 to 3.6). **Co-proxamol versus placebo:** The review identified one RCT, which found that co-proxamol (see glossary, p 1860) versus placebo significantly increased marked or moderate pain relief (72 women; 650 mg/65 mg 4 times daily; RR 3.72, 95% CI 2.13 to 6.52). **Paracetamol versus aspirin:** One RCT (35 volunteer medical, pharmacy, and dental students) identified by the review compared aspirin (500 mg 4 times daily) versus paracetamol (500 mg 4 times daily). It found no significant difference in pain relief (10 cm visual analogue scale [see glossary, p 1861]: median change from baseline 1.6 cm, 95% CI 0.4 to 3.3 with paracetamol *v* 1.2 cm, 95% CI 0 to 2.7 with aspirin). **Aspirin or paracetamol versus non-steroidal anti-inflammatory drugs:** The review identified six RCTs comparing aspirin or paracetamol versus non-steroidal anti-inflammatory drugs (313 women). Aspirin (650 mg 4 times daily) reduced pain significantly less than both naproxen (275 mg 4 times daily) (1 RCT; RR 2.29, 95% CI 1.16 to 4.29) and ibuprofen (400 mg 4 times daily) (1 RCT; RR 1.9, 95% CI 1.13 to 2.78). One RCT found no significant difference between paracetamol (1000 mg 3 times daily) versus ibuprofen (400 mg 3 times daily) in pain relief (defined as at least moderate relief) (1 RCT; RR 0.86, 95% CI 0.68 to 1.10). **Co-proxamol versus non-steroidal anti-inflammatory drugs:** The review identified three RCTs. One RCT compared co-proxamol (650 mg/65 mg 3 times daily) versus mefenamic acid (500 mg 3 times daily). The RCT found that co-proxamol versus mefenamic acid was significantly less effective in reducing dysmenorrhoea related symptoms ($P < 0.01$). Co-proxamol versus mefenamic acid also increased the need for additional medication (mean number of tablets of additional medication 2.6 with mefenamic acid *v* 6.8 with co-proxamol; no P value provided). The RCT found no significant difference between treatments in absence from work or school. Two RCTs (98 women) compared co-proxamol (650 mg/65 mg 3 times daily) versus naproxen (275 mg 3 times daily). Neither RCT found a significant difference in pain severity ($P > 0.05$), but naproxen achieved more effective pain control on some of the days measured ($P < 0.05$).

Harms: The most common adverse effects described by the review were nausea or abdominal discomfort, headaches, and dizziness.[11] Adverse effects occurred in 7–17% of women taking aspirin versus 3–17% of women taking placebo. The review found no significant difference between aspirin or paracetamol versus placebo in the frequency of adverse effects (any adverse effect for aspirin *v* placebo: RR 1.31, 95% CI 0.79 to 2.17; any adverse effect for paracetamol *v* placebo: RR 1.00, 95% CI 0.36 to 2.75). It found that co-proxamol versus naproxen significantly increased the number of women experiencing adverse effects (23–58% *v* 15–25%; RR 1.94, 95% CI 1.11 to 3.41).[11]

Comment: Most RCTs included in the systematic review were short (usually only 1 menstrual cycle on each treatment), small, and used a crossover design without a washout period. All of the RCTs (except one of co-proxamol versus naproxen) used double blinding. All the RCTs used oral administration of treatment in the form of tablets or capsules.

OPTION NON-STEROIDAL ANTI-INFLAMMATORY DRUGS (OTHER THAN ASPIRIN)

One systematic review has found that naproxen, ibuprofen, and mefenamic acid are all significantly more effective than placebo for pain relief. The review found some evidence of increased adverse effects with naproxen versus placebo.

Benefits: We found one systematic review (search date 1997) of the effects of non-steroidal anti-inflammatory drugs (NSAIDs) in primary dysmenorrhoea, which included 23 RCTs of naproxen (1728 women), 18 of ibuprofen (748 women), and five of mefenamic acid (257 women).[11] **NSAIDs versus placebo:** The systematic review found that all three NSAIDs versus placebo significantly increased pain relief (naproxen: 13 RCTs; RR 3.17, 95% CI 2.72 to 3.67, NNT 2.6, 95% CI 2 to 3.4; ibuprofen: 9 RCTs; RR 2.41, 95% CI 1.58 to 3.68, NNT 2.4, 95% CI 1.7 to 3.8; mefenamic acid: 3 RCTs; RR 2.03, 95% CI 1.65 to 2.48, NNT 2.1, 95% CI 1.6 to 4.5). The use of additional analgesics was significantly reduced for all NSAIDs versus placebo. Women taking naproxen were 60% less likely to use additional analgesics (10 RCTs; RR 0.4, 95% CI 0.3 to 0.4); those taking ibuprofen were 70% less likely (2 RCTs; RR 0.23, 95% CI 0.13 to 0.41); and those on mefenamic acid were 35% less likely (1 RCT; RR 0.65, 95% CI 0.52 to 0.80). Restriction of daily life was significantly less for naproxen (7 RCTs; RR 0.71, 95% CI 0.60 to 0.85) and ibuprofen (3 RCTs; RR 0.82, 95% CI 0.64 to 1.04). Absence from work or school was significantly reduced with naproxen (7 RCTs; RR 0.29, 95% CI 0.13 to 0.66) but not with ibuprofen (1 RCT; RR 0.14, 95% CI 0.02 to 1.10). **Comparison of NSAIDs:** The review identified five comparative RCTs. Three RCTs found no significant difference in pain relief between naproxen (550 mg loading dose followed by 275 mg) versus ibuprofen (400 mg) (RR 1.1, 95% CI 0.8 to 1.5). One RCT found that naproxen (550 mg loading dose followed by 275 mg) versus mefenamic acid (500 mg followed by 250 mg) significantly increased pain relief (RR 2.4, 95% CI 1.4 to 4.1), and another RCT found no significant difference between ibuprofen 400 mg versus mefenamic acid 250 mg (no RR or P values provided).

Harms: The most commonly reported adverse effects in the RCTs identified by the review were nausea, dizziness, and headaches.[11] Naproxen versus placebo significantly increased the number of adverse effects (number of RCTs not specified; RR 1.45, 95% CI 1.03 to 2.04). The review found no significant difference between ibuprofen versus placebo in the number of adverse effects (RR 1.12, 95% CI 0.85 to 1.47) or between mefenamic acid versus placebo (RR 0.59, 95% CI 0.28 to 1.23).[11]

Comment: All the RCTs identified by the review used oral treatment.[11] NSAIDs can be administered as suppositories, which seem to have a similar effect on overall pain relief but less effect than oral treatment for spasmodic pain.[12] Most RCTs in this systematic review used a crossover design without a washout period and were brief (usually only 1 menstrual cycle per treatment). Nine of the included RCTs did not blind the researchers to treatment allocation. Many of the trials on NSAIDs were sponsored by the pharmaceutical industry. The pain relief figures used above refer to RCTs that include women with primary dysmenorrhoea only. However, some of the figures regarding use of additional medication included data from women with undefined dysmenorrhoea. A systematic review with stricter inclusion criteria and methodological quality assessment is underway.[13]

OPTION COMBINED ORAL CONTRACEPTIVES

One systematic review found insufficient evidence of the effects of oral contraceptives in pain relief.

Benefits: We found one systematic review (search date 1999, 5 RCTs, 379 women).[14] It found no significant difference between medium dose oestrogen (> 35 μg) plus first or second generation progestogens versus placebo in pain relief at 1–3 months (4 RCTs, 320 women; 112/216 [52%] *v* 32/104 [31%]; RR 1.40, 95% CI 0.58 to 3.42). It found that oral contraceptives versus placebo reduced the number of women absent from work or school, but the difference did not quite reach significance (1 RCT; 19/49 [39%] *v* 24/40 [60%]; RR 0.65, 95% CI 0.42 to 1.00).

Harms: The review found no significant difference between combined oral contraceptives versus placebo in the number of women experiencing adverse effects, such as nausea, vomiting, depression, and abdominal pain (1 RCT, 89 women; 15/49 [31%] *v* 8/40 [20%]; RR 1.53, 95% CI 0.72 to 3.24).[14] The results of two RCTs are difficult to interpret and could not be included in the meta-analysis of adverse effects performed by the review because the RCTs randomised menstrual cycles and not women.[15,16] One small RCT (18 women) identified by the review comparing combined oral contraceptives versus placebo found that more women receiving the contraceptive pill experienced breakthrough bleeding (2/12 [17%] *v* 0/6 [0%]).[15] Another RCT (59 women) identified by the review found that combined oral contraceptives versus placebo increased weight gain, nausea, and vomiting (no further data provided).[16]

Comment: Most of the RCTs identified by the review had weak methods.[14] Because of the small number of included trials and participants, the results of the systematic review are sensitive to the statistical methods of calculation used. One of the RCTs identified by the review could not be included in the meta-analysis because of poor reporting of data.[16] All of the RCTs identified by the review used oral contraceptives that are no longer commonly prescribed, so the results may not be applicable to women today who take different preparations.[14]

QUESTION What are the effects of surgical treatments?

One small RCT found limited evidence suggesting that laparoscopic uterine nerve ablation versus diagnostic laparoscopy significantly increased pain relief. Another RCT comparing laparoscopic uterine nerve ablation versus laparoscopic presacral neurectomy found no significant difference in pain relief in the short term, but found that laparoscopic presacral neurectomy significantly reduced pain in the long term.

Benefits: We found one systematic review (search date 1998, 6 RCTs) of surgical pelvic nerve interruption for primary and secondary dysmenorrhoea.[17] Only two of the six RCTs included women with primary dysmenorrhoea. Meta-analysis was not performed because of RCT heterogeneity. One RCT identified by the review (21 women) comparing laparoscopic uterine nerve ablation (LUNA) (see glossary, p 1860) versus diagnostic laparoscopy found that LUNA significantly increased pain relief at 3 months (OR 15.5, 95% CI 2.9 to 83) and at 12 months (OR 10.9, 95% CI 1.5 to 77). The other RCT (68 women) found no significant difference between LUNA versus laparoscopic presacral neurectomy (LPSN) (see glossary, p 1860) in pain relief at 3 months' follow up (OR 0.7, 95% CI 0.2 to 2.7). However, at 12 months' follow up, the LPSN group had significantly better pain relief scores (OR 0.26, 95% CI 0.10 to 0.71).

Harms: One RCT identified by the review found that LPSN versus LUNA significantly increased constipation (31/33 [94%] with LPSN *v* 0/35 [0%] with LUNA; RR 0.01, 95% CI 0.00 to 0.24).[17]

Comment: Two larger RCTs of LUNA are underway, and data will be included in an update of the systematic review (M Proctor, personal communication, 2001). We found a second relevant systematic review but we have not included it because it includes lower levels of evidence, such as case studies.[18]

QUESTION What are the effects of complementary treatments?

OPTION TRANSCUTANEOUS ELECTRICAL NERVE STIMULATION

Two small RCTs found that high frequency transcutaneous electrical nerve stimulation versus placebo significantly increased pain relief. One RCT found no significant difference between low frequency transcutaneous electrical nerve stimulation versus placebo in pain relief. Two RCTs found conflicting evidence of the effects of transcutaneous electrical nerve stimulation versus non-steroidal anti-inflammatory drugs in pain relief.

Benefits: We found no systematic review but found three RCTs [19–21] **High frequency transcutaneous electrical nerve stimulation (TENS) versus placebo:** We found two RCTs.[19,20] The first RCT (32 women, double blind, crossover) compared three groups: high frequency TENS (see glossary, p 1861); placebo; and ibuprofen.[19] It found that TENS versus placebo significantly increased the number of women who experienced at least moderate pain relief (14/32 [44%] with TENS *v* 1/32 [3%] with placebo; OR 24, 95% CI 2.9 to 199).

The second RCT (27 women, single blind) compared high frequency TENS versus low frequency TENS versus placebo.[20] It found that high frequency TENS versus placebo significantly reduced pain (18 women: mean decrease 72% with TENS *v* 26% with placebo; WMD using fixed effects model 45, 95% CI 23 to 67). **Low frequency TENS versus placebo:** The RCT (27 women, single blind) comparing high frequency TENS versus low frequency TENS versus placebo found no significant difference between low frequency TENS versus placebo (18 women; WMD 24, 95% CI –2.9 to +51).[20] **High frequency TENS versus low frequency TENS:** One RCT found no significant difference between high frequency and low frequency TENS for pain relief (WMD 21, 95% CI –4.4 to +46).[20] **High frequency TENS versus non-steroidal anti-inflammatory drugs:** The RCT (32 women) comparing high frequency TENS, ibuprofen, and placebo found that high frequency TENS was significantly less effective than ibuprofen in achieving pain relief (14/32 [44%] with TENS *v* 24/32 [75%] using ibuprofen; OR 0.26, 95% CI 0.09 to 0.75).[19] Another unblinded RCT (12 women, crossover) found no significant difference between naproxen versus high frequency/high intensity TENS in pain relief (data were presented in graphic form but no OR or P values provided) but both significantly reduced pain from baseline ($P < 0.001$).[21]

Harms: Adverse effects of muscle vibrations, tightness, headaches, and slight burning or redness after use were experienced by four women on treatment and none on placebo (OR 10, 95% CI 0.5 to 199; $P = 0.12$).[19] In the unblinded crossover RCT, 10/12 women considered TENS to be temporarily painful but were prepared to accept this effect for the pain relief achieved.[21] None of the 12 women reported any adverse effects during treatment with naproxen.

Comment: A systematic review is underway.[22]

OPTION ACUPUNCTURE

One small RCT found limited evidence that acupuncture versus placebo acupuncture or versus no treatment significantly reduced pain.

Benefits: We found no systematic review. We found one RCT (48 women) comparing acupuncture versus placebo acupuncture (see glossary, p 1860) versus two no-treatment control groups, one of which had extra visits from a physician.[23] Treatment was for 30–40 minutes once a week for 3 weeks a month, for a total of 3 months. It found that acupuncture versus placebo acupuncture or no treatment significantly increased the proportion of women experiencing pain relief (chi squared = 13.6; $P < 0.001$). Acupuncture versus placebo acupuncture was significantly more effective in achieving pain relief (OR 17.5, 95% CI 1.6 to 192).

Harms: The RCT gave no information on adverse effects.

Comment: A systematic review is underway.[23]

OPTION BEHAVIOURAL

Two RCTs found insufficient evidence of the effects of behavioural interventions.

Benefits: We found no systematic review. We found two small RCTs on behavioural interventions (see glossary, p 1860). One involved relaxation and imagery,[24] and the other involved aerobic exercise.[25] **Relaxation treatment:** The first RCT (69 women) compared muscle relaxation plus positive imagery regarding menstruation versus self directed group discussion about menstruation versus waiting list control. The groups were divided into women with spasmodic or congestive dysmenorrhoea using the Menstrual Symptom Questionnaire. Spasmodic dysmenorrhoea was defined as spasms of pain mainly around the abdomen, and congestive dysmenorrhoea was defined as a dull aching pain in the lower abdomen and other areas of the body. It found that, in women with spasmodic or congestive dysmenorrhoea, muscle relaxation versus waiting list control significantly improved symptoms ($P < 0.01$). However, it found that only the women with spasmodic dysmenorrhoea experienced significantly less pain with relaxation versus group discussion or versus waiting list control ($P < 0.001$).[24] **Aerobic exercise:** The second RCT (36 women) comparing a training group that participated in 30 minutes of exercise 3 days a week versus a sedentary control group found that aerobic exercise significantly lowered Menstrual Distress Questionnaire scores ($P < 0.05$; results presented graphically).[25]

Harms: The RCTs gave no information on adverse effects.

Comment: Both RCTs were small and of poor methodological quality.[24,25] The classification of dysmenorrhoea into spasmodic and congestive categories is no longer commonly used and has little meaning.[25] The RCT (36 women) comparing aerobic exercise versus a sedentary control analysed results for the 26 women (72%) who completed the trial (11 in the exercise group and 15 in the control group).[25] A systematic review is underway.[26]

OPTION SPINAL MANIPULATION

Two RCTs found no significant difference in pain after one menstrual cycle with spinal manipulation versus placebo manipulationor no treatment, and two RCTs found that spinal manipulation versus placebo manipulation reduced pain after one menstrual cycle. One RCT comparing spinal manipulation versus placebo manipulation for 3 months treatment found no significant difference in in pain intensity at 3 months, but found that spinal manipulation significantly reduced pain intensity at 6 months.

Benefits: We found one systematic review (search date 2000, 5 RCTs) comparing spinal manipulation versus placebo or no treatment.[27] There was significant trial heterogeneity and the outcome of pain intensity or pain relief was reported differently by each of the trials; therefore a meta-analysis could not be performed. The first RCT (11 women) identified by the review compared high velocity, low amplitude rotation manipulation (HVLA) (see glossary, p 1860) versus no treatment versus placebo manipulation (see glossary, p 1860). It found no significant difference between HVLA versus no treatment in pain relief after 1 month (7/8 [87%] with HVLA *v* 0/2 [0%] with no treatment; RR 5.00, 95% CI 0.39 to 63.85), or HVLA versus placebo treatment (7/8 [87%] with HVLA *v* 0/1 [0%] with placebo treatment; RR 3.33, 95% CI 0.30 to 37.42). The second RCT identified by the review (44 women) comparing HVLA versus placebo manipulation found that HVLA significantly reduced pain intensity as measured by a 10 cm visual analogue scale (see glossary, p 1861) pain score after one treatment and one menstrual cycle (WMD –1.41, 95% CI –2.55 to –0.27). The third RCT (138 women) identified by the review found no significant difference between HVLA versus placebo manipulation in pain as measured by mean change in visual analogue scale pain score after one menstrual cycle (WMD +2.08, 95% CI –3.20 to +7.36). The fourth RCT (12 women) identified by the review found that HVLA versus placebo manipulation improved pain after one treatment during one menstrual cycle (no further data provided). The fifth RCT (26 women) identified by the review comparing 3 months of Toftness manipulation (see glossary, p 1861) versus placebo manipulation found that manipulation versus placebo did not significantly reduce pain intensity as measured by 10 cm visual analogue scale pain scores after 3 months (WMD 2.20, 95% CI 1.38 to 3.02), but manipulation did significantly reduce pain intensity after 6 months (WMD –1.40, 95% CI –2.21 to –0.59).[27]

Harms: One RCT identified by the review (138 women) found no significant difference between HVLA versus placebo manipulation in the number of women experiencing soreness in the lower back region within 48 hours of the intervention (3/69 [4%] *v* 2/69 [3%]; RR 1.50, 95% CI 0.26 to 8.70).[27] Soreness resolved within 24 hours. No other adverse effects were reported. The other RCTs identified by the review gave no information on adverse effects.

Comment: The overall methodological quality of the RCTs identified by the review was good: low withdrawal rate (2%), adequate randomisation method, blinding of the outcome assessor, and potential blinding of the participants as the control procedure was very similar to the treatment.

OPTION HERBAL REMEDIES

One systematic review found insufficient evidence of the effects of herbal remedies.

Benefits: We found one systematic review (search date 2000), which identified one RCT comparing a herbal remedy versus placebo.[28] It found that the Japanese herbal remedy toki-shakuyaku-san (taken 3 times daily) versus placebo remedy significantly reduced pain as measured by a visual analogue scale (see glossary, p 1861) after 6 months ($P < 0.005$), and significantly reduced the need for additional medication (diclofenac sodium) ($P < 0.01$; results presented graphically).

Harms: The RCT gave no information on adverse effects.

Comment: Toki-shakuyaku-san is a mixture of six herbs, including angelica and peony root.

OPTION DIETARY SUPPLEMENTS

Two RCTs found limited evidence that magnesium versus placebo significantly reduced pain, but one RCT found no significant difference between magnesium versus placebo in pain relief. One large RCT found that thiamine versus placebo significantly reduced pain. RCTs found insufficient evidence of the effects of fish oil, dietary change, or vitamin E.

Benefits: We found one systematic review (search date 2000, 6 RCTs)[28] and two additional RCTs.[29,30] **Fish oils versus placebo:** One RCT (42 women) identified by the review compared fish oil capsules twice daily for 1 month versus placebo. Menstrual symptom scores were significantly lower with fish oil than placebo (44 *v* 70; $P < 0.001$).[28] Less additional medication (ibuprofen 200 mg) was used in the fish oil group (mean 4.7 tablets with treatment *v* 10.1 with placebo; $P = 0.015$). One additional RCT (78 women) compared four interventions: fish oil (0.5–1 g 5 times daily); fish oil with vitamin B_{12} (0.015 mg); seal oil (higher in saturated fat than fish oil); and placebo for a minimum of 3 months.[29] It found that pain measured on a visual analogue scale (see glossary, p 1861) significantly decreased only in the fish oil with vitamin B_{12} group (reduction in mean scores: placebo –0.19; seal oil –0.2; fish oil –0.15; fish oil with vitamin B_{12} –0.73; $P = 0.015$). However, all three active treatment groups experienced significant change in the number of other menstrual symptoms and the amount of interference with daily activities ($P < 0.05$). **Magnesium versus placebo:** Three RCTs identified by the review compared magnesium versus placebo.[28] The first RCT (50 women) identified by the review compared magnesium aspartate three times daily versus placebo. It found that magnesium aspartate versus placebo significantly increased the number of women without pain after 6 months (21/25 [84%] with magnesium *v* 7/25 [28%] with placebo; RR 3.0, 95% CI 1.6 to 5.8). The second RCT (27 women) identified by the review found no significant difference between magnesium (5 mmol 3 times daily) versus placebo in reducing pain as measured by visual analogue scale pain scores, or in the number of ibuprofen tablets taken ($P = 0.07$; no further data provided). The third RCT (21 women) identified by the review found that magnesium (500 mg daily during menses) versus placebo significantly reduced pain after 5 months ($P < 0.01$).[28] **Thiamine versus placebo:** The review identified one crossover RCT (556 Indian adolescents attending school) comparing thiamine (100 mg daily for 3 months) versus placebo, which found that thiamine significantly increased the number of people with no pain before crossover after 60 days (142/277 [51%] with thiamine *v* 0/279 [0%] with placebo).[28] After completion of the RCT, 87% of all women experienced no pain. **Dietary change versus vitamin B_{12}:** One additional RCT (33 women) comparing a low fat, vegetarian diet versus a supplement placebo tablet containing vitamin B_{12} (0.02 mg) found no significant difference in the number of days with menstrual pain (WMD –0.9, 95% CI –1.8 to 0.0).[30] **Vitamin E plus ibuprofen versus ibuprofen alone:** One crossover RCT identified by the review (50 women) compared vitamin E (100 mg daily for 20 days before menses) plus ibuprofen (400 mg at the outset of painful menstruation) versus ibuprofen alone (400 mg at the onset of pain).[28] It found no significant difference between vitamin E plus ibuprofen versus ibuprofen alone in pain relief (23/26 [88%] *v* 17/24 [71%]; RR 1.25, 95% CI 0.93 to 1.67).

Harms: **Fish oils versus placebo:** One RCT identified by the review found that two women taking fish oils reported nausea and one women reported acne.[28] No adverse effects were reported in the group of women receiving placebo. **Magnesium versus placebo:** One RCT identified by the review found that magnesium versus placebo significantly increased the number of women who experienced intestinal discomfort and other minor adverse effects (5/25 [20%] with magnesium *v* 0/25 [0%] with placebo; NNH 5, 95% CI 2 to 38), although relief of these symptoms occurred when the dose was reduced from three to two tablets daily.[28] **Dietary change versus vitamin B_{12}:** One additional RCT comparing a low fat, vegetarian diet versus a supplement placebo tablet found that stomach upset, slight nausea, burping, and a bad taste in the mouth were reported by eight women across the different treatment groups.[30] No additional information was reported in the trial.

Comment: None.

GLOSSARY

Behavioural interventions Treatments that attempt modification of thought and beliefs (cognition) about symptoms and pain and/or modification of behavioural or physiological responses to symptoms and pain.

Co-proxamol Non-proprietary label for a dextropropoxyphene hydrochloride and paracetamol combination. The most common presentation is tablets containing dextropropoxyphene hydrochloride 32.5 mg and paracetamol 325 mg.

High velocity, low amplitude manipulation A technique of spinal manipulation that uses high velocity, low amplitude thrusts to manipulate vertebral joints. The technique is designed to restore motion to a restricted joint and improve function. The physician positions the patient at the barrier of restricted motion and then gives a rapid, accurate thrust in the direction of the restricted barrier to resolve the restriction and improve motion.

Laparoscopic presacral neurectomy Involves the total removal of the presacral nerves lying within the boundaries of the interiliac triangle. This procedure interrupts the majority of the cervical sensory nerve fibres and is used to diminish uterine pain.

Laparoscopic uterine nerve ablation Involves laparoscopic surgery to transect (usually they are cut and then electrocauterised) the uterosacral ligaments at their insertion into the cervix. This procedure interrupts the majority of the cervical sensory nerve fibres and is used to diminish uterine pain.

Placebo acupuncture Also known as sham acupuncture, a commonly used control intervention involving the use of acupuncture needles to stimulate non-acupuncture points in areas outside of Chinese meridians. These points can be identified by a point detector as areas of the skin that do not have skin electrical activity similar to acupuncture points. There is some disagreement over correct needle placement, as placement of a needle in any position may elicit some biological response that can complicate interpretation of results.

Placebo manipulation Also known as sham manipulation, it is a control intervention. The main principle is to use a non-therapeutic level of torque. There are two common techniques for placebo manipulation. In one, thrust is administered but the posture of the participant is such that the mechanical torque of the manipulation is substantially reduced. In the other, an activator adjusting tool is used, which can make spinal adjustments using spring recoil, where the spring is set so no force is exerted.

Toftness technique A low force technique of chiropractic adjusting that uses a sensometer to detect sites of abnormal electromagnetic radiation, and to determine which sites to adjust. Adjustment is then delivered using a metered, hand-held pressure applicator.

Transcutaneous electrical nerve stimulation (TENS) Electrodes are placed on the skin and different electrical pulse rates and intensities are used to stimulate the area. Low frequency TENS (also referred to as acupuncture-like TENS) usually consists of pulses delivered at 1–4 Hz at high intensity so they evoke visible muscle fibre contractions. High frequency TENS (conventional TENS) usually consists of pulses delivered at 50–120 Hz at a low intensity, so there are no muscle contractions.

Visual analogue scale A commonly used scale in pain assessment. It is a 10 cm horizontal or vertical line with word anchors at each end, such as "no pain" and "pain as bad as it could be". The woman is asked to make a mark on the line to represent pain intensity. This mark is converted to distance in millimetres from the "no pain" anchor to give a pain score that can range from 0–100.

REFERENCES

1. Fraser I. Prostaglandins, prostaglandin inhibitors and their roles in gynaecological disorders. *Bailliere's Clinical Obstet Gynaecol* 1992;6:829–857.
2. Zondervan KI, Yudkin PL, Vessey MP, et al. The prevalence of chronic pelvic pain in the United Kingdom: a systematic review. *Br J Obstet Gynaecol* 1998;105:93–99. Search date 1996; primary sources Medline, Embase, and Psychlit.
3. Harlow SD, Park M. A longitudinal study of risk factors for the occurrence, duration and severity of menstrual cramps in a cohort of college women. *Br J Obstet Gynaecol* 1996;103:1134–1142.
4. Campbell MA, McGrath PJ. Use of medication by adolescents for the management of menstrual discomfort. *Arch Pediatr Adolesc Med* 1997;151:905–913.
5. Robinson JC, Plichta S, Weisman CS, et al. Dysmenorrhoea and the use of oral contraceptives in adolescent women attending a family planning clinic. *Am J Obstet Gynecol* 1992;166:578–583.
6. Andersch B, Milsom I. An epidemiologic study of young women with dysmenorrhea. *Am J Obstet Gynecol* 1982;144:655–660.
7. Pedron Neuvo N, Gonzalez-Unzaga LN, De Celis-Carrillo R, et al. Incidence of dysmenorrhoea and associated symptoms in women aged 12–24 years. *Ginecologia y Obstetrica de Mexico* 1998;66:492–494.
8. Klein JR, Litt IF. Epidemiology of adolescent dysmenorrhea. *Pediatrics* 1981;68:661–664.
9. Sundell G, Milsom I, Andersch B. Factors influencing the prevalence and severity of dysmenorrhoea in young women. *Br J Obstet Gynaecol* 1990;97:588–594.
10. Chen C, Cho SI, Damokosh AI, et al. Prospective study of exposure to environmental tobacco smoke and dysmenorrhea. *Environ Health Perspect* 2000;108:1019–1022.
11. Zhang WY, Li Wan Po A. Efficacy of minor analgesics in primary dysmenorrhoea: a systematic review. *Br J Obstet Gynaecol* 1998;105:780–789. Search date 1997; primary sources Medline, Embase, and Science Citation Index.
12. Ylikorkala O, Puolakka J, Kauppila A. Comparison between naproxen tablets and suppositories in primary dysmenorrhea. *Prostaglandins* 1980;20:463–468.
13. Proctor ML, Sinclair OJ, Farquhar CM, Ivanova I, Stones W. Non-steroidal anti-inflammatory drugs for primary dysmenorrhoea (Protocol for a Cochrane Review). In: The Cochrane Library, Issue 4, 2001. Oxford: Update Software.
14. Proctor ML, Roberts H, Farquhar C. Combined oral contraceptives for primary dysmenorrhoea. In: The Cochrane Library, Issue 4, 2001. Oxford, Update Software. Search date 1999; primary sources Medline, Embase, Cinahl, Cochrane Controlled Trials Register, and hand searched citation lists.
15. Nakano R, Takemura H. Treatment of function dysmenorrhoea: a double-blind study. *Acta Obstet Gynaecol Jpn* 1971;18:41–44.
16. Matthews AE, Clarke JE. Double-blind trial of a sequential oral contraceptive (Sequens) in the treatment of dysmenorrhoea. *J Obstet Gynaecol Br Commonw* 1968;75:1117–1122.
17. Proctor ML, Farquhar CM, Sinclair OJ, et al. Surgical interruption of pelvic nerve pathways for primary and secondary dysmenorrhoea. In: The Cochrane Library, Issue 4, 2001. Oxford: Update Software. Search date 1998; primary sources Medline, Embase, Cochrane Controlled Trials Register, hand searched citation lists, and conference proceedings.
18. Khan KS, Khan SF, Nwosu CR, et al. Laparoscopic uterosacral nerve ablation in chronic pelvic pain: an overview. *Gynaecol Endosc* 1999;8:257–265. Search date 1997; primary sources Medline, Embase, and Science Citation Index.
19. Dawood MY, Ramos J. Transcutaneous electrical nerve stimulation (TENS) for the treatment of primary dysmenorrhea: a randomized crossover comparison with placebo TENS and ibuprofen. *Obstet Gynecol* 1990;75:656–660.
20. Mannheimer JS, Whalen EC. The efficacy of transcutaneous electrical nerve stimulation in dysmenorrhea. *Clin J Pain* 1985;1:75–83.

21. Hedner N, Milsom I, Eliasson T, et al. Tens bra vid smatsam mens. [TENS is effective in painful menstruation.] *Lakartidningen* 1996;93:1219–1222 [in Swedish].
22. Proctor ML, Farquhar C, Kennedy S, Jin X. Transcutaneous electrical nerve stimulation and acupuncture for the treatment of primary dysmenorrhoea (Protocol for a Cochrane Review). In: The Cochrane Library, Issue 4, 2001. Oxford: Update Software.
23. Helms JM. Acupuncture for the management of primary dysmenorrhea. *Obstet Gynecol* 1987;69:51–56.
24. Chesney MA, Tasto DL. The effectiveness of behavior modification with spasmodic and congestive dysmenorrhea. *Behav Res Ther* 1975;13:245–253.
25. Israel RG, Sutton M, O'Brien KF. Effects of aerobic training on primary dysmenorrhea symptomatology in college females. *J Am Coll Health* 1985;33:241–244.
26. Proctor ML, Murphy PA, Pattison HM, Farquhar CM. Behavioural interventions for primary and secondary dysmenorrhoea (Protocol for a Cochrane Review). In: The Cochrane Library, Issue 4, 2001. Oxford: Update Software.
27. Proctor ML, Hing W, Johnson TC, Murphy PA. Spinal manipulation for primary and secondary dysmenorrhoea. In: The Cochrane Library, Issue 4, 2001. Oxford: Update Software. Search date 2000; primary sources Medline, Embase, Cinahl, Psychlit, Bioabstracts, SPORTDiscus, Cochrane Controlled Trials Register, and hand searched citation lists.
28. Proctor ML, Murphy PA. Herbal and dietary therapies for primary and secondary dysmenorrhoea. In: The Cochrane Library, Issue 4, 2001. Oxford: Update Software. Search date 2000; Medline, Embase, Cinahl, Psychlit, Bioabstracts, Cochrane Controlled Trials Register, and hand searched citation lists.
29. Deutch B, Jorgensen EB, Hansen JC. Menstrual discomfort in Danish women reduced by dietary supplements of omega-3 PUFA and B12 (fish oil or seal oil capsules). *Nutrition Research* 2000;20:621–631.
30. Barnard ND, Scialli AR, Hurlock D, Bertron P. Diet and sex-hormone binding globulin, dysmenorrhea, and premenstrual symptoms. *Obstet Gynecol* 2000;95:245–250.

Cynthia Farquhar
Associate Professor

Michelle Proctor
Cochrane Review Group Co-ordinator

School of Medicine
University of Auckland
Auckland
New Zealand

Competing interests: None declared.

TABLE 1 **Prevalence of dysmenorrhoea: results of community and hospital surveys (see text, p 1850).[3–8]**

Study population	Population size	Location	Year	Prevalence
College students aged 17–19 years[3]	165	USA	1996	72% (13% severe)
High school students aged 14–21 years[4]	291	Canada	1997	93% (5% severe)
Adolescents attending an inner city family planning clinic[5]	308	USA	1992	80% (18% severe)
Women from an urban population aged 19 years[6]	596	Sweden	1982	73% (15% severe)
Students aged 12–24 years[7]	1066	Mexico	1998	52–64%
Adolescents aged 12–17 years[8]	2699	USA	1981	60% (14% severe)

TABLE 2 **Effects of aspirin, paracetamol, and compound analgesics for dysmenorrhoea: results of a systematic review (see text, p 1851).[11]**

Comparison	Usual dosage	Number of RCTs	Number of women	Pain relief	Adverse effects	Conclusion
Aspirin *v* placebo	650 mg four times daily	8	486	RR 1.60 (95% CI 1.12 to 2.29)	More frequent on aspirin (7–17% *v* 3–17% on placebo; RR 1.3, 95% CI 0.79 to 2.17)	Aspirin more effective than placebo (NNT 10, 95% CI 5 to 50)
Aspirin *v* paracetamol	650 mg *v* 500 mg four times daily	1	35	Median pain relief: paracetamol 1.6 (95% CI 0.4 to 3.3); aspirin 1.2 (95% CI 0 to 2.7)	NA	No significant difference
Aspirin *v* naproxen	650 mg *v* 275 mg four times daily	1	32	RR 2.29 (95% CI 1.16 to 4.29)	NA	Naproxen more effective than aspirin
Aspirin *v* ibuprofen	650 mg *v* 400 mg four times daily	1	56	RR 1.9 (95% CI 1.13 to 2.78)	NA	Ibuprofen more effective than placebo
Paracetamol *v* placebo	500 mg four times daily	1	35	RR 1.00 (95% CI 0.28 to 3.63)	No significant difference (RR 1.00, 95% CI 0.36 to 2.75)	No significant difference
Paracetamol *v* ibuprofen	1000 mg *v* 400 mg three times daily	1	67	RR 0.86 (95% CI 0.68 to 1.10)	NA	No significant difference
Co-proxamol *v* placebo	650 mg/65 mg four times daily	1	72	RR 3.72 (95% CI 2.13 to 6.52)	NA	Co-proxamol more effective than placebo
Co-proxamol *v* naproxen	650 mg/65 mg *v* 275 mg three times daily	2	98	$P > 0.05$ (no other data could be obtained from the report)	More frequent on co-proxamol (23–58% *v* 15–25% on naproxen; RR 1.94, 95% CI 1.11 to 3.41)	No significant difference
Co-proxamo *v* mefenamic acid	650 mg/65 mg *v* 500 mg three times daily	1	30	$P < 0.01$ (no other evidence can be obtained from the trial)	NA	Mefenamic acid more effective than co-proxamol

NA, not available.

Endometriosis

Search date March 2002

Cynthia Farquhar

QUESTIONS

INTERVENTIONS

See glossary, p 1872

Key Messages

In women with pain attributed to endometriosis

- **Combined ablation of endometrial deposits and uterine nerve** One RCT found that ablation of deposits plus laparoscopic uterine nerve ablation reduced pain more than diagnostic laparoscopy at 6 months.

Clin Evid 2002;8:1864–1874.

- **Cystectomy for ovarian endometrioma (better than drainage)** One RCT found that cystectomy versus drainage significantly improved pain caused by ovarian endometrioma at 2 years. Complication rates were similar.
- **Dydrogesterone** Systematic reviews have found no significant difference in pain at 6 months with dydrogesterone versus placebo given at two different doses in the luteal phase.
- **Hormonal treatment at diagnosis (danazol, medroxyprogesterone, gestrinone, gonadorelin [gonadotrophin releasing hormone] analogues)** Small systematic reviews and small RCTs have found that hormonal treatments (except for dydrogesterone) versus placebo reduce pain attributed to endometriosis, and are of similar effectiveness.
- **Laparoscopic ablation of endometrial deposits without ablation of the uterine nerve; laparoscopic uterine nerve ablation** We found insufficient evidence on the effects of these interventions. We found no RCTs comparing medical and surgical treatments.
- **Oral contraceptive pill** Two RCTs found no significant difference with combined oral contraceptives versus gonadorelin analogues in overall pain relief.
- **Postoperative hormonal treatment after conservative surgery** RCTs have found that postoperative hormonal treatment with danazol or medroxyprogesterone versus placebo for 6 months significantly reduces pain and delays the recurrence of pain at 12 and 24 months, but have found that treatment for 3 months does not seem to be effective. One RCT found no significant difference in recurrence of pain with combined oral contraceptives versus placebo at 6 months.
- **Postoperative hormonal treatment after oophorectomy** One RCT in women who previously had an oophorectomy found insufficient evidence on the effects of hormone replacement therapy versus no treatment in recurrence of endometriosis.
- **Preoperative hormonal treatment** One RCT found no significant difference in ease of surgery with preoperative treatment with gonadorelin analogues for 3 months versus no treatment.

In women with subfertility

- **Cystectomy for ovarian endometrioma (better than drainage)** One RCT found that cystectomy versus drainage significantly increased pregnancy rates in women with subfertility caused by ovarian endometrioma. Complication rates were similar.
- **Hormonal treatment at diagnosis (danazol, medroxyprogesterone, gonadorelin [gonadotrophin releasing hormone] analogues)** One systematic review and one subsequent RCT found no significant difference with hormonal treatments versus placebo in rates of pregnancy at 4–6 months.
- **Laparoscopic ablation/excision of endometrial deposits** One large RCT found that laparoscopic surgery versus diagnostic laparoscopy significantly increased cumulative pregnancy rates after 36 weeks (NNT 8, CI not available), but a subsequent smaller RCT found no significant difference with laparoscopic surgery versus diagnostic laparoscopy in pregnancy rates at 12 months. We found no RCTs comparing medical and surgical treatments.
- **Postoperative hormonal treatment (gonadorelin analogues and decapeptyl)** RCTs found no significant difference with gonadorelin analogues versus placebo after conservative surgery in rates of pregnancy or time to conception.

DEFINITION Endometriosis is characterised by ectopic endometrial tissue, which can cause dysmenorrhoea, dyspareunia, non-cyclical pelvic pain, and subfertility. Diagnosis is made by laparoscopy. Most endometrial deposits are found in the pelvis (ovaries, peritoneum, uterosacral ligaments, pouch of Douglas, and rectovaginal septum). Extrapelvic deposits, including those in the umbilicus and diaphragm, are rare. Severity of endometriosis (see glossary, p 1872) is defined by the American Fertility Society: this review uses the terms mild (stage I and II), moderate (stage III), and severe (stage IV).[1] Endometriomas are cysts of endometriosis within the ovary.

INCIDENCE/ PREVALENCE In asymptomatic women, the prevalence of endometriosis ranges from 2–22%, depending on the diagnostic criteria used and the populations studied.[2–5] In women with dysmenorrhoea, the incidence of endometriosis ranges from 40–60%, and in women with subfertility from 20–30%.[3,6,7] The severity of symptoms and the probability of diagnosis increase with age.[8] Incidence peaks at about 40 years of age.[9] Symptoms and laparoscopic appearance do not always correlate.[10]

AETIOLOGY/ RISK FACTORS The cause of endometriosis is unknown. Risk factors include early menarche and late menopause. Embryonic cells may give rise to deposits in the umbilicus, whereas retrograde menstruation may deposit endometrial cells in the diaphragm.[11,12] Use of oral contraceptives reduces the risk of endometriosis, and this protective effect persists for up to 1 year after their discontinuation.[9]

PROGNOSIS We found two RCTs in which laparoscopy was repeated in women treated with placebo.[13,14] Over 6–12 months, endometrial deposits resolved spontaneously in up to a third of women, deteriorated in nearly half, and were unchanged in the remainder.

AIMS To relieve pain (dysmenorrhoea, dyspareunia, and other pelvic pain) and to improve fertility, with minimal adverse effects.

OUTCOMES American Fertility Society scores for size and number of deposits;[1] recurrence rates; time between stopping treatment and recurrence; rate of adverse effects of treatment. **In women with pain:** Relief of pain, assessed by the Visual Analogue Scale ranging from 0–10, and subjective improvement. **In women with subfertility:** Cumulative pregnancy rate, live birth rate. **In women undergoing surgery:** Ease of surgical intervention (rated as easy, average, difficult, or very difficult).[15]

METHODS *Clinical Evidence* update search and appraisal March 2002. The authors also sought RCTs by electronic searching of databases, hand searching of 30 key journals, searching the reference lists of other RCTs, and identifying unpublished studies from abstracts, proceedings, and pharmaceutical companies. They used the search strategy and database of the Cochrane Menstrual Disorders and Subfertility Group, updated on a monthly basis, to identify RCTs on Medline and Embase. They included RCTs that used adequate diagnostic criteria for inclusion of participants (endometriosis diagnosed either by laparoscopy or laparotomy in association with dysmenorrhoea, dyspareunia, other pelvic pain, or infertility) and clinical outcomes (see outcomes above). Studies of assisted reproductive technologies were not included. Trials comparing different hormonal treatments of the same class were not included.

QUESTION What are the effects of hormonal treatments at diagnosis?

Four small systematic reviews and two additional RCTs have found that all different hormonal treatments, except for dydrogesterone, reduce pain attributed to endometriosis compared with placebo. One systematic review and one subsequent RCT found no evidence that hormonal treatments improve fertility. Adverse effects of hormonal treatments are common.

Benefits: **In women with pain attributed to endometriosis:** We found four systematic reviews (search dates 1998,[16] 2000,[17] 1997[18,19]) and two subsequent RCTs[20,21] evaluating 6 months of placebo or no treatment versus continuous ovulation suppression using danazol, gestrinone, depot medroxyprogesterone acetate (DMPA), dydrogesterone, oral contraceptives, gonadorelin analogues, or cyproterone acetate. The reviews found that when compared with placebo, all treatments were effective at reducing severe and moderate pain at 6 months, except dydrogesterone, which, given at two different dosages in the luteal phase, showed no evidence of effect. The first systematic review (search date 1998) identified seven RCTs (nearly 400 women) comparing danazol versus gonadorelin analogues.[16] It found no significant difference in pain or in resolution of endometrial deposits after 6 months of treatment. The second systematic review (search date 2000) identified one RCT (269 women) comparing danazol (200 mg/day) versus gestrinone (2.5 mg twice weekly).[22] It found no significant difference in pain reduction with danazol versus gestrinone. The first systematic review[16] included one RCT (49 women), which compared combined oral contraceptives versus gonadorelin analogues.[23] It found no significant difference in rate of relief for all types of pain, except menstrual pain for which oral contraceptives were better. A subsequent RCT (102 women) compared 12 months of combined oral contraceptive versus 4 months of combined oral contraceptive versus 8 months of gonadorelin analogues. It found no difference in pain (either menstrual or non-menstrual) at 12 months.[20] The second systematic review also included two RCTs assessing DMPA (140 women).[17] The larger RCT (80 women) compared DMPA (150 mg every 3 months) versus combined oral contraceptive plus danazol (50 mg/day). It found that DMPA was more effective at reducing dysmenorrhoea, but not any other outcomes. Long term follow up of one RCT (201 women followed for 12 months), of treatment with the gonadorelin agonist norethisterone versus oestrogen for management of painful symptoms, found that maintenance of pain relief was significantly better with norethisterone with or without oestrogen treatment.[24] One double blind RCT (48 women with verified endometriosis treated for 6 months and followed for 1 year after allocation) assessed quality of life in addition to relief of pain. It found an improvement in women treated with either gonadorelin analogues or medroxyprogesterone acetate compared to baseline measurements. No significant differences were found between groups.[21] **In women with subfertility attributed to endometriosis:** We found one systematic review (search date 1996, 4 RCTs, 244 women with "visually diagnosed" endometriosis attempting conception for more than 12 months)[25] and one subsequent RCT.[14] The trials assessed

6 months' treatment with danazol, medroxyprogesterone, or gonadorelin analogues versus placebo. The review found no significant effect on the likelihood of pregnancy with danazol (likelihood of pregnancy, danazol *v* placebo, RR 0.90, 95% CI 0.66 to 1.21). The subsequent RCT (100 infertile women) found no significant difference in pregnancy rates between medroxyprogesterone (50 mg/day) and placebo (after 16 wks: 0 pregnancies with medroxyprogesterone and 3 with placebo).[14]

Harms: **Gonadorelin (gonadotrophin releasing hormone) analogues:** The first systematic review found that gonadorelin analogues were associated with more hot flushes than placebo (about 80% *v* 30%, RR 2.7, 95% CI 1.5 to 4.8) and more headaches (33% *v* 10%, RR 3.6, 95% CI 1.1 to 11.5).[16] Gonadorelin analogues are associated with hypo-oestrogenic symptoms, such as hot flushes and vaginal dryness. RCTs have found that adding oestrogen, progestogens, or tibolone significantly relieves hot flushes caused by gonadorelin analogues (reducing symptom scores by 50% or more).[15,24,26,27] **Danazol:** In one RCT of 6 months' postoperative danazol (100 mg/day) versus no treatment, danazol was associated with more adverse effects: spotting (12% *v* 7%); bloating (16% *v* 9%); headache (21% *v* 13%); and weight gain (22% *v* 14%) (see postoperative hormonal treatment, p 1869).[28] **Gestrinone:** One RCT identified by the second systematic review[17] found a significantly higher frequency of hot flushes with gestrinone versus gonadorelin analogues; other trials found greater frequency of greasy skin and hirsutism compared with danazol, but less reduction in breast size, muscle cramps, and hunger. **Medroxyprogesterone:** The RCTs assessing hormonal treatment at diagnosis of endometriosis gave no information on adverse effects of medroxyprogesterone. One RCT (28 women with previous laparoscopic surgery) found more adverse events with DMPA versus danazol plus combined oral contraceptives: amenorrhoea (20% *v* 0%); breakthrough bleeding (15% *v* 0%); spotting (65% *v* 10%); bloating (63% *v* 28%); and weight gain (53% *v* 30%).[29]

Comment: The RCTs were mainly small with no long term follow up. Trials comparing different hormonal treatments of the same class were not included. The RCT addressing quality of life had high withdrawal rates (18/48 [38%]).[21]

QUESTION What are the effects of surgical treatments?

OPTION LAPAROSCOPIC UTERINE NERVE ABLATION

One systematic review found insufficient evidence on the effects of laparoscopic uterine nerve ablation in women with pain attributed to endometriosis.

Benefits: We found one systematic review (search date 1998, 2 RCTs, 132 women with endometriosis, stages I–III (see glossary, p 1872), age range 18–40 years).[28] It found no significant difference in pain relief between laparoscopic uterine nerve ablation (LUNA) versus laparoscopic treatment without LUNA. The largest trial (81 women) identified by the review found that satisfaction with treatment was high in both groups (73% for control *v* 68% for LUNA).

Harms: The RCTs gave no information on adverse effects.[28] Potential harms include denervation of pelvic structures and uterine prolapse.

Comment: The RCTs included in the review may have been too small to exclude a significant effect.[28]

OPTION LAPAROSCOPIC ABLATION OF ENDOMETRIAL DEPOSITS

We found no RCTs on the effects of laparoscopic ablation of deposits alone. One RCT found that combined treatment with ablation of deposits plus laparoscopic uterine nerve ablation reduced pain more than diagnostic laparoscopy at 6 months. One RCT found that laparoscopic surgery increased fertility compared with diagnostic laparoscopy; another smaller RCT found no significant difference.

Benefits: We found no systematic review. **In women with pain attributed to endometriosis:** We found no RCTs evaluating laparoscopic ablation of deposits alone. We found one RCT (63 women with mild to moderate endometriosis) comparing ablation of deposits plus laparoscopic uterine nerve ablation (LUNA) versus diagnostic laparoscopy.[30] It found that ablation plus LUNA reduced pain at 6 months (median decrease in pain score 2.85 for ablation *v* 0.05 for diagnostic laparoscopy; P = 0.01), and that 55% continued to have pain improvement 5 years later.[31] **In women with subfertility attributed to endometriosis:** We found two RCTs (in women with subfertility attributed to mild or moderate endometriosis) of laparoscopic ablation/excision of mild to moderate endometriotic deposits versus diagnostic laparoscopy.[32,33] In the larger trial (341 women) laparoscopic surgery significantly increased cumulative pregnancy rates (RR of pregnancy after 36 wks 1.7, 95% CI 1.2 to 2.6; NNT 8; raw data not provided).[32] A more recent RCT (101 women) found no significant difference in pregnancy rates at the end of 12 months' follow up (OR 0.75, 95% CI 0.31 to 1.88).[33] **Laser versus diathermy ablation:** We found no RCTs.

Harms: The RCTs gave no information on adverse effects.[30–33] Potential harms include adhesions, reduced fertility, and damage to other pelvic structures.

Comment: A further RCT of LUNA is under way in Auckland, New Zealand. One hundred and ten women were randomised and 12 months' follow up data is due by the end of 2002 (Farquhar C, personal communication, 2002).

QUESTION What are the effects of hormonal treatment after conservative surgery?

RCTs have found that 6 months of postoperative hormonal treatment with danazol or gonadorelin analogues versus placebo significantly reduces pain and delays the recurrence of pain; treatment for 3 months or treatment with combined oral contraceptives does not seem to be effective. RCTs found no evidence of an effect of postoperative hormonal treatment on fertility after conservative surgery. Adverse effects of hormonal treatment are common.

Benefits: We found no systematic review. We found seven placebo controlled RCTs, and one RCT versus expectant management of medical treatment in women who had undergone surgery for endometriosis (4 RCTs of gonadorelin analogues; 2 RCTs of danazol; 1 RCT of combined oral contraceptive; and 1 RCT comparing danazol versus depot medroxyprogesterone acetate versus expectant management).[28,34–40] We found one RCT comparing low dose continuous cyproterone acetate versus continuous monophasic oral contraceptive pill.[41] **In women with pain attributed to endometriosis:** One RCT (77 women with moderate to severe endometriosis) compared postoperative danazol (600 mg/day) versus placebo for 3 months after surgery. It found no significant difference in pain relief 6 months after finishing treatment (moderate to severe pain: 7/31 [23%] with danazol *v* 9/29 [31%] with no treatment; RR 0.73, 95% CI 0.31 to 1.70).[35] A second RCT (28 women with moderate endometriosis who had undergone conservative surgery followed by monthly injections of decapeptyl for 6 months) compared danazol (100 mg/day) for 6 months versus expectant management.[28] It found that danazol significantly reduced pain at both 12 months ($P < 0.01$) and 24 months ($P < 0.05$). Overall recurrence at 24 months was 44% with danazol versus 67% with expectant management ($P < 0.05$). A third RCT (60 women with mild to severe endometriosis) found that postoperative danazol (600 mg/day) or medroxyprogesterone (100 mg/day) for 180 days reduced pain more than placebo at 6 months.[36] Four RCTs assessed gonadorelin analogues.[34,37,38,40] The first RCT (75 women with endometriosis stages I and II) compared 3 months' treatment with nafarelin versus placebo in women who had laparotomy as part of their endometriosis treatment, and were followed for 12 months. It found no difference in pain relief at 12 months.[34] The second RCT (89 women with endometriosis stages III and IV [see glossary, p 1872]) compared monthly intramuscular leuprolide acetate depot injections for 3 months versus expectant management with 36 months' follow up in women after laparoscopic conservative surgery.[40] It found no significant difference in pain (moderate to severe pain recurrence during follow up, 10/44 [23%] with gonadorelin analogue *v* 11/45 [24%] with no treatment; cumulative pain recurrence rates at 18 months, 23% with gonadorelin analogue *v* 29% with no treatment; log rank test not significant) or fertility (pregnancies: 5/15 [33%] with gonadorelin analogue *v* 6/15 [40%] with no treatment; $P > 0.05$; cumulative pregnancy rates at 30 months presented in survival analysis graph; log rank test not significant). The two larger RCTs (109 women[37] and 269 women[38] with mild to moderate symptomatic endometriosis after conservative surgery) assessed 6 months' treatment (nafarelin 200 μg twice daily for 6 months and followed for 24 months;[37] and open label allocation of 3.6 mg of subcutaneous goserelin versus expectant management with 2 years' follow up[38]) found that gonadorelin analogues significantly reduced pain scores ($P = 0.008$)[37] and delayed the recurrence of pain by more than 12 months.[37,38] One small RCT (70 women) comparing combined oral contraceptives versus placebo postoperatively for 6 months found no reduction in the recurrence of pain associated with endometriosis (mean follow up 22 months; recurrences 2/33 [6%] with oral contraceptives v 1/35 [3%] with no treatment; RR 2.1, 95% CI 0.20 to 22.3).[39] One RCT (open label, 90 women with recurrent pelvic pain of more than 6 months' duration after complete surgical eradication of endometriosis) compared low dose continuous cyproterone acetate versus continuous monophasic oral contraceptive pill.[41] It found that both treatments were similarly effective and safe in women with modest and severe pain.[41] It found no significant difference between treatments in the proportion of women who were satisfied with treatment (33/45 [73%] with cyproterone acetate v 30/45 [67%] with oral contraceptive; RR 1.1, 95% CI 0.8 to 1.4). **In women with subfertility attributed to endometriosis:** Three of the RCTs (28, 75, and 269 women, all stages of endometriosis) assessed the effects of postoperative hormonal treatment (decapeptyl and gonadorelin analogues) versus placebo on fertility and found no difference in pregnancy rates or time to conception.[28,34,38]

Harms: See harms of hormonal treatments, p 1868.

Comment: The RCTs were mainly small with no long term follow up.

QUESTION **What are the effects of hormonal treatment on women with endometriosis who have had oophorectomy (with or without hysterectomy)** New

One RCT in women who previously had an oophorectomy found insufficient evidence on the effects of hormone replacement therapy versus no treatment.

Benefits: We found no systematic review. We found one RCT (172 women who previously had bilateral salpingo-oophorectomy for any reason with or without hysterectomy comparing HRT (115 women) versus no treatment (57 women).[42] HRT consisted of two weekly 1.5 mg estradiol (oestradiol) patches and 200 mg daily of micronised progesterone given orally during 14 days followed by a 16 day interval free of treatment. HRT was started 4 weeks after the salpingo-oophorectomy. It found no significant difference in recurrence rates at a mean of 45 months (0/57 [0%] without HRT v 4/115 [4%] with HRT; ARI +3.5%, 95% CI –3.2% to +8.6%).

Harms: The RCT found that surgical reinterventions were more frequent with HRT but this difference was not significant (2.6% with HRT v 0% with no HRT; OR 4.5, 95% CI 0.4 to 60.0).[42] The risk factors for recurrence were women who had endometriotic peritoneal involvement > 3 cm (2.4% recurrence a year with HRT v 0.3% with no HRT) and incomplete surgery (22.2% with HRT v 1.9% with no HRT).

Comment: The RCT had insufficient power to rule out clinically important differences.[42]

QUESTION **What are the effects of preoperative hormonal treatment?**

One RCT found no significant difference in ease of surgery with preoperative treatment with gonadorelin (gonadotrophin releasing hormone) analogues versus no treatment.

Benefits: We found no systematic review. We found one RCT (75 women with moderate or severe [see glossary, p 1872] endometriosis) comparing 3 months' preoperative treatment with a gonadorelin analogue versus no treatment.[43] It found no significant difference in ease of surgery, although more women with preoperative hormonal treatment were appraised as easy to treat by the surgeon (56% with treatment *v* 36% with no treatment).

Harms: See harms of hormonal treatments, p 1868.

Comment: The trial may have been too small to exclude a clinically significant effect.

QUESTION **What are the effects of treatments for ovarian endometrioma?**

OPTION **LAPAROSCOPIC DRAINAGE VERSUS LAPAROSCOPIC CYSTECTOMY**

One RCT found that pain and fertility improved more with cystectomy versus drainage, with no evidence of a difference in complication rates.

Benefits: We found no systematic review. We found one RCT (64 women) comparing laparoscopic cystectomy versus laparoscopic drainage.[44] **In women with pain attributed to endometrioma:** The RCT found that cystectomy versus drainage significantly reduced recurrence of pain at 2 years (OR 0.2, 95% CI 0.1 to 0.8) and increased the pain free interval after operation (median interval 19 months *v* 9.5 months; $P < 0.05$).[44] **In women with subfertility attributed to endometrioma:** The RCT found that compared with drainage, cystectomy significantly increased the pregnancy rate (67% with cystectomy *v* 24% with drainage; OR 8.3, 95% CI 1.2 to 59.0).[44]

Harms: The RCT reported no intraoperative or postoperative complications in either group.[44]

Comment: None.

GLOSSARY

Severity of endometriosis Determination of the stage or degree of endometrial involvement is based on a weighted point scale of arbitrary estimations, evaluating the degree of involvement of the peritoneum, ovaries, and tubes.[1] According to the allocated score, endometriosis is categorised as:

Mild (stage I and II) 1–15 points

Moderate (stage III) 16–40 points

Severe (stage IV) > 40 points

Substantive changes

Hormonal treatment at diagnosis Two new RCTs;[21,41] conclusions unchanged.

Hormonal treatment after conservative surgery One new RCT;[40] conclusions unchanged.

Hormonal treatment after oophorectomy One new RCT;[42] conclusions unchanged. The previous question addressing the effects of hormonal treatments after surgery has been split, separating conservative surgery from oophorectomy.

REFERENCES

1. American Fertility Society. Revised American Fertility Society (RAFS) classification of endometriosis. *Fertil Steril* 1985;43:351–352.
2. Mahmood TA, Templeton A. Prevalence and genesis of endometriosis. *Hum Reprod* 1991;6:544–549.
3. Gruppo Italiano per lo studio dell'endometriosi. Prevalence and anatomical distribution of endometriosis in women with selected gynaecological conditions: results from a multicentric Italian study. *Hum Reprod* 1994;9:1158–1162.
4. Moen MH, Schei B. Epidemiology of endometriosis in a Norwegian County. *Acta Obstet Gynecol Scand* 1997;76:559–562.
5. Eskenazi B, Warner ML. Epidemiology of endometriosis. *Obstet Gynecol Clin North Am* 1997;24:235–258.
6. Ajossa S, Mais V, Guerriero S, et al. The prevalence of endometriosis in premenopausal women undergoing gynecological surgery. *Clin Exp Obstet Gynecol* 1994;21:195–197.
7. Waller KG, Lindsay P, Curtis P, et al. The prevalence of endometriosis in women with infertile partners. *Eur J Obstet Gynecol Reprod Biol* 1993;48:135–139.
8. Berube S, Marcoux S, Maheux R. Characteristics related to the prevalence of minimal or mild endometriosis in infertile women. Canadian Collaborative Group on Endometriosis. *Epidemiology* 1998;9:504–510.
9. Vessey MP, Villard-Mackintosh L, Painter R. Epidemiology of endometriosis in women attending family planning clinics. *BMJ* 1993;306:182–184.
10. Vercellini P, Trespidi L, DeGiorgi O, et al. Endometriosis and pelvic pain: relation to disease stage and localization. *Fertil Steril* 1996;65:299–304.
11. Rock JA, Markham SM. Pathogenesis of endometriosis. *Lancet* 1992;340:1264–1267.
12. McLaren J, Prentice A. New aspects of pathogenesis of endometriosis. *Curr Obstet Gynaecol* 1996;6:85–91.
13. Cooke ID, Thomas EJ. The medical treatment of mild endometriosis. *Acta Obstet Gynecol Scand Suppl* 1989;150:27–30.
14. Harrison RF, Barry-Kinsella C. Efficacy of medroxyprogesterone treatment in infertile women with endometriosis: a prospective, randomized, placebo-controlled study. *Fertil Steril* 2000;74:24–30.
15. Compston JE, Yamaguchi K, Croucher PI, et al. The effects of gonadotrophin-releasing hormone agonists on iliac crest cancellous bone structure in women with endometriosis. *Bone* 1995;16:261–267.
16. Prentice A, Deary AJ, Goldbeck-Wood S, et al. Gonadotrophin releasing hormone analogues for pain associated with endometriosis. In: The Cochrane Library, Issue 2, 2001. Oxford: Update Software. Search date 1998; primary sources Medline, Embase, Cochrane Controlled Trials Register, and unpublished trials by UK distributors of GnRHAs.
17. Prentice A, Deary AJ, Bland E. Progestogens and antiprogestogens for pain associated with endometriosis. In: The Cochrane Library, Issue 2, 2001. Oxford: Update Software. Search date 2000; primary sources Medline, Embase, and Cochrane Controlled Trials Register.
18. Selak V, Farquhar C, Prentice A, et al. Danazol versus placebo for the treatment of endometriosis. In: The Cochrane Library, Issue 2, 2001. Oxford: Update Software. Search date 1997; primary sources Medline, Embase, Cochrane Controlled Trials Register, and hand searched journals and conference proceedings.
19. Moore J, Kennedy S, Prentice A. Modern combined oral contraceptives for the treatment of painful symptoms associated with endometriosis. In: The Cochrane Library, Issue 2, 2001. Oxford: Update Software. Search date 1997; primary sources Medline, Embase, and Cochrane Controlled Trials Register.
20. Parazzini F, Di Cintio E, Chatenoud L, et al. Estroprogestin vs. gonadotrophin agonists plus estroprogestin in the treatment of endometriosis-related pelvic pain: a randomized trial. Gruppo Italiano per lo Studio dell'Endometriosis. *Eur J Obstet Gynecol Reprod Biol* 2000;88:11–14.
21. Bergqvist A, Theorell T. Changes in quality of life after hormonal treatment of endometriosis. *Acta Obstet Gynecol Scand* 2001;80:628–637.
22. Bromham DR, Bookere MW, Rose R, et al. Updating the clinical experience in endometriosis: the European perspective. *B J Obstet Gynaecol* 1995(suppl);102:12–16.
23. Vercellini P, Trespidi L, Colombo A, et al. A gonadotropin-releasing hormone agonist versus a low-dose oral contraceptive for pelvic pain associated with endometriosis. *Fertil Steril* 1993;60:75–79.
24. Hornstein MD, Surrey ES, Weisberg GW, et al. Leuprolide acetate depot and hormonal add-back in endometriosis: a 12-month study. Lupron Add-Back Study Group. *Obstet Gynecol*. 1998; 91:16–24.
25. Hughes E, Fedorkow D, Collins J, et al. Ovulation suppression versus placebo in the treatment of endometriosis. In: The Cochrane Library, Issue 2, 2001. Oxford: Update Software. Search date 1996; primary sources Medline, Embase, Cochrane Controlled Trials Register, and hand searched journals and conference proceedings.
26. Gregoriou O, Konidaris S, Vitoratos N, et al. Gonadotropin-releasing hormone analogue plus hormone replacement therapy for the treatment of endometriosis: a randomized controlled trial. *Int J Fertil Womens Med* 1997;42:406–411.
27. Taskin O, Yalcinoglu AI, Kucuk S. Effectiveness of tibolone on hypoestrogenic symptoms induced by goserelin treatment in patients with endometriosis. *Fertil Steril* 1997;67:40–45.
28. Proctor M, Farquhar CM, Sinclair O, et al. Surgical interruption of pelvic nerve pathways for primary and secondary dysmenorrhoea. In: The Cochrane Library, Issue 2, 2001. Oxford: Update Software. Search date 1998; primary sources Medline, Embase, Cochrane Controlled Trials Register, and hand searched journals, conference proceedings, and references.
29. Morgante G. Low-dose danazol after combined surgical and medical therapy reduces the incidence of pelvic pain in women with moderate and severe endometriosis. *Hum Reprod* 1999;14:2371–2374.
30. Sutton CJG, Ewen SP, Whitelaw N, et al. A prospective, randomised, double-blind, controlled trial of laser laparoscopy in the treatment of pelvic pain associated with minimal, mild and moderate endometriosis. *Fertil Steril* 1994;62:696–700.
31. Sutton CJG, Pooley AS, Ewen SP. Follow-up report on a randomised, controlled trial of laser laparoscopy in the treatment of pelvic pain associated with minimal to moderate endometriosis. *Fertil Steril* 1997;68:170–174.
32. Marcoux S, Maheux R, Berube S, et al. Laparoscopic surgery in infertile women with

minimal or mild endometriosis. Canadian Collaborative Group on Endometriosis. *N Engl J Med* 1997;337:217–222.
33. Parazzini F. Ablation of lesions or no treatment in minimal-mild endometriosis in infertile women: a randomized trial. Gruppo Italiano per lo Studio dell'Endometriosis. *Hum Reprod* 1999;14:1332–1334.
34. Parazzini F, Fedele L, Busacca M, et al. Postsurgical medical treatment of advanced endometriosis: results of a randomized clinical trial. *Am J Obstet Gynecol* 1994;171:1205–1207.
35. Bianchi S, Busacca M, Agnoli B, et al. Effects of 3 month therapy with danazol after laparoscopic surgery for stage III/IV endometriosis: a randomized study. *Hum Reprod* 1999;14:1335–1337.
36. Telimaa S, Ronnberg L, Kauppila A. Placebo-controlled comparison of danazol and high-dose medroxyprogesterone acetate in the treatment of endometriosis after conservative surgery. *Gynecol Endocrinol* 1987;1:363–371.
37. Hornstein MD, Hemmings R, Yuzpe AA, et al. Use of nafarelin versus placebo after reductive laparoscopic surgery for endometriosis. *Fertil Steril* 1997;68:860–864.
38. Vercellini P, Crosignani PG, Fadini R, et al. A gonadotrophin-releasing hormone agonist compared with expectant management after conservative surgery for symptomatic endometriosis. *Br J Obstet Gynaecol* 1999;106:672–677.
39. Muzii L, Marana R, Caruana P, et al. Postoperative administration of monophasic combined oral contraceptives after laparoscopic treatment of ovarian endometriosis: a prospective, randomized trial. *Am J Obstet Gynecol* 2000;183:588–592.
40. Busacca M, Somigliana E, Bianchi S, et al. Post-operative GnRH analogue treatment after conservative surgery for symptomatic endometriosis stage III–IV: a randomized controlled trial. *Hum Reprod* 2001;16:2399–2402.
41. Audebert A, Descampes P, Marret H, et al. Pre or post operative medical treatment with nafarelin in Stage III–IV endometriosis: a French multicentered study. *Eur J Obstet Gynecol Reprod Biol* 1998;79:145–148.
42. Vercellini P, De Giorgi O, Mosconi P, et al. Cyproterone acetate versus a continuous monophasic oral contraceptive in the treatment of recurrent pelvic pain after conservative surgery for symptomatic endometriosis. *Fertil Steril* 2002;77:52–61.
43. Matorras R, Elorriaga MA, Pijoan JI, et al. Recurrence of endometriosis in women with bilateral adnexectomy (with or without total hysterectomy) who received hormone replacement therapy. *Fertil Steril* 2002;77:303–308.
44. Beretta P, Franchi M, Ghezzi F, et al. Randomised clinical trial of two laparoscopic treatments of endometriomas: cystectomy versus drainage and coagulation. *Fertil Steril* 1998;709:1176–1180.

Cynthia Cynthia Farquhar
Associate Professor
School of Medicine
University of Auckland
Auckland
New Zealand

Competing interests: None declared.

Essential vulvodynia (vulval pain)

Search date May 2002

Earlando Thomas, Damian Murphy, Charles Redman, and Bazian Ltd (temporary contributors)

QUESTIONS

INTERVENTIONS

Key Messages

- **Amitryptyline; pudendal nerve compression** We found no systematic review or RCTs on the effects of these interventions.

Essential vulvodynia (vulval pain)

DEFINITION Essential vulvodynia is characterised by a diffuse, unremitting burning sensation of the vulva, which may extend to the perineum, thigh, or buttock, and is often associated with urethral or rectal discomfort. Hyperaesthesia over a wide area is usually the only abnormal finding on physical examination. It is found primarily in postmenopausal women.

INCIDENCE/ PREVALENCE We found no data on the prevalence of essential vulvodynia.

AETIOLOGY/ RISK FACTORS The cause is unknown. The role of pudendal nerve compression is not clear; similar symptoms may be caused by pudendal nerve damage.[1–3]

PROGNOSIS Without treatment, the unremitting symptoms of essential vulvodynia may reduce the quality of life. Frequency of micturition, stress incontinence, and chronic constipation may rarely develop,[1–3] but we found no good data on prognosis without treatment.

AIMS To control symptoms and improve quality of life, with minimal adverse effects.

OUTCOMES Symptom scores for itching, burning, pain, and dyspareunia; range from 0–3 (3 represents the most severe).

METHODS *Clinical Evidence* update search and appraisal May 2002. Where we found no good RCTs, we used the best available observational studies.

QUESTION What are the effects of treatments?

OPTION AMITRIPTYLINE

We found no randomised evidence on the effects of amitriptyline in women with essential vulvodynia.

Benefits: We found no systematic review or RCTs.

Harms: In one retrospective cohort study of women with essential vulvodynia, adverse effects, mostly drowsiness and dry mouth, occurred in 9/20 (45%) women. Weight gain occurred in 10–15%. Tinnitus and palpitation were each reported by one women.[3]

Comment: There is a need for good quality research into the treatment of essential vulvodynia.

OPTION PUDENDAL NERVE DECOMPRESSION

We found no randomised evidence on the effects of pudendal nerve decompression in women with essential vulvodynia.

Benefits: We found no systematic review or RCTs.

Harms: A descriptive study (11 women with vulvodynia treated with pudendal nerve decompression) found no adverse effects.[2]

Comment: Pudendal nerve decompression may be technically challenging.

REFERENCES

1. Turner ML, Marinoff SC. Pudendal neuralgia. *Am J Obstet Gynecol* 1991;165:1233–1236.
2. Shafik A. Pudendal canal syndrome as a cause of vulvodynia and its treatment by pudendal nerve decompression. *Eur J Obstet Gynecol Reprod Biol* 1998;80:215–220.
3. McKay M. Dysesthetic ("essential") vulvodynia. Treatment with amitriptyline. *J Reprod Med* 1993;38:9–13.

Damian Murphy
Consultant Obstetrician and Gynaecologist
Department of Obstetrics and Gynaecology
New Cross Hospital
Wolverhampton
UK

Charles Redman
Consultant Obstetrician and Gynaecologist
Department of Obstetrics and Gynaecology
City General Hospital
Stoke-on-Trent
UK

Earlando Thomas
Senior Resident
Department of Obstetrics and Gynaecology
Rochester General Hospital
Rochester, New York
USA

Bazian Ltd (temporary contributors)
London
UK

Competing interests: None declared.

Fibroids (uterine myomatosis, leiomyomas)

Search date December 2001

Anne Lethaby and Beverley Vollenhoven

QUESTIONS

INTERVENTIONS

To be covered in future updates
Acupuncture/integrative medicines

Covered elsewhere in *Clinical Evidence*
Menorrhagia: many women with fibroids experience symptoms of heavy menstrual bleeding (see menorrhagia, p 1934.)

*Based on consensus.

See glossary, p 1888

Clin Evid 2002;8:1878–1891.

Key Messages

Medical treatments without surgery

- RCTs have found that gonadorelin analogues may reduce fibroid related symptoms such as heavy menstrual bleeding, and reduce uterine and fibroid volume to half the size. Adverse effects such as loss of bone density and unacceptable adverse events limit their use to 6 months. Hormone replacement therapy after initial treatment with gonadorelin analogues does not prevent bone loss but relieves some gonadorelin analogue related adverse events.
- Limited evidence from two small RCTs found no effect of non-steroidal anti-inflammatory drugs on menstrual bleeding.
- We found no RCTs on the effects of gestrinone on fibroid related symptoms. Androgenic adverse events limit its use.
- We found no good evidence on the effects of mifepristone.

Preoperative medical treatments

- One systematic review has found that gonadorelin analogues for 2–4 months prior to fibroid surgery increase haemoglobin and haematocrit, and reduce uterine and pelvic symptoms. However, women were more likely to experience adverse hypo-oestrogenic effects from preoperative treatment.
- One systematic review has found that preoperative gonadorelin analogues in women undergoing hysterectomy reduce blood loss during surgery and operating time. Women also recover more quickly from hysterectomy and have improved odds of having transverse incisions and converting from an abdominal to a vaginal procedure.
- One systematic review has found that blood counts are marginally improved postoperatively after pretreatment but there are no differences in complication rates or quality of life. However, women with pretreatment before myomectomy were more likely to have recurrence of their fibroids. We found insufficient evidence to evaluate change in fertility rates.
- One RCT found that leuprorelin (gonadorelin analogue) was superior to lynestrenol in reducing myoma size and lowering of postoperative haematocrit. There was no difference between the two treatments in clinical improvement of fibroid related symptoms.

Surgical treatments

- One RCT found that laparoscopically assisted vaginal hysterectomy resulted in less postoperative pain, shorter recovery time, and less requirements for analgesia than abdominal hysterectomy. These beneficial effects were found to be greater in women with a uterus estimated to weigh 500 g or less.
- One RCT found that laparoscopic myomectomy resulted in less postoperative pain and a shorter recovery time compared with abdominal myomectomy for fibroids.
- There is consensus that abdominal hysterectomy is superior to no treatment in improving fibroid related symptoms.

DEFINITION Fibroids (uterine leiomyomas) are benign tumours of the smooth muscle cells of the uterus. Women with fibroids can be asymptomatic or can present with menorrhagia (30%), dysmenorrhoea, pelvic pain, pressure symptoms, infertility, and recurrent pregnancy loss.[1] However, much of the data describing the relationship between the presence of fibroids and symptoms are based on uncontrolled studies that have assessed the effect of myomectomy on the presenting symptom.[2]

Fibroids (uterine myomatosis, leiomyomas)

INCIDENCE/ PREVALENCE The reported incidence of fibroids varies from 5.4%–77% depending on the method of diagnosis (the gold standard is histological evidence). A random sample of 335 Swedish women aged 25–40 years was reported to have an incidence of fibroids of 5.4% (95% CI 3.0 to 7.8%) based on transvaginal ultrasound examination. The prevalence of these tumours increased with age (age 25–32 years: 3.3%, 95% CI 0.7 to 6.0%; 33–40 years: 7.8%, 95% CI 3.6 to 12%).[3] Based on postmortem examination of women, 50% were found to have these tumours.[4] Gross serial sectioning at 2 mm intervals of 100 consecutive hysterectomy specimens revealed the presence of fibroids in 77%. These women were having hysterectomies for reasons other than fibroids.[5] The incidence of fibroids in black women is three times greater than that in white women, based on ultrasound or hysterectomy diagnosis.[6] Submucosal fibroids have been diagnosed in 6–34% of women having a hysteroscopy for abnormal bleeding, and in 2–7% of women having infertility investigations.[7]

AETIOLOGY/ RISK FACTORS The aetiology of uterine fibroids is unknown. It is known that each fibroid is of monoclonal origin and arises independently.[8,9] Factors thought to be involved include the sex steroid hormones oestrogen and progesterone as well as the insulin-like growth factors, epidermal growth factor, and transforming growth factor. Risk factors for fibroid growth include nulliparity and obesity. There is a risk reduction to a fifth with five term pregnancies, compared with nulliparous women ($P < 0.001$).[10] Obesity increases the risk of fibroid development by 21% with each 10 kg weight gain ($P = 0.008$).[10] Factors associated with reduced incidence of fibroids include cigarette smoking and hormonal contraception. Women who smoke 10 cigarettes a day have an 18% lowered risk of fibroid development compared with non-smokers ($P = 0.036$).[10] The combined oral contraceptive pill reduces the risk of fibroids with increasing duration of use compared with never users (users for 4–6 years: OR 0.8, 95% CI 0.5 to 1.2; users for ≥7 years: OR 0.5, 95% CI 0.3 to 0.9).[11] Women who have used injections containing 150 mg depot medroxyprogesterone acetate also have a reduced incidence compared with women who have never used (OR 0.44, 95% CI 0.36 to 0.55).[12]

PROGNOSIS There are little data on the long term untreated prognosis of these tumours, particularly in women who are asymptomatic at diagnosis. One small study reported that in a group of 106 women treated with observation alone over 1 year there was no significant change in symptoms and quality of life over that time.[13]

AIMS To reduce menstrual bleeding; prevent or correct iron deficiency anaemia; reduce pressure symptoms; reduce pelvic pain; and induce a change in fertility status with minimal adverse effects.

OUTCOMES Menstrual blood flow (assessed objectively [mL/cycle] or subjectively); haemoglobin concentration and haematocrit concentration; pregnancy rate; relief of pelvic pain and/or pressure (measured by a validated scale, p 1888 or subjective report); reduction in fibroid and uterine volume. Some of the outcomes relate to surgery: ease of surgery; complication rates during and after surgery; blood loss during surgery; duration of surgery; length of hospital stay; rate of blood transfusions; probability of transverse versus vertical incisions during surgery; probability of vaginal versus abdominal hysterectomy; change in quality of life; recurrence rate; satisfaction rate.

METHODS Clinical Evidence search and appraisal December 2001. We also searched the Cochrane Menstrual Disorders and Subfertility Group Register of RCTs in August 2000. This register contains published RCTs but also unpublished randomised data and conference abstracts and theses that report the results of RCTs. The register also contains the results of extensive handsearching that is coordinated by the Trials Search Coordinator and is supplemented by handsearching systematically performed by other review groups. The principal author also searched the reference lists of studies obtained from the initial search.

QUESTION What are the effects of medical treatments?

OPTION GONADORELIN ANALOGUES (GNRHA)

There is limited evidence from RCTs suggesting that gonadorelin analogues may reduce clinical symptoms associated with fibroids such as heavy menstrual bleeding. Potential side effects expected with long term treatment (e.g. hypo-oestrogenic effects) frequently limit their use to less than 6 months. RCTs have found a reduction of uterine and fibroid volume; however, this is a surrogate outcome and these benefits were not maintained after withdrawal. Hormone replacement therapy (with progestogen or combined oestrogen–progestogen) 3 months after initial gonadorelin analogue treatment reduced the rate of hot flushes but did not reverse loss of bone density.

Benefits: **Versus placebo:** We found no systematic review. We found four RCTs (154 women) comparing gonadorelin analogues without hormone replacement therapy (HRT) versus placebo.[14–17] The first RCT (13 participating centres, 128 women, 24 wks of treatment) was difficult to interpret as it had extremely high withdrawals, affecting the assessment of changes in symptoms after treatment.[14] The second RCT (38 premenopausal women) did not assess clinical outcomes.[15] The other two RCTs were too small to be evaluated (12 women[16] and 15 women[17]). Two RCTs found that fibroids return to previous size after stopping treatment.[14,15] **Versus different doses/types:** We found no systematic review. We found four small RCTs (171 women in total), two of which compared leuprolide acetate 1.88 mg with 3.75 mg,[18,19] one that compared buserelin MP 1.8 mg with leuprolide 1.88 mg by subcutaneous injection,[20] and one that compared triptorelin standard dose treatment plus three different types of dosage regimen.[21] No data were provided on clinical outcomes but one trial reported that all participants experienced partial or complete relief from symptoms throughout their treatment.[18] **Versus different modes of administration:** We found no systematic review. We found three RCTs (96 women) that compared different modes of administration of gonadorelin analogue treatment.[22–24] No results were provided in the trials for fibroid related symptoms. One RCT reported that all women had a subjective improvement in their subsequent menstrual symptoms after 6 months of treatment, especially menorrhagia and dysmenorrhoea, but no figures were provided.[22] There were no differences reported in uterine and fibroid shrinkage according to how gonadorelin analogue treatment was administered. **Versus gonadorelin analogues with HRT:** We found no systematic review. We found five RCTs that compared gonadorelin analogues treatment with gonadorelin analogues treatment plus progestogen "add-back" with HRT.[25–29] One RCT (41 women) found that leuprolide acetate plus progesterone HRT was associated with a reduction in heavy bleeding compared with leuprolide acetate followed by placebo (18/21 [86%] with progestogen HRT *v* 11/20 [55%] with placebo HRT; RR 1.6, 95% CI 1.0 to 2.4).[27] A second RCT (24 women) found that vasomotor symptoms, a common adverse event associated with gonadorelin analogue treatment, were reduced significantly in the group treated with additional medroxyprogesterone acetate ($P < 0.05$; figures not provided).[29] A third RCT (16 women) reported that progestogen HRT reduced hot flushes in women taking leuprolide (1/9 [11%] with progestogen HRT *v* 6/7 [86%] with placebo HRT; RR 0.13, 95% CI 0.02 to 0.84).[26] One RCT (50 women) compared gonadorelin analogue treatment plus placebo with gonadorelin analogue treatment plus tibolone for effects on uterine and fibroid size and fibroid related symptoms, but found no significant differences between the groups. Symptom intensity was assessed using a visual analogue scale.[30] An additional RCT compared gonadorelin analogues plus progestogen HRT with gonadorelin analogues plus combined oestrogen–progestogen HRT over a 2 year period.[31] Oestrogen–progestogen HRT prevented the regrowth of uterine size in comparison with HRT with progestogen alone. After 3 months of leuprolide treatment, there was a significant decrease in the mean uterine volume compared with baseline estimates (416 cm^3 with oestrogen–progestogen HRT *v* 440 cm^3 with progestogen alone HRT; CIs of the difference not available). After 21 months of treatment of oestrogen–progestogen, the mean uterine volume was reduced significantly (414 cm^3 with combined HRT *v* 647 cm^3 with progestogen alone; CIs not provided). Most women experienced a reduction in fibroid related symptoms and there were no differences between the HRT groups. Menorrhagia improved or resolved in 85% of all the participants, pelvic pressure in 63%, and pelvic pain in 100% of participants.

Harms: **Versus placebo:** The first RCT found that leuprolide was associated with vasomotor flushes, vaginitis, arthralgia/myalgia, asthenia, peripheral oedema, nausea, and insomnia. No significance was found in the risk of developing emotional lability/nervousness, depression, headaches, or decreased libido, although sample size may have been insufficient to rule out clinically significant differences for all these outcomes (see table 1, p 1891).[14] **With tibolone addition:** After 6 months of treatment, the mean number of hot flushes daily was reduced in the tibolone group (1.5 with tibolone *v* 4.6 with placebo; $P < 0.01$; data were read approximately from a graph).[30]

Comment: Most of the RCTs are small but there is consistent evidence from all trials about the benefits and harms of gonadorelin analogue treatment. Fibroid related symptoms are reduced by gonadorelin analogue treatment, but the treatment results in adverse events. There is not sufficient evidence to determine the optimum HRT regimen that minimises the adverse effects of gonadorelin analogues. Bone mineral density is reduced significantly after gonadorelin analogue treatment and this is not affected by HRT treatment. The RCT comparing gonadorelin analogue treatment plus placebo with gonadorelin analogue treatment plus tibolone[30] found that the significant reduction in bone mineral density after 6 months of treatment with gonadorelin plus placebo was prevented with the concurrent administration with tibolone (mean difference $P < 0.01$). The risk of fractures was not assessed.

OPTION NON-STEROIDAL ANTI-INFLAMMATORY DRUGS

We found no evidence that non-steroidal anti-inflammatory drugs effectively reduce heavy menstrual bleeding induced by fibroids. Two very small studies found no difference.

Benefits: We found two small RCTs (10 women followed for 6 months and 11 women followed for 4 months), which assessed the effects of non-steroidal anti-inflammatory drugs (ibuprofen and naproxen) on heavy menstrual bleeding in women with fibroids.[32,33] Neither study found an effect of non-steroidal anti-inflammatory drugs on heavy menstrual bleeding.

Harms: See harms under the non-steroidal anti-inflammatory drugs topic, p 1203.

Comment: Both RCTs had small numbers and may have been underpowered to assess an effect on clinical outcomes.

OPTION GESTRINONE

We found no RCT evidence on the effects of gestrinone on fibroid related symptoms. Androgenic adverse effects limit its use.

Benefits: We found no systematic review and no RCTs of the effect of gestrinone on clinical outcomes.

Harms: Two trials[34,35] found that acne and seborrhoea were common adverse events, which increased with duration of treatment. In one RCT after 1 year of treatment, seborrhoea affected 71–93% of participants and acne was reported by 31–63% of women after 2 years of treatment. Myalgia and arthralgia, mild hirsutism, hoarseness, and increased libido were also reported. Body weight also increased after 2 years of treatment, from a mean of 57.4 kg to 60.9 kg with no differences between groups. These changes reversed when treatment was discontinued.

Comment: The studies were not placebo controlled. The effects of gestrinone were assessed as comparisons with baseline values. Gestrinone needs to be adequately evaluated against other drugs or placebo. We found two uncontrolled studies (197 women) that compared the mode of administration in reducing uterine volume.[34,35] After 3 months of treatment in one trial, 76–86% of participants reported amenorrhoea. Pelvic pain was resolved in 76–98% of women. Haemoglobin increased from a mean of 12.38 g to 13.26 g and haematocrit increased from 36.9% to 38.4%.

OPTION **MIFEPRISTONE (RU486)**

We found no good evidence on mifepristone.

Benefits: We found no systematic review or clinical trials.

Harms: Mild atypical hot flushes were reported in 28–40% of women in an observational study.[36]

Comment: No conclusions can be reached on the benefits/harms of mifepristone from one observational study.

QUESTION **In women scheduled for fibroid surgery, what are the effects of preoperative medical treatments?**

OPTION **GONADORELIN ANALOGUES (GNRHA)**

One systematic review has found that gonadorelin analogues for 2–4 months prior to fibroid surgery increase haemoglobin and haematocrit, and reduce uterine and pelvic symptoms. However, women are more likely to experience adverse hypo-oestrogenic effects from preoperative treatment such as hot flushes, vaginal symptom, sweating, and withdrawal from treatment. Preoperative gonadorelin also reduces blood loss and the rate of vertical incisions during surgery. Women having hysterectomy are more likely to have a vaginal rather than an abdominal procedure after gonadorelin analogue pretreatment.

Benefits: We found one systematic review (search date 2000, 21 RCTs, 1886 women)[37] and one additional RCT.[38] The systematic review assessed gonadorelin analogue pretreatment (administered at least 3 months before surgery) compared with placebo or no treatment, in separate categories: prior to any surgery; during and after myomectomy; and during and after hysterectomy. Where possible, the overall effects were estimated by pooling the results of individual trials in the meta-analysis. One RCT that compared gonadorelin analogue pretreatment to pretreatment with lynestrenol, a progestin, was also included in the systematic review. **Versus immediate surgery or placebo treatment:** The systematic review found that pretreatment with gonadorelin analogues improved haemoglobin concentration (9 RCTs, 541 women: WMD 0.98 g/dL, 95% CI 0.74 g/dL to 1.22 g/dL) and haematocrit (4 RCTs, 138 women: 3.14%, 95% CI 1.78 to 4.51). Pelvic symptoms significantly improved when measured on a symptom scale (pelvic symptom score (see glossary, p 1888): 3 RCTs, 372 women: WMD –2.12, 95% CI –2.38 to –1.87). Women receiving gonadorelin analogue pretreatment had a lower risk of no improvement (1 RCT: OR 0.38, 95% CI 0.22 to 0.60). Intra-operative benefits were a reduction in blood loss estimated by measuring the weight of swabs and the volume of blood collected in receptacles (8 RCTs, 263 women: WMD 67 mL, 95% CI 44 to 91 mL) during myomectomy and during hysterectomy (6 RCTs, 419 women: WMD 58 mL, 95% CI 40 to 76 mL) for those who had gonadorelin analogue pretreatment. The duration of operation in gonadorelin analogue-pretreated women undergoing hysterectomy was shortened (7 RCTs: WMD 6.6 min, 95% CI 2.3 to 10.9 min) and hospital stay was shortened (4

RCTs: WMD 1 day, 95% CI 0.9 to 1.2 days). Gonadorelin analogue pretreatment was more likely to reduce the odds of vertical incision for those having laparotomy (myomectomy 1 RCT, 28 women: OR 0.11, 95% CI 0.02 to 0.75; hysterectomy 4 RCTs, 529 women: OR 0.36, 95% CI 0.23 to 0.55). There was also an indication that hysterectomy was subjectively graded by the surgeons as "not as difficult" in the pretreated women (2 RCTs: OR 0.73, 95% CI 0.25 to 0.97). These women also had improved odds of converting to a vaginal procedure (3 RCTs: OR 4.7, 95% CI 3.0 to 7.5). The systematic review found that postoperative pretreated women maintained marginally significant higher blood counts when compared with control patients (postoperative haemoglobin: 3 RCTs, 240 women: WMD 0.8 g/dL, 95% CI 0.5 g/dL to 1.1 g/dL) for both types of surgery and higher haematocrit levels after hysterectomy (2 RCTs, 173 women: WMD 1.8%, 95% CI 1.1 to 2.4), although the clinical significance of these results is unclear. One additional RCT (72 premenopausal women with symptomatic fibroids), not included in the systematic review because it did not meet inclusion criteria (see comments below), assessed whether preoperative treatment with gonadorelin analogues monthly for 4 months versus immediate surgery (hysterectomy plus bilateral oophorectomy) resulted in avoidance of scheduled hysterectomy.[38] The women in the gonadorelin analogue group were followed up for 3 years whereas those randomised to the control group had immediate surgery. If menorrhagia reoccurred during follow up, women were given another cycle of gonadorelin analogue treatment. If menorrhagia persisted after three cycles of gonadorelin analogue treatment, the participant underwent hysterectomy. After 3 years, 39% (95% CI 26 to 62) of the gonadorelin analogue treatment group had undergone hysterectomy. One second small additional RCT (24 women) assessed pregnancy rate in infertile women who had undergone myomectomy for fibroids at a mean follow up of 13 months.[39] Pregnancy rate was higher for pretreated women (AR 7/11 [64%] for pretreated women *v* 6/13 [46%] for control group; RR 1.4, 95% CI 0.7 to 2.9). **Versus other pretreatments:** One RCT (56 women) compared leuprorelin (gonadorelin analogue) with lynestrenol pretreatment.[40] Decrease in postoperative haematocrit was lower with leuprorelin (1 RCT, 42 women: WMD −7.8%, 95% CI −14% to −1.3%). The trial had a 25% withdrawal rate.

Harms: The systematic review assessed harms of gonadorelin analogue pretreatment in the categories above. Women pretreated with gonadorelin analogues were more likely to experience hypo-oestrogenic symptoms, such as hot flushes (534 women: OR 6.5, 95% CI 4.6 to 9.2), change in breast size (261 women; OR 7.7, 95% CI 2.4 to 24.9), vaginal symptoms (534 women: OR 4.0, 95% CI 2.1 to 7.6), and sweating (4 trials, 628 women: OR 8.3, 95% CI 1.0 to 5.9). Women were also more likely to withdraw from treatment because of adverse events (4 RCTs, 628 women: OR 2.5, 95% CI 1.0 to 5.9). Within the systematic review, two small RCTs (24 and 18 women) that evaluated long term follow up in women having myomectomy were identified. In one of these, 24 women were checked for fibroid recurrence at 6 months and 63% of the pretreated groups had a recurrence of their fibroids compared with 13% of the control group. Fibroid recurrence 2–3 years after surgery was over 50% in the 18 women from the second RCT, but no significant differences were found. No other harms were assessed.

Comment: The RCTs were not evaluated individually as pooled measures of effect were calculated in the systematic review. **Versus other pretreatments:** One RCT was not included in the systematic review because the outcome addressing avoidance of scheduled hysterectomy was assessed in the gonadorelin analogues group only.

QUESTION What are the effects of surgical treatments?

OPTION LAPAROSCOPICALLY ASSISTED VAGINAL HYSTERECTOMY

We found limited evidence suggesting that women having laparoscopically assisted vaginal hysterectomy had shorter recovery and less postoperative pain compared to total abdominal hysterectomy. The benefits of laparoscopically assisted vaginal hysterectomy are greater in women with uterus estimated to weigh 500 g or less.

Benefits: We found no systematic review. We found no RCTs against no intervention or sham surgery. We identified one RCT that addressed the effects of laparoscopicallly assisted hysterectomy as a surgical treatment for fibroids.[41] One RCT (62 women with symptomatic fibroids scheduled for hysterectomy) compared the effects of laparoscopically assisted vaginal hysterectomy (LAVH) and total abdominal hysterectomy (TAH) on operating time, blood loss, complications (not clearly specified), febrile morbidity, postoperative analgesic requirement, and hospital stay.[41] **In women with uterus estimated to weigh 500 g or less:** Women undergoing LAVH for uteri estimated to weigh 500 g or less in the preoperative assessment had comparable operating time (130 min on average with LAVH group *v* 120 min with TAH) but less postoperative pain and shorter recovery compared with the TAH group. Sonograms were used to estimate uterine weight. Analgesia requirement was reduced with LAVH (1/20 [5%] for the LAVH group *v* 6/11 [55%] for the TAH group; RR 0.09, 95% CI 0.01 to 0.67; NNT 2: 95% CI 1 to 6). Hospital stay was also reduced with LAVH (3.8 days, 95% CI 3.2 to 4.0 for women in the LAVH group *v* 5.8 days, 95% CI 5.0 to 6.4 with TAH; $P < 0.0001$). **In women with uterus estimated to weigh greater than 500 g:** One RCT in women undergoing LAVH with uteri weighing greater than 500 g found that those with LAVH had a shorter recovery but a longer operating time compared to TAH, and a 27% rate of conversion to laparotomy. Mean operating time was increased with LAVH (150min, 95% CI 125 to 173 min in the LAVH group *v* 108 min, 95% CI 83 to 120 min with TAH; $P = 0.002$). Mean hospital stay was reduced with LAVH (4 days, 95% CI 3.9 to 5.8 with LAVH group *v* 6 days, 95% CI 5.8 to 6.0 with TAH). Conversion to laparotomy was not significantly different between LAVH and TAH (3/11 [27%] with LAVH *v* 0/20 [20%] with TAH), although the sample size was insufficient to rule out a clinically important difference.[41]

Harms: No major complications were reported, although there was insufficient information to determine which complications were addressed.

Comment: Other RCTs have compared different types of hysterectomy in heterogeneous groups of participants but results from these RCTs are not generalisable to women with fibroids.

OPTION LAPAROSCOPIC MYOMECTOMY

Limited evidence suggests that laparoscopic myomectomy is associated with less postoperative pain and fever, and shorter recovery than abdominal myomectomy.

Benefits: We found no systematic review. We found no RCTs against no intervention or sham surgery. We found two RCTs comparing laparoscopic myomectomy with myomectomy by laparotomy.[42,43] The first RCT (40 women with < 5 myomas and the size of the largest myoma < 7 cm) found no differences in surgical time, blood loss, or postoperative complications (fever). Women undergoing laparoscopy reported a lower intensity of postoperative pain (unlabelled scale), required less analgesia, and had a shorter recovery time than women undergoing myomectomy by laparotomy. Two days after surgery, fewer women required analgesia in the laparoscopy group (analgesia free women: 17/20 [85%] with laparoscopy *v* 3/20 [15%] with laparotomy; RR 5.7, 95% CI 2.0 to 16.4; NNT 2, 95% CI 1 to 3), and by day 15 more women were fully recovered in the laparoscopy group (18/20 [90%] with laparoscopy *v* 1/20 [5%] with laparotomy; RR 18.0, 95% CI 2.7 to 122; NNT 2, 95% CI 1 to 2). The second RCT (131 women with at least 1 myoma ≥ 5 cm)[43] found no differences in surgical time. However, it also found a greater drop in haemoglobin with myomectomy by laparotomy (1.33 g/dL with laparoscopy *v* 2.17 g/dL with laparotomy; CI not provided; P < 0.001). Participants in the laparoscopy group were marginally less likely to experience postoperative fever (8/66 [12%] with laparoscopy *v* 17/65 [26%] with laparotomy; RR 0.46, 95% CI 0.22 to 1.0; NNT 9, 95% CI 4 to 116) and were more likely to have a shorter hospital stay (75.6 h with laparoscopy *v* 142.8 h with laparotomy; CI not provided; P < 0.001). Pregnancy rate after surgery did not differ between groups.

Harms: No major complications were reported in the two RCTs.[42,43] Transfusions were more frequently seen in the laparotomy group but the difference did not reach statistical significance (transfusion risk: 0/66 [0%] with laparoscopy *v* 3/65 [5%] with laparotomy; ARR –0.05, 95% CI –0.13 to +0.02).

Comment: Other RCTs have compared different types of hysterectomy in heterogeneous groups of participants but results from these RCTs are not generalisable to women with fibroids.

OPTION ABDOMINAL HYSTERECTOMY

One RCT comparing abdominal hysterectomy with laparoscopically assisted vaginal hysterectomy found limited evidence suggesting that women having total abdominal hysterectomy had longer recovery and more postoperative pain compared with laparoscopically assisted vaginal hysterectomy. Those benefits were more in women with a uterus estimated to weigh less than or equal to 500 g.

Benefits: We found no systematic review. We found no RCTs against no intervention or sham surgery. We found one RCT comparing abdominal hysterectomy with laparoscopically assisted vaginal hysterectomy (see benefits of laparoscopically assisted vaginal hysterectomy, p 1886 and benefits of laparoscopic myomectomy, p 1887).[41]

Harms: See harms under laparoscopically assisted vaginal hysterectomy, p 1887 and laparoscopic myomectomy, p 1887.

Comment: There is consensus that abdominal hysterectomy is superior to no treatment in improving fibroid related symptoms.

GLOSSARY

Pelvic score scale An ordinal scale that adds the results of pelvic pain and pelvic pressure. Each symptom is evaluated in a scale ranging from 0–3, where 0 means absence of pain, and increasing numbers represent mild, moderate, and severe pain. Because both results are added, absence of symptoms is represented by a 0 and severe pain and pelvic pressure by 6. We found no data on validation of the scale. However, it is commonly used in studies evaluating pelvic pain.

REFERENCES

1. Buttram VC, Reiter RC. Uterine leiomyomata: etiology, symptomatology and management. *Fertil Steril* 1981;6:433–445.
2. Lumsden MA, Wallace EM. Clinical presentation of uterine fibroids. *Bailliere's Clin Obstet Gynaecol (uterine fibroids)* 1998;12:177–195.
3. Borgfeldt C, Andolf E. Transvaginal ultrasonographic findings in the uterus and the endometrium: Low prevalence of leiomyoma in a random sample of women age 25–40 years. *Acta Obstet Gynecol Scand* 2000;79:202–207.
4. Thompson JD, Rock JA, eds. *Te Linde's Operative Gynecology*, 7th edition. 1992, JB Lippincott Company: London, Hagerstrom.
5. Cramer SF, Patel A. The frequency of uterine leiomyomas. *Am J Clin Pathol* 1990;90:435–438.
6. Schwartz SM, Marshall LM, Baird DD. Epidemiologic contributions to understanding the etiology of uterine leiomyomata. *Environ Health Perspect* 2000;108(suppl 5):821–827.
7. Farquhar C, Arroll B, Ekeroma A, et al. An evidence-based guideline for the management of uterine fibroids. *Aust Nzj Obstet Gynaecol* 2001;41:125–140.
8. Townsend DE, Sparkes RS, Baluda MC, McCelland G. Unicellular histogenesis of uterine leiomyomas as determined by electrophoresis of glucose-6-phosphate dehydrogenase. *Am J Obstet Gynecol* 1970;107:1168–1174.
9. Hashimoto K, Azuma C, Kamiura S, et al. Clonal determination of uterine leiomyomas by analyzing differential inactivation of the X-chromosome-linked phosphoglycerokinase gene. *Gynecol Obstet Invest* 1995;40:204–208.
10. Ross RK, Pike MC, Vessey MP, et al. Risk factors for uterine fibroids: reduced risk associated with oral contraceptives. *BMJ* 1986;293:359–363.
11. Chiaffarino F, Parazzini F, La Vecchia C, Marsico S, Surace M, Ricci E. Use of oral contraceptives and uterine fibroids: results from a case-control study. *Br J Obstet Gynaecol* 1999;106:857–860.
12. Lumbiganon P, Rugpao S, Phandhu-Fung S, Laopaiboon M, Vudhikamraksa N, Werawatakul Y. Protective effect of depot-medroxyprogesterone acetate on surgically treated uterine leiomyomas: a multicentre-case control study. *Br J Obstet Gynaecol* 1995;103:909–914.
13. Carlson KJ, Miller BA, Fowler FJ Jnr. The Maine women's health study: II. Outcomes of nonsurgical management of leiomyomas, abnormal bleeding, and chronic pelvic pain. *Obstet Gynecol* 1994;83:566–572.
14. Friedman AJ, Hoffman DI, Comite F, Browneller RW, Miller JD. Treatment of leiomyomata uteri with leuprolide acetate depot: a double-blind, placebo-controlled, multicenter study. *Obstet Gynecol* 1991;77:720.
15. Friedman AJ, Harrison-Atlas D, Barbieri RL, Benacerraf B, Gleason R, Schiff I. A randomized placebo-controlled double-blind study evaluating the efficacy of leuprolide acetate depot in the treatment of uterine leiomyomata. *Fertil Steril* 1989;51:251–254.
16. Schlaff WD, Zerhouni EA, Huth JA, Chen J, Damewood MD, Rock JA. A placebo-controlled trial of a depot gonadotropin-releasing hormone analogue (leuprolide) in the treatment of uterine leiomyomata. *Obstet Gynecol* 1989;74:856–862.

17. Espinos JJ, Marti A, Asins E, Salamero P, Lenti O, Calaf J. Efectos de dos dosis de un analogo de la GnRH (leuprorelina depot) sobre la miomatosis uterina. *Clin Invest Gin Obst* 1993;20:382–387.
18. Watanabe Y, Nakamura G, Matsuguchi H, Nozaki M, Sano M, Nakano H. Efficacy of a low-dose leuprolide acetate depot in the treatment of uterine leiomyomata in Japanese women. *Fertil Steril* 1992;58:66–71.
19. Watanabe Y, Nakamura G. Effects of two different doses of leuprolide acetate depot on uterine cavity area in patients with uterine leiomyomata. *Fertil Steril* 1995;63:487–490.
20. Takeuchi H, Kobori H, Kikuchi I, Sato Y, Mitsuhashi N. A prospective randomised study comparing endocrinological and clinical effects of two types of GnRH agonists in cases of uterine leiomyomas or endometriosis. *J Obstet Gynecol Res* 2000;26(5):325–331.
21. Broekmans FJ, Hompes PG, Heitbrink MA, et al. Two-step gonadotropin-releasing hormone agonist treatment of uterine leiomyomas: standard-dose therapy followed by reduced-dose therapy. *Am J Obstet Gynecol* 1996;175:1208–1216.
22. Vollenhoven BJ, Shekleton P, McDonald J, Healy D. Clinical predictors for buserelin acetate treatment of uterine fibroids: a prospective study of 40 women. *Fertil Steril* 1990;54:1032–1038.
23. Friedman AJ, Barbieri RL, Benacerraf BR, Schiff I. Treatment of leiomyomata with intranasal or subcutaneuous leuprolide, a gonadotropin-releasing hormone agonist. *Fertil Steril* 1987;48:560–564.
24. Costantini S, Anserini P, Valenzano M, Remorgida V, Venturini PL, De Cecco L. Luteinizing hormone-releasing hormone analog therapy of uterine fibroid: analysis of results obtained with buserelin administered intranasally and goserelin administered subcutaneously as a monthly depot. *Eur J Obstet Gynaecol Reprod Biol* 1990,37:63–69.
25. Carr BR, Marshburn PB, Weatherall PT, et al. An evaluation of the effect of gonadotropin-releasing hormone analogs and medroxyprogesterone acetate on uterine leiomyomata volume by magnetic resonance imaging: a prospective, randomized, double blind, placebo-controlled, crossover trial. *J Clin Endocrinol Metab* 1993;76:1217–1223.
26. Friedman AJ, Barbieri RL, Doubilet PM, Fine C, Schiff I. A randomized double-blind trial of a gonadotropin releasing-hormone agonist (leuprolide) with or without medroxyprogesterone acetate in the treatment of leiomyomata uteri. *Fertil Steril* 1988;49:404–409.
27. Scialli AR, Jestila KJ. Sustained benefits of leuprolide acetate with or without subsequent medroxyprogesterone acetate in the nonsurgical management of leiomyomata uteri. *Fertil Steril* 1995;64:313–320.
28. Benagiano G, Morini A, Aleandri V, et al. Sequential Gn-RH superagonist and medroxyprogesterone acetate treatment of uterine leiomyomata. *Int J Obstet Gynecol* 1990;33:333–343.
29. Caird LE, West CP, Lumsden MA, Hannan WJ, Gow SM. Medroxyprogesterone acetate with Zoladex for long-term treatment of fibroids: effects on bone density and patient acceptability. *Hum Reprod* 1997;2:436–440.
30. Palomba S, Affinito P, Giovanni MD, Tommaselli GA, Nappi C. A clinical trial of the effects of tibolone administered with gonadotropin-releasing hormone analogues for the treatment of uterine leiomyomata. *Fertil Steril* 1998;70:111–118.
31. Friedman AJ, Daly M, Juneau-Norcross M, Gleason R, Rein MS, LeBoff M. Long-term medical therapy for leiomyomata uteri: a prospective, randomized study of leuprolide acetate depot plus oestrogen-progestin or progestin 'add-back' for 2 years. *Hum Reprod* 1994;9:1618–1625.
32. Ylikorkala O, Pekonen F. Naproxen reduces idiopathic but not fibromyoma-induced menorrhagia. *Obstet Gynecol* 1986; 68:10–12.
33. Makarainen L, Ylikorkala O. Primary and myoma-associated menorrhagia: role of prostaglandins and effects of ibuprofen. *Br J Obstet Gynaecol* 1986;93:974–978.
34. Coutinho EM, Goncalves MT. Long-term treatment of leiomyomas with gestrinone. *Fertil Steril* 1989;51:939–946.
35. Coutinho EM, Boulanger GA, Goncalves MT. Regression of uterine leioyomas after treatment with gestrinone, an antiestrogen, antiprogesterone. *Am J Obstet Gynecol* 1986;155:761–767.
36. Mahajan DK, London SN. Mifepristone (RU486): a review. *Fertil Steril* 1997;68:967–976.
37. Lethaby A, Vollenhoven B, Sowter M, Healy D. Preoperative GnRH analogue therapy before hysterectomy or myomectomy for uterine fibroids. (Cochrane Review). In: The Cochrane Library, Issue 4, 2000. Oxford: Update Software. Search date 2000; primary sources the Cochrane Menstrual Disorders and Subfertility Group Register of Trials, Modline, Embase, the National Research Register, the National Library of Medicine's Clinical Trials Register, and Current Contents. Published trials were also identified from citation lists of review articles and direct contact with drug companies for unpublished trials. In most cases, the first author of each included trial was contacted for additional information.
38. Parazzini F, Bortolotti A, Chiantera V, et al. Goserelin acetate to avoid hysterectomy in pre-menopausal women with fibroids requiring surgery. *Eur J Obstet Gynecol Reprod Biol* 1999;87:31–33.
39. Campo S, Garcea N. Laparoscopic myomectomy in premenstrual women with and without preoperative treatment using gonadotrophin-releasing hormone analogues. *Hum Reprod* 1999;14:44–48.
40. Verspyck E, Marpeau L, Lucas C. Leuprorelin depot 3.75 mg versus lynestrenol in the preoperative treatment of symptomatic uterine myomas: a multicentre randomised trial. *Eur J Obstet Gynecol Reprod Biol* 2000;89:7–13.
41. Ferrari MM, Berlanda N, Mezzopane R, Ragusa G, Cavello M, Pardi G. Identifying the indications for laparoscopically assisted vaginal hysterectomy: a prospective, randomised comparison with abdominal hysterectomy in patients with symptomatic uterine fibroids. *Br J Obstet Gynaecol* 1999;107:620–625.
42. Mais V, Ajossa S, Guerriero S, Mascia M, Solla E, Melis GB. Laparoscopic versus abdominal myomectomy: a prospective, randomized trial to evaluate benefits in early outcome. *Am J Obstet Gynecol* 1996;174:654–658.
43. Seracchioli R, Rossi S, Govoni F, et al. Fertility and obstetric outcome after laparoscopic myomectomy of large myomata: a randomised comparison with abdominal myomectomy. *Hum Reprod* 2000;15:2663–2668.

Fibroids (uterine myomatosis, leiomyomas)

Anne Lethaby
Cochrane Menstrual Disorders and
Subfertility Group
Auckland
New Zealand

Beverley Vollenhoven
Department of Obstetrics and
Gynaecology Monash University
Clayton Victoria
Australia

Competing interests: None declared.

TABLE 1 Harms of gonadorelin versus placebo (see text, p 1882).[14]

	Outcome	Population	%	Outcome	Population	%	RR*	95% CI*
Vasomotor flushes	52	63	83%	5	65	8%	10.7	4.6 to 25.1
Vaginitis	11	63	17%	0	65	0%		
Arthralgia/mialgia	9	63	14%	0	65	0%		
Asthenia	10	63	16%	3	65	5%	3.4	0.97 to 996
Peripheral oedema	7	63	11%	1	65	2%	7.2	0.9 to 57
Insomnia	6	63	10%	0	65	0%		
Nausea	6	63	10%	1	65	2%	6.2	0.8 to 50
Emotional lability/nervousness	5	63	8%	1	65	2%	5.2	0.6 to 42.9
Depression	7	63	11%	2	65	3%	3.6	0.8 to 16.7
Headaches	18	63	29%	13	65	20%	1.4	0.8 to 2.7
Decreased libido	2	63	3%	0	65	0%		

*_Clinical Evidence_ recalculation.

Infertility and subfertility

Search date February 2002

Kirsten Duckitt

QUESTIONS

INTERVENTIONS

Clin Evid 2002;8:1892–1920.

Key Messages

In women with infertility caused by ovulation disorders

- **Clomifene** One systematic review has found that clomifene versus placebo significantly increases the likelihood of pregnancy in women who ovulate infrequently. Four other studies comparing clomifene versus tamoxifen have found no significant difference in ovulation rates or number of pregnancies. One RCT found that clomifene plus metformin versus clomifene alone significantly increased the pregnancy rate per person after 6 months treatment (NNT 5, 95% CI 3 to 22).
- **Cyclofenil** One RCT found no significant difference in pregnancy rates with cyclofenil versus placebo.
- **Gonadotrophins** One systematic review found no significant difference between human menopausal gonadotrophins and urofollitropin (urofollitrophin, urinary follicle stimulating hormone) in pregnancy rates. Two RCTs found no significant difference in cumulative pregnancy rates or numbers of live births with follitropin (recombinant follicle stimulating hormone) versus urofollitropin. The review found that urofollitropin versus human menopausal gonadotrophins significantly reduced the risk of ovarian hyperstimulation syndrome, although this was confined to women who were not treated with concomitant gonadotrophin releasing hormone analogues. Observational evidence suggests that gonadotrophins may be associated with an increased risk of non-invasive ovarian tumours and multiple pregnancies.
- **Laparoscopic ovarian drilling** One systematic review and one subsequent small RCT found no significant difference with laparoscopic ovarian drilling versus gonadotrophins in pregnancy rates, but found that laparoscopic ovarian drilling significantly reduced rates of multiple pregnancies.
- **Pulsatile gonadotrophin releasing hormone** One systematic review found insufficient evidence on the effects of pulsatile gonadotrophin releasing hormone treatment.

In women with tubal infertility

- **In vitro fertilisation** We found no RCTs of in vitro fertilisation versus no treatment. One RCT found that immediate versus delayed in vitro fertilisation significantly increased numbers of pregnancies and live births. Three RCTs found no significant difference in numbers of live births with in vitro fertilisation versus intracytoplasmic sperm injection. Observational evidence suggests that adverse effects associated with in vitro fertilisation include multiple pregnancies and ovarian hyperstimulation syndrome.
- **Selective salpingography plus tubal catheterisation** We found no RCTs on the effects of selective salpingography plus tubal catheterisation.
- **Tubal surgery** One systematic review in women undergoing in vitro fertilisation has found that tubal surgery versus no treatment or medical treatment significantly increases the chance of becoming pregnant and significantly increases the live birth rate. Another review found no significant difference in pregnancy rates between different types of tubal surgery. One systematic review found no significant difference in pregnancy rates with tubal surgery plus additional treatments versus tubal surgery alone to prevent adhesion formation (steroids, dextran, noxytioline).

In women with infertility caused by endometriosis

- **Drug-induced ovarian suppression** One systematic review found no significant difference in pregnancy rates between drugs that induce ovarian suppression versus placebo or danazol. The review found that ovulation suppression agents cause adverse effects that include weight gain, hot flushes, and osteoporosis, and that danazol may cause dose related weight gain and androgenic effects.
- **Intrauterine insemination plus gonadotrophins** One RCT found that intrauterine insemination plus gonadotrophins versus no treatment significantly increased live birth rates (NNT 6, 95% CI 3 to 28). A second RCT found no significant difference in birth rates with intrauterine insemination plus pituitary down regulation plus gonadotrophins versus expectant management. A third RCT found that intrauterine insemination plus gonadotrophins versus intrauterine insemination alone significantly increased pregnancy rates after the first treatment cycle (NNT 5, 95% CI 4 to 14).
- **In vitro fertilisation** We found no RCTs in women with endometriosis related infertility undergoing in vitro fertilisation treatment.
- **Laparoscopic surgical treatment** Two RCTs found inconsistent results with laparoscopic surgery versus diagnostic laparoscopy for differences in numbers of pregnancies and live births.

In couples with male factor infertility

- **Donor insemination** We found no good evidence on the effects of donor insemination.
- **Intracytoplasmic sperm injection plus in vitro fertilisation** One systematic review found insufficient evidence on the effects of intracytoplasmic sperm injection plus in vitro fertilisation versus in vitro fertilisation alone.
- **Intrauterine insemination** Two systematic reviews have found that intrauterine insemination versus intracervical insemination or natural intercourse significantly increases pregnancy rates per cycle.
- **In vitro fertilisation versus gamete intrafallopian transfer** One RCT found insufficient evidence on the effects of in vitro fertilisation versus gamete intrafallopian transfer.

In couples with unexplained infertility

- **Clomifene** One systematic review found limited evidence that clomifene versus placebo significantly increased rates of pregnancy per cycle.
- **Fallopian tube sperm perfusion** One systematic review and one subsequent RCT have found that fallopian tube sperm perfusion versus intrauterine insemination significantly increases pregnancy rates.
- **Gamete intrafallopian transfer** We found no RCTs of gamete intrafallopian transfer versus no treatment. Three RCTs found conflicting results with gamete intrafallopian transfer versus other treatments (intrauterine insemination, timed intercourse, and in vitro fertilisation, in pregnancy rates.
- **Intrauterine insemination** Two systematic reviews and one subsequent RCT in couples undergoing ovarian stimulation treatment have found that intrauterine insemination versus timed intercourse or intracervical insemination significantly increases pregnancy rates. One systematic review has found no significant difference with intrauterine insemination versus timed intercourse or intracervical insemination in pregnancy rates, but found that the addition of ovarian stimulation to any of the three interventions significantly increases pregnancy rate per cycle (NNT 11, 95% CI 7 to 58). One systematic review and

one subsequent RCT have found that fallopian tube sperm perfusion versus intrauterine insemination significantly increases pregnancy rates. One RCT found no significant difference with intrauterine insemination in natural cycles versus intrauterine insemination in stimulated cycles or versus in vitro fertilisation in pregnancy rates, but found that more couples receiving in vitro fertilisation failed to complete their six cycles of treatment.

- **In vitro fertilisation** Two small RCTs found no significant difference between in vitro fertilisation versus gamete intrafallopian transfer in pregnancy rates. One RCT found no significant difference in pregnancy rates with intrauterine insemination in natural cycles versus in vitro fertilisation, but found that more couples receiving in vitro fertilisation failed to complete their six cycles of treatment.

DEFINITION Normal fertility has been defined as achieving a pregnancy within 2 years by regular sexual intercourse.[1] However, many define infertility as the failure to conceive after 1 year of unprotected intercourse. Infertility can be primary, in couples who have never conceived, or secondary, in couples who have previously conceived. Infertile couples include those who are sterile (who will never achieve a natural pregnancy) and those who are subfertile (who could eventually achieve a pregnancy).

INCIDENCE/ PREVALENCE Although there is no evidence of a major change in the prevalence of infertility, many more couples are seeking help than previously. Currently, about 1/7 couples in industrialised countries will seek medical advice for infertility.[2] Rates of primary infertility vary widely between countries, ranging from 10% in Africa to about 6% in North America and Europe.[1] Reported rates of secondary infertility are less reliable.

AETIOLOGY/ RISK FACTORS In the UK, nearly a third of infertility cases are unexplained. The rest are caused by ovulatory failure (27%), low sperm count or quality (19%), tubal damage (14%), endometriosis (5%), and other causes (5%).[3]

PROGNOSIS In developed countries, 80–90% of couples attempting to conceive are successful after 1 year and 95% after 2 years.[3] The chances of becoming pregnant vary with the cause and duration of infertility, the woman's age, the couple's previous pregnancy history, and the availability of different treatment options.[4,5] For the first 2–3 years of unexplained infertility, cumulative conception rates remain high (27–46%) but decrease with increasing age of the woman and duration of infertility. The background rates of spontaneous pregnancy in infertile couples can be calculated from longitudinal studies of infertile couples who have been observed without treatment.[4]

AIMS To achieve the delivery of one healthy baby; to reduce the distress associated with infertility.

OUTCOMES Live births, miscarriages, multiple pregnancies, incidence of ovarian hyperstimulation syndrome (see glossary, p 1914), satisfaction with services and treatments, acceptance of childlessness if treatment is unsuccessful, and pregnancy rate. Pregnancy rate is an intermediate outcome, but one that is important in itself to many people. Ovulation is an intermediate outcome. A large number of pregnancies in infertile couples will occur spontaneously without treatment.[4] Effectiveness of treatments for infertility should be assessed on the basis of pregnancy rates over and above the spontaneous pregnancy rates, otherwise the impacts of treatments may be overestimated.

METHODS *Clinical Evidence* update search and appraisal February 2002. **Crossover design:** For infertility, RCTs with a crossover design may overestimate the treatment effect because pregnancies occurring in the first half of the trial will remove couples from the second half.[6] Crossover trials were included in some systematic reviews where no or few RCTs using a parallel group design were available. Ideally, only data from the first half of the trial, before crossover, should be used. However, a study that used a computer model to compare the results of crossover and parallel designed trials suggests that any overestimation may be clinically irrelevant.[7]

QUESTION **What are the effects of treatments for infertility caused by ovulation disorders?**

OPTION CLOMIFENE

One systematic review has found that clomifene versus placebo significantly increases the likelihood of pregnancy in women who ovulate infrequently. Four other studies comparing clomifene versus tamoxifen have found no significant difference in ovulation rates or number of pregnancies. One RCT found that clomifene plus metformin versus clomifene alone significantly increased the pregnancy rate per woman after 6 months' treatment.

Benefits: **Versus placebo:** We found one systematic review (search date not stated, 3 crossover RCTs), which compared clomifene (clomiphene) (50–200 mg) versus placebo in 217 cycles in women who ovulate infrequently (see table 1, p 1919).[8] It found that clomifene versus placebo significantly increased the chance of pregnancy (OR 3.4, 95% CI 1.2 to 9.5). **Versus tamoxifen:** We found no systematic review, but found four studies (2 RCTs, 1 quasi-randomised study, and 1 observational study; 197 anovulatory or infrequently ovulating women; see comment below).[29,35–37] The first RCT (86 anovulatory women aged < 40 years) compared tamoxifen (maximum 60 mg daily) versus clomifene (maximum 150 mg daily).[35] It found no significant difference in the overall rate of ovulation (50/113 [44%] ovulatory cycles with tamoxifen *v* 41/91 [45%] ovulatory cycles with clomifene; $P > 0.05$; see comment below) or the number of pregnancies (10/46 [22%] with tamoxifen *v* 6/40 [15%] with clomifene; RR 1.7, 95% CI 0.7 to 4.2). Three other studies found similar results.[29,36,37] **Versus other drug combinations:** We found no systematic review but found one RCT (90 infertile women with polycystic ovary syndrome, infrequent menstruation, high insulin levels, and body mass indexes > 28), which compared clomifene (at its lowest effective dose; see comment below) plus metformin (500 mg orally three times daily) versus clomifene alone (at its lowest effective dose; see comment below).[38] The RCT found that clomifene plus metformin significantly increased pregnancy rates per person after 6 months' treatment (13/45 [29%] with clomifene plus metformin *v* 4/45 [9%] with clomifene alone; RR 3.3, 95% CI 1.2 to 9.2; NNT 5, 95% CI 3 to 22).

Harms: **Ovarian cancer:** In a cohort study of 3837 infertile women, 11 women were found to have ovarian cancer.[39] In 135 women that were randomly selected as a subcohort from these 3837 women, there was an 11-fold increase in risk of ovarian cancer in women using clomifene for 12 or more cycles (RR 11.1, 95% CI 1.5 to 82.3). The association was present for both gravid and nulligravid women, and for infertile women both with ovulatory disorders and with infertility from other causes. Subsequent studies have found no association between clomifene and ovarian cancer.[40–43] **Multiple pregnancy:** Multiple pregnancy occurs in 2–13% of women with all causes of infertility taking clomifene, compared with a spontaneous multiple pregnancy rate of about 1–2% of women in North American and European populations.[44,45] In a 1 year survey in the UK, 25/44 (57%) triplet pregnancies reported were attributable to clomifene.[19] Clomifene was also implicated in two of the eight sets of quadruplets and quintuplets reported. **Ovarian hyperstimulation syndrome:** See glossary, p 1914. Clomifene tends to cause only mild ovarian hyperstimulation that does not require treatment.

Comment: Clomifene was first introduced in the 1960s and most of the trials testing its efficacy took place in the 1970s before more recent quality standards for RCTs were established. Three of the studies comparing clomifene versus tamoxifen based estimates of pregnancy rates on fewer than 30 pregnancies.[29,35,37] In the first RCT comparing tamoxifen versus clomifene, the different number of treatment cycles between groups could potentially bias the results.[35] In the RCT comparing clomifene plus metformin versus clomifene alone, the dose of clomifene was initially 50 mg daily for 5 days and only increased to 100 mg or 150 mg daily for 5 days if the lower dose was insufficient to enable ovulation to be triggered with human chorionic gonadotrophin.[38] With regard to the cohort study, 5/11 (45%) people with ovarian cancer were diagnosed with borderline epithelial tumours that had low malignant potential, and two with granulosa cell tumours that had different embryological, pathological, and epidemiological features from epithelial tumours.[39] Borderline and malignant tumours pose different risks that are not easy to combine and excluding the two granulosa cell tumours from the number of ovarian cancers found diminishes the increased risk attributed to clomifene treatment.

OPTION CYCLOFENIL

One RCT found no significant difference in pregnancy rates with cyclofenil versus placebo.

Benefits: **Versus placebo:** We found one RCT (213 women with either ovulatory disorders or unexplained infertility) comparing three cycles of cyclofenil (800 mg daily) versus placebo from days 4–8 of the ovulatory cycle.[21] It found no significant difference in cumulative pregnancy rates (26/114 [23%] with cyclofenil *v* 21/99 [21%] with placebo; RR 1.1, 95% CI 0.7 to 1.8).

Harms: The RCT did not report on adverse effects.[21]

Comment: Only 123/213 (58%) women in the RCT had ovulatory disorders and the results for these women were not presented separately.[21] Such an RCT does not exclude a possible benefit of cyclofenil.

OPTION GONADOTROPHINS

One systematic review found no significant difference between human menopausal gonadotrophins and urofollitropin (urofollitrophin, urinary follicle stimulating hormone) in pregnancy rates. Two RCTs found no significant difference in cumulative pregnancy rates or numbers of live births with follitropin (recombinant follicle stimulating hormone) versus urofollitropin. The review found that urofollitropin versus human menopausal gonadotrophins significantly reduced the risk of ovarian hyperstimulation syndrome, although this was confined to women who were not treated with concomitant gonadotrophin releasing hormone analogues. Observational evidence suggests that gonadotrophins may be associated with an increased risk of non-invasive ovarian tumours and multiple pregnancies.

Benefits: **Versus placebo:** We found no RCTs. **Versus clomifene (clomiphene):** We found no RCTs. **Human menopausal gonadotrophins versus urofollitropin:** We found one systematic review (search date not stated, 14 RCTs, 388 women with subfertility associated with polycystic ovarian syndrome), which compared human menopausal gonadotrophins versus urofollitropin.[18] It found no significant difference in pregnancy rates (OR 0.8, 95 % CI 0.4 to 1.5). **Follitropin versus urofollitropin:** We found no systematic review but found two RCTs comparing urofollitropin versus follitropin.[47,48] The first RCT (172 women with clomifene resistant, normogonadotrophic anovulation) found no significant difference with follitropin versus urofollitropin in cumulative ovulation rates (95% with follitropin *v* 96% with urofollitropin), cumulative pregnancy rates (27% with follitropin *v* 24% with urofollitropin), or miscarriage rates (31% with follitropin *v* 32% with urofollitropin).[47] A second smaller RCT (51 women with clomifene resistant, normogonadotrophic anovulation) found similar results, although a significantly lower total dose and shorter duration of follitropin was used to achieve ovulation.[48] **Versus laparoscopic ovarian drilling:** See glossary, p 1914. See benefits of laparoscopic ovarian drilling, p 1899.

Harms: **Ovarian cancer:** One case control study (200 women with ovarian cancer and 408 area matched controls) found that women with non-invasive ovarian tumours were more than three times more likely to have been exposed to an ovulation induction agent (adjusted OR 3.5, 95% CI 1.2 to 10.1), particularly to human menopausal gonadotrophins (adjusted OR 9.4, 95% CI 1.7 to 52.1).[43] Women with invasive ovarian tumours were no more likely to have been exposed to any ovulation induction agents. **Multiple pregnancy:** Multiple pregnancy occurs in 29% of women with polycystic ovaries when conventional regimens of gonadotrophins are used to induce ovulation.[28] **Ovarian hyperstimulation:** The systematic review (search date not stated, 7 RCTs) found that urofollitropin versus human menopausal gonadotrophins significantly reduced the risk of ovarian hyperstimulation (OR 0.3, 95% CI 0.2 to 0.7).[18] However, this effect was only present where no concomitant gonadotrophin releasing hormone (GnRH) analogue was used (5 RCTs; OR 0.2, 95% CI 0.1 to 0.5). The review found that concomitant use of a GnRH analogue increased the risk of ovarian hyperstimulation (2 RCTs; OR 3.2, 95% CI 1.5 to 6.7). The RCT (172 women) comparing urofollitropin versus follitropin found no significant difference in the risk of multiple pregnancy or ovarian hyperstimulation syndrome (see glossary, p 1914), although the low event rates found with either treatment limit the usefulness of the result.[47]

Comment: Despite not being placebo controlled, trials of gonadotrophins often included women who were not ovulating and, therefore, provide some evidence that treatment is effective.[18] Avoiding gonadotrophins may reduce the risk of multiple pregnancy and ovarian hyperstimulation syndrome. Follitropin is not derived from human tissues.

OPTION LAPAROSCOPIC OVARIAN DRILLING

One systematic review and one subsequent small RCT found no significant difference with laparoscopic ovarian drilling versus gonadotrophins in pregnancy rates, but found that laparoscopic ovarian drilling significantly reduced rates of multiple pregnancies.

Benefits: We found one systematic review (search date 2001, 4 RCTs, 303 women with anovulatory clomifene [chomiphene] resistant polycystic ovary syndrome)[19] (see table 1, p 1919), and one subsequent RCT (see comment below).[49] The review found no significant difference with laparoscopic ovarian drilling (see glossary, p 1914) versus gonadotrophins in pregnancy rates after 12 months' follow up (OR 1.42, 95% CI 0.84 to 2.42).[19] The subsequent RCT (18 women with polycystic ovarian syndrome who had failed to ovulate after treatment with clomifene or purified follicle stimulating hormone) compared laparoscopic ovarian drilling versus a gonadotrophin releasing hormone (GnRH) analogue plus a combined oral contraceptive.[49] All the women also received three cycles of follitropin plus intrauterine insemination. The RCT found no significant difference in the number of pregnancies (5/10 [50%] with ovarian laser drilling *v* 5/8 [63%] with GnRH plus combined oral contraceptive; RR 0.8, 95% CI 0.4 to 1.8).

Harms: The systematic review found that laparoscopic ovarian drilling versus gonadotrophins significantly reduced rates of multiple pregnancies (OR 0.16, 95% CI 0.03 to 0.98).[19] Adverse effects associated with laparoscopic ovarian drilling include the risks of general anaesthesia, postoperative adhesion formation,[50] and pelvic infection.[51] We found no evidence to support the suggestion that laparoscopic drilling increases the long term risk of premature ovarian failure. Laparoscopic drilling is thought not to increase the risk of multiple pregnancy as it usually induces spontaneous ovulation, in contrast to the multifollicular ovulation that may be induced by the use of gonadotrophins.

Comment: The trials of laparoscopic ovarian drilling included women who were not ovulating and, therefore, provide some evidence that treatment is effective despite the lack of placebo controls.[19,49]

OPTION **PULSATILE GONADOTROPHIN RELEASING HORMONE**

One systematic review found insufficient evidence on the effects of pulsatile gonadotrophin releasing hormone treatment.

Benefits: We found one systematic review (search date not stated, 3 RCTs, 29 women with subfertility and clomifene resistant polycystic ovary syndrome) that compared pulsatile gonadotrophin releasing hormone (GnRH) versus another treatment to induce ovulation.[52] The RCTs included in the review described four different comparisons, were small (each reporting 1–4 pregnancies), and of short duration (1–3 cycles), and so provided insufficient evidence to assess the value of pulsatile GnRH in polycystic ovary syndrome.

Harms: One retrospective analysis (229 cycles in 71 women) compared pulsatile GnRH versus gonadotrophins alone, and found no significant difference in multiple pregnancy rates after six cycles.[53] However, 75% of the multiple pregnancies in the gonadotrophin group were triplets or higher order multiple pregnancies, whereas all multiple pregnancies in the GnRH group were twins.

Comment: Pulsatile GnRH is used in women with anovulation caused by low serum gonadotrophins and oestrogen concentrations (hypogonadotropic hypogonadism). Hypogonadotropic hypogonadism is a well defined condition and so evidence from case series should be generalisable to most of affected women. Case series (256 anovulatory women with hypogonadotropic hypogonadism undergoing 1043 treatment cycles) found cumulative pregnancy rates of 59–73% at 6 months and 81–92% at 12 months.[54–56] Only one series reported the live birth rate; this was 65% after 12 treatment cycles.[54]

QUESTION **What are the effects of treatments for tubal infertility?**

OPTION **SELECTIVE SALPINGOGRAPHY PLUS TUBAL CATHETERISATION**

We found no RCTs on the effects of selective salpingography plus tubal catheterisation.

Benefits: We found no systematic review and no RCTs.

Harms: Observational studies have found that tubal perforation, which does not seem to be clinically important, occurred in 2%, and ectopic pregnancy in 3–9% of women undergoing selective salpingography and tubal catheterisation.[57,58]

Comment: One systematic review (search date not stated) combined data from 10 cohort and other observational studies of selective salpingography and tubal cannulation (482 women), and four observational studies of hysteroscopic cannulation for proximal tubal blockage (133 women).[57] It found that hysteroscopy versus selective salpingography and tubal catheterisation was associated with a higher pregnancy rate (pregnancies exceeding 20 weeks' gestation: 65/133 [49%] with hysteroscopy v 103/482 [21%] with salpingography). None of the observational studies included an untreated group, so it is not possible to give the treatment related pregnancy rate over and above the spontaneous pregnancy rate. Tubal patency and pregnancy without treatment have been reported in women diagnosed with bilateral proximal tube obstruction.[59]

OPTION TUBAL SURGERY

One systematic review in women undergoing in vitro fertilisation has found that tubal surgery versus no treatment or medical treatment significantly increases the chance of becoming pregnant, and significantly increases the live birth rate. Another review found no significant difference in pregnancy rates between different types of tubal surgery. One systematic review found no significant difference with tubal surgery plus additional treatments versus tubal surgery alone to prevent adhesion formation (steroids, dextran, and noxytioline) in pregnancy rates.

Benefits: **Versus no treatment or medical treatment:** We found one systematic review (search date 2000, 3 RCTs, 295 women with hydrosalpinges undergoing in vitro fertilisation [IVF]; see comment below), which found that tubal surgery versus no treatment or medical treatment (see comment below) significantly increased the chances of becoming pregnant (OR 1.75, 95% CI 1.07 to 2.86) and significantly increased the live birth rate (OR 2.13, 95% CI 1.24 to 3.65).[60] **Different types of tubal surgery versus each other:** We found three systematic reviews (search date not stated, 8 RCTs [see comment below];[61] search date not stated, 5 RCTs, 588 women;[62] search date not stated, 10 RCTs, 1086 women).[63] Two RCTs (130 women) identified by the first review found no significant difference with CO_2 laser adhesiolysis (see glossary, p 1914) versus diathermy adhesiolysis in numbers of pregnancies (16/30 [53%] with laser v 17/33 [52%] with diathermy; RR 1.04, 95% CI 0.65 to 1.67), or with CO_2 laser salpingostomy versus diathermy salpingostomy in numbers of pregnancies (26/75 [35%] with laser v 16/60 [27%] with diathermy; RR 1.30, 95% CI 0.77 to 2.19).[61] One RCT (72 women) identified by the review found no significant difference with the use of an operating microscope versus magnifying lenses (loupes) during microsurgical reversal of sterilisations in pregnancies after 2 years (26/36 [72%] with microscope v 28/36 [78%] with loupes; OR 0.75, 95% CI 0.26 to 2.15).[61] The second systematic review compared postoperative hydrotubation (see glossary, p 1914) or second look laparoscopy (see glossary, p 1914) plus adhesiolysis after tubal surgery versus control.[62] The review found that all the studies were either poor quality or under powered. It found insufficient evidence to support the routine practice of hydrotubation (1 RCT; OR 1.12, 95% CI 0.57 to 2.21) or second look laparoscopy (2 RCTs; OR 0.96 95% CI 0.44 to 2.07) after tubal surgery. The third systematic review compared tubal surgery plus additional treatments to prevent adhesion formation (steroids, dextran, and noxytioline) versus tubal surgery alone.[63] It found no significant difference in pregnancy rates with tubal surgery plus steroids (systemic or intraperitoneal) versus no steroids (4 RCTs; OR 1.10, 95% CI 0.74 to 1.64), tubal surgery plus dextran (intraperitoneal) versus no dextran (3 RCTs; OR 0.65, 95% CI 0.37 to 1.14), or tubal surgery plus noxytioline (intraperitoneal) versus no noxytioline (1 RCT; OR 0.67, 95% CI 0.30 to 1.47). **Versus IVF:** We found no RCTs (see comment below). **Proximal tubal blockage:** We found no RCTs (see comment below).

Harms: The systematic review comparing tubal surgery versus no treatment or medical treatment found no significant difference in the rate of ectopic pregnancy (OR 0.42, 95% CI 0.08 to 2.14), miscarriage per pregnancy (OR 0.49, 95% CI 0.16 to 1.52), or treatment related complications (OR 5.80, 95% CI 0.35 to 96.79).[60] Tubal surgery involves general anaesthesia and admission to hospital. There is a risk of ectopic pregnancy caused by pre-existing tubal damage; rates of 7–9% have been reported compared with 1–3% with IVF.[42,43] IVF carries the risk of multiple pregnancy and ovarian hyperstimulation syndrome (see glossary, p 1914) (see harms of IVF under treatments for infertility caused by ovulation disorders, p 1903).

Comment: Success rates with tubal surgery depend on the severity and site of disease. The best figures from surgery in women with distal tubal occlusion are live birth rates of 20–30%, with rates of up to 60% reported for the less common proximal occlusion.[11–16] **Versus no treatment or medical treatment:** In the systematic review comparing tubal surgery versus non-surgical treatment, although a variety of different surgical techniques were used, laparoscopic unilateral or bilateral salpingectomy were the most common (numerical data not provided).[60] **Different types of tubal surgery versus each other:** One systematic review (search date not stated, 7 observational studies, 279 women with proximal tubal blockage) compared microsurgery (see glossary, p 1914) (275 women) versus macrosurgery (see glossary, p 1914) (104 women).[57] It found that microsurgery significantly increased pregnancy rates (RR 2.2, 95% CI 1.5 to 3.2). One of the systematic reviews comparing different techniques for pelvic surgery versus each other included non-randomised studies if there was an appropriate control group and no RCT evidence available.[61] Of the eight RCTs included in the review, five used outdated surgical techniques, were small, and had problems relating to methods of randomisation. These data precede recent improvements in case selection and laparoscopic training. **Versus IVF:** Case series of tubal surgery have been compared with large databases of couples undergoing IVF.[11,64–68] These found that tubal surgery was as effective as IVF in women with filmy adhesions, mild distal tubal occlusion, or proximal obstruction. If successful, tubal surgery allows women to have more pregnancies without further medical intervention and without the risks associated with IVF.[69]

OPTION IN VITRO FERTILISATION

We found no RCTs of in vitro fertilisation versus no treatment. One RCT found that immediate versus delayed in vitro fertilisation significantly increased numbers of pregnancies and live births. Three RCTs found no significant difference in numbers of live births with in vitro fertilisation versus intracytoplasmic sperm injection. Observational evidence suggests that adverse effects associated with in vitro fertilisation include multiple pregnancies and ovarian hyperstimulation syndrome.

Benefits: We found no systematic review. **In vitro fertilisation (IVF) versus no treatment:** We found no RCTs. **Immediate versus delayed IVF:** We found one RCT (399 couples with any cause of infertility; the couples who received delayed IVF acted as untreated controls for at least 6 months), which found that immediate versus delayed IVF (see glossary, p 1914) significantly increased the numbers of pregnancies (33/190 [17%] with immediate IVF *v* 13/163 [8%] with delayed IVF; RR 2.18, 95% CI 1.19 to 4.0), and significantly increased the numbers of live births (22/190 [12%] with immediate IVF *v* 8/163 [5%] with delayed IVF; RR 2.36, 95% CI 1.08 to 5.16).[70] **Versus tubal surgery:** See benefits of tubal surgery, p 1901. **Versus intracytoplasmic sperm injection:** One RCT (415 couples with non-male factor infertility) found no significant difference with IVF versus intracytoplasmic sperm injection in pregnancy rates (72/224 [32%] with IVF *v* 53/211 [25%] with intracytoplasmic sperm injection; RR 1.30, 95% CI 0.95 to 1.73).[71] Two other small RCTs (167 couples in total) found similar results.[72,73]

Harms: **Multiple pregnancy:** Two RCTs did not report on multiple pregnancy rates,[70,72] and two RCTs lacked the statistical power required to detect significant differences in multiple pregnancy rates between treatments. However, of the 6450 live births following IVF in the UK in 1998–1999, 31% were multiple, including 235 (3.6%) sets of triplets and two sets of quadruplets.[54] In the UK, the number of embryos that can be replaced is restricted to three. In the USA, where there are no such restrictions, 15 367 live births included 38% multiple births, 6% of which were triplets and above.[74] **Ovarian hyperstimulation syndrome:** Severe ovarian hyperstimulation syndrome (see glossary, p 1914) occurs in 0.5–2.0% of all IVF cycles.[75] Ovarian hyperstimulation syndrome rates were not reported in the RCTs above.[70,72] **Obstetric outcome:** We found one systematic review (42 high quality observational studies) that compared obstetric outcome in mothers receiving IVF versus either a population-based control group or a selected control group matched for different variables.[76] It found that children born after IVF had a considerably higher risk of being born preterm and with a lower birth weight than children conceived naturally, although this was likely to be because of the high incidence of multiple births and maternal characteristics such as nulliparity, increased age, previous infertility, and obstetric history (absolute numbers not provided). There was no evidence of an increased overall incidence of congenital malformations in children born after conventional IVF or after embryo cryopreservation.

Comment: The success of IVF is influenced by a woman's age, duration of infertility, and pervious pregnancy history. Pregnancy rates are highest between the ages of 25 and 35 years and decline steeply after 35 years.[5] Similar clinics, which describe the same methods, report different success rates for IVF. In the UK, the live birth rate per IVF cycle varies from 0–28% with an average of 19.5% if intracytoplasmic sperm injection cycles are also taken into account.[30] The equivalent average figure in the USA is 25%, but again results vary between centres.[74,77] In the UK, larger centres (≥ 200 cycles a year) report slightly higher live birth rates than smaller centres (20% per cycle started compared with 16%).[78] Such a difference has not been consistently reported in the USA.

QUESTION What are the effects of treatment for infertility associated with endometriosis?

OPTION DRUG-INDUCED OVARIAN SUPPRESSION

One systematic review has found no significant difference in pregnancy rates between drugs that induce ovarian suppression versus either placebo or danazol. The review found that ovulation suppression agents cause adverse effects that include weight gain, hot flushes, and osteoporosis, and that danazol may cause dose related weight gain and androgenic effects.

Benefits: We found one systematic review (search date not stated, 13 RCTs).[79] **Versus placebo:** The review identified five RCTs (244 women with visually diagnosed endometriosis who had been attempting conception for < 12 months) comparing ovulation suppression agents (medroxyprogesterone, gestrinone, combined oral contraceptive pills, and gonadotrophin releasing hormone analogues) versus placebo and found no significant difference in pregnancy rates (OR 0.8, 95% CI 0.5 to 1.4).[79] **Versus danazol:** The review identified eight RCTs (658 similar women with visually diagnosed endometriosis who had been attempting conception for < 12 months), which compared ovulation suppression versus danazol and found no significant difference in pregnancy rates (OR compared with danazol 1.2, 95% CI 0.9 to 1.7).[79] **Versus surgery:** See benefits of surgical treatment, p 1906.

Harms: The review found that ovulation suppression agents caused adverse effects that included weight gain, hot flushes, and osteoporosis.[79] Adverse effects of danazol were dose related and included an average weight gain of 2–4 kg with 3 months' treatment, androgenic effects such as acne, seborrhoea, hirsutism, voice changes, and general complaints, including irritability, musculoskeletal pains, and tiredness. Hot flushes and breast atrophy were sometimes observed. Most of these adverse effects were reversible on stopping treatment.[80]

Comment: In the review, three of the trials used a combination of clomifene with other infertility drugs.[79] Treatment using ovulation suppression could waste valuable time for women who are trying to get pregnant, as the opportunity for spontaneous conceptions is lost during treatment.

OPTION INTRAUTERINE INSEMINATION PLUS GONADOTROPHINS

One RCT found that intrauterine insemination plus gonadotrophins versus no treatment significantly increased live birth rates. A second RCT found no significant difference in birth rates with intrauterine insemination plus pituitary down regulation plus gonadotrophins versus expectant management. A third RCT found that intrauterine insemination plus gonadotrophins versus intrauterine insemination alone significantly increased pregnancy rates after the first treatment cycle.

Benefits: We found no systematic review but found three RCTs.[81–83] The first RCT (104 couples) compared intrauterine insemination plus gonadotrophins (53 couples, 127 cycles) versus no treatment (50 couples, 184 cycles).[81] It found that intrauterine insemination plus gonadotrophins significantly increased live birth rates (14/53 [26%] with intrauterine insemination plus gonadotrophins *v* 4/50 [8%] with no treatment; RR 3.3, 95% CI 1.2 to 9.4; NNT 6, 95% CI 3 to 28). The second RCT (49 women with minimal or mild endometriosis) comparing three cycles of pituitary down regulation plus gonadotrophins plus intrauterine insemination versus 6 months of expectant management found no significant difference in birth rates (7/24 [29%] with intrauterine insemination *v* 5/25 [20%] with expectant management; RR 1.5, 95% CI 0.5 to 4.0).[82] When combined, these two RCTs show an overall twofold increase in live birth rates with intrauterine insemination plus gonadotrophins versus expectant management over a similar time period (RR v no treatment 2.3, 95% CI 1.1 to 4.6). The third RCT (119 couples with primary pelvic or cervical factor infertility for a mean of 3.7 years) compared alternate cycles of gonadotrophins plus intrauterine insemination versus intrauterine insemination alone.[83] It found that gonadotrophins plus intrauterine insemination versus intrauterine insemination alone significantly increased the pregnancy rate after the first treatment cycle (11/58 [19%] with gonadotrophins plus intrauterine insemination *v* 0/61 [0%] with intrauterine insemination alone; NNT 5, 95% CI 4 to 14). The 119 couples were subsequently followed up longitudinally and it was found that, in the 57 couples with a diagnosis of endometriosis, gonadotrophins plus intrauterine insemination versus intrauterine insemination alone significantly increased the probability of pregnancy over a total of 127 cycles (RR 5.1, 95% CI 1.1 to 22.5).

Harms: No cases of severe ovarian hyperstimulation or hospital admission were reported in the first or third RCTs.[81,83] In the second RCT, one severe case (1/24 [4%]), one moderate case (1/24 [4%]), and three mild cases (3/24 [13%]) of ovarian hyperstimulation syndrome (see glossary, p 1914) were reported.[82]

Comment: None.

OPTION SURGICAL TREATMENT

Two RCTs that compared laparoscopic surgery versus diagnostic laparoscopy found inconsistent results for differences in numbers of pregnancies and live births.

Benefits: **Versus placebo or ovarian suppression:** We found no RCTs (see comment below). **Laparoscopic surgery versus diagnostic laparoscopy:** We found two RCTs (in a total of 442 infertile women with minimal or mild endometriosis) comparing laparoscopic surgery (ablation or resection of endometriosis) versus diagnostic laparoscopy.[21,22] In the larger RCT (341 women), laparoscopic surgery versus diagnostic laparoscopy significantly increased the probability of pregnancy occurring within 36 weeks and lasting longer than 20 weeks (50/172 [29%] with laparoscopic surgery *v* 29/169 [17%]; RR 1.7, 95% CI 1.2 to 2.6; NNT 8, 95% CI 4 to 41; see comment below).[21] The smaller RCT (101 women) found no significant difference between laparoscopic surgery versus diagnostic laparoscopy in live birth rates after 1 year (10/51 [20%] with laparoscopic surgery *v* 10/45 [22%] with diagnostic laparoscopy; RR 0.90, 95 % CI 0.41 to 1.92).[22] See laparoscopic ablation of endometrial deposits under endometriosis, p 1864

Harms: The risks and morbidity of surgery under general anaesthesia, and of postoperative adhesion formation, should be balanced against the adverse effects of treatments involving ovarian suppression or stimulation. One multicentre series of 29 966 diagnostic and operative gynaecological laparoscopies found a mortality of 3.3/100 000 laparoscopies and a complication rate of 3.2/1000 laparoscopies.[23]

Comment: We found one systematic review (search date not stated)[24] and one non-systemic review,[25] which together identified 21 cohort studies and one quasi-randomised trial in a total of 3879 women with all stages of endometriosis. Interventions were laparoscopic or open surgery versus medical treatment or no treatment. Surgical treatment versus medical or no treatment significantly increased pregnancy rates (RR 1.4, 95% CI 1.3 to 1.5), although there was no significant difference between laparoscopic and open surgery (RR 0.9, 95% CI 0.8 to 1.0).[25] In women with mild or minimal endometriosis, analysis of pooled data found that laparoscopic surgery versus danazol or no treatment significantly increased pregnancy rates (OR 2.7, 95% CI 2.1 to 3.5).[25] In the larger RCT, comparing laparoscopic surgery versus diagnostic laparoscopy, 48/341 (14%) women who received laparoscopic surgery for their endometriosis also had peri-adnexal adhesions treated, which may have affected their fertility.[21]

OPTION IN VITRO FERTILISATION

We found no RCTs in women with endometriosis related infertility undergoing in vitro fertilisation treatment.

Benefits: We found no systematic review or RCTs.

Harms: See harms of in vitro fertilisation under treatments for tubal infertility, p 1903.

Comment: We found two retrospective cohort studies in women undergoing in vitro fertilisation comparing women with endometriosis versus women with different stages of endometriosis or other causes of infertility, which found no significant differences in pregnancy rates.[26,84] There is a need for properly controlled prospective randomised studies that present their results for different stages of endometriosis using a validated classification system. Comparisons with assisted reproductive techniques are also required.

QUESTION What are the effects of treatments for male infertility?

OPTION INTRAUTERINE INSEMINATION

Two systematic reviews have found that intrauterine insemination versus intracervical insemination or natural intercourse significantly increases pregnancy rates per cycle.

Benefits: We found two systematic reviews (search date not stated[33] and search date 1996–1997[85]). The first review (10 RCTs, 2082 treatment cycles in couples with male infertility) found that intrauterine insemination versus intracervical insemination or natural intercourse significantly increased the pregnancy rate per cycle (6.5% with intrauterine insemination *v* 3.1% with intracervical insemination or timed natural intercourse; OR 2.2, 95% CI 1.4 to 3.4).[33] The second review (17 RCTs; 3662 completed treatment cycles in couples with male subfertility) found that intrauterine insemination versus timed intercourse significantly increased pregnancy rates both in natural cycles (OR 2.4, 95% CI 1.5 to 3.8) and in controlled ovarian hyperstimulation cycles (OR 2.1, 95% CI 1.3 to 3.5).[85] The review found that intrauterine insemination in controlled cycles versus timed intercourse in natural cycles also significantly increased the probability of conception in the probability of conception (OR 6.2, 95% CI 2.4 to 16.5), but found no significant difference with intrauterine insemination in controlled cycles versus intrauterine insemination in natural cycles (OR 1.8, 95% CI 1.0 to 3.3).[77]

Harms: Apart from the risks of ovarian hyperstimulation syndrome (see glossary, p 1914) and multiple pregnancy associated with ovarian stimulation, intrauterine insemination may increase the likelihood of infection and may cause discomfort.[86] However, data from RCTs are scarce.

Comment: We found three RCTs that addressed the optimum number of inseminations in controlled ovarian stimulation cycles. Two trials found that two inseminations performed in the pre-ovulatory and peri-ovulatory periods produced significantly higher pregnancy rates than one peri-ovulatory insemination.[87,88] The other trial found a non-significant increase in pregnancy rates with two similarly timed inseminations.[89] One small crossover RCT addressed the timing of insemination in clomifene stimulated cycles. It found similar pregnancy rates per cycle whether insemination was timed with a urinary luteinising hormone kit, or whether ultrasound monitoring with human chorionic gonadotrophin induction of ovulation was used.[90]

OPTION INTRACYTOPLASMIC SPERM INJECTION PLUS IN VITRO FERTILISATION

One systematic review found insufficient evidence on the effects of intracytoplasmic sperm injections plus in vitro fertilisation versus in vitro fertilisation alone.

Benefits: **Versus in vitro fertilisation (IVF) alone:** We found one systematic review (search date not stated, 10 RCTs, 437 couples; see comment below), which compared intracytoplasmic sperm injection (ICSI) plus IVF versus IVF alone (8 RCTs compared ICSI plus IVF *v* conventional IVF; 1 RCT compared ICSI plus IVF *v* subzonal sperm injection; and 1 RCT compared ICSI plus IVF *v* additional IVF).[91] For couples with normal semen, the review found no significant difference with ICSI plus IVF versus IVF alone in fertilisation rates per retrieved oocyte or pregnancy rates, but found that ICSI plus IVF versus IVF alone significantly increased fertilisation rates per inseminated oocyte (combined OR 1.4, 95% CI 1.2 to 1.7). For couples with borderline semen (concentration 10–20 million/mL, motility 30–50%, morphology 4–14% normal forms) the review found that ICSI plus IVF versus IVF alone significantly increased fertilisation rates per oocyte retrieved (OR 3.79, 95% CI 2.97 to 4.85), and fertilisation rates per oocyte inseminated (OR 3.9, 95% CI 3.0 to 5.2). For couples with poor semen (concentration < 10 million/mL, motility < 30%, morphology < 4% normal forms), two RCTs identified by the review found that ICSI plus IVF versus subzonal sperm injection or additional IVF improved fertilisation outcomes.

Harms: Observational studies have found conflicting reports of congenital abnormalities[27,92] and sex chromosomal abnormalities in children born after ICSI (see comment below).[93,94]

Comment: The review used the proxy outcome of fertilisation rates, and eight RCTs included in the review used randomisation strategies based on oocytes or metaphase II oocytes.[91] Many couples have a strong preference for a child genetically related to both partners.[95] The data on congenital and chromosome abnormalities with ICSI are constantly being revised as experience increases.

OPTION IN VITRO FERTILISATION VERSUS GAMETE INTRAFALLOPIAN TRANSFER

One RCT found insufficient evidence on the effects of in vitro fertilisation versus gamete intrafallopian transfer.

Benefits: We found no systematic review. We found one RCT (13 couples with male infertility), which found no significant difference with in vitro fertilisation versus gamete intrafallopian transfer in numbers of pregnancies (2/7 [29%] with in vitro fertilisation *v* 2/6 [33%] with gamete intrafallopian transfer; RR 1.20, 95% CI 0.23 to 5.95).[96]

Harms: See harms of in vitro fertilisation under treatments for tubal infertility, p 1903.

Comment: None.

OPTION DONOR INSEMINATION

We found no good evidence on the effects of donor insemination.

Benefits: **Versus no treatment:** We found no systematic review or RCTs in couples with male infertility that compared donor insemination versus no treatment or other interventions.

Harms: We found no good evidence.

Comment: One systematic review (search date 1996, 12 RCTs, 2215 treatment cycles) found limited evidence that intrauterine insemination of frozen donor sperm versus intracervical insemination of donor sperm increased pregnancy rates.[86] The review included RCTs that were poor in their methodology, contained several different treatment variations making direct comparisons difficult, and included a mixture of women with and without fertility problems. Data are available from large databases, but it is sometimes unclear whether ovarian stimulation was used in addition to donor insemination. The live birth rate per cycle in the UK Human Fertilisation and Embryology Authority database (based on 7136 women) was 9%.[30] Similar rates are reported from the French donor insemination database (23 700 women over 4 years), with a mean pregnancy rate of 10.3% per cycle, and the Sheffield database (UK, 343 women, 980 treatment cycles), with an 11.3% overall live birth rate.[31,32] Comparisons of donor insemination versus no treatment or other interventions may be inappropriate as, for many couples, donor insemination is not an acceptable option. RCTs have tended to concentrate on comparisons between different techniques of donor insemination.

QUESTION What are the effects of treatment for unexplained infertility?

OPTION CLOMIFENE

One systematic review found limited evidence that clomifene versus placebo significantly increased rates of pregnancy per cycle.

Benefits: We found one systematic review (search date 2002, 5 RCTs, 4 using crossover designs; 458 cycles in women with unexplained infertility), which found that clomifene (clomiphene) versus placebo significantly increased pregnancy rates per cycle (OR 2.5, 95% CI 1.4 to 4.6; see comment below).[97] When only cycles before crossover were analysed (which was only possible with the data from 3 of these trials), the positive effect increased (OR 5.0, 95% CI 1.8 to 14.3).

Harms: See harms of clomifene under treatments for infertility caused by ovulation disorders, p 1897.

Comment: The systematic review[97] excluded a recent RCT because of the risk of selection bias with a pseudo-random allocation method based on odd or even chart numbers.[98] The other RCTs identified by the review were generally of poor quality and it is possible that, if one further medium sized RCT was performed, the direction of the overall effect found with meta-analysis could change again.[97] The review highlighted important differences between the trials: two RCTs included women with surgically treated endometriosis, one included only couples with primary infertility, and one included couples with a short duration of infertility (median of 28 months). Three of the RCTs included co-intervention with intrauterine insemination or cervicovaginal insemination. The RCTs also differed in their design (4 were crossover trials) and in the quality of randomisation (only 1 used properly concealed randomisation). The authors of the review comment that as the baseline cycle fecundity of the women included in these trials would only be about 1–2%, even with clomifene their cycle fecundity would be unlikely to exceed 5%.[97]

OPTION INTRAUTERINE INSEMINATION

Two systematic reviews and one subsequent RCT in couples undergoing ovarian stimulation treatment have found that intrauterine insemination versus timed intercourse or intracervical insemination significantly increases the rate of pregnancy. One systematic review has found no significant difference with intrauterine insemination versus timed intercourse or intracervical insemination in pregnancy rates, but has found that the addition of ovarian stimulation to any of the three interventions significantly increases pregnancy rate per cycle. One systematic review and one subsequent RCT have found that fallopian tube sperm perfusion versus intrauterine insemination significantly increases pregnancy rates. One RCT found no significant difference with intrauterine insemination in natural cycles versus intrauterine insemination in stimulated cycles or versus in vitro fertilisation in pregnancy rates, but found that more couples receiving in vitro fertilisation failed to complete their six cycles of treatment.

Benefits: **Versus timed intercourse or intracervical insemination:** We found three systematic reviews,[33,34,99] and one subsequent RCT,[100] in couples with unexplained infertility. The first review (search date not stated, 8 RCTs, number of treatment cycles not stated) compared intrauterine insemination plus ovarian stimulation with gonadotrophins versus timed intercourse plus ovarian stimulation with gonadotrophins.[99] It found that intrauterine insemination plus ovarian stimulation significantly increased the likelihood of pregnancy (OR 2.4, 95% CI 1.4 to 3.9). The second review (search date 1997, 7 RCTs, 980 treatment cycles) compared intrauterine insemination plus ovarian stimulation with gonadotrophins versus timed intercourse plus ovarian stimulation with gonadotrophins.[34] It found that intrauterine insemination plus ovarian stimulation significantly increased the pregnancy rate per cycle (110/549 [20%] with intrauterine insemination *v* 49/431 [11%] with timed intercourse; RR 0.20, 95% CI 0.08 to 0.31). The third systematic review (search date not stated, 7 RCTs, 934 treatment cycles) compared intrauterine insemination versus timed intercourse or intracervical insemination.[33] Four RCTs used gonadotrophins, two used clomifene (clomiphene), and three used no ovarian stimulation. The review found no significant difference with intrauterine insemination versus intracervical insemination or timed intercourse in pregnancy rates (OR 1.5, 95% CI 1.0 to 2.2). The review also found that the addition of ovarian stimulation with gonadotrophins to any of the three interventions significantly increased the overall pregnancy rates (45/249 [18%] with intrauterine insemination or favourable timed intracervical insemination or natural intercourse plus gonadotrophin stimulation *v* 9/108 [8%] with intrauterine insemination or favourable timed intracervical insemination or natural intercourse alone; RR 2.17, 95% CI 1.10 to 4.28; NNT 11, 95% CI 7 to 58). The subsequent RCT (932 couples) compared intracervical insemination alone, intrauterine insemination alone, intracervical insemination plus ovarian stimulation, and intrauterine insemination plus ovarian stimulation for four cycles or until pregnancy was achieved.[100] It found that intrauterine insemination plus ovarian stimulation versus intracervical insemination significantly increased the chance of becoming pregnant (OR 3.2, 95% CI 2.0 to 5.3). The RCT also found pregnancy rates of 14/233 (6%) with intracervical insemination, 35/234 (15%) with intrauterine insemination, 26/234 (11%) with ovarian stimulation plus intracervical insemination, and 54/231 (23%) with ovarian stimulation plus intrauterine insemination.[100] **Versus intrauterine insemination plus ovarian stimulation:** We found one RCT (932 couples), which found that intrauterine insemination plus ovarian stimulation versus intrauterine insemination alone significantly increased the chance of becoming pregnant (OR 1.7, 95% CI 1.2 to 2.6).[100] **Versus fallopian tube sperm perfusion:** See glossary, p 1914. See benefits of fallopian tube sperm perfusion, p 1912. **Versus gamete intrafallopian transfer:** See benefits of gamete intrafallopian transfer, p 1913. **Versus in vitro fertilisation (IVF):** We found one RCT (258 couples with either unexplained infertility or male subfertility) that compared six cycles of intrauterine insemination in natural cycles versus intrauterine insemination in stimulated cycles or versus IVF.[101] The RCT found that pregnancy rates per started treatment cycle were similar in all groups (7.4% with intrauterine insemination in natural cycles, 8.7% with intrauterine insemination in stimulated cycles, and 12.2% with IVF), with no significant differences between the different diagnostic groups. More couples in the IVF group failed to complete their six cycles of treatment, and cumulative pregnancy rates after six cycles did not differ significantly between treatment groups.

Harms: In the RCT (258 couples) comparing intrauterine insemination versus IVF, multiple pregnancy rates were 4% with intrauterine insemination in natural cycles, 29% with intrauterine insemination in stimulated cycles, and 21% with IVF (see harms of gonadotrophins, p 1898).[98] Mild ovarian hyperstimulation syndrome (see glossary, p 1914) occurred in two women in the stimulated intrauterine insemination group, and severe ovarian hyperstimulation syndrome occurred in three women in the IVF group. Apart from the risks of ovarian hyperstimulation syndrome and multiple pregnancy, intrauterine insemination may increase the likelihood of infection and may be associated with some discomfort. However, data from RCTs are scarce. One RCT (97 couples with unexplained infertility) compared low dose, step up follicle stimulating hormone (FSH) versus a conventional FSH regimen combined with intrauterine insemination.[101] There was no significant difference in pregnancy rates (7/49 [14%] with low dose FSH and intrauterine insemination *v* 7/48 [15%] with conventional FSH and intrauterine insemination;

RR 0.98, 95% CI 0.37 to 2.58), but the low dose gonadotrophins versus conventional FSH significantly reduced the number of women with ovarian hyperstimulation syndrome (4/49 [8%] with low dose FSH *v* 13/48 [27%] with conventional FSH; RR 0.30, 95% CI 0.11 to 0.86; NNT 6, 95% 3 to 28), and ovarian hyperstimulation syndrome requiring hospitalisation (0% *v* 16.7%). However, the low dose regimen did not completely prevent multiple pregnancies.

Comment: Only three of the RCTs were common to all three systematic reviews. One of the reviews scored the included studies for validity.[34] They scored from 49–70% when 100% was taken as the ideal study. The evidence from RCTs for timing and the optimum number of inseminations per cycle is conflicting (see benefits of intrauterine insemination under treatments for infertility associated with endometriosis, p 1907).

OPTION FALLOPIAN TUBE SPERM PERFUSION New

One systematic review and one subsequent RCT have found that fallopian tube sperm perfusion versus intrauterine insemination significantly increases pregnancy rates.

Benefits: **Versus intrauterine insemination:** We found one systematic review (search date not stated, 5 RCTs in couples with unexplained infertility)[102] and one subsequent RCT, which compared fallopian tube sperm perfusion (see glossary, p 1914) versus intrauterine insemination.[103] All five RCTs in the review used gonadotrophins or gonadotrophins plus clomifene, and in total 293 cycles of intrauterine insemination and 317 cycles of fallopian tube sperm perfusion were assessed. The review found that fallopian tube sperm perfusion versus intrauterine insemination significantly increased pregnancy rate per cycle (70/317 [22%] with fallopian tube sperm perfusion *v* 38/293 [13%] with intrauterine insemination; RR 1.70, 95% CI 1.19 to 2.44; NNT 11, 95% CI 7 to 33). The subsequent RCT (132 cycles in 65 couples) found that fallopian tube sperm perfusion versus intrauterine insemination significantly increased pregnancy rates per cycle (16/66 [24%] with fallopian tube sperm perfusion *v* 6/66 [9%] with intrauterine insemination; RR 2.67, 95% CI 1.11 to 6.40; NNT 7, 95% CI 4 to 38) and significantly increased pregnancy rates per person (16/33 [48%] with fallopian tube sperm perfusion *v* 6/32 [19%] with intrauterine insemination; RR 2.59, 95% CI 1.16 to 5.77; NNT 4, 95% CI 2 to 9) after a maximum of three treatment cycles.[103]

Harms: See harms of intrauterine insemination, p 1911. The systematic review did not report on harms.[102] The subsequent RCT reported that complications, including cervical bleeding, vasovagal episodes, uterine cramping, or pelvic infections, were not reported with either treatment.[103]

Comment: None.

OPTION GAMETE INTRAFALLOPIAN TRANSFER

We found no RCTs of gamete intrafallopian transfer versus no treatment. Three RCTs found conflicting results with gamete intrafallopian transfer versus other treatments (intrauterine insemination, timed intercourse, and in vitro fertilisation in pregnancy rates).

Benefits: **Versus no treatment:** We found no systematic review or RCTs. **Versus intrauterine insemination or timed intercourse:** We found no systematic review. We found three RCTs (283 couples with unexplained infertility).[104–106] The first RCT compared gamete intrafallopian transfer (GIFT) versus ovarian stimulation plus either timed intercourse or timed cervical donor insemination and found no significant difference in pregnancy rates (2/24 [8%] with GIFT cycles *v* 2/15 [13%] with ovarian stimulation; RR 0.63, 95% CI 0.10 to 3.98).[104] Of the other two RCTs, one found that GIFT versus ovarian stimulation plus intrauterine insemination increased pregnancy rates, and the other found no significant difference in pregnancy rates.[105,106] **Versus in vitro fertilisation:** See benefits of in vitro fertilisation for the treatment of unexplained infertility, p 1913.

Harms: Potential harms include the risks attributable to general anaesthesia and laparoscopy. Multiple pregnancy rates vary with the number of oocytes transferred.[106]

Comment: One prospective cohort study (99 treatment cycles, 53 couples) found that GIFT versus no treatment increased numbers of pregnancies.[107] GIFT, unlike in vitro fertilisation, gives no diagnostic information regarding fertilisation, and involves a laparoscopy and general anaesthetic, both of which are usually avoided with in vitro fertilisation. Success rates decrease with increasing age.[108,109]

OPTION IN VITRO FERTILISATION

Two small RCTs found no significant difference with in vitro fertilisation versus gamete intrafallopian transfer in pregnancy rates. One RCT found no significant difference with intrauterine insemination in natural cycles versus in vitro fertilisation in pregnancy rates, but found that more couples receiving in vitro fertilisation failed to complete their six cycles of treatment.

Benefits: We found no systematic review. **Versus gamete intrafallopian transfer:** We found two RCTs (155 couples).[96,110] Neither RCT found a significant difference between in vitro fertilisation versus gamete intrafallopian transfer in pregnancy rates. **Versus intrauterine insemination:** See benefits of intrauterine insemination for the treatment of unexplained infertility, p 1910.

Harms: See harms of in vitro fertilisation under treatments for tubal infertility, p 1903.

Comment: The RCTs were too small to rule out a significant effect of either treatment.

Infertility and subfertility

GLOSSARY

Adhesiolysis Division of adhesions, which are bands of scar tissue that form after infection or surgery.

Delayed in vitro fertilisation In vitro fertilisation treatment after 6 months of being assessed in an infertility clinic after at least 12 months of infertility.

Fallopian tube sperm perfusion Fallopian tube sperm perfusion is based on a pressure injection of 4 mL sperm suspension with an attempt to seal the cervix to prevent semen reflux. It attempts to ensure a sperm flushing of the fallopian tubes and an overflowing of the inseminate into the pouch of Douglas.

Hydrotubation Flushing of the fallopian tubes through the cervix and uterine cavity to remove surgical debris and reduce the incidence of tubal re-occlusion.

Immediate in vitro fertilisation In vitro fertilisation treatment within 6 months of being assessed in an infertility clinic after at least 12 months of infertility.

Laparoscopic ovarian drilling Ovarian drilling can be performed laparoscopically by either cautery or laser vapourisation (using CO_2, argon, or Nd:YAG lasers), which are used to create multiple perforations (about 10 holes/ovary) of the ovarian surface and stroma (inner area of the ovary). This is thought to cause ovulation by restoring the intra-ovarian hormonal environment to normal, which in turn beneficially affects the hypothalamic–pituitary–ovarian axis.

Macrosurgery Surgery without dedicated optical magnification.

Microsurgery Surgery involving optical magnification to allow the use of much finer instruments and suture material in addition to a non-touch technique, with the aim of minimising tissue handling and damage.

Ovarian hyperstimulation syndrome Can occur in mild, moderate, and severe forms. Mild ovarian hyperstimulation syndrome is characterised by fluid accumulation, as shown by weight gain, abdominal distension, and discomfort. Moderate ovarian hyperstimulation syndrome is associated with the development of nausea and vomiting in addition to ovarian enlargement, abdominal distension, discomfort, and dyspnoea. Severe ovarian hyperstimulation syndrome is a life threatening condition in which there is contraction of the intravascular volume, tense ascites, pleural and pericardial effusions, severe haemoconcentration, and the development of hepatorenal failure. Deaths have occurred, caused usually by cerebrovascular thrombosis, renal failure, or cardiac tamponade.

Second look laparoscopy Laparoscopy performed some time after tubal surgery (either open or laparoscopic) with the aim of dividing adhesions relating to the initial procedure.

Substantive changes

Clomifene (clomiphene) One new RCT;[38] conclusion unchanged.

Tubal surgery One new systematic review;[63] conclusion unchanged.

In vitro fertilisation Two new RCTs;[71,73] conclusion unchanged.

REFERENCES

1. European Society for Human Reproduction and Embryology. Guidelines to the prevalence, diagnosis, treatment and management of infertility, 1996. *Hum Reprod* 1996;11:1775–1807.
2. Schmidt L, Munster K. Infertility, involuntary infecundity, and the seeking of medical advice in industrialized countries 1970–1992: a review of concepts, measurements and results. *Hum Reprod* 1995;10:1407–1418.
3. Effective Health Care. The management of subfertility. *Effective Health Care Bulletin* 1992;3:13. Search date and primary sources not stated.
4. Collins JA, Burrows EA, Willan AR. The prognosis for live birth among untreated infertile couples. *Fertil Steril* 1995;64:22–28.
5. Templeton A, Morris JK. IVF — factors affecting outcome. In: Templeton A, Cooke ID, O'Brien PMS, eds. *35th RCOG study group evidence-based fertility treatment*. London: RCOG Press, 1998.
6. Khan KS, Daya S, Collins JA, et al. Empirical evidence of bias in infertility research: overestimation of treatment effect in crossover trials using pregnancy as the outcome measure. *Fertil Steril* 1996;65:939–945.

7. Cohlen BJ, Te Velde ER, Looman CW, et al. Crossover or parallel design in infertility trials? The discussion continues. *Fertil Steril* 1998;70:40–45.
8. Hughes E, Collins J, Vandekerckhove P. Clomiphene citrate for ovulation induction in women with oligo-amenorrhoea (Cochrane Review) In: The Cochrane Library, Issue 1, 2002. Oxford: Update Software. Search date not stated; primary source Cochrane Subfertility Group Register of Controlled Trials.
9. Holst N, Maltau JM, Forsdahl F, Handling of tubal infertility after introduction of in vitro fertilization: changes and consequences. *Fertil Steril* 1991;55:140–143.
10. Vilos GA, Verhoest CR, Martin JS, Economic evaluation of in vitro fertilization-embryo transfer and neosalpingostomy for bilateral tubal obstruction. *J Soc Obstet Gynecol Can* 1998;20:139–147.
11. Winston RM, Margara RA. Microsurgical salpingostomy is not an obsolete procedure. *Br J Obstet Gynaecol* 1991;98:637–642.
12. Singhal V, Li TC, Cooke ID. An analysis of factors influencing the outcome of 232 consecutive tubal microsurgery cases. *Br J Obstet Gynaecol* 1991;98:628–636.
13. Marana R, Quagliarello J. Distal tubal occlusion: microsurgery versus in vitro fertilization: a review. *Int J Fertil* 1988;33:107–115.
14. Meirow D, Schenker JG. Appraisal of Gift. *Eur J Obstet Gynecol Reprod* 1995;58:59–65.
15. Marana R, Quagliarello J. Proximal tubal occlusion: microsurgery versus IVF: a review. *Int J Fertil* 1988;33:338–340.
16. Patton PE, Williams TJ, Coulam CB. Results of microsurgical reconstruction in patients with combined proximal and distal occlusion: double obstruction. *Fertil Steril* 1987;47:670–674.
17. Wahab M, Li TC, Cooke ID. Reversal of sterilization versus IVF. *J Obstet Gynaecol* 1997;17:180–185.
18. Nugent D, Vandekerckhove P, Hughes E, et al. Gonadotrophin therapy for ovulation induction in subfertility associated with polycystic ovarian syndrome. In: The Cochrane Library, Issue 1, 2002. Oxford: Update Software. Search date not stated; primary sources Subfertility Register of Controlled Trials, Medline, and bibliographies of identified studies.
19. Farquhar C, Vandekerckhove P, Arnot M, et al. Laparoscopic "drilling" by diathermy or laser for ovulation induction in anovulatory polycystic ovary syndrome (Cochrane Review). In: The Cochrane Library, Issue 1, 2002. Oxford: Update Software. Search date 2001; primary source Cochrane Menstrual Disorders and Subfertility Group Register of Controlled Trials.
20. RCOG Infertility Guideline Group. *The management of infertility in secondary care*. London: RCOG, 1998.
21. Marcoux S, Maheux R, Berube S. Laparoscopic surgery in infertile women with minimal or mild endometriosis. *N Engl J Med* 1997;337:217–222.
22. Parazzini F. Ablation of lesions or no treatment in minimal-mild endometriosis in infertile women: a randomized trial. Gruppo Italiano per lo Studio dell'Endometriosi. *Hum Reprod* 1999;14:1332–1334.
23. Chapron C, Querleu D, Bruhat M, et al. Surgical complications of diagnostic and operative gynaecological laparoscopy: a series of 29 966 cases. *Hum Reprod* 1998;13:867–872.
24. Hughes EG, Fedorkow DM, Collins J. A quantitative overview of controlled trials in endometriosis-associated infertility. *Fertil Steril* 1993;59:963–970. Search date not stated; primary sources Medline, Science Citation Index, abstracts from scientific meetings, and hand searches of relevant trials and personal contacts.
25. Adamson GD, Pasta DJ. Surgical treatment of endometriosis-associated infertility: meta-analysis compared with survival analysis. *Am J Obstet Gynecol* 1994;171:1488–1504.
26. Geber S, Paraschos T, Atkinson G, et al. Results of IVF in patients with endometriosis: the severity of the disease does not affect outcome or the incidence of miscarriage. *Hum Reprod* 1995;10:1507–1511.
27. Kurinczuk J, Bower C. Birth defects in infants conceived by intracytoplasmic sperm injection: an alternative interpretation. *BMJ* 1997;315:1260–1265.
28. Wang CF, Gemzell C. The use of human gonadotrophins for the induction of ovulation in women with polycystic ovarian disease. *Fertil Steril* 1980;33:479–486.
29. Buvat J, Buvat-Herbaut M, Marcolin G, Ardaens-Boulier K. Antiestrogens as treatment of female and male infertilities. *Horm Res* 1987;28:219–229.
30. Human Fertilisation and Embryology Authority. Annual Report 2000. London: HFEA, 2000.
31. Le Lannou D, Lansac J. Artificial procreation with frozen donor sperm: the French experience of CECOS. In: Barratt CLR, Cooke ID, eds. *Donor insemination*. Cambridge: Cambridge University Press, 1993;152–169.
32. Cooke ID. Donor insemination — timing and insemination method. In: Templeton A, Cooke ID, O'Brien PMS, eds. *35th RCOG Study Group evidence-based fertility treatment*. London: RCOG Press, 1998.
33. Ford WCL, Mathur RS, Hull MGR. Intrauterine insemination: is it an effective treatment for male factor infertility? *Balliere Clin Obstet Gynecol* 1997;11:691–710. Search date not stated; primary sources Medline, BIDS, and manual scanning of leading reproductive journals.
34. Zeyneloglu HB, Arici A, Olive DL, et al. Comparison of intrauterine insemination with timed intercourse in superovulated cycles with gonadotrophins: a meta-analysis. *Fertil Steril* 1998;69:486–491. Search date 1997; primary sources Medline and hand searches of bibliographies of relevant publications and review articles.
35. Boostanfar R, Jain JK, Mishell DR Jr, et al. A prospective randomized trial comparing clomiphene citrate with tamoxifen citrate for ovulation induction. *Fertil Steril* 2001;75:1024–1026.
36. Messinis IE, Nillius SJ. Comparison between tamoxifen and clomiphene for induction of ovulation. *Acta Obstet Gynecol Scand* 1982;61:377–379.
37. Gerhard I, Runnebaum B. Comparison between tamoxifen and clomiphene therapy in women with anovulation. *Arch Gynecol* 1979;227:279–288.
38. El Biely MM, Habba M. The use of metformin to augment the induction of ovulation in obese infertile patients with polycystic ovary syndrome. *Middle East Fertil Soc J* 2001;6:43–49.
39. Rossing MA, Daling JR, Weiss NS, et al. Ovarian tumours in a cohort of infertile women. *N Engl J Med* 1994;331:771–776.
40. Venn A, Watson L, Lumley J, et al. Breast and ovarian cancer incidence after infertility and IVF. *Lancet* 1995;346:995–1000.
41. Parazzini F, Negri E, La Vecchia C, et al. Treatment for infertility and risk of invasive epithelial ovarian cancer. *Hum Reprod* 1997;12:2159–2161.

42. Mosgaard BJ, Lidegaard O, Kjaer SK, et al. Infertility, fertility drugs, and invasive ovarian cancer: a case-control study. *Fertil Steril* 1997;67:1005–1012.
43. Shushan A, Paltiel O, Iscovich J, et al. Human menopausal gonadotrophin and the risk of epithelial ovarian cancer. *Fertil Steril* 1996;65:13–18.
44. Dunn A, Macfarlane A. Recent trends in the incidence of multiple births and associated mortality in England and Wales. *Arch Dis Child Fetal Neonatal Ed* 1996;75:F10–F19.
45. State-specific variation in rates of twin births — United States, 1992–1994. *MMWR Morb Mortal Wkly Rep* 1997;46:121–125.
46. Cabau A, Krulik DR. Sterilites de cause hormonale et sterilites inexpliquees. Traitement par le cyclofenil. Etude controlee a double insu. *J Gynecol Obstet Biol Reprod* 1990;19:96–101.
47. Coelingh-Bennink HJ, Fauser BC, Out HJ. Recombinant follicle-stimulating hormone (FSH; Puregon) is more efficient than urinary follicle stimulating hormone (Metrodin) in women with clomiphene-resistant, normogonadotrophic, chronic anovulation: a prospective, multicenter, assessor-blind, randomized, clinical trial. European Puregon collaborative anovulation study group. *Fertil Steril* 1998;69:19–25.
48. Yarali H, Bukulmez O, Gurgan T. Urinary follicle stimulating hormone (FSH) versus recombinant FSH in clomiphene citrate resistant normogonadotropic, chronic anovulation: a prospective randomised study. *Fertil Steril* 1999;72:276–281.
49. Muenstermann U, Kleinstein J. Long-term GnRH analogue treatment is equivalent to laparoscopic laser diathermy in polycystic ovarian syndrome patients with severe ovarian dysfunction. *Hum Reprod* 2000;15:2526–2530.
50. Greenblatt E, Casper R. Adhesion formation after laparoscopic ovarian cautery for polycystic ovarian syndrome: lack of correlation with pregnancy rates. *Fertil Steril* 1993;60:766–770.
51. Deans A, Wayne C, Toplis P. Pelvic infection: a complication of laparoscopic ovarian drilling. *Gynaecol Endoscopy* 1997;6:301,en303.
52. Bayram N, Van Wely M, Vandekerckhove P, et al. Pulsatile luteinising hormone releasing hormone for ovulation induction in subfertility associated with polycystic ovary syndrome. In: The Cochrane Library, Issue 1, 2002. Oxford: Update Software. Search date not stated; primary sources Cochrane Menstrual Disorders and Subfertility Group Register of Controlled Trials and hand searches of reference lists of included trials.
53. Martin KA, Hall JE, Adams JM, et al. Comparison of exogenous gonadotropins and pulsatile gonadotropin-releasing hormone for induction of ovulation in hypogonadotropic amenorrhea. *J Clin Endocrinol Metab* 1993;77:125–129.
54. Balen AH, Braat DD, West C, et al. Cumulative conception and live birth rates after the treatment of anovulatory infertility: safety and efficacy of ovulation induction in 200 patients. *Hum Reprod* 1994;9:1563–1570.
55. Braat DD, Schoemaker R, Schoemaker J. Life table analysis of fecundity in intravenously gonadotropin-releasing hormone-treated patients with normogonadotropic and hypogonadotropic amenorrhea. *Fertil Steril* 1991;55:266–271.
56. Filicori M, Flamigni C, Dellai P, et al. Treatment of anovulation with pulsatile gonadotropin-releasing hormone: prognostic factors and clinical results in 600 cycles. *J Clin Endocrinol Metab* 1994;79:1215–1220.
57. Honore GM, Holden AE, Schenken RS. Pathophysiology and management of proximal tubal blockage. *Fertil Steril* 1999;71:785–795. Search date not stated; primary sources Medline and Science Citation Index.
58. Thurmond AS. Pregnancies after selective salpingography and tubal recanalization. *Radiology* 1994;190:11–13.
59. Marana R. Proximal tubal obstruction: are we overdiagnosing and overtreating? *Gynaecol Endoscopy* 1992;1:99–101.
60. Johnson NP, Mak W, Sowter MC. Surgical treatment for tubal disease in women due to undergo in vitro fertilisation. In: The Cochrane Library, Issue 1, 2002. Oxford: Update Software. Search date 2000; primary sources Cochrane Menstrual Disorders and Subfertility Group Register of Controlled Trials, Medline, Embase, Psychlit, Current Contents, Biological Abstracts, Social Sciences Index, and the National Research Register.
61. Watson A, Vandekerckhove P, Lilford R. Techniques for pelvic surgery in subfertility (Cochrane Review). In: The Cochrane Library, Issue 1, 2002. Oxford: Update Software. Search date not stated; primary source Cochrane Menstrual Disorders and Subfertility Group Register of Controlled Trials.
62. Johnson NP, Watson A. Postoperative procedures for improving fertility following pelvic reproductive surgery. In: The Cochrane Library, Issue 1, 2002. Oxford: Update Software. Search date not stated; primary source Cochrane Menstrual Disorders and Subfertility Group Register of Controlled Trials.
63. Watson A, Vandekerckhove P, Lilford R. Techniques for pelvic surgery in subfertility (Cochrane Review). In: The Cochrane Library, Issue 1, 2002. Oxford: Update Software. Search date not stated; primary source Cochrane Menstrual Disorders and Subfertility Group Register of Controlled Trials.
64. Filippini F, Darai E, Benifla JL, et al. Distal tubal surgery: a critical review of 104 laparoscopic distal tuboplasties [in French]. *J Gynecol Obstet Biol Reprod* 1996;25:471–478 (review in French).
65. Donnez J, Casanas-Roux F. Prognostic factors of fimbrial microsurgery. *Fertil Steril* 1986;46:200–204.
66. Tomazevic T, Ribic-Pucelj M, Omahen A, et al. Microsurgery and in vitro fertilization and embryo transfer for infertility resulting from pathological proximal tubal blockage. *Hum Reprod* 1996;11:2613–2617.
67. Wu CH, Gocial B. A pelvic scoring system for infertility surgery. *Int J Fertil* 1988;33:341–346.
68. Oelsner G, Sivan E, Goldenberg M, et al. Should lysis of adhesions be performed when in vitro fertilization and embryo transfer are available? *Hum Reprod* 1994;9:2339–2341.
69. Gillett WR, Clarke RH, Herbison GP. First and subsequent pregnancies after tubal surgery: evaluation of the fertility index. *Fertil Steril* 1998;68:1033–1042.
70. Jarrell J, Labelle R, Goeree R, et al. In vitro fertilization and embryo transfer: a randomized controlled trial. *Online J Curr Clin Trials* 1993;2:Doc 73.
71. Bhattacharya S, Hamilton MP, Shaaban M, et al. Conventional in-vitro fertilisation versus intracytoplasmic sperm injection for the treatment of non-male-factor infertility: a randomised controlled trial. *Lancet* 2001;357:2075–2079.
72. Bukulmez O, Yarali H, Yucel A, et al. Intracytoplasmic sperm injection versus in vitro fertilization for patients with a tubal factor as their sole cause of infertility: a prospective, randomized trial. *Fertil Steril* 2000;73:38–42.
73. Poehl M, Holagschwandtner M, Bichler K, et al. IVF-patients with nonmale factor "to ICSI" or "not to ICSI" that is the question? *J Assist Reprod Genet* 2001;18:205–208.

74. Centers for Disease Control and Prevention. US Department of Health and Human Services. 1998 Assisted Reproductive Technology Success Rates. National Summary and Clinic Reports. December 2000.
75. Brinsden PR, Wada I, Tan SL, et al. Diagnosis, prevention and management of ovarian hyperstimulation syndrome. *Br J Obstet Gynaecol* 1995;102:767–772.
76. Wennerholm U, Bergh C. Obstetric outcome and follow-up of children born after in vitro fertilization (IVF). *Hum Fertil* 2000;3:52–64.
77. Chapko KM, Weaver MR, Chapko MK, et al. Stability of in vitro fertilization-embryo transfer success rates from the 1989,1990, and 1991 clinic-specific outcome assessments. *Fertil Steril* 1995;64:757–763. Search date not stated; primary source Medline.
78. Human Fertilisation and Embryology Authority. The Patients' Guide to IVF Clinics. London: HFEA, 2000.
79. Hughes E, Fedorkow D, Collins J, et al. Ovulation suppression for endometriosis. In: The Cochrane Library, Issue 1, 2002. Oxford: Update Software. Search date not stated; primary source Cochrane Subfertility Group Register of Controlled Trials.
80. Dockeray CJ, Sheppard BL, Bonnar J. Comparison between mefenamic acid and danazol in the treatment of established menorrhagia. *Br J Obstet Gynaecol* 1989;96:840–844.
81. Tummon IS, Asher LJ, Martin JSB, et al. Randomized controlled trial of superovulation and insemination for infertility associated with minimal or mild endometriosis. *Fertil Steril* 1997;68:8–12.
82. Fedele L, Bianchi S, Marchini M, et al. Superovulation with human menopausal gonadotrophins in the treatment of infertility associated with endometriosis: a controlled randomised study. *Fertil Steril* 1992;58:28–31.
83. Nulsen JC, Walsh S, Dumez S. A randomised and longitudinal study of human menopausal gonadotrophin with intrauterine insemination in the treatment of infertility. *Obstet Gynaecol* 1993;82:780–786.
84. Olivennes F, Feldberg D, Liu H-C, et al. Endometriosis: a stage by stage analysis — the role of in vitro fertilization. *Fertil Steril* 1995;64:392–398.
85. Cohlen BJ, Vandekerckhove P, Te Velde ER, et al. Timed intercourse versus intra-uterine insemination with or without ovarian hyperstimulation for subfertility in men. In: The Cochrane Library, Issue 1, 2002. Oxford: Update Software. Search date 1996/1997; primary sources Medline, Embase, DDFU, Biosis, SciSearch, hand searching, and conference abstracts.
86. O'Brien P, Vandekerckhove P. Intra-uterine versus cervical insemination of donor sperm for subfertility. In: The Cochrane Library, Issue 1, 2002. Oxford: Update Software. Search date 1996; primary source Cochrane Subfertility Group Specialist Register of Controlled Trials.
87. Ragni G, Maggioni P, Guermandi E, et al. Efficacy of double intrauterine insemination in controlled ovarian hyperstimulation cycles. *Fertil Steril* 1999;72:619–622.
88. Silverberg KM, Johnson JV, Olive DL, et al. A prospective, randomized trial comparing two different intrauterine insemination regimens in controlled ovarian hyperstimulation cycles. *Fertil Steril* 1992;576:357–361.
89. Ransom MX, Blotner MB, Bohrer M, et al. Does increasing frequency of intrauterine insemination improve pregnancy rates significantly during superovulation cycles? *Fertil Steril* 1994;61:303–307.
90. Zreik TG, Garcia-Velasco JA, Habboosh MS, et al. Prospective, randomized, crossover study to evaluate the benefit of human chorionic gonadotrophin-timed versus urinary luteinising hormone-timed intrauterine inseminations in clomiphene citrate-stimulated treatment cycles. *Fertil Steril* 1998;71:1070–1074.
91. Van Rumste MME, Evers JLH, Farquhar CM, et al. Intra-cytoplasmic sperm injection versus partial zona dissection, subzonal insemination and conventional techniques for oocyte insemination during IVF. In: The Cochrane Library, Issue 1, 2002. Oxford: Update Software. Search date not stated; primary source Cochrane Menstrual Disorders and Subfertility Group Specialist Register of Controlled Trials.
92. Bonduelle M, Legein J, Buyesse A, et al. Prospective follow up study of 423 children born after intracytoplasmic sperm injection. *Hum Reprod* 1996;11:1558–1564.
93. Bonduelle M, Legein J, Derde M, et al. Comparative follow-up study of 130 children born after ICSI and 130 children born after IVF. *Hum Reprod* 1995;10:3327–3331.
94. Velde E, Van Baar A, Van Kooije R. Concerns about assisted reproduction. *Lancet* 1998;351: 1524–1525.
95. De Wert G. Ethics of intracytoplasmic sperm injection: proceed with care. *Hum Reprod* 1998;13(suppl 1):219–227.
96. Leeton J, Healy D, Rogers P. A controlled study between the use gamete intrafallopian transfer (GIFT) and in vitro fertilization and embryo transfer in the management of idiopathic and male infertility. *Fertil Steril* 1987;48:605–607.
97. Hughes E, Collins J, Vandekerckhove P. Clomiphene citrate for unexplained subfertility in women. In: The Cochrane Library, Issue 1, 2002. Oxford: Update Software. Search date 2000; primary sources Cochrane Menstrual Disorders and Subfertility Review Group Specialist Register of Controlled Trials, Medline, Embase, and Cinahl.
98. Fujii S, Fukui A, Fukushi Y, et al. The effects of clomiphene citrate on normally ovulatory women. *Fertil Steril* 1997;68:997–999.
99. Hughes EG. The effectiveness of ovulation induction and intrauterine insemination in the treatment of persistent infertility: a meta-analysis. *Hum Reprod* 1997;12:1865–1872. Search date not stated; primary source Cochrane Menstrual Disorders and Subfertility Group Specialist Register of Controlled Trials.
100. Guzick DS, Carson SA, Coutifaris C, et al. Efficacy of superovulation and intrauterine insemination in the treatment of infertility. National Cooperative Reproductive Medicine Network. *N Engl J Med* 1999;340:177–183.
101. Sengoku K, Tamate K, Takaoka Y, et al. The clinical efficacy of low-dose step-up follicle stimulating hormone administration for treatment of unexplained infertility. *Hum Reprod* 1999;14:349–353.
102. Trout SW, Kemmann E. Fallopian sperm perfusion versus intrauterine insemination: a randomized controlled trial and meta-analysis of the literature. *Fertil Steril* 1999;71:881–885. Search date not stated; primary source Medline.
103. Ricci G, Nucera G, Pozzobon C, et al. A simple method for fallopian tube sperm perfusion using a blocking device in the treatment of unexplained infertility. *Fertil Steril* 2001;76:1242–1248.
104. Hogerzeil HV, Spiekerman JCM, De Vries JWA, et al. A randomized trial between GIFT and ovarian stimulation for the treatment of unexplained infertility and failed artificial insemination by donor. *Hum Reprod* 1992;7:1235–1239.

105. Murdoch AP, Harris M, Mahroo M, et al. Gamete intrafallopian transfer (GIFT) compared with intrauterine insemination in the treatment of unexplained infertility. *Br J Obstet Gynaecol* 1991;98:1107–1111.

106. Wessels PHX, Cronje HS, Oosthuizen AP, et al. Cost-effectiveness of gamete intrafallopian transfer in comparison with induction of ovulation with gonadotrophins in the treatment of female infertility: a clinical trial. *Fertil Steril* 1992;57:163–167.

107. Murdoch AP, Harris M, Mahroo M, et al. Is GIFT (gamete intrafallopian transfer) the best treatment for unexplained infertility? *Br J Obstet Gynaecol* 1991;98:643–647.

108. Rombauts I, Dear M, Breheny S, et al. Cumulative pregnancy rates and live birth rates after gamete intra-fallopian transfer. *Hum Reprod* 1997;12:1338–1342.

109. Society for Assisted Reproductive Technology and the American Society for Reproductive Medicine. Assisted reproductive technology in the United States and Canada: 1995 results generated from the American Society for Reproductive Medicine/Society for Assisted Reproductive Technology Registry. *Fertil Steril* 1998;69:389–398.

110. Ranieri M, Beckett VA, Marchant S, Kinis A, Serhal P. Gamete intra-fallopian transfer or in vitro fertilization after failed ovarian stimulation and intrauterine insemination in unexplained infertility. *Hum Reprod* 1995;10:2023–2026.

Kirsten Duckitt
Consultant Obstetrician and Gynaecologist
John Radcliffe Hospital
Oxford
UK

Competing interests: None declared.

TABLE 1 **Comparative success rates of treatments for infertility: evidence from RCTs and observational studies (see text, p 1896).**

Treatment	Live birth rates	Pregnancy rates	Adverse effects
All causes of infertility			
IVF (per treated cycle)	UK 15%; US 20%[5]	59–77% (with 3–5 treatment cycles)[8]	Ectopic pregnancy: 1–3%[9,10]
GIFT (per cycle) (not including tubal infertility)	23%[14]	ND	
Infertility caused by ovulation disorders			
Clomifene to induce ovulation in amenorrhoeic women (after 2–4 cycles of treatment)		Ovulation rate 61%, pregnancy rate 14%[8]	Risk of ovarian cancer, unproved. MP: 2–13%, mostly twins.[28] OHSS: infrequent and mild
Gonadotrophins to induce ovulation in clomifene resistant PCOS (per cycle)		27–40%[3 18] FSH 27%[18]	Risk of ovarian cancer, unproved. MP: 29%[29] OHSS: 4%
Laparoscopic drilling (cumulative rate 1–2 years after treatment)		48%[19,20]	Risks of laparoscopy, general anaesthesia, and adhesions. Risk of premature ovarian failure unproved
Tubal infertility			
Tubal surgery for distal occlusion (cumulative rate 2 years after surgery)[11–13]	20–30%		Risks of general anaesthesia. Ectopic pregnancy: 7–9%[9,10]
Tubal surgery for proximal occlusion (cumulative rate)	40–60%[15,16]		
Reversal of female sterilisation (cumulative live birth rate 1–2 years after surgery)	50–90%[17] depending on method used for sterilisation		

TABLE 1 continued

Treatment	Live birth rates	Pregnancy rates	Adverse effects
Infertility associated with endometriosis			
Surgery (per cycle)		13–38%†[21–26]	Risks of surgery and general anaesthesia (for laparoscopic surgery). Mortality 3.33/100 000; complication rate 3.2/1000[23]
Male infertility			
IUI ± ovarian stimulation (per cycle)		6.5%[33]	
ICSI plus IVF (per cycle)	20%[5]		
Donor insemination* (per cycle)	9–12%[30–32]		No adverse effects if no ovarian stimulation is given, but child is not male partner's genetic offspring
Unexplained infertility			
IUI ± ovarian stimulation (per cycle)		9–12% without stimulation; 19–20% with[33,34]	

*Using frozen donor sperm in women without female factor or with corrected female factor infertility; †Over spontaneous rate.
FSH, follicle stimulating hormone; GIFT, gamete intrafallopian transfer; ICSI, intracytoplasmic sperm injection; IUI, intrauterine insemination; IVF, in vitro fertilisation; MP, multiple pregnancy; ND, no data; OHSS, ovarian hyperstimulation syndrome; PCOS, polycystic ovary syndrome.

Menopausal symptoms

Search date March 2002

Edward Morris and Janice Rymer

QUESTIONS

INTERVENTIONS

To be covered in future updates
Natural progestogen cream
Homeopathic and herbal remedies

Key Messages

- **Antidepressants** We found no RCTs on the effects of antidepressants on menopausal symptoms.
- **Clonidine** One RCT found that transdermal clonidine versus placebo for 8 weeks reduced the number of women reporting hot flushes (NNT 3, 95% CI 2 to 12), and increased the number of women reporting reductions in intensity of hot flushes (NNT 3, 95% CI 2 to 5).
- **Oestrogens** One systematic review and two subsequent RCTs have found that oestrogen versus placebo significantly improves vasomotor symptoms. Two systematic reviews and three subsequent RCTs have found that oestrogen prevents urinary tract infection and improves urogenital symptoms. One systematic review found that oestrogen reduced depressed mood. Four RCTs have found that oestrogen improves quality of life in the short term. Important adverse effects include venous thromboembolic disease, breast cancer, and endometrial cancer.
- **Phyto-oestrogens** One RCT found that soy protein versus no phyto-oestrogens reduces the severity but not the frequency of vasomotor symptoms at 6 weeks. One RCT found no significant differences in vasomotor symptoms between isoflavone and placebo after 12 weeks, and another RCT found that isoflavone versus placebo reduced the severity of vasomotor symptoms over 12 weeks. One RCT found that soy flour versus placebo significantly reduced mean number of weekly hot flushes after 12 weeks, but another RCT found no significant difference between soy protein and placebo in vasomotor symptoms. One RCT found no significant difference in vasomotor symptoms between soy flour versus wheat flour over 12 weeks. One RCT (94 women) found no significant difference between soy protein and placebo at 3 months for psychological, musculoskeletal, and genitourinary symptoms.
- **Progestogens** One systematic review and six additional RCTs have found that progestogens reduce vasomotor symptoms. We found no good quality evidence on other outcomes, including quality of life.

- **Testosterone** One RCT comparing methyltestosterone plus oestrogen versus oestrogen alone found that the addition of methyltestosterone significantly reduced hot flushes; a second RCT found no significant differences after 6 months. One crossover RCT found limited evidence that testosterone improved sexual enjoyment and libido but another RCT found no significant differences at 6 months. We found no RCTs evaluating effects of testosterone alone on other commonly experienced menopausal symptoms.
- **Tibolone** One RCT has found that tibolone versus placebo significantly reduces vasomotor symptoms. A second RCT found that tibolone versus oestrogen/progesterone replacement therapy was less effective at reducing vasomotor symptoms. A third RCT found no significant differences in vasomotor symptoms between tibolone and oestrogen/progestogen replacement therapy. One RCT found no significant differences in vaginal dryness between tibolone versus continuous hormone replacement therapy after 48 weeks, but found a significant improvement in sexual satisfaction with tibolone versus estradiol plus noresthisterone. One RCT found that tibolone versus placebo improved sexual fantasies and arousability over 3 months. One RCT found that tibolone versus conjugated oestrogen significantly improved sexual desire and coital frequency.

DEFINITION Menopause is defined as the end of the last menstrual period. A woman is deemed to be postmenopausal 1 year after her last period. For practical purposes most women are diagnosed as menopausal after 1 year of amenorrhoea. Menopausal symptoms often begin in the perimenopausal years.

INCIDENCE/PREVALENCE In the UK, the mean age for the start of the menopause is 50 years and 9 months. The median onset of the perimenopause is 45.5–47.5 years. One Scottish survey (6096 women aged 45–54 years) found that 84% of women had experienced at least one of the classic menopausal symptoms, with 45% finding one or more symptoms a problem.[1]

AETIOLOGY/RISK FACTORS Urogenital symptoms of menopause are caused by decreased oestrogen concentrations, but the cause of vasomotor symptoms and psychological effects is complex and remains unclear.

PROGNOSIS Menopause is a physiological event. Its timing may be determined genetically. Although endocrine changes are permanent, menopausal symptoms such as hot flushes, which are experienced by about 70% of women, usually resolve with time.[2] But some symptoms may remain the same or worsen, for example genital atrophy.

AIMS To reduce or prevent menopausal symptoms; and to improve quality of life, with minimum adverse effects.

OUTCOMES Frequency and severity of vasomotor, urogenital, and psychological symptoms; quality of life.

METHODS *Clinical Evidence* update search and appraisal March 2002. We included only systematic reviews and RCTs that met *Clinical Evidence* quality criteria. Many of the RCTs included were crossover trials, which may have important limitations (see *Clinical Evidence* glossary). Where results are reported only for comparisons to pretreatment values, they have been omitted, as these comparisons may be influenced in many (frequently non-quantifiable) ways by other factors apart from treatment effect.

QUESTION What are the effects of medical treatments?

OPTION OESTROGENS

One systematic review and two subsequent RCTs have found that oestrogen with or without progestogens improves vasomotor symptoms. Two systematic reviews and three subsequent RCTs have found that oestrogen significantly reduces the incidence of urinary tract infection and improves urogenital symptoms. One systematic review found that oestrogen significantly reduced depressed mood. Four RCTs have found that oestrogen improves quality of life in the short term. Important adverse effects include venous thromboembolic disease, breast cancer, and endometrial cancer.

Benefits: **Vasomotor symptoms:** We found one systematic review and two subsequent RCTs.[3–5] The systematic review (search date 2000, 21 RCTs, 2511 women) compared oral oestrogens at varying doses with or without progestogens versus placebo.[3] The review found that oestrogen versus placebo significantly reduced the occurrence of hot flushes per week and their frequency (6 RCTs, 371 women: RR 0.23, 95% CI 0.12 to 0.42; WMD −15.7, 95% CI −20.0 to −11.5 flushes/wk). It also found that oestrogen versus placebo significantly reduced the number of women with hot flushes at the end of the study (8 RCTs, 1240 women: 139/906 [15%] with oestrogen *v* 158/334 [47%] with placebo; RR 0.37, 95% CI 0.30 to 0.45; NNT 4, 95% CI 3 to 4). There was a wide variation in the frequency of hot flushes in both control and treatment groups among the RCTs (range of means for each RCT 0.9–13.8 flushes/wk with oestrogen *v* 12.6–33.5 with placebo). We found two subsequent RCTs. The first RCT (361 women) compared nasal versus transdermal oestrogen.[4] It found that both 300 μg of nasal oestrogen daily and 500 μg of transdermal oestrogen daily significantly reduced the total number of daily hot flushes and menopausal symptoms as assessed by the Kupperman index after 12 weeks. The effects were no different to the population randomised to a 50 μg patch. We found no comparisons between treatments. The second RCT (2673 women) found that daily doses of 0.3 mg, 0.45 mg or 0.625 mg of conjugated equine oestrogens (with or without medroxyprogesterone acetate 2.5 mg/day) significantly reduced vasomotor symptoms from week 3–12, assessed using diary cards to record number and severity of hot flushes ($P < 0.05$). A significant reduction from baseline frequency of hot flushes was found in all groups, including placebo ($P < 0.01$) during 12 weeks. There was no significant difference in number or severity of hot flushes between the groups taking medroxyprogesterone acetate. There were significant reductions in the number of hot flushes in the oestrogen alone groups by week 3, and in those receiving 0.625 mg of conjugated oestrogen compared with the 0.45 mg and 0.3 mg groups (data presented graphically).[5] **Urogenital system:** We found two systematic reviews (search date 1995, 6 RCTs[6] and search date 1998, 6 RCTs, 334 people[7]) and three additional RCTs.[8–10] The first systematic review found that oestrogen improved urogenital symptoms regardless of route (no figures available).[6] The second systematic review found a significant reduction in the incidence of urinary tract infection with oral or vaginal oestrogen hormone replacement therapy (HRT) versus placebo or no treatment (OR for infection when not using HRT 2.51, 95% CI 1.48 to 4.25). Vaginal oestrogens were superior to oral oestrogens in reducing urinary tract infections ($P < 0.008$).[7] One subsequent RCT (136 women) found that low dose transdermal oestrogen (25 μg/day) plus norethisterone acetate significantly reduced vaginal dryness and also dyspareunia compared with placebo over 6 months ($P < 0.001$).[8] The second subsequent RCT (145 women) found that low dose estradiol (oestradiol) versus placebo was associated with a higher number of days without vaginal dryness at weeks 9–12 (86% with 1 mg estradiol *v* 76% with 0.5 mg estradiol *v* 74% with placebo), but significance was not tested.[10] The third RCT (multicentre, 84 women treated for 24 wks, 20% withdrawals) found reported relief of dyspareunia to be significantly higher for women using a estradiol ring (90% with estradiol ring *v* 45% with placebo, $P = 0.028$).[9] **Psychological symptoms:** We found one systematic review (search date 1995, 14 RCTs including several crossover RCTs, 12 cohort studies) that found oestrogen versus placebo or no treatment reduced depressed mood (measured with different scales) among menopausal women ($P < 0.0001$).[11] Duration of treatment ranged from 1 month to 2 years. We found no RCTs of oestrogen treatment in women with clinically proven depression. We found one systematic review (search date 1996, 10 controlled trials, and 9 observational studies) of the effects of oestrogen on cognitive function in postmenopausal women and in women with Alzheimer's disease.[12] The review found that studies were too weak to allow reliable conclusions. An additional crossover RCT (62 women) found a significant reduction in subjective sleep problems compared with placebo over 7 months ($P < 0.01$).[13] **Quality of life:** We found no systematic review. We found four RCTs (639 women, 3 placebo controlled[14–16], 2 with added progestogen[16,17]) all of which found significant improvement in quality of life in women treated with oestrogen compared with baseline or placebo.[14–17] The largest RCT (223 postmenopausal women in Sweden) found a significant improvement in quality of life ($P = 0.0003$) and well-being ($P = 0.003$) with estradiol transdermal patches (50 μg/24 h) versus placebo patches after 12 weeks.[15]

Harms: Women often report an increase in weight when starting oestrogen, but we found no evidence from RCTs that oestrogen causes significant weight gain in the long term. The most important long term adverse effects are increased risk of venous thromboembolic disease (see hormone replacement therapy under prevention of ischaemic cardiac events, p 129), endometrial cancer, and breast cancer.[18–21] One systematic review (search date not stated) reanalysed 51 studies (> 160 000 women) of the relation between oestrogen (as HRT) and breast cancer. It found that the relative risk of breast cancer increased by 2.3% (95% CI 1.1% to 3.6%) each year in women using HRT.[22] Five or more years after HRT was stopped, there was no significant excess of breast cancer.[22] One systematic review of the effects of HRT (18 RCTs, 5247 women) found significant risks of endometrial hyperplasia in women taking unopposed oestrogen (RR 8.14, 95% CI 1.05 to 63.1 for 6 months' treatment; RR 37.0, 95% CI 9.3 to 147 for 36 months' treatment).[21] The review also found significant reductions in the incidence of hyperplasia when women are given progestogens, either cyclically or continuously, with continuous combined HRT having the greatest effect at 36 months (RR 0.17, 95% CI 0.02 to 1.26). One systematic review (search date 1998) of 22 studies has found no effect of either unopposed or combined HRT on body weight.[18]

Comment: Many studies used selected populations, such as women attending hospital clinics, who may be different in their behaviour, personality, and symptom profile to women of the same age seen in primary care or those who do not seek medical advice.

OPTION PROGESTOGENS

We found good evidence from one systematic review and six additional RCTs that progestogens reduce vasomotor symptoms. We found no good quality evidence on other outcomes, including quality of life.

Benefits: **Vasomotor symptoms:** We found no systematic review of progestogens alone versus placebo. We found one systematic review (search date 2000, 21 RCTs, 2511 women, follow up for 3–36 months) of oestrogen alone versus oestrogens at varying doses and routes of administration with or without progestogens, including lower dose preparations,[3] four RCTs of progestogens versus placebo[23–26] and two RCTs of progestogens versus other interventions.[27,28] The systematic review found that there was a significant reduction in severity of hot flushes in users of oestrogen alone and users of both oestrogen and progesterone, but the reduction in hot flush severity was greater in those taking progesterone and oestrogen (OR 0.1, 95% CI 0.06 to 0.19) than those taking oestrogen alone (OR 0.35, 95% CI 0.22 to 0.56). The four RCTs against placebo (three of them < 1 year in duration)[23–26] found that progestogens significantly reduced vasomotor symptoms (see table 1, p 1933). The fifth RCT (43 menopausal women), which compared oestrogen alone versus progesterone (150 mg of depot medroxyprogesterone for 25 days/month), found that, over 3 months, 18% of women taking oestrogen and 33% taking progestogen reported no vasomotor symptoms.[27] The sixth additional RCT (321 women) compared oestrogen alone versus oestrogen plus progestogen.[28] It found a reduction in hot flushes with both preparations with small differences between them (figures not provided). **Urogenital system:** We found no RCTs evaluating the effects of progestogens alone on urinary incontinence, the lower genital tract, or libido. **Psychological symptoms:** We found no RCTs. **Quality of life:** We found no studies of progestogen alone on quality of life. One RCT of cyclical progestogen plus oestrogen versus oestrogen alone for 6 months found no evidence of an effect on quality of life.[29]

Harms: We found three RCTs that evaluated harms of progestogens. The first RCT (321 women who had undergone hysterectomy and were already taking conjugated oestrogen) compared continuous progestogen (norgestrel) versus placebo. It found no difference in symptoms (including weight gain and bloating).[30] The second RCT (875 women) compared various oestrogen/progestogen combinations over 3 years.[31] It found that additional progestogen increased breast discomfort (OR 1.92, 95% CI 1.16 to 3.09). Neither RCT found evidence of an effect on cardiovascular events. The third crossover RCT (51 women receiving 2 mg estradiol) compared adverse effects of medroxyprogesterone acetate 10 mg versus norethisterone 1 mg.[32] It found that medroxyprogesterone acetate versus norethisterone induced significantly fewer negative mood symptoms, and more positive mood symptoms in women without a history of premenstrual syndrome, but medroxyprogesterone acetate induced more physical symptoms, such as breast tenderness and bloating, than norethisterone.

Comment: Progestogens are seldom given alone, which makes it hard to isolate their effects. When given without oestrogen, doses of progestogens were high, the lowest dose being 20 mg medroxyprogesterone acetate daily. We found one further RCT that compared depomedroxyprogesterone acetate versus placebo, but the disparity in size between the experimental and control groups (57 *v* 12 women) and lack of detail on randomisation strategies make the results difficult to interpret.[33] Three of the placebo controlled RCTs[23–25] had crossover comparisons, which make conclusions difficult to interpret.

OPTION TIBOLONE

One RCT has found that tibolone versus placebo significantly reduces vasomotor symptoms. A second RCT found that tibolone was less effective than oestrogen/progestogen replacement therapy in reducing vasomotor symptoms. A third RCT found no significant differences in vasomotor symptoms between tibolone and oestrogen/progestogen replacement therapy. One RCT found no significant differences in vaginal dryness between tibolone and continuous hormone replacement therapy (HRT) after 48 weeks, but found a significant improvement in sexual satisfaction with tibolone versus estradiol plus noresthisterone. One RCT found that tibolone versus placebo improved sexual fantasies and arousability over 3 months. One RCT found that tibolone versus conjugated oestrogen significantly improved sexual desire and coital frequency.

Benefits: We found no systematic review. **Vasomotor symptoms:** We found three RCTs. One RCT compared tibolone with placebo[34] and two RCTs compared tibolone with oestrogen/progestogen combinations.[35,36] The first RCT (82 women with menopausal symptoms) found tibolone versus placebo significantly reduced vasomotor symptoms at 16 weeks (39% reduction in mean score; $P = 0.001$).[34] The second RCT (437 women with menopausal symptoms) compared combined oestrogen/progestogen versus tibolone. It found that the combined oestrogen/progestogen regimen versus tibolone significantly reduced hot flushes over 48 weeks ($P = 0.01$). The third RCT (235 postmenopausal women) found no significant difference in vasomotor symptoms between combined oestrogen/progestogen and tibolone at 52 weeks (figures not available).[36] **Urogenital system:** We found three RCTs.[35,37–39] The first RCT (437 women) found that tibolone versus continuous HRT significantly improved vaginal dryness ($P < 0.0001$) after 48 weeks of treatment assessed using a five point scoring system, but found no significant difference between the treatments after 48 weeks (mean score with tibolone 1.29 *v* 1.26 with combined HRT).[35] The RCT also found that tibolone versus estradiol (oestradiol) plus norethisterone improved sexual satisfaction as measured with McCoy's Sex Scale Questionnaire ($P < 0.05$).[37] The second RCT (50 women attending a university gynaecology clinic) found that tibolone versus conjugated oestrogen significantly improved sexual desire ($P < 0.05$) and coital frequency ($P < 0.05$) as measured by a questionnaire.[38] The third RCT (crossover, 38 women) found that tibolone versus placebo significantly increased sexual fantasies ($P < 0.03$) and arousability over 3 months ($P < 0.01$).[39] We found no RCTs examining the effects on urinary incontinence. **Psychological symptoms:** We found no RCTs. **Quality of life:** We found no RCTs.

Harms: We found no evidence on adverse effects from RCTs. One non-randomised controlled trial found that the main adverse effect of tibolone was breakthrough bleeding, which occurred in about 10% of users.[40] We found no good evidence of androgenic adverse effects, such as hair growth and greasiness of the skin. Two RCTs of short term use found a 33% reduction in plasma high density lipoproteins with tibolone,[41,42] although the long term effects on cardiovascular disease are unknown.

Comment: None.

OPTION PHYTO-OESTROGENS

Onc RCT found that soy protein versus no phyto-oestrogens reduces the severity but not the frequency of vasomotor symptoms at 6 weeks. One RCT found no significant differences in vasomotor symptoms between isoflavone and placebo after 12 weeks, and another RCT found that isoflavone versus placebo reduced the severity of vasomotor symptoms over 12 weeks. One RCT found that soy flour versus placebo significantly reduced mean number of weekly hot flushes after 12 weeks, but another RCT found no significant difference between soy protein and placebo in vasomotor symptoms. One RCT found no significant difference in vasomotor symptoms between soy flour versus wheat flour over 12 weeks. One RCT (94 women) found no significant difference between soy protein and placebo at 3 months for psychological, musculoskeletal, and genitourinary symptoms.

Benefits: We found no systematic review. **Vasomotor symptoms:** We found six placebo controlled RCTs.[43–48] The first RCT (58 postmenopausal women) compared soy flour (which contains phyto-oestrogens) with wheat flour for 12 weeks.[43] It found no significant difference with soy flour versus wheat flour in reduction of hot flushes at 12 weeks (40% with soy flour *v* 25% with wheat flour, $P = 0.82$).[43] The second RCT (crossover, 51 women) compared a daily dietary supplement containing no phyto-oestrogens versus a supplement containing 34 mg soy protein. It found that soy protein reduced the severity ($P < 0.001$) but not the frequency of vasomotor symptoms at 6 weeks.[44] The third RCT (unblinded crossover, 51 women) compared isoflavone 40 mg daily versus placebo. It found no significant difference between isoflavone and placebo in vasomotor symptoms assessed after 12 weeks by flush count (mean hot flush count: 3.72 in 46 women receiving placebo *v* 4.22 in 42 women receiving isoflavone; SMD –0.5, 95% CI –8.9 to +7.9) and Greene climacteric scale (mean: 7.23 in 42 women with isoflavone *v* 6.93 in 46 women with placebo; SMD –0.3, 95% CI –19.2 to +18.6; data recalculated by *Clinical Evidence*).[45] The fourth RCT (39 women) found that soy flour reduced mean flushes per week more than placebo (45% reduction with soy flour *v* 25% with placebo tablets after 12 weeks; $P < 0.01$), although it should be noted that the women taking soy extract had a greater number of vasomotor symptoms at baseline than the placebo group.[46] The fifth RCT (94 women) found no significant difference between soy protein and placebo at 3 months for vasomotor, psychological, musculoskeletal, and genitourinary symptoms as assessed using a four point subjective rating scale.[47] The sixth RCT (177 women) found that a 50 mg daily dose of an isoflavone extract versus placebo significantly reduced hot flush severity over 12 weeks (P 0.01). There was no significant difference between groups in hot flush frequency.[48] **Other symptoms:** One RCT (94 women) found no significant difference between soy protein and placebo at 3 months for psychological, musculoskeletal, and genitourinary symptoms as assessed using a four point subjective rating scale.[47] **Quality of life:** We found no RCTs.

Harms: We found no evidence of significant adverse effects.

Comment: None.

OPTION CLONIDINE

One RCT found that transdermal clonidine versus placebo reduced the number of women reporting hot flushes, and increased the number of women reporting reductions in intensity of hot flushes after 8 weeks.

Benefits: We found no systematic reviews. **Vasomotor symptoms:** One RCT (30 women) of transdermal clonidine (3.5 cm^2 patch delivering 0.1 mg of clonidine/day for 7 days) versus placebo found a significant reduction in women reporting hot flushes at 8 weeks with clonidine (women reporting reduction in number of hot flushes: 12/15 [80%] with clonidine *v* 5/14 [35%] with placebo; RR 2.4, 95% CI 1.1 to 4.7; NNT 3, 95% CI 2 to 12) and increased the number of women perceiving a reduction in severity of the hot flushes (women reporting reduction in severity of hot flushes: 11/15 [73%] with transdermal clonidine *v* 4/14 [29%] with placebo; RR 2.7, 95% CI 1.09 to 6.6; NNT 3, 95% CI 2 to 5).[49] **Psychological symptoms:** We found no RCTs. **Quality of life:** We found no RCTs.

Harms: The RCT found no significant difference in the incidence of adverse effects between placebo and treatment groups. The analysed adverse effects included transient local skin reactions (4/15 [27%] with clonidine patch *v* 3/14 [21%] with placebo; RR 1.2, 95% CI 0.34 to 4.6). No women complained of mouth dryness or drowsiness.[49]

Comment: One RCT included in previous versions of *Clinical Evidence* has now been excluded because it failed to produce a pre-crossover analysis.[50] Transdermal patches of clonidine are not widely available. Results may not be generalisable; extrapolating results to oral clonidine is potentially misleading.

OPTION TESTOSTERONE

One RCT comparing methyltestoesterone plus oestrogen versus oestrogen alone found that the addition of methyltestosterone significantly reduced hot flushes. A second RCT found no significant differences after 6 months. One crossover RCT found limited evidence that testosterone improved sexual enjoyment and libido and another RCT found no significant differences at 6 months. We found no RCTs evaluating effects of testosterone alone on other commonly experienced menopausal symptoms.

Benefits: We found no systematic review. **Vasomotor symptoms:** We found no RCTs against placebo or evaluating testosterone alone in women with menopausal symptoms. We found two RCTs of testosterone/oestrogen combinations. The first RCT (93 postmenopausal women) compared oestrogen alone (0.625 mg or 1.25 mg/day) versus oestrogen plus methyltestosterone (1.25 mg or 2.5 mg/day). It found that the addition of a small dose of methyltestosterone significantly reduced hot flushes ($P = 0.008$) and the dose of oestrogen needed to control menopausal symptoms.[51] The second RCT (40 women) found no significant difference in vasomotor symptoms with estradiol alone versus estradiol plus testosterone after 2 and 6 months of treatment (numbers not provided).[52] **Urogenital system:** We found one RCT of a testosterone/oestrogen combination and one of testosterone alone.[52,53] The first RCT (40 women) found no significant difference in level of self reported sexual enjoyment, desire, and arousal with estradiol alone versus estradiol plus testosterone at 6 months.[52] The second RCT (crossover, 53 surgically menopausal women) compared oestrogen alone, testosterone/oestrogen, testosterone and placebo.[53] It found that, while receiving both testosterone/oestrogen and testosterone alone, women reported significantly improved levels of sexual desire ($P < 0.01$), sexual arousal ($P < 0.01$), and number of sexual fantasies ($P < 0.01$) during the treatment months. **Psychological symptoms:** We found no RCTs. **Quality of life:** We found no RCTs.

Harms: We found no evidence from RCTs or other controlled studies on the incidence of androgenic adverse effects with testosterone in women with menopausal symptoms. We found evidence of adverse effects with topical testosterone in women with premalignant vulval disorders (see topical testosterone under premalignant vulval disorders, p 1965).

Comment: The crossover RCT addressing urogenital symptoms[53] did not provide an analysis prior to crossover.

OPTION ANTIDEPRESSANTS

We found no RCTs on the effects of antidepressants on menopausal symptoms.

Benefits: We found no systematic review or RCTs that specifically addressed the effects of antidepressants on menopausal symptoms or quality of life in menopausal women.

Harms: We found no evidence on adverse effects in postmenopausal women. Antidepressants as a group can cause many central nervous system adverse effects, including sedation and agitation, as well as urinary and vision problems, liver dysfunction, and cardiac dysrhythmias (see antidepressants under depressive disorders, p 951).

Comment: None.

Substantive changes

Oestrogens One new RCT comparing the effect of different doses of oestrogen on vasomotor symptoms has been added.[5] One new systematic review evaluating the effects of hormonal replacement therapy on urinary tract infections has been added;[7] conclusions remain unchanged.
Phyto-oestrogens One new RCT comparing the effects of phyto-oestrogens versus placebo on hot flushes;[48] conclusions unchanged.
Clonidine One RCT included in previous versions of *Clinical Evidence* has now been excluded because it failed to produce a pre-crossover analysis.[50]

REFERENCES

1. Porter M, Penney G, Russell D, et al. A population based survey of women's experience of the menopause. *Br J Obstet Gynaecol* 1996;103:1025–1028.
2. Hagsta TA, Janson PO. The epidemiology of climacteric symptoms. *Acta Obstet Gynecol Scand* 1986;134(suppl.):59.
3. MacLennan A, Lester S, Moore V. Oral oestrogen replacement therapy versus placebo for hot flushes. In: The Cochrane Library, Issue 2, 2001. Oxford: Update Software. Search date 2000; primary sources Medline, Embase, Cinahl, and hand searched relevant journals and conference abstracts.
4. Lopes P, Merkus HMWM, Nauman J, et al. Randomized comparison of intranasal and transdermal estradiol. *Obstet Gynecol* 2000;96:906–912.
5. Utian WH, Shoupe D, Bachmann G, et al. Relief of vasomotor symptoms and vaginal atrophy with lower doses of conjugated equine estrogens and medroxyprogesterone acetate. *Fertil Steril* 2001;75:1065–1079.
6. Cardozo L, Bachmann G, McClish D, et al. Meta-analysis of estrogen therapy in the management of urogenital atrophy in postmenopausal women: second report of the hormones and urogenital therapy committee. *Obstet Gynecol* 1998;2:722–727. Search date 1995; primary sources Medline, Excerpta Medica, Biosis, and hand searched journals.
7. Cardozo L, Lose G, McClish D, et al. A systematic review of estrogens for recurrent urinary tract infections: third report of the hormones and urogenital therapy (HUT) committee. *Int Urogynecol J Pelvic Floor Dysfunct* 2001;12:15–20. Search date 1998; primary sources Excerpta Medica, Medline, Science Citation Index, and hand-searching relevant journals.
8. Mattsson LA. Clinical experience with continuous combined transdermal hormone replacement therapy. *J Menopause* 1999;6:25–29.
9. Casper F, Petri E. Local treatment of urogenital atrophy with an estradiol-releasing vaginal ring: a comparative and a placebo-controlled multicenter study. Vaginal Ring Study Group. *Int Urogynecol J Pelvic Floor Dysfunct* 1999;10:171–176.
10. Notelovitz M, Mattox JH. Suppression of vasomotor and vulvovaginal symptoms with continuous oral 17β-estradiol. *Menopause* 2000;7:310–317.
11. Zweifel JE, O'Brien WH. A meta-analysis of the effect of HRT upon depressed mood. *Psychoneuroendocrinology* 1997;22:189–212. Search date 1995; primary sources Psychological Abstracts, Medline, and hand searches of Dissertation Abstracts International.
12. Haskell SG, Richardson ED, Horwitz RI. The effect of ORT on cognitive function in women: a critical review of the literature. *J Clin Epidemiol* 1997;50:1249–1264. Search date 1996; primary sources Medline and hand searched reference lists.
13. Polo-Kantola P, Erkkola R, Irjala K, et al. Effect of short-term transdermal estrogen replacement therapy on sleep: a randomized, double-blind crossover trial in postmenopausal women. *Fertil Steril* 1999;71:873–880.
14. Wiklund I, Karlberg J, Mattsson L. Quality of life of postmenopausal women on a regimen of transdermal estradiol therapy: a double-blind placebo-controlled study. *Am J Obstet Gynecol* 1993;168:824–830.

15. Karlberg J, Mattsson L, Wiklund I. A quality of life perspective on who benefits from estradiol replacement therapy. *Acta Obstet Gynecol Scand* 1995;74:367–372.

16. Derman RJ, Dawood MY, Stone S. Quality of life during sequential hormone replacement therapy — a placebo-controlled study. *Int J Fertil Menopausal Stud* 1995;40:73–78.

17. Hilditch JR, Lewis J, Ross AH, et al. A comparison of the effects of oral conjugated equine estrogen and transdermal estradiol-17 β combined with an oral progestin on quality of life in postmenopausal women. *Maturitas* 1996;24:177–184.

18. Norman RJ, Flight IHK, Rees MCP. Oestrogen and progestogen hormone replacement therapy for peri-menopausal and post-menopausal women: weight and body fat distribution. In: The Cochrane Library, Issue 2, 2001. Search date 1998; primary sources Medline, Embase, Current Contents, Biological Abstracts, Cinahl, citation lists, and contact with authors of eligible trials retrieved.

19. Grady D, Sawaya G. Postmenopausal hormone therapy increases risk of deep vein thrombosis and pulmonary embolism. *Am J Med* 1998;105:41–43.

20. Barrett-Connor E. Fortnightly review: hormone replacement therapy. *BMJ* 1998;317:457–461.

21. Lethaby A, Farquhar C, Sarkis A, et al. Hormone replacement therapy in postmenopausal women: endometrial hyperplasia and irregular bleeding. In: The Cochrane Library, Issue 2, 2001. Oxford: Update Software. Search date not stated; primary sources Cochrane Menstrual Disorders and Subfertility Group Trials Register, Medline, Embase, Current Contents, Biological Abstracts, Social Sciences Index, Psychlit, Cinahl, hand searched citation lists, and contact with drug companies and trials authors.

22. Collaborative Group on Hormonal Factors in Breast Cancer. Breast cancer and hormone replacement therapy: collaborative reanalysis of data from 51 epidemiological studies of 52 705 women with breast cancer and 108 411 women without breast cancer. *Lancet* 1997;350:1047–1059. Search date and primary sources not stated; the authors collected epidemiological data on 52 705 women with breast cancer and 108 411 women without breast cancer from 51 studies identified from literature searches, review articles, and discussions with colleagues.

23. Loprinzi CL, Michalak JC, Quella SK, et al. Megestrol acetate for the prevention of hot flashes. *N Engl J Med* 1994;331:347–352.

24. Aslaksen K, Frankendal B. Effect of oral MPA on menopausal symptoms on patients with endometrial carcinoma. *Acta Obstet Gynecol Scand* 1982;61:423–428.

25. Schiff I, Tulchinsky D, Cramer D, et al. Oral medroxyprogesterone in the treatment of postmenopausal symptoms. *JAMA* 1980;244:1443–1445.

26. Leonetti HB, Longo S, Anasti JN. Transdermal progesterone cream for vasomotor symptoms and postmenopausal bone loss. *Obstet Gynecol* 1999;94:225–228.

27. Reginster JY, Zartarian M, Colau JC. Influence of nomogestrel acetate on the improvement of the quality of life induced by estrogen therapy in menopausal women. *Contracept Fertil Sex* 1996;24:847–851.

28. Lobo RA, McCormick W, Singer F, et al. DMPA compared with conjugated oestrogens for the treatment of postmenopausal women. *Obstet Gynecol* 1984;63:1–5.

29. Bullock JL, Massey FM, Gambrell RD. Use of medroxyprogesterone acetate to prevent menopausal symptoms. *Obstet Gynecol* 1975;46:165–168.

30. Medical Research Council's General Practice Research Framework. Randomised comparison of oestrogen versus oestrogen plus progesterone hormone replacement therapy in women with hysterectomy. *BMJ* 1996;312:473–478.

31. Greendale GA, Reboussin BA, Hogan P, et al. Symptom relief and side effects of postmenopausal hormones: results from the postmenopausal estrogen/progestin interventions trial. *Obstet Gynecol* 1998;92:982–988.

32. Reginster JY, Zartarian M, Colau JC. Influence of nomogestrel acetate on the improvement of the quality of life induced by estrogen therapy in menopausal women. *Contracept Fertil Sex* 1996;24:847–851.

33. Bjorn I, Bixo M, Noid KS, et al. Negative mood changes during hormone replacement therapy: a comparison between two progestogens. *Am J Obstet Gynecol* 2000;183:1419–1426.

34. Kicovic PM, Cortes-Prieto J, Luisi M, et al. Placebo-controlled cross-over study of effects of Org OD14 in menopausal women. *Reproduction* 1982;6:81–91.

35. Hammar M, Christau S, Nathorst-Boos J, et al. A double-blind, randomised trial comparing the effects of tibolone and continuous combined hormone replacement therapy in postmenopausal women with menopausal symptoms. *Br J Obstet Gynaecol* 1998;105:904–911.

36. Al Azzawi F, Wahab M, Habiba M, et al. Continuous combined hormone replacement therapy compared with tibolone. *Obstet Gynecol* 1999;93:258–264.

37. Nathorst-Boos J, Hammar M. Effect on sexual life — a comparison between tibolone and a continuous estradiol-norethisterone acetate regimen. *Maturitas* 1997;26:15–20.

38. Kokcu A, Cetinkaya MB, Yanik F, et al. The comparison of effects of tibolone and conjugated estrogen- medroxyprogesterone acetate therapy on sexual performance in postmenopausal women. *Maturitas* 2000;36:75–80.

39. Laan E, Van Lunsen RHW, Everaerd W. The effects of tibolone on vaginal blood flow, sexual desire and arousability in postmenopausal women. *Climacteric* 2001;4:28–41.

40. Morris EP, Wilson POG, Robinson J, et al. Long term effects of tibolone on the genital tract in postmenopausal women. *Br J Obstet Gynaecol* 1999;106:954–959.

41. Benedek-Jaszmann LJ. Long-term placebo-controlled efficacy and safety study of Org OD14 in climacteric women. *Maturitas* 1987;1:25–33.

42. Walker ID, Davidson JF, Richards A, et al. The effect of the synthetic steroid Org OD14 on fibrinolysis and blood lipids in postmenopausal women. *Thromb Haemost* 1985;53:303–305.

43. Murkies AL, Lombard C, Stauss BJ, et al. Dietary flour supplementation decreases postmenopausal hot flushes: effect of soy and wheat. *Maturitas* 1995;21:189–195.

44. Washburn S, Burke GL, Morgan T, et al. Effect of soy protein supplementation on serum lipoproteins, blood pressure, and menopausal symptoms in perimenopausal women. *Menopause* 1999;6:7–13.

45. Baber RJ, Templeman C, Morton T, et al. Randomized placebo-controlled trial of an isoflavone supplement and menopausal symptoms in women. *Climacteric* 1999;2:85–92.

46. Scambia G, Mango D, Signorile PG, et al. Clinical effects of a standardized soy extract in postmenopausal women: a pilot study. *Menopause* 2000;7:105–111.
47. Kotsopoulos D, Dalais FS, Liang Y-L, et al. The effects of soy protein containing phytoestrogens on menopausal symptoms in postmenopausal women. *Climacteric* 2000;3:161–167.
48. Upmalis DH, Lobo R, Bradley L, et al. Vasomotor symptom relief by soy isoflavone extract tablets in postmenopausal women: a multicenter, double-blind, randomized, placebo-controlled study. *Menopause* 2000;7:236–242.
49. Nagamani M, Kelver ME, Smith ER. Treatment of menopausal hot flashes with transdermal administration of clonidine. *Am J Obstet Gynecol* 1987;156:561–565.
50. Edington RF, Chagnon JP. Clonidine (Dixarit) for menopausal flushing. *Can Med Assoc J* 1980;123:23–26.
51. Simon J, Klaiber E, Wiita B, et al. Differential effects of estrogen-androgen and estrogen-only therapy on vasomotor symptoms, gonadotropin secretion, and endogenous androgen bioavailability in postmenopausal women. *Menopause* 1999;6:138–146.
52. Dow MG, Hart DM, Forrest CA. Hormonal treatments of sexual unresponsiveness in postmenopausal women: a comparative study. *Br J Obstet Gynaecol* 1983;90:361–366.
53. Sherwin BB, Gelfand MM, Brender W. Androgen enhances sexual motivation in females: a prospective crossover study of sex steroid administration in the surgical menopause. *Psychosom Med* 1985;47:339–351.

Edward Morris
Consultant in Obstetrics and Gynaecology
Norfolk and Norwich University Hospital
Norwich
UK

Janice Rymer
Senior Lecturer/Consultant in Obstetrics and Gynaecology
Guy's, King's and St Thomas' Medical School
London
UK

Competing interests: JR has been sponsored to attend conferences by Organon, Solvay Healthcare Ltd, Wyeth Novon, Janssen-Cilag, and Servier. JR has also received research funding from Organon and consultancy fees from Organon, Wyeth, Janssen-Cilag, and Pfizer. EM has been sponsored to attend conferences and has received speaker's fees from Eli Lilly, Organon, Novo Nordisk, and Astra Zeneca.

TABLE 1 **Placebo controlled RCTs evaluating the effect of progestogens on vasomotor symptoms (see text, p 1925).**

Trial	Total participants	Comparison	Duration	Outcome	Difference	Effect
Loprinzi [23]	163	Oral medroxyprogesterone acetate 200 mg twice daily versus placebo (crossover)	9 weeks	50% reduction in daily hot flush frequency at 4 weeks (pre-crossover)	34/48 (71%) with medroxyprogesterone acetate *v* 12/49 (24)% with placebo	RR 2.9, 95% CI 1.71 to 4.89; NNT 3, 95% CI 2 to 4
Aslaksen [24]	21	Oral medroxyprogesterone acetate 100 mg twice daily versus placebo (crossover)	24 weeks	Free from hot flushes at end of study	18/21 (86%) with medroxyprogesterone acetate *v* 7/21 (33%) with placebo	RR for no flush 2.6, 95% CI 1.37 to 4.83; NNT 2, 95 % CI 2 to 3
				Free from sweating	18/21 (86%) with medroxyprogesterone acetate *v* 3/21 (14%) with placebo	RR for no sweating 6.0, 95% CI 2.1 to 17.4; NNT 2, 95% CI 1 to 2
Schiff [25]	27	Oral medroxyprogesterone acetate 20 mg daily versus placebo (crossover)	24 weeks	% reduction in hot flushes at 12 week crossover to alternative treatment	74% with medroxyprogesterone acetate *v* 26% with placebo	$P < 0.05$
Leonetti [26]	102	Transdermal progesterone cream 20 mg versus placebo	1 year	Improvement or resolution of vasomotor symptoms as determined by review of weekly symptom diaries	25/30 (83%) with transdermal progesterone *v* 26/47 (55%) with placebo	RR 1.5, 95% CI 1.1 to 2.0; NNT 4, 95% CI 2 to 9

Menorrhagia

Search date June 2002

Kirsten Duckitt

QUESTIONS

INTERVENTIONS

See glossary, p 1948

Key Messages

Treatments

- **Combined oral contraceptives** One systematic review found insufficient evidence on the effects of oral contraceptives in the treatment of menorrhagia.
- **Danazol** One systematic review found that danazol versus placebo, luteal phase oral progestogens, mefenamic acid, naproxen, or oral contraceptives reduced blood loss but that danazol versus either non-steroidal anti-inflammatory drugs or oral progestogens significantly increased adverse effects. A second review found that danazol versus placebo significantly reduced menstrual blood loss after 2–3 months.
- **Endometrial resection versus medical treatment** One systematic review and one additional RCT compared transcervical endometrial resection versus medical treatment and found conflicting results. RCTs have found complications in 0–15% of women undergoing endometrial destruction.

- **Endometrial thinning before hysteroscopic surgery** One systematic review has found that gonadotrophin releasing hormone analogues versus placebo or versus no treatment significantly reduce the duration of surgery, operative difficulty, and the risk of continuing to have moderate or heavy periods, and significantly increase the rate of postoperative amenorrhoea after 6–12 months. The review has found that gonadotrophin releasing hormone analogues versus danazol significantly increase the rate of postoperative amenorrhoea and significantly reduce the duration of surgery, but found no significant difference in operative difficulty. One small RCT found no significant difference between perioperative depot medroxyprogesterone acetate versus no perioperative hormonal treatment in amenorrhoea after 4 years' follow up.
- **Etamsylate** One RCT found limited evidence that etamsylate versus tranexamic acid or versus mefenamic acid significantly increased menstrual blood loss.
- **Hysterectomy (*v* endometrial destruction) after medical failure** Systematic reviews have found that hysterectomy versus endometrial destruction significantly reduces menstrual blood loss, significantly increases participant satisfaction at 1 year, and significantly reduces the number of women requiring further operations within 1–4 years. RCTs have found no differences between different types of hysterectomy. One large cohort study reported major or minor complications in about a third of women undergoing hysterectomy.
- **Hysteroscopic versus non-hysteroscopic endometrial destruction after medical failure** One systematic review found that hysteroscopic methods versus non-hysteroscopic methods of endometrial destruction significantly increased amenorrhoea at 12 months, although it found no significant differences with different types of hysteroscopic procedure versus each other in amenorrhoea or satisfaction rates.
- **Intrauterine progestogens** We found no RCTs comparing intrauterine progestogens versus placebo. Two systematic reviews and two subsequent RCTs found conflicting evidence about menstrual blood loss, satisfaction rates, and quality of life scores with levonorgestrel releasing intrauterine devices versus other treatments (endometrial resection, norethisterone, medical treatment, non-steroidal anti-inflammatory drugs, and hysterectomy).
- **Non-steroidal anti-inflammatory drugs** One systematic review has found that non-steroidal anti-inflammatory drugs versus placebo significantly reduce mean menstrual blood loss. One systematic review found no significant difference in menstrual blood loss with mefenamic acid versus naproxen, or with non-steroidal anti-inflammatory drugs versus oral progestogens, oral contraceptives, or progesterone releasing intrauterine devices.
- **Oral progestogens in luteal phase only** We found no RCTs comparing oral progestogens versus placebo. One systematic review has found that luteal phase oral progestogens versus danazol, tranexamic acid, or a progesterone releasing intrauterine device significantly increase mean menstrual blood loss.
- **Oral progestogens (longer cycle)** We found no RCTs comparing oral progestogens versus placebo. One RCT found no significant difference in menstrual blood loss with 21 days per cycle of oral progestogen (oral norethisterone) versus a levonorgestrel releasing intrauterine device.

- **Tranexamic acid** Systematic reviews have found that tranexamic acid versus placebo significantly reduces menstrual blood loss. One systematic review and several additional RCTs have found that tranexamic acid versus other drugs (oral progestogens, mefenamic acid, etamsylate, flurbiprofen, and diclofenac) also significantly reduces menstrual blood loss. Adverse effects of tranexamic acid include leg cramps and nausea in around a third of women. One long term observational study found no evidence to confirm the possibility of an increased risk of thromboembolism with tranexamic acid.
- **Dilatation and curettage after medical failure; gonadorelin (GnRH; gonadotrophin releasing hormone) analogues; myomectomy after medical failure** We found no RCTs on the effects of these interventions.

DEFINITION Menorrhagia is defined as heavy but regular menstrual bleeding. Idiopathic ovulatory menorrhagia is regular heavy bleeding in the absence of recognisable pelvic pathology or a general bleeding disorder. Objective menorrhagia is taken to be a total menstrual blood loss of 80 mL or more each menstruation.[1] Subjectively, menorrhagia may be defined as a complaint of regular excessive menstrual blood loss occurring over several consecutive cycles in a woman of reproductive years.

INCIDENCE/ PREVALENCE In the UK, 5% of women (aged 30–49 years) consult their general practitioner each year with menorrhagia.[2] In New Zealand, 2–4% of primary care consultations by premenopausal women are for menstrual problems.[3]

AETIOLOGY/ RISK FACTORS Idiopathic ovulatory menorrhagia is thought to be caused by disordered prostaglandin production within the endometrium.[4] Prostaglandins may also be implicated in menorrhagia associated with uterine fibroids, adenomyosis, or the presence of an intrauterine device. Fibroids have been reported in 10% of women with menorrhagia (80–100 mL/cycle) and 40% of those with severe menorrhagia (≥ 200 mL/cycle).[5]

PROGNOSIS Menorrhagia limits normal activities and causes iron deficiency anaemia in two thirds of women proved to have objective menorrhagia.[1,6,7] One in five women in the UK and one in three women in the USA will have a hysterectomy before the age of 60 years; menorrhagia is the main presenting problem in at least 50% of these women.[8–10] About 50% of the women who have a hysterectomy for menorrhagia have a normal uterus removed.[11]

AIMS To reduce menstrual bleeding; improve quality of life; and prevent or correct iron deficiency anaemia, with minimum adverse effects.

OUTCOMES Menstrual blood flow (assessed objectively [mL/cycle] or subjectively); haemoglobin concentration; quality of life; patient satisfaction; incidence of adverse drug effects; and incidence of postoperative complications. Whether a particular percentage reduction in menstrual blood loss is considered clinically important will depend on pretreatment menstrual loss and the individual woman's perception of acceptable menstrual loss.

METHODS *Clinical Evidence* update search and appraisal June 2002. The author also handsearched reference lists of non-systematic reviews and studies obtained from the initial search, and recent issues of key journals.

QUESTION What are the effects of medical treatments?

OPTION NON-STEROIDAL ANTI-INFLAMMATORY DRUGS

One systematic review has found that non-steroidal anti-inflammatory drugs versus placebo significantly reduce mean menstrual blood loss. One systematic review found no significant difference between mefenamic acid versus naproxen, or between non-steroidal anti-inflammatory drugs versus oral progestogens, oral contraceptives, or progesterone releasing intrauterine devices in menstrual blood loss.

Benefits: **Versus placebo:** We found one systematic review (search date 1996, 12 RCTs, 313 women) comparing non-steroidal anti-inflammatory drugs (NSAIDs: mefenamic acid, naproxen, meclofenamic acid, ibuprofen, and diclofenac) versus placebo.[3] Treatment was taken only during menstruation, but doses varied depending on the drug used. The review found that NSAIDs significantly reduced mean menstrual blood loss (WMD for blood loss for all NSAIDs *v* placebo −35 mL, 95% CI −43 mL to −27 mL). **Versus other NSAIDs and other drugs:** We found one systematic review (search date not stated, 16 RCTs) comparing different NSAIDs versus each other, and NSAIDs versus other drugs.[12] It found no significant difference with mefenamic acid versus naproxen, and between NSAIDs versus oral progestogens given in the luteal phase, the combined oral contraceptive, or a progesterone releasing intrauterine device in menstrual blood loss.

Harms: The reviews found that commonly reported adverse effects included headaches and gastrointestinal disturbances, including indigestion, nausea, vomiting, and diarrhoea.[3,12] These occurred in at least 50% of women taking NSAIDs in the RCTs that reported data on adverse effects, but similar levels of adverse effects were found in placebo cycles (see NSAIDs topic, p 1203).

Comment: NSAIDs have the additional benefit of relieving dysmenorrhoea (see dysmenorrhoea, p 1849).

OPTION TRANEXAMIC ACID

Two systematic reviews have found that tranexamic acid versus placebo significantly reduces menstrual blood loss. One systematic review and several additional RCTs have found that tranexamic acid versus other drugs (oral progestogens, mefenamic acid, etamsylate, flurbiprofen, and diclofenac) also significantly reduces menstrual blood loss. Adverse effects of tranexamic acid include leg cramps and nausea, which occur in about a third of women using this drug. One long term observational study found no evidence to confirm the possibility of an increased risk of thromboembolism with tranexamic acid.

Benefits: **Versus placebo:** We found two systematic reviews.[3,13] The first review (search date 1996, 5 RCTs, 153 women) found that tranexamic acid (250–500 mg 4 times daily during menstruation) versus placebo significantly reduced mean menstrual blood loss (WMD −52 mL; other results and significance presented graphically).[3] Few studies measured patient satisfaction. The second systematic review (search date 1997, 7 RCTs) identified two RCTs that compared tranexamic acid (1 g 4 times daily) or a prodrug of tranexamic acid (Kabi 2161, 1.2 g twice daily) versus placebo.[13] It found that either active drug versus placebo significantly reduced mean menstrual blood loss (WMD –94 mL, 95% CI –151 mL to –37 mL). **Versus other drugs:** We found two systematic reviews.[3,13] One review (search date 1997) found that tranexamic acid versus luteal phase oral progestogens or mefenamic acid significantly reduced mean menstrual blood loss (WMD for tranexamic acid *v* oral progestogens –111 mL, 95% CI –179 mL to –44 mL; WMD for tranexamic acid *v* mefenamic acid –73 mL, 95% CI –123 mL to –23 mL).[13] The second review (search date 1996) did not pool data from several RCTs comparing tranexamic acid versus other drugs.[3] The RCTs consistently found that tranexamic acid versus mefenamic acid, etamsylate (ethamsylate), flurbiprofen, diclofenac, and norethisterone significantly improved outcomes. One of the RCTs (46 women) identified by the review found that tranexamic versus norethisterone acid significantly reduced limitations on social activities and sex life.[14]

Harms: Nausea and leg cramps occur in a third of women taking tranexamic acid. One systematic review (search date 1997) found no increase in gastrointestinal adverse effects compared with either placebo or other drugs.[13] Isolated case reports have suggested a risk of thromboembolism associated with tranexamic acid, but a large population based study over 19 years found no evidence that this was higher than expected in the normal population.[15]

Comment: Unlike non-steroidal anti-inflammatory drugs, tranexamic acid has no effect on dysmenorrhoea.

OPTION ETAMSYLATE

One RCT found limited evidence that etamsylate versus both tranexamic acid and mefenamic acid caused a significant increase in menstrual blood loss.

Benefits: We found one systematic review (search date not stated, 4 RCTs) comparing etamsylate (ethamsylate) versus placebo, mefenamic acid, aminocaproic acid, or tranexamic acid.[16] Most results were presented as comparison with baseline. One RCT (double blind; 81 women; see comment below) identified by the review compared three treatments: etamsylate, tranexamic acid, and mefenamic acid. The RCT found that both tranexamic acid and mefenamic acid versus etamsylate significantly reduced mean menstrual blood loss (WMD tranexamic acid *v* etamsylate –97 mL, 95% CI –140 mL to –54 mL; WMD mefenamic acid *v* etamsylate –51 mL, 95% CI –96 mL to –6 mL). The review found that etamsylate achieved an overall reduction in menstrual blood loss compared with baseline of 13% (95% CI 11% to 15%), which may not be clinically significant.

Harms: The review found no significant difference in the rate of adverse effects (i.e. nausea, headaches, and dizziness) between different drug regimens, and these adverse effects seldom caused women to withdraw from studies.[16]

Comment: The RCT reported that 27% of women had withdrawn from the study before its completion, and made no adjustment for the multiple treatment comparisons involved.[17]

OPTION DANAZOL

One systematic review found that danazol versus placebo, luteal phase oral progestogens, mefenamic acid, naproxen, or oral contraceptives reduced blood loss but that danazol versus either non-steroidal anti-inflammatory drugs or oral progestogens significantly increased adverse effects. A second review found that danazol versus placebo significantly reduced menstrual blood loss after 2–3 months.

Benefits: We found two systematic reviews (search date 2001, 9 RCTs, 353 women;[18] search date 1996, 3 RCTs, 127 women; see comment below[3]) comparing danazol versus placebo, other medical treatments, or different doses of danazol.[18] **Versus placebo:** The first review identified one RCT (66 women), which compared danazol versus placebo. It found that danazol significantly improved blood loss scores from baseline whereas placebo had no significant effect at 3 months.[18] However, it was unclear how this result was calculated. The second review found that danazol (200 mg daily continuously for 2–3 months) significantly reduced mean menstrual blood loss compared with placebo (WMD danazol *v* placebo –108 mL; CI presented graphically).[3] **Versus other drugs:** The first review found that danazol reduced blood loss more than progestogens, non-steroidal anti-inflammatory drugs, and the combined oral contraceptive pill, although confidence intervals were wide. Results were based on a small number of trials, all of which were small and may have lacked power to detect clinically important effects.[18] We found no randomised trials comparing danazol with tranexamic acid or the levonorgestrel releasing intrauterine system. **Different danazol regimens:** The first review included two small trials that compared different danazol regimens: standard dose danazol (200 mg daily); lower dose danazol (100 mg daily); and a reducing dose regimen.[18] It found no significant differences in blood loss or frequency of adverse events. However, danazol (200 mg daily) versus a reducing dose regimen reduced duration of menstruation.

Harms: The first review found that adverse events were more frequent with danazol than non-steroidal anti-inflammatory drugs (OR 7.0, 95% CI 1.7 to 28.2) or progestogens (OR 4.05, 95% CI 1.6 to 10.2). However, the review reported no significant differences in adherence to treatment.[18] RCTs included in the review reported that danazol may be associated with weight gain, androgenic effects such as acne, seborrhoea, hirsutism, voice changes, and general complaints (including irritability, musculoskeletal pains, and tiredness). Hot flushes and breast atrophy can sometimes occur. Most of these adverse effects are reversible on cessation of treatment (see harms of hormonal treatments under endometriosis, p 1864, and harms of danazol under breast pain, p 1840).

Comment: The second systematic review comparing danazol versus placebo had less rigorous inclusion criteria and included two RCTs that were excluded by the first review.[3] Women using danazol may be advised to use barrier methods of contraception because of potential virilisation of the fetus if pregnancy occurs during treatment with this drug.

OPTION COMBINED ORAL CONTRACEPTIVES

One systematic review found insufficient evidence on the effects of oral contraceptives in the treatment of menorrhagia.

Benefits: We found one systematic review (search date 1997), which identified one small RCT (38 women) comparing a combined oral contraceptive versus danazol, mefenamic acid, or naproxen.[19] It found no significant difference between any of the treatments (doses not provided) but was too small to rule out a clinically important difference.

Harms: Minor adverse effects are common and include nausea, headache, breast tenderness, changes in body weight, hypertension, changes in libido, and depression.

Comment: One non-randomised controlled trial (164 women) found that a 50 mg oral contraceptive pill led to a 53% reduction in menstrual blood loss compared with baseline.[20] The trial also found that aminocaproic acid (85 women) led to a 54% reduction and tranexamic acid (172 women) led to a 47% reduction in menstrual blood loss.[20] Two longitudinal case control studies found that women taking the contraceptive pill were less likely than those not taking the pill to experience heavy menstrual bleeding or anaemia.[21,22]

OPTION ORAL PROGESTOGENS

We found no RCTs comparing oral progestogens versus placebo. One systematic review has found that luteal phase oral progestogens versus danazol, tranexamic acid, or a progesterone releasing intrauterine device cause a significant increase in mean menstrual blood loss. One RCT identified by the review found no significant difference with a longer treatment cycle of oral progestogen versus a levonorgestrel releasing intrauterine device in menstrual blood loss.

Benefits: **Versus placebo:** We found no RCTs. **Versus other drugs:** We found one systematic review (search date not stated; 7 RCTs), which compared four treatments: luteal phase oral progestogens, danazol, tranexamic acid, and progesterone releasing intrauterine devices (IUDs).[23] It found that oral progestogens versus all of the other treatments significantly increased mean menstrual blood loss (progestogen *v* danazol WMD –56 mL, 95% CI –96 mL to –15 mL; progestogen *v* tranexamic acid WMD –111 mL, 95% CI –179 mL to –44 mL; and progestogen *v* progesterone releasing IUD WMD –51 mL, 95% CI –84 mL to –18 mL). The review also found that luteal phase oral progestogens versus danazol significantly increased the number of women who reported a greater self assessed menstrual blood loss (2 RCTs: 19/28 [68%] with luteal phase progestogens *v* 8/26 [31%] with danazol; RR 2.2, 95% CI 1.2 to 4.1; NNH 2, 95% CI 1 to 9). **Longer treatment cycle:** We found one systematic review (search date not stated).[23] One RCT (48 women) identified by the review found no significant difference with a longer regimen of oral progestogen (norethisterone, 21 days/cycle) versus a levonorgestrel releasing IUD in menstrual blood loss (94 mL with oral norethisterone *v* 104 mL with levonorgestrel IUD).

Harms: Two systematic reviews (search dates not stated) found that adverse effects (including headache, breast tenderness, premenstrual symptoms, and gastrointestinal disturbances) were reported in a third to half of the women who received oral progestogens.[16,23] In the RCT that compared longer treatment cycle with oral progestogens versus a levonorgestrel releasing IUD, 44% of women felt "well" or "very well" on the treatment and only 22% elected to continue with treatment after the 3 months of the study.[23]

Comment: None.

OPTION INTRAUTERINE PROGESTOGENS

We found no systematic review or RCTs comparing intrauterine progestogens versus placebo. Two systematic reviews and two subsequent RCTs found conflicting evidence about menstrual blood loss, satisfaction rates, and quality of life scores with levonorgestrel releasing intrauterine devices versus other treatments (endometrial resection, norethisterone, medical treatment, non-steroidal anti-inflammatory drugs, and hysterectomy).

Benefits: We found no systematic review or RCTs comparing intrauterine progestogens versus placebo. Two systematic reviews (search date 1999, 5 RCTs;[24] search date 1999, 5 RCTs[25]) and two subsequent RCTs[26,27] compared intrauterine progestogens versus other treatments. The second review identified four of the RCTs in the first review and one additional RCT.[25] **Progesterone releasing intrauterine device (IUD):** The first systematic review found one RCT that compared four different treatments: a progesterone releasing IUD (65 μg daily), danazol, mefenamic acid, or norethisterone.[24] The review did not compare treatments versus each other, but found that all treatments reduced menstrual blood loss compared with baseline values. **Levonorgestrel releasing IUD:** Both reviews found four RCTs that examined the effects of levonorgestrel releasing IUDs (20 μg daily).[24] Two RCTs (60 and 70 women) identified by the reviews compared levonorgestrel releasing IUDs versus transcervical endometrial resection (see glossary, p 1948), using the pictorial blood loss assessment chart (see glossary, p 1948).[24,25] The reviews found no significant difference between treatments in mean blood loss (endometrial resection *v* levonorgestrel IUD WMD +12.2 mL, 95% CI –1.9 mL to +26.3 mL) or satisfaction rates (satisfaction rate 94% with endometrial resection *v* 85% with levonorgestrel IUD; P = NS) after 12 months.[24] The third RCT (44 women) identified by the reviews found no significant difference between norethisterone (15 mg daily, day 5 to day 26 of cycle) versus levonorgestrel releasing IUDs in reduction of blood loss or rates of satisfaction (median reduction from baseline 6 mL/cycle with norethisterone *v* 20 mL/cycle with levonorgestrel; satisfaction data not stated).[24,25] The fourth RCT (56 women) identified by the reviews found that levonorgestrel releasing IUDs versus medical treatment significantly increased the number of women who cancelled their hysterectomy after 6 months of treatment (18/28 [64%] with levonorgestrel releasing IUD *v* 4/28 [14%] with medical treatment; RR 4.5, 95% CI 1.7 to 11.6) and improved all the quality of life scores that were assessed (details of medical treatment and results not provided).[24,25] The additional RCT (35 women) identified by the second review compared three groups: a levonorgestrel releasing IUD, flurbiprofen, and tranexamic acid (see comment below).[25] It found that a levonorgestrel releasing IUD versus both other treatments significantly reduced mean menstrual flow after 12 months (mean menstrual blood flow reduction: 96% with levonorgestrel *v* 21% with flurbiprofen, $P < 0.001$; 96% with levonorgestrel *v* 44% with tranexamic acid, $P < 0.01$). The first subsequent RCT (236 women) compared a levonorgestrel releasing IUD versus hysterectomy (see comment below).[26] It found no significant difference in health related quality of life, general health state, anxiety, depression (results presented graphically; significance data not provided), or in haemoglobin concentration (135 g/L with levonorgestrel *v* 132 g/L with hysterectomy; significance data not provided), although both treatments significantly improved these outcomes compared with baseline levels after 12 months. The second subsequent RCT (59 women) found that a levonorgestrel releasing IUD versus endometrial resection significantly increased the number of women judged to have been successfully treated after 12 months (treatment success defined as a pictorial blood loss assessment chart score of ≤ 75; 26/29 [90%] with a levonorgestrel releasing IUD *v* 20/30 [67%] with endometrial resection; RR 1.35, 95% CI 1.02 to 1.78; NNT 5, 95% CI 3 to 26).[27]

Harms: Progesterone releasing IUDs were withdrawn in the UK because of concerns about increased rates of ectopic pregnancy, although the RCTs identified by the reviews did not report this adverse effect.[24,25] The first review found that most adverse effects in women using a levonorgestrel releasing IUD were typical of progestogens (bloating, weight gain, breast tenderness).[24] One RCT included in the review found that levonorgestrel releasing IUD versus transcervical endometrial resection significantly increased the number of women reporting at least one adverse effect (56% with levonorgestrel releasing IUD *v* 26% with transcervical endometrial resection; RR 2.2, 95% CI 1.2 to 3.0).[28] One further trial found that levonorgestrel releasing IUDs versus norethisterone significantly increased the proportion of women who were amenorrhoeic after 3 months of treatment (32% with levonorgestrel releasing IUDs *v* 0% with norethisterone).[29] The other main adverse effect reported with levonorgestrel releasing IUDs was irregular, although not usually heavy, menstrual bleeding.[24] RCTs looking at the contraceptive effect of levonorgestrel releasing IUDs in younger women found that during the first few months of use the total number of bleeding days (including menstrual bleeding, intermenstrual bleeding, and spotting) increased in most women.[30] However, most women bled lightly for only 1 day a month and about 15% were amenorrhoeic after 12 months.[31]

Comment: In the additional RCT (35 women) identified by the second review, the first 20 women were given a levonorgestrel releasing IUD and the following 15 women were randomised in a crossover design to receive either flurbiprofen or tranexamic acid.[25] The first subsequent RCT (236 women) found that 24/119 (20%) women who received a levonorgestrel releasing IUD underwent a hysterectomy, 10/119 (8%) women had the IUD removed, and 3/119 (3%) women were lost to follow up after 12 months.[26] The RCT also found that women had the levonorgestrel releasing IUD removed because of intermenstrual bleeding (94%), heavy bleeding (40%), hormonal symptoms (17%), or a combination of symptoms. Long term follow up on women with menorrhagia is required to assess continuation rates, satisfaction, and whether surgical treatment is avoided or just postponed. The trials that considered long term bleeding patterns were mainly in women under 40 years of age. It is not yet known whether these results can be extrapolated to older women with menorrhagia.

OPTION GONADORELIN (GONADOTROPHIN RELEASING HORMONE) ANALOGUES

We found no good evidence on the effects of gonadorelin analogues.

Benefits: We found no systematic review or RCTs.

Harms: Adverse effects are mainly caused by reduced oestrogens. Hormone replacement to counteract hypo-oestrogenism has been tried with limited success to reduce hot flushes.[32] Bone demineralisation occurs in most women after 6 months of treatment but is reversible after treatment is stopped.[33]

Comment: A few small non-randomised studies have looked at gonadorelin analogues in menorrhagia. Others have looked at their effects in women with fibroids or on thinning the endometrium before ablation or resection. Contraception whilst using these drugs is not guaranteed.[34]

QUESTION What are the effects of surgical treatments if medical treatments fail?

OPTION DILATATION AND CURETTAGE

We found no good evidence on the effects of dilatation and curettage.

Benefits: We found no systematic review or RCTs.

Harms: Observational evidence suggest that dilatation and curettage may cause adverse effects including uterine perforation and cervical laceration as well as the usual risks of general anaesthesia.[35]

Comment: Dilatation and curettage still plays a part in the investigation of menorrhagia. We found one uncontrolled cohort study (50 women) that measured blood loss before and after dilatation and curettage.[36] It found a reduction in menstrual blood loss immediately after the procedure, but losses returned to previous levels or higher by the second menstrual period.

OPTION HYSTERECTOMY

Systematic reviews have found that hysterectomy versus endometrial destruction significantly reduces menstrual blood loss and the number of women requiring further operations, and significantly increases participant satisfaction. RCTs found no difference between different types of hysterectomy versus each other in effectiveness. One large cohort study reported major or minor complications in about a third of women undergoing hysterectomy.

Benefits: **Versus endometrial destruction:** We found two systematic reviews (search dates 1996[3] and not stated[37]). Both identified the same five RCTs (708 premenopausal women) comparing hysterectomy versus endometrial destruction (transcervical endometrial resection or laser ablation [see glossary, p 1948]). The reviews found that hysterectomy significantly reduced menstrual blood loss, and significantly increased the number of women with a reduction in menstrual blood loss after 12 months (3 RCTs; 220/220 [100%] with hysterectomy *v* 191/220 [87%] with endometrial destruction; NNT 8, 95% CI 6 to 13). However, the reviews reported that the differences in reduction in blood loss between treatments seemed to narrow, possibly because of re-treatment in the endometrial ablation group or women reaching the menopause, after longer follow up. The reviews also found that endometrial ablation versus hysterectomy significantly reduced the proportion of women who were very or moderately satisfied both after 12 months (RR 0.93, 95% CI 0.89 to 0.99) and after 2 years (RR 0.87, 95% CI 0.81 to 0.94).[3,37] Two RCTs included in the reviews found no significant difference between treatments in satisfaction rates after 3 and 4 years. The reviews found that endometrial destruction versus hysterectomy significantly increased the number of women requiring repeat surgery (after 12 months, 5 RCTs: 54/386 [14%] with endometrial destruction *v* 1/320 [0.3%] with hysterectomy; RR 44.8, 95% CI 6.2 to 321.8; after 4 years, 1 RCT: 39/102 [38%] with endometrial destruction *v* 1/95 [1%] with hysterectomy; RR 36.3, 95% CI 5.1 to 259.2), but found that endometrial destruction significantly reduced the duration of surgery (–23 min), duration of hospital stay (–5 days), and time to return to work (–4.5 wks). **Different techniques:** We found no systematic review. Five small RCTs (total of 334 women) compared abdominal, vaginal, or laparoscopic hysterectomy.[38–42] They found no evidence of a difference in effectiveness or complication rates. However, operating and recovery times varied.

Harms: Large population based analyses stratified by age have found a mortality after hysterectomy for non-malignant conditions of 1/2000 women aged under 50 years.[43] When compared with endometrial destruction, hysterectomy increased the risk of sepsis, blood transfusion, urinary retention, anaemia, pyrexia, vault and wound haematoma, and cautery of hypergranulation before hospital discharge. One large, prospective cohort study of hysterectomy for non-malignant conditions found combined major and minor complication rates (mainly fever) of 25% for vaginal hysterectomy and 43% for abdominal hysterectomy.[44]

Comment: None.

OPTION ENDOMETRIAL DESTRUCTION (RESECTION OR ABLATION)

Systematic reviews have found that hysterectomy versus endometrial destruction significantly reduces menstrual blood loss and the number of women requiring further operations, and significantly increases participant satisfaction. One systematic review found that hysteroscopic methods versus non-hysteroscopic methods of endometrial destruction significantly increased amenorrhoea at 12 months although found no significant differences with different types of hysteroscopic procedure versus each other in amenorrhoea or satisfaction rates. One systematic review and one additional RCT have compared transcervical endometrial resection versus medical treatment and found conflicting results. RCTs have found that complications occur in 0–15% of women undergoing endometrial destruction.

Benefits: **Versus hysterectomy:** See benefits of hysterectomy, p 1944. **Hysteroscopic resection or ablation versus non-hysteroscopic techniques:** We found one systematic review (search date 2001, 8 RCTs, 1595 premenopausal women) that compared different methods of endometrial ablation versus each other.[47] Hysteroscopic methods included laser ablation, rollerball ablation, transcervical endometrial resection (see glossary, p 1948), and vaporising electrode ablation. Non-hysteroscopic methods included thermal uterine balloon therapy, multielectrode balloon ablation, microwave ablation (see glossary, p 1948), and heated saline. All methods reduced menstrual blood loss compared with baseline assessment. The review found that hysteroscopic ablation versus non-hysteroscopic ablation significantly increased amenorrhoea at 12 months (OR 0.76, 95% CI 0.6 to 0.9), but that hysteroscopic versus non-hysteroscopic methods significantly increased the duration of procedure (WMD 8.4 min, 95% CI 6.8 to 10.1 min), and significantly increased the number of times general anaesthesia was required (OR 6.8, 95% CI 4.5 to 10.4), although equipment failure was more likely with non-hysteroscopic methods (OR 4.1, 95% CI 1.1 to 15.0). The review found no significant differences between hysteroscopic versus non-hysteroscopic methods for satisfaction rate, inability to work, complication rate, and subsequent requirement for additional surgery. Among hysteroscopic techniques the review found that laser ablation versus transcervical resection significantly increased procedural length (WMD 9.15 min, 95% CI 7.2 to 11.1 min), and significantly increased rates of equipment failure (OR 6.0, 95% CI 1.7 to 20.9) and fluid overload (OR 5.2, 95% CI 1.5 to 18.4), although amenorrhoea rate and satisfaction rate were similar with both methods.[45] The review found that vaporising electrode ablation versus transcervical resection reduced duration of surgery (WMD 1.5 min, 95%

CI 0.35 to 2.65 min), although it found no significant difference in amenorrhoea rate, satisfaction rate, or pictorial blood loss assessment chart (see glossary, p 1948) results after 12 months. **Resection versus medical treatment:** We found one systematic review (search date 1999, 2 RCTs, 60 and 70 women) comparing levonorgestrel releasing intrauterine devices versus transcervical endometrial resection,[24] and one additional RCT (187 women) comparing medical treatment (but not levonorgestrel intrauterine devices) versus transcervical endometrial resection.[46] The systematic review found that resection reduced the blood loss from baseline more than levonorgestrel releasing intrauterine devices, but had no significant effect on mean blood loss or satisfaction rates after 12 months (for numerical results see intrauterine progestogens, p 1941). The additional RCT (187 women) found that transcervical endometrial resection versus a variety of medical treatments (not including a levonorgestrel releasing intrauterine device) significantly increased total satisfaction at 5 years (not intention to treat analysis, 144 women followed up to 5 years; AR for total satisfaction 61% with resection *v* 39% with medical management; ARR 21%, 95% CI 4% to 37%; see comment below).[46]

Harms: Intraoperative complications include uterine perforation, haemorrhage, and fluid overload from the distension medium. Immediate postoperative complications include infection, haemorrhage, and, rarely, bowel injury. Complication rates in the RCTs included in the systematic review above ranged from 0% to 15%.[47] One large prospective survey of 10 686 women undergoing endometrial destructive procedures in the UK found an immediate complication rate of 4%.[45] Intraoperative emergency procedures were performed in 1%, and two procedure related deaths occurred. Newer non-hysteroscopic methods of endometrial destruction have been evaluated only in small numbers of women and, although complications in the RCTs seem minimal, safety data for routine use are awaited.

Comment: The additional RCT (187 women) comparing transcervical endometrial resection versus a variety of medical treatments reported that at 5 years, 90% of women had stopped medical treatment or undergone other treatments in addition. At 5 years, 77% of women in the medical group received either transcervical endometrial resection or hysterectomy and 27% of women in the transcervical resection group subsequently had repeat surgery.[46]

OPTION MYOMECTOMY

We found no good evidence on the effects of myomectomy.

Benefits: We found no systematic review. **Open versus laparoscopic myomectomy:** We found no RCTs or other studies in women with menorrhagia that measured menstrual blood loss. **Hysteroscopic myomectomy:** We found no RCTs.

Harms: Intraoperative complications for hysteroscopic myomectomy are similar to those with endometrial destructive procedures that use a hysteroscope (see harms of endometrial destruction, p 1946). The main complication of open myomectomy is haemorrhage, making a hysterectomy necessary.

Comment: One uncontrolled study (15 women, 10 with additional symptoms) reported objective measures of menstrual blood loss.[48] Mean menstrual blood loss, assessed preoperatively and at 3 and 6 months postoperatively, was significantly reduced (261 mL at baseline, 76 mL at 3 months, and 57 mL at 6 months). The study found a significant reduction in pain scores and menstrual duration, despite the fibroids removed measuring only 1–4 cm. RCTs are needed that use objective assessment of menstrual blood loss. This is especially important in the evaluation of surgical procedures because of the greater difficulty in blinding.

QUESTION What are the effects of endometrial thinning before hysteroscopic surgery?

One systematic review has found that gonadorelin (gonadotrophin releasing hormone) analogues versus placebo or no treatment significantly reduce the duration of surgery, operative difficulty, and the risk of continuing to have moderate or heavy periods, and significantly increase the rate of postoperative amenorrhoea. The review has found that gonadotrophin releasing hormone analogues versus danazol significantly increase the rate of postoperative amenorrhoea and significantly reduce the duration of surgery, but found no significant difference in operative difficulty. One small RCT found no significant difference between perioperative depot medroxyprogesterone acetate versus no perioperative hormonal treatment in amenorrhoea after 4 years follow up.

Benefits: We found one systematic review (search date not stated, 8 RCTs, 946 women) evaluating medical treatment to thin the endometrium before hysteroscopic surgery for menorrhagia.[49] **Gonadorelin (gonadotrophin releasing hormone [GnRH]) analogues versus placebo/no treatment:** Four RCTs (566 women) identified by the review found that goserelin versus placebo or no treatment significantly reduced the duration of surgery (WMD –4.7 min, 95% CI –6.1 min to –3.2 min), and significantly reduced operative difficulty (RR of encountering difficulty during procedure 0.32, 95% CI 0.22 to 0.46).[49] The review also found that goserelin versus placebo or no treatment significantly increased the rate of postoperative amenorrhoea, and significantly reduced the risk of continuing to have moderate or heavy periods (RR 0.74, 95% CI 0.59 to 0.92) after 6–12 months.[49] The review found no significant difference in patient satisfaction or the likelihood of undergoing further surgery. **GnRH analogues versus danazol:** Three RCTs (340 women) identified by the review found that gonadorelin analogues (goserelin or decapeptyl) versus danazol significantly increased the rate of postoperative amenorrhoea (RR 1.57, 95% CI 1.06 to 2.33; NNT 5.9) and significantly reduced the duration of surgery (2 RCTs: WMD –3.9 min, 95% CI –6.1 min to –1.7 min), but found no significant difference in operative difficulty (RR 0.68, 95% CI 0.31 to 1.51).[49] **Progestogens versus no treatment:** One RCT (50 women undergoing endometrial resection in the postmenstrual phase) compared depot medroxyprogesterone acetate (150 mg im 6 wks prior to surgery and immediately after surgery) versus no hormonal medication.[50] It found no significant differences between treatments for amenorrhoea or spotting of blood after 4 years' follow up (amenorrhoea: AR 28% with depot progestogen *v* 40% without, P = 0.55; spotting: AR 16% with depot progestogen *v* 24% without, P = 0.72). **Progestogens versus other medical treatments:** One RCT (40 women) compared four groups: progestogens, gonadorelin analogues, danazol, and no treatment. The trial was too small to allow firm conclusions to be drawn.[49]

Harms: The review found no significant difference with goserelin versus placebo or no treatment in the number of women with intraoperative uterine perforations (2/266 [0.8%] with goserelin *v* 1/275 [0.4%] with no treatment/placebo; RR 2.01, 95% CI 0.19 to 22.67).[49] The review found that goserelin versus danazol significantly increased the number of women reporting hot flushes, reduced libido, depression, and vaginal dryness. Oily skin, hirsutism, and weight gain were significantly more common with danazol. The review also found that danazol versus goserelin significantly increased the number of women who withdrew from RCTs because of adverse effects (11/139 [8%] with danazol *v* 1/566 [0.2%] with goserelin; RR 44.80, 95% CI 5.83 to 344).

Comment: None of the RCTs included in the review used objective measures of postoperative menstrual blood loss.[49] Rates of withdrawal or loss to follow up were low in all studies.

GLOSSARY

Laser ablation A hysteroscopic procedure in which endometrium is destroyed under direct vision by a laser beam.

Microwave endometrial ablation A procedure in which a microwave probe is passed through the cervix into the uterine cavity. When activated it is moved slowly from side to side over the whole surface of the uterine cavity in order to destroy the endometrium.

Multielectrode balloon ablation (Vesta system) A procedure in which an inflatable device with electrodes on the outside is inserted into the uterine cavity through the cervix. The electrodes make contact with the endometrium and cause necrosis.

Pictorial blood loss assessment chart (PBAC) A semi-quantitative assessment of menstrual blood loss based on women filling in the number and appearances of their sanitary protection and size of blood clots on a pictorial chart. Scores greater than or equal to 100 equate to a menstrual blood loss of greater than or equal to 80 mL.[51]

Rollerball ablation A hysteroscopic procedure in which endometrium is destroyed under direct vision by diathermy applied by a rollerball.

Thermal uterine balloon therapy A procedure in which a balloon catheter is passed through the cervix into the uterine cavity. The balloon is then filled with fluid, which is heated to about 87 °C, and left for 8 minutes. This causes necrosis of the endometrium.

Transcervical endometrial resection A hysteroscopic procedure in which endometrium is removed under direct vision by using an electrosurgical loop.

Substantive changes

Danazol One new systematic review;[18] conclusions unchanged.

Endometrial destruction (resection or ablation) One new systematic review;[47] it found that women undergoing hysteroscopic ablation were more likely to have amenorrhoea at 12 months' follow up than women having non-hysteroscopic ablation.

Endometrial resection versus medical treatment Longer term follow up of existing RCT;[46] conclusions unchanged.

Preoperative endometrial thinning One new RCT;[50] found no evidence that perioperative depot medroxyprogesterone acetate improved amenorrhoea rates compared with no hormonal therapy.

REFERENCES

1. Hallberg L, Hogdahl A, Nilsson L, et al. Menstrual blood loss – a population study: variation at different ages and attempts to define normality. *Acta Obstet Gynecol Scand* 1966;45:320–351.
2. Vessey MP, Villard-Mackintosh L, McPherson K, et al. The epidemiology of hysterectomy: findings in a large cohort study. *Br J Obstet Gynaecol* 1992;99:402–407.
3. Working Party of the National Health Committee New Zealand. *Guidelines for the management of heavy menstrual bleeding*. Wellington: Ministry of Health, 1998. (Available from The Ministry of Health, 133 Molesworth Street, PO Box 5013, Wellington, New Zealand.) Search date 1996; primary sources Medline, Embase, Current Contents, Biological Abstracts, Social Sciences Index, Psychlit, and Cinahl.
4. Smith SK, Abel MH, Kelly RW, et al. A role for prostacyclin (PGI_2) in excessive menstrual bleeding. *Lancet* 1981;1:522–524.
5. Rybo G, Leman J, Tibblin R. Epidemiology of menstrual blood loss. In: Baird DT, Michie EA, eds. *Mechanisms of menstrual bleeding*. New York: Raven Press, 1985:181–193.
6. Alexander DA, Naji AA, Pinion SB, et al. Randomised trial comparing hysterectomy with endometrial ablation for dysfunctional uterine bleeding: psychiatric and psychosocial aspects. *BMJ* 1996;312:280–284.
7. Coulter A, Peto V, Jenkinson C. Quality of life and patient satisfaction following treatment for menorrhagia. *Fam Pract* 1994;11:394–401.
8. Coulter A, McPherson K, Vessey M. Do British women undergo too many or too few hysterectomies? *Soc Sci Med* 1988;27:987–994.
9. Pokras R, Hufnagel VG. *Hysterectomy in the United States, 1965–84*. Washington, DC: Public Health Service, 1987:87–1753.
10. Coulter A, Kelland J, Long A. The management of menorrhagia. *Effective Health Care Bull* 1995;9:1–14.
11. Clarke A, Black N, Rowe P, et al. Indications for and outcome of total abdominal hysterectomy for benign disease: a prospective cohort study. *Br J Obstet Gynaecol* 1995;102:611–620.
12. Lethaby A, Augood C, Duckitt K. Nonsteroidal anti-inflammatory drugs for heavy menstrual bleeding (Cochrane review). In: The Cochrane Library, Issue 2, 2002. Oxford: Update Software. Search date not stated; primary sources Cochrane Menstrual Disorders and Subfertility Group trials register, Medline, Embase, Psychlit, Current Contents, Biological Abstracts, Social Sciences Index, Cinahl, reference lists, and drug companies.
13. Lethaby A, Farquhar C, Cooke I. Antifibrinolytics for heavy menstrual bleeding (Cochrane review). In: The Cochrane Library, Issue 2, 2002. Oxford: Update Software. Search date 1997; primary sources Cochrane Menstrual Disorders and Subfertility Group trials register, Medline, Embase, and hand searches of reference lists from experts and drug companies.
14. Preston JT, Cameron IT, Adams EJ, et al. Comparative study of tranexamic acid and norethisterone in the treatment of ovulatory menorrhagia. *Br J Obstet Gynaecol* 1995;102:401–406.
15. Rybo G. Tranexamic acid therapy is effective treatment in heavy menstrual bleeding: clinical update on safety. *Ther Adv* 1991;4:1–8.
16. Coulter A, Kelland J, Peto V, et al. Treating menorrhagia in primary care. An overview of drug trials and a survey of prescribing practice. *Int J Technol Assess Health Care* 1995;11:456–471. Search date not stated; primary sources Medline and Embase.
17. Bonnar J, Sheppard BL. Treatment of menorrhagia during menstruation: randomised controlled trial of etamsylate, mefenamic acid, and tranexamic acid. *BMJ* 1996;313:579–582.
18. Beaumont H, Augood C, Duckitt K, et al. Danazol for heavy menstrual bleeding (Cochrane Review). In: The Cochrane Library, Issue 2, 2002. Oxford: Update Software. Search date 2001; primary sources Medline, Embase, Current Contents, CINAHL, National Research Register, Menstrual Disorders and Subfertility Group's Specialised Register, reference lists and authors contacted.
19. Iyer V, Farquhar C, Jepson R. Oral contraceptive pills for heavy menstrual bleeding. In: The Cochrane Library, Issue 2, 2002. Oxford: Update Software. Search date 1997; primary source Cochrane Register of Controlled Trials.
20. Nilsson L, Rybo G. Treatment of menorrhagia. *Am J Obstet Gynecol* 1971;5:713–720.
21. Ramcharan S, Pellegrin FA, Ray MR, et al. The Walnut Creek contraceptive drug study – a prospective study of the side effects of oral contraceptives. Vol III. An interim report: a comparison of disease occurrence leading to hospitalization or death in users and nonusers of oral contraceptives. *J Reprod Med* 1980;25:345–372.
22. Royal College of General Practitioners. *Oral contraceptives and health*. London: Pitman Medical, 1974.
23. Lethaby A, Irvine G, Cameron I. Cyclical progestogens for heavy menstrual bleeding (Cochrane review). In: The Cochrane Library, Issue 2, 2002. Oxford: Update Software. Search date not stated; primary sources Cochrane Menstrual Disorders and Subfertility Group trials register, Medline, Embase, Psychlit, Current Contents, Biological Abstracts, Social Sciences Index, Cinahl, and reference lists.
24. Lethaby AE, Cooke I, Rees M. Progesterone/progestogen intrauterine releasing systems versus placebo or any other medication for heavy menstrual bleeding (Cochrane review). In: The Cochrane Library, Issue 2, 2002. Oxford: Update Software. Search date 1999; primary sources Cochrane Menstrual Disorders and Subfertility Group trials register, Medline, Embase, and experts contacted.
25. Stewart A, Cummins C, Gold L, et al. The effectiveness of the levonorgestrel-releasing intrauterine system in menorrhagia: a systematic review. *Br J Obstet Gynaecol* 2001;108:74–86. Search date 1999; primary sources Medline, Cinahl, Embase, Cochrane Library, Best Evidence, BMJ website archive facility, various internet search engines, hand searching of the *Journal of Family Planning* and *The Diplomate*, and personal

contact with Schering Health Care Ltd and the Royal College of Obstetricians and Gynaecologists Audit Unit.
26. Hurskainen R, Teperi J, Rissanen P, et al. Quality of life and cost-effectiveness of levonorgestrel-releasing intrauterine system versus hysterectomy for treatment of menorrhagia: a randomised trial. *Lancet* 2001;357:273–277.
27. Istre O, Trolle B. Treatment of menorrhagia with the levonorgestrel intrauterine system versus endometrial resection. *Fertil Steril* 2001;76:304–309.
28. Crosignani PG, Vercellini P, Mosconi P, et al. Levonorgestrel-releasing intrauterine device versus hysteroscopic endometrial resection in the treatment of dysfunctional uterine bleeding. *Obstet Gynecol* 1997;90:257–263.
29. Irvine GA, Campbell-Brown MB, Lumsden MA, et al. Randomised comparative study of the levonorgestrel intrauterine system and norethisterone for the treatment of idiopathic menorrhagia. *Br J Obstet Gynaecol* 1998;105:592–598.
30. Long-acting progestogen-only contraception. *Drug Ther Bull* 1996;34:93–96.
31. Luukkainen T. The levonorgestrel-releasing IUD. *Br J Fam Plann* 1993;19:221–224.
32. Thomas EJ, Okuda KJ, Thomas NM. The combination of a depot gonadotrophin releasing hormone agonist and cyclical hormone replacement therapy for dysfunctional uterine bleeding. *Br J Obstet Gynaecol* 1991;98:1155–1159.
33. Eldred JM, Haynes PJ, Thomas EJ. A randomized double blind placebo controlled trial of the effects on bone metabolism of the combination of nafarelin acetate and norethisterone. *Clin Endocrinol* 1992;37:354–359.
34. Pickersgill A, Kingsland CR, Garden AS, et al. Multiple gestation following gonadotrophin releasing hormone therapy for the treatment of minimal endometriosis. *Br J Obstet Gynaecol* 1994;101:260–262.
35. Smith JJ, Schulman H. Current dilatation and curettage practice: a need for revision. *Obstet Gynecol* 1985;65:516–518.
36. Haynes PJ, Hodgson H, Anderson AB, et al. Measurement of menstrual blood loss in patients complaining of menorrhagia. *Br J Obstet Gynaecol* 1977;84:763–768.
37. Lethaby A, Sheppers S, Cooke I, et al. Endometrial resection and ablation versus hysterectomy for heavy menstrual bleeding. In: The Cochrane Library, Issue 2, 2002. Oxford: Update Software. Search date not stated; primary sources Cochrane Menstrual Disorders and Subfertility Group trials register, Medline, Embase, Psychlit, Current Contents, Biological Abstracts, Social Sciences Index, and Cinahl.
38. Phipps JH, John M, Nayak S. Comparison of laparoscopically assisted vaginal hysterectomy and bilateral salpingo-oophorectomy with conventional abdominal hysterectomy and bilateral salpingo-oophorectomy. *Br J Obstet Gynaecol* 1993;100:698–700.
39. Raju KS, Auld BJ. A randomised prospective study of laparoscopic vaginal hysterectomy versus abdominal hysterectomy each with bilateral salpingo-oophorectomy. *Br J Obstet Gynaecol* 1994;101:1068–1071.
40. Richardson RE, Bournas N, Magos AL. Is laparoscopic hysterectomy a waste of time? *Lancet* 1995;345:36–41.
41. Summitt RL Jr, Stovall TG, Lipscomb GH, et al. Randomized comparison of laparoscopy-assisted vaginal hysterectomy with standard vaginal hysterectomy in an outpatient setting. *Obstet Gynecol* 1992;80:895–901.
42. Langebrekke A, Eraker R, Nesheim B, et al. Abdominal hysterectomy should not be considered as primary method for uterine removal. *Acta Obstet Gynecol Scand* 1996;75:404–407.
43. Carlson KJ. Outcomes of hysterectomy. *Clin Obstet Gynecol* 1997;40:939–946.
44. Dicker RC, Greenspan JR, Strauss LT, et al. Complications of abdominal and vaginal hysterectomy among women of reproductive age in the United States. The Collaborative Review of Sterilization. *Am J Obstet Gynecol* 1982;144:841–848.
45. Overton C, Hargreaves J, Maresh M. A national survey of the complications of endometrial destruction for menstrual disorders: the MISTLETOE study. Minimally invasive surgical techniques — laser, endothermal or endoresection. *Br J Obstet Gynaecol* 1997;104:1351–1359.
46. Cooper KG, Jack SA, Parkin DE, et al. Five-year follow up of women randomised to medical management or transcervical resection of the endometrium for heavy menstrual loss: clinical and quality of life outcomes. *Br J Obstet Gynaecol* 2001;108:1222–1228.
47. Lethaby A, Hickey M. Endometrial destruction techniques for heavy menstrual bleeding (Cochrane Review). In: The Cochrane Library, Issue 2, 2002. Oxford: Update Software. Search date 2001; primary sources Conchrane Controlled Trials Register, Medline, Embase, Current Contents, Biological Abstracts, Psyclit, Cinahl, Register of Cochrane Menstrual Disorders and Subfertility Group, reference lists of articles, contacted pharmaceutical companies, and experts in the field.
48. Broadbent JAM, Magos AL. Menstrual blood loss after hysteroscopic myomectomy. *Gynaecol Endoscop* 1995;4:41–44.
49. Sowter MC, Singla AA, Lethaby A. Pre-operative endometrial thinning agents before hysteroscopic surgery for heavy menstrual bleeding (Cochrane review). In: The Cochrane Library, Issue 2, 2002. Oxford: Update Software. Search date not stated; primary sources Cochrane Menstrual Disorders and Subfertility Group trials register, Medline, Embase, Psychlit, Biological Abstracts, Cinahl, reference lists, authors of conference abstracts, Zeneca Pharmaceuticals, and Sanofi Winthrop.
50. Kriplani A, Manchanda R, Monga D, et al. Depot medroxy progesterone acetate: a poor preparatory agent for endometrial resection *Gynecologic & Obstetric Investigation* 2001;52:180–183.
51. Higham JM, O'Brien PMS, Shaw RW. Assessment of menstrual blood loss using a pictorial chart. *Br J Obstet Gynaecol* 1990;97:734–739.

Kirsten Duckitt
Clinical Lecturer
John Radcliffe Hospital
Oxford
UK

Competing interests: None declared.

Ovarian cancer

Search date February 2002

Hani Gabra, Charles Redman, and Jennifer Byrom

QUESTIONS

INTERVENTIONS

See glossary, p 1961.

Key Messages

- We found insufficient evidence on the effects of any treatments on quality of life.

Surgical treatments for advanced ovarian cancer

- **Primary surgery plus chemotherapy versus chemotherapy alone** We found no RCTs.
- **Primary surgery versus no surgery** We found no RCTs.
- **Routine interval debulking after primary surgery plus chemotherapy** One RCT found that interval debulking after primary surgery plus chemotherapy improved overall survival over about 3.5 years. A second RCT found that interval debulking had no significant effect on survival, but it was probably underpowered to detect a clinically important effect.

- **Routine second look surgery** Two RCTs found no evidence that routine second look surgery improves overall survival compared with watchful waiting in women undergoing chemotherapy after primary surgery for advanced ovarian cancer.

Cytotoxic chemotherapy for advanced ovarian cancer

- **Adding paclitaxel to platinum regimens** One systematic review and one additional RCT have found that adding paclitaxel to platinum based chemotherapy improves progression free survival and overall survival after primary surgery for advanced ovarian cancer.
- **Adding platinum to chemotherapy regimens** One systematic review has found that adding platinum to any non-platinum regimen significantly improves survival, particularly if platinum is added to a combination regimen.
- **Carboplatin plus paclitaxel versus carboplatin plus docetaxel** We found no RCTs of sufficient quality comparing the effects of carboplatin plus paclitaxel versus carboplatin plus docetaxel.
- **Combination platinum regimens versus combination non-platinum regimens** Seven RCTs have compared combination platinum regimens versus many different non-platinum combination regimens. Most RCTs have found that platinum regimens improve outcomes, although benefits and harms depend on the regimens being compared. None have found that platinum significantly decreased progression free survival or overall survival.
- **Combination platinum regimens versus single agent platinum regimens** One systematic review and three additional RCTs found no evidence that combination platinum based regimens improved progression free or overall survival compared with single agent platinum regimens.
- **Paclitaxel plus cisplatin versus paclitaxel plus carboplatin** One RCT found no significant difference in progression free or overall survival between paclitaxel plus cisplatin versus paclitaxel plus carboplatin, although it may have lacked power to exclude clinically important effects.

DEFINITION Ovarian tumours are classified according to the assumed cell type of origin (surface epithelium, stroma, or germ cells). Most malignant ovarian tumours (85–95%) are derived from the epithelium of the ovarian surface, and are thus termed epithelial.[1] These can be further grouped into histological types (serous, mucinous, endometroid, and clear cell). Epithelial ovarian cancer is staged using the FIGO classification (see web extra table A at www.clinicalevidence.com). This review concerns only advanced epithelial ovarian cancer, which is regarded as FIGO stages II–IV.

INCIDENCE/ PREVALENCE The worldwide annual incidence of ovarian cancer exceeds 140 000.[2] Rates vary between countries. Differences in reproductive patterns, including age of menarche and menopause, gravidity, breast feeding, and use of the oral contraceptive pill may contribute to this variation. Rates are highest in Scandinavia, Northern America, and the UK, and lowest for Africa, India, China, and Japan.[3] In the UK, ovarian cancer is the fourth most common malignancy in women and is the leading cause of death from gynaecological cancers, with a lifetime risk of about 2%.[4] In the UK, the incidence was 5174 in 1988[5] and 6880 in 1998.[6] The incidence of ovarian cancer seems to be stabilising in some other countries, and in more affluent countries (Finland, Denmark, New Zealand, and the USA) rates are declining.

AETIOLOGY/ RISK FACTORS	Risk factors include increasing age, family history of ovarian cancer, low fertility, use of fertility drugs, and low parity.[7–11] Case control studies found that using the combined oral contraceptive pill for more than 5 years was associated with a 40% reduction in the risk of ovarian cancer.[3,7,12,13]
PROGNOSIS	Over 80% of women present with advanced disease, and the overall 5 year survival rates are poor (< 30%).[6] For advanced disease the major independent prognostic factors seem to be stage, and residual tumour mass after surgery.
AIMS	To prolong survival and reduce disability, and to minimise adverse effects.
OUTCOMES	Mortality; disease free survival; disease related symptoms; quality of life; adverse effects of treatment.
METHODS	*Clinical Evidence* search and appraisal February 2002. RCTs with greater than 20% withdrawal or with less than 18 month's follow up were excluded.

QUESTION What are the effects of surgery for ovarian cancer that is advanced at first presentation New

OPTION PRIMARY SURGERY

We found no RCTs in women with advanced ovarian cancer comparing the effects of primary surgery versus no surgery, or primary surgery plus chemotherapy versus chemotherapy alone.

Benefits: **Primary surgery alone versus no surgery:** We found one systematic review (search date not stated, published 1995), which found no RCTs comparing primary debulking (see glossary, p 1961) surgery versus no surgery.[1] We found no subsequent RCT. **Primary surgery plus chemotherapy versus chemotherapy alone:** We found no systematic review and no RCT.

Harms: We found no RCT.

Comment: None.

OPTION ROUTINE SECOND LOOK SURGERY

Two RCTs found no significant difference in survival with routine second look surgery versus watchful waiting in women undergoing chemotherapy after primary surgery for advanced ovarian cancer.

Benefits: **Primary surgery plus chemotherapy with or without second look surgery:** We found two RCTs in women with advanced ovarian cancer.[14,15] The first RCT (102 women in complete remission after primary debulking (see glossary, p 1961) surgery and first line chemotherapy of cisplatin plus cyclophosphamide or doxorubicin plus cyclophosphamide every 3 wks for 5 cycles) compared second look surgery (see glossary, p 1961), which included visual inspection and biopsy, versus watchful waiting.[14] Complete remission before trial entry was confirmed by clinical and biochemical assessment, computed tomography, and laparoscopy. The RCT found no significant difference between interventions for overall survival after 60 months (AR for survival 65% with second look laparotomy *v* 78% with watchful waiting; CI not provided; P = 0.14). The second RCT (166 women, after primary debulking surgery plus cisplatin every 3 wks for 5 cycles) compared three groups.[15] One group had a second look laparotomy (which included visual inspection, cytology of any free fluid, total hysterectomy, bilateral salpingo-oophorectomy, omentectomy, and multiple biopsies, followed by oral chlorambucil [12 courses of 0.2 mg/kg daily for 14 days]). The second group received second look laparotomy and pelvic irradiation. The third group received chlorambucil without second look surgery. The RCT found no significant difference among groups for overall survival after 46 months (median survival time 21 months, 95% CI 11 months to 31 months with second look laparotomy plus chlorambucil; 15 months, 95% CI 11 months to 19 months with second look laparotomy and pelvic irradiation; 17 months, 95% CI 8 months to 26 months with chlorambucil without second look surgery).

Harms: The first RCT did not report harms.[14] The second RCT reported that one woman died of a cerebrovascular accident 10 days after second look laparotomy.[15] Other reported surgical complications were ileus, wound infection, urinary and respiratory tract infection, and anaemia (rates not reported).

Comment: None.

OPTION ROUTINE INTERVAL DEBULKING

One RCT found that interval debulking after primary surgery plus chemotherapy versus continued chemotherapy without debulking significantly improved overall survival over about 3.5 years. A second RCT found that interval debulking had no significant effect on survival, but it was probably underpowered to detect a clinically important effect

Benefits: **Primary surgery plus chemotherapy with or without interval debulking:** We found two RCTs.[16,17] The first RCT (319 women with non-progressive disease after 3 cycles of cisplatin and cyclophosphamide chemotherapy after primary surgery) compared interval debulking (see glossary, p 1961) versus continued chemotherapy.[16] All women had residual tumour diameter of greater than 1 cm after primary surgery. It found that interval debulking significantly improved progression free and overall survival after a median of 3.5 years (278 women; median progression free survival 18 months with interval debulking *v* 13 months without, P = 0.01; median overall survival 26 months *v* 20 months, P = 0.01; adjusted HR for death for interval debulking *v* no interval debulking 0.77, 95% CI 0.50 to 0.90).[16] The second RCT (79 women with advanced ovarian cancer with residual tumour of at least 2 cm maximal diameter after primary surgery) compared interval debulking after primary surgery and response to chemotherapy versus continued chemotherapy without interval debulking.[17] Chemotherapy consisted of either cisplatinum plus cyclophosphamide or cisplatinum plus bleomycin plus doxorubicin followed by escalating cyclophosphamide. Of the women allocated to interval debulking, 11 had non-responsive or progressive disease after three cycles of chemotherapy and were excluded from surgery. Interval debulking (which could include hysterectomy, oophorectomy, and omentectomy) was undertaken at a median of 13 weeks after primary surgery. The RCT found no significant difference between interval debulking versus no interval debulking for overall survival after 48 months' median follow up, but may have lacked power to exclude a clinically important effect (intention to treat analysis: median survival 15 months with interval debulking *v* 12 months without; HR 0.71, 95% CI 0.44 to 1.33).

Harms: The second RCT found that among 26 women who received interval debulking, 11 received a blood transfusion, two developed intestinal fistulae, and one developed a deep vein thrombosis.[17]

Comment: None.

QUESTION **What are the effects of cytotoxic chemotherapy for ovarian cancer that is advanced at first presentation?** New

OPTION **PLATINUM BASED REGIMENS**

One systematic review has found that adding platinum to a range of non-platinum regimens significantly improves survival after surgery in women with advanced ovarian cancer. However, it found no significant benefit in the subgroup of RCTs which added platinum to single-agent non-platinum regimens. Seven additional RCTs have compared combination platinum regimens with many different non-platinum combination regimens. Most of these have found that platinum regimens improve outcomes, although benefits and harms depend on the regimens being compared. None have found that platinum significantly decreases progression free or overall survival. One systematic review and three additional RCTs found no evidence that combination platinum based regimens improved progression free or overall survival compared with single agent platinum regimens.

Benefits: **Platinum versus non-platinum chemotherapy:** We found one systematic review (search date 1998, 37 RCTs)[18] and six additional RCTs[19–24] in women with advanced ovarian cancer. The review identified 11 RCTs (1329 women with advanced ovarian cancer) comparing single agent non-platinum chemotherapy versus platinum based combination chemotherapy. It found no significant difference between these types of regimen for overall survival (9 RCTs; HR 0.93, 95% CI 0.83 to 1.05; P = 0.23; estimated ARR for 2 and 5 year survival with single agent non-platinum versus combination platinum +3%, 95% CI –2% to +7%). The review also identified nine RCTs (1704 women) assessing the effects of adding platinum to a chemotherapy regimen. Meta-analysis found that adding platinum to any regimen significantly reduced the risk of death (death with platinum added to any regimen, HR 0.88, 95% CI 0.79 to 0.98; estimated ARR of death 5%, 95% CI 1% to 8% at 2 and 5 years). Within this group, adding platinum to combination regimens also reduced risk of death (HR 0.85, 95% CI 0.74 to 0.97). However, meta-analysis of RCTs that added platinum to a single agent found no significant effect on risk of death, although results of trials were statistically heterogeneous (death with platinum added to single agent, HR 0.93, 95% CI 0.78 to 1.10).[18] The first additional RCT (171 women) compared a single platinum agent (cisplatin, 75 mg/m^2 every 28 days for 6 cycles) versus a single non-platinum agent (thiotepa, 60 mg loading dose im followed by 10 cycles of 30 mg im every 14 days).[19] It found that cisplatin versus thiotepa significantly improved progression free survival after 110 months' median follow up (median progression free survival 10.5 months with cisplatin *v* 6.3 months with thiotepa, P = 0.025; HR for thiotepa *v* cisplatin 1.64, 95% CI 1.17 to 2.30). Cisplatin versus thiotepa did not significantly improve overall survival (median overall survival 20 months with cisplatin *v* 14 months with thiotepa, P = 0.155; AR for survival at 8 years 10.6% *v* 7.4%, CI and P value not stated). The second additional RCT (228 women) found that adding cisplatin (50 mg/m^2 every 3–4 wks) to 12 cycles of doxorubicin plus cyclophosphamide with or without Bacillus Calmette-Guerin significantly improved overall survival (median survival 17.8 months with cisplatin *v* 9.9 months without cisplatin; P < 0.005).[20] The third RCT (169 women) compared 12 cycles at four weekly intervals of cisplatinum (60 mg/m^2/cycle) plus melphalan (1 mg/kg/cycle) versus hexamethylmelamine, doxorubicin, and cyclophosphamide.[21] It found no significant difference between treatments for overall survival (153 women; median survival 29.6 months with platinum *v* 26.4 months without; P value not stated) but the trial may have lacked power to exclude a clinically important difference.[21] The fourth RCT (120 women) similarly found no significant difference between hexamethylmelamine, doxorubicin, and cyclophosphamide versus cisplatin, doxorubicin, and cyclophosphamide for overall survival after 10 years (median survival 126 months without platinum *v* 138 months with platinum; P = 0.54).[22] The fifth RCT (83 women) compared 12 cycles at four weekly intervals of doxorubicin (60 mg/m^2) plus cyclophosphamide (750 mg/m^2) combined with either cisplatin (80 mg/m^2) or with vincristine (1.4 mg/m^2). It found that the platinum based regimen increased progression free and overall survival compared with the non-platinum regimen after 5 years (median progression free survival 14 months with platinum *v* 10 months without platinum, P < 0.05; median overall survival 24 months with platinum *v* 15 months without platinum, P < 0.01).[23] The sixth RCT (186 women) compared hexamethylmelamine, cyclophosphamide, methotrexate, and 5-fluorouracil versus a regimen that alternated between cyclophosphamide plus hexamethylmelamine and doxorubicin plus cisplatin.[24] It found that the platinum versus the non-platinum regimen improved progression free and overall survival after about 50 months (median progression free survival 19.5 months with platinum *v* 6.8 months without platinum, P < 0.0001; median overall survival 30.7 months with platinum *v* 19.6 months without platinum, P < 0.002). **Single agent platinum versus combined platinum chemotherapy:** We found one systematic review (search date 1998, 9 RCTs in 1095 women with advanced ovarian cancer)[18] and three additional RCTs in women with advanced ovarian cancer.[25–27] The review found no significant difference between treatments for risk of death (HR 0.91, 95% CI 0.80 to 1.05).

Separate analyses of cisplatin and carboplatin containing regimens found similar results (HR of death for single agent *v* combination cisplatin regimens 0.86, 95% CI 0.73 to 1.02; HR of death for single agent *v* combination carboplatin regimens 1.05, 95% CI 0.82 to 1.35). The first additional RCT (multicentre; 1526 women; 36% of women < 55 years old) compared six cycles of cyclophosphamide (500 mg/m^2), doxorubicin (50 mg/m^2), and cisplatin (50 mg/m^2) versus three weekly carboplatin alone ([{glomerular filtration rate multiplied by 5} + 25] mg).[26] After a median follow up of 35 months, it found no significant difference between treatments for progression free survival or overall survival (for progression free survival HR for combined treatment *v* carboplatin alone 0.92, 95% CI 0.81 to 1.04; for overall survival 1.00, 95% CI 0.86 to 1.16). The second additional RCT (611 women aged < 75 years) compared cisplatin alone (50 mg/m^2) weekly for nine cycles versus cisplatin (75 mg/m^2) plus cyclophosphamide (750 mg/m^2) three weekly for six cycles.[26] It found similar rates between groups for 3 year progression free and overall survival (3 year progression free survival 33.8% with cisplatin alone *v* 35.1% with combined treatment, CI and P values not stated; 3 year overall survival 44.1% with cisplatin alone *v* 44.6% with combined treatment, CI not provided, P = 0.96). The third RCT (176 women) compared six four weekly courses of cisplatin alone (75 mg/m^2) versus cisplatin (50 mg/m^2) plus cyclophosphamide (500 mg/m^2). It found no significant difference between treatments for progression free survival or overall survival after a median of 10 years (median progression free survival 11.9 months with single *v* 10.0 months with combination, P = 0.092; median overall survival 21.5 months with single *v* 19.4 months with combination, P = 0.1299).[27] We found one further RCT that was reported as a conference abstract (see comment below).

Harms: **Platinum versus non-platinum chemotherapy:** The first systematic review did not report adverse effects.[18] One additional RCT found that 1/85 (1%) women taking cisplatin versus thiotepa stopped cisplatin because of weakness and dizziness.[19] The RCT comparing cisplatinum and melphalan versus hexamethylmelamine, doxorubicin, and cyclophosphamide found that haematological toxicity was more common with the platinum regimen (white cells < 3000/m^3, P < 0.0001; platelets < 75 000/m^3, P < 0.0001; anaemia, P = 0.001).[9] The RCT comparing doxorubicin plus cyclophosphamide combined with either vincristine or cisplatin reported that platinum increased haematological toxicity (rates not stated).[23] One cohort analysis of two RCTs comparing platinum and non-platinum regimens found that grade 3 nausea and vomiting (see table 1, p 1964), mild renal toxicity, and neurotoxicity were significantly more common with platinum containing regimens compared with non-platinum regimens (AR grade 3 nausea and vomiting about 6–10% with platinum regimens *v* 4% with non-platinum, P = 0.004; AR any renal toxicity 17–20% with platinum *v* 4% with non-platinum, P value not stated; AR neurotoxicity 1–4% with platinum *v* 0% with non-platinum, P value not stated).[29] We found one analysis of data from two RCTs (387 women with advanced ovarian cancer) comparing hexamethylmelamine plus cyclophosphamide plus methotrexate plus 5-fluorouracil with or without cisplatin, or with cyclophosphamide plus cisplatin.[30] After median follow up of 45 months, it found that neurotoxicity was more common and more severe with regimens that included platinum versus those without platinum (AR for any neurotoxicity 47% with platinum *v* 25% without platinum; AR for grade 2–3 neurotoxicity 25% with platinum *v* 3% without platinum; CI and P values not stated). **Single agent platinum versus combined platinum chemotherapy:** The systematic review did not report adverse effects.[18] In the RCT comparing carboplatin alone versus cyclophosphamide plus doxorubicin plus cisplatin, 875 women (57%) were assessed for adverse effects.[25] Leucopenia, hair loss, and nausea and vomiting were more common with combination treatment versus carboplatin alone (AR for leucopenia 36% with combination *v* 10% with carboplatin alone; AR for hair loss 70% with combination *v* 4% with carboplatin alone; AR for nausea and vomiting 20% with combination *v* 9% with carboplatin alone). Thrombocytopenia was more common with carboplatin (AR 6% with combination *v* 16% with carboplatin alone). Renal, cardiac, and neurotoxicity were rare in both groups (1–2% in both groups for each category).

Comment: **Single agent platinum versus combined platinum chemotherapy:** We found one RCT (120 women with advanced ovarian cancer) reported as a conference abstract, which compared six cycles of cisplatin plus cyclophosphamide versus three cycles of epirubicin plus ifosfamide followed by four cycles of cisplatin.[31] It found no significant differences between treatments for relapse free or overall survival (relapse free survival at 3 years 24% with cisplatin plus cyclophosphamide *v* 41% with epirubicin plus ifosfamide plus cisplatin, CI and P values not stated; median overall survival 141 weeks with cisplatin plus cyclophosphamide *v* 172 wks with epirubicin plus ifosfamide plus cisplatin, CI and P values not stated).[31]

OPTION TAXANES

One systematic review and one additional RCT have found that adding paclitaxel to platinum based chemotherapy versus platinum based chemotherapy alone significantly improves progression free and overall survival after primary surgery in women with advanced ovarian cancer. One RCT found no significant difference in progression free or overall survival between paclitaxel plus carboplatin versus paclitaxel plus cisplatin, although it may have lacked power to exclude clinically important effects.

Benefits: **Adding paclitaxel to platinum:** We found one systematic review[32] and one additional RCT[33] in women with advanced ovarian cancer. The systematic review (search date not stated, published 2000, 3746 women) included one published RCT[34] and three unpublished RCTs, two of which have since been published.[35,36] The first included RCT (386 women) compared cisplatin (75 mg/m^2) combined with either cyclophosphamide or paclitaxel (135 mg/m^2).[34] It found that cisplatin plus paclitaxel versus cisplatin plus cyclophosphamide improved progression free survival and overall survival (median progression free survival: 18 months with cisplatin plus paclitaxel *v* 13 months with cisplatin plus cyclophosphamide,

P < 0.001; median overall survival: 38 months with cisplatin plus paclitaxel *v* 24 months with cisplatin plus cyclophosphamide, P < 0.001).[34] The second included RCT (680 women), which has since been published,[35] compared cisplatin (75 mg/m^2) combined with either cyclophosphamide or paclitaxel (175 mg/m^2). It found that cisplatin plus paclitaxel versus cisplatin plus cyclophosphamide significantly improved progression free survival and overall survival (median progression free survival 17 months with cisplatin plus paclitaxel *v* 12 months with cisplatin plus cyclophosphamide, P = 0.001; median survival 35 months with cisplatin plus paclitaxel *v* 25 months with cisplatin plus cyclophosphamide, P = 0.001). The third included RCT (614 women), which has also since been published,[36] compared three treatments: cisplatin alone (100 mg/m^2), paclitaxel alone (200 mg/m^2), and paclitaxel (135 mg/m^2) followed by cisplatin (75 mg/m^2). It found no significant difference between cisplatin alone versus cisplatin plus paclitaxel for progression free survival or overall survival after median follow up of 61 months (progression free survival: median 16 months with cisplatin alone *v* 14 months with cisplatin plus paclitaxel, HR 1.06, 95% CI 0.90 to 1.30; overall survival: median 30 months with cisplatin alone *v* 27 months with cisplatin plus paclitaxel, HR 0.99, 95% CI 0.80 to 1.23). The fourth RCT in the review, which is still unpublished (2974 women), compared three treatments: paclitaxel (175 mg/m^2) plus carboplatin, carboplatin alone, and cyclophosphamide plus doxorubicin plus cisplatin. It found no difference in progression free survival or overall survival between paclitaxel plus carboplatin versus carboplatin alone after 24 months (progression free survival: estimated RR 1.02, CI not provided; overall survival: estimated RR 1.1, CI not provided). A full report of the trial is in press (Gabra H, personal communication, 2002). We found one additional RCT[33] (45 women) comparing cisplatin (75 mg/m^2) plus either paclitaxel (175 mg/m^2) or cyclophosphamide (750 mg/m^2). It found that cisplatin plus paclitaxel versus cisplatin plus cyclophosphamide significantly increased time to relapse and increased relapse free survival after 25 months (38 women; median time to relapse 17.5 months with cisplatin plus paclitaxel *v* 9.9 months with cisplatin plus cyclophosphamide, CI and P value not stated; P value for difference in relapse free survival = 0.001, mean values and CI not provided). **Paclitaxel plus carboplatin versus paclitaxel plus cisplatin:** One RCT (208 women) compared at least six cycles of paclitaxel (175 mg/m^2 over 3 h) combined with either cisplatin (75 mg/m^2) or carboplatin ([{glomerular filtration rate multiplied by 5} + 25] mg).[37] It found that treatments had different adverse effects (see harms below), but found no significant differences between treatments for progression free survival or overall survival after a median of 37 months (median progression free survival 16 months in both groups, HR 1.07, 95% CI 0.78 to 1.48; median overall survival 30 months with paclitaxel plus cisplatin *v* 32 months with paclitaxel plus carboplatin, HR 0.85, 95% CI 0.59 to 1.24). We found several further RCTs reported as conference abstracts (see comment below). **Carboplatin plus paclitaxel or docetaxel:** We found no RCTs with sufficient follow up for inclusion (see comment below).

Harms: **Adding paclitaxel to platinum:** The systematic review found that reporting of adverse effects was not consistent among trials.[32] It presented results from two RCTs, which found that adding paclitaxel to platinum based regimens did not significantly increase haematological toxicity, fever, or anaemia (any haematological toxicity [1 RCT] RR about 1, 95% CI about 0.8 to 1.3; anaemia [1 RCT] RR 1.10, 95% CI 0.57 to 2.13; fever [1 RCT] RR 16.38 in favour of non-paclitaxel regimen, 95% CI 0.83 to 284). Compared with platinum alone, infection was more common with paclitaxel plus platinum, but less common with cyclophosphamide plus doxorubicin plus platinum (1 RCT; compared with platinum alone, RR 3.38, 95% CI 2.15 to 5.32; compared with cyclophosphamide plus doxorubicin plus platinum RR 0.59, 95% CI 0.40 to 0.86). Nausea and vomiting was reported in 7–18% of women receiving paclitaxel and hair loss was reported in 68–77% of women receiving paclitaxel. Cardiac toxicity was not reported in the included RCTs. One of the RCTs included in the review (614 women)[36] found that neutropenia, hair loss, and fever were more common with paclitaxel or paclitaxel plus cisplatin versus cisplatin alone ($P < 0.001$). Another included RCT found that grades 3 and 4 muscle pain (see table 1, p 1964), neurosensory and neuromotor symptoms, and hair loss were more common with cisplatin plus paclitaxel than cisplatin plus cyclophosphamide (AR muscle pain 6% with cisplatin plus paclitaxel *v* 0% with cisplatin plus cyclophosphamide; neurosensory symptoms 19.6% with cisplatin plus paclitaxel *v* 1% with cisplatin plus cyclophosphamide; neuromotor symptoms 5% with cisplatin plus paclitaxel *v* 0.6% with cisplatin plus cyclophosphamide; hair loss 51% with cisplatin plus paclitaxel *v* 21% with cisplatin plus cyclophosphamide; CI and P values not stated).[35] Grade 3 and 4 leucopenia (see table 1, p 1964), anaemia, and thrombocytopenia were less common with cisplatin plus paclitaxel than cisplatin plus cyclophosphamide (AR, CI, and P values not stated). Febrile neutropenia rates were similar between groups (AR 3% for both groups). **Paclitaxel plus carboplatin versus paclitaxel plus cisplatin:** The RCT comparing paclitaxel plus cisplatin versus paclitaxel plus carboplatin found no significant differences between treatments for rates of hair loss, fever, mucositis, diarrhoea, allergic reaction, cardiorespiratory complications, skin reactions, muscle or joint pain, constipation, fever, or renal toxicity. However, after six cycles of treatment, grade 4 nausea and vomiting (see table 1, p 1964) was more common with paclitaxel plus cisplatin (AR 17% with paclitaxel plus cisplatin *v* 14% with paclitaxel plus carboplatin; $P < 0.01$). Grade 3–4 thrombocytopenia and grade 4 granulocytopenia (see table 1, p 1964), were more common with paclitaxel plus carboplatin (AR for grade 3–4 thrombocytopenia 6% with paclitaxel plus carboplatin *v* 1% with paclitaxel plus cisplatin, $P < 0.01$; AR for grade 4 granulocytopenia 40% with paclitaxel plus carboplatin *v* 23% with paclitaxel plus cisplatin, $P < 0.01$).[37] We found several other RCTs reported as conference abstracts (see comment below).

Comment: **Paclitaxel plus carboplatin or paclitaxel plus cisplatin:** The first abstract reported preliminary safety data among 488 women from a trial comparing cisplatin plus paclitaxel versus carboplatin plus paclitaxel in 797 women.[38] Grade 3–4 haematological toxicity (see table 1, p 1964), was more common with the carboplatin regimen and non-haematological toxicity other than hair loss was more common with the cisplatin regimen. A second abstract from the same trial found no significant difference between treatments for progression free or overall survival after 2 years' median follow up ($P > 0.05$).[39] The third abstract reported a trial comparing paclitaxel plus carboplatin versus paclitaxel plus alternating cisplatin and carboplatin in 164 women. It found no significant differences for disease free or overall survival ($P = 0.4$ for both outcomes).[40] **Carboplatin plus paclitaxel or docetaxel:** We found one ongoing RCT (1077 women from 83 centres),[41] which will compare effects of six cycles of carboplatin ([{glomerular filtration rate multiplied by 5} + 25] mg) combined with either paclitaxel (175 mg/m^2) or docetaxel (75 mg/m^2). **Paclitaxel plus carboplatin versus carboplatin or cyclophosphamide plus doxorubicin plus cisplatin:** We found one ongoing RCT (2075 women).[42]

GLOSSARY

Debulking is removal of a major proportion of the tumour. Initial and primary debulking both refer to front line surgery (up front surgery).

Interval debulking is a second operation to remove residual tumour after a specified number of cytotoxic chemotherapy cycles, which is then followed by further chemotherapy.

Routine second look surgery is a "second look" operation to assess the response to cytotoxic chemotherapy.

REFERENCES

1. Allen DG, Heintz AP, Touw FW. A meta-analysis of residual disease and survival in stage III and IV carcinoma of the ovary. *Eur J Gynaecol Oncol* 1995;16:349–356. Search date not stated; primary sources literature search of Silver-Platter 3.1, hand searches, and personal communications.
2. Beral V. The epidemiology of ovarian cancer. In: Sharp F, Soutter WP, eds. *Proceedings of the Seventeenth Study Group of the Royal College of Obstetricians and Gynaecologists in Conjunction with the Helene Harris Memorial Trust*. London: RCOG, 1987:21–31.
3. Banks E, Beral V, Reeves G. The epidemiology of ovarian cancer: a review. *Int J Gynecol Cancer* 1997;7:425–438.
4. Parkin DM, Laara E, Muir CS. Estimates of the worldwide frequency of sixteen major cancers in 1980. *Int J Cancer* 1988;41:184–197.
5. Blake P, Lambert H, Crawford R. Cancer of the ovary and fallopian tube. In: Blake P, Lambert H, Crawford R, eds. Gynaecological oncology. A guide to clinical management. Oxford: Oxford University Press, 1998:12–44.
6. Cancer Statistics: Cancer Research Campaign, 2002. http://www.cancerresearchuk.org/aboutcancer/statistics/incidence. Last accessed 2 September 2002.
7. Whittemore AS, Harris R, Itnyre J. Characteristics relating to ovarian cancer risk: collaborative analysis of 12 US case-control studies. II. Invasive epithelial ovarian cancers in white women. Collaborative Ovarian Cancer Group. *Am J Epidemiol* 1992;136:1184–1203.
8. Yancik R. Ovarian cancer. Age contrasts in incidence, histology, disease stage at diagnosis and mortality. *Cancer* 1993;71:517–523.
9. Adami H-O, Hseih C-C, Lambe M, et al. Parity, age at first childbirth, and risk of ovarian cancer. *Lancet* 1994;344:1250–1254.
10. Rossing MA, Daling JR, Weiss NS, et al. Ovarian tumours in a cohort of infertile women. *New Engl J Med* 1994;331:771–776.
11. Venn A, Watson L, Bruinsma F, et al. Risk of cancer after use of fertility drugs with in-vitro fertilisation. *Lancet* 1999;354:1586–1590.
12. Mant JWF, Vessey MP. Ovarian and endometrial cancers. In: Doll R, Fraumeni JF Jr, Muir CS, eds. *Trends in cancer incidence and mortality*. Plainview, NY: Cold Spring Harbor Laboratory Press, 1994:287–307.
13. Booth M, Beral V, Smith P. Risk factors for ovarian cancer: a case-control study. *Br J Cancer* 1989;60:592–598.
14. Nicoletto MO, Tumolo S, Talamini R, et al. Surgical second look in ovarian cancer: a randomized study in patients with laparoscopic complete remission–a Northeastern Oncology Cooperative Group-Ovarian Cancer Cooperative Group Study. *J Clin Oncol* 1997;15:994–999.
15. Luesley D, Lawton F, Blackledge G, et al. Failure of second-look laparotomy to influence survival in epithelial ovarian cancer. *Lancet* 1988;2:599–603.
16. Van der Burg ME, van Lent M, Buyse M, et al. The effect of debulking surgery after induction chemotherapy on the prognosis in advanced epithelial ovarian cancer. Gynecological Cancer Cooperative Group of the European Organization for Research and Treatment of Cancer. *New Engl J Med* 1995;332:629–634.
17. Redman CW, Warwick J, Luesley DM, et al. Intervention debulking surgery in advanced epithelial ovarian cancer. *Br J Obstet Gynaecol* 1994;101:142–146.

18. Advanced Ovarian Cancer Trialists Group. Chemotherapy for advanced ovarian cancer. In: The Cochrane Library, Issue 1, 2002. Oxford: Update Software. Search date 1998; primary sources Medline, Cancerlit, the trial registers produced by the National Cancer Institute (Physicians Data Query) and the United Kingdom Co-ordinating Committee on Cancer Research, hand searches of relevant meeting proceedings, and contact with experts in the field and pharmaceutical companies.
19. Dorum A, Kristensen GB, Trope C. A randomised study of cisplatin versus thiotepa as induction chemotherapy in advanced ovarian carcinoma. *Eur J Cancer* 1994;30A:1470–1474.
20. Alberts DS, Mason-Liddil N, O'Toole RV, et al. Randomized Phase III trial of chemoimmunotherapy in patients with previously untreated stages III and IV suboptimal disease ovarian cancer: a Southwest Oncology Group Study. *Gynecol Oncol* 1989;32:8–15.
21. Edwards CL, Herson J, Gershenson DM, et al. A prospective randomized clinical trial of melphalan and cis-platinum versus hexamethylmelamine, adriamycin, and cyclophosphamide in advanced ovarian cancer. *Gynecol Oncol* 1983;15:261–277.
22. Sessa C, Colombo N, Bolis G, et al. Randomized comparison of hexamethylmelamine, adriamycin, cyclophosphamide (HAC) vs. cisplatin, adriamycin, cyclophosphamide (PAC) in advanced ovarian cancer: long-term results. *Cancer Treat Rev* 1991;18(suppl A):37–46.
23. Krommer CF, Szalai JP. Cyclophosphamide, adriamycin and cisplatin (CAP) versus cyclophosphamide, adriamycin and vincristin (CAV) in the treatment of advanced ovarian cancer: a randomized study. *Ann Oncol* 1992;3:37–39.
24. Neijt JP, Bokkel Huinink WW, van der Burg ME, et al. Randomised trial comparing two combination chemotherapy regimens (Hexa-CAF vs CHAP-5) in advanced ovarian carcinoma. *Lancet* 1984;2:594–600.
25. The ICON Collaborators. ICON2: randomised trial of single-agent carboplatin against three-drug combination of CAP (cyclophosphamide, doxorubicin, and cisplatin) in women with ovarian cancer. ICON Collaborators. International Collaborative Ovarian Neoplasm Study. *Lancet* 1998;352:1571–1576.
26. Bolis G, Favalli G, Danese S, et al. Weekly cisplatin given for 2 months versus cisplatin plus cyclophosphamide given for 5 months after cytoreductive surgery for advanced ovarian cancer. *J Clin Oncol* 1997;15:1938–1944.
27. Marth C, Trope C, Vergote IB, et al. Ten-year results of a randomised trial comparing cisplatin with cisplatin and cyclophosphamide in advanced, suboptimally debulked ovarian cancer. *Eur J Cancer* 1998;34:1175–1180.
28. US Food and Drug Administration. Center for Drug Evaluation and Research. http://www.fda.gov/cder/cancer/toxicityframe htm. Last accessed 13 September 2002.
29. Sevelda P, Dittrich CH, Kurz CH, et al. Prospective randomized trial of sequential alternating chemotherapy in advanced ovarian carcinoma. *Onkologie* 1992;15:288–292.
30. van der Hoop RG, van der Burg ME, Bokkel Huinink WW, et al. Incidence of neuropathy in 395 patients with ovarian cancer treated with or without cisplatin. *Cancer* 1990;66:1697–1702.
31. Bella M, Cocconi A, Mambrini A, et al. The concept of a medical debulking in advanced ovarian carcinoma before cisplatin treatment. Final results of a prospective randomized trial. *Tumori* 1998;84(supp 54): A146.
32. Lister-Sharp D, McDonagh MS, Khan KS, et al. A rapid and systematic review of the effectiveness and cost-effectiveness of the taxanes used in the treatment of advanced breast and ovarian cancer. *Health Technol Assess* 2000;4:17–115. Search date not stated; primary sources Medline, Embase, Cancerlit, Cochrane Controlled Trials Register, National Research Register, and contact with researchers and review groups.
33. Smith-Sorensen B, Kaern J, Holm R, et al. Therapy effect of either paclitaxel or cyclophosphamide combination treatment in patients with epithelial ovarian cancer and relation to TP53 gene status. Br J *Cancer* 1998;78:375–381.
34. McGuire WP, Hoskins WJ, Brady MF, et al. Cyclophosphamide and cisplatin compared with paclitaxel and cisplatin in patients with stage III and stage IV ovarian cancer. *New Engl J Med* 1996;334:1–6.
35. Piccart MJ, Bertelsen K, James K, et al. Randomized intergroup trial of cisplatin–paclitaxel versus cisplatin–cyclophosphamide in women with advanced epithelial ovarian cancer: three-year results. *J Natl Cancer Inst* 2000;92:699–708.
36. Muggia FM, Braly PS, Brady MF, et al. Phase III randomized study of cisplatin versus paclitaxel versus cisplatin and paclitaxel in patients with suboptimal stage III or IV ovarian cancer: a gynecologic oncology group study. *J Clin Oncol* 2000;18:106–115.
37. Neijt JP, Engelholm SA, Tuxen MK, et al. Exploratory Phase III study of paclitaxel and cisplatin versus paclitaxel and carboplatin in advanced ovarian cancer. *J Clin Oncol* 2000;18:3084–3092.
38. Mobus V, Schoder W, Luck HJ, et al. Cisplatin/paclitaxel vs carboplatin/paclitaxel as first-line chemotherapy in ovarian cancer: an AGO study group Phase III trial. *Ann Oncol* 1998;9:173.
39. Shröeder W, DuBois A, Kuhn W, et al. Treatment of patients with advanced ovarian cancer (FIGO IIB-IV) with cisplatin/paclitaxel or carboplatin/paclitaxel – an interim analysis of the AGO study protocol ovar-3. *Eur J Cancer* 1999; 35 supp 4: S231, abstr 908.
40. Skarlos DV, Aravantinos G, Kosmidis P, et al. Paclitaxel with carboplatin versus paclitaxel with carboplatin alternating with cisplatin as first-line chemotherapy in advanced epithelial ovarian cancer: preliminary results of a Hellenic Cooperative Oncology Group study. *Semin Oncol* 1997;24:S15.
41. Vasey PA. First results of the SCOTROC trial: a Phase III comparison of paclitaxel–carboplatin and docetaxel–carboplatin as first line chemotherapy for epithelial ovarian cancer. *Proc ASCO* 2001;84:170–178.
42. Harper P. A randomised comparison of paclitaxel (T) and carboplatin (J) versus a control arm of single agent carboplatin (J) or CAP (cyclophosphamide, doxorubicin, cisplatin): 2075 patients randomised into the 3rd International Collaborative Ovarian Neoplasm Study [abstract]. *Proc ASCO* 1999;18:A1375.

Hani Gabra
Clinical Scientist and Consultant Medical Oncologist
Cancer Research UK
Edinburgh Oncology Unit
Western General Hospital
Edinburgh
UK

Charles Redman
Consultant Gynaecological Oncologist
Department of Obstetrics and Gynaecology
City General Hospital
Stoke-on-Trent
UK

Jennifer Byrom
Lecturer in Gynaecological Oncology
Academic Department of Obstetrics and Gynaecology
Birmingham Women's Hospital
Birmingham
UK

Competing interests: HG has been reimbursed by Schering-Plough, the manufacturers of Caelyx, for attending the ASCO conference on two occasions. He has received fees for consulting from Schering-Plough. He has received funds to cover costs of the South East Scotland Gynae-Cancer network Annual Meeting from Aventis (Manufacturers of Taxotere), Bristol Myers (Manufacturers of Taxol and Carboplatin), Merck (Distributors of Hycamtin) Schering-Plough (Manufacturers of Caelyx) and Merck. He has received research support from Aventis for Scottish Gynae Cancer Trials Group clinical trials.

TABLE 1 Adverse effects of chemotherapy — Common Toxicity Criteria (see text, p 1957, 1960, 1961).[28] Published with permission.

Toxicity grade	0	1	2	3	4
Blood and bone marrow					
WBC(109/L)	≥ 4.0	3.0–3.9	2.0–2.9	1.0–1.9	< 1.0
Platelets (109/L)	WNL	75.0 normal	50.0–74.9	25.0–49.9	< 25.0
Haemoglobin (g/L)	WNL	10.0 normal	8.0–10.0	6.5–7.9	< 6.5
Granulocytes and bands (109/L)	≥ 2.0	1.5–1.9	1.0–1.4	0.5–0.9	< 0.5
Lymphocytes (109/L)	≥ 2.0	1.5–1.9	1.0–1.4	0.5–0.9	< 0.5
Nausea	None	Able to eat	Oral intake significantly decreased	No significant intake, requiring iv fluids	
Vomiting	None	1 episode in 24 h over pretreatment	≥ 6 episodes in 24 h over pretreatment; or need for iv fluids	Requiring parenteral nutrition; or physiological consequences requiring intensive care; haemodynamic collapse	
Muscle pain	None	Mild pain not interfering with function	Moderate pain: pain or analgesics interfering with function, but not interfering with activities of daily living	Severe pain: pain or analgesics severely interfering with activities of daily living	Disabling

iv, intravenous; WBC, white blood cells; WNL, within normal limits.

Premalignant vulval disorders

Search date May 2002

Damien Murphy, Charles Redman, Earlando Thomas, and Bazian Ltd (temporary contributors)

QUESTIONS

INTERVENTIONS

See glossary, p 1970

Key Messages

Lichen sclerosus

- **Oral retinoids (acitretin)** One small RCT found acitretin significantly reduced itching (NNT 5, 95% CI 3 to 84), and extent of lesions (NNT 4, 95% CI 2 to 16) compared with placebo after 20–22 weeks, but was associated with severe skin peeling and hair loss (NNH 1, 95% CI 1to 2).
- **Surgery** We found insufficient evidence on the effects of surgery in women with lichen sclerosus.
- **Topical clobetasol propionate (0.05%)** One small RCT found that topical clobetasol propionate controlled symptoms more effectively than topical testosterone propionate or petroleum jelly after 3 months' treatment. Good quality prospective observational studies reported minimal adverse effects when clobetasol propionate was used as required for maintenance treatment.
- **Topical testosterone** Two small RCTs found no evidence that testosterone propionate improved symptoms more than petroleum jelly, either as initial treatment for 12 months or after 16 weeks' treatment in women previously treated with clobetasol propionate. Testosterone propionate is associated with virilisation.

Vulval intraepithelial neoplasia

- **Surgical treatments, topical α interferon** We found insufficient evidence on the effects of surgical or topical treatments in women with vulval intraepithelial neoplasia.

Premalignant vulval disorders

DEFINITION There are two recognised premalignant conditions of the vulva. **Lichen sclerosus** is characterised by epithelial thinning, inflammation, and distinctive histological changes in the dermis. It affects all age groups but is typically found in the anogenital region in postmenopausal women. The most common presentation is severe intractable itching (pruritus vulvae) and vaginal soreness with dyspareunia. **Vulval intraepithelial neoplasia (VIN)** is dysplasia of the vulval epithelium, categorised as mild (VIN I), moderate (VIN II), or severe (VIN III). The vulval lesions are often multifocal and are usually associated with itching and pain.

INCIDENCE/ PREVALENCE We found no data on the prevalence of lichen sclerosus. The true incidence of vulval intraepithelial neoplasia is unknown, but it is being diagnosed with increased frequency in the UK and the USA. This may be because of increased recognition of the disease or a true increase in incidence.[1–3]

AETIOLOGY/ RISK FACTORS The cause is unknown. Vulval intraepithelial neoplasia is associated with human papilloma virus 16.[1]

PROGNOSIS There is currently no cure for lichen sclerosus. The risk of progression to vulval carcinoma ranges from 0–9%.[4] People with concomitant squamous cell hyperplasia are at increased risk of malignancy.[5] Malignant transformation has been reported in 2–4% of women with VIN III but the incidence seems to be lower in women with VIN I and II.[2,6] About 30% of vulval carcinomas are associated with vulval intraepithelial neoplasia.[1]

AIMS To control symptoms; to reduce the risk of malignant transformation; and to improve quality of life, with minimal adverse effects.

OUTCOMES Scores for symptoms (itching, burning, pain, and dyspareunia); gross appearance (relating to severity of lesions and extent of vulval involvement); and histological stage. Scores range from 0–3, where 3 represents the most severe. Other outcomes are rates of histological regression, recurrence, malignant transformation, and adverse effects of treatment.

METHODS *Clinical Evidence* search and appraisal May 2002. We included all RCTs that were appropriately randomised and double blinded with follow up of 80% or more participants, and with a minimum of 15 people in each study arm. Where confidence intervals were not reported but adequate information was provided, we calculated them using the software Statsdirect.[7] Where we found no good RCTs, we used the best available observational studies.

QUESTION What are the effects of treatments for lichen sclerosus?

OPTION TOPICAL CORTICOSTEROIDS

We found limited evidence from one small RCT that topical clobetasol propionate controlled symptoms more effectively than topical testosterone propionate or petroleum jelly after 3 months' treatment.

Benefits: We found no systematic review. **Short term treatment:** We found one RCT. It compared clobetasol propionate 0.05% (20 women), testosterone propionate (20 women), topical progesterone

(20 women), and petroleum jelly (19 women) for 3 months, with follow up of 3 months.[8] Clobetasol propionate was associated with significantly higher rates of symptom control and reversal of histological changes compared with any of the other treatments (AR for symptom remission 75% on clobetasol propionate, 20% on testosterone propionate, 20% on topical progesterone, and 11% on petroleum jelly). A significant difference in both gross and histological changes occurred only in the clobetasol propionate group.[8]

Harms: One RCT found no evidence that topical clobetasol propionate was associated with adverse effects,[8] and good prospective observational studies reported minimal adverse effects when clobetasol propionate was used as required for maintenance treatment for 1–3 years.[9,10]

Comment: The RCT was not double blinded and did not include a power calculation to justify sample size. Follow up was greater than 80% for assessment of treatment efficacy. The high response rate to petroleum jelly may have been more than a placebo effect: petroleum jelly has a soothing effect on the vulvar skin.

OPTION TOPICAL TESTOSTERONE

One RCT found that topical testosterone reduced symptoms less than topical clobetasol. Two small RCTs found no evidence that topical testosterone propionate was more effective than petroleum jelly. Testosterone propionate is associated with virilisation and pain.

Benefits: We found no systematic review. **Short term treatment:** We found one RCT that compared testosterone propionate 2%, clobetasol propionate 0.05%, topical progesterone, and petroleum jelly for 3 months, with follow up of 3 months (see benefits of topical steroids, p 1966).[8] A second RCT (58 women treated for 12 months) compared testosterone propionate in petroleum jelly versus petroleum jelly alone. It found no significant difference in response rates after 12 months (improvement: 20/30 [67%] with testosterone propionate in petroleum jelly *v* 21/28 [75%] with petroleum jelly; RR 0.88, 95% CI 0.64 to 1.24, calculated from data reported).[11] **Maintenance treatment:** One RCT (32 women who had previously been treated with topical clobetasol for 24 weeks) compared testosterone propionate versus petroleum jelly for a further 16 weeks. It found that recurrence of symptoms on maintenance treatment was more common with testosterone propionate than with petroleum jelly after 16 weeks (9/16 [56%] with testosterone propionate *v* 3/16 [19%] with petroleum jelly; RR 3.0, 95% CI 1.0 to 9.1; NNH 2, 95% CI 1 to 7). There was no significant difference in control of gross features between testosterone propionate and petroleum jelly (no numbers available).[12]

Harms: Topical testosterone propionate was associated with virilisation (4/20 [20%] women),[8] hypertrichosis (1/30 [3%]),[9] pruritus and pain (3/30 [10%]),[9] and burning (4/16 [25%]).[12] No harmful effects were reported with petroleum jelly.[8,9,12]

Comment: None of the RCTs were double blinded and none included a power calculation to justify sample size. All had follow up rates of greater than 80% for assessment of treatment efficacy. The high response rate to petroleum jelly may have been more than a placebo effect: petroleum jelly has a soothing effect on the vulvar skin.

OPTION ORAL RETINOIDS (ACITRETIN)

One small RCT found that acitretin was more effective than placebo. Acitretin is associated with severe peeling of palms and soles, and with hair loss.

Benefits: We found no systematic review. We found one RCT (46 eligible women) comparing acitretin versus placebo for 12–16 weeks with 4–6 weeks' follow up.[13] Acitretin versus placebo significantly improved pruritus after 20–22 weeks (0/22 [0%] with acitretin *v* 19/24 [79%] with placebo; ARR 21%, 95% CI 2% to 41%; NNT 5, 95% CI 3 to 84), atrophic features (3/22 [14%] with acitretin *v* 11/24 [46%] with placebo; RR 0.30, 95% CI 0.10 to 0.93; NNT 4, 95% CI 2 to 9), hyperkeratotic features (5/21 [24%] with acitretin *v* 16/22 [73%] with placebo; RR 0.33, 95% CI 0.15 to 0.73; NNT 3, 95% CI 2 to 4), and extent of lesions (14/22 [64%] with acitretin *v* 22/24 [92%] with placebo; RR 0.69, 95% CI 0.50 to 0.97; NNT 4, 95% CI 2 to 16). A non-significant reduction in burning sensation was also found (0/18 [0%] with acitretin *v* 3/20 [15%] with placebo; ARR +15%, 95% CI –5% to +36%).

Harms: Adverse effects were reported in 100% of women taking acitretin and 56% of those taking placebo.[13] Acitretin was associated with severe peeling of the palms and soles (11/39 [28%] women), and increased rates of hair loss (23/39 [59%] with acitretin *v* 2/39 [5%] with placebo; RR 11.5, 95% CI 2.9 to 45.5; NNH 1, 95% CI 1 to 2).[13] Acitretin was associated with congenital abnormalities in women exposed during the first trimester of pregnancy,[14,15] and therefore is contraindicated in pregnancy. Contraception has been recommended for use during treatment and for 2 years afterwards.[16]

Comment: The RCT was double blinded. Follow up rates were greater than 80% for assessment of treatment efficacy.

OPTION SURGICAL TREATMENTS

We found insufficient evidence on the effects of surgery in lichen sclerosus.

Benefits: We found no systematic review, RCTs, or good quality observational studies.

Harms: Three cohort studies reported reoperation rates after vulvectomy (33%, 23%, and 50%). The reasons for reoperating were recurrence, progression to vulval cancer, and constricted vaginal outlet.[4]

Comment: We found one non-systematic review that identified uncontrolled cohort studies of vulvectomy, cryosurgery, and laser treatment.[4] **Vulvectomy:** Five studies were reviewed. Four evaluated simple vulvectomy (see glossary, p 1970), partial vulvectomy (see glossary, p 1970), or complete vulvectomy (see glossary, p 1970) (44–120 women, 3–23 years' follow up, recurrence rates 39–59%). One study evaluated skinning vulvectomy (see glossary, p 1970) and skin graft (4 women, 4–8 years' follow up, recurrence rate 50%). **Cryosurgery:** One study was reviewed (12 women, 3 years' follow up, 2 women lost to follow up, rate of recurrence/failed treatment 42%). Complete healing took up to 3 months. **Laser treatment:** Four studies were reviewed. The largest study (62 women, 0.3–7.0 years' follow up) found a 16% recurrence rate. The other studies were small (5–7 women, 1–6 years' follow up, recurrence rates 0–14%). Complete healing took up to 6 weeks.

QUESTION **What are the effects of treatments for vulval intraepithelial neoplasia?**

OPTION **SURGICAL TREATMENTS**

We found insufficient evidence on the effects of surgical treatments in women with vulval intraepithelial neoplasia.

Benefits: We found no systematic review or RCTs.

Harms: Laser skinning vulvectomy (see glossary, p 1970) may be associated with labial fusion (14%), and in 5% of cases laser treatment of perianal lesions caused a partial transection of the anal sphincter, although continence was not evaluated. Moderate to severe postoperative pain is also common after laser vaporisation.[3,17] Vaporisation using carbon dioxide produces a plume containing carcinogenic substances, and the radiant energy can cause thermal burns, fires, and eye injuries in the operator. The risk to operators of aerosol produced during ultrasound surgical aspiration is unclear, and precautions to protect surgeons from women's body fluids may be required.[18,19] Cryosurgery may be associated with oedema, pain, and ulceration. Difficulties with precision and control may also result in vulval scarring and distortion.[18]

Comment: A minimum of 5 years' follow up would be necessary to evaluate properly the effects of treatment on rates of recurrence and malignant transformation in women with vulval intraepithelial neoplasia (VIN). One retrospective cohort study in women with VIN I, II, or III reported on rates of recurrence or persistence, at a mean of 31 months, after local excision (61 women, recurrence 25%), primary surgery including local excision, simple vulvectomy (see glossary, p 1970), knife skinning vulvectomy with grafting (103 women, recurrence 39%), and laser vaporisation (30 women, recurrence 67%). The difference between laser vaporisation and local excision was significant ($P \leq 0.001$). By 10 years, histological recurrence was seen in 79% of women treated with laser compared with 36% treated with local excision. Progression to malignant disease occurred after surgical intervention in nine women (7%).[2] A smaller cohort study found recurrence or persistence in 21% of women after simple vulvectomy (9 women, 74 months' median follow up), 44% after local excision (14 women, 74 months' median follow up), and 52% after laser skinning vulvectomy (21 women, 38 months' median follow up).[3] Other small, uncontrolled studies found recurrence rates of 8.6% with laser vaporisation (35 women, 12–36 months' follow up),[17] 22% with ultrasound surgical aspiration (9 women, 12 months' median follow up),[20] and 90% with cryosurgery (10 women, 12 months' median follow up).[6]

OPTION TOPICAL α INTERFERON

We found insufficient evidence on the effects of topical α interferon in women with vulval intraepithelial neoplasia.

Benefits: We found no systematic review and no placebo controlled or comparative RCTs. We found one small blinded crossover RCT (18 women) evaluating topical α interferon with and without 1% nonoxinol-9.[21] Outcomes were symptom control (itching, burning, and pain), reversal of histological changes, and adverse effects of treatment. Overall, 14/18 (78%) of participants had some response to α interferon (no P or CI values provided). The addition of 1% nonoxinol-9 made no significant difference to the number of complete responders, although the sample was too small to rule out a clinically important difference (complete response: 3/10 [30%] with 1% nonoxinol-9 and 6/14 [43%] without nonoxinol-9; RR 0.7, 95% CI 0.2 to 2.2).[21]

Harms: Topical α interferon was associated with transitory adverse effects, including fever (8%), mild discomfort, and mild pruritus (17%).[21]

Comment: None.

GLOSSARY

Complete vulvectomy The removal of all of the vulva with the lesion surrounded by a margin of 0.1–1.5 cm of normal tissue.

Partial vulvectomy The removal of a portion of the vulva with the lesion surrounded by a margin of 0.1–1.5 cm of normal tissue.

Simple vulvectomy The removal of the entire vulva including the labia and clitoris. The vulva is dissected free from the underlying subcutaneous tissue. It is not used for excision of invasive malignant lesions.

Skinning vulvectomy The epidermis and the underlying dermis of the vulva are removed by knife or laser. Split thickness skin graft is usually employed to cover the defect after knife excision.

REFERENCES

1. Crum CP, McLachlin CM, Tate JE, et al. Pathobiology of vulvar squamous neoplasia. *Curr Opin Obstet Gynecol* 1997;9:63–69.
2. Herod JJO, Shafi MI, Rollason TP, et al. Vulvar intraepithelial neoplasia: long term follow up treated and untreated. *Br J Obstet Gynaecol* 1996;103:446–452.
3. Shafi MI, Luesley DM, Byrne P, et al. Vulval intraepithelial neoplasia – management and outcome. *Br J Obstet Gynaecol* 1989;96:1339–1344.
4. Abramov Y, Elchalal U, Abramov D, et al. Surgical treatment of vulvar lichen sclerosus: a review. *Obstet Gynecol Surv* 1996;51:193–199.
5. Elchalal U, Gilead L, Vardy DA, et al. Treatment of vulvar lichen sclerosus in the elderly: an update. *Obstet Gynecol Surv* 1995;50:155–162.
6. Marren P, Dawber R, Wojnarowska F, et al. Failure of cryosurgery to eradicate vulval intraepithelial neoplasia: a pilot study. *J Eur Acad Dermatol Venereol* 1993;2:247–252.
7. Buchan IE. Statsdirect http://www.statsdirect.com. Cambridge (England) CamCode 2000 (last accessed 10 Sept 2002).
8. Bracco GL, Carli P, Sonni L, et al. Clinical and histologic effects of topical treatments of vulval lichen sclerosus. *J Reprod Med* 1993;38:37–40.
9. Dalziel KL, Wojnarowska F. Long-term control of vulval lichen sclerosus after treatment with a potent topical steroid cream. *J Reprod Med* 1993;38:25–27.
10. Bornstein J, Heifetz S, Kellner Y, et al. Clobetasol dipropionate 0.05% versus testosterone propionate

2% topical application for severe vulval lichen sclerosus. *Am J Obstet Gynecol* 1998;178:80–84.
11. Sideri M, Origoni L, Spinaci L, et al. Topical testosterone in the treatment of vulvar lichen sclerosus. *Int J Gynaecol Obstet* 1994;46:53–56.
12. Cattaneo A, Carli P, De Marco A, et al. Testosterone maintenance therapy. Effects on vulval lichen sclerosus treated with clobetasol propionate. *J Reprod Med* 1996;41:99–102.
13. Bousema MT, Romppanen U, Geiger J-M, et al. Acitretin in the treatment of severe lichen sclerosus or atrophicus of the vulva: a double-blind, placebo-controlled study. *J Am Acad Dermatol* 1994;30:225–231.
14. De Die-Smulders CE, Sturkenboom MC, Veraart J, et al. Severe limb defects and craniofacial anomalies in a fetus conceived during acitretin therapy. *Teratology* 1995;52:215–219.
15. Geiger JM, Baudin M, Saurat JH. Teratogenic risk with etretinate and acitretin treatment. *Dermatology* 1994;89:109–116.
16. *British National Formulary*. London: British Medical Association/Royal Pharmaceutical Society of Great Britain, September 1999;38:504.
17. Baggish MS, Dorsey JH. CO_2 laser for the treatment of vulvar carcinoma in situ. *Obstet Gynecol* 1981;57:371–374.
18. Townsend DE, Levine RU, Richart RM, et al. Management of vulvar intraepithelial neoplasia by carbon dioxide laser. *Obstet Gynecol* 1982;60:49–51.
19. Adelson MD. Ultrasonic surgical aspiration in the treatment of vulvar disease. *Obstet Gynecol* 1991;78:477–479.
20. Rader JS, Leake JF, Dillon MB, et al. Ultrasound surgical aspiration in the treatment of vulvar disease. *Obstet Gynecol* 1991;77:573–576.
21. Spirtos NM, Smith LH, Teng NNH. Prospective randomised trial of α-interferon (α-interferon gels) for the treatment of vulvar intraepithelial neoplasia III. *Gynecol Oncol* 1990;37:34–38.

Damian Murphy
Consultant Obstetrician and Gynaecologist
Department of Obstetrics and Gynaecology
New Cross Hospital
Wolverhampton
UK

Charles Redman
Consultant Obstetrician and Gynaecologist
Department of Obstetrics and Gynaecology
City General Hospital
Stoke-on-Trent
UK

Earlando Thomas
Senior Resident
Department of Obstetrics and Gynecology
Rochester, NY
USA

Bazian Ltd (temporary contributors)
London
UK

Competing interests: None declared.

Premenstrual syndrome

Search date February 2002

Katrina Wyatt

QUESTIONS

INTERVENTIONS

See glossary, p 1987

Key Messages

- Few treatments have been adequately evaluated in good quality placebo controlled RCTs.
- **Bromocriptine (breast symptoms only)** RCTs have found that bromocriptine versus placebo relieves breast tenderness, although adverse effects are common.
- **Cognitive behavioural treatment** RCTs have found that cognitive behavioural therapy versus control treatments significantly reduces premenstrual symptoms, but the evidence is insufficient to define the size of any effect.
- **Danazol** RCTs have found that danazol versus placebo significantly reduces premenstrual symptoms, but has important adverse effects associated with masculinisation when used continuously in the long term.
- **Diuretics** RCTs have found that spironactolone versus placebo improves symptoms of premenstrual syndrome including breast tenderness and bloating. Two RCTs have found that metolazone or ammonium chloride versus placebo reduce premenstrual swelling and weight gain.

Clin Evid 2002;8:1972–1991.

- **Exercise** One RCT has found that aerobic exercise versus placebo significantly improves premenstrual symptoms; another RCT has found that high intensity aerobic exercise improves symptoms significantly more than low intensity.
- **Gonadotrophin releasing hormone analogues** RCTs have found that gonadotrophin releasing hormone analogues versus placebo significantly reduce premenstrual symptoms. RCTs have found that gonadotrophin releasing hormone plus oestrogen plus progestogen (addback treatment) produces a fall in symptom scores that is intermediate between the fall produced by gonadotrophin releasing hormone analogue alone and by placebo. Treatment with gonadotrophin releasing hormone analogues for more than 6 months carries a significant risk of osteoporosis, limiting their usefulness for long term treatment.
- **Hysterectomy with or without bilateral oophorectomy** We found no RCTs. Observational studies have found that hysterectomy plus bilateral oophorectomy is curative. Hysterectomy alone may reduce symptoms, but evidence is limited because of the difficulty in providing controls. The risks are those of major surgery. Infertility is an irreversible consequence of bilateral oophorectomy.
- **Non-selective serotonin reuptake inhibitor antidepressants/anxiolytics** RCTs have found that non-selective serotonin reuptake inhibitor antidepressants and anxiolytic drugs versus placebo significantly improve at least one symptom of premenstrual syndrome, but a proportion of women stop treatment because of adverse effects.
- **Non-steroidal anti-inflammatory drugs** RCTs found that prostaglandin inhibitors versus placebo significantly improved a range of premenstrual symptoms but did not reduce premenstrual breast pain.
- **Oestrogens** Limited evidence from small RCTs suggests that estradiol versus placebo improves symptoms, but the magnitude of any effect remains unclear.
- **Oral contraceptives** RCTs found limited evidence that oral contraceptives versus placebo improved premenstrual symptoms.
- **Progesterone** One systematic review of progesterone versus placebo has found a small but significant improvement in overall premenstrual symptoms and no increase in the frequency of withdrawals caused by adverse effects. However, the improvement is unlikely to be clinically important. It remains unclear whether the route or timing of administration of progesterone is important.
- **Progestogens** RCTs found conflicting evidence about the effects of progestogens versus placebo.
- **Selective serotonin reuptake inhibitors** One systematic review and subsequent RCTs have found that selective serotonin reuptake inhibitors versus placebo significantly improve premenstrual symptoms, but cause frequent adverse events.
- **Tibolone** One small RCT found limited evidence that tibolone versus placebo (multivitamins) improved premenstrual symptom score.
- **Vitamin B6** One systematic review of poor quality RCTs found insufficient evidence about the effects of vitamin B_6. In the review, an analysis of weak RCTs suggested that vitamin B_6 versus placebo significantly reduced symptoms. Additional RCTs with weak methods found conflicting evidence on the effects of vitamin B_6.

- **Chiropractic treatment; dietary supplements; endometrial ablation; evening primrose oil; laparoscopic bilateral oophorectomy; reflexology; relaxation treatment** We found insufficient evidence about the effects of these interventions.

DEFINITION A woman has premenstrual syndrome if she complains of recurrent psychological or somatic symptoms (or both), occurring specifically during the luteal phase of the menstrual cycle, and resolving by the end of menstruation (see table 1, p 1990).[1]

INCIDENCE/ PREVALENCE Premenstrual symptoms occur in 95% of all women of reproductive age; severe, debilitating symptoms (premenstrual syndrome) occur in about 5% of those women.[1]

AETIOLOGY/ RISK FACTORS The aetiology is unknown, but hormonal and other (possibly neuroendocrine) factors probably contribute.[2,3] There may be enhanced sensitivity to progesterone, possibly caused by a deficiency of serotonin.[3]

PROGNOSIS Except after oophorectomy, symptoms usually recur when treatment is stopped.

AIMS To improve or eliminate physical and psychological symptoms; to minimise the impact on normal functioning, interpersonal relationships, and quality of life; to minimise adverse effects of treatment.

OUTCOMES **Symptom severity:** there is no consensus on how this should be assessed. One review of premenstrual syndrome outcomes found 65 different questionnaires or scales, measuring 199 different symptoms or signs.[4]

METHODS The initial search strategy was adapted from the Cochrane Collaboration's Menstrual Disorders and Subfertility Group.[5] *Clinical Evidence* search and appraisal February 2002. We aimed to include systematic reviews and subsequent RCTs that (1) diagnosed premenstrual syndrome by validated scales prior to randomisation; (2) used a pre-randomisation placebo cycle to exclude women with a non-specific response; (3) contained sufficient cycles to allow for symptom variability between cycles. Few trials fulfilled these criteria. The wide range of diagnostic scales, outcome criteria, and dosing regimens made comparison between trials difficult. We excluded reviews that systematically searched electronic databases but did not use overt criteria to appraise the results.[6]

QUESTION What are the effects of treatments for women with premenstrual syndrome?

OPTION PROGESTERONE

One systematic review of progesterone versus placebo has found a small but significant improvement in overall premenstrual symptoms and no increase in the frequency of withdrawals caused by adverse effects. However, the improvement is unlikely to be clinically important. It remains unclear whether the route or timing of administration of progesterone is important.

Benefits: We found one systematic review (search date 2000, 10 RCTs, 531 women with previously diagnosed premenstrual syndrome).[7] Six of the RCTs were crossover studies. The review found a small improvement in overall premenstrual symptoms for women taking progesterone versus control treatments over 2–6 months (standardised mean differences –0.028, 95% CI –0.017 to –0.040; no heterogeneity of pooled results). Two RCTs (116 completed) used oral progesterone and 7 RCTs (296 completed) used progesterone suppositories. One crossover RCT (25 women) compared oral progesterone versus progesterone pessaries versus placebo, and was analysed as if it was two studies. Six of the 10 RCTs administered the progesterone in the luteal phase of the menstrual cycle.

Harms: Some RCTs reported adverse effects such as abdominal pain, nausea, headache, vaginal pruritus, dizziness, drowsiness, excessive bleeding, and dysmenorrhoea.[7] Withdrawal because of adverse effects was not increased significantly by progesterone (OR 1.66, 95% CI 0.43 to 6.79).

Comment: The systematic review[7] did not specify whether results after the crossovers had been included in the analyses. The authors of the systematic review argued that the very small improvement in overall symptoms was statistically significant, but clinically unimportant. The observed change in symptoms was small compared with that produced by selective serotonin reuptake inhibitors (see selective serotonin reuptake inhibitors, p 1982). Subgroup analysis found a small but significant improvement of symptoms with oral progesterone (3 RCTs), and a small but significant deterioration of symptom suppositories or pessaries (8 RCTs). Oral micronised progesterone is not available in many countries, including the UK.[7] The systematic review tabulated the adverse effects reported with progesterone and placebo, but did not specify how many women were in the five RCTs that reported harms.

OPTION PROGESTOGENS (SYNTHETIC PROGESTERONE-LIKE DRUGS)

RCTs found conflicting evidence about the effects of progestogens versus placebo.

Benefits: We found one systematic review (search date 2000, 3 RCTs, 319 women) of progestogens versus placebo.[7] Two RCTs were crossover studies. One RCT compared medroxyprogesterone versus norethisterone versus placebo and was analysed as if it were two RCTs. The systematic review found a small but significant reduction of premenstrual symptoms with progestogens versus placebo (standardised mean differences –0.036, 95% CI –0.059 to –0.014).

Harms: None of the RCTs reported a detailed analysis of adverse effects.[7] The systematic review found no significant difference with progestogens versus placebo in the number of women who withdrew from the RCTs because of adverse events (OR 1.65, 95% CI 0.86 to 3.21).[7] The most common adverse effects associated with progestogens are nausea, breast discomfort, headache, and menstrual irregularity.

Comment: The systematic review[7] did not specify how the results of the crossover studies were analysed (in particular, whether results after the crossover were included). The review stated that it found no heterogeneity of the results from the four RCTs, but published a figure that appears to show disagreement among the studies (3 significantly favouring progestogen and 1 significantly favouring placebo).

OPTION LOW DOSE OESTROGENS

Limited evidence from three small RCTs suggests benefit from estradiol versus placebo, but the magnitude of any effect remains unclear.

Benefits: We found no systematic review but found three RCTs (71 women) of oestrogen versus placebo.[8–10] All trials diagnosed premenstrual syndrome before randomisation. The first RCT (11 women) found no significant difference in symptoms with oral conjugated equine oestrogens (0.6 mg from day 15 until menses) versus placebo over three cycles (9 women had worse symptoms with oestrogen *v* 2 women with placebo).[8] The second RCT (crossover, 40 women, 35 completed) compared estradiol (oestradiol) (200 μg transdermal patches changed every 3 days throughout the cycle) versus placebo for three cycles.[9] Oral norethisterone (5 mg daily) was added from day 19–26 for all women. Women were randomly allocated to a sequence of treatment (active for 3 cycles then placebo for 3 cycles, or the reverse). Both groups improved during the first three cycles. After the crossover, significant further improvement was seen with women switching from placebo to active treatment, but the symptoms of women switching from active treatment to placebo deteriorated to the level they were at the start of the RCT. The third RCT (crossover design, 20 women with migraine just before or during menses, 18 completed) found that estradiol (oestradiol) (estradiol gel 1.5 mg daily to the skin for 7 days over 3 cycles) versus placebo reduced the number of cycles with menstrual migraine (8/26 [31%] of the estradiol cycles *v* 26/27 [96%] of placebo cycles; $P < 0.01$).[10]

Harms: Adverse effects included mastalgia, nausea, weight gain, headache, and change in cycle length. The patch trial also reported skin irritation and skin pigmentation. Similar numbers of women withdrew on active treatment compared with placebo (3/71 [4%] with active treatment *v* 2/71 [3%] with placebo).[9]

Comment: Oestrogens may improve premenstrual symptoms. To avoid endometrial hyperplasia and adenocarcinoma, a 12 day progestogen course is needed every 28 days. Progestogen may induce premenstrual syndrome symptoms in some women. To avoid this systemic effect, progestogen may be given locally (using a levonorgestrel intrauterine device or progesterone gel). We found no RCTs evaluating this approach. We found one report of an ongoing RCT (80 women) comparing cyclical estradiol and medroxyprogesterone versus placebo in women with premenstrual syndrome and depressive symptoms.[11]

OPTION TIBOLONE

One small RCT found limited evidence of benefit from tibolone versus multivitamins.

Benefits: We found no systematic review but found one small RCT.[12] The RCT (18 women) found that tibolone for 3 months versus multivitamins (placebo) significantly improved premenstrual symptom scores (mean change in symptom score: –55% with tibolone *v* –10% with placebo; $P < 0.05$).

Harms: No adverse effects were reported.

Comment: The RCT was too small to make reliable conclusions.

OPTION DANAZOL

RCTs have found that danazol versus placebo significantly reduces premenstrual symptoms, but has important adverse effects associated with masculinisation when used continuously in the long term.

Benefits: We found no systematic review but found six RCTs.[13–18] **Continuous danazol:** Four RCTs (3 crossover, 144 women with premenstrual syndrome) found significant symptom reduction with danazol given continuously (over 3 cycles) versus placebo.[13–15,17] Many women withdrew before the trial finished (see harms of danazol below). **Luteal phase danazol:** Two RCTs gave danazol in the luteal phase only.[16,18] One RCT found that danazol versus placebo significantly reduced overall symptoms. The other, larger trial found danazol versus placebo significantly reduced only premenstrual breast pain.[16,18]

Harms: **Continuous danazol:** More people withdrew from the studies when given danazol than when given placebo (e.g. in 1 parallel RCT, withdrawals: 12/30 [40%] with danazol *v* 1/10 [10%] with placebo).[14] The initial severity of the premenstrual symptoms was higher among women who withdrew than among women who remained in the RCTs (see comment below). Observational studies have described masculinisation (deepening of the voice, hirsutism) and weight gain with long term use of danazol (see harms of danazol under breast pain, p 1843). Plasma lipid levels can change, leading to concern that the cardiovascular risk may be increased. Osteoporosis seems not to be a risk. **Luteal phase danazol:** The two RCTs did not find a significantly higher rate of short term adverse effects with danazol than with placebo. Long term adverse effects were not assessed.[16,18]

Comment: It seems clear that danazol is capable of reducing premenstrual symptoms (many women who remained in the RCTs had some types of symptom eradicated by danazol, but fewer did with placebo). However, the magnitude of the danazol effect is less certain because some of the mean improvement in symptom scores can be attributed to the withdrawal of women with worse symptoms. The RCTs did not report intention to treat analyses.

OPTION GONADOTROPHIN RELEASING HORMONE ANALOGUES (BUSERELIN, GOSERELIN, LEUPRORELIN)

RCTs have found significant reduction of symptoms with gonadotrophin releasing hormone analogues versus placebo. RCTs have found that gonadotrophin releasing hormone plus oestrogen plus progestogen (addback treatment) produced a fall in symptom scores that was intermediate between those produced by gonadotrophin releasing hormone analogue alone and placebo. Treatment with gonadotrophin releasing hormone analogues for more than 6 months carries significant risk of osteoporosis, limiting their usefulness for long term treatment.

Benefits: We found no systematic review. **Gonadotrophin releasing hormone analogues versus placebo:** We found 10 RCTs[19–28] of gonadotrophin releasing hormone (GnRH) analogues versus placebo. All 10 trials diagnosed premenstrual syndrome before randomisation. Seven of the RCTs used a crossover design. Nine of the RCTs found a significant reduction in premenstrual symptoms with GnRH analogues versus placebo (typically, by 3 months symptom scores fell to about 50% of their initial value with a GnRH analogue *v* 10% decline with placebo[27]). **GnRH analogues plus oestrogen and progestogen:** Three of the RCTs (78 women) compared GnRH analogues plus oestrogen and progestogen (addback treatment) versus placebo or GnRH analogue alone.[23,24,27] Two of the RCTs were small (8 women[23] and 10 women[24]). The largest RCT (60 women, 41 completed the 6 month study) found that GnRH plus addback treatment produced a fall in symptom scores that was intermediate between that produced by GnRH analogue alone and placebo (irritability symptom score at baseline 2 in all groups; change in score after 6 months: –0.37 with placebo *v* –0.64 with GnRH analogue plus addback *v* –1.03 with GnRH analogue alone; $P < 0.05$).[27] **GnRH analogue plus tibolone versus GnRH analogue alone:** We found one RCT (30 women with severe premenstrual syndrome (see glossary, p 1987)), which found no difference in symptom scores after 8 weeks with GnRH analogue plus tibolone versus GnRH analogue plus placebo (irritability scores: changed from 7.3 to 3.3 with GnRH analogue plus tibolone *v* from 8.4 to 4.0 with GnRH analogue alone).[29]

Harms: A large proportion of the women in the RCTs experienced adverse effects. Commonly reported adverse effects include hot flushes, night sweats, nausea, decreased libido, pruritus, bronchospasm, and headache.[19,20,22,26,28] In one typical RCT, over 6 months' withdrawals from the RCT were common (7/20 [35%] with placebo *v* 9/21 [43%] with GnRH plus addback treatment *v* 3/19 [16%] with GnRH analogue alone).[27]

Comment: A truly double blind RCT of GnRH analogues would be hard to conduct because women receiving these agents experience amenorrhoea. Treatment with gonadotrophin releasing hormone analogues for more than 6 months carries significant risk of osteoporosis, limiting their usefulness for long term treatment.

OPTION BROMOCRIPTINE

RCTs have found that bromocriptine versus placebo relieves premenstrual breast tenderness, although adverse effects are common.

Benefits: We found no systematic review. One survey of 14 trials found no evidence that bromocriptine versus placebo improved overall symptom scores in premenstrual syndrome, although it found limited evidence of improvement in premenstrual mastalgia.[30]

Harms: Bromocriptine has a high incidence of adverse effects, including nausea, dizziness, headache, weight increase, and swelling.[31–33] The survey did not include any mention of adverse effects, which on analysis of individual trials are well documented.[30] There have been very rare case reports of stroke and death following bromocriptine treatment to prevent lactation.[34]

Comment: None.

OPTION ORAL CONTRACEPTIVES

Two RCTs found limited evidence that oral contraceptives versus placebo improved premenstrual symptoms.

Benefits: We found no systematic review but found two RCTs,[35,36] which diagnosed premenstrual syndrome prior to randomisation. The first RCT (82 women) found significant reduction with triphasic oral contraceptive for three cycles versus placebo in premenstrual breast pain and bloating. Oral contraceptives were no better than placebo for mood symptoms. The second RCT (82 women with severe premenstrual syndrome (see glossary, p 1987)) found significant reduction in some premenstrual symptoms (appetite, acne, and food cravings) with an experimental oral contraception (ethinylestradiol 30 µg plus drospirenone 3 mg over 3 cycles) versus placebo.[36] Other symptom scores were improved with oral contraception, but the differences were not significant.[36]

Harms: Spotting, nausea, cramps, breast pain, and decreased libido were more commonly reported on active treatment compared with placebo. More women withdrew because of adverse effects with active treatment than with placebo (13 *v* 1).[35]

Comment: Some women develop premenstrual syndrome-like symptoms for the first time when taking the oral contraceptive pill. Anecdotal evidence suggests that oral contraceptives may be beneficial in premenstrual syndrome.[37–39] Continuous combined regimens (those without a 1 wk break) should, in theory, suppress ovulation and provide symptom relief, but we found no published trials.

OPTION DIURETICS

RCTs have found that spironactolone versus placebo improves symptoms of premenstrual syndrome including breast tenderness and bloating. Two RCTs have found that metolazone or ammonium chloride versus placebo reduce premenstrual swelling and weight gain. One RCT found insufficient evidence about the effects of chlortalidone versus placebo or lithium on premenstrual symptoms.

Benefits: **Spironolactone:** We found no systematic review but found five RCTs that compared spironolactone versus placebo.[40–44] Four RCTs (210 women) diagnosed premenstrual syndrome prior to randomisation.[40–43] Three RCTs found significant reduction of symptoms with spironolactone (100 mg daily) versus placebo, and one RCT[42] found no significant difference. Two RCTs found that significantly more women had improved irritability[43] and overall symptoms, including breast tenderness and bloating[41] with spironolactone than with placebo (20/26 [77%][43] and 14/17 [82%][41] with spironolactone *v* 11/21 [52%][43] and 9/16 [56%][41] with placebo; ARI 25%, 95% CI 5% to 45%; NNT 4). **Metolazone:** One RCT (crossover design, 46 women with premenstrual swelling or weight gain, 33 completed) found significant reduction of premenstrual symptoms with luteal phase metolazone (1, 2.5, and 5 mg daily) versus placebo.[45] There was no significant effect of dose on benefit. **Chlortalidone (chlorthalidone):** One RCT (crossover design, 25 women) found that similar numbers of women felt "much better" over 8 menstrual cycles on a global rating scale of premenstrual symptoms with chlortalidone versus placebo or lithium.[46] However, the RCT did not diagnose premenstrual syndrome prior to randomisation, and it may have been too small to detect a clinically important difference in symptoms. **Ammonium chloride:** One RCT (22 women with premenstrual weight gain) found significantly more weight loss on days 20–23 with a diuretic on sale to the general public in the USA (ammonium chloride 325 mg plus caffeine 100 mg 6 times daily for days 18–24) versus placebo.[47]

Harms: **Spironolactone:** Adverse effects were reported in only one RCT: two people reported palpitations whilst on spironolactone. **Metolazone:** Women on 5 mg metolazone complained of severe adverse effects (excessive diuresis and weakness).[45] Other adverse effects include nausea, dizziness, palpitations, excess diuresis, and weakness.[47]

Comment: Diuretics are widely used in the belief that many symptoms of premenstrual syndrome are the direct consequence of fluid retention; we found little evidence of water retention in most women with premenstrual syndrome.

OPTION NON-STEROIDAL ANTI-INFLAMMATORY DRUGS

RCTs have found benefit from prostaglandin inhibitors versus placebo for a range of premenstrual symptoms.

Benefits: We found no systematic review. **Mefenamic acid:** We found five RCTs,[48–52] but only three diagnosed premenstrual syndrome prior to randomisation.[48,49,52] One RCT (37 women) found significantly more women preferred mefenamic acid (1.5 g daily in the luteal phase for 1 cycle) than placebo (23/37 [62%] with mefenamic acid *v* 6/37 [16%] with placebo; $P < 0.002$).[48] The frequency of irritability was significantly lower with mefenamic acid than with placebo (11/36 [31%] *v* 24/33 [73%]; ARR 42%, 95% CI 19% to 66%; NNT 3).[48] The other RCT (crossover design, 19 women) found significantly improved physical and mood symptoms with three cycles of mefenamic acid versus placebo.[49] **Naproxen sodium:** Two RCTs diagnosed premenstrual syndrome before randomisation. One RCT (34 women) found significant reduction of pain symptoms with naproxen sodium (550 mg twice daily for days 21–4 in 3 cycles) versus placebo.[53] The other RCT (crossover design, 42 women randomised, 21 completed) found significant reduction of physical symptoms of premenstrual syndrome with naproxen sodium (500 mg twice daily for 6 cycles) versus placebo.[54]

Harms: Adverse effects included nausea, gastrointestinal disturbances, and rashes.[48–50]

Comment: None.

OPTION ANXIOLYTICS/NON-SELECTIVE SEROTONIN REUPTAKE INHIBITOR ANTIDEPRESSANTS

RCTs have found that non-selective serotonin reuptake inhibitor antidepressants and anxiolytic drugs versus placebo significantly improve at least one symptom of premenstrual syndrome, but a proportion of women stop treatment because of adverse effects.

Benefits: We found no systematic review. We found 13 studies covering 14 RCTs of antidepressant and anxiolytic drugs for premenstrual syndrome. Most (9/14 [64%]) reported significant improvement of one or more symptoms. **Alprazolam:** Five RCTs (150 women) compared alprazolam (0.25–2.25 mg daily) versus placebo.[55–59] The RCT using the lowest dose (0.25–0.75 mg daily) found no significant reduction in premenstrual symptoms, but four RCTs using a higher dose (≥ 0.75 mg daily) found significant reduction of symptoms. **Buspirone:** Two small RCTs (17 women,[60] 41 women[61]) found significant symptom reduction with buspirone (25 mg daily,[60] 10–20 mg daily[61]) versus placebo. **Non-selective serotonin reuptake inhibitors antidepressants:** Four small RCTs of antidepressants versus placebo (81 women) found variable results: two RCTs of clomipramine (25–75 mg daily) versus placebo found significant reduction of premenstrual symptoms, but RCTs of buproprion[62] and desipramine[63] found no significant reduction. We found no meta-analysis; it is unclear whether the difference in the results arose from the play of chance in small RCTs or because there is a difference in the effects of different antidepressants. **β blockers:** Three RCTs found variable results. Two small RCTs (27 women) found significant symptom improvement with atenolol versus placebo at lower doses (25 mg daily) but no significant difference with higher doses (100 mg daily).[64,65] The third RCT (30 women) found significant reduction of severe premenstrual headaches with propranolol (20–40 mg daily during luteal phase) versus placebo.[66] **Lithium:** One RCT (19 women) found no significant difference in premenstrual symptoms with lithium carbonate (750–1000 mg daily) versus placebo.[67]

Harms: Adverse effects such as drowsiness, nausea, anxiety, and headache led to problems with adherence to treatment in most of the trials.[55,59,68,69] **Alprazolam:** Drowsiness and sedation were found in about 50% of women, as well as lower rates of headache and nausea. **Antidepressants:** Adverse effects were frequent and more women withdrew when taking antidepressants than when taking placebo (11/81 [14%] with antidepressants v 6/81 [7%] with placebo).[62,63,68,70] Common adverse effects reported were dry mouth, fatigue, nausea, and dizziness. **Lithium:** Tremor, weakness, and gastrointestinal disturbances resulted in 4/19 (21%) withdrawals from the RCT. **Other interventions:** The other trials did not report specific adverse effects.

Comment: The evidence is limited, but is consistent with at most a small benefit from antidepressants/anxiolytics in premenstrual syndrome, which is countered by frequent adverse effects.

OPTION SELECTIVE SEROTONIN REUPTAKE INHIBITORS

One systematic review and subsequent RCTs have found that selective serotonin reuptake inhibitors versus placebo significantly improve premenstrual symptoms, but cause frequent adverse events.

Benefits: We found one systematic review,[71] one additional report of an RCT in the review,[72] and one subsequent RCT.[73] The systematic review (search date not stated, 15 RCTs, 904 women with premenstrual syndrome) found significant improvement in overall symptoms with selective serotonin reuptake inhibitors (SSRIs) versus placebo (WMD –1.07, 95% CI –1.38 to –0.75).[71] There was no significant difference in symptom improvement between continuous and intermittent dosing. The review did not report absolute proportions of women who had improved symptoms with SSRIs. A large RCT that was included in the review subsequently reported the proportion of women who had improved physical symptoms (observer rated scale of physical symptoms including breast tenderness, bloating, headache, joint and muscle pain).[72] The RCT (320 women with severe premenstrual syndrome (see glossary, p 1987) diagnosed before randomisation) found significant reduction of physical premenstrual symptoms with fluoxetine for six cycles versus placebo (substantial reduction of physical premenstrual symptoms: 11/95 [12%] with fluoxetine 20 mg v 13/85 [15%] with fluoxetine 60 mg v 4/94 [4%] with placebo; ARR fluoxetine v placebo 9.1%, 95% CI 1.5% to 16.7%; NNT 11 women treated for 6 cycles for 1 woman to have a substantial reduction in symptoms). No difference in physical premenstrual symptoms was found between the two doses of fluoxetine (20 mg v 60 mg daily; OR 0.73, 95% CI 0.31 to 1.71). The subsequent RCT (164 women with severe premenstrual syndrome diagnosed before randomisation) found significant improvement of overall premenstrual symptoms with venlafaxine (50–200 mg daily for 4 cycles) versus placebo (≥ 50% reduction in daily total symptom score: 41/68 [60%] with venlafaxine v 26/75 [35%] with placebo; ARR 25%, 95% CI 9% to 42%; NNT 4).[73]

Harms: Common adverse effects were nausea, drowsiness/fatigue, nervousness, insomnia, headache, and sexual dysfunction (see table 2, p 1991).[71] The frequency of adverse events is similar to that seen with SSRIs in other populations.[72] The systematic review found that withdrawal because of adverse effects was more likely with SSRIs than with placebo (OR 2.4, 95% CI 1.6 to 3.7).[71] Adverse effects were more likely with the higher dose of fluoxetine.[72]

Comment: SSRIs used in the trials were fluoxetine (7 trials), sertraline (5 trials), citalopram (1 trial), fluvoxamine (1 trial), and paroxetine (1 trial).[71] Venlafaxine is described as an inhibitor of serotonin and noradrenaline (norepinephrine) uptake. The systematic review found significant heterogeneity of the results ($P < 0.0001$), but the results were robust and did not depend on the type of meta-analysis (fixed effects or random effects). Many of the harms attributed to treatment were frequent, and some (nervousness, headache, insomnia) were similar to the typical symptoms of premenstrual syndrome. However, the net effect of SSRI antidepressants versus placebo was a significant reduction of total symptom scores.[71,73]

OPTION VITAMIN B_6

A systematic review of poor quality RCTs found that the evidence was insufficient to define the effects of vitamin B_6 versus placebo in women with premenstrual syndrome. In the review, an analysis of nine weak RCTs suggested a significant reduction of symptoms with vitamin B_6 versus placebo. Three additional RCTs with weak methods found conflicting evidence of the benefits of vitamin B_6.

Benefits: We found one systematic reviews[74] and three additional RCTs.[75–77] The systematic review (search date 1998, 9 RCTs, 940 women with premenstrual syndrome) found no high quality RCTs comparing vitamin B_6 (either as a single supplement or as part of a multivitamin supplement) with placebo.[74] The pooled odds ratio for relief of overall premenstrual syndrome symptoms was 2.32 (95% CI 1.95 to 2.54) with vitamin B_6 (over 2–4 months) versus placebo. There was no dose related response. One additional RCT compared vitamin B_6 with *Vitex agnus castus*; an improvement over placebo was found with both treatments.[75] Another RCT with weak methods found no improvement over placebo,[66] whereas the third additional RCT found a significant improvement.[76]

Harms: High doses (> 200 mg daily) have been associated with a reversible peripheral neuropathy.[74] The review found few reports of adverse events in the RCTs.

Comment: None of the subsequent RCTs met the criteria for inclusion in the systematic review.[74]

OPTION EVENING PRIMROSE OIL

One systematic review of poor quality RCTs found insufficient evidence about the effects of evening primrose oil.

Benefits: We found one systematic review (search date 1993, 7 RCTs, 329 women).[77] Although some trials found a small beneficial effect, the number of women included in the RCTs was low. Weak methods and different outcome measures prevented a meta-analysis. The authors concluded that there was insufficient evidence to define the effects of evening primrose oil in women with premenstrual syndrome.

Harms: Few adverse effects have been reported. There are rare reports of evening primrose oil causing seizures in people with epilepsy.

Comment: Only five of the trials in the review clearly indicated that they were randomised. Evening primrose oil is one of the most popular "self help" remedies for premenstrual syndrome, although in the UK it is licensed only for the treatment of premenstrual mastalgia.

OPTION DIETARY SUPPLEMENTS

One systematic review found insufficient evidence on the effects of calcium and magnesium supplements versus placebo in women with premenstrual syndrome.

Benefits: We found one systematic review (search date 2000).[78] **Magnesium supplements:** The systematic review (3 RCTs, 144 women) found unclear results with magnesium supplements versus placebo for premenstrual syndrome symptoms. One RCT found an improvement in overall premenstrual syndrome symptoms, one found no effect, and the third found significant improvement of bloating. The review did not perform a meta-analysis. **Calcium supplements:** The systematic review (2 RCTs, 557 women) found that calcium supplements (1–1.2 g daily for 3 cycles) versus placebo significantly reduced overall symptoms (including breast tenderness and swelling, headaches, and abdominal cramps).[78]

Harms: None reported.

Comment: **Calcium supplements:** Both RCTs were performed by the same research unit. The smaller RCT had a high withdrawal rate and compliance with treatment was poor. The second, larger RCT did not exclude other treatments of premenstrual symptoms during the RCT.[78]

OPTION COGNITIVE BEHAVIOURAL THERAPY

RCTs have found significant reduction of premenstrual symptoms with cognitive behavioural therapy versus control treatments, but the evidence is insufficient to define the size of any effect.

Benefits: **Versus control treatments:** We found no systematic review. Six RCTs compared a treatment with cognitive behavioural content versus some type of control treatment.[79–84] Four of the RCTs (112 women) found significant reduction of symptoms with cognitive behavioural therapy versus a dummy treatment (relaxation, activity through movement, or information focused treatment) or versus a waiting list group.

Harms: None reported.

Comment: It is difficult to design appropriate control treatments and to maintain blinding of allocation for cognitive behavioural therapies, but studies using both dummy and waiting list controls have found significant benefits. Several trials noted benefits of cognitive behavioural therapy over the medium to long term. Cognitive behavioural therapy may be appropriate only for a motivated subgroup of women.

OPTION EXERCISE

One RCT has found that aerobic exercise versus placebo significantly improves premenstrual symptoms; another RCT has found that high intensity aerobic exercise improves symptoms significantly more than low intensity.

Benefits: We found no systematic review, but found two RCTs.[85,86] The first RCT (32 women with premenstrual syndrome diagnosed prior to randomisation) found significantly improved symptoms with high intensity aerobic exercise versus low intensity exercise.[85] The second RCT (30 women with premenstrual syndrome) found significant reduction of premenstrual symptoms with both low intensity aerobic exercise (40% maximum effort for 45 mins, 3 times weekly, for 3 cycles) versus placebo weekly and with moderate intensity aerobic exercise (70% maximum effort for 45 mins, 3 times weekly, for 3 cycles) versus placebo.[86]

Harms: None reported.

Comment: Both reports[85,86] were available to us only as abstracts. Further details may be available in future *Clinical Evidence* updates.

OPTION CHIROPRACTIC MANIPULATION

One systematic review found insufficient evidence about the effects of chiropractic treatment in women with premenstrual syndrome.

Benefits: We found one systematic review (search date 2000, 1 RCT, 45 women).[78] The placebo controlled crossover RCT found a significant decrease in premenstrual syndrome scores with chiropractic treatment (3 sessions premenstrually over 3 cycles) versus placebo. Women who received placebo first did not experience significant additional improvement when they were switched to chiropractic treatment.

Harms: None reported.

Comment: The RCT had a high withdrawal rate (25/45 [56%] completed). Women improved most with whatever treatment they had first (real or sham treatment). The evidence is insufficient to define the effects of chiropractic treatment in women with premenstrual syndrome.

OPTION RELAXATION TREATMENT

RCTs found insufficient evidence on the effects of relaxation treatment in premenstrual syndrome.

Benefits: We found one systematic review (search date 2000, 2 RCTs, 101 women).[78] The first RCT found significant reduction of physical symptoms with muscular relaxation treatment versus reading leisure material or charting symptoms. The second RCT compared muscle relaxation versus massage, but did not compare the reduction in symptoms produced by each treatment. Both groups improved compared with baseline symptoms.

Harms: None mentioned.

Comment: Most studies of relaxation techniques have used them as an adjunct to other treatment. The evidence is insufficient to define the effects of relaxation in women with premenstrual syndrome.

OPTION REFLEXOLOGY

One systematic review of one RCT found insufficient evidence about the effects of reflexology versus sham reflexology in premenstrual syndrome.

Benefits: We found one systematic review (search date 2000, 1 RCT, 50 women).[78] The RCT found significant reduction of premenopausal symptoms with reflexology (1 weekly session over 2 cycles) versus sham reflexology.

Harms: None mentioned.

Comment: Only 35 women completed the RCT. Reflexology involved manual pressure to specific reflex areas of the body, but the sham treatment comprised uneven tactile stimulation of alternative areas (shoulder, elbow, or nose). The therapist was not blinded. The evidence is insufficient to define the effects of reflexology in women with premenstrual syndrome.

OPTION HYSTERECTOMY WITH OR WITHOUT OOPHORECTOMY

We found no RCTs. Observational studies have found that hysterectomy plus bilateral oophorectomy is curative. Hysterectomy alone may reduce symptoms, but evidence is limited because of the difficulty in providing controls. The risks are those of major surgery. Infertility is an irreversible consequence of bilateral oophorectomy.

Benefits: We found no systematic review and no RCTs.

Harms: Potential risks include those associated with major surgery.[87]

Comment: Cohort studies have described a reduction in the symptoms of premenstrual syndrome after hysterectomy.[88,89] However, without a control group, it is impossible to know how much of the observed response is attributable to the hysterectomy itself or to a non-specific placebo response that is seen in most RCTs of premenstrual syndrome. Other cohort studies have found almost complete eradication of the symptoms of premenstrual syndrome after hysterectomy plus bilateral oophorectomy.[90,91] Surgery is rarely used but may be indicated if there are coexisting gynaecological problems.

OPTION LAPAROSCOPIC BILATERAL OOPHORECTOMY

We found no RCTs on the effects of laparoscopic bilateral oophorectomy in women with premenstrual syndrome.

Benefits: We found no systematic review or RCTs.

Harms: We found insufficient evidence.

Comment: After oophorectomy, oestrogen replacement treatment and cyclical progesterone (to prevent endometrial hyperplasia and carcinoma) are often used. Progesterone may re-stimulate premenstrual syndrome.

OPTION ENDOMETRIAL ABLATION

We found no RCTs about the effects of endometrial ablation in premenstrual syndrome.

Benefits: We found no systematic review or RCTs.

Harms: We found insufficient evidence.

Comment: Studies of women with menorrhagia have claimed that endometrial ablation may relieve symptoms of premenstrual syndrome. However, it remains unclear what the benefits are in women with premenstrual syndrome.

GLOSSARY

Severe premenstrual syndrome: The definition of severe premenstrual syndrome varies among RCTs, but in recent studies[72,73] standardised criteria have been used to diagnose one variant of severe premenstrual syndrome (termed the Premenstrual Dysphoric Disorder), based on at least five symptoms, including one of four core psychological symptoms (from a list of 17 physical and psychological symptoms), being severe premenstrually and mild or absent postmenstrually. The 17 symptoms are depression, feeling hopeless or guilty, anxiety/tension, mood swings, irritability/persistent anger, decreased interest, poor concentration, fatigue, food craving or increased appetite, sleep disturbance, feeling out of control or overwhelmed, poor coordination, headache, aches, swelling/bloating/weight gain, cramps, and breast tenderness.

REFERENCES

1. O'Brien PMS. Premenstrual syndrome. London: Blackwell Science, 1987.
2. O'Brien PMS. Helping women with premenstrual syndrome. *BMJ* 1993;307:1471–1475.
3. Rapkin AJ, Morgan M, Goldman L, Brann DW, Simone D, Mahesh VB. Progesterone metabolite allopregnanolone in women with premenstrual syndrome. *Obstet Gynecol* 1997;90:709–714.
4. Budeiri DJ, Li WP, Dornan JC. Clinical trials of treatments of premenstrual syndrome: entry criteria and scales for measuring treatment outcomes. *Br J Obstet Gynaecol* 1994;101:689–695
5. Cochrane Menstrual Disorders and Subfertility Group. Search strategy for specialist registrar (Collaborative Review Groups). In: The Cochrane Library, Issue 4. Oxford: Update software, 1999.
6. Frackiewicz EJ, Shiovitz TM. Evaluation and management of premenstrual syndrome and premenstrual dysphoric disorder. *J Am Pharm Assoc* 2001;41:437–447. Search date: 2001 primary sources Medline and hand searches of bibliographies of retrieved articles.
7. Wyatt K, Dimmock P, Jones P, Obhrai M, O'Brien S. Efficacy of progesterone and progestogens in management of premenstrual syndrome: systematic review. *BMJ* 2001;323:776–780. Search date: 2000; primary sources Embase, Medline, PsychINFO, the Cochrane controlled trial register, hand searches, and pharmaceutical companies who manufacture progesterone preparations.
8. Dhar V, Murphy BE. Double-blind randomized crossover trial of luteal phase estrogens (Premarin) in the premenstrual syndrome (PMS). *Psychoneuroendocrinology* 1990;15:489–493.
9. Watson NR, Studd JW, Savvas M, Garnett T, Baber RJ. Treatment of severe premenstrual syndrome with oestradiol patches and cyclical oral norethisterone. *Lancet* 1989;2:730–732.
10. de Lignieres B, Vincens M, Mauvais-Jarvis P, Mas JL, Touboul PJ, Bousser MG. Prevention of menstrual migraine by percutaneous oestradiol. *BMJ* 1986;293:1540.
11. Panay N. Treatment of depressive symptoms in women diagnosed as having premenstrual syndrome (PMS) with long cycle hormone replacement therapy (TridestraR). National Research Register, 1999.
12. Taskin O, Gokdeniz R, Yalcinoglu A, Buhur A, Burak F, Atmaca R, Ozekici U. Placebo-controlled cross-over study of effects of tibolone on premenstrual symptoms and peripheral beta-endorphin concentrations in premenstrual syndrome. *Hum Reprod* 1998;13:2402–2405.
13. Gilmore DH, Hawthorn RJ, Hart DM. Danol for premenstrual syndrome: a preliminary report of a placebo-controlled double-blind study. *J Int Med Res* 1985;13:129–130.
14. Watts JF, Butt WR, Logan ER. A clinical trial using danazol for the treatment of premenstrual tension. *Br J Obstet Gynaecol* 1987;94:30–34.

15. Deeny M, Hawthorn R, McKay IID. Low dose danazol in the treatment of the premenstrual syndrome. *Postgrad Med J* 1991;67:450–454.
16. Sarno APJ, Miller EJJ, Lundblad EG. Premenstrual syndrome: beneficial effects of periodic, low-dose danazol. *Obstet Gynecol* 1987;70:33–36.
17. Hahn PM, Van Vugt DA, Reid RL. A randomized, placebo-controlled, crossover trial of danazol for the treatment of premenstrual syndrome. *Psychoneuroendocrinology* 1995;20:193–209.
18. O'Brien PMS, Abukhalil IEH. Randomised controlled trial of the management of premenstrual syndrome and premenstrual mastalgia using luteal phase only danazol. *Am J Obstet Gynecol* 1999;180:18–23.
19. Freeman EW, Sondheimer SJ, Rickels K. gonadotrophin-releasing hormone agonist in the treatment of premenstrual symptoms with and without ongoing dysphoria: a controlled study. *Psychopharmacol Bull* 1997;33:303–309.
20. Brown CS, Ling FW, Andersen RN, Farmer RG, Arheart KL. Efficacy of depot leuprolide in premenstrual syndrome: effect of symptom severity and type in a controlled trial. *Obstet Gynecol* 1994;84:779–786.
21. Helvacioglu A, Yeoman RR, Hazelton JM, Aksel S. Premenstrual syndrome and related hormonal changes. Long-acting gonadotrophin releasing hormone agonist treatment. *J Reprod Med* 1993;38:864–870.
22. Muse KN, Cetel NS, Futterman LA, Yen SC. The premenstrual syndrome. Effects of "medical ovariectomy". *N Engl J Med* 1984;311:1345–1349.
23. Mortola JF, Girton L, Fischer U. Successful treatment of severe premenstrual syndrome by combined use of gonadotrophin-releasing hormone agonist and estrogen/progestin. *J Clin Endocrinol Metab* 1991;72:252A–252F.
24. Mezrow G, Shoupe D, Spicer D, Lobo R, Leung B, Pike M. Depot leuprolide acetate with estrogen and progestin add-back for long-term treatment of premenstrual syndrome. *Fertil Steril* 1994;62:932–937.
25. Hammarback S, Backstrom T. Induced anovulation as treatment of premenstrual tension syndrome: a double-blind cross-over study with GnRH-agonist versus placebo. *Acta Obstet Gynecol Scand* 1988;67:159–166.
26. West CP, Hillier H. Ovarian suppression with the gonadotrophin-releasing hormone agonist goserelin (Zoladex) in management of the premenstrual tension syndrome. *Hum Reprod* 1994;9:1058–1063.
27. Leather AT, Studd JWW, Watson NR, Holland EFN. The treatment of severe premenstrual syndrome with goserelin with and without 'add-back' estrogen therapy: a placebo-controlled study. *Gynecol Endocrinol* 1999;13:48–55.
28. Sundstrom I, Nyberg S, Bixo M, Hammarback S, Backstrom T. Treatment of premenstrual syndrome with gonadotrophin-releasing hormone agonist in a low dose regimen. *Acta Obstet Gynecol Scand* 1999;78:891–899.
29. Di Carlo C, Palomba S, Tommaselli GA, Guida M, Di Spiezio SA, Nappi C. Use of leuprolide acetate plus tibolone in the treatment of severe premenstrual syndrome. *Fertil Steril* 2001;75:380–384.
30. Andersch B. Bromocriptine and premenstrual symptoms: a survey of double blind trials. *Obstet Gynecol Surv* 1983;38:643–646.
31. Ylostalo P, Kauppila A, Puolakka J, Ronnberg L, Janne O. Bromocriptine and norethisterone in the treatment of premenstrual syndrome. *Obstet Gynecol* 1982;59:292–298.
32. Graham JJ, Harding PE, Wise PH, Berriman H. Prolactin suppression in the treatment of premenstrual syndrome. *Med J Aust* 1978;2:18–20.
33. Kullander S, Svanberg L. Bromocriptine treatment of the premenstrual syndrome. *Acta Obstet Gynecol Scand* 1979;58:375–378.
34. Arrowsmith-Lowe T. Bromocriptine indications withdrawn. *FDA Med Bull* 1994;24:2.
35. Graham CA, Sherwin BB. A prospective treatment study of premenstrual symptoms using a triphasic oral contraceptive. *J Psychosom Res* 1992;36:257–266.
36. Freeman EW, Kroll R, Rapkin A, et al. Evaluation of a unique oral contraceptive in the treatment of premenstrual dysphoric disorder. *J Womens Health Gend Based Med* 2001;10:561–569.
37. Cullberg J. Mood changes and menstrual symptoms with different gestagen/estrogen combinations: a double blind comparison with a placebo. *Acta Psychiatr Scand* Suppl 1972; 236:1–86.
38. Morris NM, Udry JR. Contraceptive pills and day-by-day feelings of well-being. *Am J Obstet Gynecol* 1972;113:763–765.
39. Silbergeld S, Brast N, Noble EP. The menstrual cycle: a double blind study of symptoms, mood and behaviour and biochemical variables using Enovid and placebo. *Psychosom Med* 1971;33:411–428.
40. Hellberg D, Claesson B, Nilsson S. Premenstrual tension: a placebo-controlled efficacy study with spironolactone and medroxyprogesterone acetate. *Int J Gynaecol Obstet* 1991;34:243–248.
41. Wang M, Hammarback S, Lindhe BA, Backstrom T. Treatment of premenstrual syndrome by spironolactone: a double-blind, placebo-controlled study. *Acta Obstet Gynecol Scand* 1995;74:803–808.
42. Burnet RB, Radden HS, Easterbrook EG, McKinnon RA. Premenstrual syndrome and spironolactone. *Aust N Z J Obstet Gynaecol* 1991;31:366–368.
43. Vellacott ID, Shroff NE, Pearce MY, Stratford ME, Akbar FA. A double-blind, placebo-controlled evaluation of spironolactone in the premenstrual syndrome. *Curr Med Res Opin* 1987;10:450–456.
44. O'Brien PM, Craven D, Selby C, Symonds EM. Treatment of premenstrual syndrome by spironolactone. *Br J Obstet Gynaecol* 1979;86:142–147.
45. Werch A, Kane RE. Treatment of premenstrual tension with metolazone: a double-blind evaluation of a new diuretic. *Curr Ther Res Clin Exp* 1976;19:565–572.
46. Mattsson B, von Schoultz B. A comparison between lithium, placebo and a diuretic in premenstrual tension. *Acta Psychiatr Scand Suppl* 1974;255:75–84.
47. Hoffman JJ A double blind crossover clinical trial of an OTC diuretic in the treatment of premenstrual tension and weight gain. *Curr Ther Res* 1979;26:575–580.
48. Mira M, McNeil D, Fraser IS, Vizzard J, Abraham S. Mefenamic acid in the treatment of premenstrual syndrome. *Obstet Gynecol* 1986;68:395–398.
49. Jakubowicz DL, Godard E, Dewhurst J. The treatment of premenstrual tension with mefenamic acid: analysis of prostaglandin concentrations. *Br J Obstet Gynaecol* 1984;91:78–84.
50. Wood C, Jakubowicz D. The treatment of premenstrual symptoms with mefenamic acid. *Br J Obstet Gynaecol* 1980;87:627–630.

51. Gunston KD. Premenstrual syndrome in Cape Town. Part II: a double-blind placebo-controlled study of the efficacy of mefenamic acid. *S Afr Med J* 1986;70:159–160.
52. Budoff PW. No more menstrual cramps and other good news. New York: GP Putman and Sons, 1980.
53. Facchinetti F, Fioroni L, Sances G, Romano G, Nappi G, Genazzani AR. Naproxen sodium in the treatment of premenstrual symptoms: a placebo-controlled study. *Gynecol Obstet Invest* 1989;28:205–208.
54. Budoff PW. Use of prostaglandin inhibitors in the treatment of PMS. *Clin Obstet Gynecol* 1987;30(2):453–464.
55. Freeman EW, Rickels K, Sondheimer SJ, Polansky M. A double-blind trial of oral progesterone, alprazolam, and placebo in treatment of severe premenstrual syndrome. *JAMA* 1995;274:51–57.
56. Schmidt PJ, Grover GN, Rubinow DR. Alprazolam in the treatment of premenstrual syndrome: a double-blind, placebo-controlled trial. *Arch Gen Psychiatry* 1993;50:467–473.
57. Harrison WM, Endicott J, Rabkin JG, Nee JC, Sandberg D. Treatment of premenstrual dysphoria with alprazolam and placebo. *Psychopharmacol Bull* 1987;23:150–153.
58. Smith S, Rinehart JS, Ruddock VE, Schiff I. Treatment of premenstrual syndrome with alprazolam: results of a double-blind, placebo-controlled, randomized crossover clinical trial. *Obstet Gynecol* 1987;70:37–43.
59. Harrison WM, Endicott J, Nee J. Treatment of premenstrual dysphoria with alprazolam: a controlled study. *Arch Gen Psychiatry* 1990;47:270–275.
60. Rickels K, Freeman E, Sondheimer S. Buspirone in treatment of premenstrual syndrome. *Lancet* 1989;1:777.
61. Landen M, Eriksson O, Sundblad C, Andersch B, Naessen T, Eriksson E. Compounds with affinity for serotonergic receptors in the treatment of premenstrual dysphoria: a comparison of buspirone, nefazodone and placebo. *Psychopharmacologia* 2001;155:292–298.
62. Pearlstein TB, Stone AB, Lund SA, Scheft H, Zlotnik C, Brown WA. Comparison of fluoxetine, buproprion, and placebo in the treatment of premenstrual dysphoric disorder. *J Clin Psychopharmacol* 1997;17:261–266.
63. Sundblad C, Hedberg MA, Eriksson E. Clomipramine administered during the luteal phase reduces the symptoms of premenstrual syndrome: a placebo controlled trial. *Neuropsychopharmacology* 1993;9:133–145.
64. Rausch JL, Janowsky DS, Golshan S, Kuhn K, Risch SC. Atenolol treatment of late luteal phase dysphoric disorder. *J Affect Disord* 1988;15:141–147.
65. Parry BL, Rosebthal NE, James SP, Wehr TA. Atenolol in premenstrual syndrome: A test of the melatonin hypothesis. *Psychiatry Res* 1991;37:131–138.
66. Diegoli MSC, DaFonseca AM, Diegoli CA, Pinotti JA. A double-blind trial of four medications to treat severe premenstrual syndrome. *Int J Gynecol Obstet* 1998;62:63–67.
67. Singer K, Cheng R, Schou M. A controlled evaluation of lithium in the premenstrual tension syndrome. *Br J Psychiatry* 1974;124:50–51.
68. Sundblad C, Modigh K, Andersch B, Eriksson E. Clomipramine effectively reduces premenstrual irritability and dysphoria: a placebo-controlled trial. *Acta Psychiatr Scand* 1992;85:39–47.
69. Harrison WM, Endicott J, Nee J. Treatment of premenstrual depression with nortriptyline: a pilot study. *J Clin Psychiatry* 1989;50:136–139.
70. Freeman EW, Rickels K, Sandheimer SJ, Polansky M. Differential response to antidepressants in women with premenstrual syndrome/premenstrual dysphoric disorder. *Arch Gen Psychiatry* 1999;56;932–939.
71. Dimmock PW, Wyatt KM, Jones PW, O'Brien PMS. Efficacy of selective serotonin–reuptake inhibitors in premenstrual syndrome: A systematic. *Lancet* 2000;356:1131–1136. Search date not stated; primary sources Medline, Embase, PsychLit, Cinahl, Cochrane Controlled Trials Register, and reference lists of retrieved articles.
72. Steiner M, Romano SJ, Babcock S, et al. The efficacy of fluoxetine in improving physical symptoms associated with premenstrual dysphoric disorder. *Br J Obstet Gynaecol* 2001;108:462–468.
73. Freeman EW, Rickels K, Yonkers KA, Kunz NR, McPherson M, Upton GV. Venlafaxine in the treatment of premenstrual dysphoric disorder. *Obstet Gynecol* 2001;98:737–744.
74. Wyatt KM, Dimmock PW, O'Brien PMS. Vitamin B6 therapy: a systematic review of its efficacy in premenstrual syndrome. *BMJ* 1999;318:1375–1381. Search date 1998; primary sources Medline, Psychlit, and Cinahl.
75. Lauritzen CH, Reuter HD, Repges R, Bohnert KJ, Schmidt U. Treatment of premenstrual tension syndrome with vitex agnus castus, controlled double blind study vs pyridoxine. *Phytomedicine* 1994;4:183–189.
76. Lauritzen C. Die behandling des premenstreullen syndoms. Doppelblind studio mi hochdosertem vitamin B6 gegen placebo. *Z Allg Med* 1988;64:275–278.
77. Budciri D, Li WP, Dornan JC. Is evening primrose oil of value in the treatment of premenstrual syndrome? Control Clin Trials 1996;17:60–68. Search date 1993; primary sources Science Citation Index, Medline, Dissertation Abstracts, and companies who marketed evening primrose oil were approached for any published or unpublished trials.
78. Stevinson C, Ernst E. Complementary/alternative therapies for premenstrual syndrome: a systematic review of randomized controlled trials. *Am J Obstet Gynecol* 2001;185:227–235. Search date 2000, primary sources Medline, Embase, Biosis, Cinahl, PsycholNFO, and the Cochrane Library Ciscom.
79. Morse C, Dennerstein L, Farrell E. A comparison of hormone therapy, coping skills training and relaxation for the relief of premenstrual syndrome. *J Behav Med* 1991;14:469–489.
80. Kirkby RJ. Changes in premenstrual symptoms and irrational thinking following cognitive-behavioural coping skills training. *J Consult Clin Psychol* 1994;62.1026 1032.
81. Blake F, Salkovskis P, Gath D, Day A, Garrod A. Cognitive therapy for premenstrual syndrome: a controlled trial. *J Psychosom Res* 1998;45:307–318.
82. Corney RH, Stanton R, Newell R. Comparison of progesterone, placebo and behavioural psychotherapy in the treatment of premenstrual syndrome. *J Psychosom Obstet Gynaecol* 1990;11:211–220.
83. Christensen AP, Oei TPS. The efficacy of cognitive behaviour therapy in treating premenstrual dysphoric changes. *J Affect Disord* 1995;33:57–63.
84. Taylor D. Effectiveness of professional-peer group treatment: symptom management for women with PMS. *Res Nursing Health* 1999:22;496–511.
85. Lemos D. The effects of aerobic training on women who suffer from premenstrual syndrome. *Dissert Abstracts Int* 1991;52:563.

86. Bibi KW. The effects of acrobic exercise on premenstrual syndrome symptoms. *Dissert Abstracts Int* 1995;56:6678.
87. Shaw RW, Soutter WP, Stanton SL. Gynaecology. New York: Churchill Livingstone, 1997.
88. Metcalf MG, Braiden V, Livesey JH, Wells JE. The premenstrual syndrome: amelioration of symptoms after hysterectomy. *J Psychosom Res* 1992;36:569–584.
89. Osborn M, Gath D. Psychological and physical determinants of premenstrual symptoms before and after hysterectomy. *Psychol Med* 1990;20:565–572.
90. Casper RF, Hearn MT. The effect of hysterectomy and bilateral oophorectomy in women with severe premenstrual syndrome. *Am J Obstet Gynecol* 1990;162:105–109.
91. Casson P, Hahn PM, Van Vugt DA, Reid RL. Lasting response to ovariectomy in severe intractable premenstrual syndrome. *Am J Obstet Gynecol* 1990;162:99–105.

Katrina Wyatt
Lecture in Health Services Research
Exeter and North Devon Research and Development Support Unit
Exeter
UK

Competing interests: None declared.

TABLE 1 Commonly reported symptoms in women with premenstrual syndrome (see text, p 1974).[3]

Psychological symptoms	Irritability, depression, crying/tearfulness, anxiety, tension, mood swings, lack of concentration, confusion, forgetfulness, unsociableness, restlessness, temper outbursts/anger, sadness/blues, loneliness.
Behavioural symptoms	Fatigue, dizziness, sleep/insomnia, decreased efficiency, accident prone, sexual interest changes, increased energy, tiredness.
Physical symptoms: pain	Headache/migraine, breast tenderness/soreness/pain/swelling (collectively known as premenstrual mastalgia), back pain, abdominal cramps, general pain.
Physical symptoms: bloatedness and swelling	Weight gain, abdominal bloating or swelling, oedema of arms and legs, water retention.
Appetite symptoms	Increased appetite, food cravings, nausea.

TABLE 2 Frequency of adverse events with selective serotonin reuptake inhibitors versus placebo in women with premenstrual syndrome (see text, p 1982).[71–73]

Symptom	Systematic review[71]	RCT[73]
Nausea	66/323 (20%) *v* 13/222 (6%) NNH = 7	34/77 (45%) *v* 10/80 (13%) NNH = 3
Insomnia	56/323 (17%) *v* 17/222 (8%) NNH = 11	26/77 (34%) *v* 13/80 (16%) NNH = 6
Dizziness	32/323 (10%) *v* 46/222 (21%) NNT = 9	25/77 (32%) *v* 4/80 (4%) NNH = 4
Fatigue	46/323 (14%) *v* 24/222 (11%) NS	18/77 (23%) *v* 13/80 (16%) NS
Headache	24/323 (7%) *v* 16/222 (7%) NS	16/77 (21%) *v* 23/80 (29%) NS
Dry mouth	41/323 (13%) *v* 13/222 (6%) NNH = 15	13/77 (17%) *v* 6/80 (8%) NS
Sexual dysfunction	23/323 (7%) *v* 6/222 (3%) NNH = 23	12/77 (16%) *v* 0/80 (0%) NNH = 7

NS, not significant.

Pyelonephritis in non-pregnant women

Search date March 2002

Bruce Cooper

QUESTIONS

INTERVENTIONS

Key Messages

- **Inpatient versus outpatient management** We found no RCTs comparing inpatient versus outpatient management of women with acute uncomplicated pyelonephritis.
- **Intravenous antibiotics (ampicillin, co-trimoxazole) in women admitted to hospital with uncomplicated infection** We found no RCTs comparing intravenous antibiotics versus no antibiotics; however, it is unlikely that such an RCT would now be performed. One RCT in women admitted to hospital with uncomplicated pyelonephritis found no significant difference with intravenous ampicillin plus intravenous gentamicin versus intravenous co-trimoxazole plus intravenous gentamicin in clinical response or recurrence of bacteria in the urine. One RCT in women admitted with uncomplicated pylonephritis found no significant difference with a single dose of intravenous tobramycin plus oral ciprofloxacin versus oral ciprofloxacin plus placebo in rates of clinical success with treatment. We found no well designed trials comparing newer intravenous antibiotics versus older regimens.
- **Oral antibiotics (co-trimoxazole, co-amoxiclav, or a fluoroquinolone) for women with uncomplicated infection** We found no RCTs comparing oral antibiotics versus no antibiotics; however, it is unlikely that such an RCT would now be performed. One systematic review and one subsequent RCT in women with uncomplicated pyelonephritis have found no consistent differences between oral co-trimoxazole, co-amoxiclav, or a fluoroquinolone (ciprofloxacin, norfloxacin, levofloxacin, or lomefloxacin) in bacteriological or clinical cure rates.

Pyelonephritis in non-pregnant women

DEFINITION Acute pyelonephritis, or upper urinary tract infection, is an infection of the kidney characterised by pain when passing urine, fever, flank pain, nausea and vomiting. White blood cells are almost always present in the urine and occasionally white blood cell casts are also seen on urine microscopy. Uncomplicated infection occurs in an otherwise healthy person without any other underlying disease. Complicated infection occurs in people with structural or functional urinary tract abnormalities or additional diseases. People with acute pyelonephritis may also be divided into those able to take oral antibiotics and without signs of sepsis who may be managed at home, and those requiring treatment delivered by injection whilst in hospital.

INCIDENCE/ PREVALENCE In the USA, there are 250 000 cases of acute pyelonephritis a year.[1] Worldwide prevalence and incidence are unknown.

AETIOLOGY/ RISK FACTORS Pyelonephritis is most commonly caused when bacteria in the bladder ascend the ureters and invade the kidneys. In some cases, this may result in bacteria entering and multiplying in the bloodstream.

PROGNOSIS Complications include sepsis, infection that spreads to other organs, renal impairment, and renal abscess formation. Conditions such as underlying renal disease, diabetes mellitus, and immunosuppression may worsen prognosis with a potential increase in risk of sepsis and death, but we found no good long term evidence about such people.

AIMS To reduce the duration and severity of symptoms; to prevent or minimise potential complications, with minimum adverse effects.

OUTCOMES Urine culture after treatment; signs and symptoms of infection; rates of complications of infection; and adverse effects of treatment.

METHODS *Clinical Evidence* update search and appraisal March 2002. We excluded studies that were primarily in men, pregnant women, and people with complicated infections.

QUESTION **What are the effects of treatments for acute pyelonephritis?**

OPTION **ORAL ANTIBIOTICS (CO-TRIMOXAZOLE, CO-AMOXICLAV, OR A FLUOROQUINOLONE) FOR WOMEN WITH UNCOMPLICATED INFECTION**

We found no RCTs comparing oral antibiotics versus no antibiotics; however, it is unlikely that such an RCT would now be performed. One systematic review and one subsequent RCT in women with uncomplicated pyelonephritis have found no consistent differences between oral co-trimoxazole, co-amoxiclav, or a fluoroquinolone (ciprofloxacin, norfloxacin, levofloxacin, or lomefloxacin) in bacteriological or clinical cure rates. One RCT in women with complicated pyelonephritis comparing oral versus intravenous ciprofloxacin found no significant difference in the duration of fever or symptoms.

Pyelonephritis in non-pregnant women

Benefits: **Versus placebo:** We found no systematic review or RCTs. **Versus other oral antibiotics:** We found one systematic review (search date 1991, 9 RCTs, 470 men and non-pregnant women) (see table 1, p 1998),[2] and one subsequent RCT,[3] comparing different oral antibiotics in acute pyelonephritis. Five RCTs identified by the review were conducted in people outside hospital and four in people admitted to hospital. The studies were conducted in the USA, Europe, and Peru. All RCTs included in the review included more women than men. Most excluded people with complicating factors such as structural abnormalities of the urinary tract, additional diseases, pregnancy, or signs of possible sepsis. All RCTs in the review except one found no significant difference between different antibiotics in rates of early cure (negative urine culture within 7–10 days), and six of the nine RCTs found no significant difference in rates of late cure (negative urine culture 2–4 wks or more after stopping treatment). However, several of the individual RCTs included were too small to rule out a significant difference between antibiotic regimens. The subsequent RCT (186 people with acute uncomplicated pyelonephritis treated at home) compared levofloxacin (250 mg daily for 10 days) versus either oral ciprofloxacin (500 mg twice daily for 10 days) or oral lomefloxacin (400 mg daily for 14 days) and found similar clinical cure rates for all three antibiotics (92% with levofloxacin, 88% with ciprofloxacin, 80% with lomefloxacin; extraction of absolute numbers and significance testing not possible).[3] **Versus intravenous antibiotics:** We found no systematic review (see comment below). We found one RCT (163 people admitted to hospital with pyelonephritis or urinary tract infection associated with a structural or functional abnormality of the urinary tract or urinary tract infection acquired in hospital), which compared oral ciprofloxacin (500 mg twice daily) versus intravenous ciprofloxacin (200 mg twice daily).[4] The analysis included 83 non-pregnant women. It found no significant difference with oral versus intravenous ciprofloxacin in the mean duration of symptoms (1.7 days, 95% CI 1.5 to 1.9 with oral administration *v* 1.9 days, 95% CI 1.7 to 2.2 with iv administration; P = 0.15) or fever (1.8 days, 95% CI 1.4 to 2.2 with oral administration *v* 1.8 days, 95% CI 1.4 to 2.2 with iv administration; P = 0.85), or the median duration of hospitalisation (7 days, 95% CI 2 to 35 with oral administration *v* 8 days with iv administration, 95% CI 2 to 32; P = 0.15). There were no infection related deaths.

Harms: The subsequent RCT reported adverse effects in 3/124 (2%) people taking levofloxacin, 6/80 (8%) people taking ciprofloxacin, and 3/55 (5%) people taking lomefloxacin.[3] Gastrointestinal symptoms were common with both ciprofloxacin and levofloxacin, whereas rash was the most common adverse effect with lomefloxacin. One of the 186 people discontinued treatment (lomefloxacin) because of adverse effects.[3] In the RCT that compared oral versus intravenous ciprofloxacin, one person on oral ciprofloxacin discontinued treatment because of the development of mental confusion.[4] One person on intravenous ciprofloxacin developed pruritus, but treatment was continued until completed. No other adverse effects were reported.

Comment: We found one protocol for a systematic review which will compare oral versus intravenous antibiotic treatment for symptomatic urinary tract infections.[5] The lack of evidence in women with pyelonephritis comparing oral antibiotics versus placebo reflects the fact that RCTs in this area would be considered unethical. Calculated cure rates from the systematic review comparing the oral antibiotic regimens are likely to overestimate rates that would be achieved in clinical practice because many people were excluded, including those who experienced adverse effects, had growth of resistant bacteria on initial culture, or did not adhere to treatment.[2] The high rate of ampicillin resistance found in laboratory tests has led to a consensus view that ampicillin and amoxicillin (amoxycillin) are not recommended in pyelonephritis. We found no direct evidence to confirm or refute this view. Ampicillin and amoxicillin were found in the trials to have cure rates comparable with other antibiotics, but the studies were too small to exclude clinically important differences. The RCT comparing oral and intravenous ciprofloxacin included people with underlying structural or functional urinary abnormalities.[4]

OPTION INTRAVENOUS ANTIBIOTICS (AMPICILLIN, CO-TRIMOXAZOLE) IN WOMEN ADMITTED TO HOSPITAL WITH UNCOMPLICATED INFECTION

We found no RCTs comparing intravenous antibiotics versus no antibiotics; however, it is unlikely that such an RCT would now be performed. One RCT in women admitted to hospital with uncomplicated pyelonephritis found no significant difference with intravenous ampicillin plus intravenous gentamicin versus intravenous co-trimoxazole plus intravenous gentamicin in clinical response or recurrence of bacteria in the urine. One RCT in women admitted with uncomplicated pylonephritis found no significant difference with a single dose of intravenous tobramycin plus oral ciprofloxacin versus oral ciprofloxacin plus placebo in rates of clinical success with treatment. One RCT in women with complicated pyelonephritis comparing oral versus intravenous ciprofloxacin found no significant difference in the duration of fever or symptoms. We found no well designed trials comparing newer intravenous antibiotics versus older regimens.

Benefits: **Versus placebo:** We found no systematic review and no RCTs. **Versus other intravenous antibiotics:** We found no systematic review. We found one RCT (85 women admitted to hospital for acute uncomplicated pyelonephritis; see comment below), which compared intravenous ampicillin (1 g every 6 h) versus intravenous co-trimoxazole (160 mg/800 mg twice daily), initiated before culture results were known.[6] Both regimens were combined with intravenous gentamicin and followed by oral treatment with either ampicillin or co-trimoxazole. The RCT found that all the women who completed the trial displayed a satisfactory clinical response (defined as all symptoms related to the infection having resolved during treatment), and found no significant difference in the number of women with a recurrence of bacteria in the urine after 28 days (1/20 [5%] with ampicillin *v* 2/27 [7%] with co-trimoxazole; RR 0.7, 95% CI 0.07 to 6.94). We found no other adequately designed RCTs comparing treatments that included intravenous quinolones, cephalosporins, broad spectrum β lactams, or co-trimoxazole. **Plus oral antibiotics:** We found one RCT (118 women admitted with acute uncomplicated pylonephritis), which compared a single dose of intravenous tobramycin (2 mg/kg) plus oral ciprofloxacin (500 mg twice daily for 10 days) versus oral ciprofloxacin plus intravenous placebo (0.9% saline solution).[7] Clinical success or failure was categorised, with failure defined as the persistence of fever or pain after 48 hours of treatment. The RCT found no significant difference with intravenous tobramycin plus oral ciprofloxacin versus oral ciprofloxacin plus placebo in rates of clinical success (58/60 [97%] *v* 54/58 [93%]; RR 1.04, 95% CI 0.95 to 1.13). **Versus oral antibiotics:** See benefits of oral antibiotics, p 1994.

Harms: The RCT comparing intravenous regimes found no significant difference in the total number of possible medication related adverse effects between treatments (10/32 [32%] with ampicillin *v* 13/39 [33%] with co-trimoxazole; RR 0.9, 95% CI 0.48 to 1.85).[6] Common adverse effects with ampicillin include rash, diarrhoea, and vaginitis, and with co-trimoxazole include nausea, vomiting, and vaginitis. The RCT comparing intravenous tobramycin plus ciprofloxacin versus ciprofloxacin plus placebo reported "no undesirable side effects were observed".[7] No further details were provided.

Comment: The lack of evidence in women with pyelonephritis comparing intravenous antibiotics versus placebo reflects the fact that RCTs in this area would be considered unethical. The RCT comparing intravenous regimes reported that 47/85 (55%) women completed the trial to the 28 days follow up assessment; 14/42 (33%) women receiving ampicillin were infected with ampicillin resistant isolates and were withdrawn from the study.[6] There is a consensus view that the choice of empirical antibiotics should take into account the setting, medical history of the patient, Gram stain of the urine, previous infecting organism, and local antibiotic sensitivities.

OPTION INPATIENT VERSUS OUTPATIENT MANAGEMENT

We found no RCTs comparing inpatient versus outpatient management of women with acute uncomplicated pyelonephritis.

Benefits: We found no systematic review and no RCTs.

Harms: We found no evidence.

Comment: Hospitals might be able to provide closer monitoring and supervision of people with pyelonephritis than can be provided outside hospital. However, we found no RCTs to clarify whether treatment in hospital delivers any benefit in terms of outcomes or whether there is an increased risk of harm from hospital treatment.

Substantive changes

Intravenous antibiotics One new RCT;[7] conclusions unchanged.

REFERENCES

1. Stamm WE, Hooton TM, Johnson JR. Urinary tract infection: from pathogenesis to treatment. *J Infect Dis* 1989;15:400–406.
2. Pinson AG, Philbrick JT, Lindbeck GH, et al. Oral antibiotic therapy for acute pyelonephritis: a methodologic review of the literature. *J Gen Intern Med* 1992;7:544–553. Search date 1991; primary sources Medline and Current Contents.
3. Richard GA, Klimberg IN, Fowler CL, et al. Levofloxacin versus ciprofloxacin versus lomefloxacin in acute pyelonephritis. *Urology* 1998;52:51–55.
4. Mombelli G, Pezzoli R, Pinoja-Lutz G, et al. Oral vs intravenous ciprofloxacin in the initial empirical management of severe pyelonephritis or complicated urinary tract infections: a prospective randomized clinical trial. *Arch Intern Med* 1999;159:53–58.

5. Pohl A, Antes G, Forster J. Oral versus intravenous antibiotic therapy for symptomatic urinary tract infections (protocol for a Cochrane Review). In: The Cochrane Library, Issue 1, 2002. Oxford: Update Software.
6. Johnson JR, Lyons MF, Pearce W, et al. Therapy for women hospitalized with acute pyelonephritis: a randomized trial of ampicillin versus trimethoprim-sulfamethoxazole for 14 days. *J Infect Dis* 1991;163:325–330.
7. Le Conte P, Simon N, Bourrier P, et al. Acute pyelonephritis. Randomized multicentre double-blind study comparing ciprofloxacin with combined ciprofloxacin and tobramycin [French]. *Presse Med* 2001;30:11–15.

Bruce Cooper
Renal Research Fellow
University of Sydney
Royal North Shore Hospital St Leonards
Sydney
Australia

Competing interests: None declared.

TABLE 1 Oral antibiotic treatment for acute pyelonephritis: results of RCTs (see text, p 1994).[2]

Study number	Oral antibiotic regimens	Total number of people	Early cure* rates %	Late cure* rates %	P value
1	Amoxicillin 500 mg three times daily for 14 days	16	NA	94	NS
	Co-trimoxazole (160 mg/800 mg) twice daily for 14 days	12	NA	92	
2	Norfloxacin 400 mg twice daily for 10 days	14	100	86	NS
	Co-trimoxazole (160 mg/800 mg) twice daily for 10 days	10	100	90	
3	Ampicillin 500 mg four times daily for 10 days	8	88	NA	NS
	Cefaclor 250 mg twice daily for 10 days	6	67	NA	
4	Norfloxacin 400 mg twice daily for 7 days or longer	3	67	NA	NS
	Co-trimoxazole (160 mg/800 mg) twice daily for 7 days or longer	12	92	NA	
5	Co-amoxiclav 250 mg/125 mg three times daily for 10 days	54	94	85	P = 0.02 for late cure; NS for early cure
	Co-trimoxazole (160 mg/800 mg) twice daily for 10 days	50	82	64	
6	Ampicillin 500 mg four times daily for 2 or 6 weeks	17	100	47	P = 0.004 for late cure; NS for early cure
	Co-trimoxazole (160 mg/800 mg) twice daily for 2 or 6 weeks	22	100	91	
7	Amoxicillin 2000 mg one time dose then 1000 mg twice daily for 9 days	22	100	100	NS
	Amoxicillin 750 mg three times daily for 12 days	23	96	87	
8	Cefetamet 2000 mg daily or 1000 mg twice daily for 10–15 days	28	93	79	NS
	Cefadroxil 1000 mg twice daily for 10–15 days	22	73	52	
9	Norfloxacin 400 mg twice daily for 14 days	76	91	82	P < 0.0001 for both early and late cures
	Cefadroxil 1000 mg twice daily for 14 days	75	59	44	

*Early cure: negative urine culture within 7–10 days of starting treatment; late cure: negative urine culture 2–4 weeks or more after stopping treatment. NA, not available; NS, not significant. Pinson AG, Philbrick JT, Lindbeck GH, et al. Oral antibiotic therapy for acute pyelonephritis; a methodologic review of the literature. *J Gen Intern Med* 1992;7:544–533. Reprinted by permission of Blackwell Science, Inc.

Recurrent cystitis in non-pregnant women

Search date July 2001

Bruce Cooper and Ruth Jepson

QUESTIONS

INTERVENTIONS

Key Messages

- **Continuous antibiotic prophylaxis (trimethoprim, co-trimoxazole, nitrofurantoin, cefaclor, or a quinolone)** RCTs have found that continuous antibiotic prophylaxis lasting 6–12 months with trimethoprim, co-trimoxazole, nitrofurantoin, cefaclor, or a quinolone versus placebo significantly reduces rates of recurrent cystitis, but have found no consistent difference in the risk of infection with different regimens. One RCT comparing continuous daily antibiotic prophylaxis versus postcoital antibiotic prophylaxis found no significant difference in rates of cystitis after 1 year.
- **Cranberry juice and cranberry products** One systematic review found insufficient evidence on the effects of cranberry juice and other cranberry products on recurrent cystitis.
- **Postcoital antibiotic prophylaxis (co-trimoxazole, nitrofurantoin, or a quinolone)** Four RCTs have found that co-trimoxazole, nitrofurantoin, or a quinolone versus placebo up to 2 hours after sexual intercourse significantly reduce the rates of cystitis.
- **Prophylaxis with methenamine hippurate** We found no RCTs on the effects of methenamine hippurate (hexamine hippurate).
- **Single dose self administered co-trimoxazole** One small RCT found that continuous co-trimoxazole prophylaxis versus single dose self administered co-trimoxazole (started at the onset of cystitis symptoms) significantly reduced the number of episodes of cystitis within 1 year.

Recurrent cystitis in non-pregnant women

DEFINITION Cystitis is an infection of the lower urinary tract, which causes pain when passing urine, and causes frequency, urgency, haematuria, or suprapubic pain not associated with passing urine. White blood cells and bacteria are almost always present in the urine. The presence of fever, flank pain, nausea, or vomiting suggests pyelonephritis (upper urinary tract infection) (see pyelonephritis in non-pregnant women, p 1992). Recurrent cystitis may be either a reinfection (after successful eradication of infection) or a relapse after inadequate treatment.

INCIDENCE/ PREVALENCE The incidence of cystitis among premenopausal sexually active women is 0.5–0.7 infections per person year,[1] and 20–40% of women will experience cystitis during their lifetime. Of those, 20% will develop recurrence, almost always (90% of cases) because of reinfection rather than relapse. Rates of infection fall during the winter months.[2]

AETIOLOGY/ RISK FACTORS Cystitis is caused by uropathogenic bacteria in the faecal flora that colonise the vaginal and periurethral openings, and ascend the urethra into the bladder. Prior infection, sexual intercourse, and exposure to vaginal spermicide are risk factors for developing cystitis.[3,4]

PROGNOSIS We found little evidence on the long term effects of untreated cystitis. One study found that progression to pyelonephritis was infrequent, and that most cases of cystitis regressed spontaneously, although symptoms sometimes persisted for several months.[5] Women with a baseline rate of more than two infections a year, over many years, are likely to continue to suffer from recurrent infections.[6]

AIMS To prevent recurrent cystitis in women predisposed to frequent infections, with minimal adverse effects of treatment.

OUTCOMES Rate of infection based on symptoms and urine culture.

METHODS *Clinical Evidence* search and appraisal July 2001. We reviewed all systematic reviews and RCTs comparing different forms of prophylaxis, or comparing prophylaxis versus placebo in non-pregnant women with a history of recurrent cystitis. We excluded studies in populations consisting mainly of men or pregnant women.

QUESTION **Which interventions prevent further recurrence of cystitis in women experiencing at least two infections per year?**

OPTION **CONTINUOUS ANTIBIOTIC PROPHYLAXIS (TRIMETHOPRIM, CO-TRIMOXAZOLE, NITROFURANTOIN, CEFACLOR, OR A QUINOLONE)**

RCTs have found that continuous antibiotic prophylaxis lasting 6–12 months with trimethoprim, co-trimoxazole, nitrofurantoin, cefaclor, or a quinolone significantly reduces rates of recurrent cystitis but found no consistent difference in numbers of infections between different continuous regimens. One RCT comparing postcoital versus continuous daily antibiotic prophylaxis found no significant difference in rates of cystitis after 1 year.

Benefits: We found no systematic review. We found seven RCTs (in women with at least 2 episodes of cystitis per year) comparing different regimens for continuous antibiotic prophylaxis lasting 6–12 months (see table 1, p 2005).[7–13] **Versus placebo or no treatment:** Three of the RCTs (225 women) found that active treatment (nitrofurantoin, ciprofloxacin, norfloxacin, or co-trimoxazole) versus placebo or no treatment significantly reduced rates of cystitis.[7–9] **Versus each other:** One RCT (72 women) found that women taking oral nitrofurantoin (100 mg at night) versus oral trimethoprim (100 mg at night) had significantly fewer episodes of cystitis after 12 months ($P < 0.05$; absolute numbers not provided).[10] Four other RCTs compared different antibiotic regimens versus each other and found no significant difference in numbers of infections between treatments over 6–12 months.[7,11–13] **Versus postcoital prophylaxis:** One RCT (135 women) compared daily oral ciprofloxacin (125 mg) versus postcoital (within 2 h of sexual intercourse) oral ciprofloxacin (125 mg) (see benefits of postcoital prophylaxis, p 2002). It found no significant difference in the number of positive urine cultures after 1 year (27/239 [11%] urine cultures with daily prophylaxis *v* 32/254 [13%] urine cultures with postcoital prophylaxis; RR 0.9, 95% CI 0.55 to 1.45).[8]

Harms: Rates of adverse effects in the RCTs ranged from 7–40% for trimethoprim, 0–40% for nitrofurantoin, 5% for cefaclor, 7–21% for norfloxacin, and 13% for ciprofloxacin.[7–9,11–13] The most common adverse effects for all agents were gastrointestinal symptoms, rash, and yeast vaginitis. One cohort study (see comment below) reported no significant adverse effects in women taking trimethoprim, co-trimoxazole, or nitrofurantoin, even when treatment continued for as long as 5 years. The development of bacterial resistance from continuous antibiotic prophylaxis was rare. However, the number of co-trimoxazole resistant organisms increased during the latter part of the study.[2]

Comment: Many of the RCTs were not placebo controlled or blinded, and had small study populations. However, most of the reported rates of infection in the RCTs comparing different antibiotic regimens versus each other were much less than 0.6 per person year, suggesting that they were all effective in reducing the rate of infection in people with a history of recurrent cystitis.[7,10–13] These studies were not powered to exclude a clinically important difference between treatments and adjustments were not made for confounding factors such as frequency of sexual intercourse. We found one cohort study (51 non-pregnant women with a baseline rate of more than 2 urinary tract infections a year over many years) that compared continuous treatment with three different antibiotics (trimethoprim, co-trimoxazole, or nitrofurantoin) for more than 12 months.[2] It found that all were effective in preventing both cystitis and pyelonephritis for over 112 person years.

OPTION POSTCOITAL ANTIBIOTIC PROPHYLAXIS

RCTs have found that co-trimoxazole, nitrofurantoin or a quinolone versus placebo up to 2 hours after sexual intercourse significantly reduce the rates of cystitis. One RCT comparing postcoital versus continuous daily antibiotic prophylaxis found no significant difference in rates of cystitis after 1 year.

Benefits: We found no systematic review. **Versus placebo or no treatment:** We found four RCTs (in women with at least 2 episodes of cystitis per year) comparing postcoital (within 2 h of sexual intercourse) antibiotic regimens versus placebo or no treatment evaluated over 6–14 months.[8,14–16] All four RCTs found that active treatment (co-trimoxazole, nitrofurantoin, or a quinolone) significantly reduced rates of cystitis (see table 2, p 2006). **Versus continuous daily prophylaxis:** See benefits of continuous antibiotic prophylaxis, p 2001.

Harms: Rates of adverse effects were as follows: co-trimoxazole 18%, ciprofloxacin 6%, and nitrofurantoin less than 1%.[8,14–16] The most common adverse effects for all agents were gastrointestinal symptoms, rash, and yeast vaginitis.

Comment: Only one of the studies was placebo controlled and blinded.[14] Adjustments were not made for confounding factors such as frequency of sexual intercourse.

OPTION SINGLE DOSE SELF ADMINISTERED CO-TRIMOXAZOLE

One small RCT found that continuous co-trimoxazole prophylaxis versus single dose self administered co-trimoxazole (started at the onset of cystitis symptoms) significantly reduced rates of cystitis.

Benefits: We found no systematic review but found one RCT (38 non-pregnant women with 2 or more culture documented urinary tract infections in the previous 12 months; see comment below).[17] The RCT compared continuous oral co-trimoxazole prophylaxis (40 mg/200 mg) versus single dose self administered co-trimoxazole (40 mg/200 mg) to be taken at the onset of cystitis symptoms. It found that continuous antibiotic prophylaxis versus single dose self administered co-trimoxazole significantly reduced the number of episodes of cystitis (0.22 infections per person year with continuous prophylaxis *v* 2.2 infections per person year with self treatment; $P < 0.001$; see comment below).

Harms: The trial reported a total of eight adverse reactions; five were in women receiving continuous antibiotic prophylaxis versus three in women receiving single dose treatment (significance testing not possible).[17] Adverse reactions included mild nausea, abdominal pain, rash, mouth ulcers, and yeast vulvovaginitis.

Comment: The RCT reported that 10/38 (26%) women did not complete the full study protocol, although it is not clear whether analysis of results was by intention to treat.[17] The trial found that the women were almost always able to diagnose their own episodes of cystitis from symptoms (positive predictive value 92%). The higher rate of cystitis in women using single dose prophylaxis is to be expected because treatment was only administered after the onset of symptoms.

OPTION CRANBERRY JUICE AND CRANBERRY PRODUCTS

One systematic review found insufficient evidence on the effects of cranberry juice and other cranberry products on the prevention of recurrent cystitis.

Benefits: We found one systematic review (search date 2001, 2 RCTs, 211 women) comparing cranberry juice or other cranberry products versus placebo in the prevention of urinary tract infections (see comment below).[18] The first RCT (19 women with recurrent cystitis) included in the review compared cranberry capsules versus placebo (see comment below). The review reported 21 infections among 10 women who completed the study; six of these infections occurred in women taking cranberry capsules (the number of infections/women in the different groups was not reported; significance testing not possible). The second RCT (192 elderly women) compared cranberry juice versus placebo and found that cranberry juice significantly reduced the rate of infection (defined as ≥100 000 organisms/ml of urine plus white blood cells in the urine; OR 0.42, P = 0.004; see comment below).

Harms: No information on adverse effects was reported.

Comment: These studies were small, with high withdrawal rates (47% in the first RCT and 20% in the second RCT), and the lack of intention to treat analyses in either trial may mean that they overestimated the effectiveness of cranberry juice and products. High withdrawal rates suggest that long term adherence may be difficult to achieve.

OPTION PROPHYLAXIS WITH METHENAMINE HIPPURATE

We found no evidence on the effects of methenamine hippurate (hexamine hippurate) in women with recurrent cystitis.

Benefits: We found no systematic review and no RCTs.

Harms: We found no evidence.

Comment: None.

REFERENCES

1. Hooton TM, Scholes D, Hughes JP, et al. A prospective study of risk factors for symptomatic urinary tract infection in young women. *N Engl J Med* 1996;335:468–474.
2. Stamm WE, McKevitt M, Roberts PL, White NJ. Natural history of recurrent urinary tract infections in women. *Rev Infect Dis* 1991;13:77–84.
3. Fihn SD, Latham RH, Roberts P, Running K, Stamm WE. Association between diaphragm use and urinary tract infection. *JAMA* 1985;254:240–245.
4. Fihn SD, Boyko EJ, Normand EH, et al. Association between use of spermicide-coated condoms and *Escherichia coli* urinary tract infection in young women. *Am J Epidemiol* 1996;144:512–520.
5. Mabeck CE. Treatment of uncomplicated urinary tract infection in non-pregnant women. *Postgrad Med J* 1972;48:69–75.
6. Stamm WE, Counts GW, McKevitt M, Turck M, Holmes KK. Urinary prophylaxis with trimethoprim and trimethoprim-sulfamethoxazole: efficacy, influence on the natural history of recurrent bacteriuria and cost control. *Rev Infect Dis* 1982;4:450–455.

7. Stamm WE, Counts GW, Wagner KF, et al. Antimicrobial prophylaxis of recurrent urinary tract infections: a double-blind placebo-controlled trial. *Ann Intern Med* 1980;92:770–775.
8. Melekos MD, Asbach HW, Gerharz E, Zarakovitis IE, Weingaertner K, Naber KG. Post-intercourse versus daily ciprofloxacin prophylaxis for recurrent urinary tract infections in premenopausal women. *J Urol* 1997;157:935–939.
9. Nicolle LE, Harding GKM, Thompson M, Kennedy J, Urias B, Ronald AR. Prospective, randomized, placebo-controlled trial of norfloxacin for the prophylaxis of recurrent urinary tract infection in women. *Antimicrob Agents Chemother* 1989;33:1032–1035.
10. Brumfitt W, Smith GW, Hamilton-Miller JMT, Gargan RA. A clinical comparison between macrodantin and trimethoprim for prophylaxis in women with recurrent urinary infection. *J Antimicrob Chemother* 1985;16:111–120.
11. Raz R, Boger S. Long-term prophylaxis with norfloxacin versus nitrofurantoin in women with recurrent urinary tract infection. *Antimicrob Agents Chemother* 1991;35:1241–1242.
12. Brumfitt W, Hamilton-Miller JMT, Smith GW, Al-Wali W. Comparative trial of norfloxacin and macrocrystalline nitrofurantoin (Macrodantin) in the prophylaxis of recurrent urinary tract infection in women. *Q J Med* 1991;81:811–820.
13. Brumfitt W, Hamilton-Miller JMT. A comparative trial of low-dose cefaclor and macrocrystalline nitrofurantoin in the prevention of recurrent urinary tract infection. *Infection* 1995;23:98–102.
14. Stapleton A, Latham RH, Johnson C, Stamm WE. Postcoital antimicrobial prophylaxis for recurrent urinary tract infection: a randomized, double-blind placebo-controlled trial. *JAMA* 1990;264:703–706.
15. Pfau A, Sacks TG. Effective postcoital quinolone prophylaxis of recurrent urinary tract infection in women. *J Urol* 1994;152:136–138.
16. Pfau A, Sacks T, Englestein D. Recurrent urinary tract infections in premenopausal women: prophylaxis based on an understanding of the pathogenesis. *J Urol* 1983;129:1153–1156.
17. Wong ES, McKevitt M, Running K, Counts GW, Turck M, Stamm WE. Management of recurrent urinary tract infections with patient-administered single-dose therapy. *Ann Intern Med* 1985;102:302–307.
18. Jepson RG, Mihaljevic L, Craig J. Cranberries for preventing urinary tract infections (Cochrane Review). In: The Cochrane Library, Issue 3, 2001. Oxford: Update Software. Search date January 2001; primary sources Cochrane Collaboration Field in Complementary Medicine Registry of randomised trials, Cochrane Controlled Trials Register (CCTR) and CENTRAL, Psychlit, LILACS, Cinahl, Medline, Embase, Biological Abstracts, Current Contents, the Internet, hand searches of reference lists of review articles and relevant trials, conference abstracts from relevant meetings, and personal contact with companies involved with the manufacture of cranberry preparations.

Bruce Cooper
Renal Research Fellow
University of Sydney
Royal North Shore Hospital
St Leonards
Australia

Ruth Jepson
Research Training Fellow
Department of General Practice
University of Edinburgh
Edinburgh
UK

Competing interests: None declared.

TABLE 1 **Continuous antimicrobial prophylactic regimens for recurrent urinary tract infections: results of RCTs** **(see text, p 2001).**

Study design	Total number of people	Regimen	Duration of prophylaxis (months)	Infections per patient year	P value
Placebo controlled RCT[7]	60	Placebo	6	2.80	< 0.001 (placebo *v* drug treatment)
		Co-trimoxazole (40 mg/200 mg) at bedtime		0.15	
		Nitrofurantoin 100 mg at bedtime		0.14	
		Nitrofurantoin 100 mg at bedtime		0	
Open RCT[8]	135	Without prophylaxis	12	3.62–3.66	< 0.001
		Ciprofloxacin 125 mg postcoital		0.043	
		Ciprofloxacin 125 mg daily		0.031	
Placebo controlled RCT[9]	30	Placebo	12	1.6	< 0.001
		Norfloxacin 200 mg at bedtime		0	
Open RCT[10]	72	Trimethoprim 100 mg at bedtime	12	1.00	< 0.05
		Nitrofurantoin 100 mg bedtime		0.17	
Open RCT[11]	94	Norfloxacin 200 mg at bedtime	6	0.04	= 0.05
		Nitrofurantoin 50 mg at bedtime		0.60	
Open RCT[12]	88	Norfloxacin 200 mg at bedtime	12	0.002	Not reported
		Nitrofurantoin 100 mg at bedtime		0.003	
Open RCT[13]	97	Cefaclor 250 mg at bedtime	12	0.006	Not reported
		Nitrofurantoin 50 mg at bedtime		0.006	

TABLE 2 Postcoital regimens for recurrent urinary tract infections: results of RCTs (see text, p 2002).

Study design	Total number of people	Regimen	Duration of prophylaxis (months)	Infections per patient year	P value
Placebo controlled RCT[14]	27	Placebo	6	3.6	= 0.0001
		Postcoital co-trimoxazole (40 mg/20 mg)		0.3	
Open RCT[15]	33	Without prophylaxis	14	6.13	= 0.0000
		Postcoital prophylaxis with either ofloxacin 100 mg, norfloxacin 200 mg, or ciprofloxacin 125 mg		0.02	
Open RCT[8]	135	Without prophylaxis	12	3.62–3.66	< 0.0001
		Ciprofloxacin 125 mg daily		0.031	
		Ciprofloxacin 125 mg postcoital		0.043	
Open RCT[16]	56	Without prophylaxis	12	4.6	< 0.001
		Postcoital prophylaxis with either			
		Co-trimocazole 80 mg/400 mg		0	
		Nitrofurantoin 50–100 mg		0.1	

Vulvovaginal candidiasis

Search date November 2001

Jeanne Marrazzo

QUESTIONS

INTERVENTIONS

To be covered in future updates

Treatments in pregnant women

Treatments in women with HIV infection

Treatments in women with diabetes mellitus

Treatment in postmenopausal women

Complementary and alternative treatments (*Lactobacilli*, tea tree oil, *Solanum nigriscens*, stockings *v* tights)

See glossary, p 2017

Key Messages

Acute vulvovaginal candidiasis

- **Intravaginal imidazoles** RCTs have found that intravaginal imidazoles (e.g. clotrimazole) versus placebo significantly reduce persistent symptoms of vulvovaginal candidiasis after 1 month. RCTs found no clear evidence that effects differ significantly among the various intravaginal imidazoles. RCTs found no clear evidence of any difference between shorter and longer durations of treatment (1–14 days).
- **Intravaginal nystatin** One RCT found that intravaginal nystatin versus placebo significantly reduced the proportion of women with a poor symptomatic response after 14 days (NNT 3, 95% CI 2 to 12).

- **Oral itraconazole** One RCT found that oral itraconazole versus placebo significantly reduced persistent symptoms at 1 week after treament (NNT 4, 95% CI 2 to 31). One systematic review has found no significant difference in persistant symptoms at 7– days or 28–35 days with oral itraconazole versus intravaginal imidazoles.
- **Oral fluconazole** We found no RCTs of oral fluconazole versus placebo or no treatment. A systematic review has found no significant difference with oral fluconazole versus intravaginal imidazoles in the symptoms of vulvovaginal candidiasis. RCTs have found that fluconazole versus intravaginal imidazoles is associated with increased frequency of mild nausea, headache, and abdominal pain (NNH 11, 95% CI 6 to 54 after 14 days).
- **Oral ketoconazole** We found no RCTs of oral ketoconazole versus placebo or versus no treatment. Four RCTs have found no significant difference with oral ketoconazole versus intravaginal imidazoles in the reduction of persistent symptoms, but found that ketoconazole significantly increased the frequency of minor adverse events (mainly nausea). Case reports have associated ketoconazole with a low risk of fulminant hepatitis (1/12 000 courses of treatment with oral ketoconazole).
- **Treating a male sexual partner** RCTs found no significant difference with treating versus not treating a woman's male sexual partner in the resolution of the woman's acute vulvovaginal candidiasis symptoms, or in the rate of symptomatic relapse.

Recurrent vulvovaginal candidiasis

- **Oral itraconazole** One RCT found that oral itraconazole versus placebo significantly reduced the rate of recurrence over 6 months (NNT 4, 95% CI 3 to 11).
- **Prophylaxis with intermittent or continuous ketoconazole** One RCT found that oral ketoconazole (given either intermittently or continuously at a lower dose) versus placebo significantly reduced symptomatic recurrences over 6 months. Ketoconazole is associated with an increased frequency of gastrointestinal adverse effects, and case reports have associated ketoconazole with a low risk of serious fulminant hepatitis (1/12 000 courses of treatment with oral ketoconazole).
- **Regular prophylaxis with oral fluconazole** We found no RCTs about the effects of fluconazole in preventing recurrence of vulvovaginal candidiasis.
- **Regular prophylaxis with intravaginal imidazole** RCTs comparing regular prophylaxis with intravaginal imidazole versus placebo found inconsistent effects on the proportion of women with symptomatic relapse. One RCT found that regular prophylactic intravaginal imidazole versus treatment at the onset of symptoms reduced the frequency of episodes of symptomatic vaginitis, but the difference was not significant. The RCTs were too small to exclude a clinically important benefit.

DEFINITION Vulvovaginal candidiasis is symptomatic vaginitis (inflammation of the vagina), which often involves the vulva, caused by infection with a *Candida* yeast. Predominant symptoms are vulvar itching and abnormal vaginal discharge (which may be minimal, a "cheese like" material, or a watery secretion). Differentiation from other forms of vaginitis requires the presence of yeast on microscopy of vaginal fluid. The definition of recurrent vulvovaginal candidiasis varies among RCTs, but is commonly defined as four or more symptomatic episodes a year.[1] This summary excludes studies of asymptomatic women with vaginal colonisation by *Candida* species.

INCIDENCE/ PREVALENCE Vulvovaginal candidiasis is the second most common cause of vaginitis (after bacterial vaginosis). Estimates of its incidence are limited, and often derived from women attending hospital clinics. At least one episode of vulvovaginal candidiasis occurs during the lifetime of 50–75% of all women. About half of the women who have an episode develop recurrent vulvovaginal candidiasis.[2] Vulvovaginal candidiasis is diagnosed in 5–15% of women attending sexually transmitted disease and family planning clinics.[1]

AETIOLOGY/ RISK FACTORS *Candida albicans* accounts for 85–90% of vulvovaginal candidiasis infections. Development of symptomatic vulvovaginal candidiasis probably represents increased growth of yeast that previously colonised the vagina without causing symptoms. Risk factors for vulvovaginal candidiasis include pregnancy (RR 2–10), diabetes mellitus, and systemic antibiotics. The evidence that different types of contraceptives are risk factors is contradictory. The incidence of vulvovaginal candidiasis rises with initiation of sexual activity, but we found no direct evidence that vulvovaginal candidiasis is sexually transmitted.[3–5]

PROGNOSIS We found few descriptions of the natural history of untreated vulvovaginal candidiasis. Discomfort is the main complication, and can include pain while passing urine, or during sexual intercourse. Balanitis (see glossary, p 2017) in male partners of women with vulvovaginal candidiasis can occur, but it is rare.

AIMS To alleviate symptoms with minimal adverse effects from treatment.

OUTCOMES Clinical cure rates, either measured in the short term (5–15 days) or medium term (3–6 wks) after treatment. The definition of clinical cure varies among RCTs but often includes both complete resolution of symptoms and negative culture of *Candida*.

METHODS *Clinical Evidence* search and appraisal November 2001. We included only those studies in which most recruits were from the target population (e.g. to answer the question for non-pregnant women we sought RCTs that excluded pregnant women or RCTs in which pregnant women represented $< 20\%$ of the recruits). Studies of women with HIV infection were excluded. Many RCTs excluded women with diabetes mellitus. Studies were included only if recruitment included only women with both symptoms of vaginal candidiasis and laboratory confirmation of candidal infection.

QUESTION **What are the effects of treatments for symptomatic vulvovaginal candidiasis in non-pregnant women**

OPTION **INTRAVAGINAL NYSTATIN**

One RCT found that intravaginal nystatin versus placebo significantly reduced the proportion of women with a poor symptomatic response after 14 days treatment. One RCT found that intravaginal boric acid may reduce persistent symptoms more than intravaginal nystatin, but old case reports have described systemic toxicity from the use of intravaginal

boric acid. We found limited evidence that intravaginal nystatin was less effective than intravaginal imidazoles at reducing persistent symptoms. We found no comparison of intravaginal nystatin versus oral fluconazole, itraconazole, or ketoconazole.

Benefits: **Versus placebo or no treatment:** We found no systematic review but found one RCT of nystatin versus placebo.[6] The RCT (double blind, 50 women) found that intravaginal nystatin (500 000 IU twice daily for 14 days) versus placebo significantly reduced the proportion of women with a symptomatic response categorised as "poor" (2/25 [8%] with nystatin *v* 10/25 [40%] with placebo; ARR 32%, 95% CI 8% to 56%; OR 0.18, 95% CI 0.05 to 0.65; NNT 3, 95% CI 2 to 12). **Versus antiseptics:** We found one RCT,[8] intravaginal boric acid (600 mg capsule once daily) versus intravaginal nystatin (100 000 IU capsule once daily) for 14 days significantly reduced the proportion of women with persistent symptoms or a positive culture 30 days after finishing treatment (14/50 [28%] with boric acid *v* 26/52 [50%] with nystatin; OR 0.40, 95% CI 0.18 to 0.89). **Versus intravaginal imidazoles:** See intravaginal imidazoles, p 2010.

Harms: One RCT found no reports of adverse effects among 52 women using intravaginal nystatin.[8]

Comment: The *Clinical Evidence* search found no RCTs of nystatin versus placebo; the single RCT cited above[6] is the only published RCT supplied by the Medical Information Department of Bristol Myers Squibb after searching their internal database. We found no RCTs versus other antiseptics, such as gentian violet. The RCT of nystatin versus boric acid found minimal absorption of boric acid, but old case reports have described boron toxicity after intravaginal use.[9]

OPTION INTRAVAGINAL IMIDAZOLES (CLOTRIMAZOLE, MICONAZOLE, ECONAZOLE, TIOCONAZOLE, BUTOCONAZOLE, TERCONAZOLE, FENTICONAZOLE, AND SERTACONAZOLE)

Six RCTs have found that intravaginal imidazoles versus placebo reduce persistent symptoms of vulvovaginal candidiasis after 1 month. Numerous RCTs found no clear evidence that effects differ significantly among the various intravaginal imidazoles. RCTs found no clear evidence of any difference in persistent symptoms between shorter and longer durations of treatment (1–14 days). RCTs have found an increased frequency of mild vulvar irritation with intravaginal imidazoles compared with oral treatments.

Benefits: **Versus placebo:** We found one systematic review (search date 1993[7], 3 RCTs[10–12]) and 3 additional RCTs (see web extra table A at www.clinicalevidence.com).[13–15] Four of the six RCTs found significant reduction of persistent symptoms of vaginal candidiasis 4 weeks after treatment with topical imidazoles versus placebo. One RCT found a non-significant reduction. The sixth RCT (99 women, performed in family practice in Denmark) found no benefit versus placebo, but the follow up rate was low (62/99 [64%]). Overall, we found that intravaginal imidazoles versus placebo significantly reduced persistent symptoms of vaginal candidiasis in the medium term (6 RCTs: 131/392 [33%] with imidazoles *v* 98/141 [70%] with placebo; OR 0.16, 95% CI 0.04 to 0.60 calculated with a random effects model; see comment below (see web extra figure A at www.clinicalevidence.com). **Versus nystatin:** We found one systematic review (search date 1993, no RCTs)[7] and two additional small RCTs that reported clinical outcomes.[16,17] The first RCT (212 women) compared intravaginal miconazole, clotrimazole, econazole, and nystatin.[16] It found significantly lower symptomatic relapse over 6 months with intravaginal imidazoles versus nystatin (52/167 [31%] with imidazoles *v* 26/45 [58%] with nystatin; OR 0.32, 95% CI 0.16 to 0.63; NNT 4). The second RCT[17] (70 women) found no significant difference in the proportion of women with persistent symptoms with clotrimazole (100 mg for 14 days) versus high strength nystatin vaginal cream (1 million IU, once daily for 7 days) after 4 weeks (2/33 [6%] with nystatin v 1/37 [3%] with clotrimazole; OR 2.24, 95% CI 0.23 to 22.40). **Versus other imidazoles:** We found one systematic review[7] (search date 1993, 12 RCTs [10,11,18–27]) and 22 additional RCTs (see web extra table B at www.clinicalevidence.com).[17,28–48] Many of the RCTs were too small to exclude clinically important differences. Pooling of the results is difficult because the outcomes vary among the RCTs. The populations selected by each RCTs vary considerably in the prevalence of prognostic risk factors (such as diabetes mellitus or a history of recurrent attacks in the previous year). Together, these RCTs provide no clear evidence of any consistent difference in effectiveness among the different imidazoles. **Duration of treatment:** We found one systematic review (search date 1993, 13 RCTs)[7] and 9 additional RCTs that compared regimens using the same imidazole but for different durations.[11,18,20,24,49–64] These RCTs found no consistent differences in the proportion of women with persistent symptoms, but they were also too small to establish or exclude clinically important differences.

Harms: In the RCTs of intravaginal imidazoles versus placebo, most women did not report any adverse events.[10–15] The commonest adverse event was vulvar irritation. Most RCTs did not report frequencies of specific adverse events with placebo. In one RCT, adverse events were more common in the group of women taking a placebo tablet than among the group using intravaginal imidazole (1 episode of irritation in 23 women using imidazole *v* 9 adverse events [mainly nausea and headache] in 22 women receiving oral placebo).[12]

Comment: Most RCTs were small and many had weak methods (poorly described randomisation, inadequate concealment and blinding, definitions of cure based on mycology results rather than symptoms). We excluded all RCTs that defined cure only on the basis of mycology results. The RCT that found no benefit with intravaginal clotrimazole versus placebo caused significant heterogeneity of the results (see web extra figure A at www.clinicalevidence.com).

OPTION ORAL FLUCONAZOLE

We found no RCTs of oral fluconazole versus placebo or no treatment. A systematic review has found no significant difference with oral fluconazole versus intravaginal imidazoles in the symptoms of vulvovaginal candidiasis. RCTs have found that fluconazole versus intravaginal imidazoles is associated with increased frequency of mild nausea, headache, and abdominal pain.

Benefits: **Oral fluconazole versus placebo:** We found no systematic review and no RCTs. **Versus intravaginal nystatin:** We found no RCTs. **Versus intravaginal imidazoles:** We found one systematic review (search date 2000, 6 RCTs, 947 women), which found no significant difference with oral fluconazole versus intravaginal imidazoles (clotrimazole, miconazole, econazole) in persistent symptoms in the short term (124/627 [20%] with oral fluconazole *v* 121/620 [20%] with intravaginal imidazole; OR 1.00, 95% CI 0.75 to 1.33) or in the medium term (74/432 [17%] *v* 71/404 [18%]; OR 0.96, 95% CI 0.67 to 1.37).[65] Subgroup analyses found no significant difference in persistent symptoms with different imidazoles, or with single or multiple doses of treatment. For example, three RCTs of oral fluconazole versus intravaginal clotrimazole found no reduction in the persistence of symptoms in the medium term (43/220 [20%] with fluconazole *v* 40/218 [18%] with topical clotrimazole; OR 1.10, 95% CI 0.68 to 1.79).

Harms: Large RCTs have found that oral fluconazole versus intravaginal imidazoles may be associated with increased nausea, headache, and abdominal pain.[66–69] In one RCT (429 women) of oral fluconazole versus intravaginal clotrimazole, adverse events were more common with fluconazole (59/217 [27%] with fluconazole *v* 37/212 [17%] with intravaginal clotrimazole; OR 1.75, 95% CI 1.11 to 2.75; NNH 11, 95% CI 6 to 54 after 14 days).[66] The individual events that were more common with fluconazole were headache (12% *v* 9%), abdominal pain (7% *v* 3%), and nausea (4% *v* 0%). Another RCT (235 women) found that nausea and other gastrointestinal symptoms were significantly more common with fluconazole than with intravaginal econazole (9/121 [7%] *v* 2/114 [2%]; OR 3.55, 95% CI 1.06 to 11.90) but local vulvar burning and increased vaginal discharge were significantly more common with intravaginal econazole (3/121 [2%] *v* 25/114 [22%]; OR 0.16, 95% CI 0.07 to 0.35).[67] A third RCT (369 women) found very few adverse events with either fluconazole or clotrimazole (8/188 [4%] *v* 9/181 [5%]).[68] A fourth RCT (183 women) found that nausea was reported by similar proportions with oral fluconazole versus oral ketoconazole (9/92 [10%] with fluconazole *v* 13/91 [14%] with ketoconazole).[69]

Comment: We found no evidence of a difference in symptom reduction with oral fluconazole versus intravaginal imidazole, but found evidence that gastrointestinal adverse events are significantly more likely with fluconazole. This is insufficient evidence to conclude that fluconazole is effective compared with placebo. Indirect evidence of the likely effectiveness of oral fluconazole versus placebo can be derived by convoluting the effects for fluconazole versus imidazoles with the effect for imidazoles versus placebo: this gives an indirect estimate, which suggests that fluconazole versus placebo is likely to be effective (calculated OR 0.11, 95% CI 0.03 to 0.41).

OPTION ORAL ITRACONAZOLE

One RCT found that oral itraconazole versus placebo significantly reduced persistent symptoms at 1 week after treament. One systematic review has found no significant difference in persistant symptoms at 7– days or 28–35 days with oral itraconazole versus intravaginal imidazoles.

Benefits: **Versus oral placebo:** We found one systematic review (search date 2000, 1 RCT[12], 90 women).[65] The RCT found that oral itraconazole (200 mg daily for 3 days) versus placebo significantly reduced the proportion of women with persistent symptoms at 1 week after treatment (13/48 [27%] with itraconazole *v* 12/22 [55%] with placebo; ARR 27%, 95% CI 3% to 49%; OR 0.31, 95% CI 0.11 to 0.88; NNT 4, 95% CI 2 to 31).[12] **Versus intravaginal nystatin:** We found no RCTs. **Versus intravaginal imidazoles:** We found one systematic review (search date 2000, 3 RCTs, 300 women), which found no significant difference with oral itraconazole versus intravaginal imidazoles (clotrimazole, econazole) in persistent symptoms at 7–10 days (3 RCTs: 39/162 [24%] with itraconazole *v* 36/138 [26%] with imidazoles; OR 0.83, 95% CI 0.49 to 1.43) or at 28–35 days (2 RCTs: 15/74 with itraconazole *v* 12/54 with imidazoles; OR 0.81, 95% CI 0.34 to 1.94).[65]

Harms: One RCT found that itraconazole versus clotrimazole significantly increased adverse events (17/50 [34%] with itraconazole *v* 1/23 [4%] with clotrimazole; OR 4.83, 95% CI 1.55 to 15.1); the events with increased frequency were nausea (14%), headache (12%), dizziness (6%), and bloating (6%).[12] However, a second RCT (double blind, 81 women) found similar numbers of adverse events with oral itraconazole versus intravaginal econazole (4/40 [10%] with itraconazole *v* 8/41 [20%] with econazole; OR 0.48, 95% CI 0.14 to 1.61).[70]

Comment: The evidence suggests that oral itraconazole and intravaginal imidazoles have similar effects on the symptoms of vaginal candidiasis, but itraconazole has more gastrointestinal adverse effects.

OPTION ORAL KETOCONAZOLE

We found no RCTs of oral ketoconazole versus placebo or versus no treatment. Four RCTs have found no significant difference with oral ketoconazole versus intravaginal imidazoles in the reduction of persistent symptoms, but found that ketoconazole significantly increased the frequency of minor adverse events (mainly nausea). Case reports have associated ketoconazole with a low risk of fulminant hepatitis (1/12 000 courses of treatment with oral ketoconazole).

Benefits: **Versus oral placebo:** We found no systematic review or RCT. **Versus intravaginal nystatin:** We found no RCTs. **Versus intravaginal imidazoles:** We found one systematic review (search date 1993, 4 RCTs, 280 women)[7] and three additional RCTs (see web extra table C at www.clinicalevidence.com).[71–73] The systematic review concluded that oral treatment is as effective as topical treatment at eliminating *Candida*, but did not compare clinical outcomes. One additional RCT (140 women) found that oral ketoconazole (400 mg daily for 5 days) versus intravaginal isoconazole (600 mg daily for 5 days) significantly increased persistent symptoms 1 week after treatment (34/64 [53%] with ketoconazole *v* 11/68 [16%] with isoconazole; ARI 37%, 95% CI 21% to 53%; OR 5.11, 95% CI 2.50 to 10.50) and 1 month after treatment (17/59 [29%] with ketoconazole *v* 8/61 [13%] with isoconazole; ARI 16%, 95% CI 12% to 30%; OR 2.60, 95% 1.07 to 6.18). Another additional RCT (unblinded, 151 women) recruited women with acute vulvovaginal candidiasis and a history of recurrent attacks (3 or more acute attacks in the previous year).[73] It found that oral ketoconazole (400 mg daily for 14 days) versus intravaginal clotrimazole (100 mg daily for 7 days) had similar rates of recurrent symptomatic relapse after 4 weeks (11/55 [20%] with ketoconazole *v* 15/57 [26%] with clotrimazole; OR 0.70, 95% CI 0.29 to 1.69). On pooling the results of the 5 RCTs[71–75] that report the number of women with persistent symptoms 1–5 weeks after treatment, we found no significant difference with ketoconazole versus intravaginal imidazole in the proportion of women with persistent symptoms (41/268 [15%] with ketoconazole *v* 30/211 [14%] with intravaginal imidazoles; OR 1.26, 95% CI 0.52 to 3.05) (see web extra figure B at www.clinicalevidence.com). **Versus oral itraconazole:** We found no systematic review and no RCT. **Versus oral fluconazole:** We found one systematic review (search date 1993[7], 1 RCT[69], 183 women). The RCT found no significant difference with ketoconazole (400 mg daily for 5 days) versus fluconazole (1 dose of 150 mg) in the proportion of women with persistent symptoms after 5–16 days (17/72 [24%] with ketoconazole *v* 17/80 [21%] with fluconazole; OR 1.15, 95% CI 0.53 to 2.45) or after 27–62 days (14/72 [19%] with ketoconazole *v* 14/76 [18%] with fluconazole; OR 1.07, 95% CI 0.47 to 2.43).

Harms: In the RCTs, mild adverse effects (nausea, fatigue, headaches, or abdominal pain) were more common with oral ketoconazole than with intravaginal imidazole (3/70 [4%] *v* 0/70[72]; 0/25 *v* 0/25[71]; 5/20 [25%] *v* 1/20 [5%][75]; 3/56 [5%] *v* 2/47 [4%][76]; overall OR 3.21, 95% CI 1.08 to 9.55) (see web extra figure C at www.clinicalevidence.com). One RCT (151 women) found that ketoconazole versus intravaginal clotrimazole increased rates of headache (23% *v* 4%), nausea (22% *v* 1%), abdominal discomfort (14% *v* 7%), and fatigue (7% *v* 2%).[73] Minor adverse events were not increased with ketoconazole versus fluconazole (13/91 [14%] *v* 9/92 [10%]).[69] Observational studies have found that asymptomatic elevation of liver enzymes is common, and fulminant hepatitis was observed in about 1/12 000 courses of treatment with oral ketoconazole.[77]

Comment: In women with uncomplicated vulvovaginal candidiasis, ketoconazole and intravaginal imidazoles have similar effects on persistent symptoms. The possibility of rare but serious hepatitis has led to a consensus that the risks associated with oral ketoconazole may outweigh its benefits in this group of women.

OPTION EFFECTS OF TREATING A MALE SEXUAL PARTNER

Two RCTs found no significant difference with treating versus not treating a woman's male sexual partner in the resolution of the woman's acute vulvovaginal candidiasis symptoms, or in the rate of symptomatic relapse.

Benefits: We found no systematic review but found two RCTs.[78,79] In the first RCT (40 women with acute vulvovaginal candidiasis and their male partners), all the women received itraconazole (100 mg daily for 5 days). Their male partners were randomised to itraconazole (100 mg daily for 5 days) versus placebo. Participants and clinicians were blind to treatment allocation. The RCT found no difference between treating the male partner with itraconazole versus placebo in the number of women with persistent symptoms after 30 days (2/19 [11%] with itraconazole *v* 4/18 [22%] with placebo; OR 0.43, 95% CI 0.08 to 2.43).[78] The second RCT (117 women with vaginal candidiasis, and their male partners) treated the women with ketoconazole (200–600 mg daily for 3 days) and the male partners were randomised to ketoconazole (400 mg daily) versus placebo for 3 days. The participants and clinicians were blind to treatment allocation. The RCT found no difference in the proportion of women cured 1 week after treatment (48/57 [84%] with partners receiving ketoconazole *v* 53/60 [88%] with partners receiving placebo; OR 0.71, 0.25 to 2.02; see comment below, or the proportion of initially cured women who relapsed by 4 weeks after treatment (13/48 [27%] with ketoconazole *v* 19/53 [36%] with placebo; OR 0.67, 95% CI 0.29 to 1.54).[79]

Harms: The RCTs did not report evidence about harms.[78,79]

Comment: The women recruited in the RCTs were not selected because of a history of recurrent vulvovaginal candidiasis. The definition of "cured" and "relapsed" in the second RCT is not clear, but seems to be some combination of improved symptoms and negative cultures. Only a small number of men had any penile symptoms, and these were distributed equally between the ketoconazole and placebo groups. We found no clear evidence that treating male sexual partners influences the recovery of women's vulvovaginal candidiasis. However, the confidence intervals are wide even after pooling the 30 day outcomes from both RCTs (OR 0.85, 95% CI 0.40 to 1.80);[78,79] therefore the evidence is insufficient to establish or to exclude clinically important benefits or harms.

QUESTION What are the effects of treatments in non-pregnant women with recurrent vulvovaginal candidiasis

OPTION INTRAVAGINAL IMIDAZOLE

Two RCTs of regular prophylaxis with intravaginal imidazole versus placebo found inconsistent effects on the proportion of women with symptomatic relapse. Another RCT found that regular prophylactic intravaginal imidazole versus treatment only at the onset of symptoms reduced the frequency of episodes of symptomatic vaginitis, but the difference was not significant. The RCTs were too small to exclude a clinically important reduction.

Benefits: **Versus placebo:** We found one systematic review (search date 1993, 2 RCTs, 89 women with recurrent vulvovaginal candidiasis).[7] The RCTs compared intravaginal clotrimazole (500 mg each month) versus intravaginal placebo (monthly). Both RCTs found that prophylaxis versus placebo reduced the proportion of women with symptomatic relapse, although in one RCT the difference was significant and in the other RCT it was not. On pooling the results, we found no difference with regular prophylaxis versus placebo in the proportion of women with symptomatic relapse (18/48 [38%] with prophylaxis *v* 31/41 [76%] with placebo; OR [random effects meta-analysis] 0.23, 95% CI 0.05 to 1.12). **Regular prophylactic treatment versus as required treatment:** We found one crossover RCT (unblinded, 23 women with recurrent vaginal candidiasis), which found that regular intravaginal clotrimazole (500 mg each month) versus empirical treatment (clotrimazole 500 mg at the onset of symptoms) reduced the number of symptomatic episodes of vaginitis over 6 months, but the result was not significant (2.2 episodes per person with regular treatment *v* 3.7 with empirical treatment; $P = 0.05$).[80] Women used significantly more clotrimazole during the 6 month prophylactic period (7.3 doses of clotrimazole per woman *v* 3.6 doses of empirical treatment; $P < 0.001$). In the RCT, significantly more women preferred empirical treatment than prophylactic treatment (74% *v* 17%).

Harms: see harms of intravaginal imidazoles, p 2010.

Comment: One RCT defined recurrent vaginal candidiasis as greater than four proven episodes of candidal vaginitis in the previous year.[80] All three RCTs found that prophylaxis reduces the risk of symptomatic recurrence, but the RCTs were too small to establish or exclude a clinically important reduction.

OPTION ORAL FLUCONAZOLE

We found no RCTs about the effects of fluconazole in preventing of recurrent vulvovaginal candidiasis.

Benefits: We found no systematic review or RCTs.

Harms: We found no RCTs.

Comment: None.

OPTION ORAL ITRACONAZOLE

One RCT in women with vulvovaginal candidiasis found that oral itraconazole versus placebo significantly reduced the rate of recurrence over 6 months. One RCT found insufficient evidence about the effects of oral itraconazole versus intravaginal clotrimazole.

Benefits: We found no systematic review. **Oral itraconazole versus placebo:** One RCT (single blind, 114 women with recurrent vulvovaginal candidiasis)[81] found that oral itraconazole (400 mg monthly) versus placebo significantly reduced recurrence of vulvovaginal candidiasis symptoms (recurrence during 6 months' follow up: 20/55 [36%] with itraconazole *v* 34/53 [64%] with placebo; ARR 28%, 95% CI 9% to 47%; OR 0.33, 95% CI 0.16 to 0.71;

NNT 4, 95% CI 3 to 11). After discontinuation of itraconazole, recurrence rates were similar.[81] **Intermittent oral itraconazole versus intravaginal imidazoles:** We found one RCT (unblinded, 44 women)[82] comparing weekly itraconazole (200 mg twice weekly) versus intravaginal clotrimazole (200 mg twice weekly) for 6 months. One woman withdrew from itraconazole treatment and five withdrew from clotrimazole treatment. It found that oral itraconazole versus intravaginal clotrimazole increased the proportion of women with symptomatic recurrences over 6 months (see comment below); 7/21 [33%] with itraconazole *v* 0/17 with clotrimazole).[82]

Harms: The first RCT did not report details of any adverse events (see oral itraconazole, p 2013).[81]

Comment: The evidence of one RCT suggests that, compared with placebo, oral itraconazole is likely to reduce recurrent symptomatic vaginitis. The results of the comparison between oral itraconazole and intravaginal clotrimazole are difficult to interpret because the study was unblinded, and because the unbalanced withdrawal from the RCT could explain the observed difference between groups.

OPTION ORAL KETOCONAZOLE

One RCT found that oral ketoconazole, given intermittently or continuously at a lower dose versus placebo significantly reduced the rate of symptomatic recurrence. This benefit is associated with an increased risk of harms, including rare cases of fulminant hepatitis.

Benefits: **Versus placebo or no treatment:** We found one systematic review (search date 1993, 1 RCT, 63 women).[7] The RCT (74 women) compared intermittent oral ketoconazole (400 mg daily for 5 days of each menstrual cycle) versus low dose ketoconazole (100 mg daily for 6 months) versus placebo over 6 months.[83] The RCT found that intermittent oral ketoconazole versus placebo reduced symptomatic recurrence of vulvovaginal candidiasis over 6 months (6/21 [29%] with intermittent ketoconazole *v* 15/21 [71%] with placebo; OR 0.19, 95% CI 0.06 to 0.62; NNT 3, 95% CI 2 to 8 I). It also found that continuous ketoconazole versus placebo reduced symptomatic recurrence of vulvovaginal candidiasis over 6 months (1/21 [5%] with continuous ketoconazole; OR 0.06, 95% CI 0.02 to 0.22; NNT 2). **Versus intravaginal imidazoles:** We found no systematic review and no RCTs.

Harms: Ketoconazole is associated with an increased frequency of gastrointestinal adverse effects and case reports of rare fulminant hepatitis (see ketoconazole, p 2013).

Comment: The adverse effects of ketoconazole and no good evidence of increased benefit compared with safer alternatives, has led to a consensus that ketoconazole is likely to be harmful compared with those alternatives.

GLOSSARY

Balanitis Balanitis is inflammation of the glans of the penis. The foreskin is often involved (balanoposthitis).

REFERENCES

1. Sobel JD. Vulvovaginal candidiasis. In: Holmes KK MP-A, Sparling PF, Lemon SM, Stamm WE, Piot P, Wasserheit JN, eds. *Sexually transmitted diseases*. 3rd ed. New York: McGraw-Hill, 1999: 629–639.
2. Sobel JD, Faro S, Force RW, et al. Vulvovaginal candidiasis: epidemiologic, diagnostic, and therapeutic considerations. *Am J Obstet Gynecol* 1998;178:203–211.
3. Foxman B. The epidemiology of vulvovaginal candidiasis: risk factors. *Am J Public Health* 1990;80:329–331.
4. Geiger AM, Foxman B, Sobel JD. Chronic vulvovaginal candidiasis: characteristics of women with *Candida albicans*, *C glabrata* and no *Candida*. *Genitourin Med* 1995;71:304–307.
5. Geiger AM, Foxman B, Gillespie BW. The epidemiology of vulvovaginal candidiasis among university students. *Am J Public Health* 1995;85:1146–1148.
6. Isaacs JH. Nystatin vaginal cream in monilial vaginitis. *Illinois Med J* 1973;3:240–241.
7. Reef SE, Levine WC, McNeil MM, et al. Treatment options for vulvovaginal candidiasis, 1993. *Clin Infect Dis* 1995;20:S80–S90. Search date 1993; primary sources Medline and hand search of two textbooks.
8. Van Slyke KK, Michel VP, Rein MF. Treatment of vulvovaginal candidiasis with boric acid powder. *Am J Obstet Gynecol* 1981;141:145–148.
9. Valdes-Dapena MA, Arey JB. Boric acid poisoning: three fatal cases and a review of the literature. *J Paediatr* 1962;61:531.
10. Thomason JL, Gelbart SM, Kellett AV, Scaglione NJ, Gotwalt KT, Broekhuizen FF. Terconazole for the treatment of vulvovaginal candidiasis. *J Reprod Med* 1990;35:992–994.
11. Brown D Jr, Henzl MR, LePage ME, et al. Butoconazole vaginal cream in the treatment of vulvovaginal candidiasis: comparison with miconazole nitrate and placebo. *J Reprod Med* 1986;31:1045–1048.
12. Stein GE, Mummaw N. Placebo-controlled trial of itraconazole for treatment of acute vaginal candidiasis. *Antimicrob Agents Chemother* 1993;37:89–92.
13. Bro F. Single-dose 500-mg clotrimazole vaginal tablets compared with placebo in the treatment of *Candida vaginitis*. *J Fam Pract* 1990;31:148–152.
14. Fleury F, Hodgson C. Single-dose treatment of vulvovaginal candidiasis with a new 500mg clotrimazole vaginal tablet. *Adv Ther* 1984;1:349–356.
15. Guess EA, Hodgson C. Single-dose topical treatment of vulvovaginal candidiasis with a new 500mg clotrimazole vaginal tablet. *Adv Ther* 1984;1:137–145.
16. Dennerstein GJ, Langley R. Vulvovaginal candidiasis: treatment and recurrence. *Aust N Z J Obstet Gynaecol* 1982;22:231–233.
17. Cassar NL. High-potency nystatin cream in the treatment of vulvovaginal candidiasis. *Curr Ther Res* 1983;34:305–310.
18. Franklin R. Seven-day clotrimazole therapy for vulvovaginal candidiasis. *South Med J* 1978;71:141–143.
19. Corson SL, Kapikian RR, Nehring R. Terconazole and miconazole cream for treating vulvovaginal candidiasis. *J Reprod Med* 1991;36:561–567.
20. Kjaeldgaard A. Comparison of terconazole and clotrimazole vaginal tablets in the treatment of vulvovaginal candidosis. *Pharmatherapeutica* 1986;4:525–531.
21. Stein GE, Gurwith D, Mummaw N, Gurwith M. Single-dose tioconazole compared with 3-day clotrimazole treatment in vulvovaginal candidiasis. *Antimicrob Agents Chemother* 1986;29:969–971.
22. Kaufman RH, Henzl MR, Brown D Jr, et al. Comparison of three-day butoconazole treatment with seven-day miconazole treatment for vulvovaginal candidiasis. *J Reprod Med* 1989;34:479–483.
23. Droegemueller W, Adamson D G, Brown D. Three-day treatment with butoconazole nitrate for vulvovaginal candidiasis. *Obstet Gynecol* 1984;64:530–534.
24. Jacobson JB, Hajman AJ, Wiese J. A new vaginal antifungal agent – butoconazole nitrate. *Acta Obstet Gynecol Scand* 1985;64:241–244.
25. Hajman AJ. Vulvovaginal candidosis: comparison of 3-day treatment with 2% butoconazole nitrate cream and 6-day treatment of 1% clotrimazole cream. *J Int Med Res* 1988;16:367–375.
26. Adamson GD, Brown D Jr, Standard JV, Henzl MR. Three-day treatment with butoconazole vaginal suppositories for vulvovaginal candidiasis. *J Reprod Med Obstet Gynecol* 1986;31:131–132.
27. Bradbeer CS, Mayhew SR, Barlow D. Butaconazole and miconazole in treating vaginal candidiasis. *Genitourin Med* 1985;61:270–272.
28. Glasser A. Single-dose treatment of vaginal mycoses. Effectiveness of clotrimazole and econazole. *Fortschr Med* 1986;104:259–262.
29. Gastaldi A. Treatment of vaginal candidiasis with fenticonazole and miconazole. *Curr Ther Res Clin Exp* 1985;38:489–493.
30. Gabriel G, Thin RN. Clotrimazole and econazole in the treatment of vaginal candidosis. A single-blind comparison. *Br J Ven Dis* 1983;59:56–58.
31. Amrouni B, Pereiro M, Florez A, Pontes C, Izquierdo I, Toribio J. A phase III comparative study of the efficacies of flutrimazole versus clotrimazole for the treatment of vulvovaginal candidiasis. *J Mycol Med* 2000;10:62–65.
32. Arendt J. Terconazole versus clotrimazole cream in vulvovaginal candidiasis. *Adv Ther* 1989;6:287–294.
33. Gouveia DC, Jones Da Silva C. Oxiconazole in the treatment of vaginal candidiasis: single dose versus 3-day treatment with econazole. *Pharmatherapeutica* 1984;3:682–685.
34. Brewster E, Preti PM, Ruffmann R, Studd J. Effect of fenticonazole in vaginal candidiasis: a double-blind clinical trial versus clotrimazole. *J Int Med Res* 1986;14:306–310.
35. Balsdon M-J. Comparison of miconazole-coated tampons with clotrimazole vaginal tablets in the treatment of vaginal candidosis. *Br J Ven Dis* 1981;57:275–278.
36. Bradbeer CS, Thin RN. Comparison of econazole and isoconazole as single dose treatment for vaginal candidosis. *Genitourin Med* 1985;61:396–398.
37. Brown D Jr, Binder CL, Gardner HL, Wells J. Comparison of econazole and clotrimazole in the treatment of vulvovaginal candidiasis. *Obstet Gynecol* 1980;56:121–123.
38. Brown D, Henzl MR, Kaufman RH, et al. Butoconazole nitrate 2% for vulvovaginal candidiasis. *J Reprod Med* 1999;44:933–938.
39. Cohen L. Single dose treatment of vaginal candidosis: comparison of clotrimazole and isoconazole. *Br J Ven Dis* 1984;60:42–44.
40. Dellenbach P, Thomas J-L, Guerin V, Ochsenbein E, Contet-Audonneau N. Topical treatment of vaginal candidosis with sertaconazole and econazole sustained-release suppositories. *Int J Gynecol Obstet* 2000;71:S47–S42.
41. Wiest W, Azzollini E, Ruffmann R. Comparison of single administration with an ovule of 600 mg

fenticonazole versus a 500 mg clotrimazole vaginal pessary in the treatment of vaginal candidiasis. *J Int Med Res* 1989;17:369–372.

42. Palacio-Hernanz A, Sanz-Sanz F, Rodriquez-Noriega A. Double-blind investigation of R-42470 (terconazole cream 0.4%) and clotrimazole (cream 1%) for the topical treatment of mycotic vaginitis. *Chemioterapia* 1984;3:192–195.
43. Lolis D, Kanellopoulos N, Liappas I, Xyngakis A, Zissis NP. Double-blind evaluation of miconazole tampons, compared with clotrimazole vaginal tablets, in vaginal candidiasis. *Clin Ther* 1981;4:212–216.
44. Studd JW, Dooley MM, Welch CC, et al. Comparative clinical trial of fenticonazole ovule (600 mg) versus clotrimazole vaginal tablet (500 mg) in the treatment of symptomatic vaginal candidiasis. *Curr Med Res Opin* 1989;11:477–484.
45. Herbold H. Comparative studies to the clinical efficacy of two 1-dose-therapies of vaginal candidosis. *Med Welt* 1985;36:255–257.
46. Lappin MA, Brooker DC, Francisco CA, Dorfman J. Effect of butoconazole nitrate 2% vaginal cream and miconazole nitrate 2% vaginal cream treatments in patients with vulvovaginal candidiasis. *Infect Dis Obstet Gynecol* 1996;4:323–328
47. Lebherz TB, Goldman L, Wiesmeier E, Mason D, Ford LC. A comparison of the efficacy of two vaginal creams for vulvovaginal candidiasis, and correlations with the presence of *Candida* species in the perianal area and oral contraceptive use. *Clin Ther* 1983;5:409–416.
48. Stettendorf S, Benijts G, Vignali M, Kreysing W. Three-day therapy of vaginal candidiasis with clotrimazole vaginal tablets and econazole ovules: a multicenter comparative study. *Chemotherapy* 1982;28:87–91.
49. Wolfson N, Samuels B, Hodgson C, Graves K. One-day management of vulvovaginal candidiasis. *J La State Med Soc* 1987;139:27–29.
50. Lebherz T, Guess E, Wolfson N. Efficacy of single- versus multiple-dose clotrimazole therapy in the management of vulvovaginal candidiasis. *Am J Obstet Gynecol* 1985;152:965–968.
51. Fleury F, Hughes D, Floyd, R. Therapeutic results obtained in vaginal mycoses after single-dose treatment with 500 mg clotrimazole vaginal tablets. *Am J Obstet Gynecol* 1985;152:968–970.
52. Loendersloot EW, Goormans E, Wiesenhaan PE, Barthel PJ, Branolte JH. Efficacy and tolerability of single-dose versus six-day treatment of candidal vulvovaginitis with vaginal tablets of clotrimazole. *Am I Obstet Gynecol* 1985;152:953–955.
53. Wolfson N, Samuels B, Riley J. A three-day treatment regimen for vulvovaginal candidiasis. *J La State Med Soc* 1982;134:28–31.
54. Oates JK, Davidson F. Treatment of vaginal candidiasis with clotrimazole. *Postgrad Med J* 1974;50:99–102.
55. Lebherz TB, Ford LC, Kleinkopf V. A comparison of a three-day and seven-day clotrimazole regimen for vulvovaginal candidiasis. *Clin Ther* 1981;3:344–348.
56. Robertson WH. Vulvovaginal candidiasis treated with clotrimazole cream in seven days compared with fourteen day treatment with miconazole cream. *Am J Obstet Gynecol* 1978;132:321–323.
57. Pasquale SA, Lawson J, Sargent EC Jr, Newdeck JP. A dose–response study with Monistat cream. *Obstet Gynecol* 1979;53:250–253.
58. Floyd R, Hodgson C. One-day treatment of vulvovaginal candidiasis with a 500-mg clotrimazole vaginal tablet compared with a three-day regimen of two 100-mg vaginal tablets daily. *Clin Ther* 1986;8:181–186.
59. Hughes D, Kriedman T, Hodgson C. Treatment of vulvovaginal candidiasis with a single 500-mg clotrimazole vaginal tablet compared with two 100-mg tablets daily for three days. *Curr Ther Res Clin Exp* 1986;39:773–777.
60. Mizuno S, Cho N. Clinical evaluation of three-day treatment of vaginal mycosis with clotrimazole vaginal tablets. *J Int Med Res* 1983;11:179–185.
61. Milsom I, Forssman L. Treatment of vaginal candidosis with a single 500-mg clotrimazole pessary. *Br J Ven Dis* 1982;58:124–126.
62. Westphal J. Treatment of *Candida mycoses* of the vulva and vagina with clotrimazole. Comparison of single-dose and six-day therapy. *Fortschr Med* 1988;106:445–448.
63. Upmalis DH, Cone FL, Lamia CA, et al. Single-dose miconazole nitrate vaginal ovule in the treatment of vulvovaginal candidiasis: two single-blind, controlled studies versus miconazole nitrate 100mg cream for 7 days. *J Women's Health Gender-based Medicine*. 2000;9:421–429.
64. Wiest W, Ruffmann R. Short-term treatment of vaginal candidiasis with fenticonazole ovules: a three dose schedule comparative trial. *J Int Med Res* 1987;15:319–325.
65. Watson MC, Grimshaw JM, Bond CM, Mollison J, Ludbrook A. Oral versus intra-vaginal imidazole and triazole anti-fungal treatment of uncomplicated vulvovaginal candidiasis (thrush). In: The Cochrane Library, Issue 4, 2001. Oxford: Update Software. Search date 2000, primary sources Cochrane Library, Medline, Embase, Cochrane Collaboration Sexually Transmitted Disease Group Specialised Register of Controlled Trials, hand search of reference lists, UK manufacturers of anti-fungals.
66. Sobel JD, Brooker D, Stein GE, et al. Single oral dose fluconazole compared with conventional clotrimazole topical therapy of *Candida vaginitis*. *Am J Obstet Gynecol* 1995;172:1263–1268.
67. Osser S, Haglund A, Westström L. Treatment of vaginal candidiasis: a prospective randomized investigator-blind multicenter study comparing topically applied econazole with oral fluconazole. *Acta Obstet Gynecol Scand* 1991;70:73–78.
68. Anon. A comparison of single-dose oral fluconazole with 3-day intravaginal clotrimazole in the treatment of vaginal candidiasis. *Br J Obstet Gynaecol* 1989;96:226–232.
69. Kutzer E, Oittner R, Leodolter S, Brammer KW. A comparison of fluconazole and ketoconazole in the oral treatment of vaginal candidiasis; report of a double-blind multicentre trial. *Eur J Obstet Gynecol Reprod Biol* 1988;29:305–313.
70. Timonen H, Hartikainen-Vahtera P, Kivijarvi A, et al. A double-blind comparison of the effectiveness of itraconazole oral capsules with econazole vaginal capsules in the treatment of vaginal candidosis. *Drug Invest* 1992;4:515–520.
71. Comninos A, Kapellakis I, Pikouli-Giannopoulou P, Manafi Th. Double-blind evaluation of ketoconazole comparatively with clotrimazole in vaginal candidiasis. *Curr Ther Res* 1984;36:100–104.
72. Farkas B, Simon N. Ergebnisse einer Vergleichsstudie mit einem oral und einem lokal zu applizierenden Antimykotikum bei Vaginalmykosen. *Mykosen* 1984;27:554–561.
73. Sobel JD, Schmitt C, Stein G, Mummaw N, Christensen S, Meriwether C. Initial management of recurrent vulvovaginal candidiasis with oral ketoconazole and topical clotrimazole. *J Reprod Med* 1994;39:517–520.

74. Puolakka J, Tuimala R. Comparison between oral ketoconazole and topical miconazole in the treatment of vaginal candidiasis. *Acta Obstet Gynecol Scand* 1983;62:575–577.

75. Rohde-Werner H. Topical tioconazole versus systemic ketoconazole treatment of vaginal candidiasis. *J Int Med Res* 1984;12:298–302.

76. Bingham JS. Single blind comparison of ketoconazole 200 mg oral tablets and clotrimazole 100 mg vaginal tablets and 1% cream in treating acute vaginal candidosis. *Br J Ven Dis* 1984;60:175–177.

77. Lake-Bakaar G. Scheuer PJ. Sherlock S. Hepatic reactions associated with ketoconazole in the United Kingdom. *BMJ* 1987;294:419–422.

78. Calderon-Marquez JJ. Itraconazole in the treatment of vaginal candidosis and the effect of treatment of the sexual partner. *Rev Inf Dis* 1987;9:S143–S145.

79. Bisschop MP, Merkus JM, Scheygrond H, van Cutsem J. Co-treatment of the male partner in vaginal candidosis: a double-blind randomized control study. *Br J Obstet Gynaecol* 1986;93:79–81.

80. Fong IW. The value of prophylactic (monthly) clotrimazole versus empiric self-treatment in recurrent vaginal candidiasis. *Genitourin Med* 1994;70:124–126.

81. Spinillo A, Colonna L, Piazzi G, Baltaro F, Monaco A, Ferrari A. Managing recurrent vulvovaginal candidiasis. Intermittent prevention with itraconazole. *J Reprod Med* 1997;42:83–87.

82. Fong IW. The value of chronic suppressive therapy with itraconazole versus clotrimazole in women with recurrent vaginal candidiasis. *Genitourin Med* 1992;68:374–377.

83. Sobel JD. Recurrent vulvovaginal candidiasis. A prospective study of the efficacy of maintenance ketoconazole therapy. *N Engl J Med* 1986;315:1455–1458.

84. Miller PI, Humphries M, Grassick K. A single-blind comparison of oral and intravaginal treatments in acute and recurrent vaginal candidosis in general practice. *Pharmatherapeutica* 1984;3:582–587.

Jeanne Marrazzo
Assistant Professor, Medicine
University of Washington
Seattle
USA

Competing interests: JM has received research funding from Pfizer Pharmaceutical, the makers of Diflucan.

Pressure sores

Search date February 2002

Nicky Cullum, E Andrea Nelson, and Jane Nixon

QUESTIONS

INTERVENTIONS

PREVENTION

Beneficial

Foam alternatives (compared with standard foam mattresses) .2023

Pressure relieving overlays on operating tables. 2023

Likely to be beneficial

Low air loss beds in intensive care (compared with standard beds) 2023

Medical sheepskin overlays . .2025

Unknown effectiveness

Electric profiling beds 2023

Different seat cushions 2023

Low tech constant low pressure supports 2023

Alternating pressure surfaces .2023

Low air loss hydrotherapy beds. 2023

Repositioning (regular "turning") 2025

Topical lotions and dressings .2025

Likely to be ineffective or harmful

Air filled vinyl boots with foot cradle 2023

TREATMENT

Likely to be beneficial

Air fluidised supports (compared with standard care) 2026

Unknown effectiveness

Low tech constant low pressure supports 2026

Alternating pressure surfaces .2026

Low air loss beds 2026

Seat cushions. 2026

Hydrocolloid dressings (compared with gauze soaked in saline or hypochlorite) 2027

Other dressings. 2027

Debridement 2027

Topical phenytoin 2027

Surgery 2027

Nutritional supplements. 2027

Electrotherapy. 2027

Therapeutic ultrasound 2027

Low level laser therapy 2027

Topical negative pressure. . . .2027

See glossary, p 2028

Key Messages

Prevention

- **Air filled vinyl boots with foot cradle** One small RCT found that air filled vinyl boots with foot cradles versus hospital pillows were associated with a significantly faster rate of development of pressure sores.
- **Foam alternatives (*v* standard foam mattresses)** A meta-analysis of five RCTs has found that foam alternatives versus standard hospital foam mattresses significantly reduce the incidence of pressure sores after 10–14 days in people at high risk (NNT 5, 95% CI 4 to 7).
- **Low air loss beds in intensive care (*v* standard beds)** One RCT found that low air loss beds versus standard beds significantly reduced the risk of new pressure sores over the duration of the trial, which was not specified (NNT 3, 95% CI 2 to 5).

Pressure sores

- **Medical sheepskin overlays** One RCT in people aged 60 years or over undergoing orthopaedic surgery has found that medical sheepskins versus standard treatment significantly reduces the incidence of pressure sores after an unstated period (NNT 5, 95% CI 4 to 9).
- **Pressure relieving overlays on operating tables** One systematic review has found that the use of pressure relieving overlays on operating tables significantly reduces the incidence of pressure sores.
- **Alternating pressure surfaces; different seat cushions; electric profiling beds; low air loss hydrotherapy beds; low tech constant low pressure supports; repositioning (regular "turning"); topical lotions and dressings** We found insufficient evidence about the effects of these interventions in preventing pressure sores.

Treatment

- **Air fluidised supports (*v* standard care)** Two RCTs in people in hospital found that air fluidised supports versus standard care healed more established sores. One RCT in people cared for at home found no significant difference with air fluidised supports versus standard care in healing; this trial had a high withdrawal rate.
- **Alternating pressure surfaces; debridement; electrotherapy; hydrocolloid dressings (*v* gauze soaked in saline or hypochlorite); low air loss beds; low level laser therapy; low tech constant low pressure supports; nutritional supplements; other dressings; seat cushions; surgery; topical negative pressure; topical phenytoin; therapeutic ultrasound** We found insufficient evidence on the effects of these interventions in healing pressure sores.

DEFINITION Pressure sores (also known as pressure ulcers, bed sores, and decubitus ulcers) may present as persistently hyperaemic, blistered, broken, or necrotic skin, and may extend to underlying structures, including muscle and bone. Whether blanching and non-blanching erythema constitute pressure sores remains controversial.

INCIDENCE/ PREVALENCE The most comprehensive data on prevalence and incidence come from hospital populations. Studies have found a prevalence of 6–10% in National Health Service hospitals in the UK,[1] and 8% in a teaching hospital in the USA.[2]

AETIOLOGY/ RISK FACTORS Pressure sores are caused by unrelieved pressure, shear, or friction, and are most common below the waist and at bony prominences such as the sacrum, heels, and hips. They occur in all healthcare settings. Increased age, reduced mobility, and impaired nutrition emerge consistently as risk factors.[3] However, the relative importance of these and other factors is uncertain.

PROGNOSIS The presence of pressure sores has been associated with a two to fourfold increased risk of death in elderly people and people in intensive care.[4,5] However, pressure sores are a marker for underlying disease severity and other comorbidities rather than an independent predictor of mortality.[4] Pressure sores vary considerably in size and severity.

AIMS To prevent pressure sore formation; to heal existing pressure sores; and to improve quality of life.

OUTCOMES Incidence and severity of pressure sores; rate of change of area and volume; time to heal. Interface pressure recorded at various anatomical sites is a surrogate outcome sometimes used in studies of preventive interventions; it has not yet been linked to clinical outcomes.

METHODS *Clinical Evidence* update search and appraisal February 2002, following a search of the Specialist Trials Register of the Cochrane Wounds Group (compiled by searching 19 electronic databases, including Medline, Cinahl, BIDS, and Embase, and hand searching journals and conference proceedings). We reviewed all RCTs that used objective clinical outcome measures. For many trials, we could not be sure that pressure sore size was evenly distributed between groups at baseline. Unequal distribution of wound size at baseline will impact on all measures of wound healing. Ideally, studies of treatment should stratify randomisation by initial wound area and be of sufficient size to ensure even distribution of baseline wound size. Many of the studies performed by manufacturers were in healthy people who are not representative of clinical subjects, and these studies have been excluded.

QUESTION What are the effects of preventive interventions?

OPTION PRESSURE RELIEVING SURFACES

A meta-analysis of five RCTs has found that foam alternatives to the standard hospital foam mattress significantly reduce the incidence of pressure sores over 10–14 days in people at high risk. We found no evidence of a "best" foam alternative. We found insufficient evidence on the effects of electric profiling beds, different seat cushions, and constant low pressure supports. The relative merits of alternating and constant low pressure, and of the different alternating pressure surfaces, are unclear. One RCT found that low air loss beds versus standard beds significantly reduced the risk of new pressure sores over the duration of the trial. One systematic review has found that the use of pressure relieving overlays on operating tables significantly reduces the incidence of pressure sores. One RCT found that air filled vinyl boots with foot cradles versus hospital pillows were associated with more rapid development of pressure sores.

Benefits: We found one systematic review (search date 2000).[6] **Foam alternatives versus standard hospital mattress:** The systematic review[6] identified four RCTs, and we found one subsequent RCT,[7] all undertaken primarily in elderly people in orthopaedic hospital wards. A meta-analysis of the five RCTs (N Cullum, EA Nelson, and J Nixon, personal communication, 2002) found that foam alternatives to the standard hospital mattress significantly reduced the incidence of sores over 10–14 days (RR 0.31, 95% CI 0.22 to 0.46; NNT 5, 95% CI 4 to 7).[6,7] **Different foam alternatives:** The systematic review identified five RCTs comparing different foam alternatives.[6] One RCT found that a five section foam and fibre replacement versus a 4 inch (10 cm) thick dimpled foam overlay reduced the risk of developing a pressure sore (RR 0.42, 95% CI 0.18 to 0.90; NNT for 10–21 days' treatment 3, 95% CI 2 to 25).

The other RCTs were too small to detect a difference between the foam alternatives. **Electric profiling beds:** One RCT (70 people in medical or surgical hospital wards) comparing an electrically operated four section profiling bed plus pressure relieving foam mattress versus a standard hospital bed with pressure relieving mattress (foam or alternating pressure) found no significant difference in the incidence of pressure sores (no one receiving either intervention developed a sore).[8] The RCT may have been underpowered to detect a clinically important difference. **Different seat cushions:** The systematic review identified two RCTs (194 people).[6] One RCT compared slab foam versus bespoke contoured foam cushions (53 people) and the other RCT compared the Jay gel and foam wheelchair cushion versus a foam cushion (141 people).[6] The RCTs found no significant difference in the incidence of pressure sores with different types of cushions, but they may have been too small to detect a clinically important difference.[6] **Low tech constant low pressure supports:** See glossary, p 2029. The systematic review identified seven RCTs, which were too small or flawed to allow conclusions.[6] **Alternating pressure surfaces:** See glossary, p 2028. The systematic review identified nine RCTs that compared alternating pressure surfaces versus standard foam or constant low pressure supports.[6] Most RCTs were too small to rule out a clinically important difference in the prevention of pressure sores. One RCT found that an alternating pressure surface versus a standard foam mattress significantly reduced the incidence of pressure sores (RR 0.32, 95% CI 0.14 to 0.72; NNT for 10 days' treatment 11, 95% CI 6 to 34). Another RCT found that a range of alternating pressure surfaces versus a range of constant low pressure supports significantly reduced the incidence of pressure sores. The other RCTs found no significant difference between alternating pressure devices and constant low pressure supports. **Low air loss beds:** See glossary, p 2028. The systematic review identified one RCT.[6] It found that low air loss beds versus standard beds in intensive care significantly reduced the risk of new pressure sores over the duration of the trial, which was not stated (RR 0.24, 95% CI 0.11 to 0.51; NNT 3, 95% CI 2 to 5).[6] **Low air loss hydrotherapy beds:** See glossary, p 2028. The systematic review identified one RCT in incontinent people admitted to acute and long stay hospital wards.[6] It found that low air loss hydrotherapy beds versus a range of support surfaces significantly increased the risk of developing a pressure sore (RR 3.6, 95% CI 6.7 to 11.3). **Pressure relieving overlays on the operating table:** The systematic review identified three RCTs.[6] The first RCT (446 people having elective major general, gynaecological, or vascular surgery) found that a pressure relieving viscoelastic polymer pad versus a standard table significantly reduced the incidence of postoperative pressure sores (RR 0.52, 95% CI 0.32 to 0.83; NNT for intraoperative use 11, 95% CI 6 to 36). Meta-analysis of results from the two other RCTs (N Cullum, EA Nelson, and J Nixon, personal communication, 2001) found that an alternating pressure surface (used during and for 7 days after surgery) versus a gel pad (used during surgery) plus a standard mattress (used for 7 days after surgery) significantly reduced the incidence of pressure sores over 7 days (RR 0.20, 95% CI 0.06 to 0.65; NNT for 7 days' treatment 16, 95% 9 to 48). It is unclear whether the reduced incidence of pressure sores was because of intraoperative or postoperative pressure relief, or both.[6] **Air filled vinyl boot with foot cradle:** The systematic review identified one small RCT, which found hospital pillows versus a vinyl boot (air filled with a built in foot cradle) significantly reduced the rate of developing pressure sores (mean time to skin breakdown 10 days *v* 13 days; P < 0.036 log rank test).[6]

Harms: The systematic review noted that hypothermia was found in a few people using low air loss hydrotherapy beds.[6]

Comment: Most RCTs were small and of poor quality, and few performed the same comparison. Alternative foam mattresses used foam of varying densities, often within the same mattress, and were sometimes sculptured.

OPTION OTHER PREVENTIVE INTERVENTIONS

Systematic reviews found insufficient evidence about the effects of repositioning (regular "turning"), topical lotions, or dressings. One RCT has found that medical sheepskin overlays versus standard treatment significantly reduce the incidence of pressure sores in people aged 60 years or over undergoing orthopaedic surgery.

Benefits: **Repositioning (regular "turning"):** We found one systematic review (search date 1995, 3 small RCTs, 56 people [see comment below]), which found no significant difference in the incidence of pressure sores with regular manual repositioning versus control treatment.[9] We found no RCTs evaluating placing people in different positions. **Topical lotions and dressings:** We found one systematic review (search date 2000), which identified two RCTs of topical lotions.[10] One RCT (319 people) comparing hexachlorophene (hexachlorophane) lotion versus cetrimide lotion found no significant difference in the incidence of new pressure sores over 3 weeks (OR 0.97, 95% CI 0.46 to 1.65; no raw data provided). These results must be interpreted with caution as they are based on a completer analysis of 167 people. The other RCT compared hexachlorophene lotion versus an inert lotion and found no significant difference in the proportion of people with changes in skin condition over 3 weeks.[10] **Medical sheepskin overlays:** We found one systematic review (search date 2000, 1 small, poor quality RCT)[6] and one subsequent RCT[11] of sheepskin overlays versus standard treatment. The systematic review found no conclusive evidence.[6] The subsequent RCT (297 people aged ≥ 60 years undergoing orthopaedic surgery) found that medical sheepskin overlays plus standard pressure area care versus standard care alone significantly reduced the incidence of pressure sores over the duration of the trial, which was unstated (RR 0.30, 95% CI 0.17 to 0.51; NNT 5, 95% CI 4 to 9).[11]

Harms: We found no direct or indirect evidence of harm arising from repositioning, topical lotions or dressings, or medical sheepskin overlays.

Comment: The RCTs identified by the reviews were small, of poor quality, and few comparisons have been undertaken more than once.[9,10] In one of the RCTs of regular repositioning identified by the review,[9] 23 people were randomised to repositioning but only 10 people were actually repositioned regularly.

Pressure sores

QUESTION What are the effects of treatments?

OPTION PRESSURE RELIEVING SURFACES

Two RCTs in people in hospital found that air fluidised supports versus standard care healed more established sores. One RCT in people cared for at home found no significant difference with air fluidised supports versus standard care in healing; this trial had a high withdrawal rate. We found insufficient evidence on the effects of other types of pressure supporting bed or mattress, or seat cushions.

Benefits: We found one systematic review (search date 2000).[6] **Air fluidised supports:** See glossary, p 2028. The systematic review identified four RCTs comparing air fluidised supports versus standard care.[6] Two RCTs (people in hospital) found that air fluidised supports versus standard care (alternating pressure mattresses, regular changes of position, sheepskin, gel pads, or limb protectors) healed more established sores. The third RCT (97 people being cared for at home) found no significant difference; this RCT had a high withdrawal rate. The fourth RCT (people who had undergone plastic surgery to repair pressure sores) found no significant difference in pressure sore healing rates between air fluidised supports and dry flotation. **Low tech constant low pressure supports:** See glossary, p 2029. The systematic review identified one RCT (in elderly people with pressure sores in a nursing home), which found no significant difference in pressure sore healing rates between a layered foam replacement mattress and a water mattress. **Alternating pressure surfaces:** See glossary, p 2028. The systematic review[6] identified three RCTs. Two RCTs (in older people with pressure sores in hospital) found no statistically significant differences in rates of pressure sore healing with different alternating pressure mattresses. The third RCT (32 older people in hospital and nursing homes) found no significant difference in pressure sore healing between an alternating pressure mattress replacement and standard care. **Low air loss beds:** See glossary, p 2028. The systematic review (2 RCTs) found that low air loss beds versus convoluted foam had no significant effect on the number of sores healed.[6] We found no RCTs comparing low air loss beds versus alternating pressure or air fluidised supports. **Seat cushions:** The systematic review identified one RCT (25 people) comparing seat cushions using dry flotation versus alternating pressure, which found no significant difference in healing rates.[6]

Harms: The systematic review[6] noted that, in one of the RCTs identified,[12] hypothermia was found in a few people using low air loss hydrotherapy beds.

Comment: **Air fluidised support:** People are unable to move into and out of bed independently while using an air fluidised bed, and this limits the type of people for whom it is suitable. Air fluidised support has been evaluated in a range of settings, including surgical and medical wards and home care. **Low air loss beds:** These have been evaluated in a range of acute and elderly care settings.

OPTION OTHER TREATMENTS

Evidence on the effects of dressings is inconclusive. A meta-analysis of RCTs found that hydrocolloid versus gauze dressings soaked in saline or hypochlorite had no significant effect on pressure sore healing. Systematic reviews and subsequent RCTs found insufficient evidence on the effects of other types of dressings, debridement, topical phenytoin, surgery, nutritional supplements, electrotherapy, therapeutic ultrasound, low level laser therapy, or topical negative pressure on healing rates of pressure sores.

Benefits: **Hydrocolloid dressings (compared with gauze soaked in saline or hypochlorite):** We found one systematic review (search date 1997, 6 RCTs)[13] and one subsequent RCT[14] of dressings or topical agents for pressure sores. Most RCTs were small, poor quality, and inconclusive. A meta-analysis within the review and the subsequent RCT found a significant effect, but a subsequent meta-analysis (N Cullum, EA Nelson, and J Nixon, personal communication, 2001) using a more conservative statistical technique found no significant difference in healing of pressure sores (RR 1.63, 95% CI 0.97 to 2.75).[14–19] **Other dressings:** We found one systematic review (search date 1997, 12 RCTs comparing hydrocolloid *v* other dressings, 11 RCTs comparing other dressing types)[13] and four subsequent RCTs.[20–23] The RCTs had weak methods and were too small to draw reliable conclusions. **Debridement:** We found one systematic review (search date 1998)[24] and four subsequent RCTs.[25–28] The systematic review found no RCTs comparing debridement versus no debridement.[24] It identified 32 RCTs comparing different debriding agents, but these were small, included a range of wounds, and few comparisons were undertaken in more than one RCT. The review concluded that there was insufficient evidence to promote the use of any particular debriding agent over another.[24] The first subsequent RCT (23 people with 30 ulcers) comparing dextranomer paste (see glossary, p 2028) versus saline soaked gauze found no significant difference in the proportion of sores prepared for skin grafting within 15 days (5/15 [33%] with dextranomer paste *v* 4/15 [27%] with saline; ARI 7%, 95% CI −26% to 38%).[25] The second subsequent RCT (43 people) comparing collagenase versus hydrocolloid dressings found no significant difference in healing (3 people in each group healed, no denominator provided).[26] The third subsequent RCT (24 women) comparing collagenase versus hydrocolloid for full thickness heel sores found that sores treated with collagenase healed significantly more quickly, but no data demonstrating baseline equivalence for wound size were presented.[27] The fourth subsequent RCT (21 people) comparing papain plus urea with collagenase found no significant difference in healing rates over 4 weeks.[28] **Topical phenytoin:** We found one RCT (48 patients) comparing topical phenytoin suspension (100 mg capsule in 5 mL saline) versus hydrocolloid dressings or antibiotic ointment as a treatment for partial thickness pressure sores. It found that topical phenytoin versus hydrocolloid dressings or antibiotic ointment significantly increased the healing rate (mean time to healing 35.3 ± 14.3 days with phenytoin *v* 51.8 ± 19.6 days with hydrocolloid *v* 53.8 ± 8.5 days with antibiotic; $P < 0.005$ for both comparisons), but no data demonstrating baseline equivalence for wound size were presented.[29] **Surgery:** We found no RCTs of surgical treatments for pressure sores. **Nutritional supplements:** We found two RCTs of ascorbic acid supplementation for healing pressure sores.[30,31] One small RCT in people undergoing surgery who had pressure sores found that ascorbic acid supplementation (500 mg twice daily) versus placebo improved healing rates.[30] A larger RCT (88 people) found no significant difference in healing rates between those receiving ascorbic acid 500 mg twice daily and those receiving 10 mg twice daily.[31] We found no RCTs of the effects of parenteral nutrition or hyperalimentation on wound healing. **Electrotherapy:** See glossary, p 2028. We found four RCTs comparing electrotherapy versus sham treatment.[32–35] They were of varying quality. Overall, they suggested that electrotherapy improved healing of pressure sores, but confirmatory studies are needed. **Therapeutic ultrasound:** See glossary, p 2029. We found one systematic review (search date 1999, 3 RCTs).[36] All three RCTs found no evidence of improved pressure sore healing with ultrasound therapy versus no ultrasound therapy.[36] **Low level laser therapy:** See glossary, p 2028. We found one systematic review (search date 1998, 1 RCT, 18 people) of low level laser therapy in pressure sores. It found no evidence of benefit.[37] **Topical negative pressure:** See glossary, p 2029. We found one systematic review (search date 2000, 2 small RCTs, 1 of which included some people with pressure sores).[38] The review found no clear evidence of improved pressure sore healing with topical negative pressure versus no topical negative pressure.[38]

Harms: We found no reports on harms with these treatments.

Comment: Overall, the evidence relating to these treatments is poor.

GLOSSARY

Air fluidised supports Membranes covering a layer of particles, which are fluidised by having air forced through them. The air flow can be turned off, making the surface solid again, to allow the person to be moved. It is difficult for people to get in and out of these beds independently; therefore, they are usually reserved for people who spend most of the day in bed.

Alternating pressure surfaces Mattresses or overlays made of one or two layers of parallel air sacs. Alternate sacs are inflated and deflated, providing alternating pressure and then release for each area of skin.

Dextranomer paste Anhydrous, porous beads 0.1–0.3 mm in diameter. These beads are hydrophilic and absorb/adsorb exudate, wound debris, and bacteria depending on particle size.

Electrotherapy The application of electrical fields by placing electrodes near a wound. Treatments include pulsed electromagnetic therapy, low intensity direct current, negative polarity and positive polarity electrotherapy, and alternating polarity electrotherapy.

Low air loss beds A mattress comprising inflatable upright sacs made of semi-permeable fabric. Inflating the sacs increases the area of contact between the individual and the support surface and reduces the pressure on the skin. It is difficult for people to get in and out of these beds independently; therefore, they are usually reserved for people who spend most of the day in bed.

Low air loss hydrotherapy beds A mattress comprising cushions covered by a permeable, fast drying filter sheet, through which air is circulated. The bed also contains a urine collecting device.

Low level laser therapy Also known as low intensity or low power therapy. It is thought to work by inducing a photochemical response to laser light, resulting in biochemical alterations in cells and physiological changes.

Low or high tech constant low pressure supports Mattresses, overlays, and cushions made of high density or contoured foam, or filled with fibre, gel, water, beads, or air. They increase the area of contact between the person and the support surface; therefore, they reduce the interface pressure. See also air fluidised supports, low air loss beds, and low air loss hydrotherapy beds.

Therapeutic ultrasound The application of ultrasound to a wound, using a transducer and a water based gel. The power of ultrasound waves used in wound healing is low in order to avoid heating the tissues.

Topical negative pressure: Negative pressure (suction) applied to a wound through an open cell dressing (e.g. foam, felt).

Substantive changes

Prevention

Pressure relieving surfaces; foam alternatives versus standard hospital mattress One new RCT;[7] conclusions unchanged.

Pressure relieving surfaces; electric profiling beds One RCT found no significant difference in pressure sores with an electrically operated four section profiling bed plus pressure relieving foam mattress versus a standard hospital bed with pressure relieving mattress, but it may have been underpowered to detect a clinically important difference.[8]

Treatment

Other treatments; debridement Two new RCTs;[27,28] conclusions unchanged.

Other treatments; topical phenytoin One new RCT found that sores treated with topical phenytoin healed significantly more quickly than those treated with hydrocolloid dressings or antibiotic ointment.[29]

REFERENCES

1. O'Dea K. Prevalence of pressure damage in hospital patients in the UK. *J Wound Care* 1993;2:221–225.
2. Granick MS, Solomon MP, Wind S, et al. Wound management and wound care. *Adv Plastic Reconstruct Surg* 1996;12:99–121.
3. Allman RM. Pressure ulcer prevalence, incidence, risk factors, and impact. *Clin Geriatr Med* 1997;13:421–436.
4. Thomas DR, Goode PS, Tarquine PH, et al. Hospital acquired pressure ulcers and risk of death. *J Am Geriatr Soc* 1996;44:1435–1440.
5. Clough NP. The cost of pressure area management in an intensive care unit. *J Wound Care* 1994;3:33–35.
6. Cullum N, Nelson EA, Flemming K, et al. Systematic reviews of wound care management: (5) beds; (6) compression; (7) laser therapy, therapeutic ultrasound, electrotherapy and electromagnetic therapy. *Health Technol Assess* 2001;5(9):1–221. Search date 2000; primary sources 19 electronic databases, including Medline, Cinahl, Embase, and Cochrane Controlled Trials Register, and hand searches.
7. Gunningberg L, Lindholm C, Carlsson M, et al. Effect of viscoelastic foam mattresses on the development of pressure ulcers in patients with hip fractures. *J Wound Care* 2000;9:455–460.
8. Keogh A, Dealey C. Profiling beds versus standard hospital beds: effects on pressure ulcer incidence outcomes. *J Wound Care* 2001;10:15–19.
9. Cullum N, Deeks JJ, Fletcher AW, et al. Preventing and treating pressure sores. *Qual Health Care* 1995;4:289–297. Search date 1995; primary sources Medline, Cinahl, and hand searching of five journals.
10. O'Meara SM, Cullum NA, Majid M, et al. Systematic review of antimicrobial agents used for chronic wounds. *Br J Surg* 2001;88:4–21. Search date 2000; primary sources 19 electronic databases, including Medline and Cinahl, hand searches, and a panel of experts.
11. McGowan S, Montgomery K, Jolley D, et al. The role of sheepskins in preventing pressure ulcers in elderly orthopaedic patients. *Primary Intention* 2000;8:1–8.
12. Bennett RG, Baran PJ, DeVone L, et al. Low airloss hydrotherapy versus standard care for incontinent hospitalized patients. *J Am Geriatr Soc* 1998;46:569–576.
13. Bradley M, Cullum N, Nelson EA, et al. Systematic reviews of wound care management: (2). Dressings and topical agents used in the healing of chronic wounds. *Health Technol Assess* 1999;3(17 pt 2):1–35. Search date 1997; primary source Medline.
14. Matzen S, Peschardt A, Alsbjø rn B. A new amorphous hydrocolloid for the treatment of pressure sores: a randomised controlled study. *Scand J Plast Reconstr Hand Surg* 1999;33:13–15.
15. Barrois B. Comparison of Granuflex and medicated paraffin gauze in pressure sores. *Proceedings of the 2nd European Conference on Advances in Wound Management*. London: Macmillan, 1993:209.

Pressure sores

16. Alm A, Hornmark AM, Fall PA, et al. Care of pressure sores: a controlled study of the use of a hydrocolloid dressing compared with wet saline gauze compresses. *Acta Derm Venereol Suppl (Stockh)* 1989;149:1–10.
17. Colwell JC, Foreman MD, Trotter JP. A comparison of the efficacy and cost-effectiveness of two methods of managing pressure ulcers. *Decubitus* 1993;6:28–36.
18. Xakellis GC, Chrischilles EA. Hydrocolloid versus saline-gauze dressings in treating pressure ulcers: a cost-effectiveness analysis. *Arch Phys Med Rehabil* 1992;73:463–469.
19. Gorse GJ, Messner RL. Improved pressure sore healing with hydrocolloid dressings. *Arch Dermatol* 1987;123:766–771.
20. Thomas DR, Goode PS, LaMaster K, et al. Acemann hydrogel dressing versus saline dressing for pressure ulcers. A randomized, controlled trial. *Adv Wound Care* 1998;11:273–276.
21. Rees RS, Robson MC, Smiell JM, et al. Becaplermin gel in the treatment of pressure ulcers: a phase II randomized, double-blind, placebo controlled study. *Wound Repair Regen* 1999;7:141–147.
22. Seaman S, Herbster S, Muglia J, et al. Simplifying modern wound management for nonprofessional caregivers. *Ostomy Wound Manage* 2000;46:18–27.
23. Price P, Bale S, Crook Het al. The effect of a radiant heat dressing on pressure ulcers. *J Wound Care* 2000;9:201–205.
24. Bradley M, Cullum N, Sheldon T. The debridement of chronic wounds: a systematic review. *Health Technol Assess* 1999;3(17 pt 1). Search date 1998; primary sources 19 electronic databases, including Medline and Embase.
25. Ljunberg S. Comparison of dextranomer paste and saline dressings for the management of decubital ulcers. *Clin Ther* 1998;20:737–743.
26. Burgos A, Gimenez J, Moreno E, et al. Cost, efficacy, efficiency and tolerability of collagenase ointment versus hydrocolloid occlusive dressing in the treatment of pressure sores. A comparative, randomised, multicentre study. *Clin Drug Invest* 2000;19:357–365.
27. Müller E, Van Leen MWF, Bergemann R. Economic evaluation of collagenase containing ointment and hydrocolloid dressing in the treatment of pressure ulcers. *Pharmacoeconomics* 2001;19:1209–1216.
28. Alvarez OM, Fernandez OA, Rogers Rset al. Chemical debridement of pressure ulcers: a prospective randomized comparative trial of collagenase and papain/urea formulations. *Wounds*;12:15–25.
29. Rhodes RS, Heyneman CA, Culbertson VL, et al. Topical phenytoin treatment of stage II decubitus ulcers in the elderly. *Ann Pharmacother* 2001;35:675–681.
30. Taylor TV, Rimmer S, Day B, et al. Ascorbic acid supplementation in the treatment of pressure sores. *Lancet* 1974;2:544–546.
31. Ter Riet G, Kessels AG, Knipschild PG. Randomized clinical trial of ascorbic acid in the treatment of pressure ulcers. *J Clin Epidemiol* 1995;48:1453–1460.
32. Salzberg CA, Cooper Vastola SA, Perez F, et al. The effects of non-thermal pulsed electromagnetic energy on wound healing of pressure ulcers in spinal cord-injured patients: a randomized, double-blind study. *Ostomy Wound Manage* 1995;41:42–48.
33. Wood JM, Evans PE 3rd, Schallreuter KU, et al. A multicenter study on the use of pulsed low-intensity direct current for healing chronic stage II and stage III decubitus ulcers. *Arch Dermatol* 1993;129:999–1009.
34. El-Zeky F. Efficacy of high voltage pulsed current for healing of pressure ulcers in patients with spinal cord injury. *Phys Ther* 1991;71:433–442.
35. Kloth LC, Feedar JA. Acceleration of wound healing with high voltage, monophasic, pulsed current. *Phys Ther* 1988;68:503–508.
36. Flemming K, Cullum N. Therapeutic ultrasound for pressure sores (Cochrane Review). In: The Cochrane Library, Issue 1, 2001. Oxford: Update Software. Search date 1999; primary sources 19 electronic databases, including Medline, Cinahl, Embase, and Cochrane Controlled Trials Register, hand searches, and contact with companies and experts in the field.
37. Lucas C, Stanborough RW, Freeman CL, et al. Efficacy of low level laser therapy on wound healing in human subjects. A systematic review. *Lasers Med Sci* 2000;15:84–93. Search date 1998; primary sources Medline, Embase, and Cinahl.
38. Evans D, Land L. Topical negative pressure for treating chronic wounds (Cochrane Review). In: The Cochrane Library, Issue 1, 2001. Oxford: Update Software. Search date 2000; primary sources Cochrane Wounds Group Specialised Trials Register, hand searches of reference lists, and contact with relevant companies and a panel of experts.

Nicky Cullum

E Andrea Nelson
Research Fellow
Centre for Evidence Based Nursing
Department of Health Sciences
University of York
York
UK

Jane Nixon
Senior Research Fellow
Centre for Evidence Based Healthcare
University of Huddersfield
Huddersfield
UK

Competing interests: EAN and NC are co-investigators on a trial for which Beiersdorf provided trial related education. EAN, NC, and JN are co-investigators on a trial of pressure relieving surfaces for which Huntleigh Healthcare Ltd has provided trial related education. EAN has been reimbursed for attending symposia by Smith & Nephew, Huntleigh Healthcare Ltd, and ConvaTec. JN has received lecture fees and has been reimbursed for attending symposia by Central Medical Supplies, Huntleigh Healthcare Ltd, and HillRom. JN has also undertaken consultancy work for Huntleigh Healthcare Ltd.

Venous leg ulcers

Search date February 2002

E Andrea Nelson, Nicky Cullum, and June Jones

QUESTIONS

INTERVENTIONS

See glossary, p 2043

Key Messages

Treatment

- **Compression** One systematic review has found that compression versus no compression significantly increases the proportion of venous leg ulcers healed.
- **Cultured allogenic bilayer skin replacement** One RCT found that cultured allogenic bilayer skin replacement versus a non-adherent dressing significantly increased the proportion of ulcers healed after 6 months (NNT 7, 95% CI 4 to 41).
- **Flavonoids** Two RCTs have found that flavonoids versus placebo or versus standard care significantly increase the proportion of ulcers healed.

Clin Evid 2002;8:2031–2045.

Venous leg ulcers

- **Hydrocolloid (occlusive) dressings versus simple low adherent dressings in the presence of compression** One systematic review found that, in the presence of compression, hydrocolloid dressings did not heal more venous leg ulcers than simple, low adherent dressings.
- **Pentoxifylline** One systematic review has found that oral pentoxifylline versus placebo significantly increases the proportion of ulcers healed at 6 months (NNT 6, 95% CI 4 to 14).
- **Peri-ulcer injection of granulocyte–macrophage colony stimulating factor (GM-CSF)** One RCT found that peri-ulcer injection of GM-CSF versus placebo significantly increased the proportion of ulcers healed after 13 weeks' treatment (NNT 2, 95 % CI 1 to 7).
- **Sulodexide** One RCT found limited evidence that sulodexide plus compression versus compression alone significantly increased the proportion of ulcers healed after 60 days' treatment.
- **Systemic mesoglycan** One RCT found that systemic mesoglycan plus compression versus compression alone significantly increased the proportion of ulcers healed after 24 weeks' treatment.
- **Topically applied autologous platelet lysate** One RCT found no difference after 9 months in time to healing of ulcers with topically applied autologous platelet lysate versus placebo.
- **Antimicrobial agents; aspirin; debriding agents; foam, film, or alginate (semi-occlusive) dressings versus simple dressings in the presence of compression; intermittent pneumatic compression; low level laser treatment; oral zinc; skin grafting; thromboxane α_2 antagonists; topical calcitonin gene related peptide plus vasoactive intestinal polypeptide; topical mesoglycan; topical negative pressure; therapeutic ultrasound; vein surgery** We found insufficient evidence about the effects of these interventions on ulcer healing.

Preventing recurrence

- **Compression** One RCT found that compression stockings versus no stockings significantly reduced the risk of ulcer recurrence after 6 months (NNT 2, 95% CI 2 to 5).
- **Rutoside; stanozolol; vein surgery** We found insufficient evidence about the effects of these interventions on ulcer recurrence.

DEFINITION Definitions of leg ulcers vary, but the following is widely used: loss of skin on the leg or foot that takes more than 6 weeks to heal. Some definitions exclude ulcers confined to the foot, whereas others include ulcers on the whole of the lower limb. This review deals with ulcers of venous origin in people without concurrent diabetes mellitus, arterial insufficiency, or rheumatoid arthritis.

INCIDENCE/ PREVALENCE Between 1.5 and 3/1000 people have active leg ulcers. Prevalence increases with age to about 20/1000 in people aged over 80 years.[1]

AETIOLOGY/ RISK FACTORS Leg ulceration is strongly associated with venous disease. However, about a fifth of people with leg ulceration have arterial disease, either alone or in combination with venous problems, which may require specialist referral.[1] Venous ulcers (also known as varicose or stasis ulcers) are caused by venous reflux or obstruction, both of which lead to poor venous return and venous hypertension.

PROGNOSIS People with leg ulcers have a poorer quality of life than age matched controls because of pain, odour, and reduced mobility.[2] In the UK, audits have found wide variation in the types of care (hospital inpatient care, hospital clinics, outpatient clinics, home visits), in the treatments used (topical agents, dressings, bandages, stockings), in healing rates, and in recurrence rates (26–69% in 1 year).[3,4]

AIMS To promote healing; to reduce recurrence; to improve quality of life, with minimal adverse effects.

OUTCOMES Ulcer area; number of ulcers healed; number of ulcer free limbs; recurrence rates; number of new ulcer episodes; number of ulcer free weeks or months; number of people who are ulcer free; frequency of dressing/bandage changes; quality of life; adverse effects of treatment.

METHODS *Clinical Evidence* search and appraisal February 2002. We included RCTs with clinically important and objective outcomes: proportion of wounds healed, healing rates, incidence of new or recurring wounds, infection, and quality of life.

QUESTION What are the effects of treatments?

OPTION COMPRESSION

One systematic review has found that compression (elastomeric multilayer high compression bandages, Unna's boot, high compression hosiery, or short stretch bandages) heals venous leg ulcers more effectively than no compression. RCTs found insufficient evidence to compare different methods of compression. Meta-analysis of four RCTs found no significant difference in the proportion of people whose ulcers healed with 12–26 weeks of high compression versus non-high compression bandages. Small RCTs found insufficient evidence of the effects of multilayer high compression versus short stretch bandages. One systematic review found a significant increase in the proportion of ulcers healed with multilayer compression versus single layer bandages.

Benefits: **Compression versus no compression:** We found one systematic review (search date 2000, 6 RCTs, 260 people) comparing compression versus no compression.[5] It found that compression (e.g. elastomeric multilayer high compression bandages, short stretch bandages, double layer bandages, compression hosiery, or Unna's boot — see glossary, p 2044) healed venous leg ulcers more effectively than no compression (e.g. dressing alone). The RCTs were heterogeneous, using different forms of compression in different settings and populations. The results were not pooled. The results of individual RCTs consistently favoured compression. **Elastomeric versus non-elastomeric multilayer compression:** The systematic review[5] identified three RCTs (273 people), and we found one subsequent RCT (112 people)[6] comparing elastomeric multilayer high compression bandages versus non-elastomeric multilayer compression. Meta-analysis of all four RCTs (Nelson EA, Cullum N, Jones J, personal communication, 2002) found no significant difference in the proportion of people whose ulcers healed with 12–26 weeks of high compression versus non-high compression bandages (RR 1.30, 95% CI 0.94 to 1.82). **Multilayer high compression versus short stretch bandages:** The systematic review[5] identified four small RCTs (167 people), and we identified one subsequent RCT (112 people).[7] Meta-analysis of all five RCTs (Nelson EA, Cullum N, Jones J, personal communication, 2002) found no significant difference in healing rates between multilayer high compression and short stretch bandages (RR for healing 0%, 95% CI 0.81 to 1.24). The lack of power in these small studies means that a clinically important difference cannot be excluded. **Multilayer high compression versus single layer bandage:** The systematic review identified four RCTs (280 people) comparing multilayer high compression versus a single layer of bandage.[5] It found a significant increase in the proportion of ulcers healed with multilayer compression versus single layer bandages (82/139 [59%] *v* 59/141 [42%]; RR 1.41, 95% CI 1.12 to 1.77; NNT for variable periods of treatment 6, 95% CI 4 to 18) (see table 1, p 2046).

Harms: High levels of compression applied to limbs with insufficient arterial supply, or inexpert application of bandages, can lead to tissue damage and, at worst, amputation.[12] Complication rates were rarely reported in RCTs. One observational study (194 people) found that four layer compression bandaging for several months was associated with toe ulceration in 12 (6%) people.[13]

Comment: People found to be suitable for high compression are those with clinical signs of venous disease (ulcer in the gaiter region, from the upper margin of the malleolus to the bulge of the gastrocnemius; staining of the skin around an ulcer; or eczema), no concurrent diabetes mellitus or rheumatoid arthritis, and adequate arterial supply to the foot as determined by ankle/brachial pressure index. The precise ankle/brachial pressure index below which compression is contraindicated is often quoted as 0.8; however, many RCTs used the higher cut off of 0.9.[5] Effectiveness is likely to be influenced by the ability of those applying the bandage to generate safe levels of compression. Bandages may be applied by the person with the leg ulcer, their carer, nurse, or doctor. We found no comparisons of healing rates between specialist and non-specialist application of compression. Training improves bandaging technique among nurses.[14] Bandages containing elastomeric fibres can be applied weekly as they maintain their tension over time. Bandages made of wool or cotton, or both, such as short stretch bandages, may need to be reapplied more frequently as they do not maintain their tension.

OPTION INTERMITTENT PNEUMATIC COMPRESSION

One small RCT found no significant difference in the proportion of people with healed ulcers over 2–3 months with intermittent pneumatic compression versus compression bandages, but it may have been too small to exclude a clinically important difference. One RCT found improved healing at 3 months with intermittent pneumatic compression plus compression bandaging versus compression bandaging alone, but two RCTs found no significant difference in healing at 6 months.

Benefits: **Intermittent pneumatic compression versus compression bandaging:** We found one systematic review (search date 2001), which identified one small RCT (16 people).[15] It found no difference in the proportion of people with healed ulcers over 2–3 months with intermittent pneumatic compression (see glossary, p 2043) versus compression (0/10 v 0/6), but the RCT may have been too small to exclude a clinically important difference.[15] **Intermittent pneumatic compression plus compression bandaging versus compression bandaging alone:** We found one systematic review (search date 2001), which identified three small RCTs (115 people).[15] The systematic review could not perform a meta-analysis because of clinical and methodological heterogeneity between the trials. The first RCT (45 people) found that intermittent pneumatic compression plus graduated compression stockings versus graduated compression stockings alone significantly increased the proportion of people with healed ulcers at 3 months (10/21 [48%] v 1/24 [4%]; RR 11.4, 95% CI 1.6 to 82). The second RCT (53 people) comparing intermittent pneumatic compression plus elastic stockings versus Unna's boot (see glossary, p 2044) found no significant difference in the proportion of people healed at 6 months (20/28 [71%] v 15/20 [75%]; RR 0.95, 95% CI 0.67 to 1.34). The third RCT (22 people) found no significant difference in healing at 6 months with intermittent pneumatic compression plus Unna's boot versus Unna's boot alone (12/12 [100%] v 8/10 [80%]; RR 1.25, 95% CI 0.92 to 1.70).[15]

Harms: The RCTs identified by the review gave no information on adverse effects.[15]

Comment: Availability may vary widely between healthcare settings. Treatment can be delivered in the home, in outpatient clinics, or in the hospital ward. Clinical RCTs have evaluated the use of intermittent pneumatic pressure for 1 hour twice weekly and 3–4 hours daily. Treatment requires resting for 1–4 hours daily, which may reduce quality of life.

OPTION DRESSINGS AND TOPICAL AGENTS

One systematic review found insufficient evidence on the effects of semi-occlusive dressings (foam, film, or alginate) versus simple dressings, in the presence of compression. The review found that, in the presence of compression, hydrocolloid dressings did not heal more venous leg ulcers than simple, low adherent dressings. The review found insufficient evidence from small, heterogeneous RCTs about the effects of topical agents, such as growth factors, versus inert comparators. One small RCT found no significant difference in the proportion of people with healed ulcers after 12 weeks' treatment with calcitonin gene related peptide plus vasoactive intestinal polypeptide versus placebo. One RCT found that cultured allogenic bilayer skin replacement versus simple dressings significantly increased complete ulcer healing over 6 months. One RCT found no difference after 9 months in time to healing with topical autologous platelet lysate versus placebo. Another systematic review found insufficient evidence on the effects of topical negative

pressure. A third systematic review found insufficient evidence on the effects of antimicrobial agents versus placebo or standard care. A fourth systematic review found insufficient evidence on the effects of debriding agents versus traditional dressings.

Benefits: **Foam, film, or alginate (semi-occlusive) dressings compared with simple dressings, in the presence of compression:** We found one systematic review (search date 1997, 5 RCTs) comparing semi-occlusive dressings (foam, film, alginates) versus simple dressings (such as paraffin-tulle or knitted viscose dressings).[16] Two comparisons of foam dressings versus simple dressings; two of film dressings versus simple dressings; and one comparing an alginate versus a simple dressing found no evidence of benefit. However, the RCTs were too small (10–132 people, median 60) to detect anything but a very large difference in effectiveness. **Hydrocolloid (occlusive) dressings compared with simple low adherent dressings, in the presence of compression:** We found one systematic review (search date 1997), which identified nine RCTs comparing hydrocolloid dressings versus simple dressings in the presence of compression.[16] A pooled analysis of seven RCTs (714 people) found no evidence of benefit. **Comparisons between occlusive or semi-occlusive dressings:** The same systematic review identified 12 small RCTs comparing different occlusive or semi-occlusive dressings.[16] It found no significant difference in healing rates between dressings, or insufficient data were provided to calculate their significance. We found one subsequent RCT comparing hydrocolloid versus hydrocellular dressings, which found no difference in healing rates.[17] **Topical agents (e.g. growth factors) versus inert comparators:** The same systematic review identified 16 RCTs comparing topical agents (such as growth factors, cell suspensions, oxygen free-radical scavengers) versus either placebo or standard care in the treatment of venous leg ulcers.[16] It found insufficient evidence to recommend any topical agent. The studies were small (9–233 people, median 45) and heterogeneous; therefore, results could not be pooled. We found four subsequent RCTs, which are described below.[10,18–20] **Cultured allogenic bilayer skin replacement versus non-adherent dressing:** The first subsequent RCT (293 people) comparing a cultured allogenic bilayer skin replacement (see glossary, p 2043), which contained both epidermal and dermal components versus a non-adherent dressing, found a significantly greater proportion of ulcers healed completely in 6 months with the skin replacement (92/146 [63%] *v* 63/129 [49%]; RR 1.29, 95% CI 1.04 to 1.60; NNT for 6 months' treatment 7, 95% CI 4 to 41) (see table 1, p 2046).[10] **Topical calcitonin gene related peptide plus vasoactive intestinal polypeptide versus placebo:** The second subsequent RCT (66 people) of calcitonin (salcatonin) gene related peptide plus vasoactive intestinal polypeptide administered by iontophoresis (see glossary, p 2043) versus placebo iontophoresis found no significant difference in the proportion of people with healed ulcers after 12 weeks' treatment (11/33 [37%] *v* 6/33 [28%]; RR 1.83, 95% CI 0.77 to 4.38), but may have been too small to exclude a clinically important difference.[18] **Topical mesoglycan:** The third subsequent RCT (40 people) of topically applied mesoglycan, a profibrinolytic agent, found no evidence of benefit.[19] **Topically applied autologous platelet lysate:** The fourth subsequent RCT (86 people) found no difference after 9 months in time to healing with topical autologous platelet lysate versus placebo.[20] **Topical negative pressure**: We found one systematic review (search date 2000, 2 small RCTs, 34 people).[21] One of the RCTs included some people with venous leg ulcers. It found no clear evidence of benefit of topical negative pressure (see glossary, p 2044), but the RCTs may have been too small to exclude a clinically important difference in outcomes. **Antimicrobial agents versus placebo or standard care:** We found one systematic review (search date 1997, 14 RCTs) comparing antimicrobial agents versus either placebo agents or standard care.[22] The RCTs were small (25–153 people, median 56), of poor quality, and no firm conclusions could be drawn. **Debriding agents:** We found one systematic review (search date 1997) comparing debriding agents versus traditional agents.[23] The review did not perform a meta-analysis specifically in people with venous leg ulcers.[23] Six RCTs (277 people) identified by the review compared dextranomer polysaccharide bead dressings versus traditional dressings, but only two RCTs reported complete ulcer healing. Data pooling of these RCTs (137 ulcers) found no significant difference in the proportion of ulcers completely healed over 3 weeks (RR 2.15, 95% CI 0.34 to 13.3), but the size of the trials meant that a clinically important difference cannot be excluded (Nelson EA, Cullum N, Jones J, personal communication, 2002). Seven RCTs (451 people) identified by the review compared cadexomer iodine versus traditional dressings, but only three RCTs reported complete ulcer healing. Data pooling of these RCTs (181 ulcers) found that cadexomer iodine versus traditional dressings healed significantly more ulcers (31/60 *v* 15/75; RR 2.03, 95% CI 1.21 to 3.43), but the ulcers were smaller in people treated with cadexomer iodine, and results must be treated with caution as four RCTs could not be included in the data pooling. Two RCTs identified by the review compared enzymatic preparations versus traditional dressings (52 ulcers) and found no evidence of benefit.[23] Four RCTs identified by the review compared debriding agents versus each other, two compared cadexomer iodine versus dextranomer (69 people), one compared cadexomer iodine versus hydrogel (95 people), and one compared dextranomer versus hyaluronic acid (50 people). The RCTs found no significant difference in ulcer healing with different debriding agents, but may have been too small to detect a clinically important difference.[23]

Harms: It is unlikely that low adherent primary wound dressings cause harm, although dressings containing iodine may affect thyroid function if used over large surface areas for extended periods.[24] Many people (50–85%) with venous leg ulcers have contact sensitivity to preservatives, perfumes, or dyes.[25]

Comment: Simple primary dressings maintain a moist environment beneath compression bandages by preventing loss of moisture from the wound.[26]

OPTION **THERAPEUTIC ULTRASOUND**

One systematic review found insufficient evidence about the effects of therapeutic ultrasound in the treatment of venous leg ulcers.

Benefits: We found one systematic review (search date 1999, 7 RCTs, 470 people) comparing therapeutic ultrasound (see glossary, p 2044) versus no ultrasound or sham ultrasound for venous leg ulcers.[27] Ultrasound improved ulcer healing in all studies, but a significant difference was found in only four of the seven RCTs, and heterogeneity precluded pooling the seven RCTs.

Harms: Mild erythema, local pain, and small areas of bleeding have been reported in some trials.

Comment: None.

OPTION **SYSTEMIC DRUG TREATMENTS**

One systematic review has found good evidence that oral pentoxifylline versus placebo significantly increases ulcer healing over 6 months in people receiving compression. Two RCTs have found that flavonoids versus placebo or standard care significantly increase the proportion of ulcers healed. One RCT found that injections of granulocyte macrophage–colony stimulating factor versus placebo significantly increased complete healing. One RCT found limited evidence that sulodexide plus compression versus compression alone significantly increased the proportion of ulcers healed after 60 days' treatment. One RCT found that systemic mesoglycan plus compression versus compression alone significantly increased the proportion of ulcers healed after 24 weeks treatment. RCTs found insufficient evidence on the effects of oral thromboxane α_2 antagonists, aspirin, or oral zinc supplements.

Benefits: **Pentoxifylline:** We found one systematic review (search date 2001, 9 RCTs, 572 people) comparing pentoxifylline (oxpentifylline) (1200 mg or 2400 mg daily) versus placebo or versus other treatments in the presence or absence of compression.[8] It found that, in the presence of compression, pentoxifylline versus placebo significantly increased the proportion of people with healed ulcers over 8–24 weeks (5 RCTs: 155/243 [64%] *v* 96/204 [47%]; RR 1.30, 95% CI 1.10 to 1.54; NNT for 6 months' treatment 6, 95% CI 4 to 14) (see table 1, p 2046). One RCT identified by the review found no evidence of benefit for pentoxifylline compared with defibrotide in people receiving compression.[8] **Flavonoids:** We found two RCTs (245 people) comparing a flavonoid 1000 mg daily (900 mg diosmin and 100 mg hesperidin) versus placebo or standard care.[28,29] These RCTs had different lengths of follow up but were similar in other respects. When pooled in a random effects model (Nelson EA, Cullum N, Jones J, personal communication, 2001), flavonoids healed more ulcers than placebo (100/206 [48%] with flavonoids *v* 53/189 [28%] with placebo; RR 1.80, 95% CI 1.20 to 2.70). **Peri-ulcer injection of granulocyte macrophage–colony stimulating factor versus placebo:** One RCT (60 people) compared a 4 week course of injections around the ulcer of granulocyte–macrophage colony stimulating factor (400 μg) versus placebo and found a significantly increased proportion of people whose ulcers had completely healed after 13 weeks' treatment (23/39 [59%] v 4/21 [19%]; RR 3.21, 95% CI 1.23 to 8.34; NNT for 13 weeks' treatment 2, 95% CI 1 to 7) (see table 1, p 2046).[9] **Sulodexide:** We found one RCT (94 people). It found that significantly more ulcers healed after 60 days' treatment with sulodexide (daily im injection for 30 days and then orally for 30 days) in addition to compression treatment than with compression alone (35% v 58%; RR 1.61, 95% CI 1.03 to 2.63; NNT 4, 95% CI 2 to 64) (see table 1, p 2046).[11] **Systemic mesoglycan:** We found one RCT (183 people) comparing systemic mesoglycan (daily im injection for 21 days and then orally for 21 wks) plus compression versus placebo plus compression.[30] It found that systemic mesoglycan versus placebo significantly increased the proportion of people with healed ulcers after 24 weeks' treatment (82/92 [89%] v 69/91 [76%]; RR 1.17, 95% CI 1.03 to 1.35). **Thromboxane α_2 antagonists:** We found one RCT (165 people) of an oral thromboxane α_2 antagonist versus placebo. It found no significant difference in the proportion of ulcers healed (54% v 55%).[31] **Oral zinc:** We found one systematic review (search date 1997, 5 RCTs, 151 people) comparing daily doses of 440–660 mg oral zinc sulphate versus placebo. The review found no evidence of benefit for oral zinc.[32] **Aspirin:** We found one small RCT of aspirin (300 mg daily, enteric coated) versus placebo. It found that more ulcers healed with aspirin versus placebo (38% v 0%), but the RCT had several methodological weaknesses so the result should be treated with caution.[33]

Harms: The systematic review of pentoxifylline found more adverse effects with pentoxifylline than with placebo, although the difference was not significant (RR 1.25, 95% CI 0.87 to 1.80).[8] Nearly half of the adverse effects were gastrointestinal (dyspepsia, vomiting, or diarrhoea). Adverse effects of flavonoids, such as gastrointestinal disturbance, were reported in 10% of people.

Comment: Sulodexide is not widely available, and daily injections may be unacceptable to some people.

OPTION VEIN SURGERY

One RCT found insufficient evidence of the effects of vein surgery on ulcer healing.

Benefits: We found no systematic review. We found one RCT (47 people) comparing vein surgery (perforator ligation) versus no surgery or surgery plus skin grafting.[34] It found no difference in the proportion of ulcers healed after 1 year, or in the rate of ulcer healing. The RCT may have been too small to rule out a beneficial effect.

Harms: Vein surgery carries the usual risks of surgery and anaesthesia.

Comment: Several operative approaches are commonly used, including perforator ligation, saphenous vein stripping, and a combination of both procedures.

OPTION SKIN GRAFTING

One systematic review found insufficient evidence of the effects of skin grafting on ulcer healing.

Benefits: We found one systematic review (search date 1999, 6 RCTs, 197 people) of skin grafts (autografts or allografts) for venous leg ulcers.[35] In five RCTs people also received compression bandaging; two RCTs (98 people) evaluated split thickness autografts; three RCTs (92 people) evaluated cultured keratinocyte allografts; and one RCT (7 people, 13 ulcers) compared tissue engineered skin (artificial skin) with split thickness skin grafts. We found insufficient evidence to determine whether skin grafting increased the healing of venous ulcers.[35]

Harms: Taking a skin graft leaves a wound that itself requires management and may cause pain. We found no evidence of harm from tissue engineered skin.

Comment: None.

OPTION LOW LEVEL LASER TREATMENT

Systematic reviews found insufficient evidence of the effects of low level laser treatment on ulcer healing.

Benefits: We found two systematic reviews.[36,37] The first review (search date 1998) identified four RCTs (139 people).[36] Two RCTs compared low level laser treatment (see glossary, p 2044) versus sham treatment and found no significant difference in healing rates over 12 weeks (17/44 [39%] *v* 14/44 [32%]; RR 1.21, 95% CI 0.73 to 2.03). One three-arm RCT (30 people) identified by the review compared laser treatment versus laser treatment plus infrared light or versus non-coherent, unpolarised red light. It found that significantly more ulcers healed completely after 9 months' treatment in the group receiving a combination of laser and infrared light compared with non-coherent, unpolarised red light (12/15 [80%] *v* 5/15 [33%]; RR 2.4, 95% CI 1.12 to 5.13). The fourth RCT identified by the review compared laser and ultraviolet light and found no significant difference in healing over 4 weeks.[36] The second review (search date 1999, 5 RCTs)[37] identified but did not fully describe the four RCTs identified by the first review. The review did not perform a meta-analysis. The additional RCT identified by the review (9 people, 12 venous leg ulcers) compared low level laser treatment versus sham treatment and found limited evidence that ulcer area reduction was greater with laser over 10 weeks (25% of ulcers remained unhealed in people receiving laser *v* 85% in people receiving sham treatment).[37] The RCT did not assess complete ulcer healing.

Harms: Eye protection is required when using some types of laser as the high energy beam may lead to damage of the retina.

Comment: The laser power, wavelength, frequency, duration, and follow up of treatment were different for all of the studies.

QUESTION **What are the effects of interventions to prevent recurrence?**

OPTION **COMPRESSION**

We found limited evidence that compression reduced recurrence but non-compliance with compression is a risk factor for recurrence.

Benefits: **Versus no compression:** We found one systematic review of compression hosiery versus no compression (search date 2000, no identified RCTs),[38] and one subsequent RCT.[39] The RCT (153 people) found that compression stockings worn versus compression stockings not worn significantly reduced recurrence at 6 months (21% *v* 46%; RR 0.46, 95% CI 0.28 to 0.76; NNT for 6 months' treatment 2, 95% CI 2 to 5).[39] **Versus other forms of compression:** We found one systematic review (search date 2000, 2 RCTs).[38] One RCT (166 people) compared two brands of UK Class 2 stockings (see comment below) and found no difference in recurrence. The larger RCT (300 people) compared Class 2 and Class 3 stockings (see comment below). With intention to treat analysis, the RCT found no significant reduction in recurrence after 5 years with high compression hosiery (UK Class 3) compared with moderate compression hosiery (UK Class 2). This analysis may underestimate the effectiveness of the Class 3 hosiery because a significant proportion of people changed from Class 3 to Class 2. Both RCTs found that non-compliance with compression hosiery was associated with recurrence.

Harms: The application of high compression to limbs with reduced arterial supply may result in ischaemic tissue damage and, at worst, amputation.[8]

Comment: Compression hosiery is classified according to the magnitude of pressure exerted at the ankle; the UK classification states that Class 2 hosiery is capable of applying 18–24 mm Hg pressure and Class 3 is capable of applying 25–35 mm Hg pressure at the ankle. Other countries use different classification systems. Hosiery reduces venous reflux by locally increasing venous pressure in the legs relative to the rest of the body. This effect only takes place while hosiery is worn. The association between non-compliance with compression and recurrence of venous ulceration provides some indirect evidence of the benefit of compression in prevention. People are advised to wear compression hosiery for life and may be at risk of pressure necrosis from their compression hosiery if they subsequently develop arterial disease. Regular reassessment of the arterial supply is considered good practice, but we found no evidence about the optimal frequency of assessment. Other measures designed to reduce leg oedema, such as resting with the leg elevated, may be useful.

OPTION SYSTEMIC DRUG TREATMENT

One systematic review found insufficient evidence on the effects of rutoside or stanozolol on ulcer recurrence.

Benefits: We found one systematic review (search date 1997, 2 RCTs, 198 people) comparing stanozolol or rutoside versus placebo in the prevention of leg ulcer recurrence.[40] **Rutoside:** The first RCT (139 people) identified by the review comparing rutoside versus placebo found no significant difference in recurrence at 18 months (32% *v* 34%; P = 0.93; no raw data available to calculate CI). **Stanozolol:** The second RCT (60 people) identified by the review comparing stanozolol versus placebo for 6 months found no significant difference in recurrence at the end of the study (length of follow up not specified; recurrence in 7/25 [28%] legs with stanozolol *v* 4/23 [17%]; RR 1.61, 95% CI 0.54 to 4.79).[40]

Harms: Stanozolol is an anabolic steroid; adverse effects included acne, hirsutism, amenorrhoea, oedema, headache, dyspepsia, rash, hair loss, depression, jaundice, and changes in liver enzymes. Tolerance of rutoside was reported to be good; adverse effects included headache, flushing, rashes, and mild gastrointestinal disturbances.[41]

Comment: None.

OPTION VEIN SURGERY

One RCT identified by a systematic review found insufficient evidence on the effects of vein surgery on ulcer recurrence.

Benefits: We found one systematic review (search date 1997, 1 RCT, 30 people).[40] The identified RCT, which was poorly controlled, compared surgery plus compression hosiery versus compression hosiery alone for prevention of recurrence. It found a reduced rate of recurrence when surgery was carried out in addition to the use of compression hosiery (5% *v* 24%; RR 0.21, 95% CI 0.03 to 0.80).

Harms: Vein surgery has the usual risks of surgery and anaesthesia.

Comment: The results of the RCT should be interpreted with caution because it was small and poorly controlled.[40] The RCT randomised legs rather than people.

GLOSSARY

Cultured allogenic bilayer skin replacement Also called human skin equivalent. This is made of a lower (dermal) layer of bovine collagen containing living human dermal fibroblasts and an upper (epidermal) layer of living human keratinocytes.

Elastomeric multilayer high compression bandages Usually a layer of padding material followed by one to three additional layers of elastomeric bandages.

Intermittent pneumatic compression External compression applied by inflatable leggings or boots either over, or instead of, compression hosiery or bandages. A pump successively inflates and deflates the boots to promote the return of blood from the tissues. Newer systems have separate compartments in the boots so that the foot is inflated before the ankle, which is inflated before the calf.

Iontophoresis The delivery of an ionic substance by application of an electrical current.

Low level laser treatment Application of treatment energy (< 10 J/cm^2) using lasers of 50 mW or less.

Short stretch bandages Minimally extensible bandages usually made of cotton with few or no elastomeric fibres. They are applied at near full extension to form a semi-rigid bandage.

Therapeutic ultrasound Application of ultrasound to a wound, using a transducer and a water based gel. Prolonged application can lead to heating of the tissues, but when used in wound healing the power used is low and the transducer is constantly moved by the therapist so that the tissue is not significantly heated.

Topical negative pressure Negative pressure (suction) applied to a wound through an open cell dressing (e.g. foam, felt).

Unna's boot An inner layer of zinc oxide impregnated bandage, which hardens as it dries to form a semi-rigid layer against which the calf muscle can contract. It is usually covered in an elastomeric bandage.

Substantive changes

Compression: elastomeric versus non-elastomeric multilayer compression One new RCT;[6] conclusions unchanged.

Compression: multilayer high compression versus short stretch bandages One new RCT;[7] conclusions unchanged.

Intermittent pneumatic compression One new systematic review;[15] conclusions unchanged.

Dressings and topical agents: debriding agents One systematic review found insufficient evidence on the effects of debriding agents versus traditional dressings.[23]

Low level laser treatment One new systematic review;[37] conclusions unchanged.

Drug treatments: systemic mesoglycan One new RCT found that systemic mesoglycan plus compression versus compression alone significantly increased the proportion of ulcers healed after 24 weeks' treatment.[30]

REFERENCES

1. Callam MJ, Ruckley CV, Harper DR, et al. Chronic ulceration of the leg: extent of the problem and provision of care. *BMJ* 1985;290:1855–1856.
2. Roe B, Cullum N, Hamer C. Patients' perceptions of chronic leg ulceration. In: Cullum N, Roe B, eds. *Leg ulcers: nursing management*. Harrow: Scutari, 1995:125–134.
3. Roe B, Cullum N. The management of leg ulcers: current nursing practice. In: Cullum N, Roe B, eds. *Leg ulcers: nursing management*. Harrow: Scutari, 1995:113–124.
4. Vowden KR, Barker A, Vowden P. Leg ulcer management in a nurse-led, hospital-based clinic. *J Wound Care* 1997;6:233–236.
5. Cullum N, Nelson EA, Fletcher AW, et al. Compression bandages and stockings in the treatment of venous leg ulcers. In: The Cochrane Library, Issue 1, 2002. Oxford: Update Software. Search date 2000; primary sources 19 electronic databases, hand searches, and personal contacts.
6. Meyer F, Burnand KG, McGuiness C, et al. Randomized clinical RCT comparing the efficacy of two bandaging regimens in the treatment of venous leg ulcer. *Br J Surg* 2002;89:40–44.
7. Partsch H, Damstra RJ, Tazelaar DJ, et al. Multicentre, randomised controlled RCT of four-layer bandaging versus short-stretch bandaging in the treatment of venous leg ulcers. *VASA* 2001;30:108–113.
8. Jull AB, Waters J, Arroll B. Oral pentoxifylline for treatment of venous leg ulcers. In: The Cochrane Library, Issue 1, 2002. Oxford: Update Software. Search date 2001; primary sources Cochrane Peripheral Vascular Diseases and Wounds Group, specialised registers, hand searches of reference lists, relevant journals and conference proceedings, personal contact with manufacturer of pentoxifylline, and experts in the field.
9. Da Costa RM, Ribeiro Jesus FM, Aniceto C, et al. Randomized, double-blind, placebo-controlled, dose-ranging study of granulocyte–macrophage colony stimulating factor in patients with chronic venous leg ulcers. *Wound Repair Regen* 1999;7:17–25.
10. Falanga V, Margolis D, Alvarez O, et al. Rapid healing of venous ulcers and lack of clinical rejection with an allogeneic cultured human skin equivalent. Human Skin Equivalent Investigators Group. *Arch Dermatol* 1998;134:293–300.
11. Scondotto G, Aloisi D, Ferrari P, et al. Treatment of venous leg ulcers with sulodexide. *Angiology* 99;50:883–889.
12. Callam MJ, Ruckley CV, Dale JJ, et al. Hazards of compression treatment of the leg: an estimate from Scottish surgeons. *BMJ* 1987;295:1382.
13. Chan CLH, Meyer FJ, Hay RJ, et al. Toe ulceration associated with compression bandaging: observational study. *BMJ* 2001;323;1099.
14. Nelson EA, Ruckley CV, Barbenel J. Improvements in bandaging technique following training. *J Wound Care* 1995;4:181–184.
15. Mani R, Vowden K, Nelson EA. Intermittent pneumatic compression for treating venous leg ulcers. In: The Cochrane Library, Issue 1, 2002. Oxford: Update Software. Search date 2001; primary sources The Cochrane Wound Group Trials

Register and hand searches of journals, relevant conference proceedings and citations within obtained reviews and papers and personal contact with relevant companies
16. Bradley M, Cullum N, Nelson EA, et al. Dressings and topical agents for healing of chronic wounds: a systematic review. *Health Technol Assess* 1999;3 No17(Pt2). Search date 1997; primary sources Cochrane Library, Medline, Embase, and Cinahl.
17. Seeley J, Jensen JL, Hutcherson J. A randomised clinical study comparing a hydrocellular dressing to a hydrocolloid dressing in the management of pressure ulcers. *Ostomy Wound Manage* 1999;45:39–47.
18. Gherardini G, Gurlek A, Evans GRD, et al. Venous ulcers: improved healing by iontophoretic administration of calcitonin gene-related peptide and vasoactive intestinal polypeptide. *Plast Reconstr Surg* 1998;101:90–93.
19. La Marc G, Pumilia G, Martino A. Effectiveness of mesoglycan topical treatment of leg ulcers in subjects with chronic venous insufficiency. *Minerva Cardioangiol* 1999;47:315–319.
20. Stacey MC, Mata SD, Trengove NJ, et al. Randomised double-blind placebo controlled RCT of autologous platelet lysate in venous ulcer healing. *Eur J Vasc Endovasc Surg* 2000;20:296–301.
21. Evans D, Land L. Topical negative pressure for treating chronic wounds. In: The Cochrane Library, Issue 1, 2002. Oxford: Update Software. Search date 2000; primary sources Cochrane Wounds Group specialised register, experts, relevant companies, and a hand search.
22. O'Meara S, Cullum N, Majid M, et al. Systematic reviews of wound care management: (3) antimicrobial agents for chronic wounds. *Health Technol Assess* 2000;4(No 21):1–237. Search date 1997; primary sources Cochrane Library, Medline, Embase, and Cinahl.
23. Bradley M, Cullum N, Sheldon T. The debridement of chronic wounds: a systematic review. *Health Technol Assess*, 1999; 3 (17 Pt 1). Search date 1997; primary sources 19 electronic databases (including the Cochrane Wounds Group Specialised Register) and hand searches of specialist wound care journals, conference proceedings and bibliographies of retrieved relevant publications and personal contact with appropriate companies and an advisory panel of experts.
24. Thomas S. *Wound management and dressings.* London: Pharmaceutical Press, 1990.
25. Cameron J, Wilson C, Powell S, et al. Contact dermatitis in leg ulcer patients. *Ostomy Wound Manage* 1992;38:10–11.
26. Wu P, Nelson EA, Reid WH, et al. Water vapour transmission rates in burns and chronic leg ulcers: influence of wound dressings and comparison with in vitro evaluation. *Biomaterials* 1996;17:1373–1377.
27. Flemming K, Cullum N. Therapeutic ultrasound for venous leg ulcers. In: The Cochrane Library, Issue 1, 2002. Oxford: Update Software. Search date 1999; primary sources Cochrane Wounds Group specialised register, and hand searches of citation lists.
28. Guilhou JJ, Dereure O, Marzin L, et al. Efficacy of Daflon 500 mg in venous leg ulcer healing: a double-blind, randomized, controlled versus placebo RCT in 107 patients. *Angiology* 1997;48:77–85.
29. Glinski W, Chodynicka B, Roszkiewicz J, et al. The beneficial augmentative effect of micronised purified flavonoid fraction (MPFF) on the healing of leg ulcers: an open, multicentre, controlled randomised study. *Phlebology* 1999;14:151–157.
30. Arosio E, Ferrari G, Santoro F, et al. A placebo-controlled, double blind study of mesoglycan in the treatment of chronic venous ulcers. *Eur J Vasc Endovas Surg* 2001;22:365–372.
31. Lyon RT, Veith FJ, Bolton L, et al. Clinical benchmark for healing of chronic venous ulcers. Venous Ulcer Study Collaborators. *Am J Surgery* 1998;176:172–175.
32. Wilkinson EAJ, Hawke CI. Does oral zinc aid the healing of chronic leg ulcers? A systematic literature review. *Arch Dermatol* 1998;134:1556–1560. Search date 1997; primary sources Medline, Embase, Cinahl, Science Citation Index, Biosis, British Diabetic Association Database, Ciscom, Cochrane Controlled Register of Clinical RCTs, Dissertation Abstracts, Royal College of Nursing Database, electronic databases of ongoing research, hand searches of wound care journals and conference proceedings, and contact with manufacturer of zinc sulphate tablets.
33. Layton AM, Ibbotson SH, Davies JA, et al. Randomised RCT of oral aspirin for chronic venous leg ulcers. *Lancet* 1994;344:164–165.
34. Warburg FE, Danielsen L, Madsen SM, et al. Vein surgery with or without skin grafting versus conservative treatment for leg ulcers. *Acta Dermatol Vereol* 1994;74:307–309.
35. Jones JE, Nelson EA. Skin grafting for venous leg ulcers. In: The Cochrane Library, Issue 1, 2002. Oxford: Update Software. Search date 1999; primary sources Cochrane Wounds Group specialised register, hand searches of reference lists, relevant journals, conference proceedings, and personal contact with experts in the field.
36. Flemming K, Cullum N. Laser therapy for venous leg ulcers. In: The Cochrane Library, Issue 1, 2002. Oxford: Update Software. Search date 1998; primary sources 19 electronic databases, hand searches of journals, conference proceedings, and bibliographies.
37. Schneider WL, Hailey D. Low level laser therapy for wound healing. Alberta Heritage Foundation Report 1999. Search date 1999; primary sources Medline, HealthStar, Embase, Dissertation Abstracts, Current Contents, Cinahl, Cochrane Library, the internet.
38. Cullum N, Nelson EA, Flemming K, et al. Systematic reviews of wound care management: (5) beds; (6) compression; (7) laser therapy, therapeutic ultrasound, electrotherapy and electromagnetic therapy. *Health Technol Assess* 2001;5(9). Search date 2000; primary sources Cochrane Wounds Group specialised register, 19 electronic databases (up to December 1999), and hand searches of relevant journals, conferences and bibliographies of retrieved publications, and personal contact with manufacturers and an advisory panel of experts.
39. Vandongen YK, Stacey MC. Graduated compression elastic stockings reduce lipodermatosclerosis and ulcer recurrence. *Phlebology* 2000;15:33–37.
40. Cullum N, Fletcher A, Semlyen A, et al. Compression therapy for venous leg ulcers. *Qual Health Care* 1997;6:226–231. Search date 1997; primary sources 18 databases, including Medline, Embase, Cinahl with no restriction on date, hand searches of relevant journals, conference proceedings, and correspondence with experts to obtain unpublished papers.
41. Taylor HM, Rose KE, Twycross RG. A double-blind clinical RCT of hydroxyethylrutosides in obstructive arm lymphoedema. *Phlebology* 1993;8(suppl 1):22–28

Venous leg ulcers

E Andrea Nelson
Research Fellow

Nicky Cullum
Centre for Evidence Based Nursing
Department of Health Sciences
University of York
York
UK

June Jones
Clinical Nurse Specialist
North Sefton and West Lancashire
Community Services NHS Trust
Southport
UK

Competing interests: EAN has been reimbursed for attending symposia by Smith and Nephew, Johnson & Johnson, and Huntleigh Healthcare Ltd, and Convatec. EAN and NC are applicants on a RCT of compression bandages for which Beiersdorf UK Ltd is providing RCT related education. JJ has been reimbursed for attending symposia by 3M and Convatec.

TABLE 1 **NNTs for healing of leg ulcers (see text, p 2033).**

Intervention	NNT (95% CI)
Elastomeric multilayer compression *v* non-elastomeric multilayer compression bandages	5 (3 to 12)[5]
Multilayer high compression *v* single layer compression bandages	6 (4 to 18)[5]
Pentoxifylline 400 mg three times a day *v* placebo (concurrent use of compression)	6 (4 to 14)[8]
Peri-ulcer injection of GM–CSF* (400 μg) *v* placebo	2 (1 to 17)[9]
Cultured allogenic bilayer skin equivalent *v* non-adherent dressing	7 (4 to 41)[10]
Sulodexide plus compression *v* compression alone	4 (2 to 64)[11]

*GM–CSF, granulocyte–macrophage colony stimulating factor.

Note

When looking up a class of drug, the reader is advised to also look up specific examples of that class of drug where additional entries may be found. The reverse situationalso applies. Abbreviations used: CVD, cardiovasculardisease; HRT, hormone replacement the rapy; IVF, in vitro fertilisation; MI, myocardial infarction; NSAIDs, non-steroidal anti-inflammatory drugs; STD, sexually transmitted disease.

INDEX

Subject index

Estimating cardiovascular risk and treatment benefit

Adapted from the New Zealand guidelines on management of dyslipidaemia[1] and raised blood pressure[2] by Rod Jackson

How to use these colour charts

The charts help the estimation of a person's absolute risk of a cardiovascular event and the likely benefit of drug treatment to lower cholesterol or blood pressure. For these charts cardiovascular events include: new angina, myocardial infarction, coronary death, stroke or transient ischaemic attack (TIA), onset of congestive cardiac failure or peripheral vascular syndrome.

There is a group of patients in whom risk can be assumed to be high (>20% in 5 years) without using the charts. They include those with symptomatic cardiovascular disease (angina, myocardial infarction, congestive heart failure, stroke, TIA, and peripheral vascular disease), or left ventricular hypertrophy on ECG.

To estimate a person's absolute five-year risk:

- Find the table relating to their sex, diabetic status (on insulin, oral hypoglycaemics or fasting blood glucose over 8 mmol/L), smoking status and age. The age shown in the charts is the mean for that category, i.e. age 60 = 55 to 65 years.
- Within the table find the cell nearest to the person's blood pressure and total cholesterol : HDL ratio. For risk assessment it is enough to use a mean blood pressure based on two readings on each of two occasions, and cholesterol measurements based on one laboratory or two non-fasting Reflotron measurements. More readings are needed to establish the pre-treatment baseline.
- The colour of the box indicates the person's five-year cardiovascular disease risk (see below).

Notes: (1) People with a strong history of CVD (first degree male relatives with CVD before 55 years, female relatives before 65 years) or obesity (body mass index above 30 kg/m^2) are likely to be at greater risk than the tables indicate. The magnitude of the independent predictive value of these risk factors remains unclear—their presence should influence treatment decisions for patients at borderline treatment levels. (2) If total cholesterol or total cholesterol:HDL ratio is greater than 8 then the risk is at least 15%. (3) Nearly all people aged 75 years or over also have an absolute cardiovascular risk over 15%.

REFERENCES

1. Dyslipidaemia Advisory Group. 1996 National Heart Foundation clinical guidelines for the assessment and management of dyslipidaemia. *NZ Med J* 1996;109:224–232.
2. National Health Committee. Guidelines for the management of mildly raised blood pressure in New Zealand: Ministry of Health National Health Committee Report, Wellington, 1995.

RISK LEVEL Five-year CVD risk (non-fatal and fatal)		**BENEFIT (1)** CVD events prevented per 100 treated for five years*	**BENEFIT (2)** Number needed to treat for five years to prevent one event*
Very High	>30%	>10 per 100	<10
	25–30%	9 per 100	11
	20–25%	7.5 per 100	13
High	15–20%	6 per 100	16
Moderate	10–15%	4 per 100	25
Mild	5–10%	2.5 per 100	40
	2.5–5%	1.25 per 100	80
	<2.5%	<0.8 per 100	>120

*Based on a 20% reduction in total cholesterol or a reduction in blood pressure of 10–15 mmHg systolic or 5–10 mm Hg diastolic, which is estimated to reduce CVD risk by about one third over 5 years.

RISK LEVEL: MEN

NO DIABETES

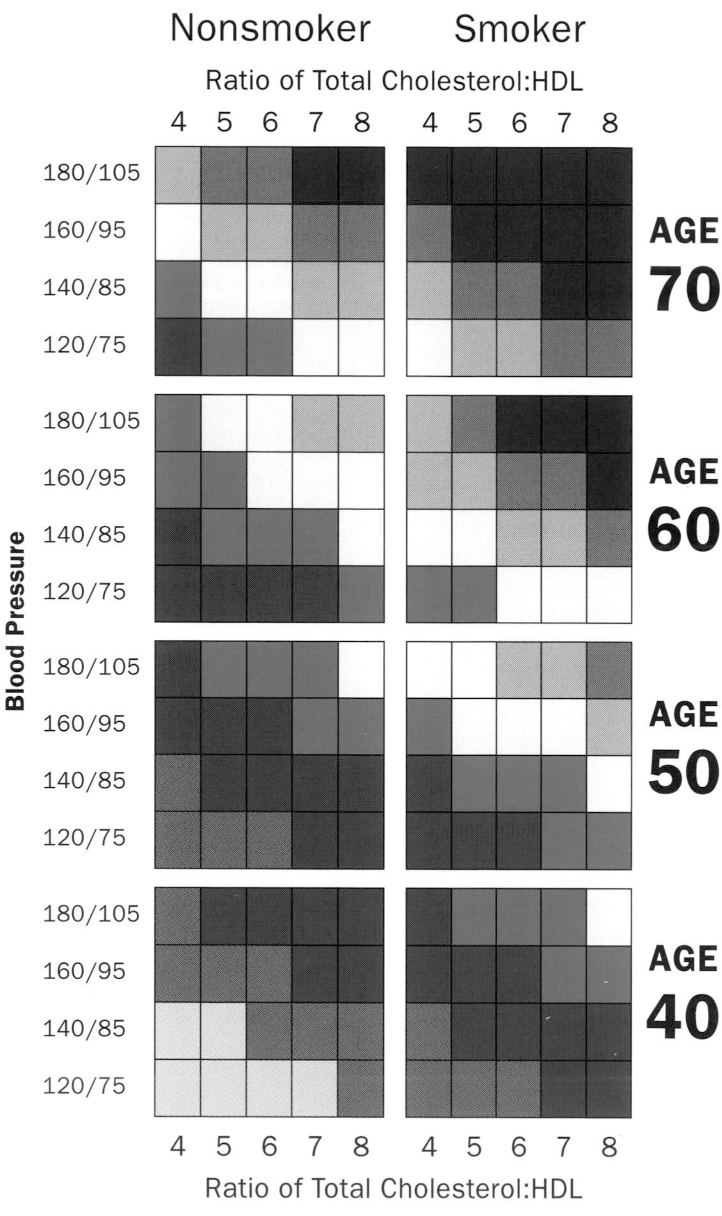

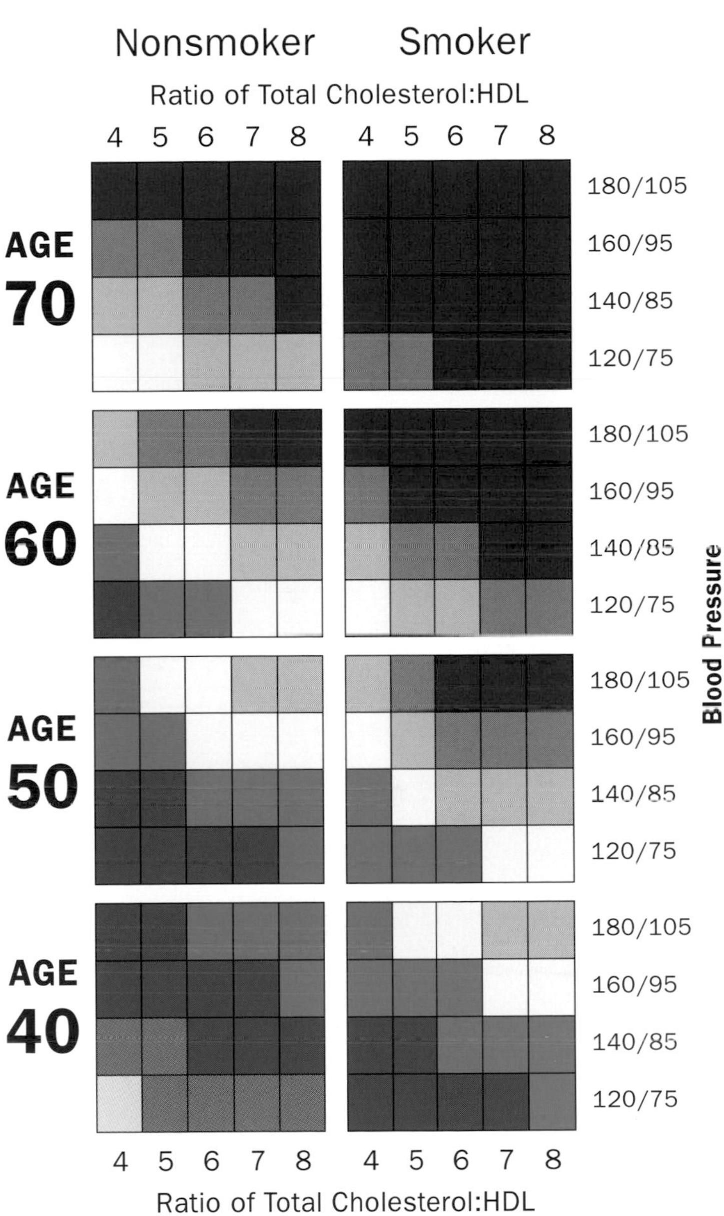
DIABETES
Nonsmoker
Smoker
Ratio of Total Cholesterol:HDL
4 5 6 7 8 4 5 6 7 8
AGE 70
AGE 60
AGE 50
AGE 40
180/105
160/95
140/85
120/75
Blood Pressure
4 5 6 7 8 4 5 6 7 8
Ratio of Total Cholesterol:HDL

Appendix 1

Estimating cardiovascular risk and treatment benefit

RISK LEVEL: WOMEN

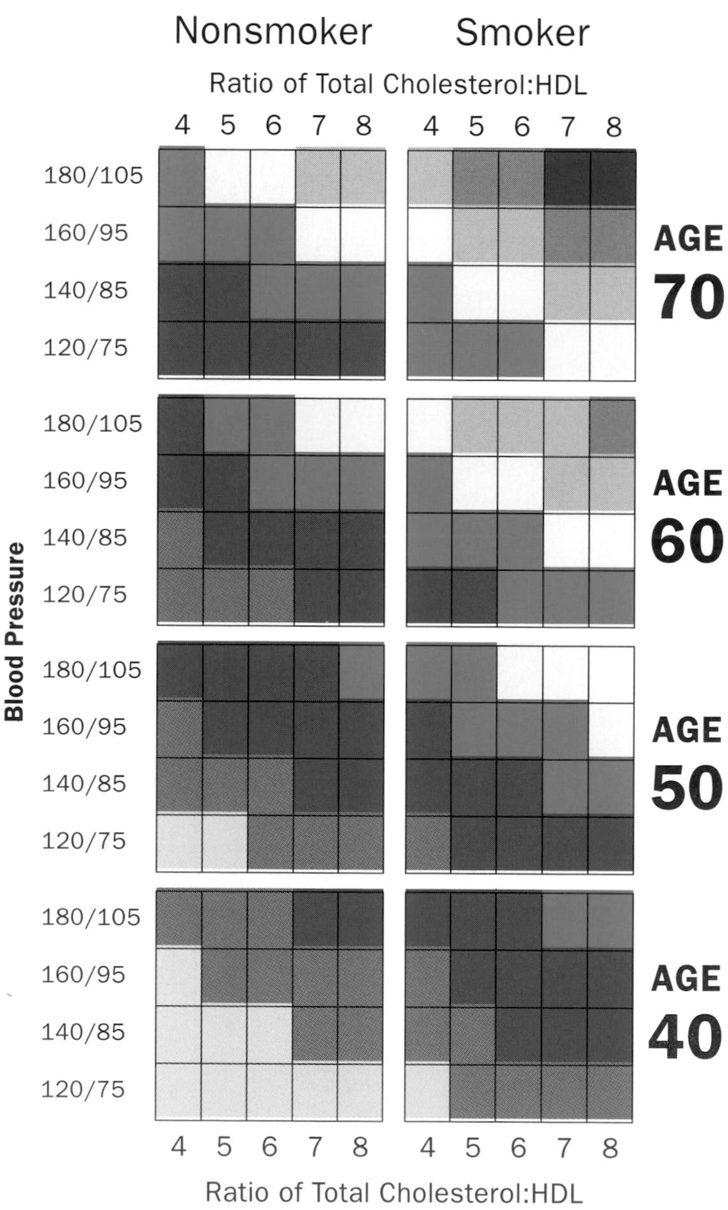

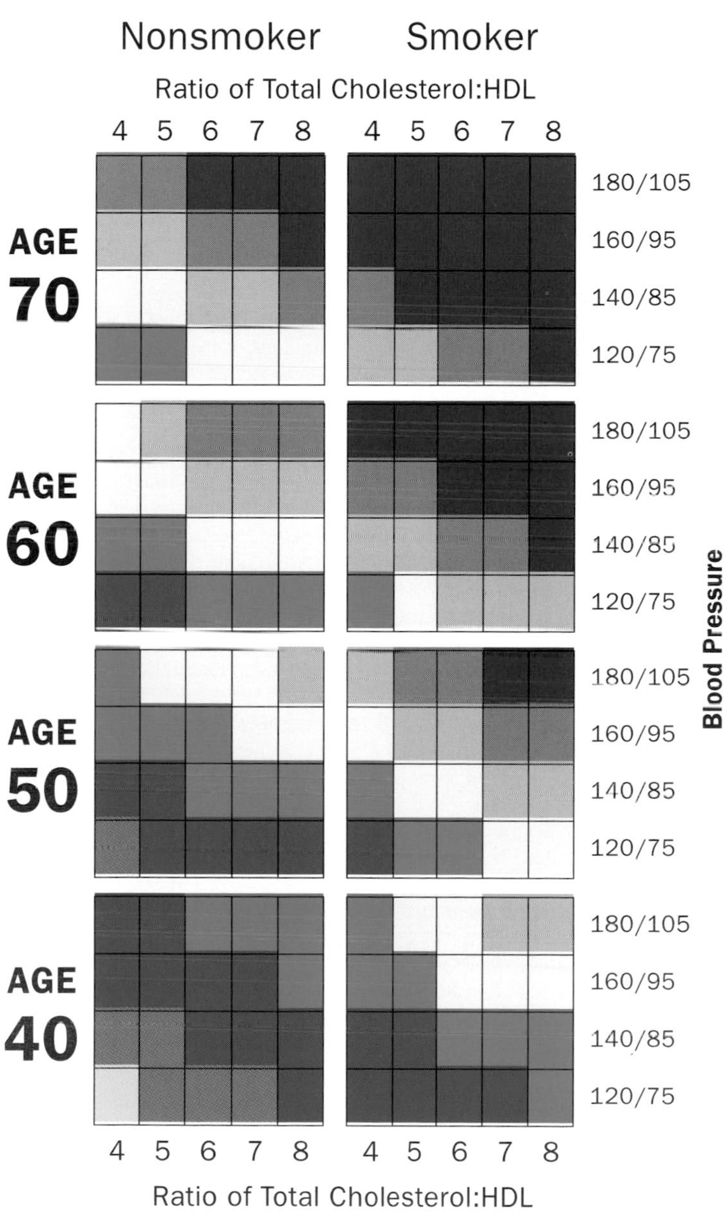

DIABETES
Nonsmoker
Smoker
Ratio of Total Cholesterol:HDL
4 5 6 7 8
4 5 6 7 8
AGE 70
AGE 60
AGE 50
AGE 40
180/105
160/95
140/85
120/75
Blood Pressure
Ratio of Total Cholesterol:HDL

The number needed to treat: adjusting for baseline risk

Adapted with permission from Chatellier et al, 1996[1]

BACKGROUND

The number needed to treat (NNT) to avoid a single additional adverse outcome is a meaningful way of expressing the benefit of an active treatment over a control. It can be used both to summarise the results of a therapeutic trial or series of trials and to help medical decision making about an individual patient.

If the absolute risk of adverse outcomes in a therapeutic trial is ARC in the control group and ART in the treatment group, then the absolute risk reduction (ARR) is defined as (ARC – ART). The NNT is defined as the inverse of the ARR:

$$\text{NNT} = 1/(\text{ARC} - \text{ART})$$

Since the Relative Risk Reduction (RRR) is defined as (ARC – ART)/ARC, it follows that NNT, RRR and ARC are related by their definitions in the following way:

$$\text{NNT} \times \text{RRR} \times \text{ARC} = 1$$

This relationship can be used to estimate the likely benefits of a treatment in populations with different levels of baseline risk (that is different levels of ARC). This allows extrapolation of the results of a trial or meta-analysis to people with different baseline risks. Ideally, there should be experimental evidence of the RRR in each population. However, in many trials, subgroup analyses show that the RRR is approximately constant in groups of patients with different characteristics. Cook and Sackett therefore proposed that decisions about individual patients could be made by using the NNT calculated from the RRR measured in trials and the baseline risk in the absence of treatment estimated for the individual patient.[2]

The method may not apply to periods of time different to that studied in the original trials.

USING THE NOMOGRAM

The nomogram shown on the next page allows the NNT to be found directly without any calculation: a straight line should be drawn from the point corresponding to the estimated absolute risk for the patient on the left hand scale to the point corresponding to the relative risk reduction stated in a trial or meta-analysis on the central scale. The intercept of this line with the right hand scale gives the NNT. By taking the upper and lower limits of the confidence interval of the RRR, the upper and lower limits of the NNT can be estimated.

REFERENCES

1. Chatellier G, Zapletal E, Lemaitre D, *et al*. The number needed to treat: a clinically useful nomogram in its proper context. *BMJ* 1996;321:426–429.
2. Cook RJ, Sackett DL. The number needed to treat: a clinically useful measure of treatment effect. *BMJ* 1995;310:452–454.

The number needed to treat

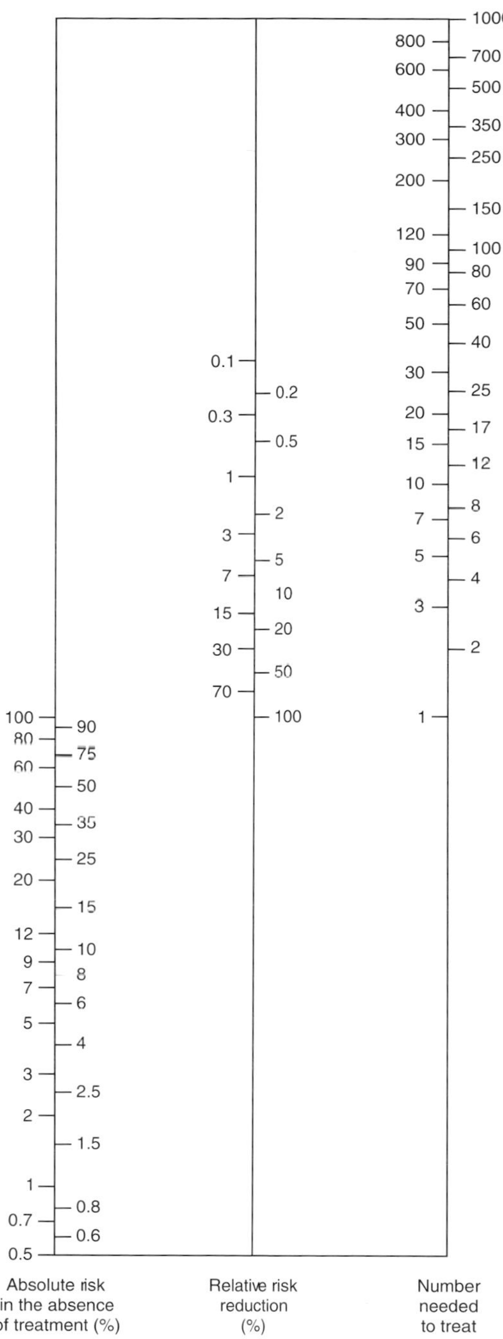

FIGURE **Nomogram for calculating the number needed to treat. Published with permission[1]**

Appendix 3

Clinical Evidence mini CD-ROM

The *Clinical Evidence* mini CD-ROM allows you to:

- Refer to the full *Clinical Evidence* content including clinical questions, summary and background information, evidence detail, figures, tables and appendices
- Choose the method of navigation you prefer, through the table of contents, topic sections or the search engine
- Hyperlink references to abstracts where they appear on PubMed and Cochrane (Internet access required)
- Hyperlink to the glossary, figures, tables and references
- Print the full text of any of the 158 topics

To access *Clinical Evidence* help:

- From within the *Clinical Evidence* CD-ROM, simply click on the link at the top of the screen or from within Windows, select Programs > Clinical Evidence > Help (if you have already installed *Clinical Evidence*)
- For technical help, please go to the FAQs at www.clinicalevidence.com
- For damaged CD-ROMs please contact:
  BMJ Publishing Group • Tel: +44(0) 207 383 6270 • subscriptions@bmjgroup.com (UK/ROW)
  For individual subscriptions • Tel: +1 800 373 2897/+1 240 646 7000 • clinevid@pmds.com (USA)
  For individuals receiving *Clinical Evidence* courtesy of UnitedHealth Foundation: ce@unitedhealthfoundation.org

To install *Clinical Evidence*

(i) Exit from any Windows programs you have running.
(ii) Insert the *Clinical Evidence* Installation CD-ROM into the CD-ROM drive. The installation starts automatically (if it does not, select Run from the Start menu and enter d:\setup (where d: is your CD-ROM drive letter).
(iii) Follow the on-screen instructions. As part of this process, you can install Adobe Acrobat Reader so you can efficiently print *Clinical Evidence* topics — this can also be installed later by following the instructions below. An additional 20 Mbytes of hard disk space is required for this.

Minimum system requirements

An IBM compatible PC with at least this specification:

- 60 Mbytes hard disk space
- 90 MHz processor
- 32 MBytes of RAM
- CD-ROM drive
- Modem, if you want to access the Internet for updates, etc.
- SVGA monitor recommended

Operating systems

This software has been tested with the following operating systems:

- Microsoft Windows 95
- Microsoft Windows 98
- Microsoft Windows 2000 Professional
- Microsoft Windows XP Professional
- Microsoft Windows NT SP6
- Microsoft Windows 2000 Server

Please note

Windows XP Home Edition is not a supported operating system. However, please refer to the Windows XP Home section in the Readme file, which is located:
Start > Programs > Clinical Evidence > Readme (if you have already installed *Clinical Evidence*) or contact technical help.

Browsers

Microsoft Internet Explorer 5.5 is the recommended browser, and should be your default browser when installing *Clinical Evidence*.
This software has been tested with the following browsers:

- Microsoft Internet Explorer 5.0 (English)
- Microsoft Internet Explorer 5.5 (English)
- Microsoft Internet Explorer 6.0 (English)
- Netscape 4.7 (English)
- Netscape 6.0 (English)

Please note

Microsoft Internet Explorer 4 is not a supported browser.
Microsoft Internet Explorer 6 is not compatible with Windows 95.
Internet Explorer 5.5 and 6.0 are available on the installation CD-ROM — see below for details.

To install Microsoft Internet Explorer v5.5

(i) With the *Clinical Evidence* Installation CD-ROM in the CD-ROM drive, select Run from the Start menu.
(ii) Type d:\other\ie5.5\ie5setup and click OK (where d: is your CD-ROM drive letter).
(iii) Follow the on-screen instructions. The typical installation requires approximately 17 Mbytes of hard disk space.

To install Microsoft Internet Explorer v6.0

(i) With the *Clinical Evidence* Installation CD-ROM in the CD-ROM drive, select Run from the Start menu.
(ii) Type d:\other\ie6.0\ie6setup and click OK (where d: is your CD-ROM drive letter).
(iii) Follow the on-screen instructions. The typical installation requires approximately 25 Mbytes of hard disk space.

To install Adobe Acrobat Reader v5.0.5

(i) With the *Clinical Evidence* Installation CD-ROM in the CD-ROM drive, select Run from the Start menu.
(ii) Type d:\Adobe\ar505enu and click OK (where d: is your CD-ROM drive letter).
(iii) Follow the on-screen instructions.